MONTGOMERY COLLEGE
ROCKVILLE CAMPUS LIBRARY
ROCKVILLE, MARYLAND

AMERICA'S
TOP DOCTORS®

A CASTLE CONNOLLY GUIDE

9th Edition

America's trusted source for identifying Top Doctors

All Rights Reserved

Terms of Use

The selection of medical providers for inclusion in this book was based in part on opinions solicited from physicians, nurses, and other health care professionals. The author and publishers cannot assure the accuracy of information provided to them by third parties, since such opinions are necessarily subjective and may be incomplete. The omission from this book of particular health care providers does not mean that such providers are not competent or reputable.

The purpose of this book is educational and informational. It is not intended to replace the advice of your physician or to assist the layman in diagnosing or treating illness, disease, or injury. Following the advice or recommendations set forth in this book is entirely at the reader's own risk. The author and publishers cannot ensure accuracy of, or assume responsibility for, the information in the book as such information is affected by constant change. Liability to any person or organization for any loss or damage caused by errors or omissions in this book is hereby disclaimed. Whenever possible, readers should consult their own primary care physician when selecting health care providers, including any selection based upon information contained in this book. In order to protect patient privacy the names of patients cited in anecdotes throughout the book have been omitted.

The book purchaser acknowledges and agrees that breach of these Terms of Use (including without limitation if you use data obtained via this publication for any commercial purpose, or otherwise in contravention of these Terms of Use), Castle Connolly for all such damages. Furthermore, you acknowledge and agree that you will reimburse any and all legal fees incurred by Castle Connolly in connection with such breach.

The confidence of our readers in our editorial integrity is crucial to the success of the Castle Connolly Guides. Any use of the Castle Connolly name, or of any list or listing (or portion of either) from any Castle Connolly Guide, for advertising or for any commercial purpose, without prior written consent, is strictly prohibited and may result in legal action.

For more information, please contact:

Castle Connolly Medical Ltd., 42 West 24th St, New York, New York 10010
212-367-8400x10
E-mail: info@castleconnolly.com
Web site: http://www.castleconnolly.com.

Library of Congress Control Number: 2009934821
ISBN   1-883769-85-X;   978-1-883769-85-7   (softcover)
ISBN   1-883769-83-3;   978-1-883769-83-3   (hardcover)
Printed in the United States of America

Table of Contents

Table of Contents

Table of Contents

Table of Contents

Table of Contents

Table of Contents

Table of Contents

Table of Contents

Table of Contents

Table of Contents

Table of Contents

Table of Contents

Table of Contents

Appendices

Indices

About The Publishers

John K. Castle, the Chairman of Castle Connolly Medical Ltd., has spent much of the last three decades involved with healthcare institutions and issues. Mr. Castle served as Chairman of the Board of New York Medical College for eleven years, an institution where he served on the Board of Trustees for twenty-two years.

Mr. Castle has been extensively involved in other healthcare and voluntary activities as well. He served for five years as a commissioner and officer of the Joint Commission formerly known as (JCAHO), the body which accredits most public and private hospitals throughout the United States. Mr. Castle has also served as a trustee of five different hospitals in the metropolitan New York region, including NewYork Presbyterian Hospital, where he continues to serve.

Mr. Castle has also served as the Chairman of the Columbia Presbyterian Science Advisory Council and as a Director of the Whitehead Institute for Biomedical Research. He is a Fellow of New York Academy of Medicine and has served as a Trustee of the Academy. He was Chairman of the United Hospital Fund of New York's Capital Campaign and continues as Director Emeritus of the United Hospital Fund. He is a Life Member of the MIT Corporation, the governing body of the Massachusetts Institute of Technology.

Mr. Castle's goal, as is the goal of Dr. John Connolly and all the Castle Connolly team, is to publish *America's Top Doctors*®, *America's Top Doctors*® *for Cancer*, *Top Doctors: New York Metro Area*, and other materials as well as build websites to help the public identify the very best in healthcare resources.

Mr. Castle received his bachelor's degree from the Massachusetts Institute of Technology, his MBA as a Baker Scholar with High Distinction from Harvard, and two Honorary Doctorate degrees.

John J. Connolly, Ed.D. is the President & CEO of Castle Connolly Medical Ltd., and is the nation's foremost authority on identifying top physicians. Dr. Connolly's experience in healthcare is extensive.

For more than a decade he served as President of New York Medical College, the nation's second largest private medical college. He is a Fellow of the New York Academy of Medicine, a Fellow of the New York Academy of Sciences, a Director of the New York Business Group on Health, a member of the President's Council of the United Hospital Fund, and a member of the Board of Advisors of Funding First, a Lasker Foundation initiative. Dr. Connolly has served as a trustee of two hospitals and as Chairman of the Board of one. He is extensively involved in healthcare and community activities and has served on a number of voluntary and corporate boards including the Board of the American Lyme Disease Foundation, of which he is a founder and past chairman, and the Board of Advisors of the Whitehead Institute for Biomedical Research. He is also a Director and Chairman of the Professional Examination Service. He holds a Bachelor of Science degree from Worcester State College, a Master's degree from the University of Connecticut, and a Doctor of Education degree in College and University Administration from Teacher's College, Columbia University.

Dr. Connolly has appeared on or been interviewed by over 100 television and radio stations nationwide including *"Good Morning America"* (ABC-TV), *"The Today Show"* (NBC-TV), *"20/20"* (ABC-TV), *"48 Hours"* (CBS-TV), *"Fox Cable News"* (national), *"Morning News"* (CNN) and *"Weekend Today in New York"* (WNBC-TV). The *New York Times*, the *Chicago Tribune*, the *Daily News* (New York), the *Boston Herald* and other newspapers, as well as many national and regional magazines, have featured Castle Connolly Guides and/or Dr. Connolly in stories.

Medical Advisory Board

Castle Connolly Medical Ltd. is pleased to have associated with a distinguished group of medical leaders who offer invaluable advice and wisdom in our efforts to assist consumers in making good healthcare choices. We thank each member of the Medical Advisory Board for their valuable contributions.

Jeremiah A. Barondess, M.D.
President Emeritus
New York Academy of Medicine,
Professor of Clinical Medicine Emeritus,
Weill-Cornell Medical College

Roger Bulger, M.D.
National Institutes of Health (ret.)

Menard M. Gertler, M.D., D. Sc.
Clinical Professor of Medicine
Cornell University Medical School

Arthur Hull Hayes, M.D.
Former President,
E.M. Pharmaceuticals
Former Commissioner,
U.S. Food & Drug Administration

Leo Henikoff, M.D.
President and CEO (Ret.)
Rush Presbyterian-St. Luke's
Medical Center

Yutaka Kikkawa, M.D.
Professor and Chairman (Emeritus)
Department of Pathology
University of California, Irvine
College of Medicine

David Paige, M.D.
Professor
Bloomberg School of Public Health
Johns Hopkins University

Ronald Pion, M.D.
Chairman and CEO
Medical Telecommunications Associates

Richard L. Reece, M.D.
Editor
Physician Practice Options

Leon G. Smith, M.D.
Chairman of Medicine
St. Michael's Medical Center, NJ

Helen Smits, M.D.
Former Deputy Director
HealthCare Financing Administration (HCFA)

Ralph Snyderman, M.D.
Former President and CEO
Duke University Health System

Foreword

The challenge of finding the best healthcare is a formidable one for most Americans and for others who seek medical care in the United States. While this country offers the best medical care in the world, many people are overwhelmed by its complexity and bureaucracy.

While most of us are fortunate and never need to venture beyond our local communities to find medical specialists able to meet our healthcare needs, the needs of many patients cannot be met in their local areas. For them, the search for the top specialists can be as important as life itself!

This great nation is fortunate in possessing some of the world's leading medical centers and specialty hospitals where cutting edge research is conducted and innovative new therapies are practiced daily. These health centers employ and train many of the world's most skilled physicians. The organization which I formerly headed, the Association of Academic Health Centers, serves as a forum of exchange for these centers of medical excellence and, therefore, I know them well. However, I also know well the difficulty and challenges that patients and their families face in identifying and locating the tremendous wealth of medical talent and dedication that lies within the walls of these outstanding facilities.

Castle Connolly Medical Ltd. has dedicated extensive time and resources to identify-ing the best healthcare this nation has to offer. They have done this not to serve physicians or hospitals, but to serve healthcare consumers. Their efforts will be vital and important resources to Americans and others who seek the best medical care available in this country—wherever it is being practiced.

Roger Bulger, M.D.
National Institutes of Health (ret.)
Washington DC

Introduction

There are times in life when the nature of a disease or medical condition that afflicts you or a loved one warrants identifying the top doctor—the very best specialist anywhere in the nation—to diagnose or treat that particular medical problem. At times like these, you need Castle Connolly *America's Top Doctors*®, the national guide designed to assist you under just these circumstances.

While the overall quality of medical care throughout the United States is generally of very high quality and in many places is superb, there are still those rare, complex or extremely difficult problems that demand resources beyond the ordinary or that require talents that are exceptional.

This guide identifies those top medical specialists throughout the country who possess the skill and experience to address these problems. Top specialists who provide excellent care tend to be located predominantly, although not exclusively, at major medical centers, specialty hospitals and leading teaching hospitals. These exceptional physicians are acknowledged as such by their peers and are recognized for their expertise by the medical profession.

The top specialists we have identified are not the only excellent physicians who are caring for patients in this nation. Since there are more than 720,000 doctors in the United States, we cannot identify every top specialist. Therefore, we have included narrative to assist those using this guide who may not find the specialist they need within its listings. Clearly, there are many primary care physicians and other well-trained specialists in communities and hospitals throughout the United States.

Most physicians in this guide are board certified not only in a specialty, but also in a subspecialty or in multiple subspecialties. Board or subspecialty certification alone, however, does not distinguish them from excellent specialists at hospitals in your community, many of whom are also board certified in both a specialty and a subspecialty.

However, the majority of physicians included in this guide have trained at the top medical centers under medical pioneers who possess state-of-the-art knowledge in a specific disease or problem and have often devised new techniques and therapeutic approaches, many of which are life-saving procedures or cures. These doctors most often practice their science and art at leading hospitals and, more specifically, in programs at hospitals that are recognized for their excellence in a given field. Many others have been trained at leading centers in other nations since the U.S. is not alone in pioneering new medical knowledge, although its position as the leader in "high-tech" medicine is generally acknowledged.

Introduction

Another major characteristic distinguishing the majority of physicians in this guide from those at local hospitals is their continued focus and training. Rather than practicing at a community hospital (or even at a leading regional hospital) and developing a general, broad-based practice, these physicians continued their training in a particular disease, syndrome or subspecialty to such a degree that they developed extensive knowledge and unique skills in treating that particular problem.

Often that focused, advanced training is accompanied by active involvement in clinical research. This is an additional reason why the physicians listed in this guide are located at only a few hundred of the more than six thousand hospitals in the United States. It is difficult, although not impossible, to conduct important clinical research in isolation or without an environment supportive of research. It takes time, money, residents, research associates, technicians, equipment and more to produce significant clinical research. Certainly there have been individuals who have made important and lasting contributions to research with little or none of this support, but those instances are rare. Today, for the most part, major advances in medicine occur in the labs and on the floors of major medical centers and specialty hospitals, in medical schools and in clinical labs created and financed for that purpose by commercial enterprises.

How Physicians Were Selected For Inclusion In This Guide

Castle Connolly's Top Doctors™ selection process begins with surveys of physicians and healthcare professionals. Each year, Castle Connolly surveys thousands of physicians and other healthcare professionals and asks them to identify excellent doctors in every specialty in their region and throughout the nation. When we began the research for the first edition of America's Top Doctors®, we surveyed over 230,000 of the nation's leading medical specialists, department chairs, residency program directors, vice presidents of medical affairs and presidents of the nation's leading medical centers and specialty hospitals.

In addition to mail and online surveys, the Castle Connolly physician-led research team makes thousands of phone calls each year, talking with leading specialists, chairs of clinical departments and vice presidents of medical affairs, seeking to identify top specialists for every diseases and procedures.

The Castle Connolly physician-led research team carefully reviews the credentials of every physician being considered for inclusion in Castle Connolly Guides, magazine articles and website. The review includes, among other factors, scrutiny of medical education, training, hospital appointments, administrative posts, professional achievements, and malpractice and disciplinary history.

Information on outcomes, procedure volume and malpractice is becoming increasingly available, but the public disclosure varies from state to state. Castle Connolly uses its best efforts to gather the information that is available and use it effectively. Ultimately, however, it is the professional judgment of the Castle Connolly editors, the Chief Medical and Research Officer and the research staff, which determines Castle Connolly Top Doctor™ selection.

Physicians may also be removed from the Castle Connolly lists if, in the judgment of the selection team, that is warranted. Some of the reasons physicians are removed include retirement, change in practice (taking a full time administrative post, for example), unavailability to patients, malpractice or disciplinary issues, negative physician or patient feedback, professional demeanor or a change in the "mix" of specialists Castle Connolly will present for a given community. Being removed from a Castle Connolly list does not necessarily indicate something negative about the physician. At the same time, Castle Connolly does not claim to identify every excellent physician in the nation or a region. The physicians identified through the Castle Connolly research process are clearly among the very best, but there are always other very good physicians not identified by Castle Connolly and that is why our guides, websites and other distribution channels for this critical information describe a process whereby consumers can identify excellent physicians using their own efforts.

How do we accomplish this enormous task? Over the years, the Castle Connolly physician-led research team developed its extensive database of physicians across the nation through periodic mail, telephone and email surveys. This cumulative database is systematically maintained and continuously updated. Surveyed physicians nominate top doctors in both their own and related specialties – especially those to whom they would refer their own patients. Each year this database is supplemented by further mail surveys and telephone interviews with leaders in the various medical specialties and leading physicians at major medical centers. In our research for the first edition of this guide, online surveys also were conducted with members of Physicians' Online (POL), the country's largest community of physicians connected through the Internet.

To augment our large mail, telephone and online samplings, additional surveys are conducted among the following carefully selected groups: directors of graduate medical programs; directors of clinical services at member hospitals of the Council of Teaching Hospitals (COTH); board members of medical specialty academies, associations and societies; and deans and chairs of departments at medical schools.

Building on years of prior research, thousands of top doctors included in earlier editions of our guides, as well as a random sample of physicians not listed, are invited to offer their nominations for Castle Connolly *America's Top Doctors*®.

Over 25,000 physicians have been nominated through this process. Extensive biographical forms were sent to those physicians most frequently nominated for completion. After careful review of their professional backgrounds, the Castle Connolly research staff conducted further research to check disciplinary and license histories.

The result is a carefully researched and highly selective list of the top specialists in the nation. This select group of physicians, identified through our extensive research process, constitutes a list of physicians recognized by their peers for their excellence in providing care for specific diseases and problems.

Introduction

Undoubtedly, there will be comments that we have missed some fine doctors who should be included. That is inevitable, since this guide is designed to identify only those doctors noted for excellence in diagnosing or treating a specific problem or disease.

We do not intentionally include physicians simply because they have important titles. While a position as a chief of service or a department head at a teaching hospital is an important post, such positions are achieved through a combination of many talents including administrative skills, seniority and factors that are not as important for inclusion in this guide as is skill in clinical care. The same is true of leaders of county medical societies, professional associations or even specialty groups. While these are significant positions and acknowledge a leadership among peers, these titles are not essential to clinical skill recognition.

The same perspective applies to research expertise. Many physicians listed in the Guide are engaged in clinical research and make significant contributions to their fields, with some devoting a substantial portion of their time to research. However, we avoided including those physicians who solely conduct research and who do not provide patient care.

The result of this extensive research effort is a list of outstanding, highly skilled physicians who are recognized as among the best in their specialties and in the nation; a list which consumers/patients can use to find the very best specialists to meet their particular needs.

Lastly, this book differs from the regional Castle Connolly Guides in two important ways. First, Castle Connolly *America's Top Doctors* *9th Edition* is national, not regional, in scope. Second, the regional Guides are based on the generally accurate premise that healthcare is local and most people find their healthcare where they live and work. However, Castle Connolly *America's Top Doctors* *9th Edition* is designed to meet the needs of those people who cannot find the right specialists locally but who can and will travel anywhere in the country to be cared for by a top specialist at an outstanding hospital. This guide will assist readers in that important search and, for that reason, does not include primary care physicians.

Using This Guide To Find Top Specialists

This guide is organized and planned to be as user-friendly as possible. Still, as with anything as complex as medical specialties, subspecialties and the myriad of diseases and problems that specialists treat, there needs to be a system to organize the physicians' names, the diseases and problems they manage and their special expertise.

To organize the specialists in this guide, we have followed the American Board of Medical Specialties (ABMS) format. The ABMS is the authoritative body for the recognition of medical specialties. Without the ABMS as the official controlling body there would be hundreds of unregulated medical specialties.

The ABMS recognizes twenty-five specialties and more than ninety subspecialties. The listing of ABMS specialties and subspecialties can be found in Appendix A. In addition to ABMS recognized specialties, there are at least one hundred other groups calling themselves "medical specialists" that are not recognized by the ABMS. Some of these groups are working toward recognition and have exams and other standards for membership. Others are organizations of physicians interested in a particular problem or area of medicine that exist to exchange information but have no intention of seeking ABMS recognition. Some groups calling themselves "boards" really have little authority or meaningful standards. Thus, while a physician may state he/she is, for example, a specialist in cosmetic surgery, there is no ABMS recognized specialty by that name. Therefore, you have no idea whether this physician has any special training and expertise or is simply trying to recruit paying patients to a lucrative aspect of surgical practice.

You can get information on a doctor's credentials from the doctor, from the doctor's hospital (Medical Affairs Office) or from your health plan if a doctor is in the network. You can also get this information from numerous Web sites, including www.castleconnolly.com. You can check on a physician's board certification by calling the ABMS at (866) 275-2267 or by logging on to its Web site at www.abms.org.

If you seek a particular type of specialist or subspecialist, turn to the section of this guide covering that medical specialty or subspecialty. There you will be able to further restrict your search to a specific geographic region or, if you prefer, to search throughout the nation.

Using This Guide To Find Top Specialists

To make your search easier, we have organized the specialties and subspecialties into the following regions: New England, Mid Atlantic, Midwest, Southeast, Southwest, Great Plains and Mountains, and West Coast and Pacific. To find an outstanding cardiologist in St. Louis, for example, look under Cardiovascular Disease and then under the Midwest region. (See Pages 38-39 for geographical regions and states.)

A second way to use this guide is to look at the Special Expertise Index, which lists the areas of special expertise of included physicians. This list of special expertise indicates more than 2,000 medical topics including diseases, therapeutic approaches and techniques. You can look up the particular disease, problem or technique you are interested in and locate a physician in that manner. We assume that many people using this guide will know what their particular problem is and will begin their exploration with this index. However, we encourage you to read the entire text since it will help you to better understand how to find the right physician for yourself or a family member, especially if one is not found in this guide.

Choosing An Appropriate Specialist

It may seem that choosing the correct specialist to treat a particular medical problem is simply a matter of finding a top doctor in a specific medical specialty. For treatment of a problem with your vision, you would choose an ophthalmologist. A skin or hair problem would require treatment by a dermatologist and a broken bone would need the care of an orthopaedic surgeon.

Sometimes, however, the type of specialist needed may not be obvious. For example, back surgery may be performed by either an orthopaedic surgeon or a neurosurgeon. Different aspects of sports medicine, as another example, are practiced by orthopaedic surgeons who treat sports-related injuries in both adults and children, pediatricians who treat only children or internists and family practitioners whose focus is on prevention of injuries.

In some cases, several specialists with expertise in different areas of medical practice all become involved in treating the same patient's health problem. For example, a person with diabetes might need care from an endocrinologist, a cardiologist and an ophthalmologist. In other situations, doctors trained in different specialties may use varied approaches or differing therapies to manage a disease or condition. Such is the case, for example, with prostate cancer: a patient could be treated by a urologist, a medical oncologist, or a radiation oncologist. The urologist might provide the patient with a surgical treatment option, while the medical oncologist would treat the patient with chemotherapy and the radiotherapist would use radiation therapy and/or radioactive seed implantation. All approaches could be successful, or one might be preferable to another, depending on the patient and his condition. Therefore, a wise patient will thoroughly explore all options before making a choice.

Finding the right specialist is also important in terms of the quality of your care. For example, many orthopaedic surgeons will operate on hands, but it is clearly preferable to have someone trained and certified specifically in hand surgery (a subspecialty of both orthopaedic surgery and plastic surgery) to perform that delicate surgery. Similarly, a dermatologist may indicate that his/her practice includes cosmetic surgery; however, there is no approved ABMS dermatology subspecialty or fellowship training in cosmetic surgery. While many dermatologists do pursue additional training in cosmetic surgery, it should be understood that dermatologic practice is limited to cutaneous procedures ranging from the removal of skin tumors to laser resurfacing. On the other hand, some board certified otolaryngologists have additional training that enables them to perform cosmetic surgery procedures on the head and neck.

Choosing the right type of specialist is as important as selecting the right doctor. For example, the diagnosis of melanoma, a very serious, potentially life threatening form of skin cancer, is missed in many cases. Therefore, if you have a skin lesion that might possibly be melanoma, you should be certain that the pathologist reading your slides is board certified in the subspecialty of dermatopathology.

These examples illustrate this important principle: always seek the best healthcare. Look for the best-trained doctors, not those who simply can do the job. That doesn't mean that you need to consult a doctor listed in this guide every time you have a health problem. It does mean you should be certain that the physicians who care for you, whether in your community or at a world-class medical center, are trained appropriately and are qualified to provide the care you require. Remember, when it comes to healthcare no one wants second best!

Given this complexity, how do you find the right specialist to provide your care? The first and most important person to look to for guidance is your primary care physician. He/she will assess your medical condition, determine the appropriate type of specialist to recommend and perhaps refer you to a specific doctor or doctors. You should always ask your primary care physician why a particular specialist is being recommended, since that specialist may be a colleague in your doctor's medical group or may be the only (or the most conveniently located) specialist of the type in your health plan. Ask how well your primary care physician knows the specialist, whether they have a long-standing professional relationship and if other patients referred to the specialist had successful outcomes. Be sure to ask for several recommendations, if possible, to provide you with some choice among specialists.

If you do not have a primary care doctor, try to learn as much as you can about your medical problem and the type of specialist best suited to treat it. However, keep in mind that many diseases or conditions present with symptoms that often are indistinguishable from those of other diseases or conditions, making them difficult to diagnose precisely even for physicians armed with the results of diagnostic tests.

Judging The Qualifications Of A Physician

The specialists listed in Castle Connolly *America's Top Doctors*® are clearly among the best in the nation and have been identified through a rigorous research process and thorough screening by the Castle Connolly research team. Through our extensive surveys and research we have done much of the work in finding a top referral specialist for you. But how do you judge the qualifications of a physician who may not be listed in this Guide? If you are trying to find a specialist on your own, how should you go about it? How can you tell when a physician has the appropriate training in a specialty and how do you distinguish what is meaningful and what is not from among all those plaques and certificates on a doctor's wall?

The following pages will outline that process for you. In fact, what is written here reflects much of the logic that underlies the selection of physicians for this book.

The following material will help you not only in finding a top specialist in this Guide, but it also should be helpful to you in choosing among the many specialists, primary care doctors and other physicians that you will need to consult throughout your life.

The reality is that few of us see only one doctor in our lifetime. Each of us may be cared for by a primary care physician, an ophthalmologist, an orthopaedic surgeon, a dermatologist, a surgeon or a number of other specialists. The choices can be many and they can be among the most important choices that we make in our lives.

Education

Your review of your prospective doctor's education and training should begin with medical school. While you may feel that the institution at which someone earned a bachelor's degree could be an indication of the quality of the doctor, most people in the medical field do not believe it plays a major role. A degree from a highly selective undergraduate college or university will help an aspiring doctor gain admission to a medical school, but once there, all students are peers. However, the information on undergraduate colleges, if important to you, is available in *The Official ABMS Directory of Board Certified Medical Specialists*® and other medical directories.

American medical schools are highly standardized, at least in terms of basic quality. A group known as the Liaison Committee for Medical Education (LCME) accredits all U.S. medical schools that grant medical degrees (MDs) and osteopathic degrees (DOs). Most also are accredited by the appropriate state agency, if one exists, and by regional accrediting agencies that accredit colleges and universities of all kinds.

Furthermore, U.S. medical schools have universally high standards for admission, including success on the undergraduate level and on the Medical College Admissions Tests (MCATs). Although frequently criticized for being slow to change and for training too many specialists, the system of medical education in the United States has insured high quality in medical practice. One recent positive change is a strong effort in most medical schools to diversify the composition of the student body. While these schools have been less successful in enrolling racial minorities, the number of women in U.S. medical schools has increased to the point that women now make up about 50 percent of most classes. In certain specialties preferred by women medical graduates (pediatrics, for example) it is possible that in coming years the majority of specialists will be female.

Most doctors practicing in the United States are graduates of U.S. medical schools, but there are two other groups of doctors who make up a relatively small portion of the total physician population. They are (1) foreign nationals who graduated from foreign schools and (2) U.S. nationals who graduated from foreign schools. (Canadian medical schools are not considered foreign).

Foreign Medical Graduates

Foreign medical schools vary greatly in quality. Even some of the oldest and finest European schools have become virtually "open door," with huge numbers of unscreened students making teaching and learning difficult. Others are excellent and provided the model for our system of medical education.

The fact that someone graduated from a foreign school does not mean that he/she is a poor doctor. Foreign schools, like U.S. schools, produce good doctors and poor doctors. Foreign medical graduates must pass the same exam taken by U.S. graduates for licensure, but the failure rate for foreign graduates is significantly higher. In the first year of using the new United States Medical Licensing Exam (USMLE), 93 percent of U.S. medical school graduates passed Step II, the clinical exam, as compared with 39 percent of the foreign graduates. It is clear that the quality of foreign schools, if not individual doctors, is not the same as U.S. medical schools, at least as measured by our standards. Nonetheless, many communities and patients have been well served by foreign medical graduates practicing in this country—often in areas where it has been difficult to attract graduates of American schools.

In addition, many foreign medical schools and their teaching hospitals are world renowned for their leadership in medical care, research and teaching and many of the technologies and techniques we utilize in the U.S. today have been developed and perfected in foreign countries.

Residency

Most doctors practicing today have at least three years of postgraduate training (following the MD or DO) in an approved residency program. This not only is an important step in the process of becoming a competent doctor, but it is also a requirement for board (specialty) certification. Most people assume that a prospective doctor needs to complete a three-year residency program to obtain a medical license. That is not an accurate assumption! New York State, for example, requires only one postgraduate year. However, since all approved residencies last at least three years and some, such as those in neurosurgery, general surgery, orthopaedic surgery and urology, may extend for five or more years, it is important to know the details of a doctor's training. Licensure alone is not enough of a basis upon which to make a decision.

Without undertaking extensive and detailed research on every residency program, the best assessment you can make of a doctor's residency program is to see if it took place in a large medical center whose name you recognize. The more prestigious institutions tend to attract the best medical students, sometimes regardless of the quality of the individual residency program. If in doubt about a doctor's training, ask the doctor if the residency he/she completed was in the specialty of the practice; if not, ask why not.

It is also important to be certain that a doctor completed a residency that has been approved by the appropriate governing board of the specialty, such as the American Board of Surgery, the American Board of Radiology, or the American Osteopathic Board of Pediatrics. These board groups are listed in Appendix A. If you are really concerned about a doctor's training, you should call the hospital that offered the residency and ask if the residency program was approved by the appropriate specialty group. If still in doubt, consult the publication *Directory of Graduate Medical Education Programs*, often called the "green book," found in medical school or hospital libraries, which lists all approved residencies.

Board Certification

With an MD or DO degree and a license, an individual may practice in any medical specialty with or without additional training. For example, doctors with a license but no special training may call themselves cardiologists, pediatricians or gynecologists. This is why board certification is such an important factor. The American Board of Medical Specialties (ABMS) recognizes 25 specialties and more than 90 subspecialties. Visit www.abms.org or call 866-275-2267 for more information. Eighteen boards certify in 106 specialties under the aegis of the American Osteopathic Association (AOA). Visit www.osteopathic.org or call 800-621-1773 for more information. Doctors who have qualified for such specialization are called board certified; they have completed an approved residency and passed the board's exam. (See Appendix A for the approved ABMS and AOA lists). While many doctors who are not board certified do call themselves "specialists," board certification is the best standard by which to measure competence and training. Throughout this Guide a description of each specialty and subspecialty is provided as an introduction to the listing of physicians in that specialty.

You can be confident that doctors who are board certified have, at a minimum, the proper training in their specialty and have demonstrated their proficiency through supervision and testing. While there are many non-board certified doctors who are highly competent, it is more difficult to assess the level of their training. While board certification alone does not guarantee competence, it is a standard that reflects successful completion of an appropriate training program. If it is impossible to find a doctor in your area who is board certified in a particular subspecialty, for example, geriatric medicine or sports medicine, at least be certain the physician is board certified in a related specialty such as internal medicine or orthopaedic surgery.

Board certified doctors are referred to as Diplomates of the Board. Some of the colleges of medical specialties (e.g., the American College of Radiology, the American College of Surgeons) have multiple levels of recognition. The first is basic membership and the second, more prestigious and difficult to obtain, is status as a Fellow. Fellowship status in the colleges is meaningful and is based on experience, professional achievement and recognition by one's peers, including extensive experience in patient care. It should be viewed as a significant professional qualification.

Board Eligibility

Many doctors who have been more recently trained are waiting to take the boards. They are sometimes described as "board eligible," a common term that the ABMS advocates abandoning because of its ambiguity. Board eligible means that the doctor has completed an approved residency and is qualified to sit for the related board's exam.

Each member board of the ABMS has its own policy regarding the use and recognition of the board eligible term. Therefore, the description "board eligible" should not be viewed as a genuine qualification, especially if a doctor has been out of medical school long enough to have taken the certification exam. To the boards, a doctor is either board certified or not. Furthermore, most of the specialty boards permit unlimited attempts to pass the exam and, in some cases, doctors who have failed the exam twice or even ten times continue to call themselves board eligible. In osteopathic medicine, the board eligible status is recognized only for the first six years after completion of a residency.

Using This Guide To Find Top Specialists

In addition to the approved lists of specialties and subspecialties of the ABMS and AOA, there are a wide variety of other doctors and groups of doctors who call themselves specialists. At present there are at least 100 such groups called "self-designated medical specialties." They range from doctors who are working to create a recognized body of knowledge and subspecialty training to less formal groups interested in a particular approach to the practice of medicine. These groups may or may not have standards for membership. There is no way to determine the true extent of their members' training and neither the ABMS or the AOA recognizes them. While you should be cautious of doctors who claim they are specialists in these areas, many do have advanced training and the groups at least offer a listing of people interested in a particular approach to medical care. Rely on board certification to assure yourself of basic competence, and use membership in one of these groups to indicate strong interest and possible additional training in a particular aspect of medicine. A list of these self-designated medical specialties may be found in Appendix B.

Recertification

A relatively new focus of the specialty boards is the area of recertification. Until recently, board certification lasted for an unlimited time. Now, almost all the boards have put time limits on the certification period. For example, in Internal Medicine and Anesthesiology, the time limit is ten years; in Family Practice, six, and under some circumstances, seven years. These more stringent standards reflect an increasing emphasis on recertification by both the medical boards and state agencies responsible for licensing doctors.

Since the policies of the boards vary widely, it is a good procedure to ask a doctor if certification was awarded and when. If the date was seven to ten years ago, ask if he/she has been recertified. Unfortunately, many boards permit "grandfathering," whereby already certified doctors do not have to be recertified, and recertification requirements apply only to newly certified doctors. Appendix A contains a list of the names and addresses of the boards and the certification period for each board specialty. Even if recertification is not required, it is good professional practice for doctors to undertake the process. It assures you, the patient, that they are attempting to stay current.

Many states have a continuing medical education requirement for doctors. These states typically require a minimum number of continuing medical education (CME) credits for a doctor to maintain a medical license. Seven states require 150 CME credits over a three-year period. Osteopathic doctors are required to take 120 hours of CME credits within three years to maintain certification.

Fellowships

The purpose of a fellowship is to provide advanced training in the clinical techniques and research of a particular specialty. Fellowships usually, but not always, are designed to lead to board certification in a subspecialty such as cardiology, which is a subspecialty of internal medicine. Many physicians listed in this Guide have had fellowship training. In the U.S. there are a variety of fellowship programs available to doctors, which fall into two broad categories: approved and unapproved. Approved fellowships are those that are approved by the appropriate medical specialty board (e.g., the American Board of Radiology) and lead to subspecialty certificates. Fellowship programs that are unapproved are often in the same areas of training as those that are approved, but they do not lead to subspecialty certificates. Unfortunately, all too often, an unapproved fellowship exists only to provide relatively inexpensive labor for the research and/or patient care activities of a clinical department in a medical school or hospital. In such cases, the learning that takes place is secondary and may be a good deal less than in an approved fellowship. On the other hand, any fellowship is better than none at all and some unapproved fellowships have that status for a valid reason that should not reflect negatively on the program. For example, the fellowship may have been recently created, with approval being sought. To check that a fellowship is an approved one, call the hospital where the training took place or call the medical board for that specialty.

Some physicians may have completed more than one fellowship and may be boarded in two or more subspecialties. Also, some physicians may pursue fellowship training and subspecialty certification, but then choose to practice in their primary field of certification. For example, a doctor who is board certified in internal medicine also may have obtained board certification in cardiology, but may choose to practice primarily internal medicine rather than cardiology. For the most part, the physicians in this Guide practice in their subspecialties.

Professional Reputation

There are doctors who meet every professional standard on paper, but who are simply not good doctors. In all probability the medical community has ascertained that and, while the individual may still practice medicine, his/her reputation will reflect that collective assessment. There are also doctors who are outstanding leaders in their fields because of research or professional activities but who are not particularly strong, or perhaps even active, in patient care. It is important to distinguish that kind of professional reputation from a reputation as a competent, caring doctor in delivering patient care, or in the case of this Guide, as an outstanding practitioner in a given specialty.

Using This Guide To Find Top Specialists

Hospital Appointment

Most doctors are on the medical staff of one or more hospitals and are known as "attendings;" some are not. If a doctor does not have admitting privileges or is not on the attending staff of a hospital, you may wish to consider choosing a different doctor. It can be very difficult to ascertain whether or not the lack of hospital appointment is for a good reason. For example, it is understandable that some doctors who are raising families or heading toward retirement choose not to meet the demands (meetings, committees, etc.) of being an attending. However, if you need care in a hospital, the lack of such an appointment means that another doctor will have to oversee that care. In some specialties, such as dermatology and psychiatry, doctors may conduct their entire practice in the office and a hospital appointment is not as essential, or as good a criterion for assessment, as in other specialties.

While mistakes are made, most hospitals are quite careful about admissions to their medical staffs. The best hospitals are highly selective, so a degree of screening (or "credentialing") has been done for you. In other words, the best doctors practice at the best hospitals. Since caring for a patient in a hospital is often a team effort involving a number of specialists, the reputation of the hospital to which the doctor admits patients carries special weight. Hospital medical staffs review their colleagues' credentials and authorize performance of specific procedures. In addition, they typically review and reappoint their medical staff every two or three years. In effect, this is an additional screening to protect patients. It is especially true of hospitals that have what are known as closed staffs, where it is impossible to obtain admitting privileges unless there is a vacancy that the administration and medical staff deem necessary to fill. If you are having a surgical procedure and are concerned about the doctor's skill or experience, it may be worthwhile to call the Medical Affairs office at the doctor's hospital to see if he/she is authorized to perform that procedure in that hospital.

The reasons for a hospital's selectivity are easy to understand: no hospital wishes to expose itself to liability and every hospital wants to have the best reputation possible in order to attract patients. Obviously, the quality of the medical staff is immensely important in creating that reputation.

Physicians listed in this guide are primarily on the staffs of major medical centers, usually teaching hospitals, and leading specialty hospitals, e.g. children's, cancer, heart, psychiatric, etc. There are many excellent physicians on the staffs of community hospitals that call themselves "medical centers," but they are not physicians who typically attract complex cases and referrals from outside their area.

To learn about a hospital visit its website. It is also useful to review a hospital's accreditation status under the Joint Commission on the Accreditation of Healthcare Organizations at www.JCAHO.com. A new website created by the federal government, www.hospitalcompare.com, offers some measures of comparative hospital quality and may be of interest as well.

A last and very important reason why a hospital appointment is an essential requirement in your choice of doctor is that some states permit doctors to practice without malpractice insurance. If you are injured as a result of a doctor's poor care, you could be without recourse. However, few hospitals permit doctors to practice in them unless they carry malpractice insurance. This not only protects the hospital, but the patient as well.

Medical School Faculty Appointment

Many doctors have appointments on the faculties of medical schools. There is a range of categories from "straight" appointments, meaning full-time appointment as professor, associate professor, assistant professor or instructor, to clinical ranks that may reflect lesser degrees of involvement in teaching or research. If someone carries what is known as a straight academic rank (i.e. "professor of surgery," without clinical in the title), this usually means that the individual is engaged full-time in medical school research, teaching activities and patient care. The title "clinical professor of surgery" usually indicates a less direct involvement in medical school activities such as teaching and research.

Doctors who are full-time academicians may be in the forefront of new techniques and research, but they are not necessarily better doctors. Nonetheless, you would be assured that they have the support of other faculty, residents and medical students.

When you are seeking a subspecialist, a doctor's relationship to a medical school becomes more meaningful since medical school faculties tend to be made up of subspecialists. You are less likely to find large numbers of general or primary care practitioners engaged full-time on a medical school faculty. The newest approaches and techniques in medicine, for the most part, are explored and developed by medical school faculties in their laboratories and clinical practice settings. This is where they practice their subspecialties, as well as teach and conduct research. Such leading specialists are not necessarily better doctors than community doctors; rather, they are trained to provide a different kind of medical care. Obviously the type of medical care users of this guide are seeking is that different kind of care available primarily from top subspecialists at leading hospitals and medical centers.

Medical Society Membership

Most medical society memberships sound very prestigious and some are; however, there are many societies that are not selective and which virtually any doctor can join. In addition, membership in many of the more prestigious societies is based on research and publication or on leadership in the field and may have little to do with direct patient care. While it is clearly an honor to be invited to join these groups, membership may be less than helpful in discerning whether a doctor can deliver the excellent clinical care you require.

Using This Guide To Find Top Specialists

Experience

Experience is difficult to assess. Obviously, in most cases, an older doctor has more experience; on the other hand, a younger doctor has been more recently immersed in the challenge of medical school, residency, or even a fellowship, and may be the most up-to-date. If a doctor is board certified, you may assume that assures at least a minimal amount of experience, but since it could be as little as a year, check the date of graduation from medical school or completion of residency to know precisely how long a doctor has been in practice.

There is a good deal of evidence that there is a positive relationship between quantity of experience and quality of care. It may be that, the more a doctor performs a procedure, the better he/she becomes at it. That is why it is important to ask a doctor about his or her experience with the procedure that you need. Does the doctor see and treat similar cases every day, every week or only rarely? Of course, with some rare diseases, rarely is the only possible answer, but it is relative frequency that is critical. Major metropolitan areas, especially New York and San Francisco, became leaders in the treatment of AIDS because of the number of patients seen in those metropolitan areas. Doctors in the suburbs of New York City (especially in New York's Westchester, Nassau and Suffolk counties) and in Fairfield County, Connecticut became leaders in the research and treatment of Lyme disease because that region is the epicenter of the disease.

In some states, data is available on volume or numbers of certain procedures performed at hospitals. For this information in New York you can call the Center for Medical Consumers, a non-profit advocacy organization, or visit its web site at www.medicalconsumers.org. For volume and outcome information in other states, visit the web site of Health Care Choices at www.healthcarechoices.org. The federal government has posted outcome data for hospitals, but for a limited number of procedures, on a website www.healthcarecompare.com. There is a good deal of controversy, however, on the validity and usefulness of such data. Opponents cite the fact that some of the data is produced from Medicare patient records only and, thus, is based solely on an elderly population that does not represent the total activity of a hospital or doctor. Proponents of the use of such volume data agree that it is not perfect, but suggest it can be one useful criterion in selecting the best places to receive care for these specific problems

The one type of experience you should specifically want to know about is that dealing with any special procedure, particularly a surgical one, that has recently been developed and introduced into practice. For example, in the 1980's many doctors using laparoscopic cholecystectomy, a then new surgical technique for removing gallbladders, experienced a high percentage of problems because they were not properly trained. This prompted the American Board of Surgery to announce new standards for the training of surgeons using this technique. Do not hesitate to ask about your doctor's training in a procedure and how frequently and with what degree of success he/she has performed it. Practice may not lead to perfection, but it does improve skills and enhance the probability of success.

In some cases, relatively young doctors have recently completed residency or fellowship training under recognized leaders who have developed new approaches or techniques for dealing with a particular problem. They may have learned the new techniques from their mentors and may be far ahead of the field (and ahead of more senior and distinguished colleagues) in using those approaches. So age and experience must be considered and weighed along with other factors when choosing a physician.

Second Opinions

Second opinions are a valuable medical tool, too infrequently used in many instances and overused in others. Clearly, you do not want to seek another doctor's opinion on every ailment or problem that you face, but a second opinion should be pursued in the following situations:

• before major surgery

• if the diagnosis is serious or life threatening

• if a rare disease is diagnosed

• if a diagnosis is uncertain

• if the number of tests or procedures recommended might be excessive

• if a test result has serious implications (e.g., a positive Pap smear)

• if the treatment suggested is risky or expensive

• if you are uncomfortable with the diagnosis and/or treatment

• if a course of treatment is not successful

• if you question your doctor's competence

• if your insurance company requires it

Most doctors will be supportive if you request a second opinion and many will recommend it. In many cases, insurance companies will pay for second opinions, but check ahead of time to make sure your insurance plan does cover them. In an HMO you may have to be more assertive because one way HMOs control costs is by limiting second opinions. Often, the opinion of a second doctor will confirm the opinion of the first, but the reassurance may be worth the time and extra cost. On the other hand, if the second opinion differs from the first, you have two alternatives: seek the opinion of a third doctor, or educate yourself as much as possible by talking to both doctors, reading up on the problem, and trusting your instincts about which diagnosis is correct.

Office And Practice Arrangements

Although clearly not as important as training or reputation, a specialist's office and practice arrangements often are of significance to patients. Practice arrangements include office hours, office location, billing procedures and accessibility among the many factors that result in how well the office is run.

Some specialists only will see new patients who are referred to them by another doctor. Therefore, you may need to have your treating physician contact the specialist's office to arrange for your initial visit. Your health plan may also require that your primary care doctor provide a referral.

If English is not your first language, it may be advisable to determine whether someone in the specialist's office speaks your primary language or if a translator can be present during appointments. This will ease communication and assure that all questions, responses and instructions are understood.

Accessibility of the specialist's office may be a concern if you are wheelchair-bound, are elderly or cannot climb stairs or negotiate narrow corridors. Convenient parking may also be important to you.

Other arrangements that may need to be made in advance of your first visit or discussed with the specialist's office staff concern payment. You may wish to ask the following:

- Does the specialist accept your health insurance coverage?

- Is the specialist within your plan's network and will you need to pay a co-payment? Or, is the specialist out-of-network and will you have to pay for your care out-of-pocket, meet a deductible or submit a form for reimbursement?

- Are credit cards an acceptable mode of payment?

- Does the specialist accept Medicare, Medicaid or no-fault insurance? Does the specialist treat workers' compensation cases?

- If you are a non-resident of the United States, will you need to arrange for the transfer or exchange of currency to pay the specialist's fee?

When you are choosing a top specialist, these issues may be of lesser or greater importance, depending on the problem and type of care warranted. If you are traveling a great distance to have a specific procedure performed by a top specialist at a major medical center, continuing long-term monitoring or follow-up care by that physician may not be required or may not be feasible and such things as office practice arrangements are of less importance. On the other hand, if you have a chronic problem that needs to be monitored with follow-up care provided by the same top specialist, then such issues as accessibility of the doctor's office, appointment hours, waiting times and courtesy and professionalism of the staff become more significant.

Personal Chemistry

One element of the doctor-patient relationship that we stress in our guides is chemistry between doctor and patient, a part of which is often referred to as a doctor's "bedside manner." While this factor is of major import in a long-term relationship such as one you would have with your primary care physician, it is of less importance when you see a specialist only once or twice. However, since many people using this book may have chronic conditions that require ongoing care, it is important to give the matter some consideration.

It is vital that there is a sense of mutual trust and respect between patient and doctor; a judgment that individuals must make for themselves. Among the many talented doctors listed in this guide, there are very likely some to whom you would relate well and others with whom you may not feel as comfortable.

Patients prefer doctors who listen, demonstrate concern, are responsive to patient needs and spend sufficient time with them. The qualities of physicians in this regard, even the excellent ones in this guide, vary immensely.

You, the patient, are the only one who can assess these qualities because individuals react differently to various personalities. It is important for you to carefully judge your feelings towards a physician, especially if you are embarking on a long-term relationship. You should feel you can be open, trusting and responsive to your physician and that your relationship will be a positive one. Otherwise, find another doctor, since not doing so could adversely affect your care.

Once you have used this guide to identify the top specialist(s) best suited to treat your condition, there is much you can do to maximize the value of your first visit.

Maximizing Your First Appointment With A Top Doctor

After your research is done and you've secured an appointment for an initial consultation with a top doctor known for his/her expertise in the diagnosis or treatment of your particular medical condition, what should you do?

Whether your visit to the specialist's office is a car ride or a plane trip away, there undoubtedly will be arrangements to make before your appointment. You may have to take time off from work, arrange for childcare while you are away and make travel plans and hotel reservations, but there are a number of other important steps to take to assure that you and the specialist make the best use of the time you spend together.

Have you done everything you can to prepare yourself and the specialist for the consultation? The following checklist will help you maximize the value of your visit to the specialist and will go a long way toward focusing you on the task at hand—getting the best advice or treatment for your health problem from one of the top doctors in the medical specialty related to your condition.

Gathering The Facts

- Does the specialist have all the information needed to make a diagnosis of or treatment plan for your condition?

- Have your medical records, test results and X-rays been sent ahead of time to allow for their review by the specialist in advance of your first appointment?

- Have you written out your medical history, including that of your siblings, parents and grandparents, emphasizing the particular problem for which you are visiting this specialist?

- Are you prepared with a written list of questions?

- Do you understand the answers?

A specialist becoming newly involved in your care needs to learn as much as possible about the state of your health in a very limited time. Since top doctors are extremely busy people with many demands on their time, you should make certain that all relevant records and case summaries are obtained and sent to the specialist well in advance of your appointment.

Obtaining Your Records

All healthcare providers, including hospitals, doctors and their staffs, are under legal obligation to maintain the privacy of your medical records. In order to obtain release of those records, you must make a request in writing. If you need to obtain records from a number of providers, you should write one clear and concise letter authorizing release of your records and including your name, address, telephone number, date of birth, identification number and any other identifying information such as a hospital chart number. You then can make photocopies of this letter, but be sure to sign and date each copy as if it were an original. You also may want to specifically name those test results (e.g., pathology slides) or X-ray films (not just written reports or summaries) that must be included in addition to making a general request for your records. It's also a good idea to indicate the date of your appointment so the office staff can respond in a timely manner.

Although state laws require the timely release of medical records, hospital medical records departments and doctors' offices often take several weeks to pull and review patient charts and get them in the mail either to you or to another doctor. In addition to written authorization, you may be asked to pay the costs involved in copying your records, test results and X-ray films because many doctors' offices will not release the originals. Consider placing a call in advance to determine the procedure for releasing your records, how long you can expect it to take and the costs involved so that you can save time by including payment with your release authorization letter. Be sure to allow sufficient time in advance of your consultation appointment for your request to be processed. Since you often must wait several weeks for an appointment with a specialist, allow at least that amount of time to obtain your records.

Even after making your written requests, you should follow up each letter with a telephone call to be sure that your records actually are sent. You should not assume that your request for records will be promptly fulfilled by an often overburdened, although well-intentioned, office staff.

Remember, the more information the specialist has about your condition, the fewer repeat or additional tests or procedures you will need to undergo, the lower the costs of your consultation and, most important, the more expeditiously the specialist will be able to render an opinion.

The Facts And Only The Facts

Be thorough and organized in documenting your personal and familial medical histories, the medications you take and in relaying information about your condition. Even seemingly minor bits of information may provide subtle clues to the nature of your medical problem and the optimal way in which to treat it. It's also advisable to bring a list with you of names, addresses and telephone numbers of all physicians who have cared for you, especially those you have seen regarding your current medical problem.

Even though thoroughness is essential to presenting a clear picture of your medical condition, bear in mind that the specialist needs to get to your core health concerns as quickly as possible. Therefore, if you have a complex medical history, you may want to ask your current doctors to provide treatment summaries in addition to copies of your medical records. Hospital records should include your admission history and physical exam, dictated consultation and operation notes and discharge summaries for all hospitalizations. You may also be able to get a cumulative lab and X-ray summary for your hospital stays.

Unlike X-rays, which can be copied at reasonable cost, original pathology slides must be transported by mail or hand-carried. Your specialist may wish to have the pathologist with whom he/she works speak directly with the pathologist who initially interpreted your slides as part of the process of evaluating your case.

Being Prepared

You are likely to be a bit nervous when you meet with the specialist you have chosen. Anxiety about your health and concern about your future care may cause you to forget information you should provide or miss hearing or understanding important information that the specialist communicates. Therefore, you may want to write down all relevant information so that you do not leave out anything of importance when you meet with the specialist or complete forms in the office. You also may want to write out your questions in advance so you don't forget anything.

To avoid leaving out important details of your condition or past treatment, prepare a concise, chronological summary before your consultation takes place. You may wish to type it and provide a copy to the specialist for inclusion in your chart. Highlight major medical results or significant events in the course of an illness or treatment if these will enlighten the doctor about your condition. Your personal perspective on the state of your health is vital to a full understanding of your medical problem.

It is possible that the specialist will use language that you do not understand or may speak quickly assuming certain knowledge on your part about your condition or its treatment. Don't hesitate to ask for clarification as often or repeatedly as you may need to in order to fully comprehend what you are being told. If you are concerned that you may forget what the doctor tells you, ask the doctor's permission to take notes or ask if you might bring along a tape recorder so you can later replay what was said, especially any instructions you are given. You may prefer to bring along a relative or close friend to serve as a "second set of ears," but, again, seek the doctor's permission to do so in advance of your appointment.

Following this process will assure that you and the specialist you are consulting get the most from your appointment. After all, you both have the same goal: restoring you to optimal health and well being.

What To Do If You Can't Get An Appointment

At times it may be difficult, perhaps even impossible, to secure an appointment with the specific specialist you have identified. There are a number of reasons why this may occur. For example, the specialist may not be taking any new patients or may have such a busy schedule that it takes several weeks or months to get an appointment. He/she may only see patients during very limited hours because of teaching, research or other responsibilities or currently may have other limitations related to the acceptance of new patients.

However, bear in mind that the doctors in this guide are the leaders in their specialties and therefore they work with and train the very best and brightest in their specialties. So, if you are unable to consult with a particular doctor, consider making an appointment with one of his/her outstanding colleagues. You can do this by asking a member of the doctor's office staff to refer you to an associate who is a member of the practice group or to another excellent physician who is specially trained to address your particular medical issue.

You can be comfortable knowing that you will receive high quality care from another specialist who practices in the same top setting.

Utilizing Special Resources

The following information on special resources has been included to meet the needs of healthcare consumers who have extraordinarily difficult or unique health problems, and have been unable to identify the resources to address their problems. These patients and their doctors may need to search for very new, cutting-edge, perhaps even experimental and not yet approved therapies. In such cases the search may lead to clinical trials; tests of new drugs and new medical devices or innovative therapeutic approaches. Fortunately, these situations are rare, but when they do occur, they are critical.

In addition to the outstanding private and public hospitals recognized in this guide, the U.S. government maintains its own unique, expert source of patient care and clinical research at the National Institutes of Health (NIH). In fact, the NIH operates its own hospital at which the care provided is usually related to clinical studies its researchers are undertaking.

In addition to those at the NIH, clinical trials also are conducted at leading medical centers and other organizations throughout the country. These facilities may be testing a new drug therapy, a new use for an existing medication or a medical device to deal with a problem that is not being resolved through the use of more traditional approaches.

This section will guide you in utilizing these special resources.

The Clinical Trial As A Treatment Option

For some patients the best medical treatment may only be available through clinical trials (also called treatment studies), which are designed to develop improved ways to use current medical treatments or to find new medical treatments by studying their effects on humans. Treatments are studied to determine if they are safe, effective and better treatments than conventional or standard therapies. Only if they meet all three of these criteria are they made available to the general public.

Many people are frightened by the term "clinical trial" because it conveys the notion of being a "guinea pig" in an experiment. Contrary to popular belief, however, most new treatments are extensively studied by scientists in the laboratory before they are ever tested by physicians in clinical settings. Among the factors that keep patients from participating in clinical trials are: lack of awareness about clinical trials as a treatment option; fear of side effects or adverse reactions to treatment; refusal of insurance companies to pay for experimental treatments; failure of a physician to inform the patient about clinical trials; difficulty finding suitable clinical trials; unavailability of clinical trials for certain medical problems; distance of the patient from major medical centers conducting clinical trials; disruption of personal and family life; and the decision to stop medical treatment altogether.

Despite these and other obstacles, many people do seek out clinical trials. One of the most pressing reasons to participate is the opportunity to obtain treatment that might not be available otherwise. New medical treatments can offer participants hope for a cure, an extended lifespan, or an improvement in how they feel. Some participants also take comfort in knowing that others may benefit from their contribution to medical knowledge.

Deciding if a clinical trial is the right treatment option for you is no simple matter. Certainly, you will want to talk about it with your doctor(s) and other professionals involved in your care, as well as with family members and friends. But in order to fully benefit from what others have to say — based on either their professional knowledge or personal experience — you need to understand exactly what a clinical trial is and what your role as a volunteer will be.

Understanding Clinical Trials

Clinical trials are conducted for just about every medical condition, including life-threatening diseases such as AIDS or cancer; chronic illnesses such as diabetes and asthma; psychiatric disorders such as depression or anxiety; behavioral problems such as smoking and substance abuse; and even common ailments such as hair loss and acne. Chances are, there is at least one trial (and probably more) that may be appropriate for you.

With more than 100 different types of cancer, it is understandable that a large number of clinical trials are cancer-related. Extensive information about clinical trials for cancer can be found on www.cancer.gov, the Web site of the National Cancer Institute (NCI). NCI is part of the NIH. CenterWatch, an online clinical trials listing service, identifies over 14,000 clinical trials that are actively recruiting patients. Veritas Medicine, another useful online organization, allows individuals to perform personalized searches of its clinical trials database. See Appendix D for "Selected Resources" for more information on clinical trials.

Most clinical trials study new medical treatments, combinations of treatments, or improvements in conventional treatments using drugs, surgery and other medical procedures, medical devices, radiation or other therapies. Newer types of clinical trials, called screening or prevention trials, study how to prevent the incidence or recurrence of disease through the use of medicines, vitamins, minerals or other supplements; and how to screen for disease, especially in its early stages. Another type of trial studies how to improve the quality of life for patients, including both their physical and emotional well-being.

Clinical trials are sponsored both by the federal government (through the National Institutes of Health, the National Cancer Institute and many others) and by private industry through pharmaceutical and biotechnology companies, and through healthcare institutions (hospitals or health maintenance organizations) and community-based physician-investigators. The National Cancer Institute sponsors clinical trials at more than 1000 sites in the United States. Trials are carried out in major medical research centers such as teaching hospitals as well as in community hospitals, specialized medical clinics (for example, those for the treatment of AIDS or Alzheimer's disease) and in doctors' offices.

Though clinical trials often involve hospitalized patients, a fair number of trials are conducted on an outpatient basis. Many trials are part of a cooperative network which may include as few as one or two sites or hundreds of locations, although one center generally assumes responsibility for overall coordination of the research. More than 45 research-oriented institutions, recognized for their scientific excellence, have been designated by the NCI as comprehensive or clinical cancer centers. See Appendix D "Selected Resources" to find out how to locate these centers.

Clinical research is based on a protocol (established rules or procedures) describing who will be studied, how and when medications, procedures and/or treatments will be administered and how long the study will last. Trials that are conducted simultaneously at different sites use the same protocol to ensure that all patients are treated identically and all data are collected uniformly so that study findings can be compared.

Clinical trials generally are conducted in three phases, as outlined in the study protocol. The first phase begins testing of the treatment on a small group of human subjects after rigorous and successful animal testing has been concluded. The interim phase varies, but usually involves a broader test group and is designed to further evaluate the treatment's safety and more accurately determine appropriate dosage, application methods and side effects. In some trials there may be a fourth phase, conducted after the treatment is in widespread use, to monitor the results of long-term use and the occurrence of any serious side effects.

Some clinical trials test one treatment on one group of subjects, while others compare two or more groups of subjects. In such comparison studies participants are divided into two groups: the control group that receives the standard treatment and the experimental or treatment group which receives the new treatment. For example, the control group may undergo a surgical procedure while the experimental or treatment group undergoes a surgical procedure plus radiation to determine which treatment modality is more effective. To ensure that patient characteristics do not unduly influence the study findings, patients may be randomly assigned to either the control or the experimental group, meaning that each patient's assignment is based purely on chance. In cases in which a standard treatment does not exist for a particular disease, the experimental group of patients receives the new treatment and the control group receives no treatment at all, or receives a placebo, an inactive medicine or procedure that has no treatment value and is sometimes called a "dummy" pill or a "sugar" pill. It is important to keep in mind that patients are never put into a control group without any treatment if there is a known treatment that could help them. Also, whether a patient is receiving an investigational drug or a placebo, he/she receives the same level and quality of medical care as those receiving the investigational treatment.

Questions to ask your doctor and the trial's research team if you are considering participating in a clinical trial:

- Who is sponsoring the trial?

- How many patients will be involved?

- Will the trial be testing a single treatment or a combination of treatments?

- Will there be one treatment group or more than one treatment group?

- If more than one treatment group, how are patients assigned to each group?

- Has this treatment been studied in previous clinical trials? What were the findings?

Protecting the Rights of Participants

The safety of those who participate in clinical trials is a serious matter and is the number one priority of medical investigators. All clinical research, regardless of type of sponsorship, is guided by the same ethical and legal codes that govern the medical profession and the practice of medicine. Most clinical research is federally funded or federally regulated (at least in part) with built-in safeguards for patients. According to federal government regulations (and some state laws), every clinical trial in the United States must be approved and monitored by an Institutional Review Board (IRB), which is an independent committee of physicians, statisticians, community advocates and others (representing at least five distinct disciplines) to ensure that the protocol is being followed.

Government regulations require researchers to fully inform participants about all aspects of a clinical trial before they agree to participate through a process called informed consent. To be sure that you understand your role in a clinical trial, you should jot down any questions beforehand so as not to forget them. You should also consider bringing along a friend or family member for support and additional input, and perhaps even tape recording the conversation (after asking permission to do so) to make sure you do not forget or misunderstand anything. Each participant in a clinical trial must be given a written consent form, which should be available in English and other languages. The consent form explains the following:

- Why the research is being done.

- What the researchers hope to accomplish.

- What types of treatment interventions (and other tests or procedures) will be performed.

- How long the study will continue.

- What the expected benefits and the possible risks are.

- What other treatments are available.

- What costs will be covered by the study, by the patient or by third-party payers such as Medicare, Medicaid or private insurance.

Patients also are informed that they may leave the trial, or exclude themselves from any part of it, at any time. Informed consent means exactly what the term implies: you agree to join a clinical trial only after you completely understand exactly what your participation will involve for the duration of the study. By law, each patient must be provided with a copy of the signed consent form, which also must include the name and telephone number of a contact person for questions or additional information. Informed consent is a continuous process, so do not hesitate to ask questions before, during or after the trial.

The investigators must protect the privacy of each participant in a clinical trial by ensuring that all medical records are kept confidential except for inspection by the sponsoring agency, the Food and Drug Administration and other agencies involved in regulating the drug or treatment, and all data are collected anonymously by assigning a numeric code or initials to each individual.

During the course of the trial, participants are regularly seen by members of the research team to monitor their health and well-being. Participants also should be responsible for their own health by following the treatment plan (such as taking the proper dosage of medications on time), keeping all scheduled visits and informing members of the healthcare team about any symptoms that occur. If during the course of the trial, the treatment proves to be ineffective or harmful, the patient is free to leave the study and still obtain conventional care. Conversely, as soon as there is evidence that one treatment modality is better than another, all patients in the trial are given the benefit of the new information.

Questions to ask the sponsors about your rights as a participant in a clinical trial:

- Who is responsible for approving and monitoring this research?
  Is there an IRB?

- Who informs me about the trial process? Do I sign a consent form? Will I receive a copy?

- May I leave the trial at any time? Have previous patients dropped out? Why?

- Whom do I contact if I am experiencing any difficulty with this trial?

Enrolling In Clinical Trials

Each clinical trial has its own guidelines, called eligibility criteria, for determining who can participate. Treatment studies recruit participants who have a disease or other medical condition, while screening and prevention studies generally recruit healthy volunteers. Inclusion criteria (those that allow you to participate in a study) and exclusion criteria (those that keep you from participating in a study) ensure that the study will answer the research questions posed in the research protocol while maintaining the safety of participants. The disease being studied is a primary factor in selecting suitable patients, but other factors such as the patient's gender, age, treatment history and other diagnosed medical conditions may also be important. Unfortunately, eligibility also may depend upon ability to pay. Many health plans do not cover all of the costs associated with clinical trials because they define these trials as experimental procedures. However, trials sometimes pay volunteers for their time and/or reimburse them for travel, childcare, meals and lodging.

To prevent people who qualify from being excluded from clinical trials for financial reasons, agencies such as the National Cancer Institute are working with health plans to find solutions and a growing number of states require insurance companies to pay for all routine patient care costs in cancer trials. To encourage more senior citizens to participate in cancer trials, Medicare plans to revise its payment policy to cover those trials.

When choosing a clinical trial you should determine the factors that are most important to you. For instance, patients generally prefer to participate in trials near their homes so that they can maintain their usual day-to-day activities, be surrounded by family and friends and avoid travel and lodging costs. If travel or temporary relocation becomes necessary, try to find a trial site that is near to some family member or friend or one that is in a locale similar to your own city or town. Many organizations, such as the National Cancer Institute, will work with patients and their families to identify support networks for them wherever they participate.

Questions to ask the trial's sponsor about eligibility criteria:

- What are the inclusion and exclusion criteria for the clinical trial(s) I am considering?

- How can I improve my chances of being accepted?
  Can I change my health plan to one that will cover the trial's costs?
  Can I relocate to another city or state?

- If I am not eligible for one trial, what other trials are being conducted for my condition?

- Will I be paid for my time or reimbursed for my out-of-pocket expenses?

Participating In A Clinical Trial

Clinical trials are conducted by a research team led by a principal investigator (usually a physician) and are comprised of physicians, nurses and other health professionals such as social workers, psychologists and nutritionists. As a participant you may be required to commit a fair amount of time to a clinical trial, often more than with standard treatment. Initially, you will probably be given a physical examination and asked for your medical history. During the trial, you will have regular or periodic visits to the trial site which may include diagnostic and laboratory tests. You also may be asked to follow fixed schedules for medications and other interventions and to keep detailed records of your symptoms and health condition. Generally, clinical trials last from six to twenty-six weeks, though some (called maintenance trials) can last up to a year to determine if a treatment will prevent the relapse of a medical condition.

Participants in clinical trials should remain under the care of their regular physician(s) since clinical trials tend to provide short-term treatment for a specific medical condition and do not generally provide comprehensive primary care. In fact, some trials require that a patient's regular physician sign a consent form before the patient is enrolled. In addition, your regular physician can collaborate with the research team to make sure there are no adverse reactions between your other medications or treatments and the investigational treatment.

Questions to ask the research team or your physician about your role in a clinical trial:

- Who are the members of the health team?
  Who will be in charge of my care?

- How long will the trial last?

- How does treatment in the trial compare with or differ from the standard treatment?

- Will I be hospitalized? How often? For how long a period of time?

- What will occur during each visit?
  What treatments or procedures will I be given?

- Will I still be able to see my regular physician(s)?
  Will my doctor and the research team collaborate?

- Can I be put in touch with other patients who have participated in this trial?

Weighing The Benefits And Risks Of A Clinical Trial

If you are considering participation in a clinical trial, you need to consider the medical, emotional and financial ramifications of participation. Of course, the obvious benefit of a clinical trial is the chance that a new treatment may improve your health and prognosis. You will have access to drugs and other medical interventions before they are widely available to the public and you will obtain expert and specialized medical care at leading healthcare facilities. Many patients receive an added psychological benefit by taking an active role in their treatment.

It is important to bear in mind that some medical interventions used in clinical trials may carry potential risks depending upon the type of treatment and the patient's condition. While many side effects or adverse reactions are temporary (such as hair loss and nausea caused by some anti-cancer drugs), other more serious reactions can be permanent and even life-threatening (for example, heart, liver or kidney damage).

Deciding whether or not to participate in a clinical trial is often a matter of determining if the trial's potential benefits outweigh its possible risks. This is a highly personal decision that may be difficult to make in situations involving experimental treatment in which limited medical information may be available.

Questions to ask the research team about the benefits and risks of a clinical trial:

- What other treatment option(s) do I have at this time?
  Is there any chance that a more promising treatment may be available soon?

- What are the short and long-term benefits and risks as compared with standard treatment?

- Will I experience any known side effects or adverse reactions?
  Will these be temporary, long-term or permanent?
  Relatively minor or perhaps life-threatening?

- If I am harmed in any way by the new treatment, what other treatments will I be entitled to?
  Who will pay for subsequent treatment?

Getting Information On Clinical Trials

The more information you have about a clinical trial, the easier it will be to make a decision about whether or not it is right for you, and the more confident you will be that you made an appropriate decision. In addition to the "Selected Resources" appendix in this guide, the staff at your local public library, community hospital, or major medical center can assist you in locating the information you need from books, consumer organizations and on the Internet.

Learning About The National Institutes Of Health(NIH)

The National Institutes of Health (NIH) comprise one of the world's leading medical research centers and the Federal government's principal agency for biomedical research. An agency of the United States Department of Health, United States Public Health Service, NIH encompasses 25 separate institutions and centers with its main campus located in Bethesda, Maryland. Research is also conducted at several field units across the country and abroad.

Patient Care At The NIH

The Warren Grant Magnuson Clinical Center, NIH's principal medical research center and hospital located in Bethesda, Maryland, provides medical care only to patients participating in clinical research programs. Two categories of patients participate in the Clinical Center studies: children and adults who wish to improve their own health, such as those with newly diagnosed medical problems, ongoing medical problems or family history of disease; and healthy volunteers wishing to advance knowledge about the causes, progress and treatment of disease. The patient's case must fit into an ongoing NIH research project for which the patient has the precise kind or stage of illness under investigation. General diagnostic and treatment services common to community hospitals are not available.

The Magnuson Clinical Center is the world's largest biomedical research hospital and ambulatory care facility, housing 1,600 laboratories conducting basic and clinical research. There are 1,200 tenured physicians, dentists and researchers on staff along with 660 nurses and 570 allied healthcare professionals (dieticians, imaging technologists, medical technologists, medical records and clerical staff, pharmacists and therapists).

The Center's hospital is specially designed for medical research and accommodates 540 carefully selected patients who are participating in clinical research programs. Its 350-bed facility has 24 inpatient care units to which 7,000 patients are admitted annually. The Center also has an Ambulatory Care Research Facility (ACRF) that serves 68,000 outpatient visits each year. A new facility, called the Mark O. Hatfield Clinical Research Center, which began accepting patients in early 2005, has 242 beds for inpatient care and 90 day-hospital stations for outpatient care. The Mark O. Hatfield Center carries out the latest biomedical research that results in new forms of disease diagnosis, prevention and treatment, which is then incorporated into improved methods of patient care.

This is a fine example of Translational Medicine where excellent research discoveries are translated into new and improved methods of clinical treatment. In other words, the laboratory discoveries are brought to the bedside.

The Clinical Center also maintains a Children's Inn for pediatric outpatients and their families. This family-centered residence operates 24 hours a day, 7 days a week, 365 days a year.

In an effort to bring clinical research to the community, NIH supports approximately 80 General Clinical Research Centers (GCRCs) around the country, located within hospitals of major academic medical centers.

It is important to note that, as part of the federal government, the Warren Grant Magnuson Clinical Center provides treatment in clinical trials at no cost to its patients. In some cases, patients receive a stipend to help cover the costs of traveling to Bethesda for treatment and follow-up care. Travel costs for the initial screening visit, however, are not covered.

Areas Of Clinical Study At The NIH

At the Magnuson Clinical Center alone, NIH physician-scientists conduct nearly 1,000 studies each year. Among the areas of study are cancer and related diseases.

Not all of these clinical areas are under investigation at any given time, however. The Patient Recruitment and Public Liaison Office (PRPL) at the NIH Clinical Center assists patients, their families and their physicians in obtaining information about participation in NIH clinical trials. Trained nurses are available to answer questions about the research programs and admission procedures.

Cancer Care At The Warren Grant Magnuson Clinical Center

The National Cancer Institute (NCI) is the largest of the biomedical research institutes and centers at NIH. There, clinical studies are designed to evaluate new and promising ways to prevent, detect, diagnose and treat cancer. The Warren Grant Magnuson Clinical Center provides a separate outpatient division for cancer patients and also has several designated inpatient units.

If you are interested in entering a cancer study at the Magnuson Clinical Center (or at the General Clinical Research Centers), you should first discuss treatment options with a physician. As a general rule, patients interested in participating in clinical studies must be referred by a physician. However, in some instances, self-referral may be permitted.

Patients with medical problems other than cancer or healthy volunteers who wish to participate in a clinical study should contact the particular NIH institute responsible for the clinical area involved.

Cancer Care At The NCI Clinical Centers And Comprehensive Cancer Centers

You may also obtain clinical oncology services (education, screening, diagnosis or treatment) or participate in clinical trials at one of the 22 Cancer Centers or 39 Comprehensive Cancer Centers designated by the NCI for their scientific excellence and extensive resources devoted to cancer and cancer-related problems. Centers are located in 32 states, with the majority of sites in California, New York and Pennsylvania. You can find out about clinical trials at the NCI-designated centers by contacting NCI's Clinical Studies Support Center (CSSC) or by calling each center directly. Information about other cancer-related services at these centers also may be obtained from the center itself. For more information, you can visit the National Cancer Institute's website at www.cancer.gov.

How To Use This Guide

Locating A Specialist

This guide is organized to make finding the right specialists for you or your loved ones as simple as possible. Physicians' biographies are presented by specialty and are organized by geographic region within each specialty or subspecialty. Thus, you may search for a particular type of specialist or subspecialist in one or more regions or throughout the nation.

A second way to locate the right specialist is to use the "**Special Expertise Index**" beginning on page 1163. This index is organized according to diseases, conditions and procedures or techniques. For example, you can locate a top specialist for diabetes or for Mohs' surgery by looking for those terms in the "**Special Expertise Index.**"

If you already know a specialist's name, you can find his/her listing by using the "**Alphabetical Listing of Doctors**" beginning on page 1249.

SAMPLE PHYSICIAN LISTING

Smith, John MD [Ped] - **Spec Exp:** Asthma Allergy; **Hospital:** Children's Hosp (page 120);
Name [Specialty]   Special Expertise(s)   Admitting Hospital & Hospital
                                            Information Page

Address: 300 Ridge Road Boston, MA 12345; **Phone:** (617) 555-2343; **Board Cert:** Ped 75;
       Office Address   Office Phone   Board Certification(s)

Med School: Harvard Med Sch 70; **Resid:** Ped, Children's Hosp 73;
       Medical School   Residency(ies)

Fellow: AM, Children's Hosp 74; **Fac Appt:** Assoc Prof Ped, The Med Sch
       Fellowship(s)   Faculty Appointment

Geographic Regions And States

To assist you in using Castle Connolly *America's Top Doctors*® in the most efficient and effective manner, the Guide is divided into seven geographic regions. This will help you to locate a specialist in your local or neighboring region. For example, if you live in Mississippi in the Southeast region and you are willing and able to travel to Louisiana in the Southwest region to consult with a specialist in neurology, you can review just those two regions, under the section headed "NEUROLOGY." However, if you prefer to review the information on neurologists throughout the country, you can search the entire neurology section. Or, you can consult the "SPECIAL EXPERTISE INDEX" in the back of this Guide and choose a neurologist who has specific expertise to meet your particular needs.

The geographic regions are as follows:

New England

Mid Atlantic

Southeast

Midwest

Great Plains and Mountains

Southwest

West Coast and Pacific

The states that are included in each region are listed on the following page and a map of the regions is also provided. Please note that not all regions are represented in all specialties. For example, in "Geriatric Psychiatry" there are no listings in the Southwest region.

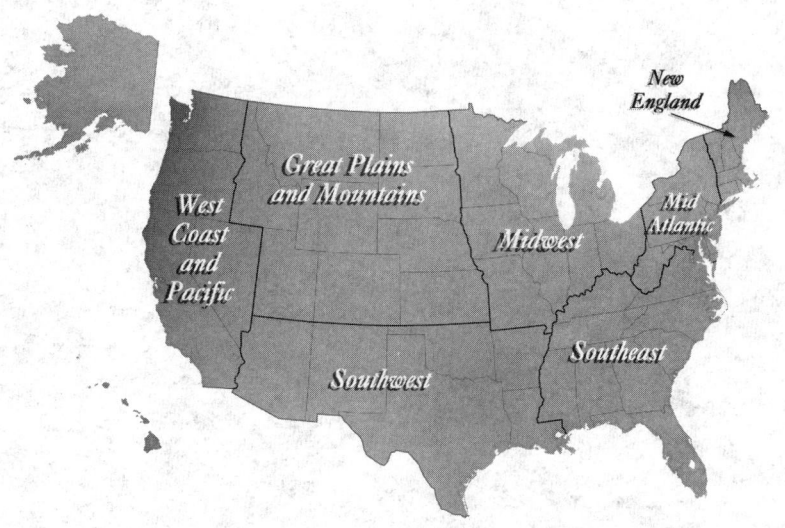

West Coast and Pacific:
Alaska
California
Hawaii
Nevada
Oregon
Washington

Great Plains and Mountains:
Colorado
Idaho
Kansas
Montana
Nebraska
North Dakota
South Dakota
Utah
Wyoming

Southwest:
Arizona
Arkansas
Louisiana
New Mexico
Oklahoma
Texas

Midwest:
Illinois
Indiana
Iowa
Michigan
Minnesota
Missouri
Ohio
Wisconsin

New England:
Connecticut
Maine
Massachusetts
New Hampshire
Rhode Island
Vermont

Mid Atlantic:
Delaware
Maryland
New Jersey
New York
Pennsylvania
Washington, DC
West Virginia

Southeast:
Alabama
Florida
Georgia
Kentucky
Mississippi
North Carolina
South Carolina
Tennessee
Virginia

Medical Specialties

In the pages that follow, each list of doctors in a medical specialty or subspecialty is preceded by a brief description of that specialty (or subspecialty) and the training required for board certification.

Critical Care Medicine has been excluded because in emergency situations there is neither time nor opportunity for choice. A number of other specialities not relevant to most patients (e.g., Forensic Psychiatry) have not been included as well.

The following descriptions of medical specialties and subspecialties were provided by the American Board of Medical Specialties (ABMS), an organization comprised of the 24 medical specialty boards that provide certification in 25 medical specialties. A complete listing of all specialists certified by the ABMS can be found in *The Official ABMS Directory of Board Certified Medical Specialists*, and is published by *Marquis Who's Who*. It is available (either in a multi-volume directory or on CD-ROM) in most public libraries, hospital libraries, university libraries and medical libraries. The ABMS also operates a toll-free phone line at 1-866-275-2267 and a website at www.abms.org to verify the certification status of individual doctors.

The following important policy statement, approved by the ABMS Assembly on March 19, 1987, remains valid.

The Purpose Of Certification

The intent of the certification process, as defined by the member boards of the American Board of Medical Specialties, is to provide assurance to the public that a certified medical specialist has successfully completed an approved educational program and an evaluation, including an examination process designed to assess the knowledge, experience and skills requisite to the provision of high quality patient care in that specialty.

Medical Specialties

Medical Specialty and Subspecialty Descriptions and Abbreviations

The following medical specialties and subspecialties are indicated in the doctors' listings by their abbreviations. Specialties are indicated in bold, subspecialties in italics, and the four primary care specialties in bold capitals. To review the official American Board of Medical Specialties (ABMS) organization of specialties, refer to Appendix A.

Addiction Psychiatry *AdP*

Deals with habitual psychological and physiological dependence on a substance or practice which is beyond voluntary control.

Adolescent Medicine *AM*

Involves the primary care treatment of adolescents and young adults.

Allergy & Immunology **A&I**

Diagnosis and treatment of allergies, asthma, and skin problems such as hives and contact dermatitis.

Anesthesiology **Anes**

Provides pain relief in maintenance or restoration of a stable condition during and following an operation. Anesthesiologists also diagnose and treat acute and long standing pain problems.

Cardiac Electrophysiology (Clinical) *CE*

Involves complicated technical procedures to evaluate heart rhythms and determine appropriate treatment for them.

Cardiovascular Disease *Cv*

Involves the diagnosis and treatment of disorders of the heart, lungs, and blood vessels.

Child & Adolescent Psychiatry *ChAP*

Deals with the diagnosis and treatment of mental diseases in children and adolescents.

Child Neurology *ChiN*

Diagnosis and medical treatment of disorders of the brain, spinal cord, and nervous system in children.

Clinical Genetics **CG**

Deals with identifying the genetic causes of inherited diseases and ailments and preventing, when possible, their occurrence.

Colon and Rectal Surgery **CRS**

Surgical treatment of diseases of the intestinal tract, colon and rectum, anal canal, and perianal area.

Critical Care Medicine *CCM*

Involves diagnosing and taking immediate action to prevent death or further injury of a patient. Examples of critical injuries include shock, heart attack, drug overdose, and massive bleeding.

Dermatology   **D**

Diagnosis and treatment of benign and malignant disorders of the skin, mouth, external genitalia, hair and nails, as well as a number of sexually transmitted diseases.

Diagnostic Radiology   *DR*

Involves the study of all modalities of radiant energy in medical diagnoses and therapeutic procedures utilizing radiologic guidance.

Endocrinology, Diabetes & Metabolism   *EDM*

Involves the study and treatment of patients suffering from hormonal and chemical disorders.

FAMILY MEDICINE   **FP**

Deals with and oversees the total healthcare of individual patients and their family members. Family practitioners are more common in rural areas and may perform procedures more commonly performed by specialists (e.g., minor surgery).

Forensic Psychiatry   *FPsy*

Concerns the evaluation of certain diagnostic groups of patients that include those with sexual disorders, antisocial personality disorders, paranoid disorders, and addictive disorders.

Gastroenterology   *Ge*

The study, diagnosis and treatment of diseases of the digestive organs including the stomach, bowels, liver, and gallbladder.

Geriatric Medicine   *Ger*

Deals with diseases of the elderly and the problems associated with aging.

Geriatric Psychiatry   *GerPsy*

Involves the diagnosis, prevention, and treatment of mental illness in the elderly.

Gynecologic Oncology   *GO*

Deals with cancers of the female genital tract and reproductive systems.

Hand Surgery   *HS*

Involves the treatment of injury to the hand through surgical techniques.

Hematology   *Hem*

Involves the diagnosis and treatment of diseases and disorders of the blood, bone marrow, spleen, and lymph glands.

Infectious Disease   *Inf*

The study and treatment of diseases caused by a bacterium, virus, fungus, or animal parasite.

INTERNAL MEDICINE   **IM**

Diagnosis and nonsurgical treatment of diseases, especially those of adults. Internists may act as primary care specialists, highly trained family doctors, or they may subspecialize in specialties such as cardiology or nephrology.

Maternal & Fetal Medicine   *MF*

Involves the care of women with high-risk pregnancies and their unborn fetuses.

Medical Specialties

Medical Oncology   *Onc*

Refers to the study and treatment of tumors and other cancers.

Neonatal-Perinatal Medicine   *NP*

Involves the diagnosis and treatments of infants prior to, during, and one month beyond birth.

Nephrology   *Nep*

Concerned with disorders of the kidneys, high blood pressure, fluid and mineral balance, dialysis of body wastes when the kidneys do not function, and consultation with surgeons about kidney transplantation.

Neurological Surgery   **NS**

Involves surgery of the brain, spinal cord, and nervous system.

Neurology   **N**

Diagnosis and medical treatment of disorders of the brain, spinal cord, and nervous system.

Neuroradiology   *NRad*

Involves the utilization of imaging procedures during diagnosis as they relate to the brain, spine and spinal cord, head, neck, and organs of special sense in adults and children.

Nuclear Medicine   **NuM**

Evaluation of the functions of all the organs in the body and treatment of thyroid disease, benign and malignant tumors, and radiation exposure through the use of radioactive substances.

Nuclear Radiology   *NR*

Involves the use of radioactive substances to diagnose and treat certain functions and diseases of the body.

OBSTETRICS & GYNECOLOGY   **ObG**

Deals with the medical aspects of and intervention in pregnancy and labor and the overall health of the female reproductive system.

Occupational Medicine   *OM*

Concentrates on the effect of the work environment on the health of employees.

Ophthalmology   **Oph**

Diagnosis and treatment of diseases of and injuries to the eye.

Orthopaedic Surgery   **OrS**

Involves operations to correct injuries which interfere with the form and function of the extremities, spine, and associated structures.

Otolaryngology   **Oto**

Explores and treats diseases in the interrelated areas of the ears, nose and throat.

Otology/Neurotology   *ON*

Concentrates on the management, prevention, cure and care of patients with diseases of the ear and temporal bone, including disorders of hearing and balance.

Pain Medicine   *PM*

Involves providing a high level of care for patients experiencing problems with acute or chronic pain in both hospital and ambulatory settings.

Pediatric Cardiology   *PCd*

Involves the diagnosis and treatment of heart disease in children.

Pediatric Critical Care Medicine   *PCCM*

Involves the care of children who are victims of life threatening disorders such as severe accidents, shock, and diabetes acidosis.

Pediatric Dermatology   *PD*

Diagnosis and treatment of benign and malignant disorders of the skin, mouth, external genitalia, hair and nails in children.

Pediatric Endocrinology   *PEn*

Involves the study and treatment of children with hormonal and chemical disorders.

Pediatric Gastroenterology   *PGe*

The study, diagnosis, and treatment of diseases of the digestive tract in children.

Pediatric Hematology-Oncology   *PHO*

The study and treatment of cancers of the blood and blood-forming parts of the body in children.

Pediatric Infectious Disease   *PInf*

The study and treatment of diseases caused by a virus, bacterium, fungus, or animal parasite in children.

Pediatric Nephrology   *PNep*

Deals with the diagnosis and treatment of disorders of the kidneys in children.

Pediatric Otolaryngology   *POto*

Involves the diagnosis and treatment of disorders of the ear, nose, and throat which affect children.

Pediatric Pulmonology   *PPul*

Involves the diagnosis and treatment of diseases of the chest, lungs, and chest tissue in children.

Pediatric Radiology   *PR*

Involves diagnostic imaging as it pertains to the newborn, infant, child, and adolescent.

Pediatric Rheumatology   *PRhu*

Involves the treatment of diseases of the joints and connective tissues in children.

Pediatric Surgery   *PS*

Treatment of disease, injury, or deformity in children through surgical techniques.

PEDIATRICS   **Ped**

Diagnosis and treatment of diseases of childhood and monitoring of the growth, development, and well-being of preadolescents.

Medical Specialties

Physical Medicine & Rehabilitation   **PMR**

The use of physical therapy and physical agents such as water, heat, light electricity, and mechanical manipulations in the diagnosis, treatment, and prevention of disease and body disorders.

Plastic Surgery   **PlS**

Involves reconstructive and cosmetic surgery of the face and other body parts.

Preventive Medicine   **PrM**

A specialty focusing on the prevention of illness and on the health of groups rather than individuals.

Psychiatry   **Psyc**

Examination, treatment, and prevention of mental illness through the use of psychoanalysis and/or drugs.

Public Health & General Preventive Medicine   *PHGPM*

Involves the investigation of the causes of epidemic disease and the prevention of a wide variety of acute and chronic illness.

Pulmonary Disease   *Pul*

Involves the diagnosis and treatment of diseases of the chest, lungs, and airways.

Radiation Oncology   *RadRo*

Involves the use of radiant energy and isotopes in the study and treatment of disease, especially malignant cancer.

Reproductive Endocrinology   *RE*

Deals with the endocrine system (including the pituitary, thyroid, parathyroid, adrenal glands, placenta, ovaries, and testes) and how its failure relates to infertility.

Rheumatology   *Rhu*

Involves the treatment of diseases of the joints, muscles, bones and associated structures.

Sleep Medicine   *Sleep Med*

Involves the investigation and treatment of patients with sleep disorders.

Spinal Cord Injury Medicine   *SpCdInj*

Involves the prevention, diagnosis, treatment and management of traumatic spinal cord injuries.

Sports Medicine   *SM*

Refers to the practice of an orthopaedist or other physician who specializes in injuries to the bone or other soft tissues (muscles, tendons, ligaments) caused by participation in athletic activity.

Surgery   **S**

Treatment of disease, injury, and deformity by surgical procedures.

Surgery of the Hand   *SHd*

Involves providing appropriate care for all structures in the upper extremity directly affecting the hand and wrist function.

Surgical Critical Care   *SCC*

Involves specialized care in the management of the critically ill patient, particularly the trauma victim and postoperative patient in the emergency department, intensive care unit, trauma unit, burn unit, and other similar settings.

Thoracic Surgery (includes open heart surgery)   **TS**

Involves surgery on the heart, lungs, and chest area.

Urology   **U**

Diagnosis and treatment of diseases of the genitals in men and disorders of the urinary tract and bladder in both men and women.

Vascular & Interventional Radiology   *VIR*

Involves diagnosing and treating diseases by percutaneous methods guided by various radiologic imaging modalities.

Vascular Surgery   *VascS*

Involves the operative treatment of disorders of the blood vessels excluding those to the heart, lungs, or brain.

The Training Of A Specialist

Excerpted from "Which Medical Specialist For You?" American Board of Medical Specialties, Evanston, IL, Revised 2000

Everyone knows that a "medical doctor" is a physician who has had years of training to understand the diagnosis, treatment and prevention of disease. The basic training for a physician specialist includes four years of premedical education in a college or university, four years of medical school, and after receiving the M.D. degree, at least three years of specialty training under supervision (called a "residency"). Training in subspecialties can take an additional one to three years.

Some specialists are primary care doctors such as family physicians, general internists and general pediatricians. Other specialists concentrate on certain body systems, specific age groups, or complex scientific techniques developed to diagnose or treat certain types of disorders. Specialties in medicine developed because of the rapidly expanding body of knowledge about health and illness and the constantly evolving new treatment techniques for disease.

A subspecialist is a physician who has completed training in a general medical specialty and then takes additional training in a more specific area of that specialty called a subspecialty. This training increases the depth of knowledge and expertise of the specialist in that particular field. For example, cardiology is a subspecialty of internal medicine, pediatric surgery is a subspecialty of surgery and pediatrics, and child and adolescent psychiatry is a subspecialty of psychiatry. The training of a subspecialist within a specialty requires an additional one or more years of full-time education.

The training, or residency, of a specialist begins after the doctor has received the M.D. degree from a medical school. Resident physicians dedicate themselves for three to seven years to full-time experience in hospital and/or ambulatory care settings, caring for patients under the supervision of experienced specialists. Educational conferences and research experience are often part of that training. In years past, the first year of post-medical school training was called an internship, but is now called residency.

Licensure

The legal privilege to practice medicine is governed by state law and is not designed to recognize the knowledge and skills of a trained specialist. A physician is licensed to practice general medicine and surgery by a state board of medical examiners after passing a state or national licensure examination. Each state or territory has its own procedures to license physicians and sets the general standards for all physicians in that state or territory.

Who Credentials A Specialist And Subspecialist?

Specialty boards certify physicians as having met certain published standards. There are 24 specialty boards that are recognized by the American Board of Medical Specialties (ABMS) and the American Medical Association (AMA). All of the specialties and subspecialties recognized by the ABMS and the AMA are listed in the brief descriptions that follow. Remember, a subspecialist first must be trained and certified as a specialist.

In order to be certified as a medical specialist by one of these recognized boards a physician must complete certain requirements. Generally, these include:

1 Completion of a course of study leading to the M.D. or D.O. (Doctor of Osteopathy) degree from a recognized school of medicine.

2 Completion of three to seven years of full-time training in an accredited residency program designed to train specialists in the field.

3 Many specialty boards require assessments and documentation of individual performance from the residency training director, or from the chief of service in the hospital where the specialist has practiced.

4 All of the ABMS Member Boards require that a person seeking certification have an unrestricted license to practice medicine in order to take the certification examination.

5 Finally, each candidate for certification must pass a written examination given by the specialty board. Fifteen of the 24 specialty boards also require an oral examination conducted by senior specialists in that field. Candidates who have passed the exams and other requirements are then given the status of "Diplomate" and are certified as specialists. A similar process is followed for specialists who want to become subspecialists.

All of the ABMS Member Boards now, or will soon, issue only time-limited certificates which are valid for six to ten years. In order to retain certification, diplomates must become "recertified," and must periodically go through an additional process involving continuing education in the specialty, review of credentials and further examination. Boards that may not yet require recertification have provided voluntary recertification with similar requirements.

How To Determine If A Physician Is A Certified Specialist

Certified specialists are listed in *The Official ABMS Directory of Board Certified Medical Specialists* published by *Marquis Who's Who*. The ABMS Directory can be found in most public libraries, hospital libraries, university libraries and medical libraries, and is also available on CD-ROM. Alternatively, you could ask for that information from your county medical society, the American Board of Medical Specialties, or one of the specialty boards.

The ABMS operates a toll free number (1-866-275-2267) to verify the certification status of individual physicians. Additionally, information about the ABMS organization and links to an electronic directory of certified specialists can be accessed through the ABMS Web site at www.abms.org.

Almost all board certified specialists also are members of their medical specialty societies. These societies are dedicated to furthering standards, practice and professional and public education within individual medical specialties. Some, such as the American College of Surgeons and the American College of Obstetricians and Gynecologists, require board certification for full membership. A physician who has attained full membership is called a "Fellow" of the society and is entitled to use this designation in all formal communications such as certificates, publications, business cards, stationery and signage. Thus, "John Doe, M.D., F.A.C.S." (Fellow of the American College of Surgeons) is a board certified surgeon. Similarly, F.A.A.D. (Fellow of the American Academy of Dermatology) following the M.D. or D.O. in a physician's title would likely indicate board certification in that specialty.

The Partnership For Excellence Program

Among the more than 6,000 acute care and specialty hospitals in the United States, many have extraordinary capabilities for superior patient care. These hospitals, renowned for their use of state-of-the-art equipment and up-to-the-minute technology, also attract outstanding physicians and other healthcare professionals. Many of their physicians are among those in the listings in this Guide.

To assist you in your search for top specialists and to supplement the information contained in the physician listings that follow, we invited a select group of these fine institutions to profile their services, special programs and centers of excellence in the *Partnership for Excellence* program. This special section contains pages sponsored by the included hospitals. This paid sponsorship program is totally separate from the physician selection process, which is based upon nominations by physicians and a completely independent review by our physician led research team.

The *Partnership for Excellence* program provides an overview of the programs and services offered by the included hospitals with information related to their accreditation and sponsorship. Most also provide their physician referral numbers, should you wish to ask the hospitals for recommendations of doctors not listed in Castle Connolly *America's Top Doctors* ® 9th Edition.

In addition to the *Partnership for Excellence* program, profiled hospitals were also invited to highlight their special programs or services that focus on a particular disease or medical condition. These can be found in the "Centers of Excellence" sections that are interspersed throughout this book following the medical specialties and/or subspecialties to which they relate. Sponsored pages in the centers of excellence sections reflect the depth of commitment of these hospitals, which provide the staff, resources and financial support necessary to develop these special programs.

By visiting our website **www.CastleConnolly.com**, you may also link to the websites of these outstanding hospitals for even more detailed information on their cancer programs. We believe you will find this informaton helpful in your search for the best healthcare—from both physicians and hospitals—through out the United States!

Participating Hospitals

- Bascom Palmer Eye Institute

- Cleveland Clinic

- Continuum Health Partners

- Fox Chase Cancer Center

- Hospital for Special Surgery

- Hospital of the University of Pennsylvania - UPHS

- The Johns Hopkins Hospital

- Lenox Hill Hospital

- Maimonides Medical Center

- Mount Sinai Medical Center

- New York Eye & Ear Infirmary

- New York-Presbyterian Hospital

- NYU Cancer Institute

- NYU Langone Medical Center

- NYU Hospital for Joint Diseases

- Rusk Institute of Rehabilitation Medicine

- St. Francis Hospital -The Heart Center

- UHealth University of Miami Health System

- UHealth University of Miami Hospital

- Wake Forest University Baptist Medical Center

INTERNATIONALLY ACCLAIMED

Bascom Palmer Eye Institute is committed to the protection and preservation of the treasured gift of sight and is recognized as one of the world's finest and most progressive centers for ophthalmic care, vision research, and education. Each of our 65 clinical faculty members specializes in a specific area of ophthalmology and is board-certified by the American Board of Ophthalmology. In addition to providing care to more than 250,000 patients annually, all clinical faculty members have research and teaching responsibilities at the University of Miami Miller School of Medicine.

BASCOM PALMER EYE INSTITUTE RANKED #1 IN USA

Bascom Palmer continues to be ranked the nation's best ophthalmic hospital by board-certified ophthalmologists from across the United States. In 2009, it was ranked #1 in ophthalmology by *U.S. News & World Report* for the sixth consecutive year; and #1 in the nation for Clinical (Patient Care) and its Residency program by *Ophthalmology Times*.

BASCOM PALMER RESEARCHERS ADVANCE OPHTHALMIC CARE AND TREATMENT

Consistent with its mission to resolve diseases and disorders of the eye, the physicians and scientists of Bascom Palmer Eye Institute develop new theories, therapeutic techniques, and surgical instruments. Many of the institute's innovations have advanced the course of ophthalmic practices worldwide, including:

- Discovering a new treatment for wet macular degeneration and introducing the use of bevacizumab (Avastin) as a remarkable breakthrough therapy.
- Performing the nation's first modified osteo-odonto-keratoprosthesis using a blind patient's eyetooth to restore sight.
- Alerting ophthalmologists around the world of fungal infections affecting contact lens users, significantly reducing the number of new infections.
- Performing the first successful vitreous surgery – and inventing miniature surgical instrumentation required for this procedure.
- Unraveling the mystery of normal tension glaucoma.
- Establishing predictive tests and new treatments for complicated retinal detachments.

To schedule an appointment please call (800) 329-7000 or visit www.bascompalmer.org.

Miami:	Palm Beach Gardens:	Naples:	Plantation:
900 NW 17th Street	7101 Fairway Drive,	311 9th Street North	1000 South Pine Island Road
Miami, FL 33136	Palm Beach Gardens, FL 33418	Naples, FL 34102	Plantation, FL 33324
(305) 326-6000	(561) 515-1500	(239) 659-3937	(954) 465-2700

Cleveland Clinic

Hospital Overview

One of the largest and busiest health centers in America. Number one in heart care. National leaders in urology, rheumatology and digestive diseases. Treating all illnesses and disorders of the body. Second opinions a specialty.

General Overview

Founded in 1921, Cleveland Clinic is a 1,000-staffed-bed hospital that integrates clinical and hospital care with research and education in a private, non-profit group practice. This group practice model provides an environment that allows our physicians to stay at the cutting edge of medical technology. They pool their expertise and their wisdom for the benefit of the patient and the community.

Vital Statistics

In 2008, more than 1,800 full-time physicians and scientists, representing 120 medical specialties and subspecialties, provided for more than 3 million outpatient visits, 50,000 hospital admissions and 73,500 surgeries for patients from throughout the United States and more than 80 countries.

One of America's Best

In 2009, Cleveland Clinic was ranked one of the top 4 hospitals in America in the *U.S. News & World Report* annual "America's Best Hospitals" survey. In cardiology and cardiac surgery, we lead the nation. Our heart program has been ranked number one in America for 15 years in a row. Cleveland Clinic's Urology, Rheumatology and Digestive Disease programs are ranked second in the nation. Additional specialties rated among America's best include Cancer, Endocrinology, Geriatric Care, Gynecology, Nephrology, Neurology and Neurological Surgery, Ophthalmology, Orthopaedics, Otolaryngology and Pulmonary.

Global Patient Services

Global Patient Services is a full-service department dedicated to meeting the needs of both our out-of-state and international patients. The National Center and the International Center, which make up Global Patient Services, provide personalized concierge programs and services to welcome patients and add to their comfort before, during and after their stay.

For more information about Cleveland Clinic, to schedule a second opinion or to learn about assistance for out-of-town patients, call 800.890.2467 or visit www.clevelandclinic.org/topdocs.

Cleveland Clinic | 9500 Euclid Avenue / AC311 | Cleveland OH 44195

"Better care of the sick, investigation of their problems and further education of those who serve."

"Patients First"

"Patients First" is the guiding principle of Cleveland Clinic. It declares the primacy of patient care, patient comfort and patient communication in every activity we undertake. It affirms the importance of research and education for their contributions to clinical medicine and the improvement of patient care. At the same time, "Patients First" demands a relentless focus on measurable quality. By setting standards, collecting data and analyzing the results, Cleveland Clinic puts patients first through improved outcomes and better service, providing a healthier future for all.

Beth Israel · **Roosevelt Hospital** · **St. Luke's Hospital** · **Long Island College Hospital** · **NY Eye & Ear Infirmary**

Sponsorship: Voluntary Not-for-profit   **Beds:** 2,727 certified beds
Accreditation: Joint Commission of Accreditation of Healthcare Organizations (JCAHO), Accreditation Council for Graduate Medical Education, Medical Society of New York, in conjunction with the Accreditation Council for Continuing Medical Education

A STRONG PARTNERSHIP WITH A PROUD HERITAGE

Continuum Health Partners is a partnership of six venerable health care providers: Beth Israel Medical Center-Milton and Carroll Petrie Division, Beth Israel Medical Center-Kings Highway Division, St. Luke's Hospital, Roosevelt Hospital, Long Island College Hospital of Brooklyn, and The New York Eye and Ear Infirmary. Each of the six partner institutions was established more than a century ago by individuals committed to improving health and health care in their communities. Today, the system represents over 4,000 physicians and dentists and is superbly equipped to respond to the health care needs of the populations we serve. Our providers also see patients in group and private practice settings and in ambulatory centers in New York City and Westchester County.

LOCATIONS

Continuum Health Partners has campuses throughout Manhattan and Brooklyn. Beth Israel Medical Center has two divisions: the Milton and Caroll Petrie Division on the East Side, and the Kings Highway Division in Brooklyn. The Phillips Ambulatory Care Center, a state-of-art outpatient center, is located at Union Square. St. Luke's Hospital is in Morningside Heights and Roosevelt Hospital is in the Columbus Circle and Lincoln Center neighborhoods on the West Side. Long Island College Hospital of Brooklyn is located in the Brooklyn Heights/Cobble Hill section of Brooklyn. The New York Eye and Ear Infirmary is located on Second Avenue and 14th street.

ACADEMIC AFFILIATIONS

Beth Israel Medical Center is the University Hospital and Manhattan Campus for the Albert Einstein College of Medicine. St. Luke's-Roosevelt Hospital Center is an Academic Affiliate of Columbia University College of Physicians and Surgeons. Long Island College Hospital of Brooklyn is the primary teaching affiliate of the SUNY-Health Science Center in Brooklyn. The New York Eye and Ear Infirmary is the primary teaching center of the New York Medical College and affiliated teaching hospitals in the areas of ophthalmology and otolaryngology.

For a referral to a great doctor in your neighborhood, call (800) 420-4004. Our Physician Referral Service can help you find a primary care physician or specialist affiliated with Beth Israel, St. Luke's, Roosevelt, Long Island College Hospital, or The New York Eye and Ear Infirmary. Visit our Website at www.chpnyc.org

FOX CHASE
CANCER CENTER

333 Cottman Avenue
Philadelphia, PA 19111-2497
Phone: 1-888-FOX CHASE
www.fccc.edu

Sponsorship	Independent Nonprofit
Beds	100 licensed beds
Accreditation	The Joint Commission; American Hospital Association; American College of Surgeons Commission on Cancer; College of American Pathology; American College of Radiology

U.S. News & World Report consistently ranks Fox Chase Cancer Center among the nation's best. Fox Chase is also the first hospital in Pennsylvania and the nation's first cancer hospital to earn the Magnet Award for Nursing Excellence from the American Nurses Credentialing Center.

Overview

Fox Chase Cancer Center is one of the leading cancer research and treatments centers in the United States. Founded in 1904 in Philadelphia as one of the nation's first cancer hospitals, Fox Chase was also among the first institutions to be designated a National Cancer Institute Comprehensive Cancer Center in 1974. Fox Chase researchers have won the highest awards in their fields, including two Nobel Prizes. Fox Chase physicians are also routinely recognized in national rankings, and the Center's nursing program has received the Magnet status for excellence three consecutive times. Today, Fox Chase conducts a broad array of nationally competitive basic, translational, and clinical research, with special programs in cancer prevention, detection, survivorship, and community outreach.

- Fox Chase's 100-bed hospital is one of the few in the country devoted entirely to adult cancer care.
- Annual hospital admissions exceed 4,500 and outpatient visits to physicians total more than 75,000 a year.
- Fox Chase's board-certified specialists are recognized nationally and internationally in medical, radiation and surgical oncology, diagnostic imaging, diagnostic pathology, pain management, oncology nursing and oncology social work.
- The staff provides a coordinated approach to meet the treatment needs of each patient. Special multidisciplinary centers provide consultations and treatment recommendations for specific types of cancer.
- The nursing staff of specially trained oncology nurses provides one of the best nurse-to-patient ratios in the area.
- Fox Chase investigators have received numerous awards and honors, including Nobel Prizes in medicine and chemistry; a Kyoto Prize, a Lasker Clinical Research Award, memberships in the National Academy of Sciences and General Motors Cancer Research Foundation Prizes.
- Fox Chase is a founding member of the National Comprehensive Cancer Network, an alliance of the nation's leading academic cancer centers, and the hub of Fox Chase Cancer Center Partners, a select group of more than 22 community hospitals with Fox Chase-affiliated cancer programs.

For more about Fox Chase physicians and services, visit our web site, www.fccc.edu, or call 1-888-FOX CHASE.

HOSPITAL FOR SPECIAL SURGERY

HOSPITAL
FOR
SPECIAL
SURGERY

535 East 70th Street • New York, NY 10021
Physician Referral: 800.854.0071 • www.HSS.edu

Specialists in Mobility

Sponsorship: Private, Non-Profit
Beds: 162
Accreditation: The Joint Commission
Web Site: HSS.edu

FIRST IN ITS FIELD
Founded in 1863, Hospital for Special Surgery is a leading specialty
hospital for orthopedics and rheumatology.

FIRST IN JOINT REPLACEMENTS
HSS performs more knee replacements and more hip surgeries than
any other hospital in the nation. HSS pioneered designs and surgical
techniques for the first modern total knee replacement in the 1970's
and has been leading total knee replacement ever since.

PIONEERING MINIMALLY INVASIVE SURGERY
HSS surgeons pioneered the techniques, special instruments, and
smaller implants that made minimally invasive total hip and knee
replacements possible. HSS also pioneered minimally invasive spine surgery techniques that reduce
the need for spinal fusion. With 28 state-of-the-art Musculoskeletal Operating Rooms, HSS is a world
leader in orthopedic surgery, performing over 22,000 procedures per year. HSS anesthesiologists, world
leaders in regional anesthesia, developed special pain blocks required for minimally invasive surgery.
HSS surgeons are innovators in hand, elbow, shoulder, and spine surgery techniques and are leading
experts in arthroscopy and hip preservation.

GLOBAL LEADERS IN RHEUMATOLOGY
HSS rheumatologists are international authorities and pioneering researchers in all rheumatological
and autoimmune conditions and treatments, including lupus, rheumatoid arthritis, juvenile
rheumatoid arthritis, osteoarthritis, scleroderma, gout, uveitis, and Antiphospholipid Syndrome.
Cutting edge research and treatment centers include the Mary Kirkland Center for Lupus Research,
the Barbara Volcker Center for Women and Rheumatic Diseases, the Scleroderma Center, and the
Gosden Robinson Inflammatory Arthritis Center.

WORLD'S MOST EXPERIENCED MUSCULOSKELETAL RADIOLOGISTS
HSS is the world's largest academic center dedicated to musculoskeletal imaging. HSS developed
the landmark MRI pulse-sequencing techniques that reveal early degenerative changes in cartilage.
HSS innovations in Ultrasound and MRI allow earlier diagnosis of autoimmune conditions, arthritis,
and joint implant loosening.

HSS.edu

Every
Musculoskeletal
Specialty.

One Innovative
Web Site.

Top Ranked in the Northeast in Orthopedics & Rheumatology by *U.S.News & World Report* **for 19 Consecutive Years**	**A National Institutes of Health Core Center for Musculoskeletal Repair and Regeneration**
Two Time Recipient of Nursing's Highest Honor: Magnet Status	**Team Physicians and Athletic Trainers for: NY Mets, NY Giants, NY Knicks, NY Liberty, NY Red Bulls, Nets Basketball, St. John's Athletics, CUNY Athletic Conference, Association of Tennis Professionals, US Rowing, USA Swimming and other Professional and College Teams**
#1 Hospital in NYC in a Study on Patient Satisfaction by *Consumer Reports*	

Penn Medicine

OVERVIEW

For more than two centuries, Penn physicians and scientists have been committed to the highest standards of patient care, education and research. That commitment has been recognized throughout the greater Philadelphia region and across the nation.

Penn Medicine received $390 million in research grant funding from the National Institutes of Health in 2008, with several departments ranking first nationally. Overall, Penn has more individual departments ranked in the top five than any other academic medical center. *U.S.News & World Report* also consistently ranks Penn Medicine, the University of Pennsylvania Schools of Medicine and Nursing among the nation's best.

What Sets Penn Apart?

Penn's physicians and scientists are united in the health system's mission to expand the frontiers of medicine through new discoveries in the detection, treatment and prevention of human disease. Because they develop and test new treatments through clinical trials, their patients gain access to the very latest advances and future generations will benefit from the work they do today.

Penn continues to lead the way in discovering new treatment methods for diseases once considered incurable, including groundbreaking research in cancer, cardiac, neurosciences, orthopaedics, genetics and imaging.
Over the past 30 years, Penn physicians and scientists have participated in many important discoveries, including:

- The first general vaccine against pneumonia.

- The introduction of total intravenous feeding.

- The development of cognitive therapy.

- The development of magnetic resonance imaging and other imaging technologies.

- The discovery of the Philadelphia chromosome, which revolutionized cancer research by making the connection between genetic abnormalities and cancer.

- The development of a cure for atrial fibrillation.

- Pioneering new procedures in robotic-assisted surgery.

Locations

Patients are seen at:

- Hospital of the University of Pennsylvania
- Penn Presbyterian Medical Center
- Pennsylvania Hospital
- Penn Medicine at Bucks County
- Penn Medicine at Cherry Hill
- Penn Medicine at Radnor
- Penn Medicine at Rittenhouse
- PennCare, a primary care physician network, provides services in the local communities in Bucks, Chester, Delaware, Montgomery and Philadelphia counties in Pennsylvania and in Southern New Jersey.
- Hospice and home care services are provided by Penn Home Care and Hospice Services.

On the Web

Visit PennMedicine.org for the latest patient education with explanation of surgical procedures and follow-up care, screening tools, drug interactions and descriptions as well as an encyclopedia of health information.

To learn more about Penn physicians or services, call 800.789.PENN or visit PennMedicine.org

JOHNS HOPKINS
MEDICINE

600 North Wolfe Street, Baltimore Maryland 21287
www.hopkinsmedicine.org

Johns Hopkins Medicine unites physicians and scientists of the Johns Hopkins University School of Medicine with the organizations, health professionals and facilities of the Johns Hopkins Health System, including the world-renowned Johns Hopkins Hospital. All share a single mission: to improve the health of the community and the world by setting the standard of excellence in medical education, research and clinical care.

We heal. Ranked as America's top hospital year after year by *U.S. News & World Report*, The Johns Hopkins Hospital and its related facilities serve as beacons of hope for thousands of patients in our community, in our nation and throughout the world.

We discover. Research is the foundation of clinical care. Johns Hopkins physicians and researchers consistently receive more research grants from the National Institutes of Health than faculty at any other institution. Johns Hopkins has been home to four Nobel laureates, 11 Lasker awardees, 12 National Academy of Sciences members and 32 members of the Institute of Medicine.

We teach. The Johns Hopkins University School of Medicine educates and trains medical students, graduate students and postdoctoral fellows from around the world.

Our Centers of Excellence include
- Asthma & Allergy Center
- Brady Urologic Institute
- Children's Center
- Sidney Kimmel Comprehensive Cancer Center
- Comprehensive Transplant Center
- Heart and Vascular Institute
- Institute for Basic Biomedical Sciences
- Solomon H. Snyder Department of Neuroscience
- McKusick-Nathans Institute of Genetic Medicine
- Wilmer Eye Institute

The Marburg Pavilion, a special group of patient rooms offering five-star hotel-like accommodations and amenities, is available at The Johns Hopkins Hospital. An executive physical program also is available that offers comprehensive and expedited examinations.

To find a physician or make an appointment at Johns Hopkins, call 410-735-7575 in Baltimore. For calls outside Baltimore, call 410-735-4872. For calls outside the United States, call +01-410-955-8032.

Lenox Hill Hospital

100 East 77th Street, New York, NY 10075
Telephone: 212-434-2000
www.lenoxhillhospital.org

Beds: 652
Sponsorship: Voluntary Not-for-Profit
Accreditation: Joint Commission, College of American Pathologists, American Association of Blood Banks, Accreditation Council for Graduate Medical Education, Accreditation Council for Continuing Medical Education, Commission on Accreditation of Allied Health Education Programs, American College of Radiology

GENERAL PROFILE

Lenox Hill Hospital is a fully accredited, acute care hospital with a national reputation for providing the highest quality care, training new physicians, and contributing to progress in research. The hospital is ranked among the top 50 hospitals in Heart and Heart Surgery, Digestive Disorders, and Neurology & Neurosurgery by *U.S.News & World Report*.

MEDICAL STAFF AND TEACHING PROGRAMS

Lenox Hill Hospital's 1,400 physicians have national and international reputations in their fields. The Hospital independently sponsors 17 accredited residency and fellowship programs.

CENTERS OF EXCELLENCE
LENOX HILL HEART AND VASCULAR INSTITUTE OF NEW YORK (LHHVI)

LHHVI is one of the only centers in Manhattan to offer the full complement of minimally invasive heart surgery. LHH surgeons are able to perform coronary artery bypass surgery, valve repair and replacement, atrial fibrillation ablation, and remodeling of the heart, all minimally invasively. The first totally endoscopic coronary artery bypss surgery to be performed on a beating heart in New York was performed by LHH surgeons in 2009. LHH is one of the few hospitals in the nation to offer integrated care of aortic disease, which involves collaboration between cardiothoracic surgery, vascular surgery, interventional radiology, structural cardiology and internal medicine. This is in keeping with a tradition of excellence begun in 1938, when Lenox Hill Hospital cardiologists performed the first angiogram in the U.S. In 1978, Hospital cardiologists performed the first ever coronary angioplasty. In 1991, they implanted one of the first coronary stents in NYC, and in 1994 performed the nation's first minimally invasive direct coronary artery bypass surgery.

Maimonides Medical Center
MAIMONIDES CARDIAC INSTITUTE

Maimonides
Medical Center

4802 Tenth Avenue • Brooklyn, New York 11219
Phone: 800.682.5558/718.283.8902 • Fax: 718.635.7505
www.maimonidesmed.org/cardiac

Having pioneered numerous heart care innovations through the years, the Cardiac Institute offers diagnostic studies and therapeutic treatments, procedures and surgeries. It has been ranked by the Centers for Medicare and Medicaid Services among those hospitals achieving excellent ratings in both heart attack and heart failure patient outcomes.

Cardiology
Among the most published and respected in the field, the Maimonides cardiology team continuously sets higher standards for patient care. Edgar Lichstein, MD, Chair of Medicine, has been chief investigator of NIH-sponsored cardiac drug trials, and our Congestive Heart Failure (CHF) Program is among the most effective in the nation.

Interventional Cardiology
Led by Cardiac Institute Chair Jacob Shani, MD, numerous therapeutic devices were developed and implemented here. Our Electrophysiology Lab has a superb record of achievement in diagnosing and treating arrhythmias. A close collaboration with the Department of Emergency Medicine ensures that chest pain patients are evaluated immediately and that interventional procedures are used to stop heart attacks in progress whenever necessary.

Cardiothoracic Surgery
The Maimonides Cardiothoracic Surgery program has an illustrious history, setting the national standard for advances in service. Under the direction of Stephen Lahey, MD, minimally invasive and robotic heart surgeries are offered in state-of-the-art facilities. In collaboration with Electrophysiology, Cardiothoracic Surgery has established an Atrial Fibrillation Center of Excellence. Maimonides provides one of the most prestigious cardiothoracic residency programs in the US.

Historic Moments
- In 1967, the first successful human heart transplant in the nation was performed at Maimonides.
- The intra-aortic balloon pump was developed here in 1970.
- Surgical techniques that protect the spine during cardiothoracic surgery were perfected here in 1982.
- Revolutionary cardiac catheterization devices were invented here in 1992 and 1997.
- Maimonides was the first hospital in US to implement fully automatic external cardiac defibrillators in 2001.

Physicians at Maimonides are among the small percentage in the US who use computers to enter patient orders, thereby reducing the risk of errors, increasing efficiency, and speeding the healing process. Maimonides has appeared on the American Hospital Association's "Most Wired" and "Most Wireless" lists more often than any other health care institution in the metropolitan area. Advanced technology allows our doctors to focus more attention on caring for their patients.

**Maimonides Medical Center
Passionate about medicine.
Compassionate about people.**

www.maimonidesmed.org/cardiac

MOUNT SINAI
SCHOOL OF
MEDICINE

THE MOUNT SINAI MEDICAL CENTER

One Gustave L. Levy Place
Fifth Avenue and 100th Street
New York, NY 10029-6574
Physician Referral: 1-800-MD-SINAI (637-4624)
www.mountsinai.org

Sponsorship: Voluntary Not-for-Profit
Beds: 1,171
Accreditation: The Joint Commission;
Commission for Accreditation of Rehabilitation Facilities;
Magnet Award for Nursing Excellence

Since its founding over 150 years ago, The Mount Sinai Medical Center has been a leader in patient care and translational research. Generations of our patients have benefited as teams of physicians and scientists have always worked together to rapidly translate laboratory research into new treatments.

Located between the Upper East Side and East and Central Harlem—New York City's most and least affluent communities—Mount Sinai provides a broad range of services that meet the needs of every patient we treat. The Medical Center consists of The Mount Sinai Hospital and Mount Sinai School of Medicine, both which continue to be ranked by *U.S. News & World Report* as premier institutions in the nation.

In 2009, Mount Sinai earned Honor Roll status and was ranked 19th in the nation in *America's Best Hospitals*, published by *U.S. News & World Report*. Mount Sinai was also ranked in 11 specialties: geriatric care; digestive disorders; neurology and neurosurgery; ear, nose and throat; heart and heart surgery; kidney disorders; gynecology; cancer; orthopedics; psychiatry; and rehabilitation. In addition, the School of Medicine was ranked 22nd by the *Best Graduate Schools* edition.

Mount Sinai Heart, under the direction of Valentin Fuster, MD, PhD, combines Mount Sinai's world-class resources with innovative thinking, comprehensive and interdisciplinary programs, and an unwavering commitment to the prevention and treatment of cardiovascular disease. Mount Sinai became the first hospital in the country to successfully perform left atrial appendage occlusion, an innovative procedure that can help patients with atrial fibrillation obviate the need for lifelong anticoagulant treatment. Capitalizing on the talent and expertise of internationally renowned Mount Sinai physicians David H. Adams, MD; Michael L. Marin, MD; Samin K. Sharma, MD; Eric A. Rose, MD; Vivek Y. Reddy, MD; and a host of other highly regarded cardiac surgeons, interventionalists, and cardiologists, Mount Sinai Heart provides patients with the most advanced approach to their care.

The Tisch Cancer Institute coordinates a full-service diagnostic and treatment program for cancer patients. Current clinical programs include those in cancer of the liver, breast, prostate, head and neck—which includes Transoral Robotic Surgery as a treatment option—as well as hematological malignancies, such as myeloproliferative disorders.

Recognized as a national leader in organ transplantation, **The Recanati/Miller Transplantation Institute** is one of the few places in the country that provides multi-organ transplantation. Mount Sinai surgeons were the first in New York State to perform many combined transplant procedures, including liver and kidney transplantation, pediatric liver transplantation, and living adult- and pediatric-donor liver transplantation.

Geriatrics and Palliative Medicine specialists at Mount Sinai promote healthy aging and provide a balanced and integrated approach to improving the quality of life for New York's elderly. Consistently ranked third in the country for geriatrics by *U.S. News & World Report*, Mount Sinai remains a national pioneer in geriatric medicine.

NY Eye & Ear Infirmary

Continuum Health Partners, Inc.

THE NEW YORK EYE AND EAR INFIRMARY

310 East 14th Street
New York, New York 10003
Tel. 212.979.4000   Fax. 212.228.0664
www.nyee.edu

BEDS:	69; Operating Rooms: 17; Surgical Cases: 25,000+ a year
Sponsorship:	Voluntary Not-for-Profit
Accreditation:	The Joint Commission
	College of American Pathologists

GENERAL OVERVIEW

The New York Eye and Ear Infirmary is one of the world's leading facilities for the diagnosis and treatment of diseases of the eyes, ears, nose, throat and related conditions. Founded in 1820, it is the first and most historic specialty hospital in the nation, as well as one of the busiest.

ACADEMIC AND CLINICAL AFFILIATIONS

A voluntary, not-for-profit institution, the Infirmary is a member of Continuum Health Partners, Inc. and an affiliated teaching hospital of New York Medical College. There are highly regarded residency programs in ophthalmology and otolaryngology, plus some two dozen post-graduate fellowship positions.

THE MEDICAL STAFF

The Medical Staff includes more than 500 board-certified attending physicians and surgeons throughout the metropolitan area. Many are renowned for their breakthrough research introducing widely practiced techniques.

SPECIALTIES

Ophthalmology: Within this area are subspecialties of cataract, glaucoma, retina, cornea and external disease, ocular plastic surgery, pediatric ophthalmology and strabismus, neuro-ophthalmology. ocular tumor and uveitis. Laser, photography, fluorescein angiography and electrophysiological testing are among the most advanced services available anywhere.

Otolaryngology: The department is in the forefront of treatment modalities using highly sophisticated endoscopic and laser equipment. Subspecialties include rhinology, laryngology, head & neck surgery, otology/neurotology, facial plastic surgery, pediatric otolaryngology, audiology, speech therapy and hearing aid dispensing.

Plastic & Reconstructive Surgery: Microsurgical capabilities and premium patient accommodations provide an optimum environment for facial plasty, liposuction and repair of defects from disease or trauma.

RELATED SERVICES

New York Eye Trauma Center: An advanced program for emergency treatment of eye injuries, it also is the Eye Injury Registry of New York State and leading collector of data which will help develop preventative strategies.

Ambulatory Surgery: A comprehensive Ambulatory Surgery Center is designed to expedite admission testing, pre-op preparation and post-op recovery in an efficient and comfortable setting.

Pediatric Specialty Care: Services of eye and ear, nose and throat specialists are coordinated with other professional and support staff especially sensitive to the youngest patients.

RESEARCH AND EDUCATION

The New York Eye and Ear Infirmary is a national and international leader in research in its specialties, achieving many "firsts" in successful surgical procedures and medical treatments. Laboratories include Cell Culture, Ocular Imaging, and Microsurgical Education. Over a hundred studies and clinical trials are currently being conducted.

Physician Referral: Call 1.800.449.HOPE (4673)

NewYork-Presbyterian
The University Hospital of Columbia and Cornell

Affiliated with Columbia University College of Physicians and Surgeons and Weill Medical College of Cornell University

NewYork-Presbyterian Hospital
Weill Cornell Medical Center
525 East 68th Street
New York, NY 10021

NewYork-Presbyterian Hospital
Columbia University Medical Center
622 West 168th Street
New York, NY 10032

Sponsorship: Voluntary Not-for-Profit
Beds: 2,335
Accreditation: Joint Commission on Accreditation of Healthcare Organizations (JCAHO), Commission on Accreditation of Rehabilitation Facilities (CARF) and College of American Pathologists (CAP)

The *U.S. News & World Report* has ranked NewYork-Presbyterian Hospital higher in more specialties than any other hospital in the New York area. NewYork-Presbyterian Hospital was named to the *Honor Roll of America's Best Hospitals*.

OVERVIEW:

NewYork-Presbyterian Hospital is the largest hospital in New York and one of the most comprehensive healthcare institutions in the world with 5,500 physicians, approximately 96,000 discharges and nearly 1 million outpatient visits annually, and with its affiliated medical schools, more than $330 million in research support.

AMONG ITS RENOWNED CENTERS OF EXCELLENCE ARE:

Morgan Stanley Children's Hospital and the Komansky Center for Children's Health – One of the largest, most comprehensive children's hospitals in the world providing highly sophisticated pediatric medical, surgical and intensive care, including a pediatric cardiovascular center, in a compassionate environment.

NewYork-Presbyterian Cancer Centers – Coordinated, multidisciplinary care and the latest therapeutic options and clinical trials available for all types of cancer.

NewYork-Presbyterian Heart – Expert diagnostic capabilities and medical and surgical innovations for simple to complex heart conditions.

NewYork-Presbyterian Neuroscience Centers – Latest research, diagnosis and treatment capabilities in Alzheimer's disease, Multiple Sclerosis, Parkinson's disease, aneurysms, epilepsy, brain tumors, stokes and other neurological disorders.

NewYork-Presbyterian Psychiatry – World-renowned center of excellence in psychiatric treatment, research and education.

NewYork-Presbyterian Transplant Institute – Adult and pediatric heart, liver, and kidney and adult pancreas and lung transplantation and cutting-edge research.

NewYork-Presbyterian Vascular Care Center – Comprehensive and integrated preventive, diagnostic and treatment program for diverse problems related to arteries and veins throughout the body.

NewYork-Presbyterian Digestive Disease Services – Expert capabilities in the broad range of conditions that affect the organs as well as other components of the digestive system.

William Randolph Hearst Burn Center – Largest and busiest burn center in the nation which also conducts research to improve survival and enhance quality of life for burn victims.

In addition, the Hospital offers extraordinary expertise, comprehensive programs and specialized resources in the fields of AIDS, Complementary Medicine, Gene Therapy, Reproductive Medicine and Infertility, Trauma Center and Women's Health Care.

ACADEMIC AFFILIATIONS:

NewYork-Presbyterian is the only hospital in the world affiliated with two Ivy League medical schools; The Joan and Sanford I Weill Medical College of Cornell University and the Columbia University College of Physicians and Surgeons.

Physician Referral: To find a NewYork-Presbyterian Hospital affiliated physician to meet your needs, call toll free 1-877-NYP-WELL (1-877-697-9355) or visit our website at www.nyp.org

NYU Langone Medical Center

550 First Avenue (at 31St Street)
New York, NY 10016
Physician Referral:
(888)7-NYU-MED (888-769-8633)
www.med.nyu.edu

NYU Langone Medical Center is one of the nation's premier centers of excellence in health care, biomedical research, and medical education. For over 168 years, NYU physicians and researchers have made countless contributions to the practice and science of health care.

Today the Medical Center consists of the three hospitals of NYU Hospitals Center: Tisch Hospital, a 705-bed acute-care general hospital, Rusk Institute of Rehabilitation Medicine, the first and largest facility of its kind, and NYU Hospital for Joint Diseases, a leader in musculoskeletal care; and NYU School of Medicine, which includes the Smilow Research Center, the Skirball Institute of Biomolecular Medicine, and the Sackler Institute of Graduate Biomedical Sciences.

NYU Langone Medical Center is internationally renowned for excellence in areas such as cancer, cardiac and vascular surgery, cardiovascular disease, dermatology, infertility, minimally invasive surgery, neurology and neurosurgery, pediatrics, radiology, rehabilitation medicine and urology.

As an integral part of an academic medical center, NYU's clinical services are continually informed and enhanced by hundreds of basic and clinical research projects, as well as by major initiatives in translational research that promise to speed the transfer of laboratory discoveries to the patient's bedside.

NYU Langone Medical Center has brought together some of our most outstanding basic and translational scientists with clinicians to create six Centers of Excellence focusing on: Addiction, Brain Aging, Cancers of the Skin, Multiple Sclerosis, Musculoskeletal Disease, and Center of Urologic Disease. By applying the expertise and resources of multiple disciplines to focus on specific health problems, our Centers of Excellence are having a transformative effect, both on the productivity of our research and the quality of our patient care.

Additionally, the strengths of NYU Langone Medical Center include the talents of affiliates and partners, such as Bellevue Hospital Center and the Manhattan Veterans Affairs Medical Center.

Looking for information on our expert physicians? 1-888-769-8633

Additional Areas of Expertise:

Adult Cardiovascular Services	Internal Medicine	Pediatric Infectious Diseases
Behavioral Health	Maternal and Fetal Medicine	Pediatric Pulmonology
Cardiac Surgery	Minimally Invasive Surgery	Pediatric Rheumatology
Child and Adolescent Psychiatry	Neonatal-Perinatal Medicine	Pediatric Surgery
Clinical Genetics	Nuclear Medicine	Program for IVF Reproductive
Colon and Rectal Surgery	Obstetrics and Gynecology	Psychiatry
Dermatology	Orthopaedic Services	Pulmonology
Gastroenterology	Otolaryngology	Radiology
Geriatric Medicine	Pediatric Cardiology	Rheumatology
Hand Surgery	Pediatric Critical Care	Thoracic Surgery
Hematology/Oncology	Pediatric Gastroenterology	Urology
Infectious Diseases	Pediatric Hematology	Vascular Surgery
		Wound Care

NYU — Rusk Institute of Rehabilitation Medicine
NYU LANGONE MEDICAL CENTER

400 East 34th Street
(between 1st Avenue and FDR Drive)
New York, NY 10016
At NYU Hospital for Joint Diseases
301 East 17th Street (at 2nd Avenue):
New York, NY 10003
(212) 598-6252: www.ruskinstitute.org

About the Institute:

The Rusk Institute of Rehabilitation Medicine at NYU Langone Medical Center is the world's first university-affiliated facility devoted entirely to rehabilitation medicine. The Institute is the largest center of its kind for the treatment of adults and children with disabilities. Founded in 1948 by Dr. Howard Rusk, it has been voted as the best rehabilitation hospital in New York and among the top ten in the country since 1989, when *U.S. News & World Report.*

We specialize in the following areas:

The Rusk Institute of Rehabilitation provides patients with access to a continuum rehabilitation care depending on their individual medical needs, including acute hospital-based inpatient programs, outpatient programs and specialty clinics.

INPATIENT FACILITIES:

The Brain Injury Program provides a structured therapeutic program tailored to meet the medical and rehabilitative needs of patients who have sustained a brain injury or neurological illness. Specialized limb deficiency programs are available to patients who have undergone amputations.

The Medically Complex Conditions Unit offers individualized treatment programs for patients with a variety of medically complex conditions such as spinal cord injuries, multiple sclerosis, Parkinson's disease, amputations and pain syndrome.

Specialized pediatric therapy programs are available to newborns, children and young adults, including communication programs, educational services, occupational therapy, physical therapy, psychology and speech-language pathology services.

The Joan and Joel Smilow Cardiac Rehabilitation & Prevention Center provides personalized cardiac rehabilitation.

The NYUHJD Orthopaedic Rehabilitation Unit provides rehabilitation of musculoskeletal disorders and injuries.

The William Randolph Hearst Foundation Stroke Rehabilitation Unit treats all aspects of stroke rehabilitation.

OUTPATIENT FACILITIES:

The Adult Physical Therapy Outpatient Unit offers evaluation and treatment for musculoskeletal and neurological disorders through individual and group programs.

The Chest Physical Therapy Program provides programs to individuals with lung congestion, secretion retention or areas of lung collapse.

Occupational therapists work with individuals to devise a comprehensive treatment program to help them regain their independence in daily tasks.

The Outpatient Rehabilitation Psychology Service is the largest of its kind on the East coast, providing care to patients with neurological and medical conditions on an outpatient basis.

The Physical Therapy Department provides an array of outpatient programs designed to address concerns associated with pregnancy, osteoporosis, pelvic floor dysfunction and some cancers.

The Speech-Language Pathology Department offers rehabilitation services to patients with communication disorders due to neurological problems.

The Swallowing Disorders Center is dedicated to the diagnosis and therapeutic management of swallowing and feeding disorders.

The Vestibular Rehabilitation Program is the first program of its kind in the tri-state area, providing diagnosis and treatment for patients suffering from dizziness and imbalance.

The Vocational Services Department provides individuals with disabilities with the competencies needed to return to school, work and to lead a productive lifestyle.

SPECIALTY CLINICS:

The Adult Spasticity Clinic provides examination and treatment to patients with spasticity, resulting from cerebral palsy, traumatic brain injury, spinal cord injury, multiple sclerosis and stroke.

Patients with **neuromuscular disease** receive physical and occupational therapies, vocational counseling, equipment and seating and mobility services.

St. Francis Hospital The Heart Center®

100 Port Washington Blvd.
Roslyn, New York 11576
www.stfrancisheartcenter.com
(516) 562-6000   1-888-HEARTNY
A member of Catholic Health Services of Long Island

St. Francis Hospital, The Heart Center® is New York State's only specialty designated cardiac center, offering one of the leading cardiac care programs in the nation. Founded in 1922 by the Franciscan Missionaries of Mary, the Hospital is recognized as an innovator in the delivery of specialized cardiovascular services in an environment where excellence and compassion are emphasized. St. Francis also offers a superb program in non-cardiac surgery, including some of the most advanced technology and minimally invasive techniques available for vascular, prostate, ear-nose-throat (ENT), abdominal, oncologic, and orthopedic surgery.

Cardiac Diagnostics and Treatment

St. Francis Hospital performs more cardiac procedures than any other hospital in New York State and has been consistently recognized for its outstanding quality of care. In 2009, St. Francis Hospital was ranked as one of America's best hospitals by *U.S. News & World Report*.

Cardiac surgery: In 2008, 1,568 open-heart surgeries were performed at St. Francis Hospital. The Hospital's seven cardiothoracic surgeons have the combined experience of over 20,000 open-heart procedures in the last 10 years alone and are experts in all types of heart surgery, from conventional, open-heart bypass to off-pump coronary artery bypass (OPCAB) to the newest, minimally invasive valve procedures, including surgical techniques designed to treat certain cardiac arrhythmias or irregular heart rhythms.

Cardiac catheterization: In 2008, St. Francis interventional cardiologists performed 8,759 cardiac catheterizations and 3,544 percutaneous coronary interventions (angioplasty and insertion of stents). The Hospital is also recognized as one of the East Coast's highest volume centers for catheter-based techniques to close atrial septal defects (ASDs) and patent foramen ovale (PFO).

Arrhythmia and Pacemaker Center: St. Francis has a leading national program for pacemaker implantation and the diagnosis and treatment of cardiac rhythm abnormalities. The Center has unparalleled expertise in radiofrequency cardiac ablation, including treatment of atrial fibrillation.

Research and Technology: At the St. Francis Cardiac Research Institute, a team of world-renowned researchers is working with the latest non-invasive imaging technology, including advanced techniques and world class expertise in cardiac CT angiography, cardiac magnetic resonance imaging, cardiac PET/CT and three-dimensional echocardiography. This multimodality approach to investigating the heart's function and disease processes is aimed at improving methods of diagnosing heart disease.

Prevention and Education

St. Francis Hospital's satellite campus, The DeMatteis Center for Cardiac Research and Education, in Greenvale, New York, is one of the few freestanding campuses in the U.S. dedicated to the prevention of heart disease. It is the site of community health lectures, as well as the largest medically staffed cardiac fitness and rehabilitation program on Long Island.

Physician referral:	**1-888-HEARTNY**
Sponsorship:	Voluntary not-for-profit
Beds:	364
Accreditation:	Awarded accreditation from the Joint Commission.

UHEALTH: HEALTH CARE FOR THE 21ST CENTURY

UHealth's physicians and health care professionals provide care and conduct research at more than 30 facilities, including:

- University of Miami Hospital
- Sylvester Comprehensive Cancer Center
- Bascom Palmer Eye Institute
- Diabetes Research Institute
- The Miami Project to Cure Paralysis
- Mailman Center for Child Development
- John P. Hussman Institute for Human Genetics

In affiliation with:

- Jackson Memorial Hospital
- Holtz Children's Hospital
- Miami VA Medical Center

For more than 56 years, the University of Miami has been a vital part of South Florida's health care landscape. Now, known by the name UHealth – University of Miami Health System, we continue our leading role as South Florida's source for breakthrough medicine and the region's unequivocal health care leader. Backed by up-to-the-minute research, award-winning community service, and top-ranked physicians practicing in more than 100 medical specialties and subspecialties, UHealth provides health care for the 21st Century.

LEONARD M. MILLER SCHOOL OF MEDICINE

The University of Miami's Leonard M. Miller School of Medicine serves as the "engine" driving UHealth. Driven by the vision of University President Donna Shalala, (the former U.S. Secretary of Health and Human Services,) and Dean Pascal J. Goldschmidt, the Miller School of Medicine has attracted international leaders from dozens of fields. Moreover, this renowned team is transforming thousands of lives by helping our patients – and the beneficiaries of our research – live longer and live healthier.

TOP DOCTORS

UHealth doctors are among the nation's most respected. Our more than 2,000 physicians have been recognized by their peers as among the best in South Florida and the nation. In fact, more than 400 are listed as "best doctors" in regional and national rankings.* Providing care to one of the most diverse patient populations in the world and delivering services in five counties stretching from the Atlantic to the Gulf of Mexico, UHealth physicians keep Florida healthy.

*Based on listings provided by Best Doctors®, Castle Connolly Medical Ltd., and Florida Super Doctors.

INNOVATIVE RESEARCH

Currently, UHealth physicians and scientists are involved in more than 1,500 ongoing studies, many of which lead to clinical trials that directly change the standard for care. They work every day to uncover new information, build better understanding, and develop new cures.

A HOSPITAL FOR THE 21ST CENTURY

University of Miami Hospital is the only university-owned, multi-specialty, acute care hospital in South Florida and part of UHealth – University of Miami Health System. Here, physicians on the faculty of the Miller School of Medicine and community physicians, plan and provide care, investigate new treatments still in the clinical research phase, and utilize the most advanced technologies available.

BREAKTHROUGH MEDICINE HAPPENS HERE

UHealth physicians participate in hundreds of ongoing studies, many of which culminate in clinical trials underway at University of Miami Hospital. These studies give our patients access to up-to-the-minute breakthroughs straight from the laboratory. Currently, our physicians are investigating new approaches to prevention, diagnosis, and treatment in a number of areas, including: cardiology, sports medicine, orthopaedics, neurology, urology, gynecology, and otolaryngology.

TOP TECHNOLOGY

To provide better diagnoses, deliver more effective treatments, and promote faster recoveries, University of Miami Hospital has invested in the latest technology. At our new cardiac catheterization and electrophysiology labs, we use the Stereoaxis Magnetic Navigation System and the Siemens Artis Zeego Robot to accurately and safely guide catheters through the most delicate vessels. Surgeons representing multiple specialties at University of Miami Hospital use the da Vinci Surgical System® to increase the speed and precision of their procedures. And our 128-slice CT scanner produces the highest-resolution 3D images available.

PRIORITIZING THE PATIENT EXPERIENCE

In addition to all-private rooms and a team of nurses trained to deliver high quality, compassionate care, University of Miami Hospital offers 24-hour access to personal patient representatives; physical, occupational, and speech therapists; and an on-site pharmacy. We even have a specially outfitted ambulance for transferring patients from other facilities.

To make an appointment, please call 305-689-5511.

University of Miami Hospital Services

- Bariatric Center of Excellence
- Cardiac Services
- Critical Care (46 beds)
- Dermatology
- Emergency Room
- Endocrinology
- Gastrointestinal Center
- Gynecology/Women's Services
- Hepatology
- Hyperbaric Medicine
- Infertility Center
- International Medicine
- Laser and Laparoscopic Surgery
- Minimally Invasive Robotic Surgery
- Nephrology
- Neurology and Neurosurgery
- Orthopaedics – Joint Center
- Otolaryngology (ENT)
- Outpatient Rehabilitation
- Pain Management Center
- Plastic and Reconstructive Surgery
- Podiatry
- Progressive Care Unit
- Psychiatry
- Pulmonary Medicine
- Radiation Oncology
- Sports Medicine Program
- Urology
- Vascular Surgery
- Wound Healing Center

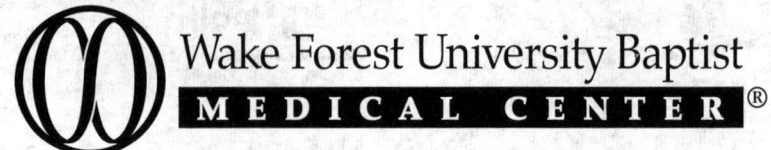

Medical Center Boulevard • Winston-Salem, NC 27157 • 336-716-2011
Health On-Call® (Patient Access) 1-800-446-2255
Physician-To-Physician Calls (PAL®) 1-800-277-7654
wfubmc.edu • brennerchildrens.org • besthealth.com

OVERVIEW

Wake Forest University Baptist Medical Center encompasses **Wake Forest University School of Medicine**, whose reputation attracts some of the nation's top doctors to its Wake Forest University Physicians faculty practice, and **North Carolina Baptist Hospital**, a nationally ranked, academic tertiary care facility. Internationally known for state-of-the-art treatment and technology, research leadership and teaching excellence, Wake Forest University Baptist Medical Center is ranked a top hospital by *U.S.News & World Report* since 1993. More than 600 physicians offer preventive and highly specialized care.

COMPREHENSIVE SPECIALTY CENTERS AND SERVICES

Brenner Children's Hospital . . . the highest levels of neonatal and pediatric care in a state-of-the-art setting; **Heart Center** . . . groundbreaking research, technology and treatment, region's only transplant service; **Comprehensive Cancer Center of WFU** . . . NCI-designated for research, advanced technologies, treatments such as Gamma Knife, Intensity Modulated Radiation Therapy; **Neurosciences** . . . Stroke, ALS , Epilepsy, and Brain Tumor Centers, expertise in deep brain stimulation; the region's most comprehensive, advanced services in **Digestive Health, Nephrology, Orthopaedics, Otolaryngology, Reproductive Medicine and Urology.**

RESEARCH EXCELLENCE

Wake Forest Baptist has more than 1,000 research and clinical trials under way, and its Translational Science Institute is accelerating discovery that will benefit patients. At the **Wake Forest Institute for Regenerative Medicine**, doctors are applying tissue engineering to build more than 22 organs and tissues and have successfully implanted human, laboratory-grown bladders. The **Center for Genomics and Personalized Medicine Research** is advancing the possibilities of diagnosis and treatment of disease based on individuals' genetic and environmental factors. The **Brain Tumor Center** is at the forefront of molecular medicine therapies and radiation-induced brain injury research. The **Center for Biomolecular Imaging** is creating new ways to view the brain, heart and cancers.

TECHNOLOGY LEADERSHIP

Committed to serving our patients with the most advanced technology, Wake Forest Baptist is home to one of North America's first **Integrated Brachytherapy Units**, a faster, extremely precise cancer treatment using radioactive seed implants . . . one of the nation's first **Bioanatomic Imaging and Treatment Programs**, allowing for new levels of accuracy in tumor identification and treatment . . . North Carolina's only **MEG** (magnetoencephalography), brain-function imaging that enables highly precise neurosurgical planning . . . **Leksell Gamma Knife® Perfexion™**, the latest upgrade to the gold standard technology for non-invasive brain surgeries, and the new **Elekta Axesse™** whole body radiotherapy linear accelerator for tumor treatment . . . one of North Carolina's most innovative robotic-assisted surgery programs using the **da Vinci® robot**.

OUTSTANDING NURSING

Outstanding nursing earned Wake Forest Baptist one of the nation's first 15 Magnet Awards for nursing excellence, awarded by the American Nurses Credentialing Center and twice recertified. Patient-centered care is the driving goal of Wake Forest Baptist caregivers.

To make an appointment or find a specialist call Health On-Call® at **1-800-446-2255**.

Physician
Listings

Adolescent Medicine

a subspecialty of Pediatrics

An internist or pediatrician who specializes in adolescent medicine is a multidiciplinary healthcare specialist trained in the unique physical, psychological and social characteristics of adolescents, their healthcare problems and needs.

Training Required: Three years in internal medicine OR three years in pediatrics *plus* additional training and examination for certification in adolescent medicine

ADOLESCENT MEDICINE

New England

Emans, Sarah Jean H MD [AM] - **Spec Exp:** Pediatric Gynecology; Adolescent Gynecology; **Hospital:** Children's Hospital - Boston; **Address:** Childrens Hosp, Dept Adolescent Med, 300 Longwood Ave, Boston, MA 02115-5724; **Phone:** 617-355-7181; **Board Cert:** Pediatrics 1993; Adolescent Medicine 2002; **Med School:** Harvard Med Sch 1970; **Resid:** Pediatrics, Chldns Hosp 1973; **Fellow:** Adolescent Medicine, Chldns Hosp 1974; **Fac Appt:** Prof Ped, Harvard Med Sch

Mid Atlantic

Diaz, Angela MD [AM] - **Spec Exp:** Adolescent Reproductive Health; Abuse/Neglect; **Hospital:** Mount Sinai Med Ctr; **Address:** 320 E 94th St Fl 2, New York, NY 10128-5604; **Phone:** 212-423-2900; **Board Cert:** Pediatrics 1987; Adolescent Medicine 2004; **Med School:** Columbia P&S 1981; **Resid:** Pediatrics, Mt Sinai Med Ctr 1984; **Fellow:** Adolescent Medicine, Mt Sinai Med Ctr 1985; **Fac Appt:** Prof Ped, Mount Sinai Sch Med

Ginsburg, Kenneth R MD [AM] - **Hospital:** Chldns Hosp of Philadelphia, The; **Address:** 3550 Market St Fl 4, Blvd, Philadelphia, PA 19104; **Phone:** 215-590-3537; **Board Cert:** Pediatrics 1998; Adolescent Medicine 2002; **Med School:** Albert Einstein Coll Med 1987; **Resid:** Pediatrics, Chldns Hosp 1990; **Fac Appt:** Assoc Prof Ped, Univ Pennsylvania

Murray, Pamela J MD [AM] - **Spec Exp:** Adolescent Gynecology; **Hospital:** Chldns Hosp of Pittsburgh - UPMC; **Address:** Children's Hosp Pittsburgh, Addolescent Medicine, 3705 Fifth Ave at DeSoto St, Pittsburgh, PA 15213; **Phone:** 412-692-8504; **Board Cert:** Pediatrics 1983; Adolescent Medicine 2002; **Med School:** Med Coll PA 1978; **Resid:** Pediatrics, Children's Hosp 1981; **Fellow:** Public Health, Univ New South Wales 1987; **Fac Appt:** Assoc Prof Ped, Univ Pittsburgh

Southeast

Ford, Carol Ann MD [AM] - **Hospital:** Univ NC Hosps; **Address:** UNC-Chapel Hill, Dept Ped Adol Med, 231 Macnider Bldg Ave, Box 7225, Chapel Hill, NC 27599-7225; **Phone:** 919-966-2504; **Board Cert:** Internal Medicine 1987; Pediatrics 1998; Adolescent Medicine 1994; **Med School:** Univ Fla Coll Med 1983; **Resid:** Internal Medicine, North Carolina Meml Hosp 1987; Pediatrics, North Carolina Meml Hosp 1987; **Fellow:** Adolescent Medicine, UCSF Med Ctr 1995; **Fac Appt:** Asst Prof Ped, Univ NC Sch Med

Midwest

Fortenberry, J Dennis MD [AM] - **Spec Exp:** Sexually Transmitted Diseases; **Hospital:** Riley Hosp for Children; **Address:** Dept Adolescent Medicine, 410 W 10th, rm 1001, Indianapolis, IN 46202; **Phone:** 317-274-8812; **Board Cert:** Internal Medicine 1983; Adolescent Medicine 2004; **Med School:** Univ Okla Coll Med 1979; **Resid:** Internal Medicine, Univ OK Hlth Sci Ctr 1982; **Fellow:** Adolescent Medicine, Univ OK Hlth Sci Ctr 1983; **Fac Appt:** Prof Med, Indiana Univ

Kokotailo, Patricia K MD [AM] - **Spec Exp:** Adolescent Gynecology; Substance Abuse; **Hospital:** Univ WI Hosp & Clins; **Address:** Univ Wisc Chldns Hosp, Dept Peds-Adol Med, 2800 University Ave, Ste 200, Madison, WI 53705; **Phone:** 608-263-6421; **Board Cert:** Pediatrics 1987; Adolescent Medicine 2002; **Med School:** Northwestern Univ 1982; **Resid:** Pediatrics, Johns Hopkins Hosp 1985; **Fellow:** Adolescent Medicine, Johns Hopkins Hosp 1989; **Fac Appt:** Prof Ped, Univ Wisc

Great Plains and Mountains

Kaplan, David W MD [AM] - **Spec Exp:** Eating Disorders; Depression; Headache; **Hospital:** Chldn's Hosp - Aurora, The; **Address:** Chldns Hosp, 13123 E 16th Ave, Box B025, Aurora, CO 80045; **Phone:** 720-777-6131; **Board Cert:** Pediatrics 1975; Public Health & Genl Preventive Med 1980; Adolescent Medicine 2009; **Med School:** Case West Res Univ 1970; **Resid:** Pediatrics, Univ Colorado Med Ctr 1972; Pediatrics, Chldns Hosp Med Ctr 1975; **Fellow:** Public Health & Genl Preventive Med, Harvard Sch Pub Hlth 1976; **Fac Appt:** Prof Ped, Univ Colorado

Southwest

Bermudez, Ovidio B MD [AM] - **Spec Exp:** Eating Disorders; Obesity; **Hospital:** Laureate Psyc Clinic & Hosp, St Francis Hosp - Tulsa; **Address:** Eating Disorders Clinic, 6655 S Yale Ave, Tulsa, OK 74136; **Phone:** 918-491-3702; **Board Cert:** Pediatrics 2005; Adolescent Medicine 2002; **Med School:** Dominican Republic 1985; **Resid:** Pediatrics, Med Coll Penn 1988; **Fellow:** Adolescent Medicine, Univ Alabama 1990; **Fac Appt:** Clin Prof Ped, Univ Okla Coll Med

Hergenroeder, Albert C MD [AM] - **Spec Exp:** Pediatric & Adolescent Sports Medicine; Eating Disorders; Adolescent Reproductive Health; **Hospital:** Texas Chldns Hosp; **Address:** Texas Chldns Hosp, Adol Med, 6701 Fannin St, Clinical Care Ctr, 1710.00 Fl 11, Houston, TX 77030; **Phone:** 832-822-3660; **Board Cert:** Pediatrics 1993; Sports Medicine 2004; Adolescent Medicine 2002; **Med School:** Univ Pittsburgh 1980; **Resid:** Pediatrics, Duke Univ Med Ctr 1983; **Fellow:** Adolescent Medicine, Univ Wash 1985; **Fac Appt:** Prof Ped, Baylor Coll Med

West Coast and Pacific

Anderson, Martin M MD [AM] - **Hospital:** UCLA Ronald Reagan Med Ctr; **Address:** UCLA Med Ctr, Dept Pediatrics, 10833 Le Conte Ave, 12-476 MDcc, Los Angeles, CA 90095; **Phone:** 310-825-9346; **Board Cert:** Pediatrics 1986; Adolescent Medicine 2002; **Med School:** UC Davis 1980; **Resid:** Pediatrics, Mott Chldns Hosp 1983; **Fellow:** Adolescent Medicine, UCSF Med Ctr 1986; **Fac Appt:** Prof Ped, UCLA

Irwin Jr, Charles E MD [AM] - **Spec Exp:** Eating Disorders; Adolescent Gynecology; **Hospital:** UCSF Med Ctr; **Address:** UCSF Chldns Hosp, 400 Parnassus Ave Fl 2, Box 0503, San Francisco, CA 94143; **Phone:** 415-353-2002; **Board Cert:** Pediatrics 1993; Adolescent Medicine 2002; **Med School:** UCSF 1971; **Resid:** Pediatrics, UCSF Med Ctr 1974; **Fellow:** Adolescent Medicine, UCSF Med Ctr 1977; **Fac Appt:** Prof Ped, UCSF

MacKenzie, Richard G MD [AM] - **Spec Exp:** Eating Disorders; Menstrual Disorders; **Hospital:** Chldns Hosp - Los Angeles; **Address:** 5000 Sunset Blvd, Fl 4, Los Angeles, CA 90027-5861; **Phone:** 323-361-2112; **Med School:** McGill Univ 1966; **Resid:** Internal Medicine, Royal Victoria Hosp-Montreal 1969; **Fellow:** Adolescent Medicine, Chidrens Hosp 1970; **Fac Appt:** Assoc Prof Ped, USC Sch Med

Adolescent Medicine

Morris, Robert E MD [AM] - **Spec Exp:** Chronic Illness; Teen Behavior Evaluation-High Risk; Juvenile Correctional Health Care; **Hospital:** Santa Monica - UCLA Med Ctr & Ortho Hosp, UCLA Ronald Reagan Med Ctr; **Address:** UCLA Sch Med, Dept Peds, 10833 Le Conte Ave, Los Angeles, CA 90095-1752; **Phone:** 310-825-9346; **Board Cert:** Pediatrics 1986; Adolescent Medicine 2005; **Med School:** Temple Univ 1971; **Resid:** Pediatrics, Univ Wash 1974; Pediatric Gastroenterology, UCLA Med Ctr 1982; **Fac Appt:** Prof Ped, UCLA

Staggers, Barbara C MD [AM] - **Spec Exp:** Teen Behavior Evaluation-High Risk; **Hospital:** Chldns Hosp - Oakland; **Address:** 5400 Telegraph Ave, Oakland, CA 94618; **Phone:** 510-428-3129; **Board Cert:** Pediatrics 1999; Adolescent Medicine 2003; **Med School:** UCSF 1980; **Resid:** Pediatrics, Chldns Hosp 1983; **Fellow:** Adolescent Medicine, UCSF Med Ctr 1985

NYU Child Study Center

NYU LANGONE MEDICAL CENTER

577 First Avenue
New York, NY 10016
212-263-6622
www.aboutourkids.org

NYU CHILD STUDY CENTER

About the Child Study Center, Department of Child and Adolescent Psychiatry:

The Child Study Center at NYU Langone Medical Center is dedicated to increasing the awareness of child and adolescent psychiatric and learning disorders and improving the prevention, identification and treatment of these disorders. For over a decade, the Child Study Center has been providing hope and care to children and their families. Its expert clinicians treat thousands of children from around the globe by providing diagnostic consultations and a wide variety of medication and evidence-based psychotherapeutic treatments for all conditions, in addition to the areas highlighted below. Through its website, www.AboutOurKids.org, and professional education programs, parents are provided with the tools and knowledge needed to promote children's mental health. The Department was also designated as the only New York State Center of Excellence in Mental Health.

We specialize in the following areas:

ANXIETY AND MOOD DISORDERS

The Anita Saltz Institute for Anxiety and Mood Disorders at NYU Langone Medical Center offers the most current and effective treatment for children, adolescents, and young adults, including thorough evaluation. Our psychopharmacologists are experts in understanding the issues of treating children with bipolar disorder and our researchers are studying treatments for children with severe temper outbursts and adolescent depression. We offer several programs including The Selective Mutism Service, providing specialized care for children who cannot speak in public; Dialectical Behavior Therapy (DBT) for adolescents with self-destructive behaviors; and Cognitive Behavior Therapy (CBT) for anxiety and mood disorders, including obsessive-compulsive disorder.

ATTENTION DEFICIT HYPERACTIVITY AND BEHAVIOR DISORDERS

The Institute for Attention Deficit Hyperactivity and Behavior Disorders focuses on the treatment of ADHD. Our Parent-Child Interaction Therapy Program (PCIT) is a state-of-the-art treatment for behavioral problems in young children and is the largest program of its kind in the northeast. The Institute is also developing new treatments for preschool children with ADHD and for children with severe organizational difficulties. We also offer a summer-long program for school-age children with ADHD.

AUTISM, ASPERGER'S SYNDROME AND COMMUNICATION DISORDERS

The Autism Spectrum programs at the Child Study Center provide extensive evaluations for toddlers and preschoolers having social and communication difficulties. Our Early Social Interaction treatment is a home-based intervention for children identified with symptoms of autism. Our specialists are also experienced at supporting the needs of teens and young adults who have been diagnosed with Asperger.

LEARNING DISORDERS

The Institute for Learning and Academic Achievement evaluates children with suspected learning weaknesses or poor academic achievement using a multidisciplinary team-based approach. We provide a carefully crafted, personalized set of recommendations that gives parent-, educator-, and child-friendly integrated strategies for improvement to help children achieve their academic potential.

TICS AND TOURETTE'S DISORDER

The Tics and Tourette's Clinical and Research programs are dedicated to the evaluation and treatment of individuals with tics, Tourette's disorder and related problems. Comprehensive evaluation and state-of-the-art treatment is provided including Habit Reversal Therapy (HRT) as well as opportunities for participation in research studies that include new treatments.

Allergy & Immunology

An allergist-immunologist is trained in evaluation, physical and laboratory diagnosis and management of disorders involving the immune system. Selected examples of such conditions include asthma, anaphylaxis, rhinitis, eczema and adverse reactions to drugs, foods and insect stings as well as immune deficiency diseases (both acquired and congenital), defects in host defense and problems related to autoimmune disease, organ transplantation or malignancies of the immune system. As our understanding of the immune system develops, the scope of this specialty is widening.

Training programs are available at some medical centers to provide individuals with expertise in both allergy/immunology and adult rheumatology, or in both allergy/immunology and pediatric pulmonology. Such individuals are candidates for dual certification.

Training Required: Two years in allergy/immunology OR prior certification in internal medicine or pediatrics *plus* additional training and examination

ALLERGY & IMMUNOLOGY

New England

MacLean, James A MD [A&I] - **Spec Exp:** Asthma; Allergy; Urticaria; **Hospital:** Mass Genl Hosp, N Shore Med Ctr - Salem Hosp; **Address:** Mass General Hosp, 55 Fruit St, Cox 201, Boston, MA 02114-2621; **Phone:** 617-726-3850; **Board Cert:** Internal Medicine 1988; Allergy & Immunology 2001; **Med School:** McGill Univ 1985; **Resid:** Internal Medicine, Royal Victoria Hosp 1989; **Fellow:** Allergy & Immunology, Mass Genl Hosp 1991; Immunopathology, Mass Genl Hosp 1994; **Fac Appt:** Asst Prof A&I, Harvard Med Sch

Umetsu, Dale T MD/PhD [A&I] - **Spec Exp:** Asthma; Immune Deficiency; Eczema; Food Allergy; **Hospital:** Children's Hospital - Boston; **Address:** Div Immunology, Children's Hosp, 1 Blackfan Cir, Karp Labs, rm 10127, Boston, MA 02115; **Phone:** 617-919-2439; **Board Cert:** Pediatrics 1984; Allergy & Immunology 1985; **Med School:** NYU Sch Med 1979; **Resid:** Pediatrics, Chldns Hosp 1982; **Fellow:** Allergy & Immunology, Chldns Hosp 1984; **Fac Appt:** Prof Ped, Harvard Med Sch

Wong, Johnson T MD [A&I] - **Spec Exp:** Asthma; Rhinosinusitis; Urticaria; Immune Deficiency; **Hospital:** Mass Genl Hosp, Newton - Wellesley Hosp; **Address:** 8 Hawthorne Pl, Ste 104, Boston, MA 02114; **Phone:** 617-742-5730; **Board Cert:** Internal Medicine 1983; Allergy & Immunology 1985; **Med School:** UCSF 1980; **Resid:** Internal Medicine, UCLA-Wadsworth VA Hosp 1983; **Fellow:** Allergy & Immunology, Mass Genl Hosp 1986; **Fac Appt:** Asst Prof Med, Harvard Med Sch

Mid Atlantic

Buchbinder, Ellen MD [A&I] - **Spec Exp:** Asthma & Allergy; Rhinitis; Hives; Eczema; **Hospital:** Mount Sinai Med Ctr (page 64); **Address:** 111B E 88th St, New York, NY 10128; **Phone:** 212-410-3246; **Board Cert:** Internal Medicine 1981; Allergy & Immunology 1983; **Med School:** Tulane Univ 1978; **Resid:** Internal Medicine, New England Deaconess Hosp 1981; **Fellow:** Allergy & Immunology, Mass Genl Hosp 1983; **Fac Appt:** Asst Clin Prof Med, Mount Sinai Sch Med

Chandler, Michael MD [A&I] - **Spec Exp:** Asthma; Sinus Disorders; Airway Disorders; **Hospital:** Mount Sinai Med Ctr (page 64); **Address:** 115 E 61st St Fl 12, New York, NY 10021-8183; **Phone:** 212-486-6715; **Board Cert:** Internal Medicine 1984; Allergy & Immunology 1987; **Med School:** Wayne State Univ 1981; **Resid:** Internal Medicine, Northwestern Meml Hosp 1984; **Fellow:** Allergy & Immunology, Northwestern Meml Hosp 1986; **Fac Appt:** Asst Clin Prof Med, Mount Sinai Sch Med

Cohn, John R MD [A&I] - **Spec Exp:** Asthma; Allergic Rhinitis; Voice Disorders & Allergies; **Hospital:** Thomas Jefferson Univ Hosp; **Address:** 1015 Chestnut St, Ste 1300, Asthma, Allergy & Pulmonary Assocs, Philadelphia, PA 19107; **Phone:** 215-923-7685; **Board Cert:** Internal Medicine 1979; Allergy & Immunology 1981; Pulmonary Disease 1982; **Med School:** Thomas Jefferson Univ 1976; **Resid:** Internal Medicine, Thomas Jefferson Univ Hosp 1979; **Fellow:** Allergy & Immunology, Duke Univ Med Ctr 1982; Pulmonary Disease, Duke Univ Med Ctr 1982; **Fac Appt:** Prof Med, Thomas Jefferson Univ

Cunningham-Rundles, Charlotte MD/PhD [A&I] - **Spec Exp:** Immunotherapy; Immunodeficiency Disorders; **Hospital:** Mount Sinai Med Ctr (page 64); **Address:** 5 E 98th St, New York, NY 10029; **Phone:** 212-659-9268; **Board Cert:** Internal Medicine 1972; **Med School:** Columbia P&S 1969; **Resid:** Internal Medicine, Bellevue Hosp Ctr 1972; **Fellow:** Allergy & Immunology, NYU Med Ctr 1974; **Fac Appt:** Prof Med, Mount Sinai Sch Med

Ein, Daniel MD [A&I] - **Spec Exp:** Asthma & Allergy; Sinus Disorders; Chemical Exposure; Immune Deficiency; **Hospital:** G Washington Univ Hosp; **Address:** 2150 Pennsylvania Ave NW, Ste G400, Washington, DC 20037; **Phone:** 202-741-2770; **Board Cert:** Internal Medicine 1980; Allergy & Immunology 1989; **Med School:** Albert Einstein Coll Med 1964; **Resid:** Internal Medicine, Mass Genl Hosp 1969; **Fellow:** Immunology, Natl Cancer Inst 1968; **Fac Appt:** Clin Prof Med, Geo Wash Univ

Fishman, Henry J MD [A&I] - **Spec Exp:** Asthma & Allergy; Chemical Exposure; **Hospital:** G Washington Univ Hosp; **Address:** 2141 K St NW, Ste 206, Washington, DC 20037; **Phone:** 202-833-3500; **Board Cert:** Internal Medicine 1982; Allergy & Immunology 1985; **Med School:** Univ Rochester 1979; **Resid:** Internal Medicine, Geo Wash Med Ctr 1982; **Fellow:** Allergy & Immunology, Georgetown Univ Hosp 1984; **Fac Appt:** Asst Clin Prof Med, Georgetown Univ

Kaliner, Michael A MD [A&I] - **Spec Exp:** Asthma & Allergy; Sinusitis; Rhinitis; **Hospital:** W MD Hosp Ctr; **Address:** Institute for Asthma and Allergy, 5454 Wisconsin Ave, Ste 700, Chevy Chase, MD 20815; **Phone:** 301-986-9262; **Board Cert:** Internal Medicine 1974; Allergy & Immunology 1993; **Med School:** Univ MD Sch Med 1967; **Resid:** Internal Medicine, UCSF Med Ctr 1970; **Fellow:** Allergy & Immunology, Harvard Univ 1973; **Fac Appt:** Clin Prof Med, Geo Wash Univ

Mazza, David S MD [A&I] - **Spec Exp:** Asthma; Sinus Disorders; Eczema; **Hospital:** St Luke's - Roosevelt Hosp Ctr - Roosevelt Div (page 57), St Vincent Cath Med Ctrs - Manhattan; **Address:** 7 Lexington Ave, Ste 3, New York, NY 10010-5517; **Phone:** 212-677-7170; **Board Cert:** Pediatrics 1983; Allergy & Immunology 1999; **Med School:** Univ VT Coll Med 1977; **Resid:** Pediatrics, NYU-Bellevue Hosp 1980; **Fellow:** Pediatrics, Bellevue Hosp 1982; Allergy & Immunology, St Luke's-Roosevelt Hosp Ctr 1989; **Fac Appt:** Assoc Prof Ped, Columbia P&S

Metcalfe, Dean D MD [A&I] - **Spec Exp:** Mast Cell Diseases; Food Allergy; Anaphylaxis; **Hospital:** Natl Inst of Hlth - Clin Ctr; **Address:** Natl Inst Allergy & Infectious Disease, Allergic Disease Lab, 10 Center Drive Bldg 10 - rm 11C205, Bethesda, MD 20892-1881; **Phone:** 301-496-2165; **Board Cert:** Internal Medicine 1975; Allergy & Immunology 1977; Rheumatology 1980; **Med School:** Univ Tenn Coll Med, Memphis 1972; **Resid:** Internal Medicine, Univ Mich Hosps 1974; Allergy & Immunology, Natl Inst Allergy & Infectious Dis-NIH 1977; **Fellow:** Rheumatology, Peter Bent Brigham Hosp 1979

Reisman, Robert E MD [A&I] - **Spec Exp:** Anaphylaxis; Asthma; Insect Allergies; **Hospital:** Buffalo General Hosp, Women's & Chldn's Hosp of Buffalo, The; **Address:** Buffalo Medical Group, 295 Essjay Rd, Williamsville, NY 14221-8216; **Phone:** 716-630-1130; **Board Cert:** Internal Medicine 1969; Allergy & Immunology 1972; **Med School:** SUNY Buffalo 1956; **Resid:** Internal Medicine, Buffalo Genl Hosp 1959; **Fellow:** Allergy & Immunology, Buffalo Genl Hosp 1961; **Fac Appt:** Clin Prof Med, SUNY Buffalo

Shepherd, Gillian M MD [A&I] - **Spec Exp:** Food & Drug Allergy; Rhinosinusitis & Asthma; Urticaria; Insect Allergies; **Hospital:** NY-Presby Hosp/Weill Cornell (page 66), Meml Sloan-Kettering Cancer Ctr; **Address:** 235 E 67th St, Ste 203, New York, NY 10021-6040; **Phone:** 212-288-9300; **Board Cert:** Internal Medicine 1979; Allergy & Immunology 1981; **Med School:** NY Med Coll 1976; **Resid:** Internal Medicine, Lenox Hill Hosp 1979; **Fellow:** Allergy & Immunology, New York Hosp-Cornell 1981

Slankard, Marjorie MD [A&I] - **Spec Exp:** Sinus Disorders; Asthma; Food Allergy; **Hospital:** NY-Presby Hosp/Columbia (page 66), Valley Hosp; **Address:** 16 E 60th St, Ste 321, New York, NY 10022-1002; **Phone:** 212-326-8410; **Board Cert:** Internal Medicine 1974; Allergy & Immunology 1977; **Med School:** Univ MO-Columbia Sch Med 1971; **Resid:** Internal Medicine, New York Hosp 1974; Internal Medicine, Rockefeller Univ Hosp 1974; **Fellow:** Immunology, New York Hosp-Cornell 1976; Immunology, Mount Sinai Med Ctr 1980; **Fac Appt:** Clin Prof Med, Columbia P&S

Allergy & Immunology

Strober, Warren MD [A&I] - **Spec Exp:** Immune Deficiency; Inflammatory Bowel Disease/Crohn's; **Hospital:** Natl Inst of Hlth - Clin Ctr; **Address:** NIH-Laboratory of Host Defense, Bldg 10-CRC, rm 5W-3940, Bethesda, MD 20892-1890; **Phone:** 301-496-6810; **Board Cert:** Internal Medicine 1974; Allergy & Immunology 1977; **Med School:** Univ Rochester 1962; **Resid:** Internal Medicine, Strong Meml Hosp 1964; Allergy & Immunology, Natl Inst Hlth 1972

Southeast

Benenati, Susan V MD [A&I] - **Spec Exp:** Asthma; Latex Allergy; Sinus Disorders; Nasal Allergy; **Hospital:** Baptist Hosp of Miami, South Miami Hosp; **Address:** 7000 SW 62nd Ave, Ste 510, South Miami, FL 33143-4721; **Phone:** 305-665-1623; **Board Cert:** Internal Medicine 1988; Allergy & Immunology 1999; **Med School:** Univ S Fla Coll Med 1984; **Resid:** Internal Medicine, Indiana Univ Med Ctr 1988; **Fellow:** Allergy & Immunology, Johns Hopkins Hosp 1990

Bonner, James R MD [A&I] - **Spec Exp:** Asthma; Urticaria; Sinusitis; **Hospital:** Univ of Ala Hosp at Birmingham, VA Med Ctr; **Address:** Univ Alabama Hosp, Allergy/Immunology, 2000 Sixth Ave S, Birmingham, AL 35233-2110; **Phone:** 205-801-8100; **Board Cert:** Internal Medicine 1974; Infectious Disease 1976; Allergy & Immunology 1979; **Med School:** Univ Mich Med Sch 1971; **Resid:** Internal Medicine, Univ Ala Med Ctr 1974; **Fellow:** Allergy & Immunology, Univ Ala Med Ctr 1977; **Fac Appt:** Prof Med, Univ Alabama

DeShazo, Richard D MD [A&I] - **Spec Exp:** Immunodeficiency Disorders; Allergy; Rheumatology; **Hospital:** Univ Mississippi Med Ctr, VA Med Ctr; **Address:** Univ Mississippi Med Ctr, Dept Med, 2500 N State St, Jackson, MS 39216; **Phone:** 601-984-5600; **Board Cert:** Internal Medicine 1974; Allergy & Immunology 1977; Rheumatology 1982; Geriatric Medicine 2005; **Med School:** Univ Alabama 1971; **Resid:** Internal Medicine, Walter Reed Genl Hosp 1974; **Fellow:** Microbiology, Walter Reed Army Inst Rsch 1975; Clinical Immunology, Walter Reed Genl Hosp 1977; **Fac Appt:** Prof Med, Univ Miss

Friedman, Stuart A MD [A&I] - **Spec Exp:** Asthma; Sinus Disorders; Allergy; **Hospital:** Boca Raton Comm Hosp, Delray Med Ctr; **Address:** 5162 Linton Blvd, Ste 201, Delray Beach, FL 33484-6567; **Phone:** 561-495-2580; **Board Cert:** Internal Medicine 1980; Allergy & Immunology 1983; **Med School:** Spain 1976; **Resid:** Internal Medicine, Winthrop Univ Hosp 1980; **Fellow:** Immunology, Univ Cincinnati Med Ctr 1982; **Fac Appt:** Asst Clin Prof Med, Univ Miami Sch Med

Ledford, Dennis K MD [A&I] - **Spec Exp:** Asthma; **Hospital:** University Comm Hosp, Tampa Genl Hosp; **Address:** Univ So Florida Coll Med, Dept Allergy & Immunology, 13801 Bruce B Downs Blvd, Ste 502, Tampa, FL 33613-4745; **Phone:** 813-971-9743; **Board Cert:** Internal Medicine 1980; Rheumatology 1984; Allergy & Immunology 1985; Clinical & Laboratory Immunology 1986; **Med School:** Univ Tenn Coll Med, Memphis 1976; **Resid:** Internal Medicine, City of Memphis Hosp 1980; **Fellow:** Rheumatology, NYU Hosp-Bellevue 1982; Allergy & Immunology, Univ S Florida Coll Med 1985; **Fac Appt:** Assoc Prof A&I, Univ S Fla Coll Med

Lieberman, Phillip L MD [A&I] - **Spec Exp:** Asthma; Rhinitis; Anaphylaxis; **Hospital:** Baptist Memorial Hospital - Memphis, Methodist Univ Hosp - Memphis; **Address:** 7205 Wolf River Blvd, Ste 200, Germantown, TN 38138; **Phone:** 901-757-6100; **Board Cert:** Internal Medicine 1970; Allergy & Immunology 2003; **Med School:** Univ Tenn Coll Med, Memphis 1965; **Resid:** Internal Medicine, Memphis City Hosps 1969; **Fellow:** Allergy & Immunology, Northwestern Univ Affil Hosp 1971; **Fac Appt:** Clin Prof A&I, Univ Tenn Coll Med, Memphis

Lockey, Richard F MD [A&I] - **Spec Exp:** Allergy; Asthma; Rhinitis; Immune Deficiency; **Hospital:** University Comm Hosp, Tampa Genl Hosp; **Address:** 13001 Bruce B Downs Blvd, Ste 111D, Tampa, FL 33613-3946; **Phone:** 813-972-7631; **Board Cert:** Internal Medicine 1970; Allergy & Immunology 1974; **Med School:** Temple Univ 1965; **Resid:** Internal Medicine, Univ Mich Hosp 1968; **Fellow:** Allergy & Immunology, Univ Mich Hosp 1970; **Fac Appt:** Prof Med, Univ S Fla Coll Med

Pacin, Michael P MD [A&I] - **Spec Exp:** Insect Allergies; Asthma; Rhinitis; **Hospital:** Baptist Hosp of Miami, South Miami Hosp; **Address:** Florida Ctr Asthma & Allergy, 9035 Sunset Drive, Ste 202, Miami, FL 33173; **Phone:** 305-279-3366; **Board Cert:** Internal Medicine 1974; Allergy & Immunology 1979; **Med School:** Washington Univ, St Louis 1969; **Resid:** Internal Medicine, Jewish Hosp 1971; Internal Medicine, Jackson Meml Hosp 1972; **Fellow:** Allergy & Immunology, Long Beach VA Hosp 1974

Sullivan, Timothy J MD [A&I] - **Spec Exp:** Drug Allergy; Anaphylaxis; Asthma; **Hospital:** Northside Hosp, St Joseph's Hosp - Atlanta; **Address:** 5555 Peachtree Dunwoody Rd, Ste 125, Atlanta, GA 30342; **Phone:** 404-255-2918; **Board Cert:** Allergy & Immunology 1979; **Med School:** Univ Miami Sch Med 1966; **Resid:** Internal Medicine, Barnes Hosp 1971; **Fellow:** Allergy & Immunology, Barnes Hosp 1973

Midwest

Baker Jr, James Russell MD [A&I] - **Spec Exp:** Immune Deficiency-Thyroid; **Hospital:** Univ Michigan Hlth Sys; **Address:** UM Allergy Specialty Clinic, 24 Frank Lloyd Wright Drive, Ste H-2100, P.O.Box 442, Ann Arbor, MI 48106; **Phone:** 734-647-2777; **Board Cert:** Internal Medicine 1981; Allergy & Immunology 1983; Clinical & Laboratory Immunology 1986; **Med School:** Loyola Univ-Stritch Sch Med 1978; **Resid:** Internal Medicine, Walter Reed Army Med Ctr 1981; **Fellow:** Allergy & Immunology, Walter Reed Army Med Ctr/NIAID 1984; **Fac Appt:** Prof A&I, Univ Mich Med Sch

Berger, Melvin MD/PhD [A&I] - **Spec Exp:** Immune Deficiency; Asthma & Allergy; **Hospital:** Rainbow Babies & Chldns Hosp, Univ Hosps Case Med Ctr; **Address:** Pediatric Immunology, 11100 Euclid Ave, MC 6008B, Cleveland, OH 44106-1736; **Phone:** 216-844-3237; **Board Cert:** Pediatrics 1981; Allergy & Immunology 1981; **Med School:** Case West Res Univ 1976; **Resid:** Pediatrics, Chldns Hosp Med Ctr 1978; **Fellow:** Allergy & Immunology, Natl Inst Allergy & Infect Dis (NIH) 1981; **Fac Appt:** Prof Ped, Case West Res Univ

Bernstein, David Isaac MD [A&I] - **Spec Exp:** Occupational Asthma; Asthma; Rhinosinusitis; **Hospital:** Univ Hosp - Cincinnati; **Address:** U Cincinnatti Med Ctr, 231 Bethesda Ave, ML 0563, Cincinnati, OH 45229-0563; **Phone:** 513-558-4701; **Board Cert:** Internal Medicine 1980; Allergy & Immunology 1983; Diagnostic Lab Immunology 1988; **Med School:** Univ Cincinnati 1977; **Resid:** Internal Medicine, Cleveland Clinic 1980; **Fellow:** Allergy & Immunology, Northwestern Univ 1982; **Fac Appt:** Clin Prof Med, Univ Cincinnati

Bernstein, Jonathan A MD [A&I] - **Spec Exp:** Asthma; Occupational Asthma; Drug Allergy; Eczema; **Hospital:** Univ Hosp - Cincinnati; **Address:** U Cincinnatti Med Ctr, 231 Albert Sabin Way, ML 0563, Cincinnati, OH 45267-0563; **Phone:** 513-558-4701; **Board Cert:** Internal Medicine 1988; Allergy & Immunology 2001; **Med School:** Univ Cincinnati 1985; **Resid:** Internal Medicine, Cleveland Clinic 1988; **Fellow:** Allergy & Immunology, Northwestern Univ 1990; **Fac Appt:** Assoc Prof Med, Univ Cincinnati

Busse, William MD [A&I] - **Spec Exp:** Asthma; Autoimmune Disease; Rhinitis; **Hospital:** Univ WI Hosp & Clins; **Address:** 600 Highland Ave, rm B6-242, Madison, WI 53792; **Phone:** 608-263-6180; **Board Cert:** Internal Medicine 1972; Allergy & Immunology 1974; **Med School:** Univ Wisc 1966; **Resid:** Internal Medicine, Cincinnati Genl Hosp 1968; Internal Medicine, Cincinnati Genl Hosp 1971; **Fellow:** Allergy & Immunology, Univ Wisconsin 1973; **Fac Appt:** Prof Med, Univ Wisc

Allergy & Immunology

Gewurz, Anita T MD [A&I] - Spec Exp: Immune Deficiency; Asthma; **Hospital:** Rush Univ Med Ctr; **Address:** Univ Consultants, 1725 W Harrison St, Ste 117, Chicago, IL 60612; **Phone:** 312-942-6296; **Board Cert:** Pediatrics 1976; Allergy & Immunology 1977; **Med School:** Albany Med Coll 1970; **Resid:** Pediatrics, Univ Illinois Med Ctr 1973; Allergy & Immunology, Rush-Presby-St Lukes Hosp 1976; **Fellow:** Allergy & Immunology, Grant Hosp 1977; Allergy & Immunology, Northwestern Univ Med Sch 1985; **Fac Appt:** Prof Med, Rush Med Coll

Grammer, Leslie C MD [A&I] - Spec Exp: Asthma; Sinusitis; Drug Allergy; **Hospital:** Northwestern Meml Hosp, Rehab Inst of Chicago; **Address:** Northwestern Med Faculty Fdn, Amb Care Ctr, 675 N St Clair Fl 18 - Ste 18-250, Chicago, IL 60611-5975; **Phone:** 312-695-8624; **Board Cert:** Internal Medicine 1979; Allergy & Immunology 1981; Diagnostic Lab Immunology 1986; Occupational Medicine 1989; **Med School:** Northwestern Univ 1976; **Resid:** Internal Medicine, Northwestern Meml Hosp 1979; **Fellow:** Allergy & Immunology, Northwestern Meml Hosp 1981; **Fac Appt:** Prof Med, Northwestern Univ

Greenberger, Paul A MD [A&I] - Spec Exp: Asthma; Anaphylaxis; Drug Allergy; Hypersensitivity Pneumonitis; **Hospital:** Northwestern Meml Hosp, Jesse A Brown VA Med Ctr; **Address:** Northwestern Medical Faculty Fdn, Ambulatory Care Center, 675 N St Clair Fl 18 - Ste 18-250, Chicago, IL 60611; **Phone:** 312-695-8624; **Board Cert:** Internal Medicine 1976; Allergy & Immunology 1979; Diagnostic Lab Immunology 1986; **Med School:** Indiana Univ 1973; **Resid:** Internal Medicine, Jewish Hosp 1976; **Fellow:** Allergy & Immunology, Northwestern Meml Hosp 1978; **Fac Appt:** Prof Med, Northwestern Univ

Korenblat, Phillip E MD [A&I] - Spec Exp: Allergy; Asthma; Anaphylaxis; **Hospital:** Barnes-Jewish West County Hosp, Missouri Baptist Med Ctr; **Address:** 1040 N Mason Rd, Ste 115, St Louis, MO 63141-6361; **Phone:** 314-542-0606; **Board Cert:** Internal Medicine 1971; Allergy & Immunology 1974; **Med School:** Univ Ark 1960; **Resid:** Internal Medicine, Jewish Hosp 1965; **Fellow:** Allergy & Immunology, Scripps Clin Rsch Fdn 1966; **Fac Appt:** Clin Prof Med, Washington Univ, St Louis

Routes, John M MD [A&I] - Spec Exp: Immunodeficiency Disorders; Asthma; Allergy; **Hospital:** Chldns Hosp - Wisconsin; **Address:** Children's Hosp Wisconsin, 9000 W Wisconsin Ave, Ste 440, Milwaukee, WI 53226; **Phone:** 414-266-6840; **Board Cert:** Internal Medicine 1984; Allergy & Immunology 1987; **Med School:** Indiana Univ 1981; **Resid:** Internal Medicine, Univ Utah Affil Hosps 1984; **Fellow:** Allergy & Immunology, Natl Jewish Hosp 1989; Infectious Disease, Natl Jewish Hosp 1990; **Fac Appt:** Prof Ped, Univ Colorado

Sanders, Georgiana MD [A&I] - Spec Exp: Asthma; Food Allergy & Eczema; Rhinitis; **Hospital:** Univ Michigan Hlth Sys, St Joseph Mercy Hosp - Ann Arbor; **Address:** Domino's Farms Allergy Specialy Clin, 24 Frank Lloyd Wright Dr, Ste H-2100, PO Box 442, Ann Arbor, MI 48106; **Phone:** 734-936-5634; **Board Cert:** Pediatrics 1982; Allergy & Immunology 1985; **Med School:** Univ Cincinnati 1975; **Resid:** Pediatrics, Chldns Hosp Mich 1978; Pediatrics, Boston City Hosp 1979; **Fellow:** Allergy & Immunology, Univ of Michigan Hosp 1984; **Fac Appt:** Asst Clin Prof Med, Univ Mich Med Sch

Wood, John A MD [A&I] - Spec Exp: Asthma; **Hospital:** St Luke's Hosp - Chesterfield, MO; **Address:** 224 S Woodsmill Rd, Ste 500S, Chesterfield, MO 63017; **Phone:** 314-878-6260; **Board Cert:** Internal Medicine 1972; Pulmonary Disease 1978; Allergy & Immunology 1979; **Med School:** Univ Okla Coll Med 1968; **Resid:** Internal Medicine, Univ Hosp 1970; Internal Medicine, Barnes Hosp-Wash Univ Sch Med 1971; **Fellow:** Pulmonary Disease, Wash Univ Sch Med 1977; Allergy & Immunology, Wash Univ Sch Med 1977; **Fac Appt:** Asst Prof Med, Washington Univ, St Louis

Southwest

Freeman, Theodore M MD [A&I] - **Spec Exp:** Insect Allergies; Asthma; Rhinitis; **Hospital:** SW TX Meth Hosp; **Address:** 8285 Fredericksberg Rd, San Antonio, TX 78229; **Phone:** 210-614-3923; **Board Cert:** Internal Medicine 1983; Allergy & Immunology 1987; Clinical & Laboratory Immunology 1988; **Med School:** Univ S Fla Coll Med 1980; **Resid:** Internal Medicine, Keesler Med Ctr 1983; **Fellow:** Allergy & Immunology, Wilford Hall Med Ctr 1986; Diagnostic Lab Immunology, Mass Genl Hosp 1987; **Fac Appt:** Assoc Prof Med, Uniformed Srvs Univ, Bethesda

Gruchalla, Rebecca S MD/PhD [A&I] - **Spec Exp:** Asthma & Allergy; Drug Allergy; Immunodeficiency Disorders; **Hospital:** UT Southwestern Med Ctr at Dallas, Chldns Med Ctr of Dallas; **Address:** Div Allergy & Immunology, 5323 Harry Hines Blvd, Dallas, TX 75390-8872; **Phone:** 214-645-2800; **Board Cert:** Internal Medicine 1988; Allergy & Immunology 2001; **Med School:** Univ Tex SW, Dallas 1985; **Resid:** Internal Medicine, Hosp Univ Penn 1988; **Fellow:** Allergy & Immunology, Univ Tex SW Med Ctr 1990; **Fac Appt:** Prof Med, Univ Tex SW, Dallas

Lewis, John C MD [A&I] - **Spec Exp:** Autoimmune Disease; **Hospital:** Mayo Clinic - Scottsdale; **Address:** Mayo Clinic, Div Allergy & Immunology, 13400 E Shea Blvd, ALRG-2B, Scottsdale, AZ 85259-5404; **Phone:** 480-301-8227; **Board Cert:** Internal Medicine 1985; Allergy & Immunology 2001; **Med School:** Loyola Univ-Stritch Sch Med 1982; **Resid:** Internal Medicine, Wilford Hall USAF Med Ctr 1985; **Fellow:** Allergy & Immunology, Mayo Clinic 1990; **Fac Appt:** Prof Med, Mayo Med Sch

Schubert, Mark S MD/PhD [A&I] - **Spec Exp:** Asthma & Allergy; Sinus Disorders; **Hospital:** Banner Good Samaritan Regl Med Ctr - Phoenix, St Joseph's Hosp & Med Ctr - Phoenix; **Address:** Asthma Allergy Clinic, 300 W Clarendon Rd, Ste 120, Phoenix, AZ 85013-2517; **Phone:** 602-277-3337; **Board Cert:** Internal Medicine 1987; Allergy & Immunology 1999; **Med School:** Univ Ariz Coll Med 1983; **Resid:** Neurological Surgery, Barrow Neurological Inst 1985; Internal Medicine, Good Samaritan Med Ctr 1987; **Fellow:** Allergy Immunology & Rheumatology, Stanford Univ Med Ctr 1989; **Fac Appt:** Assoc Clin Prof Med, Univ Ariz Coll Med

West Coast and Pacific

Altman, Leonard C MD [A&I] - **Spec Exp:** Urticaria; Asthma; Sinusitis; Allergy; **Hospital:** Univ Wash Med Ctr, Chldns Hosp and Regl Med Ctr - Seattle; **Address:** 4540 Sand Point Way NE, Ste 200, Seattle, WA 98105-3941; **Phone:** 206-527-1200; **Board Cert:** Internal Medicine 1975; Allergy & Immunology 1979; **Med School:** Harvard Med Sch 1969; **Resid:** Internal Medicine, Univ Wash Affil Hosps 1971; Internal Medicine, Univ Wash Affil Hosps 1975; **Fellow:** Allergy & Immunology, Natl Inst Hlth 1974; **Fac Appt:** Clin Prof Med, Univ Wash

Henderson Jr, William R MD [A&I] - **Spec Exp:** Asthma; Allergic Rhinitis; **Hospital:** Univ Wash Med Ctr; **Address:** 1959 NE Pacific St, Ste EA 300, Seattle, WA 98195; **Phone:** 206-543-3780; **Board Cert:** Internal Medicine 1976; Allergy & Immunology 1979; **Med School:** UCSF 1973; **Resid:** Internal Medicine, Stanford Med Ctr 1975; Internal Medicine, Natl Inst Hlth 1976; **Fellow:** Allergy & Immunology, Natl Inst Hlth 1978; **Fac Appt:** Prof Med, Univ Wash

Meltzer, Eli O MD [A&I] - **Spec Exp:** Asthma & Allergy; Sinus Disorders; Rhinitis; **Hospital:** Rady Children's Hosp - San Diego, Sharp Meml Hosp; **Address:** Allergy & Asthma Medical & Research Ctr, 9610 Granite Ridge Drive, Ste B, San Diego, CA 92123-2661; **Phone:** 858-292-1144; **Board Cert:** Pediatrics 1969; Allergy & Immunology 1972; Pediatric Allergy & Immunology 1969; **Med School:** Jefferson Med Coll 1964; **Resid:** Pediatrics, St Christophers Hosp Chldn 1967; **Fellow:** Pediatric Allergy & Immunology, National Jewish Hosp 1969; **Fac Appt:** Clin Prof Ped, UCSD

Allergy & Immunology

Montanaro, Anthony MD [A&I] - **Spec Exp:** Asthma; Allergy; Anaphylaxis; Immunodeficiency Disorders; **Hospital:** OR Hlth & Sci Univ; **Address:** OHSU Div Allergy & Clin Immunology, 3181 SW Sam Jackson Park Rd, MC OP-34, Portland, OR 97239-2098; **Phone:** 503-494-4300; **Board Cert:** Internal Medicine 1981; Allergy & Immunology 1993; Rheumatology 1984; **Med School:** Univ Wash 1978; **Resid:** Internal Medicine, Mercy Med Ctr 1981; **Fellow:** Allergy Immunology & Rheumatology, Oregon Hlth Sci Univ 1983; **Fac Appt:** Prof Med, Oregon Hlth & Sci Univ

Ostrom, Nancy K MD [A&I] - **Spec Exp:** Asthma & Allergy; **Hospital:** Rady Children's Hosp - San Diego; **Address:** 9610 Granite Ridge Drive, Ste B, San Diego, CA 92123; **Phone:** 858-292-1144; **Board Cert:** Pediatrics 1984; Allergy & Immunology 1987; **Med School:** Mayo Med Sch 1980; **Resid:** Pediatrics, Mayo Clinic 1983; **Fellow:** Allergy & Immunology, Mayo Clinic 1985; **Fac Appt:** Assoc Clin Prof Ped, UCSD

Tamaroff, Marc A MD [A&I] - **Spec Exp:** Sinus Disorders; Asthma; Rhinitis; **Hospital:** Long Beach Meml Med Ctr, Lakewood Reg Med Ctr; **Address:** 3816 Woodruff Ave, Ste 209, Long Beach, CA 90808-2145; **Phone:** 562-496-4749; **Board Cert:** Internal Medicine 1979; Allergy & Immunology 1983; **Med School:** Univ Ariz Coll Med 1974; **Resid:** Internal Medicine, St Mary Med Ctr 1977; **Fellow:** Allergy & Immunology, UCLA Med Ctr 1979; **Fac Appt:** Assoc Clin Prof Med, UCLA

Wasserman, Stephen I MD [A&I] - **Spec Exp:** Asthma; Rhinitis; Sinus Disorders; Urticaria; **Hospital:** UCSD Med Ctr; **Address:** UCSD, MC 0637, Stein Bldg-rm 244, 9500 Gilman Drive, La Jolla, CA 92093-0637; **Phone:** 858-822-4261; **Board Cert:** Internal Medicine 1973; Allergy & Immunology 1975; **Med School:** UCLA 1968; **Resid:** Internal Medicine, Peter Bent Brigham Hosp 1970; **Fellow:** Allergy & Immunology, R Breck-PB Brigham Hosps 1974; **Fac Appt:** Prof Med, UCSD

Cleveland Clinic

Pulmonary, Allergy and Critical Care Medicine

The Section of Allergy/Immunology at Cleveland Clinic is one of the largest allergy and immunology groups in the United States with a national reputation for excellence. Patients have access not only to state-of-the-art medical therapies but also to investigational protocols.

Allergy/immunology diagnosis and treatment takes place in a multidisciplinary fashion that includes close coordination with specialists in other areas.

Asthma

We provide state-of-the-art management for patients whose asthma is not well controlled. This includes assessments of coexisting conditions that make asthma difficult to treat or unresponsive to standard treatment. We offer new medications that may not be available in primary care settings and interventions that may not be provided by asthma specialists in the community.

Aspirin Sensitivity and Desensitization

Individuals who are sensitive to aspirin often experience respiratory reactions, including wheezing, shortness of breath, or skin reactions, such as hives or swelling. We offer a special desensitization program for aspirin-sensitive patients who have respiratory reactions but require aspirin for cardiovascular or rheumatic conditions. This procedure, available at only a few centers in the United States, can permit such patients to take aspirin safely.

Areas of Expertise

- Asthma
- Rhinitis, allergic and non-allergic
- Sinusitis
- Chronic cough
- Aspirin sensitivity
- Urticaria/angioedema
- Atopic dermatitis
- Adverse reactions to medicine, food and bee stings
- Anaphylaxis
- Systemic mastocytosis
- Immunodeficiency

For more information about the Cleveland Clinic Department of Pulmonary, Allergy and Critical Care Medicine, to schedule a second opinion or to learn about assistance for out-of-town patients, call 800.890.2467 or visit www. clevelandclinic.org/allergytopdocs.

Department of Pulmonology, Allergy and Critical Care Medicine
9500 Euclid Avenue / AC311 | Cleveland OH 44195

Cardiovascular Disease

a subspecialty of Internal Medicine

Cardiovascular Disease: An internist specializing in diseases of the heart, lungs and blood vessels and manages complex cardiac conditions such as heart attacks and life-threatening, abnormal heartbeat rhythms.

Cardiac Electrophysiology: A field of special interest within the subspecialty of cardiovascular disease which involves intricate technical procedures to evaluate heart rhythms and determine appropriate treatment for them.

Interventional Cardiology: An area of medicine within the subspecialty of cardiology which uses specialized imaging and other diagnostic techniques to evaluate blood flow and pressure in the coronary arteries and chambers of the heart, and uses technical procedures and medications to treat abnormalities that impair the function of the heart.

Training Required: Three years in internal medicine *plus* additional training and examination for certification in cardiovascular disease, clinical electrophysiology or interventional cardiology

CARDIOVASCULAR DISEASE

New England

Balady, Gary MD [Cv] - **Spec Exp:** Preventive Cardiology; **Hospital:** Boston Med Ctr; **Address:** Boston Med Ctr, Dept Cardiology, 88 East Newton St, Preston 4 Cardiovascular Ctr, Boston, MA 02118; **Phone:** 617-638-7490; **Board Cert:** Internal Medicine 1982; Cardiovascular Disease 1985; **Med School:** UMDNJ-Rutgers Med Sch 1979; **Resid:** Internal Medicine, Boston Univ Med Ctr 1982; **Fellow:** Cardiovascular Disease, Boston Univ Med Ctr 1985; **Fac Appt:** Prof Med, Boston Univ

Baughman, Kenneth MD [Cv] - **Spec Exp:** Congestive Heart Failure; Heart Valve Disease; Coronary Artery Disease; **Hospital:** Brigham & Women's Hosp; **Address:** Brigham & Womens Hosp, Shapiro Cardiovascular Ctr, 75 Francis St, Office 05-154, Boston, MA 02115; **Phone:** 857-307-1964; **Board Cert:** Internal Medicine 1975; Cardiovascular Disease 1979; **Med School:** Univ MO-Columbia Sch Med 1972; **Resid:** Internal Medicine, Johns Hopkins Hosp 1977; **Fellow:** Cardiovascular Disease, Mass Genl Hosp 1979; **Fac Appt:** Prof Med, Harvard Med Sch

Cabin, Henry S MD [Cv] - **Spec Exp:** Interventional Cardiology; Cardiac Catheterization; **Hospital:** Yale-New Haven Hosp; **Address:** 333 Cedar St, PO Box 208017, New Haven, CT 06520-8017; **Phone:** 203-785-4129; **Board Cert:** Internal Medicine 1978; Cardiovascular Disease 1983; Interventional Cardiology 2000; **Med School:** Yale Univ 1975; **Resid:** Internal Medicine, Yale-New Haven Hosp 1978; **Fellow:** Internal Medicine, Natl Heart Lung and Blood Inst 1981; Cardiovascular Disease, Yale New Haven Hosp 1982; **Fac Appt:** Prof Med, Yale Univ

Catherwood, Edward MD [Cv] - **Hospital:** Dartmouth - Hitchcock Med Ctr; **Address:** Dartmouth-Hitchcock Medical Ctr, Div Cardiology, 1 Medical Center Drive, Lebanon, NH 03756; **Phone:** 603-650-3540; **Board Cert:** Internal Medicine 1978; Cardiovascular Disease 1981; Critical Care Medicine 1999; **Med School:** Jefferson Med Coll 1975; **Resid:** Internal Medicine, Hahnemann Univ Hosp 1978; **Fellow:** Cardiovascular Disease, Hahnemann Univ Hosp 1980; **Fac Appt:** Asst Prof Med, Dartmouth Med Sch

Hutter Jr, Adolph M MD [Cv] - **Hospital:** Mass Genl Hosp; **Address:** 55 Fruit St, Yawkey Ctr, rm 5B, Boston, MA 02114-3139; **Phone:** 617-726-2884; **Board Cert:** Internal Medicine 1969; Cardiovascular Disease 1971; **Med School:** Univ Wisc 1963; **Resid:** Internal Medicine, Strong Meml Hosp 1968; **Fellow:** Cardiovascular Disease, Mass Genl Hosp 1970; **Fac Appt:** Prof Med, Harvard Med Sch

Johnson, Paula A MD [Cv] - **Spec Exp:** Heart Disease in Women; Preventive Cardiology; Congestive Heart Failure; **Hospital:** Brigham & Women's Hosp; **Address:** Brigham & Womens Hosp, 75 Francis St, PB5-534, Boston, MA 02115; **Phone:** 617-732-5500; **Board Cert:** Internal Medicine 1988; Cardiovascular Disease 2001; **Med School:** Harvard Med Sch 1985; **Resid:** Internal Medicine, Brigham & Womens Hosp 1988; **Fellow:** Cardiovascular Disease, Brigham & Womens Hosp 1991; **Fac Appt:** Assoc Prof Med, Harvard Med Sch

Kirshenbaum, James M MD [Cv] - **Spec Exp:** Cardiac Catheterization; Coronary Artery Disease; Congestive Heart Failure; **Hospital:** Brigham & Women's Hosp; **Address:** Brigham & Womens Hosp, Div Cardiology, 75 Francis St, Boston, MA 02115-6110; **Phone:** 857-307-1967; **Board Cert:** Internal Medicine 1982; Cardiovascular Disease 1985; Interventional Cardiology 1999; **Med School:** Harvard Med Sch 1979; **Resid:** Internal Medicine, Peter Bent Brigham Hosp 1982; **Fellow:** Cardiovascular Disease, Brigham & Womens Hosp 1985; **Fac Appt:** Assoc Prof Med, Harvard Med Sch

Konstam, Marvin A MD [Cv] - **Spec Exp:** Transplant Medicine-Heart; Heart Failure; Coronary Angioplasty/Stents; **Hospital:** Tufts Med Ctr; **Address:** New England Med Ctr, Div Cardiology, 750 Washington St, Box 108, Boston, MA 02111; **Phone:** 617-636-6293; **Board Cert:** Internal Medicine 1979; Cardiovascular Disease 1981; Diagnostic Radiology 1980; **Med School:** Columbia P&S 1975; **Resid:** Diagnostic Radiology, Mass Genl Hosp 1978; Internal Medicine, Mass Genl Hosp 1979; **Fellow:** Cardiovascular Disease, Brigham & Women's Hosp 1981; **Fac Appt:** Prof Med, Tufts Univ

Liang, Bruce T MD [Cv] - **Spec Exp:** Ischemic Heart Disease; Congestive Heart Failure; **Hospital:** Univ of Conn Hlth Ctr, John Dempsey Hosp; **Address:** Univ Connecticut Health Ctr, Cardiopulmonary & Hypertension Service, 263 Farmington Ave, Farmington, CT 06030-2202; **Phone:** 860-679-3343; **Board Cert:** Internal Medicine 1985; Cardiovascular Disease 1987; **Med School:** Harvard Med Sch 1982; **Resid:** Internal Medicine, Hosp Univ Penn 1985; **Fellow:** Cardiovascular Disease, Brigham & Womens Hosp 1987; **Fac Appt:** Prof Med, Univ Conn

Libby, Peter MD [Cv] - **Spec Exp:** Preventive Cardiology; Coronary Artery Disease; Cholesterol/Lipid Disorders; **Hospital:** Brigham & Women's Hosp; **Address:** Brigham & Women's Hosp, Cardiovasc Div, 75 Francis St, Boston, MA 02115-5822; **Phone:** 617-732-8086; **Board Cert:** Internal Medicine 1976; Cardiovascular Disease 1981; **Med School:** UCSD 1973; **Resid:** Internal Medicine, Peter Bent Brigham Hosp 1976; **Fellow:** Physiology, Harvard Med Sch 1979; Cardiovascular Disease, Brigham & Woman's Hosp 1980; **Fac Appt:** Prof Med, Harvard Med Sch

Loscalzo, Joseph MD/PhD [Cv] - **Spec Exp:** Coronary Artery Disease; Peripheral Vascular Disease; **Hospital:** Brigham & Women's Hosp; **Address:** Brigham & Women's Hosp, Div Cardiology, 75 Francis St, Boston, MA 02115; **Phone:** 617-732-6340; **Board Cert:** Internal Medicine 1981; Cardiovascular Disease 1983; **Med School:** Univ Pennsylvania 1978; **Resid:** Internal Medicine, Peter Bent Brigham Hosp 1981; **Fellow:** Cardiovascular Disease, Brigham & Women's Hosp 1983; **Fac Appt:** Prof Med, Harvard Med Sch

Manning, Warren MD [Cv] - **Spec Exp:** Heart Valve Disease; Echocardiography; **Hospital:** Beth Israel Deaconess Med Ctr - Boston; **Address:** BIDMC, Dept Non-Invasive Cardiology, 330 Brookline Ave, Boston, MA 02215-5400; **Phone:** 617-667-2192; **Board Cert:** Internal Medicine 1986; Cardiovascular Disease 1989; **Med School:** Harvard Med Sch 1983; **Resid:** Internal Medicine, Beth Israel Hosp 1986; **Fellow:** Cardiovascular Disease, Beth Israel Hosp 1989; **Fac Appt:** Prof Med, Harvard Med Sch

O'Gara, Patrick T MD [Cv] - **Spec Exp:** Heart Valve Disease; Coronary Artery Disease; Aortic Diseases & Dissection; **Hospital:** Brigham & Women's Hosp; **Address:** Brigham & Womens Hosp, Cardiovascular Div, 75 Francis St, Boston, MA 02115-6106; **Phone:** 857-307-1990; **Board Cert:** Internal Medicine 1981; Cardiovascular Disease 1983; **Med School:** Northwestern Univ 1978; **Resid:** Internal Medicine, Mass Genl Hosp 1981; **Fellow:** Cardiovascular Disease, Mass Genl Hosp 1983; **Fac Appt:** Assoc Prof Med, Harvard Med Sch

Palacios, Igor F MD [Cv] - **Spec Exp:** Interventional Cardiology; **Hospital:** Mass Genl Hosp; **Address:** Mass Genl Hosp, Cardiac Unit, 55 Fruit St, GRB 800, Boston, MA 02114; **Phone:** 617-726-8424; **Board Cert:** Internal Medicine 1979; Cardiovascular Disease 1981; Interventional Cardiology 1999; **Med School:** Venezuela 1969; **Resid:** Cardiovascular Disease, Hosp Univ de Caracas 1973; **Fellow:** Cardiovascular Disease, Mass Genl Hosp-Harvard 1980; **Fac Appt:** Assoc Prof Med, Harvard Med Sch

Pfeffer, Marc Alan MD [Cv] - **Hospital:** Brigham & Women's Hosp; **Address:** Brigham & Women's Hospital, 75 Francis St, Boston, MA 02115; **Phone:** 617-732-5681; **Board Cert:** Internal Medicine 1979; Cardiovascular Disease 1981; **Med School:** Univ Okla Coll Med 1976; **Resid:** Internal Medicine, Peter Bent Brigham Hosp 1979; **Fellow:** Cardiovascular Disease, Peter Bent Brigham Hosp 1980; **Fac Appt:** Prof Med, Harvard Med Sch

Cardiovascular Disease

Phillips, Robert A MD/PhD [Cv] - **Spec Exp:** Hypertension; Coronary Artery Disease; Heart Valve Disease; **Hospital:** UMass Memorial Med Ctr; **Address:** U Mass Memorial, 55 Lake Ave North, S3-836, Worcester, MA 01655; **Phone:** 508-334-3747; **Board Cert:** Internal Medicine 1983; Cardiovascular Disease 1985; **Med School:** Mount Sinai Sch Med 1980; **Resid:** Internal Medicine, Columbia Presby Med Ctr 1983; **Fellow:** Cardiovascular Disease, Mt Sinai Med Ctr 1985; Hypertension, Mt Sinai Med Ctr 1986; **Fac Appt:** Prof Med, Univ Mass Sch Med

Ridker, Paul M MD [Cv] - **Spec Exp:** Coronary Artery Disease; Preventive Cardiology; Cholesterol/Lipid Disorders; **Hospital:** Brigham & Women's Hosp; **Address:** Brigham & Women's Hospital, Div Preventive Medicine, 640 Center St, Jamaica Plains, MA 02130; **Phone:** 617-983-4100; **Board Cert:** Internal Medicine 1989; **Med School:** Harvard Med Sch 1986; **Resid:** Internal Medicine, Brigham & Women's Hosp 1989; **Fellow:** Cardiovascular Disease, Brigham & Women's Hosp 1991; **Fac Appt:** Assoc Prof Med, Harvard Med Sch

Roberts, Barbara H MD [Cv] - **Spec Exp:** Heart Disease in Women; Preventive Cardiology; **Hospital:** Miriam Hosp; **Address:** The Miriam Hosp - Women's Cardiac Ctr, 164 Summit Ave, Fain Hlth Ctrs Fl 2, Providence, RI 02906; **Phone:** 401-793-7870; **Board Cert:** Internal Medicine 1975; Cardiovascular Disease 1975; **Med School:** Case West Res Univ 1968; **Resid:** Internal Medicine, Yale-New Haven Hosp 1971; **Fellow:** Cardiovascular Disease, PB Brigham Hosp-Harvard 1975; **Fac Appt:** Assoc Clin Prof Med, Brown Univ

Simons, Michael MD [Cv] - **Spec Exp:** Ischemic Heart Disease; Nuclear Cardiology; **Hospital:** Yale-New Haven Hosp; **Address:** 333 Cedar St - FMP, rm 316, New Haven, CT 06520; **Phone:** 203-785-5790; **Board Cert:** Internal Medicine 1987; Cardiovascular Disease 2001; **Med School:** Yale Univ 1984; **Resid:** Internal Medicine, New England Med Ctr 1986; **Fellow:** Cardiology Research, Natl Inst Hlth 1989; Cardiovascular Disease, Beth Israel Hosp 1991; **Fac Appt:** Prof Med, Dartmouth Med Sch

Stevenson, Lynne W MD [Cv] - **Spec Exp:** Heart Failure; Transplant Medicine-Heart; **Hospital:** Brigham & Women's Hosp; **Address:** Brigham & Women's Hospital, 75 Francis St, Boston, MA 02115; **Phone:** 857-307-4000; **Board Cert:** Internal Medicine 1982; Cardiovascular Disease 1985; **Med School:** Stanford Univ 1979; **Resid:** Internal Medicine, UCLA Med Ctr 1982; **Fellow:** Cardiovascular Disease, UCLA Med Ctr 1984; **Fac Appt:** Prof Med, Harvard Med Sch

Zaret, Barry L MD [Cv] - **Spec Exp:** Nuclear Cardiology; Heart Failure; Coronary Artery Disease; **Hospital:** Yale-New Haven Hosp; **Address:** 333 Cedar St, 3-FMP, New Haven, CT 06520-8017; **Phone:** 203-785-4127; **Board Cert:** Internal Medicine 1973; Cardiovascular Disease 1973; **Med School:** NYU Sch Med 1966; **Resid:** Internal Medicine, Bellevue Hosp Ctr 1969; **Fellow:** Cardiovascular Disease, Johns Hopkins Hosp 1971; **Fac Appt:** Prof Med, Yale Univ

Zusman, Randall M MD [Cv] - **Spec Exp:** Hypertension; Cholesterol/Lipid Disorders; Atrial Fibrillation; Coronary Artery Disease; **Hospital:** Mass Genl Hosp; **Address:** Massachusettes Hospital, Yawkey Ctr, 55 Fruit St, Ste 5928, Boston, MA 02114; **Phone:** 617-726-7790; **Board Cert:** Internal Medicine 1976; Cardiovascular Disease 1983; **Med School:** Yale Univ 1973; **Resid:** Internal Medicine, Mass General Hosp 1978; Internal Medicine, Natl Heart, Lung, & Blood Inst (NHBLI) 1977; **Fellow:** Cardiovascular Disease, Mass General Hosp 1979; **Fac Appt:** Assoc Prof Med, Harvard Med Sch

Mid Atlantic

Blumenthal, David S MD [Cv] - **Spec Exp:** Heart Valve Disease; Preventive Cardiology; Coronary Artery Disease; **Hospital:** NY-Presby Hosp/Weill Cornell (page 66); **Address:** 407 E 70th St, Fl 1, New York, NY 10021-5302; **Phone:** 212-861-3222; **Board Cert:** Internal Medicine 1978; Cardiovascular Disease 1981; **Med School:** Cornell Univ-Weill Med Coll 1975; **Resid:** Internal Medicine, NY Hosp 1978; Internal Medicine, NY Hosp 1981; **Fellow:** Cardiovascular Disease, Johns Hopkins Hosp 1980; **Fac Appt:** Clin Prof Med, Cornell Univ-Weill Med Coll

Blumenthal, Roger S MD [Cv] - **Spec Exp:** Preventive Cardiology; Hypertension; Cardiovascular Disease/Young Adult; **Hospital:** Johns Hopkins Hosp (page 61); **Address:** Johns Hopkins Hospital, Div Cardiology, 600 N Wolfe St Blalock Bldg - rm 524C, Baltimore, MD 21287; **Phone:** 410-955-7376; **Board Cert:** Internal Medicine 1988; Cardiovascular Disease 2003; **Med School:** Cornell Univ-Weill Med Coll 1985; **Resid:** Internal Medicine, Johns Hopkins Hosp 1988; **Fellow:** Cardiovascular Disease, Johns Hopkins Hosp 1992; **Fac Appt:** Assoc Prof Med, Johns Hopkins Univ

Borer, Jeffrey S MD [Cv] - **Spec Exp:** Heart Valve Disease; Heart Failure; Nuclear Cardiology; **Hospital:** SUNY Downstate Med Ctr, NY-Presby Hosp/Weill Cornell (page 66); **Address:** SUNY Downstate Med Ctr, Div Cardiology, 445 Lenox Rd, Brooklyn, NY 11226; **Phone:** 212-289-7777; **Board Cert:** Internal Medicine 1973; Cardiovascular Disease 1975; **Med School:** Cornell Univ-Weill Med Coll 1969; **Resid:** Internal Medicine, Mass Genl Hosp 1971; **Fellow:** Cardiovascular Disease, Natl Heart, Lung & Blood Inst 1974; Cardiovascular Disease, Guy's Hosp 1975; **Fac Appt:** Prof Med, SUNY Downstate

Bove, Alfred A MD/PhD [Cv] - **Spec Exp:** Diving Medicine; Heart Failure; Sports Medicine; **Hospital:** Temple Univ Hosp; **Address:** Temple Univ Hosp, Div Cardiology, 3401 N Broad St, Parkinson Pavillon, Philadelphia, PA 19140; **Phone:** 215-707-5757; **Board Cert:** Internal Medicine 1971; Cardiovascular Disease 1983; Undersea & Hyperbaric Medicine 2000; **Med School:** Temple Univ 1966; **Resid:** Internal Medicine, Temple Univ Hosp 1970; **Fellow:** Physiology, Temple Univ Hosp 1970; Physiology, Mayo Clinic 1971; **Fac Appt:** Prof Emeritus Med, Temple Univ

Brozena, Susan C MD [Cv] - **Spec Exp:** Transplant Medicine-Heart; Congestive Heart Failure; Heart Disease in Women; **Hospital:** Hosp Univ Penn - UPHS (page 60); **Address:** Hosp Univ Penn, Div Cardiovascular Med, 3400 Spruce St, 6 Penn Tower, Philadelphia, PA 19104-4283; **Phone:** 215-615-0800; **Board Cert:** Internal Medicine 1984; Cardiovascular Disease 1987; **Med School:** Temple Univ 1981; **Resid:** Internal Medicine, Temple Univ Hosp 1984; **Fellow:** Cardiovascular Disease, Temple Univ Hosp 1986; **Fac Appt:** Assoc Prof Med, Univ Pennsylvania

Cohen, Howard A MD [Cv] - **Spec Exp:** Interventional Cardiology; Carotid Artery Stent Placement; **Hospital:** Lenox Hill Hosp (page 62); **Address:** Lenox Hill Hospital, Interventional Cardiology, 130 E 77th St Fl 9, New York, NY 10021; **Phone:** 212-434-6401; **Board Cert:** Internal Medicine 1976; Cardiovascular Disease 1977; **Med School:** NYU Sch Med 1970; **Resid:** Internal Medicine, Bellevue Hosp Ctr 1974; **Fellow:** Cardiovascular Disease, Johns Hopkins Hosp 1976

Coppola, John T MD [Cv] - **Spec Exp:** Cardiac Catheterization; Angioplasty; **Hospital:** St Vincent Cath Med Ctrs - Manhattan; **Address:** 275 7th Ave Fl 3, New York, NY 10001; **Phone:** 646-660-9999; **Board Cert:** Internal Medicine 1981; Cardiovascular Disease 1983; Interventional Cardiology 1999; **Med School:** NY Med Coll 1978; **Resid:** Internal Medicine, St Vincent Catholic Med Ctr 1981; **Fellow:** Cardiovascular Disease, St Vincent Catholic Med Ctr 1983

Devereux, Richard B MD [Cv] - **Spec Exp:** Marfan's Syndrome; **Hospital:** NY-Presby Hosp/Weill Cornell (page 66); **Address:** 525 E 68th St, rm K-415, New York, NY 10065; **Phone:** 212-746-4655; **Board Cert:** Internal Medicine 1974; Cardiovascular Disease 1977; **Med School:** Univ Pennsylvania 1971; **Resid:** Internal Medicine, New York Hosp 1974; **Fellow:** Cardiovascular Disease, Hosp Univ Penn 1976; **Fac Appt:** Prof Med, Cornell Univ-Weill Med Coll

Cardiovascular Disease

Edmundowicz, Daniel MD [Cv] - **Spec Exp:** Preventive Cardiology; Cholesterol/Lipid Disorders; **Hospital:** UPMC Passavant, UPMC Presby, Pittsburgh; **Address:** Cardiovascular Inst at Univ Center, 120 Lytton Ave, Ste 302, Pittsburgh, PA 15213; **Phone:** 412-802-3014; **Board Cert:** Internal Medicine 2005; Cardiovascular Disease 1998; **Med School:** Hahnemann Univ 1990; **Resid:** Internal Medicine, Temple Univ Hosp 1993; **Fellow:** Cardiovascular Disease, Univ Pittsburgh Med Ctr 1996; **Fac Appt:** Assoc Prof Med, Univ Pittsburgh

Eisen, Howard J MD [Cv] - **Spec Exp:** Transplant Medicine-Heart; Congestive Heart Failure; **Hospital:** Hahnemann Univ Hosp; **Address:** Drexel Univ Coll Med, Div Cardiology, 245 N 15th St, MS 1012, Philadelphia, PA 19102; **Phone:** 215-762-3829; **Board Cert:** Internal Medicine 1984; Cardiovascular Disease 1987; **Med School:** Univ Pennsylvania 1981; **Resid:** Internal Medicine, Hosp Univ Penn 1984; **Fellow:** Cardiovascular Disease, Barnes Jewish Hosp 1987; **Fac Appt:** Prof Med, Drexel Univ Coll Med

Follansbee, William P MD [Cv] - **Spec Exp:** Nuclear Cardiology; **Hospital:** UPMC Presby, Pittsburgh; **Address:** UPMC Cardiovascular Inst, 200 Lothrop St, Ste 5B, Pittsburgh, PA 15213; **Phone:** 412-647-3437; **Board Cert:** Internal Medicine 1977; Cardiovascular Disease 1981; **Med School:** Univ Pennsylvania 1974; **Resid:** Internal Medicine, Hosp Univ Penn 1979; **Fellow:** Cardiovascular Disease, Hosp Univ Penn 1978; **Fac Appt:** Prof Med, Univ Pittsburgh

Friedman, Sanford MD [Cv] - **Spec Exp:** Preventive Cardiology; **Hospital:** Mount Sinai Med Ctr (page 64); **Address:** 103 E 81st St, New York, NY 10028; **Phone:** 212-988-3772; **Board Cert:** Internal Medicine 1980; Cardiovascular Disease 1977; **Med School:** Tufts Univ 1971; **Resid:** Internal Medicine, Mt Sinai Med Ctr 1974; **Fellow:** Cardiovascular Disease, Mt Sinai Med Ctr 1976; **Fac Appt:** Assoc Clin Prof Med, Mount Sinai Sch Med

Fuster, Valentin MD/PhD [Cv] - **Spec Exp:** Coronary Artery Disease; Heart Valve Disease; Congenital Heart Disease; Preventive Cardiology; **Hospital:** Mount Sinai Med Ctr (page 64); **Address:** One Gustave L Levy Pl, Box 1030, New York, NY 10029-6500; **Phone:** 212-241-7911; **Board Cert:** Internal Medicine 1976; Cardiovascular Disease 1977; **Med School:** Spain 1967; **Resid:** Internal Medicine, Mayo Clinic 1972; Cardiovascular Disease, Mayo Clinic 1974; **Fellow:** Cardiovascular Disease, Univ Edinburgh 1971; **Fac Appt:** Prof Med, Mount Sinai Sch Med

Gliklich, Jerry MD [Cv] - **Spec Exp:** Heart Valve Disease; Arrhythmias; **Hospital:** NY-Presby Hosp/Columbia (page 66); **Address:** 161 Fort Washington Ave, Ste 535, New York, NY 10032-3713; **Phone:** 212-305-5588; **Board Cert:** Internal Medicine 1978; Cardiovascular Disease 1981; **Med School:** Columbia P&S 1975; **Resid:** Internal Medicine, NY Hosp 1978; **Fellow:** Cardiovascular Disease, Columbia-Presby Med Ctr 1981; **Fac Appt:** Clin Prof Med, Columbia P&S

Goldberg, Nieca MD [Cv] - **Spec Exp:** Heart Disease in Women; Preventive Cardiology; Echocardiography; **Hospital:** NYU Langone Med Ctr (page 67), Lenox Hill Hosp (page 62); **Address:** 177 E 87th St, New York, NY 10128; **Phone:** 212-289-2045; **Board Cert:** Internal Medicine 1987; Cardiovascular Disease 2005; **Med School:** SUNY Downstate 1984; **Resid:** Internal Medicine, St Lukes Roosevelt Hosp Ctr 1987; **Fellow:** Cardiovascular Disease, SUNY Hlth Sci Ctr 1990; **Fac Appt:** Asst Clin Prof Med, NYU Sch Med

Gottdiener, John S MD [Cv] - **Spec Exp:** Echocardiography; **Hospital:** Univ of MD Med Ctr; **Address:** 22 S Greene St, rm S3B08, Baltimore, MD 21201; **Phone:** 410-328-6190; **Board Cert:** Internal Medicine 1975; Cardiovascular Disease 1979; **Med School:** Georgetown Univ 1970; **Resid:** Internal Medicine, Univ NC Hosp 1972; **Fellow:** Cardiovascular Disease, Georgetown Univ Hosp 1976; **Fac Appt:** Prof Med, Univ MD Sch Med

Gottlieb, Stephen Scott MD [Cv] - **Spec Exp:** Heart Failure; Transplant Medicine-Heart; **Hospital:** Univ of MD Med Ctr; **Address:** Univ Maryland Med Ctr, Cardiology, 22 S Greene St, rm S3B08, Baltimore, MD 21201; **Phone:** 410-328-8788; **Board Cert:** Internal Medicine 1984; Cardiovascular Disease 1987; **Med School:** Brown Univ 1981; **Resid:** Internal Medicine, Univ Chicago Hosps 1984; **Fellow:** Cardiovascular Disease, Mt Sinai Hosp 1985; **Fac Appt:** Prof Med, Univ MD Sch Med

Greenberg, Mark A MD [Cv] - **Spec Exp:** Interventional Cardiology; Cardiac Catheterization; Heart Valve Disease; **Hospital:** Montefiore Med Ctr - Div. Moses; **Address:** 111 E 210th St, Division of Cardiology, Bronx, NY 10467; **Phone:** 718-920-4212; **Board Cert:** Internal Medicine 1973; Cardiovascular Disease 1979; Interventional Cardiology 1999; **Med School:** Univ IL Coll Med 1973; **Resid:** Internal Medicine, Montefiore Hosp Med Ctr 1976; **Fellow:** Cardiovascular Disease, Montefiore Hosp Med Ctr 1978; **Fac Appt:** Clin Prof Med, Albert Einstein Coll Med

Halperin, Jonathan L MD [Cv] - **Spec Exp:** Peripheral Vascular Disease; Atrial Fibrillation; **Hospital:** Mount Sinai Med Ctr (page 64); **Address:** 1190 5th Ave, New York, NY 10029; **Phone:** 212-241-7243; **Board Cert:** Internal Medicine 1980; Cardiovascular Disease 1981; **Med School:** Boston Univ 1975; **Resid:** Internal Medicine, Mass Genl Hosp 1977; **Fellow:** Vascular Medicine, Boston Univ Med Ctr 1978; Cardiovascular Disease, Boston Univ Med Ctr 1980; **Fac Appt:** Prof Med, Mount Sinai Sch Med

Herling, Irving M MD [Cv] - **Spec Exp:** Cholesterol/Lipid Disorders; Preventive Cardiology; Heart Valve Disease; **Hospital:** Hosp Univ Penn - UPHS (page 60); **Address:** Hosp Univ Penn, Div Cardiology, East Pavilion Fl 2 - Ste 2-218E, 3400 Spruce St, 800 Penn Tower, Philadelphia, PA 19104-4206; **Phone:** 215-662-7700; **Board Cert:** Internal Medicine 1977; Cardiovascular Disease 1979; **Med School:** Univ Pennsylvania 1974; **Resid:** Internal Medicine, Hosp Univ Penn 1977; **Fellow:** Cardiovascular Disease, Hosp Univ Penn 1979; **Fac Appt:** Assoc Prof Med, Univ Pennsylvania

Horn, Evelyn M MD [Cv] - **Spec Exp:** Pulmonary Hypertension; Heart Failure; Ventricular Assist Device (LVAD); Heart Conditions-Complex; **Hospital:** NY-Presby Hosp/Weill Cornell (page 66); **Address:** Perkins Heart Failure Ctr-Weill Cornell, 1305 York Ave Fl 8, New York, NY 10021; **Phone:** 212-746-2381; **Board Cert:** Internal Medicine 1983; Cardiovascular Disease 1985; **Med School:** Mount Sinai Sch Med 1980; **Resid:** Internal Medicine, Mt Sinai Hosp 1983; **Fellow:** Cardiovascular Disease, Cedars- Mt Sinai Med Ctr 1985; **Fac Appt:** Clin Prof Med, Columbia P&S

Inra, Lawrence A MD [Cv] - **Spec Exp:** Coronary Artery Disease; Heart Valve Disease; Cholesterol/Lipid Disorders; Hypertension; **Hospital:** NY-Presby Hosp/Weill Cornell (page 66), Hosp For Special Surgery (page 59); **Address:** 407 E 70th St, New York, NY 10021; **Phone:** 212-249-1011; **Board Cert:** Internal Medicine 1979; Cardiovascular Disease 1981; **Med School:** Johns Hopkins Univ 1976; **Resid:** Internal Medicine, NY Hosp 1979; **Fellow:** Cardiovascular Disease, Mt Sinai Hosp 1981; **Fac Appt:** Assoc Clin Prof Med, Cornell Univ-Weill Med Coll

Kostis, John B MD [Cv] - **Spec Exp:** Hypertension; Coronary Artery Disease; Cholesterol/Lipid Disorders; **Hospital:** Robert Wood Johnson Univ Hosp - New Brunswick; **Address:** UMDNJ-Robert Wood Johnson Med School, 1 Robert Wood Johnson Pl, Box 19, New Brunswick, NJ 08903-0019; **Phone:** 732-235-7685; **Board Cert:** Internal Medicine 1973; Cardiovascular Disease 1973; **Med School:** Greece 1960; **Resid:** Internal Medicine, Evanglismos Hosp 1964; Internal Medicine, Cumberland Med Ctr 1967; **Fellow:** Cardiovascular Disease, Philadelphia Genl Hosp 1969; **Fac Appt:** Prof Med, UMDNJ-RW Johnson Med Sch

Mather, Paul J MD [Cv] - **Spec Exp:** Heart Failure; Transplant Medicine-Heart; **Hospital:** Thomas Jefferson Univ Hosp; **Address:** Jefferson Heart Inst, 925 Chestnut St, Mezzanine Level, Philadelphia, PA 19107; **Phone:** 215-955-4194; **Board Cert:** Internal Medicine 2002; Cardiovascular Disease 1995; **Med School:** Temple Univ 1988; **Resid:** Internal Medicine, Temple Univ 1991; **Fellow:** Cardiovascular Disease, Temple Univ 1994; **Fac Appt:** Assoc Prof Med, Temple Univ

Meller, Jose MD [Cv] - **Spec Exp:** Cardiac Catheterization; Hypertension; Angioplasty; **Hospital:** Mount Sinai Med Ctr (page 64); **Address:** 941 Park Ave, New York, NY 10028; **Phone:** 212-988-3772; **Board Cert:** Internal Medicine 1973; Cardiovascular Disease 1975; **Med School:** Chile 1969; **Resid:** Internal Medicine, Elmhurst Hosp 1971; Internal Medicine, Mt Sinai Med Ctr 1972; **Fellow:** Cardiovascular Disease, Mt Sinai Med Ctr 1974; **Fac Appt:** Prof Med, Mount Sinai Sch Med

Mieres, Jennifer H MD [Cv] - **Spec Exp:** Nuclear Cardiology; Heart Disease in Women; **Hospital:** NYU Langone Med Ctr (page 67); **Address:** NYU Medical Ctr, Div Cardiology, 560 1st Ave, New York, NY 10016; **Phone:** 212-263-5667; **Board Cert:** Internal Medicine 1991; Cardiovascular Disease 1997; Nuclear Cardiology 1996; **Med School:** Boston Univ 1986; **Resid:** Internal Medicine, St Lukes Roosevelt Hosp 1990

Mosca, Lori J MD/PhD [Cv] - **Spec Exp:** Preventive Cardiology; **Hospital:** NY-Presby Hosp/Columbia (page 66); **Address:** NY Presbyterian Med Ctr, Div Preventive Cardiology, 622 W 168th St, PH10-203D, New York, NY 10032; **Phone:** 212-305-4866; **Board Cert:** Internal Medicine 1989; **Med School:** SUNY Upstate Med Univ 1984; **Resid:** Internal Medicine, SUNYHealth Sci Ctr 1987; **Fellow:** Cardiovascular Disease, Columbia Presby Med Ctr 1991; Epidemiology, Columbia Presby Med Ctr 1992; **Fac Appt:** Assoc Prof Med, Columbia P&S

Naccarelli, Gerald V MD [Cv] - **Spec Exp:** Pacemakers; Arrhythmias; **Hospital:** Penn State Milton S Hershey Med Ctr; **Address:** Heart & Vascular Institute, 500 University Drive, rm H1511, PO Box 850, MC HO47, Hershey, PA 17033; **Phone:** 717-531-3907; **Board Cert:** Internal Medicine 1979; Cardiovascular Disease 1981; **Med School:** Penn State Univ-Hershey Med Ctr 1976; **Resid:** Internal Medicine, NC Bapt Hosp 1978; Internal Medicine, Hershey Med Ctr 1979; **Fellow:** Cardiovascular Disease, Indiana Univ Med Ctr 1982; **Fac Appt:** Prof Med, Penn State Univ-Hershey Med Ctr

Parrillo, Joseph E MD [Cv] - **Spec Exp:** Septic Shock; Heart Failure; **Hospital:** Cooper Univ Hosp; **Address:** Cooper Medical Ctr, Div Cardiology, 1 Cooper Plaza, Dorrance Bldg, Ste D384, Camden, NJ 08103; **Phone:** 856-968-8349; **Board Cert:** Internal Medicine 1975; Allergy & Immunology 1977; Cardiovascular Disease 1981; Critical Care Medicine 2005; **Med School:** Cornell Univ-Weill Med Coll 1972; **Resid:** Internal Medicine, Mass General Hosp 1975; Allergy & Immunology, Natl Inst Hlth 1978; **Fellow:** Cardiovascular Disease, Mass General Hosp 1980; **Fac Appt:** Prof Med, UMDNJ-RW Johnson Med Sch

Plehn, Jonathan MD [Cv] - **Spec Exp:** Echocardiography; Congestive Heart Failure; Heart Valve Disease; **Hospital:** Natl Naval Med Ctr, Natl Inst of Hlth - Clin Ctr; **Address:** Natl Naval Med Ctr, Div of Cardiology, 8901 Wisconsin Ave, Bethesda, MD 20889; **Phone:** 301-295-4484; **Board Cert:** Internal Medicine 1981; Cardiovascular Disease 1983; **Med School:** NYU Sch Med 1977; **Resid:** Internal Medicine, Montefiore Hosp 1980; Cardiovascular Disease, Montefiore Hosp 1981; **Fellow:** Cardiovascular Disease, Rush Presby-St Lukes Hosp 1983

Poon, Michael MD [Cv] - **Spec Exp:** Coronary Artery Disease; Pulmonary Hypertension; Cardiac CT Angiography; Cardiac Imaging; **Hospital:** Stony Brook Univ Med Ctr; **Address:** Stony Brook Health Science Ctr, Level 4, rm 120, Stony Brook, NY 11794; **Phone:** 631-444-5400; **Board Cert:** Cardiovascular Disease 2007; **Med School:** Mount Sinai Sch Med 1987; **Resid:** Internal Medicine, Mount Sinai Med Ctr 1991; **Fellow:** Cardiovascular Disease, Mount Sinai Med Ctr 1993; **Fac Appt:** Prof Med, SUNY Stony Brook

Reis, Steven E MD [Cv] - **Spec Exp:** Heart Disease in Women; Congestive Heart Failure; Syndrome X; Preventive Cardiology; **Hospital:** UPMC Presby, Pittsburgh, Magee-Womens Hosp - UPMC; **Address:** UPMC Cardiovascular Inst at Univ Ctr, 120 Lytton Ave, Ste 100B, Pittsburgh, PA 15213; **Phone:** 412-802-3000; **Board Cert:** Internal Medicine 2000; Cardiovascular Disease 2000; **Med School:** Harvard Med Sch 1987; **Resid:** Internal Medicine, Brigham & Womens Hosp 1990; **Fellow:** Cardiovascular Disease, Johns Hopkins Hosp 1994; **Fac Appt:** Assoc Prof Med, Univ Pittsburgh

Russell, Stuart D MD [Cv] - **Spec Exp:** Heart Failure; **Hospital:** Johns Hopkins Hosp (page 61); **Address:** Johns Hopkins Hosp, Carnegie 568, 600 N Wolfe St, Baltimore, MD 21287; **Phone:** 410-955-5708; **Board Cert:** Internal Medicine 2006; Cardiovascular Disease 2007; **Med School:** Univ Wash 1991; **Resid:** Internal Medicine, Johns Hopkins Hosp 1994; **Fellow:** Cardiovascular Disease, Duke Univ Med Ctr 1997; **Fac Appt:** Assoc Prof Med, Johns Hopkins Univ

Sacchi, Terrence J MD [Cv] - **Spec Exp:** Arrhythmias; Cardiac Catheterization; Coronary Angioplasty/Stents; Percutaneous Coronary Baloon Angioplasty; **Hospital:** New York Methodist Hosp; **Address:** NY Methodist Hospital, Buckley 2, 506 6th St, Brooklyn, NY 11215; **Phone:** 718-780-7830; **Board Cert:** Internal Medicine 1979; Cardiovascular Disease 1981; Interventional Cardiology 1999; **Med School:** Albany Med Coll 1976; **Resid:** Internal Medicine, St Vincents Hosp 1979; **Fellow:** Cardiovascular Disease, Georgetown Univ Hosp 1981; Interventional Cardiology, Mercy Hosp 1987; **Fac Appt:** Assoc Clin Prof Med, SUNY Downstate

Saunders, Elijah MD [Cv] - **Spec Exp:** Hypertension-Complex; Coronary Disease in Black Populations; **Hospital:** Univ of MD Med Ctr; **Address:** Univ MD Med Sch, Div Hypertension, 419 W Redwood St, Ste 620, Baltimore, MD 21201; **Phone:** 410-328-4366; **Med School:** Univ MD Sch Med 1960; **Resid:** Internal Medicine, Univ Maryland Med Ctr; **Fellow:** Cardiovascular Disease, Univ Maryland Med Ctr; **Fac Appt:** Prof Med, Univ MD Sch Med

Schulman, Steven P MD [Cv] - **Hospital:** Johns Hopkins Hosp (page 61); **Address:** 600 N Wolfe St, Carnegie 568, Baltimore, MD 21287; **Phone:** 410-955-7378; **Board Cert:** Internal Medicine 1986; Cardiovascular Disease 1989; **Med School:** Johns Hopkins Univ 1981; **Resid:** Internal Medicine, Johns Hopkins Hosp 1984; **Fellow:** Cardiovascular Disease, Johns Hopkins Hosp 1988; **Fac Appt:** Assoc Prof Med, Johns Hopkins Univ

Schwartz, Allan MD [Cv] - **Spec Exp:** Interventional Cardiology; Cardiac Catheterization; Mitral Valve Disease; **Hospital:** NY-Presby Hosp/Columbia (page 66); **Address:** 161 Ft Washington Ave, Ste 551, New York, NY 10032-3713; **Phone:** 212-305-5367; **Board Cert:** Internal Medicine 1977; Cardiovascular Disease 1979; **Med School:** Columbia P&S 1974; **Resid:** Internal Medicine, Columbia-Presby Med Ctr 1976; **Fellow:** Cardiovascular Disease, Mass Genl Hosp 1978; **Fac Appt:** Clin Prof Med, Columbia P&S

Schwartz, William J MD [Cv] - **Spec Exp:** Coronary Artery Disease; Cardiac Catheterization; Congestive Heart Failure; **Hospital:** Lenox Hill Hosp (page 62), Mount Sinai Med Ctr (page 64); **Address:** Broadway Cardioplmonary, 150 E 77th St, Ste 1E, New York, NY 10075; **Phone:** 212-439-6000; **Board Cert:** Internal Medicine 1978; Cardiovascular Disease 1981; **Med School:** Albert Einstein Coll Med 1975; **Resid:** Internal Medicine, Bronx Municipal Hosp 1978; **Fellow:** Cardiovascular Disease, Bronx Municipal Hosp 1979

Shlofmitz, Richard A MD [Cv] - **Spec Exp:** Interventional Cardiology; Cardiac Catheterization; **Hospital:** St Francis Hosp - The Heart Ctr (page 69); **Address:** 100 Port Washington Blvd, Ste 105, Roslyn, NY 11576; **Phone:** 516-390-9640; **Board Cert:** Internal Medicine 1984; Cardiovascular Disease 1987; **Med School:** NYU Sch Med 1980; **Resid:** Internal Medicine, North Shore Univ Hosp 1984; **Fellow:** Cardiovascular Disease, Columbia Presby Med Ctr 1987

Smart, Frank W MD [Cv] - **Spec Exp:** Congestive Heart Failure; Transplant Medicine-Heart; Ventricular Assist Device (LVAD); **Hospital:** Morristown Mem Hosp, Overlook Hosp; **Address:** Morristown Meml Hosp, Dept Cardiology, 100 Madison Ave, Box 5, Gagnon C Level, Morristown, NJ 07962; **Phone:** 973-971-4179; **Board Cert:** Internal Medicine 1988; Cardiovascular Disease 2001; **Med School:** Louisiana State U, New Orleans 1985; **Resid:** Internal Medicine, Ochsner Fdn Hosp 1988; **Fellow:** Cardiovascular Disease, Baylor Coll Med 1991

Cardiovascular Disease

Steingart, Richard MD [Cv] - **Spec Exp:** Heart Failure; Nuclear Cardiology; Heart Disease in Cancer Patients; Cardiac Effects of Cancer/Cancer Therapy; **Hospital:** Meml Sloan-Kettering Cancer Ctr; **Address:** 1275 York Avenue, New York, NY 10065; **Phone:** 800-525-2225; **Board Cert:** Internal Medicine 1977; Cardiovascular Disease 1979; **Med School:** Mount Sinai Sch Med 1974; **Resid:** Internal Medicine, Yale-New Haven Hosp 1977; **Fellow:** Cardiovascular Disease, Mt Sinai Med Ctr 1979; **Fac Appt:** Prof Med, Cornell Univ-Weill Med Coll

Tenenbaum, Joseph MD [Cv] - **Spec Exp:** Heart Valve Disease; Coronary Artery Disease; Atrial Fibrillation; **Hospital:** NY-Presby Hosp/Columbia (page 66); **Address:** 161 Ft Washington Ave, Ste 535, Irving Pavilion, New York, NY 10032-3713; **Phone:** 212-305-5288; **Board Cert:** Internal Medicine 1977; Cardiovascular Disease 1979; **Med School:** Harvard Med Sch 1974; **Resid:** Internal Medicine, Columbia-Presby Med Ctr 1977; **Fellow:** Cardiovascular Disease, Mt Sinai Hosp 1979; **Fac Appt:** Prof Med, Columbia P&S

Waxman, Harvey L MD [Cv] - **Spec Exp:** Arrhythmias; Cardiac Catheterization; Heart Valve Disease; **Hospital:** Penn Presby Med Ctr - UPHS (page 60); **Address:** Penn Presby Med Ctr, Philadelphia Heart Institute, 39th & Market Sts, 4PHI, Philadelphia, PA 19104; **Phone:** 215-662-9000; **Board Cert:** Internal Medicine 1977; Cardiovascular Disease 1979; Cardiac Electrophysiology 2002; **Med School:** Mount Sinai Sch Med 1974; **Resid:** Internal Medicine, Bellevue Hosp 1977; **Fellow:** Cardiovascular Disease, Jackson Meml Hosp 1979; Cardiac Electrophysiology, Hosp Univ Penn 1980; **Fac Appt:** Clin Prof Med, Univ Pennsylvania

Webb, Gary D MD [Cv] - **Spec Exp:** Congenital Heart Disease-Adult; **Hospital:** Hosp Univ Penn - UPHS (page 60); **Address:** Pearlman Center Fl 2, 3400 Civic Center Blvd, East Pavilion, Philadelphia, PA 19104-4283; **Phone:** 215-615-3388; **Board Cert:** Internal Medicine ; Cardiovascular Disease ; **Med School:** McGill Univ 1967; **Resid:** Internal Medicine, Royal Victoria Hosp 1972; **Fellow:** Cardiovascular Disease, Toronto Genl Hosp 1974

Weitz, Howard H MD [Cv] - **Spec Exp:** Preventive Cardiology; **Hospital:** Thomas Jefferson Univ Hosp; **Address:** Jefferson Heart Institute, 925 Chestnut St, Mezzanine Level, Philadelphia, PA 19107; **Phone:** 215-955-4194; **Board Cert:** Internal Medicine 1981; Cardiovascular Disease 1985; **Med School:** Thomas Jefferson Univ 1978; **Resid:** Internal Medicine, Thos Jefferson Univ Hosp 1982; **Fellow:** Cardiovascular Disease, Thos Jefferson Univ Hosp 1984; **Fac Appt:** Prof Med, Thomas Jefferson Univ

Southeast

Bashore, Thomas M MD [Cv] - **Spec Exp:** Heart Valve Disease; Pulmonary Hypertension; Congenital Heart Disease-Adult; **Hospital:** Duke Univ Med Ctr; **Address:** Duke Univ Med Ctr, PO Box 3012, Durham, NC 27710-0001; **Phone:** 919-684-2407; **Board Cert:** Internal Medicine 1975; Cardiovascular Disease 1977; **Med School:** Ohio State Univ 1972; **Resid:** Internal Medicine, NC Meml Hosp 1975; **Fellow:** Cardiovascular Disease, Duke Univ Med Ctr 1977; **Fac Appt:** Prof Med, Duke Univ

Bass, Theodore A MD [Cv] - **Spec Exp:** Interventional Cardiology; Coronary Artery Disease; **Hospital:** Shands Jacksonville; **Address:** Shands Jacksonville Cardiovascular Ctr, 655 W 8th St ACC Bldg Fl 5, Jacksonville, FL 32209; **Phone:** 904-244-2655; **Board Cert:** Internal Medicine 1979; Cardiovascular Disease 1981; Interventional Cardiology 2001; **Med School:** Brown Univ 1976; **Resid:** Internal Medicine, Mayo Clinic 1979; **Fellow:** Cardiovascular Disease, University Hosp 1981; **Fac Appt:** Prof Med, Univ Fla Coll Med

Beller, George A MD [Cv] - **Spec Exp:** Coronary Artery Disease; Nuclear Cardiology; **Hospital:** Univ Virginia Med Ctr; **Address:** UVA Hlth Systems, Cardiology Dept, Box 800158, Charlottesville, VA 22908-0158; **Phone:** 434-924-2134; **Board Cert:** Internal Medicine 1971; Cardiovascular Disease 1977; **Med School:** Univ VA Sch Med 1966; **Resid:** Internal Medicine, Univ Wisconsin Hosps 1968; Cardiovascular Disease, Boston City Hosp 1970; **Fellow:** Cardiovascular Disease, Mass Genl Hosp 1974; **Fac Appt:** Prof Med, Univ VA Sch Med

Borzak, Steven MD [Cv] - **Spec Exp:** Coronary Artery Disease; Arrhythmias; Heart Failure; Cholesterol/Lipid Disorders; **Hospital:** JFK Med Ctr - Atlantis, Bethesda Memorial Hosp; **Address:** 110 JFK Drive, Ste 110, Atlantis, FL 33462-1146; **Phone:** 561-641-9541; **Board Cert:** Internal Medicine 1987; Cardiovascular Disease 2001; **Med School:** Univ IL Coll Med 1984; **Resid:** Internal Medicine, Michael Reese Hosp 1988; **Fellow:** Cardiovascular Disease, Brigham & Womens Hosp 1991; **Fac Appt:** Prof Med, Nova SE Univ, Coll Osteo Med

Bourge, Robert C MD [Cv] - **Spec Exp:** Heart Failure; Transplant Medicine-Heart; Pulmonary Hypertension; **Hospital:** Univ of Ala Hosp at Birmingham; **Address:** UAB Div Cardiovascular Disease, 311 THT, 1900 University Blvd, Birmingham, AL 35294-0001; **Phone:** 205-934-3624; **Board Cert:** Internal Medicine 1982; Cardiovascular Disease 1985; Nuclear Medicine 1987; **Med School:** Louisiana State U, New Orleans 1979; **Resid:** Internal Medicine, Univ Alabama Hosps 1982; Nuclear Medicine, Univ Alabama Hosps 1985; **Fellow:** Cardiovascular Disease, Univ Alabama Hosps 1984; **Fac Appt:** Prof Med, Univ Alabama

Byrd III, Benjamin F MD [Cv] - **Spec Exp:** Congenital Heart Disease; Echocardiography; **Hospital:** Vanderbilt Univ Med Ctr; **Address:** Vanderbilt Heart Inst, 1215 21st Ave, MCE S Tower, Ste 5209, Nashville, TN 37232; **Phone:** 615-322-2318; **Board Cert:** Internal Medicine 1981; Cardiovascular Disease 1983; **Med School:** Vanderbilt Univ 1977; **Resid:** Psychiatry, Harvard Univ 1979; Internal Medicine, Vanderbilt Univ Hosp 1981; **Fellow:** Cardiovascular Disease, Vanderbilt Univ Hosp 1983; Cardiovascular Disease, UCSF 1984; **Fac Appt:** Assoc Prof Med, Vanderbilt Univ

Califf, Robert M MD [Cv] - **Spec Exp:** Coronary Artery Disease; Cholesterol/Lipid Disorders; Heart Failure; **Hospital:** Duke Univ Med Ctr; **Address:** 2400 Pratt St, Ste 0311, Durham, NC 27705; **Phone:** 919-668-8820; **Board Cert:** Internal Medicine 1984; Cardiovascular Disease 1985; **Med School:** Duke Univ 1978; **Resid:** Internal Medicine, UCSF Med Ctr 1980; **Fellow:** Cardiovascular Disease, Duke Univ Med Ctr 1983; **Fac Appt:** Prof Med, Duke Univ

Chizner, Michael A MD [Cv] - **Spec Exp:** Preventive Cardiology; Coronary Artery Disease; Cardiac Catheterization; Coronary Angioplasty/Stents; **Hospital:** Broward General Med Ctr, Imperial Point Med Ctr; **Address:** 1625 SE 3rd Ave, Ste 300, Fort Lauderdale, FL 33316; **Phone:** 954-355-5001; **Board Cert:** Internal Medicine 1977; Cardiovascular Disease 1979; **Med School:** Cornell Univ-Weill Med Coll 1974; **Resid:** Internal Medicine, New York Hosp 1977; **Fellow:** Cardiovascular Disease, Georgetown Affil Hosps 1979; **Fac Appt:** Clin Prof Med, Univ Miami Sch Med

Clements Jr, Stephen MD [Cv] - **Spec Exp:** Cardiac Catheterization; Echocardiography; **Hospital:** Emory Univ Hosp; **Address:** Emory Clinic, 1365 Clifton Rd NE Bldg A, Atlanta, GA 30322; **Phone:** 404-778-3468; **Board Cert:** Internal Medicine 1971; Cardiovascular Disease 1975; **Med School:** Med Coll GA 1966; **Resid:** Internal Medicine, Grady Meml Hosp 1970; **Fellow:** Cardiovascular Disease, Emory Univ Hosp 1971; **Fac Appt:** Prof Med, Emory Univ

Corrigan, Victor E MD [Cv] - **Spec Exp:** Cardiac Catheterization; Interventional Cardiology; Transplant Medicine-Heart; **Hospital:** Piedmont Hosp, St Joseph's Hosp - Atlanta; **Address:** Piedmont Heart Inst, 95 Collier Rd, Ste 5015, Atlanta, GA 30309; **Phone:** 404-851-5400; **Board Cert:** Internal Medicine 1986; Cardiovascular Disease 1989; Interventional Cardiology 1999; **Med School:** Med Coll GA 1983; **Resid:** Internal Medicine, Emory Univ Hosp 1986; **Fellow:** Cardiovascular Disease, Emory Univ Hosp 1988

Cardiovascular Disease

Gandy Jr, Winston MD [Cv] - **Spec Exp:** Echocardiography; Invasive Cardiology; **Hospital:** Piedmont Hosp; **Address:** Atlanta Cardiology Group, 95 Collier Rd, Ste 5015, Atlanta, GA 30309; **Phone:** 404-605-5100; **Board Cert:** Internal Medicine 1989; Cardiovascular Disease 2002; **Med School:** Howard Univ 1986; **Resid:** Internal Medicine, Emory Univ 1989; **Fellow:** Cardiovascular Disease, Univ Alabama 1992

Hare, Joshua M MD [Cv] - **Spec Exp:** Heart Failure; Stem Cell Therapy in Heart Failure; **Hospital:** Univ of Miami Hosp & Clins/Sylvester Comp Canc Ctr (page 70); **Address:** University of Miami, Miller School, 1120 NW 14th St, Ste 1124, Miami, FL 33136; **Phone:** 305-243-4813; **Board Cert:** Cardiovascular Disease 2006; **Med School:** Johns Hopkins Univ 1988; **Resid:** Internal Medicine, Johns Hopkins Hosp 1991; **Fellow:** Cardiovascular Disease, Brigham & Women's Hosp 1993

Harrison, J Kevin MD [Cv] - **Spec Exp:** Interventional Cardiology; Heart Valve Disease; **Hospital:** Duke Univ Med Ctr; **Address:** Duke Univ Med Ctr, PO Box 3331, Durham, NC 27710; **Phone:** 919-681-3763; **Board Cert:** Internal Medicine 1988; Cardiovascular Disease 2001; Interventional Cardiology 2003; **Med School:** NYU Sch Med 1984; **Resid:** Internal Medicine, Johns Hopkins Hosp 1987; **Fellow:** Cardiovascular Disease, Duke Univ Med Ctr 1990; **Fac Appt:** Prof Med, Duke Univ

Iskandrian, Ami E MD [Cv] - **Spec Exp:** Nuclear Cardiology; Coronary Artery Disease; Heart Valve Disease; **Hospital:** Univ of Ala Hosp at Birmingham; **Address:** Univ Alabama-Birmingham, 318 LHRB, 1900 University Blvd, Birmingham, AL 35294-0006; **Phone:** 205-934-0545; **Board Cert:** Internal Medicine 1974; Cardiovascular Disease 1975; **Med School:** Iraq 1965; **Resid:** Internal Medicine, Univ Baghdad Affil Hosp 1971; Internal Medicine, Hahnemann Univ Hosp 1973; **Fellow:** Cardiovascular Disease, Hahnemann Univ Hosp 1975; **Fac Appt:** Prof Med, Univ Alabama

Linton, MacRae F MD [Cv] - **Spec Exp:** Cholesterol/Lipid Disorders; Preventive Cardiology; **Hospital:** Vanderbilt Univ Med Ctr; **Address:** Vanderbilt Heart Inst, 1215 21st Ave, MCE S Tower, Ste 2509, Nashville, TN 37232-8802; **Phone:** 615-322-2318; **Board Cert:** Internal Medicine 1988; **Med School:** Univ Tenn Coll Med, Memphis 1985; **Resid:** Internal Medicine, Vanderbilt Univ Med Ctr 1988; **Fellow:** Endocrinology, UCSF Med Ctr 1991; **Fac Appt:** Prof Med, Vanderbilt Univ

Miller, D Douglas MD [Cv] - **Spec Exp:** Heart Disease in Women; Nuclear Cardiology; **Hospital:** Med Coll of GA Hosp and Clin (MCG Health Inc); **Address:** MCG Health System, 1003 Chafee Ave, Augusta, GA 30912; **Phone:** 706-721-2426; **Med School:** McGill Univ 1978; **Resid:** Internal Medicine, Montreal Genl Hosp 1981; Cardiovascular Disease, Montreal Heart Inst 1982; **Fellow:** Cardiovascular Disease, Emory Univ Med Ctr 1984; Nuclear Cardiology, Mass Genl Hosp-Harvard 1986; **Fac Appt:** Prof Med, St Louis Univ

Myerburg, Robert J MD [Cv] - **Spec Exp:** Arrhythmias; Pacemakers; Heart Attack; **Hospital:** Jackson Meml Hosp (page 70); **Address:** Univ Miami School Med, Div Cardiology, PO Box 016960 (D-39), Miami, FL 33101-6960; **Phone:** 305-585-5523; **Board Cert:** Internal Medicine 1968; Cardiovascular Disease 1970; **Med School:** Univ MD Sch Med 1961; **Resid:** Internal Medicine, Charity Hosp 1966; **Fellow:** Cardiovascular Disease, Grady Meml Hosp 1968; Cardiac Electrophysiology, Columbia P&S 1970; **Fac Appt:** Prof Med, Univ Miami Sch Med

Nocero Jr, Michael A MD [Cv] - **Spec Exp:** Nuclear Cardiology; **Hospital:** Florida Hosp - Orlando; **Address:** 1745 N Mills Ave, Orlando, FL 32803; **Phone:** 407-841-7151; **Board Cert:** Internal Medicine 1972; Cardiovascular Disease 1976; **Med School:** NYU Sch Med 1966; **Resid:** Internal Medicine, Bellevue Hosp Ctr NYU 1971; **Fellow:** Cardiovascular Disease, Bellevue Hosp Ctr NYU 1973

O'Connor, Christopher M MD [Cv] - **Spec Exp:** Heart Failure; **Hospital:** Duke Univ Med Ctr; **Address:** Duke University Med Ctr, P.O. Box 3356, Durham, NC 27710; **Phone:** 919-681-6195; **Board Cert:** Internal Medicine 1988; Cardiovascular Disease 1989; **Med School:** Univ MD Sch Med 1983; **Resid:** Internal Medicine, Duke Univ Med Ctr 1986; Cardiovascular Disease, Duke Univ Med Ctr 1989

O'Neill, William W MD [Cv] - **Spec Exp:** Interventional Cardiology; Heart Valve Disease; **Hospital:** Univ of Miami Hosp & Clins/Sylvester Comp Canc Ctr (page 70); **Address:** Univ Miami Dept Medicine, 1600 NW 10 Ave, R-MSB 1122A, Miami, FL 33136; **Phone:** 305-243-9483; **Board Cert:** Internal Medicine 1980; Cardiovascular Disease 1983; Interventional Cardiology 1999; **Med School:** Wayne State Univ 1977; **Resid:** Internal Medicine, Wayne State Univ Affil Hosps 1980; **Fellow:** Cardiovascular Disease, Univ Mich Med Ctr 1982; **Fac Appt:** Prof Med, Univ Miami Sch Med

Ohman, E Magnus MD [Cv] - **Spec Exp:** Interventional Cardiology; Coronary Artery Disease; Preventive Cardiology; Acute Coronary Syndromes; **Hospital:** Duke Univ Med Ctr; **Address:** Duke Univ Med Ctr, Box 3126, Durham, NC 27710; **Phone:** 919-681-5816; **Med School:** Ireland 1981; **Resid:** Internal Medicine, St Laurences Hosp/St Vicents Hosp 1984; **Fellow:** Research, St Laurences Hosp 1987; Cardiovascular Disease, Duke Univ Med Ctr 1991; **Fac Appt:** Prof Med, Duke Univ

Oparil, Suzanne MD [Cv] - **Spec Exp:** Hypertension; Heart Disease in Women; **Hospital:** Univ of Ala Hosp at Birmingham; **Address:** Hypertension Program, 933 19 St S, Birmingham, AL 35294; **Phone:** 205-934-9281; **Board Cert:** Internal Medicine 1970; **Med School:** Columbia P&S 1965; **Resid:** Internal Medicine, Columbia Presby Med Ctr 1967; Internal Medicine, Mass Genl Hosp 1968; **Fellow:** Cardiovascular Disease, Mass Genl Hosp 1971; **Fac Appt:** Prof Med, Univ Alabama

Pepine, Carl J MD [Cv] - **Spec Exp:** Coronary Artery Disease; Hypertension; Heart Disease in Women; **Hospital:** Shands at Univ of FL; **Address:** Univ Florida, Div Cardiovascular Med, 1600 SW Archer Rd, Box 100277, Gainesville, FL 32610-0277; **Phone:** 352-265-0820; **Board Cert:** Internal Medicine 1971; Cardiovascular Disease 1973; **Med School:** UMDNJ-NJ Med Sch, Newark 1966; **Resid:** Internal Medicine, Jefferson Univ Hosp 1968; Internal Medicine, Naval Hosp-Thomas Jefferson Univ 1969; **Fellow:** Cardiovascular Disease, Naval Hosp-Thomas Jeff Univ 1971; **Fac Appt:** Prof Med, Univ Fla Coll Med

Phillips III, Harry R MD [Cv] - **Spec Exp:** Angioplasty; Cardiac Catheterization; **Hospital:** Duke Univ Med Ctr; **Address:** Duke Univ Med Ctr, Box 3126, Durham, NC 27710; **Phone:** 919-681-4804; **Board Cert:** Internal Medicine 1978; Cardiovascular Disease 1979; Interventional Cardiology 2001; **Med School:** Duke Univ 1975; **Resid:** Internal Medicine, Mass Genl Hosp 1977; **Fellow:** Cardiovascular Disease, Mass Genl Hosp 1979

Powers, Eric R MD [Cv] - **Spec Exp:** Heart Valve Disease; Interventional Cardiology; Coronary Artery Disease; **Hospital:** MUSC Med Ctr; **Address:** MUSC Heart & Vascular Ctr, 25 Courtenay Drive, ART 7052, MSC 592, Charleston, SC 29425-5920; **Phone:** 843-792-1952; **Board Cert:** Internal Medicine 1977; Cardiovascular Disease 1979; Interventional Cardiology 2000; **Med School:** Harvard Med Sch 1974; **Resid:** Internal Medicine, Mass Genl Hosp 1976; **Fellow:** Cardiovascular Disease, Mass Genl Hosp 1979; **Fac Appt:** Prof Med, Med Univ SC

Rogers, Joseph Gordon MD [Cv] - **Spec Exp:** Congestive Heart Failure; Transplant Medicine-Heart; **Hospital:** Duke Univ Med Ctr; **Address:** DUMC, Box 3034, Durham, NC 27710; **Phone:** 919-681-3398; **Board Cert:** Cardiovascular Disease 2005; **Med School:** Univ Nebr Coll Med 1988; **Resid:** Internal Medicine, Univ Nebraska Med Ctr 1991; **Fellow:** Cardiovascular Disease, Wash Univ Med Ctr 1995; **Fac Appt:** Assoc Prof Med, Duke Univ

Cardiovascular Disease

Smith Jr, Sidney C MD [Cv] - **Spec Exp:** Cholesterol/Lipid Disorders; Coronary Artery Disease; Invasive Cardiology; **Hospital:** Univ NC Hosps; **Address:** 300 Meadowmont Village Cir, Ste 313, Chapel Hill, NC 27517; **Phone:** 919-966-7244; **Board Cert:** Internal Medicine 1972; Cardiovascular Disease 1973; **Med School:** Yale Univ 1967; **Resid:** Internal Medicine, Peter Bent Brigham Hosp 1969; **Fellow:** Cardiovascular Disease, Peter Bent Brigham Hosp 1971; Research, Harvard Med Sch 1971; **Fac Appt:** Prof Med, Univ NC Sch Med

Vetrovec, George MD [Cv] - **Spec Exp:** Interventional Cardiology; **Hospital:** Med Coll of VA Hosp; **Address:** 1200 E Broad St, rm 607, Box 980036, West Hospital, Richmond, VA 23298; **Phone:** 804-828-8885; **Board Cert:** Internal Medicine 1974; Cardiovascular Disease 1977; Interventional Cardiology 1999; **Med School:** Univ VA Sch Med 1970; **Resid:** Internal Medicine, Med Coll Virginia Hosp 1974; **Fellow:** Cardiovascular Disease, Med Coll Virginia Hosp 1976; **Fac Appt:** Prof Med, Med Coll VA

Vignola, Paul MD [Cv] - **Spec Exp:** Interventional Cardiology; **Hospital:** Aventura Hosp & Med Ctr; **Address:** Aventura Hosp, Cardiac Cath Lab, 20900 Biscayne Blvd, Aventura, FL 33180; **Phone:** 305-682-7379; **Board Cert:** Internal Medicine 1974; Cardiovascular Disease 1977; Interventional Cardiology 1999; **Med School:** Yale Univ 1971; **Resid:** Internal Medicine, Yale-New Haven Hosp 1974; **Fellow:** Cardiovascular Disease, Mass Genl Hospital-Harvard 1976; **Fac Appt:** Assoc Clin Prof Med, Univ Miami Sch Med

Wells, Gretchen L MD/PhD [Cv] - **Spec Exp:** Heart Valve Disease; Congenital Heart Disease-Adult; Heart Disease in Pregnancy; Cardiac Effects of Chemotherapy; **Hospital:** Wake Forest Univ Baptist Med Ctr (page 72); **Address:** Wake Forest Baptist Med Ctr, Dept Cardiology, Medical Center Blvd, Winston-Salem, NC 27157-1045; **Phone:** 336-716-6674; **Board Cert:** Cardiovascular Disease 2000; **Med School:** Univ Alabama 1994; **Resid:** Internal Medicine, NC Baptist Hosp 1997; **Fellow:** Cardiovascular Disease, Wake Forest Univ 2000; **Fac Appt:** Assoc Prof Med, Wake Forest Univ

Midwest

Armstrong, William F MD [Cv] - **Spec Exp:** Echocardiography; Non-Invasive Cardiology; **Hospital:** Univ Michigan Hlth Sys; **Address:** 1500 E Med Ctr Drive, rm L3119, Women's/0273, Ann Arbor, MI 48109; **Phone:** 734-647-7321; **Board Cert:** Internal Medicine 1979; Cardiovascular Disease 1981; **Med School:** Med Coll VA 1976; **Resid:** Internal Medicine, Med Coll Va Hosp 1979; **Fellow:** Cardiovascular Disease, Indiana Univ Hosp 1982; **Fac Appt:** Prof Med, Univ Mich Med Sch

Bonow, Robert O MD [Cv] - **Spec Exp:** Heart Valve Disease; Coronary Artery Disease; Nuclear Cardiology; **Hospital:** Northwestern Meml Hosp; **Address:** Northwestern Cardiovascular Inst, 675 N St Clair St, Galter 19-100, Chicago, IL 60611; **Phone:** 312-695-4965; **Board Cert:** Internal Medicine 1976; Cardiovascular Disease 1981; **Med School:** Univ Pennsylvania 1973; **Resid:** Internal Medicine, Hosp Univ Penn 1976; **Fellow:** Cardiovascular Disease, NIH-NHLBI 1979; **Fac Appt:** Prof Med, Northwestern Univ

Braverman, Alan C MD [Cv] - **Spec Exp:** Marfan's Syndrome; Aortic Diseases & Dissection; **Hospital:** Barnes-Jewish Hosp; **Address:** Wash Univ Med Sch, Div Cardiovascular Disease, 660 S Euclid Ave, Box 8086, St Louis, MO 63110; **Phone:** 314-362-1291; **Board Cert:** Internal Medicine 1988; Cardiovascular Disease 2001; **Med School:** Univ MO-Kansas City 1985; **Resid:** Internal Medicine, Brigham & Womens Hosp 1988; Internal Medicine, Brigham & Womens Hosp 1991; **Fellow:** Cardiovascular Disease, Brigham & Womens Hosp/Harvard 1990; **Fac Appt:** Prof Med, Washington Univ, St Louis

Burket, Mark W MD [Cv] - **Spec Exp:** Peripheral Vascular Disease; Coronary Artery Disease; Percutaneous Vascular Interventions; **Hospital:** Univ of Toledo Med Ctr; **Address:** 3000 Arlington Ave, Ste 1192, Toledo, OH 43614; **Phone:** 419-383-3697; **Board Cert:** Internal Medicine 1982; Cardiovascular Disease 1985; Interventional Cardiology 1999; **Med School:** Ohio State Univ 1979; **Resid:** Internal Medicine, Ohio State Univ 1982; **Fellow:** Cardiovascular Disease, Med Coll Ohio 1985; **Fac Appt:** Prof Med, Med Univ Ohio at Toledo

Cerqueira, Manuel MD [Cv] - **Spec Exp:** Cardiac Imaging; Nuclear Cardiology; Coronary Artery Disease; **Hospital:** Cleveland Clin Fdn (page 56); **Address:** Cleveland Clinic, 9500 Euclid JB3, MC JB3, Cleveland, OH 44195; **Phone:** 216-444-2665; **Board Cert:** Internal Medicine 1981; Nuclear Medicine 1984; Cardiovascular Disease 1989; **Med School:** NYU Sch Med 1976; **Resid:** Internal Medicine, Bellevue Hosp Ctr 1980; Cardiovascular Disease, Yale-New Haven Hosp 1982; **Fellow:** Nuclear Medicine, Yale-New Haven Hosp 1983; **Fac Appt:** Prof Med, Cleveland Cl Coll Med/Case West Res

Chaitman, Bernard R MD [Cv] - **Spec Exp:** Nuclear Cardiology; Echocardiography; **Hospital:** St Louis Univ Hosp; **Address:** Univ Club Tower, 1034 S Brentwood Blvd, Ste 1550, St Louis, MO 63117; **Phone:** 314-725-4668; **Board Cert:** Internal Medicine 1973; Cardiovascular Disease 1975; Echocardiography 2001; **Med School:** McGill Univ 1969; **Resid:** Internal Medicine, Royal Victoria Hosp 1972; **Fellow:** Cardiovascular Disease, Univ Oregon Hosps 1974; Cardiovascular Disease, Univ of Montreal 1975; **Fac Appt:** Prof Med, St Louis Univ

Connolly, Heidi M MD [Cv] - **Spec Exp:** Congenital Heart Disease; Heart Disease in Pregnancy; **Hospital:** Mayo Med Ctr & Clin - Rochester; **Address:** Mayo Clin, 200 First St SW, Gonda 6-207, Rochester, MN 55905; **Phone:** 507-284-1226; **Board Cert:** Internal Medicine 1989; Cardiovascular Disease 2001; **Med School:** Ireland 1986; **Resid:** Internal Medicine, Mayo Clinic 1989; **Fellow:** Cardiovascular Disease, Mayo Clinic 1991; **Fac Appt:** Assoc Prof Med, Mayo Med Sch

Cooper, Christopher J MD [Cv] - **Spec Exp:** Interventional Cardiology; **Hospital:** Univ of Toledo Med Ctr; **Address:** University of Toledo, Cardiovascular Medicine, 28442 E River Rd, Toledo, OH 43551; **Phone:** 419-931-0030; **Board Cert:** Internal Medicine 2004; Cardiovascular Disease 2005; Interventional Cardiology 1999; **Med School:** Univ Cincinnati 1988; **Resid:** Internal Medicine, Brigham & Womens Hosp 1991; **Fellow:** Cardiovascular Disease, Brigham & Women's Hosp-Harvard Med Sch 1994; **Fac Appt:** Prof Med, Univ Toledo, Med Univ OH

Eagle, Kim A MD [Cv] - **Spec Exp:** Aortic Diseases & Dissection; Acute Coronary Syndromes; Heart Attack; Peripheral Vascular Disease; **Hospital:** Univ Michigan Hlth Sys; **Address:** Dominos Farms, 24 Frank Lloyd Wright Drive, Ann Arbor, MI 48106-0363; **Phone:** 734-998-7400; **Board Cert:** Internal Medicine 1982; Cardiovascular Disease 1987; **Med School:** Tufts Univ 1979; **Resid:** Internal Medicine, Yale New Haven Hosp 1983; **Fellow:** Cardiovascular Disease, Mass Genl Hosp-Harvard 1986; **Fac Appt:** Asst Prof Med, Univ Mich Med Sch

Geltman, Edward M MD [Cv] - **Spec Exp:** Congestive Heart Failure; Transplant Medicine-Heart; Non-Invasive Cardiology; **Hospital:** Barnes-Jewish Hosp, Barnes-Jewish West County Hosp; **Address:** Washington Univ Sch of Med, Cardiovascular Division, 660 S Euclid Ave, Box 8086, St Louis, MO 63110; **Phone:** 314-362-1291; **Board Cert:** Internal Medicine 1974; Cardiovascular Disease 1979; **Med School:** NYU Sch Med 1971; **Resid:** Internal Medicine, Bellevue Hosp 1974; **Fellow:** Cardiovascular Disease, Barnes Jewish Hosp 1978; **Fac Appt:** Prof Med, Washington Univ, St Louis

Cardiovascular Disease

Gibbons, Raymond J MD [Cv] - **Spec Exp:** Nuclear Cardiology; Heart Attack; **Hospital:** Mayo Med Ctr & Clin - Rochester; **Address:** Mayo Clinic, Div Cardiovascular Disease, 200 First St SW, Rochester, MN 55905; **Phone:** 507-284-2541; **Board Cert:** Internal Medicine 1979; Cardiovascular Disease 1981; **Med School:** Harvard Med Sch 1976; **Resid:** Internal Medicine, Mass Genl Hosp 1978; **Fellow:** Cardiovascular Disease, Duke Univ Med Ctr 1981; **Fac Appt:** Prof Med, Mayo Med Sch

Grubb, Blair P MD [Cv] - **Spec Exp:** Autonomic Disorders; **Hospital:** Univ of Toledo Med Ctr, St Vincent's Mercy Med Ctr - Toledo; **Address:** 3000 Arlington Rd, Ste 1192, Toledo, OH 43614-2598; **Phone:** 419-383-3697; **Board Cert:** Internal Medicine 1985; Cardiovascular Disease 1987; **Med School:** Dominican Republic 1980; **Resid:** Internal Medicine, Grtr Baltimore Med Ctr 1985; **Fellow:** Cardiovascular Disease, MS Hershey Med Ctr/Penn State 1987; Cardiac Electrophysiology, MS Hershey Med Ctr/Penn State 1988; **Fac Appt:** Prof Med, Univ SD Sch Med

Hauptman, Paul J MD [Cv] - **Spec Exp:** Heart Failure; **Hospital:** St Louis Univ Hosp; **Address:** SLUCare Cardiology, University Club Tower, 1034 S Brentwood Blvd, Ste 1120, Saint Louis, MO 63117; **Phone:** 314-977-4663; **Board Cert:** Cardiovascular Disease 2003; **Med School:** Cornell Univ 1987; **Resid:** Internal Medicine, Brigham & Womens Hosp 1990; **Fellow:** Cardiovascular Disease, Mt Sinai Hosp 1992; Cardiovascular Disease, Brigham & Womens Hosp 1993; **Fac Appt:** Prof Med, St Louis Univ

Hayes, Sharonne N MD [Cv] - **Spec Exp:** Heart Disease in Women; Preventive Cardiology; Cholesterol/Lipid Disorders; Echocardiography; **Hospital:** Mayo Med Ctr & Clin - Rochester; **Address:** Mayo Clin Women's Heart Clin, 200 First St SW Gonda 5 Bldg - rm 368, Rochester, MN 55905; **Phone:** 507-284-3683; **Board Cert:** Internal Medicine 1986; Cardiovascular Disease 1989; **Med School:** Northwestern Univ 1983; **Resid:** Internal Medicine, Mayo Clin 1986; **Fellow:** Cardiovascular Research, Mayo Clin 1987; Cardiovascular Disease, Mayo Clin 1990; **Fac Appt:** Assoc Prof Med, Mayo Med Sch

Heroux, Alain MD [Cv] - **Spec Exp:** Transplant Medicine-Heart; Heart Failure; **Hospital:** Loyola Univ Med Ctr; **Address:** 2160 S 1st Ave Bldg 111 - rm 1110, Maywood, IL 60153; **Phone:** 708-327-2738; **Med School:** Canada 1981; **Resid:** Internal Medicine, Laval Univ Med Ctr 1985; Cardiovascular Disease, Royal Victory Hosp 1987; **Fellow:** Univ Virginia Med Coll 1989; **Fac Appt:** Asst Prof Med, Rush Med Coll

Jaffe, Allan S MD [Cv] - **Spec Exp:** Ischemic Heart Disease; Heart Disease & Depression; **Hospital:** Mayo Med Ctr & Clin - Rochester; **Address:** Mayo Clinic, Div Cardiovascular Disease, 200 First St SW, Gonda 5-468, Rochester, MN 55905; **Phone:** 507-284-3680; **Board Cert:** Internal Medicine 1976; Cardiovascular Disease 1979; **Med School:** Univ MD Sch Med 1973; **Resid:** Internal Medicine, Barnes Hosp 1975; Internal Medicine, Wash Univ 1976; **Fellow:** Cardiovascular Disease, Barnes Hosp 1978; **Fac Appt:** Prof Med, Mayo Med Sch

Johnson, Maryl R MD [Cv] - **Spec Exp:** Congestive Heart Failure; Transplant Medicine-Heart; **Hospital:** Univ WI Hosp & Clins; **Address:** Univ Wisconsin Hosp/Clinics - Cardiology, 600 Highland Ave, Madison, WI 53792-0001; **Phone:** 608-263-0080; **Board Cert:** Internal Medicine 1981; Cardiovascular Disease 1983; **Med School:** Univ Iowa Coll Med 1977; **Resid:** Internal Medicine, Univ Iowa Hosp 1981; **Fellow:** Cardiovascular Disease, Univ Iowa Hosp 1982; **Fac Appt:** Prof Med, Univ Wisc

Kereiakes, Dean J MD [Cv] - **Spec Exp:** Coronary Angioplasty/Stents; Congestive Heart Failure; Interventional Cardiology; **Hospital:** Christ Hospital; **Address:** 2123 Auburn Ave, Ste 136, Cincinnati, OH 45219-2966; **Phone:** 513-721-8881; **Board Cert:** Internal Medicine 1981; Cardiovascular Disease 1985; **Med School:** Univ Cincinnati 1978; **Resid:** Internal Medicine, UCSF Med Ctr 1982; Internal Medicine, Mass Genl Hosp 1981; **Fellow:** Cardiovascular Disease, UCSF 1984; Coronary Angioplasty, Sequoia Hosp 1984; **Fac Appt:** Clin Prof Med, Ohio State Univ

Klein, Lloyd W MD [Cv] - **Spec Exp:** Coronary Artery Disease; Angiography-Coronary; Interventional Cardiology; Coronary Syndrome-Acute; **Hospital:** Gottlieb Meml Hosp, Rush Univ Med Ctr; **Address:** Clinical Cardiology Assocs, 675 W North Ave, POB Bldg Fl 2 - Ste 202, Melrose Park, IL 60160; **Phone:** 708-681-7862; **Board Cert:** Internal Medicine 1980; Cardiovascular Disease 1983; Interventional Cardiology 1999; **Med School:** Univ Cincinnati 1977; **Resid:** Internal Medicine, Einstein-Bronx Muni Hosp 1980; **Fellow:** Cardiovascular Disease, Mt Sinai Hosp 1982; **Fac Appt:** Prof Med, Rush Med Coll

Mehlman, David J MD [Cv] - **Spec Exp:** Echocardiography; Heart Valve Disease; Coronary Artery Disease; **Hospital:** Northwestern Meml Hosp; **Address:** Northwestern Cardiovascular Inst, 675 N St Clair St, Galter Bldg Fl 19 - Ste 100, Chicago, IL 60611; **Phone:** 312-695-4965; **Board Cert:** Internal Medicine 1976; Cardiovascular Disease 1979; **Med School:** Johns Hopkins Univ 1973; **Resid:** Internal Medicine, Johns Hopkins Hosp 1976; **Fellow:** Cardiovascular Disease, Univ Chicago Hosps 1978; **Fac Appt:** Assoc Prof Med, Northwestern Univ

Moran, John F MD [Cv] - **Spec Exp:** Coronary Artery Disease; Congestive Heart Failure; Cholesterol/Lipid Disorders; **Hospital:** Loyola Univ Med Ctr; **Address:** 2160 S 1st Ave, Bldg 110 - Ste 6210, Maywood, IL 60153; **Phone:** 708-327-2784; **Board Cert:** Internal Medicine 1971; Cardiovascular Disease 1973; **Med School:** Loyola Univ-Stritch Sch Med 1964; **Resid:** Internal Medicine, Univ Illinois Med Ctr 1967; **Fellow:** Cardiovascular Disease, Univ Chicago Hosps 1969; **Fac Appt:** Prof Med, Loyola Univ-Stritch Sch Med

Nemickas, Rimgaudas MD [Cv] - **Spec Exp:** Coronary Artery Disease; Heart Valve Disease; Cholesterol/Lipid Disorders; **Hospital:** Adv Illinois Masonic Med Ctr, Holy Cross Hosp - Chicago; **Address:** 4901 W 79th St, Ste 7, Burbank, IL 60459; **Phone:** 708-424-2024; **Board Cert:** Internal Medicine 1969; Cardiovascular Disease 1973; **Med School:** Loyola Univ-Stritch Sch Med 1961; **Resid:** Internal Medicine, Univ Illinois Hosp 1967; **Fellow:** Cardiovascular Disease, Cook County Hosp 1963; Cardiovascular Disease, Univ Chicago Hosps 1969; **Fac Appt:** Clin Prof Med, Loyola Univ-Stritch Sch Med

Nishimura, Rick A MD [Cv] - **Spec Exp:** Echocardiography; Pericardial Disease; **Hospital:** Mayo Med Ctr & Clin - Rochester, St Mary's Hosp - Rochester; **Address:** Mayo Clin, 200 First St SW Gonda 5 Bldg - rm 368, Rochester, MN 55905; **Phone:** 507-284-8342; **Board Cert:** Internal Medicine 1981; Cardiovascular Disease 1983; **Med School:** Rush Med Coll 1978; **Resid:** Internal Medicine, Mayo Clin 1980; **Fellow:** Cardiovascular Disease, Mayo Clin 1983; **Fac Appt:** Prof Med, Mayo Med Sch

Nissen, Steven E MD [Cv] - **Spec Exp:** Cholesterol/Lipid Disorders; Intravascular Ultrasound; Coronary Intensive Care; **Hospital:** Cleveland Clin Fdn (page 56); **Address:** 9500 Euclid Ave, MC J2-3, Cleveland, OH 44195; **Phone:** 216-445-6852; **Board Cert:** Internal Medicine 1981; Cardiovascular Disease 1983; **Med School:** Univ Mich Med Sch 1978; **Resid:** Internal Medicine, UC Davis Medical Ctr 1981; **Fellow:** Cardiovascular Disease, Univ Kentucky-Chandler Med Ctr 1983; **Fac Appt:** Prof Med, Cleveland Cl Coll Med/Case West Res

Rahko, Peter S MD [Cv] - **Spec Exp:** Congestive Heart Failure; Heart Valve Disease; Echocardiography; Echocardiography - Transesophageal; **Hospital:** Univ WI Hosp & Clins, Meriter Hosp; **Address:** 600 Highland Ave, rm G7-343 CSC, MC 3248, Madison, WI 53792-3248; **Phone:** 608-263-1530; **Board Cert:** Internal Medicine 1982; Cardiovascular Disease 1985; **Med School:** Univ Minn 1979; **Resid:** Internal Medicine, Indiana Univ Med Ctr 1982; **Fellow:** Cardiovascular Disease, Univ Pittsburgh 1985; **Fac Appt:** Prof Med, Univ Wisc

Cardiovascular Disease

Reiss, Craig MD [Cv] - **Spec Exp:** Ischemic Heart Disease; Heart Valve Disease; Preventive Cardiology; Coronary Artery Disease; **Hospital:** Barnes-Jewish Hosp, Barnes-Jewish West County Hosp; **Address:** Wash Univ Med Sch, Div Cardiovascular Disease, 1020 N Mason Rd, Ste 106, St Louis, MO 63141; **Phone:** 314-362-1291; **Board Cert:** Internal Medicine 1986; Cardiovascular Disease 1989; **Med School:** Univ MO-Kansas City 1983; **Resid:** Internal Medicine, Brigham & Women's Hosp 1989; **Fellow:** Cardiovascular Disease, Brigham & Women's Hosp 1988; **Fac Appt:** Assoc Prof Med, Washington Univ, St Louis

Rich, Stuart MD [Cv] - **Spec Exp:** Pulmonary Hypertension; Heart Failure; **Hospital:** Univ of Chicago Med Ctr; **Address:** 5841 S Maryland Ave, MC 2016, Chicago, IL 60637; **Phone:** 773-702-6049; **Board Cert:** Internal Medicine 1978; Cardiovascular Disease 1981; **Med School:** Loyola Univ-Stritch Sch Med 1974; **Resid:** Internal Medicine, Barnes-Jewish Hosp 1978; **Fellow:** Cardiovascular Disease, Univ Chicago Hosp 1980; **Fac Appt:** Prof Med, Rush Med Coll

Rosenbush, Stuart W MD [Cv] - **Spec Exp:** Cardiac Catheterization; Coronary Angioplasty/Stents; Coronary Artery Disease; Heart Failure; **Hospital:** Rush Univ Med Ctr, Skokie/North Shore Univ Htlh Syst; **Address:** Assocs In Cardiology Ltd, 1725 W Harrison St, Ste 1138, Chicago, IL 60612-3835; **Phone:** 312-563-3233; **Board Cert:** Internal Medicine 1979; Cardiovascular Disease 1981; Interventional Cardiology 2000; **Med School:** Univ IL Coll Med 1976; **Resid:** Internal Medicine, Michael Reese Hosp 1979; **Fellow:** Cardiovascular Disease, Rush Presby-St Lukes Med Ctr 1981; **Fac Appt:** Asst Prof Med, Rush Med Coll

Safian, Robert D MD [Cv] - **Spec Exp:** Interventional Cardiology; **Hospital:** William Beaumont Hosp; **Address:** Beaumont Heart Ctr, 3601 W 13 Mile Rd Fl 3, Royal Oak, MI 48073; **Phone:** 248-898-4163; **Board Cert:** Internal Medicine 1983; Cardiovascular Disease 1987; Interventional Cardiology 1999; **Med School:** Univ Fla Coll Med 1979; **Resid:** Pathology, Univ Miami Med Ctr 1981; Internal Medicine, UCSD Med Ctr 1983; **Fellow:** Cardiovascular Disease, Beth Israel Hosp-Harvard 1987

Sanborn, Timothy MD [Cv] - **Spec Exp:** Interventional Cardiology; Gene Therapy-Cardiac Angiogenesis; Heart Valve Disease; Carotid Artery Stent Placement; **Hospital:** Evanston/Northshore Univ Hlth Syst, Glenbrook/NorthShore Univ Hlth Syst; **Address:** 2650 Ridge Ave, Walgreen Bldg Fl 3, Evanston, IL 60201; **Phone:** 847-570-2250; **Board Cert:** Internal Medicine 1980; Cardiovascular Disease 2003; Interventional Cardiology 1999; **Med School:** Northwestern Univ 1977; **Resid:** Internal Medicine, Boston City Hosp 1980; **Fellow:** Cardiovascular Disease, Boston Univ Med Ctr 1983; **Fac Appt:** Prof Med, Northwestern Univ

Shapiro, Jerrold MD [Cv] - **Spec Exp:** Echocardiography; Preventive Cardiology; **Hospital:** Swedish Covenant Hosp; **Address:** 4801 W Peterson Ave, Ste 610, Chicago, IL 60646-5713; **Phone:** 773-283-5900; **Board Cert:** Internal Medicine 1976; Cardiovascular Disease 1977; **Med School:** Univ IL Coll Med 1968; **Resid:** Internal Medicine, Ill Masonic Med Ctr 1972; **Fellow:** Cardiovascular Disease, Northwestern Meml Hosp 1974

Sorrentino, Matthew MD [Cv] - **Spec Exp:** Preventive Cardiology; Hypertension; **Hospital:** Univ of Chicago Med Ctr; **Address:** 5841 S Maryland Ave, MC 6080, Chicago, IL 60637; **Phone:** 773-702-9461; **Board Cert:** Internal Medicine 1987; Cardiovascular Disease 2001; **Med School:** Univ Chicago-Pritzker Sch Med 1984; **Resid:** Internal Medicine, Univ Chicago Hosps 1989; **Fellow:** Cardiovascular Disease, Univ Chicago Hosps 1991; **Fac Appt:** Assoc Prof Med, Univ Chicago-Pritzker Sch Med

Stein, James H MD [Cv] - **Spec Exp:** Preventive Cardiology; Echocardiography; Cholesterol/Lipid Disorders; **Hospital:** Univ WI Hosp & Clins; **Address:** Univ WI Hosp, Clinic Sci Center, 600 Highland Ave, Ste G7341, MC 3248, Madison, WI 53792; **Phone:** 608-263-9648; **Board Cert:** Internal Medicine 2003; Cardiovascular Disease 2007; **Med School:** Yale Univ 1990; **Resid:** Internal Medicine, Univ Chicago Hosps 1993; **Fellow:** Cardiovascular Disease, Rush-Presby St Lukes Med Ctr 1996; **Fac Appt:** Prof Med, Univ Wisc

Stewart, William J MD [Cv] - **Spec Exp:** Heart Valve Disease; Echocardiography; **Hospital:** Cleveland Clin Fdn (page 56); **Address:** Div Cardiovascular Medicine, 9500 Euclid Ave, Desk J1-5, Cleveland, OH 44195; **Phone:** 216-444-5923; **Board Cert:** Internal Medicine 1980; Cardiovascular Disease 1983; **Med School:** Univ Cincinnati 1977; **Resid:** Internal Medicine, Univ Mich Hosp 1980; **Fellow:** Cardiovascular Disease, Boston Univ Med Ctr 1982; Cardiovascular Disease, Mass Genl Hosp 1984; **Fac Appt:** Assoc Prof Med, Cleveland Cl Coll Med/Case West Res

Volgman, Annabelle S MD [Cv] - **Spec Exp:** Heart Disease in Women; Arrhythmias; Atrial Fibrillation; Preventive Cardiology; **Hospital:** Rush Univ Med Ctr, Rush Oak Park Hosp; **Address:** Rush Heart Ctr for Women, 1725 W Harrison St, Professional Bldg, Ste 1159, Chicago, IL 60612; **Phone:** 312-942-5020; **Board Cert:** Cardiovascular Disease 2006; **Med School:** Columbia P&S 1984; **Resid:** Internal Medicine, Univ Chicago Hosps 1987; **Fellow:** Cardiovascular Disease, Northwestern Meml Hosp 1989; Cardiac Electrophysiology, Northwestern Meml Hosp 1990; **Fac Appt:** Assoc Prof Med, Rush Med Coll

von der Lohe, Elisabeth MD [Cv] - **Spec Exp:** Heart Disease in Women; Interventional Cardiology; **Hospital:** Indiana Univ Hosp, Methodist Hosp - Indianapolis; **Address:** Krannert Inst Cardiology, Womens Heart Clinic, 1800 N Capital Blvd, Ste E400, Indianapolis, IN 46202; **Phone:** 317-962-0561; **Board Cert:** Internal Medicine 2000; Cardiovascular Disease 2001; Interventional Cardiology 2003; **Med School:** Germany 1978; **Resid:** Internal Medicine, Marien Hosp 1981; **Fellow:** Cardiovascular Disease, Klinikum Aachen 1986; **Fac Appt:** Clin Prof Med, Indiana Univ

Wagoner, Lynne E MD [Cv] - **Spec Exp:** Congestive Heart Failure; Heart Disease in Women; Transplant Medicine-Heart; Pulmonary Hypertension; **Hospital:** Mercy Hosp - Fairfield, Christ Hospital; **Address:** 2123 Auburn Ave, Ste 624, Cincinnati, OH 45219; **Phone:** 513-751-4222; **Board Cert:** Internal Medicine 1989; Cardiovascular Disease 2003; **Med School:** E Carolina Univ 1986; **Resid:** Internal Medicine, Pitt Co Meml Hosp 1989; **Fellow:** Cardiovascular Disease, Univ Utah 1994

Walsh, Mary N MD [Cv] - **Spec Exp:** Heart Disease in Women; Nuclear Cardiology; Congestive Heart Failure; **Hospital:** St Vincent Indianapolis Hosp; **Address:** The Care Group at St Vincent, 8333 Naab Rd, Ste 400, Indianapolis, IN 46260; **Phone:** 317-338-6666; **Board Cert:** Internal Medicine 1986; Cardiovascular Disease 2001; **Med School:** Univ Minn 1983; **Resid:** Internal Medicine, Univ Tex SW Med Ctr 1986; **Fellow:** Cardiovascular Disease, Wash Univ 1989; **Fac Appt:** Asst Clin Prof Med, Indiana Univ

Weaver, W Douglas MD [Cv] - **Spec Exp:** Heart Attack; Angioplasty; Cholesterol/Lipid Disorders; **Hospital:** Henry Ford Hosp; **Address:** Henry Ford Hosp, 2799 W Grand Blvd, Cardiology K-14, Detroit, MI 48202-2689; **Phone:** 313-916-4420; **Board Cert:** Internal Medicine 1974; Cardiovascular Disease 1977; **Med School:** Tufts Univ 1971; **Resid:** Internal Medicine, Univ Wash Hosps 1974; **Fellow:** Cardiovascular Disease, Univ Wash Hosps 1976

Wilkoff, Bruce L MD [Cv] - **Spec Exp:** Defibrillator Cable Extraction; **Hospital:** Cleveland Clin Fdn (page 56); **Address:** Cleveland Clinic, 9500 Euclid Ave, Desk J2-2, Cleveland, OH 44195; **Phone:** 216-444-4975; **Board Cert:** Internal Medicine 1982; Cardiovascular Disease 1985; **Med School:** Ohio State Univ 1979; **Resid:** Internal Medicine, Univ Hosps 1982; **Fellow:** Cardiovascular Disease, Univ Hosps 1984; Cerebrovascular Disease, Ohio State Univ 1986

Cardiovascular Disease

Williams, Kim A MD [Cv] - **Spec Exp:** Nuclear Cardiology; Coronary Artery Disease; **Hospital:** Univ of Chicago Med Ctr; **Address:** 5758 S Maryland Ave, MC 9015, Chicago, IL 60637; **Phone:** 773-702-9461; **Board Cert:** Internal Medicine 1982; Cardiovascular Disease 1985; Nuclear Medicine 1986; **Med School:** Univ Chicago-Pritzker Sch Med 1979; **Resid:** Internal Medicine, Emory Univ 1982; **Fellow:** Cardiovascular Disease, Univ Chicago 1984; Nuclear Medicine, Univ Chicago 1986; **Fac Appt:** Assoc Prof Med, Univ Chicago-Pritzker Sch Med

Young, James B MD [Cv] - **Spec Exp:** Transplant Medicine-Heart; Heart Failure; Ventricular Assist Device (LVAD); **Hospital:** Cleveland Clin Fdn (page 56); **Address:** 9500 Euclid Ave Desk J3-4, Cleveland, OH 44195; **Phone:** 216-444-2270; **Board Cert:** Internal Medicine 1977; Cardiovascular Disease 1979; **Med School:** Baylor Coll Med 1974; **Resid:** Internal Medicine, Baylor Affil Hosp 1977; Internal Medicine, Methodist Hosp 1980; **Fellow:** Cardiovascular Disease, Baylor Affl Hosp 1979; **Fac Appt:** Prof Med, Cleveland Cl Coll Med/Case West Res

Great Plains and Mountains

Anderson, Jeffrey L MD [Cv] - **Spec Exp:** Arrhythmias; Cholesterol/Lipid Disorders; Cardiac MRI; **Hospital:** LDS Hosp, Salt Lake Regional Med Ctr; **Address:** Intermountain Med Ctr, 5121 S Cottonwood St, Murray, UT 84107; **Phone:** 801-507-4757; **Board Cert:** Internal Medicine 1975; Cardiovascular Disease 1979; Cardiac Electrophysiology 2002; **Med School:** Harvard Med Sch 1972; **Resid:** Internal Medicine, Mass Genl Hosp 1974; **Fellow:** Research, Natl Inst Hlth 1976; Cardiovascular Disease, Stanford Univ Med Ctr 1978; **Fac Appt:** Prof Med, Univ Utah

Benjamin, Ivor J MD [Cv] - **Spec Exp:** Arrhythmias; **Hospital:** Univ Utah Hosps and Clins; **Address:** Div Cardiology, 30 N 1900 E, rm 4A100, Salt Lake City, UT 84132; **Phone:** 801-581-7715; **Board Cert:** Internal Medicine 1985; Cardiovascular Disease 1989; **Med School:** Johns Hopkins Univ 1982; **Resid:** Internal Medicine, Yale-New Haven Hosp 1985; **Fellow:** Cardiology Research, Yale-New Haven Hosp 1988; Echocardiography, Michael Reese Hosp 1989; **Fac Appt:** Prof Med, Univ Utah

Lindenfeld, JoAnn MD [Cv] - **Spec Exp:** Congestive Heart Failure; Transplant Medicine-Heart; Heart Disease in Women; **Hospital:** Univ Colorado Hosp; **Address:** 1635 Aurora Ct, rm 7083, Aurora, CO 80045; **Phone:** 720-848-0850; **Board Cert:** Internal Medicine 1976; Cardiovascular Disease 1979; **Med School:** Univ Mich Med Sch 1973; **Resid:** Internal Medicine, UCSD Med Ctr 1977; **Fellow:** Cardiovascular Disease, Univ Tex Hlth Sci Ctr 1979; **Fac Appt:** Prof Med, Univ Colorado

Southwest

Carabello, Blase A MD [Cv] - **Spec Exp:** Heart Valve Disease; **Hospital:** DeBakey VA Med Ctr-Houston; **Address:** Houston VA Medical Ctr, 2002 Holcombe Blvd, MS 111MCL, Houston, TX 77030; **Phone:** 713-794-7070; **Board Cert:** Internal Medicine 1977; Cardiovascular Disease 1979; **Med School:** Temple Univ 1973; **Resid:** Internal Medicine, Mass General Hosp 1976; **Fellow:** Cardiovascular Disease, Peter Bent Brigham Hosp 1978; **Fac Appt:** Prof Med, Baylor Coll Med

Freeman, Gregory L MD [Cv] - **Spec Exp:** Interventional Cardiology; Angioplasty; **Hospital:** Univ Hlth Syst-San Antonio; **Address:** Cardiology Clinical Associates, 4411 Medical Drive, Ste 300, San Antonio, TX 78229; **Phone:** 210-614-5400; **Board Cert:** Internal Medicine 1979; Cardiovascular Disease 1983; **Med School:** Loyola Univ-Stritch Sch Med 1976; **Resid:** Internal Medicine, Cook County Hosp 1979; **Fellow:** Cardiovascular Disease, Loyola Univ Med Ctr 1981; Research, UCSD Sch Med 1983; **Fac Appt:** Prof Med, Univ Tex, San Antonio

Gould, K Lance MD [Cv] - **Spec Exp:** Preventive Cardiology; PET Imaging; Cholesterol/Lipid Disorders; **Hospital:** Meml Hermann Hosp - Texas Med Ctr; **Address:** Univ Texas - PET Imaging Ctr, 6431 Fannin, Rm 4.256 MSB, Houston, TX 77030-1501; **Phone:** 713-500-6611; **Med School:** Case West Res Univ 1964; **Resid:** Internal Medicine, Univ Wash Med Ctr 1967; Cardiovascular Disease, Univ Wash Med Ctr 1964; **Fellow:** Cardiovascular Disease, Univ Wash Med Ctr 1971; **Fac Appt:** Prof Med, Univ Tex, Houston

Krajcer, Zvonimir MD [Cv] - **Spec Exp:** Peripheral Vascular Disease; **Hospital:** St Luke's Episcopal Hosp-Houston; **Address:** 6624 Fannin St, Ste 2780, Houston, TX 77030; **Phone:** 713-791-4158; **Board Cert:** Internal Medicine 1975; Cardiovascular Disease 1977; **Med School:** Slovenia 1970; **Resid:** Internal Medicine, Northwestern Medical Ctr 1974; **Fellow:** Cardiovascular Disease, St Luke's Episcopal Hosp 1977; **Fac Appt:** Clin Prof Med, Baylor Coll Med

Massin, Edward Krauss MD [Cv] - **Spec Exp:** Congestive Heart Failure; Transplant Medicine-Heart; Coronary Artery Disease; **Hospital:** St Luke's Episcopal Hosp-Houston; **Address:** Cardiology Consultants Houston, 6624 Fannin St, Ste 2310, Houston, TX 77030-2335; **Phone:** 713-796-2668; **Board Cert:** Internal Medicine 1973; Cardiovascular Disease 1973; **Med School:** Washington Univ, St Louis 1965; **Resid:** Internal Medicine, Barnes Hosp 1967; **Fellow:** Cardiovascular Disease, Univ Colo Med Ctr 1971; **Fac Appt:** Clin Prof Med, Baylor Coll Med

McPherson, David D MD [Cv] - **Spec Exp:** Echocardiography; Congenital Heart Disease-Adult; Heart Valve Disease; **Hospital:** Univ Hlth Syst-San Antonio; **Address:** 6431 Fannin St, MSB 1252, Houston, TX 77030; **Phone:** 713-500-6553; **Board Cert:** Internal Medicine 2005; Cardiovascular Disease 2007; **Med School:** Univ Alberta 1978; **Resid:** Internal Medicine, Dalhousie Univ 1981; **Fellow:** Cardiovascular Disease, Dalhousie Univ 1983; Cardiovascular Disease, Iowa Univ Med 1984; **Fac Appt:** Prof Med, Northwestern Univ

Nagueh, Sherif F MD [Cv] - **Spec Exp:** Echocardiography; Heart Failure; **Hospital:** Methodist Hosp - Houston; **Address:** Methodist DeBakey Heart & Vascular Ctr, 6550 Fannin, Ste 1901, Smith Tower, Houston, TX 77030; **Phone:** 713-441-1100; **Board Cert:** Internal Medicine 2003; Cardiovascular Disease 2007; **Med School:** Egypt 1986; **Resid:** Internal Medicine, Baylor Coll Med 1993; **Fellow:** Cardiovascular Disease, Baylor Coll Med 1996; **Fac Appt:** Prof Med, Cornell Univ-Weill Med Coll

Quinones, Miguel A MD [Cv] - **Spec Exp:** Echocardiography; Heart Valve Disease; **Hospital:** Methodist Hosp - Houston; **Address:** Methodist DeBakey Cardiology Assocs, 6550 Fannin St Smith Bldg - rm 1901, Houston, TX 77030; **Phone:** 713-441-1100; **Board Cert:** Internal Medicine 1972; Cardiovascular Disease 1974; **Med School:** Puerto Rico 1968; **Resid:** Internal Medicine, Harlem Hosp 1971; **Fellow:** Cardiovascular Disease, Baylor Coll Med 1974; **Fac Appt:** Prof Med, Univ Tex, Houston

Ramee, Stephen Robert MD [Cv] - **Spec Exp:** Angiography-Coronary; Interventional Cardiology; **Hospital:** Ochsner Fdn Hosp; **Address:** Ochsner Clinic, Cath Lab, 1514 Jefferson Hwy, New Orleans, LA 70121; **Phone:** 504-842-3724; **Board Cert:** Internal Medicine 1983; Cardiovascular Disease 1985; Interventional Cardiology 1999; **Med School:** Geo Wash Univ 1980; **Resid:** Internal Medicine, Letterman Army Med Ctr 1983; **Fellow:** Cardiovascular Disease, Letterman Army Med Ctr 1985

Stainback III, Raymond F MD [Cv] - **Spec Exp:** Stroke; Coronary Artery Disease; Heart Valve Disease; Echocardiography-Transesophageal; **Hospital:** St Luke's Episcopal Hosp-Houston; **Address:** Hall-Garcia Cardiology Assoc, 6624 Fannin St Ste 2480, Houston, TX 77030-2309; **Phone:** 713-529-5530; **Board Cert:** Cardiovascular Disease 2007; Echocardiography 2008; **Med School:** Baylor Coll Med 1987; **Resid:** Internal Medicine, Vanderbilt Univ Med Ctr 1990; **Fellow:** Cardiovascular Disease, Vanderbilt Univ Med Ctr 1993; Echocardiography, UCSF Med Ctr 1995; **Fac Appt:** Asst Clin Prof Med, Baylor Coll Med

Cardiovascular Disease

Tajik, A Jamil MD [Cv] - **Spec Exp:** Echocardiography; Heart Valve Disease; **Hospital:** Mayo Clinic - Scottsdale; **Address:** 13400 E Shea Blvd, Scottsdale, AZ 85259; **Phone:** 480-301-4876; **Board Cert:** Internal Medicine 1973; Cardiovascular Disease 1973; **Med School:** Pakistan 1965; **Resid:** Internal Medicine, Mayo Clinic 1970; **Fellow:** Cardiovascular Disease, Mayo Clinic 1972

Thames, Marc D MD [Cv] - **Spec Exp:** Coronary Artery Disease; Congestive Heart Failure; **Hospital:** Scottsdale Hlthcare - Shea; **Address:** Cardiovascular Consultants, 3805 E Bell Rd, Ste 3100, Phoenix, AZ 85032-3356; **Phone:** 602-867-8644; **Board Cert:** Internal Medicine 1974; Cardiovascular Disease 1979; **Med School:** Med Coll VA 1970; **Resid:** Internal Medicine, Peter Bent Brigham Hosp 1974; **Fellow:** Cardiology Research, Peter Bent Brigham Hosp 1975; Cardiovascular Disease, Mayo Clinic 1977

Wilansky, Susan MD [Cv] - **Spec Exp:** Heart Disease in Women; Heart Disease in Pregnancy; Echocardiography; **Hospital:** Mayo Clinic - Scottsdale; **Address:** Mayo Clinic, Dept Cardiology, 13400 E Shea Blvd, Scottsdale, AZ 85259; **Phone:** 480-301-8200; **Board Cert:** Cardiovascular Disease 1989; **Med School:** McMaster Univ 1979; **Resid:** Internal Medicine, Univ Toronto Hosp 1983; **Fellow:** Cardiovascular Disease, Univ Toronto Hosp 1985; Echocardiography, Univ Toronto Hosp 1986; **Fac Appt:** Assoc Prof Med, Mayo Med Sch

Willerson, James T MD [Cv] - **Spec Exp:** Ischemic Heart Disease; Stem Cell Therapy in Heart Failure; **Hospital:** St Luke's Episcopal Hosp-Houston; **Address:** 7000 Fannin St, Ste 1700, Houston, TX 77030; **Phone:** 832-355-3942; **Board Cert:** Internal Medicine 1972; Cardiovascular Disease 1974; **Med School:** Baylor Coll Med 1965; **Resid:** Internal Medicine, Mass Genl Hosp 1967; **Fellow:** Cardiovascular Disease, Mass Genl Hosp 1967; **Fac Appt:** Prof Med, Univ Tex, Houston

Zoghbi, William A MD [Cv] - **Spec Exp:** Echocardiography; **Hospital:** Methodist Hosp - Houston; **Address:** SM-677 6550 Fannin, Houston, TX 77030; **Phone:** 713-790-4342; **Board Cert:** Internal Medicine 1982; Cardiovascular Disease 1985; **Med School:** Meharry Med Coll 1979; **Resid:** Internal Medicine, Baylor Coll Affil Hosps 1982; **Fellow:** Cardiovascular Disease, Baylor Coll Med 1985

West Coast and Pacific

Bairey-Merz, C Noel MD [Cv] - **Spec Exp:** Preventive Cardiology; Heart Disease in Women; **Hospital:** Cedars-Sinai Med Ctr; **Address:** Cedars-Sinai Women's Hlth Program, 444 S San Vicente Blvd, Ste 600, Los Angeles, CA 90048; **Phone:** 310-423-9680; **Board Cert:** Internal Medicine 1984; Cardiovascular Disease 1987; **Med School:** Harvard Med Sch 1981; **Resid:** Internal Medicine, UCSF Med Ctr 1984; **Fellow:** Cardiovascular Disease, Cedars-Sinai Med Ctr 1986; **Fac Appt:** Assoc Clin Prof Med, UCLA

Blanchard, Daniel G MD [Cv] - **Spec Exp:** Echocardiography; Hypertension; **Hospital:** UCSD Med Ctr; **Address:** Perlman Medical Office, 9350 Campus Point Dr, Box 0986, La Jolla, CA 92037; **Phone:** 858-657-8530; **Board Cert:** Internal Medicine 1988; Cardiovascular Disease 2002; **Med School:** UCSD 1985; **Resid:** Internal Medicine, UCSD Med Ctr 1988; **Fellow:** Cardiovascular Disease, USCD Med Ctr 1991; **Fac Appt:** Prof Med, UCSD

Brindis, Ralph G MD [Cv] - **Spec Exp:** Acute Coronary Syndromes; Interventional Cardiology; **Hospital:** Kaiser Permanente Oakland Med Ctr, Alta Bates Summit Med Ctr-Oakland; **Address:** Hospital Bldg Fl 2, 280 W MacArthur Blvd, Oakland, CA 94611; **Phone:** 510-752-7109; **Board Cert:** Internal Medicine 1980; Cardiovascular Disease 1983; Interventional Cardiology 1999; **Med School:** Emory Univ 1977; **Resid:** Internal Medicine, Herbert C Moffitt Hosp 1980; Internal Medicine, Fort Miley VA Hosp 1981; **Fellow:** Cardiovascular Disease, Herbert C Moffitt Hosp 1983; **Fac Appt:** Prof Med, UCSF

Budoff, Matthew J MD [Cv] - **Spec Exp:** Cholesterol/Lipid Disorders; Preventive Cardiology; Cardiac Imaging; **Hospital:** LAC - Harbor - UCLA Med Ctr, Little Co of Mary-Torrance Hosp; **Address:** 1124 W Carson St, Torrance, CA 90502; **Phone:** 310-222-4107; **Board Cert:** Internal Medicine 2003; Cardiovascular Disease 2007; **Med School:** Geo Wash Univ 1990; **Resid:** Internal Medicine, UCLA/Harbor Med Ctr 1993; **Fellow:** Cardiovascular Disease, UCLA/Harbor Med Ctr 1997; **Fac Appt:** Assoc Prof Med, UCLA

Chatterjee, Kanu MD [Cv] - **Spec Exp:** Coronary Artery Disease; Congestive Heart Failure; **Hospital:** UCSF Med Ctr; **Address:** 1182 Moffitt Hosp, 505 Parnassus Ave Fl 11th, Box 0124, San Francisco, CA 94143-0327; **Phone:** 415-476-1326; **Board Cert:** Internal Medicine 1973; Cardiovascular Disease 1975; **Med School:** India 1956; **Resid:** Internal Medicine, Coventry & Warwickshire Hosps 1966; **Fellow:** Cardiovascular Disease, St George's Hosp 1969; Research, Brompton Hosp 1971; **Fac Appt:** Prof Med, UCSF

Dichek, David A MD [Cv] - **Spec Exp:** Gene Therapy; Coronary Artery Disease; **Hospital:** Univ Wash Med Ctr; **Address:** University of Washington, Dept Cardiology, 1959 NE Pacific St, Box 357710, Seattle, WA 98195; **Phone:** 206-598-4300; **Board Cert:** Internal Medicine 1987; Cardiovascular Disease 2004; **Med School:** UCLA 1984; **Resid:** Internal Medicine, Mass Genl Hosp 1987; **Fellow:** Cardiovascular Disease, NIH/Johns Hopkins Hosp 1992; **Fac Appt:** Prof Med, Univ Wash

Elkayam, Uri MD [Cv] - **Spec Exp:** Congestive Heart Failure; Heart Disease in Pregnancy; Heart Valve Disease; **Hospital:** LAC & USC Med Ctr, USC Univ Hosp; **Address:** LAC & USC Med Ctr, Div Cardiology, 1200 N State St, rm 7621, Los Angeles, CA 90033; **Phone:** 323-226-7541; **Board Cert:** Internal Medicine 1989; **Med School:** Israel 1973; **Resid:** Internal Medicine, Ichilov Hosp 1976; **Fellow:** Cardiovascular Disease, Albert Einstein Hosp 1978; Cardiovascular Disease, Cedars Sinai Med Ctr 1979; **Fac Appt:** Prof Med, USC Sch Med

Fishbein, Daniel P MD [Cv] - **Spec Exp:** Congestive Heart Failure; Transplant Medicine-Heart; **Hospital:** Univ Wash Med Ctr; **Address:** Univ Wash, Div Cardiology, 1959 NE Pacific St, Box 356422, Seattle, WA 98195-6422; **Phone:** 206-221-4507; **Board Cert:** Internal Medicine 1983; Cardiovascular Disease 1987; **Med School:** Albert Einstein Coll Med 1980; **Resid:** Internal Medicine, Univ Wash Med Ctr 1983; **Fellow:** Cardiovascular Disease, Univ Wash Med Ctr 1987; Interventional Cardiology, Univ Wash Med Ctr 1989; **Fac Appt:** Assoc Prof Med, Univ Wash

Fonarow, Gregg C MD [Cv] - **Spec Exp:** Preventive Cardiology; Heart Failure; Cholesterol/Lipid Disorders; **Hospital:** UCLA Ronald Reagan Med Ctr; **Address:** 200 UCLA Medical Plaza, Ste 224, Los Angeles, CA 90095; **Phone:** 310-825-8816; **Board Cert:** Cardiovascular Disease 2003; **Med School:** UCLA 1987; **Resid:** Internal Medicine, UCLA Med Ctr 1990; **Fellow:** Cardiovascular Disease, UCLA Med Ctr 1993; **Fac Appt:** Prof Med, UCLA

Hunt, Sharon Ann MD [Cv] - **Spec Exp:** Transplant Medicine-Heart; **Hospital:** Stanford Univ Med Ctr; **Address:** 300 Pasteur Drive CVRB 265 Bldg, Stanford, CA 94305; **Phone:** 650-498-6605; **Board Cert:** Internal Medicine 1977; Cardiovascular Disease 1979; **Med School:** Stanford Univ 1972; **Resid:** Internal Medicine, Stanford Univ Hosp 1974; **Fellow:** Cardiovascular Disease, Stanford Univ Hosp 1976; **Fac Appt:** Prof Med, Stanford Univ

Johnson, Allen D MD [Cv] - **Spec Exp:** Coronary Artery Disease; Heart Valve Disease; Congenital Heart Disease-Adult; Congestive Heart Failure; **Hospital:** Scripps Green Hosp; **Address:** Scripps Clinic-Torrey Pines, 10666 N Torrey Pines Rd, rm SW206, La Jolla, CA 92037; **Phone:** 858-554-8836; **Board Cert:** Internal Medicine 1973; Cardiovascular Disease 1973; **Med School:** Johns Hopkins Univ 1965; **Resid:** Internal Medicine, Johns Hopkins Hosp 1970; **Fellow:** Cardiovascular Disease, UCSD Med Ctr 1972; **Fac Appt:** Clin Prof Med, Univ SD Sch Med

Cardiovascular Disease

Judelson, Debra R MD [Cv] - **Spec Exp:** Hypertension; Cholesterol/Lipid Disorders; Heart Disease in Women; **Hospital:** Cedars-Sinai Med Ctr, Brotman Med Ctr; **Address:** Women's Heart Institute, Cardiovascular Med Group Southern CA, 414 N Camden Drive, Ste 1100, Beverly Hills, CA 90210-4532; **Phone:** 310-278-3400 x155; **Board Cert:** Internal Medicine 1979; Cardiovascular Disease 1981; **Med School:** Harvard Med Sch 1976; **Resid:** Internal Medicine, Kaiser Foundation Hosp 1979; **Fellow:** Cardiovascular Disease, Kaiser Foundation Hosp 1981

Kaul, Sanjiv MD [Cv] - **Spec Exp:** Cardiac Imaging; Echocardiography; Coronary Artery Disease; Preventive Cardiology; **Hospital:** OR Hlth & Sci Univ; **Address:** OHSU Cardiovascular Med, 3181 SW Sam Jackson Park Rd, MC UHN62, Portland, OR 97239; **Phone:** 503-494-8750; **Board Cert:** Internal Medicine 1980; Cardiovascular Disease 1983; **Med School:** India 1975; **Resid:** Internal Medicine, Univ Vermont Med Ctr 1980; Cardiovascular Disease, Wadsworth VA Hosp-UCLA 1982; **Fellow:** Cardiovascular Disease, Mass Genl Hosp 1984; **Fac Appt:** Prof Med, Oregon Hlth & Sci Univ

Kobashigawa, Jon Akira MD [Cv] - **Spec Exp:** Transplant Medicine-Heart; **Hospital:** UCLA Ronald Reagan Med Ctr; **Address:** 100 UCLA Med Plaza, Ste 630, Los Angeles, CA 90095-6988; **Phone:** 310-794-1200; **Board Cert:** Internal Medicine 1983; Cardiovascular Disease 1987; **Med School:** Mount Sinai Sch Med 1980; **Resid:** Internal Medicine, UCLA Med Ctr 1983; **Fellow:** Cardiovascular Disease, UCLA Med Ctr 1986; **Fac Appt:** Clin Prof Med, UCLA

Lewis, Sandra J MD [Cv] - **Spec Exp:** Heart Disease in Women; Preventive Cardiology; Congestive Heart Failure; **Hospital:** Legacy Good Samaritan Hosp and Med Ctr, Legacy Emanuel Hospitals; **Address:** Northwest Cardiovascular Inst, 2222 NW Lovejoy St, Ste 606, Portland, OR 97210; **Phone:** 503-229-7554; **Board Cert:** Internal Medicine 1980; Cardiovascular Disease 1985; **Med School:** Stanford Univ 1977; **Resid:** Internal Medicine, Stanford Univ Med Ctr 1980; **Fellow:** Cardiovascular Disease, Stanford Univ Med Ctr 1983; **Fac Appt:** Assoc Clin Prof Med, Oregon Hlth & Sci Univ

Redberg, Rita F MD [Cv] - **Spec Exp:** Echocardiography; Heart Disease in Women; Preventive Cardiology; **Hospital:** UCSF Med Ctr; **Address:** UCSF Cardiology, 350 Parnassus Ave, Ste 300, San Francisco, CA 94143; **Phone:** 415-353-2873; **Board Cert:** Internal Medicine 1985; Cardiovascular Disease 1989; **Med School:** Univ Pennsylvania 1982; **Resid:** Internal Medicine, Columbia-Presby Med Ctr 1985; **Fellow:** Cardiovascular Disease, Columbia-Presby Med Ctr 1988; **Fac Appt:** Prof Med, UCSF

Schnittger, Ingela MD [Cv] - **Spec Exp:** Cardiovascular Imaging; Cardiac Imaging; **Hospital:** Stanford Univ Med Ctr; **Address:** 300 Pasteur Drive, rm H2157, Stanford, CA 94305-5233; **Phone:** 650-723-5196; **Board Cert:** Internal Medicine 1980; Cardiovascular Disease 1983; **Med School:** Sweden 1975; **Resid:** Internal Medicine, Stanford Univ Hosp 1980; **Fellow:** Cardiovascular Disease, Stanford Univ Hosp 1983; **Fac Appt:** Assoc Prof Med, Stanford Univ

Shah, Prediman K MD [Cv] - **Spec Exp:** Coronary Artery Disease; Cholesterol/Lipid Disorders; **Hospital:** Cedars-Sinai Med Ctr; **Address:** Cedars-Sinai Med Ctr, 8700 Beverly Blvd, Ste 5531, Los Angeles, CA 90048-1865; **Phone:** 310-423-3884; **Board Cert:** Internal Medicine 1975; Cardiovascular Disease 1977; **Med School:** India 1969; **Resid:** Internal Medicine, All India Inst Med Scis 1971; Internal Medicine, Montefiore Hosp 1974; **Fellow:** Cardiovascular Disease, Montefiore Hosp 1976; **Fac Appt:** Prof Med, UCLA

CARDIAC ELECTROPHYSIOLOGY

New England

Batsford, William P MD [CE] - **Spec Exp:** Arrhythmias; **Hospital:** Yale-New Haven Hosp; **Address:** Yale Univ School Medicine, Section Cardiovascular Medicine, 333 Cedar St, 3 FMP, Box 208017, New Haven, CT 06520-8017; **Phone:** 203-785-4126; **Board Cert:** Internal Medicine 1972; Cardiovascular Disease 1977; **Med School:** Albany Med Coll 1969; **Resid:** Internal Medicine, Hosp Univ Penn 1972; **Fac Appt:** Prof Med, Yale Univ

Buxton, Alfred E MD [CE] - **Spec Exp:** Arrhythmias; **Hospital:** Rhode Island Hosp, Miriam Hosp; **Address:** 2 Dudley St, Ste 360, Providence, RI 02905; **Phone:** 401-444-3020; **Board Cert:** Internal Medicine 1977; Cardiovascular Disease 1981; Cardiac Electrophysiology 2002; **Med School:** Univ Pennsylvania 1973; **Resid:** Internal Medicine, Hosp Univ Penn 1977; **Fellow:** Cardiovascular Disease, Hosp Univ Penn 1980; Cardiac Electrophysiology, Hosp Univ Penn 1981; **Fac Appt:** Prof Med, Brown Univ

Josephson, Mark Eric MD [CE] - **Spec Exp:** Arrhythmias; **Hospital:** Beth Israel Deaconess Med Ctr - Boston; **Address:** 185 Pilgrim Rd Baker Bldg Fl 4, Boston, MA 02215; **Phone:** 617-667-8800; **Board Cert:** Internal Medicine 1973; Cardiovascular Disease 1975; Cardiac Electrophysiology 2002; **Med School:** Columbia P&S 1969; **Resid:** Internal Medicine, Mt Sinai Med Ctr 1971; **Fellow:** Cardiovascular Disease, Hosp Univ Penn 1975; **Fac Appt:** Prof Med, Harvard Med Sch

Ruskin, Jeremy N MD [CE] - **Spec Exp:** Arrhythmias; **Hospital:** Mass Genl Hosp; **Address:** Mass General Hosp, Arrhythmia Service, 55 Fruit St, Boston, MA 02114; **Phone:** 617-726-8514; **Board Cert:** Internal Medicine 1974; Cardiovascular Disease 1975; Cardiac Electrophysiology 2003; **Med School:** Harvard Med Sch 1971; **Resid:** Internal Medicine, Beth Israel Hosp 1974; Cardiovascular Disease, Mass Genl Hosp 1977; **Fac Appt:** Assoc Prof Med, Harvard Med Sch

Stevenson, William G MD [CE] - **Spec Exp:** Arrhythmias; **Hospital:** Brigham & Women's Hosp; **Address:** Brigham & Womens Hosp, Cardiology, 75 Francis St, Boston, MA 02115; **Phone:** 857-307-1948; **Board Cert:** Internal Medicine 1982; Cardiovascular Disease 1985; Cardiac Electrophysiology 2005; **Med School:** Tulane Univ 1979; **Resid:** Internal Medicine, UCLA Med Ctr 1982; **Fellow:** Cardiovascular Disease, UCLA Med Ctr 1984; Cardiac Electrophysiology, UCLA Med Ctr 1985; **Fac Appt:** Prof Med, Harvard Med Sch

Mid Atlantic

Callans, David J MD [CE] - **Spec Exp:** Arrhythmias; Pacemakers; **Hospital:** Hosp Univ Penn - UPHS (page 60); **Address:** 3400 Spruce St, 9 Founders, Philadelphia, PA 19104; **Phone:** 215-662-6052; **Board Cert:** Internal Medicine 1989; Cardiovascular Disease 2005; Cardiac Electrophysiology 2005; **Med School:** Johns Hopkins Univ 1986; **Resid:** Internal Medicine, Hosp Univ Penn 1989; Cardiovascular Disease, Hosp Univ Penn 1999; **Fac Appt:** Prof Med, Univ Pennsylvania

Chinitz, Larry MD [CE] - **Spec Exp:** Arrhythmias; Pacemakers; Defibrillators; Atrial Fibrillation; **Hospital:** NYU Langone Med Ctr (page 67); **Address:** 403 E 34th St Fl 2, New York, NY 10016-6402; **Phone:** 212-263-7149; **Board Cert:** Internal Medicine 1982; Cardiovascular Disease 1985; Cardiac Electrophysiology 1998; **Med School:** NYU Sch Med 1979; **Resid:** Internal Medicine, Bellevue Hosp 1983; **Fellow:** Cardiovascular Disease, NYU Med Ctr/Bellevue 1985; Cardiac Electrophysiology, Montefiore/NYU 1985; **Fac Appt:** Assoc Prof Med, NYU Sch Med

Cardiovascular Electrophysiology

Cohen, Martin B MD [CE] - **Spec Exp:** Interventional Cardiology; Pacemakers; Defibrillators; Coronary Angioplasty/Stents; **Hospital:** Westchester Med Ctr, White Plains Hosp Ctr; **Address:** 19 Bradhurst Ave, Ste 700, Hawthorne, NY 10532-2140; **Phone:** 914-593-7800; **Board Cert:** Internal Medicine 1983; Cardiovascular Disease 1985; Cardiac Electrophysiology 2006; Interventional Cardiology 2004; **Med School:** SUNY Downstate 1980; **Resid:** Internal Medicine, Univ Hosp 1983; **Fellow:** Cardiovascular Disease, Univ Hosp 1985; Interventional Cardiology, Westchester Co Med Ctr 1986; **Fac Appt:** Assoc Clin Prof Med, NY Med Coll

Lerman, Bruce MD [CE] - **Spec Exp:** Catheter Ablation; Defibrillators; Arrhythmias; **Hospital:** NY-Presby Hosp/Weill Cornell (page 66); **Address:** NY Weill Cornell Med Ctr, 520 E 70th St, Starr 4, New York, NY 10021-9800; **Phone:** 212-746-2169; **Board Cert:** Internal Medicine 1980; Cardiovascular Disease 1985; Cardiac Electrophysiology 2002; **Med School:** Loyola Univ-Stritch Sch Med 1977; **Resid:** Internal Medicine, Northwestern Univ Hosp 1980; Internal Medicine, Univ Michigan Med Ctr 1981; **Fellow:** Cardiovascular Disease, Hosp Univ Penn 1982; Cardiovascular Disease, Johns Hopkins Hosp 1983; **Fac Appt:** Prof Med, Cornell Univ-Weill Med Coll

Levine, Joseph H MD [CE] - **Spec Exp:** Arrhythmias; Sudden Death Prevention; Atrial Fibrillation; Pacemakers; **Hospital:** St Francis Hosp - The Heart Ctr (page 69), Good Samaritan Hosp Med Ctr - West Islip; **Address:** 100 Port Washington Blvd, Roslyn, NY 11576; **Phone:** 516-622-1011; **Board Cert:** Internal Medicine 1983; Cardiovascular Disease 1987; Cardiac Electrophysiology 2003; **Med School:** Univ Rochester 1980; **Resid:** Internal Medicine, Yale-New Haven Hosp 1983; **Fellow:** Cardiovascular Disease, Johns Hopkins Hosp 1986; Cardiac Electrophysiology, Hosp Univ Penn 1986

Marchlinski, Francis E MD [CE] - **Spec Exp:** Pacemakers; Arrhythmias; **Hospital:** Hosp Univ Penn - UPHS (page 60); **Address:** Hosp University Penn, Div Cardiology, 3400 Spruce St Founders Bldg Fl 9, Philadelphia, PA 19104-4206; **Phone:** 215-662-6005; **Board Cert:** Internal Medicine 1979; Cardiovascular Disease 1981; Cardiac Electrophysiology 2002; **Med School:** Univ Pennsylvania 1976; **Resid:** Internal Medicine, Hosp Univ Penn 1979; **Fellow:** Cardiovascular Disease, Hosp Univ Penn 1982; **Fac Appt:** Prof Med, Univ Pennsylvania

Mehta, Davendra MD/PhD [CE] - **Spec Exp:** Arrhythmias; Congenital Heart Disease-Adult; Atrial Fibrillation; Heart Failure; **Hospital:** Mount Sinai Med Ctr (page 64); **Address:** One Gustave L Levy Pl Fl 3, New York, NY 10029-6501; **Phone:** 212-427-1540; **Board Cert:** Cardiovascular Disease 2009; Cardiac Electrophysiology 1998; **Med School:** India 1979; **Resid:** Internal Medicine, Leicester Royal Infirmary 1983; **Fellow:** Cardiovascular Disease, Groby Road Hosp 1986; Electrocardiography, St George's Hosp 1989; **Fac Appt:** Assoc Prof Med, Mount Sinai Sch Med

Southeast

Curtis, Anne B MD [CE] - **Spec Exp:** Pacemakers; Arrhythmias; Defibrillators; **Hospital:** Tampa Genl Hosp, University Comm Hosp; **Address:** S Tampa Ctr for Advanced Health Care, 2A Columbia Drive Fl 3, Tampa, FL 33606; **Phone:** 813-259-0600; **Board Cert:** Internal Medicine 1982; Cardiovascular Disease 1985; Cardiac Electrophysiology 2002; **Med School:** Columbia P&S 1979; **Resid:** Internal Medicine, Columbia- Presby Hosp 1982; **Fellow:** Cardiovascular Disease, Duke Univ Med Ctr 1985; Cardiac Electrophysiology, Duke Univ Med Ctr 1986; **Fac Appt:** Prof Med, Univ S Fla Coll Med

Del Negro, Albert A MD [CE] - **Spec Exp:** Arrhythmias; **Hospital:** Inova Fairfax Hosp, Inova Alexandria Hosp; **Address:** 3020 Hamaker Ct, Ste 401, Fairfax, VA 22031; **Phone:** 703-849-0770; **Board Cert:** Internal Medicine 1979; Cardiovascular Disease 1981; **Med School:** Georgetown Univ 1969; **Resid:** Internal Medicine, DC Genl Hosp 1972; **Fellow:** Cardiovascular Disease, Georgetown Univ Med Ctr 1973; Cardiovascular Disease, VA Med Ctr 1974; **Fac Appt:** Asst Clin Prof Med, Georgetown Univ

DeLurgio, David B MD [CE] - **Spec Exp:** Arrhythmias; Atrial Fibrillation; Sudden Death Prevention; Heart Failure; **Hospital:** Emory Univ Hosp Midtown; **Address:** Emory Univ Hosp Midtown, 550 Peachtree St NE Fl 6, Atlanta, GA 30308; **Phone:** 404-686-2504; **Board Cert:** Cardiovascular Disease 2007; Cardiac Electrophysiology 1998; **Med School:** UCLA 1990; **Resid:** Internal Medicine, Emory Univ Med Ctr 1993; **Fellow:** Cardiovascular Disease, UCLA Med Ctr 1995; **Fac Appt:** Assoc Prof Med, Emory Univ

DiMarco, John P MD/PhD [CE] - **Spec Exp:** Arrhythmias; Pacemakers; Defibrillators; **Hospital:** Univ Virginia Med Ctr; **Address:** Univ Virginia Hlth Scis Ctr, PO Box 800158, Charlottesville, VA 22908-0158; **Phone:** 434-924-2031; **Board Cert:** Internal Medicine 1978; Cardiovascular Disease 1981; Cardiac Electrophysiology 2005; **Med School:** Case West Res Univ 1975; **Resid:** Internal Medicine, Mass Genl Hosp 1977; Critical Care Medicine, Case West Res Univ 1978; **Fellow:** Cardiovascular Disease, Mass Genl Hosp 1980; Cardiac Electrophysiology, Mass Genl Hosp 1981; **Fac Appt:** Prof Med, Univ VA Sch Med

Ellenbogen, Kenneth A MD [CE] - **Spec Exp:** Arrhythmias; Pacemakers; Defibrillators; **Hospital:** Med Coll of VA Hosp, Henrico Doctors Hosp; **Address:** Dept Electrophysiology, PO Box 980053, Richmond, VA 23298; **Phone:** 804-828-7565; **Board Cert:** Internal Medicine 1983; Cardiovascular Disease 1985; Cardiac Electrophysiology 2005; **Med School:** Johns Hopkins Univ 1980; **Resid:** Internal Medicine, Johns Hopkins Hosp 1983; **Fellow:** Cardiovascular Disease, Duke Univ Med Ctr 1986; **Fac Appt:** Prof Med, Med Coll VA

Interian Jr, Alberto MD [CE] - **Spec Exp:** Arrhythmias; **Hospital:** Mercy Hosp, Jackson Meml Hosp (page 70); **Address:** Mercy Arrhythmia & Syncope Ctr, 3641 S Miami Ave, Ste 221, Miami, FL 33133; **Phone:** 305-285-2685; **Board Cert:** Internal Medicine 1985; Cardiovascular Disease 1987; Cardiac Electrophysiology 2000; **Med School:** Univ Miami Sch Med 1982; **Resid:** Internal Medicine, Univ Miami Hosps 1985; **Fellow:** Cardiovascular Disease, Univ Miami Hosps 1988; **Fac Appt:** Prof Med, Univ Miami Sch Med

Kay, G Neal MD [CE] - **Spec Exp:** Arrhythmias; Pacemakers; **Hospital:** Univ of Ala Hosp at Birmingham; **Address:** UAB, Div Cardiovascular Disease, 321-J THT, 1530 3rd Ave South, Birmingham, AL 35294; **Phone:** 205-934-1335; **Board Cert:** Internal Medicine 1983; Cardiovascular Disease 1989; Cardiac Electrophysiology 2006; **Med School:** Univ Mich Med Sch 1979; **Resid:** Internal Medicine, Univ Alabama Hosp 1983; **Fellow:** Cardiovascular Disease, Duke Univ Med Ctr 1986; **Fac Appt:** Prof Med, Univ Alabama

Sorrentino, Robert A MD [CE] - **Spec Exp:** Arrhythmias; Defibrillators; Pacemakers; Heart Failure; **Hospital:** Med Coll of GA Hosp and Clin (MCG Health Inc); **Address:** Medical College of Georgia, 1120 15th St BBR Bldg - rm 6518, Augusta, GA 30912-0004; **Phone:** 706-721-4997; **Board Cert:** Internal Medicine 1988; Cardiovascular Disease 2002; Cardiac Electrophysiology 2008; **Med School:** Albany Med Coll 1985; **Resid:** Internal Medicine, Duke Univ Med Ctr 1988; **Fellow:** Cardiovascular Disease, Duke Univ Med Ctr 1991; **Fac Appt:** Prof Med, Med Coll GA

Midwest

Anderson, Mark E MD/PhD [CE] - **Spec Exp:** Arrhythmias; **Hospital:** Univ Iowa Hosp & Clinics; **Address:** 200 Hawkins Drive, E315, GH, Iowa City, IA 52242-1081; **Phone:** 319-353-7101; **Board Cert:** Internal Medicine 2005; Cardiovascular Disease 2005; **Med School:** Univ Minn 1989; **Resid:** Internal Medicine, Stanford Univ Med Ctr 1991; **Fellow:** Cardiovascular Disease, Stanford Univ Sch Med 1994; Cardiac Electrophysiology, Stanford Univ Sch Med 1996; **Fac Appt:** Prof Med, Univ Iowa Coll Med

Cardiovascular Electrophysiology

Hammill, Stephen C MD [CE] - **Spec Exp:** Pacemakers; Arrhythmias; **Hospital:** Mayo Med Ctr & Clin - Rochester; **Address:** Mayo Clin, 200 First St SW, Rochester, MN 55905; **Phone:** 507-284-4888; **Board Cert:** Internal Medicine 1978; Cardiovascular Disease 1981; Cardiac Electrophysiology 2005; **Med School:** Univ Colorado 1974; **Resid:** Internal Medicine, Univ Colo Hlth Sci Ctr 1977; **Fellow:** Cardiovascular Disease, Duke Univ Med Ctr 1981; **Fac Appt:** Prof Med, Mayo Med Sch

Hayes, David L MD [CE] - **Spec Exp:** Pacemakers; **Hospital:** Mayo Med Ctr & Clin - Rochester; **Address:** Mayo Clinic, 200 1st St SW Gonda 5 Bldg - rm 200, Rochester, MN 55905; **Phone:** 507-284-3684; **Board Cert:** Internal Medicine 1980; Cardiovascular Disease 1981; **Med School:** Univ MO-Kansas City 1977; **Resid:** Internal Medicine, Mayo Clin 1980; **Fellow:** Cardiovascular Disease, Mayo Clin 1982; **Fac Appt:** Prof Med, Mayo Med Sch

Lindsay, Bruce MD [CE] - **Spec Exp:** Arrhythmias; **Hospital:** Barnes-Jewish Hosp; **Address:** Cleveland Clinic, Desk J2-2, 9500 Euclid Ave, Cleveland, OH 44195; **Phone:** 216-444-4293; **Board Cert:** Internal Medicine 1980; Cardiovascular Disease 1987; Cardiac Electrophysiology 2002; **Med School:** Jefferson Med Coll 1976; **Resid:** Internal Medicine, Univ Michigan Medical Ctr 1980; **Fellow:** Cardiovascular Disease, Barnes-Jewish Hosp 1985; **Fac Appt:** Assoc Prof Med, Univ Wash

Love, Charles J MD [CE] - **Spec Exp:** Defibrillator Cable Extraction; Pacemakers; **Hospital:** Ohio St Univ Med Ctr; **Address:** Heart & Lung Inst Fl 2, 473 W 12 Ave, Columbus, OH 43210; **Phone:** 614-293-4947; **Board Cert:** Internal Medicine 1986; Cardiovascular Disease 1989; Cardiac Electrophysiology 2004; **Med School:** Univ Pittsburgh 1983; **Resid:** Internal Medicine, Ohio State Univ Hosp 1986; **Fellow:** Cardiac Electrophysiology, Ohio State Univ Hosp 1988; **Fac Appt:** Prof Med, Ohio State Univ

Morady, Fred MD [CE] - **Spec Exp:** Arrhythmias; WPW Syndrome; **Hospital:** Univ Michigan Hlth Sys; **Address:** Specialty Electrophysiology, 1500 E Med Ctr Drive, 2394 CVC/5853, Ann Arbor, MI 48109; **Phone:** 734-647-7321; **Board Cert:** Internal Medicine 1978; Cardiovascular Disease 1981; Cardiac Electrophysiology 2005; **Med School:** UCSF 1975; **Resid:** Internal Medicine, UCSF Med Ctr 1978; **Fellow:** Cardiovascular Disease, UCSF Med Ctr 1980; **Fac Appt:** Prof Med, Univ Mich Med Sch

Prystowsky, Eric N MD [CE] - **Spec Exp:** Arrhythmias; Catheter Ablation; Atrial Fibrillation; **Hospital:** St Vincent Indianapolis Hosp; **Address:** 8333 Naab Rd, Ste 400, Indianapolis, IN 46260; **Phone:** 317-338-6024; **Board Cert:** Internal Medicine 1976; Cardiovascular Disease 1979; Cardiac Electrophysiology 2005; **Med School:** Mount Sinai Sch Med 1973; **Resid:** Internal Medicine, Mt Sinai Hosp 1976; **Fellow:** Cardiovascular Disease, Duke Univ Med Ctr 1979

Schuger, Claudio D MD [CE] - **Spec Exp:** Arrhythmias; Defibrillators; **Hospital:** Henry Ford Hosp; **Address:** Henry Ford Hosp, Div Cardiology, 2799 W Grand Blvd, Detroit, MI 48202; **Phone:** 313-916-2417; **Board Cert:** Cardiac Electrophysiology 1998; Cardiovascular Disease 2007; **Med School:** Argentina 1977; **Resid:** Internal Medicine, Hacarmel Hosp 1982; **Fellow:** Cardiovascular Disease, Bikur Cholim Hosp 1985; Cardiac Electrophysiology, Harper Hosp 1990; **Fac Appt:** Assoc Prof Med, Wayne State Univ

Tchou, Patrick J MD [CE] - **Spec Exp:** Arrhythmias; **Hospital:** Cleveland Clin Fdn (page 56); **Address:** Dept Cardiology, 9500 Euclid Ave, Ste J2-2, Cleveland, OH 44195; **Phone:** 216-444-6792; **Board Cert:** Internal Medicine 1982; Cardiovascular Disease 1985; Cardiac Electrophysiology 2002; **Med School:** Case West Res Univ 1979; **Resid:** Internal Medicine, Metro Genl Hosp 1982; **Fellow:** Cardiovascular Disease, Metro Genl Hosp 1984; Cardiac Electrophysiology, Mt Sinai Med Ctr 1985; **Fac Appt:** Prof Med, Ohio State Univ

Waldo, Albert MD [CE] - **Spec Exp:** Arrhythmias; Syncope; Atrial Fibrillation; **Hospital:** Univ Hosps Case Med Ctr; **Address:** Univ Hosps Case Med Ctr-Cardiology, 11100 Euclid Ave, MS LKS-5038, Cleveland, OH 44106-1736; **Phone:** 216-844-7690; **Board Cert:** Internal Medicine 1971; Cardiovascular Disease 1975; **Med School:** SUNY Downstate 1962; **Resid:** Internal Medicine, Baltimore City Hosp 1965; Internal Medicine, Kings Co Hosp 1966; **Fellow:** Cardiovascular Disease, Columbia Presby Med Ctr 1968; Cardiac Electrophysiology, Columbia Presby Med Ctr 1969; **Fac Appt:** Prof Med, Case West Res Univ

Wilber, David James MD [CE] - **Spec Exp:** Atrial Fibrillation; Catheter Ablation; Sudden Death Prevention; **Hospital:** Loyola Univ Med Ctr; **Address:** Loyola Univ Med Ctr, Cardiovascular Inst, 2160 S First Ave Bldg 110 - rm 6232, Maywood, IL 60153; **Phone:** 708-216-2642; **Board Cert:** Internal Medicine 1980; Cardiovascular Disease 1985; Cardiac Electrophysiology 2002; **Med School:** Northwestern Univ 1977; **Resid:** Internal Medicine, Northwestern Meml Hosp 1980; **Fellow:** Cardiovascular Disease, Univ Mich Med Sch 1984; Cardiac Electrophysiology, Mass Genl Hosp 1986; **Fac Appt:** Prof Med, Loyola Univ-Stritch Sch Med

Great Plains and Mountains

Lewkowiez, Laurent MD [CE] - **Spec Exp:** Arrhythmias; Ventricular Tachycardia Ablation; Atrial Fibrillation; **Hospital:** Denver Health Med Ctr; **Address:** Denver Hlth Med Ctr, Div Cardiology, 777 Bannock St, Denver, CO 80204; **Phone:** 303-436-5499; **Board Cert:** Cardiovascular Disease 2000; Cardiac Electrophysiology 2003; **Med School:** Univ SC Sch Med 1992; **Resid:** Internal Medicine, Univ Colorado Hlth Sci Ctr 1996; **Fellow:** Nuclear Cardiology, Univ Colorado Hlth Sci Ctr 1998; Cardiac Electrophysiology, Univ Colorado Hlth Sci Ctr 2001; **Fac Appt:** Asst Prof Med, Univ Colorado

West Coast and Pacific

Cannom, David S MD [CE] - **Spec Exp:** Arrhythmias; **Hospital:** Good Samaritan Hosp - LA; **Address:** 1245 Wilshire Blvd, Ste 703, Los Angeles, CA 90017; **Phone:** 213-977-0419; **Board Cert:** Internal Medicine 1980; Cardiovascular Disease 1975; **Med School:** Univ Minn 1967; **Resid:** Internal Medicine, Yale-New Haven Hosp 1969; **Fellow:** Cardiovascular Disease, Stanford Unv 1973; **Fac Appt:** Clin Prof Med, UCLA

Feld, Gregory K MD [CE] - **Hospital:** UCSD Med Ctr; **Address:** 4168 Front St, MC 8649, San Diego, CA 92103-8649; **Phone:** 619-543-5428; **Board Cert:** Internal Medicine 1980; Cardiovascular Disease 1983; Cardiac Electrophysiology 2002; **Med School:** Dartmouth Med Sch 1977; **Resid:** Internal Medicine, Wadsworth VA Hosp 1981; **Fellow:** Cardiothoracic Research, Wadsworth VA Hosp 1984; **Fac Appt:** Prof Med, UCSD

Gang, Eli Shimshon MD [CE] - **Spec Exp:** Arrhythmias; **Hospital:** Cedars-Sinai Med Ctr, Brotman Med Ctr; **Address:** 414 N Camden Drive, Ste 1100, Beverly Hills, CA 90210; **Phone:** 310-278-3400; **Board Cert:** Internal Medicine 1978; Cardiovascular Disease 1981; **Med School:** Columbia P&S 1975; **Resid:** Internal Medicine, Roosevelt Hosp 1978; **Fellow:** Cardiovascular Disease, Columbia Presby Hosp 1979; **Fac Appt:** Clin Prof Med, UCLA

Swerdlow, Charles D MD [CE] - **Spec Exp:** Defibrillators; Arrhythmias; **Hospital:** Cedars-Sinai Med Ctr, UCLA Ronald Reagan Med Ctr; **Address:** 8635 W 3rd St, Ste 1190W, Los Angeles, CA 90048-6101; **Phone:** 310-652-4600; **Board Cert:** Internal Medicine 1979; Cardiovascular Disease 1981; Cardiac Electrophysiology 2004; **Med School:** Harvard Med Sch 1976; **Resid:** Internal Medicine, LA Co- Harbor Genl Hosp 1979; **Fellow:** Cardiovascular Disease, Stanford Univ Med Ctr 1981; **Fac Appt:** Clin Prof Med, UCLA

INTERVENTIONAL CARDIOLOGY

New England

Diver, Daniel J MD [IC] - **Spec Exp:** Angioplasty; Coronary Artery Disease; **Hospital:** St Francis Hosp & Med Ctr; **Address:** St Francis Hosp - Div Cardiology, 114 Woodland St, Hartford, CT 06105; **Phone:** 860-714-4019; **Board Cert:** Internal Medicine 1984; Cardiovascular Disease 1989; Interventional Cardiology 1999; **Med School:** Johns Hopkins Univ 1981; **Resid:** Internal Medicine, Johns Hopkins Hosp 1984; **Fellow:** Cardiovascular Disease, Beth Israel Hosp/Harvard 1987; **Fac Appt:** Prof Med, Univ Conn

Gibson, C Michael MD [IC] - **Spec Exp:** Acute Coronary Syndromes; Clinical Trials; **Hospital:** Beth Israel Deaconess Med Ctr - Boston; **Address:** Beth Israel Deaconess Med Ctr, Interventional Cardiology, 185 Pilgrim Rd, Baker 4, Boston, MA 02215; **Phone:** 617-667-8800; **Board Cert:** Internal Medicine 1989; Cardiovascular Disease 2002; Interventional Cardiology 2002; **Med School:** Univ Chicago-Pritzker Sch Med 1986; **Resid:** Internal Medicine, Brigham & Womens Hosp 1989; Internal Medicine, Brigham & Womens Hosp 1993; **Fellow:** Cardiovascular Disease, Beth Israel Deaconess Med Ctr 1992; **Fac Appt:** Assoc Prof Med, Harvard Med Sch

Jacobs, Alice K MD [IC] - **Spec Exp:** Cardiac Catheterization; Heart Disease in Women; Interventional Cardiology; **Hospital:** Boston Med Ctr; **Address:** Boston Univ Med Ctr, Dept Cardiology, 88 E Newton St, rm C822, Boston, MA 02118; **Phone:** 617-638-8707; **Board Cert:** Internal Medicine 1978; Endocrinology 1979; Cardiovascular Disease 1985; Interventional Cardiology 1999; **Med School:** St Louis Univ 1975; **Resid:** Internal Medicine, St Louis Univ Hosp 1977; **Fellow:** Endocrinology, UCSD Med Ctr 1980; Cardiovascular Disease, Boston Univ Med Ctr 1982; **Fac Appt:** Prof Med, Boston Univ

Laham, Roger MD [IC] - **Spec Exp:** Angioplasty; **Hospital:** Beth Israel Deaconess Med Ctr - Boston; **Address:** Beth Israel Deaconess Med Ctr, 185 Pilgrim Rd, Baker 4, Boston, MA 02215; **Phone:** 617-667-8800; **Board Cert:** Internal Medicine 2004; Cardiovascular Disease 2005; Interventional Cardiology 1999; **Med School:** Amer Univ Beirut 1989; **Resid:** Internal Medicine, Duke Univ Med Ctr 1992; **Fellow:** Cardiovascular Disease, Harvard Med Sch 1995; **Fac Appt:** Assoc Prof Med, Harvard Med Sch

Rosenfield, Kenneth MD [IC] - **Spec Exp:** Angioplasty & Stent Placement; **Hospital:** Mass Genl Hosp, Anna Jaques Hosp; **Address:** Mass Genl Hosp, 55 Fruit St, Ste GRB800, Boston, MA 02114; **Phone:** 617-724-1935; **Board Cert:** Internal Medicine 1985; Cardiovascular Disease 1989; Interventional Cardiology 2002; **Med School:** Univ Mass Sch Med 1982; **Resid:** Internal Medicine, Kaiser Fdn Hosp 1985; **Fellow:** Cardiovascular Disease, New Eng Med Ctr 1988; Interventional Cardiology, St Elizabeth's Med Ctr 1989

Williams, David O MD [IC] - **Hospital:** Brigham & Women's Hosp; **Address:** Brigham & Women's Hosp, Cardiovascular Div, 75 Francis St PBB Bldg Fl 1st, Boston, MA 02115; **Phone:** 617-732-5089; **Board Cert:** Internal Medicine 1972; Cardiovascular Disease 1975; Interventional Cardiology 1999; **Med School:** Hahnemann Univ 1969; **Resid:** Internal Medicine, Hahnemann Univ Hosp 1972; **Fellow:** Cardiovascular Disease, UC Davis Med Ctr 1974; **Fac Appt:** Prof Med, Brown Univ

Mid Atlantic

Gray, William A MD [IC] - **Spec Exp:** Percutaneous Valve Repair; Peripheral Vascular Disease; Patent Foramen Ovale; **Hospital:** NY-Presby Hosp/Columbia (page 66); **Address:** Ctr for Interventional Vascular Therapy, 161 Fort Washington Ave Fl 5, New York, NY 10032; **Phone:** 212-305-7060; **Board Cert:** Internal Medicine 1987; Cardiovascular Disease 2002; Interventional Cardiology 1999; **Med School:** Temple Univ 1984; **Resid:** Internal Medicine, Rhode Island Hosp 1988; **Fellow:** Cardiovascular Disease, Brown Univ 1992; **Fac Appt:** Assoc Clin Prof Med, Columbia P&S

Herrmann, Howard C MD [IC] - **Spec Exp:** Cardiac Catheterization; Angioplasty & Stent Placement; Heart Valve Disease; Atrial Septal Defect Closure; **Hospital:** Hosp Univ Penn - UPHS (page 60), Penn Presby Med Ctr - UPHS (page 60); **Address:** Hosp Univ Penn, Div Cardiovascular Med, 3400 Spruce St, 9.120 Founders Bldg, Philadelphia, PA 19104-4283; **Phone:** 215-662-2180; **Board Cert:** Internal Medicine 1984; Cardiovascular Disease 1987; Interventional Cardiology 1999; **Med School:** Harvard Med Sch 1981; **Resid:** Internal Medicine, Mass General Hosp 1984; **Fellow:** Cardiovascular Disease, Mass General Hosp 1987; **Fac Appt:** Prof Med, Univ Pennsylvania

Leon, Martin MD [IC] - **Hospital:** NY-Presby Hosp/Columbia (page 66); **Address:** 161 Ft Washington Ave Fl 5, New York, NY 10032; **Phone:** 212-305-7060; **Board Cert:** Internal Medicine 1979; Cardiovascular Disease 1983; Interventional Cardiology 1999; **Med School:** Yale Univ 1975; **Resid:** Internal Medicine, Yale-New Haven Hosp 1978; **Fellow:** Cardiovascular Disease, Yale-New Haven Hosp 1980

Moses, Jeffrey W MD [IC] - **Spec Exp:** Angiography-Coronary; Angioplasty & Stent Placement; Heart Valve Disease; **Hospital:** NY-Presby Hosp/Columbia (page 66); **Address:** 161 Fort Washington Fl 5, New York, NY 10032; **Phone:** 212-305-7060; **Board Cert:** Internal Medicine 1977; Cardiovascular Disease 1981; Interventional Cardiology 1999; **Med School:** Univ Pennsylvania 1974; **Resid:** Internal Medicine, Penn Presby Med Ctr 1977; **Fellow:** Cardiovascular Disease, Penn Presby Med Ctr 1980

Petrossian, George A MD [IC] - **Spec Exp:** Carotid Artery Stent Placement; Peripheral Vascular Disease; Coronary Angioplasty/Stents; Renovascular Disease; **Hospital:** St Francis Hosp - The Heart Ctr (page 69), South Nassau Comm Hosp; **Address:** New York Cardiology Group, 1405 Old Northern Blvd Fl 1st, Roslyn, NY 11576-1353; **Phone:** 516-484-6777; **Board Cert:** Internal Medicine 1986; Cardiovascular Disease 1989; Interventional Cardiology 2000; **Med School:** Mount Sinai Sch Med 1983; **Resid:** Internal Medicine, Columbia-Presby Med Ctr 1987; **Fellow:** Cardiovascular Disease, Columbia -Presby Med Ctr 1989; Interventional Cardiology, Mass Genl Hosp 1990

Pichard, Augusto MD [IC] - **Spec Exp:** Angioplasty & Stent Placement; Cardiac Catheterization; **Hospital:** Washington Hosp Ctr; **Address:** 110 Irving St NW, Ste 4B1, Washington, DC 20010; **Phone:** 202-877-5975; **Board Cert:** Internal Medicine 1975; Cardiovascular Disease 1977; Interventional Cardiology 1999; **Med School:** Chile 1969; **Resid:** Internal Medicine, Univ Chile 1970; Internal Medicine, Catholic Univ 1971; **Fellow:** Cardiovascular Disease, Cleveland Clinic 1973; **Fac Appt:** Clin Prof Med, Geo Wash Univ

Reiner, Jonathan S MD [IC] - **Spec Exp:** Angioplasty & Stent Placement; **Hospital:** G Washington Univ Hosp; **Address:** MFA, Dept Cardiology, 2150 Pennsylvania Ave NW, Washington, DC 20037; **Phone:** 202-741-3333; **Board Cert:** Internal Medicine 1989; Cardiovascular Disease 2004; Interventional Cardiology 1999; **Med School:** Georgetown Univ 1986; **Resid:** Internal Medicine, North Shore Univ Hosp 1989; **Fellow:** Cardiovascular Disease, George Wash Univ Sch Med 1993; **Fac Appt:** Asst Prof Med, Geo Wash Univ

Interventional Cardiology

Resar, Jon R MD [IC] - **Spec Exp:** Percutaneous Coronary Intervention; Percutaneous Valve Repair; Percutaneous ASD/PFO closure; **Hospital:** Johns Hopkins Hosp (page 61); **Address:** Johns Hopkins Hosp, Dept Cardiology, 600 N Wolfe St, Blalock 524, Baltimore, MD 21287; **Phone:** 410-614-1132; **Board Cert:** Internal Medicine 1988; Cardiovascular Disease 2000; Interventional Cardiology 1999; **Med School:** Med Coll Wisc 1985; **Resid:** Internal Medicine, Johns Hopkins Hosp 1988; **Fellow:** Cardiovascular Disease, Johns Hopkins Hosp 1990; Interventional Cardiology, Johns Hopkins Hosp; **Fac Appt:** Assoc Prof Med, Johns Hopkins Univ

Roubin, Gary MD/PhD [IC] - **Spec Exp:** Coronary Angioplasty/Stents; Carotid Artery Stent Placement; Peripheral Vascular Disease; **Hospital:** Lenox Hill Hosp (page 62); **Address:** 130 E 77th St Fl 9th, New York, NY 10021; **Phone:** 212-434-2606; **Med School:** Australia 1975; **Resid:** Internal Medicine, Royal Prince Albert Hosp 1979; Cardiovascular Disease, Hallstrom Inst of Cardiology 1981; **Fellow:** Cardiology Research, Natl Heart Fdn 1983; Interventional Cardiology, Emory Univ 1985; **Fac Appt:** Clin Prof Med, NYU Sch Med

Shani, Jacob MD [IC] - **Spec Exp:** Cardiac Catheterization; Angioplasty & Stent Placement; Percutaneous Valve Repair; **Hospital:** Maimonides Med Ctr (page 63); **Address:** Maimonides Med Ctr, Cardiac Cath Lab, 4802 10th Ave, Brooklyn, NY 11219-2844; **Phone:** 718-283-7480; **Board Cert:** Internal Medicine 1981; Cardiovascular Disease 1983; Interventional Cardiology 1999; **Med School:** Israel 1977; **Resid:** Internal Medicine, Maimonides Med Ctr 1981; **Fellow:** Cardiovascular Disease, Beth Israel Hosp 1983; **Fac Appt:** Prof Med, SUNY Downstate

Shorofsky, Stephen R MD/PhD [IC] - **Spec Exp:** Arrhythmias; **Hospital:** Univ of MD Med Ctr; **Address:** Univ Maryland Med Ctr, Div Cardiology, 22 S Greene St, rm N3W77, Baltimore, MD 21201; **Phone:** 410-328-6056; **Board Cert:** Internal Medicine 1988; Cardiovascular Disease 2001; Cardiac Electrophysiology 2004; **Med School:** Univ Chicago-Pritzker Sch Med 1985; **Resid:** Internal Medicine, Univ Chicago Hosps 1988; **Fellow:** Cardiovascular Disease, Univ Chicago Hosps 1991; **Fac Appt:** Assoc Prof Med, Univ MD Sch Med

Stone, Gregg W MD [IC] - **Spec Exp:** Angioplasty & Stent Placement; Coronary Artery Disease; **Hospital:** NY-Presby Hosp/Columbia (page 66); **Address:** Columbia Univ Med Ctr, 161 Fort Washington Ave Fl 5, New York, NY 10032; **Phone:** 212-851-9304; **Board Cert:** Internal Medicine 1985; Cardiovascular Disease 1987; Interventional Cardiology 1999; **Med School:** Johns Hopkins Univ 1982; **Resid:** Internal Medicine, NY Hosp-Cornell Medical Ctr 1985; **Fellow:** Cardiovascular Disease, Cedars-Sinai Medical Ctr 1988; Coronary Angioplasty, Mid-America Heart Inst 1989

Southeast

Applegate, Robert J MD [IC] - **Spec Exp:** Cardiac Catheterization; Angioplasty; **Hospital:** Wake Forest Univ Baptist Med Ctr (page 72); **Address:** Wake Forest, Div Cardiology, Medical Center Blvd, Winston-Salem, NC 27157-1045; **Phone:** 336-716-6674; **Board Cert:** Internal Medicine 1983; Cardiovascular Disease 1987; Interventional Cardiology 1999; **Med School:** Univ VA Sch Med 1980; **Resid:** Internal Medicine, Oregon Hlth Sci Univ Hosp 1983; **Fellow:** Pharmacology, Univ Texas Hlth Sci Ctr 1984; Cardiovascular Disease, Univ Texas Hlth Sci Ctr 1986; **Fac Appt:** Prof Med, Wake Forest Univ

Douglas Jr, John S MD [IC] - **Spec Exp:** Angioplasty & Stent Placement; Cardiac Catheterization; Coronary Artery Disease; **Hospital:** Emory Univ Hosp; **Address:** Emory Univ Hosp-Div Cardiology, 1364 Clifton Rd, rm F606, Atlanta, GA 30322; **Phone:** 404-727-7040; **Board Cert:** Internal Medicine 1972; Cardiovascular Disease 1975; Interventional Cardiology 1999; **Med School:** Washington Univ, St Louis 1967; **Resid:** Internal Medicine, NC Memorial Hosp 1969; Internal Medicine, Grady Memorial Hosp 1972; **Fellow:** Cardiovascular Disease, Emory Affil Hosps 1974; **Fac Appt:** Prof Med, Emory Univ

Heldman, Alan W MD [IC] - **Spec Exp:** Cardiomyopathy-Hypertrophic; Coronary Restenosis; Stem Cell Therapy in Heart Failure; **Hospital:** Univ of Miami Hosp (page 71); **Address:** Univ Miami Dept Cardiology, 1321 NW 14th St, Ste 606, Miami, FL 33136; **Phone:** 305-243-5554; **Board Cert:** Interventional Cardiology 1999; **Med School:** Univ Alabama 1988; **Resid:** Internal Medicine, Johns Hopkins Hosp 1991; **Fellow:** Cardiovascular Disease, Johns Hopkins 1994; Interventional Cardiology, Johns Hopkins 1995; **Fac Appt:** Prof Med, Univ Miami Sch Med

Khawaja, Shazib N MD [IC] - **Spec Exp:** Peripheral Vascular Disease; Vascular Medicine; Echocardiography; Nuclear Cardiology; **Hospital:** Tanner Med Ctr; **Address:** 100 Professional Park, Ste 310, Carrollton, GA 30117; **Phone:** 770-836-9326; **Board Cert:** Internal Medicine 1998; Cardiovascular Disease 2001; Interventional Cardiology 2003; Vascular Medicine 2007; **Med School:** Univ S Ala Coll Med 1995; **Resid:** Internal Medicine, Albany Med Ctr 1998; **Fellow:** Cardiovascular Disease, Dartmouth Hitchcock Med Ctr 2000; Interventional Cardiology, Univ Minnesota Med Ctr 2002; **Fac Appt:** Asst Clin Prof Med, Univ S Ala Coll Med

Knopf, William D MD [IC] - **Spec Exp:** Coronary Angioplasty/Stents; Angioplasty; Carotid Artery Stent Placement; Angiogenesis; **Hospital:** Piedmont Hosp; **Address:** Piedmont Heart Inst, 95 Collier Rd, Ste 2035, Atlanta, GA 30309; **Phone:** 404-605-5161; **Board Cert:** Internal Medicine 1982; Cardiovascular Disease 1985; Interventional Cardiology 1999; **Med School:** Emory Univ 1979; **Resid:** Internal Medicine, Univ TX SW=Parkland Hosp 1982; **Fellow:** Cardiovascular Disease, Emory Univ Hosp 1985; **Fac Appt:** Assoc Clin Prof Med, Med Coll GA

Margolis, James MD [IC] - **Spec Exp:** Cardiac Catheterization; Invasive Cardiology; Angioplasty; **Hospital:** Univ of Miami Hosp (page 71), Baptist Hosp of Miami; **Address:** Miami Intl Cardiac Consultants, 3801 Biscayne Blvd Fl 3, Miami, FL 33137; **Phone:** 305-571-0620; **Board Cert:** Internal Medicine 1973; Cardiovascular Disease 1975; Interventional Cardiology 1999; **Med School:** Univ IL Coll Med 1968; **Resid:** Internal Medicine, Barnes Hosp 1972; **Fellow:** Cardiovascular Disease, Duke Med Ctr 1974; **Fac Appt:** Clin Prof Med, Univ Miami Sch Med

Matar, Fadi MD [IC] - **Spec Exp:** Angioplasty; **Hospital:** Tampa Genl Hosp, St Joseph's Hosp - Tampa; **Address:** 509 S Armenia Ave, Ste 200, Tampa, FL 33609; **Phone:** 813-353-1515; **Board Cert:** Interventional Cardiology 1999; Cardiovascular Disease 2007; **Med School:** Amer Univ Beirut 1987; **Resid:** Internal Medicine, Maryland Genl Hosp 1990; **Fellow:** Cardiovascular Disease, Wash Hosp Ctr 1994; **Fac Appt:** Asst Prof Med, Univ S Fla Coll Med

Morris, Douglas C MD [IC] - **Spec Exp:** Angioplasty; Cardiac Catheterization; Heart Valve Disease; **Hospital:** Emory Univ Hosp, Emory Univ Hosp Midtown; **Address:** Emory Heart Center, 1365A Clifton Rd NE, Ste A2205, Atlanta, GA 30322; **Phone:** 404-778-5310; **Board Cert:** Internal Medicine 1973; Cardiovascular Disease 1975; Interventional Cardiology 1999; **Med School:** Baylor Coll Med 1968; **Resid:** Internal Medicine, Vanderbilt Univ Med Ctr 1970; Internal Medicine, Vanderbilt Univ Med Ctr 1973; **Fellow:** Cardiovascular Disease, Emory Univ Hosps 1975; **Fac Appt:** Prof Med, Emory Univ

Reddy, Bhagat K MD [IC] - **Spec Exp:** Angioplasty & Stent Placement; Carotid Artery Stent Placement; Peripheral Vascular Disease; **Hospital:** Piedmont Hosp; **Address:** Piedmont Heart Inst, 275 Collier Rd NW, Ste 300, Atlanta, GA 30309; **Phone:** 404-355-9815; **Board Cert:** Internal Medicine 1999; Cardiovascular Disease 2002; Interventional Cardiology 2003; Vascular Medicine 2004; **Med School:** India 1995; **Resid:** Internal Medicine, Robert Packer Hosp 1999; **Fellow:** Cardiovascular Disease, Med Univ Ohio 2002; Interventional Cardiology, Vanderbilt Univ Med Ctr 2003

Interventional Cardiology

Midwest

Ellis, Stephen G MD [IC] - **Spec Exp:** Angioplasty & Stent Placement; Angiogenesis; **Hospital:** Cleveland Clin Fdn (page 56); **Address:** Cleveland Clinic, Div Cardiovasc Med, 9500 Euclid Ave, Desk J2-3, Cleveland, OH 44195; **Phone:** 216-445-6712; **Board Cert:** Internal Medicine 1981; Cardiovascular Disease 1985; Interventional Cardiology 1999; **Med School:** UCLA 1978; **Resid:** Internal Medicine, Cedars-Sinai Med Ctr 1981; **Fellow:** Cardiovascular Disease, Stanford Univ Med Ctr 1985; Interventional Cardiology, Emory Univ Hosp 1986; **Fac Appt:** Prof Med, Cleveland Cl Coll Med/Case West Res

Feldman, Ted E MD [IC] - **Spec Exp:** Angioplasty; **Hospital:** Evanston/Northshore Univ Hlth Syst; **Address:** ENH Med Group, Cardiology, 2650 Ridge Ave Walgreen Bldg Fl 3, Evanston, IL 60201; **Phone:** 847-570-2250; **Board Cert:** Internal Medicine 1981; Cardiovascular Disease 1985; Interventional Cardiology 1999; **Med School:** Indiana Univ 1978; **Resid:** Internal Medicine, Rush-Presby-St Lukes Hosp 1982; **Fellow:** Cardiovascular Disease, Univ Chicago 1985; **Fac Appt:** Prof Med, Northwestern Univ

Henry, Timothy D MD [IC] - **Spec Exp:** Acute Coronary Syndromes; Angiogenesis; **Hospital:** Abbott - Northwestern Hosp; **Address:** Minneapolis Heart Inst, 920 E 28th St, Ste 40, Minneapolis, MN 55407; **Phone:** 612-863-3900; **Board Cert:** Internal Medicine 1985; Cardiovascular Disease 1989; Interventional Cardiology 2000; **Med School:** UCSF 1982; **Resid:** Internal Medicine, Univ Colorado Hosp 1985; **Fellow:** Cardiovascular Disease, Univ Minnesota 1990; Interventional Cardiology, Univ Minnesota 1991; **Fac Appt:** Prof Med, Univ Minn

Holmes Jr, David R MD [IC] - **Spec Exp:** Heart Attack; Acute Coronary Syndromes; Angioplasty & Restenosis; **Hospital:** Mayo Med Ctr & Clin - Rochester; **Address:** Mayo Clinic, Div Cardiovasc Dis, 200 First St SW, Rochester, MN 55905; **Phone:** 507-255-2504; **Board Cert:** Internal Medicine 1974; Cardiovascular Disease 1977; Interventional Cardiology 1999; **Med School:** Med Coll Wisc 1971; **Resid:** Internal Medicine, Mayo Clinic 1974; **Fellow:** Cardiovascular Disease, Mayo Clinic 1977; **Fac Appt:** Prof Med, Mayo Med Sch

Losordo, Douglas W MD [IC] - **Spec Exp:** Stem Cell Therapy in Heart Failure; Angiogenesis; Angioplasty & Stent Placement; Heart Attack; **Hospital:** Northwestern Meml Hosp; **Address:** 675 N St Clair St, Galter Bldg Fl 11 - Ste 240, Chicago, IL 60611; **Phone:** 312-695-0072; **Board Cert:** Internal Medicine 1986; Cardiovascular Disease 1989; Interventional Cardiology 2002; **Med School:** Univ VT Coll Med 1983; **Resid:** Internal Medicine, St Elizabeth's Med Ctr 1986; **Fellow:** Cardiovascular Disease, St Elizabeth's Med Ctr 1989; **Fac Appt:** Prof Med, Northwestern Univ-Feinberg Sch Med

Schreiber, Theodore L MD [IC] - **Spec Exp:** Coronary Angioplasty/Stents; Carotid Artery Disease; **Hospital:** Harper Univ Hosp; **Address:** Harper University Hospital, 3990 John R St, Webber Bldg - Ste 9370, Detroit, MI 48201; **Phone:** 313-745-7025; **Board Cert:** Internal Medicine 1981; Cardiovascular Disease 1983; Interventional Cardiology 2000; **Med School:** Cornell Univ-Weill Med Coll 1978; **Resid:** Internal Medicine, NY Hosp-Cornell Med Ctr 1981; **Fellow:** Cardiovascular Disease, NY Hosp-Cornell Med Ctr 1983; **Fac Appt:** Assoc Prof Med, Wayne State Univ

Whitlow, Patrick MD [IC] - **Spec Exp:** Cardiac Catheterization; **Hospital:** Cleveland Clin Fdn (page 56); **Address:** Dept Cardiology, 9500 Euclid Ave, Desk F25, Cleveland, OH 44195; **Phone:** 216-444-1746; **Board Cert:** Internal Medicine 1979; Cardiovascular Disease 1981; Interventional Cardiology 1999; **Med School:** Duke Univ 1976; **Resid:** Internal Medicine, Parkland Meml Hosp 1979; **Fellow:** Cardiovascular Disease, Univ Alabama Hosp 1981

Southwest

Bailey, Steven R MD [IC] - **Spec Exp:** Coronary Artery Disease; Coronary Angioplasty/Stents; Congenital Heart Disease; Heart Valve Disease; **Hospital:** Univ Hlth Syst-San Antonio, Christus Santa Rosa Med Ctr Hosp; **Address:** 7703 Floyd Curl Drive, MC 7872, San Antonio, TX 78229-3900; **Phone:** 210-567-4601; **Board Cert:** Internal Medicine 1981; Cardiovascular Disease 1983; Interventional Cardiology 1999; **Med School:** Oregon Hlth & Sci Univ 1978; **Resid:** Internal Medicine, Fitzsimmons AMC 1981; **Fellow:** Cardiovascular Disease, Fitzsimmons AMC 1983; **Fac Appt:** Prof Med, Univ Tex, San Antonio

Kleiman, Neal Stephen MD [IC] - **Spec Exp:** Angioplasty; **Hospital:** Methodist Hosp - Houston; **Address:** 6550 Fannin, Smith Tower St, Ste 1901, Houston, TX 77030; **Phone:** 713-441-1100; **Board Cert:** Internal Medicine 1984; Cardiovascular Disease 1987; Interventional Cardiology 1999; **Med School:** Columbia P&S 1981; **Resid:** Internal Medicine, Baylor Coll Med 1984; **Fellow:** Interventional Cardiology, Baylor Coll Med 1987; **Fac Appt:** Assoc Prof Med, Baylor Coll Med

Perin, Emerson C MD [IC] - **Spec Exp:** Stem Cell Therapy in Heart Failure; Angiogenesis; **Hospital:** St Luke's Episcopal Hosp-Houston; **Address:** Southwest Cardiology Consultants, 6624 Fannin St, Ste 2220, St Lukes Medical Tower Fl 22, Houston, TX 77030-2334; **Phone:** 713-791-9400; **Board Cert:** Internal Medicine 1988; Interventional Cardiology 1999; **Med School:** Brazil 1983; **Resid:** Internal Medicine, Jackson Meml Hosp 1988; **Fellow:** Cardiovascular Disease, St Luke's Episcopal Hosp 1991; **Fac Appt:** Asst Prof Med, Baylor Coll Med

Smalling, Richard Warren MD/PhD [IC] - **Spec Exp:** Coronary Artery Disease; Peripheral Vascular Disease; Heart Valve Disease; Congenital Heart Disease; **Hospital:** Meml Hermann Hosp - Texas Med Ctr; **Address:** 6431 Fannin St, MS 1246, Houston, TX 77030-1501; **Phone:** 713-500-6559; **Board Cert:** Internal Medicine 1978; Cardiovascular Disease 1981; Interventional Cardiology 1999; **Med School:** Univ Tex, Houston 1975; **Resid:** Internal Medicine, UCSD Med Ctr 1978; **Fellow:** Cardiovascular Disease, UCSD Med Ctr 1980; **Fac Appt:** Prof Med, Univ Tex, Houston

West Coast and Pacific

Mahmud, Ehtisham MD [IC] - **Spec Exp:** Cardiac Catheterization; Carotid Artery Stent Placement; Stem Cell Therapy in Heart Failure; Gene Therapy; **Hospital:** UCSD Med Ctr; **Address:** UCSD Med Ctr, 200 W Arbor Drive, San Diego, CA 92037; **Phone:** 619-543-5990; **Board Cert:** Cardiovascular Disease 2000; Interventional Cardiology 2001; **Med School:** Univ Alberta 1989; **Resid:** Internal Medicine, UC San Diego 1995; **Fellow:** Cardiovascular Disease, UC San Diego 1999; Interventional Cardiology, Emory Univ 2000; **Fac Appt:** Asst Prof Med, UCSD

Teirstein, Paul S MD [IC] - **Spec Exp:** Coronary Angioplasty/Stents; Coronary Radiation Therapy; **Hospital:** Scripps Green Hosp; **Address:** Scripps Clinic, 10666 N Torrey Pines Rd, Mail Drop S1056, La Jolla, CA 92037; **Phone:** 858-554-9905; **Board Cert:** Internal Medicine 1983; Cardiovascular Disease 1987; Interventional Cardiology 1999; **Med School:** Mount Sinai Sch Med 1980; **Resid:** Internal Medicine, Brigham & Womens Hosp 1983; **Fellow:** Cardiovascular Disease, Stanford Univ 1986; Interventional Cardiology, Mid-Amer Heart Inst 1987

Yeung, Alan MD [IC] - **Spec Exp:** Mitral Valve Disease; Coronary Artery Disease; **Hospital:** Stanford Univ Med Ctr; **Address:** Stanford Univ Medical Ctr, Dept Interventional Cardiology, 300 Pasteur Drive, rm H2103, MC 5218, Stanford, CA 94305-5218; **Phone:** 650-723-0180; **Board Cert:** Internal Medicine 1987; Cardiovascular Disease 1989; Interventional Cardiology 2000; **Med School:** Harvard Med Sch 1984; **Resid:** Internal Medicine, Mass General Hosp 1987; **Fellow:** Cardiovascular Disease, Brigham & Women's Hosp 1990; **Fac Appt:** Prof Med, Stanford Univ

Cleveland Clinic

Heart and Vascular Institute

America's Best Care

Cleveland Clinic's Heart and Vascular Institute is one of the largest and most experienced cardiovascular specialty groups in the world, providing patients with expert medical management and a full range of therapies. Our areas of expertise combine research, education and clinical practice to provide innovative and scientifically based treatments for cardiovascular disease. *U.S.News & World Report* has ranked the Cleveland Clinic best in the nation for heart care every year since 1995.

Patients come to the Heart and Vascular Institute from every state in the country and from around the world. In 2008, our staff recorded 300,000 patient visits, completed more than 13,000 procedures and performed more than 3,600 open heart surgeries. This experience, along with our outcomes, distinguishes the Cleveland Clinic Heart and Vascular Institute from all other institutions.

Clinical Trials and Research

Our Heart and Vascular Institute is a recognized leader in the multicenter and international trials. An outstanding clinical infrastructure and strong commitment to basic science allow Cleveland Clinic to remain on the cutting edge of treatment and research in cardiovascular disease. More than 200 clinical research project and trials currently are under way here, ranging from cardiac stem therapies to new generations of heart assist devices. Cleveland Clinic researchers are investigating new alternative treatment options for patients with severe aortic valve stenosis and are researching non-invasive repair of the mitral and tricuspid valves.

History of Innovations

Cleveland Clinic doctors have helped define the modern era of cardiovascular care, having pioneered coronary angiography and saphenous vein bypass surgery. Today, our staff continues this proud tradition of innovation and discovery to shape the future of the field.

For more information about the Cleveland Clinic Heart and Vascular Institute, to schedule a second opinion or to learn about assistance for out-of-town patients, call 800.890.2467 or visit www.clevelandclinic.org/hearttopdocs.

Heart and Vascular Institute | 9500 Euclid Avenue / AC311 | Cleveland OH 44195

New Home to the Heart and Vascular Institute

The #1 heart program in America now has a new home in the Sydell and Arnold Miller Family Pavilion. The one million-square-foot building, the country's largest single-use facility for heart and vascular care, features 16 state-of-the-art operating rooms, 12 new catheterization labs, five electrophysiology labs and four dedicated intensive care units.

This patient-centered facility also features private patient rooms, comfortable accommodations for family members, a light-filled central lobby and an extraordinary rooftop plaza, making the building as beautiful as it is efficient.

Beth Israel Medical Center
Roosevelt Hospital
St. Luke's Hospital
Long Island College Hospital of Brooklyn

Cardiac Services

(800) 420-4004

Continuum Health Partners offers outstanding cardiac programs at its member hospitals—Beth Israel Medical Center, Roosevelt Hospital, St. Luke's Hospital and Long Island College Hospital of Brooklyn—with a constant dedication to clinical excellence.

The Continuum hospitals offer the full array of clinical expertise needed to diagnose and treat the many conditions that can affect the heart, including coronary artery disease, heart valve insufficiencies, congenital and non-congenital structural abnormalities, hypertension, heart failure, heart rhythm abnormalities and hypertrophic cardiomyopathy.

We are strong believers in prevention and early detection, and our experts provide complete cardiac diagnostic testing, utilizing state-of-the-art echocardiography, nuclear and non-nuclear stress testing, angiography, PET scanning and more. We also offer programs for coronary artery disease prevention, smoking cessation, treatment centers for obesity and diabetes, and complementary techniques for relaxation and stress reduction, such as massage therapy and therapeutic touch.

Our state-of-the-art cardiac catheterization labs are available around the clock for emergency cardiac cases—when every minute counts—offering life-saving angioplasty to patients arriving in our emergency departments with acute heart attack conditions.

Our cardiac surgery outcomes have been recognized by the New York State Department of Health as having some of the lowest mortality rates in New York City, and our programs have maintained a consistent level of performance since their inception.

Some of the unique features in the cardiac programs at the Continuum hospitals include robotic surgical capabilities for minimally invasive cardiac surgery, a nationally recognized arrhythmia service, CT angiography for non-invasive cardiac angiograms, minimally invasive radial artery harvesting for bypass surgery, nationally and internationally recognized experts in heart failure and hypertension, and a commitment to research to find the cures of tomorrow.

Continuum Health Partners, Inc.

Beth Israel **Roosevelt Hospital** **St. Luke's Hospital** **Long Island College Hospital** **NY Eye & Ear Infirmary**

www.chpnyc.org

Penn Medicine

PENN HEART AND VASCULAR

Penn Heart and Vascular combines the renowned expertise of its clinicians, researchers and educators to provide comprehensive, high quality care to all patients, no matter how "high risk" their condition.

In February 2009, the outpatient services of nine Penn Medicine practices moved into the Perelman Center for Advanced Medicine to form the Penn Heart and Vascular Center. The Heart and Vascular Center provides patient-centered care, provided by the highest caliber of physicians and nurses, using the most advanced treatment options.

World-Class Heart and Vascular Care

Penn Heart and Vascular is recognized as one of the nation's leading heart and vascular programs offering patients a wide range of diagnostic, medical and surgical treatment options available no where else in the region, including but not limited to:

- Consultations and 2nd opinions
- Cholesterol management
- Heart failure management
- Cardiac interventions
- Implantable defibrillators and pacemakers
- Ablation therapy for heart rhythm disorders
- Congenital heart repair
- Minimally invasive valve repair and replacement
- Endovascular stent graft repair for thoracic aortic aneurysms
- Mechanical assist devices
- Heart transplantation

Advancing Technology and Research

- Among the few surgical institutions in the nation with a fully incorporated research facility, ensuring the future progress of cardiovascular research at Penn.

- Pioneering the most advanced techniques and devices, such as ablation therapy for ventricular tachycardia and atrial fibrillation.
- Offering a full-range of surgical options including transcatheter, minimally invasive, robotic, off-pump, port access, and bloodless techniques.
- Conducting numerous clinical studies, such as mechanical assist devices and percutaneous approaches to treating heart valve disease.
- Serving as the lead national site for several trials, including endovascular stent graft repair for thoracic aortic aneurysms, being conducted in collaboration with Penn vascular surgeons.
- Implanting the first temporary total artificial heart in the region, Penn continues to bring a new generation of ventricular assist devices to the treatment of late-stage heart failure.

A National and Regional Referral Center

- Penn Heart and Vascular is among the nation's top 5 adult heart transplant centers, performing more adult heart transplants than all other Philadelphia area hospitals combined.
- Penn offers the most advanced mechanical assist device options for patients with end-stage heart failure and for those patients awaiting heart transplantation.
- The Hospital of the University of Pennsylvania is a world leader in corrective therapies that cure complex heart rhythm disorders and has 5 times more experience than any other regional cardiac center.

- Penn has the largest valve program in the region with a nationally recognized team of physicians who perform more minimally invasive valve repairs and replacements with better patient outcomes.
- Penn is one of the largest valve centers in the U.S. for advanced port access surgery for mitral valve repair or replacement.
- Penn's Thoracic Aortic Surgery Program was the first in the region fully dedicated to the timely recognition, treatment and long-term management of patients with severe aortic disease. Hundreds of aortic surgeries and more thoracic aortic procedures are performed each year than at any other hospital in the Philadelphia region.

Nationally Recognized Expertise

- Penn Heart and Vascular at the Hospital of the University of Pennsylvania is ranked 9th in the nation, and best in the Philadelphia region, for heart care and heart surgery by *U.S.News & World Report*
- Penn Presbyterian Medical Center was among Thomson Reuter's "100 Top Cardiovascular Hospitals" for six years.
- *Best Doctors in America*® lists more doctors from Penn Medicine than any other academic medical center or health system in the Philadelphia region.

JOHNS HOPKINS
M E D I C I N E

Heart and Vascular Institute
600 North Wolfe Street, Baltimore, Maryland 21287

For patient appointments: 410-502-0550
hopkinsmedicine.org/heart

At the Johns Hopkins Heart and Vascular Institute, we are recognized by peers worldwide for pioneering research, advanced treatments, effective use of technology and our focus on patient care.

Our mission has always been to advance the scientific understanding of cardiovascular disease and to translate that knowledge to better care for patients. Ranked among the top heart and heart surgery programs in the nation every year by *U.S. News & World Report*, our physicians are clinical scientists who, in addition to taking care of patients, are leaders in improving outcomes and quality of life for heart and vascular patients all over the world.

Our team includes both adult and pediatric cardiologists, electrophysiologists, endovascular specialists, interventional radiologists and heart and vascular surgeons. Believing that no case is routine, we collaborate to ensure that every patient receives the full benefit of the collective expertise and compassionate touch so widely available here.

Our expertise spans every aspect of heart and vascular care, from arrhythmias and congenital and inherited heart disease to cardiomyopathy, heart failure, aortic and valve disease, aneurysms, peripheral arterial disease, venous disease and stroke prevention.

Our Centers of Excellence include
- Center for the Prevention of Heart Disease
- Center for Aortic Diseases
- Center for Inherited Heart Diseases
- Hypertrophic Cardiomyopathy Center
- Comprehensive Marfan Center
- Comprehensive Cardiothoracic Transplant Center
- Cardiomyopathy and Heart Failure Center
- Electrophysiology and Arrhythmia Service
- Ventricular Assist Device Service
- Endovascular Interventions
- Limb Salvage and Revascularization
- Noninvasive Vascular Evaluation

Innovation and Discovery
- In addition to diagnosing and treating a range of inherited heart diseases, our cardiologists and scientists are engaged in path-breaking research aimed at earlier detection of and intervention for sudden cardiac death.
- Not only does our heart and vascular team have the world's longest experience treating people with Marfan syndrome, we have translated our research on the condition's genetic underpinnings to help launch a large clinical trial of a drug that may slow or prevent the aortic aneurysms the syndrome causes.
- Building on research launched here, we are helping to lead the first clinical trial that's using stem cells from a person's own heart to help repair the damage done by a heart attack.
- Our vascular specialists have been leaders in discovering the potential benefits of statin medications for the medical and surgical management of people undergoing vascular surgery.

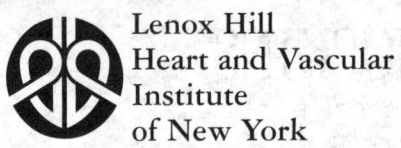

Lenox Hill Heart and Vascular Institute of New York

Lenox Hill Hospital
100 East 77th Street, New York, NY 10075
Telephone: 212-434-2000
www.lenoxhillhospital.org

SETTING THE WORLD STANDARD FOR COMPLEX CARDIAC CARE

The Lenox Hill Heart and Vascular Institute is among the leading cardiovascular care programs nationwide. From diagnosis to treatment and recovery, the Institute provides comprehensive care through its distinguished team of cardiologists, interventional cardiologists, electrophysiologists, cardiothoracic and vascular surgeons, and radiologists.

DEPTH OF EXPERIENCE

Lenox Hill Hospital has been a leader in cardiovascular care for decades, developing groundbreaking techniques to minimize heart damage and speed recovery:

1938 — Lenox Hill Hospital cardiologists performed first angiogram in U.S.

1978 — first coronary angioplasty in the U.S. performed at Lenox Hill Hospital

1991 — Lenox Hill Hospital doctors implanted first coronary stent in NYC

1994 — Lenox Hill Hospital surgeons introduced minimally invasive direct coronary artery bypass surgery to nation

2003 — First FDA approved drug coated stent in the nation was implanted at Lenox Hill Hospital in a procedure our doctors now perform over 3,000 times each year

2004 — Largest carotid stent program in U.S.

2005 — Largest minimally invasive heart assist program in tri-state area; second largest nationally

2008—First 256 Slice Computer Tomographic (CT) Scanner in the Northeastern U.S., and only one of three in the country, was installed at Lenox Hill Hospital

2009— Ranked among the nation's top hospitals in Heart and Heart Surgery by *U.S. News & World Report*

2009— Lenox Hill Hospital surgeons performed New York's first totally endsocopic coronary artery bypass surgery on a beating heart

A WIDE RANGE OF TREATMENTS

Physicians at the Institute constantly seek to broaden the understanding of heart and vascular disease and expand the boundaries of care through research and clinical trials. The interventional cardiology team is recognized for leadership in the use of angioplasty to clear clogged arteries. The endovascular specialists are involved in groundbreaking research involving the use of carotid stents to provide lower-risk treatment of arterial blockages without surgery, and also perform minimally invasive procedures to treat complex abdominal aneurysms. The Institute's cardiothoracic surgeons are pioneers in "beating heart" surgery, and the use of robotics and minimally invasive procedures including coronary bypass, valve repair, atrial fibrillation surgery, and heart failure surgery. Surgeons specializing in vascular surgery perform surgery on the aorta, and the carotid and lower extremity arteries, including aneurysms. The Institute's electrophysiology specialists perform diagnostic, treatment and curative procedures for abnormal heart rhythms.

Lenox Hill Hospital was ranked among the nation's top 50 hospitals in Heart and Heart Surgery by *U.S. News & World Report*. LHH surgeons are able to perform coronary artery bypass surgery, valve repair and replacement, atrial fibrillation ablation, and remodeling of the heart, all minimally invasively. LHH is one of the few hospitals in the nation to offer integrated care of aortic disease, which involves collaboration between cardiothoracic surgery, vascular surgery, interventional radiology, structural cardiology and internal medicine. On March 2, 2009, an LHH multidisciplinary cardiac and vascular team pioneered an important new technique to repair para-valvular leaks with greater patient safety. Physicians used collagen and coil devices together to close the ventricular puncture site in a transapical catheter-based repair. This procedural breathrough can significantly reduce the risks and increase the success rate of leaky valve repair in as many as 10,000 patients a year.

Maimonides
Medical Center

Having pioneered numerous heart care innovations through the years, the Cardiac Institute offers diagnostic studies and therapeutic treatments, procedures and surgeries. It has been ranked by the Centers for Medicare and Medicaid Services among those hospitals achieving excellent ratings in both heart attack and heart failure patient outcomes.

Cardiology
Among the most published and respected in the field, the Maimonides cardiology team continuously sets higher standards for patient care. Edgar Lichstein, MD, Chair of Medicine, has been chief investigator of NIH-sponsored cardiac drug trials, and our Congestive Heart Failure (CHF) Program is among the most effective in the nation.

Interventional Cardiology
Led by Cardiac Institute Chair Jacob Shani, MD, numerous therapeutic devices were developed and implemented here. Our Electrophysiology Lab has a superb record of achievement in diagnosing and treating arrhythmias. A close collaboration with the Department of Emergency Medicine ensures that chest pain patients are evaluated immediately and that interventional procedures are used to stop heart attacks in progress whenever necessary.

Cardiothoracic Surgery
The Maimonides Cardiothoracic Surgery program has an illustrious history, setting the national standard for advances in service. Under the direction of Stephen Lahey, MD, minimally invasive and robotic heart surgeries are offered in state-of-the-art facilities. In collaboration with Electrophysiology, Cardiothoracic Surgery has established an Atrial Fibrillation Center of Excellence. Maimonides provides one of the most prestigious cardiothoracic residency programs in the US.

Historic Moments
- In 1967, the first successful human heart transplant in the nation was performed at Maimonides.
- The intra-aortic balloon pump was developed here in 1970.
- Surgical techniques that protect the spine during cardiothoracic surgery were perfected here in 1982.
- Revolutionary cardiac catheterization devices were invented here in 1992 and 1997.
- Maimonides was the first hospital in US to implement fully automatic external cardiac defibrillators in 2001.

Physicians at Maimonides are among the small percentage in the US who use computers to enter patient orders, thereby reducing the risk of errors, increasing efficiency, and speeding the healing process. Maimonides has appeared on the American Hospital Association's "Most Wired" and "Most Wireless" lists more often than any other health care institution in the metropolitan area. Advanced technology allows our doctors to focus more attention on caring for their patients.

Maimonides Medical Center
Passionate about medicine.
Compassionate about people.

www.maimonidesmed.org/cardiac

MOUNT SINAI
SCHOOL OF
MEDICINE

THE MOUNT SINAI MEDICAL CENTER
MOUNT SINAI HEART—CARDIOVASCULAR HEALTH
One Gustave L. Levy Place
Fifth Avenue and 100th Street
New York, NY 10029-6574
Physician Referral: 1-800-MD-SINAI (637-4624)
www.mountsinai.org/heart

At **MOUNT SINAI HEART**, we take both a personal and a global view of cardiovascular health. Our system of integrated care combines the world's most accomplished physicians, research scientists, and educators with innovative thinking, creative programs, and an unwavering commitment to the prevention and treatment of cardiovascular disease. With access to the latest discoveries and the most experienced minds, our doctors bring a diversity of views to ensure that patients receive the perfect treatments for their individual needs. The rapid translation of innovative research concepts into prevention, diagnosis, and therapy means that patients receive multidisciplinary treatment of unprecedented quality. Our programs span the care of patients from the earliest stages of life (our pediatric cardiologists can detect cardiac disease in the unborn fetus) well into the advanced elderly years (through specialized geriatric cardiology).

In addition to consultative cardiology, cardiac catheterization, heart and lung transplantation, cardiovascular surgery, heart failure, pulmonary hypertension, lipid management, and hypertension, we provide the following in these specialties:

Noninvasive diagnostic imaging – State-of-the-art echocardiography, nuclear cardiology, PET, CT, and MRI technology;

Coronary artery disease – We are ranked as New York State's safest center for coronary angioplasty and other catheter-based procedures;

Cardiac rhythm disturbances – Expert management of all aspects of heart rhythm disorders, such as atrial fibrillation and tachycardias, and implantable devices such as pacemakers and defibrillators;

Valvular heart disease – A wide range of medical and surgical options, including a leading program for valve repair and long-term follow-up care;

Aortic diseases – Pioneering techniques for stent-graft repair of thoracic and abdominal aortic aneurysms and for surgical correction of the most complex aortic pathology;

Congenital heart disease – Expertise in pediatric cardiology and in minimally invasive approaches to the correction of congenital heart defects in children and adults;

Cardiac failure and transplantation – A multidisciplinary team approach to comprehensive, compassionate care for patients with the most advanced forms of heart failure and cardiomyopathy;

Comprehensive cardiac disease prevention and rehabilitation – A unique synergism that provides unparalleled patient care while yielding breakthroughs in the prevention and treatment of cardiovascular disease;

LEADING SURGEONS, INNOVATIVE TREATMENTS
Under the direction of internationally renowned cardiologist Valentin Fuster, MD, PhD, Mount Sinai Heart is recognized worldwide for expertise in evaluating, managing, and preventing cardiovascular disease through the integration of patient care, education, and research. Mount Sinai Heart encompasses the Zena and Michael A. Wiener Cardiovascular Institute and the Marie-Josée and Henry R. Kravis Center for Cardiovascular Health at Mount Sinai, both preeminent resources for the study and treatment of heart and blood vessel diseases.

Vascular medicine and surgery – Noninvasive diagnostic procedures and an interdisciplinary approach to disease management, from medical, surgical, catheter-based, and gene therapy techniques for arterial obstruction, limb salvage, venous, and lymphatic diseases.

Mount Sinai's Cardiac Catheterization Laboratory – Offers leading-edge technologies of all kinds to study the heart with the greatest precision available, including diagnostic angiography, angioplasty, and biopsy. The Cardiac Catheterization Laboratory increased its best safety rate of percutaneous coronary interventions in 2008 by over 25 percent.

NewYork-Presbyterian

The University Hospital of Columbia and Cornell

NewYork-Presbyterian Heart

Affiliated with Columbia University College of Physicians and Surgeons and Weill Medical College of Cornell University

NewYork-Presbyterian Hospital
Columbia University Medical Center
622 West 168th Street
New York, NY 10032

NewYork-Presbyterian Hospital
Weill Cornell Medical Center
525 East 68th Street
New York, NY 10021

OVERVIEW:

The NewYork-Presbyterian Heart has a reputation for treating some of the highest risk cases in the world – healing those patients who cannot be helped anywhere else. We are committed to delivering the finest possible care to adult and pediatric patients by:

- combining the finest minds and cutting-edge technology with the most compassionate care
- helping patients make sense of the complex steps involved in treating their heart condition;
- providing them with a full set of appropriate treatment options for consideration after a complete diagnosis;
- listening, guiding and fully informing patients so that together we can confidently choose the best treatment.

The NewYork-Presbyterian Heart has:

- A well-deserved reputation for clinical excellence – the only heart center in the New York area ranked among the nation's best by *U.S. News & World Report*;
- World-renowned expertise in all areas of cardiac care, including transplantation, open-heart surgery, arrhythmia control, left ventricular assist devices (LVAD) and robotics;
- One of the country's largest and most successful pediatric cardiology, cardiology interventional and cardiac surgery programs.
- The latest heart-imaging technology, including such innovative tools as advanced digital equipment for stress echocardiography SPECT, state-of-the-art MRI, intravascular/intracoronary ultrasound, electrophysiologic studies, nuclear scanning and an outstanding cardiac catheterization laboratory;
- A state-of-the-art Interventional Cardiology Center to diagnose and treat heart disease without surgery, on an inpatient or outpatient basis, including: angioplasty, balloon valvuloplasty, stenting, and intracoronary radiation for restenosis.

Physician Referral: For a physician referral or to learn more about the NewYork-Presbyterian Heart call toll free **1-877-NYP-WELL** (1-877-697-9355) visit our website at **www.nypheart.org**

HIGHLIGHTS INCLUDE:

- Performed more heart transplants than any other hospital in the world over the last two decades.

- First Robotics-Assisted Coronary Artery Bypass Surgery in the U.S.

- One of the principal investigators (12 institutions throughout the United States) involved in ongoing FDA clinical trials to explore the use and effectiveness of robotics in cardiac surgery.

- Lead medical center in a three-year landmark study of 129 patients – REMATCH (Randomized Evaluation of Mechanical Assistance for the Treatment of Congestive Heart Failure) — which found that implanted heart pumps can extend and improve the quality of life of terminally ill heart failure patients.

- Participating in FDA-approved randomized clinical trial to evaluate use of drug-coated stents versus regular stents on incidence of reoccurrence of renarrowing inside stent.

NYU Cardiac and Vascular Institute

NYU LANGONE MEDICAL CENTER

550 First Avenue (at 31St Street)
New York, NY 10016
Physician Referral:
(888)7-NYU-MED (888-769-8633)
www.med.nyu.edu

CARDIAC SURGERY

About the Division of Cardiac Surgery:

The Division of Cardiac Surgery is a nationally recognized leader in advanced treatments and technologies for both adult and congenital heart disease. Our team's multidisciplinary approach to high quality patient-centered care and commitment to research are just a few of the many factors that set us apart. NYU Langone Medical Center is one of the tri-state area's largest cardiac surgery centers and our world renowned surgeons are true pioneers in minimally invasive heart surgery and mitral valve repair. We have performed over 4,750 minimally invasive heart surgery procedures since pioneering the technique in 1996 and offer over 30 years of experience in mitral valve repair. We also perform state-of-the-art surgical procedures for heart valve replacement and aortic aneurysm repair and specialize in high-risk and elderly patients.

We specialize in the following areas:

AORTIC ANEURYSM REPAIR
NYU Langone Medical Center was one of the first centers in the U.S. to adopt the minimally invasive approach to thoracic aneurysm repair. We have participated in numerous FDA clinical trials to determine the efficacy of endovascular repair. Our approach to endovascular repair includes a catheter-based intervention with insertion of a stent graft into the aorta to the site of the aneurysm. The Department of Cardiothoracic Surgery also treats hundreds of patients with aneurysms each year with traditional surgical techniques.

HIGH-RISK CARDIAC SURGERY
Our cardiac surgery team also specializes in the surgical care of high-risk patients. Surgical procedures for high-risk patients include, but are not limited to, coronary revascularization for severe left main disease, heart valve repair or replacement, surgical ventricular restoration, ventricular assist device implantations, and thoracic aortic dissection repair.

MINIMALLY INVASIVE CARDIAC SURGERY
Over 4,750 minimally invasive heart surgery procedures have been performed at NYU Langone Medical Center since 1996. Benefits include dramatic reduction in pain, lower risk of bleeding and infection and an accelerated recovery. Most patients are candidates for minimally invasive procedures which have become the preferred approach for the majority of our heart surgery patients, including mitral valve repair and replacement, aortic valve replacement and coronary artery bypass.

MITRAL VALVE REPAIR
Our heart surgeons introduced mitral valve repair into the U.S., and have refined the technique over the last 30 years. We have performed the most mitral valve repair procedures in the country, avoiding the need to replace the mitral valve, which would require future reoperations. The 3,500 mitral valve repair procedures performed at NYU Langone Medical Center since 1979 have demonstrated that repair is preferable over replacement and that surgery should be performed as early as possible when the risks of treatment are the lowest. We are a leader in the field of mitral valve repair, training visiting surgeons from around the world.

NYU Cardiac and Vascular Institute
NYU LANGONE MEDICAL CENTER

550 First Avenue (at 31St Street)
New York, NY 10016
Physician Referral:
(888)7-NYU-MED (888-769-8633)
www.med.nyu.edu

CARDIOVASCULAR DISEASES

About the Cardiac and Vascular Institute:

The heart and vascular specialists at the Cardiac and Vascular Institute at NYU Langone Medical Center continue to lead in developing new techniques for repairing heart valves, curing heart rhythm disorders, treating aortic diseases and congestive heart failure. The Institute is recognized as a leader in cardiovascular care, ranking 11th in the nation for cardiology in *U.S. News & World Report's* annual 'Best Hospitals' ranking and is a service in which top quality patient care, cutting-edge research and world-renowned training programs all come together. Cardiac and vascular physicians work collaboratively with the cardiac rehabilitation team to move patients seamlessly from treatment into the recovery and maintenance phase of their care.

We specialize in the following:

CARDIAC CATHETERIZATION

At the leading edge of interventional cardiology, the Cardiac Catheterization Laboratory offers superior catheter-based diagnosis and evaluation of cardiac health. The lab provides a full range of procedures to evaluate how well the heart muscle and valves are working, to detect and measure any narrowing of the coronary arteries, and to recommend appropriate treatment as needed.

CARDIAC REHABILITATION AND PREVENTION

The Joan and Joel Smilow Cardiac Rehabilitation and Prevention Center focuses on individualized patient care and takes place in a state-of-the-art facility where patients work on building both aerobic capacity and strength to help patients return rehabilitated to their everyday lives.

CARDIAC SURGERY

The Division of Cardiac Surgery is a nationally recognized leader in advanced treatments and technologies for adult and congenital heart disease. Our team's multidisciplinary approach to high quality patient-centered care and commitment to research are just a few of the many factors that set us apart. We have performed over 4,750 minimally invasive heart surgery procedures since pioneering the technique in 1996 and offer over 30 years of experience in mitral valve repair. We also perform state-of-the-art surgical procedures for heart valve replacement and aortic aneurysm repair and specialize in high-risk and elderly patients.

CARDIOLOGY

The Leon H. Charney Division of Cardiology is an exceptional leader in cardiovascular biomedical research, patient care and education. Clinicians and researchers at the Medical Center are advancing the field of cardiovascular medicine, contributing to the reputation of NYU Langone Medical Center as a comprehensive cardiovascular center of excellence.

HEART FAILURE

The cardiologists and surgeons at the Heart Failure Center offer the most advanced echocardiograms, pacemaker or defibrillator implantations and open heart surgeries (including promising new procedures to reshape the hearts of patients with chronic heart failure).

NUCLEAR CARDIOLOGY/STRESS

The Nuclear Cardiology/Stress Laboratory performs a range of tests that assist cardiologists in the diagnosis and assessment of many forms of heart disease.

VASCULAR SURGERY

Treating thousands of patients, with conditions ranging from arterial aneurysms to deep vein thrombosis, as well as carotid stenosis and limb salvage, the Division of Vascular and Endovascular Surgery offers expert patient care with an emphasis on minimally invasive diagnostic and treatment approaches. The Medical Center also offers minimally invasive vein surgery, endovascular aortic surgery, thoracic aneurysm correction and abdominal aneurysm interventions.

550 First Avenue (at 31St Street)
New York, NY 10016
Physician Referral:
(888)7-NYU-MED (888-769-8633)
www.med.nyu.edu

CARDIAC AND VASCULAR INSTITUTE

About the Cardiac and Vascular Institute:

The heart and vascular specialists at the Cardiac and Vascular Institute at NYU Langone Medical

Center continue to lead in developing new techniques for repairing heart valves, curing heart rhythm disorders, treating aortic diseases and congestive heart failure. The Institute is recognized as a leader in cardiovascular care, ranking 11th in the nation for cardiology in *U.S. News & World Report's* annual 'Best Hospitals' ranking and is a service in which top quality patient care, cutting-edge research and world-renowned training programs all come together. Cardiac and vascular physicians work collaboratively with the cardiac rehabilitation team to move patients seamlessly from treatment into the recovery and maintenance phase of their care.

We specialize in the following:

CARDIAC CATHETERIZATION

At the leading edge of interventional cardiology, the Cardiac Catheterization Laboratory offers superior catheter-based diagnosis and evaluation of cardiac health. The lab provides a full range of procedures to evaluate how well the heart muscle and valves are working, to detect and measure any narrowing of the coronary arteries, and to recommend appropriate treatment as needed.

CARDIAC REHABILITATION AND PREVENTION

The Joan and Joel Smilow Cardiac Rehabilitation and Prevention Center focuses on individualized patient care and takes place in a state-of-the-art facility where patients work on building both aerobic capacity and strength to help patients return rehabilitated to their everyday lives.

CARDIAC SURGERY

The Division of Cardiac Surgery is a nationally recognized leader in advanced treatments and technologies for adult and congenital heart disease. Our team's multidisciplinary approach to high quality patient-centered care and commitment to research are just a few of the many factors that set us apart. We have performed over 4,750 minimally invasive heart surgery procedures since pioneering the technique in 1996 and offer over 30 years of experience in mitral valve repair. We also perform state-of-the-art surgical procedures for heart valve replacement and aortic aneurysm repair and specialize in high-risk and elderly patients.

CARDIOLOGY

The Leon H. Charney Division of Cardiology is an exceptional leader in cardiovascular biomedical research, patient care and education. Clinicians and researchers at the Medical Center are advancing the field of cardiovascular medicine, contributing to the reputation of NYU Langone Medical Center as a comprehensive cardiovascular center of excellence.

HEART FAILURE

The cardiologists and surgeons at the Heart Failure Center offer the most advanced echocardiograms, pacemaker or defibrillator implantations and open heart surgeries (including promising new procedures to reshape the hearts of patients with chronic heart failure).

NUCLEAR CARDIOLOGY/STRESS

The Nuclear Cardiology/Stress Laboratory performs a range of tests that assist cardiologists in the diagnosis and assessment of many forms of heart disease.

VASCULAR SURGERY

Treating thousands of patients, with conditions ranging from arterial aneurysms to deep vein thrombosis, as well as carotid stenosis and limb salvage, the Division of Vascular and Endovascular Surgery offers expert patient care with an emphasis on minimally invasive diagnostic and treatment approaches. The Medical Center also offers minimally invasive vein surgery, endovascular aortic surgery, thoracic aneurysm correction and abdominal aneurysm interventions.

St. Francis Hospital The Heart Center®
100 Port Washington Blvd.
Roslyn, New York 11576
www.stfrancisheartcenter.com
(516) 562-6000   1-888-HEARTNY
A member of Catholic Health Services of Long Island

Non-Invasive Cardiac Imaging

Using the latest in non-invasive cardiac imaging technology, St. Francis Hospital's physicians have immediate access to information regarding blood flow, heart muscle strength, anatomy, and coronary artery blockages that allows them to more effectively guide a patient's course of treatment.

Among the most recent advances in St. Francis Hospital's range of services are:

Coronary CT Angiography

St. Francis Hospital was the first hospital on Long Island to offer Multidetector Computed Tomography (MDCT) for non-invasive coronary artery imaging and helped pioneer a new Cardiac Imaging Specialist network which has exclusive rights to perform MDCT for several leading health insurers. This technology provides previously unobtainable non-invasive visualization of the coronary arteries and plaque buildup in the walls of the arteries.

Cardiac MRI

The only center on Long Island with world-class expertise in cardiac MRI, St. Francis Hospital has the ability to non-invasively evaluate heart anatomy, function, scarring, blood flow and inflammation using advanced techniques on two state-of-the-art scanners. Cardiac MRI allows physicians to evaluate effects of heart attack, effects of coronary artery blockages and the causes of heart failure to determine whether or not patients will benefit from heart surgery or other therapies. World-renowned cardiac MRI authority Nathaniel Reichek, M.D., leads St. Francis Hospital's clinical and research applications with cardiac MRI.

Three-Dimensional Echocardiography

St. Francis Hospital is an internationally recognized leader in three-dimensional echocardiography for quantifying the effects of heart disease and the leading center in the New York metropolitan area in this field. By creating three-dimensional reconstructions of the heart and blood flow within it, this technology provides diagnostic information that far surpasses that available with conventional echocardiography in many patients.

Nuclear Imaging

Nuclear imaging, which involves the injection of nuclear isotopes and continuous imaging by a gamma camera that circles the patient's body, improves the accuracy of stress testing. St. Francis Hospital offers the latest advances in nuclear cardiology, such as single-photon emission computed tomography with CT image correction (SPECT/CT). The nuclear cardiology laboratory at St. Francis Hospital is also a leader in developing new types of computer analysis to improve the value of SPECT imaging, and was among the first facilities in the U.S. to receive accreditation from The Intersocietal Commission for the Accreditation of Nuclear Medicine Laboratories. In 2009, St. Francis became the only Long Island hospital offering cardiac positron emission tomography with CT, or PET/CT, a new advanced approach which can further enhance diagnostic assessment and clinical decision making.

Non-Invasive Imaging at St. Francis Hospital

Non-invasive imaging services at St. Francis Hospital include:
- multidetector computed tomographic coronary angiography
- cardiac MRI
- SPECT/CT nuclear imaging
- transesophageal echocardiography
- three-dimensional echocardiography
- Stress testing with nuclear, echocardiographic or MRI imaging

St. Francis Hospital's cutting-edge non-invasive imaging technology is also being applied in its research programs on cardiovascular disease. Applying its depth of experience with various imaging modalities, the Hospital has launched a multi-disciplinary effort at its St. Francis Cardiac Research Institute to improve methods for the diagnosis and treatment of cardiac disease. Past research efforts at the Hospital include The St. Francis Heart Study–the largest study on coronary risk factors to be conducted at any single center—which supported the use of CT scanning for atherosclerotic plaque detection as a tool for cardiac risk evaluation.

St. Francis Hospital The Heart Center®

100 Port Washington Blvd.
Roslyn, New York 11576
www.stfrancisheartcenter.com
(516) 562-6000 1-888-HEARTNY
A member of Catholic Health Services of Long Island

A Leader in Cardiac Care

St. Francis Hospital, The Heart Center® is New York State's only specialty designated cardiac center and is the busiest heart center in the Northeast. Located in Roslyn, New York, on Long Island's North Shore, St. Francis Hospital has been ranked among the best hospitals in the United States by *U.S. News & World Report* in heart and heart surgery, digestive disorders and geriatrics for three consecutive years.

St. Francis:

• Performs more open-heart surgeries and cardiac interventional procedures than any other hospital in New York State

• Offers innovative approaches to cardiac surgery, including minimally invasive procedures and off-pump coronary artery bypass surgery, designed to minimize trauma and reduce surgical complications

• Performs one of the region's highest volumes of catheter-based techniques to close atrial septal defects (ASDs) and patent foramen ovale (PFO)

• Operates a nationally recognized Arrhythmia and Pacemaker Center staffed with electrophysiologists with over a decade of experience in radiofrequency ablation, a permanent cure for certain arrhythmias, including atrial fibrillation

• Maintains a high volume center for the implantation of cardiac pacemakers and defibrillators

• Offers the only world-class program in cardiac imaging that fully integrates all technologies including advanced methods in cardiac MRI, coronary CT angiography, PET/CT and three-dimensional echocardiography

• Has received the Magnet Award for excellence in nursing services

• Is a premier center for clinical trials and studies of the application of image-guided methods of diagnosis and treatment of heart disease

St. Francis Hospital has near-perfect patient satisfaction ratings, with over 99 percent of patients saying they would recommend the Hospital to family and friends.

"Our large cardiac caseload and our growing research program put us in an excellent position to introduce new techniques that can benefit thousands of people in need each year."

–Alan D. Guerci,M.D.
President and Chief Executive Officer
St. Francis Hospital, The Heart Center®

Child Neurology

a subspecialty of Neurology

A neurologist specializes in the diagnosis and treatment of all types of disease or impaired function of the brain, spinal cord, peripheral nerves, muscles and autonomic nervous system, as well as the blood vessels that relate to these structures. A child neurologist has special skills in the diagnosis and management of neurologic disorders of the neonatal period, infancy, early childhood and adolescence.

Training Required: Four years

CHILD NEUROLOGY

New England

Darras, Basil T MD [ChiN] - **Spec Exp:** Neuromuscular Disorders; Cerebral Palsy; **Hospital:** Children's Hospital - Boston; **Address:** 300 Longwood Ave, Childrens Hosp, Neurology, Fegan 11, Boston, MA 02115; **Phone:** 617-355-8235; **Board Cert:** Clinical Genetics 1987; Pediatrics 1988; Child Neurology 1992; Neuromuscular Medicine 2008; **Med School:** Greece 1977; **Resid:** Pediatrics, Nassau County Med Ctr 1982; Child Neurology, Tufts-New England Med Ctr 1985; **Fellow:** Clinical Genetics, Yale Univ Sch Med 1988; **Fac Appt:** Prof N, Harvard Med Sch

Holmes, Gregory L MD [ChiN] - **Spec Exp:** Epilepsy/Seizure Disorders; **Hospital:** Dartmouth - Hitchcock Med Ctr; **Address:** Dartmouth-Hitchcock Med Ctr, Dept Neurology, 1 Medical Center Drive, Lebanon, NH 03756; **Phone:** 603-650-8586; **Board Cert:** Pediatrics 1979; Neurology 1980; **Med School:** Univ VA Sch Med 1974; **Resid:** Pediatrics, Yale-New Haven Hosp 1976; **Fellow:** Pediatric Neurology, Univ Virginia 1979; **Fac Appt:** Prof N, Dartmouth Med Sch

Mandelbaum, David E MD/PhD [ChiN] - **Spec Exp:** Epilepsy/Seizure Disorders; Brain Tumors-Pediatric; Neonatal Neurology; Autism; **Hospital:** Rhode Island Hosp, Women & Infants Hosp of RI; **Address:** Dept of Neurology, 593 Eddy St George Bldg, Providence, RI 02903; **Phone:** 401-444-5685; **Board Cert:** Child Neurology 1987; Pediatrics 1987; Clinical Neurophysiology 2003; Neurodevelopmental Disabilities 2001; **Med School:** Columbia P&S 1980; **Resid:** Pediatrics, Yale-New Haven Hosp 1982; Neurology, Neuro Inst-Columbia 1983; **Fellow:** Child Neurology, Neuro Inst-Columbia 1985; **Fac Appt:** Prof Ped, Brown Univ

Novotny, Edward MD [ChiN] - **Spec Exp:** Epilepsy/Seizure Disorders; Neurologic Imaging; Neurophysiology; **Hospital:** Yale-New Haven Hosp; **Address:** Dept of Pediatrics, Yale Sch of Med, PO Box 208064, New Haven, CT 06520-8064; **Phone:** 203-785-5730; **Board Cert:** Pediatrics 1986; Child Neurology 1986; Clinical Neurophysiology 2004; **Med School:** St Louis Univ 1979; **Resid:** Pediatrics, Univ CA Daivs Med Ctr 1981; Neurology, Stanford Univ Med Ctr 1984; **Fellow:** Epilepsy, Stanford Univ Med Ctr 1986; Magnetic Resonance Imaging, Yale Univ 1989; **Fac Appt:** Assoc Prof Ped, Yale Univ

Pomeroy, Scott L MD/PhD [ChiN] - **Spec Exp:** Neuro-Oncology; Brain Tumors; **Hospital:** Children's Hospital - Boston, Dana-Farber Cancer Inst; **Address:** Chldns Hosp, Dept Neurology-Fegan 11, 300 Longwood Ave, Boston, MA 02115; **Phone:** 617-355-6386; **Board Cert:** Pediatrics 2003; Child Neurology 1988; **Med School:** Univ Conn 1982; **Resid:** Pediatrics, Chldns Hosp 1984; Neurology, Barnes Hosp/Washington Univ 1985; **Fellow:** Pediatric Neurology, St Louis Chldns Hosp 1987; Neurological Biology, Washington Univ 1989; **Fac Appt:** Prof N, Harvard Med Sch

Sahin, Mustafa MD/PhD [ChiN] - **Spec Exp:** Tuberous Sclerosis; Brain Vascular Malformations; Sturge-Weber Syndrome; Cortical Malformations; **Hospital:** Children's Hospital - Boston; **Address:** Childrens Hospital Boston, 300 Longwood Ave, Fegan 11, Boston, MA 02115; **Phone:** 617-355-2711; **Board Cert:** Child Neurology 2001; **Med School:** Yale Univ 1995; **Resid:** Pediatrics, Chldns Hosp 1997; Child Neurology, Chldns Hosp 2000; **Fac Appt:** Asst Prof N, Harvard Med Sch

Shaywitz, Bennett A MD [ChiN] - **Spec Exp:** Learning Disorders; Dyslexia; Headache; **Hospital:** Yale-New Haven Hosp; **Address:** Yale Univ Sch Med, Dept Peds, 333 Cedar St, Box 208064, New Haven, CT 06520-8064; **Phone:** 203-785-4641; **Board Cert:** Pediatrics 1968; Child Neurology 1973; **Med School:** Washington Univ, St Louis 1963; **Resid:** Pediatrics, Bronx Muni Hosp Ctr 1967; **Fellow:** Child Neurology, Albert Einstein Coll Med 1970; **Fac Appt:** Prof Ped, Yale Univ

Volpe, Joseph J MD [ChiN] - **Spec Exp:** Neonatal Neurology; Cerebral Palsy; **Hospital:** Children's Hospital - Boston, Mass Genl Hosp; **Address:** 300 Longwood Ave, Fegan 11, Boston, MA 02115-5724; **Phone:** 617-355-8994; **Board Cert:** Pediatrics 1970; Child Neurology 1974; **Med School:** Harvard Med Sch 1964; **Resid:** Pediatrics, Mass Genl Hosp 1966; Neurology, Mass Genl Hosp 1971; **Fellow:** Research, Natl Inst Child Hlth Human Dev 1968; **Fac Appt:** Prof N, Harvard Med Sch

Mid Atlantic

Allen, Jeffrey MD [ChiN] - **Spec Exp:** Neuro-Oncology; Brain Tumors; **Hospital:** NYU Langone Med Ctr (page 67); **Address:** Hassenfeld Childrens Ctr, 160 E 32nd St, Ste L3, New York, NY 10016; **Phone:** 212-263-9907; **Board Cert:** Child Neurology 1977; **Med School:** Harvard Med Sch 1969; **Resid:** Pediatrics, Montreal Chldns Hosp 1973; Pediatric Neurology, Montreal Neur Inst/McGill 1976; **Fac Appt:** Prof Ped, NYU Sch Med

Bergman, Ira MD [ChiN] - **Spec Exp:** Complex Diagnosis; Neuro-Oncology; **Hospital:** Chldns Hosp of Pittsburgh - UPMC; **Address:** Chldns Hospital of Pittsburgh, 3705 Fifth Ave, Pittsburgh, PA 15213; **Phone:** 412-692-5520; **Board Cert:** Pediatrics 1981; Child Neurology 1980; **Med School:** Univ Chicago-Pritzker Sch Med 1974; **Resid:** Pediatrics, Mass Genl Hosp 1976; **Fellow:** Neurology, Mass Genl Hosp 1979; **Fac Appt:** Assoc Prof Ped, Univ Pittsburgh

Comi, Anne M MD [ChiN] - **Spec Exp:** Sturge-Weber Syndrome; **Hospital:** Kennedy Krieger Inst, Johns Hopkins Hosp (page 61); **Address:** Kennedy-Krieger Institute, 707 N Broadway, Baltimore, MD 21215; **Phone:** 443-923-9150; **Board Cert:** Child Neurology 2000; **Med School:** SUNY Buffalo 1993; **Resid:** Pediatrics, Childrens Hosp Buffalo 1996; Pediatric Neurology, Johns Hopkins Hospital 1999; **Fac Appt:** Assoc Prof N, Johns Hopkins Univ

Crawford, Thomas O MD [ChiN] - **Spec Exp:** Neuromuscular Disorders; Muscular Dystrophy; Ataxia Telangiectasia; **Hospital:** Johns Hopkins Hosp (page 61); **Address:** Pediatric Neurology, 200 N Wolfe St, Ste 2158, Baltimore, MD 21287; **Phone:** 410-955-4259; **Board Cert:** Pediatrics 1986; Child Neurology 1990; **Med School:** USC Sch Med 1980; **Resid:** Pediatrics, LAC-USC Med Ctr 1984; Child Neurology, Chldns Hosp 1987; **Fellow:** Neuromuscular Medicine, Johns Hopkins Hosp 1988; **Fac Appt:** Assoc Prof N, Johns Hopkins Univ

De Vivo, Darryl C MD [ChiN] - **Spec Exp:** Metabolic Disorders; Neuromuscular Disorders; Spinal Muscular Atrophy (SMA); **Hospital:** NY-Presby Hosp/Columbia (page 66); **Address:** Neurological Institute, 710 W 168th St, rm 201, New York, NY 10032; **Phone:** 212-305-5244; **Board Cert:** Child Neurology 1972; **Med School:** Univ VA Sch Med 1964; **Resid:** Pediatrics, Mass Genl Hosp 1966; Neurology, Mass Genl Hosp 1967; **Fellow:** Neurology, Natl Inst Hlth 1969; Child Neurology, Children's Hosp 1970; **Fac Appt:** Prof N, Columbia P&S

Duffner, Patricia K MD [ChiN] - **Spec Exp:** Brain Tumors; Krabbe Disease; Cancer Survivors-Late Effects of Therapy; **Hospital:** Women's & Chldn's Hosp of Buffalo, The; **Address:** Women & Childrens Hosp, Dept Neurology, 219 Bryant St, Buffalo, NY 14222-2006; **Phone:** 716-878-7819; **Board Cert:** Pediatrics 1977; Child Neurology 1979; **Med School:** SUNY Buffalo 1972; **Resid:** Pediatrics, Buffalo Chldns Hosp 1975; **Fellow:** Child Neurology, SUNY Buffalo 1978; **Fac Appt:** Prof N, SUNY Buffalo

Eviatar, Lydia MD [ChiN] - **Spec Exp:** Headache; Balance Disorders; Tourette's Syndrome; Cerebral Palsy; **Hospital:** Schneider Chldn's Hosp, Blythedale Children's Hosp; **Address:** 410 Lakeville Rd, Ste 105, New Hyde Park, NY 11042-1433; **Phone:** 516-465-5255; **Board Cert:** Pediatrics 1969; Child Neurology 1977; **Med School:** Israel 1961; **Resid:** Pediatrics, Tel Hashomer Hosp 1966; **Fellow:** Child Neurology, UCLA Med Ctr 1967; Neurology, UCLA Med Ctr 1969; **Fac Appt:** Prof N, Albert Einstein Coll Med

Child Neurology

Finkel, Richard S MD [ChiN] - **Spec Exp:** Neuromuscular Disorders; **Hospital:** Chldns Hosp of Philadelphia, The; **Address:** Children's Hosp of Philadelphia, Neurology Division, 34th St & Civic Ctr Blvd, Philadelphia, PA 19104; **Phone:** 215-590-2763; **Board Cert:** Pediatrics 1984; Child Neurology 1986; **Med School:** Washington Univ, St Louis 1978; **Resid:** Pediatrics, Chldn's Hosp 1980; **Fellow:** Neurology, Chldn's Hosp/ Brigham & Women's Hosp 1983; **Fac Appt:** Clin Prof N, Univ Pennsylvania

Maytal, Joseph MD [ChiN] - **Spec Exp:** Epilepsy/Seizure Disorders; Migraine; **Hospital:** Schneider Chldn's Hosp; **Address:** Dept Pediatric Neurology, Schneider Children's Hospital, 410 Lakeville Rd, Ste 105, New Hyde Park, NY 11042; **Phone:** 516-465-5255; **Board Cert:** Pediatrics 1986; Child Neurology 1988; **Med School:** Israel 1979; **Resid:** Pediatrics, Brookdale Hosp 1983; Child Neurology, Montefiore Med Ctr 1986; **Fellow:** Neurological Physiology, Albert Einstein Med Coll 1987; **Fac Appt:** Clin Prof N, Albert Einstein Coll Med

Mink, Jonathan W MD [ChiN] - **Spec Exp:** Movement Disorders; Tourette's Syndrome; Dystonia; **Hospital:** Univ of Rochester Strong Meml Hosp; **Address:** Univ Rochester, Dept Child Neurology, 601 Elmsood Ave, Box 631, Rochester, NY 14642; **Phone:** 585-275-2971; **Board Cert:** Child Neurology 2007; **Med School:** Washington Univ, St Louis 1989; **Resid:** Pediatrics, St Louis Chldns Hosp 1991; Child Neurology, Barnes Hosp/St Louis Chldns Hosp 1994; **Fellow:** Movement Disorders, Washington Univ 1995; **Fac Appt:** Prof N, Univ Rochester

Packer, Roger J MD [ChiN] - **Spec Exp:** Brain Tumors; Neurofibromatosis; **Hospital:** Chldns Natl Med Ctr; **Address:** Chldns Natl Med Ctr, Dept Neurology, 111 Michigan Ave NW, Washington, DC 20010-2978; **Phone:** 202-476-6230; **Board Cert:** Child Neurology 1982; Pediatrics 1982; **Med School:** Northwestern Univ 1976; **Resid:** Pediatrics, Chldns Med Ctr 1978; Neurology, Chldns Hosp-Univ Penn 1981; **Fac Appt:** Prof N, Geo Wash Univ

Phillips, Peter C MD [ChiN] - **Spec Exp:** Brain Tumors; Neuro-Oncology; **Hospital:** Chldns Hosp of Philadelphia, The; **Address:** Childrens Hosp Philadelphia, 34th St & Civic Center Blvd, Philadelphia, PA 19104; **Phone:** 215-590-5188; **Board Cert:** Pediatrics 1985; Child Neurology 1986; **Med School:** Univ Conn 1978; **Resid:** Pediatrics, Chldns Hosp 1980; Pediatric Neurology, Neuro Inst 1983; **Fellow:** Neuro-Oncology, Meml Sloan Kettering Cancer Ctr 1986; **Fac Appt:** Prof N, Univ Pennsylvania

Shinnar, Shlomo MD/PhD [ChiN] - **Spec Exp:** Epilepsy/Seizure Disorders; Headache; **Hospital:** Montefiore Med Ctr - Div. Moses; **Address:** Montefiore Medical Ctr, Children's Hospital, 111 E 210th St Fl 4, Bronx, NY 10467-2401; **Phone:** 718-920-4378; **Board Cert:** Neurology 1984; Pediatrics 1984; Clinical Neurophysiology 2005; **Med School:** Albert Einstein Coll Med 1978; **Resid:** Pediatrics, Johns Hopkins Hosp 1980; Neurology, Johns Hopkins Hosp 1983; **Fac Appt:** Prof N, Albert Einstein Coll Med

Southeast

Fenichel, Gerald M MD [ChiN] - **Spec Exp:** Neuromuscular Disorders; Muscular Dystrophy; **Hospital:** Vanderbilt Univ Med Ctr, Vanderbilt Children's Hosp; **Address:** Vanderbilt Childrens Hosp, Dept Neurology, 2200 Childrens Way, DOT, rm 11244, Nashville, TN 37232-9559; **Phone:** 615-936-5536; **Board Cert:** Neurology 1966; Child Neurology 1968; **Med School:** Yale Univ 1959; **Resid:** Neurology, Natl Inst Neuro Disorders-NIH 1963; Neurology, Yale-New Haven Hosp 1964; **Fac Appt:** Prof N, Vanderbilt Univ

Goldstein, Edward M MD [ChiN] - **Spec Exp:** Muscular Dystrophy; Movement Disorders; Botox Therapy; Headache; **Hospital:** Chldns Hlthcare Atlanta - Scottish Rite; **Address:** 5505 Peachtree Dunwoody Rd, Ste 500, Atlanta, GA 30342; **Phone:** 404-256-3535; **Board Cert:** Child Neurology 1994; **Med School:** Johns Hopkins Univ 1985; **Resid:** Pediatrics, Johns Hopkins Univ 1987; Neurology, Johns Hopkins Univ 1990; **Fellow:** Neuromuscular Disease, Emory Univ 1993

Greenwood, Robert S MD [ChiN] - **Spec Exp:** Neurofibromatosis; Epilepsy; **Hospital:** Univ NC Hosps; **Address:** 101 Manning Drive, Chapel Hill, NC 27599; **Phone:** 919-966-1401; **Board Cert:** Pediatrics 1974; Child Neurology 1979; **Med School:** Univ Tex Med Br, Galveston 1968; **Resid:** Pediatrics, Chldns Hosp 1971; Child Neurology, Chldns Hosp 1975; **Fellow:** Child Neurology, Chldns Hosp 1977; **Fac Appt:** Prof N, Univ NC Sch Med

Lavenstein, Bennett L MD [ChiN] - **Spec Exp:** Movement Disorders; Neuromuscular Disorders; **Hospital:** Chldns Natl Med Ctr, Inova Fairfax Hosp for Chldn; **Address:** 8501 Arlington Blvd, Fairfax, VA 22031; **Phone:** 571-226-8368; **Board Cert:** Pediatrics 1977; Child Neurology 1979; **Med School:** Univ MD Sch Med 1974; **Resid:** Pediatrics, Univ of MD Hlth System 1977; Neurology, Georgetown Univ Hosp 1979; **Fellow:** Neuromuscular Medicine, Natl Inst Hlth; **Fac Appt:** Assoc Clin Prof N, Univ VA Sch Med

Santos, Cesar C MD [ChiN] - **Spec Exp:** Epilepsy; Sleep Disorders; Stroke in Children; Clinical Trials; **Hospital:** Wake Forest Univ Baptist Med Ctr (page 72); **Address:** Wake Forest Univ Baptist Med Ctr, Dept Pediatric Neurology, Medical Center Blvd, Winston-Salem, NC 27157; **Phone:** 336-716-4101; **Board Cert:** Pediatrics 2004; Child Neurology 2004; Clinical Neurophysiology 2005; **Med School:** Philippines 1982; **Resid:** Pediatrics, St Lukes Roosevelt Hosp 1988; **Fellow:** Neurology, Duke Univ Med Ctr 1991; Neurological Physiology, Duke Univ 1992; **Fac Appt:** Prof N, Wake Forest Univ

Wheless, James W MD [ChiN] - **Spec Exp:** Epilepsy/Seizure Disorders; **Hospital:** Le Bonheur Chldns Med Ctr, St Jude Children's Research Hosp; **Address:** 777 Washington Ave, Ste 240, Memphis, TN 38105; **Phone:** 901-287-5060; **Board Cert:** Pediatrics 1987; Child Neurology 1989; Clinical Neurophysiology 2007; **Med School:** Univ Okla Coll Med 1982; **Resid:** Pediatrics, Univ Oklahoma Med Ctr 1985; **Fellow:** Pediatric Neurology, Chldns Meml Hosp 1988; Epilepsy, Med Coll Georgia Affil Hosp 1989; **Fac Appt:** Prof N, Univ Tenn Coll Med, Memphis

Midwest

Brunstrom, Janice MD [ChiN] - **Spec Exp:** Cerebral Palsy; **Hospital:** St Louis Chldns Hosp; **Address:** Washington Univ Sch Med, Dept Ped Neuro, 660 S Euclid Ave, Box 8111, St Louis, MO 63110; **Phone:** 314-454-6120; **Board Cert:** Pediatrics 2003; Child Neurology 2005; **Med School:** Med Coll VA 1987; **Resid:** Neurology, St Louis Chldns Hosp 1989; Neurology, Barnes Jewish Hosp 1990; **Fellow:** Child Neurology, St Louis Chldns Hosp 1995; **Fac Appt:** Asst Prof N, Washington Univ, St Louis

Cohen, Bruce H MD [ChiN] - **Spec Exp:** Brain Tumors; Epilepsy; Neurometabolic Disorders; Pain Management; **Hospital:** Cleveland Clin Fdn (page 56); **Address:** Cleveland Clinic, 9500 Euclid Ave, Desk S71, Cleveland, OH 44195; **Phone:** 216-444-9182; **Board Cert:** Pediatrics 2004; Child Neurology 1990; **Med School:** Albert Einstein Coll Med 1982; **Resid:** Pediatrics, Chldns Hosp 1984; Child Neurology, Neurologic Inst-Columbia 1987; **Fellow:** Pediatric Neuro-Oncology, Chldns Hosp 1989

Child Neurology

Edgar, Terence MD [ChiN] - **Spec Exp:** Neuromuscular Disorders; Cerebral Palsy; Epilepsy; **Hospital:** St Vincent Hosp - Green Bay; **Address:** Prevea Health, 1821 S Webster Fl 3rd, Green Bay, WI 54301; **Phone:** 920-272-1270; **Board Cert:** Pediatrics 2003; Child Neurology 2006; **Med School:** South Africa 1984; **Resid:** Pediatrics, Univ Wisconsin Hosp & Clin 1995; **Fellow:** Pediatrics, Univ Wisconsin Hosp & Clin 1993; Child Neurology, Univ Wisconsin Hosp & Clin 1996

Epstein, Leon G MD [ChiN] - **Spec Exp:** AIDS/HIV; Migraine; **Hospital:** Children's Mem Hosp; **Address:** Chldns Meml Hosp, Div Neurology, 2300 Childrens Plaza, Box 51, Chicago, IL 60614; **Phone:** 773-880-4352; **Board Cert:** Child Neurology 1979; **Med School:** Wayne State Univ 1973; **Resid:** Neurology, St Josephs Mercy Hosp 1974; Neurology, Univ Arizona Med Ctr 1976; **Fellow:** Neurology, Columbia Presby Med Ctr 1978; **Fac Appt:** Prof Ped, Northwestern Univ

Kotagal, Suresh MD [ChiN] - **Spec Exp:** Sleep Disorders/Apnea; **Hospital:** Mayo Med Ctr & Clin - Rochester, St Mary's Hosp - Rochester; **Address:** Mayo Clinic, 200 First St SW, Rochester, MN 55905-0002; **Phone:** 507-266-0774; **Board Cert:** Pediatrics 1979; Child Neurology 1982; **Med School:** India 1974; **Resid:** Child Neurology, Chldns Hosp Mich 1976; Pediatrics, St Louis Univ 1979; **Fellow:** Sleep Medicine, Stanford Univ 1982; **Fac Appt:** Prof N, Mayo Med Sch

Kovnar, Edward H MD [ChiN] - **Spec Exp:** Epilepsy/Seizure Disorders; Neurophysiology; Developmental Disorders; **Hospital:** Chldns Hosp - Wisconsin; **Address:** Advanced Healthcare, SC, 3003 W Good Hope Rd, Milwaukee, WI 53209-0996; **Phone:** 414-352-8828; **Board Cert:** Pediatrics 1984; Child Neurology 1984; Neurodevelopmental Disabilities 2005; **Med School:** Washington Univ, St Louis 1977; **Resid:** Pediatrics, Chldns Hosp 1979; Neurology, Barnes Hosp 1980; **Fellow:** Pediatric Neurology, Chldns Hosp 1982; Clinical Neurophysiology, Chldns Hosp 1991

Noetzel, Michael MD [ChiN] - **Spec Exp:** Cerebral Palsy; Brain Injury; Movement Disorders; **Hospital:** St Louis Chldns Hosp; **Address:** 660 S Euclid Ave, Box 8111, St Louis, MO 63110; **Phone:** 314-454-6120; **Board Cert:** Child Neurology 1984; Pediatrics 1984; **Med School:** Univ VA Sch Med 1977; **Resid:** Pediatrics, St Louis Chldns Hosp 1979; Neurology, Barnes Hosp 1980; **Fellow:** Child Neurology, St Louis Chldns Hosp 1982; **Fac Appt:** Prof Ped, Washington Univ, St Louis

Nordli Jr, Douglas R MD [ChiN] - **Spec Exp:** Epilepsy; Rasmussen's Syndrome; **Hospital:** Children's Mem Hosp; **Address:** Children's Memorial Hospital, Epilepsy Ctr, 2300 Children's Plaza, Box 29, Chicago, IL 60614-3394; **Phone:** 773-883-6159; **Board Cert:** Child Neurology 1990; **Med School:** Columbia P&S 1984; **Resid:** Pediatrics, Babies Hosp 1986; Child Neurology, Neuro Inst/Columbia-Presby Med Ctr 1989; **Fellow:** Clinical Neurophysiology, Neuro Inst/Columbia-Presby Med Ctr 1990; **Fac Appt:** Assoc Prof N, Northwestern Univ

Patterson, Marc C MD [ChiN] - **Spec Exp:** Neurogenetics; Developmental Delay; Metabolic Disorders; **Hospital:** Mayo Med Ctr & Clin - Rochester; **Address:** Mayo Clinic, Dept Neurology, 200 First St SW, Rochester, MN 55905; **Phone:** 507-284-9974; **Board Cert:** Child Neurology 2004; Neurodevelopmental Disabilities 2001; **Med School:** Australia 1981; **Resid:** Neurology, Univ Queenland 1988; Child Neurology, Mayo Clinic 1990; **Fellow:** Metabolic Neurology, Natl Inst Health 1992; Pediatrics, Mayo Cilnic 1993; **Fac Appt:** Prof N, Mayo Med Sch

Wiznitzer, Max MD [ChiN] - **Hospital:** Rainbow Babies & Chldns Hosp; **Address:** Rainbow Babies & Chldns Hosp, 11100 Euclid Ave, Ste 585, MS RBC6090, Cleveland, OH 44106; **Phone:** 216-844-3691; **Board Cert:** Pediatrics 1982; Child Neurology 1986; Neurodevelopmental Disabilities 2004; **Med School:** Northwestern Univ 1977; **Resid:** Pediatrics, Chldns Hosp Med Ctr 1980; **Fellow:** Developmental-Behavioral Pediatrics, Cincinnati Med Ctr 1981; Pediatric Neurology, Chldns Hosp 1984; **Fac Appt:** Assoc Prof Ped, Case West Res Univ

Wyllie, Elaine MD [ChiN] - **Spec Exp:** Epilepsy/Seizure Disorders; **Hospital:** Cleveland Clin Fdn (page 56); **Address:** Div Ped Neurology, 9500 Euclid Ave, Desk S51, Cleveland, OH 44195; **Phone:** 216-444-2095; **Board Cert:** Pediatrics 1982; Child Neurology 1986; **Med School:** Indiana Univ 1978; **Resid:** Pediatrics, Indiana Univ Med Ctr 1980; Pediatrics, Case West Med Ctr 1981; **Fellow:** Child Neurology, Cleveland Clinic 1984; Clinical Neurophysiology, Cleveland Clinic 1985; **Fac Appt:** Prof Ped, Cleveland Cl Coll Med/Case West Res

Great Plains and Mountains

Bale Jr, James F MD [ChiN] - **Spec Exp:** Infections-Neurologic; Infections-Congenital; **Hospital:** Primary Children's Med Ctr, Univ Utah Hosps and Clins; **Address:** Primary Chldns Med Ctr, 100 N Mario Capecchi Drive, Salt Lake City, UT 84113; **Phone:** 801-587-7575; **Board Cert:** Pediatrics 2002; Child Neurology 1982; **Med School:** Univ Mich Med Sch 1975; **Resid:** Pediatrics, Univ Utah Hosps 1977; Neurology, Univ Utah Hosps 1980; **Fellow:** Infectious Disease, Univ Utah 1981; Neurovirology, UCSF-VA Med Ctr 1982; **Fac Appt:** Prof N, Univ Utah

Southwest

Iannaccone, Susan T MD [ChiN] - **Spec Exp:** Neuromuscular Disorders; **Hospital:** Chldns Med Ctr of Dallas, UT Southwestern Med Ctr at Dallas; **Address:** Division of Pediatric Neurology, Ambulatory Care Pavilion in Dallas, 2350 Stemmons Frwy., Ste 5074, Dallas, TX 75207; **Phone:** 214-456-2768; **Board Cert:** Pediatrics 1975; Child Neurology 1976; **Med School:** SUNY Hlth Sci Ctr 1969; **Resid:** Pediatrics, St Louis Chldns Hosp 1972; Neurology, Strong Meml Hosp 1975; **Fellow:** Neurology, Strong Meml Hosp 1975

Riviello Jr, James J MD [ChiN] - **Spec Exp:** Epilepsy/Seizure Disorders; Epilepsy in Tuberous Sclerosis; **Hospital:** Texas Chldns Hosp; **Address:** 6621 Fannin, CC1250, Dept Neurology, Houston, TX 77030; **Phone:** 832-822-1750; **Board Cert:** Pediatrics 1984; Child Neurology 1985; Clinical Neurophysiology 2006; **Med School:** Tulane Univ 1978; **Resid:** Pediatrics, St Christopher Hosp Chldn 1981; Neurology, Temple Univ Hosp 1982; **Fellow:** Pediatric Neurology, St Christopher Hosp Chldn 1983; **Fac Appt:** Prof N, Baylor Coll Med

Sharp, Gregory B MD [ChiN] - **Spec Exp:** Epilepsy; **Hospital:** UAMS Med Ctr, Arkansas Chldns Hosp; **Address:** 1 Children's Way, Little Rock, AR 72202; **Phone:** 501-364-1100; **Board Cert:** Pediatrics 2004; Child Neurology 1993; **Med School:** Univ Ark 1984; **Resid:** Pediatrics, Univ Ark Chldns Hosp 1987; **Fellow:** Pediatric Neurology, Mayo Clinic 1990; **Fac Appt:** Asst Prof Ped, Univ Ark

West Coast and Pacific

Ashwal, Stephen MD [ChiN] - **Spec Exp:** Metabolic Disorders; **Hospital:** Loma Linda Univ Med Ctr; **Address:** Pediatric Neurosciences Ctr, 2195 Club Ctr Drive, Ste A, San Bernadino, CA 92408; **Phone:** 909-835-1810; **Board Cert:** Pediatrics 1975; Child Neurology 1978; **Med School:** NYU Sch Med 1970; **Resid:** Pediatrics, Bellevue Hosp 1973; **Fellow:** Child Neurology, Univ Minn Med Ctr 1976; **Fac Appt:** Prof Ped, Loma Linda Univ

Chamberlain, Marc C MD [ChiN] - **Spec Exp:** Brain Tumors; Neuro-Oncology; Clinical Trials; **Hospital:** Univ Wash Med Ctr; **Address:** Seattle Cancer Care Alliance, 825 Eastlake Ave E, POB 10923, MS G4940, Seattle, WA 98109-1023; **Phone:** 206-288-8280; **Board Cert:** Pediatrics 1985; Child Neurology 1989; **Med School:** Columbia P&S 1977; **Resid:** Pediatrics, Montefiore Med Ctr 1981; Neurology, UCLA Med Ctr 1983; **Fellow:** Neuro-Oncology, UCSF Med Ctr 1986; **Fac Appt:** Prof N, Univ Wash

Child Neurology

Ferriero, Donna MD [ChiN] - **Spec Exp:** Neuroendocrinology; **Hospital:** UCSF Med Ctr; **Address:** UCSF, Box 0410, 350 Parnassus Ave, Ste 609, San Francisco, CA 94143-0663; **Phone:** 415-353-2525; **Board Cert:** Pediatrics 1986; Child Neurology 1987; **Med School:** UCSF 1979; **Resid:** Pediatrics, Mass Genl Hosp 1982; Child Neurology, UCSF Med Ctr 1985; **Fellow:** Neurological Endocrinology, UCSF Med Ctr 1987; **Fac Appt:** Prof N, UCSF

Fisher, Paul G MD [ChiN] - **Spec Exp:** Neuro-Oncology; Brain Tumors; **Hospital:** Lucile Packard Chldn's Hosp; **Address:** Stanford Cancer Ctr-Dept Neurology, 875 Blake Wilbur Drive, rm 2220, Stanford, CA 94305; **Phone:** 650-725-8630; **Board Cert:** Pediatrics 2003; Child Neurology 2008; **Med School:** UCSF 1989; **Resid:** Pediatrics, Johns Hopkins Univ Hosp 1991; Neurology, Johns Hopkins Univ Hosp 1994; **Fellow:** Neuro-Oncology, Children's Hosp 1994; **Fac Appt:** Assoc Prof Ped, Stanford Univ

Haas, Richard H MD [ChiN] - **Spec Exp:** Mitochondrial Disorders; Neurometabolic Disorders; **Hospital:** UCSD Med Ctr, Rady Children's Hosp - San Diego; **Address:** UCSD Sch Med, Div Ped Neuro, 9500 Gilman Drive, MC 0935, La Jolla, CA 92093-0935; **Phone:** 858-822-6700; **Board Cert:** Child Neurology 1983; Pediatrics 1985; **Med School:** England, UK 1972; **Resid:** Pediatrics, Univ London 1979; Child Neurology, Univ Colo Hlth Sci Ctr 1981; **Fellow:** Biochemical Mental Retardation, Univ Colo Hlth Sci Ctr 1981; **Fac Appt:** Prof Ped, UCSD

Lott, Ira T MD [ChiN] - **Spec Exp:** Down Syndrome; **Hospital:** Chldns Hosp Orange Co, UC Irvine Med Ctr; **Address:** UC Irvine Med Ctr, Dept Ped Neur, 101 City Drive S, Orange, CA 92868; **Phone:** 714-532-7554; **Board Cert:** Pediatrics 1975; Child Neurology 1977; **Med School:** Ohio State Univ 1967; **Resid:** Pediatrics, Mass Genl Hosp 1969; **Fellow:** Research, Natl Inst Hlth 1971; Neurology, Harvard-Mass Genl Hosp 1974; **Fac Appt:** Prof N, UC Irvine

Mitchell, Wendy G MD [ChiN] - **Spec Exp:** Epilepsy/Seizure Disorders; Opsoclonus-Ataxia in Children; **Hospital:** Chldns Hosp - Los Angeles; **Address:** Chldns Hosp Los Angeles, Dept Neuro, 4650 Sunset Blvd, Box 82, Los Angeles, CA 90027-6062; **Phone:** 323-361-2498; **Board Cert:** Pediatrics 1978; Child Neurology 1983; **Med School:** UCSF 1973; **Resid:** Pediatrics, Moffit Hosp-UCSF 1975; Child Neurology, Univ North Carolina 1981; **Fellow:** Behavioral Pediatrics, Mt Zion Hosp 1976; Univ North Carolina 1978; **Fac Appt:** Prof N, USC Sch Med

Roddy, Sarah M MD [ChiN] - **Spec Exp:** Tourette's Syndrome; **Hospital:** Loma Linda Chldns Hosp; **Address:** Pediatric Neuroscience Center, 2195 Club Center Drive, Ste A, San Bernadino, CA 92408; **Phone:** 909-835-1810; **Board Cert:** Child Neurology 1987; Pediatrics 1987; **Med School:** Loma Linda Univ 1980; **Resid:** Pediatrics, Loma Linda Univ Med Ctr 1983; **Fellow:** Pediatric Neurology, Loma Linda Univ Med Ctr 1986; **Fac Appt:** Assoc Prof N, Loma Linda Univ

Rosser, Tena L MD [ChiN] - **Spec Exp:** Neurocutaneous Disorders; Neurofibromatosis; Tuberous Sclerosis; **Hospital:** Chldns Hosp - Los Angeles; **Address:** Chldns Hosp Los Angeles, Dept Neurology, 4650 Sunset Blvd, #82, Los Angeles, CA 90027; **Phone:** 323-361-2471; **Board Cert:** Pediatrics 2007; Child Neurology 2003; **Med School:** Univ NC Sch Med 1996; **Resid:** Pediatrics, Chldn's Natl Med Ctr 1999; **Fellow:** Child Neurology, Chldn's Natl Med Ctr 2003; **Fac Appt:** Asst Prof N, USC-Keck School of Medicine

Sankar, Raman MD/PhD [ChiN] - **Spec Exp:** Epilepsy/Seizure Disorders; Headache; Migraine; **Hospital:** Mattel Chldns Hosp at UCLA, UCLA Ronald Reagan Med Ctr; **Address:** UCLA Sch Med-Div Ped Neurology, 22-474 MDCC, Box 951752, Los Angeles, CA 90095-1752; **Phone:** 310-825-6196; **Board Cert:** Child Neurology 2005; **Med School:** Tulane Univ 1986; **Resid:** Pediatrics, Chldns Hosp 1988; Neurology, UCLA Med Ctr 1989; **Fellow:** Child Neurology, UCLA Med Ctr 1991; **Fac Appt:** Prof Ped, UCLA

Shields, William Donald MD [ChiN] - **Spec Exp:** Epilepsy/Seizure Disorders; **Hospital:** UCLA Ronald Reagan Med Ctr; **Address:** UCLA Med Ctr, Dept Ped Neurology, 10833 Le Conte Ave, Los Angeles, CA 90095-1752; **Phone:** 310-825-6196; **Board Cert:** Child Neurology 1977; Pediatrics 1978; **Med School:** Univ Utah 1971; **Resid:** Pediatrics, USC Med Ctr 1973; Neurology, Univ Utah Med Ctr 1976; **Fac Appt:** Prof Ped, UCLA

Trauner, Doris A MD [ChiN] - **Spec Exp:** Autism; Speech Disorders; **Hospital:** Rady Children's Hosp - San Diego; **Address:** UCSD Med Ctr, Div Ped Neurology, 9500 Gilman Drive, Dept 0935, La Jolla, CA 92093-0935; **Phone:** 858-966-5819; **Board Cert:** Pediatrics 1978; Child Neurology 1979; Neurodevelopmental Disabilities 2001; **Med School:** Med Coll VA 1972; **Resid:** Pediatrics, UCSD Med Ctr 1974; Neurology, UCSD Med Ctr 1975; **Fellow:** Child Neurology, Univ Chicago 1977; **Fac Appt:** Prof Ped, UCSD

Clinical Genetics

A specialist trained in diagnostic and therapeutic procedures for patients with genetically-linked diseases. This specialist uses modern cytogenetic, radiologic and biochemical testing to assist in specialized genetic counseling, implements needed therapeutic interventions and provides prevention through prenatal diagnosis.

A clinical geneticist demonstrates competence in providing comprehensive diagnostic, management and counseling services for genetic disorders.

A medical geneticist plans and coordinates large scale screening programs for inborn errors of metabolism, hemoglobinopathies, chromosome abnormalities and neural tube defects.

Training Required: Two or four years

CLINICAL GENETICS

New England

Bale, Allen E MD [CG] - **Spec Exp:** Cancer Genetics; **Hospital:** Yale-New Haven Hosp; **Address:** 333 Cedar St, SHM Bldg - rm 1321, New Haven, CT 06519; **Phone:** 203-785-5745; **Board Cert:** Internal Medicine 1983; Clinical Genetics 1987; Clinical Molecular Genetics 2006; **Med School:** Univ Mass Sch Med 1979; **Resid:** Internal Medicine, Western Penn Hosp 1983; **Fellow:** Medical Genetics, NIH 1987; **Fac Appt:** Assoc Prof CG, Yale Univ

Bianchi, Diana MD [CG] - **Spec Exp:** Twin to Twin Transfusion Syndrome (TTTS); Fetal Abnormalities; **Hospital:** Tufts Med Ctr; **Address:** New Engl Med Ctr/Div Med Genetics, 800 Washington St, Box 394, Boston, MA 02111; **Phone:** 617-636-1468; **Board Cert:** Pediatrics 1985; Clinical Genetics 1987; Neonatal-Perinatal Medicine 1987; **Med School:** Stanford Univ 1980; **Resid:** Pediatrics, Chldns Hosp 1983; **Fellow:** Neonatology, Chldns Hosp 1986; Clinical Genetics, Harvard Med Sch 1987; **Fac Appt:** Prof Ped, Tufts Univ

Holmes, Lewis B MD [CG] - **Spec Exp:** Birth Defects; Inherited Disorders; Prenatal Diagnosis; **Hospital:** Mass Genl Hosp, Brigham & Women's Hosp; **Address:** Mass Genl Hosp, Dept Pediatrics, 175 Cambridge St Fl 5 - rm 504, Boston, MA 02114; **Phone:** 617-726-1742; **Board Cert:** Pediatrics 1968; Clinical Genetics 1982; **Med School:** Duke Univ 1963; **Resid:** Pediatrics, Mass Genl Hosp 1965; **Fellow:** Pediatric Endocrinology, Mass Genl Hosp 1966; **Fac Appt:** Prof Ped, Harvard Med Sch

Mahoney, Maurice J MD [CG] - **Spec Exp:** Fetal Therapy; Prenatal Diagnosis; **Hospital:** Yale-New Haven Hosp; **Address:** Yale Genetics Consultation Serv, 333 Cedar St, rm WWW330, New Haven, CT 06520-8005; **Phone:** 203-785-2661; **Board Cert:** Pediatrics 1967; Clinical Genetics 1982; Clinical Biochemical Genetics 1982; **Med School:** Univ Pittsburgh 1962; **Resid:** Pediatrics, Johns Hopkins Hosp 1965; Pediatrics, Childrens Hosp 1966; **Fellow:** Clinical Genetics, Yale Univ Sch Med 1970; **Fac Appt:** Prof CG, Yale Univ

Seashore, Margretta MD [CG] - **Spec Exp:** Inherited Metabolic Disorders; **Hospital:** Yale-New Haven Hosp; **Address:** Yale Univ Sch Med, Dept Genetics, 333 Cedar St, rm 305, Box 208005, New Haven, CT 06520-8005; **Phone:** 203-785-2660; **Board Cert:** Pediatrics 1970; Clinical Biochemical Genetics 1982; Clinical Genetics 1982; **Med School:** Yale Univ 1965; **Resid:** Pediatrics, Yale-New Haven Hosp 1968; **Fellow:** Clinical Genetics, Yale-New Haven Hosp 1970; **Fac Appt:** Prof CG, Yale Univ

Mid Atlantic

Anyane-Yeboa, Kwame MD [CG] - **Spec Exp:** Dysmorphology; Prenatal Diagnosis; **Hospital:** NYPresby-Morgan Stanley Children's Hosp (page 66), St Luke's - Roosevelt Hosp Ctr - Roosevelt Div (page 57); **Address:** Morgan Stanley Children's Hospital of NY, 3959 Broadway Fl 6N - rm 601A, New York, NY 10032; **Phone:** 212-305-6731; **Board Cert:** Pediatrics 1979; Clinical Genetics 1982; **Med School:** Ghana 1972; **Resid:** Pediatrics, Harlem Hosp 1977; **Fellow:** Clinical Genetics, Babies Hosp-Columbia Presby 1980; **Fac Appt:** Assoc Prof Ped, Columbia P&S

Bialer, Martin G MD/PhD [CG] - **Spec Exp:** Marfan's Syndrome; Neurofibromatosis; Metabolic Genetic Disorders; Cancer Genetics; **Hospital:** Schneider Chldn's Hosp, NS-LIJ Hlth Sys; **Address:** 1554 Northern Blvd, Ste 204, Manhasset, NY 11030; **Phone:** 516-365-3996; **Board Cert:** Pediatrics 1987; Clinical Biochemical Genetics 1990; Clinical Genetics 1990; **Med School:** Med Univ SC 1983; **Resid:** Pediatrics, N Shore Univ Hosp 1986; **Fellow:** Clinical Genetics, Univ VA Hlth Sci Ctr 1989; **Fac Appt:** Clin Prof Ped, NYU Sch Med

Davis, Jessica G MD [CG] - **Spec Exp:** Marfan's Syndrome; Mental Retardation; Neurofibromatosis; Ehlers-Danlos Syndrome; **Hospital:** NY-Presby Hosp/Weill Cornell (page 66), Hosp For Special Surgery (page 59); **Address:** 525 E 68th St, Box 128, New York, NY 10021-4870; **Phone:** 646-962-2205; **Board Cert:** Clinical Genetics 1984; **Med School:** Columbia P&S 1959; **Resid:** Pediatrics, St Luke's Hosp 1962; Clinical Genetics, Albert Einstein Coll Med 1965; **Fellow:** Cytogenetics, Albert Einstein Coll Med 1966; Pediatrics, Albert Einstein Col Med 1968; **Fac Appt:** Assoc Clin Prof Ped, Cornell Univ-Weill Med Coll

Desnick, Robert J MD/PhD [CG] - **Spec Exp:** Inherited Metabolic Disorders; Fabry's Disease; Gaucher Disease; Porphyria; **Hospital:** Mount Sinai Med Ctr (page 64), Beth Israel Med Ctr- Kings Hwy Div (page 57); **Address:** Mt Sinai Sch Med, Box 1498, Fifth Ave @ 100th St, New York, NY 10029; **Phone:** 212-241-6947; **Board Cert:** Clinical Genetics 1982; Clinical Molecular Genetics 1999; Clinical Biochemical Genetics 1982; **Med School:** Univ Minn 1971; **Resid:** Pediatrics, Univ Minn Hosps 1973; **Fac Appt:** Prof CG, Mount Sinai Sch Med

Desposito, Franklin MD [CG] - **Spec Exp:** Birth Defects; Genetic Disorders; **Hospital:** UMDNJ-Univ Hosp-Newark, St Barnabas Med Ctr; **Address:** 90 Bergen St, Ste 5400, Newark, NJ 07103; **Phone:** 973-972-3300; **Board Cert:** Pediatrics 1986; Clinical Genetics 1982; Clinical Cytogenetics 1990; Clinical Molecular Genetics 2006; **Med School:** Ros Franklin Univ/Chicago Med Sch 1957; **Resid:** Pediatrics, Long Island Jewish Hosp 1961; **Fellow:** Hematology, Univ Wisc Sch Med 1963; **Fac Appt:** Prof Ped, UMDNJ-NJ Med Sch, Newark

Driscoll, Deborah A MD [CG] - **Spec Exp:** Prenatal Genetic Diagnosis; Fetal Abnormalities; Adolescent Gynecology; **Hospital:** Hosp Univ Penn - UPHS (page 60); **Address:** Chldns Hosp of Philadelphia, Clin Genetics Ctr, 34th St and Civic Ctr Blvd, rm 9S20, Philadelphia, PA 19104; **Phone:** 215-662-3232; **Board Cert:** Obstetrics & Gynecology 2007; Clinical Genetics 1990; **Med School:** NYU Sch Med 1983; **Resid:** Obstetrics & Gynecology, Hosp Univ Penn 1987; **Fellow:** Clinical Genetics, Hosp Univ Penn 1989; **Fac Appt:** Assoc Prof ObG, Univ Pennsylvania

Marion, Robert W MD [CG] - **Spec Exp:** Spina Bifida; Williams Syndrome; Marfan's Syndrome; Down Syndrome; **Hospital:** Montefiore Med Ctr - Div. Moses, Blythedale Children's Hosp; **Address:** 3415 Bainbridge Ave, Bronx, NY 10467; **Phone:** 718-741-2323; **Board Cert:** Pediatrics 1985; Clinical Genetics 1987; **Med School:** Albert Einstein Coll Med 1979; **Resid:** Pediatrics, Montefiore Med Ctr 1982; **Fellow:** Clinical Genetics, Montefiore Med Ctr 1984; **Fac Appt:** Prof Ped, Albert Einstein Coll Med

Ostrer, Harry MD [CG] - **Spec Exp:** Genetic Disorders; Hereditary Cancer; **Hospital:** NYU Langone Med Ctr (page 67); **Address:** NYU Medical Ctr, 550 1st Ave, rm MSB136, New York, NY 10016; **Phone:** 212-263-5746; **Board Cert:** Clinical Genetics 1984; Pediatrics 1985; Clinical Cytogenetics 1990; Clinical Molecular Genetics 2006; **Med School:** Columbia P&S 1976; **Resid:** Pediatrics, Johns Hopkins Hosp 1978; Clinical Genetics, Natl Inst Health 1981; **Fellow:** Molecular Genetics, Johns Hopkins Hosp 1983; **Fac Appt:** Prof Ped, NYU Sch Med

Clinical Genetics

Pyeritz, Reed E MD/PhD [CG] - **Spec Exp:** Marfan's Syndrome; Hereditary Hemorrhagic Telangiectasia; Inherited Disorders; **Hospital:** Hosp Univ Penn - UPHS (page 60), Chldns Hosp of Philadelphia, The; **Address:** Univ Penn, Div Medical Genetics, 3400 Spruce St, 538 Maloney Bldg, Philadelphia, PA 19104; **Phone:** 215-662-4740; **Board Cert:** Internal Medicine 1978; Clinical Genetics 2004; **Med School:** Harvard Med Sch 1975; **Resid:** Internal Medicine, Peter Bent Brigham Hosp 1977; Clinical Genetics, Johns Hopkins Hosp 1978; **Fac Appt:** Prof Med, Univ Pennsylvania

Rosenbaum, Kenneth MD [CG] - **Spec Exp:** Birth Defects; **Hospital:** Chldns Natl Med Ctr; **Address:** Chldns Natl Med Ctr, Dept Med Genetics, 111 Michigan Ave NW, rm 1950, Washington, DC 20010; **Phone:** 202-476-2187; **Board Cert:** Pediatrics 1976; Clinical Genetics 1982; Clinical Cytogenetics 1982; **Med School:** Univ Louisville Sch Med 1971; **Resid:** Pediatrics, Childrens Natl Med Ctr 1974; **Fellow:** Clinical Genetics, Johns Hopkins Hosp 1977; **Fac Appt:** Assoc Prof Ped, Geo Wash Univ

Shapiro, Lawrence R MD [CG] - **Spec Exp:** Dysmorphology; Prenatal Diagnosis; Hereditary Cancer; Developmental Disorders; **Hospital:** Westchester Med Ctr; **Address:** Regional Med Genetics Ctr, Children/Women's Physicians of Westchester, 503 Grasslands Ave, Ste 200, Valhalla, NY 10595; **Phone:** 914-304-5300; **Board Cert:** Pediatrics 1967; Clinical Genetics 1982; Clinical Cytogenetics 1982; **Med School:** NYU Sch Med 1962; **Resid:** Pediatrics, Chldns Hosp 1964; Pediatrics, Bellevue Hosp 1965; **Fellow:** Clinical Genetics, Mount Sinai Med Ctr 1968; **Fac Appt:** Prof Ped, NY Med Coll

Zackai, Elaine MD [CG] - **Spec Exp:** Craniosynostosis; Cytogenetic Disorders; **Hospital:** Chldns Hosp of Philadelphia, The; **Address:** Childrens Hosp Philadelphia, Dept Clinical Genetics, 34th St & Civic Center Blvd, rm 2NE004, Philadelphia, PA 19104; **Phone:** 215-590-2920; **Board Cert:** Pediatrics 1977; Clinical Genetics 1982; Clinical Cytogenetics 1982; **Med School:** NYU Sch Med 1968; **Resid:** Pediatrics, Chldns Hosp 1970; **Fellow:** Clinical Genetics, Chldns Hosp 1971; Clinical Genetics, Yale Univ Med Sch 1972; **Fac Appt:** Prof Ped, Univ Pennsylvania

Southeast

Driscoll, Daniel J MD/PhD [CG] - **Spec Exp:** Prader-Willi Syndrome; Obesity-Pediatric; Angelman Syndrome; **Hospital:** Shands at Univ of FL; **Address:** Pediatric Genetics & Metabolism, Univ FL Hlth Sicence Ctr, PO Box 100296, Gainesville, FL 32610-0296; **Phone:** 352-392-4104; **Board Cert:** Pediatrics 1987; Clinical Genetics 1990; Clinical Cytogenetics 1990; **Med School:** Albany Med Coll 1983; **Resid:** Pediatrics, Johns Hopkins Hosp 1986; **Fellow:** Clinical Genetics, Johns Hopkins Hosp 1989; **Fac Appt:** Prof Ped, Univ Fla Coll Med

Fernhoff, Paul M MD [CG] - **Spec Exp:** Birth Defects; Metabolic Genetic Disorders; **Hospital:** Chldns Hlthcare Atlanta - Scottish Rite, Emory Univ Hosp; **Address:** Emory Univ Sch Med, Div Med Genetics, 2165 N Decatur Rd, Decatur, GA 30033-5307; **Phone:** 404-778-8500; **Board Cert:** Pediatrics 1976; Clinical Genetics 1982; **Med School:** Jefferson Med Coll 1971; **Resid:** Pediatrics, Children's Hosp 1974; **Fellow:** Clinical Genetics, Emory Univ Hosp 1979; **Fac Appt:** Assoc Prof Ped, Emory Univ

Korf, Bruce R MD/PhD [CG] - **Spec Exp:** Inherited Disorders; Neuro-Genetics; Neurofibromatosis; **Hospital:** Univ of Ala Hosp at Birmingham; **Address:** Univ Alabama Birmingham-KAUL 230, 720 20th St S, Birmingham, AL 35294-0024; **Phone:** 205-934-4983; **Board Cert:** Clinical Genetics 1984; Child Neurology 1986; Pediatrics 1988; Clinical Molecular Genetics 2006; **Med School:** Cornell Univ-Weill Med Coll 1980; **Resid:** Pediatrics, Chldns Hosp 1982; Child Neurology, Chldns Hosp 1985; **Fellow:** Clinical Genetics, Chldns Hosp 1985; **Fac Appt:** Prof CG, Univ Alabama

Saul, Robert MD [CG] - **Spec Exp:** Birth Defects; Neurofibromatosis; **Hospital:** Self Regional Healthcare; **Address:** Greenwood Genetic Ctr, 101 Gregor Mendel Cir, Greenwood, SC 29646-2307; **Phone:** 864-941-8100; **Board Cert:** Pediatrics 1981; Clinical Genetics 1982; **Med School:** Univ Colorado 1976; **Resid:** Pediatrics, Duke Med Ctr 1979; **Fellow:** Clinical Genetics, Greenwood Genetics Ctr 1981; **Fac Appt:** Clin Prof Ped, Univ SC Sch Med

Stevenson, Roger E MD [CG] - **Spec Exp:** Birth Defects; Mental Retardation; **Hospital:** Self Regional Healthcare; **Address:** Greenwood Genetic Ctr, 101 Gregor Mendel Circle, Research Bldg, Greenwood, SC 29646; **Phone:** 864-941-8100; **Board Cert:** Pediatrics 1971; Clinical Genetics 1982; Clinical Cytogenetics 1984; **Med School:** Wake Forest Univ 1966; **Resid:** Pediatrics, Johns Hopkins Hosp 1969; **Fellow:** Clinical Genetics, Johns Hopkins Hosp 1972

Sutphen, Rebecca MD [CG] - **Spec Exp:** Genetic Disorders; Hereditary Cancer; Cancer Risk Assessment; **Hospital:** H Lee Moffitt Cancer Ctr & Research Inst; **Address:** H Lee Moffitt Cancer Ctr, 12902 Magnolia Drive, Tampa, FL 33612; **Phone:** 800-456-3434; **Board Cert:** Clinical Molecular Genetics 2007; Clinical Cytogenetics 2007; Clinical Genetics 2007; **Med School:** Temple Univ 1990; **Resid:** Pediatrics, All Children's Hosp 1993; **Fellow:** Clinical Genetics, Univ S Fla Coll Med 1995; **Fac Appt:** Assoc Prof CG, Univ S Fla Coll Med

Midwest

Burton, Barbara MD [CG] - **Spec Exp:** Marfan's Syndrome; Phenylketonuria (PKU); Lysosomal Diseases; Inborn Errors of Metabolism; **Hospital:** Children's Mem Hosp, Northwestern Meml Hosp; **Address:** Chldns Meml Hosp, Dept Genetics, 2300 Children's Plaza, Box 59, Chicago, IL 60614-3363; **Phone:** 773-880-4462; **Board Cert:** Pediatrics 1978; Clinical Genetics 1982; Clinical Biochemical Genetics 1982; **Med School:** Northwestern Univ 1973; **Resid:** Pediatrics, Chldns Meml Hosp 1975; **Fellow:** Clinical Genetics, Chldns Meml Hosp 1977; **Fac Appt:** Prof Ped, Northwestern Univ

Charrow, Joel MD [CG] - **Spec Exp:** Biochemical Genetics; Lysosomal Diseases; Neurofibromatosis; **Hospital:** Children's Mem Hosp; **Address:** Chldns Meml Hosp-Div Genetics, 2300 Chldn Plaza, Box 59, Chicago, IL 60614-3318; **Phone:** 773-880-4462; **Board Cert:** Pediatrics 1980; Clinical Genetics 1982; Clinical Biochemical Genetics 1987; **Med School:** Mount Sinai Sch Med 1976; **Resid:** Pediatrics, Chldns Meml Hosp 1979; **Fellow:** Clinical Genetics, Chldns Meml Hosp-Northwestern Univ 1981; **Fac Appt:** Prof Ped, Northwestern Univ

Elias, Sherman MD [CG] - **Spec Exp:** Prenatal Diagnosis; Reproductive Genetics; **Hospital:** Northwestern Meml Hosp; **Address:** 250 E Superior, Ste 03-2306, Chicago, IL 60611-2914; **Phone:** 312-472-3636; **Board Cert:** Obstetrics & Gynecology 1996; Clinical Genetics 2004; **Med School:** Univ KY Coll Med 1972; **Resid:** Obstetrics & Gynecology, Univ Louisville Hosp 1976; **Fellow:** Clinical Genetics, Yale Univ 1975; Clinical Genetics, Northwestern Univ 1978; **Fac Appt:** Prof ObG, Northwestern Univ

Pergament, Eugene MD/PhD [CG] - **Spec Exp:** Prenatal Genetic Diagnosis; Down Syndrome; Genetic Preimplantation Diagnosis; **Hospital:** Northwestern Meml Hosp; **Address:** 680 N Lake Shore Drive, Ste 1230, Chicago, IL 60611; **Phone:** 312-981-4360; **Board Cert:** Clinical Genetics 1982; Clinical Cytogenetics 1984; **Med School:** Univ Chicago-Pritzker Sch Med 1970; **Resid:** Pediatrics, Univ Chicago 1972; **Fac Appt:** Prof ObG, Northwestern Univ

Clinical Genetics

Rubinstein, Wendy S MD/PhD [CG] - **Spec Exp:** Breast Cancer; Colon Cancer; Pancreatic Cancer; **Hospital:** Evanston/Northshore Univ Hlth Syst; **Address:** Ctr for Medical Genetics, 1000 Central St, Ste 620, Evanston, IL 60201; **Phone:** 847-570-1029; **Board Cert:** Internal Medicine 2003; Clinical Genetics 2007; Clinical Molecular Genetics 2007; **Med School:** Mount Sinai Sch Med 1989; **Resid:** Internal Medicine, Strong Meml Hosp 1992; **Fellow:** Clinical Genetics, Univ Pittsburgh 1996; Clinical Molecular Genetics, Univ Pittsburgh 1996; **Fac Appt:** Asst Prof Med, Northwestern Univ

Saal, Howard M MD [CG] - **Spec Exp:** Craniofacial Disorders; Cleft Palate/Lip; Neurofibromatosis; **Hospital:** Cincinnati Chldns Hosp Med Ctr; **Address:** Chldns Hosp Med Ctr, Div Human Genetics, 3333 Burnet Ave Bldg E5 - rm 5430, MC 4006, Cincinnati, OH 45229-3039; **Phone:** 513-636-4760; **Board Cert:** Clinical Genetics 1984; Clinical Cytogenetics 1984; Pediatrics 1985; **Med School:** Wayne State Univ 1979; **Resid:** Pediatrics, Univ Conn Hlth Ctr 1982; **Fellow:** Medical Genetics, Univ Washington 1984; **Fac Appt:** Prof Ped, Univ Cincinnati

Weaver, David D MD [CG] - **Spec Exp:** Bone Disorders-Inherited; Genetic Disorders; Inherited Disorders; Birth Defects; **Hospital:** Riley Hosp for Children, Indiana Univ Hosp; **Address:** 975 W Walnut St IB Bldg - Ste 130, Indianapolis, IN 46202-5251; **Phone:** 317-274-1057; **Board Cert:** Pediatrics 1978; Clinical Genetics 1982; **Med School:** Oregon Hlth & Sci Univ 1966; **Resid:** Pediatrics, Oregon Hlth Scis Univ Sch Med 1972; **Fellow:** Clinical Genetics, Univ Washington Sch Med 1974; Metabolic Diseases, Oregon Health Scis Med Ctr 1976; **Fac Appt:** Prof Emeritus CG, Indiana Univ

Whelan, Alison MD [CG] - **Spec Exp:** Gynecologic Cancer Risk; Colon & Rectal Cancer Risk; Hereditary Cancer; **Hospital:** Barnes-Jewish Hosp, St Louis Chldns Hosp; **Address:** Washington Univ Sch Med, 660 S Euclid Ave, Campus Box 8116, St Louis, MO 63110; **Phone:** 314-454-6093; **Board Cert:** Internal Medicine 1989; Clinical Genetics 2007; **Med School:** Washington Univ, St Louis 1986; **Resid:** Internal Medicine, Barnes Hosp 1989; Pediatrics, Wash Univ Sch Med 1994; **Fellow:** Research, Wash Univ Sch Med 1991; Clinical Genetics, Wash Univ Sch Med 1994; **Fac Appt:** Prof Med, Washington Univ, St Louis

Great Plains and Mountains

Carey, John C MD [CG] - **Spec Exp:** Neurofibromatosis; Birth Defects; Hearing Loss; **Hospital:** Primary Children's Med Ctr, Univ Utah Hosps and Clins; **Address:** Div Medical Genetics, 50 N Med Drive Bldg SOM - rm 2C412, Salt Lake City, UT 84132; **Phone:** 801-581-8943; **Board Cert:** Pediatrics 1979; Clinical Genetics 1982; **Med School:** Georgetown Univ 1972; **Resid:** Pediatrics, UCSF Med Ctr 1975; **Fellow:** Clinical Genetics, UCSF Med Ctr 1979; **Fac Appt:** Prof Ped, Univ Utah

Hoyme, H Eugene MD [CG] - **Spec Exp:** Fetal Alcohol Syndrome; Cytogenetic Disorders; Dysmorphology; **Hospital:** Sanford Health SD; **Address:** PO Box 5039, 1305 W 18th St, Sioux Falls, SD 57117-5039; **Phone:** 605-333-6447; **Board Cert:** Pediatrics 1980; Clinical Genetics 1984; Clinical Cytogenetics 1987; **Med School:** Univ Chicago-Pritzker Sch Med 1976; **Resid:** Pediatrics, UCSD Med Ctr 1979; **Fellow:** Dysmorphology, UCSD Med Ctr 1981; **Fac Appt:** Prof Ped, Univ SD Sch Med

Opitz, John MD [CG] - **Spec Exp:** Skeletal Dysplasia; Sexual Differentiation Disorders; Mental Retardation; **Hospital:** Univ Utah Hosps and Clins; **Address:** Univ Utah, Div Med Genetics, 2C412 SOM, 50 N Medical Drive, Salt Lake City, UT 84132; **Phone:** 801-581-8943; **Board Cert:** Pediatrics 1964; Clinical Genetics 1982; **Med School:** Univ Iowa Coll Med 1959; **Resid:** Pediatrics, SUI Hosp 1961; Pediatrics, Univ Wisc Hosps 1962; **Fellow:** Clinical Genetics, Univ Wisc Hosps 1964; **Fac Appt:** Prof Ped, Univ Utah

Southwest

Beaudet, Arthur L MD [CG] - **Spec Exp:** Genetic Biochemical Disorders; **Hospital:** Texas Chldns Hosp; **Address:** Texas Children's Hosp, 6621 Fannin St, MC CC1560, Houston, TX 77030; **Phone:** 832-822-4280; **Board Cert:** Pediatrics 1973; Clinical Genetics 1982; Clinical Biochemical Genetics 1982; Clinical Molecular Genetics 2006; **Med School:** Yale Univ 1967; **Resid:** Pediatrics, Johns Hopkins Hosp 1969; **Fellow:** Biochemical Genetics, Natl Inst Hlth 1971; **Fac Appt:** Prof CG, Baylor Coll Med

Craigen, William MD/PhD [CG] - **Spec Exp:** Biochemical Genetics; Mitochondrial Disorders; **Hospital:** Texas Chldns Hosp, Ben Taub Genl Hosp; **Address:** Texas Children's Hosp, 6621 Fannin St, MC CC1560, Houston, TX 77030; **Phone:** 832-822-4280; **Board Cert:** Pediatrics 2002; Clinical Genetics 2006; Clinical Biochemical Genetics 2006; **Med School:** Baylor Coll Med 1988; **Resid:** Pediatrics, Baylor Coll Med 1990; Pediatrics, Baylor Coll Med 1992; **Fellow:** Clinical Genetics, Baylor Coll Med 1990; **Fac Appt:** Assoc Prof CG, Baylor Coll Med

Cunniff, Christopher M MD [CG] - **Spec Exp:** Birth Defects; **Hospital:** Univ Med Ctr - Tucson; **Address:** Univ Ariz Coll Med, Dept Ped Genetics, 1501 N Campbell Ave, Tucson, AZ 85724; **Phone:** 520-626-5175; **Board Cert:** Pediatrics 2003; Clinical Genetics 1990; **Med School:** Univ Alabama 1984; **Resid:** Pediatrics, MC Hosp Vermont 1987; **Fellow:** Dysmorphology, UCSD 1989; **Fac Appt:** Assoc Prof Ped, Univ Ariz Coll Med

Mulvihill, John J MD [CG] - **Spec Exp:** Genetic Disorders; Neurofibromatosis; Fertility in Cancer Survivors; **Hospital:** Chldns Hosp OU Med Ctr; **Address:** Childrens Hosp, 940 NE 13th St, rm 2B2418, Oklahoma City, OK 73104; **Phone:** 405-271-8685; **Board Cert:** Pediatrics 1975; Clinical Genetics 1982; **Med School:** Univ Wash 1969; **Resid:** Pediatrics, Johns Hopkins Hosp 1974; **Fellow:** Research, NCI-Natl Inst Hlth 1972; **Fac Appt:** Prof CG, Univ Okla Coll Med

Northrup, Hope MD [CG] - **Spec Exp:** Biochemical Genetics; Neuro-Genetics; Dysmorphology; **Hospital:** Meml Hermann Hosp - Texas Med Ctr, LBJ General Hosp; **Address:** Univ TX Med Sch, Dept Peds-Div Med Genetics, rm MSB-3.144, Box 20708, Houston, TX 77225-0708; **Phone:** 713-500-5760; **Board Cert:** Pediatrics 1988; Clinical Genetics 1990; Clinical Biochemical Genetics 1990; **Med School:** Med Univ SC 1983; **Resid:** Pediatrics, Chldns Med Ctr-Univ Tex SW 1986; **Fellow:** Medical Genetics, Inst Molec Gene-Baylor Coll Med 1989; **Fac Appt:** Prof Ped, Univ Tex, Houston

Plon, Sharon E MD/PhD [CG] - **Spec Exp:** Hereditary Cancer; Cancer Risk Assessment; Breast Cancer Risk Assessment; Ovarian Cancer Genetics; **Hospital:** Texas Chldns Hosp, St Luke's Episcopal Hosp-Houston; **Address:** Kleberg Genetics Ctr, Texas Chldn's Hosp, 6621 Fannin St, MC 3-3320, Houston, TX 77030; **Phone:** 832-824-4251; **Board Cert:** Clinical Genetics 2006; **Med School:** Harvard Med Sch 1987; **Resid:** Internal Medicine, Univ Washington Affil Hosp 1988; **Fellow:** Molecular Genetics, National Cancer Inst 1990; Medical Genetics, Fred Hutchinson Cancer Research Ctr 1993; **Fac Appt:** Prof CG, Baylor Coll Med

West Coast and Pacific

Boles, Richard G MD [CG] - **Spec Exp:** Mitochondrial Disorders; Vomiting-Cyclic; **Hospital:** Chldns Hosp - Los Angeles; **Address:** 4650 Sunset Blvd, MS 90, Los Angeles, CA 90027; **Phone:** 323-361-2178; **Board Cert:** Clinical Genetics 2006; Clinical Biochemical Genetics 2006; Pediatrics 2002; **Med School:** UCLA 1987; **Resid:** Pediatrics, Harbor-UCLA Med Ctr 1990; **Fellow:** Genetics and Metabolism, Yale Univ Sch Med 1993; **Fac Appt:** Assoc Prof Ped, USC Sch Med

Clinical Genetics

Cassidy, Suzanne MD [CG] - **Spec Exp:** Prader-Willi Syndrome; Connective Tissue Disorders; Neurocutaneous Disorders; **Hospital:** UCSF Med Ctr; **Address:** 533 Parnassus Ave, rm U-100A, Box 0706, San Francisco, CA 94143; **Phone:** 415-476-2757; **Board Cert:** Pediatrics 1982; Clinical Genetics 1983; **Med School:** Vanderbilt Univ 1976; **Resid:** Pediatrics, Univ Wash Affil Prgms 1979; **Fellow:** Clinical Genetics, Univ Wash 1981; **Fac Appt:** Prof Ped, UC Irvine

Cederbaum, Stephen D MD [CG] - **Spec Exp:** Inborn Errors of Metabolism; **Hospital:** UCLA Ronald Reagan Med Ctr; **Address:** 635 Charles E Young Drive S, rm 347, Los Angeles, CA 90095-7332; **Phone:** 310-825-0402; **Board Cert:** Clinical Genetics 1982; Clinical Biochemical Genetics 1982; **Med School:** NYU Sch Med 1964; **Resid:** Internal Medicine, Barnes Hosp 1966; **Fellow:** Clinical Genetics, Univ Wash 1970; **Fac Appt:** Prof Ped, UCLA

Curry, Cynthia J MD [CG] - **Hospital:** Chldns Hosp Central CA, Comm Regl Med Ctr - Fresno; **Address:** Genetic Medicine Central California, 351 E Barstow, Ste 106, Fresno, CA 93710-6073; **Phone:** 559-227-4472; **Board Cert:** Pediatrics 1973; Clinical Genetics 1982; **Med School:** Yale Univ 1967; **Resid:** Pediatrics, Univ Wash Orth Chldns Hosp 1969; Pediatrics, Univ Minn Hosp 1970; **Fellow:** Dysmorphology, UCSF Med Ctr 1976; **Fac Appt:** Prof CG, UCSF

Falk, Rena MD [CG] - **Spec Exp:** Prenatal Diagnosis; Mental Retardation; Prenatal Genetic Diagnosis; **Hospital:** Cedars-Sinai Med Ctr; **Address:** 8700 Beverly Blvd, MOT West 1150, Los Angeles, CA 90048; **Phone:** 310-423-9914; **Board Cert:** Pediatrics 1976; Clinical Genetics 1982; Clinical Cytogenetics 1984; **Med School:** UCLA 1971; **Resid:** Pediatrics, Cedars-Sinai Med Ctr 1973; **Fellow:** Clinical Genetics, UCLA Med Schl 1975; UCLA 1977; **Fac Appt:** Prof Ped, UCLA

Graham Jr, John M MD [CG] - **Spec Exp:** Dysmorphology; Craniofacial Disorders; Mental Retardation; **Hospital:** Cedars-Sinai Med Ctr; **Address:** 8700 Beverly Blvd, MOT West 1150, Los Angeles, CA 90048; **Phone:** 310-423-9914; **Board Cert:** Pediatrics 1982; Clinical Genetics 1982; **Med School:** Med Univ SC 1975; **Resid:** Pediatrics, Boston Chldns Hosp-Harvard 1977; **Fellow:** Developmental-Behavioral Pediatrics, Boston Chldns Hosp 1978; Dysmorphology, Univ Wash 1980; **Fac Appt:** Prof Ped, UCLA

Grody, Wayne W MD/PhD [CG] - **Spec Exp:** Genetic Disorders; Hereditary Cancer; **Address:** UCLA School Medicine, Div, Med Genetic & Molecular Pathology, 10833 Le Conte Ave, Los Angeles, CA 90095-1732; **Phone:** 310-825-5648; **Board Cert:** Clinical Genetics 1990; Anatomic & Clinical Pathology 1987; Clinical Biochemical Genetics 1990; Molecular Genetic Pathology 2001; **Med School:** Baylor Coll Med 1977; **Resid:** Pathology, UCLA Med Ctr 1986; **Fellow:** Clinical Genetics, UCLA Med Ctr 1987; **Fac Appt:** Prof CG, UCLA

Hudgins, Louanne MD [CG] - **Spec Exp:** Congenital Anomalies-Limb; **Hospital:** Stanford Univ Med Ctr; **Address:** Stanford Univ Med Ctr, Dept Pediatrics-Medical Genetics, 300 Pasteur Drive, rm H315, Stanford, CA 94305; **Phone:** 650-723-6858; **Board Cert:** Pediatrics 2004; Clinical Genetics 2006; **Med School:** Univ Kans 1984; **Resid:** Pediatrics, Univ Conn Hlth Ctr 1987; **Fellow:** Clinical Genetics, Univ Conn Hlth Ctr 1990; **Fac Appt:** Assoc Prof Ped, Stanford Univ

Jonas, Adam J MD [CG] - **Spec Exp:** Biochemical Genetics; Inherited Disorders; **Hospital:** LAC - Harbor - UCLA Med Ctr; **Address:** Harbor-UCLA Med Ctr, Div Med Genetics, 1000 W Carson St, Box 17, Torrance, CA 90509-2910; **Phone:** 310-222-2301; **Board Cert:** Pediatrics 1982; Clinical Biochemical Genetics 1987; Clinical Genetics 1990; **Med School:** UCSD 1976; **Resid:** Pediatrics, Chldns Ortho Hosp 1978; Pediatrics, Univ Hosp 1979; **Fellow:** Genetics and Metabolism, UCSD Sch Med 1982; **Fac Appt:** Prof Ped, UCLA

Jones, Marilyn MD [CG] - **Spec Exp:** Dysmorphology; Craniofacial Disorders; **Hospital:** Rady Children's Hosp - San Diego, UCSD Med Ctr; **Address:** 3020 Children's Way, MC 5031, San Diego, CA 92123-2746; **Phone:** 858-966-5840; **Board Cert:** Pediatrics 1979; Clinical Genetics 2006; **Med School:** Columbia P&S 1974; **Resid:** Internal Medicine, UCSD Med Ctr 1977; Pediatrics, UCSD Med Ctr 1978; **Fellow:** Dysmorphology, UCSD Med Ctr 1979

Morris, Colleen A MD [CG] - **Spec Exp:** Williams Syndrome; Inherited Disorders; Fetal Alcohol Syndrome; **Hospital:** Univ Med Ctr - Las Vegas; **Address:** Univ Nevada Sch Medicine, Dept Pediatrics/Genetics, 2040 W Charleston Blvd, Ste 401, Las Vegas, NV 89102; **Phone:** 702-671-2200; **Board Cert:** Pediatrics 1986; Clinical Genetics 1987; **Med School:** Loyola Univ-Stritch Sch Med 1981; **Resid:** Pediatrics, Phoenix Hosp 1984; **Fellow:** Clinical Genetics, Univ Utah Sch Med 1986; **Fac Appt:** Prof Ped, Univ Nevada

Nussbaum, Robert MD [CG] - **Spec Exp:** Genetic Disorders; **Hospital:** UCSF Med Ctr; **Address:** Inst Human Genetics, 513 Parnassus Ave, rm HSE901E, San Francisco, CA 94143-0794; **Phone:** 415-476-1127; **Board Cert:** Internal Medicine 1978; Clinical Genetics 1982; Clinical Molecular Genetics 2004; **Med School:** Harvard Med Sch 1975; **Resid:** Internal Medicine, Barnes Hosp 1978; **Fellow:** Clinical Genetics, Baylor Univ 1983

Pagon, Roberta A MD [CG] - **Spec Exp:** Eye Diseases-Hereditary; Sexual Differentiation Disorders; **Hospital:** Chldns Hosp and Regl Med Ctr - Seattle; **Address:** Chldns Hosp Med Ctr, 4800 Sand Point Way, Box 5371, MS A7937, Seattle, WA 98105; **Phone:** 206-987-2056; **Board Cert:** Pediatrics 1978; Clinical Genetics 1982; **Med School:** Harvard Med Sch 1972; **Resid:** Pediatrics, Univ Wash Affil Hosp 1975; **Fellow:** Clinical Genetics, Univ Wash 1979; **Fac Appt:** Prof Ped, Univ Wash

Randolph, Linda MD [CG] - **Spec Exp:** Dysmorphology; Skeletal Dysplasia; Prenatal Genetic Diagnosis; Neurofibromatosis; **Hospital:** Chldns Hosp - Los Angeles, Hollywood Comm Hosp - Van Nuys; **Address:** 4650 Sunset Blvd, MS 90, Los Angeles, CA 90027; **Phone:** 323-361-2178; **Board Cert:** Pediatrics 1987; Clinical Genetics 1987; Clinical Cytogenetics 1990; **Med School:** Geo Wash Univ 1982; **Resid:** Pediatrics, Chldns Natl Med Ctr 1985; **Fellow:** Clinical Molecular Genetics, Harbor-UCLA Med Ctr & Cedar-Sinai Med Ctr 1989; **Fac Appt:** Asst Prof Ped, USC-Keck School of Medicine

Rimoin, David L MD/PhD [CG] - **Spec Exp:** Skeletal Dysplasia; Marfan's Syndrome; Birth Defects; **Hospital:** Cedars-Sinai Med Ctr; **Address:** 8700 Beverly Blvd, MOT West 1150, Los Angeles, CA 90048; **Phone:** 310-423-9914; **Board Cert:** Internal Medicine 1968; Clinical Genetics 1984; **Med School:** McGill Univ 1961; **Resid:** Internal Medicine, Royal Victoria Hosp 1963; Internal Medicine, Johns Hopkins Hosp 1964; **Fellow:** Clinical Genetics, Johns Hopkins Hosp 1967; **Fac Appt:** Prof Ped, UCLA

Seaver, Laurie H MD [CG] - **Spec Exp:** Birth Defects; Fetal Alcohol Syndrome; Dysmorphology; **Hospital:** Kapiolani Med Ctr for Women & Chldn, Queen's Med Ctr - Honolulu; **Address:** Hawaii Community Genetics, 1441 Kapiolani Blvd, Ste 1800, Honolulu, HI 96814; **Phone:** 808-973-3403; **Board Cert:** Pediatrics 2005; Clinical Genetics 2006; **Med School:** Univ Ariz Coll Med 1987; **Resid:** Pediatrics, Univ Ariz 1990; **Fellow:** Clinical Genetics, Univ Ariz Coll Med 1993

Weitzel, Jeffrey N MD [CG] - **Spec Exp:** Breast Cancer; Ovarian Cancer; Hereditary Cancer; **Hospital:** City of Hope Natl Med Ctr & Beckman Rsch; **Address:** City of Hope Cancer Ctr, 1500 E Duarte Rd, Duarte, CA 91010; **Phone:** 626-256-8662; **Board Cert:** Internal Medicine 1986; Medical Oncology 1989; Clinical Genetics 1996; **Med School:** Univ Minn 1983; **Resid:** Internal Medicine, Univ Minn Hosps 1986; Hematology, Hammersmith Hosp 1987; **Fellow:** Hematology & Oncology, Tufts -New England Med Ctr 1992; Clinical Genetics, Tufts-New England Med Ctr 1996; **Fac Appt:** Assoc Clin Prof Med, USC Sch Med

Clinical Genetics

Wilcox Jr, William R MD [CG] - **Spec Exp:** Inborn Errors of Metabolism; Skeletal Dysplasia; **Hospital:** Cedars-Sinai Med Ctr; **Address:** Cedars Sinai Med Ctr, Dept Med Genetics, 8700 Beverly Blvd, Ste 1150 West, Los Angeles, CA 90048; **Phone:** 310-423-9914; **Board Cert:** Clinical Genetics 2006; Clinical Biochemical Genetics 2007; Clinical Molecular Genetics 2007; **Med School:** UCLA 1988; **Resid:** Pediatrics, UCLA Med Ctr 1991; **Fellow:** Clinical Genetics, Cedars-Sinai Med Ctr 1994; **Fac Appt:** Prof Ped, UCLA

THE MOUNT SINAI MEDICAL CENTER
GENETICS AND GENOMIC SCIENCES

One Gustave L. Levy Place
Fifth Avenue and 100th Street
New York, NY 10029-6574
Physician Referral: 1-800-MD-SINAI (637-4624)
www.mountsinai.org

THE DEPARTMENT OF GENETICS AND GENOMIC SCIENCES at The Mount Sinai Medical Center is one of the largest medical genetics centers in the nation, providing expert diagnostic, therapeutic, and counseling services for patients and families with genetic disorders, birth defects, and pregnancy loss. The Department performs sophisticated diagnostic tests in its state-of-the-art DNA, biochemical, and cytogenetics laboratories.

The Department has more than 50 internationally recognized physician and scientist faculty members, 10 experienced genetic counselors, and a full support and research staff of more than 150 people who provide expert clinical services.

Programs and services offered by the Department include:

- Cardiovascular Genetics Program
- Comprehensive genetic diagnostic and counseling services
- Clinical and laboratory evaluation of patients with genetic disorders, birth defects, and reproductive loss
- Ethnicity-based carrier screening programs
- Prenatal diagnostic services
- Cancer genetic counseling program
- The Center for Jewish Genetic Disease
- Program for Inherited Metabolic Diseases
- The Comprehensive Gaucher Disease Treatment Program
- The International Center for Fabry Disease
- The International Center for Types A and B Niemann-Pick Disease
- Cleft and Craniofacial Program

GROUNDBREAKING RESEARCH AND NEW FORMS OF TREATMENT Diseases and conditions run in families. In fact, there are more than 10,000 known genetic disorders, and current research is identifying the genetic susceptibilities or predispositions for many common diseases and cancers. The Department of Genetics and Genomic Sciences at Mount Sinai is performing research to develop new and improved methods for the diagnosis, prevention, and treatment of rare and common diseases. The Human Genome Project and advances in gene therapy and stem cell biology have accelerated this research.

Advances In Diagnosis And Disease Treatment – In the past several years, Mount Sinai researchers have had remarkable success in identifying the genes responsible for genetic diseases and in developing new treatments for inherited disorders. The following are some examples and results of this important work:

- Research pioneered by the Department of Genetics and Genomic Sciences resulted in the development of a safe, effective, FDA-approved treatment for Fabry disease, an inherited metabolic disorder that can cause kidney failure, heart disease, stroke, and premature death.

- Departmental faculty have developed a treatment for Niemann-Pick Type B disease, a hereditary disorder that results in death in childhood or early adulthood.

- We have identified the genes responsible for several diseases, including a debilitating juvenile arthritis, dystonia, and an inherited form of obesity. The identification of these genes may lead to greater understanding of and new treatments for these diseases. We have also recently identified a gene linked to prostate cancer.

- Our researchers have identified three genes causing Noonan syndrome, a common genetic disorder that causes congenital heart defects. Affected families can now receive early diagnosis and prevention.

Colon & Rectal Surgery

A colon and rectal surgeon is trained to diagnose and treat various diseases of the intestinal tract, colon, rectum, anal canal and perianal area by medical and surgical means. This specialist also deals with other organs and tissues (such as the liver and gallbladder) involved with primary
intestinal disease.

Colon and rectal surgeons have the expertise to diagnose and often manage anorectal conditions such as hemorrhoids, fissures (painful tears in the anal lining), abscesses and fistulae (infections located around the anus and rectum) in the office setting. They also treat problems of the intestine and colon and perform endoscopic procedures to evaluate and treat problems such as cancer, polyps (precancerous growths) and inflammatory conditions.

Training Required: Six years (including general surgery)

COLON & RECTAL SURGERY

New England

Bleday, Ronald MD [CRS] - **Spec Exp:** Colon & Rectal Cancer; **Hospital:** Brigham & Women's Hosp, Dana-Farber Cancer Inst; **Address:** Brigham & Women's Hosp, Dept Genl Surg, 75 Francis St, ASB II, Boston, MA 02115; **Phone:** 617-732-8460; **Board Cert:** Surgery 1999; Colon & Rectal Surgery 2003; **Med School:** McGill Univ 1982; **Resid:** Surgery, Rhode Island Hosp 1989; Surgical Oncology, Brigham & Womens Hosp 1986; **Fellow:** Endoscopy, Mass Genl Hosp 1990; Colon & Rectal Surgery, Univ Minn 1991; **Fac Appt:** Assoc Prof S, Harvard Med Sch

Harnsberger, Jeffrey R MD [CRS] - **Spec Exp:** Inflammatory Bowel Disease; Colon & Rectal Cancer; **Hospital:** Dartmouth - Hitchcock Med Ctr, Elliot Hosp; **Address:** Dartmouth-Hitchcock Manchester, 100 Hitchcock Way, Manchester, NH 03104; **Phone:** 603-695-2840; **Board Cert:** Surgery 2001; Colon & Rectal Surgery 2005; **Med School:** Med Coll OH 1987; **Resid:** Surgery, Dartamouth-Hitchcock Med Ctr 1992; **Fellow:** Colon & Rectal Surgery, St Louis Univ Med Ctr 1993; **Fac Appt:** Asst Prof S, Dartmouth Med Sch

Hyman, Neil H MD [CRS] - **Spec Exp:** Inflammatory Bowel Disease; Colon & Rectal Cancer; **Hospital:** Fletcher Allen Health Care- Med Ctr Campus; **Address:** FAHC 111 Colchester Ave, 111 Colchester Ave, Burlington, VT 05401; **Phone:** 802-847-3339; **Board Cert:** Surgery 1998; Colon & Rectal Surgery 2003; **Med School:** Univ VT Coll Med 1984; **Resid:** Surgery, Mt Sinai Med Ctr 1989; **Fellow:** Colon & Rectal Surgery, Cleveland Clinic 1990; **Fac Appt:** Prof S, Univ VT Coll Med

Longo, Walter E MD [CRS] - **Spec Exp:** Colon & Rectal Cancer; Gastrointestinal Surgery; Inflammatory Bowel Disease; **Hospital:** Yale-New Haven Hosp; **Address:** Yale Univ School Medicine, Dept Surgery/Gastroenterology, Box 208062, New Haven, CT 06520-8062; **Phone:** 203-785-2616; **Board Cert:** Surgery 2001; Colon & Rectal Surgery 2006; **Med School:** NY Med Coll 1984; **Resid:** Surgery, Yale-New Haven Hosp 1990; **Fellow:** Research, Yale-New Haven Hosp 1988; Colon & Rectal Surgery, Cleveland Clinic 1991; **Fac Appt:** Prof S, Yale Univ

Nagle, Deborah A MD [CRS] - **Spec Exp:** Colon & Rectal Cancer; Anal Cancer; Laparoscopic Surgery; **Hospital:** Beth Israel Deaconess Med Ctr - Boston; **Address:** Beth Israel Deaconess Med Ctr, 330 Brookline Ave Stoneman Bldg - rm 932, Boston, MA 02215; **Phone:** 617-667-4159; **Board Cert:** Colon & Rectal Surgery 2006; Surgery 2004; **Med School:** Univ Pennsylvania 1988; **Resid:** Surgery, Graduate Hosp 1993; Colon & Rectal Surgery, Thos Jefferson Univ Hosp 1994

Read, Thomas E MD [CRS] - **Spec Exp:** Colon & Rectal Cancer; Inflammatory Bowel Disease; Laparoscopic Surgery; **Hospital:** Lahey Clin; **Address:** Lahey Clinic, 41 Mall Rd, 6 West, Burlington, MA 01805; **Phone:** 781-744-8971; **Board Cert:** Surgery 2005; Colon & Rectal Surgery 2006; **Med School:** UCSF 1988; **Resid:** Surgery, UCSF Med Ctr 1995; **Fellow:** Colon & Rectal Surgery, Lahey Clinic 1996; **Fac Appt:** Assoc Prof S, Tufts Univ

Roberts, Patricia L MD [CRS] - **Spec Exp:** Diverticulitis; Colon & Rectal Cancer; Inflammatory Bowel Disease; **Hospital:** Lahey Clin; **Address:** 41 Mall Rd, Burlington, MA 01805; **Phone:** 781-744-8243; **Board Cert:** Surgery 1996; Colon & Rectal Surgery 2003; **Med School:** Boston Univ 1981; **Resid:** Surgery, Boston City Hosp 1986; **Fellow:** Colon & Rectal Surgery, Lahey Clinic 1988; **Fac Appt:** Prof S, Tufts Univ

Schoetz Jr, David J MD [CRS] - **Spec Exp:** Inflammatory Bowel Disease/Crohn's; Colon & Rectal Cancer; Incontinence-Fecal; Anorectal Disorders; **Hospital:** Lahey Clin; **Address:** Lahey Clin Med Ctr, Dept Colon & Rectal Surg, 41 Mall Rd, Burlington, MA 01805-0001; **Phone:** 781-744-8889; **Board Cert:** Surgery 2001; Colon & Rectal Surgery 1983; **Med School:** Med Coll Wisc 1974; **Resid:** Surgery, Boston Univ Med Ctr 1981; Surgery, Boston Univ Med Ctr 1978; **Fellow:** Colon & Rectal Surgery, Lahey Clin 1982; **Fac Appt:** Prof S, Tufts Univ

Shellito, Paul C MD [CRS] - **Spec Exp:** Colon & Rectal Cancer; Ulcerative Colitis; Anorectal Disorders; **Hospital:** Mass Genl Hosp; **Address:** 15 Parkman St, Ste 460, Boston, MA 02114-3117; **Phone:** 617-724-0365; **Board Cert:** Surgery 2002; Colon & Rectal Surgery 1994; **Med School:** Harvard Med Sch 1977; **Resid:** Surgery, Mass Genl Hosp 1983; Surgery, Auckland Univ Med Sch 1981; **Fellow:** Colon & Rectal Surgery, Univ Minn 1985; **Fac Appt:** Asst Prof S, Harvard Med Sch

Mid Atlantic

Caushaj, Fillor Philip MD [CRS] - **Spec Exp:** Colon & Rectal Cancer; Inflammatory Bowel Disease; Laparoscopic Surgery; **Hospital:** Montefiore Med Ctr - Div. Moses, Montefiore Med Ctr - Div. Weiler; **Address:** 1575 Blondell Ave Fl 2 - Ste 125, Bronx, NY 10461; **Phone:** 718-405-8240; **Board Cert:** Colon & Rectal Surgery 1986; Surgery 2004; **Med School:** Johns Hopkins Univ 1979; **Resid:** Surgery, Columbia-Presby Med Ctr 1984; **Fellow:** Colon & Rectal Surgery, Lahey Clinic 1985; **Fac Appt:** Prof S, Albert Einstein Coll Med

Eisenstat, Theodore E MD [CRS] - **Spec Exp:** Colon Cancer; Inflammatory Bowel Disease; Anorectal Disorders; Hemorrhoids; **Hospital:** Robert Wood Johnson Univ Hosp - New Brunswick, JFK Med Ctr - Edison; **Address:** 3900 Park Ave, Ste 101, Edison, NJ 08820-3032; **Phone:** 732-494-6640; **Board Cert:** Surgery 1974; Colon & Rectal Surgery 1994; **Med School:** NY Med Coll 1968; **Resid:** Surgery, Thomas Jefferson Univ Hosp 1971; Surgery, Pennsylvania Hosp 1973; **Fellow:** Colon & Rectal Surgery, Muhlenberg Med Ctr 1978; **Fac Appt:** Clin Prof S, UMDNJ-RW Johnson Med Sch

Fry, Robert D MD [CRS] - **Spec Exp:** Colon & Rectal Cancer; Inflammatory Bowel Disease/Crohn's; Anal Cancer; Hemorrhoids; **Hospital:** Pennsylvania Hosp (page 60), Hosp Univ Penn - UPHS (page 60); **Address:** Pennsylvania Hospital, Div Colon & Rectal Surgery, 700 Spruce St, Ste 305, Philadelphia, PA 19106-4023; **Phone:** 215-829-5333; **Board Cert:** Surgery 2006; Colon & Rectal Surgery 1998; **Med School:** Washington Univ, St Louis 1972; **Resid:** Surgery, Barnes Jewish Hosp 1977; **Fellow:** Colon & Rectal Surgery, Cleveland Clinic 1978; **Fac Appt:** Prof S, Univ Pennsylvania

Gingold, Bruce S MD [CRS] - **Spec Exp:** Colostomy Avoidance; Inflammatory Bowel Disease/Crohn's; Anorectal Disorders; Colon & Rectal Cancer; **Hospital:** St Vincent Cath Med Ctrs - Manhattan; **Address:** 36 7th Ave, Ste 522, New York, NY 10011-6600; **Phone:** 212-675-2997; **Board Cert:** Colon & Rectal Surgery 1976; **Med School:** Jefferson Med Coll 1970; **Resid:** Surgery, St Vincent's Hosp & Med Ctr 1975; **Fellow:** Colon & Rectal Surgery, Cleveland Clinic 1976; **Fac Appt:** Assoc Clin Prof S, NY Med Coll

Goldstein, Scott D MD [CRS] - **Spec Exp:** Colon & Rectal Cancer; Inflammatory Bowel Disease; Laparoscopic Surgery; **Hospital:** Thomas Jefferson Univ Hosp; **Address:** 1100 Walnut St, Ste 500, Philadelphia, PA 19107; **Phone:** 215-955-5869; **Board Cert:** Surgery 1984; Colon & Rectal Surgery 1985; **Med School:** SUNY Buffalo 1978; **Resid:** Surgery, Lenox Hill Hosp 1983; Colon & Rectal Surgery, UMDNJ Med Ctr 1984; **Fac Appt:** Assoc Prof S, Thomas Jefferson Univ

Colon & Rectal Surgery

Gorfine, Stephen R MD [CRS] - **Spec Exp:** Anal Disorders & Reconstruction; Hemorrhoids; Rectal Cancer; Anal Cancer; **Hospital:** Mount Sinai Med Ctr (page 64), Lenox Hill Hosp (page 62); **Address:** 25 E 69th St, New York, NY 10021-4925; **Phone:** 212-517-8600; **Board Cert:** Internal Medicine 1981; Surgery 2007; Colon & Rectal Surgery 1988; **Med School:** Univ Mass Sch Med 1978; **Resid:** Internal Medicine, Mt Sinai Hosp 1981; Surgery, Mt Sinai Hosp 1985; **Fellow:** Colon & Rectal Surgery, Ferguson Hosp 1987; **Fac Appt:** Clin Prof S, Mount Sinai Sch Med

Guillem, Jose MD [CRS] - **Spec Exp:** Colon & Rectal Cancer; Rectal Cancer/Sphincter Preservation; Colon & Rectal Cancer-Hereditary; Peritoneal Mucinous Carcinomatosis; **Hospital:** Meml Sloan-Kettering Cancer Ctr; **Address:** 1275 York Avenue, New York, NY 10065; **Phone:** 212-639-8278; **Board Cert:** Colon & Rectal Surgery 2005; Surgery 2004; **Med School:** Yale Univ 1983; **Resid:** Surgery, Columbia-Presby Med Ctr 1990; **Fellow:** Colon & Rectal Surgery, Lahey Clinic 1991; **Fac Appt:** Prof CRS, Cornell Univ-Weill Med Coll

Medich, David MD [CRS] - **Spec Exp:** Colon & Rectal Cancer; Ulcerative Colitis; Inflammatory Bowel Disease/Crohn's; **Hospital:** Allegheny General Hosp; **Address:** Allegheny General Hosp, South Tower, 320 E North Ave Fl 5, Pittsburgh, PA 15212; **Phone:** 412-359-3901; **Board Cert:** Surgery 2004; Colon & Rectal Surgery 2006; **Med School:** Ohio State Univ 1987; **Resid:** Surgery, Univ Pittsburgh 1990; **Fellow:** Research, Univ Pittsburgh 1993; Colon & Rectal Surgery, Cleveland Clinic 1994; **Fac Appt:** Assoc Prof CRS, Drexel Univ Coll Med

Milsom, Jeffrey W MD [CRS] - **Spec Exp:** Inflammatory Bowel Disease; Laparoscopic Surgery; Colon & Rectal Cancer; Crohn's Disease; **Hospital:** NY-Presby Hosp/Weill Cornell (page 66); **Address:** NY Cornell Med Ctr, Div Colorectal Surgery, 1315 York Ave Fl 2, New York, NY 10065-5304; **Phone:** 212-746-6030; **Board Cert:** Colon & Rectal Surgery 1986; **Med School:** Univ Pittsburgh 1979; **Resid:** Surgery, Roosevelt Hosp 1981; Surgery, Univ Virginia Med Ctr 1984; **Fellow:** Colon & Rectal Surgery, Ferguson Hosp 1985; **Fac Appt:** Prof S, Cornell Univ-Weill Med Coll

Rombeau, John L MD [CRS] - **Spec Exp:** Colon & Rectal Cancer; Inflammatory Bowel Disease/Crohn's; Ulcerative Colitis; Rectal Cancer/Sphincter Preservation; **Hospital:** Temple Univ Hosp; **Address:** Department of Surgery, 3401 N Broad St, Parkinson Pavilion Fl 4, Philadelphia, PA 19104-5103; **Phone:** 215-707-3133; **Board Cert:** Colon & Rectal Surgery 1977; **Med School:** Loma Linda Univ 1967; **Resid:** Surgery, Good Samaritan Hosp 1971; Surgery, LAC-USC Med Ctr 1975; **Fellow:** Colon & Rectal Surgery, Cleveland Clinic 1976; Nutrition & Metabolism, Brigham & Women's Hosp 1977; **Fac Appt:** Prof S, Temple Univ

Stein, David E MD [CRS] - **Spec Exp:** Colon & Rectal Cancer & Surgery; Laparoscopic Surgery; Inflammatory Bowel Disease; Anorectal Disorders; **Hospital:** Hahnemann Univ Hosp; **Address:** 245 N 15th St, #4013, Philadelphia, PA 19102; **Phone:** 215-762-1545; **Board Cert:** Surgery 2004; Colon & Rectal Surgery 2004; **Med School:** SUNY Downstate 1997; **Resid:** Surgery, T Jefferson Univ Hosp 2002; **Fellow:** Colon & Rectal Surgery, Cleveland Clinic 2003; **Fac Appt:** Asst Prof S, Drexel Univ Coll Med

Steinhagen, Randolph MD [CRS] - **Spec Exp:** Colostomy Avoidance; Colon & Rectal Cancer; Inflammatory Bowel Disease/Crohn's; **Hospital:** Mount Sinai Med Ctr (page 64); **Address:** Div Colon & Rectal Surgery, 5 E 98th St Fl 14, Box 1259, New York, NY 10029-6501; **Phone:** 212-241-3547; **Board Cert:** Surgery 2002; Colon & Rectal Surgery 1985; **Med School:** Wayne State Univ 1977; **Resid:** Surgery, Mount Sinai Hosp 1982; **Fellow:** Colon & Rectal Surgery, Cleveland Clinic 1983; **Fac Appt:** Assoc Prof S, Mount Sinai Sch Med

Whelan, Richard L MD [CRS] - **Spec Exp:** Laparoscopic Surgery; Colon & Rectal Cancer; **Hospital:** St Luke's - Roosevelt Hosp Ctr - Roosevelt Div (page 57); **Address:** 425 W 59th St, Ste 7B, New York, NY 10019; **Phone:** 212-523-8172; **Board Cert:** Surgery 1997; Colon & Rectal Surgery 1989; **Med School:** Columbia P&S 1982; **Resid:** Surgery, Columbia Presby Hosp 1987; **Fellow:** Colon & Rectal Surgery, Univ Minn Med Ctr 1988; **Fac Appt:** Assoc Clin Prof S, Columbia P&S

Wong, W Douglas MD [CRS] - **Spec Exp:** Rectal Cancer/Sphincter Preservation; Colon & Rectal Cancer; Anal Disorders & Reconstruction; **Hospital:** Meml Sloan-Kettering Cancer Ctr; **Address:** 1275 York Ave, Ste C-1067, New York, NY 10065; **Phone:** 212-639-5117; **Board Cert:** Surgery 1997; Colon & Rectal Surgery 2004; **Med School:** Univ Manitoba 1972; **Resid:** Surgery, Univ Manitoba Hosp 1977; **Fellow:** Colon & Rectal Surgery, Univ Minn Med Ctr 1984; **Fac Appt:** Prof S, Cornell Univ-Weill Med Coll

Southeast

Galandiuk, Susan MD [CRS] - **Spec Exp:** Colon & Rectal Cancer; Inflammatory Bowel Disease/Crohn's; **Hospital:** Univ of Louisville Hosp, Norton Hosp; **Address:** 401 E Chestnut St, Ste 710, Louisville, KY 40202; **Phone:** 502-583-8303; **Board Cert:** Surgery 2008; Colon & Rectal Surgery 2002; **Med School:** Germany 1982; **Resid:** Surgery, Cleveland Clinic Fdtn 1988; **Fellow:** Research, Univ Louisville Hosp 1989; Colon & Rectal Surgery, Mayo Clinic 1990; **Fac Appt:** Prof CRS, Univ Louisville Sch Med

Golub, Richard W MD [CRS] - **Spec Exp:** Colon & Rectal Cancer; Laparoscopic Surgery; Hemorrhoids; **Hospital:** Sarasota Meml Hosp, Doctors Hosp - Sarasota; **Address:** Surgical Specialists, 3333 Cattlemen Rd, Ste 206, Sarasota, FL 34232; **Phone:** 941-341-0042; **Board Cert:** Surgery 2000; Colon & Rectal Surgery 2003; **Med School:** Albert Einstein Coll Med 1984; **Resid:** Surgery, Univ Hosp 1990; **Fellow:** Colon & Rectal Surgery, Grant Medical Center 1991

Hartmann, Rene F MD [CRS] - **Spec Exp:** Laparoscopic Surgery; Rectovaginal Fistula; Colon Cancer; Inflammatory Bowel Disease; **Hospital:** Mercy Hosp, Baptist Hosp of Miami; **Address:** Laparoscopic Ctr of S Florida, 9195 Sunset Drive, Ste 230, Miami, FL 33173; **Phone:** 305-271-0300; **Board Cert:** Colon & Rectal Surgery 1994; **Med School:** Venezuela 1971; **Resid:** Surgery, Jackson Meml Hosp 1976; Surgery, Orange Meml Hosp 1977; **Fellow:** Colon & Rectal Surgery, Grant Hosp 1978; **Fac Appt:** Assoc Clin Prof S, Univ Miami Sch Med

Mantyh, Christopher MD [CRS] - **Spec Exp:** Inflammatory Bowel Disease; Colon & Rectal Cancer & Surgery; Rectal Cancer/Sphincter Preservation; Incontinence-Fecal; **Hospital:** Duke Univ Med Ctr; **Address:** 200 Trent Drive, Durham, NC 27710; **Phone:** 919-681-3977; **Board Cert:** Surgery 1999; Colon & Rectal Surgery 2000; **Med School:** Univ Wisc 1991; **Resid:** Surgery, Duke Univ Med Ctr 1998; **Fellow:** Colon & Rectal Surgery, Cleveland Clinic 1999

Marcet, Jorge MD [CRS] - **Spec Exp:** Colon & Rectal Cancer; **Hospital:** Tampa Genl Hosp; **Address:** 1 Tampa General Cir, Ste F145, Tampa, FL 33606; **Phone:** 813-844-4545; **Board Cert:** Surgery 2001; Colon & Rectal Surgery 2003; **Med School:** Cornell Univ-Weill Med Coll 1985; **Resid:** Surgery, St Luke's-Roosevelt Med Ctr 1990; **Fellow:** Colon & Rectal Surgery, Columbia Presby Med Ctr 1990; Colon & Rectal Surgery, St Luke's-Roosevelt Med Ctr 1991; **Fac Appt:** Assoc Prof S, Univ S Fla Coll Med

Nogueras, Juan J MD [CRS] - **Spec Exp:** Colon & Rectal Cancer; Inflammatory Bowel Disease/Crohn's; Incontinence-Fecal; **Hospital:** Cleveland Clin - Weston; **Address:** Cleveland Clinic, Dept Colorectal Surgery, 2950 Cleveland Clinic Blvd, Weston, FL 33331; **Phone:** 954-659-5251; **Board Cert:** Surgery 2007; Colon & Rectal Surgery 2003; **Med School:** Jefferson Med Coll 1982; **Resid:** Surgery, Columbia Presby Med Ctr 1987; **Fellow:** Colon & Rectal Surgery, Univ Minn Med Ctr 1991

Colon & Rectal Surgery

Vernava III, Anthony M MD [CRS] - **Spec Exp:** Colon & Rectal Cancer; Incontinence-Fecal; Inflammatory Bowel Disease; **Hospital:** Physicians Regl Med Ctr; **Address:** Medical Surgical Specialists, 6101 Pine Ridge Rd, Naples, FL 34119; **Phone:** 239-348-4400; **Board Cert:** Surgery 2007; Colon & Rectal Surgery 1989; **Med School:** St Louis Univ 1982; **Resid:** Surgery, St Louis Univ Med Ctr 1988; Colon & Rectal Surgery, Univ Minnesota Med Ctr 1989; **Fellow:** Colon & Rectal Surgery, St Marks Hosp 1990

Wexner, Steven MD [CRS] - **Spec Exp:** Colon & Rectal Cancer; Inflammatory Bowel Disease/Crohn's; Laparoscopic Surgery; **Hospital:** Cleveland Clin - Weston; **Address:** 2950 Cleveland Clinic Blvd, Weston, FL 33331-3609; **Phone:** 954-659-5278; **Board Cert:** Surgery 2005; Colon & Rectal Surgery 2006; **Med School:** Cornell Univ-Weill Med Coll 1982; **Resid:** Surgery, Roosevelt Hosp 1987; **Fellow:** Colon & Rectal Surgery, Univ Minn 1988; **Fac Appt:** Prof S, Cleveland Cl Coll Med/Case West Res

Midwest

Abcarian, Herand MD [CRS] - **Spec Exp:** Rectal Cancer/Sphincter Preservation; Inflammatory Bowel Disease; Anorectal Disorders; Incontinence-Fecal; **Hospital:** Univ of IL Med Ctr at Chicago, Gottlieb Meml Hosp; **Address:** 675 W North Ave, Ste 406, Melrose Park, IL 60160; **Phone:** 708-450-5075; **Board Cert:** Surgery 1972; Colon & Rectal Surgery 1972; **Med School:** Iran 1965; **Resid:** Surgery, Cook County Hosp 1971; Colon & Rectal Surgery, Cook County Hosp 1972; **Fac Appt:** Prof S, Univ IL Coll Med

Delaney, Conor P MD/PhD [CRS] - **Spec Exp:** Laparoscopic Surgery; Colon & Rectal Cancer; Inflammatory Bowel Disease/Crohn's; **Hospital:** Univ Hosps Case Med Ctr; **Address:** 11100 Euclid Ave, MS 5047, Cleveland, OH 44106-5047; **Phone:** 216-844-8087; **Board Cert:** Surgery 1998; Colon & Rectal Surgery 1998; **Med School:** Ireland 1989; **Resid:** Surgery, Univ Hosp 1993; Surgery, Univ Hosp 1999; **Fellow:** Research, Univ of Pittsburgh 1995; Colon & Rectal Surgery, Cleveland Clinic 2000; **Fac Appt:** Prof S, Cleveland Cl Coll Med/Case West Res

Fleshman, James MD [CRS] - **Spec Exp:** Colon & Rectal Cancer; Laparoscopic Surgery; Inflammatory Bowel Disease; **Hospital:** Barnes-Jewish Hosp, Barnes-Jewish West County Hosp; **Address:** Wash Univ Sch Med, Div Col Rectal Surgery, 660 S Euclid Ave, Box 8109, St Louis, MO 63110; **Phone:** 314-454-7177; **Board Cert:** Colon & Rectal Surgery 1988; Surgery 1996; **Med School:** Washington Univ, St Louis 1980; **Resid:** Surgery, Jewish Hospital 1986; **Fellow:** Colon & Rectal Surgery, Univ Toronto 1987; **Fac Appt:** Prof S, Washington Univ, St Louis

Foley, Eugene F MD [CRS] - **Spec Exp:** Colon & Rectal Cancer; Ulcerative Colitis; **Hospital:** Univ WI Hosp & Clins; **Address:** Univ WI Hosp & Clins, 600 Highland Ave, Madison, WI 53792-7375; **Phone:** 608-263-7502; **Board Cert:** Surgery 2003; Colon & Rectal Surgery 2005; **Med School:** Harvard Med Sch 1985; **Resid:** Surgery, New England Deaconess Hosp 1991; **Fellow:** Colon & Rectal Surgery, Lahey Clinic 1993; **Fac Appt:** Prof S, Univ Wisc

Geisler, Daniel P MD [CRS] - **Spec Exp:** Colon & Rectal Cancer & Surgery; Minimally Invasive Surgery; Rectal Cancer/Sphincter Preservation; Anal Cancer; **Hospital:** Cleveland Clin Fdn (page 56); **Address:** Cleveland Clinic, 9500 Euclid Ave, MC A30, Cleveland, OH 44195; **Phone:** 216-445-7616; **Board Cert:** Surgery 2003; Colon & Rectal Surgery 2005; **Med School:** St Louis Univ 1996; **Resid:** Surgery, Univ Oklahoma Hlth Sci Ctr 2001; **Fellow:** Colon & Rectal Surgery, Lankenau Hosp 2002; Minimally Invasive Surgery, Saint Vincent Hlth Ctr 2003; **Fac Appt:** Assoc Prof S, Cleveland Cl Coll Med/Case West Res

Kodner, Ira J MD [CRS] - **Spec Exp:** Colon & Rectal Cancer; Inflammatory Bowel Disease/Crohn's; Laparoscopic Surgery; **Hospital:** Barnes-Jewish Hosp; **Address:** Wash Univ Sch Med, Div Col Rectal Surgery, 660 S Euclid Ave, Box 8109, St Louis, MO 63110; **Phone:** 314-454-7177; **Board Cert:** Surgery 1975; Colon & Rectal Surgery 1975; **Med School:** Washington Univ, St Louis 1967; **Resid:** Surgery, Barnes-Jewish Hosp 1974; **Fellow:** Colon & Rectal Surgery, Cleveland Clinic 1975; **Fac Appt:** Prof S, Washington Univ, St Louis

Lavery, Ian C MD [CRS] - **Spec Exp:** Colon & Rectal Cancer; Inflammatory Bowel Disease; Pediatric Gastrointestinal Surgery; **Hospital:** Cleveland Clin Fdn (page 56); **Address:** 9500 Euclid Ave, Desk A30, Cleveland, OH 44195; **Phone:** 216-444-6930; **Board Cert:** Colon & Rectal Surgery 1998; **Med School:** Australia 1967; **Resid:** Surgery, Princess Alexandra Hosp 1974; Colon & Rectal Surgery, Cleveland Clinic 1977; **Fac Appt:** Prof S, Case West Res Univ

Lowry, Ann C MD [CRS] - **Spec Exp:** Anal Sphincter Repair; Rectovaginal Fistula; Inflammatory Bowel Disease; **Hospital:** Abbott - Northwestern Hosp, Fairview Southdale Hosp; **Address:** 6363 France Ave S, Ste 212, Edina, MN 55435; **Phone:** 651-312-1700; **Board Cert:** Colon & Rectal Surgery 1988; **Med School:** Tufts Univ 1977; **Resid:** Surgery, New Eng Med Ctr Hosps 1982; **Fellow:** Colon & Rectal Surgery, Univ Minn Affil Hosps 1987; **Fac Appt:** Clin Prof S, Univ Minn

Ludwig, Kirk A MD [CRS] - **Spec Exp:** Colon & Rectal Cancer & Surgery; Pelvic Organ Prolapse; Rectal Cancer/Sphincter Preservation; Incontinence-Fecal; **Hospital:** Froedtert Meml Lutheran Hosp; **Address:** 9200 W Wisconsin Ave, Dept Surgery, Milwaukee, WI 53226; **Phone:** 414-805-5800; **Board Cert:** Surgery 2005; Colon & Rectal Surgery 2007; **Med School:** Univ Cincinnati 1988; **Resid:** Surgery, Med Coll Wisc 1994; **Fellow:** Colon & Rectal Surgery, Cleveland Clinic 1996; **Fac Appt:** Assoc Prof S, Med Coll Wisc

Madoff, Robert D MD [CRS] - **Spec Exp:** Colon & Rectal Cancer; Inflammatory Bowel Disease; Incontinence/Pelvic Floor Disorders; **Hospital:** Univ Minn Med Ctr, Fairview - Univ Campus; **Address:** 516 Delaware St SE, Phillips-Wangensteen Bldg, MMC 88, Minneapolis, MN 55455; **Phone:** 612-624-9708; **Board Cert:** Colon & Rectal Surgery 2002; **Med School:** Columbia P&S 1979; **Resid:** Surgery, Univ Minn Hosps 1987; **Fellow:** Colon & Rectal Surgery, Univ Minn Hosps 1988; **Fac Appt:** Prof S, Univ Minn

Nelson, Heidi MD [CRS] - **Spec Exp:** Colon & Rectal Cancer; Gastrointestinal Cancer; **Hospital:** Mayo Med Ctr & Clin - Rochester, Rochester Methodist Hosp; **Address:** Mayo Clinic, Gonda 9 South, 200 First St SW, Rochester, MN 55905; **Phone:** 507-284-3329; **Board Cert:** Surgery 2007; Colon & Rectal Surgery 1989; **Med School:** Univ Wash 1981; **Resid:** Surgery, Oregon Hlth Sci Univ Hosp 1987; Colon & Rectal Surgery, Oregon Hlth Sci Univ Hosp 1985; **Fellow:** Colon & Rectal Surgery, Mayo Clinic 1988; **Fac Appt:** Prof S, Mayo Med Sch

Pemberton, John H MD [CRS] - **Spec Exp:** Inflammatory Bowel Disease/Crohn's; Colon & Rectal Cancer; **Hospital:** St Mary's Hosp - Rochester, Rochester Methodist Hosp; **Address:** Mayo Clinic, Div Colon & Rectal Surg, 200 First St SW, Gonda 9-S, Rochester, MN 55905; **Phone:** 507-284-2359; **Board Cert:** Surgery 2001; Colon & Rectal Surgery 1985; **Med School:** Tulane Univ 1976; **Resid:** Surgery, Mayo Clinic 1983; **Fellow:** Colon & Rectal Surgery, Mayo Clinic 1984; **Fac Appt:** Prof S, Mayo Med Sch

Rafferty, Janice F MD [CRS] - **Spec Exp:** Colon & Rectal Cancer; Ulcerative Colitis; Crohn's Disease; Anal Disorders & Reconstruction; **Hospital:** Univ Hosp - Cincinnati, Christ Hospital; **Address:** U of Cincinnati, Colon & Rectal Surgery, 2123 Auburn Ave, Ste 524, Cincinnati, OH 45219; **Phone:** 513-929-0104; **Board Cert:** Colon & Rectal Surgery 2008; Surgery 2004; **Med School:** Ohio State Univ 1988; **Resid:** Surgery, Univ CincinnatiHosp 1995; Colon & Rectal Surgery, Barnes Jewish Hosp 1996; **Fac Appt:** Assoc Prof S, Univ Cincinnati

Colon & Rectal Surgery

Remzi, Feza H MD [CRS] - **Spec Exp:** Colon & Rectal Cancer & Surgery; Inflammatory Bowel Disease; **Hospital:** Cleveland Clin Fdn (page 56); **Address:** Cleveland Clinic, 9500 Euclid Ave, MC A30, Cleveland, OH 44195; **Phone:** 216-445-5020; **Board Cert:** Surgery 2002; Colon & Rectal Surgery 2007; **Med School:** Turkey 1989; **Resid:** Colon & Rectal Surgery, Cleveland Clinic 1996; Colon & Rectal Surgery, Cleveland Clinic 1997

Rothenberger, David A MD [CRS] - **Spec Exp:** Colon & Rectal Cancer; **Hospital:** Univ Minn Med Ctr, Fairview - Univ Campus; **Address:** Univ Minnesota Med Ctr, Dept Surg, 516 Delaware St SE MMC 88, Minneapolis, MN 55455; **Phone:** 612-624-9708; **Board Cert:** Colon & Rectal Surgery 2006; **Med School:** Tufts Univ 1973; **Resid:** Surgery, St Paul-Ramsey Med Ctr 1978; **Fellow:** Colon & Rectal Surgery, Univ Minnesota Hosps 1979; **Fac Appt:** Prof S, Univ Minn

Saclarides, Theodore J MD [CRS] - **Spec Exp:** Rectal Cancer/Sphincter Preservation; Laparoscopic Surgery; Inflammatory Bowel Disease; **Hospital:** Rush Univ Med Ctr, Skokie/North Shore Univ Htlh Syst; **Address:** University Surgeons, 1725 W Harrison St, Ste 810, Chicago, IL 60612-3832; **Phone:** 312-942-6543; **Board Cert:** Surgery 2007; Colon & Rectal Surgery 1989; **Med School:** Univ Miami Sch Med 1982; **Resid:** Surgery, Rush Univ Med Ctr 1987; **Fellow:** Colon & Rectal Surgery, Mayo Clinic 1988; **Fac Appt:** Prof S, Rush Med Coll

Senagore, Anthony MD [CRS] - **Spec Exp:** Laparoscopic Surgery; Colon & Rectal Cancer; Anorectal Disorders; Inflammatory Bowel Disease/Crohn's; **Hospital:** Spectrum Hlth Blodgett Campus; **Address:** Spectrum Health, 100 Michigan St NE, MC 005, Grand Rapids, MI 49503; **Phone:** 616-391-2467; **Board Cert:** Surgery 2006; Colon & Rectal Surgery 2001; Surgical Critical Care 2006; **Med School:** Mich State Univ 1981; **Resid:** Surgery, Butterworth Hosp 1987; Colon & Rectal Surgery, Ferguson Hosp 1989; **Fac Appt:** Prof S, Med Univ Ohio at Toledo

Stryker, Steven J MD [CRS] - **Spec Exp:** Colon & Rectal Cancer; Inflammatory Bowel Disease; Laparoscopic Surgery; **Hospital:** Northwestern Meml Hosp; **Address:** 676 N Saint Clair St, Ste 1525A, Chicago, IL 60611-2862; **Phone:** 312-943-5427; **Board Cert:** Surgery 2004; Colon & Rectal Surgery 1986; **Med School:** Northwestern Univ 1978; **Resid:** Surgery, Northwestern Meml Hosp 1983; **Fellow:** Colon & Rectal Surgery, Mayo Clinic 1985; **Fac Appt:** Clin Prof S, Northwestern Univ

Trudel, Judith L MD [CRS] - **Spec Exp:** Colon & Rectal Cancer; Anorectal Disorders; **Hospital:** St. John's Hosp, St Joseph's Hosp; **Address:** Colon & Rectal Surgery Assoc, 1055 Westgate Drive, Ste 190, Saint Paul, MN 55114; **Phone:** 651-312-1620; **Board Cert:** Surgery 2007; Colon & Rectal Surgery 2006; **Med School:** Canada 1979; **Resid:** Surgery, Montreal Genl Hosp 1985; **Fellow:** Colon & Rectal Surgery, Cleveland Clinic 1986; **Fac Appt:** Assoc Prof S, Univ Minn

Wolff, Bruce G MD [CRS] - **Spec Exp:** Inflammatory Bowel Disease; Crohn's Disease; Colon & Rectal Cancer; **Hospital:** Mayo Med Ctr & Clin - Rochester; **Address:** Mayo Clinic, Gonda 9 South, 200 First St SW, Rochester, MN 55905; **Phone:** 507-284-3329; **Board Cert:** Surgery 2000; Colon & Rectal Surgery 2001; **Med School:** Duke Univ 1973; **Resid:** Surgery, NY Hosp-Cornell Med Ctr 1981; **Fellow:** Colon & Rectal Surgery, Mayo Clinic 1982; **Fac Appt:** Prof S, Mayo Med Sch

Great Plains and Mountains

Schatz, Lisa Shawn MD [CRS] - **Hospital:** Rose Med Ctr; **Address:** Western Surgical Care, 4500 E 9th Ave, Ste 710, Denver, CO 80220; **Phone:** 303-320-7826; **Board Cert:** Surgery 2001; Colon & Rectal Surgery 2002; **Med School:** Case West Res Univ 1995; **Resid:** Surgery, Univ Hosps of Cleveland 2000; Colon & Rectal Surgery, Ochsner Clinic 2001; **Fac Appt:** Assoc Clin Prof CRS, Univ Colorado

Thorson, Alan G MD [CRS] - **Spec Exp:** Colon & Rectal Cancer; Laparoscopic Surgery; Incontinence-Fecal; Ileal Pouch Anal Anastomosis; **Hospital:** Nebraska Meth Hosp, Archbishop Bergan Mercy Med Ctr; **Address:** 9850 Nicholas St, Ste 100, Omaha, NE 68114-2191; **Phone:** 402-343-1122; **Board Cert:** Colon & Rectal Surgery 1999; **Med School:** Univ Nebr Coll Med 1979; **Resid:** Surgery, Univ Nebraska Affil Hosp 1984; Colon & Rectal Surgery, Univ Minn Affil Hosp 1985; **Fac Appt:** Assoc Clin Prof S, Creighton Univ

Williams, Shauna Tseu MD [CRS] - **Hospital:** St. Luke's Reg Med Ctr - Boise, St Alphonsus Regl Med Ctr; **Address:** 901 N Curtis Rd, Ste 303, Boise, ID 83706; **Phone:** 208-377-2273; **Board Cert:** Surgery 1998; Colon & Rectal Surgery 2003; **Med School:** Univ Hawaii JA Burns Sch Med 1984; **Resid:** Surgery, Univ Oregon Hlth Sci Ctr 1990; **Fellow:** Colon & Rectal Surgery, Mayo Clinic 1991

Southwest

Adkins, Terrance P MD [CRS] - **Spec Exp:** Colon & Rectal Cancer; Inflammatory Bowel Disease; **Hospital:** Tucson Med Ctr; **Address:** Southwestern Surgery Assoc, 1951 N Wilmot Rd Bldg 2, Tucson, AZ 85712; **Phone:** 520-795-5845; **Board Cert:** Surgery 2001; Colon & Rectal Surgery 2004; **Med School:** Univ Tex SW, Dallas 1985; **Resid:** Surgery, Univ Utah Med Ctr 1991; **Fellow:** Colon & Rectal Surgery, Univ Texas Med Ctr 1992; **Fac Appt:** Asst Clin Prof S, Univ Ariz Coll Med

Bailey, H Randolph MD [CRS] - **Spec Exp:** Rectal Cancer/Sphincter Preservation; Inflammatory Bowel Disease; Incontinence-Fecal; Endometriosis-Intestine; **Hospital:** Methodist Hosp - Houston, St Luke's Episcopal Hosp-Houston; **Address:** Colon & Rectal Clinic, Smith Twr, 6550 Fannin St, Ste 2307, Houston, TX 77030-2717; **Phone:** 713-790-9250; **Board Cert:** Surgery 1974; Colon & Rectal Surgery 2004; **Med School:** Univ Tex SW, Dallas 1968; **Resid:** Surgery, Hermann Hosp-Univ Tex Med Sch 1973; **Fellow:** Colon & Rectal Surgery, Ferguson-Droste Hosp 1974; **Fac Appt:** Clin Prof S, Univ Tex, Houston

Beck, David E MD [CRS] - **Spec Exp:** Colon & Rectal Cancer; Minimally Invasive Surgery; Inflammatory Bowel Disease; **Hospital:** Ochsner Fdn Hosp, Summit Hosp-Baton Rouge; **Address:** Ochsner Clinic Fdn, Colorectal Surgery, 1514 Jefferson Hwy, 4th Fl, rm 04 East, New Orleans, LA 70121-2429; **Phone:** 504-842-4060; **Board Cert:** Colon & Rectal Surgery 1987; **Med School:** Univ Miami Sch Med 1979; **Resid:** Surgery, Wilford Hall USAF Med Ctr 1984; **Fellow:** Colon & Rectal Surgery, Cleveland Clinic Fdn 1986; **Fac Appt:** Assoc Clin Prof S, Louisiana State U, New Orleans

Efron, Jonathan E MD [CRS] - **Spec Exp:** Colon & Rectal Cancer; Incontinence-Fecal; Inflammatory Bowel Disease; Anorectal Disorders; **Hospital:** Mayo Clinic - Scottsdale; **Address:** Mayo Clinic, Concourse B, 13400 E Shea Blvd, Scottsdale, AZ 85259; **Phone:** 480-342-2697; **Board Cert:** Surgery 1999; Colon & Rectal Surgery 2000; **Med School:** Univ MD Sch Med 1993; **Resid:** Surgery, LIJ Medical Ctr 1999; **Fellow:** Colon & Rectal Surgery, Cleveland Clinic 2000; Research, Cleveland Clinic 2001; **Fac Appt:** Assoc Prof S, Mayo Med Sch

Heppell, Jacques P MD [CRS] - **Spec Exp:** Colon & Rectal Cancer; Inflammatory Bowel Disease; Anorectal Disorders; **Hospital:** Mayo Clinic - Phoenix; **Address:** Mayo Clinic, GENS/CB/Distribution 13, 5777 E Mayo Blvd, Phoenix, AZ 85054; **Phone:** 480-342-2697; **Board Cert:** Surgery 2004; Colon & Rectal Surgery 1995; **Med School:** Univ Montreal 1974; **Resid:** Surgery, Univ Montreal Med Ctr 1979; **Fellow:** Colon & Rectal Surgery, Mayo Clinic 1983; **Fac Appt:** Prof S, Mayo Med Sch

Colon & Rectal Surgery

Huber Jr, Philip J MD [CRS] - **Spec Exp:** Colon & Rectal Cancer; Inflammatory Bowel Disease; **Hospital:** Med City Dallas Hosp, Presby Hosp of Dallas; **Address:** 7777 Forest Lane, Ste C-204, Dallas, TX 75230; **Phone:** 972-566-6115; **Board Cert:** Surgery 1997; Colon & Rectal Surgery 1993; **Med School:** Columbia P&S 1972; **Resid:** Surgery, Parkland Hosp 1977; Colon & Rectal Surgery, Presby Hosp 1978

West Coast and Pacific

Beart Jr, Robert W MD [CRS] - **Spec Exp:** Colon & Rectal Cancer; Inflammatory Bowel Disease/Crohn's; **Hospital:** USC Norris Cancer Hosp, USC Univ Hosp; **Address:** USC Comprehensive Cancer Center, Topping Tower Suite 7418, 1441 Eastlake Ave, Los Angeles, CA 90033; **Phone:** 323-865-3690; **Board Cert:** Colon & Rectal Surgery 1995; **Med School:** Harvard Med Sch 1971; **Resid:** Surgery, Univ Colo Med Ctr 1976; Colon & Rectal Surgery, Mayo Clinic 1978; **Fellow:** Transplant Surgery, Univ Colo Med Ctr 1975; **Fac Appt:** Prof S, USC Sch Med

Chiu, Yanek S MD [CRS] - **Hospital:** CA Pacific Med Ctr - Pacific Campus; **Address:** 3838 California St, Ste 616, San Francisco, CA 94118; **Phone:** 415-668-0411; **Board Cert:** Colon & Rectal Surgery 1997; **Med School:** Boston Univ 1971; **Resid:** Surgery, Boston Med Ctr 1976; **Fellow:** Colon & Rectal Surgery, Mayo Clinic 1978; **Fac Appt:** Assoc Clin Prof CRS, UCSF

Coutsoftides, Theodore MD [CRS] - **Spec Exp:** Laparoscopic Surgery; Inflammatory Bowel Disease; Anal Sphincter Repair; **Hospital:** St Joseph's Hosp - Orange; **Address:** 1310 W Stewart Drive, Ste 605, Orange, CA 92868-3857; **Phone:** 714-532-2544; **Board Cert:** Colon & Rectal Surgery 1977; **Med School:** Israel 1970; **Resid:** Surgery, Cleveland Clinic 1973; Surgery, Royal Victoria Hosp 1976; **Fellow:** Colon & Rectal Surgery, Cleveland Clinic 1977; **Fac Appt:** Assoc Prof S, UC Irvine

Lee, Patrick Y H MD [CRS] - **Hospital:** Providence Portland Med Ctr, Legacy Health System; **Address:** Surgical Specialty Group, Colon & Rectal Clinic, 511 SW 10th Ave, Ste 714, Portland, OR 97219; **Phone:** 503-222-1615; **Board Cert:** Surgery 2004; Colon & Rectal Surgery 2007; **Med School:** Northwestern Univ-Feinberg Sch Med 1988; **Resid:** Surgery, Oregon Hlth Sci Ctr 1994; **Fellow:** Colon & Rectal Surgery, Cleveland Clinic 1995

Ramamoorthy, Sonia L MD [CRS] - **Spec Exp:** Colon & Rectal Cancer; Diverticulitis; Incontinence/Pelvic Floor Disorders; Inflammatory Bowel Disease; **Hospital:** UCSD Med Ctr; **Address:** UCSD, Dept Surgery, 200 W Arbor Drive, MC 8400, San Diego, CA 92103-8400; **Phone:** 619-471-9640; **Board Cert:** Surgery 2002; Colon & Rectal Surgery 2005; **Med School:** Boston Univ 1996; **Resid:** Surgery, UCSD Med Ctr 2001; **Fellow:** Colon & Rectal Surgery, Barnes-Jewish Hosp 2002; Research, UCSD Med Ctr 2006; **Fac Appt:** Asst Prof S, UCSD

Sokol, Thomas P MD [CRS] - **Spec Exp:** Colon & Rectal Cancer & Surgery; Incontinence-Fecal; **Hospital:** Cedars-Sinai Med Ctr, Century City Hosp; **Address:** 8737 Beverly Blvd, Ste 402, Los Angeles, CA 90048-1828; **Phone:** 310-854-3580; **Board Cert:** Colon & Rectal Surgery 2008; **Med School:** Ros Franklin Univ/Chicago Med Sch 1980; **Resid:** Surgery, Habor UCLA Med Ctr 1985; **Fellow:** Colon & Rectal Surgery, Carle Fdn Hosp/Univ Ill 1986; **Fac Appt:** Assoc Clin Prof S, UCLA

Stamos, Michael J MD [CRS] - **Spec Exp:** Rectal Cancer/Sphincter Preservation; Laparoscopic Surgery; Inflammatory Bowel Disease; Colon & Rectal Cancer; **Hospital:** UC Irvine Med Ctr; **Address:** UC Irvine Med Ctr, Div Colon & Rectal Surg, 333 City Blvd W, Ste 850, Orange, CA 92868-2993; **Phone:** 888-717-4463; **Board Cert:** Surgery 2000; Colon & Rectal Surgery 2003; **Med School:** Case West Res Univ 1985; **Resid:** Surgery, Jackson Meml Hosp 1990; Colon & Rectal Surgery, Ochsner Clinic 1991; **Fac Appt:** Prof S, UC Irvine

Welton, Mark L MD [CRS] - **Spec Exp:** Ulcerative Colitis; Crohn's Disease; Colon & Rectal Cancer; Anal Cancer; **Hospital:** Stanford Univ Med Ctr; **Address:** Advanced Medical Center, 875 Blake Wilbur Drive, Stanford, CA 94305-5655; **Phone:** 650-723-5461; **Board Cert:** Surgery 2000; Colon & Rectal Surgery 2005; **Med School:** UCLA 1984; **Resid:** Surgery, UCLA Med Ctr 1992; **Fellow:** Colon & Rectal Surgery, Barnes Jewish Hosp 1993; **Fac Appt:** Assoc Prof S, Stanford Univ

Wong, Ronald J MD [CRS] - **Spec Exp:** Laparoscopic Surgery; **Hospital:** Queen's Med Ctr - Honolulu; **Address:** Queen's Physicians' Office Bldg 1, 1380 Lusitana St, Ste 614, Honolulu, HI 96813; **Phone:** 808-524-1856; **Board Cert:** Surgery 1997; **Med School:** Univ Hawaii JA Burns Sch Med 1981; **Resid:** Surgery, Univ Hawaii 1985; Surgery, Catholic Med Ctr 1987; **Fellow:** Colon & Rectal Surgery, Suburban Hosp 1989; Research, Cornell Univ Med Ctr 1988; **Fac Appt:** Clin Prof S, Univ Hawaii JA Burns Sch Med

Worsey, Michael J MD [CRS] - **Spec Exp:** Colon & Rectal Cancer; Inflammatory Bowel Disease; **Hospital:** Scripps Meml Hosp - La Jolla; **Address:** Advanced Surgical Associates, 9834 Genesee Ave, Ste 201, La Jolla, CA 92037; **Phone:** 858-558-2272; **Board Cert:** Surgery 1998; Colon & Rectal Surgery 1999; **Med School:** England, UK 1985; **Resid:** Surgery, Bristol Royal Infirm & Royal Gwent Hosp 1989; Surgery, Univ Pittsburgh Med Ctr 1997; **Fellow:** Colon & Rectal Surgery, Cleveland Clin 1998

Cleveland Clinic

Digestive Disease Institute

A National Leader in Digestive Disease

Cleveland Clinic's Digestive Disease Institute is one of the largest digestive programs in the country and the first to fully integrate its departments of Colorectal Surgery, Gastroenterology & Hepatology, Hepato-pancreato-biliary and Transplant Surgery, and Nutrition. Combining these disciplines in one location facilitates unprecedented patient care, multidisciplinary education and collaborative research.

In 2008, Cleveland Clinic Digestive Disease Institute physicians saw over 100,000 patients and performed over 5,000 surgical cases and 33,000 endoscopic cases. Our advanced endoscopists performed 1,077 ERCP procedures, and consistently perform these procedures and a wide range of advanced endoscopy services efficiently and safely with complication rates at or below national averages. Transplant surgeons completed 182 digestive disease-related organ transplants – including liver transplantation, pancreas transplantation, and intestinal transplantation, achieving outstanding outcomes.

The Digestive Disease Institute is a recognized world leader in J-Pouch surgeries, and nationally the largest referral center for repairing failed pelvic pouches. Over the years, our staff has pioneered many new technologies and procedures for treating digestive disorders, and has developed key specialties in:

- Colon & Rectal Cancer
- Crohn's & Ulcerative Colitis
- Ostomy Avoidance
- Familial Adenomatous Polyposis
- Diverticulitis
- Laparoscopic Surgery
- Robotic Liver and Pancreas Surgery
- Anorectal Disease (Fistulas, Hemorrhoids)
- Functional Bowel Disorders/Incontinence
- Enterostomal Therapy/Ostomy Reversal
- Hepatobiliary Surgery
- Liver Transplant

- Pancreatic Disease
- Therapeutic Endoscopy
- Esophageal Disorders
- Liver Disease
- Deep Enteroscopy
- Capsule Endoscopy
- Abdominal Fistulas
- Nutrition Therapy
- IBD/Pouchitis
- Clinical Trials

Cleveland Clinic's Digestive Disease Institute is ranked #2 in the nation by *U.S.News and World Report's* 2009 "America's Best Hospitals" Survey.

For more information about Cleveland Clinic's Digestive Disease Institute, or to schedule a second opinion or learn about assistance for out-of-state patients, call 800.890.2467 or visit www.clevelandclinic.org/gastrotopdocs.

Digestive Disease Institute
Cleveland Clinic | 9500 Euclid Avenue / AC311 | Cleveland OH 44195

NYU Langone Medical Center

550 First Avenue (at 31St Street)
New York, NY 10016
Physician Referral:
(888)7-NYU-MED (888-769-8633)
www.med.nyu.edu

COLON AND RECTAL SURGERY

About Colon and Rectal Surgery of Manhattan:

The surgeons at Colon and Rectal Surgery of Manhattan at NYU, an affiliated practice of Langone Medical Center, perform more than 5,000 outpatient and inpatient procedures each year using laser, laparoscopic, endoscopic and other minimally invasive techniques. Candidates for surgery receive same-day care that includes imaging, radiation and nutritional support. The program provides an integrated team approach, resulting in an environment that offers complete, patient-centered care.

We specialize in the following areas:

ADRENALECTOMIES

Surgeons at NYU Langone Medical Center are skilled at performing adrenalectomies, the surgical removal of one or both of the adrenal glands. This procedure is usually advised for patients with tumors of the adrenal glands. Adrenal gland tumors may be malignant or benign, but all typically excrete excessive amounts of one or more hormones. Adrenalectomy is usually performed by conventional (open) surgery, but in selected patients surgeons may use laparoscopy. With laparoscopy, adrenalectomy can be accomplished through four very small incisions.

COLORECTAL CANCER

NYU Langone Medical Center offers the most advanced screening options available for the diagnosis of colon cancer, the second leading cause of cancer death in the U.S. Additionally, the Medical Center continues to investigate colorectal cancer screenings in special populations such as women, veterans, immigrants, minorities and patients with HIV, and offer the use of virtual colonoscopy for the detection of colorectal polyps and cancer.

LAPAROSCOPIC TECHNIQUES

Surgeons at NYU Langone Medical Center use tiny incisions to remove a segment of the colon, which dramatically speeds recovery and reduces the need for pain medication. In addition treating colon cancer laparoscopically, this technique is used to treat pancreatic tumors, splenic conditions, hiatus hernias, small bowel tumors and adrenalectomies.

LIVER LESIONS

At Colon and Rectal Surgery of Manhattan at NYU Langone Medical Center, surgeons effectively treat liver lesions with painless radiofrequency ablation.

ROBOTIC SURGERY

NYU Langone Medical Center is the first hospital in New York City to use the minimally invasive da Vinci Si HD robotic surgical system. Used in several procedures, this technology is also used in operations of the colon. The machine allows for a 40 percent higher definition view of the surgical field as well as an additional surgical arm to hold surgical instruments. The device also allows physicians to import and display medical test results from any computer or diagnostic medical device.

VIRTUAL COLONOSCOPY

NYU Langone Medical Center offers the latest developments in colon cancer detection, including virtual colonoscopy. The noninvasive procedure makes use of sophisticated imaging techniques to generate a 3-D reconstruction of the inner surface of the colon, which can then be evaluated for abnormalities by specially trained radiologists.

Dermatology

A dermatologist is trained to diagnose and treat pediatric and adult patients with benign and malignant disorders of the skin, mouth, external genitalia, hair and nails, as well as a number of sexually transmitted diseases. The dermatologist may have additional training and experience in the diagnosis and treatment of skin cancers, melanomas, moles and other tumors of the skin, the management of contact dermatitis and other allergic and nonallergic skin disorders, and in the recognition of the skin manifestations of systemic (including internal malignancy) and infectious diseases. Dermatologists may have special training in dermatopathology and in the surgical techniques used in dermatology. They also have expertise in the management of cosmetic disorders of the skin such as hair loss and scars, and the skin changes associated with aging.

Training Required: Four years.

Certification in the following subspecialties requires additional training and examination.

Dermatopathology: A dermatopathologist has the expertise to diagnose and monitor diseases of the skin including infectious, immunologic, degenerative and neoplastic diseases. This entails the examination and interpretation of specially prepared tissue sections, cellular scrapings and smears of skin lesions by means of routine and special (electron and fluorescent) microscopes.

Pediatric Dermatology: A dermatologist trained to diagnose and treat pediatric patients with dermatologic diseases.

DERMATOLOGY

New England

Anderson, Richard Rox MD [D] - **Spec Exp:** Cosmetic Dermatology; **Hospital:** Mass Genl Hosp; **Address:** Dermatology Laser Center, 50 Staniford St, Ste 250, Boston, MA 02114; **Phone:** 617-724-6960; **Board Cert:** Dermatology 2001; **Med School:** Harvard Med Sch 1984; **Resid:** Dermatology, Mass Genl Hosp 1991; **Fellow:** Dermatologic Research, Mass Genl Hosp 1988; **Fac Appt:** Assoc Prof D, Harvard Med Sch

Arndt, Kenneth MD [D] - **Spec Exp:** Skin Laser Surgery; Cosmetic Dermatology; **Hospital:** Beth Israel Deaconess Med Ctr - Boston, New England Bapt Hosp; **Address:** Skincare Phys of Chestnut Hill, 1244 Boylston St, Ste 302, Chestnut Hill, MA 02467; **Phone:** 617-731-1600; **Board Cert:** Dermatology 1966; **Med School:** Yale Univ 1961; **Resid:** Dermatology, Mass Genl Hosp 1965; **Fellow:** Dermatology, Harvard Med Sch 1965; **Fac Appt:** Clin Prof D, Harvard Med Sch

Bolognia, Jean L MD [D] - **Spec Exp:** Melanoma; Skin Cancer; **Hospital:** Yale-New Haven Hosp; **Address:** 2 Church St S, Ste 305, New Haven, CT 06519; **Phone:** 203-789-1249; **Board Cert:** Dermatology 2005; **Med School:** Yale Univ 1980; **Resid:** Internal Medicine, Yale-New Haven Hosp 1982; Dermatology, Yale-New Haven Hosp 1985; **Fellow:** Dermatology, Yale-New Haven Hosp 1987; **Fac Appt:** Prof D, Yale Univ

Del Giudice, Stephen M MD [D] - **Spec Exp:** Skin Cancer; Phototherapy; Psoriasis; Acne; **Hospital:** Concord Hospital; **Address:** Dartmouth Hitchcock Concord-Dermatology, 253 Pleasant St, Concord, NH 03301; **Phone:** 603-226-6119; **Board Cert:** Dermatology 1987; **Med School:** Tufts Univ 1981; **Resid:** Dermatology, Yale-New Haven Hosp 1987

Dover, Jeffrey MD [D] - **Spec Exp:** Cosmetic Dermatology; **Hospital:** Beth Israel Deaconess Med Ctr - Boston, New England Bapt Hosp; **Address:** 1244 Boylston St, Ste 302, Chesnut Hill, MA 02467; **Phone:** 617-731-1600; **Board Cert:** Dermatology 1985; **Med School:** Univ Ottawa 1981; **Resid:** Dermatology, Univ Toronto 1984; Dermatology, St Johns Hosp 1985; **Fellow:** Dermatology, Mass Genl Hosp-Harvard 1987; **Fac Appt:** Assoc Prof D, Yale Univ

Edelson, Richard L MD [D] - **Spec Exp:** Cutaneous Lymphoma; Immune Deficiency-Skin Disorders; **Hospital:** Yale-New Haven Hosp; **Address:** 2 Church St S, Ste 305, New Haven, CT 06519; **Phone:** 203-789-1249; **Board Cert:** Dermatology 1977; **Med School:** Yale Univ 1970; **Resid:** Dermatology, Mass Genl Hosp 1972; Dermatology, Natl Inst Hlth 1975; **Fac Appt:** Prof D, Yale Univ

Falanga, Vincent MD [D] - **Spec Exp:** Wound Healing/Care; Collagen Vascular Diseases; Scleroderma; **Hospital:** Roger Williams Hosp; **Address:** Roger Williams Med Ctr, Dept Dermatology, 50 Maude St Elmhurst Bldg, Providence, RI 02908; **Phone:** 401-456-2521; **Board Cert:** Internal Medicine 1980; Dermatology 1982; **Med School:** Harvard Med Sch 1977; **Resid:** Internal Medicine, Univ Miami 1980; **Fellow:** Dermatology, Univ Penn 1982; **Fac Appt:** Prof D, Boston Univ

Fewkes, Jessica L MD [D] - **Spec Exp:** Mohs' Surgery; Skin Cancer-Head & Neck; Melanoma-Head & Neck; **Hospital:** Mass Eye & Ear Infirmary, Mass Genl Hosp; **Address:** Mass Eye & Ear Infirmary, 243 Charles St Fl 9, Boston, MA 02114; **Phone:** 617-573-3789; **Board Cert:** Dermatology 1982; **Med School:** UCSF 1978; **Resid:** Dermatology, Mass Genl Hosp 1982; **Fellow:** Chemosurgery, Duke Univ Med Ctr 1983; **Fac Appt:** Asst Prof D, Harvard Med Sch

Gilchrest, Barbara MD [D] - **Spec Exp:** Photoaging; Melanoma; Skin Cancer; **Hospital:** Boston Med Ctr; **Address:** Boston Med Ctr- Dermatolgy Dept, 720 Harrison Ave, Boston, MA 02118-2394; **Phone:** 617-638-7420; **Board Cert:** Internal Medicine 1975; Dermatology 1978; **Med School:** Harvard Med Sch 1971; **Resid:** Internal Medicine, Boston City Hosp 1973; Dermatology, Harvard Med Sch 1976; **Fellow:** Photo Biology, Harvard Med Sch 1975; **Fac Appt:** Prof D, Boston Univ

Gottlieb, Alice MD/PhD [D] - **Spec Exp:** Psoriasis; Psoriatic Arthritis; **Hospital:** Tufts Med Ctr; **Address:** 800 Washington St, Box 114, Boston, MA 02111; **Phone:** 617-636-5370; **Board Cert:** Internal Medicine 1982; Dermatology 2001; Rheumatology 1984; **Med School:** Cornell Univ-Weill Med Coll 1980; **Resid:** Internal Medicine, New York Hosp 1982; Dermatology, New York Hosp 1993; **Fellow:** Rheumatology, Hosp Special Surgery 1984; **Fac Appt:** Prof D, Tufts Univ

Kane, Kay S MD [D] - **Spec Exp:** Pediatric Dermatology; **Hospital:** Children's Hospital - Boston; **Address:** 1244 Boylston St, Route 9, Chestnut Hill, MA 02467; **Phone:** 617-731-1600; **Board Cert:** Dermatology 2005; **Med School:** Harvard Med Sch 1993; **Resid:** Dermatology, Mass General Hosp 1997; **Fac Appt:** Prof D, Harvard Med Sch

Kupper, Thomas S MD [D] - **Spec Exp:** Melanoma; Cutaneous Lymphoma; Skin Cancer; **Hospital:** Brigham & Women's Hosp, Dana-Farber Cancer Inst; **Address:** Brigham & Women's Hosp, Dept Dermatology, 77 Avenue Louis Pasteur, Ste 671, Boston, MA 02115; **Phone:** 617-525-5550; **Board Cert:** Dermatology 1989; **Med School:** Yale Univ 1981; **Resid:** Surgery, Yale-New Haven Hosp 1983; Dermatology, Yale-New Haven Hosp 1989; **Fac Appt:** Prof D, Harvard Med Sch

Leffell, David J MD [D] - **Spec Exp:** Mohs' Surgery; Melanoma; Skin Cancer; Skin Laser Surgery; **Hospital:** Yale-New Haven Hosp; **Address:** Yale New Haven Hosp-Dept Dermatology, 40 Temple St, Ste 5A, PO Box 208059, New Haven, CT 06520; **Phone:** 203-785-3466; **Board Cert:** Internal Medicine 1984; Dermatology 1987; **Med School:** McGill Univ 1981; **Resid:** Internal Medicine, New York Hosp 1984; Dermatology, Yale-New Haven Hosp 1986; **Fellow:** Dermatology, Yale-New Haven Hosp 1987; Dermatologic Surgery, Univ Michigan Med Ctr 1988; **Fac Appt:** Prof D, Yale Univ

Maloney, Mary MD [D] - **Spec Exp:** Mohs' Surgery; Skin Laser Surgery; **Hospital:** UMass Memorial Med Ctr; **Address:** Univ Mass Med Ctr, Dept Derm, 281 Lincoln St Fl 4, Worcester, MA 01605-2138; **Phone:** 508-334-5962; **Board Cert:** Dermatology 1982; **Med School:** Univ VT Coll Med 1977; **Resid:** Internal Medicine, Hartford Hospital 1979; Dermatology, Dartmouth-Hitchcock Med Ctr 1982; **Fellow:** Dermatologic Surgery, UCSF Med Ctr 1983; **Fac Appt:** Prof D, Univ Mass Sch Med

McDonald, Charles J MD [D] - **Spec Exp:** Cutaneous Lymphoma; Autoimmune Disease; Melanoma; Psoriasis; **Hospital:** Rhode Island Hosp, Miriam Hosp; **Address:** Rhode Island Hosp, Dept Dermatology, 593 Eddy St, APC-10, Providence, RI 02903-4923; **Phone:** 401-444-7959; **Board Cert:** Dermatology 1966; **Med School:** Howard Univ 1960; **Resid:** Internal Medicine, Hosp St Raphael 1963; Dermatology, Yale New Haven Hosp 1965; **Fellow:** Clinical Oncology, Yale New Haven Hosp 1966; **Fac Appt:** Prof D, Brown Univ

Mihm Jr, Martin C MD [D] - **Spec Exp:** Melanoma; Vascular Birthmarks; Dermatopathology; **Hospital:** Mass Genl Hosp; **Address:** Mass General Hosp, 55 Fruit St, Warren Bldg 825, Boston, MA 02114-2926; **Phone:** 617-724-1350; **Board Cert:** Dermatology 1969; Dermatopathology 1974; Anatomic Pathology 1974; **Med School:** Univ Pittsburgh 1961; **Resid:** Internal Medicine, Mt Sinai Hosp 1964; Dermatology, Mass Genl Hosp 1967; **Fellow:** Anatomic Pathology, Mass Genl Hosp 1972; **Fac Appt:** Clin Prof Path, Harvard Med Sch

Dermatology

Neel, Victor A MD/PhD [D] - **Spec Exp:** Mohs' Surgery; Skin Cancer; **Hospital:** Mass Genl Hosp; **Address:** 50 Staniford St, Ste 270, Boston, MA 02114; **Phone:** 617-726-1869; **Board Cert:** Dermatology 2000; **Med School:** Cornell Univ-Weill Med Coll 1995; **Resid:** Pediatrics, Rhode Island Hosp 1997; Dermatology, Rhode Island Hosp 2000; **Fellow:** Mohs Surgery, UCLA Med Ctr 2001

Olbricht, Suzanne M MD [D] - **Spec Exp:** Skin Cancer; Mohs' Surgery; **Hospital:** Lahey Clin; **Address:** Lahey Clinic, 41 Mall Rd, Burlington, MA 01805; **Phone:** 781-744-8348; **Board Cert:** Dermatology 1983; Internal Medicine 1979; **Med School:** Baylor Coll Med 1976; **Resid:** Internal Medicine, Mass General Hosp 1979; Dermatology, Mass General Hosp 1983; **Fellow:** Mohs Surgery, Mass General Hosp 1991; **Fac Appt:** Assoc Prof D, Harvard Med Sch

Sober, Arthur MD [D] - **Spec Exp:** Melanoma; Skin Cancer; **Hospital:** Mass Genl Hosp; **Address:** Mass General Hospital, 50 Staniford St, Ste 200, Boston, MA 02114; **Phone:** 617-726-2914; **Board Cert:** Dermatology 1975; Internal Medicine 1974; **Med School:** Geo Wash Univ 1968; **Resid:** Internal Medicine, Beth Israel Hosp 1970; Dermatology, Mass General Hosp 1974; **Fellow:** Immunology, Peter Bent Brigham Hosp 1976; **Fac Appt:** Prof D, Harvard Med Sch

Stern, Robert S MD [D] - **Spec Exp:** Psoriasis; Drug Allergy; Skin Cancer; **Hospital:** Beth Israel Deaconess Med Ctr - Boston; **Address:** Beth Israel Deaconess Med Ctr, Dept Derm, 330 Brookline Ave, Boston, MA 02215-5400; **Phone:** 617-667-3689; **Board Cert:** Dermatology 1977; **Med School:** Yale Univ 1970; **Resid:** Dermatology, Mass Genl Hosp 1976; **Fac Appt:** Prof D, Harvard Med Sch

Mid Atlantic

Alster, Tina MD [D] - **Spec Exp:** Cosmetic Dermatology; Scar Revision; Hemangiomas/Birthmarks; **Hospital:** Georgetown Univ Hosp; **Address:** 1430 K St NW, Ste 200, Washington Inst of Derm Laser Surgery, Washington, DC 20005; **Phone:** 202-628-8855; **Board Cert:** Dermatology 1990; **Med School:** Duke Univ 1986; **Resid:** Dermatology, Yale Univ 1989; **Fellow:** Dermatologic Laser Surgery, Boston Univ Hosp 1990; **Fac Appt:** Clin Prof D, Georgetown Univ

Anhalt, Grant J MD [D] - **Spec Exp:** Blistering Diseases; Pemphigus; Autoimmune Disease; **Hospital:** Johns Hopkins Hosp (page 61); **Address:** 7401 Osler Drive, Ste 107, Towson, MD 21204; **Phone:** 410-321-5900; **Board Cert:** Dermatology 1980; Clinical & Laboratory Dermatologic Immunology 1987; **Med School:** Canada 1975; **Resid:** Internal Medicine, Hlth Scis Ctr 1977; Dermatology, Univ Mich Med Ctr 1980; **Fellow:** Immunology, Univ Mich Med Ctr 1981; **Fac Appt:** Prof D, Johns Hopkins Univ

Bernstein, Robert M MD [D] - **Spec Exp:** Hair Restoration/Transplant; Hair Loss in Women; **Hospital:** NY-Presby Hosp/Columbia (page 66); **Address:** 110 E 55th St, New York, NY 10022; **Phone:** 212-826-2400; **Board Cert:** Dermatology 1982; Hair Restoration Surgery 1998; **Med School:** UMDNJ-NJ Med Sch, Newark 1978; **Resid:** Dermatology, Montefiore Med Ctr 1982; **Fac Appt:** Clin Prof D, Columbia P&S

Bickers, David MD [D] - **Spec Exp:** Skin Cancer; Photodynamic Therapy; Psoriasis; Phototherapy; **Hospital:** NY-Presby Hosp/Columbia (page 66); **Address:** 16 E 60th St, Ste 300, New York, NY 10022-1002; **Phone:** 212-326-8465; **Board Cert:** Dermatology 1974; **Med School:** Univ VA Sch Med 1967; **Resid:** Dermatology, NYU Med Ctr 1973; **Fellow:** Pharmacology, Rockefeller Univ Hosp 1974; **Fac Appt:** Prof D, Columbia P&S

Brandt, Fredric S MD [D] - **Spec Exp:** Botox Therapy; Cosmetic Dermatology; **Address:** Laser & Skin Surgery Ctr, 317 E 34th St Fl 6, New York, NY 10016; **Phone:** 212-889-7096; **Board Cert:** Internal Medicine 1978; Dermatology 1981; **Med School:** Hahnemann Univ 1975; **Resid:** Internal Medicine, VA Hosp 1981; Dermatology, Univ Miami Hosps 1983

Braun III, Martin MD [D] - **Spec Exp:** Mohs' Surgery; Skin Cancer; **Hospital:** G Washington Univ Hosp; **Address:** 2112 F St NW, Ste 701, Washington, DC 20037; **Phone:** 202-293-7618; **Board Cert:** Dermatology 1977; Dermatopathology 1982; **Med School:** Univ MD Sch Med 1970; **Resid:** Dermatology, Univ Mich Med Ctr 1976; **Fellow:** Mohs Surgery, Precept w/ Dr Frederic Mohs 1975; **Fac Appt:** Clin Prof D, Geo Wash Univ

Brodland, David MD [D] - **Spec Exp:** Mohs' Surgery; Skin Cancer; Reconstructive Surgery-Skin; **Hospital:** UPMC Shadyside, Jefferson Hosp - Pittsburgh; **Address:** South Hills Med Bldg, 575 Coal Valley Rd, Ste 360, Clairton, PA 15025; **Phone:** 412-466-9400; **Board Cert:** Dermatology 1989; **Med School:** Southern IL Univ 1985; **Resid:** Dermatology, Mayo Grad Sch Med 1989; **Fellow:** Mohs Surgery, John A Zitelli MD 1990; **Fac Appt:** Asst Clin Prof D, Univ Pittsburgh

Bystryn, Jean-Claude MD [D] - **Spec Exp:** Melanoma; Blistering Diseases; Skin Cancer; Hair Loss; **Hospital:** NYU Langone Med Ctr (page 67); **Address:** 530 1st Ave, Ste 7F, New York, NY 10016; **Phone:** 212-889-3846; **Board Cert:** Dermatology 1970; Clinical & Laboratory Dermatologic Immunology 1985; **Med School:** NYU Sch Med 1962; **Resid:** Internal Medicine, Montefiore Hosp 1964; Dermatology, NYU Med Ctr 1969; **Fellow:** Immunology, New York Univ 1972; **Fac Appt:** Prof D, NYU Sch Med

Cohen, Bernard A MD [D] - **Spec Exp:** Pediatric Dermatology; Skin Laser Surgery; Hemangiomas; Vascular Malformations; **Hospital:** Johns Hopkins Hosp (page 61); **Address:** Johns Hopkins Div Ped Dermatology, Rubenstein Child Health Bldg, 200 N Wolfe St, Ste 2107, Baltimore, MD 21287; **Phone:** 410-955-2049; **Board Cert:** Pediatrics 1982; Dermatology 1984; Pediatric Dermatology 2004; **Med School:** Johns Hopkins Univ 1977; **Resid:** Pediatrics, Johns Hopkins Hosp 1980; Dermatology, Johns Hopkins Hosp 1984; **Fac Appt:** Prof D, Johns Hopkins Univ

Cotsarelis, George MD [D] - **Spec Exp:** Hair loss; Scalp Disorders; Hair Restoration/Transplant; **Hospital:** Hosp Univ Penn - UPHS (page 60); **Address:** Penn Medicine at Radnor, Dermatology, 250 King of Prussia Rd, Radnor, PA 19087; **Phone:** 610-902-2400; **Board Cert:** Dermatology 2001; **Med School:** Univ Pennsylvania 1987; **Resid:** Dermatology, Hosp Univ Penn 1992; **Fellow:** Dermatology, Hosp Univ Penn; **Fac Appt:** Asst Prof D, Univ Pennsylvania

Deleo, Vincent A MD [D] - **Spec Exp:** Photosensitive Skin Diseases; Contact Dermatitis; Facial Rejuvenation; Eczema; **Hospital:** St Luke's - Roosevelt Hosp Ctr - Roosevelt Div (page 57), Beth Israel Med Ctr - Petrie Division (page 57); **Address:** 1090 Amsterdam Ave Fl 11, New York, NY 10025; **Phone:** 212-523-5898; **Board Cert:** Dermatology 1976; **Med School:** Louisiana State U, New Orleans 1969; **Resid:** Dermatology, Columbia-Presby Med Ctr 1976; **Fac Appt:** Clin Prof D, Columbia P&S

Dzubow, Leonard M MD [D] - **Spec Exp:** Mohs' Surgery; Skin Cancer; **Address:** 101 Chesley Drive, Media, PA 19063; **Phone:** 484-621-0082; **Board Cert:** Internal Medicine 1978; Dermatology 2006; **Med School:** Univ Pennsylvania 1975; **Resid:** Internal Medicine, Hosp Univ Penn 1978; Dermatology, NYU-Skin Cancer Unit 1980; **Fellow:** Mohs Surgery, NYU-Skin Cancer Unit 1981; **Fac Appt:** Prof D, Univ Pennsylvania

Dermatology

Franks Jr, Andrew G MD [D] - **Spec Exp:** Lupus/SLE; Raynaud's Disease; Scleroderma; Dermatomyositis; **Hospital:** NYU Langone Med Ctr (page 67); **Address:** NYU Dermatologic Assocs, Faculty Practice Tower, 530 First Ave Fl 7 - Ste 7R, New York, NY 10016; **Phone:** 212-263-5889; **Board Cert:** Internal Medicine 1975; Dermatology 1977; Rheumatology 1978; **Med School:** NY Med Coll 1971; **Resid:** Internal Medicine, Beth Israel Med Ctr 1974; Dermatology, Columbia-Presby Med Ctr 1975; **Fellow:** Rheumatology, Columbia-Presby Med Ctr 1977; **Fac Appt:** Prof D, NYU Sch Med

Geronemus, Roy MD [D] - **Spec Exp:** Skin Laser Surgery; Cosmetic Dermatology; Mohs' Surgery; Skin Cancer; **Hospital:** NYU Langone Med Ctr (page 67), New York Eye & Ear Infirm (page 65); **Address:** 317 E 34 St, Ste 11N, New York, NY 10016-4974; **Phone:** 212-686-7306; **Board Cert:** Dermatology 1983; **Med School:** Univ Miami Sch Med 1979; **Resid:** Dermatology, NYU-Skin Cancer Unit 1983; **Fellow:** Mohs Surgery, NYU-Skin Cancer Unit 1984; **Fac Appt:** Clin Prof D, NYU Sch Med

Gordon, Marsha MD [D] - **Spec Exp:** Cosmetic Dermatology; Botox Therapy; Skin Cancer; **Hospital:** Mount Sinai Med Ctr (page 64); **Address:** 5 E 98th St Fl 5, New York, NY 10029-6501; **Phone:** 212-241-9728; **Board Cert:** Dermatology 1988; **Med School:** Univ Pennsylvania 1984; **Resid:** Dermatology, Mt Sinai Hosp 1988; **Fac Appt:** Clin Prof D, Mount Sinai Sch Med

Granstein, Richard D MD [D] - **Spec Exp:** Autoimmune Disease; Skin Cancer; Psoriasis; **Hospital:** NY-Presby Hosp/Weill Cornell (page 66); **Address:** 1305 York Ave Fl 9, New York, NY 10021; **Phone:** 646-962-7546; **Board Cert:** Dermatology 1983; Clinical & Laboratory Dematologic Immunology 1985; **Med School:** UCLA 1978; **Resid:** Dermatology, Mass Genl Hosp 1981; **Fellow:** Research, Natl Cancer Inst 1982; Dermatology, Mass Genl Hosp 1983; **Fac Appt:** Prof D, Cornell Univ-Weill Med Coll

Grossman, Melanie MD [D] - **Spec Exp:** Skin Laser Surgery; Tattoo Removal; Laser Resurfacing; Facial Rejuvenation; **Hospital:** NY-Presby Hosp/Columbia (page 66); **Address:** 161 Madison Ave, Ste 4NW, New York, NY 10016-5405; **Phone:** 212-725-8600; **Board Cert:** Dermatology 1999; **Med School:** NYU Sch Med 1988; **Resid:** Internal Medicine, Yale-New Haven Hosp 1989; Dermatology, Columbia-Presby Med Ctr 1992; **Fellow:** Laser Surgery, Mass Genl Hosp 1995; **Fac Appt:** Asst Clin Prof D, Columbia P&S

Halpern, Allan C MD [D] - **Spec Exp:** Skin Cancer; Melanoma; Melanoma Early Detection/Prevention; **Hospital:** Meml Sloan-Kettering Cancer Ctr; **Address:** 1275 York Avenue, New York, NY 10065; **Phone:** 212-610-0766; **Board Cert:** Internal Medicine 1984; Dermatology 1988; **Med School:** Albert Einstein Coll Med 1981; **Resid:** Internal Medicine, Montefiore Hosp 1985; Dermatology, Hosp Univ Penn 1989; **Fellow:** Epidemiology, Hosp Univ Penn 1989; **Fac Appt:** Assoc Prof Med, Cornell Univ-Weill Med Coll

James, William D MD [D] - **Spec Exp:** Contact Dermatitis; Acne; Rosacea; **Hospital:** Hosp Univ Penn - UPHS (page 60); **Address:** Univ Penn Dept Dermatology, 3600 Spruce St, 2 Maloney, Philadelphia, PA 19104; **Phone:** 215-662-4282; **Board Cert:** Dermatology 1981; Diagnostic Lab Immunology 1985; **Med School:** Indiana Univ 1977; **Resid:** Dermatology, Letterman Army Med Ctr 1981; **Fac Appt:** Prof D, Univ Pennsylvania

Katz, Stephen MD [D] - **Spec Exp:** Immune Deficiency-Skin Disorders; **Hospital:** Natl Inst of Hlth - Clin Ctr; **Address:** NIH-Dermatology Branch, 31 Center Drive, MSC 2350, Bldg 31 - rm 4C32, Bethesda, MD 20892; **Phone:** 301-496-2481; **Board Cert:** Dermatology 1971; Clinical & Laboratory Dematologic Immunology 1985; **Med School:** Tulane Univ 1966; **Resid:** Dermatology, Jackson Meml Hosp 1970; **Fellow:** Research 1974

Kress, Douglas W MD [D] - **Spec Exp:** Pediatric Dermatology; **Hospital:** Chldns Hosp of Pittsburgh - UPMC; **Address:** Children's Dermatology Ctr, 11279 Perry Hwy, Ste 108, Wexford, PA 15090; **Phone:** 724-933-9190; **Board Cert:** Dermatology 1996; Pediatric Dermatology 2004; **Med School:** Jefferson Med Coll 1992; **Resid:** Dermatology, Univ Pittsburgh Med Ctr 1996; **Fellow:** Pediatric Dermatology, Children's Hosp 2003; **Fac Appt:** Assoc Clin Prof D, Univ Pittsburgh

Kriegel, David MD [D] - **Spec Exp:** Mohs' Surgery; Botox Therapy; Skin Laser Surgery; Cosmetic Dermatology; **Hospital:** Mount Sinai Med Ctr (page 64); **Address:** 250 W 57th St, Ste 825, New York, NY 10107-0809; **Phone:** 212-489-6669; **Board Cert:** Dermatology 2003; **Med School:** Boston Univ 1987; **Resid:** Dermatology, New England Med Ctr 1991; **Fellow:** Mohs Surgery, Stony Brook Univ Hosp 1993; **Fac Appt:** Assoc Prof D, Mount Sinai Sch Med

Lebwohl, Mark MD [D] - **Spec Exp:** Skin Cancer; Cutaneous Lymphoma; Psoriasis; Pseudoxanthoma Elasticum; **Hospital:** Mount Sinai Med Ctr (page 64); **Address:** 5 E 98th St Fl 5, New York, NY 10029-6501; **Phone:** 212-241-9728; **Board Cert:** Internal Medicine 1981; Dermatology 1983; **Med School:** Harvard Med Sch 1978; **Resid:** Internal Medicine, Mt Sinai Hosp 1981; **Fellow:** Dermatology, Mt Sinai Hosp 1983; **Fac Appt:** Prof D, Mount Sinai Sch Med

Lessin, Stuart R MD [D] - **Spec Exp:** Melanoma; Skin Cancer; Cutaneous Lymphoma; Melanoma Risk Assessment; **Hospital:** Fox Chase Cancer Ctr (page 58); **Address:** Fox Chase Cancer Ctr, Dept Dermatology, 333 Cottman Ave, Philadelphia, PA 19111; **Phone:** 215-728-2570; **Board Cert:** Dermatology 1986; **Med School:** Temple Univ 1982; **Resid:** Dermatology, Hosp Univ Penn 1986; **Fellow:** Molecular Biology, Wistar Inst 1987; **Fac Appt:** Prof D, Temple Univ

Miller, Stanley J MD [D] - **Spec Exp:** Skin Cancer; Mohs' Surgery; Melanoma; **Hospital:** Johns Hopkins Hosp (page 61); **Address:** Charles Towson Bldg, 1104 Kenilworth Drive, Ste 201, Towson, MD 21204; **Phone:** 443-279-0340; **Board Cert:** Dermatology 1989; **Med School:** Univ VT Coll Med 1984; **Resid:** Dermatology, UCSD Med Ctr 1989; **Fellow:** Dermatologic Surgery, Univ Penn 1991; **Fac Appt:** Prof D, Johns Hopkins Univ

Nigra, Thomas P MD [D] - **Spec Exp:** Hair Loss; Psoriasis; Skin Cancer; Vitiligo; **Hospital:** Washington Hosp Ctr, Natl Rehab Hosp; **Address:** Dermatology Assocs, 110 Irving St NW, 2B44, Washington, DC 20010; **Phone:** 202-877-6227; **Board Cert:** Dermatology 1973; **Med School:** Univ Pennsylvania 1967; **Resid:** Dermatology, Mass Genl Hosp 1973; Dermatology, Natl Insts of Health 1971; **Fac Appt:** Clin Prof D, Geo Wash Univ

Orlow, Seth J MD/PhD [D] - **Spec Exp:** Pediatric Dermatology; Hemangiomas/Birthmarks; Psoriasis/Eczema; **Hospital:** NYU Langone Med Ctr (page 67); **Address:** 530 1st Ave, Ste 7R, New York, NY 10016-6402; **Phone:** 212-263-5889; **Board Cert:** Dermatology 1990; Pediatric Dermatology 2004; **Med School:** Albert Einstein Coll Med 1986; **Resid:** Pediatrics, Mt Sinai Hosp 1987; Dermatology, Yale-New Haven Hosp 1989; **Fellow:** Pediatric Dermatology, Yale-New Haven Hosp 1990; **Fac Appt:** Prof D, NYU Sch Med

Ramsay, David L MD [D] - **Spec Exp:** Cutaneous Lymphoma; Skin Cancer; **Hospital:** NYU Langone Med Ctr (page 67); **Address:** 530 1st Ave, Ste 7G, New York, NY 10016-6402; **Phone:** 212-683-6283; **Board Cert:** Dermatology 1974; **Med School:** Indiana Univ 1969; **Resid:** Dermatology, NYU Med Ctr 1973; **Fellow:** Dermatology, Univ Ill Hosp 1973; **Fac Appt:** Clin Prof D, NYU Sch Med

Rigel, Darrell S MD [D] - **Spec Exp:** Melanoma; Skin Cancer; Cosmetic Dermatology; **Hospital:** NYU Langone Med Ctr (page 67), Mount Sinai Med Ctr (page 64); **Address:** 35 E 35th Street, Ste 208, New York, NY 10016-3823; **Phone:** 212-684-5964; **Board Cert:** Dermatology 1983; **Med School:** Geo Wash Univ 1978; **Resid:** Dermatology, NYU Med Ctr 1982; **Fellow:** Dermatologic Surgery, NYU Med Ctr 1983; **Fac Appt:** Clin Prof D, NYU Sch Med

Dermatology

Robins, Perry MD [D] - **Spec Exp:** Mohs' Surgery; Skin Cancer; Melanoma; **Hospital:** NYU Langone Med Ctr (page 67), Bellevue Hosp Ctr; **Address:** 345 E 37 St, Ste 209, New York, NY 10016; **Phone:** 212-263-7222; **Med School:** Germany 1961; **Resid:** Dermatology, VA Med Ctr 1964; **Fellow:** Dermatology, NYU Med Ctr 1967; **Fac Appt:** Prof Emeritus D, NYU Sch Med

Rook, Alain H MD [D] - **Spec Exp:** Cutaneous Lymphoma; Immune Deficiency-Skin Disorders; Mycosis Fungoides; **Hospital:** Hosp Univ Penn - UPHS (page 60); **Address:** Dept Dermatology, 3400 Spruce St Maloney Bldg Fl 2, Philadelphia, PA 19104; **Phone:** 215-662-7610; **Board Cert:** Internal Medicine 1979; Nephrology 1980; Dermatology 2001; **Med School:** Univ Mich Med Sch 1975; **Resid:** Internal Medicine, McGill Univ Med Ctr 1977; Dermatology, Hosp Univ Penn 1989; **Fellow:** Nephrology, McGill Univ Med Ctr 1979; Immunology, NIH 1986; **Fac Appt:** Prof D, Univ Pennsylvania

Sarnoff, Deborah S MD [D] - **Spec Exp:** Skin Laser Surgery; Cosmetic Dermatology; Mohs' Surgery; Skin Cancer; **Hospital:** NYU Langone Med Ctr (page 67); **Address:** 625 Park Ave, New York, NY 10065; **Phone:** 212-794-4000; **Board Cert:** Dermatology 1984; **Med School:** Geo Wash Univ 1980; **Resid:** Dermatology, NYU Med Ctr 1984; **Fellow:** Dermatologic Surgery, NYU Med Ctr 1986; **Fac Appt:** Clin Prof D, NYU Sch Med

Schultz, Neal MD [D] - **Spec Exp:** Cosmetic Dermatology; Melanoma Early Detection/Prevention; Skin Laser Surgery; Tattoo Removal; **Hospital:** Mount Sinai Med Ctr (page 64), Lenox Hill Hosp (page 62); **Address:** 1130 Park Ave, New York, NY 10128; **Phone:** 212-369-9600; **Board Cert:** Dermatology 1978; **Med School:** Columbia P&S 1973; **Resid:** Internal Medicine, Mt Sinai Hosp 1975; Dermatology, Mt Sinai Hosp 1978; **Fac Appt:** Asst Clin Prof D, Mount Sinai Sch Med

Shalita, Alan MD [D] - **Spec Exp:** Acne; Rosacea; **Hospital:** SUNY Downstate Med Ctr, Kings County Hosp Ctr; **Address:** SUNY Downstate Med Ctr, 450 Clarkson Ave, Dermatology, Box 46, Brooklyn, NY 11203-2012; **Phone:** 718-270-1230; **Board Cert:** Dermatology 1971; **Med School:** Wake Forest Univ 1964; **Resid:** Dermatology, NYU Med Ctr 1970; **Fellow:** Dermatologic Research, NYU Med Ctr 1973; **Fac Appt:** Prof D, SUNY Downstate

Shupack, Jerome L MD [D] - **Spec Exp:** Rare Skin Disorders; Psoriasis; Geriatric Dermatology; **Hospital:** NYU Langone Med Ctr (page 67); **Address:** 530 1st Ave, HCC 7F, New York, NY 10016-6402; **Phone:** 212-263-7344; **Board Cert:** Dermatology 1970; **Med School:** Columbia P&S 1963; **Resid:** Internal Medicine, Mt Sinai Hosp 1965; Dermatology, NYU Med Ctr 1970; **Fac Appt:** Prof D, NYU Sch Med

Soter, Nicholas A MD [D] - **Spec Exp:** Urticaria; Psoriasis; Vasculitis; **Hospital:** NYU Langone Med Ctr (page 67); **Address:** 530 1st Ave, Ste 7R, Dermatology Assocs-Langone, New York, NY 10016-6402; **Phone:** 212-263-5889; **Board Cert:** Dermatology 1970; Diagnostic Lab Immunology 1985; **Med School:** Univ Tex SW, Dallas 1965; **Resid:** Dermatology, Baylor Med Ctr 1968; Dermatology, Mass Genl Hosp 1969; **Fac Appt:** Prof D, NYU Sch Med

Stanley, John R MD [D] - **Spec Exp:** Blistering Diseases; Pemphigus; **Hospital:** Hosp Univ Penn - UPHS (page 60); **Address:** Univ of Pennsylvania, Dept Dermatology, 3400 Spruce St, 2 Rhoads Pavilion, Philadelphia, PA 19104; **Phone:** 215-662-2737; **Board Cert:** Dermatology 1978; Clinical & Laboratory Dematologic Immunology 1985; **Med School:** Harvard Med Sch 1974; **Resid:** Dermatology, NYU Med Ctr 1978; **Fac Appt:** Prof D, Univ Pennsylvania

Werth, Victoria P MD [D] - **Spec Exp:** Autoimmune Disease; Lupus/SLE; Connective Tissue Disorders; Blistering Diseases; **Hospital:** Hosp Univ Penn - UPHS (page 60); **Address:** Univ Penn Health Services, 3600 Spruce St, 2 Rhoads Pavilion, Philadelphia, PA 19104; **Phone:** 215-662-2737; **Board Cert:** Internal Medicine 1983; Dermatology 1986; Diagnostic Lab Immunology 1989; **Med School:** Johns Hopkins Univ 1980; **Resid:** Internal Medicine, Northwestern Meml Hosp 1983; Dermatology, NYU Med Ctr 1986; **Fellow:** Immunological Dermatology, NYU Sch Med 1988; **Fac Appt:** Assoc Prof D, Univ Pennsylvania

Yan, Albert C MD [D] - **Spec Exp:** Pediatric Dermatology; Vascular Malformations; Genetic Disorders-Skin; Atopic Dermatitis; **Hospital:** Chldns Hosp of Philadelphia, The, Hosp Univ Penn - UPHS (page 60); **Address:** Children's Hosp of Philadelphia, Dept Dermatology, 34th & Civic Ctr Blvd, Philadelphia, PA 19104; **Phone:** 215-590-2169; **Board Cert:** Dermatology 2008; Pediatrics 2004; Pediatric Dermatology 2004; **Med School:** Univ Pennsylvania 1993; **Resid:** Pediatrics, Children's Hosp 1996; Dermatology, Hosp Univ Penn 1999; **Fac Appt:** Asst Prof Ped, Univ Pennsylvania

Zitelli, John MD [D] - **Spec Exp:** Mohs' Surgery; Skin Cancer; Melanoma; **Hospital:** UPMC Shadyside, Jefferson Hosp - Pittsburgh; **Address:** Shadyside Med Ctr, 5200 Centre Ave, Ste 303, Pittsburgh, PA 15232-1312; **Phone:** 412-681-9400; **Board Cert:** Dermatology 1980; **Med School:** Univ Pittsburgh 1976; **Resid:** Dermatology, Univ Hlth Ctr Hosp 1979; **Fellow:** Mohs Surgery, Univ Wisconsin 1980; **Fac Appt:** Assoc Clin Prof D, Univ Pittsburgh

Southeast

Amonette, Rex A MD [D] - **Spec Exp:** Skin Cancer; Mohs' Surgery; **Address:** Memphis Dermatology Clinic, 1455 Union Ave, Memphis, TN 38104-6727; **Phone:** 901-726-6655; **Board Cert:** Dermatology 1974; **Med School:** Univ Ark 1966; **Resid:** Dermatology, Univ Tenn Med Ctr 1971; **Fellow:** Mohs Surgery, NYU Med Ctr 1972; **Fac Appt:** Clin Prof D, Univ Tenn Coll Med, Memphis

Brody, Harold J MD [D] - **Spec Exp:** Cosmetic Dermatology; Cosmetic Surgery; **Hospital:** Emory Univ Hosp Midtown; **Address:** 1218 W Paces Ferry Rd NE, Ste 200, Atlanta, GA 30327; **Phone:** 404-525-7409; **Board Cert:** Dermatology 1978; **Med School:** Med Univ SC 1974; **Resid:** Dermatology, Emory Affil Hosps 1978; **Fac Appt:** Clin Prof D, Emory Univ

Burton III, Claude S MD [D] - **Spec Exp:** Leg Ulcers; Wound Healing/Care; Hemangiomas; Laser Surgery; **Hospital:** Duke Univ Med Ctr; **Address:** DUMC, Box 3511, Durham, NC 27710; **Phone:** 919-684-3432; **Board Cert:** Internal Medicine 1982; Dermatology 1984; **Med School:** Duke Univ 1979; **Resid:** Internal Medicine, Duke Univ Med Ctr 1982; Dermatology, Duke Univ Med Ctr 1984; **Fac Appt:** Prof D, Duke Univ

Callen, Jeffrey P MD [D] - **Spec Exp:** Lupus/SLE; Dermatomyositis; Vasculitis; Skin Signs of Int Disease/Cancer; **Hospital:** Univ of Louisville Hosp, Norton Hosp; **Address:** 310 E Broadway, Ste 200, Louisville, KY 40202; **Phone:** 502-583-1749; **Board Cert:** Internal Medicine 1975; Dermatology 1999; **Med School:** Univ Mich Med Sch 1972; **Resid:** Internal Medicine, Univ Mich Med Ctr 1975; Dermatology, Univ Mich Med Ctr 1977; **Fac Appt:** Prof Med, Univ Louisville Sch Med

Camisa, Charles MD [D] - **Spec Exp:** Psoriasis; Oral Dermatology; Lichen Planus; **Hospital:** Physicians Regl Med Ctr; **Address:** Riverchase Dermatology, 1015 Crosspointe Drive, Naples, FL 34110; **Phone:** 239-596-9075; **Board Cert:** Dermatology 1981; Clinical & Laboratory Dermatologic Immunology 1987; **Med School:** Mount Sinai Sch Med 1977; **Resid:** Dermatology, NYU Med Ctr 1981; **Fac Appt:** Assoc Prof D, Univ S Fla Coll Med

Dermatology

Cohen, Bernard H MD [D] - **Spec Exp:** Hair Restoration/Transplant; Hair Loss; **Hospital:** Jackson Meml Hosp (page 70); **Address:** 4425 Ponce de Leon Blvd, Ste 230, Coral Gables, FL 33146; **Phone:** 305-476-9544; **Board Cert:** Dermatology 1972; Hair Restoration Surgery ; **Med School:** Columbia P&S 1967; **Resid:** Dermatology, NYU Med Ctr 1971; **Fac Appt:** Clin Prof D, Univ Miami Sch Med

Cook, Jonathan L MD [D] - **Spec Exp:** Skin Cancer; Mohs' Surgery; Reconstructive Surgery-Skin; Laser Surgery; **Hospital:** Duke Univ Med Ctr; **Address:** Duke Univ Med Ctr, Box 3915, Durham, NC 27710; **Phone:** 919-684-6805; **Board Cert:** Dermatology 2005; **Med School:** Med Univ SC 1992; **Resid:** Dermatology, Emory Univ Hosp 1996; **Fellow:** Dermatologic Surgery, Hosp Univ Penn 1997; **Fac Appt:** Prof D, Duke Univ

Eichler, Craig J MD [D] - **Spec Exp:** Skin Cancer; Dermatologic Surgery; **Hospital:** Physicians Regl Med Ctr; **Address:** 6101 Pine Ridge Rd, Naples, FL 34119-3900; **Phone:** 239-348-4335; **Board Cert:** Dermatology 2003; **Med School:** Univ Fla Coll Med 1989; **Resid:** Dermatology, Univ Texas Med Branch 1993

Elmets, Craig A MD [D] - **Spec Exp:** Psoriasis/Eczema; Phototherapy; Skin Cancer; Photodynamic Therapy; **Hospital:** Univ of Ala Hosp at Birmingham, VA Med Ctr; **Address:** Univ of Alabama-Birmingham-Derm Dept, 1530 3 Ave S EFH Bldg - rm 414, Birmingham, AL 35294; **Phone:** 205-996-7546; **Board Cert:** Internal Medicine 1978; Dermatology 1980; Clinical & Laboratory Dermatologic Immunology 1989; **Med School:** Univ Iowa Coll Med 1975; **Resid:** Internal Medicine, Kansas Med Ctr 1978; Dermatology, Univ Iowa Hosps 1980; **Fellow:** Immunological Dermatology, Univ Texas Hlth Sci Ctr 1982; **Fac Appt:** Prof D, Univ Alabama

Epstein, Jeffrey S MD [D] - **Spec Exp:** Hair Restoration/Transplant; Facial Plastic Surgery; **Hospital:** South Miami Hosp; **Address:** 6280 Sunset Drive, Ste 504, Miami, FL 33143; **Phone:** 305-666-1774; **Board Cert:** Otolaryngology 1994; Facial Plastic & Reconstr Surgery 1995; Hair Restoration Surgery 1998; **Med School:** Univ VT Coll Med 1988; **Resid:** Otolaryngology, Jackson Meml Hosp 1993; **Fellow:** Facial Plastic Surgery, Sheldon S Kabaker MD 1994; **Fac Appt:** Clin Prof Oto, Univ Miami Sch Med

Fenske, Neil A MD [D] - **Spec Exp:** Skin Cancer; Melanoma; Psoriasis; **Hospital:** H Lee Moffitt Cancer Ctr & Research Inst, Tampa Genl Hosp; **Address:** 12901 Bruce B Downs Blvd, MDC-33, Tampa, FL 33612-4742; **Phone:** 813-974-2920; **Board Cert:** Dermatology 1977; Dermatopathology 1984; **Med School:** St Louis Univ 1973; **Resid:** Dermatology, Wisc Hlth Sci Ctr 1977; **Fac Appt:** Prof Med, Univ S Fla Coll Med

Flowers, Franklin P MD [D] - **Spec Exp:** Mohs' Surgery; Dermatopathology; **Hospital:** Shands at Univ of FL; **Address:** Shands Healthcare, PO Box 100383, Gainesville, FL 32610-0383; **Phone:** 352-265-8001; **Board Cert:** Dermatology 1976; Dermatopathology 1981; **Med School:** Univ Fla Coll Med 1971; **Resid:** Dermatology, Ohio State Univ 1975; **Fellow:** Mohs Surgery, Univ Alabama 1993; **Fac Appt:** Prof Med, Univ Fla Coll Med

Garrett, Algin MD [D] - **Spec Exp:** Skin Cancer; Mohs' Surgery; **Hospital:** Med Coll of VA Hosp; **Address:** Stonypoint Medical Park, 9000 Stonypoint Pkwy Fl 2, Richmond, VA 23235; **Phone:** 804-560-8991; **Board Cert:** Dermatology 1983; **Med School:** Penn State Univ-Hershey Med Ctr 1978; **Resid:** Internal Medicine, VA Med Ctr 1980; Dermatology, Med Col VA 1983; **Fellow:** Mohs Surgery, Cleveland Clinic Found 1988; **Fac Appt:** Prof D, Va Commonwealth Univ Sch Med

Green, Howard A MD [D] - **Spec Exp:** Mohs' Surgery; Skin Cancer; **Hospital:** St Mary's Med Ctr - W Palm Bch; **Address:** 120 Butler St, Ste A, West Palm Beach, FL 33407-6106; **Phone:** 561-659-1510; **Board Cert:** Internal Medicine 1988; Dermatology 2004; **Med School:** Boston Univ 1985; **Resid:** Internal Medicine, Jefferson Univ Hosp 1988; Dermatology, Harvard Affil Hosps 1992; **Fellow:** Mohs Surgery, Boston Univ Med Ctr 1993

Grichnik, James M MD/PhD [D] - **Spec Exp:** Melanoma; Skin Cancer; **Hospital:** Univ of Miami Hosp & Clins/Sylvester Comp Canc Ctr (page 70); **Address:** Univ Miami, UMHC-Sylvester CCC, 1475 NW 12th Ave, D1, Miami, FL 33136; **Phone:** 305-243-6045; **Board Cert:** Dermatology 2003; **Med School:** Harvard Med Sch 1990; **Resid:** Dermatology, Duke Univ Med Ctr 1994; **Fac Appt:** Assoc Prof D, Duke Univ

Johr, Robert MD [D] - **Spec Exp:** Pigmented Lesions; Melanoma; Pediatric Dermatology; **Hospital:** Univ of Miami Hosp & Clins/Sylvester Comp Canc Ctr (page 70), Boca Raton Comm Hosp; **Address:** 1050 NW 15th St, Ste 201A, Boca Raton, FL 33486-1341; **Phone:** 561-368-4545; **Board Cert:** Dermatology 1981; **Med School:** Mexico 1975; **Resid:** Dermatology, Roswell Park Cancer Ctr 1977; Dermatology, Metro Med Ctr/Case Western Reserve 1979; **Fac Appt:** Clin Prof D, Univ Miami Sch Med

Jorizzo, Joseph L MD [D] - **Spec Exp:** Rheumatologic Dermatology; Immune Deficiency-Skin Disorders; **Hospital:** Wake Forest Univ Baptist Med Ctr (page 72); **Address:** Wake Forest Univ Sch Med, Dept Derm, Med Ctr Blvd, Winston-Salem, NC 27157-0001; **Phone:** 336-716-3926; **Board Cert:** Dermatology 1979; **Med School:** Boston Univ 1975; **Resid:** Dermatology, Univ North Carolina Hosps 1979; **Fellow:** Dermatology, Dermatology Inst 1980; **Fac Appt:** Prof D, Wake Forest Univ

Kirsner, Robert S MD/PhD [D] - **Spec Exp:** Wound Healing/Care; Leg Ulcers; **Hospital:** Univ of Miami Hosp (page 71), Jackson Meml Hosp (page 70); **Address:** Univ Miami, Dept Dermatology, 1444 NW 9th Ave, Miami, FL 33136-1406; **Phone:** 305-243-6704; **Board Cert:** Dermatology 2005; **Med School:** Univ Miami Sch Med 1988; **Resid:** Internal Medicine, Univ Miami-Jackson Meml Hosp 1990; Dermatology, Univ Miami-Jackson Meml Hosp 1995; **Fellow:** Wound Healing, Univ Miami-Jackson Meml Hosp 1992; **Fac Appt:** Prof D, Univ Miami Sch Med

Leshin, Barry MD [D] - **Spec Exp:** Skin Cancer; Mohs' Surgery; **Address:** 125 Sunnynoll Ct, Ste 100, Winston-Salem, NC 27106; **Phone:** 336-724-2434; **Board Cert:** Dermatology 1985; **Med School:** Univ Tex, Houston 1981; **Resid:** Dermatology, Univ Iowa Hosp 1985; **Fellow:** Dermatologic Surgery, Univ Iowa Hosp 1986; **Fac Appt:** Clin Prof PlS, Wake Forest Univ

McMichael, Amy J MD [D] - **Spec Exp:** Hair loss; Ethnic Skin Disorders; Pigmented Lesions; Skin Cancer; **Hospital:** Wake Forest Univ Baptist Med Ctr (page 72); **Address:** Medical Center Drive, Winston-Salem, NC 27157; **Phone:** 336-716-3926; **Board Cert:** Dermatology 2004; **Med School:** Univ Pennsylvania 1990; **Resid:** Dermatology, Univ Mich Hosps 1994

Olsen, Elise A MD [D] - **Spec Exp:** Hair loss; Hirsutism; Cutaneous Lymphoma; **Hospital:** Duke Univ Med Ctr; **Address:** Duke Univ Med Ctr, Box 3294, Durham, NC 27710; **Phone:** 919-684-3432; **Board Cert:** Dermatology 1983; **Med School:** Baylor Coll Med 1978; **Resid:** Internal Medicine, Univ NC Meml Hosp 1980; Dermatology, Duke Univ Med Ctr 1983; **Fac Appt:** Prof D, Duke Univ

Sherertz, Elizabeth F MD [D] - **Spec Exp:** Eczema; Contact Dermatitis; Occupational Skin Diseases; **Address:** 1400 West Gate Ctr Drive, Ste 200, Winston-Salem, NC 27103; **Phone:** 336-774-8636; **Board Cert:** Dermatology 1982; **Med School:** Univ VA Sch Med 1978; **Resid:** Dermatology, Duke Univ Med Ctr 1982; **Fac Appt:** Clin Prof D, Wake Forest Univ

Dermatology

Sobel, Stuart MD [D] - **Spec Exp:** Skin Cancer; Cosmetic Dermatology; **Hospital:** Meml Regl Hosp, Joe Di Maggio Chldns Hosp; **Address:** 4340 Sheridan St, Ste 101, Hollywood, FL 33021-3511; **Phone:** 954-983-5533; **Board Cert:** Dermatology 1977; **Med School:** Tufts Univ 1972; **Resid:** Dermatology, Mt Sinai Hosp 1976

Sokoloff, Daniel O MD [D] - **Spec Exp:** Skin Cancer; Cosmetic Dermatology; **Hospital:** St Mary's Med Ctr - W Palm Bch, Good Sam Med Ctr - W Palm Beach; **Address:** 4475 Med Ctr Way, Ste 2, 1000 45th St, Ste 1, West Palm Beach, FL 33407-2416; **Phone:** 561-863-1000; **Board Cert:** Dermatology 1982; **Med School:** Geo Wash Univ 1977; **Resid:** Dermatology, Baylor Coll Med 1982

Thiers, Bruce H MD [D] - **Spec Exp:** Cutaneous Lymphoma; Skin Cancer; Psoriasis; **Hospital:** MUSC Med Ctr; **Address:** MUSC Dept Dermatology, 135 Rutledge Ave Fl 11, MS 578, Charleston, SC 29425; **Phone:** 843-792-9784; **Board Cert:** Dermatology 1978; **Med School:** SUNY Buffalo 1974; **Resid:** Dermatology, SUNY Buffalo Med Ctr 1978; **Fac Appt:** Prof D, Med Univ SC

Midwest

Arpey, Christopher J MD [D] - **Spec Exp:** Mohs' Surgery; **Hospital:** Univ Iowa Hosp & Clinics; **Address:** UIHC Dept Dermatology, 200 Hawkins Drive, 300 EMRB, Iowa City, IA 52242-1009; **Phone:** 319-356-2856; **Board Cert:** Dermatology 2001; Internal Medicine 1989; **Med School:** Univ Rochester 1986; **Resid:** Internal Medicine, Univ Iowa Hosps & Clinics 1989; Dermatology, Univ Hosps 1992; **Fellow:** Mohs Surgery, Univ Iowa Hosps & Clinics 1994; **Fac Appt:** Prof D, Univ Iowa Coll Med

Bailin, Philip L MD [D] - **Spec Exp:** Mohs' Surgery; Skin Laser Surgery; Skin Cancer; **Hospital:** Cleveland Clin Fdn (page 56); **Address:** Cleveland Clinic, Dept Dermatology, 9500 Euclid Ave, Desk A61, Cleveland, OH 44195-5032; **Phone:** 216-444-2115; **Board Cert:** Dermatology 1975; **Med School:** Northwestern Univ 1968; **Resid:** Dermatology, Cleveland Clin Fdn 1974; **Fellow:** Dermatopathology, Armed Forces Inst Pathology 1975; Mohs Surgery, Univ Wisc Hosp & Clin

Cornelius, Lynne A MD [D] - **Spec Exp:** Melanoma; **Hospital:** Barnes-Jewish Hosp; **Address:** Washington Univ Dept Dermatology, 660 S Euclid, Box 8123, St Louis, MO 63110; **Phone:** 314-362-2643; **Board Cert:** Dermatology 1989; **Med School:** Univ MO-Columbia Sch Med 1984; **Resid:** Dermatology, Barnes Jewish Hosp-Wash Univ 1989; **Fellow:** Immunological Dermatology, Emory Univ Med Ctr 1992; **Fac Appt:** Assoc Prof D, Washington Univ, St Louis

Crutchfield III, Charles Edward MD [D] - **Spec Exp:** Skin Cancer; Psoriasis; Eczema; Cosmetic Dermatology; **Address:** Crutchfield Dermatology, 1185 Town Centre Drive, Ste 101, Saint Paul, MN 55123; **Phone:** 651-209-3600; **Board Cert:** Dermatology 2008; **Med School:** Mayo Med Sch 1994; **Resid:** Dermatology, Univ Minnesota Affil Hosp 1998; **Fac Appt:** Assoc Clin Prof D, Univ Minn

Fivenson, David MD [D] - **Spec Exp:** Blistering Diseases; Wound Healing/Care; Lupus/SLE; **Hospital:** St Joseph Mercy Hosp - Ann Arbor; **Address:** 3001 Miller Rd, Ann Arbor, MI 48103; **Phone:** 734-222-9630; **Board Cert:** Dermatology 1989; Clinical & Laboratory Dematologic Immunology 1991; **Med School:** Univ Mich Med Sch 1984; **Resid:** Dermatology, Univ Cincinnati Med Ctr 1989; **Fellow:** Immunological Dermatology, UCSD Med Ctr 1986

Garden, Jerome M MD [D] - **Spec Exp:** Skin Laser Surgery; Facial Rejuvenation; Vascular Birthmarks; **Hospital:** Northwestern Meml Hosp, Children's Mem Hosp; **Address:** 150 E Huron St, Ste 1200, Chicago, IL 60611-2946; **Phone:** 312-280-0890; **Board Cert:** Dermatology 1984; **Med School:** Northwestern Univ 1980; **Resid:** Internal Medicine, Northwestern Univ Affil Hosp 1981; Dermatology, Northwestern Univ Affil Hosp 1984; **Fac Appt:** Prof D, Northwestern Univ

Hanke, C William MD [D] - **Spec Exp:** Mohs' Surgery; Skin Laser Surgery; Cosmetic Dermatology; Photodynamic Therapy; **Hospital:** St Vincent Carmel Hosp, Clarian Hlth Ptrs; **Address:** Laser & Skin Surgery Ctr of Indiana, 13400 N Meridian St, Ste 290, Carmel, IN 46032-1486; **Phone:** 317-660-4900; **Board Cert:** Dermatology 1978; Dermatopathology 1982; **Med School:** Univ Iowa Coll Med 1971; **Resid:** Dermatology, Cleveland Clinic 1978; Dermatopathology, Indiana Univ 1982; **Fellow:** Cutaneous Oncology, Cleveland Clinic 1979; **Fac Appt:** Clin Prof D, Indiana Univ

Hruza, George J MD [D] - **Spec Exp:** Skin Laser Surgery; Mohs' Surgery; Cosmetic Surgery; **Hospital:** St Luke's Hosp - Chesterfield, MO, St Louis Univ Hosp; **Address:** Laser & Derm Surg Ctr, 1001 Chesterfield Pkwy E, Ste 101, St Louis, MO 63017; **Phone:** 314-878-3839; **Board Cert:** Dermatology 1986; **Med School:** NYU Sch Med 1982; **Resid:** Dermatology, NYU Med Ctr-Skin Cancer Unit 1986; **Fellow:** Laser Surgery, Mass Genl Hosp-Harvard 1987; Mohs Surgery, Univ Wisc Affil Hosp 1988; **Fac Appt:** Assoc Clin Prof D, St Louis Univ

Johnson, Timothy M MD [D] - **Spec Exp:** Melanoma; Mohs' Surgery; **Hospital:** Univ Michigan Hlth Sys; **Address:** Univ Michigan Dermatology, 1910 Taubman Ctr, 1500 E Medical Center Drive, Ann Arbor, MI 48109-5314; **Phone:** 734-936-4190; **Board Cert:** Dermatology 1988; **Med School:** Univ Tex, Houston 1984; **Resid:** Dermatology, Univ Texas Med Ctr 1988; **Fellow:** Cutaneous Oncology, Univ Mich Med Ctr 1989; Mohs Surgery, Univ Oregon Hlth Sci Ctr 1990; **Fac Appt:** Prof D, Univ Mich Med Sch

Lim, Henry W MD [D] - **Spec Exp:** Phototherapy; Vitiligo; Cutaneous Lymphoma; Skin Cancer; **Hospital:** Henry Ford Hosp; **Address:** Henry Ford Hosp, Dept Derm, 3031 W Grand Blvd, Ste 800, Detroit, MI 48202-3141; **Phone:** 313-916-4060; **Board Cert:** Dermatology 2005; Clinical & Laboratory Dermatologic Immunology 1985; **Med School:** SUNY Downstate 1975; **Resid:** Dermatology, NYU Med Ctr 1979; **Fellow:** Immunological Dermatology, NYU Med Ctr 1980; **Fac Appt:** Prof Path, Wayne State Univ

Lowe, Lori MD [D] - **Spec Exp:** Dermatopathology; Skin Cancer; **Hospital:** Univ Michigan Hlth Sys; **Address:** Univ Michigan Dept Pathology, 1301 Catherine Rd, M3261-Med Sci I, Ann Arbor, MI 48109-5602; **Phone:** 734-764-4460; **Board Cert:** Dermatology 1990; Dermatopathology 1991; **Med School:** Univ Tex, Houston 1985; **Resid:** Dermatology, Univ Tex Hlth Sci Ctr 1990; **Fellow:** Dermatopathology, Univ Colo Hlth Sci Ctr 1991; **Fac Appt:** Prof D, Univ Mich Med Sch

Lucky, Anne W MD [D] - **Spec Exp:** Pediatric Dermatology; Acne; **Hospital:** Cincinnati Chldns Hosp Med Ctr; **Address:** Derm Assocs Cincinnati, 7691 Five Mile Rd, Ste 312, Cincinnati, OH 45230; **Phone:** 513-232-3332; **Board Cert:** Pediatrics 1975; Pediatric Endocrinology 1978; Dermatology 1981; Pediatric Dermatology 2004; **Med School:** Yale Univ 1970; **Resid:** Pediatrics, Boston Chldns Hosp 1973; Dermatology, Yale-New Haven Hosp 1981; **Fellow:** Pediatric Endocrinology, Natl Inst Hlth 1976; **Fac Appt:** Prof D, Univ Cincinnati

Neuburg, Marcelle MD [D] - **Spec Exp:** Mohs' Surgery; Skin Cancer; Pigmented Lesions; **Hospital:** Froedtert Meml Lutheran Hosp; **Address:** Dept Dermatology, 9200 W Wisconsin Ave, Milwaukee, WI 53226; **Phone:** 414-805-5300; **Board Cert:** Internal Medicine 1985; Dermatology 1988; **Med School:** Oregon Hlth & Sci Univ 1982; **Resid:** Internal Medicine, Georgetown Univ Hosp 1985; Dermatology, Boston Univ Sch Med Ctr 1988; **Fellow:** Mohs Surgery, Tufts New England Med Ctr 1990; **Fac Appt:** Prof D, Med Coll Wisc

Otley, Clark C MD [D] - **Spec Exp:** Mohs' Surgery; Skin Cancer; Skin Cancer in Transplant Patients; Dermatologic Surgery; **Hospital:** Mayo Med Ctr & Clin - Rochester; **Address:** Mayo Clinic, 200 First St SW, Rochester, MN 55905; **Phone:** 507-284-3579; **Board Cert:** Dermatology 2004; **Med School:** Duke Univ 1991; **Resid:** Dermatology, Mass Genl Hosp 1995; **Fellow:** Dermatologic Surgery, Mayo Clinic 1996; **Fac Appt:** Assoc Prof D, Mayo Med Sch

Dermatology

Paller, Amy S MD [D] - **Spec Exp:** Genetic Disorders-Skin; Immune Deficiency-Skin Disorders; Atopic Dermatitis; Pediatric Dermatology; **Hospital:** Children's Mem Hosp; **Address:** 676 N St Clair St, Chicago, IL 60611-2997; **Phone:** 773-327-3446; **Board Cert:** Pediatrics 1982; Pediatric Dermatology 2004; Dermatology 2007; **Med School:** Stanford Univ 1978; **Resid:** Pediatrics, Chldns Meml Hosp 1981; Dermatology, Northwestern Meml Hosp 1983; **Fellow:** Research, Univ NC Hosp 1984; **Fac Appt:** Prof D, Northwestern Univ

Rhodes, Arthur R MD [D] - **Spec Exp:** Melanoma; Melanoma Risk Assessment; Melanoma Early Detection/Prevention; Pediatric Dermatology; **Hospital:** Rush Univ Med Ctr; **Address:** Rush University Dermatology, 1725 W Harrison St, Ste 264, Chicago, IL 60612; **Phone:** 312-942-2195; **Board Cert:** Internal Medicine 1972; Dermatology 1978; **Med School:** Columbia P&S 1969; **Resid:** Internal Medicine, Beth Israel Hosp 1972; Dermatology, Mass Genl Hosp 1978; **Fac Appt:** Prof D, Rush Med Coll

Treadwell, Patricia A MD [D] - **Spec Exp:** Pediatric Dermatology; Vascular Birthmarks; **Hospital:** Riley Hosp for Children, Wishard Hlth Srvs; **Address:** 1001 W 10th St Bryce Bldg, Fl 2 - rm B2100, Indianapolis, IN 46202; **Phone:** 317-630-7396; **Board Cert:** Pediatrics 1982; Dermatology 1983; **Med School:** Cornell Univ-Weill Med Coll 1977; **Resid:** Pediatrics, James Whitcomb Riley Hosp 1980; Dermatology, Indiana Univ Med Ctr 1983; **Fac Appt:** Prof D, Indiana Univ

Voorhees, John MD [D] - **Spec Exp:** Psoriasis; Photoaging; **Hospital:** Univ Michigan Hlth Sys; **Address:** Univ Michigan, Dept Dermatology, 1500 E Med Ctr Drive, rm 1910 Taubman Ctr, Ann Arbor, MI 48109-5314; **Phone:** 734-936-4054; **Board Cert:** Dermatology 1970; **Med School:** Univ Mich Med Sch 1963; **Resid:** Dermatology, Univ Mich Hosp 1969; **Fac Appt:** Prof D, Univ Mich Med Sch

Wheeland, Ronald MD [D] - **Spec Exp:** Skin Laser Surgery; Mohs' Surgery; Cosmetic Dermatology; **Hospital:** Univ of Missouri Hosp & Clins; **Address:** Univ Missouri, Dept Dermatology, One Hospital Drive, Columbia, MO 65212; **Phone:** 573-882-4800 x2; **Board Cert:** Dermatology 1977; Dermatopathology 1978; **Med School:** Univ Ariz Coll Med 1973; **Resid:** Dermatology, Univ Ok Hlth Sci Ctr 1977; **Fellow:** Dermatopathology, Univ Ok Hlth Sci Ctr 1978; Dermatologic Surgery, Cleveland Clin Fnd 1984; **Fac Appt:** Prof D, Univ MO-Columbia Sch Med

Wood, Gary S MD [D] - **Spec Exp:** Cutaneous Lymphoma; Melanoma; Skin Cancer; **Hospital:** Univ WI Hosp & Clins, VA Hospital, Madison; **Address:** Univ Wisconsin Health, Dept Dermatology, 1 S Park St Fl 7, Madison, WI 53715-1375; **Phone:** 608-287-2620; **Board Cert:** Anatomic Pathology 1983; Dermatology 1986; Dermatopathology 1987; **Med School:** Univ IL Coll Med 1979; **Resid:** Anatomic Pathology, Stanford Univ Med Ctr 1983; Dermatology, Stanford Univ Med Ctr 1985; **Fellow:** Immunopathology, Stanford Univ Med Ctr 1981; **Fac Appt:** Prof D, Univ Wisc

Zelickson, Brian D MD [D] - **Spec Exp:** Skin Laser Surgery; **Hospital:** Abbott - Northwestern Hosp, Fairview Southdale Hosp; **Address:** 825 Nicollet Mall, Med Arts Bldg - Ste 1002, Minneapolis, MN 55402; **Phone:** 612-338-0711; **Board Cert:** Dermatology 1999; **Med School:** Mayo Med Sch 1986; **Resid:** Dermatology, Mayo Clinic 1990; **Fac Appt:** Asst Prof D, Univ Minn

Great Plains and Mountains

Belsito, Donald V MD [D] - **Spec Exp:** Contact Dermatitis; Cutaneous Lymphoma; Immune Deficiency-Skin Disorders; Skin Cancer; **Hospital:** Shawnee Mission Med Ctr, Overland Pk Regl Med Ctr; **Address:** American Dermatology Assocs, 6333 Long Ave, Shawnee, KS 66216; **Phone:** 913-631-6330; **Board Cert:** Internal Medicine 1979; Dermatology 1983; Clinical & Laboratory Dermatologic Immunology 1985; **Med School:** Cornell Univ-Weill Med Coll 1976; **Resid:** Internal Medicine, Case West Res Univ Hosps 1979; Dermatology, NYU Med Ctr 1982; **Fac Appt:** Clin Prof D, Univ MO-Kansas City

Bowen, Glen M MD [D] - **Spec Exp:** Melanoma; Cutaneous Lymphoma; Clinical Trials; Mohs' Surgery; **Hospital:** Univ Utah Hosps and Clins, Cottonwood Hosp & Med Ctr; **Address:** Huntsman Cancer Inst, 500 N Medical Drive, rm 4A330, Salt Lake City, UT 84132; **Phone:** 801-585-0197; **Board Cert:** Dermatology 2005; **Med School:** Univ Utah 1990; **Resid:** Dermatology, Univ Michigan Med Ctr 1993; **Fellow:** Immunological Dermatology, Univ Michigan Med Ctr 1995; Mohs Surgery, Univ Utah 2001; **Fac Appt:** Assoc Prof D, Univ Utah

Krueger, Gerald MD [D] - **Spec Exp:** Psoriasis; **Hospital:** Univ Utah Hosps and Clins; **Address:** Univ Utah Hlth Sci Ctr, Dept Derm, 30 N 1900 E, Ste 4A330, Salt Lake City, UT 84132; **Phone:** 801-581-6465; **Board Cert:** Dermatology 1973; **Med School:** Loma Linda Univ 1966; **Resid:** Dermatology, Univ Colorado Med Ctr 1972; **Fac Appt:** Prof D, Univ Utah

Sontheimer, Richard D MD [D] - **Spec Exp:** Immune Deficiency-Skin Disorders; Lupus/SLE; Dermatomyositis; **Hospital:** Univ Utah Hosps and Clins; **Address:** Univ Health Care, Dept Dermatology, 30 North 1900 East, 4A330 School of Medicine, Salt Lake City, UT 84132; **Phone:** 801-581-6465; **Board Cert:** Internal Medicine 1976; Dermatology 1979; Clinical & Laboratory Dermatologic Immunology 1985; **Med School:** Univ Tex SW, Dallas 1972; **Resid:** Internal Medicine, Univ Utah Affil Hosps 1976; Dermatology, Parkland Meml Hosp 1979; **Fellow:** Research, Southwestern Med Sch 1978; **Fac Appt:** Prof D, Univ Utah

Southwest

Butler, David F MD [D] - **Spec Exp:** Skin Cancer; **Hospital:** Scott & White Mem Hosp; **Address:** Scott White Meml Hosp, Dept Dermatology, 409 W Adams St, Temple, TX 76501; **Phone:** 254-742-3724; **Board Cert:** Dermatology 1985; **Med School:** Univ Tex Med Br, Galveston 1980; **Resid:** Dermatology, Walter Reed Army Med Ctr 1985; **Fac Appt:** Assoc Prof D, Texas Tech Univ

Carney, John M MD [D] - **Spec Exp:** Mohs' Surgery; Skin Cancer; **Hospital:** UAMS Med Ctr; **Address:** Southwest Med Arts Bldg, 11321 Interstate 30, Ste 201, Little Rock, AR 72209; **Phone:** 501-455-4700; **Board Cert:** Dermatology 1984; **Med School:** Northwestern Univ 1979; **Resid:** Dermatology, Univ Hosps 1984; **Fellow:** Physiology, Harvard Med Sch 1985; Dermatologic Surgery, Univ Tenn Med Ctr 1986

Cockerell, Clay J MD [D] - **Spec Exp:** Dermatopathology; **Hospital:** UT Southwestern Med Ctr at Dallas; **Address:** Dermatopath Labs, 2330 Butler St, Ste 115, Dallas, TX 75235; **Phone:** 214-638-2222; **Board Cert:** Dermatology 2008; Dermatopathology 1986; **Med School:** Baylor Coll Med 1981; **Resid:** Dermatology, NYU Med Ctr 1985; **Fellow:** Dermatopathology, NYU Med Ctr 1986; **Fac Appt:** Prof DP, Univ Tex SW, Dallas

Connolly, Suzanne MD [D] - **Spec Exp:** Connective Tissue Disorders; Skin Cancer; **Hospital:** Mayo Clinic - Scottsdale; **Address:** Mayo Clinic, Dept Dermatology, 13400 E Shea Blvd, Scottsdale, AZ 85259; **Phone:** 480-301-6479; **Board Cert:** Dermatology 1979; Diagnostic Lab Immunology 1985; **Med School:** UCSF 1975; **Resid:** Dermatology, Mayo Clinic 1979; **Fac Appt:** Assoc Prof D, Mayo Med Sch

Duvic, Madeleine MD [D] - **Spec Exp:** Cutaneous Lymphoma; Skin Cancer; Alopecia Areata; **Hospital:** UT MD Anderson Cancer Ctr, St Luke's Episcopal Hosp-Houston; **Address:** MD Anderson Cancer Ctr, Dept Dermatology, 1515 Holcombe Blvd, Unit 434, Houston, TX 77030; **Phone:** 713-745-1113; **Board Cert:** Dermatology 1981; Internal Medicine 1982; **Med School:** Duke Univ 1977; **Resid:** Dermatology, Duke Univ Med Ctr 1980; Internal Medicine, Duke Univ Med Ctr 1982; **Fellow:** Geriatric Medicine, Duke Univ Med Ctr 1984; **Fac Appt:** Prof D, Univ Tex, Houston

Dermatology

Hansen, Ronald C MD [D] - **Spec Exp:** Pediatric Dermatology; **Hospital:** Phoenix Children's Hosp; **Address:** Phoenix Childrens Hosp, Dept Dermatology, 1920 E Cambridge Ave, Ste E200, Phoenix, AZ 85006; **Phone:** 602-546-0895; **Board Cert:** Pediatrics 1974; Dermatology 1980; **Med School:** Univ Iowa Coll Med 1968; **Resid:** Pediatrics, Childrens Hosp 1970; Pediatrics, Stanford Univ Med Ctr 1972; **Fellow:** Dermatology, Univ Medical Ctr 1980; **Fac Appt:** Prof D, Univ Ariz Coll Med

Levy, Moise L MD [D] - **Spec Exp:** Pediatric Dermatology; Vascular Malformations; **Hospital:** Children's Hospital - Austin; **Address:** 1301 Barbara Jordan Blvd, Austin, TX 78723; **Phone:** 512-628-1920; **Board Cert:** Pediatrics 1985; Dermatology 1986; **Med School:** Univ Tex, Houston 1979; **Resid:** Pediatrics, Univ Tex Affil Hosp 1983; Dermatology, Baylor Coll Med 1986; **Fac Appt:** Prof D, Baylor Coll Med

Lim, Katherine MD [D] - **Spec Exp:** Mohs' Surgery; Skin Cancer; **Address:** Mayo Clinic, Dept Dermatology, 13400 E Shea Blvd, Scottsdale, AZ 85259-5499; **Phone:** 480-301-6479; **Board Cert:** Dermatology 1996; **Med School:** Northwestern Univ 1992; **Resid:** Dermatology, Mayo Clinic 1996; **Fellow:** Mohs Surgery, Mayo Clinic 1997

Menter, M Alan MD [D] - **Spec Exp:** Psoriasis; Cosmetic Dermatology; Eczema; **Hospital:** Baylor Univ Medical Ctr, UT Southwestern Med Ctr at Dallas; **Address:** 3900 Junius St, Ste 145, Dallas, TX 75246; **Phone:** 972-386-7546 x400; **Board Cert:** Dermatology 1978; **Med School:** South Africa 1966; **Resid:** Dermatology, Pretoria Genl Hosp 1971; Dermatology, Guys Hosp 1972; **Fellow:** Dermatology, St Johns Hosp 1973; Dermatology, Univ Texas SW 1979; **Fac Appt:** Clin Prof D, Univ Tex SW, Dallas

Orengo, Ida F MD [D] - **Spec Exp:** Melanoma; Mohs' Surgery; **Hospital:** St Luke's Episcopal Hosp-Houston, DeBakey VA Med Ctr-Houston; **Address:** Baylor College of Medicine, 6620 Main St, Ste 1425, Houston, TX 77030; **Phone:** 713-798-6925; **Board Cert:** Dermatology 2001; **Med School:** Harvard Med Sch 1988; **Resid:** Dermatology, Baylor Coll Med 1991; **Fac Appt:** Assoc Prof D, Baylor Coll Med

Taylor, R Stan MD [D] - **Spec Exp:** Mohs' Surgery; Melanoma; Skin Cancer; **Hospital:** UT Southwestern Med Ctr at Dallas, Parkland Hlth & Hosp Sys; **Address:** Univ Tex SW Med Sch, Dept Derm, 5323 Harry Hines Blvd, MC 9192, Dallas, TX 75390-7208; **Phone:** 214-645-8950; **Board Cert:** Dermatology 1989; **Med School:** Univ Tex Med Br, Galveston 1985; **Resid:** Dermatology, Univ Mich Med Ctr 1989; **Fellow:** Immunological Dermatology, Univ Mich 1990; Mohs Surgery, Oregon Hlth Sci Univ 1991; **Fac Appt:** Prof D, Univ Tex SW, Dallas

West Coast and Pacific

Bennett, Richard G MD [D] - **Spec Exp:** Mohs' Surgery; Skin Cancer; **Hospital:** UCLA Ronald Reagan Med Ctr, USC Univ Hosp; **Address:** 1301 20th St, Ste 570, Santa Monica, CA 90404-2080; **Phone:** 310-315-0171; **Board Cert:** Dermatology 1975; **Med School:** Case West Res Univ 1970; **Resid:** Dermatology, Hosp Univ Penn 1974; **Fellow:** Chemosurgery, NYU Med Ctr 1977; **Fac Appt:** Clin Prof D, UCLA

Berg, Daniel MD [D] - **Spec Exp:** Skin Cancer; Mohs' Surgery; Skin Laser Surgery; Cosmetic Dermatology; **Hospital:** Univ Wash Med Ctr; **Address:** 4225 Roosevelt Way NE, Seattle, WA 98105; **Phone:** 206-598-6647; **Board Cert:** Dermatology 1999; **Med School:** Univ Toronto 1985; **Resid:** Internal Medicine, Sunnybrook Med Ctr 1988; Dermatology, Duke Univ Med Ctr 1991; **Fellow:** Dermatologic Surgery, Univ Toronto 1992; Dermatologic Surgery, Univ British Columbia 1994; **Fac Appt:** Prof D, Univ Wash

Eichenfield, Lawrence F MD [D] - **Spec Exp:** Eczema; Acne; Vascular Birthmarks; Pediatric Dermatology; **Hospital:** Rady Children's Hosp - San Diego, UCSD Med Ctr; **Address:** Chldns Hosp, Ped & Adolescent Dermatology, 8010 Frost St, Ste 602, San Diego, CA 92123-4204; **Phone:** 858-966-6795; **Board Cert:** Dermatology 1999; Pediatric Dermatology 2004; **Med School:** Mount Sinai Sch Med 1984; **Resid:** Pediatrics, Chldns Hosp 1987; Dermatology, Hosp Univ Penn 1991; **Fac Appt:** Prof Ped, UCSD

Fitzpatrick, Richard E MD [D] - **Spec Exp:** Cosmetic Dermatology; Skin Laser Surgery-Resurfacing; Hair Restoration/Transplant; **Hospital:** Scripps Meml Hosp - La Jolla; **Address:** 9850 Genesee St, Ste 480, La Jolla, CA 90237; **Phone:** 858-452-2066; **Board Cert:** Dermatology 2003; **Med School:** Emory Univ 1970; **Resid:** Dermatology, UCLA Med Ctr 1978; **Fac Appt:** Assoc Clin Prof D, UCSD

Frieden, Ilona J MD [D] - **Spec Exp:** Pediatric Dermatology; Vascular Birthmarks; Hemangiomas; **Hospital:** UCSF - Mt Zion Med Ctr; **Address:** UCSF, Dept Dermatology, 1701 Divisadero St, Fl 3, Box 0316, San Francisco, CA 94115-0316; **Phone:** 415-353-7800; **Board Cert:** Dermatology 2005; Pediatrics 1983; Pediatric Dermatology 2004; **Med School:** UCSF 1977; **Resid:** Pediatrics, UCSF Med Ctr 1980; Dermatology, UCSF Med Ctr 1983; **Fac Appt:** Clin Prof D, UCSF

Friedlander, Sheila Fallon MD [D] - **Spec Exp:** Pediatric Dermatology; Infectious Disease; Vascular Malformations; Hemangiomas; **Hospital:** Rady Children's Hosp - San Diego; **Address:** 8010 Frost St, Ste 602, San Diego, CA 92123; **Phone:** 858-966-6795; **Board Cert:** Pediatrics 1984; Dermatology 1990; Pediatric Dermatology 2004; **Med School:** Univ Chicago-Pritzker Sch Med 1979; **Resid:** Pediatrics, Bronx Municipal Hosp 1983; Dermatology, UCLA Med Ctr 1990; **Fellow:** Infectious Disease, Montefiore Med Ctr 1986; **Fac Appt:** Clin Prof Ped, UCSD

Glogau, Richard G MD [D] - **Spec Exp:** Cosmetic Dermatology; Skin Laser Surgery; Mohs' Surgery; Botox Therapy; **Hospital:** UCSF Med Ctr; **Address:** 350 Parnassus Ave, Ste 400, San Francisco, CA 94117; **Phone:** 415-564-1261; **Board Cert:** Dermatology 1978; Dermatopathology 1982; **Med School:** Harvard Med Sch 1973; **Resid:** Dermatology, UCSF Med Ctr 1977; **Fellow:** Chemosurgery, UCSF Med Ctr 1978; **Fac Appt:** Clin Prof D, UCSF

Greenway, Hubert T MD [D] - **Spec Exp:** Skin Cancer; Mohs' Surgery; Melanoma; **Hospital:** Scripps Green Hosp; **Address:** Scripps Clinic, Div Mohs' Surgery, 10666 N Torrey Pines Rd, MS 112A, La Jolla, CA 92037; **Phone:** 858-554-8646; **Board Cert:** Dermatology 1982; **Med School:** Med Coll GA 1974; **Resid:** Dermatology, Naval Hosp 1982; **Fellow:** Mohs Surgery, Univ Wisconsin Med Ctr 1981

Grimes, Pearl E MD [D] - **Spec Exp:** Pigmented Lesions; Ethnic Skin Disorders; **Hospital:** UCLA Ronald Reagan Med Ctr; **Address:** 5670 Wilshire Blvd, Ste 650, Los Angeles, CA 90036; **Phone:** 323-467-4389; **Board Cert:** Dermatology 1979; **Med School:** Washington Univ, St Louis 1974; **Resid:** Dermatology, Howard Univ 1979; **Fac Appt:** Clin Prof D, UCLA

Hanifin, Jon M MD [D] - **Spec Exp:** Atopic Dermatitis; **Hospital:** OR Hlth & Sci Univ; **Address:** OHSU, Dept Dermatology, 3303 SW Bond Ave, MC CH16D, Portland, OR 97239; **Phone:** 503-418-3376; **Board Cert:** Dermatology 1970; **Med School:** Univ Wisc 1965; **Resid:** Dermatology, UCSF Med Ctr 1969; **Fellow:** Clinical & Laboratory Immunology, UCSF Med Ctr; **Fac Appt:** Prof D, Oregon Hlth & Sci Univ

Kilmer, Suzanne L MD [D] - **Spec Exp:** Skin Laser Surgery-Resurfacing; Facial Rejuvenation; Cosmetic Dermatology; **Hospital:** Mercy General Hosp - Sacramento; **Address:** The Laser & Skin Surgery Center, 3835 J St, Sacramento, CA 95816-5520; **Phone:** 916-456-0400; **Board Cert:** Dermatology 1999; **Med School:** UC Davis 1987; **Resid:** Dermatology, UC Davis Med Ctr 1991; **Fellow:** Laser Surgery, Mass Genl Hosp 1992; **Fac Appt:** Asst Clin Prof D, UC Davis

Dermatology

Kim, Youn-Hee MD [D] - **Spec Exp:** Cutaneous Lymphoma; Skin Cancer; **Hospital:** Stanford Univ Med Ctr; **Address:** Stanford Outpatient Med Ctr, 450 Broadway, Redwood City, CA 94063; **Phone:** 650-723-6316; **Board Cert:** Dermatology 1989; **Med School:** Stanford Univ 1984; **Resid:** Dermatology, Metropolitan Hospital 1989

Koo, John Ying Ming MD [D] - **Spec Exp:** Psoriasis/Eczema; Photosensitive Skin Diseases; Psychodermatology; **Hospital:** UCSF Med Ctr; **Address:** Psoriasis Day Treatment Ctr, 515 Spruce St, San Francisco, CA 94118; **Phone:** 415-476-4701; **Board Cert:** Dermatology 1988; Psychiatry 1988; **Med School:** Harvard Med Sch 1981; **Resid:** Psychiatry, UCLA Neur Psyc Inst 1985; Dermatology, UCSF Med Ctr 1988; **Fac Appt:** Prof D, UCSF

Lask, Gary P MD [D] - **Spec Exp:** Skin Laser Surgery-Resurfacing; Cosmetic Dermatology; **Hospital:** UCLA Ronald Reagan Med Ctr; **Address:** 16260 Ventura Blvd, Ste 530, Encino, CA 91436; **Phone:** 818-788-4022; **Board Cert:** Dermatology 1983; **Med School:** Mexico 1977; **Resid:** Dermatology, Martin Luther King Jr Hosp 1983; **Fac Appt:** Clin Prof D, UCLA

Rubin, Mark G MD [D] - **Spec Exp:** Skin Laser Surgery; Cosmetic Dermatology; **Hospital:** UCSD Med Ctr; **Address:** 153 S Lasky Drive, Ste 1, Beverly Hills, CA 90212; **Phone:** 310-556-0119; **Board Cert:** Dermatology 1985; **Med School:** Jefferson Med Coll 1981; **Resid:** Dermatology, Henry Ford Hosp 1985; **Fac Appt:** Assoc Prof D, UCSD

Swanson, Neil A MD [D] - **Spec Exp:** Skin Cancer; Cosmetic Dermatology; **Hospital:** OR Hlth & Sci Univ, VA Medical Center - Portland; **Address:** Oregon HSU, Center for Health & Healing, 3303 SW Bond Ave, CH16D, Portland, OR 97239; **Phone:** 503-418-3376; **Board Cert:** Dermatology 1980; **Med School:** Univ Rochester 1976; **Resid:** Dermatology, Univ Michigan Med Ctr 1979; **Fellow:** Dermatology, UCSF Med Ctr 1980; **Fac Appt:** Prof D, Oregon Hlth & Sci Univ

Swetter, Susan M MD [D] - **Spec Exp:** Melanoma; Melanoma Early Detection/Prevention; Skin Cancer; **Hospital:** Stanford Univ Med Ctr, VA Hlth Care Sys - Palo Alto; **Address:** Stanford Univ Med Ctr, Dept Dermatology, 900 Blake Wilbur Dr, W0069, MC 5334, Stanford, CA 94305; **Phone:** 650-723-0119; **Board Cert:** Dermatology 2001; **Med School:** Univ Pennsylvania 1990; **Resid:** Dermatology, Stanford Univ Med Ctr 1994; **Fac Appt:** Assoc Prof D, Stanford Univ

Cleveland Clinic

Dermatology

Cleveland Clinic Department of Dermatology, part of the Dermatology and Plastic Surgery Institute, offers a full array of subspecialized care for adult and pediatric patients. Our physicians diagnose and treat all disorders of the skin, hair and nails, whether primary or related to an underlying systemic illness, including industrial-related conditions.

Dermatologic Surgery

The department offers a full range of procedures in the subspecialty area of dermatologic surgery. These include Mohs micrographic surgery for high-risk skin cancers (including local tissue reconstruction), laser surgery, chemical peels, soft tissue augmentation, botox injections, hair transplant and liposuction. Additionally, our Cutaneous Care Center provides outpatient treatment, rather than hospitalization, for patients with extensive, severe or chronic skin diseases utilizing phototherapy and excimer laser treatment.

Staff dermatologists and residents are involved in research, either institutionally or through industrial support of clinical trials.

Cleveland Clinic dermatologists offer expert diagnostic and management options including:
- Skin Cancer and Mohs Surgery
- Psoriasis
- Varicose Veins and Spider Veins
- Phototherapy
- Pediatric Dermatology
- Industrial Dermatology
- Cosmetic Dermatology
- Laser Surgery

For more information about the Cleveland Clinic Department of Dermatology, to schedule a second opinion or to learn about assistance for out-of-town patients, call 800.890.2467 or visit www.clevelandclinic.org/dermtopdocs.

Department of Dermatology
9500 Euclid Avenue / AC311 | Cleveland OH 44195

NYU **Langone Medical Center**

550 First Avenue (at 31St Street)
New York, NY 10016
Physician Referral:
(888)7-NYU-MED (888-769-8633)
www.med.nyu.edu

DERMATOLOGY

About the Ronald O. Perelman Department of Dermatology:

With a history dating back to 1882, the Ronald O. Perelman Department of Dermatology at NYU Langone Medical Center is a national and international leader in dermatology, utilizing the most up-to-date breakthroughs in medicine and science. The Department provides dermatologic care for more than 100,000 patients each year. In addition, faculty members conduct research focused on the most significant dermatologic problems including the prevention, detection and treatment of melanoma and other skin cancers. Our services include medical, surgical, pediatric and cosmetic dermatology as well as laser and Mohs micrographic surgery for skin cancers.

We specialize in the following areas:

DERMATOLOGIC SURGERY AND COSMETIC DERMATOLOGY

Dermatologic Surgery Associates at NYU Langone Medical Center provide patients with specialized care for the treatment of malignant and benign skin lesions and offers cutting-edge therapies for aesthetic and cosmetic concerns. Mohs surgery represents an advanced technique for the removal of the most common forms of skin cancer to minimize the chance of recurrence. This microscopically controlled tissue-sparing procedure is performed by a specially-trained dermatologic surgeon.

DERMATOPATHOLOGY

Highly trained dermatopathologists at the Medical Center examine skin tissues submitted by physicians from biopsies and surgeries to diagnose skin diseases and malignancies. One of the busiest academic skin pathology units in the country, the Dermatopathology Section also provides consultative services for the review of skin pathology specimens performed elsewhere.

DERMATOPHARMACOLOGY

The Dermatopharmacology Unit in the Charles C. Harris Skin and Cancer Unit at NYU Langone Medical Center is one of the nation's most distinguished clinical research centers in dermatology. It is primarily responsible for carrying out clinical trials relating to inflammatory skin diseases such as psoriasis, skin cancer, infections, and autoimmune illnesses.

GENERAL DERMATOLOGY

Dermatologic Associates at NYU Langone Medical Center is a professional practice providing consultations and continuing care in a private office setting. Dermatologic Associates is a multi-subspecialty facility that provides care for all patients with disorders of the skin, hair, and nails as well as for patients with complex illnesses, difficult to diagnose conditions or those experiencing treatment dilemmas. Examples include inflammatory skin diseases such as psoriasis and lupus, cancers and other skin tumors, infections and allergic skin diseases such as eczema, contact dermatitis and hives.

PEDIATRIC DERMATOLOGY

Pediatric Dermatology Associates at NYU Langone Medical Center is a professional practice dedicated to the treatment of diseases affecting the skin, hair, nails and mucous membranes of children and adolescents such as acne, eczema, hemangiomas, moles and genetic and congenital disorders affecting the skin.

SKIN CANCER

The Charles C. Harris Skin and Cancer Unit at Tisch Hospital at NYU Langone Medical Center is an outpatient dermatology teaching center, combining unique patient care with superior medical education. The resident and attending physicians provide diagnostic and treatment services for skin diseases for patients of all ages, including common conditions such as acne, eczema and warts as well as complex medical conditions such as connective tissue disorders, pigmented lesions, skin allergies and skin cancers.

Endocrinology, Diabetes & Metabolism

a subspecialty of Internal Medicine

An internist who concentrates on disorders of the internal (endocrine) glands such as the thyroid and adrenal glands. This specialist also deals with disorders such as diabetes, metabolic and nutritional disorders, pituitary diseases, menstrual and sexual problems.

Training Required: Three years in internal medicine *plus* additional training and examination for certification in endocrinology, diabetes and metabolism.

ENDOCRINOLOGY, DIABETES & METABOLISM

New England

Abrahamson, Martin J MD [EDM] - **Spec Exp:** Diabetes; **Hospital:** Beth Israel Deaconess Med Ctr - Boston; **Address:** Joslin Diabetes Clinic, 1 Joslin Pl, Boston, MA 02215; **Phone:** 617-732-2501; **Board Cert:** Internal Medicine 2005; Endocrinology, Diabetes & Metabolism 2005; **Med School:** South Africa 1977; **Resid:** Internal Medicine, Groote Schuuer Hosp-Univ Cape Town 1983; **Fellow:** Endocrinology, Diabetes & Metabolism, Groote Schuuer Hosp-Univ Cape Town 1985; Research, Univ Cape Town 1987; **Fac Appt:** Assoc Prof Med, Harvard Med Sch

Axelrod, Lloyd MD [EDM] - **Spec Exp:** Diabetes; Geriatric Endocrinology; **Hospital:** Mass Genl Hosp; **Address:** 50 Stanford St Fl 3 - Ste 340, Boston, MA 02114; **Phone:** 617-726-8722; **Board Cert:** Internal Medicine 1973; Endocrinology, Diabetes & Metabolism 1973; **Med School:** Harvard Med Sch 1967; **Resid:** Internal Medicine, Peter Bent Brigham Hosp 1969; Internal Medicine, Mass Genl Hosp 1971; **Fellow:** Endocrinology, Diabetes & Metabolism, Peter Bent Brigham Hosp 1970; Endocrinology, Diabetes & Metabolism, Mass Genl Hosp 1972; **Fac Appt:** Assoc Prof Med, Harvard Med Sch

Beaser, Richard S MD [EDM] - **Spec Exp:** Diabetes; **Hospital:** Beth Israel Deaconess Med Ctr - Boston; **Address:** Joslin Clinic, 1 Joslin Pl, Boston, MA 02215; **Phone:** 617-732-2665; **Board Cert:** Internal Medicine 1980; **Med School:** Boston Univ 1977; **Resid:** Internal Medicine, Mass Med Ctr 1980; **Fellow:** Endocrinology, Diabetes & Metabolism, Joslin Clinic 1981; **Fac Appt:** Assoc Clin Prof Med, Harvard Med Sch

Biller, Beverly M K MD [EDM] - **Spec Exp:** Pituitary Disorders; Cushing's Syndrome; Acromegaly; **Hospital:** Mass Genl Hosp; **Address:** Neuroendocrine Clinic Center, Zero Emerson Pl, Ste 112, Boston, MA 02114-3117; **Phone:** 617-726-3870; **Board Cert:** Internal Medicine 1986; Endocrinology 1989; **Med School:** Univ Okla Coll Med 1983; **Resid:** Internal Medicine, Beth Israel Deaconness Hosp 1986; **Fellow:** Endocrinology, Diabetes & Metabolism, Mass Genl Hosp 1989; **Fac Appt:** Assoc Prof Med, Harvard Med Sch

Comi, Richard J MD [EDM] - **Spec Exp:** Diabetes; Hypoglycemia; Thyroid Disorders; Pituitary Disorders; **Hospital:** Dartmouth - Hitchcock Med Ctr; **Address:** Dartmouth-Hitchcock Med Ctr, Endocrinology, One Medical Ctr Drive, Lebanon, NH 03756; **Phone:** 603-650-8630; **Board Cert:** Internal Medicine 1983; Endocrinology 1987; **Med School:** Harvard Med Sch 1980; **Resid:** Internal Medicine, Mass Genl Hosp 1983; **Fellow:** Endocrinology & Diabetes, Natl Inst Hlth 1986

Daniels, Gilbert MD [EDM] - **Spec Exp:** Thyroid Disorders; Parathyroid Disease; Adrenal Disorders; **Hospital:** Mass Genl Hosp; **Address:** 15 Parkman St, Bldg WACC - Ste 730, Boston, MA 02114; **Phone:** 617-726-8430; **Board Cert:** Internal Medicine 1972; Endocrinology, Diabetes & Metabolism 1975; **Med School:** Harvard Med Sch 1966; **Resid:** Internal Medicine, Mass Genl Hosp 1972; **Fellow:** Biochemistry, Natl Inst Hlth 1970; Endocrinology, Diabetes & Metabolism, UCSF Med Ctr 1971; **Fac Appt:** Prof Med, Harvard Med Sch

Godine, John E MD/PhD [EDM] - **Spec Exp:** Diabetes; **Hospital:** Mass Genl Hosp; **Address:** 50 Staniford St Fl 3 - Ste 340, Boston, MA 02114; **Phone:** 617-726-8722; **Board Cert:** Internal Medicine 1979; Endocrinology, Diabetes & Metabolism 1981; **Med School:** Harvard Med Sch 1976; **Resid:** Internal Medicine, Mass Genl Hosp 1978; **Fellow:** Endocrinology, Diabetes & Metabolism, Mass Genl Hosp 1981; **Fac Appt:** Asst Prof Med, Harvard Med Sch

Inzucchi, Silvio E MD [EDM] - **Spec Exp:** Diabetes; Pituitary Disorders; Growth Hormone Disorder-Adult; Cholesterol/Lipid Disorders; **Hospital:** Yale-New Haven Hosp; **Address:** Yale Univ Sch Med, Div Endocrinology, Box 208020, New Haven, CT 06520-8020; **Phone:** 203-737-1932; **Board Cert:** Internal Medicine 1988; Endocrinology, Diabetes & Metabolism 2006; **Med School:** Harvard Med Sch 1985; **Resid:** Internal Medicine, Yale-New Haven Hosp 1988; **Fellow:** Endocrinology, Diabetes & Metabolism, Yale-New Haven Hosp 1994; **Fac Appt:** Prof Med, Yale Univ

Kahn, Barbara B MD [EDM] - **Spec Exp:** Obesity; Nutrition; **Hospital:** Beth Israel Deaconess Med Ctr - Boston; **Address:** Beth Israel Deaconess Medical Ctr, 330 Brookline Ave, rm RN380-6, Boston, MA 02215; **Phone:** 617-667-2151; **Board Cert:** Internal Medicine 1980; Endocrinology, Diabetes & Metabolism 1985; **Med School:** Stanford Univ 1977; **Resid:** Internal Medicine, UC Davis Med Ctr 1980; **Fellow:** Endocrinology, Diabetes & Metabolism, Natl Inst Hlth 1982; **Fac Appt:** Prof Med, Harvard Med Sch

Klibanski, Anne MD [EDM] - **Spec Exp:** Pituitary Disorders; Prolactin Disorders; Acromegaly; **Hospital:** Mass Genl Hosp; **Address:** Neuroendocrine Clinic Ctr, Zero Emerson Pl, Ste 112, Boston, MA 02114; **Phone:** 617-726-7948; **Board Cert:** Internal Medicine 1978; Endocrinology, Diabetes & Metabolism 1981; **Med School:** NYU Sch Med 1975; **Resid:** Internal Medicine, Bellevue Hosp Ctr 1978; **Fellow:** Endocrinology, Mass Genl Hosp 1981; **Fac Appt:** Prof Med, Harvard Med Sch

LeBoff, Meryl S MD [EDM] - **Spec Exp:** Osteoporosis; Metabolic Bone Disease; **Hospital:** Brigham & Women's Hosp; **Address:** 221 Longwood Ave, Boston, MA 02115; **Phone:** 617-732-5666; **Board Cert:** Internal Medicine 1979; Endocrinology, Diabetes & Metabolism 1981; **Med School:** UMDNJ-NJ Med Sch, Newark 1975; **Resid:** Internal Medicine, USC Med Ctr 1979; **Fellow:** Endocrinology, Brigham & Womens Hosp 1982; **Fac Appt:** Assoc Prof Med, Harvard Med Sch

Lechan, Ronald MD/PhD [EDM] - **Spec Exp:** Pituitary Disorders; Hypothalamic Dysfunction; Islet Cell Tumors; **Hospital:** Tufts Med Ctr; **Address:** New England Med Ctr, 750 Washington St, Box 268, Boston, MA 02111; **Phone:** 617-636-5689; **Board Cert:** Internal Medicine 1979; Endocrinology, Diabetes & Metabolism 1981; **Med School:** Univ VT Coll Med 1976; **Resid:** Internal Medicine, Beth Israel Hosp 1978; **Fellow:** Endocrinology, Diabetes & Metabolism, Tufts-New England Med Ctr 1981; **Fac Appt:** Prof Med, Tufts Univ

Levine, Robert A MD [EDM] - **Spec Exp:** Thyroid Cancer; Growth/Development Disorders; Metabolic Bone Disease; Thyroid Disorders; **Hospital:** St Joseph Hosp; **Address:** Thyroid Center of New Hampshire, 5 Coliseum Ave, Nashua, NH 03060; **Phone:** 603-881-7141; **Board Cert:** Internal Medicine 1984; Endocrinology, Diabetes & Metabolism 1987; **Med School:** Univ Conn 1981; **Resid:** Internal Medicine, Mt Auburn Hosp 1984; **Fellow:** Endocrinology, Yale Univ 1987

Seely, Ellen Wells MD [EDM] - **Spec Exp:** Pregnancy & Endocrine Disorders; Diabetes in Pregnancy; Diabetes in Women; Thyroid Disorders in Pregnancy; **Hospital:** Brigham & Women's Hosp; **Address:** Brigham & Womens Hosp, Endocrine Div, 221 Longwood Ave, rm 277, Boston, MA 02115-5804; **Phone:** 617-732-5661; **Board Cert:** Internal Medicine 1984; Endocrinology, Diabetes & Metabolism 1987; **Med School:** Columbia P&S 1981; **Resid:** Internal Medicine, Brigham & Womens Hosp 1984; **Fellow:** Endocrinology, Diabetes & Metabolism, Brigham & Womens Hosp 1987; **Fac Appt:** Assoc Prof Med, Harvard Med Sch

Sherwin, Robert MD [EDM] - **Spec Exp:** Diabetes; **Hospital:** Yale-New Haven Hosp; **Address:** Yale Univ Sch Med, Sect Endocrinology, 333 Cedar St, Box 208020, New Haven, CT 06520-8020; **Phone:** 203-785-4183; **Board Cert:** Internal Medicine 1972; **Med School:** Albert Einstein Coll Med 1967; **Resid:** Internal Medicine, Mt Sinai Hosp 1969; Internal Medicine, Mt Sinai Hosp 1972; **Fellow:** Metabolism, Yale-New Haven Hosp 1973; **Fac Appt:** Prof Med, Yale Univ

Endocrinology, Diabetes & Metabolism

Mid Atlantic

Ball, Douglas W MD [EDM] - **Spec Exp:** Thyroid Cancer; **Hospital:** Johns Hopkins Hosp - Baltimore (page 61); **Address:** Sidney Kimmel Cancer Ctr, 1830 E Monument St, Ste 333, Baltimore, MD 21287; **Phone:** 410-955-8964; **Board Cert:** Internal Medicine 1987; **Med School:** Geo Wash Univ 1984; **Resid:** Internal Medicine, Univ Pittsburgh 1987; **Fellow:** Endocrinology, Diabetes & Metabolism, Johns Hopkins Hosp 1991; **Fac Appt:** Assoc Prof Med, Johns Hopkins Univ

Bergman, Donald MD [EDM] - **Spec Exp:** Osteoporosis; Thyroid Disorders; Calcium Disorders; **Hospital:** Mount Sinai Med Ctr (page 64); **Address:** 1199 Park Ave, Ste 1F, New York, NY 10128; **Phone:** 212-876-7333; **Board Cert:** Internal Medicine 1975; Endocrinology, Diabetes & Metabolism 1977; **Med School:** Jefferson Med Coll 1971; **Resid:** Obstetrics & Gynecology, Mount Sinai Hosp 1972; Internal Medicine, Mount Sinai Hosp 1975; **Fellow:** Endocrinology, Diabetes & Metabolism, Mount Sinai Hosp 1977; **Fac Appt:** Clin Prof Med, Mount Sinai Sch Med

Bilezikian, John P MD [EDM] - **Spec Exp:** Osteoporosis; Bone Disorders-Metabolic; Parathyroid Disease; **Hospital:** NY-Presby Hosp/Columbia (page 66); **Address:** Columbia Med Ctr, Metabolic Bone Diseases, Harkness Pavilion, 180 Ft Washington Ave Fl 9 - Ste 904, New York, NY 10032; **Phone:** 212-305-2663; **Board Cert:** Internal Medicine 1975; Endocrinology, Diabetes & Metabolism 1977; **Med School:** Columbia P&S 1969; **Resid:** Internal Medicine, Columbia-Presby Hosp 1975; **Fellow:** Endocrinology, Diabetes & Metabolism, Natl Inst Health 1977; **Fac Appt:** Prof Med, Columbia P&S

Blum, Conrad B MD [EDM] - **Spec Exp:** Cholesterol/Lipid Disorders; Thyroid Disorders; Diabetes; **Hospital:** NY-Presby Hosp/Columbia (page 66); **Address:** 16 E 60th St, Ste 320, New York, NY 10022-1002; **Phone:** 212-326-8421; **Board Cert:** Internal Medicine 1976; Endocrinology, Diabetes & Metabolism 1977; **Med School:** Northwestern Univ 1971; **Resid:** Internal Medicine, Brigham Hosp 1976; **Fellow:** Endocrinology, Diabetes & Metabolism, Northwestern Univ Med Sch 1977; **Fac Appt:** Clin Prof Med, Columbia P&S

Bockman, Richard MD/PhD [EDM] - **Spec Exp:** Bone Disorders-Metabolic; Osteoporosis; Thyroid Disorders; **Hospital:** Hosp For Special Surgery (page 59), NY-Presby Hosp/Weill Cornell (page 66); **Address:** 519 E 72nd St, New York, NY 10021; **Phone:** 212-606-1458; **Board Cert:** Internal Medicine 1975; **Med School:** Yale Univ 1968; **Resid:** Internal Medicine, NYU Med Ctr 1975; **Fellow:** Internal Medicine, NY-Cornell Med Ctr 1973; **Fac Appt:** Prof Med, Cornell Univ-Weill Med Coll

Calvi, Laura MD [EDM] - **Spec Exp:** Osteoporosis; Parathyroid Disease; **Hospital:** Univ of Rochester Strong Meml Hosp; **Address:** 601 Elmwood Ave, Box 693, Rochester, NY 14642; **Phone:** 585-275-2901; **Board Cert:** Internal Medicine 1998; Endocrinology, Diabetes & Metabolism 2000; **Med School:** Harvard Med Sch 1995; **Resid:** Internal Medicine, Mass Genl Hosp 1998; **Fac Appt:** Asst Prof Med, Univ Rochester

Cooper, David S MD [EDM] - **Spec Exp:** Thyroid Disorders; **Hospital:** Johns Hopkins Hosp - Baltimore (page 61); **Address:** Div Endocrinology & Metabolism, 1830 E Monument St, Ste 333, Baltimore, MD 21287; **Phone:** 410-955-3663; **Board Cert:** Internal Medicine 1987; Endocrinology, Diabetes & Metabolism 1979; **Med School:** Tufts Univ 1973; **Resid:** Internal Medicine, Barnes Hosp 1976; **Fellow:** Endocrinology, Mass Genl Hosp 1978; **Fac Appt:** Prof Med, Johns Hopkins Univ

Davies, Terry MD [EDM] - **Spec Exp:** Thyroid Disorders in Pregnancy; Graves' Disease; Hashimoto's Disease; Thyroid Cancer; **Hospital:** Mount Sinai Med Ctr (page 64), VA Med Ctr - Manhattan; **Address:** 5 E 98th St, Box 1055, New York, NY 10029-6500; **Phone:** 212-241-7975; **Med School:** England 1971; **Resid:** Internal Medicine, Univ Newcastle 1975; **Fellow:** Endocrinology, Diabetes & Metabolism, Univ Newcastle 1977; Endocrinology, Diabetes & Metabolism, Natl Inst Hlth 1979; **Fac Appt:** Prof Med, Mount Sinai Sch Med

Dobs, Adrian S MD [EDM] - **Spec Exp:** Hormonal Disorders; Hypogonadism-Male; Metabolic Disorders; Complementary Medicine; **Hospital:** Johns Hopkins Hosp - Baltimore (page 61); **Address:** Johns Hopkins Hosp, 1830 E Monument St, Fl 3 - Ste 328, Baltimore, MD 21287; **Phone:** 410-955-2130; **Board Cert:** Internal Medicine 1981; Endocrinology 1987; **Med School:** Albany Med Coll 1978; **Resid:** Internal Medicine, Montefiore Hosp 1982; **Fellow:** Endocrinology, Johns Hopkins Hosp 1984; **Fac Appt:** Prof Med, Johns Hopkins Univ

Felig, Philip MD [EDM] - **Spec Exp:** Diabetes; Thyroid Disorders; Osteoporosis; **Hospital:** Lenox Hill Hosp (page 62), Beth Israel Med Ctr - Petrie Division (page 57); **Address:** 1056 5th Ave, New York, NY 10028-0112; **Phone:** 212-534-5900; **Board Cert:** Internal Medicine 1968; **Med School:** Yale Univ 1961; **Resid:** Internal Medicine, Yale-New Haven Hosp 1967; **Fellow:** Endocrinology, Diabetes & Metabolism, Peter Bent Brigham Hosp 1969

Fleischer, Norman MD [EDM] - **Spec Exp:** Thyroid Disorders; Adrenal Disorders; Pituitary Disorders; **Hospital:** Montefiore Med Ctr - Weiler-Einstein Div; **Address:** 1575 Blondell Ave, Ste 200, Bronx, NY 10461-2601; **Phone:** 866-633-8253; **Board Cert:** Internal Medicine 1968; Endocrinology, Diabetes & Metabolism 1973; **Med School:** Vanderbilt Univ 1961; **Resid:** Internal Medicine, Bronx Muni Hosp Ctr 1964; **Fellow:** Endocrinology, Diabetes & Metabolism, Vanderbilt Univ 1966; **Fac Appt:** Prof Med, Albert Einstein Coll Med

Greene, Loren Wissner MD [EDM] - **Spec Exp:** Thyroid Disorders; Osteoporosis; Pituitary Disorders; Diabetes; **Hospital:** NYU Med Ctr (page 68), NY Downtown Hosp; **Address:** 530 1st Ave, Ste 4B, New York, NY 10016-6402; **Phone:** 212-263-7449; **Board Cert:** Internal Medicine 1978; Endocrinology, Diabetes & Metabolism 1981; **Med School:** NYU Sch Med 1975; **Resid:** Internal Medicine, Bellevue Hosp Ctr-NYU 1978; **Fellow:** Endocrinology, Bellevue Hosp Ctr-NYU 1980; **Fac Appt:** Assoc Clin Prof Med, NYU Sch Med

Greenspan, Susan L MD [EDM] - **Spec Exp:** Osteoporosis; **Hospital:** UPMC Presby, Pittsburgh; **Address:** Univ Pittsburgh, Osteoporosis Ctr, 3471 Fifth Ave, Kaufmann Bldg - Ste 1110, Pittsburgh, PA 15213; **Phone:** 412-692-2472; **Board Cert:** Internal Medicine 1982; Endocrinology, Diabetes & Metabolism 1987; Geriatric Medicine 1998; **Med School:** Harvard Med Sch 1979; **Resid:** Internal Medicine, Beth Israel Hosp 1982; **Fellow:** Endocrinology, Mass Genl Hosp 1985; **Fac Appt:** Prof Med, Univ Pittsburgh

Jacobs, Thomas MD [EDM] - **Spec Exp:** Adrenal Disorders; Pituitary Disorders; Calcium Disorders; **Hospital:** NY-Presby Hosp/Columbia (page 66); **Address:** 161 Fort Washington Ave, rm 210, New York, NY 10032-3713; **Phone:** 212-305-5578; **Board Cert:** Internal Medicine 1973; Endocrinology, Diabetes & Metabolism 1975; **Med School:** Johns Hopkins Univ 1968; **Resid:** Internal Medicine, Columbia Presby Hosp 1973; **Fellow:** Endocrinology, Diabetes & Metabolism, Univ Wash Med Ctr 1975; **Fac Appt:** Clin Prof Med, Columbia P&S

Kleinberg, David MD [EDM] - **Spec Exp:** Neuroendocrinology; Pituitary Disorders; **Hospital:** NYU Med Ctr (page 68); **Address:** 530 1st Ave, Ste 4C, New York, NY 10016; **Phone:** 212-263-6772; **Board Cert:** Internal Medicine 1972; Endocrinology 1975; **Med School:** Univ Miami Sch Med 1966; **Resid:** Internal Medicine, Maimonides Med Ctr 1968; Internal Medicine, Columbia-Presby Med Ctr 1971; **Fellow:** Endocrinology, Diabetes & Metabolism, Columbia-Presby Med Ctr 1970; **Fac Appt:** Prof Med, NYU Sch Med

Korytkowski, Mary T MD [EDM] - **Spec Exp:** Diabetes; Polycystic Ovarian Syndrome; Thyroid Disorders; Diabetic Vascular Disease; **Hospital:** UPMC Presby, Pittsburgh; **Address:** Center for Diabetes & Endocrinology, 3601 Fifth Ave, Falk Med Bldg, Ste 562, Pittsburgh, PA 15213-3403; **Phone:** 412-586-9714; **Board Cert:** Internal Medicine 1985; Endocrinology 1989; **Med School:** Univ NC Sch Med 1982; **Resid:** Internal Medicine, Francis Scott Key Med Ctr 1985; **Fellow:** Endocrinology, Diabetes & Metabolism, Sinai Hosp/Johns Hopkins Hosp 1988; **Fac Appt:** Prof Med, Univ Pittsburgh

Endocrinology, Diabetes & Metabolism

Ladenson, Paul W MD [EDM] - **Spec Exp:** Thyroid Disorders; Thyroid Cancer; **Hospital:** Johns Hopkins Hosp - Baltimore (page 61); **Address:** Johns Hopkins-Div Endocrinology & Metabolism, 1830 E Monument St, rm 333, Baltimore, MD 21287; **Phone:** 410-955-3663; **Board Cert:** Internal Medicine 1978; Endocrinology, Diabetes & Metabolism 1981; **Med School:** Harvard Med Sch 1975; **Resid:** Internal Medicine, Mass Genl Hosp 1978; **Fellow:** Endocrinology, Diabetes & Metabolism, Mass Genl Hosp 1980; **Fac Appt:** Prof Med, Johns Hopkins Univ

Mahler, Richard J MD [EDM] - **Spec Exp:** Thyroid Disorders; Diabetes; **Hospital:** NY-Presby Hosp/Weill Cornell (page 66); **Address:** 220 E 69th St, New York, NY 10021-5737; **Phone:** 212-879-4073; **Board Cert:** Internal Medicine 1987; **Med School:** NY Med Coll 1959; **Resid:** Internal Medicine, NY Med-Metro Med 1962; Endocrinology, Diabetes & Metabolism, NY Med Coll 1963; **Fellow:** Endocrinology, Diabetes & Metabolism, Univ Durham/Univ New Castle 1964; **Fac Appt:** Assoc Clin Prof Med, Cornell Univ-Weill Med Coll

Mandel, Susan J MD [EDM] - **Spec Exp:** Thyroid Disorders; Calcium Disorders; **Hospital:** Hosp Univ Penn - UPHS (page 60); **Address:** Hosp Univ Penn, Div Endocrinology, 3400 Spruce St, 1 Maloney, Philadelphia, PA 19104; **Phone:** 215-662-2300; **Board Cert:** Internal Medicine 1989; Endocrinology 2001; **Med School:** Columbia P&S 1986; **Resid:** Internal Medicine, Columbia Presby Med Ctr 1989; **Fellow:** Endocrinology, Brigham & Womens Hosp 1992; **Fac Appt:** Assoc Prof Med, Univ Pennsylvania

McConnell, Robert John MD [EDM] - **Spec Exp:** Thyroid Disorders; Thyroid Ultrasound; **Hospital:** NY-Presby Hosp/Columbia (page 66); **Address:** 161 Fort Washington Ave, Ste 210, New York, NY 10032-3713; **Phone:** 212-305-5579; **Board Cert:** Internal Medicine 1978; Endocrinology, Diabetes & Metabolism 1981; **Med School:** Columbia P&S 1973; **Resid:** Internal Medicine, Barnes Hosp 1975; **Fellow:** Endocrinology, Diabetes & Metabolism, Columbia-Presby Hosp 1978; **Fac Appt:** Prof Med, Columbia P&S

Mersey, James H MD [EDM] - **Spec Exp:** Diabetes; **Hospital:** Greater Baltimore Med Ctr, St Joseph Med Ctr; **Address:** 6535 N Charles St, Ste 400, Towson, MD 21204; **Phone:** 410-828-7417; **Board Cert:** Internal Medicine 1975; Endocrinology, Diabetes & Metabolism 1977; **Med School:** Johns Hopkins Univ 1972; **Resid:** Internal Medicine, Johns Hopkins Hosp 1977; **Fellow:** Endocrinology, Diabetes & Metabolism, Peter Bent Brigham Hosp 1976; **Fac Appt:** Asst Prof Med, Johns Hopkins Univ

Roberts, Michelle M MD [EDM] - **Spec Exp:** Osteoporosis; Diabetes; **Hospital:** UPMC Presby, Pittsburgh; **Address:** Falk Medical Bldg, 3601 Fifth Ave, Ste 3B, Pittsburgh, PA 15213; **Phone:** 412-586-9714; **Board Cert:** Internal Medicine 1986; Endocrinology, Diabetes & Metabolism 1989; **Med School:** Duke Univ 1983; **Resid:** Internal Medicine, Univ Pittsburgh Med Ctr 1986; **Fellow:** Endocrinology, Diabetes & Metabolism, Univ Pittsburgh Med Ctr 1989; **Fac Appt:** Assoc Clin Prof Med, Univ Pittsburgh

Saudek, Christopher D MD [EDM] - **Spec Exp:** Diabetes; **Hospital:** Johns Hopkins Hosp - Baltimore (page 61); **Address:** 600 N Wolfe St, Osler 575, Baltimore, MD 21287; **Phone:** 410-955-2132; **Board Cert:** Internal Medicine 1972; **Med School:** Cornell Univ-Weill Med Coll 1967; **Resid:** Internal Medicine, Presby-St Lukes Hosp 1969; Internal Medicine, Boston City Hosp 1970; **Fellow:** Endocrinology, Diabetes & Metabolism, Thorndale Lab-Harvard 1972; **Fac Appt:** Prof Med, Johns Hopkins Univ

Schwartz, Stanley S MD [EDM] - **Spec Exp:** Diabetes; **Hospital:** Hosp Univ Penn - UPHS (page 60); **Address:** Hosp Univ Penn, EDM Div, 3400 Spruce St, 9-Penn Twr, Philadelphia, PA 19104; **Phone:** 215-662-2518; **Board Cert:** Internal Medicine 1976; Endocrinology, Diabetes & Metabolism 1979; **Med School:** Univ Chicago-Pritzker Sch Med 1973; **Resid:** Internal Medicine, Hosp Univ Penn 1976; **Fellow:** Endocrinology, Diabetes & Metabolism, Univ Chicago Hosps 1978; **Fac Appt:** Assoc Clin Prof Med, Univ Pennsylvania

Shuldiner, Alan R MD [EDM] - **Spec Exp:** Diabetes; Eating Disorders/Obesity; **Hospital:** Univ of MD Med Sys; **Address:** Univ MD Sch Med, Div Endocrinology, 660 W Redwood St, rm HH-494, Baltimore, MD 21201; **Phone:** 410-706-1623; **Board Cert:** Internal Medicine 1988; Endocrinology 1989; **Med School:** Harvard Med Sch 1984; **Resid:** Internal Medicine, Columbia-Presby Hosp 1986; **Fellow:** Endocrinology, Diabetes & Metabolism, Natl Inst Hlth 1990; **Fac Appt:** Prof Med, Univ MD Sch Med

Siris, Ethel MD [EDM] - **Spec Exp:** Osteoporosis; Paget's Disease of Bone; Bone Disorders-Metabolic; **Hospital:** NY-Presby Hosp/Columbia (page 66); **Address:** 180 Ft Washington Ave, Harkness Bldg - Ste 904, New York, NY 10032-3710; **Phone:** 212-305-9531; **Board Cert:** Internal Medicine 1974; Endocrinology, Diabetes & Metabolism 1977; **Med School:** Columbia P&S 1971; **Resid:** Internal Medicine, Columbia-Presby Med Ctr 1974; **Fellow:** Endocrinology, Diabetes & Metabolism, Natl Inst Hlth 1976; Endocrinology, Diabetes & Metabolism, Columbia-Presby Med Ctr 1977; **Fac Appt:** Prof Med, Columbia P&S

Snyder, Peter J MD [EDM] - **Spec Exp:** Pituitary Tumors; Reproductive Endocrinology-Male; **Hospital:** Hosp Univ Penn - UPHS (page 60); **Address:** Univ Pennsylvania Med Group, 3400 Spruce St, Philadelphia, PA 19104; **Phone:** 215-898-0208; **Board Cert:** Internal Medicine 1972; Endocrinology, Diabetes & Metabolism 1972; **Med School:** Harvard Med Sch 1965; **Resid:** Internal Medicine, Beth Israel Hosp 1967; Internal Medicine, Beth Israel Hosp 1970; **Fellow:** Endocrinology, Diabetes & Metabolism, Hosp Univ Penn 1971; **Fac Appt:** Prof Med, Univ Pennsylvania

Surks, Martin MD [EDM] - **Spec Exp:** Thyroid Disorders; **Hospital:** Montefiore Med Ctr, N Central Bronx Hosp; **Address:** 3400 Bainbridge Ave Fl 2, Bronx, NY 10467; **Phone:** 866-633-8255; **Board Cert:** Internal Medicine 1967; Endocrinology, Diabetes & Metabolism 1977; **Med School:** NYU Sch Med 1960; **Resid:** Internal Medicine, Montefiore Hosp Med Ctr 1962; Internal Medicine, VA Hosp 1964; **Fellow:** Research, Natl Inst Arthritis-Metabolic Disease 1964; **Fac Appt:** Prof Med, Albert Einstein Coll Med

Tuttle, R Michael MD [EDM] - **Spec Exp:** Thyroid Cancer; **Hospital:** Meml Sloan-Kettering Cancer Ctr; **Address:** 1275 York Avenue, New York, NY 10065; **Phone:** 800-525-2225; **Board Cert:** Endocrinology, Diabetes & Metabolism 2004; **Med School:** Univ Louisville Sch Med 1987; **Resid:** Internal Medicine, DD Eisenhower Army Med Ctr 1990; **Fellow:** Endocrinology, Diabetes & Metabolism, Madigan Army Med Ctr 1993; **Fac Appt:** Assoc Prof Med, Cornell Univ-Weill Med Coll

Wartofsky, Leonard MD [EDM] - **Spec Exp:** Thyroid Cancer; Thyroid Disorders; **Hospital:** Washington Hosp Ctr; **Address:** 110 Irving St NW, Ste 2A62, Washington, DC 20010-2975; **Phone:** 202-877-3109; **Board Cert:** Internal Medicine 1971; Endocrinology, Diabetes & Metabolism 1972; **Med School:** Geo Wash Univ 1964; **Resid:** Internal Medicine, Barnes Jewish Hosp 1966; Internal Medicine, Montefiore Med Ctr 1967; **Fellow:** Endocrinology, Diabetes & Metabolism, Boston City Hosp 1969; **Fac Appt:** Prof Med, Georgetown Univ

Young, Iven MD [EDM] - **Spec Exp:** Thyroid Disorders; Osteoporosis; Pituitary Disorders; **Hospital:** St Vincent Cath Med Ctrs - Manhattan; **Address:** 130 W 12th St, Ste 7D, New York, NY 10011-8250; **Phone:** 212-675-9332; **Board Cert:** Internal Medicine 1966; Endocrinology, Diabetes & Metabolism 1973; **Med School:** NYU Sch Med 1959; **Resid:** Internal Medicine, VA Med Ctr 1963; **Fellow:** Endocrinology, NYU Med Ctr 1966; **Fac Appt:** Assoc Clin Prof Med, NY Med Coll

Endocrinology, Diabetes & Metabolism

Southeast

Ain, Kenneth B MD [EDM] - **Spec Exp:** Thyroid Cancer; Thyroid Disorders; **Hospital:** Univ of Kentucky Chandler Hosp, VA Med Ctr - Lexington; **Address:** Markey Cancer Center, 800 Rose St, rm CC455, Lexington, KY 40536-0001; **Phone:** 859-323-3778; **Board Cert:** Internal Medicine 1984; Endocrinology, Diabetes & Metabolism 1987; **Med School:** Brown Univ 1981; **Resid:** Internal Medicine, Hahnemann Univ 1984; **Fellow:** Endocrinology, Univ Chicago 1986; Thyroid Oncology, NIDDK, Natl Inst Hlth 1990; **Fac Appt:** Prof Med, Univ KY Coll Med

Barrett, Eugene J MD [EDM] - **Spec Exp:** Diabetes; Cholesterol/Lipid Disorders; **Hospital:** Univ Virginia Med Ctr; **Address:** Univ Virginia, Div Endocrinology, PO Box 801410, Charlottesville, VA 22908; **Phone:** 434-924-1175; **Board Cert:** Internal Medicine 1978; Endocrinology, Diabetes & Metabolism 1995; **Med School:** Univ Rochester 1975; **Resid:** Internal Medicine, Strong Meml Hosp 1977; **Fellow:** Endocrinology, Diabetes & Metabolism, Yale Univ 1980; **Fac Appt:** Prof Med, Univ VA Sch Med

Bell, David S H MD [EDM] - **Spec Exp:** Diabetes; Diabetes-Insulin Pump Therapy; Diabetic Vascular Diaease; **Hospital:** Univ of Ala Hosp at Birmingham; **Address:** 1020 26th St S, Birmingham, AL 35205; **Phone:** 205-933-2667; **Board Cert:** Internal Medicine 1987; Endocrinology, Diabetes & Metabolism 1981; **Med School:** Ireland 1970; **Resid:** Internal Medicine, Royal Victoria Hosp 1973; Endocrinology, Diabetes & Metabolism, Univ Saskatchewan Hosp 1975; **Fellow:** Endocrinology, Diabetes & Metabolism, Greater Baltimore Med Ctr 1976; **Fac Appt:** Prof Med, Univ Ala

Clore, John MD [EDM] - **Spec Exp:** Diabetes; Hypoglycemia; **Hospital:** Med Coll of VA Hosp; **Address:** PO Box 980155, Richmond, VA 23298; **Phone:** 804-828-2161; **Board Cert:** Internal Medicine 1985; Endocrinology, Diabetes & Metabolism 1989; **Med School:** Med Coll VA 1982; **Resid:** Internal Medicine, Med Coll Virginia 1985; **Fellow:** Endocrinology, Diabetes & Metabolism, Med Coll Virginia 1988; **Fac Appt:** Assoc Prof Med, Va Commonwealth Univ Sch Med

Dalkin, Alan Craig MD [EDM] - **Spec Exp:** Bone Disorders-Metabolic; Osteoporosis; **Hospital:** Univ Virginia Med Ctr; **Address:** Univ VA Hlth Sys, Div Endocrinology, PO Box 801412, Charlottesville, VA 22908; **Phone:** 434-243-2603; **Board Cert:** Internal Medicine 1987; Endocrinology 1989; **Med School:** Univ Mich Med Sch 1984; **Resid:** Internal Medicine, Univ Chicago Hosps 1987; **Fellow:** Endocrinology, Diabetes & Metabolism, Univ Mich Med Ctr 1990; **Fac Appt:** Assoc Prof Med, Univ VA Sch Med

Earp III, H Shelton MD [EDM] - **Spec Exp:** Cancer-Hormonal Influences; **Hospital:** Univ NC Hosps; **Address:** UNC Lineberger Comprehensive Cancer Center, 450 West Drive, Fl 1 - rm 10-012, Chapel Hill, NC 27599; **Phone:** 919-966-3036; **Board Cert:** Internal Medicine 1976; Endocrinology, Diabetes & Metabolism 1977; **Med School:** Univ NC Sch Med 1970; **Resid:** Internal Medicine, NC Memorial Hosp 1975; **Fellow:** Endocrinology, Diabetes & Metabolism, Univ North Carolina Hosp 1977; **Fac Appt:** Prof Med, Univ NC Sch Med

Feinglos, Mark MD [EDM] - **Spec Exp:** Diabetes; Thyroid Disorders; **Hospital:** Duke Univ Med Ctr; **Address:** Duke Univ Med Ctr, Box 3921, Durham, NC 27710-0001; **Phone:** 919-684-4005; **Board Cert:** Internal Medicine 1976; Endocrinology, Diabetes & Metabolism 1977; **Med School:** McGill Univ 1973; **Resid:** Internal Medicine, Duke Univ Med Ctr 1975; **Fellow:** Endocrinology, Diabetes & Metabolism, Duke Univ Med Ctr 1977; **Fac Appt:** Prof Med, Duke Univ

Koch, Christian A MD [EDM] - **Spec Exp:** Endocrine Cancers; Thyroid Cancer; Growth Hormone Disorder-Adult; Hypertension; **Hospital:** Univ Hosps & Clins - Jackson; **Address:** 2500 N State St, Jackson, MS 39216; **Phone:** 601-984-5525; **Board Cert:** Internal Medicine 1999; Endocrinology, Diabetes & Metabolism 2000; **Med School:** Germany 1991; **Resid:** Internal Medicine, Ohio State Univ Hosp 1997; **Fellow:** Endocrinology, Natl Inst Hlth 2001; **Fac Appt:** Prof Med, Univ Miss

Marshall, John C MD/PhD [EDM] - **Spec Exp:** Pituitary Disorders; Neuroendocrinology; Polycystic Ovarian Syndrome; **Hospital:** Univ Virginia Med Ctr; **Address:** Univ VA Hlth System, Hospital Dr, Box 800612, Charlottesville, VA 22908-0001; **Phone:** 434-924-2431; **Board Cert:** Internal Medicine 1978; Endocrinology, Diabetes & Metabolism 1981; **Med School:** England 1965; **Resid:** Neurology, Natl Hosp Queen Square 1968; Cardiovascular Disease, Natl Heart Hosp 1969; **Fellow:** Endocrinology, Diabetes & Metabolism, Hammersmith Hosp 1972; Endocrinology, Diabetes & Metabolism, UCLA 1974; **Fac Appt:** Prof Med, Univ VA Sch Med

Nestler, John E MD [EDM] - **Spec Exp:** Polycystic Ovarian Syndrome; Diabetes; **Hospital:** Med Coll of VA Hosp; **Address:** Med Coll Va, Div Endocrinology, Box 980111, Richmond, VA 23298-0111; **Phone:** 804-828-2161; **Board Cert:** Internal Medicine 1982; Endocrinology 1985; **Med School:** Univ Pennsylvania 1979; **Resid:** Internal Medicine, Med Coll Virginia 1983; **Fellow:** Endocrinology, Hosp Univ Penn 1985; **Fac Appt:** Prof Med, Med Coll VA

Ontjes, David A MD [EDM] - **Spec Exp:** Osteoporosis; Thyroid Disorders; Adrenal Disorders; Pituitary Disorders; **Hospital:** Univ NC Hosps; **Address:** UNC-Chapel Hill, 257 MacNider Bldg, Chapel Hill, NC 27599-7527; **Phone:** 919-966-3336; **Board Cert:** Internal Medicine 1980; Endocrinology, Diabetes & Metabolism 1972; **Med School:** Harvard Med Sch 1964; **Resid:** Internal Medicine, Boston City Hosp 1966; **Fac Appt:** Prof Med, Univ NC Sch Med

Ovalle, Fernando MD [EDM] - **Spec Exp:** Diabetes; Polycystic Ovarian Syndrome; Hypoglycemia; **Hospital:** Univ of Ala Hosp at Birmingham; **Address:** UAB Sch Med, 510 20th St S FOT Bldg Fl 7 - Ste 702, Birmingham, AL 35294; **Phone:** 205-975-2422; **Board Cert:** Endocrinology, Diabetes & Metabolism 1997; **Med School:** Mexico 1989; **Resid:** Internal Medicine, Henry Ford Hosp 1995; **Fellow:** Endocrinology, Diabetes & Metabolism, Barnes Jewish Hosp 1997; **Fac Appt:** Assoc Prof Med, Univ Ala

Powers, Alvin C MD [EDM] - **Spec Exp:** Diabetes; Thyroid Disorders; **Hospital:** Vanderbilt Univ Med Ctr; **Address:** Vanderbilt Univ Med Ctr, Div Endocrinology, 2213 Garland Ave, MRB#4, Nashville, TN 37232-0475; **Phone:** 615-936-1653; **Board Cert:** Internal Medicine 1982; Endocrinology, Diabetes & Metabolism 1985; **Med School:** Univ Tenn Coll Med, Memphis 1979; **Resid:** Internal Medicine, Duke Univ Med Ctr 1982; **Fellow:** Endocrinology, Diabetes & Metabolism, Joslin Diabetes Ctr 1983; Endocrinology, Diabetes & Metabolism, Mass Genl Hosp 1985; **Fac Appt:** Prof Med, Vanderbilt Univ

Quinn, Suzanne L MD [EDM] - **Hospital:** Shands at Univ of FL, Malcolm Randall VA Med Ctr; **Address:** Shands Univ Florida, Dept Endocrinology, 2000 SW Archer Rd, Gainesville, FL 32610; **Phone:** 352-265-8230; **Board Cert:** Internal Medicine 1988; Endocrinology, Diabetes & Metabolism 2003; **Med School:** Univ Fla Coll Med 1985; **Resid:** Internal Medicine, Univ Fla Coll Med 1988; **Fellow:** Endocrinology, Diabetes & Metabolism, Univ Fla Coll Med 1992; **Fac Appt:** Assoc Prof Med, Univ Fla Coll Med

Skyler, Jay S MD [EDM] - **Spec Exp:** Diabetes; **Hospital:** Jackson Meml Hosp, Univ of Miami Hosp & Clins/Sylvester Comp Canc Ctr; **Address:** Diabetes Research Inst, 1450 NW 10th Ave, Ste 3054, Miami, FL 33136; **Phone:** 305-243-6146; **Board Cert:** Internal Medicine 1972; Endocrinology, Diabetes & Metabolism 1973; **Med School:** Jefferson Med Coll 1969; **Resid:** Internal Medicine, Duke Univ Med Ctr 1971; **Fellow:** Endocrinology, Diabetes & Metabolism, Duke Univ Med Ctr 1973; **Fac Appt:** Prof Med, Univ Miami Sch Med

Vance, Mary Lee MD [EDM] - **Spec Exp:** Pituitary Disorders; Adrenal Disorders; **Hospital:** Univ Virginia Med Ctr; **Address:** Univ Virginia Hlth Sys, PO Box 800601, Charlottesville, VA 22908-0601; **Phone:** 434-924-2284; **Board Cert:** Internal Medicine 1980; **Med School:** Louisiana State U, New Orleans 1977; **Resid:** Internal Medicine, Baylor Univ Med Ctr 1980; **Fellow:** Endocrinology, Univ Virginia Med Ctr 1983; **Fac Appt:** Prof Med, Univ VA Sch Med

Endocrinology, Diabetes & Metabolism

Weissman, Peter MD [EDM] - **Spec Exp:** Diabetes; **Hospital:** Baptist Hosp of Miami; **Address:** 7867 N Kendall Drive, Ste 80, Miami, FL 33156; **Phone:** 305-595-0777; **Board Cert:** Internal Medicine 1972; Endocrinology, Diabetes & Metabolism 1972; **Med School:** NYU Sch Med 1966; **Resid:** Internal Medicine, Barnes Hosp/Wash Univ 1968; **Fellow:** Geriatric Medicine, Gerontology Rsch Ctr 1970; Endocrinology, Diabetes & Metabolism, Univ Mich Hosp 1972; **Fac Appt:** Assoc Clin Prof Med, Univ Miami Sch Med

Midwest

Bahn, Rebecca S MD [EDM] - **Spec Exp:** Graves' Disease; Graves' Disease-Eye; **Hospital:** Mayo Med Ctr & Clin - Rochester; **Address:** Mayo Clinic, Div Endocrinology, 200 First St SW, Rochester, MN 55905; **Phone:** 507-284-1600; **Board Cert:** Internal Medicine 1985; Endocrinology, Diabetes & Metabolism 1987; **Med School:** Mayo Med Sch 1981; **Resid:** Internal Medicine, Mayo Clinic 1984; **Fellow:** Endocrinology, Diabetes & Metabolism, Mayo Clinic 1986; **Fac Appt:** Prof Med, Mayo Med Sch

Brennan, Michael D MD [EDM] - **Spec Exp:** Thyroid Disorders; Diabetes; **Hospital:** Mayo Med Ctr & Clin - Rochester; **Address:** Mayo Clinic, Div Endocrinology, 200 First St SW, Rochester, MN 55905; **Phone:** 507-266-5247; **Board Cert:** Internal Medicine 1975; Endocrinology, Diabetes & Metabolism 1977; **Med School:** Ireland 1969; **Resid:** Internal Medicine, Mayo Clinic 1975; Internal Medicine, Henry Ford Hosp 1972; **Fellow:** Endocrinology, Diabetes & Metabolism, Mayo Clinic 1977; **Fac Appt:** Assoc Prof Med, Mayo Med Sch

Clutter, William E MD [EDM] - **Spec Exp:** Endocrine Cancers; Calcium Disorders; Metabolic Bone Disease; **Hospital:** Barnes-Jewish Hosp, Washington Univ Med Ctr; **Address:** Washington Univ, Dept Internal Medicine, 4921 Parkview Pl Fl 5 - Ste C, St Louis, MO 63110; **Phone:** 314-362-3500; **Board Cert:** Internal Medicine 1978; Endocrinology, Diabetes & Metabolism 1981; **Med School:** Ohio State Univ 1975; **Resid:** Internal Medicine, Barnes Jewish Hosp 1978; **Fellow:** Endocrinology, Diabetes & Metabolism, Barnes Jewish Hosp 1980; **Fac Appt:** Prof Med, Washington Univ, St Louis

Cryer, Philip E MD [EDM] - **Spec Exp:** Diabetes; Hypoglycemia; **Hospital:** Barnes-Jewish Hosp, St Louis Chldns Hosp; **Address:** Wash Univ Sch Med, Div Endo, Metab & Lipid Rsch, 660 S Euclid Ave, Box 8127, St Louis, MO 63110-1093; **Phone:** 314-362-7635; **Board Cert:** Internal Medicine 1972; Endocrinology, Diabetes & Metabolism 1972; **Med School:** Northwestern Univ 1965; **Resid:** Internal Medicine, Barnes Jewish Hosp 1972; **Fellow:** Endocrinology, Diabetes & Metabolism, Wash Univ Sch Med 1968; **Fac Appt:** Prof Med, Washington Univ, St Louis

Econs, Michael J MD [EDM] - **Spec Exp:** Osteoporosis; Paget's Disease of Bone; Metabolic Bone Disease; **Hospital:** Indiana Univ Hosp; **Address:** 541 N Clinical Dr, CL 459, Indianapolis, IN 46202; **Phone:** 317-274-1339; **Board Cert:** Internal Medicine 1986; Endocrinology, Diabetes & Metabolism 1989; **Med School:** UCSF 1983; **Resid:** Internal Medicine, Univ Maryland Hosp 1986; **Fellow:** Endocrinology, Duke Univ Med Ctr 1989; **Fac Appt:** Prof Med, Indiana Univ

Ehrmann, David A MD [EDM] - **Spec Exp:** Polycystic Ovarian Syndrome; Diabetes; **Hospital:** Univ of Chicago Hosps; **Address:** Univ Chicago, Div Endocrinology, 5758 S Maryland Ave, Ste 5A, MC 1027, Chicago, IL 60637; **Phone:** 773-702-6138; **Board Cert:** Internal Medicine 1985; Endocrinology, Diabetes & Metabolism 1987; **Med School:** Univ Mich Med Sch 1982; **Resid:** Internal Medicine, Univ Mich Med Ctr 1985; **Fellow:** Endocrinology, Diabetes & Metabolism, Univ Chicago Hosps 1987; **Fac Appt:** Assoc Prof Med, Univ Chicago-Pritzker Sch Med

Emanuele, Mary Ann MD [EDM] - **Spec Exp:** Diabetes; **Hospital:** Loyola Univ Med Ctr; **Address:** Loyola Univ Med Ctr, Dept Endocrinology, 2160 S 1st Ave Bldg 54 - rm 137A, Maywood, IL 60153-3304; **Phone:** 708-216-0160; **Board Cert:** Internal Medicine 1978; Endocrinology, Diabetes & Metabolism 1983; **Med School:** Loyola Univ-Stritch Sch Med 1975; **Resid:** Internal Medicine, Univ Hawaii Med Ctr 1978; **Fellow:** Endocrinology, Edward Hines Jr VA Hosp 1980; **Fac Appt:** Prof Med, Loyola Univ-Stritch Sch Med

Emanuele, Nicholas V MD [EDM] - **Hospital:** Hines VA Hosp; **Address:** Hines VA Hosp Bldg 200 - rm 1426, PO Box 5000, Hines, IL 60141; **Phone:** 708-202-8387 x21415; **Board Cert:** Internal Medicine 1975; Endocrinology 1979; **Med School:** Northwestern Univ 1967; **Resid:** Internal Medicine, Hines VA Hosp 1974; **Fellow:** Endocrinology, Northwestern Univ 1976

Herman, William H MD [EDM] - **Spec Exp:** Diabetes; Diabetes in Pregnancy; **Hospital:** Univ Michigan Hlth Sys; **Address:** A Alfred Taubman Health Care Ctr, 1500 E Medical Ctr Dr, 3920 TC, SPC5334, Ann Arbor, MI 48109-0354; **Phone:** 734-647-5922; **Board Cert:** Internal Medicine 1982; Endocrinology, Diabetes & Metabolism 1989; **Med School:** Boston Univ 1979; **Resid:** Internal Medicine, Univ Mich Med Ctr 1982; Preventive Medicine, Ctrs Dis Control 1985; **Fellow:** Endocrinology, Diabetes & Metabolism, Univ Mich Med Ctr 1988; **Fac Appt:** Prof Med, Univ Mich Med Sch

Hoogwerf, Byron J MD [EDM] - **Spec Exp:** Diabetes; Cholesterol/Lipid Disorders; Clinical Trials; Preventive Cardiology; **Hospital:** Cleveland Clin Fdn (page 56); **Address:** Cleveland Clinic, Div Endocrinology, 9500 Euclid Ave, Desk A-53, Cleveland, OH 44195-0001; **Phone:** 216-444-8347; **Board Cert:** Internal Medicine 1978; Endocrinology, Diabetes & Metabolism 1981; **Med School:** Univ Minn 1971; **Resid:** Internal Medicine, Hennepin Co Med Ctr 1978; **Fellow:** Endocrinology, Diabetes & Metabolism, Univ Minn Hosps 1981; **Fac Appt:** Prof Med, Ohio State Univ

Jensen, Michael D MD [EDM] - **Spec Exp:** Eating Disorders/Obesity; Nutrition; **Hospital:** Mayo Med Ctr & Clin - Rochester; **Address:** Mayo Clinic, Div Endocrinology, 200 First St SW, Rochester, MN 55905; **Phone:** 507-284-2462; **Board Cert:** Internal Medicine 1982; Endocrinology, Diabetes & Metabolism 1985; **Med School:** Univ MO-Kansas City 1979; **Resid:** Internal Medicine, Mayo Clinic 1982; **Fellow:** Endocrinology, Diabetes & Metabolism, Mayo Clinic 1985; **Fac Appt:** Prof Med, Mayo Med Sch

Khosla, Sundeep MD [EDM] - **Spec Exp:** Osteoporosis; Bone Disorders-Metabolic; **Hospital:** Mayo Med Ctr & Clin - Rochester; **Address:** Mayo Clinic, Div Endocrinology, 200 First St SW, Rochester, MN 55905; **Phone:** 507-284-1600; **Board Cert:** Internal Medicine 1985; Endocrinology 1987; **Med School:** Harvard Med Sch 1982; **Resid:** Internal Medicine, Mass Genl Hosp 1985; **Fellow:** Endocrinology, Diabetes & Metabolism, Mass Genl Hosp 1988; **Fac Appt:** Asst Prof Med, Mayo Med Sch

Kloos, Richard MD [EDM] - **Spec Exp:** Thyroid Cancer; **Hospital:** Ohio St Univ Med Ctr; **Address:** 446 McCampbell Hall, 1581 Dodd Drive, Columbus, OH 43210; **Phone:** 614-292-3800; **Board Cert:** Nuclear Medicine 2005; Internal Medicine 2002; Endocrinology, Diabetes & Metabolism 2005; **Med School:** Case West Res Univ 1989; **Resid:** Internal Medicine, MetroHealth MC 1992; **Fellow:** Endocrinology, Diabetes & Metabolism, Univ Michigan 1995; Nuclear Medicine, Univ Michigan 1996; **Fac Appt:** Assoc Prof Med, Ohio State Univ

Kopp, Peter A MD [EDM] - **Spec Exp:** Thyroid Cancer; Pituitary Disorders; Parathyroid Disease; Diabetes; **Hospital:** Northwestern Meml Hosp; **Address:** Northwestern Meml Hospital, 675 N St Clair St, Ste 14-100, Chicago, IL 60611; **Phone:** 312-695-7970; **Board Cert:** Internal Medicine 2003; Endocrinology, Diabetes & Metabolism 2004; **Med School:** Switzerland 1985; **Resid:** Internal Medicine, Regl Hosp 1992; Endocrinology, Diabetes & Metabolism, Univ Berne 1990; **Fellow:** Endocrinology, Diabetes & Metabolism, Northwestern Univ Hosp 1997; **Fac Appt:** Assoc Prof Med, Northwestern Univ-Feinberg Sch Med

Endocrinology, Diabetes & Metabolism

Licata, Angelo A MD [EDM] - **Spec Exp:** Bone Disorders-Metabolic; Osteoporosis; Calcium Disorders; **Hospital:** Cleveland Clin Fdn (page 56); **Address:** Div Endocrinology, 9500 Euclid Ave, Desk A53, Cleveland, OH 44195; **Phone:** 216-444-6248; **Board Cert:** Internal Medicine 1983; **Med School:** Univ Rochester 1973; **Resid:** Internal Medicine, Washington Univ Hosp 1974; Internal Medicine, Georgetown Univ Hosp 1978; **Fellow:** Endocrinology, Diabetes & Metabolism, Natl Inst Hlth 1976; **Fac Appt:** Asst Clin Prof Med, Case West Res Univ

Mazzone, Theodore MD [EDM] - **Spec Exp:** Cholesterol/Lipid Disorders; Diabetes; **Hospital:** Univ of IL Med Ctr at Chicago; **Address:** Univ Illinois Chicago, Div Diabetes & Metabolism, 1819 W Polk St, Chicago, IL 60612-7333; **Phone:** 312-355-4426; **Board Cert:** Internal Medicine 1980; Endocrinology, Diabetes & Metabolism 1983; **Med School:** Northwestern Univ 1977; **Resid:** Internal Medicine, UCLA Med Ctr 1980; **Fellow:** Endocrinology, Diabetes & Metabolism, Univ Wash Med Ctr 1983; **Fac Appt:** Prof Med, Univ IL Coll Med

McGill, Janet B MD [EDM] - **Spec Exp:** Diabetes; **Hospital:** Barnes-Jewish Hosp; **Address:** 4921 Parkview Pl, Box 8127, St Louis, MO 63110-1010; **Phone:** 314-747-7300; **Board Cert:** Internal Medicine 1983; Endocrinology, Diabetes & Metabolism 1987; **Med School:** Mich State Univ 1979; **Resid:** Internal Medicine, William Beaumont Hosp 1984; Endocrinology, Diabetes & Metabolism, William Beaumont Hosp 1985; **Fellow:** Diabetes, Washington Univ 1987; **Fac Appt:** Assoc Prof Med, Washington Univ, St Louis

McMahon, M Molly MD [EDM] - **Spec Exp:** Nutrition; Diabetes; **Hospital:** Mayo Med Ctr & Clin - Rochester; **Address:** Mayo Clinic, Div Endocrinology, 200 First St SW, Rochester, MN 55905; **Phone:** 507-284-2463; **Board Cert:** Internal Medicine 1985; Endocrinology, Diabetes & Metabolism 1987; **Med School:** Univ Wisc 1981; **Resid:** Internal Medicine, Med Coll Wisc 1984; **Fellow:** Endocrinology, Diabetes & Metabolism, Mayo Clinic 1987; Nutrition, New Eng Deaconess Hosp 1988

Polonsky, Kenneth S MD [EDM] - **Spec Exp:** Diabetes; **Hospital:** Barnes-Jewish Hosp; **Address:** Wash Univ School Medicine, Div Endo, Metab, & Lipid Rsch, 660 S Euclid Ave, Campus Box 8066, St Louis, MO 63110-1010; **Phone:** 314-362-8061; **Board Cert:** Internal Medicine 1978; **Med School:** South Africa 1973; **Resid:** Internal Medicine, Michael Reese Hosp & Med Ctr 1976; Internal Medicine, VA Hosp 1976; **Fellow:** Internal Medicine, Univ Chicago 1978; **Fac Appt:** Prof Med, Washington Univ, St Louis

Rizza, Robert Alan MD [EDM] - **Spec Exp:** Diabetes; Cholesterol/Lipid Disorders; **Hospital:** St Mary's Hosp - Rochester, Rochester Methodist Hosp; **Address:** Mayo Clinic - Div Endo, 200 First St SW, Fl W18B, Rochester, MN 55905-0002; **Phone:** 507-284-1600; **Board Cert:** Internal Medicine 1976; Endocrinology, Diabetes & Metabolism 1979; **Med School:** Univ Fla Coll Med 1971; **Resid:** Internal Medicine, Johns Hopkins Hosp 1973; **Fellow:** Endocrinology, Mayo Clinic 1979; **Fac Appt:** Prof Med, Mayo Med Sch

Semenkovich, Clay F MD [EDM] - **Spec Exp:** Cholesterol/Lipid Disorders; Diabetes; Endocrinology; **Hospital:** Barnes-Jewish Hosp; **Address:** Wash Univ Sch Med, Div Endo, Metab & Lipid Rsch, 660 S Euclid Ave, Box 8127, St Louis, MO 63110; **Phone:** 314-362-7617; **Board Cert:** Internal Medicine 1984; Endocrinology, Diabetes & Metabolism 1987; **Med School:** Washington Univ, St Louis 1981; **Resid:** Internal Medicine, Barnes Hosp 1984; **Fellow:** Endocrinology, Diabetes & Metabolism, Wash Univ 1986; **Fac Appt:** Prof Med, Washington Univ, St Louis

Service, Frederick J MD/PhD [EDM] - **Spec Exp:** Hypoglycemia; Diabetes; **Hospital:** Mayo Med Ctr & Clin - Rochester; **Address:** Mayo Clinic, Div Endocrinology, 200 First St SW, Rochester, MN 55905-0001; **Phone:** 507-284-5643; **Board Cert:** Internal Medicine 1977; Endocrinology, Diabetes & Metabolism 1972; **Med School:** McGill Univ 1962; **Resid:** Internal Medicine, Royal Victoria Hosp 1965; **Fellow:** Endocrinology, Diabetes & Metabolism, Mayo Grad Sch 1969; **Fac Appt:** Prof Med, Mayo Med Sch

Sowers, James R MD [EDM] - **Spec Exp:** Diabetes; Hypertension; Cholesterol/Lipid Disorders; **Hospital:** Univ of Missouri Hosp & Clins; **Address:** UMC, Dept Internal Med, One Hospital Drive, rm D109, Columbia, MO 65212; **Phone:** 573-882-2573; **Board Cert:** Internal Medicine 1974; Endocrinology, Diabetes & Metabolism 1977; **Med School:** Univ MO-Columbia Sch Med 1971; **Resid:** Internal Medicine, St Johns Mercy Med Ctr 1974; **Fellow:** Endocrinology, Wadsworth VA Hosp Ctr-UCLA 1976; **Fac Appt:** Prof Med, Univ MO-Columbia Sch Med

Veldhuis, Johannes D MD [EDM] - **Spec Exp:** Reproductive Endocrinology; Pituitary Disorders; Adrenal Disorders; Hypogonadism; **Hospital:** Mayo Med Ctr & Clin - Rochester; **Address:** Mayo Clinic, Div Endocrinology, 200 First St Sw, Joseph 5-194, Rochester, MN 55905; **Phone:** 507-284-3915; **Board Cert:** Internal Medicine 1977; Endocrinology 1979; **Med School:** Penn State Univ-Hershey Med Ctr 1974; **Resid:** Internal Medicine, Mayo Grad Sch Med 1977; **Fellow:** Endocrinology, Diabetes & Metabolism, Penn State Univ Hosp 1978; **Fac Appt:** Prof Med, Mayo Med Sch

Watts, Nelson B MD [EDM] - **Spec Exp:** Osteoporosis; Metabolic Bone Disease; Paget's Disease of Bone; **Hospital:** Univ Hosp - Cincinnati; **Address:** Univ Bone Health & Osteoporosis Ctr, 222 Piedmont Ave, Ste 6300, Cincinnati, OH 45219; **Phone:** 513-475-7400; **Board Cert:** Internal Medicine 1972; Endocrinology, Diabetes & Metabolism 1985; **Med School:** Univ NC Sch Med 1969; **Resid:** Internal Medicine, Charlotte Meml Hosp 1972; **Fellow:** Endocrinology, Diabetes & Metabolism, NC Meml Hosp 1971; **Fac Appt:** Prof Med, Univ Cincinnati

Werner, Phillip L MD [EDM] - **Spec Exp:** Diabetes; **Hospital:** Adv Luth Genl Hosp; **Address:** 1775 Ballard Rd, Nesset Pavilion, Park Ridge, IL 60068; **Phone:** 847-318-2400; **Board Cert:** Internal Medicine 1975; Endocrinology 1977; **Med School:** Univ IL Coll Med 1972; **Resid:** Internal Medicine, Univ Illinois Affl Hosp 1975; **Fellow:** Endocrinology, Diabetes & Metabolism, Univ Wash 1977; **Fac Appt:** Prof Med, Ros Franklin Univ/Chicago Med Sch

Great Plains and Mountains

Eckel, Robert H MD [EDM] - **Spec Exp:** Cholesterol/Lipid Disorders; Eating Disorders/Obesity; Diabetes; **Hospital:** Univ Colorado Hosp; **Address:** Univ Colorado Hlth Scis Ctr, PO Box 6510, MS F732, Aurora, CO 80045; **Phone:** 720-848-2650; **Board Cert:** Internal Medicine 1976; Endocrinology, Diabetes & Metabolism 1979; **Med School:** Univ Cincinnati 1973; **Resid:** Internal Medicine, Univ Wisconsin Hosps 1976; **Fellow:** Endocrinology, Diabetes & Metabolism, Univ Washington 1979; **Fac Appt:** Prof Med, Univ Colorado

Recker, Robert Roy MD [EDM] - **Spec Exp:** Osteoporosis; Diabetes; Endocrinology; **Hospital:** Creighton Univ Med Ctr, VA Medical Ctr - Omaha; **Address:** Creighton Univ Osteoporosis, Div Endocrinology, 601 N 30th St, Ste 4820, Omaha, NE 68131; **Phone:** 402-280-4470; **Board Cert:** Internal Medicine 1971; **Med School:** Creighton Univ 1963; **Resid:** Internal Medicine, Creighton Affil Hosps 1969; **Fellow:** Endocrinology, Diabetes & Metabolism, Creighton Univ 1971; **Fac Appt:** Prof Med, Creighton Univ

Ridgway, E Chester MD [EDM] - **Spec Exp:** Thyroid Cancer; Thyroid Disorders; Pituitary Disorders; **Hospital:** Univ Colorado Hosp, VA Med Ctr; **Address:** UCHSC at Fitzsimons, Endocrinology, 1635 N Ursula St, Box 6510, MS F732, Aurora, CO 80045; **Phone:** 720-848-2650; **Board Cert:** Internal Medicine 1972; Endocrinology 1973; **Med School:** Univ Colorado 1968; **Resid:** Internal Medicine, Mass Genl Hosp 1970; **Fellow:** Endocrinology, Mass Genl Hosp 1972; **Fac Appt:** Prof Med, Univ Colorado

Endocrinology, Diabetes & Metabolism

Southwest

Cunningham, Glenn R MD [EDM] - **Spec Exp:** Diabetes; Hypogonadism; Erectile Dysfunction; **Hospital:** St Luke's Episcopal Hosp - Houston; **Address:** 6624 Fannin St, Ste 1180, Houston, TX 77030; **Phone:** 832-355-7208; **Board Cert:** Internal Medicine 1972; Endocrinology, Diabetes & Metabolism 1972; **Med School:** Univ Okla Coll Med 1966; **Resid:** Internal Medicine, Duke Univ Med Ctr 1970; **Fellow:** Endocrinology, Duke Univ Med Ctr 1971; **Fac Appt:** Prof Med, Baylor Coll Med

Lavis, Victor Ralph MD [EDM] - **Spec Exp:** Diabetes; **Hospital:** UT MD Anderson Cancer Ctr, Meml Hermann Hosp - Texas Med Ctr; **Address:** MD Anderson Cancer Ctr, 1515 Holcombe Blvd, Ste 435, Houston, TX 77050; **Phone:** 713-792-2841; **Board Cert:** Internal Medicine 1969; Endocrinology, Diabetes & Metabolism 1998; **Med School:** Stanford Univ 1962; **Resid:** Internal Medicine, Boston Cty Hosp 1964; Internal Medicine, UCLA Med Ctr 1967; **Fellow:** Endocrinology, Diabetes & Metabolism, Univ Washington 1970; **Fac Appt:** Prof Med, Univ Tex, Houston

Raskin, Philip MD [EDM] - **Spec Exp:** Diabetes; **Hospital:** Parkland Meml Hosp - Dallas, UT Southwestern Med Ctr - Dallas; **Address:** Univ Tex SW Med Ctr, 5323 Harry Hines Blvd, Ste G5.238, Dallas, TX 75390-8858; **Phone:** 214-645-2800; **Board Cert:** Internal Medicine 1972; Endocrinology 1973; **Med School:** Univ Pittsburgh 1966; **Resid:** Internal Medicine, Hlth Ctr Hosps-Univ Pittsburgh 1968; **Fellow:** Endocrinology, Diabetes & Metabolism, UT SW Med Sch 1972; **Fac Appt:** Prof Med, Univ Tex SW, Dallas

Reasner II, Charles A MD [EDM] - **Spec Exp:** Thyroid Disorders; **Hospital:** Univ Hlth Sys - Univ Hosp (San Antonio, TX); **Address:** Texas Diabetes Inst, 701 S Zarzamora St, MS 12-5, San Antonio, TX 78207; **Phone:** 210-358-7402; **Board Cert:** Internal Medicine 1983; Endocrinology 1985; **Med School:** Loma Linda Univ 1979; **Resid:** Internal Medicine, USAF Med Ctr 1983; **Fellow:** Endocrinology, Diabetes & Metabolism, Wilford Hall Med Ctr 1985; **Fac Appt:** Assoc Prof Med, Univ Tex, San Antonio

Robbins, Richard MD [EDM] - **Spec Exp:** Thyroid Cancer; Pituitary Tumors; Pituitary Disorders; **Hospital:** Methodist Hosp - Houston; **Address:** The Methodist Hosp, 6550 Fannin St, Ste 1001, Houston, TX 77030; **Phone:** 713-441-6640; **Board Cert:** Internal Medicine 1978; Endocrinology, Diabetes & Metabolism 1983; **Med School:** Creighton Univ 1975; **Resid:** Internal Medicine, New York Hosp-Cornell Med Ctr 1978; **Fellow:** Endocrinology, New England Med Ctr 1981; **Fac Appt:** Prof Med, Cornell Univ-Weill Med Coll

Rubenfeld, Sheldon MD [EDM] - **Spec Exp:** Thyroid Cancer; Thyroid Disorders; Diabetes; **Hospital:** St Luke's Episcopal Hosp - Houston, Methodist Hosp - Houston; **Address:** 7515 S Main St, Ste 690, Houston, TX 77030; **Phone:** 713-795-5750; **Board Cert:** Internal Medicine 1976; Endocrinology, Diabetes & Metabolism 1979; **Med School:** Georgetown Univ 1971; **Resid:** Internal Medicine, Baylor Affil Hosps 1976; **Fellow:** Endocrinology, Baylor Affil Hosps 1978; **Fac Appt:** Clin Prof Med, Baylor Coll Med

Sherman, Steven I MD [EDM] - **Spec Exp:** Thyroid Cancer; Endocrine Cancers; **Hospital:** UT MD Anderson Cancer Ctr; **Address:** MD Anderson Cancer Ctr, 1515 Holcombe Blvd, Unit 435, Houston, TX 77030; **Phone:** 713-792-2840; **Board Cert:** Internal Medicine 1988; Endocrinology, Diabetes & Metabolism 2007; **Med School:** Johns Hopkins Univ 1985; **Resid:** Internal Medicine, Johns Hopkins Hosp 1988; **Fellow:** Endocrinology, Diabetes & Metabolism, Johns Hopkins Hosp 1991

Waguespack, Steven G MD [EDM] - **Spec Exp:** Thyroid Cancer; Pituitary Tumors; Adrenal Tumors & Disorders; **Hospital:** UT MD Anderson Cancer Ctr; **Address:** MD Anderson Cancer Ctr, Dept Endocrine Neoplasia, 1400 Holcombe Blvd, Unit 435, Houston, TX 77030; **Phone:** 713-563-4400; **Board Cert:** Internal Medicine 1998; Endocrinology, Diabetes & Metabolism 2002; Pediatric Endocrinology 2003; **Med School:** Univ Tex, Houston 1994; **Resid:** Internal Medicine & Pediatrics, Indiana Univ Hosp 1998; **Fellow:** Endocrinology, Indiana Univ Hosp 2002; **Fac Appt:** Assoc Prof Med, Univ Tex, Houston

West Coast and Pacific

Berkson, Richard A MD [EDM] - **Spec Exp:** Diabetes; Thyroid Disorders; **Hospital:** St Mary Med Ctr - Long Beach, CA, Long Beach Meml Med Ctr; **Address:** 1868 Pacific Ave, Long Beach, CA 90806-6113; **Phone:** 562-595-4718; **Board Cert:** Internal Medicine 1975; Endocrinology, Diabetes & Metabolism 1977; **Med School:** SUNY Buffalo 1972; **Resid:** Internal Medicine, SUNY Buffalo Affil Hosp 1975; **Fellow:** Endocrinology, Diabetes & Metabolism, Joslin Clinic 1976; Endocrinology, Diabetes & Metabolism, UCLA Med Ctr 1977; **Fac Appt:** Assoc Clin Prof Med, UCLA

Braunstein, Glenn D MD [EDM] - **Spec Exp:** Hormonal Disorders; **Hospital:** Cedars-Sinai Med Ctr; **Address:** Cedars Sinai Med Ctr, 8700 Beverly Blvd, Ste 2119, Los Angeles, CA 90048; **Phone:** 310-423-5140; **Board Cert:** Internal Medicine 1973; Endocrinology, Diabetes & Metabolism 1975; **Med School:** UCSF 1968; **Resid:** Internal Medicine, Peter Bent Bringham Hosp 1970; Endocrinology, Diabetes & Metabolism, Natl Inst Hlth-NICHHD 1972; **Fellow:** Endocrinology, Diabetes & Metabolism, LA Co Harbor Genl Hosp 1973; **Fac Appt:** Prof Med, UCLA

Chopra, Inder J MD [EDM] - **Spec Exp:** Thyroid Disorders; Endocrine Disorders; **Hospital:** Ronald Reagan UCLA Med Ctr; **Address:** UCLA Sch Med, Div Endocrinology, 900 Veteran Ave, Ste 24-130, Los Angeles, CA 90095-7073; **Phone:** 310-825-2346; **Board Cert:** Internal Medicine 1972; Endocrinology, Diabetes & Metabolism 1973; **Med School:** India 1961; **Resid:** Internal Medicine, All India Inst Med Sci 1965; Internal Medicine, Queens Med Ctr 1968; **Fellow:** Endocrinology, Diabetes & Metabolism, LAC-Harbor-UCLA Med Ctr 1971; **Fac Appt:** Prof Med, UCLA

Darwin, Christine H MD [EDM] - **Spec Exp:** Pituitary Tumors; Diabetes; **Hospital:** Ronald Reagan UCLA Med Ctr; **Address:** 200 UCLA Medical Plaza, Ste 365A, Box 951693, Los Angeles, CA 90095-7065; **Phone:** 310-794-5584; **Board Cert:** Geriatric Medicine 1994; Endocrinology, Diabetes & Metabolism 1997; **Med School:** India 1980; **Resid:** Internal Medicine, UC Irvine Med Ctr 1987; **Fellow:** Endocrinology, VA Hosp 1988; Endocrinology, USC Med Ctr 1993; **Fac Appt:** Assoc Prof Med, UCLA

Fitzgerald, Paul A MD [EDM] - **Spec Exp:** Diabetes; Thyroid Cancer; Pituitary Tumors; Thyroid Disorders; **Hospital:** UCSF Med Ctr; **Address:** 350 Parnassus Ave, Ste 710, San Francisco, CA 94117; **Phone:** 415-665-1136; **Board Cert:** Internal Medicine 1975; Endocrinology, Diabetes & Metabolism 1981; **Med School:** Jefferson Med Coll 1972; **Resid:** Internal Medicine, Presby Med Ctr-Univ Colo 1975; **Fellow:** Endocrinology, Diabetes & Metabolism, UCSF Med Ctr 1978; **Fac Appt:** Clin Prof Med, UCSF

Heber, David MD [EDM] - **Spec Exp:** Nutrition & Cancer Prevention; Nutrition & Disease Prevention/Control; Nutrition & Obesity; **Hospital:** Ronald Reagan UCLA Med Ctr; **Address:** 900 Veteran Ave, Rm 12-217, UCLA Center for Human Nutrition, Los Angeles, CA 90095-1742; **Phone:** 310-206-1987; **Board Cert:** Internal Medicine 1976; Endocrinology, Diabetes & Metabolism 1977; **Med School:** Harvard Med Sch 1973; **Resid:** Internal Medicine, LA Co Harbor Genl Hosp 1975; **Fellow:** Endocrinology, Diabetes & Metabolism, LA Co Harbor Genl Hosp 1978; **Fac Appt:** Prof Med, UCLA

Endocrinology, Diabetes & Metabolism

Hirsch, Irl B MD [EDM] - **Spec Exp:** Diabetes; **Hospital:** Univ Wash Med Ctr; **Address:** Univ Wash Med Ctr, Diabetes Care Ctr, 4225 Roosevelt Way NE, Ste 101, Seattle, WA 98105; **Phone:** 206-548-4882; **Board Cert:** Internal Medicine 1987; Endocrinology, Diabetes & Metabolism 1989; **Med School:** Univ MO-Columbia Sch Med 1984; **Resid:** Internal Medicine, Mt Sinai Med Ctr 1987; **Fellow:** Metabolism, Washington Univ Sch Med 1989; **Fac Appt:** Prof Med, Univ Wash

Hoffman, Andrew R MD [EDM] - **Spec Exp:** Pituitary Disorders; Pituitary Tumors; Neuroendocrinology; **Hospital:** Stanford Univ Med Ctr, VA Hlth Care Sys - Palo Alto; **Address:** 300 Pastur Drive Boswell Bldg - rm A-175, Stanford, CA 94305; **Phone:** 650-723-6961; **Board Cert:** Internal Medicine 1979; Endocrinology 1981; **Med School:** Stanford Univ 1976; **Resid:** Internal Medicine, Mass Genl Hosp 1978; **Fellow:** Pharmacology, Mass Genl Hosp 1980; Endocrinology, Diabetes & Metabolism, Mass Genl Hosp 1982; **Fac Appt:** Prof Med, Stanford Univ

Hsueh, Willa Ann MD [EDM] - **Spec Exp:** Diabetes; Hypertension; **Hospital:** Ronald Reagan UCLA Med Ctr; **Address:** 900 Veteran Ave, Ste 24-130, Los Angeles, CA 90095; **Phone:** 310-794-5403; **Board Cert:** Internal Medicine 1976; Endocrinology, Diabetes & Metabolism 1977; **Med School:** Ohio State Univ 1973; **Resid:** Internal Medicine, Johns Hopkins Hosp 1975; **Fellow:** Endocrinology, Diabetes & Metabolism, Johns Hopkins Hosp 1976; **Fac Appt:** Prof Med, UCLA

Ipp, Eli MD [EDM] - **Spec Exp:** Diabetes; **Hospital:** LAC - Harbor - UCLA Med Ctr; **Address:** 21840 S Normandy Ave, Ste 700, Torrance, CA 90502; **Phone:** 310-222-5101; **Board Cert:** Internal Medicine 1979; Endocrinology, Diabetes & Metabolism 1981; **Med School:** South Africa 1968; **Resid:** Internal Medicine, Tel Hashomer Hosp 1974; **Fellow:** Endocrinology, Diabetes & Metabolism, Univ Tex SW Med Ctr 1978; **Fac Appt:** Prof Med, UCLA

Kamdar, Vikram V MD [EDM] - **Spec Exp:** Diabetes; Diabetic Leg/Foot; Thyroid Disorders; **Hospital:** Santa Monica - UCLA Med Ctr, Ronald Reagan UCLA Med Ctr; **Address:** 1801 Wilshire Blvd, Ste 100, Santa Monica, CA 90403; **Phone:** 310-828-7172; **Board Cert:** Internal Medicine 1978; Endocrinology, Diabetes & Metabolism 1979; **Med School:** India 1971; **Resid:** Internal Medicine, Lemuel Shattuck Hosp 1972; Endocrinology, Diabetes & Metabolism, Cedars-Sinai Med Ctr 1977; **Fellow:** Endocrinology, Diabetes & Metabolism, LA Co-USC Med Ctr 1975; **Fac Appt:** Assoc Clin Prof Med, UCLA

Kandeel, Fouad MD/PhD [EDM] - **Spec Exp:** Thyroid Cancer; Endocrine Cancers; Neuroendocrinology; **Hospital:** City of Hope Natl Med Ctr & Beckman Rsch; **Address:** City of Hope, Diabetes Department, 1500 E Duarte Rd, Duarte, CA 91010; **Phone:** 626-256-4673 x62251; **Med School:** Egypt 1969; **Fac Appt:** Assoc Clin Prof Med, UCLA

Melmed, Shlomo MD [EDM] - **Spec Exp:** Pituitary Tumors; Acromegaly; Pituitary Disorders; **Hospital:** Cedars-Sinai Med Ctr; **Address:** Cedars Sinai Med Ctr, 8700 Beverly Blvd, Ste 2015, Los Angeles, CA 90048; **Phone:** 310-423-4691; **Board Cert:** Internal Medicine 1979; Endocrinology, Diabetes & Metabolism 1983; **Med School:** South Africa 1970; **Resid:** Internal Medicine, Sheba Med Ctr 1976; **Fellow:** Endocrinology, Diabetes & Metabolism, Wadsworth VA Hosp 1980; **Fac Appt:** Prof Med, UCLA

Orwoll, Eric S MD [EDM] - **Spec Exp:** Osteoporosis; Osteoporosis in Men; **Hospital:** OR Hlth & Sci Univ; **Address:** Oregon Hlth & Sci Univ, Bone/Mineral Unit, 3181 SW Sam Jackson Park Rd, MC PPV05, Portland, OR 97239; **Phone:** 503-494-3273; **Board Cert:** Internal Medicine 1977; Endocrinology, Diabetes & Metabolism 1979; **Med School:** Univ MD Sch Med 1974; **Resid:** Internal Medicine, Providence Med Ctr 1977; **Fellow:** Endocrinology, Diabetes & Metabolism, Univ Oregon Hlth Sci Ctr 1979; **Fac Appt:** Prof Med, Oregon Hlth Sci Univ

Riddle, Matthew C MD [EDM] - **Spec Exp:** Diabetes; Clinical Trials; **Hospital:** OR Hlth & Sci Univ; **Address:** Oregon Hlth & Sci Univ, Div Endo, 3181 SW Sam Jackson Park Rd, MC L-345, Portland, OR 97239-3011; **Phone:** 503-494-3273; **Board Cert:** Internal Medicine 1972; Endocrinology, Diabetes & Metabolism 1972; **Med School:** Harvard Med Sch 1964; **Resid:** Internal Medicine, Rush-Presby-St Lukes Hosp 1969; **Fellow:** Endocrinology, Diabetes & Metabolism, Rush Presby-St Lukes Hosp 1971; Endocrinology, Diabetes & Metabolism, Univ Washington 1973; **Fac Appt:** Prof Med, Oregon Hlth Sci Univ

Singer, Peter A MD [EDM] - **Spec Exp:** Thyroid Disorders; **Hospital:** USC Univ Hosp - R K Eamer Med Plz; **Address:** 1520 San Pablo St Fl 1 - Ste 1000, Los Angeles, CA 90033; **Phone:** 323-442-5100; **Board Cert:** Internal Medicine 1972; Endocrinology, Diabetes & Metabolism 1973; **Med School:** UCSF 1965; **Resid:** Internal Medicine, LAC-USC Med Ctr 1971; **Fellow:** Endocrinology, Diabetes & Metabolism, LAC-USC Med Ctr 1973; **Fac Appt:** Clin Prof Med, USC Sch Med

Swerdloff, Ronald S MD [EDM] - **Spec Exp:** Reproductive Endocrinology-Male; Pituitary Disorders; **Hospital:** LAC - Harbor - UCLA Med Ctr; **Address:** 1000 W Carson St, Box 446, Torrance, CA 90509-2910; **Phone:** 310-222-1867; **Board Cert:** Internal Medicine 1968; Endocrinology 1972; **Med School:** UCSF 1962; **Resid:** Internal Medicine, Univ Washington Hosp 1964; Endocrinology, Diabetes & Metabolism, NIH Gerontology Branch 1966; **Fellow:** Endocrinology, Diabetes & Metabolism, Harbor-UCLA Med Ctr 1969; **Fac Appt:** Prof Med, UCLA

Woeber, Kenneth A MD [EDM] - **Spec Exp:** Thyroid Disorders; **Hospital:** UCSF Med Ctr; **Address:** 2200 Post St, rm C-432, Box 1640, San Francisco, CA 94143; **Phone:** 415-885-7574; **Board Cert:** Internal Medicine 1980; Endocrinology, Diabetes & Metabolism 1973; **Med School:** South Africa 1957; **Resid:** Internal Medicine, Jackson Meml Hosp 1962; **Fellow:** Endocrinology, Diabetes & Metabolism, Harvard/Boston City Hosp 1964; **Fac Appt:** Prof Med, UCSF

Cleveland Clinic

Endocrinology, Diabetes and Metabolism

Cleveland Clinic Department of Endocrinology treats patients in all the major disease categories such as diabetes, thyroid disorders, sexual hormone disorders, metabolism, pituitary disorders and more. In addition, the department has several specialty clinics dedicated to:

- Cardiovascular risk reduction
- Type 1 Diabetes
- Pituitary
- Thyroid
- Transition Clinic (Pediatrics to Adult)
- Intensive Diabetic Care- DM2 Clinic

Patients with difficult-to-control diabetes or high risk patients with diabetes (i.e. diabetics who recently experienced a heart attack or underwent bypass surgery) can be treated at the Diabetes Mellitus Disease Management (DM2) Clinic for seamless, intensive management of their disease. The goal is to stabilize patients within six months, and return them back to their primary care providers within twelve months.

Thyroid Biopsy

The department has been a leader in incorporating fine needle aspirations and ultrasounds into the realm of endocrinology. Our fellowship program was one of the first in the nation to train fellows in ultrasound-guided biopsy techniques of the thyroid.

Pituitary Clinic

Pituitary care at Cleveland Clinic is a collaborative approach between endocrinologists, neurosurgeons and radiation oncologists, resulting in national recognition. Cleveland Clinic is one of the top centers in the U.S. for volume of pituitary surgeries at an institution.

Center for Osteoporosis and Metabolic Bone Disease

A joint effort between the Departments of Endocrinology and Rheumatology, and the Center for Osteoporosis and Metabolic Bone Disease is devoted to the evaluation and treatment of patients with osteoporosis and other forms of diseases that affect bones. The Center's goal is to evaluate patients at an early stage to prevent complications and treat patients at the earliest possible stage to prevent additional disease manifestations.

For more information about the Cleveland Clinic Department of Endocrinology, Diabetes and Metabolism, to schedule a second opinion or to learn about assistance for out-of-town patients, call call 800.890.2467 or visit www.clevelandclinic.org/endotopdocs.

Department of Endocrinology, Diabetes and Metabolism
9500 Euclid Avenue / AC311 | Cleveland OH 44195

Gastroenterology

a subspecialty of Internal Medicine

An internist who specializes in diagnosis and treatment of diseases of the digestive organs including the stomach, bowels, liver and gallbladder. This specialist treats conditions such as abdominal pain, ulcers, diarrhea, cancer and jaundice and performs complex diagnostic and therapeutic procedures using endoscopes to see internal organs.

Training Required: Three years in internal medicine *plus* additional training and examination for certification in gastroenterology.

GASTROENTEROLOGY

New England

Carr-Locke, David L MD [Ge] - **Spec Exp:** Pancreatic/Biliary Endoscopy (ERCP); Pancreatic & Biliary Disease; Endoscopy; **Hospital:** Brigham & Women's Hosp; **Address:** 620 Tremont Ave, Boston, MA 02120; **Phone:** 617-732-7414; **Board Cert:** Internal Medicine 1974; **Med School:** England, UK 1972; **Resid:** Obstetrics & Gynecology, Orsett Hosp 1974; Internal Medicine, Leicester Hosp 1976; **Fellow:** Gastroenterology, Leicester Hosp 1978; Research, New Eng Baptist Hosp 1979; **Fac Appt:** Assoc Prof Med, Harvard Med Sch

Dienstag, Jules L MD [Ge] - **Spec Exp:** Liver Disease; Hepatitis; Transplant Medicine-Liver; **Hospital:** Mass Genl Hosp; **Address:** Mass Genl Hosp, GI Unit, 55 Fruit St Warren Bldg Fl 10, Boston, MA 02114-2622; **Phone:** 617-724-7562; **Board Cert:** Internal Medicine 1975; **Med School:** Columbia P&S 1972; **Resid:** Internal Medicine, Univ Chicago-Billings Hosp 1974; **Fellow:** Infectious Disease, Natl Inst Hlth 1976; Gastroenterology, Mass Genl Hosp 1978; **Fac Appt:** Prof Med, Harvard Med Sch

Friedman, Lawrence S MD [Ge] - **Spec Exp:** Liver Disease; **Hospital:** Newton - Wellesley Hosp, Mass Genl Hosp; **Address:** Newton-Wellesley Hospital, Dept Medicine, 2014 Washington St, Newton, MA 02462; **Phone:** 617-243-5480; **Board Cert:** Internal Medicine 1981; Gastroenterology 2005; **Med School:** Johns Hopkins Univ 1978; **Resid:** Internal Medicine, Johns Hopkins Hosp 1981; **Fellow:** Gastroenterology, Mass Genl Hosp 1984; **Fac Appt:** Prof Med, Harvard Med Sch

Levine, Joel B MD [Ge] - **Spec Exp:** Colon & Rectal Cancer Detection; Colonoscopy; Gastroesophageal Reflux Disease (GERD); **Hospital:** Univ of Conn Hlth Ctr, John Dempsey Hosp; **Address:** Univ Connecticut Health Center, Colon Cancer Prevention Program, 263 Farmington Ave, Farmington, CT 06030-2813; **Phone:** 860-679-4567; **Board Cert:** Internal Medicine 1973; Gastroenterology 1977; **Med School:** SUNY Downstate 1969; **Resid:** Internal Medicine, Univ Chicago Hosps 1971; Internal Medicine, Mass Genl Hosp 1974; **Fellow:** Gastroenterology, Mass Genl Hosp 1977; **Fac Appt:** Prof Med, Univ Conn

Mason, Joel B MD [Ge] - **Spec Exp:** Nutrition in Acute Illness; Nutrition in Bowel Disorders; Nutrition & Cancer Prevention; Inflammatory Bowel Disease; **Hospital:** Tufts Med Ctr; **Address:** Tufts Med Ctr #239, 800 Washington St, Boston, MA 02111-1513; **Phone:** 617-636-5623; **Board Cert:** Internal Medicine 1984; Gastroenterology 1987; **Med School:** Univ Chicago-Pritzker Sch Med 1981; **Resid:** Internal Medicine, Univ Iowa Hosps 1984; **Fellow:** Gastroenterology, Univ Chicago Hosps 1986; Nutrition, Univ Chicago Hosps 1986; **Fac Appt:** Assoc Prof Med, Tufts Univ

Rothstein, Richard I MD [Ge] - **Spec Exp:** Gastroesophageal Reflux Disease (GERD); Swallowing Disorders; Barrett's Esophagus; Endoscopy; **Hospital:** Dartmouth - Hitchcock Med Ctr; **Address:** Dartmouth-Hitchcock Medical Center, Div Gastroenterology, 1 Medical Center Drive, Lebanon, NH 03756; **Phone:** 603-650-8343; **Board Cert:** Internal Medicine 1983; Gastroenterology 1987; **Med School:** Boston Univ 1980; **Resid:** Internal Medicine, Univ Mass Med Ctr 1983; **Fellow:** Gastroenterology, Dartmouth-Hitchcock Med Ctr 1985; **Fac Appt:** Prof Med, Dartmouth Med Sch

Siegel, Corey A MD [Ge] - **Spec Exp:** Inflammatory Bowel Disease; Crohn's Disease; Colonoscopy; Ulcerative Colitis; **Hospital:** Dartmouth - Hitchcock Med Ctr; **Address:** Dartmouth-Hitchcock Med Ctr, Gastroenterology & Hepatology Div, 1 Medical Ctr Drive, Lebanon, NH 03756; **Phone:** 603-650-8101; **Board Cert:** Internal Medicine 2001; Gastroenterology 2005; **Med School:** Tufts Univ 1998; **Resid:** Internal Medicine, Dartmouth-Hitchcock Med Ctr 2002; **Fellow:** Gastroenterology, Dartmouth-Hitchcock Med Ctr 2004; Inflammatory Bowel Disease, Mass Genl Hosp 2005

Wolfe, M Michael MD [Ge] - **Hospital:** Boston Med Ctr; **Address:** 650 Albany St, Ste 504, Boston, MA 02118; **Phone:** 617-638-8330; **Board Cert:** Internal Medicine 1979; Gastroenterology 1981; **Med School:** Ohio State Univ 1976; **Resid:** Internal Medicine, Med Coll Penn Hosp 1979; **Fellow:** Gastroenterology, Univ Florida Hosps 1982; **Fac Appt:** Prof Med, Boston Univ

Mid Atlantic

Albert, Michael B MD [Ge] - **Spec Exp:** Inflammatory Bowel Disease; Ulcerative Colitis; **Hospital:** G Washington Univ Hosp; **Address:** 2141 K St NW, Ste 208, Washington, DC 20037; **Phone:** 202-223-5544; **Board Cert:** Internal Medicine 1985; Gastroenterology 1987; **Med School:** Johns Hopkins Univ 1982; **Resid:** Internal Medicine, Mayo Clinic 1984; Internal Medicine, Duke Univ Med Ctr 1985; **Fellow:** Gastroenterology, G Washington Univ Med Ctr 1987; **Fac Appt:** Prof Med, Geo Wash Univ

Aronchick, Craig A MD [Ge] - **Spec Exp:** Colonoscopy; Colon Cancer Screening; **Hospital:** Pennsylvania Hosp (page 60); **Address:** 230 W Washington Square, Farm Journal Bldg, Fl 4, Philadelphia, PA 19106; **Phone:** 215-829-3561; **Board Cert:** Internal Medicine 1981; Gastroenterology 1983; **Med School:** Temple Univ 1978; **Resid:** Internal Medicine, Temple Univ Hosp 1981; **Fellow:** Gastroenterology, Hosp Univ Penn 1983; **Fac Appt:** Assoc Clin Prof Med, Univ Pennsylvania

Bayless, Theodore MD [Ge] - **Spec Exp:** Inflammatory Bowel Disease/Crohn's; Ulcerative Colitis; Malabsorption Syndrome; **Hospital:** Johns Hopkins Hosp (page 61); **Address:** 600 N Wolfe St, Blalock Bldg - Ste 461, C/O Johns Hopkins Hosp, Baltimore, MD 21287-0005; **Phone:** 410-955-4166; **Board Cert:** Internal Medicine 1966; **Med School:** Ros Franklin Univ/Chicago Med Sch 1957; **Resid:** Internal Medicine, Cornell-Bellevue Hosp 1958; Internal Medicine, Meml Sloan Kettering Hosp 1960; **Fellow:** Gastroenterology, Johns Hopkins Hosp 1962; **Fac Appt:** Prof Med, Johns Hopkins Univ

Bodenheimer Jr, Henry C MD [Ge] - **Spec Exp:** Hepatitis; Liver & Biliary Disease; Transplant Medicine-Liver; Toxicology; **Hospital:** Beth Israel Med Ctr - Petrie Division (page 57); **Address:** Beth Israel Med Ctr Dept of Med, 1st Ave @ 16th St, New York, NY 10003; **Phone:** 212-420-4077; **Board Cert:** Internal Medicine 1978; Gastroenterology 1981; Transplant Hepatology 2006; **Med School:** Tufts Univ 1975; **Resid:** Internal Medicine, Mount Sinai Hosp 1978; **Fellow:** Gastroenterology, Mount Sinai Hosp 1979; Gastroenterology, Rhode Island Hosp 1981; **Fac Appt:** Prof Med, Albert Einstein Coll Med

Borum, Marie L MD [Ge] - **Spec Exp:** Colon Cancer Screening; AIDS/HIV-Gastrointestinal Complications; Women's Health; Liver Disease; **Hospital:** G Washington Univ Hosp; **Address:** MFA Dept Medicine, 2150 Pennsylvania Ave NW, Ste 3-405, Washington, DC 20037; **Phone:** 202-741-3333; **Board Cert:** Internal Medicine 1988; Gastroenterology 2001; **Med School:** UMDNJ-Rutgers Med Sch 1985; **Resid:** Internal Medicine, G Washington Univ Med Ctr 1988; **Fellow:** Gastroenterology, G Washington Univ Med Ctr 1991; **Fac Appt:** Prof Med, Geo Wash Univ

Brandt, Lawrence MD [Ge] - **Spec Exp:** Geriatric Gastroenterology; Inflammatory Bowel Disease; **Hospital:** Montefiore Med Ctr - Div. Moses, Montefiore Med Ctr - Div. Weiler; **Address:** 3400 Bainbridge Ave Fl 2, Bronx, NY 10467-2401; **Phone:** 866-633-8255; **Board Cert:** Internal Medicine 1972; Gastroenterology 2006; **Med School:** SUNY Downstate 1968; **Resid:** Internal Medicine, Mt Sinai Hosp 1972; **Fellow:** Gastroenterology, Mt Sinai Hosp 1972; **Fac Appt:** Prof Med, Albert Einstein Coll Med

Gastroenterology

Brown Jr, Robert S MD [Ge] - **Spec Exp:** Hepatitis; Liver Disease; Transplant Medicine-Liver; Transplant Medicine-Kidney; **Hospital:** NY-Presby Hosp/Columbia (page 66); **Address:** Ctr for Liver Disease & Transplantation, 622 W 168th St Fl 14 - rm 105, New York, NY 10032; **Phone:** 212-305-0914; **Board Cert:** Internal Medicine 2002; Gastroenterology 2005; **Med School:** NYU Sch Med 1989; **Resid:** Internal Medicine, Beth Israel Deaconess Med Ctr 1992; **Fellow:** Gastroenterology, UCSF Med Ctr 1994; Hepatology, UCSF Med Ctr 1995; **Fac Appt:** Prof Med, Columbia P&S

Canto, Marcia MD [Ge] - **Spec Exp:** Endoscopy; Endoscopic Ultrasound; Pancreatic Cancer-Early Detection; **Hospital:** Johns Hopkins Hosp (page 61); **Address:** Dept of Med, Gastroenterology, 1830 E Monument St, rm 426, Baltimore, MD 21205; **Phone:** 410-614-5388; **Board Cert:** Internal Medicine 1989; **Med School:** Philippines 1985; **Resid:** Internal Medicine, SUNY Hlth Sci Ctr 1991; **Fellow:** Gastroenterology, SUNY Hlth Sci Ctr 1993; **Fac Appt:** Assoc Prof Med, Johns Hopkins Univ

Cohen, Jonathan MD [Ge] - **Spec Exp:** Pancreatic/Biliary Endoscopy (ERCP); Pancreatic Disease; Liver Disease; Colonoscopy; **Hospital:** NYU Langone Med Ctr (page 67); **Address:** 232 E 30th St, New York, NY 10016-8202; **Phone:** 212-889-5544; **Board Cert:** Gastroenterology 2005; **Med School:** Harvard Med Sch 1990; **Resid:** Internal Medicine, Beth Israel Hosp 1993; **Fellow:** Gastroenterology, UCLA Med Ctr 1995; Endoscopy, Wellesley Hosp 1995; **Fac Appt:** Clin Prof Med, NYU Sch Med

Cohen, Lawrence B MD [Ge] - **Spec Exp:** Gastroesophageal Reflux Disease (GERD); Esophageal Disorders; Colon & Rectal Cancer; Endoscopy; **Hospital:** Mount Sinai Med Ctr (page 64); **Address:** 311 E 79th St, Ste 2A, New York, NY 10021-0903; **Phone:** 212-996-6633; **Board Cert:** Internal Medicine 1981; Gastroenterology 1983; **Med School:** Hahnemann Univ 1978; **Resid:** Internal Medicine, Mt Sinai Hosp 1981; **Fellow:** Gastroenterology, Mt Sinai Hosp 1983; **Fac Appt:** Assoc Clin Prof Med, Mount Sinai Sch Med

Di Marino Jr, Anthony J MD [Ge] - **Spec Exp:** Celiac Disease; Gastroesophageal Reflux Disease (GERD); Ulcerative Colitis; Irritable Bowel Syndrome; **Hospital:** Thomas Jefferson Univ Hosp; **Address:** Thomas Jefferson Univ, Div Gastroenterology, 132 S 10th St, Ste 480, Philadelphia, PA 19107; **Phone:** 215-955-2728; **Board Cert:** Internal Medicine 1977; Gastroenterology 1972; **Med School:** Hahnemann Univ 1968; **Resid:** Internal Medicine, Hahnemann Univ Hosp 1970; Internal Medicine, Hosp Univ Penn 1971; **Fellow:** Gastroenterology, Hosp Univ Penn 1973; **Fac Appt:** Prof Med, Thomas Jefferson Univ

Dieterich, Douglas T MD [Ge] - **Spec Exp:** Hepatitis; AIDS/HIV-Gastrointestinal Complications; Liver Disease; Endoscopy; **Hospital:** Mount Sinai Med Ctr (page 64), NYU Langone Med Ctr (page 67); **Address:** 5 E 98th St Fl 8, New York, NY 10029; **Phone:** 212-241-7270; **Board Cert:** Internal Medicine 1981; Gastroenterology 1987; **Med School:** NYU Sch Med 1978; **Resid:** Internal Medicine, Bellevue Hosp Ctr-NYU 1981; **Fellow:** Gastroenterology, Bellevue Hosp Ctr-NYU 1983; **Fac Appt:** Prof Med, Mount Sinai Sch Med

Farmer, Richard G MD [Ge] - **Spec Exp:** Inflammatory Bowel Disease/Crohn's; **Hospital:** Univ of Rochester Strong Meml Hosp; **Address:** Univ Rochester Med Ctr, 601 Elmwood Ave, Box 646, Rochester, NY 14642; **Phone:** 585-275-7432; **Board Cert:** Internal Medicine 1963; Gastroenterology 1968; **Med School:** Univ MD Sch Med 1956; **Resid:** Internal Medicine, Mayo Clinic 1960; **Fellow:** Gastroenterology, Mayo Clinic 1960; **Fac Appt:** Prof Med, Univ Rochester

Fisher, Robert S MD [Ge] - **Spec Exp:** Gastrointestinal Motility Disorders; Peptic Acid Disorders; Gastrointestinal Functionional Disorders; **Hospital:** Temple Univ Hosp; **Address:** 3401 N Broad St, Philadelphia, PA 19140; **Phone:** 215-707-9922; **Board Cert:** Internal Medicine 1971; Gastroenterology 1973; **Med School:** Univ Pennsylvania 1964; **Resid:** Internal Medicine, Temple Univ Med Ctr 1970; **Fellow:** Gastroenterology, Hosp Univ Penn 1972; **Fac Appt:** Prof Med, Temple Univ

Freiman, Hal MD [Ge] - **Spec Exp:** Gastroesophageal Reflux Disease (GERD); Biliary Disease; Pancreatic/Biliary Endoscopy (ERCP); Hepatitis; **Hospital:** St Vincent Cath Med Ctrs - Manhattan; **Address:** 59 W 12th St, Ste 1D, New York, NY 10011-8520; **Phone:** 212-206-0074; **Board Cert:** Internal Medicine 1981; Gastroenterology 1983; **Med School:** Albany Med Coll 1978; **Resid:** Internal Medicine, St Vincent's Hosp 1981; **Fellow:** Gastroenterology, Westchester Co Med Ctr 1983; **Fac Appt:** Asst Clin Prof Med, NY Med Coll

Gerdes, Hans MD [Ge] - **Spec Exp:** Endoscopy; Endoscopic Ultrasound; Barrett's Esophagus; Gastrointestinal Cancer; **Hospital:** Meml Sloan-Kettering Cancer Ctr; **Address:** 1275 York Avenue, New York, NY 10065; **Phone:** 800-525-2225; **Board Cert:** Internal Medicine 1987; Gastroenterology 1989; **Med School:** Cornell Univ-Weill Med Coll 1983; **Resid:** Internal Medicine, New York Hosp 1986; **Fellow:** Gastroenterology, Meml Sloan Kettering Cancer Ctr 1989

Giardiello, Francis MD [Ge] - **Spec Exp:** Colon Cancer; Colon & Rectal Cancer-Familial Polyposis; Cancer Risk Assessment; **Hospital:** Johns Hopkins Hosp (page 61); **Address:** 1830 E Mounument St, rm 431, Baltimore, MD 21205; **Phone:** 410-955-2635; **Board Cert:** Internal Medicine 1983; Gastroenterology 1985; **Med School:** Tufts Univ 1980; **Resid:** Internal Medicine, Univ Michigan 1983; **Fellow:** Gastroenterology, Johns Hopkins 1985; **Fac Appt:** Prof Med, Johns Hopkins Univ

Ginsberg, Gregory G MD [Ge] - **Spec Exp:** Pancreatic/Biliary Endoscopy (ERCP); Endoscopy; Endoscopic Ultrasound; Barrett's Esophagus; **Hospital:** Hosp Univ Penn - UPHS (page 60); **Address:** Univ Pennsylvania, Gastroenterology Div, 3400 Spruce St 3 Ravdin Bldg, Philadelphia, PA 19104; **Phone:** 215-349-8222; **Board Cert:** Internal Medicine 2000; Gastroenterology 2000; **Med School:** Jefferson Med Coll 1987; **Resid:** Internal Medicine, Georgetown Univ Med Ctr 1990; **Fellow:** Gastroenterology, Georgetown Univ Med Ctr 1992; **Fac Appt:** Prof Med, Univ Pennsylvania

Goggins, Michael MD [Ge] - **Spec Exp:** Pancreatic Cancer-Early Detection; **Hospital:** Johns Hopkins Hosp (page 61); **Address:** Johns Hopkins Univ Sch Med, 1550 Orleans St, CRB-2 St, rm 342, Baltimore, MD 21231; **Phone:** 410-955-3511; **Med School:** Ireland 1988; **Resid:** Internal Medicine, St Jame's Hosp 1990; **Fellow:** Gastroenterology, St Jame's Hosp 1992; **Fac Appt:** Assoc Prof Med, Johns Hopkins Univ

Green, Peter MD [Ge] - **Spec Exp:** Celiac Disease; Endoscopy; Colonoscopy; Malabsorption Syndrome; **Hospital:** NY-Presby Hosp/Columbia (page 66); **Address:** Celiac Disease Ctr, Harkness Bldg, 180 Fort Washington Ave, rm 956, New York, NY 10032-3713; **Phone:** 212-305-5590; **Med School:** Australia 1970; **Resid:** Internal Medicine, North Shore Med Ctr 1974; **Fellow:** Gastroenterology, North Shore Med Ctr 1976; Gastroenterology, Beth Israel Hosp 1977; **Fac Appt:** Clin Prof Med, Columbia P&S

Greenwald, Bruce D MD [Ge] - **Spec Exp:** Endoscopic Ultrasound; Barrett's Esophagus; Esophageal Cancer; Clinical Trials; **Hospital:** Univ of MD Med Ctr; **Address:** Univ of Maryland Hosp, Gastroenterology, 22 S Greene St Fl 3 - rm N3W62, Baltimore, MD 21201-1544; **Phone:** 410-328-8731; **Board Cert:** Internal Medicine 2000; Gastroenterology 2000; **Med School:** Univ MD Sch Med 1987; **Resid:** Internal Medicine, Univ of Virginia Hosp 1990; **Fellow:** Gastroenterology, Univ of Maryland Hosp 1992; **Fac Appt:** Assoc Prof Med, Univ MD Sch Med

Haber, Gregory B MD [Ge] - **Spec Exp:** Endoscopy; Pancreatic/Biliary Endoscopy (ERCP); Endoscopic Ultrasound; Barrett's Esophagus; **Hospital:** Lenox Hill Hosp (page 62); **Address:** 100 E 77th St, New York, NY 10075; **Phone:** 212-434-6279; **Med School:** Univ Toronto 1970; **Resid:** Internal Medicine, Univ Toronto Med Ctr 1975; **Fellow:** Gastroenterology, Univ Toronto Med Ctr 1978

Gastroenterology

Haluszka, Oleh MD [Ge] - **Spec Exp:** Pancreatic/Biliary Endoscopy (ERCP); Gastrointestinal Cancer; Endoscopic Ultrasound; Endoscopy; **Hospital:** Fox Chase Cancer Ctr (page 58); **Address:** Fox Chase Cancer Ctr, 333 Cottman Ave, Ste C307, Philadelphia, PA 19111; **Phone:** 215-214-1424; **Board Cert:** Internal Medicine 1987; Gastroenterology 2001; **Med School:** Uniformed Srvs Univ, Bethesda 1982; **Resid:** Internal Medicine, US Naval Hosp 1987; **Fellow:** Gastroenterology, US Naval Hosp 1990; Endoscopy, Med Coll Wisconsin 1993; **Fac Appt:** Assoc Clin Prof Med, Temple Univ

Hoops, Timothy C MD [Ge] - **Spec Exp:** Esophageal Disorders; Endoscopy; Colonoscopy; **Hospital:** Penn Presby Med Ctr - UPHS (page 60); **Address:** Penn Presbyterian Medical Ctr, 51 N 39th St, Ste 218, Philadelphia, PA 19104; **Phone:** 215-662-8900; **Board Cert:** Internal Medicine 1984; Gastroenterology 1987; **Med School:** Univ IL Coll Med 1981; **Resid:** Internal Medicine, Univ Colorado Hlth Sci Ctr 1984; **Fellow:** Gastroenterology, Univ Colorado Hlth Sci Ctr 1986; **Fac Appt:** Assoc Clin Prof Med, Univ Pennsylvania

Itzkowitz, Steven H MD [Ge] - **Spec Exp:** Colon & Rectal Cancer; Colon & Rectal Cancer Detection; Inflammatory Bowel Disease; **Hospital:** Mount Sinai Med Ctr (page 64); **Address:** 5 E 98th St, Box 1625, New York, NY 10029-6501; **Phone:** 212-241-4299; **Board Cert:** Internal Medicine 1982; Gastroenterology 1985; **Med School:** Mount Sinai Sch Med 1979; **Resid:** Internal Medicine, Bellevue Hosp/NYU Med Ctr 1982; **Fellow:** Gastroenterology, UCSF Med Ctr 1984; **Fac Appt:** Prof Med, Mount Sinai Sch Med

Jacobson, Ira MD [Ge] - **Spec Exp:** Liver & Biliary Disease; Pancreatic Disease; Colonoscopy; Hepatitis; **Hospital:** NY-Presby Hosp/Weill Cornell (page 66); **Address:** 1305 York Ave Fl 4, New York, NY 10021-5016; **Phone:** 646-962-4040; **Board Cert:** Internal Medicine 1982; Gastroenterology 1985; Transplant Hepatology 2006; **Med School:** Columbia P&S 1979; **Resid:** Internal Medicine, UCSF Med Ctr 1982; **Fellow:** Gastroenterology, Mass Genl Hosp 1984; **Fac Appt:** Prof Med, Cornell Univ-Weill Med Coll

Kalloo, Anthony N MD [Ge] - **Spec Exp:** Endoscopy; Pancreatic Disease; **Hospital:** Johns Hopkins Hosp (page 61); **Address:** Cancer Research Bldg II, 1550 Orleans St, 1-M12, Baltimore, MD 21231; **Phone:** 410-955-9697; **Board Cert:** Internal Medicine 1985; Gastroenterology 1987; **Med School:** Jamaica 1979; **Resid:** Internal Medicine, Howard Univ Hosp 1985; **Fellow:** Gastroenterology, VA Med Ctr/Georgetown Univ Hosp 1987; **Fac Appt:** Assoc Prof Med, Johns Hopkins Univ

Kantsevoy, Sergey V MD/PhD [Ge] - **Spec Exp:** Pancreatic Disease; Endoscopic Ultrasound; Pancreatic/Biliary Endoscopy (ERCP); **Hospital:** Mercy Med Ctr; **Address:** 301 St Paul Pl, Baltimore, MD 21202; **Phone:** 410-332-9356; **Board Cert:** Gastroenterology 2000; **Med School:** Russia 1983; **Resid:** Internal Medicine, Bronx-Lebanon Hosp Ctr 1995; Internal Medicine, Washington Hosp Ctr 1997; **Fellow:** Gastroenterology, Johns Hopkins Hosp 2000; **Fac Appt:** Asst Prof Med, Johns Hopkins Univ

Kastenberg, David M MD [Ge] - **Spec Exp:** Gastrointestinal Cancer; Colon & Rectal Cancer Detection; Nutrition & Cancer Prevention; **Hospital:** Thomas Jefferson Univ Hosp; **Address:** Jefferson Univ Hosps, 132 S 10th St Main Bldg - Ste 480, Dept Gastroenterology, Phildelphia, PA 19107; **Phone:** 215-955-8900; **Board Cert:** Internal Medicine 2000; Gastroenterology 2000; **Med School:** NYU Sch Med 1987; **Resid:** Internal Medicine, Temple Univ Hosp 1990; **Fellow:** Gastroenterology, Thomas Jefferson Univ Hosp 1992; **Fac Appt:** Asst Clin Prof Med, Jefferson Med Coll

Katz, Philip O MD [Ge] - **Spec Exp:** Gastroesophageal Reflux Disease (GERD); Swallowing Disorders; Barrett's Esophagus; Esophageal Disorders; **Hospital:** Albert Einstein Med Ctr; **Address:** 5501 Old York Rd, Klein Bldg - Ste 363, Philadelphia, PA 19141; **Phone:** 215-456-8210; **Board Cert:** Internal Medicine 1981; Gastroenterology 1987; **Med School:** Bowman Gray 1978; **Resid:** Internal Medicine, NC Baptist Hosp 1981; **Fellow:** Gastroenterology, NC Baptist Hosp 1986; **Fac Appt:** Clin Prof Med, Thomas Jefferson Univ

Kochman, Michael L MD [Ge] - **Spec Exp:** Endoscopy; Pancreatic/Biliary Endoscopy (ERCP); Gastrointestinal Cancer; **Hospital:** Hosp Univ Penn - UPHS (page 60); **Address:** Hosp Univ Penn, Div Gastroenterology, 3400 Spruce St, 3 Dulles, Philadelphia, PA 19104-4206; **Phone:** 215-349-8222; **Board Cert:** Internal Medicine 1989; Gastroenterology 2003; **Med School:** Univ IL Coll Med 1986; **Resid:** Internal Medicine, Univ Illinois Med Ctr 1990; **Fellow:** Gastroenterology, Univ Michigan Med Ctr 1993; **Fac Appt:** Prof Med, Univ Pennsylvania

Korsten, Mark A MD [Ge] - **Spec Exp:** Constipation; Gastrointestinal Motility Disorders; Spinal Cord Injury & Colonic Motility; Liver Disease; **Hospital:** Mount Sinai Med Ctr (page 64), VA Med Ctr - Bronx; **Address:** 130 W Kingsbridge Rd, Bronx, NY 10468-3904; **Phone:** 718-584-9000 x6753; **Board Cert:** Internal Medicine 1973; Gastroenterology 1975; **Med School:** Yale Univ 1970; **Resid:** Internal Medicine, Mt Sinai Hosp 1973; **Fellow:** Gastroenterology, Mt Sinai Hosp 1975; **Fac Appt:** Prof Med, Mount Sinai Sch Med

Kotler, Donald P MD [Ge] - **Spec Exp:** Esophageal Disorders; Nutrition & AIDS; **Hospital:** St Luke's - Roosevelt Hosp Ctr - St Luke's Hosp (page 57); **Address:** 1111 Amsterdam Ave, SR 12, New York, NY 10025; **Phone:** 212-523-3670; **Board Cert:** Internal Medicine 1976; Gastroenterology 1979; **Med School:** Albert Einstein Coll Med 1973; **Resid:** Internal Medicine, Jacobi Med Ctr 1976; **Fellow:** Gastroenterology, Hosp Univ Penn 1978; **Fac Appt:** Assoc Prof Med, Columbia P&S

Kowalski, Thomas E MD [Ge] - **Spec Exp:** Pancreatic Disease; Biliary Disease; Pancreatic/Biliary Endoscopy (ERCP); Endoscopic Ultrasound; **Hospital:** Thomas Jefferson Univ Hosp; **Address:** 132 S 10th St Main Bldg - Ste 480, Philadelphia, PA 19107; **Phone:** 215-955-9936; **Board Cert:** Internal Medicine 2003; Gastroenterology 2003; **Med School:** SUNY Buffalo 1988; **Resid:** Internal Medicine, Johns Hopkins Hosp 1991; **Fellow:** Gastroenterology, Hosp Univ Penn 1993; Advanced Endoscopy, Hosp Univ Penn 1994; **Fac Appt:** Assoc Prof Med, Thomas Jefferson Univ

Kurtz, Robert C MD [Ge] - **Spec Exp:** Pancreatic Cancer(Familial); Gastrointestinal Cancer; Endoscopy; Nutrition & Cancer Prevention/Control; **Hospital:** Meml Sloan-Kettering Cancer Ctr; **Address:** 1275 York Avenue, New York, NY 10065; **Phone:** 800-525-2225; **Board Cert:** Internal Medicine 1971; Gastroenterology 1977; **Med School:** Jefferson Med Coll 1968; **Resid:** Internal Medicine, NY Hosp/Meml Sloan Kettering Cancer Ctr 1971; **Fellow:** Gastroenterology, Meml Sloan Kettering Cancer Ctr 1973; **Fac Appt:** Prof Med, Cornell Univ-Weill Med Coll

Lebwohl, Oscar MD [Ge] - **Spec Exp:** Endoscopy; Inflammatory Bowel Disease/Crohn's; Ulcerative Colitis; Gastrointestinal Cancer; **Hospital:** NY-Presby Hosp/Columbia (page 66); **Address:** 161 Fort Washington Ave, rm 420, New York, NY 10032-3713; **Phone:** 212-305-5363; **Board Cert:** Internal Medicine 1975; Gastroenterology 1977; **Med School:** Harvard Med Sch 1972; **Resid:** Internal Medicine, Mt Sinai Med Ctr 1975; **Fellow:** Gastroenterology, Columbia-Presby Med Ctr 1976; Hepatology, Mt Sinai Med Ctr 1977; **Fac Appt:** Clin Prof Med, Columbia P&S

Lewis, Blair MD [Ge] - **Spec Exp:** Endoscopy; Capsule Endoscopy; **Hospital:** Mount Sinai Med Ctr (page 64); **Address:** 1067 5th Ave, New York, NY 10128-0101; **Phone:** 212-369-6600; **Board Cert:** Internal Medicine 1985; Gastroenterology 1987; **Med School:** Albert Einstein Coll Med 1982; **Resid:** Internal Medicine, Montefiore Med Ctr 1985; **Fellow:** Gastroenterology, Mt Sinai Med Ctr 1987; **Fac Appt:** Clin Prof Med, Mount Sinai Sch Med

Gastroenterology

Lichtenstein, Gary R MD [Ge] - **Spec Exp:** Inflammatory Bowel Disease; **Hospital:** Hosp Univ Penn - UPHS (page 60); **Address:** Div Gastroenterology, 3400 Civic Center Blvd, Pearl Center, 4 South Pavilion, Philadelphia, PA 19104-4283; **Phone:** 215-349-8222; **Board Cert:** Internal Medicine 1987; Gastroenterology 1989; **Med School:** Mount Sinai Sch Med 1984; **Resid:** Internal Medicine, Duke Univ Med Ctr 1987; **Fellow:** Gastroenterology, Hosp Univ Penn 1990; **Fac Appt:** Prof Med, Univ Pennsylvania

Lightdale, Charles J MD [Ge] - **Spec Exp:** Barrett's Esophagus; Gastrointestinal Cancer; Endoscopic Ultrasound; **Hospital:** NY-Presby Hosp/Columbia (page 66); **Address:** Columbia-Presby Med Ctr, Irving Pavilion, 161 Fort Washington Ave, rm 812, New York, NY 10032-3713; **Phone:** 212-305-3423; **Board Cert:** Internal Medicine 1972; Gastroenterology 1973; **Med School:** Columbia P&S 1966; **Resid:** Internal Medicine, Yale-New Haven Hosp 1968; Internal Medicine, NY Hosp-Cornell 1969; **Fellow:** Gastroenterology, NY Hosp-Cornell 1973; **Fac Appt:** Clin Prof Med, Columbia P&S

Lipshutz, William H MD [Ge] - **Spec Exp:** Inflammatory Bowel Disease/Crohn's; Colonoscopy; Esophageal Disorders; Gastroesophageal Reflux Disease (GERD); **Hospital:** Pennsylvania Hosp (page 60); **Address:** 230 W Washington Sq, Farm Journal Bldg Fl 4, Philadelphia, PA 19106; **Phone:** 215-829-3561; **Board Cert:** Internal Medicine 1972; Gastroenterology 1973; **Med School:** Univ Pennsylvania 1967; **Resid:** Internal Medicine, Pennsylvania Hosp 1972; **Fellow:** Gastroenterology, Hosp Univ Penn 1971; **Fac Appt:** Clin Prof Med, Univ Pennsylvania

Magun, Arthur M MD [Ge] - **Spec Exp:** Hepatitis; Ulcerative Colitis; Endoscopy; Inflammatory Bowel Disease/Crohn's; **Hospital:** NY-Presby Hosp/Columbia (page 66); **Address:** 161 Fort Washington Ave, rm 338, New York, NY 10032-3713; **Phone:** 212-305-5287; **Board Cert:** Internal Medicine 1980; Gastroenterology 1983; **Med School:** Mount Sinai Sch Med 1977; **Resid:** Internal Medicine, Columbia-Presby Med Ctr 1980; **Fellow:** Gastroenterology, Columbia-Presby Med Ctr 1983; **Fac Appt:** Clin Prof Med, Columbia P&S

Markowitz, David D MD [Ge] - **Spec Exp:** Gastroesophageal Reflux Disease (GERD); Esophageal Disorders; Endoscopy; **Hospital:** NY-Presby Hosp/Columbia (page 66); **Address:** 161 Ft Washington Ave, Ste 853, New York, NY 10032; **Phone:** 212-305-1024; **Board Cert:** Internal Medicine 1988; Gastroenterology 2001; **Med School:** Columbia P&S 1985; **Resid:** Internal Medicine, Columbia-Presby Hosp 1988; **Fellow:** Gastroenterology, Columbia-Presby Hosp 1991; **Fac Appt:** Assoc Prof Med, Columbia P&S

Mayer, Lloyd MD [Ge] - **Spec Exp:** Inflammatory Bowel Disease/Crohn's; Ulcerative Colitis; **Hospital:** Mount Sinai Med Ctr (page 64); **Address:** 1425 Madison Ave, rm 11-20, Box 1089, New York, NY 10029; **Phone:** 212-659-9266; **Board Cert:** Internal Medicine 1979; Gastroenterology 1981; **Med School:** Mount Sinai Sch Med 1976; **Resid:** Internal Medicine, Bellevue Hosp 1979; **Fellow:** Gastroenterology, Mt Sinai Hosp 1981; **Fac Appt:** Prof Med, Mount Sinai Sch Med

Metz, David C MD [Ge] - **Spec Exp:** Peptic Acid Disorders; Neuroendocrine Tumors; Gastroesophageal Reflux Disease (GERD); Gastrointestinal Motility Disorders; **Hospital:** Hosp Univ Penn - UPHS (page 60); **Address:** Hosp Univ Penn, Div Gastroenterology, 3400 Spruce St, 3 Ravdin, Philadelphia, PA 19104; **Phone:** 215-662-4279; **Board Cert:** Internal Medicine 1989; Gastroenterology 2001; **Med School:** South Africa 1982; **Resid:** Internal Medicine, Albert Einstein Med Ctr 1988; **Fellow:** Gastroenterology, Natl Inst Hlth 1991; **Fac Appt:** Prof Med, Univ Pennsylvania

Miskovitz, Paul MD [Ge] - **Spec Exp:** Endoscopy; Liver Disease; **Hospital:** NY-Presby Hosp/Weill Cornell (page 66); **Address:** 635 Madison Ave Fl 17, New York, NY 10022; **Phone:** 212-717-4966; **Board Cert:** Internal Medicine 1978; Gastroenterology 1981; **Med School:** Cornell Univ-Weill Med Coll 1975; **Resid:** Internal Medicine, NY Hosp 1978; **Fellow:** Gastroenterology, NY Hosp 1980; **Fac Appt:** Clin Prof Med, Cornell Univ-Weill Med Coll

Munoz, Santiago J MD [Ge] - **Spec Exp:** Liver Disease; Transplant Medicine-Liver; Hepatitis; **Hospital:** Temple Univ Hosp; **Address:** Temple University Hospital, Div Gasteoenterology & Transplantation, 3401 N Broad St, Philadelphia, PA 19150; **Phone:** 215-707-6732; **Board Cert:** Internal Medicine 1985; Gastroenterology 1989; **Med School:** Chile 1978; **Resid:** Internal Medicine, Jefferson Hosp 1985; **Fellow:** Pharmacology, Johns Hopkins Hosp 1983; Gastroenterology, Jefferson Hosp 1987; **Fac Appt:** Assoc Prof Med, Temple Univ

Okolo III, Patrick I MD [Ge] - **Spec Exp:** Liver Cancer; Pancreatic Cancer; Gastrointestinal Cancer; Clinical Trials; **Hospital:** Johns Hopkins Hosp (page 61); **Address:** 3001 S Hanover St, Ste Gruehn 300, Baltimore, MD 21225; **Phone:** 410-350-8209; **Board Cert:** Internal Medicine 2004; Gastroenterology 2008; **Med School:** Nigeria 1988; **Resid:** Internal Medicine, Indiana Univ Med Ctr 1994; **Fellow:** Gastroenterology, John Hopkins Hosp 1997; **Fac Appt:** Assoc Prof Med, Johns Hopkins Univ

Peikin, Steven MD [Ge] - **Spec Exp:** Endoscopy; **Hospital:** Cooper Univ Hosp; **Address:** 501 Fellowship Rd, Ste 101, Mt Laurel, NJ 08054; **Phone:** 856-642-2133; **Board Cert:** Internal Medicine 1977; Gastroenterology 1979; **Med School:** Jefferson Med Coll 1974; **Resid:** Internal Medicine, Moffit Hosps 1977; **Fellow:** Gastroenterology, Mass Genl Hosp 1980; **Fac Appt:** Prof Med, Robert W Johnson Med Sch

Pezzone, Michael A MD/PhD [Ge] - **Spec Exp:** Irritable Bowel Syndrome; Inflammatory Bowel Disease; Pain-Pelvic; **Hospital:** UPMC Presby, Pittsburgh, UPMC Shadyside; **Address:** UPMC Presbyterian Medical Ctr, Digestive Disorders Ctr, 200 Lothrop St, Pittsburgh, PA 15213; **Phone:** 412-647-8666; **Board Cert:** Internal Medicine 2007; Gastroenterology 2000; **Med School:** Univ Pittsburgh 1994; **Resid:** Internal Medicine, Univ Pittsburgh Med Ctr 1997; **Fellow:** Gastroenterology, Univ Pittsburgh Med Ctr 2000; **Fac Appt:** Assoc Prof Med, Univ Pittsburgh

Pochapin, Mark B MD [Ge] - **Spec Exp:** Pancreatic Cancer; Endoscopic Ultrasound; Colon & Rectal Cancer Detection; Diarrheal Diseases; **Hospital:** NY-Presby Hosp/Weill Cornell (page 66); **Address:** The Jay Monahan Ctr for GI Hlth, 1315 York Ave, New York, NY 10021; **Phone:** 212-746-4014; **Board Cert:** Gastroenterology 2004; **Med School:** Cornell Univ-Weill Med Coll 1988; **Resid:** Internal Medicine, NY Hosp-Cornell Med Ctr 1991; **Fellow:** Gastroenterology, Montefiore Med Ctr 1993; **Fac Appt:** Assoc Clin Prof Med, Cornell Univ-Weill Med Coll

Ravich, William J MD [Ge] - **Spec Exp:** Swallowing Disorders; Gastroesophageal Reflux Disease (GERD); Barrett's Esophagus; **Hospital:** Johns Hopkins Hosp (page 61), Greater Baltimore Med Ctr; **Address:** 10751 Falls Rd, Ste 401, Lutherville, MD 21093; **Phone:** 410-616-2840; **Board Cert:** Internal Medicine 1978; Gastroenterology 1981; **Med School:** Ros Franklin Univ/Chicago Med Sch 1975; **Resid:** Internal Medicine, Montefiore Hosp 1978; **Fellow:** Gastroenterology, Johns Hopkins Hosp 1981; **Fac Appt:** Assoc Prof Med, Johns Hopkins Univ

Reddy, K Rajender MD [Ge] - **Spec Exp:** Liver Disease; Hepatitis; Transplant Medicine-Liver; **Hospital:** Hosp Univ Penn - UPHS (page 60); **Address:** Div Gastroenterology, 3400 Civic Center Blvd, 4 South Pavilion, Philadelphia, PA 19104; **Phone:** 215-349-8222; **Board Cert:** Internal Medicine 1980; Gastroenterology 1983; Transplant Hepatology 2006; **Med School:** India 1972; **Resid:** Internal Medicine, NY Med Coll Hosps 1980; Gastroenterology, E Tenn State Univ 1982; **Fellow:** Hepatology, Univ Miami Hosps 1983; **Fac Appt:** Prof Med, Univ Pennsylvania

Reynolds, James C MD [Ge] - **Spec Exp:** Gastroesophageal Reflux Disease (GERD); Gastrointestinal Motility Disorders; Barrett's Esophagus; **Hospital:** Hahnemann Univ Hosp; **Address:** Drexel Gastroenterology Assocs, 219 N Broad St Fl 5, Philadelphia, PA 19107; **Phone:** 215-965-6000; **Board Cert:** Internal Medicine 1980; Gastroenterology 1985; **Med School:** Univ Fla Coll Med 1977; **Resid:** Internal Medicine, New York Hosp 1980; **Fellow:** Gastroenterology, Hosp U Penn 1983; **Fac Appt:** Prof Med, Drexel Univ Coll Med

Gastroenterology

Richter, Joel E MD [Ge] - **Spec Exp:** Gastroesophageal Reflux Disease (GERD); Esophageal Disorders; Barrett's Esophagus; Swallowing Disorders; **Hospital:** Temple Univ Hosp; **Address:** Temple Univ Hospital, Parkinson Pavilion, 3401 N Broad St, Fl 8 - Ste 801, Philadelphia, PA 19140; **Phone:** 215-707-5069; **Board Cert:** Internal Medicine 1978; Gastroenterology 1981; **Med School:** Univ Tex SW, Dallas 1975; **Resid:** Internal Medicine, Natl Naval Med Ctr 1978; **Fellow:** Gastroenterology, Natl Naval Med Ctr 1980; **Fac Appt:** Prof Med, Temple Univ

Schiano, Thomas D MD [Ge] - **Spec Exp:** Liver Disease; Transplant Medicine-Liver; Liver Failure; Transplant Medicine-Bowel; **Hospital:** Mount Sinai Med Ctr (page 64); **Address:** Mount Sinai Medical Ctr, One Gustave L Levy Pl, Box 1104, New York, NY 10029; **Phone:** 212-241-0034; **Board Cert:** Internal Medicine 2000; Gastroenterology 2005; Transplant Hepatology 2006; **Med School:** Mexico 1987; **Resid:** Internal Medicine, Maimonides Med Ctr 1992; Gastroenterology, Temple Univ 1995; **Fellow:** Nutrition, Meml Sloan-Kettering Cancer Ctr 1993; Hepatology, Mt Sinai Med Ctr 1996; **Fac Appt:** Prof Med, Mount Sinai Sch Med

Shike, Moshe MD [Ge] - **Spec Exp:** Gastrointestinal Cancer; Nutrition & Cancer Prevention; Endoscopy; **Hospital:** Meml Sloan-Kettering Cancer Ctr; **Address:** 1275 York Avenue, New York, NY 10065; **Phone:** 800-525-2225; **Board Cert:** Internal Medicine 1977; Gastroenterology 1981; **Med School:** Israel 1975; **Resid:** Internal Medicine, Mt Auburn Hosp 1977; **Fellow:** Gastroenterology, Toronto Genl Hosp 1981; **Fac Appt:** Prof Med, Cornell Univ-Weill Med Coll

Slivka, Adam MD/PhD [Ge] - **Spec Exp:** Pancreatic & Biliary Disease; Pancreatic Cancer; **Hospital:** UPMC Presby, Pittsburgh; **Address:** Digestive Disorders Center, 200 Lothrop St, 3rd Fl-PUH, Pittsburgh, PA 15213; **Phone:** 412-647-8666; **Board Cert:** Internal Medicine 2002; Gastroenterology 1995; **Med School:** Mount Sinai Sch Med 1988; **Resid:** Internal Medicine, Brigham & Womens Hosp 1991; **Fellow:** Gastroenterology, Brigham & Womens Hosp 1994; **Fac Appt:** Assoc Prof Med, Univ Pittsburgh

Smoot, Duane Thomas MD [Ge] - **Spec Exp:** Colon & Rectal Cancer Detection; Gastrointestinal Cancer; Peptic Acid Disorders; **Hospital:** Howard Univ Hosp; **Address:** Howard Univ Hosp, Med, Div Gastroenterology, Ste 5100, 2041 Georgia Ave NW Tower Bldg, Washington, DC 20060; **Phone:** 202-865-6620; **Board Cert:** Internal Medicine 1987; Gastroenterology 2003; **Med School:** Howard Univ 1983; **Resid:** Internal Medicine, Univ MD Hosp 1986; **Fellow:** Gastroenterology, Univ MD Hosp 1989; **Fac Appt:** Prof Med, Howard Univ

Stevens, Peter D MD [Ge] - **Spec Exp:** Endoscopy; Pancreatic Disease; Pancreatic/Biliary Endoscopy (ERCP); **Hospital:** NY-Presby Hosp/Columbia (page 66); **Address:** NY Presby-Columbia Presbyterian Med Ctr, 161 Fort Washington St, Ste 864, New York, NY 10032; **Phone:** 212-305-1909; **Board Cert:** Gastroenterology 2003; **Med School:** Columbia P&S 1987; **Resid:** Internal Medicine, Columbia Presby Med Ctr 1991; **Fellow:** Gastroenterology, Columbia Presby Med Ctr 1993; Endoscopy, Columbia Presby Med Ctr 1994; **Fac Appt:** Asst Clin Prof Med, Columbia P&S

Tobias, Hillel MD [Ge] - **Spec Exp:** Liver Disease; Hepatitis B & C; Liver & Biliary Disease; **Hospital:** NYU Langone Med Ctr (page 67); **Address:** 232 E 30th St, New York, NY 10016-8202; **Phone:** 212-889-5544; **Board Cert:** Internal Medicine 1967; Gastroenterology 1979; **Med School:** Washington Univ, St Louis 1960; **Resid:** Internal Medicine, Bellevue Hosp 1963; **Fellow:** Hepatology, Royal Free Hosp 1965; Hepatology, Mount Sinai Hosp 1967; **Fac Appt:** Prof Med, NYU Sch Med

Waye, Jerome MD [Ge] - **Spec Exp:** Endoscopy; Colon Cancer; Colonoscopy; **Hospital:** Mount Sinai Med Ctr (page 64), Lenox Hill Hosp (page 62); **Address:** 650 Park Ave, New York, NY 10021-6115; **Phone:** 212-439-7779; **Board Cert:** Internal Medicine 1965; Gastroenterology 1970; **Med School:** Boston Univ 1958; **Resid:** Internal Medicine, Mt Sinai Hosp 1961; **Fellow:** Gastroenterology, Mt Sinai Hosp 1962; **Fac Appt:** Clin Prof Med, Mount Sinai Sch Med

Weinberg, David Seth MD [Ge] - **Spec Exp:** Colonoscopy; Cancer Risk Assessment; Cancer Prevention; Endoscopy; **Hospital:** Fox Chase Cancer Ctr (page 58); **Address:** Fox Chase Cancer Ctr-Dept GI, 333 Cottman Ave, Ste P3047, Philadelphia, PA 19111; **Phone:** 215-214-1424; **Board Cert:** Gastroenterology 2006; **Med School:** Cornell Univ-Weill Med Coll 1989; **Resid:** Internal Medicine, Beth Israel Hosp 1992; **Fellow:** Gastroenterology, Hosp U Penn 1995; Epidemiology, Hosp U Penn 1995

Winawer, Sidney J MD [Ge] - **Spec Exp:** Colon Cancer; Cancer Prevention; **Hospital:** Meml Sloan-Kettering Cancer Ctr; **Address:** 1275 York Avenue, New York, NY 10065; **Phone:** 800-525-2225; **Board Cert:** Internal Medicine 1965; Gastroenterology 1973; **Med School:** SUNY Downstate 1956; **Resid:** Internal Medicine, VA Hosp 1961; Internal Medicine, Maimonides Hosp 1962; **Fellow:** Gastroenterology, Boston City Hosp 1964; **Fac Appt:** Prof Med, Cornell Univ-Weill Med Coll

Southeast

Abreu, Maria T MD [Ge] - **Spec Exp:** Inflammatory Bowel Disease; Ulcerative Colitis; Crohn's Disease; **Hospital:** Univ of Miami Hosp (page 71); **Address:** Univ Miami Miller Sch Med, PO Box 016960 (D-49), Miami, FL 33101; **Phone:** 305-243-8644; **Board Cert:** Gastroenterology 2005; **Med School:** Univ Miami Sch Med 1990; **Resid:** Internal Medicine, Brigham & Women's Hosp 1992; **Fellow:** Gastroenterology, UCLA Med Ctr 1995; **Fac Appt:** Prof Med, Univ Miami Sch Med

Barkin, Jamie S MD [Ge] - **Spec Exp:** Pancreatic & Biliary Disease; Gastrointestinal Cancer; Endoscopy; **Hospital:** Mount Sinai Med Ctr - Miami, Univ of Miami Hosp & Clins/Sylvester Comp Canc Ctr (page 70); **Address:** Mount Sinai Medical Center, Gumenick Bldg, 4300 Alton Rd, Ste 2522, Miami Beach, FL 33140-2800; **Phone:** 305-674-2240; **Board Cert:** Internal Medicine 1973; Gastroenterology 1975; **Med School:** Univ Miami Sch Med 1970; **Resid:** Internal Medicine, Univ Miami Hosp 1973; **Fellow:** Gastroenterology, Univ Miami Hosp 1975; **Fac Appt:** Prof Med, Univ Miami Sch Med

Bloomer, Joseph R MD [Ge] - **Spec Exp:** Porphyria; Liver Disease; Transplant Medicine-Liver; **Hospital:** Univ of Ala Hosp at Birmingham, UAB Highlands Hosp; **Address:** UAB, Div Gastroenterology/ Hepatology, 1918 University Blvd, 395 MCLM, Birmingham, AL 35294-0005; **Phone:** 205-975-9699; **Board Cert:** Internal Medicine 1972; **Med School:** Case West Res Univ 1966; **Resid:** Internal Medicine, UCSF Med Ctr 1968; **Fellow:** Hepatology, Yale Univ 1972; **Fac Appt:** Prof Med, Univ Alabama

Brazer, Scott R MD [Ge] - **Spec Exp:** Gastroesophageal Reflux Disease (GERD); Chest Pain-Non Cardiac; Colon Cancer Screening; **Hospital:** Univ NC Hosps; **Address:** 249 E Highway 54, Ste 200, Durham, NC 27713; **Phone:** 919-806-8322; **Board Cert:** Internal Medicine 1984; Gastroenterology 1987; **Med School:** Case West Res Univ 1981; **Resid:** Internal Medicine, Duke Univ Med Ctr 1984; Internal Medicine, Duke Univ Med Ctr 1988; **Fellow:** Gastroenterology, Duke Univ 1987

Castell, Donald O MD [Ge] - **Spec Exp:** Esophageal Disorders; Gastroesophageal Reflux Disease (GERD); Gastrointestinal Motility Disorders; **Hospital:** MUSC Med Ctr; **Address:** MUSC Digestive Disease Ctr, 96 Jonathan Lucas St, Box 250327, Charleston, SC 29425; **Phone:** 843-792-7522; **Board Cert:** Internal Medicine 1977; Gastroenterology 1970; **Med School:** Geo Wash Univ 1960; **Resid:** Internal Medicine, US Naval Hosp 1965; **Fellow:** Gastroenterology, Tufts Univ 1969; **Fac Appt:** Prof Med, Univ SC Sch Med

Gastroenterology

Cotton, Peter MD [Ge] - **Spec Exp:** Pancreatic Disease; Biliary Disease; Pancreatic/Biliary Endoscopy (ERCP); **Hospital:** MUSC Med Ctr; **Address:** MUSC, Digestive Disease Center - 210 CSB, 96 Jonathan Lucas St, Box 250327, Charleston, SC 29425; **Phone:** 843-792-6865; **Med School:** England, UK 1963; **Resid:** Internal Medicine, St Thomas' Hosp 1970; Gastroenterology, St Thomas' Hosp 1973; **Fac Appt:** Prof Med, Med Univ SC

DeVault, Kenneth MD [Ge] - **Spec Exp:** Gastroesophageal Reflux Disease (GERD); **Hospital:** Mayo - Jacksonville; **Address:** Mayo Clinic, Davis Bldg, 6th Fl, 4500 San Pablo Rd S, Jacksonville, FL 32224-1865; **Phone:** 904-953-2254; **Board Cert:** Internal Medicine 1989; Gastroenterology 2003; **Med School:** Bowman Gray 1986; **Resid:** Internal Medicine, Vanderbilt Univ Med Ctr 1989; **Fellow:** Gastroenterology, T Jefferson Univ Med Ctr 1992; **Fac Appt:** Prof Med, Mayo Med Sch

Drossman, Douglas A MD [Ge] - **Spec Exp:** Gastrointestinal Motility Disorders; Pain-Abdominal/Functional; Gastrointestinal Functional Disorders; **Hospital:** Univ NC Hosps; **Address:** Univ NC, Div Digestive Diseases, 4150 Bio Informatics Bldg, Campus Box 7080, Chapel Hill, NC 27599-7080; **Phone:** 919-966-0141; **Board Cert:** Internal Medicine 1973; Gastroenterology 1979; **Med School:** Albert Einstein Coll Med 1970; **Resid:** Internal Medicine, NC Meml Hosp 1972; Internal Medicine, Bellevue Hosp Ctr-NYU 1973; **Fellow:** Psychiatry, Univ Rochester 1976; Gastroenterology, NC Meml Hosp-UNC 1978; **Fac Appt:** Prof Med, Univ NC Sch Med

Elliott, Norman L MD [Ge] - **Spec Exp:** Enteroscopy-Small Bowel; Endoscopy; **Hospital:** Emory Univ Hosp Midtown; **Address:** Atlanta Gastroenterology Assocs, 550 Peachtree St NE, Ste 1600, Atlanta, GA 30308; **Phone:** 404-881-1094; **Board Cert:** Internal Medicine 1982; Gastroenterology 1985; **Med School:** Yale Univ 1979; **Resid:** Internal Medicine, Emory Univ Hosp 1982; **Fellow:** Gastroenterology, Univ Alabama 1985; **Fac Appt:** Asst Clin Prof Med, Emory Univ

Eloubeidi, Mohamad A MD [Ge] - **Spec Exp:** Gastrointestinal Cancer; Colon & Rectal Cancer; Pancreatic Cancer; Endoscopic Ultrasound; **Hospital:** Univ of Ala Hosp at Birmingham; **Address:** 1530 3rd Ave S, Ste LHRB-406, Birmingham, AL 35294-0007; **Phone:** 205-934-7955; **Board Cert:** Internal Medicine 2006; Gastroenterology 2000; **Med School:** Lebanon 1993; **Resid:** Internal Medicine, Duke Univ Med Ctr 1996; **Fellow:** Gastroenterology, Duke Univ Med Ctr 1999; Advanced Endoscopy, Med Univ South Carolina 2000; **Fac Appt:** Assoc Prof Med, Univ Alabama

Estores, David MD [Ge] - **Spec Exp:** Barrett's Esophagus; Swallowing Disorders; **Hospital:** H Lee Moffitt Cancer Ctr & Research Inst; **Address:** Ctr for Swallowing Disorders, 12901 Bruce B Downs Blvd, MDC 72, Tampa, FL 33612-4742; **Phone:** 813-974-3374; **Board Cert:** Internal Medicine 1989; Gastroenterology 2001; **Med School:** Philippines 1985; **Resid:** Internal Medicine, St Lukes Hosp 1989; **Fellow:** Gastroenterology, Univ Pittsburgh-Presby Hosp 1992

Forsmark, Christopher MD [Ge] - **Spec Exp:** Pancreatic/Biliary Endoscopy (ERCP); Celiac Disease; Pancreatic Disease; Endoscopy; **Hospital:** Shands at Univ of FL; **Address:** University of Florida, 1600 SW Archer Rd, Box 100214, Gainesville, FL 32610; **Phone:** 352-392-2877; **Board Cert:** Internal Medicine 1986; Gastroenterology 2006; **Med School:** Johns Hopkins Univ 1983; **Resid:** Internal Medicine, UCSF Med Ctr 1987; **Fellow:** Gastroenterology, USCF Med Ctr 1990; **Fac Appt:** Prof Med, Univ Fla Coll Med

Hawes, Robert H MD [Ge] - **Spec Exp:** Endoscopic Ultrasound; Pancreatic/Biliary Endoscopy (ERCP); Pancreatic Disease; **Hospital:** MUSC Med Ctr; **Address:** 96 Jonathan Lucas St, Ste 210, Box 250327, Charleston, SC 29425; **Phone:** 843-792-6865; **Board Cert:** Internal Medicine 1985; Gastroenterology 1987; **Med School:** Indiana Univ 1980; **Fac Appt:** Prof Med, Med Univ SC

Hoffman, Brenda J MD [Ge] - **Spec Exp:** Liver & Biliary Disease; Endoscopic Ultrasound; Gastrointestinal Cancer; Colon & Rectal Cancer-Familial Polyposis; **Hospital:** MUSC Med Ctr; **Address:** MUSC Digestive Disease Center, 25 Courteney Drive, rm MS7100A, MSC290, Charleston, SC 29425; **Phone:** 843-792-6999; **Board Cert:** Internal Medicine 1986; Gastroenterology 1989; **Med School:** Univ KY Coll Med 1983; **Resid:** Internal Medicine, MUSC Med Ctr 1987; **Fellow:** Gastroenterology, MUSC Med Ctr 1989; **Fac Appt:** Prof Med, Univ SC Sch Med

Isaacs, Kim MD/PhD [Ge] - **Spec Exp:** Inflammatory Bowel Disease; Crohn's Disease; Ulcerative Colitis; **Hospital:** Univ NC Hosps; **Address:** Univ NC, Div Digestive Disease/Nutrition, CB# 7080, Bioinformatics Bldg, 130 Mason Farm Rd Fl 1, Chapel Hill, NC 27599-7080; **Phone:** 919-966-0140; **Board Cert:** Internal Medicine 1987; Gastroenterology 2001; **Med School:** SUNY Stony Brook 1984; **Resid:** Internal Medicine, Univ NC Hosps 1987; **Fellow:** Gastroenterology, Univ NC Hosps 1989; **Fac Appt:** Assoc Prof Med, Univ NC Sch Med

Lambiase, Louis R MD [Ge] - **Spec Exp:** Pancreatic Disease; Endoscopic Ultrasound; Pain-Abdominal/Functional; Liver Disease; **Hospital:** Shands Jacksonville, Naval Hosp - Jacksonville; **Address:** Univ Florida Gastroenterology, 4555 Emerson St, Ste 300, Jacksonville, FL 32207; **Phone:** 904-633-0797; **Board Cert:** Internal Medicine 2002; Gastroenterology 2003; **Med School:** Univ Miami Sch Med 1987; **Resid:** Internal Medicine, Presbyterian/ VA Hosps 1990; **Fellow:** Gastroenterology, Univ Fla 1993; **Fac Appt:** Assoc Prof Med, Univ Fla Coll Med

Liddle, Rodger A MD [Ge] - **Spec Exp:** Inflammatory Bowel Disease; Pancreatic Disease; Hormone Secreting Tumors; **Hospital:** Duke Univ Med Ctr, VA Med Ctr - Durham; **Address:** Duke Univ Med Ctr, Div Gastroenterology, Box 3913, Durham, NC 27710; **Phone:** 919-681-6380; **Board Cert:** Internal Medicine 1981; Gastroenterology 1983; **Med School:** Vanderbilt Univ 1978; **Resid:** Internal Medicine, UCSF Med Ctr 1981; **Fellow:** Gastroenterology, UCSF Med Ctr 1984; **Fac Appt:** Prof Med, Duke Univ

Lind, Christopher D MD [Ge] - **Spec Exp:** Gastroesophageal Reflux Disease (GERD); Swallowing Disorders; Biliary Disease; Achalasia; **Hospital:** Vanderbilt Univ Med Ctr; **Address:** Vanderbilt Univ Med Ctr, Div GI, 1660 TVC GI Clin, Nashville, TN 37232-5280; **Phone:** 615-322-0128; **Board Cert:** Internal Medicine 1984; Gastroenterology 1987; **Med School:** Vanderbilt Univ 1981; **Resid:** Internal Medicine, Univ Virginia Hosps 1985; **Fellow:** Gastroenterology, Shands/Univ Florida 1986; Gastroenterology, Univ Virginia Hosps 1988; **Fac Appt:** Prof Med, Vanderbilt Univ

Martin, Paul MD [Ge] - **Spec Exp:** Liver Disease; Hepatitis; Transplant Medicine-Liver; **Hospital:** Univ of Miami Hosp (page 71), Jackson Meml Hosp (page 70); **Address:** Schiff Liver Inst/Ctr for Liver Diseases, 1500 NW 12 Ave, Jackson Medical Tower E-1101, Miami, FL 33136; **Phone:** 305-243-4615; **Board Cert:** Internal Medicine 1984; Gastroenterology 1987; Transplant Hepatology 2006; **Med School:** Ireland 1978; **Resid:** Internal Medicine, St Vincent's Hosp 1982; Internal Medicine, Univ Alberta 1984; **Fellow:** Gastroenterology, Queen Univ 1986; Hepatology, Natl Inst Hlth 1989; **Fac Appt:** Prof Med, Univ Miami Sch Med

Mertz, Howard MD [Ge] - **Spec Exp:** Irritable Bowel Syndrome; Endoscopic Ultrasound; Inflammatory Bowel Disease; **Hospital:** Saint Thomas Hosp - Nashville; **Address:** 4230 Harding Rd, Ste 309W, Nashville, TN 37205; **Phone:** 615-383-0165; **Board Cert:** Internal Medicine 1989; Gastroenterology 2002; **Med School:** Baylor Coll Med 1986; **Resid:** Internal Medicine, Johns Hopkins Hosp 1989; **Fellow:** Gastroenterology, UCLA Med Ctr 1991; **Fac Appt:** Assoc Prof Med, Vanderbilt Univ

Gastroenterology

Plevy, Scott MD [Ge] - **Spec Exp:** Inflammatory Bowel Disease; **Hospital:** Univ NC Hosps; **Address:** 4100 Bioinformatics Bldg, 130 Mason Farm Rd, GI Clinic, CB 7080, Chapel Hill, NC 27599; **Phone:** 919-966-6000; **Board Cert:** Gastroenterology 2007; **Med School:** Columbia P&S 1988; **Resid:** Internal Medicine, Brigham-Womens Hosp 1991; **Fellow:** Gastroenterology, Univ of California 1992; Inflammatory Bowel Disease, Cedars-Sinai Med CTR 1994; **Fac Appt:** Assoc Prof Med, Univ NC Sch Med

Porayko, Michael K MD [Ge] - **Spec Exp:** Liver Disease; Transplant Medicine-Liver; Hepatitis C; **Hospital:** Vanderbilt Univ Med Ctr; **Address:** GI Clinic, 1301 Medical Center Drive, Ste 1660, Nashville, TN 37232; **Phone:** 615-322-0128; **Board Cert:** Internal Medicine 1984; Gastroenterology 1987; Transplant Hepatology 2006; **Med School:** Univ IL Coll Med 1981; **Resid:** Internal Medicine, Michigan State Univ affil Hosps 1984; **Fellow:** Gastroenterology, Lahey Clin & New England Deaconess Hosp 1987; Hepatology, Mayo Clinic 1988; **Fac Appt:** Assoc Prof Med, Vanderbilt Univ

Raiford, David S MD [Ge] - **Spec Exp:** Autoimmune Liver Disease; Steatohepatitis; Liver Disease; Transplant Medicine-Liver; **Hospital:** Vanderbilt Univ Med Ctr; **Address:** Vanderbilt Hepatology, 1660 The Vanderbilt Clin, Nashville, TN 37232-5280; **Phone:** 615-322-0128; **Board Cert:** Internal Medicine 1989; Gastroenterology 2001; Transplant Hepatology 2006; **Med School:** Johns Hopkins Univ 1985; **Resid:** Internal Medicine, Johns Hopkins Hosp 1988; **Fellow:** Hepatology, Johns Hopkins Hosp 1991; **Fac Appt:** Prof Med, Vanderbilt Univ

Rubin, Raymond A MD [Ge] - **Spec Exp:** Liver Disease; Transplant Medicine-Liver; **Hospital:** Piedmont Hosp; **Address:** Digestive Healthcare of Georgia, 95 Collier Rd NW, Ste 4085, Atlanta, GA 30309; **Phone:** 404-355-3200; **Board Cert:** Internal Medicine 1989; Gastroenterology 2003; Transplant Hepatology 2006; **Med School:** Cornell Univ-Weill Med Coll 1986; **Resid:** Internal Medicine, Hosp Univ Penn 1990; **Fellow:** Gastroenterology, Hosp Univ Penn 1992

Sartor, R Balfour MD [Ge] - **Spec Exp:** Inflammatory Bowel Disease; **Hospital:** Univ NC Hosps; **Address:** Univ NC Sch Medicine, Div Gastroenterology/Hepatology, Biomolecular Bldg- rm 7309, Box 7032, Chapel Hill, NC 27599-7032; **Phone:** 919-966-6000; **Board Cert:** Internal Medicine 1978; Gastroenterology 1981; **Med School:** Baylor Coll Med 1974; **Resid:** Internal Medicine, Baylor Affil Hosp 1977; **Fellow:** Gastroenterology, Univ NC Hosps 1981; **Fac Appt:** Prof Med, Univ NC Sch Med

Schiff, Eugene MD [Ge] - **Spec Exp:** Hepatitis C; Liver Disease; **Hospital:** Univ of Miami Hosp (page 71), Jackson Meml Hosp (page 70); **Address:** Ctr for Liver Disease, 1500 NW 12th Ave, Ste 1101 ET, Miami, FL 33136; **Phone:** 305-243-5787; **Board Cert:** Internal Medicine 1980; Gastroenterology 1972; **Med School:** Columbia P&S 1962; **Resid:** Internal Medicine, Cincinnati Genl Hosp 1964; Internal Medicine, Parkland Meml Hosp 1967; **Fellow:** Gastroenterology, Univ Tex SW Med Ctr 1969; **Fac Appt:** Prof Med, Univ Miami Sch Med

Scudera, Peter L MD [Ge] - **Spec Exp:** Colon & Rectal Cancer Detection; Pancreatic/Biliary Endoscopy (ERCP); Hepatitis-Chronic; **Hospital:** Inova Fair Oaks Hosp, Inova Fairfax Hosp; **Address:** 3700 Joseph Siewick Dr, Ste 308, Fairfax, VA 22033; **Phone:** 703-716-8700; **Board Cert:** Internal Medicine 1987; Gastroenterology 1989; **Med School:** Cornell Univ-Weill Med Coll 1984; **Resid:** Internal Medicine, New York Hosp 1987; **Fellow:** Gastroenterology, New York Hosp-Cornell 1989

Seidner, Douglas L MD [Ge] - **Spec Exp:** Nutrition; Inflammatory Bowel Disease; Endoscopy; **Hospital:** Vanderbilt Univ Med Ctr; **Address:** Vanderbilt Center for Human Nutrition, 1211 21st Ave S, 514 Medical Arts Building, Nashville, TN 37232; **Phone:** 615-936-1288; **Board Cert:** Internal Medicine 1986; Gastroenterology 2000; **Med School:** SUNY Upstate Med Univ 1983; **Resid:** Internal Medicine, Beth Israel Deaconess Med Ctr 1986; **Fellow:** Nutrition & Metabolism, Beth Israel Deaconess Med Ctr 1987; Gastroenterology, George Washington Univ Med Ctr 1989

Shiffman, Mitchell MD [Ge] - **Spec Exp:** Transplant Medicine-Liver; Hepatitis C; Liver Disease; **Hospital:** Med Coll of VA Hosp; **Address:** Hepatology Section, Box 980341, Richmond, VA 23298-0341; **Phone:** 804-828-4060; **Board Cert:** Internal Medicine 1986; Gastroenterology 1989; **Med School:** SUNY Upstate Med Univ 1983; **Resid:** Internal Medicine, Med Coll Va Hosp 1986; **Fellow:** Gastroenterology, Med Coll Va Hosp 1988; **Fac Appt:** Prof Med, Med Coll VA

Toskes, Phillip MD [Ge] - **Spec Exp:** Nutrition; Malabsorption Syndrome; Pancreatic Disease; **Hospital:** Shands at Univ of FL; **Address:** Univ Florida, Div Gastroenterolgy, P.O. Box 100214, Gainesville, FL 32610-0214; **Phone:** 352-392-2877; **Board Cert:** Internal Medicine 1970; Gastroenterology 1973; **Med School:** Univ MD Sch Med 1965; **Resid:** Internal Medicine, Univ Maryland Hosp 1968; **Fellow:** Gastroenterology, Hosp Univ Penn 1970; **Fac Appt:** Prof Med, Univ Fla Coll Med

Vaezi, Michael F MD/PhD [Ge] - **Spec Exp:** Gastroesophageal Reflux Disease (GERD); Esophageal Disorders; Achalasia; **Hospital:** Vanderbilt Univ Med Ctr; **Address:** 1301 Med Ctr Drive, Ste 1660, Nashville, TN 37232; **Phone:** 615-322-0128; **Board Cert:** Internal Medicine 2007; Gastroenterology 1999; **Med School:** Univ Alabama 1992; **Resid:** Internal Medicine, Univ AL-Birmingham Med Ctr 1995; **Fellow:** Gastroenterology, Cleveland Clin 1996; **Fac Appt:** Prof Med, Vanderbilt Univ

Wilcox, C Mel MD [Ge] - **Spec Exp:** AIDS/HIV-Gastrointestinal Complications; Endoscopy; Pancreatic & Biliary Disease; **Hospital:** Univ of Ala Hosp at Birmingham; **Address:** UAB-Div Gastroenterology, 703 S 19th St, ZRB 633, Birmingham, AL 35294-0007; **Phone:** 205-975-4958; **Board Cert:** Internal Medicine 1986; Gastroenterology 2007; **Med School:** Med Coll GA 1983; **Resid:** Internal Medicine, Univ Alabama Hosps 1986; **Fellow:** Gastroenterology, UCSF 1990; **Fac Appt:** Prof Med, Univ Alabama

Yanda, Randy Joseph MD [Ge] - **Spec Exp:** Endoscopy; Pancreatic/Biliary Endoscopy (ERCP); Colon Cancer Screening; **Hospital:** Piedmont Hosp; **Address:** Digestive Healthcare of Georgia, 95 Collier Rd NW, Ste 4055, Atlanta, GA 30309; **Phone:** 404-355-3200; **Board Cert:** Internal Medicine 1987; Gastroenterology 2001; **Med School:** Univ Iowa Coll Med 1984; **Resid:** Internal Medicine, UCSF Med Ctr 1987; **Fellow:** Gastroenterology, UCSF Med Ctr 1990

Younossi, Zobair MD [Ge] - **Spec Exp:** Liver Disease; **Hospital:** Inova Fairfax Hosp; **Address:** Ctr for Liver Diseases, Fairfax Hosp, 3300 Gallows Rd, Claude Moore Bldg, Falls Church, VA 22042; **Phone:** 703-776-3182; **Board Cert:** Gastroenterology 2005; Transplant Hepatology 2006; **Med School:** Univ Rochester 1989; **Resid:** Gastroenterology, Scripps Clin & Rsch Fdn 1993; **Fellow:** Hepatology, Scripps Clin & Rsch Fdn 1995; **Fac Appt:** Prof Med, Va Commonwealth Univ Sch Med

Midwest

Achkar, Edgar MD [Ge] - **Spec Exp:** Esophageal Disorders; Gastrointestinal Motility Disorders; **Hospital:** Cleveland Clin Fdn (page 56); **Address:** 9500 Euclid Ave, Desk A31, Cleveland, OH 44195; **Phone:** 216-444-6523; **Board Cert:** Internal Medicine 1978; Gastroenterology 1979; **Med School:** Lebanon 1964; **Resid:** Internal Medicine, Lahey Clin 1967; **Fellow:** Gastroenterology, Lahey Clin 1968; Gastroenterology, Clevland Clin 1969; **Fac Appt:** Prof Med, Cleveland Cl Coll Med/Case West Res

Gastroenterology

Bacon, Bruce MD [Ge] - **Spec Exp:** Hepatitis C; Hepatic Iron Metabolism; Liver Disease; **Hospital:** St Louis Univ Hosp, SSM St Mary's Hlth Ctr - St Louis; **Address:** 3660 Vista Ave, Ste 308, St Louis, MO 63110-2540; **Phone:** 314-977-6150; **Board Cert:** Internal Medicine 1978; Gastroenterology 2008; Transplant Hepatology 2006; **Med School:** Case West Res Univ 1975; **Resid:** Internal Medicine, Metro Genl Hosp 1979; **Fellow:** Gastroenterology, Metro Genl Hosp 1982; **Fac Appt:** Prof Med, St Louis Univ

Baron, Todd H MD [Ge] - **Spec Exp:** Endoscopy; Pancreatic/Biliary Endoscopy (ERCP); **Hospital:** Mayo Med Ctr & Clin - Rochester; **Address:** Mayo Clin, 200 First St SW, Charleton 8, Rochester, MN 55905; **Phone:** 507-266-6931; **Board Cert:** Internal Medicine 1989; Gastroenterology 2003; **Med School:** Univ Fla Coll Med 1986; **Resid:** Internal Medicine, Univ Alabama Med Ctr 1990; **Fellow:** Gastroenterology, Univ Alabama Med Ctr 1993; **Fac Appt:** Assoc Prof Med, Univ Ariz Coll Med

Brown, Kimberly A MD [Ge] - **Spec Exp:** Liver Disease; Transplant Medicine-Liver; Hepatitis C; Liver Cancer; **Hospital:** Henry Ford Hosp; **Address:** Henry Ford Hosp, Dept Gastroenterology, 2799 W Grand Blvd K-747 Bldg Fl 7, Detroit, MI 48202-2608; **Phone:** 313-916-8632; **Board Cert:** Internal Medicine 1988; Gastroenterology 2002; Transplant Hepatology 2006; **Med School:** Wayne State Univ 1985; **Resid:** Internal Medicine, Univ Michigan Med Ctr 1989; **Fellow:** Gastroenterology, Univ Michigan Med Ctr 1992

Chari, Suresh T MD [Ge] - **Spec Exp:** Pancreatic Disease; **Hospital:** Mayo Med Ctr & Clin - Rochester; **Address:** Mayo Clinic, 200 First St SW Mayo Bldg Fl 9, Rochester, MN 55905; **Phone:** 507-266-4347; **Board Cert:** Gastroenterology 1999; **Med School:** India 1982; **Resid:** Internal Medicine, Univ Arizona Hlth Sci Ctr 1996; **Fellow:** Gastroenterology, Mayo Clinic 1999; **Fac Appt:** Prof Med, Mayo Med Sch

Chey, William D MD [Ge] - **Spec Exp:** Gastrointestinal Motility Disorders; Gastrointestinal Functional Disorders; Inflammatory Bowel Disease; Gastroesophageal Reflux Disease (GERD); **Hospital:** Univ Michigan Hlth Sys; **Address:** Taubman Health Care Ctr, 1500 E Medical Center Drive, Ste 3912, Ann Arbor, MI 48109; **Phone:** 734-936-4772; **Board Cert:** Internal Medicine 1989; Gastroenterology 2003; **Med School:** Emory Univ 1986; **Resid:** Internal Medicine, Emory Univ Med Ctr 1989; **Fellow:** Gastroenterology, Univ Mich Hosps 1993; **Fac Appt:** Prof Med, Univ Mich Med Sch

Cominelli, Fabio MD/PhD [Ge] - **Spec Exp:** Inflammatory Bowel Disease/Crohn's; Ulcerative Colitis; **Hospital:** Univ Hosps Case Med Ctr; **Address:** Univ Hosps Case Medical Ctr, Div Gastroenterology, 11100 Euclid Ave, Cleveland, OH 44106-5066; **Phone:** 216-844-7344; **Med School:** Italy 1983; **Resid:** Gastroenterology, Careggi Hosp-Univ Italy 1986; **Fellow:** Gastroenterology, Harbor-UCLA Med Ctr 1989; **Fac Appt:** Prof Med, Case West Res Univ

Craig, Robert M MD [Ge] - **Spec Exp:** Inflammatory Bowel Disease/Crohn's; Liver Disease; Swallowing Disorders; Diarrheal Diseases; **Hospital:** Northwestern Meml Hosp; **Address:** 233 E Erie St, Ste 206, Chicago, IL 60611-5938; **Phone:** 312-908-9644; **Board Cert:** Internal Medicine 1972; Gastroenterology 1975; **Med School:** Northwestern Univ 1967; **Resid:** Internal Medicine, VA Rsch Hosp 1969; Internal Medicine, VA Rsch Hosp 1972; **Fellow:** Gastroenterology, Northwestern Meml Hosp 1974; **Fac Appt:** Prof Med, Northwestern Univ

Crippin, Jeffrey S MD [Ge] - **Spec Exp:** Transplant Medicine-Liver; Liver Disease; Liver Failure; Gastrointestinal Cancer; **Hospital:** Barnes-Jewish Hosp; **Address:** Barnes Jewish Hosp, Div Gastroenterology, 660 S Euclid Ave Campus Box 8124, St Louis, MO 63110; **Phone:** 314-454-8160; **Board Cert:** Internal Medicine 1987; Gastroenterology 2001; Transplant Hepatology 2006; **Med School:** Univ Kans 1984; **Resid:** Internal Medicine, Kansas Univ Med Ctr 1988; **Fellow:** Gastroenterology, Mayo Clinic 1991; **Fac Appt:** Assoc Prof Med, Washington Univ, St Louis

Di Bisceglie, Adrian M MD [Ge] - **Spec Exp:** Hepatitis C; Hepatitis; Liver Cancer; **Hospital:** St Louis Univ Hosp; **Address:** St Louis Univ Hosp, Dept. Gastroenterology, 3635 Vista Ave, PO Box 15250, St Louis, MO 63110-0250; **Phone:** 314-577-8764; **Board Cert:** Internal Medicine 2002; Gastroenterology 2002; **Med School:** South Africa 1977; **Resid:** Internal Medicine, Baragwanath Hosp 1984; **Fellow:** Hepatology, Natl Inst Hlth 1988; **Fac Appt:** Prof Med, St Louis Univ

Edmundowicz, Steven A MD [Ge] - **Spec Exp:** Endoscopy; Biliary Disease; Pancreatic Disease; Pancreatic Cancer; **Hospital:** Barnes-Jewish Hosp; **Address:** Washington Univ Sch Med, Div Gastroenterology, 660 S Euclid Ave, Box 8124, St Louis, MO 63110; **Phone:** 314-747-2066; **Board Cert:** Internal Medicine 1986; Gastroenterology 1989; **Med School:** Jefferson Med Coll 1983; **Resid:** Internal Medicine, Barnes Hosp 1986; **Fellow:** Gastroenterology, Barnes Hosp/Wash Univ 1989; **Fac Appt:** Prof Med, Washington Univ, St Louis

Elliott, David MD/PhD [Ge] - **Spec Exp:** Celiac Disease; Inflammatory Bowel Disease/Crohn's; Intestinal Parasites; **Hospital:** Univ Iowa Hosp & Clinics; **Address:** Univ Iowa Hosp, Digestive Disease, 200 Hawkins Drive, rm 4611-JCP, Iowa City, IA 52242; **Phone:** 319-356-4060; **Board Cert:** Internal Medicine 1991; Gastroenterology 1993; **Med School:** Wayne State Univ 1988; **Resid:** Internal Medicine, Johns Hopkins Hosp 1991; **Fellow:** Gastroenterology, Univ Iowa Hosps 1993; **Fac Appt:** Assoc Prof Med, Univ Iowa Coll Med

Elta, Grace H MD [Ge] - **Spec Exp:** Biliary Disease; **Hospital:** Univ Michigan Hlth Sys; **Address:** Univ Michigan Hlth Sys, 1500 E Med Ctr Drive, 3912 Taubman Ctr, Ann Arbor, MI 48109-0362; **Phone:** 888-229-7408; **Board Cert:** Internal Medicine 1980; Gastroenterology 1983; **Med School:** Univ Mich Med Sch 1977; **Resid:** Internal Medicine, New England Med Ctr 1980; **Fellow:** Gastroenterology, New England Med Ctr 1982; **Fac Appt:** Prof Med, Univ Mich Med Sch

Falk, Gary W MD [Ge] - **Spec Exp:** Swallowing Disorders; Esophageal Disorders; Chest Pain-Non Cardiac; Barrett's Esophagus; **Hospital:** Cleveland Clin Fdn (page 56); **Address:** Cleveland Clinic, 9500 Euclid Ave, MS A30, Cleveland, OH 44195; **Phone:** 216-444-1762; **Board Cert:** Internal Medicine 1983; Gastroenterology 1985; **Med School:** Univ Rochester 1980; **Resid:** Internal Medicine, George Washington Univ Hosp 1983; **Fellow:** Gastroenterology, Univ Michigan Med Ctr 1986; **Fac Appt:** Prof Med, Case West Res Univ

Goldberg, Michael J MD [Ge] - **Spec Exp:** Colon Cancer; Inflammatory Bowel Disease; Pancreatic & Biliary Disease; Pancreatic/Biliary Endoscopy (ERCP); **Hospital:** Evanston/Northshore Univ Hlth Syst, Glenbrook/NorthShore Univ Hlth Syst; **Address:** 2650 Ridge Ave, Ste G-208, Evanston, IL 60201; **Phone:** 847-657-1900; **Board Cert:** Internal Medicine 1978; Gastroenterology 1981; **Med School:** Univ IL Coll Med 1975; **Resid:** Internal Medicine, Univ Illinois Hosp 1978; **Fellow:** Gastroenterology, Tufts-New England Med Ctr 1980; **Fac Appt:** Assoc Clin Prof Med, Northwestern Univ

Gostout, Christopher MD [Ge] - **Spec Exp:** Gastroscopy; Endoscopy; **Hospital:** Mayo Med Ctr & Clin - Rochester; **Address:** Mayo Clin, Div GI, 200 First St SW Mayo Bldg Fl 9, Rochester, MN 55905; **Phone:** 507-266-6932; **Board Cert:** Internal Medicine 1979; Gastroenterology 1981; **Med School:** SUNY Downstate 1976; **Resid:** Internal Medicine, Mayo Clin 1979; **Fellow:** Gastroenterology, Mayo Clin 1981

Hanauer, Stephen B MD [Ge] - **Spec Exp:** Inflammatory Bowel Disease; Crohn's Disease; Ulcerative Colitis; Clinical Trials; **Hospital:** Univ of Chicago Med Ctr; **Address:** Univ Chicago Hosps, 5841 S Maryland Ave, MC 4076, Chicago, IL 60637-1426; **Phone:** 773-702-1466; **Board Cert:** Internal Medicine 1980; Gastroenterology 1983; **Med School:** Univ IL Coll Med 1977; **Resid:** Internal Medicine, Univ Chicago Hosps 1980; **Fellow:** Gastroenterology, Univ Chicago Hosps 1982; **Fac Appt:** Prof Med, Univ Chicago-Pritzker Sch Med

Gastroenterology

Jensen, Donald M MD [Ge] - **Spec Exp:** Transplant Medicine-Liver; Hepatitis C; Liver & Biliary Disease; Liver Cancer; **Hospital:** Univ of Chicago Med Ctr; **Address:** Univ of Chicago, Ctr for Liver Disease, 5841 S Maryland Ave, MC 7120, Chicago, IL 60637; **Phone:** 773-702-2300; **Board Cert:** Internal Medicine 1975; Gastroenterology 1981; **Med School:** Univ IL Coll Med 1972; **Resid:** Internal Medicine, Rush Presby St Lukes Hosp 1975; Gastroenterology, Rush Presby St Lukes Hosp 1976; **Fellow:** Gastroenterology, King's Coll Hosp 1978; **Fac Appt:** Prof Med, Univ Chicago-Pritzker Sch Med

Kahrilas, Peter J MD [Ge] - **Spec Exp:** Esophageal Disorders; Swallowing Disorders; **Hospital:** Northwestern Meml Hosp; **Address:** 675 N St Clair Fl 17 - Ste 250, Chicago, IL 60611; **Phone:** 312-695-5620; **Board Cert:** Internal Medicine 1982; Gastroenterology 1987; **Med School:** Univ Rochester 1979; **Resid:** Internal Medicine, Univ Hosp 1982; **Fellow:** Gastroenterology, Northwestern Meml Hosp 1984; Research, Med Coll Wisconsin 1986; **Fac Appt:** Prof Med, Northwestern Univ

Konicek, Frank J MD [Ge] - **Spec Exp:** Endoscopy; Inflammatory Bowel Disease/Crohn's; Pancreatic Disease; Liver Disease; **Hospital:** Swedish Covenant Hosp, Adv Illinois Masonic Med Ctr; **Address:** 3004 N Ashland Ave, Chicago, IL 60657-3012; **Phone:** 773-871-4600; **Board Cert:** Internal Medicine 1977; Gastroenterology 1975; **Med School:** Loyola Univ-Stritch Sch Med 1963; **Resid:** Internal Medicine, St Francis Hosp 1965; Internal Medicine, Hines VA Hosp 1969; **Fellow:** Gastroenterology, Hines VA Hosp 1971; **Fac Appt:** Clin Prof Med, Loyola Univ-Stritch Sch Med

Kwo, Paul Y MD [Ge] - **Spec Exp:** Hepatitis B & C; Transplant Medicine-Liver; **Hospital:** Indiana Univ Hosp; **Address:** 975 W Walnut St, IB327, Indianapolis, IN 46202-5181; **Phone:** 317-274-3090; **Board Cert:** Gastroenterology 2005; Transplant Hepatology 2006; **Med School:** Wayne State Univ 1988; **Resid:** Internal Medicine, Univ Maryland Med Ctr 1991; **Fellow:** Gastroenterology, Mayo Clinic 1995; **Fac Appt:** Clin Prof Med, Indiana Univ

La Russo, Nicholas F MD [Ge] - **Spec Exp:** Transplant Medicine-Liver; Liver & Biliary Disease; **Hospital:** Mayo Med Ctr & Clin - Rochester; **Address:** Mayo Clinic, Div Gastroenterology, 200 First St SW, Rochester, MN 55905-0001; **Phone:** 507-284-3917; **Board Cert:** Internal Medicine 1972; Gastroenterology 1979; **Med School:** NY Med Coll 1969; **Resid:** Internal Medicine, Mayo Clinic 1972; **Fellow:** Gastroenterology, Mayo Clinic 1975; **Fac Appt:** Prof Med, Mayo Med Sch

Lashner, Bret A MD [Ge] - **Spec Exp:** Inflammatory Bowel Disease; **Hospital:** Cleveland Clin Fdn (page 56); **Address:** 9500 Euclid Ave, Desk A31, Cleveland, OH 44195; **Phone:** 216-444-6524; **Board Cert:** Internal Medicine 1983; Gastroenterology 1985; **Med School:** NYU Sch Med 1980; **Resid:** Internal Medicine, Temple Univ Hosp 1983; **Fellow:** Gastroenterology, Univ Chicago Hosps 1986; **Fac Appt:** Assoc Prof Med, Case West Res Univ

Lindor, Keith MD [Ge] - **Spec Exp:** Liver Disease; Biliary Disease; **Hospital:** Mayo Med Ctr & Clin - Rochester; **Address:** Mayo Clinic, Div Gastroenterology, 200 First St SW, Rochester, MN 55905; **Phone:** 507-284-4313; **Board Cert:** Internal Medicine 1982; Gastroenterology 1987; **Med School:** Mayo Med Sch 1979; **Resid:** Internal Medicine, N Carolina Baptist Hosp 1982; **Fellow:** Gastroenterology, Mayo Clin 1986; **Fac Appt:** Prof Med, Mayo Med Sch

Loftus Jr, Edward V MD [Ge] - **Spec Exp:** Inflammatory Bowel Disease; Crohn's Disease; Ulcerative Colitis; Microscopic Colitis; **Hospital:** Mayo Med Ctr & Clin - Rochester; **Address:** Mayo Clinic, Div Gastroenterology, E 1 9B, 200 First St SW, Rochester, MN 55905; **Phone:** 507-266-0873; **Board Cert:** Internal Medicine 2003; Gastroenterology 2005; **Med School:** Univ Pennsylvania 1988; **Resid:** Internal Medicine, Temple Univ Hosp 1991; **Fellow:** Gastroenterology, Mayo Clinic 1995; **Fac Appt:** Prof Med, Mayo Med Sch

Lucey, Michael R MD [Ge] - **Spec Exp:** Liver Disease; Transplant Medicine-Liver; **Hospital:** Univ WI Hosp & Clins; **Address:** Univ Wisc Hosps & Clins, 600 Highland Ave, H6-516 CSC, Madison, WI 53792; **Phone:** 608-263-7322; **Board Cert:** Internal Medicine 2001; Gastroenterology 2001; Transplant Hepatology 2006; **Med School:** Ireland 1980; **Resid:** Internal Medicine, Fed Dublin Vol Hosps 1979; Gastroenterology, St Bartholomews Hosp/Kings Coll Hosp 1985; **Fellow:** Gastroenterology, Univ Michigan Med Ctr 1987; **Fac Appt:** Prof Med, Univ Wisc

Luxon, Bruce MD/PhD [Ge] - **Spec Exp:** Liver Disease; Hepatitis C; Autoimmune Liver Disease; **Hospital:** Univ Iowa Hosp & Clinics; **Address:** 200 Hawkins Drive, rm 4687 JCP, Iowa City, IA 52242; **Phone:** 319-356-4060; **Board Cert:** Internal Medicine 1989; Gastroenterology 2001; Transplant Hepatology 2006; **Med School:** Univ MO-Columbia Sch Med 1985; **Resid:** Internal Medicine, Univ MO-Columbia Sch Med 1989; **Fellow:** Gastroenterology, UCSF Med Ctr 1992; **Fac Appt:** Prof Med, St Louis Univ

Meiselman, Mick S MD [Ge] - **Spec Exp:** Colonoscopy; Pancreatic & Biliary Disease; Gastroesophageal Reflux Disease (GERD); **Hospital:** Glenbrook/NorthShore Univ Hlth Syst, Evanston/Northshore Univ Hlth Syst; **Address:** 506 Green Bay Rd, Kenilworth, IL 60043-1002; **Phone:** 847-256-3495; **Board Cert:** Internal Medicine 1982; Gastroenterology 1985; **Med School:** Northwestern Univ 1979; **Resid:** Internal Medicine, Cedars-Sinai/UCLA 1982; **Fellow:** Gastroenterology, UCSF Med Ctr 1984; **Fac Appt:** Assoc Clin Prof Med, Northwestern Univ

Murray, Joseph A MD [Ge] - **Spec Exp:** Celiac Disease; Esophageal Disorders; **Hospital:** Mayo Med Ctr & Clin - Rochester; **Address:** Mayo Clinic, Div Gastroenterology, 200 First St SW, Rochester, MN 55905; **Phone:** 507-284-2631; **Board Cert:** Internal Medicine 1999; Gastroenterology 2000; **Med School:** Ireland 1983; **Resid:** Internal Medicine, St Laurences Hosp 1986; Gastroenterology, Beaumont Hosp 1988; **Fellow:** Gastroenterology, Univ Iowa Hosps & Clins 1990; **Fac Appt:** Prof Med, Mayo Med Sch

O'Brien, John J MD [Ge] - **Spec Exp:** Esophageal Disorders; Liver Disease; **Hospital:** Providence Hosp - Southfield; **Address:** Providence Hosp, 16001 W 9 Mile Rd, Southfield, MI 48075; **Phone:** 248-849-3152; **Board Cert:** Internal Medicine 1988; Gastroenterology 2005; **Med School:** Univ MO-Columbia Sch Med 1981; **Resid:** Internal Medicine, St Lukes Hosp 1984; Gastroenterology, Univ KY Med Ctr 1986; **Fellow:** Gastroenterology, Johns Hopkins Hosp 1989; **Fac Appt:** Prof Med, Univ Mich Med Sch

Owyang, Chung MD [Ge] - **Spec Exp:** Gastrointestinal Motility Disorders; Digestive Disorders; **Hospital:** Univ Michigan Hlth Sys; **Address:** Univ Mich, Div Gastroenterology, 1500 E Med Ctr Dr, Rm 3912 Taubman Ctr, Ann Arbor, MI 48109-0362; **Phone:** 734-936-4785; **Board Cert:** Internal Medicine 1976; Gastroenterology 1981; **Med School:** McGill Univ 1972; **Resid:** Internal Medicine, Montreal Genl Hosp 1975; **Fellow:** Gastroenterology, Mayo Grad Med Sch 1978; **Fac Appt:** Prof Med, Univ Mich Med Sch

Rao, Satish S C MD/PhD [Ge] - **Spec Exp:** Constipation; Incontinence-Fecal; Chest Pain-Non Cardiac; Gastroesophageal Reflux Disease (GERD); **Hospital:** Univ Iowa Hosp & Clinics; **Address:** Univ Iowa Hosp & Clinics, Div Gastro, 200 Hawkins Drive, rm 4612 JCP, Iowa City, IA 52242; **Phone:** 319-356-4060; **Board Cert:** Gastroenterology 1998; **Med School:** India 1978; **Resid:** Internal Medicine, Sunderland Hosps 1982; Internal Medicine, York Dist Hosp 1984; **Fellow:** Royal Hallamshire Hosp 1986; Gastroenterology, Royal Liverpool Hosp 1988; **Fac Appt:** Prof Med, Univ Iowa Coll Med

Reichelderfer, Mark MD [Ge] - **Spec Exp:** Endoscopy; Inflammatory Bowel Disease; **Hospital:** Univ WI Hosp & Clins; **Address:** 600 Highland Ave, MC 2451, Madison, WI 53792-5124; **Phone:** 608-263-8094; **Board Cert:** Internal Medicine 1977; Gastroenterology 1979; **Med School:** Columbia P&S 1974; **Resid:** Internal Medicine, Mary Imogene Bassett Hosp 1977; **Fellow:** Gastroenterology, Univ Wisc Hosps & Clin 1979; **Fac Appt:** Prof Med, Univ Wisc

Gastroenterology

Rex, Douglas K MD [Ge] - **Spec Exp:** Endoscopy; Endoscopic Ultrasound; Colon & Rectal Cancer Detection; **Hospital:** Indiana Univ Hosp; **Address:** 550 N University Blvd, Ste 4100, Indianapolis, IN 46202; **Phone:** 317-278-9763; **Board Cert:** Internal Medicine 1985; Gastroenterology 1987; **Med School:** Indiana Univ 1980; **Resid:** Internal Medicine, Indiana Univ Med Ctr 1982; Internal Medicine, Indiana Univ Hosp 1985; **Fellow:** Gastroenterology, Indiana Univ Med Ctr 1984; **Fac Appt:** Prof Med, Indiana Univ

Sandborn, William J MD [Ge] - **Spec Exp:** Inflammatory Bowel Disease/Crohn's; Ulcerative Colitis; Crohn's Disease; **Hospital:** Mayo Med Ctr & Clin - Rochester; **Address:** Mayo Clin, Div GI, 200 First St SW, Rochester, MN 55905; **Phone:** 507-284-0959; **Board Cert:** Gastroenterology 2003; **Med School:** Loma Linda Univ 1987; **Resid:** Internal Medicine, Loma Linda Univ 1990; **Fellow:** Gastroenterology, Mayo Clin 1993; **Fac Appt:** Assoc Prof Med, Mayo Med Sch

Schulze, Konrad S MD [Ge] - **Spec Exp:** Gastroesophageal Reflux Disease (GERD); Peptic Acid Disorders; Gastroparesis; **Hospital:** Univ Iowa Hosp & Clinics; **Address:** UIHC, Dept Gastroenterology, 200 Hawkins Drive, rm 4551 JCP, Iowa City, IA 52242; **Phone:** 319-356-4060; **Board Cert:** Internal Medicine 1987; Gastroenterology 1975; **Med School:** Germany 1968; **Resid:** Psychiatry, Boston City Hosp 1971; Internal Medicine, Montreal Genl Hosp 1974; **Fellow:** Gastroenterology, Univ Iowa 1977; **Fac Appt:** Prof Med, Univ Iowa Coll Med

Semrad, Carol E MD [Ge] - **Spec Exp:** Celiac Disease; Diarrheal Diseases; Malabsorption Syndrome; Nutrition; **Hospital:** Univ of Chicago Med Ctr; **Address:** 5841 S Maryland Ave, MC 4080.S401, Chicago, IL 60637; **Phone:** 773-702-6921; **Board Cert:** Internal Medicine 1985; Gastroenterology 1987; **Med School:** Columbia P&S 1982; **Resid:** Internal Medicine, Columbia-Presby Med Ctr 1985; **Fellow:** Gastroenterology, Columbia-Presby Med Ctr 1986; **Fac Appt:** Assoc Prof Med, Univ Chicago-Pritzker Sch Med

Shaker, Reza MD [Ge] - **Spec Exp:** Swallowing Disorders; Gastrointestinal Motility Disorders; Gastroesophageal Reflux Disease (GERD); Pancreatic/Biliary Endoscopy (ERCP); **Hospital:** Froedtert Meml Lutheran Hosp, VA Hospital, Madison; **Address:** Med Coll Wisconsin/Gastroenterology, 9200 W Wisconsin Ave, rm E4510, Milwaukee, WI 53226; **Phone:** 414-955-6840; **Med School:** Iran 1975; **Resid:** Internal Medicine, Kingsbrook Jewish Med Ctr 1985; **Fellow:** Gastroenterology, Med Coll Wisconsin 1988; **Fac Appt:** Prof Med, Univ Wisc

Sherman, Stuart MD [Ge] - **Spec Exp:** Pancreatic & Biliary Disease; Endoscopy; Pancreatic/Biliary Endoscopy (ERCP); **Hospital:** Indiana Univ Hosp; **Address:** Indiana Univ Med Ctr, 550 N University Blvd, Ste 4100, Indianapolis, IN 46202; **Phone:** 317-274-0925; **Board Cert:** Internal Medicine 1985; Gastroenterology 1989; **Med School:** Washington Univ, St Louis 1982; **Resid:** Internal Medicine, Presby Univ Hosp 1985; **Fellow:** Gastroenterology, UCLA Med Ctr 1989; **Fac Appt:** Clin Prof Med, Indiana Univ

Silverman, William B MD [Ge] - **Spec Exp:** Pancreatic/Biliary Endoscopy (ERCP); **Hospital:** Univ Iowa Hosp & Clinics; **Address:** UIHC, Div GI/Hepatology, 200 Hawkins Drive, rm 4553 JCP, Iowa City, IA 52242; **Phone:** 319-356-4060; **Board Cert:** Internal Medicine 1988; Gastroenterology 2008; **Med School:** Belgium 1984; **Resid:** Internal Medicine, Lutheran General Hosp 1987; **Fellow:** Gastroenterology, Case Western Res Univ 1989; Gastroenterology, Indiana Univ Hosp 1990; **Fac Appt:** Prof Med, Univ Iowa Coll Med

Tremaine, William J MD [Ge] - **Spec Exp:** Inflammatory Bowel Disease/Crohn's; Ulcerative Colitis; Irritable Bowel Syndrome; **Hospital:** Mayo Med Ctr & Clin - Rochester, St Mary's Hosp - Rochester; **Address:** Mayo Clin, Div Gastroenterology, 200 First St SW, Rochester, MN 55905-0002; **Phone:** 507-284-2468; **Board Cert:** Internal Medicine 1979; Gastroenterology 1981; **Med School:** Univ Miss 1976; **Resid:** Internal Medicine, Mayo Clin 1980; **Fellow:** Gastroenterology, Mayo Clin 1981; **Fac Appt:** Prof Med, Mayo Med Sch

Van Thiel, David H MD [Ge] - **Spec Exp:** Transplant Medicine-Liver; Hepatitis; Liver Disease; **Hospital:** Rush Univ Med Ctr; **Address:** Rush Univ Hepatologists, 1725 W Harrison Rd, Ste 158, Chicago, IL 60612; **Phone:** 312-942-8910; **Board Cert:** Internal Medicine 1972; Gastroenterology 1975; **Med School:** UCLA 1967; **Resid:** Internal Medicine, NY Hosp 1969; Internal Medicine, Univ Hosp 1972; **Fellow:** Gastroenterology, Univ Hosp 1974; Research, NIH 1976; **Fac Appt:** Prof Med, Loyola Univ-Stritch Sch Med

Vargo, John J MD [Ge] - **Spec Exp:** Endoscopy; Capsule Endoscopy; Pancreatc/Biliary Endoscopy (ERCP); Pancreatic Disease; **Hospital:** Cleveland Clin - Weston; **Address:** Cleveland Clinic, 9500 Euclid Ave, MC A30, Cleveland, OH 44195; **Phone:** 216-445-5012; **Board Cert:** Internal Medicine 1988; Gastroenterology 2001; **Med School:** Univ Rochester 1985; **Resid:** Internal Medicine, Montefiore Hosp 1988; **Fellow:** Gastroenterology, Cleveland Clinic 2000; **Fac Appt:** Assoc Prof Med, Case West Res Univ

Vege, Santhi S MD [Ge] - **Spec Exp:** Pancreatic Disease; **Hospital:** Mayo Med Ctr & Clin - Rochester; **Address:** Mayo Clin, 200 First St SW Gonda Bldg Fl 9, Rochester, MN 55905; **Phone:** 507-284-2478; **Board Cert:** Internal Medicine 2007; **Med School:** India 1975; **Resid:** Internal Medicine, Govt Genl Hosp 1978; Internal Medicine, Mayo Clin 1997; **Fellow:** Gastroenterology, Post Grad Inst 1981; Gastroenterology, Mayo Clin 1998; **Fac Appt:** Prof Med, Mayo Med Sch

Wald, Arnold MD [Ge] - **Spec Exp:** Constipation; Gastrointestinal Motility Disorders; Irritable Bowel Syndrome; Incontinence-Fecal; **Hospital:** Univ WI Hosp & Clins; **Address:** Univ Wisconsin Hosp & Clinics, 600 Highland Ave, H6/516 CSC, Madison, WI 57392-2451; **Phone:** 608-263-1995; **Board Cert:** Internal Medicine 1972; Gastroenterology 1975; **Med School:** SUNY Downstate 1968; **Resid:** Internal Medicine, SUNY - Downstate Med Ctr 1971; **Fellow:** Gastroenterology, Johns Hopkins Hosp 1975; **Fac Appt:** Prof Med, Univ Wisc

Waxman, Irving MD [Ge] - **Spec Exp:** Gastrointestinal Cancer; Pancreatic Cancer; Endoscopy; **Hospital:** Univ of Chicago Med Ctr; **Address:** University of Chicago Hospitals, 5758 S Maryland Ave, MC 9028, Chicago, IL 60637; **Phone:** 773-702-1459; **Board Cert:** Internal Medicine 1988; Gastroenterology 2003; **Med School:** Mexico 1985; **Resid:** Internal Medicine, New Eng Deaconess Hosp 1988; **Fellow:** Gastroenterology, Georgetown Univ Med Ctr 1991; Endoscopy, Univ Academic Med Ctr 1991; **Fac Appt:** Prof Med, Univ Chicago-Pritzker Sch Med

Wiesner, Russell H MD [Ge] - **Spec Exp:** Transplant Medicine-Liver; **Hospital:** Mayo Med Ctr & Clin - Rochester; **Address:** Mayo Clin, Div GI, 200 First St SW, Rochester, MN 55905; **Phone:** 507-284-8714; **Board Cert:** Internal Medicine 1978; Gastroenterology 1981; **Med School:** Med Coll Wisc 1975; **Resid:** Internal Medicine, Mayo Clin 1978

Great Plains and Mountains

Bjorkman, David MD [Ge] - **Spec Exp:** Peptic Acid Disorders; Endoscopy; **Hospital:** Univ Utah Hosps and Clins; **Address:** 30 N 1900 East, Salt Lake City, UT 84132; **Phone:** 801-581-6436; **Board Cert:** Internal Medicine 1983; Gastroenterology 1985; **Med School:** Univ Utah 1980; **Resid:** Internal Medicine, Brigham & Women's Harvard 1983; **Fellow:** Gastroenterology, Brigham & Women's Harvard 1985; **Fac Appt:** Prof Med, Univ Utah

Burt, Randall W MD [Ge] - **Spec Exp:** Colon Cancer; Colon & Rectal Cancer-Familial Polyposis; **Hospital:** Univ Utah Hosps and Clins; **Address:** Huntsman Cancer Institute, 2000 Circle of Hope, Salt Lake City, UT 84112; **Phone:** 801-585-3281; **Board Cert:** Internal Medicine 1977; Gastroenterology 1979; **Med School:** Univ Utah 1974; **Resid:** Internal Medicine, Barnes Hosp 1977; **Fellow:** Gastroenterology, Univ Utah Med Ctr 1979; **Fac Appt:** Prof Med, Univ Utah

Gastroenterology

Everson, Gregory T MD [Ge] - **Spec Exp:** Liver Disease; Hepatitis; Transplant Medicine-Liver; **Hospital:** Univ Colorado Hosp; **Address:** Univ Colorado Hlth Sci Ctr, 1635 NE Aurora Ct, Box B-154, Aurora, CO 80045; **Phone:** 720-848-2245; **Board Cert:** Internal Medicine 1979; Gastroenterology 1983; Transplant Hepatology 2006; **Med School:** Cornell Univ-Weill Med Coll 1976; **Resid:** Internal Medicine, Creighton Univ Med Ctr 1979; **Fellow:** Gastroenterology, Univ Colorado Health Sci Ctr 1982; **Fac Appt:** Prof Med, Univ Colorado

Fang, John C MD [Ge] - **Spec Exp:** Endoscopy; Esophageal Disorders; Irritable Bowel Syndrome; Barrett's Esophagus; **Hospital:** Univ Utah Hosps and Clins; **Address:** 1525 W 2100 S, Salt Lake City, UT 84119; **Phone:** 801-213-9900; **Board Cert:** Gastroenterology 1998; **Med School:** Washington Univ, St Louis 1989; **Resid:** Internal Medicine, Temple Univ Hosp 1992; **Fellow:** Gastroenterology, Univ VA Hlth Sci Ctr 1995; **Fac Appt:** Assoc Prof Med, Univ Utah

Hunter, Ellen B MD [Ge] - **Spec Exp:** Hepatitis; **Hospital:** St. Luke's Reg Med Ctr - Boise; **Address:** 425 W Vannock St, Boise, ID 83702; **Phone:** 208-343-6458; **Board Cert:** Internal Medicine 1986; Gastroenterology 1989; **Med School:** Georgetown Univ 1983; **Resid:** Internal Medicine, Vanderbilt Univ Med Ctr 1986; **Fellow:** Gastroenterology, Mayo Clinic 1989

Sorrell, Michael MD [Ge] - **Spec Exp:** Transplant Medicine-Liver; Hepatitis; Liver Tumors; Liver Disease; **Hospital:** Nebraska Med Ctr; **Address:** 983285 Nebraska Medical Ctr, Omaha, NE 68198-3285; **Phone:** 402-559-7912; **Board Cert:** Internal Medicine 1972; **Med School:** Univ Nebr Coll Med 1959; **Resid:** Internal Medicine, Univ Nebraska Hosp 1968; Gastroenterology, Univ Nebraska Hosp 1969; **Fellow:** Hepatology, New Jersey Coll Med 1971; **Fac Appt:** Prof Med, Univ Nebr Coll Med

Young, Renee L MD [Ge] - **Spec Exp:** Inflammatory Bowel Disease; Crohn's Disease; **Hospital:** Nebraska Med Ctr; **Address:** Univ Nebraskaed Ctr, 982000 NE Med Ctr, Omaha, NE 68198; **Phone:** 404-559-4015; **Board Cert:** Internal Medicine 1986; Gastroenterology 2001; **Med School:** Univ Nebr Coll Med 1983; **Resid:** Internal Medicine, Univ Nebraska Med Ctr 1986; **Fellow:** Gastroenterology, Univ Nebraska Med Ctr 1990; **Fac Appt:** Assoc Prof Med, Univ Nebr Coll Med

Southwest

Anderson, Karl MD [Ge] - **Spec Exp:** Porphyria; Liver Disease; **Hospital:** UT Med Br Hosp at Galveston; **Address:** 800 Harborside Drive, Galveston, TX 77555-1109; **Phone:** 281-337-5134; **Board Cert:** Internal Medicine 1972; Gastroenterology 1972; **Med School:** Johns Hopkins Univ 1965; **Resid:** Internal Medicine, Vanderbilt Univ Hosp 1967; Internal Medicine, New York Hosp-Cornell Med Ctr 1968; **Fellow:** Gastroenterology, New York Hosp-Cornell Med Ctr 1970; **Fac Appt:** Prof Med, Univ Tex Med Br, Galveston

Balart, Luis A MD [Ge] - **Spec Exp:** Hepatitis C; **Hospital:** Tulane Univ Hosp & Clin; **Address:** 1415 Tulane Ave, New Orleans, LA 70112; **Phone:** 504-988-5800; **Board Cert:** Internal Medicine 1976; Gastroenterology 1981; **Med School:** Cuba 1973; **Resid:** Internal Medicine, Naval Regl Med Ctr 1976; **Fac Appt:** Assoc Clin Prof Med, Louisiana State U, New Orleans

Boland, C Richard MD [Ge] - **Spec Exp:** Colon & Rectal Cancer Detection; Cancer Genetics; **Hospital:** Baylor Univ Medical Ctr; **Address:** GI Cancer Research Lab H-250, 3500 Gaston Ave, Dallas, TX 75246; **Phone:** 214-820-2692; **Board Cert:** Internal Medicine 1978; Gastroenterology 1981; **Med School:** Yale Univ 1973; **Resid:** Internal Medicine, USPHS Hosp 1978; **Fellow:** Gastroenterology, UCSF Med Ctr 1981; **Fac Appt:** Clin Prof Med, Univ Tex SW, Dallas

Boyer, Thomas D MD [Ge] - **Spec Exp:** Liver Disease; Hepatitis; Transplant Medicine-Liver; **Hospital:** Univ Med Ctr - Tucson; **Address:** Arizona Liver Institute, 1501 N Campbell Ave, Box 245136, Tucson, AZ 85724; **Phone:** 520-626-5952; **Board Cert:** Internal Medicine 1975; Gastroenterology 1977; **Med School:** USC Sch Med 1969; **Resid:** Internal Medicine, LAC-USC Med Ctr 1974; **Fellow:** Hepatology, John Wesley Co Hosp-USC Med Ctr 1976; **Fac Appt:** Prof Med, Univ Ariz Coll Med

Brady III, Charles E MD [Ge] - **Spec Exp:** Esophageal Disorders; Endoscopy; **Hospital:** Univ Hlth Syst-San Antonio, Audie L Murphy Meml Vets Hosp; **Address:** Univ Tex Hlth Sci Ctr, Div GI, 7703 Floyd Curl Drive, MC 7878, San Antonio, TX 78229-3900; **Phone:** 210-567-4879; **Board Cert:** Internal Medicine 1974; Gastroenterology 1977; **Med School:** Med Coll VA 1971; **Resid:** Internal Medicine, Wilford Hall Med Ctr 1974; **Fellow:** Gastroenterology, Univ Tex 1976; **Fac Appt:** Assoc Prof Med, Univ Tex, San Antonio

Bresalier, Robert MD [Ge] - **Spec Exp:** Gastrointestinal Cancer; Peptic Acid Disorders; **Hospital:** UT MD Anderson Cancer Ctr; **Address:** MD Anderson Canc Ctr, GI Med & Nutrition, 1515 Holcombe Blvd - Unit 436, Houston, TX 77030-4009; **Phone:** 713-745-4340; **Board Cert:** Internal Medicine 1981; Gastroenterology 1983; **Med School:** Univ Chicago-Pritzker Sch Med 1978; **Resid:** Internal Medicine, Barnes Hosp-Washington Univ 1981; **Fellow:** Gastroenterology, UCSF Med Ctr 1983; **Fac Appt:** Prof Med, Univ Tex, Houston

Cunningham, John T MD [Ge] - **Spec Exp:** Biliary Disease; Pancreatic Disease; **Hospital:** Univ Med Ctr - Tucson; **Address:** Univ Medical Ctr, Div Gastroenterology, 1501 N Campbell Ave, PO Box 245028, Tucson, AZ 85724-5028; **Phone:** 520-626-6119; **Board Cert:** Internal Medicine 1975; Gastroenterology 1977; **Med School:** Med Coll VA 1970; **Resid:** Internal Medicine, Med Univ S Carolina 1975; **Fellow:** Gastroenterology, Med Univ S Carolina 1977; **Fac Appt:** Prof Med, Univ Ariz Coll Med

Das, Ananya MD [Ge] - **Spec Exp:** Endoscopy; Endoscopic Ultrasound; Pancreatic/Biliary Endoscopy (ERCP); **Hospital:** Mayo Clinic - Scottsdale; **Address:** Mayo Clinic, Div Gastroenterology, 13400 E Shea Blvd, Scottsdale, AZ 85259; **Phone:** 480-301-6990; **Board Cert:** Gastroenterology 1998; **Med School:** India 1987; **Resid:** Internal Medicine, SUNY Hlth Sci Ctr 1996; **Fellow:** Gastroenterology, Cleveland Clinic 1998; Endoscopy, Cleveland Clinic 2000; **Fac Appt:** Assoc Prof Med, Mayo Med Sch

Davis, Gary L MD [Ge] - **Spec Exp:** Liver Disease; Hepatitis; Transplant Medicine-Liver; **Hospital:** Baylor Univ Medical Ctr; **Address:** 3500 Gaston Ave, 4 Roberts, Transplant Services Department, Dallas, TX 75246; **Phone:** 214-820-8500; **Board Cert:** Internal Medicine 1979; Gastroenterology 1983; **Med School:** Univ Minn 1976; **Resid:** Internal Medicine, Mayo Clinic 1979; **Fellow:** Gastroenterology, Mayo Clinic 1981; Hepatology, Natl Inst Hlth 1984; **Fac Appt:** Prof Med, Baylor Coll Med

Fallon, Michael B MD [Ge] - **Spec Exp:** Liver Disease; Hepatitis C; **Hospital:** Meml Hermann Meml City Hosp; **Address:** UT Physicians-Genl Med, 6410 Fannin, Ste 600, Houston, TX 77030; **Phone:** 832-325-7100; **Board Cert:** Internal Medicine 1988; Gastroenterology 2001; **Med School:** Univ VA Sch Med 1984; **Resid:** Internal Medicine, Yale-New Haven Hosp 1988; **Fellow:** Gastroenterology, Yale-New Haven Hosp 1990; **Fac Appt:** Assoc Prof Med, Univ Alabama

Feldman, Mark MD [Ge] - **Spec Exp:** Peptic Acid Disorders-Consultation; **Hospital:** Presby Hosp of Dallas; **Address:** 8200 Walnut Hill Ln, Dept Internal Med, Dallas, TX 75231; **Phone:** 214-345-7881; **Board Cert:** Internal Medicine 1976; Gastroenterology 1989; **Med School:** Temple Univ 1972; **Resid:** Internal Medicine, Temple Univ 1977; **Fellow:** Gastroenterology, Univ SW Texas 1976; **Fac Appt:** Prof Med, Univ Tex SW, Dallas

Gastroenterology

Fleischer, David MD [Ge] - **Spec Exp:** Barrett's Esophagus; Esophageal Cancer; **Hospital:** Mayo Clinic - Scottsdale; **Address:** Mayo Clinic - Scottsdale, 13400 E Shea Blvd, Div Gastroenterology 2A, Scottsdale, AZ 85259; **Phone:** 480-301-8484; **Board Cert:** Internal Medicine 1975; Gastroenterology 1977; **Med School:** Vanderbilt Univ 1970; **Resid:** Internal Medicine, Metro General Hosp 1975; **Fellow:** Gastroenterology, LA Co Harbor-UCLA Med Ctr 1977; **Fac Appt:** Prof Med, Mayo Med Sch

Galati, Joseph Steven MD [Ge] - **Spec Exp:** Liver Disease; Transplant Medicine-Liver; Hepatitis C; **Hospital:** St Luke's Episcopal Hosp-Houston, Meml Hermann Hosp - Texas Med Ctr; **Address:** 6624 Fannin St, Ste 1990, Houston, TX 77030; **Phone:** 713-794-0700; **Board Cert:** Gastroenterology 2005; **Med School:** Grenada 1987; **Resid:** Internal Medicine, SUNY Hlth Sci Ctr-Kings Co Hosp 1991; **Fellow:** Gastroenterology, Univ Nebraska 1994; **Fac Appt:** Asst Prof Med, Univ Tex, Houston

Glombicki, Alan Paul MD [Ge] - **Spec Exp:** Hepatitis; Transplant Medicine-Liver; Digestive Disorders; **Hospital:** St Luke's Episcopal Hosp-Houston, Meml Hermann Hosp - Texas Med Ctr; **Address:** 7737 SW Freeway, Ste 840, Houston, TX 77074; **Phone:** 713-777-2555; **Board Cert:** Internal Medicine 1986; Gastroenterology 1987; **Med School:** Univ IL Coll Med 1981; **Resid:** Internal Medicine, Baylor Coll Med 1984; Hepatology, Baylor Coll Med 1987; **Fellow:** Gastroenterology, Baylor Coll Med 1986; **Fac Appt:** Asst Clin Prof Med, Univ Tex, Houston

Hodges, David S MD [Ge] - **Spec Exp:** Inflammatory Bowel Disease/Crohn's; Irritable Bowel Syndrome; Gastrointestinal Functional Disorders; **Hospital:** Univ Med Ctr-Lubbock; **Address:** Tex Tech Med Ctr, Dept Int Med, 3601 4th St, MS 9410, Lubbock, TX 79430; **Phone:** 806-743-3150; **Board Cert:** Internal Medicine 1986; Gastroenterology 1989; **Med School:** Texas Tech Univ 1983; **Resid:** Internal Medicine, Lubbock Genl Hosp 1986; **Fellow:** Gastroenterology, Lubbock Genl Hosp 1989; **Fac Appt:** Assoc Prof Med, Texas Tech Univ

Leighton, Jonathan A MD [Ge] - **Spec Exp:** Capsule Endoscopy; Inflammatory Bowel Disease/Crohn's; Ulcerative Colitis; **Hospital:** Mayo Clinic - Scottsdale; **Address:** Mayo Clin-Scottsdale, 13400 E Shea Blvd, Gastro.Div-2A, Scottsdale, AZ 85259; **Phone:** 480-301-8000; **Board Cert:** Internal Medicine 1984; Gastroenterology 2001; **Med School:** Univ Ariz Coll Med 1981; **Resid:** Internal Medicine, Univ Texas Hlth Sci Ctr 1984; **Fellow:** Gastroenterology, Univ Texas Hlth Sci Ctr; **Fac Appt:** Assoc Prof Med, Mayo Med Sch

Schiller, Lawrence R MD [Ge] - **Spec Exp:** Diarrheal Diseases; Gastrointestinal Functional Disorders; Gastrointestinal Motility Disorders; **Hospital:** Baylor Univ Medical Ctr; **Address:** Digestive Associates of Texas, 712 N Washington Ave, Ste 200, Dallas, TX 75246; **Phone:** 214-545-3990; **Board Cert:** Internal Medicine 1976; Gastroenterology 1981; **Med School:** Jefferson Med Coll 1972; **Resid:** Internal Medicine, Temple Univ Hosp 1976; **Fellow:** Gastroenterology, Univ Texas Hlth Sci Ctr 1980; **Fac Appt:** Clin Prof Med, Univ Tex SW, Dallas

Speeg, Kermit V MD/PhD [Ge] - **Spec Exp:** Transplant Medicine-Liver; **Hospital:** Univ Hlth Syst-San Antonio; **Address:** Dept Gastroenterology, 7703 Floyd Curl Drive, MC 7878, San Antonio, TX 78229-3900; **Phone:** 210-567-4879; **Board Cert:** Internal Medicine 1976; **Med School:** Univ Tex SW, Dallas 1972; **Resid:** Internal Medicine, Vanderbilt Univ Hosp 1974; **Fellow:** Gastroenterology, Vanderbilt Univ Hosp 1977; **Fac Appt:** Prof Med, Univ Tex, San Antonio

Stump, David L MD [Ge] - **Hospital:** Methodist Hosp-San Antonio; **Address:** Gastroenterology Clinic SA, 8550 Datapoint Drive, Ste LL100, San Antonio, TX 78229-3436; **Phone:** 210-615-8308; **Board Cert:** Internal Medicine 1983; Gastroenterology 1985; **Med School:** Indiana Univ 1980; **Resid:** Internal Medicine, Indiana Univ Med Ctr 1983; **Fellow:** Gastroenterology, UT San Antonio 1985

Vierling, John M MD [Ge] - **Spec Exp:** Liver Disease; Transplant Medicine-Liver; Autoimmune Liver Disease; Hepatitis B & C; **Hospital:** St Luke's Episcopal Hosp-Houston; **Address:** Dept of Med, Baylor College of Med, 1709 Dryden, Ste 500, Houston, TX 77030; **Phone:** 713-798-8070; **Board Cert:** Internal Medicine 1975; Gastroenterology 1979; Transplant Hepatology 2006; **Med School:** Stanford Univ 1972; **Resid:** Internal Medicine, Strong Meml Hosp 1974; Hepatology, Natl Inst Hlth 1977; **Fellow:** Gastroenterology, UCSF Med Ctr 1978; **Fac Appt:** Prof Med, Baylor Coll Med

West Coast and Pacific

Cello, John P MD [Ge] - **Spec Exp:** Endoscopy; Colonoscopy; Capsule Endoscopy; Pancreatic/Biliary Endoscopy (ERCP); **Hospital:** San Francisco Genl Hosp, UCSF Med Ctr; **Address:** San Francisco Genl Hosp-Univ California, 1001 Potrero Ave, Ste NH3D, San Francisco, CA 94110; **Phone:** 415-206-4746; **Board Cert:** Internal Medicine 1972; Gastroenterology 1977; **Med School:** Harvard Med Sch 1969; **Resid:** Internal Medicine, Peter Bent Brigham Hosp 1972; **Fellow:** Gastroenterology, UCSF Med Ctr 1977; **Fac Appt:** Prof Med, UCSF

Chang, Kenneth J MD [Ge] - **Spec Exp:** Gastrointestinal Cancer; Endoscopic Ultrasound; **Hospital:** UC Irvine Med Ctr; **Address:** UC Irvine Med Ctr, 101 The City Drive 22C Bldg, Orange, CA 92868; **Phone:** 714-456-6187; **Board Cert:** Internal Medicine 1988; Gastroenterology 2001; **Med School:** Brown Univ 1985; **Resid:** Internal Medicine, Rhode Island Hosp 1988; **Fellow:** Gastroenterology, UC-Irvine Med Ctr 1990

Ellis, Jonathan C MD [Ge] - **Hospital:** Cedars-Sinai Med Ctr; **Address:** 9090 Wilshire Blvd, Ste 101, Beverly Hills, CA 90211; **Phone:** 310-550-0400; **Board Cert:** Internal Medicine 1985; Gastroenterology 1989; **Med School:** Stanford Univ 1982; **Resid:** Internal Medicine, Cedars Sinai Med Ctr 1986; **Fellow:** Gastroenterology, UCLA 1988; **Fac Appt:** Assoc Prof Med, UCLA

Fennerty, Brian MD [Ge] - **Spec Exp:** Gastroesophageal Reflux Disease (GERD); **Hospital:** OR Hlth & Sci Univ; **Address:** Digestive Hlth, Ctr for Hlth & Healing, 3303 SW Bond Ave Fl 6, Portland, OR 97239; **Phone:** 503-494-4373; **Board Cert:** Internal Medicine 1984; Gastroenterology 2008; **Med School:** Creighton Univ 1980; **Resid:** Internal Medicine, Naval Hospital 1984; **Fellow:** Gastroenterology, Arizona Hlth Sci Ctr 1989; **Fac Appt:** Prof Med, Oregon Hlth & Sci Univ

Gerson, Lauren B MD [Ge] - **Spec Exp:** Gastroesophageal Reflux Disease (GERD); Barrett's Esophagus; Esophageal Disorders; Capsule Endoscopy; **Hospital:** Stanford Univ Med Ctr; **Address:** Stanford Univ Med Ctr, Gastroenterology, 300 Pasteur Drive, rm A149, MC 5202, Stanford, CA 94305; **Phone:** 650-723-6961; **Board Cert:** Gastroenterology 2002; **Med School:** SUNY Buffalo 1990; **Resid:** Internal Medicine, California Pacific Med Ctr 1993; **Fellow:** Gastroenterology, Stanford Univ Med Ctr 1995; **Fac Appt:** Assoc Prof Med, Stanford Univ

Gish, Robert MD [Ge] - **Spec Exp:** Liver Cancer; Transplant Medicine-Liver; Hepatitis; Clinical Trials; **Hospital:** CA Pacific Med Ctr - Pacific Campus; **Address:** 2340 Clay St Fl 3, San Francisco, CA 94115; **Phone:** 415-600-1020; **Board Cert:** Internal Medicine 1984; Gastroenterology 1987; Transplant Hepatology 2006; **Med School:** Univ Kans 1980; **Resid:** Internal Medicine, UCSD Med Ctr 1983; **Fellow:** Gastroenterology, UCLA Med Ctr 1988; **Fac Appt:** Assoc Clin Prof Med, UCSF

Han, Steven-Huy B MD [Ge] - **Spec Exp:** Transplant Medicine-Liver; Hepatitis B & C; Liver Disease; **Hospital:** UCLA Ronald Reagan Med Ctr; **Address:** UCLA Medical Ctr, 200 UCLA Medical Plaza, Ste 214, Los Angeles, CA 90095; **Phone:** 310-794-7788; **Board Cert:** Gastroenterology 1998; Transplant Hepatology 2006; **Med School:** Albany Med Coll 1990; **Resid:** Internal Medicine, Santa Clara Valley Med Ctr 1993; **Fellow:** Gastroenterology, USC Med Ctr 1996; Hepatology, UCLA Med Ctr 1996; **Fac Appt:** Assoc Prof Med, UCLA

Gastroenterology

Hillebrand, Donald J MD [Ge] - **Spec Exp:** Transplant Medicine-Liver; Liver Failure; **Hospital:** Scripps Green Hosp; **Address:** Scripps Green Hosp, 10666 N Torrey Pines Rd, MC 203N, La Jolla, CA 92037; **Phone:** 858-455-9100; **Board Cert:** Internal Medicine 2004; Gastroenterology 2006; Transplant Hepatology 2006; **Med School:** Univ Iowa Coll Med 1990; **Resid:** Internal Medicine, Univ Iowa Hosps 1993; **Fellow:** Gastroenterology, Univ Iowa Hosps 1994

Kimmey, Michael B MD [Ge] - **Spec Exp:** Pancreatic/Biliary Endoscopy (ERCP); Endoscopy; Endoscopic Ultrasound; **Hospital:** St Joseph Med Ctr - Tacoma, Tacoma Genl Hosp; **Address:** 1112 6th Ave, Ste 200, Tacoma, WA 98405; **Phone:** 253-272-8664; **Board Cert:** Internal Medicine 1982; Gastroenterology 1987; **Med School:** Washington Univ, St Louis 1979; **Resid:** Internal Medicine, Univ Wash Med Ctr 1982; **Fellow:** Gastroenterology, Univ Wash Med Ctr 1987; **Fac Appt:** Clin Prof Med, Univ Wash

Kozarek, Richard MD [Ge] - **Spec Exp:** Pancreatic/Biliary Endoscopy (ERCP); Inflammatory Bowel Disease; Pancreatic Disease; **Hospital:** Virginia Mason Med Ctr, Swedish Med Ctr - Seattle; **Address:** 1100 9th Ave, Seattle, WA 98101-2756; **Phone:** 206-223-6934; **Board Cert:** Internal Medicine 1977; Gastroenterology 1979; **Med School:** Univ Wisc 1973; **Resid:** Internal Medicine, Good Samaritan Hosp 1976; **Fellow:** Gastroenterology, Univ Arizona/ VA Hosp 1978; **Fac Appt:** Clin Prof Med, Univ Wash

Lenz, Heinz J MD [Ge] - **Spec Exp:** Gastrointestinal Cancer; Colon & Rectal Cancer; **Hospital:** USC Univ Hosp; **Address:** 1441 East Lake Ave, NOR 3456, Los Angeles, CA 90033; **Phone:** 323-865-3955; **Board Cert:** Internal Medicine 2000; Gastroenterology 2000; **Med School:** Germany 1981; **Resid:** Internal Medicine, Univ Hamburg Affil Hosp 1987; Internal Medicine, UC San Diego Med Ctr 1989; **Fellow:** Gastroenterology, UC San Diego Med Ctr 1990; **Fac Appt:** Prof Med, USC-Keck School of Medicine

Ostroff, James W MD [Ge] - **Spec Exp:** Pancreatic/Biliary Endoscopy (ERCP); Colonoscopy; **Hospital:** UCSF Med Ctr, UCSF - Mt Zion Med Ctr; **Address:** 350 Parnassus Ave, Ste 410, San Francisco, CA 94117-3608; **Phone:** 415-502-2112; **Board Cert:** Internal Medicine 1980; Gastroenterology 1983; **Med School:** Cornell Univ-Weill Med Coll 1977; **Resid:** Internal Medicine, NY Hosp-Cornell Med Ctr 1980; **Fellow:** Gastroenterology, UCSF Hosps 1982; **Fac Appt:** Prof Med, UCSF

Pasricha, Pankaj MD [Ge] - **Spec Exp:** Swallowing Disorders-Botox Therapy; Gastrointestinal Motility Disorders; Pancreatic Disease; **Hospital:** Stanford Univ Med Ctr; **Address:** 300 Pasteur Drive, rm A175, MC 5309, Stanford, CA 94305; **Phone:** 650-723-6961; **Board Cert:** Internal Medicine 1988; Gastroenterology 2006; **Med School:** India 1983; **Resid:** Internal Medicine, DC Genl Hosp 1988; **Fellow:** Pulmonary Disease, New England Med Ctr 1990; Gastroenterology, Johns Hopkins Hosp 1992; **Fac Appt:** Prof Med, Univ Tex Med Br, Galveston

Poordad, Fred F MD [Ge] - **Spec Exp:** Liver Disease; Hepatitis B & C; Transplant Medicine-Liver; **Hospital:** Cedars-Sinai Med Ctr; **Address:** Cedars Sinai Medical Ctr, Liver Diseases, West Tower, 8635 W 3rd St, Ste 590, Los Angeles, CA 90048; **Phone:** 310-423-2641; **Board Cert:** Gastroenterology 2005; Transplant Hepatology 2006; **Med School:** Canada 1990; **Resid:** Internal Medicine, St Thomas Med Ctr/Ohio State Univ Med Ctr 1993; **Fellow:** Gastroenterology, Univ S Carolina Med Ctr 1995; Hepatology, Johns Hopkins Hosp 2005; **Fac Appt:** Assoc Prof Med, UCLA-David Geffen Sch Med

Roth, Bennett E MD [Ge] - **Spec Exp:** Gastroesophageal Reflux Disease (GERD); Inflammatory Bowel Disease/Crohn's; Irritable Bowel Syndrome; **Hospital:** UCLA Ronald Reagan Med Ctr; **Address:** 200 UCLA Med Plaza, Ste 365A, Los Angeles, CA 90095; **Phone:** 310-825-1597; **Board Cert:** Internal Medicine 1972; Gastroenterology 1975; **Med School:** Hahnemann Univ 1968; **Resid:** Internal Medicine, Hosp Univ Penn 1971; **Fellow:** Gastroenterology, UCLA Med Ctr 1974; **Fac Appt:** Prof Med, UCLA

Surawicz, Christina MD [Ge] - **Spec Exp:** Clostridium Difficile Disease; Infectious Diarrhea; **Hospital:** Harborview Med Ctr, Univ Wash Med Ctr; **Address:** 325 9th Ave, Box 359773, Seattle, WA 98104-2420; **Phone:** 206-731-5021; **Board Cert:** Internal Medicine 1976; Gastroenterology 1979; **Med School:** Univ KY Coll Med 1973; **Resid:** Internal Medicine, Univ Washington Med Ctr 1976; **Fellow:** Gastroenterology, Univ Washington Med Ctr 1979; **Fac Appt:** Prof Med, Univ Wash

Targan, Stephan R MD [Ge] - **Spec Exp:** Inflammatory Bowel Disease; Crohn's Disease; **Hospital:** Cedars-Sinai Med Ctr; **Address:** Cedars-Sinai IBD Ctr, 8723 Alden Drive, Ste 3, Los Angeles, CA 90048; **Phone:** 310-423-4100; **Board Cert:** Internal Medicine 1974; Infectious Disease 1976; Gastroenterology 1979; **Med School:** Johns Hopkins Univ 1971; **Resid:** Internal Medicine, Harbor-UCLA Med Ctr 1976; **Fellow:** Infectious Disease, Harbor-UCLA Med Ctr 1976; Gastroenterology, UCLA Med Ctr 1978; **Fac Appt:** Prof Med, UCLA

THE MOUNT SINAI MEDICAL CENTER
GASTROINTESTINAL AND SURGICAL SPECIALTIES

One Gustave L. Levy Place
Fifth Avenue and 100th Street
New York, NY 10029-6574
Physician Referral: 1-800-MD-SINAI (637-4624)
www.mountsinai.org

MOUNT SINAI
SCHOOL OF
MEDICINE

Mount Sinai's **DIVISIONS OF GASTROENTEROLOGY, COLON AND RECTAL SURGERY, LIVER DISEASES, AND PEDIATRIC GASTROENTEROLOGY, NUTRITION, AND LIVER DISEASES** are renowned for their delivery of patient care, research, and education in diseases of the gastrointestinal (GI) tract. In 2000, the National Institutesof Health (NIH) recognized the importance of Mount Sinai as a research center with a grant forGI/Liver fellowship training. Mount Sinai is the only medical school in New York City to earn this prestigious award.

Division of Gastroenterology – Successes within the Division include breakthroughs in the medical and surgical management of inflammatory bowel disease (IBD), ulcerative colitis, and Crohn's disease. Mount Sinai spearheaded novel therapies for treating severe IBD and helped establish the role of colonoscopy in preventing colon cancer by removing precancerous polyps. More recent innovations include employing a tiny camera within a swallowable capsule to capture images in the stomach and intestines. Mount Sinai's IBD Center, Women's GI Health Center, and GI Cancer Center offer patients the latest comprehensive, interdisciplinary care; newer agents through clinical trials; and services of such specialists as psychologists and nutritionists.

Division of Colon and Rectal Surgery – Mount Sinai surgeons have a distinguished history in the surgical treatment of gastrointestinal disorders, and surgeons in the Division continue that tradition today, focusing on surgical therapies for all diseases involving the colon, rectum, and anus. With expertise in the treatment of Crohn's disease (which was first described at Mount Sinai in 1932), ulcerative colitis, colon and rectal cancer, and diverticulitis, we specialize in the newer techniques of rectal surgery with an emphasis on colostomy avoidance. The newest minimally invasive techniques are offered as well as other cutting-edge technologies for the treatment of such disorders as hemorrhoids, fistulas, and rectal tumors.

Division of Liver Diseases – With a steadily growing research budget, Mount Sinai carries out a diverse portfolio of research projects. These projects feature both clinical care and scientific investigations, including liver transplantation; diagnosis and treatment of viral hepatitis; treatment of scarring, or fibrosis; management of primary biliary cirrhosis, an autoimmune disease of bile ducts; treatment of liver cancer; and diagnosis and treatment of genetic liver diseases, including Wilson's disease (copper overload) and hemachromatosis (iron overload).

Division of Pediatric Gastroenterology, Nutrition, and Liver Diseases – The Division provides consultative services and treatment for the full range of children's digestive and nutritional diseases. The Children's IBD Center is the only multidisciplinary center for pediatric patients with Crohn's disease and ulcerative colitis in the New York metropolitan area and receives referrals from across the country. The Transplant Program is one of the largest in the nation and was the first program in New York to perform liver transplants and, later, small bowel transplants. The Division is active in clinical research in IBD, focusing on issues of genetic factors, psychosocial interactions, and drug trials. Several NIH grants support research in the areas of biliary atresia, bile salt absorption, and outcome analysis in children with liver failure.

Surgical Programs for Gastrointestinal Disorders – Mount Sinai provides a comprehensive center, uniting the medical disciplines of gastroenterology and its related surgical specialties, as well as an array of minimally invasive surgical programs. The center houses renowned programs for the treatment of IBD and colorectal diseases, as well as Reconstructive and Laparoscopic Surgery Programs through the Division of Laparoscopic Surgery, which is internationally known for pioneering a number of minimally invasive procedures for the treatment of Crohn's disease and ulcerative colitis.

NYU Langone Medical Center

550 First Avenue (at 31St Street)
New York, NY 10016
Physician Referral:
(888)7-NYU-MED (888-769-8633)
www.med.nyu.edu

GASTROENTEROLOGY

About the Division of Gastroenterology, Department of Medicine:

The Division of Gastroenterology at NYU Langone Medical Center is dedicated to the diagnosis and treatment of patients with diseases of the gastrointestinal tract. Its physicians offer a rich body of knowledge in the diagnosis and management of inflammatory bowel disease, peptic ulcer disease, esophageal disorders, gastrointestinal cancer, and liver, biliary and pancreatic diseases.

We specialize in the following areas:

COLORECTAL CANCER

NYU Langone Medical Center offers the most advanced screening options available for the diagnosis of colon cancer, the second leading cause of cancer death in the U.S. Additionally, members of the Division continue to investigate colorectal cancer screenings in special populations such as women, veterans, immigrants, minorities and patients with HIV, and offer the use of virtual colonoscopy for the detection of colorectal polyps and cancer.

ESOPHAGEAL DISEASES

The Esophageal Disease Center at NYU Langone Medical Center offers patients state-of-the-art diagnosis and treatment of esophageal disorders and an ongoing program of translational and clinical research. The Center focuses on gastroesophageal reflux disease, esophageal motility disorders, Barrett's esophagus, adenocarcinoma of the esophagus and swallowing disorders. The Center offers diagnostic studies, such as esophageal manometry, impedance testing for swallowing, pH catheter and impedance testing for reflux and BRAVO capsule pH testing, as well as therapies, such Barrett's ablation and esophageal dilations, including those for achalasia.

GASTROINTESTINAL CANCERS

Gastrointestinal cancers are the most common group of cancers in the United States, accounting for approximately 20 percent of all non-skin cancers. They include cancers of the esophagus, stomach, colon/rectum, small intestine, liver, pancreas, gallbladder, and biliary tract. NYU Cancer Institute physicians treat patients with all types of gastrointestinal cancers, including those with complex cases such as those with recurrent disease or those whose disease persists despite treatments received elsewhere. Patients have the opportunity to participate in numerous clinical trials.

NATIONALLY RECOGNIZED LEADERS

Members of the Division of Gastroenterology are nationally recognized and are involved in numerous studies focusing on gastroenterology and hepatology, including clinical research in liver diseases (especially hepatitis C), colon cancer screenings, acute and chronic GI bleeding, and Helicobacter pylori (bacterial inflammation of the stomach).

COMPLEX TREATMENTS AND DIAGNOSIS

Members of the Division have specific interest and expertise in the diagnosis of gastrointestinal bleeding of obscure origin, including the use of enteroscopy and capsule endoscopy. They have specific interest in diagnosis and treatment of patients with complex pancreatic-biliary diseases, including the use of ERCP and endoscopic ultrasound.

VIRTUAL COLONOSCOPY

NYU Langone Medical Center offers the latest developments in colon cancer detection, including virtual colonoscopy. The noninvasive procedure makes use of sophisticated imaging techniques to generate a 3-D reconstruction of the colon, which can then be evaluated for abnormalities by specially trained radiologists. The study gives a complete evaluation of the entire surface of the colon and can be performed more quickly, with little discomfort and extremely accurate readings.

Geriatric Medicine

a subspecialty of Internal Medicine or Family Practice

An internist or family physician with special knowledge of the aging process and special skills in the diagnostic, therapeutic, preventive and rehabilitative aspects of illness in the elderly. This specialist cares for geriatric patients in the patient's home, the office, long-term care settings such as nursing homes and the hospital.

Family Medicine

A family physician is concerned with the total healthcare of the individual and the family, and is trained to diagnose and treat a wide variety of ailments in patients of all ages. The family physician receives a broad range of training that includes internal medicine, pediatrics, obstetrics and gynecology, psychiatry and geriatrics. Special emphasis is placed on prevention and the primary care of entire families, utilizing consultations and community resources when appropriate.

Training Required: Three years in internal medicine or family practice *plus* additional training and examination for certification in geriatric medicine.

GERIATRIC MEDICINE

New England

Cooney Jr, Leo M MD [Ger] - **Spec Exp:** Geriatric Functional Assessment; Rheumatology; Mobility Evaluation & Treatment; **Hospital:** Yale-New Haven Hosp; **Address:** Yale-New Haven Hosp, Adler Geriatric Ctr, 20 York St, New Haven, CT 06510; **Phone:** 203-688-2204; **Board Cert:** Internal Medicine 1974; Rheumatology 1978; Geriatric Medicine 2000; **Med School:** Yale Univ 1969; **Resid:** Internal Medicine, Boston City Hosp 1971; Internal Medicine, Boston City Hosp 1974; **Fellow:** Rheumatology, Boston Med Ctr 1975; **Fac Appt:** Prof Med, Yale Univ

Lipsitz, Lewis Arnold MD [Ger] - **Spec Exp:** Falls in the Elderly; Hypertension; Hypotension; Syncope; **Hospital:** Beth Israel Deaconess Med Ctr - Boston, Hebrew Rehab Ctr for the Aged; **Address:** Beth Israel Med Ctr, Gerontology, 110 Francis St, LMOB 1B, Boston, MA 02215; **Phone:** 617-632-8696; **Board Cert:** Internal Medicine 1980; Geriatric Medicine 1999; **Med School:** Univ Pennsylvania 1977; **Resid:** Internal Medicine, Beth Israel Hosp 1980; **Fellow:** Geriatric Medicine, Harvard Med School Affil Hosp 1983; **Fac Appt:** Prof Med, Harvard Med Sch

Minaker, Kenneth MD [Ger] - **Spec Exp:** Aging; Neuroendocrinology; Cardiovascular Disease; **Hospital:** Mass Genl Hosp, Brigham & Women's Hosp; **Address:** Charles River Plaza, Ste 502, 165 Cambridge St, Boston, MA 02114-2723; **Phone:** 617-726-4600; **Med School:** Univ Toronto 1972; **Resid:** Internal Medicine, Univ Toronto 1981; **Fellow:** Geriatric Medicine, Mass Gen Hosp 1983; **Fac Appt:** Assoc Prof Med, Harvard Med Sch

Tinetti, Mary E MD [Ger] - **Spec Exp:** Falls in the Elderly; Geriatric Functional Assessment; **Hospital:** Yale-New Haven Hosp; **Address:** Yale-New Haven Hosp, Adler Geriatric Ctr, 20 York St, New Haven, CT 06510; **Phone:** 203-688-6361; **Board Cert:** Internal Medicine 1981; **Med School:** Univ Mich Med Sch 1978; **Resid:** Internal Medicine, Univ Minnesota 1981; **Fellow:** Geriatric Medicine, Univ Rochester 1984; **Fac Appt:** Prof Med, Yale Univ

Mid Atlantic

Bloom, Patricia A MD [Ger] - **Spec Exp:** Dementia; Geriatric Functional Assessment; Osteoporosis; **Hospital:** Mount Sinai Med Ctr (page 64); **Address:** 1440 Madison Ave, New York, NY 10029-6542; **Phone:** 212-659-8552; **Board Cert:** Internal Medicine 1978; Geriatric Medicine 1998; **Med School:** Univ Minn 1975; **Resid:** Internal Medicine, Montefiore Med Ctr 1978; **Fac Appt:** Assoc Prof Med, Mount Sinai Sch Med

Burton, John R MD [Ger] - **Hospital:** Johns Hopkins Bayview Med Ctr (page 61); **Address:** Division of Geriatric Medicine, 5505 Hopkins Bayview Cir, Baltimore, MD 21224; **Phone:** 410-550-0520; **Board Cert:** Internal Medicine 1980; Geriatric Medicine 2005; Nephrology 1974; **Med School:** McGill Univ 1965; **Resid:** Internal Medicine, Baltimore City Hosp 1971; **Fellow:** Nephrology, Mass Genl Hosp 1972; **Fac Appt:** Prof Med, Johns Hopkins Univ

Finucane, Thomas E MD [Ger] - **Spec Exp:** Pain Management; Swallowing Disorders; Ethics; Palliative Care; **Hospital:** Johns Hopkins Bayview Med Ctr (page 61), Johns Hopkins Hosp (page 61); **Address:** 5505 Hopkins Bayview Cir, Level 01, Baltimore, MD 21224; **Phone:** 410-550-0925; **Board Cert:** Internal Medicine 1982; Geriatric Medicine 1998; **Med School:** Emory Univ 1978; **Resid:** Internal Medicine, George Washington Univ Hosp 1982; **Fac Appt:** Prof Med, Johns Hopkins Univ

Freedman, Michael L MD [Ger] - **Spec Exp:** Alzheimer's Disease; Anemia; Nutrition; **Hospital:** NYU Langone Med Ctr (page 67), Bellevue Hosp Ctr; **Address:** 530 First Ave, Ste 4J, New York, NY 10016-6402; **Phone:** 212-263-7043; **Board Cert:** Internal Medicine 1971; Hematology 1974; Geriatric Medicine 1998; **Med School:** Tufts Univ 1963; **Resid:** Internal Medicine, Bellevue Hosp 1965; Internal Medicine, Bellevue Hosp 1969; **Fellow:** Hematology, Natl Inst Hlth-NCI 1968; **Fac Appt:** Prof Med, NYU Sch Med

Gambert, Steven R MD [Ger] - **Spec Exp:** Endocrinology; Osteoporosis; Aging; **Hospital:** Univ of MD Med Ctr; **Address:** Univ Maryland, Dept Medicine, 22 S Greene St, rm N3E09, Baltimore, MD 21201; **Phone:** 410-328-2454; **Board Cert:** Internal Medicine 1978; **Med School:** Columbia P&S 1975; **Resid:** Internal Medicine, Dartmouth Affl Hosp 1977; **Fellow:** Geriatric Medicine, Beth Israel Hosp-Harvard 1979; Endocrinology, Beth Israel Hosp-Harvard 1979; **Fac Appt:** Prof Med, Univ MD Sch Med

Lachs, Mark S MD [Ger] - **Spec Exp:** Abuse/Neglect; **Hospital:** NY-Presby Hosp/Weill Cornell (page 66); **Address:** Irving Sherwood Wright Center on Aging, 1484 First Ave, New York, NY 10075; **Phone:** 212-746-7000; **Board Cert:** Internal Medicine 1988; Geriatric Medicine 2002; **Med School:** NYU Sch Med 1985; **Resid:** Internal Medicine, Hosp Univ Penn 1988; **Fellow:** Geriatric Medicine, Yale Univ 1990; **Fac Appt:** Prof Med, Cornell Univ-Weill Med Coll

Meier, Diane E MD [Ger] - **Spec Exp:** Palliative Care; **Hospital:** Mount Sinai Med Ctr (page 64); **Address:** Mt Sinai School Medicine, Box 1070, New York, NY 10029-6501; **Phone:** 212-241-1446; **Board Cert:** Internal Medicine 1981; Geriatric Medicine 1999; Hospice & Palliative Medicine 2008; **Med School:** Northwestern Univ 1977; **Resid:** Internal Medicine, Oregon Hlth Sci Univ 1981; **Fellow:** Geriatric Medicine, VA Med Ctr 1983; **Fac Appt:** Prof Med, Mount Sinai Sch Med

Palmer, Robert M MD [Ger] - **Spec Exp:** Geriatric Functional Assessment; Dementia; **Hospital:** UPMC Presby, Pittsburgh; **Address:** 3471 5th Ave Kaufmann Bldg - Ste 500, Pittsburgh, PA 15213; **Phone:** 412-692-4200; **Board Cert:** Internal Medicine 1975; Geriatric Medicine 1998; **Med School:** Univ Mich Med Sch 1971; **Resid:** Internal Medicine, LA County Med Ctr 1975; **Fellow:** Geriatric Medicine, UCLA Med Ctr 1986

Resnick, Neil M MD [Ger] - **Spec Exp:** Voiding Dysfunction; Incontinence; **Hospital:** UPMC Presby, Pittsburgh, UPMC Shadyside; **Address:** 3471 5th Ave, Kaufmann Bldg, Ste 500, Pittsburgh, PA 15213-3313; **Phone:** 412-692-2364; **Board Cert:** Internal Medicine 1980; Geriatric Medicine 1998; **Med School:** Stanford Univ 1977; **Resid:** Internal Medicine, Beth Israel Hosp 1980; **Fellow:** Geriatric Medicine, Harvard Univ 1982; Urodynamics, Harvard Univ 1984; **Fac Appt:** Prof Med, Univ Pittsburgh

Studenski, Stephanie A MD [Ger] - **Spec Exp:** Balance Disorders; Mobility Evaluation & Treatment; Falls in the Elderly; **Hospital:** UPMC Presby, Pittsburgh; **Address:** 4 East Montifiore, 200 Lothrop St, Pittsburgh, PA 15213; **Phone:** 412-692-4200; **Board Cert:** Internal Medicine 1982; Rheumatology 1984; Geriatric Medicine 2002; **Med School:** Univ Kans 1979; **Resid:** Internal Medicine, Duke Univ Med Ctr 1982; **Fellow:** Rheumatology, Duke Univ Med Ctr 1984; Geriatric Medicine, Duke Univ Med Ctr 1986; **Fac Appt:** Prof Med, Univ Pittsburgh

Southeast

Boling, Peter A MD [Ger] - **Spec Exp:** Frail Elderly; Home Care; **Hospital:** VCU Med Ctr; **Address:** VCU Medical Center, Div General Internal Medicine, PO Box 980102, Richmond, VA 23298-0102; **Phone:** 804-828-9357; **Board Cert:** Internal Medicine 1984; Geriatric Medicine 2000; **Med School:** Univ Rochester 1981; **Resid:** Internal Medicine, Med Coll Va Hosp Hosp 1984; **Fac Appt:** Prof Med, Med Coll VA

Geriatric Medicine

Ciocon, Jerry O MD [Ger] - **Spec Exp:** Chronic Fatigue-Elderly; Pain-Musculoskeletal; Memory Disorders; **Hospital:** Cleveland Clin - Weston; **Address:** Cleveland Clinic, Div Geriatrics, 2950 Cleveland Clinic Blvd, Weston, FL 33331-3609; **Phone:** 954-659-5867; **Board Cert:** Internal Medicine 1985; Geriatric Medicine 2000; **Med School:** Philippines 1980; **Resid:** Internal Medicine, Mercy Hosp 1985; **Fellow:** Geriatric Medicine, LI Jewish Med Ctr 1987; **Fac Appt:** Asst Clin Prof Med, Ohio State Univ

Greganti, Mac A MD [Ger] - **Spec Exp:** Diagnostic Problems; Dementia; **Hospital:** Univ NC Hosps; **Address:** Univ North Carolina Hosp, Dept Med, 125 MacNider Bldg CB#7005, Chapel Hill, NC 27599-7005; **Phone:** 919-966-3063; **Board Cert:** Internal Medicine 1987; **Med School:** Univ Miss 1972; **Resid:** Internal Medicine, Strong Meml Hosp 1975; **Fac Appt:** Prof Med, Univ NC Sch Med

Groene, Linda A MD [Ger] - **Spec Exp:** Osteoporosis; Sleep Disorders/Apnea; Dementia; **Hospital:** Imperial Point Med Ctr, Holy Cross Hosp - Fort Lauderdale; **Address:** 6405 N Federal Hwy, Ste 102, Ft Lauderdale, FL 33308; **Phone:** 954-772-0062; **Board Cert:** Internal Medicine 1986; Geriatric Medicine 2000; **Med School:** Louisiana State U, New Orleans 1981; **Resid:** Pathology, Jackson Meml Hosp 1983; Internal Medicine, Mt Sinai Med Ctr 1986

Hanson, Laura C MD [Ger] - **Spec Exp:** Frailty Syndrome; Palliative Care; **Hospital:** Univ NC Hosps; **Address:** UNC Sch Med, MacNider Bldg - rm 262, CB 7550, Chapel Hill, NC 27599; **Phone:** 919-966-5945 x251; **Board Cert:** Internal Medicine 1989; Geriatric Medicine 2002; **Med School:** Harvard Med Sch 1986; **Resid:** Internal Medicine, Brigham & Womens Hosp 1988; Internal Medicine, Univ North Carolina Hosp 1989; **Fellow:** Geriatric Medicine, Univ North Carolina Hosp 1991; **Fac Appt:** Assoc Prof Med, Univ NC Sch Med

Lyles, Kenneth W MD [Ger] - **Spec Exp:** Bone Disorders-Metabolic; Tumoral Calcinosis; Parathyroid Disease; **Hospital:** Duke Univ Med Ctr, VA Med Ctr - Durham; **Address:** Duke Univ Med Center, Box 3881, Durham, NC 27710; **Phone:** 919-660-7520; **Board Cert:** Internal Medicine 1977; Endocrinology 1979; Geriatric Medicine 2000; **Med School:** Med Coll VA 1974; **Resid:** Internal Medicine, Med Coll VA 1977; **Fellow:** Endocrinology, Diabetes & Metabolism, Duke Univ Med Ctr 1979; Geriatric Medicine, Duke Univ/VA Med Ctr 1981; **Fac Appt:** Prof Med, Duke Univ

Ritchie, Christine S MD [Ger] - **Spec Exp:** Palliative Care; **Hospital:** Univ of Ala Hosp at Birmingham; **Address:** UAB Hospital, 1521 11th Ave S, Birmingham, AL 35294; **Phone:** 205-975-8190; **Board Cert:** Internal Medicine 2002; Geriatric Medicine 2006; Hospice & Palliative Medicine 2003; **Med School:** Univ NC Sch Med 1988; **Resid:** Internal Medicine, Univ Ala Sch Med 1992; **Fellow:** Geriatric Medicine, Univ Ala Sch Med 1994; **Fac Appt:** Assoc Prof Med, Univ Alabama

Midwest

Carr, David B MD [Ger] - **Spec Exp:** Polypharmacology (Excess Medications); Alzheimer's Disease; **Hospital:** Barnes-Jewish Hosp; **Address:** Wash Univ Sch Med, Div Geriatrics, 4488 Forest Park, Ste 160, St Louis, MO 63108; **Phone:** 314-286-1967; **Board Cert:** Internal Medicine 1989; Geriatric Medicine 2000; **Med School:** Univ MO-Columbia Sch Med 1985; **Resid:** Internal Medicine, Mich State Assoc Hosps 1988; **Fellow:** Geriatric Medicine, Duke Univ 1990; **Fac Appt:** Prof Med, Washington Univ, St Louis

Dale, Lowell C MD [Ger] - **Spec Exp:** Tobacco Abuse; Nutrition; **Hospital:** Mayo Med Ctr & Clin - Rochester; **Address:** Mayo Clinic, 200 First St SW, Colonial 3-10, Rochester, MN 55905; **Phone:** 507-284-2439; **Board Cert:** Internal Medicine 1984; **Med School:** Univ Minn 1981; **Resid:** Internal Medicine, Mayo Clin 1984; **Fellow:** Internal Medicine, Mayo Clin 1985; **Fac Appt:** Asst Prof Med, Mayo Med Sch

Duthie, Edmund H MD [Ger] - **Spec Exp:** Geriatric Functional Assessment; **Hospital:** Froedtert Meml Lutheran Hosp, Clement J Zablocki VA Med Ctr; **Address:** 9200 W Wisconsin Ave, Milwaukee, WI 53226; **Phone:** 262-253-2455; **Board Cert:** Internal Medicine 1979; Geriatric Medicine 1998; **Med School:** Georgetown Univ 1976; **Resid:** Internal Medicine, Med Coll Wisc Hosps 1979; **Fellow:** Geriatric Medicine, Jewish Inst Geri Care-SUNY 1980; **Fac Appt:** Prof Med, Med Coll Wisc

Gorbien, Martin J MD [Ger] - **Spec Exp:** Dementia; Alzheimer's Disease; Geriatric Functional Assessment; Palliative Care; **Hospital:** Rush Univ Med Ctr; **Address:** 1725 W Harrison St, Ste 955, Chicago, IL 60612; **Phone:** 312-942-7030; **Board Cert:** Geriatric Medicine 2008; **Med School:** Mexico 1983; **Resid:** Internal Medicine, Mercy Hosp & Med Ctr 1987; **Fellow:** Geriatric Medicine, UCLA Med Ctr 1989; **Fac Appt:** Assoc Prof Med, Rush Med Coll

Morley, John MD [Ger] - **Spec Exp:** Endocrinology; Menopause-Male; Alzheimer's Disease; Frailty Syndrome; **Hospital:** St Louis Univ Hosp; **Address:** St Louis Univ Hlth Sci Ctr, Div Ger Med, 3660 Vista, Ste 204, St Louis, MO 63104-1004; **Phone:** 314-977-6055; **Board Cert:** Internal Medicine 1978; Geriatric Medicine 1998; Endocrinology 1981; **Med School:** South Africa 1972; **Resid:** Internal Medicine, Johannesburg Genl Hosp 1974; Internal Medicine, Baragwanath Hosp 1976; **Fellow:** Endocrinology, Diabetes & Metabolism, Wadsworth VA Hosp-UCLA 1979; **Fac Appt:** Prof Med, St Louis Univ

Olson Jr, Jack C MD [Ger] - **Spec Exp:** Dementia; Depression; **Hospital:** Rush Univ Med Ctr; **Address:** Senior Care, Rush Univ Professional Bldg 3, 1725 W Harrison St, Ste 955, Chicago, IL 60612-3836; **Phone:** 312-942-7030; **Board Cert:** Internal Medicine 1987; Geriatric Medicine 2000; **Med School:** Univ Mich Med Sch 1984; **Resid:** Internal Medicine, Univ Wisconsin Affil Hosp 1987; **Fellow:** Geriatric Medicine, Univ Wisconsin Affil Hosp 1989; **Fac Appt:** Asst Prof Med, Univ Chicago-Pritzker Sch Med

Sachs, Greg A MD [Ger] - **Spec Exp:** Memory Disorders; Alzheimer's Disease; **Hospital:** Indiana Univ Hosp; **Address:** Indiana Univ Hospital, Dept Medicine & Geriatrics, 1001 W 10th St, rm M200, Indianapolis, IN 46202; **Phone:** 317-630-2557; **Board Cert:** Internal Medicine 1988; Geriatric Medicine 2000; **Med School:** Yale Univ 1985; **Resid:** Internal Medicine, Univ Chicago Hosps 1987; **Fellow:** Geriatric Medicine, Univ Chicago Hosps 1990; **Fac Appt:** Assoc Prof Med, Indiana Univ

Sheehan, Myles MD [Ger] - **Spec Exp:** Dementia; Geriatric Functional Assessment; **Hospital:** Loyola Univ Med Ctr; **Address:** Loyola Univ Med Ctr, 2160 S 1st Ave , Bldg 120 - rm 310, Maywood, IL 60153; **Phone:** 708-216-8887; **Board Cert:** Internal Medicine 1984; Geriatric Medicine 2002; **Med School:** Dartmouth Med Sch 1981; **Resid:** Internal Medicine, Beth Israel Deaconess Med Ctr 1984; **Fellow:** Geriatric Medicine, Beth Israel Deaconess Med Ctr 1991; **Fac Appt:** Assoc Prof Med, Loyola Univ-Stritch Sch Med

Great Plains and Mountains

Kutner, Jean S MD [Ger] - **Spec Exp:** Palliative Care; Preventive Medicine; Women's Health; **Hospital:** Univ Colorado Hosp; **Address:** 360 S Garfield St, Ste 500, Denver, CO 80209; **Phone:** 303-493-8333; **Board Cert:** Internal Medicine 2004; Geriatric Medicine 1998; Hospice & Palliative Medicine 2003; **Med School:** UCSF 1991; **Resid:** Internal Medicine, UCSF Med Ctr 1994; **Fellow:** Internal Medicine, Univ Colorado Sch Med 1996; Geriatric Medicine, Univ Colorado Sch Med 1997; **Fac Appt:** Assoc Prof Med, Univ Colorado

Geriatric Medicine

Schwartz, Robert S MD [Ger] - **Spec Exp:** Diabetes; Exercise Therapy; Hormonal Disorders; **Hospital:** Univ Colorado Hosp, VA Med Ctr; **Address:** Univ Colorado at Denver & Health Sci Ctr, 12631 E 17th Ave Bldg 15 Fl 8111, Box B179, Denver, CO 80262-0001; **Phone:** 303-319-7891; **Board Cert:** Internal Medicine 1977; Endocrinology 1981; Geriatric Medicine 2000; **Med School:** Ohio State Univ 1974; **Resid:** Internal Medicine, Univ Wash Med Ctr 1977; **Fellow:** Endocrinology, Diabetes & Metabolism, Univ Wash Med Ctr 1980; **Fac Appt:** Prof Med, Univ Colorado

Supiano, Mark A MD [Ger] - **Spec Exp:** Hypertension; Geriatric Functional Assessment; **Hospital:** Univ Utah Hosps and Clins; **Address:** Univ Utah, Geriatrics Div, 30 N 1900 E, SOM AB 193, Salt Lake City, UT 84132; **Phone:** 801-587-9103; **Board Cert:** Internal Medicine 1985; Geriatric Medicine 1998; **Med School:** Univ Wisc 1982; **Resid:** Internal Medicine, Univ Mich Med Ctr 1985; **Fellow:** Geriatric Medicine, Univ Mich Med Ctr 1987; **Fac Appt:** Prof Med, Univ Utah

Southwest

Carter, William Jerry MD [Ger] - **Spec Exp:** Geriatric Endocrinology; **Hospital:** John L McClellan VA Med Ctr; **Address:** 2200 Fort Roots Drive, Geriatric Clinic 3B, North Little Rock, AR 72114; **Phone:** 501-257-2061; **Board Cert:** Internal Medicine 1974; Endocrinology, Diabetes & Metabolism 1975; Geriatric Medicine 2005; **Med School:** Univ Ark 1963; **Resid:** Internal Medicine, Univ Ark Med Scis 1967; **Fellow:** Endocrinology, Diabetes & Metabolism, Univ Ark Med Scis 1971; **Fac Appt:** Prof Med, Univ Ark

Dyer, Carmel B MD [Ger] - **Spec Exp:** Elder Abuse; Dementia; Delirium; Geriatric Functional Assessment; **Hospital:** Meml Hermann Hosp - Texas Med Ctr, LBJ General Hosp; **Address:** 6431 Fannin St, rm MSB-4.200, Houston, TX 77030; **Phone:** 713-500-6290; **Board Cert:** Internal Medicine 2000; Geriatric Medicine 2000; **Med School:** Baylor Coll Med 1988; **Resid:** Internal Medicine, Baylor Affil Hosps 1991; **Fellow:** Geriatric Medicine, Baylor Affil Hosps 1993; **Fac Appt:** Prof Med, Univ Tex, Houston

Liem, Pham MD [Ger] - **Spec Exp:** Dementia; Alzheimer's Disease; Delirium; **Hospital:** UAMS Med Ctr, Cent Ark Vet Hlthcare Sys; **Address:** Univ Hosp Arkansas Med Sci, 4301 W Markham, Slot #748, Little Rock, AR 72205-7101; **Phone:** 501-257-2673; **Board Cert:** Family Medicine 2006; Geriatric Medicine 1998; **Med School:** Vietnam 1973; **Resid:** Family Medicine, Univ Ark Med Sch 1980; **Fellow:** Geriatric Medicine, Univ Ark Med Sch 1982; **Fac Appt:** Prof Med, Univ Ark

Lipschitz, David A MD/PhD [Ger] - **Spec Exp:** Preventive Medicine; Nutrition; **Hospital:** St Vincent Med Ctr; **Address:** Longevity Center-St Vincent Senior Hlth, One St Vincent Circle, Ste 210, Little Rock, AR 72205; **Phone:** 501-552-4777; **Board Cert:** Internal Medicine 1975; Hematology 1976; **Med School:** South Africa 1966; **Resid:** Internal Medicine, Johannesburg Genl Hosp 1972; **Fellow:** Hematology, Univ Washington 1974; Internal Medicine, Montefiore Hosp 1975; **Fac Appt:** Prof Med, Univ Ark

Wei, Jeanne MD/PhD [Ger] - **Spec Exp:** Cardiovascular Disease; **Hospital:** UAMS Med Ctr, John L McClellan VA Med Ctr; **Address:** Donald W Reynolds Ctr on Aging, 4301 W Markham St, Slot 748, Little Rock, AR 72205; **Phone:** 501-296-1000; **Board Cert:** Internal Medicine 1978; Cardiovascular Disease 1979; Geriatric Medicine 2001; **Med School:** Univ IL Coll Med 1975; **Resid:** Internal Medicine, Johns Hopkins Hosp 1977; **Fellow:** Cardiovascular Disease, Johns Hopkins Hosp 1979; Research, Natl Inst Aging 1979; **Fac Appt:** Prof Med, Univ Ark

West Coast and Pacific

Abrass, Itamar B MD [Ger] - **Spec Exp:** Geriatric Endocrinology; Endocrine Disorders; Diabetes; **Hospital:** Harborview Med Ctr, Univ Wash Med Ctr; **Address:** Harborview Medical Ctr, 325 9th Ave, Box 359755, Seattle, WA 98101; **Phone:** 206-744-9100; **Board Cert:** Internal Medicine 1974; Endocrinology, Diabetes & Metabolism 1975; Geriatric Medicine 1988; **Med School:** UCSF 1966; **Resid:** Internal Medicine, Columbia-Pesby Med Ctr 1968; **Fellow:** Endocrinology, Diabetes & Metabolism, UCSD Med Ctr 1971; **Fac Appt:** Prof Med, Univ Wash

Landefeld, Charles S MD [Ger] - **Spec Exp:** Cardiovascular Disease; Incontinence; **Hospital:** UCSF Med Ctr, VA Med Ctr - San Francisco; **Address:** 3333 California St, Ste 380, San Francisco, CA 94118; **Phone:** 415-750-6625; **Board Cert:** Internal Medicine 1982; **Med School:** Yale Univ 1979; **Resid:** Internal Medicine, UCSF Med Ctr 1983; **Fellow:** Geriatric Medicine, Brigham-Womens Hosp 1985; **Fac Appt:** Prof Med, UCSF

McCormick, Wayne MD [Ger] - **Spec Exp:** Dementia; AIDS/HIV; **Hospital:** Univ Wash Med Ctr, Harborview Med Ctr; **Address:** Harborview Medical Ctr, 325 9th Ave Fl 4, Box 359860, Seattle, WA 98104; **Phone:** 206-744-4191; **Board Cert:** Internal Medicine 1986; Geriatric Medicine 2002; Public Health & Genl Preventive Med 1992; **Med School:** Washington Univ, St Louis 1983; **Resid:** Internal Medicine, Michael Reese Hosp 1987; **Fellow:** Geriatric Medicine, Univ Wash Med Ctr 1990; **Fac Appt:** Asst Prof Med, Univ Wash

Reuben, David B MD [Ger] - **Spec Exp:** Geriatric Functional Assessment; **Hospital:** UCLA Ronald Reagan Med Ctr, Santa Monica - UCLA Med Ctr & Ortho Hosp; **Address:** UCLA Sch Med, Div Geriatrics, 10945 Le Conte Ave, Ste 2339, Los Angeles, CA 90095; **Phone:** 310-206-8272; **Board Cert:** Internal Medicine 1980; Geriatric Medicine 2005; **Med School:** Emory Univ 1977; **Resid:** Internal Medicine, Rhode Island Hosp 1980; **Fellow:** Geriatric Medicine, UCLA Med Ctr 1987; **Fac Appt:** Prof Med, UCLA

Tenover, Joyce S MD/PhD [Ger] - **Spec Exp:** Menopause-Male; Prostate Disease; Polypharmacology (Excess Medications); Hormonal Disorders; **Hospital:** VA Hlth Care Sys - Palo Alto; **Address:** VA Palo Alto HCS, GRECC (182B), 3801 Miranda Ave, Palo Alto, CA 94304; **Phone:** 650-493-5000 x66946; **Board Cert:** Internal Medicine 1983; Geriatric Medicine 1997; **Med School:** Geo Wash Univ 1980; **Resid:** Internal Medicine, Univ Wash Affil Hosps 1983; Internal Medicine, VA Med Ctr 1984; **Fellow:** Geriatric Medicine, VA Med Ctr 1987; **Fac Appt:** Prof Med, Emory Univ

Cleveland Clinic

Geriatric Medicine

Cleveland Clinic's Center for Geriatric Medicine, part of the Medicine Institute at Cleveland Clinic, specializes in diagnosing and treating frail, elderly patients with complex medical conditions and social problems.

Cleveland Clinic's Center for Geriatric Medicine consists of an interdisciplinary team of health care professionals dedicated to creating comprehensive, coordinated care plans for all patients. The Center for Geriatric Medicine fulfills its "patients first" mission through clinical, educational and research activities with an emphasis on improving the quality of life of older patients. The Center for Geriatric Medicine is an integral part of Cleveland Clinic, a not-for-profit multispecialty academic medical center.

Cleveland Clinic's Center for Geriatric Medicine offer several specialized programs to help ensure older patients receive the full scope of care necessary for optimal outcomes. These programs include:

Geriatric Evaluation and Management (GEM) Program

Cleveland Clinic's GEM Program is the cornerstone of the comprehensive care offered to older patients and their families. It takes an in-depth look at a patient's physical and psychological health, including the person's medical history, current status, recent changes and special concerns. Older adults appropriate for geriatric assessments include those with cognitive or physical decline; falls; weight loss; depression; social isolation and polypharmacy. Cleveland Clinic specialists from all disciplines are consulted as needed. After the evaluation is complete, the patient and invited family meet with the assessment team to discuss how best to care for the patient, using the most appropriate medications, therapies, community programs and other resources. The Center for Geriatric Medicine also operates a similar comprehensive Geriatric Assessment Program at Euclid Hospital and Cleveland Clinic Independence Family Health Center.

Aging Brain Clinic

Cleveland Clinic's Aging Brain Clinic brings together a medical team that includes physicians who specialize in geriatric medicine, neurology and neurosurgery. Patients appropriate for these clinics are older adults with ventriculomegaly (hydrocephalus) and cognitive, gait and urological problems. Experts in other medical specialties, such as urology and vascular medicine, as well as professionals in social work, nutrition, psychiatry and neuropsychology are involved as needed.

Inpatient Consultations

One of the special features that Cleveland Clinic offers older adults hospitalized for acute medical or surgical problems is an inpatient geriatrics assessment. These assessments can be requested by the attending physician for specific geriatric concerns, including: depression, delirium (acute confusion), dementia, falls, concerns about medications or other geriatric issues.

For more information about Cleveland Clinic Center for Geriatric Medicine, to schedule a second opinion or learn about assistance for out-of-state patients, call 800.890.2467 or visit www.clevelandclinic.org/geriatrictopdocs.

Center for Geriatric Medicine | 9500 Euclid Avenue / AC311 | Cleveland OH 44195

Maimonides
Medical Center

Maimonides serves one of the oldest populations in New York City, with one quarter of our patients over the age of 75. The Geriatrics Program at Maimonides is fully equipped to meet the special needs of this growing segment of the population. Directed by Barbara Paris, MD, the program encompasses inpatient and outpatient services, featuring the Acute Care for Elderly (ACE) Unit and the Safe at Home program. The staff is focused on the continuity, coordination, quality and dignity of care provided.

Patient Evaluation
ACE Unit services focus on acute medical care and account for the complex needs of hospitalized elderly patients. Special attention is given to the assessment of memory loss and understanding the underlying causes of geriatric syndromes that result in falls, incontinence and frailty. Psychosocial issues affecting elderly patients such as loneliness and end-of-life care are also addressed.

Wound Care
Because patients can have wounds that do not heal easily, we provide special attention through our wound care team.

Safe at Home Program
The Safe at Home program actively manages the care of the frail elderly to keep them in their homes and within their communities. The program is designed to identify inpatients, aged 75 years and older, who are at high risk during the transitional period from hospital to home; provide them with coordinated comprehensive care after the transition from hospital to home; actively engage family caregivers and community support networks; increase patient satisfaction with their care during this transitional period; and reduce re-hospitalizations, emergency room visits, and nursing home placements.

Outpatient Geriatric Services
Our geriatric team offers comprehensive assessment and primary care services throughout Southern Brooklyn.

Physicians at Maimonides are among the small percentage in the US who use computers to enter patient orders, thereby reducing the risk of errors, increasing efficiency, and speeding the healing process. Maimonides has appeared on the American Hospital Association's "Most Wired" and "Most Wireless" lists more often than any other health care institution in the metropolitan area. Advanced technology allows our doctors to focus more attention on caring for their patients.

**Maimonides Medical Center
Passionate about medicine.
Compassionate about people.**

www.maimonidesmed.org/geriatrics

MOUNT SINAI
SCHOOL OF
MEDICINE

THE MOUNT SINAI MEDICAL CENTER
THE BROOKDALE DEPARTMENT OF
GERIATRICS AND PALLIATIVE MEDICINE
One Gustave L. Levy Place
Fifth Avenue and 100th Street
New York, NY 10029-6574
Physician Referral: 1-800-MD-SINAI (637-4624)
www.mountsinai.org

The Best in Clinical Care

In recognition of the care offered to older patients, the Mount Sinai **BROOKDALE DEPARTMENT OF GERIATRICS AND PALLIATIVE MEDICINE** is cited time and time again as the finest in the nation. In its 2009 *Best Graduate Schools* issue, *U.S. News & World Report* ranked Mount Sinai School of Medicine 22nd in research. *America's Best Hospitals* guide has also ranked Mount Sinai's geriatrics specialty third for several years running.

We offer a full spectrum of patient care, including a specialized inpatient care team for the elderly to minimize complications sometimes associated with an older person's hospital stay, a primary care geriatrics practice for older adults living in the community, a hospital-based consultation service for patients throughout Mount Sinai, a number of community-linked programs and partnerships, and a palliative care team dedicated to ensuring the highest quality care and support for patients and families facing serious illnesses.

The Martha Stewart Center for Living, a new modern facility designed by renowned architect C.C. Pei, provides clinical care and education for patients and serves as a training ground for physicians.

Groundbreaking Research – Mount Sinai's researchers continue to advance the understanding, prevention, and treatment of age-related disorders. The extensive research on aging conducted by the Brookdale Department of Geriatrics and Palliative Medicine includes studies on health services, medical decision making and ethical dilemmas, palliative care, the neurobiology of aging, and clinical interventions to promote independence in old age. The Department's expertise serves as a renowned educational resource for all Mount Sinai affiliates and other institutions in teaching geriatrics and gerontology to medical students, medical residents, geriatrics fellows, established physicians, and health profession trainees in other disciplines.

History Of Excellence – The Mount Sinai Medical Center is a pioneer in geriatric medicine. In 1909, a Mount Sinai physician coined the term "geriatrics," and in 1914, he wrote the first textbook on medical care for older adults. Today, the Brookdale Department of Geriatrics and Palliative Medicine continues to break new ground, offering comprehensive care, disease prevention, and the promotion of healthy and productive aging. The Department's enhanced expertise in assessing and managing patients with dementia greatly complements its established, interdisciplinary approach to patient care, in which medical staff and social workers address each patient's needs as a team.

THE FIRST FREESTANDING DEPARTMENT OF GERIATRICS AT A U.S. MEDICAL SCHOOL
Mount Sinai's Brookdale Department of Geriatrics and Palliative Medicine was the first freestanding department of geriatrics established by a U.S. medical school, and it continues to be one of the very best. It offers unparalleled inpatient and outpatient care, as well as numerous treatment programs designed to meet the unique needs of older adults. Mount Sinai is also home to world-class researchers dedicated to advancing our understanding of Alzheimer's disease and other common geriatric conditions. At the Department's heart are its patients. The geriatricians of The Mount Sinai Medical Center work hard to improve life and longevity for New York's elderly.

NYU Langone Medical Center

550 First Avenue (at 31St Street)
New York, NY 10016
Physician Referral:
(888)7-NYU-MED (888-769-8633)
www.med.nyu.edu

GERIATRIC MEDICINE

About the Section of Geriatrics, Division of General Internal Medicine, Department of Medicine:

The goal of geriatric medicine at NYU Langone Medical Center is to keep us all — for as long as possible — healthy, functional and vital members of our families and communities. NYU Langone Medical Center has a distinguished history in this vital specialty as a federally designated research center and leader in the care of geriatrics. Finding new answers and applying them to patient care are equally important.

We specialize in the following areas:

THE BELFER GERIATRICS CENTER

The Center takes a comprehensive approach to the care of people over the age of 65. Geriatrics, home care, neurology, orthopaedics, dentistry, geropsychiatry, and many other disciplines are available to patients here.

INPATIENT GERIATRICS SERVICES

Using a team approach, a senior geriatrician leads nurses, pharmacists, geropsychiatrists, rehabilitation experts, and fellowship trainees in caring for geriatric patients with complex conditions. NYU Langone Medical Center has also just started a new service to improve the care delivered to all older patients. If screening reveals a hospitalized patient is suffering from a geriatric problem (such as cognitive impairment), special consultation is offered to the patient's health care team.

THE NYU HEALTHY AGING INITIATIVE

The Section of Geriatric Medicine has a strong interest in healthy aging – assessing older individuals and advising them on what they can do to avoid developing problems such as cognitive or functional impairment. This is a fundamental part of the care provided by geriatricians within NYU Langone Medical Center's faculty group practice. In addition, we are currently piloting a Healthy Aging Clinic, with plans to expand it to NYU in the near future.

THE WILLIAM AND SYLVIA SILBERSTEIN AGING AND DEMENTIA RESEARCH CENTER

The Silberstein Aging and Dementia Research Center is a National Institute on Aging-designated Center of Excellence in Alzheimer's treatment. The facility provides comprehensive diagnostic evaluations to determine if memory loss is "normal" or more serious; a memory enhancement program for age-related memory decline; clinical trials for mild memory loss and for Alzheimer's treatment; state-of-the-art brain imaging techniques; methods to minimize disability in Alzheimer's patients; and comprehensive counseling and support groups for patients, caregivers and family members.

Gynecologic Oncology

a subspecialty of
Obstetrics & Gynecology

An obstetrician/gynecologist who provides consultation and comprehensive management of patients with gynecologic cancer, including those diagnostic and therapeutic procedures necessary
for the total care of the patient with gynecologic cancer and resulting complications.

Training Required: Four years *plus* two years in clinical practice before certification in obstetrics and gynecology is complete *plus* additional training and examination in gynecologic oncology.

GYNECOLOGIC ONCOLOGY

New England

Azodi, Masoud MD [GO] - **Spec Exp:** Laparoscopic Surgery; Ovarian Cancer-Early Detection; Uterine Cancer; **Hospital:** Yale-New Haven Hosp; **Address:** Yale Surgical Oncology, 800 Howard Ave Fl 3, New Haven, CT 06519-1369; **Phone:** 203-785-4013; **Board Cert:** Gynecologic Oncology 2002; Obstetrics & Gynecology 2000; **Med School:** Wright State Univ 1992; **Resid:** Obstetrics & Gynecology, Aultman Hospital 1996; **Fellow:** Obstetrics & Gynecology, Yale-New Haven Hosp 1999; **Fac Appt:** Assoc Prof ObG, Yale Univ

Berkowitz, Ross S MD [GO] - **Spec Exp:** Gynecologic Cancer; **Hospital:** Brigham & Women's Hosp, Dana-Farber Cancer Inst; **Address:** Div OB/GYN Oncology, 75 Francis St, Boston, MA 02115-6110; **Phone:** 617-732-8843; **Board Cert:** Obstetrics & Gynecology 1981; Gynecologic Oncology 1982; **Med School:** Boston Univ 1973; **Resid:** Surgery, Peter Bent Brigham Hosp 1975; Obstetrics & Gynecology, Boston Hosp for Women 1978; **Fellow:** Gynecologic Oncology, Boston Hosp for Women 1980; **Fac Appt:** Prof ObG, Harvard Med Sch

Brewer, Molly A MD [GO] - **Spec Exp:** Ovarian Cancer; **Hospital:** Univ of Conn Hlth Ctr, John Dempsey Hosp; **Address:** Univ Conn Hlth Ctr, Div Gyn Oncology, 263 Farmington Ave, MC2875, Farmington, CT 06032-2875; **Phone:** 860-679-2100; **Board Cert:** Obstetrics & Gynecology 2008; Gynecologic Oncology 2008; **Med School:** SUNY Upstate Med Univ 1991; **Resid:** Obstetrics & Gynecology, Oregon Hlth Scis Ctr 1995; **Fellow:** Gynecologic Oncology, MD Anderson Cancer Ctr 1997

Cain, Joanna M MD [GO] - **Spec Exp:** Ovarian Cancer; Breast Cancer Risk Assessment; Uterine Cancer; Ovarian Cancer-Early Detection; **Hospital:** Women & Infants Hosp of RI; **Address:** Women & Infants Hospital, 101 Dudley St, Providence, RI 02905; **Phone:** 401-274-1122 x1575; **Board Cert:** Obstetrics & Gynecology 2007; Gynecologic Oncology 2007; **Med School:** Creighton Univ 1978; **Resid:** Obstetrics & Gynecology, Univ Washington Med Ctr 1981; **Fellow:** Gynecologic Oncology, Meml Sloan Kettering Cancer Ctr 1983; **Fac Appt:** Prof ObG, Brown Univ

Currie, John L MD [GO] - **Spec Exp:** Gynecologic Cancer; Pelvic Reconstruction; Gynecologic Problems of Obesity; **Hospital:** Hartford Hosp; **Address:** Hartford Hospital, 85 Seymour St Fl 7 - Ste 705, Box 5037, Hartford, CT 06106-5501; **Phone:** 860-545-4341; **Board Cert:** Obstetrics & Gynecology 1991; Gynecologic Oncology 1982; **Med School:** Univ NC Sch Med 1967; **Resid:** Gynecologic Oncology, Hosp Univ Penn 1972; **Fellow:** Gynecologic Oncology, Duke Univ Med Ctr 1980; **Fac Appt:** Prof ObG, Univ Conn

DeMars, Leslie R MD [GO] - **Spec Exp:** Gynecologic Cancer; Colposcopy; Laparoscopic Surgery; **Hospital:** Dartmouth - Hitchcock Med Ctr; **Address:** Dartmouth-Hitchcock Med Ctr, Gyn-Oncology, 1 Medical Center Drive, Lebanon, NH 03756; **Phone:** 603-653-3530; **Board Cert:** Obstetrics & Gynecology 2007; Gynecologic Oncology 2007; **Med School:** Univ VT Coll Med 1987; **Resid:** Obstetrics & Gynecology, Univ N Carolina Hosps 1991; **Fellow:** Gynecologic Oncology, Univ N Carolina Hosps 1994; **Fac Appt:** Asst Prof ObG, Dartmouth Med Sch

Granai, Cornelius O MD [GO] - **Spec Exp:** Gynecologic Cancer; Complementary Medicine; International Health; **Hospital:** Women & Infants Hosp of RI, Rhode Island Hosp; **Address:** Womens & Infants Hosp, 101 Dudley St, GYN Oncology Department, Providence, RI 02905; **Phone:** 401-453-7520; **Board Cert:** Obstetrics & Gynecology 2007; Gynecologic Oncology 2007; **Med School:** Univ VT Coll Med 1977; **Resid:** Obstetrics & Gynecology, Hershey Med Ctr 1981; **Fellow:** Gynecologic Oncology, Tufts Univ 1984; **Fac Appt:** Assoc Prof ObG, Brown Univ

Muto, Michael G MD [GO] - **Spec Exp:** Ovarian Cancer; Cervical Cancer; Vulvar & Vaginal Cancer; Robotic Surgery; **Hospital:** Dana-Farber Cancer Inst, Brigham & Women's Hosp; **Address:** Dana Farber Cancer Inst, 44 Binney St Fl 9, Boston, MA 02115; **Phone:** 617-582-7931; **Board Cert:** Gynecologic Oncology 2007; Obstetrics & Gynecology 2007; **Med School:** Univ Mass Sch Med 1983; **Resid:** Obstetrics & Gynecology, Brigham & Women's Hosp 1987; **Fellow:** Gynecologic Oncology, Brigham & Women's Hosp 1990; **Fac Appt:** Assoc Prof ObG, Harvard Med Sch

Rutherford, Thomas J MD [GO] - **Spec Exp:** Ovarian Cancer; Uterine Cancer; Ovarian Cancer-Early Detection; Cervical Cancer; **Hospital:** Yale-New Haven Hosp; **Address:** Yale Univ Sch Med Dept Ob-Gyn, 333 Cedar St, Box 208063, New Haven, CT 06520; **Phone:** 203-785-6301; **Board Cert:** Obstetrics & Gynecology 2007; Gynecologic Oncology 2007; **Med School:** Med Coll OH 1989; **Resid:** Obstetrics & Gynecology, Cooper Hosp 1993; **Fellow:** Gynecologic Oncology, Yale-New Haven Hosp 1995; **Fac Appt:** Assoc Prof ObG, Yale Univ

Santin, Alessandro MD [GO] - **Spec Exp:** Immunotherapy; Ovarian Cancer; Vulvar & Vaginal Cancer; **Hospital:** Yale-New Haven Hosp; **Address:** Yale Gynecologic Oncology, 800 Howard Ave, New Haven, CT 06519; **Phone:** 203-737-2280; **Med School:** Italy 1989; **Resid:** Obstetrics & Gynecology, Univ Brescia Sch Med 1993; **Fellow:** Gynecologic Oncology, UC Irvine 1995; Gynecologic Oncology, UAMS Med Ctr 2000; **Fac Appt:** Prof ObG, Yale Univ

Schwartz, Peter E MD [GO] - **Spec Exp:** Ovarian Cancer; Uterine Cancer; Gynecologic Surgery-Complex; Cervical Cancer; **Hospital:** Yale-New Haven Hosp, Hosp of St Raphael; **Address:** Yale Univ Sch Med, Dept Ob/Gyn, 333 Cedar St, rm FMB-316, New Haven, CT 06510-3289; **Phone:** 203-785-4014; **Board Cert:** Obstetrics & Gynecology 1973; Gynecologic Oncology 1979; **Med School:** Albert Einstein Coll Med 1966; **Resid:** Obstetrics & Gynecology, Yale-New Haven Hosp 1970; **Fellow:** Gynecologic Oncology, MD Anderson Cancer Ctr 1975; **Fac Appt:** Prof ObG, Yale Univ

Tarraza, Hector M MD [GO] - **Spec Exp:** Gynecologic Cancer; **Hospital:** Maine Med Ctr; **Address:** 102 Campus Drive, rm 116, Scarborough, ME 04074; **Phone:** 207-883-0069; **Board Cert:** Obstetrics & Gynecology 1998; Gynecologic Oncology 1998; **Med School:** Harvard Med Sch 1981; **Resid:** Obstetrics & Gynecology, Mass Genl Hosp 1985; **Fellow:** Gynecologic Oncology, Mass Genl Hosp 1987; **Fac Appt:** Prof ObG, Univ VT Coll Med

Mid Atlantic

Abbas, Fouad M MD [GO] - **Spec Exp:** Gynecologic Cancer; Ovarian Cancer; Cervical Cancer; **Hospital:** Sinai Hosp - Baltimore; **Address:** Sinai Hosp Baltimore, 2411 W Belvedere Ave, Ste 206, Baltimore, MD 21215; **Phone:** 410-601-9030; **Board Cert:** Obstetrics & Gynecology 2007; Gynecologic Oncology 2007; **Med School:** Univ MD Sch Med 1986; **Resid:** Obstetrics & Gynecology, John Hopkins Hosp 1990; **Fellow:** Gynecologic Oncology, John Hopkins Hosp 1992; **Fac Appt:** Asst Prof ObG, Univ MD Sch Med

Abu-Rustum, Nadeem R MD [GO] - **Spec Exp:** Ovarian Cancer; Uterine Cancer; Cervical Cancer; Vulvar Disease/Cancer; **Hospital:** Meml Sloan-Kettering Cancer Ctr; **Address:** 1275 York Avenue, New York, NY 10065; **Phone:** 800-525-2225; **Board Cert:** Obstetrics & Gynecology 1998; Gynecologic Oncology 2000; **Med School:** Lebanon 1990; **Resid:** Obstetrics & Gynecology, Greater Baltimore Med Ctr 1994; **Fellow:** Gynecologic Oncology, Meml Sloan-Kettering Cancer Ctr 1997; **Fac Appt:** Assoc Prof ObG, Cornell Univ-Weill Med Coll

Gynecologic Oncology

Barakat, Richard R MD [GO] - **Spec Exp:** Laparoscopic Surgery; Ovarian Cancer; Uterine Cancer; **Hospital:** Meml Sloan-Kettering Cancer Ctr; **Address:** 1275 York Avenue, New York, NY 10065; **Phone:** 800-525-2225; **Board Cert:** Obstetrics & Gynecology 2006; Gynecologic Oncology 2006; **Med School:** SUNY Hlth Sci Ctr 1985; **Resid:** Obstetrics & Gynecology, Bellevue Hosp 1989; **Fellow:** Gynecologic Oncology, Meml Sloan Kettering Cancer Ctr 1991; **Fac Appt:** Assoc Prof ObG, Cornell Univ-Weill Med Coll

Barnes, Willard MD [GO] - **Spec Exp:** Pelvic Tumors; Gynecologic Cancer; **Hospital:** Georgetown Univ Hosp, Virginia Hosp Ctr - Arlington; **Address:** Georgetown Univ Hosp, Lombardi Cancer Ctr, Dept Gyn Oncology, 3800 Reservoir Rd NW, Washington, DC 20007-2194; **Phone:** 202-444-2114; **Board Cert:** Obstetrics & Gynecology 2007; Gynecologic Oncology 2007; **Med School:** Univ Miss 1979; **Resid:** Obstetrics & Gynecology, Univ Miss Med Ctr 1983; **Fellow:** Gynecologic Oncology, Georgetown Univ Med Ctr 1985; **Fac Appt:** Assoc Prof ObG, Georgetown Univ

Barter, James MD [GO] - **Spec Exp:** Laparoscopic Surgery; Ovarian Cancer; Gynecologic Cancer; **Hospital:** Holy Cross Hospital - Silver Spring, Suburban Hosp; **Address:** 6301 Executive Blvd, Montros Rd, Rockville, MD 20852; **Phone:** 301-770-4967; **Board Cert:** Obstetrics & Gynecology 1997; Gynecologic Oncology 1997; **Med School:** Univ VA Sch Med 1977; **Resid:** Internal Medicine, Univ Kentucky Med Ctr 1979; Obstetrics & Gynecology, Duke Univ Med Ctr 1983; **Fellow:** Gynecologic Oncology, Univ Alabama 1985; **Fac Appt:** Clin Prof ObG, Georgetown Univ

Boice, Charles R MD [GO] - **Spec Exp:** Gynecologic Cancer; Ovarian Cancer; Cervical Cancer; **Hospital:** Univ Wash Med Ctr, Columbia Hosp for Women Med Ctr; **Address:** 10301 Georgia Ave, Ste 205, Silver Springs, MD 20902; **Phone:** 301-592-1600; **Board Cert:** Obstetrics & Gynecology 1981; Gynecologic Oncology 1982; **Med School:** Loma Linda Univ 1973; **Resid:** Obstetrics & Gynecology, Los Angeles Med Ctr 1973; Surgery, City Hope Natl Med Ctr 1978; **Fellow:** Oncology, Univ Texas-MD Anderson Cancer Ctr 1980; **Fac Appt:** Assoc Clin Prof ObG, Univ Wash

Bristow, Robert E MD [GO] - **Spec Exp:** Ovarian Cancer; Cervical Cancer; Uterine Cancer; **Hospital:** Johns Hopkins Hosp (page 61); **Address:** Johns Hopkins Hosp, 600 N Wolfe St, Phipps 281, Baltimore, MD 21287; **Phone:** 410-955-8240; **Board Cert:** Obstetrics & Gynecology 1999; Gynecologic Oncology 2003; **Med School:** USC Sch Med 1991; **Resid:** Obstetrics & Gynecology, Johns Hopkins Hosp 1995; **Fellow:** Gynecologic Oncology, UCLA Med Ctr 1998; **Fac Appt:** Assoc Prof ObG, Johns Hopkins Univ

Caputo, Thomas A MD [GO] - **Spec Exp:** Cervical Cancer; Ovarian Cancer; Uterine Cancer; Vulvar Disease/Cancer; **Hospital:** NY-Presby Hosp/Weill Cornell (page 66); **Address:** NY Presby Hosp-Weill Cornell, 525 E 68th St, Ste J130, New York, NY 10021; **Phone:** 212-746-3179; **Board Cert:** Obstetrics & Gynecology 1993; Gynecologic Oncology 1977; **Med School:** UMDNJ-NJ Med Sch, Newark 1965; **Resid:** Obstetrics & Gynecology, Martland Hosp 1969; **Fellow:** Gynecologic Oncology, Emory Univ Hosp 1974; **Fac Appt:** Clin Prof ObG, Cornell Univ-Weill Med Coll

Carlson, John A MD [GO] - **Spec Exp:** Gynecologic Cancer; Ovarian Cancer; Gynecologic Surgery-Complex; **Hospital:** St Peter's Univ Hosp; **Address:** St Peter's Univ Hosp, 254 Easton Ave Cares Bldg, New Brunswick, NJ 08901; **Phone:** 732-937-6003; **Board Cert:** Obstetrics & Gynecology 1981; Gynecologic Oncology 1982; **Med School:** Georgetown Univ 1974; **Resid:** Obstetrics & Gynecology, Hosp Univ Penn 1978; **Fellow:** Gynecologic Oncology, MD Anderson Hosp 1980; **Fac Appt:** Prof ObG, Drexel Univ Coll Med

Coukos, George MD/PhD [GO] - **Spec Exp:** Ovarian Cancer; Gynecologic Cancer; Vaccine Therapy; Clinical Trials; **Hospital:** Hosp Univ Penn - UPHS (page 60); **Address:** Perelman Ctr, Jordan Gynecologic Ctr, 3400 Civic Center Blvd Fl 3 W, Philadelphia, PA 19104; **Phone:** 215-662-3318; **Board Cert:** Obstetrics & Gynecology 2004; Gynecologic Oncology 2004; **Med School:** Italy 1987; **Resid:** Obstetrics & Gynecology, Hosp Univ Penn 1997; **Fellow:** Gynecologic Oncology, Hosp Univ Penn 2000; **Fac Appt:** Assoc Prof ObG, Univ Pennsylvania

Curtin, John P MD [GO] - **Spec Exp:** Uterine Cancer; Ovarian Cancer; Laparoscopic Surgery; **Hospital:** NYU Langone Med Ctr (page 67); **Address:** NYU Clin Cancer Ctr, 160 E 34th St Fl 4, New York, NY 10016-6402; **Phone:** 212-731-5345; **Board Cert:** Obstetrics & Gynecology 2007; Gynecologic Oncology 2007; **Med School:** Creighton Univ 1979; **Resid:** Obstetrics & Gynecology, Univ Minn Med Ctr 1984; **Fellow:** Gynecologic Oncology, Meml Sloan-Kettering Cancer Ctr 1988; **Fac Appt:** Prof ObG, NYU Sch Med

Dottino, Peter R MD [GO] - **Spec Exp:** Laparoscopic Surgery; Gynecologic Cancer; **Hospital:** Mount Sinai Med Ctr (page 64), Hackensack Univ Med Ctr; **Address:** 800-A 5th Ave, Ste 405, New York, NY 10021-7215; **Phone:** 212-888-8439; **Board Cert:** Obstetrics & Gynecology 2007; Gynecologic Oncology 2007; **Med School:** Georgetown Univ 1979; **Resid:** Obstetrics & Gynecology, SUNY Downstate Med Ctr 1983; **Fellow:** Gynecologic Oncology, Mt Sinai Hosp 1985

Dunton, Charles J MD [GO] - **Spec Exp:** Ovarian Cancer; Uterine Cancer; Cervical Cancer; Pap Smear Abnormalities; **Hospital:** Lankenau Hosp; **Address:** 100 E Lancaster Ave, Med Office Bldg East, Ste 661, Wynnewood, PA 19096; **Phone:** 610-649-8085; **Board Cert:** Obstetrics & Gynecology 2007; Gynecologic Oncology 2007; **Med School:** Jefferson Med Coll 1980; **Resid:** Obstetrics & Gynecology, Lankenau Hosp 1984; **Fellow:** Gynecologic Oncology, Hosp Univ Penn 1989; **Fac Appt:** Prof ObG, Jefferson Med Coll

Edwards, Robert P MD [GO] - **Spec Exp:** Ovarian Cancer; Gynecologic Cancer; Cervical Cancer; Clinical Trials; **Hospital:** Magee-Womens Hosp - UPMC; **Address:** UPP-Dept Women's Health, 300 Halket St, Ste 0610, Pittsburgh, PA 15213; **Phone:** 412-641-5411; **Board Cert:** Obstetrics & Gynecology 2007; Gynecologic Oncology 2007; **Med School:** Univ Pittsburgh 1984; **Resid:** Obstetrics & Gynecology, Magee WomensHosp-UPMC 1989; **Fellow:** Gynecologic Oncology, Univ Alabama Med Ctr 1993; **Fac Appt:** Prof ObG, Univ Pittsburgh

Fields, Abbie L MD [GO] - **Spec Exp:** Fertility Preservation in Cancer; Robotic Surgery; Cancer Genetics; Pelvic Reconstruction; **Hospital:** Washington Hosp Ctr; **Address:** Washington Hospital Center, 110 Irving St NW, rm 5B-33B, Washington, DC 20010; **Phone:** 202-877-2391; **Board Cert:** Obstetrics & Gynecology 2007; Gynecologic Oncology 2007; **Med School:** Ohio State Univ 1987; **Resid:** Obstetrics & Gynecology, Northwestern Univ 1991; **Fellow:** Gynecologic Oncology, Johns Hopkins Hosp 1993

Fishman, David A MD [GO] - **Spec Exp:** Ovarian Cancer; Ovarian Cancer-Early Detection; Gynecologic Cancer; **Hospital:** Mount Sinai Med Ctr (page 64); **Address:** 1190 Fifth Ave, New York, NY 10029; **Phone:** 212-241-1111; **Board Cert:** Obstetrics & Gynecology 2005; Gynecologic Oncology 2005; **Med School:** Texas Tech Univ 1988; **Resid:** Obstetrics & Gynecology, Yale-New Haven Hosp 1992; **Fellow:** Gynecologic Oncology, Yale-New Haven Hosp 1994; **Fac Appt:** Prof ObG, NYU Sch Med

Giuntoli II, Robert Lawrence MD [GO] - **Spec Exp:** Gynecologic Cancer; Ovarian Cancer; Gestational Trophoblastic Disease; Immunotherapy; **Hospital:** Johns Hopkins Hosp (page 61); **Address:** Johns Hopkins Hosp, Div Gyn Onc, 600 N Wolfe St, Phipps #281, Baltimore, MD 21287-1281; **Phone:** 410-502-4245; **Board Cert:** Obstetrics & Gynecology 2005; Gynecologic Oncology 2005; **Med School:** Univ Pennsylvania 1994; **Resid:** Obstetrics & Gynecology, Duke Univ Med Ctr 1998; **Fellow:** Gynecologic Oncology, Mayo Clinic 2002; **Fac Appt:** Asst Prof ObG, Johns Hopkins Univ

Herzog, Thomas J MD [GO] - **Spec Exp:** Cervical Cancer; Gynecologic Cancer; Laparoscopic Surgery; Ovarian Cancer; **Hospital:** NY-Presby Hosp/Columbia (page 66); **Address:** Herbert Irving Pavilion, 161 Fort Washington Ave, 8-837, New York, NY 10032; **Phone:** 212-305-3410; **Board Cert:** Obstetrics & Gynecology 2008; Gynecologic Oncology 2008; **Med School:** Univ Cincinnati 1986; **Resid:** Obstetrics & Gynecology, Good Samaritan Hosp 1990; **Fellow:** Gynecologic Oncology, Barnes Jewish Hosp 1993; **Fac Appt:** Prof ObG, Columbia P&S

Gynecologic Oncology

Kelley III, Joseph L MD [GO] - **Spec Exp:** Breast Cancer; Ovarian Cancer; Cervical Cancer; Gynecologic Cancer; **Hospital:** Magee-Womens Hosp - UPMC; **Address:** UPP-Dept Women's Health, 300 Halket St, Ste 0610, Pittsburgh, PA 15213; **Phone:** 412-641-5411; **Board Cert:** Obstetrics & Gynecology 2007; Gynecologic Oncology 2007; **Med School:** St Louis Univ 1985; **Resid:** Obstetrics & Gynecology, Magee-Womens Hosp 1989; **Fellow:** Gynecologic Oncology, MD Anderson Cancer Ctr 1991; **Fac Appt:** Assoc Prof ObG, Univ Pittsburgh

Koulos, John MD [GO] - **Spec Exp:** Cervical Cancer; Uterine Cancer; Ovarian Cancer; **Hospital:** Beth Israel Med Ctr - Petrie Division (page 57); **Address:** Beth Israel Hosp Cancer Ctr, 10 Union Square E, Ste 4C, New York, NY 10003; **Phone:** 212-844-5729; **Board Cert:** Obstetrics & Gynecology 2006; Gynecologic Oncology 2006; **Med School:** Northwestern Univ 1978; **Resid:** Obstetrics & Gynecology, Northwestern Univ Med Sch 1982; **Fellow:** Gynecologic Oncology, Meml Sloan Kettering Cancer Ctr 1984; **Fac Appt:** Assoc Prof ObG, NY Med Coll

Lele, Shashikant B MD [GO] - **Spec Exp:** Ovarian Cancer; Reconstructive Surgery; Pelvic Surgery-Complex; **Hospital:** Roswell Park Cancer Inst, Buffalo General Hosp; **Address:** Roswell Park Cancer Inst, Dept Gynecology, Elm & Carlton Sts, Buffalo, NY 14263; **Phone:** 716-845-5776; **Board Cert:** Obstetrics & Gynecology 1976; Gynecologic Oncology 1979; **Med School:** India 1968; **Resid:** Obstetrics & Gynecology, JJ Hosp-Grant Med Ctr 1970; Obstetrics & Gynecology, Mt Sinai Hosp 1973; **Fellow:** Gynecologic Oncology, Roswell Park Cancer Inst 1976; **Fac Appt:** Clin Prof ObG, SUNY Buffalo

Morgan, Mark A MD [GO] - **Spec Exp:** Laparoscopic Surgery; Gynecologic Surgery-Complex; Gynecologic Cancer; Uro-Gynecology; **Hospital:** Fox Chase Cancer Ctr (page 58); **Address:** Fox Chase Cancer Ctr-Gyn Oncology, 333 Cottman Ave, Philadelphia, PA 19111; **Phone:** 215-214-1430; **Board Cert:** Obstetrics & Gynecology 2007; Gynecologic Oncology 2007; **Med School:** SUNY Downstate 1982; **Resid:** Obstetrics & Gynecology, Hosp Univ Penn 1986; **Fellow:** Gynecologic Oncology, Hosp Univ Penn 1988

Odunsi, Adekunle O MD/PhD [GO] - **Spec Exp:** Ovarian Cancer; Immunotherapy; Clinical Trials; **Hospital:** Roswell Park Cancer Inst; **Address:** Roswell Park Cancer Inst, Gyn Oncology, Elm and Carlton Streets, Buffalo, NY 14263; **Phone:** 716-845-2300; **Board Cert:** Obstetrics & Gynecology 2004; Gynecologic Oncology 2004; **Med School:** Nigeria 1984; **Resid:** Obstetrics & Gynecology, Rosie Maternity & Addenbrookes Hosps 1990; Obstetrics & Gynecology, Yale-New Haven Hosp 1999; **Fellow:** Gynecologic Oncology, Roswell Park Cancer Inst 2001; **Fac Appt:** Prof ObG, SUNY Buffalo

Randall, Thomas C MD [GO] - **Spec Exp:** Gynecologic Cancer; Pelvic Reconstruction; Robotic Surgery; **Hospital:** Pennsylvania Hosp (page 60); **Address:** Pennsylvania Hospital, Dept OB/GYN, 801 Spruce St Fl 7, Philadelphia, PA 19107; **Phone:** 215-829-2345; **Board Cert:** Obstetrics & Gynecology 2001; Gynecologic Oncology 2002; **Med School:** Johns Hopkins Univ 1987; **Resid:** Obstetrics & Gynecology, Johns Hopkins Hosp 1991; **Fellow:** Gynecologic Oncology, Hosp Univ Penn 1992; **Fac Appt:** Assoc Prof ObG, Univ Pennsylvania

Rosenblum, Norman G MD/PhD [GO] - **Spec Exp:** Ovarian Cancer; Uterine Cancer; Vulvar Disease/Cancer; **Hospital:** Thomas Jefferson Univ Hosp; **Address:** 834 Chesnut St, Ste 300, Philadelphia, PA 19107-5127; **Phone:** 215-955-6200; **Board Cert:** Obstetrics & Gynecology 2007; Gynecologic Oncology 2007; **Med School:** Jefferson Med Coll 1978; **Resid:** Obstetrics & Gynecology, Hosp Univ Penn 1982; **Fellow:** Gynecologic Oncology, Hosp Univ Penn 1984; **Fac Appt:** Prof ObG, Jefferson Med Coll

Rubin, Stephen C MD [GO] - **Spec Exp:** Gynecologic Cancer; Ovarian Cancer; Cervical Cancer; Uterine Cancer; **Hospital:** Hosp Univ Penn - UPHS (page 60); **Address:** Perelman Center, Jordan Gynecologic Ctr, 3400 Civic Center Blvd Fl 3 W, Philadelphia, PA 19104-4283; **Phone:** 215-662-3318; **Board Cert:** Obstetrics & Gynecology 2005; Gynecologic Oncology 2005; **Med School:** Univ Pennsylvania 1976; **Resid:** Obstetrics & Gynecology, Hosp Univ Penn 1980; **Fellow:** Gynecologic Oncology, Hosp Univ Penn 1982; **Fac Appt:** Prof ObG, Univ Pennsylvania

Southeast

Alvarez, Ronald D MD [GO] - **Spec Exp:** Gynecologic Cancer; Ovarian Cancer; **Hospital:** Univ of Ala Hosp at Birmingham, Brookwood Med Ctr; **Address:** Univ Alabama, Div Gyn Oncology, 619 19th St S, OHB 538, Birmingham, AL 35249-7333; **Phone:** 205-934-4986; **Board Cert:** Obstetrics & Gynecology 2007; Gynecologic Oncology 2007; **Med School:** Louisiana State U, New Orleans 1983; **Resid:** Obstetrics & Gynecology, Univ Alabama Hosp 1987; **Fellow:** Gynecologic Oncology, Univ Alabama Hosp 1990; **Fac Appt:** Assoc Prof ObG, Univ Alabama

Berchuck, Andrew MD [GO] - **Spec Exp:** Ovarian Cancer; Uterine Cancer; **Hospital:** Duke Univ Med Ctr; **Address:** Duke Univ Med Center, DUMC Box 3079, Durham, NC 27710; **Phone:** 919-684-3765; **Board Cert:** Obstetrics & Gynecology 1998; Gynecologic Oncology 1998; **Med School:** Case West Res Univ 1980; **Resid:** Obstetrics & Gynecology, Case Western Resrv 1984; **Fellow:** Gynecology, UT Southwestern 1985; Gynecologic Oncology, Meml Sloan-Kettering 1987; **Fac Appt:** Prof ObG, Duke Univ

Clarke-Pearson, Daniel L MD [GO] - **Spec Exp:** Pelvic Reconstruction; Gynecologic Surgery-Complex; Gynecologic Cancer; **Hospital:** Univ NC Hosps, Wesley Long Comm Hosp; **Address:** Univ of North Carolina, CB #7570, Chapel Hill, NC 27599; **Phone:** 919-966-5280; **Board Cert:** Obstetrics & Gynecology 2006; Gynecologic Oncology 2006; **Med School:** Case West Res Univ 1975; **Resid:** Obstetrics & Gynecology, Duke Univ Med Ctr 1979; **Fellow:** Gynecologic Oncology, Duke Univ Med Ctr 1981; **Fac Appt:** Prof ObG, Univ NC Sch Med

Creasman, William T MD [GO] - **Spec Exp:** Uterine Cancer; Ovarian Cancer; Cervical Cancer; **Hospital:** MUSC Med Ctr; **Address:** Med Univ S Carolina-Dept ObGyn, Charleston, SC 29425; **Phone:** 843-792-4509; **Board Cert:** Obstetrics & Gynecology 1991; Gynecologic Oncology 1974; **Med School:** Baylor Coll Med 1960; **Resid:** Obstetrics & Gynecology, Rochester Med Ctr 1967; **Fellow:** Gynecologic Oncology, Anderson Hosp Tumor Inst 1969; **Fac Appt:** Prof ObG, Med Univ SC

DePriest, Paul D MD [GO] - **Spec Exp:** Ovarian Cancer-Early Detection; Cervical Cancer; Pap Smear Abnormalities; **Hospital:** Univ of Kentucky Chandler Hosp; **Address:** Univ Kentucky Gynecologic Oncology, Whiteney Hendrickson Bldg, 800 Rose St, rm 331E1, Lexington, KY 40536; **Phone:** 859-323-5277; **Board Cert:** Obstetrics & Gynecology 2007; Gynecologic Oncology 2007; **Med School:** Univ KY Coll Med 1985; **Resid:** Obstetrics & Gynecology, Univ Kentucky Med Ctr 1989; **Fellow:** Gynecologic Oncology, Univ Kentucky Med Ctr 1991; **Fac Appt:** Prof ObG, Univ KY Coll Med

Finan, Michael A MD [GO] - **Spec Exp:** Ovarian Cancer; Cervical Cancer; Uterine Cancer; **Hospital:** Univ of S AL Med Ctr, USA Children & Women's Hospital; **Address:** 1660 Springhill Ave, Mobile, AL 36604; **Phone:** 251-665-8000; **Board Cert:** Obstetrics & Gynecology 2007; Gynecologic Oncology 2007; **Med School:** Louisiana State U, New Orleans 1986; **Resid:** Obstetrics & Gynecology, Univ South Fla Affil Hosps 1990; **Fellow:** Gynecologic Oncology, H Lee Moffitt Cancer Ctr 1992; **Fac Appt:** Prof ObG, Univ S Ala Coll Med

Gynecologic Oncology

Fiorica, James V MD [GO] - **Spec Exp:** Gynecologic Cancer; Breast Cancer; Cervical Cancer; **Hospital:** Sarasota Meml Hosp; **Address:** 1888 Hillview St, Sarasota, FL 34239; **Phone:** 941-917-8383; **Board Cert:** Obstetrics & Gynecology 2007; Gynecologic Oncology 2007; **Med School:** Tufts Univ 1982; **Resid:** Obstetrics & Gynecology, Univ South Fla Affil Hosp 1986; **Fellow:** Gynecologic Oncology, Univ South Fla Affil Hosp 1989; Breast Disease, Tufts Univ 1990; **Fac Appt:** Clin Prof ObG, Univ S Fla Coll Med

Fowler Jr, Wesley C MD [GO] - **Spec Exp:** Vulvar Disease/Cancer; DES-Exposed Females; Cancer Prevention; Gynecologic Cancer; **Hospital:** Univ NC Hosps; **Address:** UNC Chapel Hill, Div Ob/Gyn, Campus Box 7572, Chapel Hill, NC 27599-7572; **Phone:** 919-966-7822; **Board Cert:** Obstetrics & Gynecology 1991; Gynecologic Oncology 1979; **Med School:** Univ NC Sch Med 1966; **Resid:** Obstetrics & Gynecology, NC Memorial Hosp 1971; **Fellow:** Gynecologic Oncology, NC Memorial Hosp 1971; **Fac Appt:** Prof ObG, Univ NC Sch Med

Ghamande, Sharad A MD [GO] - **Spec Exp:** Ovarian Cancer; Clinical Trials; **Hospital:** Med Coll of GA Hosp and Clin (MCG Health Inc); **Address:** MCG Health System, 1120 15th St, Augusta, GA 30912; **Phone:** 706-721-6744; **Board Cert:** Obstetrics & Gynecology 2003; Gynecologic Oncology 2003; **Med School:** India 1990; **Resid:** Obstetrics & Gynecology, Boston Univ Hosp 1997; **Fellow:** Gynecologic Oncology, Roswell Park Canc Inst 2000; **Fac Appt:** Assoc Prof ObG, Med Coll GA

Horowitz, Ira R MD [GO] - **Spec Exp:** Laparoscopic Surgery; Ovarian Cancer; Cervical Cancer; **Hospital:** Emory Univ Hosp, Emory Univ Hosp Midtown; **Address:** Emory Clinic, 1365A Clifton Rd NE Fl 4, Atlanta, GA 30322; **Phone:** 404-778-4416; **Board Cert:** Obstetrics & Gynecology 2007; Gynecologic Oncology 2007; **Med School:** Baylor Coll Med 1980; **Resid:** Obstetrics & Gynecology, Baylor Affil Hosp 1984; **Fellow:** Gynecologic Oncology, Johns Hopkins Hosp 1987; **Fac Appt:** Prof ObG, Emory Univ

Kohler, Matthew F MD [GO] - **Spec Exp:** Pelvic Reconstruction; **Hospital:** MUSC Med Ctr; **Address:** MUSC Med Ctr- Women's Hlth Ob/Gyn, 86 Jonathan Lucas St, MS 957, Charleston, SC 29425; **Phone:** 843-792-9300; **Board Cert:** Obstetrics & Gynecology 2007; Gynecologic Oncology 2007; **Med School:** Duke Univ 1987; **Resid:** Obstetrics & Gynecology, Duke Univ Med Ctr 1991; **Fellow:** Gynecologic Oncology, Duke Univ Med Ctr 1994; **Fac Appt:** Assoc Prof ObG, Med Univ SC

Lancaster, Johnathan M MD/PhD [GO] - **Spec Exp:** Ovarian Cancer; Cancer Genetics; Gene Therapy; **Hospital:** H Lee Moffitt Cancer Ctr & Research Inst; **Address:** H Lee Moffitt Cancer Ctr - Gyn Oncology, 12902 Magnolia Drive, MC CGYNPROG, Tampa, FL 33612; **Phone:** 813-745-7272; **Board Cert:** Obstetrics & Gynecology 2008; Gynecologic Oncology 2008; **Med School:** Wales, UK 1997; **Resid:** Obstetrics & Gynecology, Duke Univ Med Ctr 2000; **Fellow:** Gynecologic Oncology, Duke Univ Med Ctr 2003; **Fac Appt:** Asst Prof ObG, Univ S Fla Coll Med

Lentz, Samuel S MD [GO] - **Spec Exp:** Gynecologic Cancer; Pelvic Reconstruction; Incontinence; Incontinence-Fecal; **Hospital:** Wake Forest Univ Baptist Med Ctr (page 72), Forsyth Med Ctr; **Address:** Wake Forest Univ Sch Med, Div Gyn Oncology, Medical Center Blvd, Winston-Salem, NC 27157; **Phone:** 336-716-6673; **Board Cert:** Obstetrics & Gynecology 2007; Gynecologic Oncology 2007; **Med School:** Wake Forest Univ 1978; **Resid:** Obstetrics & Gynecology, NC Baptist Hosp 1982; **Fellow:** Gynecologic Oncology, Mayo Clinic 1989; **Fac Appt:** Prof ObG, Wake Forest Univ

Lucci, Joseph A MD [GO] - **Spec Exp:** Cervical Cancer; **Hospital:** Univ of Miami Hosp (page 71), Jackson Meml Hosp (page 70); **Address:** Univ Miami Dept Ob/Gyn, 1611 NW 12th Ave, Ste 3003, Miami, FL 33136; **Phone:** 305-243-2233; **Board Cert:** Obstetrics & Gynecology 2007; Gynecologic Oncology 2007; **Med School:** Univ Tex, Houston 1984; **Resid:** Obstetrics & Gynecology, St Josephs Hosp 1988; **Fellow:** Gynecologic Oncology, UC Irvine 1992; **Fac Appt:** Clin Prof ObG, Univ Miami Sch Med

Makhija, Sharmila K MD [GO] - **Spec Exp:** Ovarian Cancer; Cervical Cancer; **Hospital:** Emory Univ Hosp; **Address:** The Emory Clinic Bldg A, 1365 Clifton Rd NE Fl 4, Atlanta, GA 30322; **Phone:** 404-778-3401; **Board Cert:** Obstetrics & Gynecology 2007; Gynecologic Oncology 2007; **Med School:** Univ Alabama 1992; **Resid:** Obstetrics & Gynecology, Univ Louisville Hosp 1996; **Fellow:** Gynecologic Oncology, Meml Sloan Kettering Cancer Ctr 1999; **Fac Appt:** Assoc Prof ObG, Emory Univ

Penalver, Manuel A MD [GO] - **Spec Exp:** Gynecologic Cancer; Cervical Cancer; Pelvic Tumors; **Hospital:** Doctors' Hosp, Baptist Hosp of Miami; **Address:** South Florida Gyn Oncology, 5000 University Drive, Ste 3300, Coral Gables, FL 33146; **Phone:** 305-663-7001; **Board Cert:** Obstetrics & Gynecology 2007; Gynecologic Oncology 2007; **Med School:** Univ Miami Sch Med 1977; **Resid:** Obstetrics & Gynecology, Univ Miami/Jackson Meml Hosp 1982; **Fellow:** Gynecologic Oncology, Univ Miami/Jackson Meml Hosp 1984

Poliakoff, Steven R MD [GO] - **Spec Exp:** Ovarian Cancer; Minimally Invasive Surgery; Cancer Genetics; Robotic Surgery; **Hospital:** Mount Sinai Med Ctr - Miami, South Miami Hosp; **Address:** 6280 Sunset Dr, Ste 502, South Miami, FL 33143-4870; **Phone:** 305-596-0870; **Board Cert:** Obstetrics & Gynecology 1983; **Med School:** Univ NC Sch Med 1975; **Resid:** Obstetrics & Gynecology, Johns Hopkins Hosp 1979; **Fellow:** Gynecologic Oncology, Jackson Meml Hosp/Univ Miami 1981

Soper, John T MD [GO] - **Spec Exp:** Gynecologic Cancer; **Hospital:** Univ NC Hosps; **Address:** Univ North Carolina, Dept OB/GYN, Physicians Office Bldg, 101 Manning Drive, Ste B-103, Chapel Hill, NC 27599-7572; **Phone:** 919-966-1195; **Board Cert:** Obstetrics & Gynecology 2007; Gynecologic Oncology 2007; **Med School:** Univ Iowa Coll Med 1978; **Resid:** Obstetrics & Gynecology, Univ Utah Med Ctr 1982; **Fellow:** Gynecologic Oncology, Duke Univ Med Ctr 1985; **Fac Appt:** Prof ObG, Univ NC Sch Med

Spann Jr, Cyril O MD [GO] - **Spec Exp:** Gynecologic Cancer; Ovarian Cancer; **Hospital:** Grady Hlth Sys, Emory Univ Hosp Midtown; **Address:** Dept Gynecology & Obstetrics, 69 Jesse Hill Jr Drive Fl 4, Atlanta, GA 30303; **Phone:** 404-686-8121; **Board Cert:** Obstetrics & Gynecology 2005; Gynecologic Oncology 2005; **Med School:** Meharry Med Coll 1981; **Resid:** Obstetrics & Gynecology, Emory Univ Med Ctr 1985; **Fellow:** Gynecologic Oncology, Univ NC Meml Hosp 1989; **Fac Appt:** Prof ObG, Emory Univ

Taylor Jr, Peyton T MD [GO] - **Spec Exp:** Gynecologic Surgery-Complex; Gynecologic Cancer; **Hospital:** Univ Virginia Med Ctr; **Address:** Univ VA Hlth Sys, Dept Ob/Gyn, PO Box 800712, Charlottesville, VA 22908; **Phone:** 434-924-9933; **Board Cert:** Obstetrics & Gynecology 1994; Gynecologic Oncology 1981; **Med School:** Univ Alabama 1968; **Resid:** Obstetrics & Gynecology, Univ VA Hosp 1970; Obstetrics & Gynecology, Univ VA Hosp 1975; **Fellow:** Surgical Oncology, Natl Cancer Inst 1972; Gynecologic Oncology, Univ Va Hosp 1977; **Fac Appt:** Prof ObG, Univ VA Sch Med

Van Nagell Jr, John R MD [GO] - **Spec Exp:** Ovarian Cancer; Cervical Cancer; **Hospital:** Univ of Kentucky Chandler Hosp; **Address:** UKMC, Dept Ob/Gyn, 800 Rose St, Lexington, KY 40536-0001; **Phone:** 859-323-5553; **Board Cert:** Obstetrics & Gynecology 1973; Gynecologic Oncology 1976; **Med School:** Univ Pennsylvania 1967; **Resid:** Obstetrics & Gynecology, Kentucky Med Ctr 1971; **Fac Appt:** Prof ObG, Univ KY Coll Med

Gynecologic Oncology

Midwest

Belinson, Jerome L MD [GO] - **Spec Exp:** Ovarian Cancer; Cervical Cancer; **Hospital:** Cleveland Clin Fdn (page 56); **Address:** 9500 Euclid Ave, Desk A81, Cleveland, OH 44195; **Phone:** 216-444-7933; **Board Cert:** Obstetrics & Gynecology 1998; Gynecologic Oncology 1980; **Med School:** Univ MO-Columbia Sch Med 1968; **Resid:** Obstetrics & Gynecology, Columbia Presby Med Ctr 1973; **Fellow:** Gynecologic Oncology, Jackson Meml Hosp 1977; **Fac Appt:** Prof ObG, Ohio State Univ

Cliby, William A MD [GO] - **Spec Exp:** Ovarian Cancer; **Hospital:** Mayo Med Ctr & Clin - Rochester; **Address:** Mayo Clinic, 200 First St SW, Rochester, MN 55905; **Phone:** 507-266-9323; **Board Cert:** Obstetrics & Gynecology 2007; Gynecologic Oncology 2007; **Med School:** Univ VT Coll Med 1987; **Resid:** Obstetrics & Gynecology, Duke Univ Med Ctr 1991; **Fellow:** Gynecologic Oncology, Mayo Clinic 1994; Research, Fred Hutchinson Cancer Rsch Ctr; **Fac Appt:** Prof ObG, Mayo Med Sch

Copeland, Larry J MD [GO] - **Spec Exp:** Ovarian Cancer; Uterine Cancer; Gynecologic Cancer; **Hospital:** Arthur G James Cancer Hosp & Research Inst, Ohio St Univ Med Ctr; **Address:** 1654 Upham Drive, Ste 505, Columbus, OH 43210-1250; **Phone:** 614-293-8697; **Board Cert:** Obstetrics & Gynecology 1991; Gynecologic Oncology 1981; **Med School:** Univ Western Ontario 1973; **Resid:** Obstetrics & Gynecology, McMaster Univ Affil Hosps 1977; **Fellow:** Gynecologic Oncology, MD Anderson Cancer Ctr-Univ Tex 1979; **Fac Appt:** Prof ObG, Ohio State Univ

De Geest, Koen MD [GO] - **Spec Exp:** Ovarian Cancer; Uterine Cancer; Clinical Trials; **Hospital:** Univ Iowa Hosp & Clinics; **Address:** Univ Iowa, Div Gynecological Oncology, 200 Hawkins Drive, rm 4630 JCP, Iowa City, IA 52242; **Phone:** 319-356-2015; **Board Cert:** Obstetrics & Gynecology 2007; Gynecologic Oncology 2007; **Med School:** Belgium 1977; **Resid:** Obstetrics & Gynecology, Univ Ghent 1982; **Fellow:** Gynecologic Oncology, Penn State/Hershey Med Ctr 1990; **Fac Appt:** Prof ObG, Univ Iowa Coll Med

Fowler, Jeffrey M MD [GO] - **Spec Exp:** Laparoscopic Surgery; Gynecologic Cancer; Robotic Surgery; Pelvic Reconstruction; **Hospital:** Ohio St Univ Med Ctr; **Address:** Ohio State Univ, Div Gynecologic Oncology, 320 W Tenth Ave, M-210 SLH, Columbus, OH 43210; **Phone:** 614-293-8737; **Board Cert:** Obstetrics & Gynecology 2007; Gynecologic Oncology 2007; **Med School:** Northwestern Univ 1985; **Resid:** Obstetrics & Gynecology, Ohio State Univ Hosp 1989; **Fellow:** Gynecologic Oncology, Cedars-Sinai Med Ctr 1991; **Fac Appt:** Prof ObG, Ohio State Univ

Johnston, Carolyn M MD [GO] - **Spec Exp:** Gynecologic Surgery-Complex; Cervical Cancer; **Hospital:** Univ Michigan Hlth Sys; **Address:** Womens Hosp-Div Gyn Oncology, 1500 E Med Ctr Drive, rm L4510, Ann Arbor, MI 48109-0276; **Phone:** 734-647-8906; **Board Cert:** Obstetrics & Gynecology 2000; Gynecologic Oncology 2000; **Med School:** Yale Univ 1984; **Resid:** Obstetrics & Gynecology, Univ Chicago Hosp 1988; **Fellow:** Gynecologic Oncology, Mt Sinai Hosp 1990; **Fac Appt:** Assoc Clin Prof ObG, Univ Mich Med Sch

Lurain, John R MD [GO] - **Spec Exp:** Gestational Trophoblastic Disease; Uterine Cancer; Ovarian Cancer; Cervical Cancer; **Hospital:** Northwestern Meml Hosp; **Address:** Northwestern Univ Feinberg Sch Med, 250 E Superior St, Ste 05-2168, Chicago, IL 60611-3056; **Phone:** 312-695-0990; **Board Cert:** Obstetrics & Gynecology 1977; Gynecologic Oncology 1981; **Med School:** Univ NC Sch Med 1972; **Resid:** Obstetrics & Gynecology, Univ Pittsburgh Med Ctr 1975; **Fellow:** Gynecologic Oncology, Roswell Park Cancer Inst 1979; **Fac Appt:** Prof ObG, Northwestern Univ

Mutch, David G MD [GO] - **Spec Exp:** Gynecologic Cancer; Pelvic Reconstruction; **Hospital:** Barnes-Jewish Hosp; **Address:** 4911 Barnes Jewish Hospital Plaza, St Louis, MO 63110; **Phone:** 314-362-3181; **Board Cert:** Obstetrics & Gynecology 2006; Gynecologic Oncology 2006; **Med School:** Washington Univ, St Louis 1980; **Resid:** Obstetrics & Gynecology, Barnes Hosp-Wash Univ 1984; **Fellow:** Gynecologic Oncology, Duke Univ Med Ctr 1987; **Fac Appt:** Prof ObG, Washington Univ, St Louis

Potkul, Ronald MD [GO] - **Spec Exp:** Ovarian Cancer; Cervical Cancer; **Hospital:** Loyola Univ Med Ctr; **Address:** Loyola Univ Med Ctr, 2160 S 1st Ave Bldg 112 - rm 267, Maywood, IL 60153; **Phone:** 708-327-3500; **Board Cert:** Obstetrics & Gynecology 1997; Gynecologic Oncology 1997; **Med School:** Univ Chicago-Pritzker Sch Med 1981; **Resid:** Obstetrics & Gynecology, Univ Chicago Hosps 1985; **Fellow:** Gynecologic Oncology, Georgetown Univ Hosp 1988; **Fac Appt:** Prof ObG, Loyola Univ-Stritch Sch Med

Rader, Janet S MD [GO] - **Spec Exp:** Cervical Cancer; Ovarian Cancer; Uterine Cancer; **Hospital:** Barnes-Jewish Hosp, Missouri Baptist Med Ctr; **Address:** 660 S Euclid Ave, Box 8064, St Louis, MO 63110; **Phone:** 314-362-3181; **Board Cert:** Obstetrics & Gynecology 2007; Gynecologic Oncology 2007; **Med School:** Univ MO-Columbia Sch Med 1983; **Resid:** Obstetrics & Gynecology, Michael Reese Hosp 1987; **Fellow:** Gynecologic Oncology, Johns Hopkins Hosp 1990; **Fac Appt:** Prof ObG, Washington Univ, St Louis

Reynolds, R Kevin MD [GO] - **Hospital:** Univ Michigan Hlth Sys; **Address:** Women's Hosp, Div Gyn Onc, 1500 E Med Ctr Drive, rm L4510, Ann Arbor, MI 48109-0276; **Phone:** 734-764-9106; **Board Cert:** Obstetrics & Gynecology 2007; Gynecologic Oncology 2007; **Med School:** Univ New Mexico 1982; **Resid:** Obstetrics & Gynecology, Univ Vt Hosp 1986; **Fellow:** Gynecologic Oncology, Univ Mich Med Ctr 1991; **Fac Appt:** Asst Prof ObG, Univ Mich Med Sch

Rice, Laurel W MD [GO] - **Spec Exp:** Ovarian Cancer; Uterine Cancer; Cervical Cancer; **Hospital:** Univ WI Hosp & Clins; **Address:** 1 S Park St, Ste 555, Madison, WI 53715; **Phone:** 608-263-3194; **Board Cert:** Obstetrics & Gynecology 2006; Gynecologic Oncology 2006; **Med School:** Univ Colorado 1983; **Resid:** Obstetrics & Gynecology, Brigham-Womens Hosp 1987; **Fellow:** Obstetrics & Gynecology, Brigham-Womens Hosp 1989; **Fac Appt:** Assoc Prof ObG, Univ VA Sch Med

Rose, Peter G MD [GO] - **Spec Exp:** Cervical Cancer; Ovarian Cancer; Uterine Cancer; **Hospital:** Cleveland Clin Fdn (page 56), MetroHealth Med Ctr; **Address:** Cleveland Clinic Fdn, 9500 Euclid Ave A-81, Cleveland, OH 44195; **Phone:** 216-444-1712; **Board Cert:** Obstetrics & Gynecology 2007; Gynecologic Oncology 2007; **Med School:** Boston Univ 1981; **Resid:** Surgery, Vanderbilt Univ Med Ctr 1983; Obstetrics & Gynecology, Ohio State Univ Med Ctr 1986; **Fellow:** Gynecologic Oncology, Roswell Park Med Ctr 1988; **Fac Appt:** Prof ObG, Case West Res Univ

Rotmensch, Jacob MD [GO] - **Spec Exp:** Gynecologic Cancer; Ovarian Cancer; Cervical Cancer; **Hospital:** Rush Univ Med Ctr; **Address:** University Gynecologic Oncology Assocs, 1725 W Harrison St, Ste 829, Chicago, IL 60612; **Phone:** 312-942-6300; **Board Cert:** Obstetrics & Gynecology 2007; Gynecologic Oncology 2007; **Med School:** Meharry Med Coll 1977; **Resid:** Obstetrics & Gynecology, Johns Hopkins Hosp 1981; **Fellow:** Gynecologic Oncology, Johns Hopkins Hosp 1984; **Fac Appt:** Prof ObG, Rush Med Coll

Schink, Julian C MD [GO] - **Spec Exp:** Ovarian Cancer; **Hospital:** Northwestern Meml Hosp; **Address:** 675 N St Clair St, Fl 21 - Ste 100, Chicago, IL 60611; **Phone:** 312-695-0990; **Board Cert:** Obstetrics & Gynecology 2000; Gynecologic Oncology 2000; **Med School:** Univ Tex, San Antonio 1982; **Resid:** Obstetrics & Gynecology, Northwestern Univ Med Sch 1986; **Fellow:** Gynecologic Oncology, UCLA Med Ctr 1988; **Fac Appt:** Prof ObG, Northwestern Univ

Gynecologic Oncology

Smith, Donna M MD [GO] - **Spec Exp:** Cervical Cancer; Ovarian Cancer; **Hospital:** Loyola Univ Med Ctr; **Address:** Cardinal Bernardin Cancer Ctr, Clinic A, 2160 S 1st Ave Bldg 112 - rm 267, Maywood, IL 60153; **Phone:** 708-327-3500; **Board Cert:** Obstetrics & Gynecology 2007; Gynecologic Oncology 2007; **Med School:** Univ MO-Kansas City 1980; **Resid:** Obstetrics & Gynecology, Emory Univ Hosp 1984; **Fellow:** Gynecologic Oncology, Georgetown Univ Med Ctr 1987; **Fac Appt:** Assoc Prof ObG, Loyola Univ-Stritch Sch Med

Stehman, Frederick B MD [GO] - **Spec Exp:** Clinical Trials; Gynecologic Cancer; **Hospital:** Indiana Univ Hosp, Wishard Hlth Srvs; **Address:** Indiana Univ Hosp, Dept ObGyn, 535 Barnhill, Rt 433, Indianapolis, IN 46202; **Phone:** 317-274-7241; **Board Cert:** Obstetrics & Gynecology 2005; Gynecologic Oncology 2003; **Med School:** Univ Mich Med Sch 1972; **Resid:** Obstetrics & Gynecology, Univ Kansas Med Ctr 1975; Surgery, Univ Kansas Med Ctr 1977; **Fellow:** Gynecologic Oncology, UCLA Med Ctr 1979; **Fac Appt:** Prof ObG, Indiana Univ

Waggoner, Steven MD [GO] - **Spec Exp:** Ovarian Cancer; Cervical Cancer; Uterine Cancer; **Hospital:** Univ Hosps Case Med Ctr; **Address:** Dept Ob/Gyn, Div Gyn Oncology, 11100 Euclid Ave, rm 7136, Cleveland, OH 44106; **Phone:** 216-844-3954; **Board Cert:** Obstetrics & Gynecology 2007; Gynecologic Oncology 2007; **Med School:** Univ Wash 1984; **Resid:** Obstetrics & Gynecology, Univ Chicago Hosps 1988; **Fellow:** Gynecologic Oncology, Georgetown Univ 1991; **Fac Appt:** Prof ObG, Case West Res Univ

Great Plains and Mountains

Davidson, Susan MD [GO] - **Spec Exp:** Gynecologic Cancer; **Hospital:** Univ Colorado Hosp; **Address:** Univ Colorado Hosp, Dept OB/GYN, 12631 E 17th Ave B198-4 Bldg, Box 6511, Denver, CO 80262; **Phone:** 720-848-1060; **Board Cert:** Obstetrics & Gynecology 2007; Gynecologic Oncology 2007; **Med School:** Univ Tex, San Antonio 1984; **Resid:** Obstetrics & Gynecology, Univ Texas Med Ctr 1988; **Fellow:** Gynecologic Oncology, Meml Sloan Kettering Cancer Ctr 1990; **Fac Appt:** Assoc Prof ObG, Univ Colorado

Remmenga, Steven W MD [GO] - **Spec Exp:** Ovarian Cancer; Cervical Cancer; Gynecologic Cancer; **Hospital:** Nebraska Med Ctr; **Address:** Univ Nebraska Med Ctr, Gyne Oncology, 983255 Nebraska Med Ctr, Omaha, NE 68198-3255; **Phone:** 402-559-5068; **Board Cert:** Obstetrics & Gynecology 1998; Gynecologic Oncology 1998; **Med School:** Univ Nebr Coll Med 1981; **Resid:** Obstetrics & Gynecology, Naval Hospital 1986; **Fellow:** Gynecologic Oncology, Walter Reed Army Med Ctr 1990; **Fac Appt:** Assoc Prof ObG, Univ Nebr Coll Med

Soisson, Andrew P MD [GO] - **Spec Exp:** Cervical Cancer; **Hospital:** LDS Hosp, Univ Utah Hosps and Clins; **Address:** Univ Hosp, Div Gyn Oncology, 30 N 1900 E, rm 2B200, Salt Lake City, UT 84132; **Phone:** 801-587-4399; **Board Cert:** Obstetrics & Gynecology 2006; Gynecologic Oncology 2006; **Med School:** Georgetown Univ 1981; **Resid:** Obstetrics & Gynecology, Madigan AMC 1985; **Fellow:** Gynecologic Oncology, Duke Univ Med Ctr 1990; **Fac Appt:** Assoc Prof ObG, Univ Utah

Southwest

Burnett, Alexander F MD [GO] - **Spec Exp:** Laparoscopic Surgery; Fertility Preservation in Cancer; Gynecologic Cancer; **Hospital:** UAMS Med Ctr; **Address:** 4301 W Markham St, Slot 793, Little Rock, AR 72205; **Phone:** 501-296-1099; **Board Cert:** Obstetrics & Gynecology 2007; Gynecologic Oncology 2007; **Med School:** Georgetown Univ 1986; **Resid:** Obstetrics & Gynecology, Georgetown Univ Affil Hosp 1990; **Fellow:** Gynecologic Oncology, Georgetown Univ Affil Hosp 1993; **Fac Appt:** Assoc Prof ObG, Univ Ark

Chambers, Setsuko K MD [GO] - **Spec Exp:** Gynecologic Cancer; Breast Cancer; Ovarian Cancer; **Hospital:** Univ Med Ctr - Tucson; **Address:** 1515 N Campbell Ave, Arizona Cancer Center, Tucson, AZ 85724; **Phone:** 520-626-9285; **Board Cert:** Obstetrics & Gynecology 2007; Gynecologic Oncology 2007; **Med School:** Brown Univ 1980; **Resid:** Obstetrics & Gynecology, Yale-New Haven Hosp 1984; **Fellow:** Gynecologic Oncology, Yale-New Haven Hosp 1986; **Fac Appt:** Prof ObG, Univ Ariz Coll Med

Follen, Michele MD/PhD [GO] - **Spec Exp:** Gynecologic Cancer; Clinical Trials; Cervical Cancer; **Hospital:** UT MD Anderson Cancer Ctr; **Address:** MD Anderson Cancer Ctr, 1515 Holcombe Blvd, Unit 1362, Houston, TX 77030; **Phone:** 713-745-2564; **Board Cert:** Obstetrics & Gynecology 1999; Gynecologic Oncology 1999; **Med School:** Univ Mich Med Sch 1980; **Resid:** Obstetrics & Gynecology, Columbia-Presby Med Ctr 1983; **Fellow:** Gynecologic Oncology, MD Anderson Cancer Ctr 1986; **Fac Appt:** Prof ObG, Univ Tex, Houston

Fromm, Geri-Lynn MD [GO] - **Spec Exp:** Cervical Cancer; Ovarian Cancer; Gestational Trophoblastic Disease; **Hospital:** St Luke's Episcopal Hosp-Houston, Woman's Hosp TX; **Address:** 2223 Dorrington St, Houston, TX 77030; **Phone:** 713-665-0404; **Board Cert:** Obstetrics & Gynecology 2007; Gynecologic Oncology 2007; **Med School:** Northwestern Univ 1981; **Resid:** Obstetrics & Gynecology, Magee Womens Hosp 1985; **Fellow:** Gynecologic Oncology, MD Anderson Cancer Ctr 1987; **Fac Appt:** Assoc Clin Prof ObG, Baylor Coll Med

Gershenson, David M MD [GO] - **Spec Exp:** Ovarian Rare & Borderline Tumors; Uterine Cancer-Serous Carcinoma; Fertility Preservation in Cancer; Sex Cord-Stromal Tumors; **Hospital:** UT MD Anderson Cancer Ctr, St Luke's Episcopal Hosp-Houston; **Address:** Univ Tex MD Anderson Cancer Ctr, PO Box 301439, Houston, TX 77030-1439; **Phone:** 713-745-2565; **Board Cert:** Obstetrics & Gynecology 1991; Gynecologic Oncology 1981; **Med School:** Vanderbilt Univ 1971; **Resid:** Obstetrics & Gynecology, Yale-New Haven Hosp 1975; **Fellow:** Gynecologic Oncology, MD Anderson Cancer Ctr 1979; **Fac Appt:** Prof ObG, Univ Tex, Houston

Hatch, Kenneth MD [GO] - **Spec Exp:** Cervical Cancer; Uro-Gynecology; Pelvic Organ Prolapse Repair; **Hospital:** Univ Med Ctr - Tucson, NW Med Ctr; **Address:** Univ Arizona College of Medicine, 1515 N Campbell Ave, rm 1968, Tucson, AZ 85724; **Phone:** 520-626-9285; **Board Cert:** Obstetrics & Gynecology 1993; Gynecologic Oncology 1981; **Med School:** Univ Nebr Coll Med 1971; **Resid:** Obstetrics & Gynecology, Univ AL Med Ctr Birmingham 1976; **Fellow:** Gynecologic Oncology, Univ AL Med Ctr Birmingham 1978; **Fac Appt:** Prof ObG, Univ Ariz Coll Med

Levenback, Charles MD [GO] - **Spec Exp:** Vulvar Disease/Cancer; Cervical Cancer; Gynecologic Cancer; **Hospital:** UT MD Anderson Cancer Ctr; **Address:** PO Box 301439 - Unit 1362, Houston, TX 77230; **Phone:** 713-745-2563; **Board Cert:** Obstetrics & Gynecology 2007; Gynecologic Oncology 2007; **Med School:** Mount Sinai Sch Med 1983; **Resid:** Obstetrics & Gynecology, Albert Einstein Coll Med 1987; **Fellow:** Gynecologic Oncology, Meml Sloan Kettering Cancer Ctr 1989; **Fac Appt:** Prof ObG, Univ Tex, Houston

Lu, Karen Hsieh MD [GO] - **Spec Exp:** Ovarian Cancer; Ovarian Cancer-Early Detection; Uterine Cancer; Cancer Genetics; **Hospital:** UT MD Anderson Cancer Ctr; **Address:** Univ of Texas MD Anderson Cancer Ctr, 1515 Holcombe Blvd, Houston, TX 77030; **Phone:** 713-745-8902; **Board Cert:** Obstetrics & Gynecology 2003; Gynecologic Oncology 2003; **Med School:** Yale Univ 1991; **Resid:** Obstetrics & Gynecology, Brigham & Women's Hosp 1994; **Fellow:** Gynecologic Oncology, Brigham & Women's Hosp 1999; **Fac Appt:** Prof ObG, Univ Tex SW, Dallas

Gynecologic Oncology

Magrina, Javier MD [GO] - **Spec Exp:** Gynecologic Cancer; Endometriosis; Hysterectomy Alternatives; Robotic Surgery; **Hospital:** Mayo Clinic - Scottsdale; **Address:** Mayo Clinic, 5779 E Mayo Blvd, Phoenix, AZ 85054; **Phone:** 480-342-2668; **Board Cert:** Obstetrics & Gynecology 1994; Gynecologic Oncology 1982; **Med School:** Spain 1972; **Resid:** Obstetrics & Gynecology, Mayo Clinic 1977; **Fellow:** Gynecologic Oncology, Kansas Med Ctr 1980; **Fac Appt:** Prof ObG, Mayo Med Sch

Sood, Anil K MD [GO] - **Hospital:** UT MD Anderson Cancer Ctr; **Address:** Univ Texas MD Anderson Cancer Ctr, 1515 Holcombe Blvd Ste 440, Houston, TX 77030-4000; **Phone:** 713-745-5266; **Board Cert:** Obstetrics & Gynecology 1999; Gynecologic Oncology 2001; **Med School:** Univ NC Sch Med 1991; **Resid:** Obstetrics & Gynecology, Univ FL 1995; **Fellow:** Gynecologic Oncology, Univ NC Sch Med 1998

Walker, Joan L MD [GO] - **Spec Exp:** Ovarian Cancer; Cervical Cancer; Uterine Cancer; **Hospital:** OU Med Ctr; **Address:** OU Health Science Ctr, Dept Ob/Gyn, PO Box 26901, Oklahoma City, OK 73126; **Phone:** 405-271-8707; **Board Cert:** Obstetrics & Gynecology 2007; Gynecologic Oncology 2007; **Med School:** UCLA 1982; **Resid:** Obstetrics & Gynecology, Hosp Univ Penn 1986; **Fellow:** Gynecologic Oncology, UC-Irvine 1990; **Fac Appt:** Assoc Prof ObG, Univ Okla Coll Med

West Coast and Pacific

Berek, Jonathan S MD [GO] - **Spec Exp:** Ovarian Cancer; Uterine Cancer; Cervical Cancer; Vulvar & Vaginal Cancer; **Hospital:** Stanford Univ Med Ctr; **Address:** Stanford Univ School of Medicine, 300 Pasteur Dr, HH333, Stanford, CA 94305-2296; **Phone:** 650-498-6000; **Board Cert:** Obstetrics & Gynecology 2008; Gynecologic Oncology 2008; **Med School:** Johns Hopkins Univ 1975; **Resid:** Obstetrics & Gynecology, Brigham & Womans Hosp 1979; **Fellow:** Gynecologic Oncology, UCLA Sch Med 1981; **Fac Appt:** Prof ObG, Stanford Univ

Berman, Michael L MD [GO] - **Spec Exp:** Gynecologic Cancer; Cervical Cancer; **Hospital:** UC Irvine Med Ctr, Long Beach Meml Med Ctr; **Address:** Cho Family Comprehensive Cancer Ctr, 101 The City Drive Bldg 56 - Ste 260, Orange, CA 92868-3201; **Phone:** 714-456-8020; **Board Cert:** Obstetrics & Gynecology 2005; Gynecologic Oncology 2005; **Med School:** Geo Wash Univ 1967; **Resid:** Obstetrics & Gynecology, GW Univ Hosp 1969; Obstetrics & Gynecology, LAC-Harbor Hosp 1974; **Fellow:** Gynecologic Oncology, UCLA Med Ctr 1976; **Fac Appt:** Prof ObG, UC Irvine

Carney, Michael E MD [GO] - **Spec Exp:** Gynecologic Cancer; Pelvic Surgery-Complex; Minimally Invasive Surgery; **Hospital:** Kapiolani Med Ctr for Women & Chldn; **Address:** Kapiolani Med Ctr for Women & Children, 1319 Punahou St, Ste 640, Honolulu, HI 96826; **Phone:** 808-983-6090; **Board Cert:** Obstetrics & Gynecology 2002; Gynecologic Oncology 2002; **Med School:** Loyola Univ-Stritch Sch Med 1990; **Resid:** Obstetrics & Gynecology, Duke Univ Med Ctr 1994; **Fellow:** Gynecologic Oncology, Duke Univ Med Ctr 1999; **Fac Appt:** Asst Prof ObG, Univ Hawaii JA Burns Sch Med

Chan, John K MD [GO] - **Spec Exp:** Ovarian Cancer; Pelvic Surgery-Complex; Gene Therapy; Clinical Trials; **Hospital:** UCSF Med Ctr; **Address:** UCSF Medical Center, 1600 Divisidaro St, Box 1702, San Francisco, CA 94143; **Phone:** 415-353-9600; **Board Cert:** Obstetrics & Gynecology 2006; Gynecologic Oncology 2006; **Med School:** UCLA 1995; **Resid:** Obstetrics & Gynecology, UC Irvine Med Ctr 1999; **Fellow:** Gynecologic Oncology, MD Anderson Cancer Ctr 1999; Gynecologic Oncology, UC Irvine 2003; **Fac Appt:** Asst Prof ObG, UCSF

Di Saia, Philip J MD [GO] - **Spec Exp:** Ovarian Cancer; Gynecologic Cancer; Cervical Cancer; **Hospital:** UC Irvine Med Ctr; **Address:** 101 The City Drive Bldg 56 - rm 800, Route 80, Orange, CA 92668; **Phone:** 714-456-8000; **Board Cert:** Obstetrics & Gynecology 1983; Gynecologic Oncology 1974; **Med School:** Tufts Univ 1963; **Resid:** Obstetrics & Gynecology, Yale-New Haven Hosp 1967; **Fellow:** Gynecologic Oncology, MD Anderson Hosp 1971; **Fac Appt:** Prof ObG, UC Irvine

Goff, Barbara A MD [GO] - **Spec Exp:** Ovarian Cancer; Uterine Cancer; Cervical Cancer; Gynecologic Surgery-Complex; **Hospital:** Univ Wash Med Ctr; **Address:** Univ Washington, Dept ObGyn, Box 356460, Seattle, WA 98195; **Phone:** 206-288-2273; **Board Cert:** Obstetrics & Gynecology 2007; Gynecologic Oncology 2007; **Med School:** Univ Pennsylvania 1986; **Resid:** Obstetrics & Gynecology, Mass Genl Hosp/Brigham & Womens Hosp 1990; **Fellow:** Gynecologic Oncology, Mass Genl Hosp 1993; **Fac Appt:** Prof ObG, Univ Wash

Greer, Benjamin E MD [GO] - **Spec Exp:** Gynecologic Cancer; **Hospital:** Univ Wash Med Ctr; **Address:** Univ Wash, Dept OB/GYN, Box 356460, Seattle, WA 98195; **Phone:** 206-288-2273; **Board Cert:** Obstetrics & Gynecology 2002; Gynecologic Oncology 2002; **Med School:** Univ Pennsylvania 1966; **Resid:** Obstetrics & Gynecology, Univ Colorado Med Ctr 1970; **Fac Appt:** Prof ObG, Univ Wash

Karlan, Beth Y MD [GO] - **Spec Exp:** Ovarian Cancer; Gynecologic Cancer; **Hospital:** Cedars-Sinai Med Ctr; **Address:** 8700 Beverly Blvd, Ste 290W, Los Angeles, CA 90048; **Phone:** 310-423-3302; **Board Cert:** Obstetrics & Gynecology 1998; Gynecologic Oncology 1998; **Med School:** Harvard Med Sch 1982; **Resid:** Obstetrics & Gynecology, Yale-New Haven Hosp 1986; **Fellow:** Gynecologic Oncology, UCLA 1989; **Fac Appt:** Prof ObG, UCLA

Monk, Bradley J MD [GO] - **Spec Exp:** Gynecologic Surgery-Complex; Cervical Cancer; Ovarian Cancer; Gynecologic Cancer; **Hospital:** UC Irvine Med Ctr; **Address:** UC Irvine Comprehensive Cancer Ctr, 101 The City Drive Bldg 56 - rm 260, Irvine, CA 92868; **Phone:** 714-456-6570; **Board Cert:** Obstetrics & Gynecology 2007; Gynecologic Oncology 2007; **Med School:** Univ Ariz Coll Med 1988; **Resid:** Obstetrics & Gynecology, UCLA Med Ctr 1992; **Fellow:** Gynecologic Oncology, UC Irvine Med Ctr 1995; **Fac Appt:** Assoc Prof ObG, UC Irvine

Muntz, Howard G MD [GO] - **Spec Exp:** Gynecologic Cancer; Ovarian Cancer; Clinical Trials; Gynecologic Surgery-Complex; **Hospital:** Northwest Hosp; **Address:** Women's Cancer Care of Seattle, 1560 N 115th St, Ste 101, Seattle, WA 98133; **Phone:** 206-368-6806; **Board Cert:** Obstetrics & Gynecology 2007; Gynecologic Oncology 2007; **Med School:** Harvard Med Sch 1984; **Resid:** Obstetrics & Gynecology, Brigham & Womens Hosp 1988; **Fellow:** Gynecologic Oncology, Mass General Hosp 1991; **Fac Appt:** Assoc Clin Prof ObG, Univ Wash

Plaxe, Steven C MD [GO] - **Spec Exp:** Ovarian Cancer; Uterine Cancer; Gestational Trophoblastic Disease; **Hospital:** UCSD Med Ctr; **Address:** Moores Cancer Center, 3855 Health Sciences Drive, MC 0987, La Jolla, CA 92093-0987; **Phone:** 858-822-6199; **Board Cert:** Obstetrics & Gynecology 2008; Gynecologic Oncology 2008; **Med School:** Mount Sinai Sch Med 1981; **Resid:** Obstetrics & Gynecology, Yale-New Haven Hosp 1985; **Fellow:** Gynecologic Oncology, Mt Sinai Med Ctr 1988; **Fac Appt:** Prof ObG, UCSD

Powell, Catherine Bethan MD [GO] - **Spec Exp:** Gynecologic Cancer; Cancer Genetics; **Hospital:** Kaiser Permanente S San Francisco Med Ctr; **Address:** Kaiser Permanente Medical Group Inc, 2238 Geary Blvd Fl 5, San Francisco, CA 94115; **Phone:** 415-833-4199; **Board Cert:** Obstetrics & Gynecology 2007; Gynecologic Oncology 2007; **Med School:** Univ Pennsylvania 1982; **Resid:** Obstetrics & Gynecology, Pennsylvania Hosp 1987; **Fellow:** Gynecologic Oncology, Wash Univ 1990

Gynecologic Oncology

Smith, Lloyd H MD [GO] - **Spec Exp:** Ovarian Cancer; Uterine Cancer; Vulvar Disease/Cancer; Vaginal Cancer; **Hospital:** UC Davis Med Ctr, Sutter Mem Hospital-Sacramento; **Address:** UC Davis Med Ctr, Dept Ob/Gyn, 4860 Y St, Ste 2500, Sacramento, CA 95817-2307; **Phone:** 916-734-6946; **Board Cert:** Obstetrics & Gynecology 1998; Gynecologic Oncology 1998; **Med School:** UC Davis 1981; **Resid:** Obstetrics & Gynecology, UC Davis Med Ctr 1985; **Fellow:** Gynecologic Oncology, Stanford Univ Hosp 1988; **Fac Appt:** Prof ObG, UC Davis

Spirtos, Nicola Michael MD [GO] - **Spec Exp:** Gynecologic Cancer; Ovarian Cancer; **Hospital:** Univ Med Ctr - Las Vegas; **Address:** 3131 La Canada St, Ste 110, Las Vegas, NV 89169; **Phone:** 702-693-6870; **Board Cert:** Obstetrics & Gynecology 1998; Gynecologic Oncology 1998; **Med School:** Northwestern Univ 1980; **Resid:** Obstetrics & Gynecology, Women's Hosp LAC-USC Med Ctr 1984; **Fellow:** Gynecologic Oncology, Stanford Univ Affil Hosp 1987

Stern, Jeffrey L MD [GO] - **Spec Exp:** Laparoscopic Surgery; Vulvar Disease/Cancer; **Hospital:** Alta Bates Summit Med Ctr-Alta Bates Campus; **Address:** Womens Cancer Ctr Northern Calif, 2001 Dwight Way, Berkley, CA 94704; **Phone:** 510-204-5770; **Board Cert:** Obstetrics & Gynecology 1983; Gynecologic Oncology 1984; **Med School:** SUNY Upstate Med Univ 1976; **Resid:** Obstetrics & Gynecology, Johns Hopkins Hosp 1980; **Fellow:** Gynecologic Oncology, USC Med Ctr 1982

Teng, Nelson NH MD/PhD [GO] - **Spec Exp:** Ovarian Cancer; Clinical Trials; **Hospital:** Stanford Univ Med Ctr; **Address:** Dept Gyn Oncology, 875 Blake Wilbur Drive, Stanford, CA 94305-5317; **Phone:** 650-498-8080; **Board Cert:** Obstetrics & Gynecology 2003; Gynecologic Oncology 2003; **Med School:** Univ Miami Sch Med 1977; **Resid:** Obstetrics & Gynecology, UCLA Med Ctr 1981; **Fellow:** Gynecologic Oncology, Stanford Univ Sch Med 1984; **Fac Appt:** Assoc Prof ObG, Stanford Univ

NYU **Cancer Institute**
NYU LANGONE MEDICAL CENTER

NYU Clinical Cancer Institute
160 East 34th Street
New York, NY 10016
www.nyuci.org/atcd

NYU Langone Medical Center
505 First Avenue (at 31st Street)
New York, NY 10016
www.med.nyu.edu

Stephen D. Hassenfeld
Children's CenterFor Cancer and Blood Disorders
160 East 32nd Street, New York, NY 10016
www.nyumc.org/hassenfeld

NYU CANCER INSTITUTE

About the Cancer Institute:

The NYU Cancer Institute is an NCI-designated cancer center and provides personalized patient care that is both compassionate and state of the art. The doctors and researchers work together to develop innovative therapies for patients. The Institute is world-renowned for excellence in cancer-focused research, personalized care, education and community outreach. Its mission is to discover the origins of human cancer and to use that knowledge to eradicate the personal and societal burden of cancer in our community, the nation and the world. The center and its multidisciplinary team of experts provide access to the latest treatment options and clinical trials along with a variety of programs in cancer prevention, screening, diagnostics, genetic counseling and supportive services.

We specialize in the following areas:

PATIENT-FOCUSED SETTING

The NYU Clinical Cancer Center is the principal outpatient facility of The Cancer Institute and serves as home to our patients and their caregivers. The center and its multidisciplinary team of experts provide access to the latest treatment options and clinical trials along with a variety of programs in cancer prevention, screening, diagnostics, genetic counseling and supportive services. In addition the NYUCI emphasizes the importance of a holistic approach to management services in complementary medicine, psychosocial support, survivorship and palliative care.

RENOWNED EXPERTISE

The NYU Cancer Institute brings together experts from a variety of disciplines to create collaborative research endeavors and clinical care teams. The Institute offers a full continuum of personalized care, from prevention through diagnosis, treatment and post-treatment support. The compassion and expertise of our team members helps patients better manage the symptoms of their diseases as well as meet their special needs. Additionally, we have created special emphasis programs in diseases such as breast cancer, melanoma, GI cancer, prostate cancer, hematologic malignancies and lung cancer among others, as well as, translational programs in cancer healthcare disparities, molecularly-targeted therapy, and the cell signaling pathways involved in cancer.

A TRANSLATIONAL APPROACH

NYU Langone Medical Center scientists and other researchers excel in uncovering how cancer develops at the molecular level, and how we can harness that knowledge to reduce the risk of cancer and treat the disease. The Medical Center constantly seeks to create new opportunities for collaboration between investigators within our own institution, those located elsewhere in the NYU network of campuses, and researchers at other institutions.

THE STEPHEN D. HASSENFELD CHILDREN'S CENTER FOR CANCER AND BLOOD DISORDERS

The center is a leading pediatric outpatient facility for the treatment of childhood cancers and blood diseases. Its unique interdisciplinary and family-centered approach combines the most advanced medical treatments with psychosocial and emotional support services for young patients and their families.

Hand Surgery

a subspecialty of Orthopaedics, Surgery or Plastic Surgery

A specialist trained in the investigation, preservation and restoration by medical, surgical and rehabilitative means of all structures of the upper extremity directly affecting the form and function of the hand and wrist.

For more information about the mentioned specialties or those physicians, see **Orthopaedic Surgery, Surgery** or **Plastic Surgery** section(s).

Training Required: Five years (including general surgery) in orthopaedics *plus* two years in clinical practice before final certification is achieved *plus* additional training and examination in hand surgery OR five to seven years in plastic surgery *plus* additional training and examination in hand surgery.

HAND SURGERY

New England

Akelman, Edward MD [HS] - **Spec Exp:** Carpal Tunnel Syndrome; Arthritis; Wrist/Hand Injuries; **Hospital:** Rhode Island Hosp; **Address:** 2 Dudley St, Ste 200, Rhode Island Hosp, Providence, RI 02905; **Phone:** 401-457-1510; **Board Cert:** Orthopaedic Surgery 2008; Hand Surgery 2008; **Med School:** Dartmouth Med Sch 1978; **Resid:** Surgery, Peter Bent Brigham Hosp 1980; Orthopaedic Surgery, Yale-New Haven Hosp 1984; **Fellow:** Hand Surgery, Roosevelt Hosp 1985; **Fac Appt:** Prof OrS, Brown Univ

Belsky, Mark R MD [HS] - **Spec Exp:** Arthritis; Nerve Disorders/Surgery; Elbow Surgery; **Hospital:** Newton - Wellesley Hosp; **Address:** 2000 Washington St, Green - Ste 563, Newton, MA 02462-1629; **Phone:** 617-965-4263; **Board Cert:** Orthopaedic Surgery 1982; Hand Surgery 2001; **Med School:** Tufts Univ 1974; **Resid:** Surgery, Peter Bent Brigham Hosp 1976; Orthopaedic Surgery, Tufts-New England Med Ctr 1979; **Fellow:** Hand Surgery, Roosevelt Hosp 1980; **Fac Appt:** Clin Prof OrS, Tufts Univ

Sampson, Christian E MD [HS] - **Spec Exp:** Hand Injuries; Hand & Fingers Vascular Surgery; **Hospital:** Brigham & Women's Hosp; **Address:** Brigham & Women's Hosp, Div Plastic Surg, 75 Francis St, Boston, MA 02115; **Phone:** 617-732-6297; **Board Cert:** Plastic Surgery 2004; Hand Surgery 2003; **Med School:** Boston Univ 1986; **Resid:** Surgery, Boston Univ Med Ctr 1991; Plastic Surgery, Brigham & Women's Hosp 1993; **Fellow:** Hand Surgery, Roosevelt Hosp 1994

Waters, Peter Michael MD [HS] - **Spec Exp:** Brachial Plexus Palsy; Hand-Congenital Anomaly; **Hospital:** Children's Hospital - Boston; **Address:** Chldns Hosp, Dept Ortho Surgery, 300 Longwood Ave, Hunnewell - 2, Boston, MA 02115-5724; **Phone:** 617-355-6021; **Board Cert:** Orthopaedic Surgery 2002; Hand Surgery 2004; **Med School:** Tufts Univ 1981; **Resid:** Pediatrics, Mass Genl Hosp 1983; Orthopaedic Surgery, Harvard Combined Prog 1988; **Fellow:** Hand Surgery, Brigham/Chldns Hosp 1989; **Fac Appt:** Assoc Prof OrS, Harvard Med Sch

Weiss, Arnold P MD [HS] - **Spec Exp:** Carpal Tunnel Syndrome; Wrist Surgery; Elbow Replacement; **Hospital:** Rhode Island Hosp; **Address:** Univ Orthopedics, 2 Dudley St, Ste 200, Providence, RI 02905-3248; **Phone:** 401-457-1520; **Board Cert:** Orthopaedic Surgery 2004; Hand Surgery 2004; **Med School:** Johns Hopkins Univ 1985; **Resid:** Orthopaedic Surgery, Johns Hopkins Hosp 1990; **Fellow:** Hand Surgery, Indiana Hand Ctr 1991; **Fac Appt:** Prof OrS, Brown Univ

Mid Atlantic

Athanasian, Edward MD [HS] - **Spec Exp:** Bone & Soft Tissue Tumors; Hand & Upper Extremity Tumors; Hand & Upper Extremity Surgery; **Hospital:** Hosp For Special Surgery (page 59), Meml Sloan-Kettering Cancer Ctr; **Address:** Hospital for Special Surgery, 535 E 70th St, New York, NY 10021; **Phone:** 212-606-1962; **Board Cert:** Orthopaedic Surgery 1997; Hand Surgery 1999; **Med School:** Columbia P&S 1988; **Resid:** Surgery, Beth Israel Hosp 1989; Orthopaedic Surgery, Hosp Special Surgery 1993; **Fellow:** Hand Surgery, Mayo Clinic 1994; Orthopaedic Oncology, Meml Sloan Kettering Cancer Ctr 1995; **Fac Appt:** Asst Prof OrS, Cornell Univ-Weill Med Coll

Baratz, Mark E MD [HS] - **Spec Exp:** Hand Surgery; Upper Extremity Surgery; Elbow Reconstruction; **Hospital:** Allegheny General Hosp; **Address:** 1307 Federal St Fl 2, Pittsburgh, PA 15212; **Phone:** 412-359-4263; **Board Cert:** Orthopaedic Surgery 2004; Hand Surgery 2004; **Med School:** Univ Pittsburgh 1984; **Resid:** Orthopaedic Surgery, Univ Hlth Ctr 1990; **Fellow:** Orthopaedic Surgery, Univ Hlth Ctr 1987; Hand Surgery, Med Coll Penn 1991; **Fac Appt:** Prof OrS, Drexel Univ Coll Med

Culp, Randall MD [HS] - **Spec Exp:** Microsurgery; Hand & Upper Extremity Surgery; Elbow Surgery; **Hospital:** Thomas Jefferson Univ Hosp, Lankenau Hosp; **Address:** Philadelphia Hand Center, 700 S Henderson Rd, Ste 200, King of Prussia, PA 19406; **Phone:** 610-768-5959; **Board Cert:** Orthopaedic Surgery 2001; Hand Surgery 2001; **Med School:** Penn State Univ-Hershey Med Ctr 1982; **Resid:** Orthopaedic Surgery, Hosp Univ Penn 1987; **Fellow:** Hand Surgery, Hosp Univ Penn 1988; **Fac Appt:** Prof OrS, Jefferson Med Coll

Glickel, Steven MD [HS] - **Spec Exp:** Hand & Wrist Surgery; Elbow Surgery; Peripheral Nerve Surgery; **Hospital:** St Luke's - Roosevelt Hosp Ctr - Roosevelt Div (page 57); **Address:** 1000 10th Ave Fl 3, New York, NY 10019-1147; **Phone:** 212-523-7590; **Board Cert:** Orthopaedic Surgery 1985; Hand Surgery 2000; **Med School:** Harvard Med Sch 1976; **Resid:** Surgery, Columbia Presby Hosp 1978; Orthopaedic Surgery, Harvard Comb Ortho 1981; **Fellow:** Hand Surgery, St Luke's-Roosevelt Hosp Ctr 1983; Research, Columbia Presby Hosp 1982; **Fac Appt:** Assoc Clin Prof OrS, Columbia P&S

Graham, Thomas J MD [HS] - **Spec Exp:** Hand & Wrist Surgery; Elbow Surgery; Sports Injuries; Wrist/Hand Injuries; **Hospital:** Union Meml Hosp-Baltimore; **Address:** Curtis National Hand Ctr, 3333 N Calvert St Fl 2, Baltimore, MD 21218; **Phone:** 410-235-3869; **Board Cert:** Orthopaedic Surgery 2007; Hand Surgery 2007; **Med School:** Univ Cincinnati 1988; **Resid:** Orthopaedic Surgery, Univ Michigan Med Ctr 1993; **Fellow:** Hand Surgery, Indiana Hand Ctr 1994; Elbow Surgery, Mayo Clinic 1994; **Fac Appt:** Assoc Clin Prof OrS, Johns Hopkins Univ

Imbriglia, Joseph E MD [HS] - **Spec Exp:** Arthritis; Carpal Tunnel Syndrome; Shoulder Surgery; Rotator Cuff Surgery; **Hospital:** UPMC Passavant-Cranberry, UPMC Passavant; **Address:** 6001 Stonewood Drive, Wexford, PA 15090-7380; **Phone:** 724-933-3850; **Board Cert:** Orthopaedic Surgery 1977; Hand Surgery 2000; **Med School:** Hahnemann Univ 1970; **Resid:** Surgery, Univ Pittsburgh Med Ctr 1972; Orthopaedic Surgery, Columbia Presby Med Ctr 1975; **Fellow:** Hand Surgery, Columbia Presby Med Ctr 1976; **Fac Appt:** Clin Prof OrS, Univ Pittsburgh

Kozin, Scott H MD [HS] - **Spec Exp:** Congenital Hand Deformities; Brachial Plexus Palsy-Pediatric; Spinal Cord Injury-Pediatric; Hand Surgery; **Hospital:** Philadelphia Shriners Hosp; **Address:** Shriners Hosp for Children, 3551 N Broad St, Philadelphia, PA 19140; **Phone:** 215-430-4074; **Board Cert:** Orthopaedic Surgery 2005; Hand Surgery 2005; **Med School:** Hahnemann Univ 1986; **Resid:** Orthopaedic Surgery, Albert Einstein Med Ctr 1991; **Fellow:** Hand Surgery, Mayo Clinic 1992; **Fac Appt:** Assoc Prof OrS, Temple Univ

Kulick, Roy G MD [HS] - **Spec Exp:** Carpal Tunnel Syndrome; Arthritis; Tendon Surgery; **Hospital:** Montefiore Med Ctr - Div. Weiler; **Address:** The Tower at Montefiore Medical Park, 1695 Eastchester Rd Fl 2, Bronx, NY 10461; **Phone:** 718-920-2060; **Board Cert:** Orthopaedic Surgery 1980; Hand Surgery 2001; **Med School:** Cornell Univ-Weill Med Coll 1973; **Resid:** Surgery, St Lukes-Roosevelt Hosp 1975; Orthopaedic Surgery, Columbia-Presby ed tr 1978; **Fellow:** Hand Surgery, Hosp for Special Surgery 1979; **Fac Appt:** Assoc Prof OrS, Albert Einstein Coll Med

Hand Surgery

Lane, Lewis B MD [HS] - **Spec Exp:** Carpal Tunnel Syndrome; Arthritis; Sports Injuries; Hand Reconstruction; **Hospital:** N Shore Univ Hosp, St Francis Hosp - The Heart Ctr (page 69); **Address:** 600 Northern Blvd, Ste 300, Great Neck, NY 11021; **Phone:** 516-627-8717; **Board Cert:** Orthopaedic Surgery 1981; Hand Surgery 2000; **Med School:** Columbia P&S 1974; **Resid:** Surgery, NY Hosp 1975; Orthopaedic Surgery, Hosp for Special Surg 1979; **Fellow:** Research, Hosp for Special Surg 1976; Hand Surgery, St Luke's-Roosevelt Hosp Ctr 1980; **Fac Appt:** Assoc Clin Prof OrS, Albert Einstein Coll Med

Lee, W P Andrew MD [HS] - **Spec Exp:** Reconstructive Surgery; Cartilage Damage; Transplant-Hand; Pediatric Hand Surgery; **Hospital:** UPMC Presby, Pittsburgh, Chldns Hosp of Pittsburgh - UPMC; **Address:** Univ Pittsburgh, Scaife Hall 6B, 3601 Terrace St, Ste 6B, Pittsburgh, PA 15261; **Phone:** 412-648-9670; **Board Cert:** Hand Surgery 2005; Plastic Surgery 2005; **Med School:** Johns Hopkins Univ 1983; **Resid:** Surgery, Johns Hopkins Univ Hosp 1989; Plastic Surgery, Mass Genl Hosp 1991; **Fellow:** Microsurgery, Johns Hopkins Hosp 1987; Hand Surgery, Indiana Hand Ctr 1993; **Fac Appt:** Prof S, Univ Pittsburgh

Lubahn, John D MD [HS] - **Spec Exp:** Microsurgery; **Hospital:** Hamot Med Ctr, St Vincent Hlth Ctr; **Address:** 300 State St, Ste 205, Erie, PA 16507; **Phone:** 814-456-6022; **Board Cert:** Orthopaedic Surgery 2000; Hand Surgery 2000; **Med School:** Case West Res Univ 1975; **Resid:** Surgery, Univ Rochester Med Ctr 1977; Orthopaedic Surgery, Univ Rochester Med Ctr 1980; **Fellow:** Hand Surgery, Univ Louisville Hosp 1981

Melone Jr, Charles P MD [HS] - **Spec Exp:** Arthritis; Wrist Surgery; Fractures; **Hospital:** Beth Israel Med Ctr - Petrie Division (page 57); **Address:** 321 E 34th St, New York, NY 10016; **Phone:** 212-340-0000; **Board Cert:** Orthopaedic Surgery 1976; Hand Surgery 2004; **Med School:** Georgetown Univ 1969; **Resid:** Surgery, Nassau Co Med Ctr 1971; Orthopaedic Surgery, Nassau Co Med Ctr 1974; **Fellow:** Hand Surgery, NYU Med Ctr 1975; **Fac Appt:** Clin Prof OrS, Albert Einstein Coll Med

Osterman Jr, A Lee MD [HS] - **Spec Exp:** Upper Extremity Surgery; Wrist Surgery; Neuromuscular Disorders; **Hospital:** Thomas Jefferson Univ Hosp, Chldns Hosp of Philadelphia, The; **Address:** Philadelphia Hand Ctr, 700 S Henderson Rd, Ste 200, King of Prussia, PA 19406-4207; **Phone:** 610-265-3135; **Board Cert:** Orthopaedic Surgery 1980; Hand Surgery 2001; **Med School:** Univ Pennsylvania 1973; **Resid:** Orthopaedic Surgery, Hosp Univ Penn 1978; **Fellow:** Hand Surgery, Hosp Univ Penn 1979; Microvascular Surgery, Duke Univ Med Ctr 1980; **Fac Appt:** Prof OrS, Jefferson Med Coll

Raskin, Keith MD [HS] - **Spec Exp:** Wrist/Hand Injuries; Arthritis; Carpal Tunnel Syndrome; Elbow Surgery; **Hospital:** NYU Langone Med Ctr (page 67), Hosp For Joint Diseases (page 67); **Address:** 317 E 34th St, Fl 3, New York, NY 10016; **Phone:** 212-263-4263; **Board Cert:** Orthopaedic Surgery 2002; Hand Surgery 2002; **Med School:** Geo Wash Univ 1983; **Resid:** Orthopaedic Surgery, NYU Med Ctr 1988; **Fellow:** Hand Surgery, Union Mem Hosp 1989; **Fac Appt:** Assoc Clin Prof OrS, NYU Sch Med

Rosenwasser, Melvin P MD [HS] - **Spec Exp:** Carpal Tunnel Syndrome; Sports Injuries; Elbow Surgery; Trauma; **Hospital:** NY-Presby Hosp/Columbia (page 66); **Address:** 622 W 168th St, PH 11, New York, NY 10032; **Phone:** 212-305-4565; **Board Cert:** Orthopaedic Surgery 1999; Hand Surgery 1999; **Med School:** Columbia P&S 1976; **Resid:** Surgery, Roosevelt Hosp 1979; Orthopaedic Surgery, Columbia Presby Hosp 1982; **Fellow:** Hand Surgery, Columbia Presby Hosp 1983; **Fac Appt:** Prof OrS, Columbia P&S

Sotereanos, Dean G MD [HS] - **Spec Exp:** Hand & Upper Extremity Surgery; Elbow Surgery; **Hospital:** UPMC Mercy, Pittsburgh; **Address:** 1307 Federal St Fl 2, Pittsburgh, PA 15212; **Phone:** 412-359-8571; **Board Cert:** Orthopaedic Surgery 2003; Hand Surgery 2003; **Med School:** Hahnemann Univ 1984; **Resid:** Surgery, Univ Pittsburgh Med Ctr 1986; Orthopaedic Surgery, Univ Pittsburgh Med Ctr 1989; **Fellow:** Hand Surgery, Duke Univ Med Ctr 1990; **Fac Appt:** Assoc Prof OrS, Univ Pittsburgh

Strauch, Robert MD [HS] - **Spec Exp:** Hand Reconstruction; Hand & Elbow Nerve Disorders; Hand & Wrist Surgery; Elbow Surgery; **Hospital:** NY-Presby Hosp/Columbia (page 66); **Address:** 622 W 168th St, rm PH-11, New York, NY 10032; **Phone:** 212-305-4272; **Board Cert:** Orthopaedic Surgery 2005; Hand Surgery 2005; **Med School:** Columbia P&S 1986; **Resid:** Orthopaedic Surgery, Columbia-Presby Hosp 1991; **Fellow:** Hand Surgery, Indiana Hand Center 1992; **Fac Appt:** Prof OrS, Columbia P&S

Weiland, Andrew J MD [HS] - **Spec Exp:** Wrist/Hand Injuries; Hand Reconstruction; **Hospital:** Hosp For Special Surgery (page 59), NY-Presby Hosp/Weill Cornell (page 66); **Address:** Hospital for Special Surgery, 535 E 70th St, New York, NY 10021-4872; **Phone:** 212-606-1575; **Board Cert:** Orthopaedic Surgery 1992; **Med School:** Wake Forest Univ 1968; **Resid:** Surgery, Univ Michigan Med Ctr 1970; Orthopaedic Surgery, Johns Hopkins Hosp 1975; **Fellow:** Hand Surgery, Kleinert Hosp 1975; **Fac Appt:** Prof OrS, Cornell Univ-Weill Med Coll

Wolfe, Scott W MD [HS] - **Spec Exp:** Wrist Surgery; Nerve Disorders/Surgery; Fractures; **Hospital:** Hosp For Special Surgery (page 59); **Address:** Hospital for Special Surgery, 523 E 72 St Fl 4, New York, NY 10021; **Phone:** 212-606-1529; **Board Cert:** Orthopaedic Surgery 2003; Hand Surgery 2003; **Med School:** Cornell Univ-Weill Med Coll 1984; **Resid:** Orthopaedic Surgery, Hosp Special Surg 1989; **Fellow:** Hand & Microvascular Surgery, Columbia Presby Med Ctr 1990; **Fac Appt:** Prof OrS, Cornell Univ-Weill Med Coll

Southeast

Breidenbach, Warren C MD [HS] - **Spec Exp:** Transplant-Hand; **Hospital:** Jewish Hosp HlthCre Svcs Inc; **Address:** 225 Abraham Flexner Way, Ste 700, Louisville, KY 40202; **Phone:** 502-561-4263; **Board Cert:** Plastic Surgery 1988; Hand Surgery 2003; **Med School:** Univ Calgary 1975; **Resid:** Plastic Surgery, McGill Univ 1982; **Fellow:** Microsurgery, Eastern Va Med Sch 1982; Hand Surgery, Univ Med Ctr 1983; **Fac Appt:** Asst Clin Prof PlS, Univ Louisville Sch Med

Carneiro, Ronaldo D S MD [HS] - **Spec Exp:** Carpal Tunnel Syndrome; Wrist Surgery; Arthritis; **Hospital:** Physicians Regl Med Ctr; **Address:** 8340 Collier Blvd, Ste 303, Naples, FL 34114; **Phone:** 239-348-4040; **Board Cert:** Plastic Surgery 1990; Hand Surgery 1994; **Med School:** Brazil 1970; **Resid:** Surgery, Union Meml Hosp 1975; Plastic Surgery, Allentown & Sacred Heart Hosp Ctr 1977; **Fellow:** Hand Surgery, Jackson Meml Hosp-Univ Miami Hosp 1977; Plastic Surgery, Univ Miami Sch Med 1978; **Fac Appt:** Assoc Clin Prof PlS, Univ S Fla Coll Med

Greene, Thomas L MD [HS] - **Spec Exp:** Arthritis; Peripheral Nerve Surgery; Arthroscopic Surgery; Tendon Surgery; **Hospital:** Tampa Genl Hosp, St Joseph's Hosp - Tampa; **Address:** 2727 W Dr Martin Luther King Jr Blvd, Ste 560, Tampa, FL 33607-6009; **Phone:** 813-873-0337; **Board Cert:** Orthopaedic Surgery 1983; Hand Surgery 2000; **Med School:** Ohio State Univ 1975; **Resid:** Surgery, Univ Michigan Med Ctr 1977; Orthopaedic Surgery, Univ Michigan Med Ctr 1980; **Fellow:** Hand Surgery, St Vincent's Hosp 1981

Hand Surgery

Hunt III, Thomas R MD [HS] - **Spec Exp:** Hand & Wrist Surgery; Arthritis; Trauma; Hand Reconstruction; **Hospital:** Univ of Ala Hosp at Birmingham; **Address:** UAB, Div Orthopaedic Surgery, 1313 13th St S, Ste 201, Birmingham, AL 35205-5327; **Phone:** 205-930-8339; **Board Cert:** Orthopaedic Surgery 2006; Hand Surgery 2006; **Med School:** Vanderbilt Univ 1986; **Resid:** Orthopaedic Surgery, Univ Kansas Med Ctr 1992; **Fellow:** Hand Surgery, Hosp Univ Penn 1993; **Fac Appt:** Prof S, Univ Alabama

Koman, L Andrew MD [HS] - **Spec Exp:** Pediatric Hand Surgery; Vascular Disorders-Upper Extremity; Pain-Nerve Injury; **Hospital:** Wake Forest Univ Baptist Med Ctr (page 72); **Address:** Wake Forest Univ Baptist Med Ctr, Dept Orthopaedic Surgery, Medical Center Blvd, Winston-Salem, NC 27157-1070; **Phone:** 336-716-8094; **Board Cert:** Orthopaedic Surgery 1981; Hand Surgery 2000; **Med School:** Duke Univ 1974; **Resid:** Surgery, Duke Univ Med Ctr 1975; Orthopaedic Surgery, Duke Univ Med Ctr 1979; **Fellow:** Hand Surgery, Duke Univ Med Ctr 1980; **Fac Appt:** Prof OrS, Wake Forest Univ

Midwest

Bishop, Allen T MD [HS] - **Spec Exp:** Microsurgery; Brachial Plexus Palsy; **Hospital:** Mayo Med Ctr & Clin - Rochester; **Address:** Mayo Clin, Div Hand Surgery, 200 First St SW, Rochester, MN 55905; **Phone:** 507-284-4149; **Board Cert:** Orthopaedic Surgery 2000; Hand Surgery 2000; **Med School:** Mayo Med Sch 1981; **Resid:** Orthopaedic Surgery, Mayo Clin 1986; **Fellow:** Hand Surgery, St Vincent Hosp 1987; **Fac Appt:** Prof OrS, Mayo Med Sch

Carroll, Charles MD [HS] - **Spec Exp:** Carpal Tunnel Syndrome; Dupuytren's Contracture; Elbow Surgery; Shoulder Surgery; **Hospital:** Northwestern Meml Hosp, NorthShore Univ HlthSys; **Address:** Northwest Orthopaedic Inst, 680 N Lakeshore Drive, Ste 924, Chicago, IL 60611; **Phone:** 312-664-6848; **Board Cert:** Orthopaedic Surgery 2001; Hand Surgery 2001; **Med School:** Univ MD Sch Med 1982; **Resid:** Surgery, Johns Hopkins Hosp 1984; Orthopaedic Surgery, Johns Hopkins Hosp 1987; **Fellow:** Hand Surgery, Indiana Univ Med Ctr 1988; Shoulder Surgery, Univ Western Ontario 1988; **Fac Appt:** Assoc Clin Prof OrS, Northwestern Univ

Chung, Kevin Chi MD [HS] - **Spec Exp:** Reconstructive Surgery; Hand & Microvascular Surgery; Upper Extremity Trauma; Nail Surgery; **Hospital:** Univ Michigan Hlth Sys; **Address:** University of Michigan, TC 2130-SPC 5340, 1500 E Medical Ctr Drive, Ann Arbor, MI 48109; **Phone:** 734-936-5885; **Board Cert:** Hand Surgery 2007; Plastic Surgery 2007; **Med School:** Emory Univ 1987; **Resid:** Plastic Surgery, Univ Michigan Hosp & Hlth Ctr 1994; Hand Surgery, Union Meml Hosp 1995; **Fac Appt:** Assoc Prof S, Univ Mich Med Sch

Cohen, Mark S MD [HS] - **Spec Exp:** Hand Surgery; Wrist Surgery; Elbow Surgery; **Hospital:** Rush Univ Med Ctr; **Address:** Midwest Orthopedics at Rush, 1725 W Harrison St, Ste 1042, Chicago, IL 60612-3841; **Phone:** 312-432-2346; **Board Cert:** Orthopaedic Surgery 2006; Hand Surgery 2006; **Med School:** Harvard Med Sch 1986; **Resid:** Orthopaedic Surgery, UCSD Med Ctr 1992; **Fellow:** Hand Surgery, Indiana Hand Ctr 1993; **Fac Appt:** Prof OrS, Rush Med Coll

Derman, Gordon H MD [HS] - **Spec Exp:** Carpal Tunnel Syndrome; Tendon Surgery; Repetitive Motion Injuries; Nerve Disorders/Surgery; **Hospital:** Rush Univ Med Ctr, NorthShore Univ HlthSys; **Address:** 1725 W Harrison St, Ste 740, Chicago, IL 60612; **Phone:** 312-432-9200; **Board Cert:** Plastic Surgery 1984; Hand Surgery 1996; **Med School:** Rush Med Coll 1975; **Resid:** Surgery, Loyola Univ Med Ctr 1981; Plastic Surgery, Univ Mich Hosp 1983; **Fellow:** Microsurgery, Rush/Presby St Luke's Med Ctr 1976; **Fac Appt:** Asst Prof S, Rush Med Coll

DeSilva, Stephen P MD [HS] - **Hospital:** Henry Ford Hosp; **Address:** Henry Ford Hospital, 2799 West Grand Blvd Fl 12, Detroit, MI 48202; **Phone:** 313-916-4481; **Board Cert:** Orthopaedic Surgery 2002; Hand Surgery 2002; **Med School:** Johns Hopkins Univ 1983; **Resid:** Orthopaedic Surgery, Mayo Clinic 1988; **Fellow:** Hand Surgery, Union Meml Hosp 1989; **Fac Appt:** Prof OrS, Wayne State Univ

Failla, Joseph M MD [HS] - **Spec Exp:** Hand Surgery; Hand Reconstruction; **Hospital:** Providence Hosp - Southfield, Huron Valley-Sinai Hosp; **Address:** Farmbrook Med Complex One Bldg - Ste 201, 29829 Telegraph Rd, Southfield, MI 48034; **Phone:** 248-352-4263; **Board Cert:** Orthopaedic Surgery 2001; Hand Surgery 2001; **Med School:** SUNY Buffalo 1982; **Resid:** Orthopaedic Surgery, SUNY-Buffalo 1987; **Fellow:** Hand Surgery, Mayo Clinic 1988

Fischer, Thomas J MD [HS] - **Spec Exp:** Microsurgery; Elbow Reconstruction; **Hospital:** St Vincent Indianapolis Hosp, Methodist Hosp - Indianapolis; **Address:** 8501 Harcourt Rd, Indianapolis, IN 46280-0434; **Phone:** 317-875-9105; **Board Cert:** Orthopaedic Surgery 2000; Hand Surgery 2000; **Med School:** Indiana Univ 1979; **Resid:** Orthopaedic Surgery, Univ Wash Affil Hosp 1984; **Fellow:** Hand Surgery, Hand Surg Assocs 1985; Hand Surgery, Duke Univ Med Ctr 1986; **Fac Appt:** Assoc Clin Prof OrS, Indiana Univ

Gelberman, Richard H MD [HS] - **Spec Exp:** Tendon Surgery; Peripheral Nerve Surgery; **Hospital:** Barnes-Jewish Hosp; **Address:** Wash Univ Sch Med, Dept Ortho Surg, 660 S Euclid Ave, Box 8233, St Louis, MO 63110; **Phone:** 314-747-2500; **Board Cert:** Orthopaedic Surgery 2007; Hand Surgery 2007; **Med School:** Univ Tenn Coll Med, Memphis 1969; **Resid:** Surgery, Univ Wisc Med Ctr 1975; **Fellow:** Hand Surgery, Duke Univ Med Ctr 1977; Pediatric Orthopaedic Surgery, Chldns Hosp-Harvard 1986; **Fac Appt:** Prof OrS, Washington Univ, St Louis

Harris, Gerald D MD [HS] - **Spec Exp:** Reconstructive Microvascular Surgery; **Hospital:** Northwestern Meml Hosp; **Address:** 737 N Michigan Ave, Ste 700, Chicago, IL 60611; **Phone:** 312-337-6960; **Board Cert:** Plastic Surgery 1980; Hand Surgery 1998; **Med School:** Univ IL Coll Med 1973; **Resid:** Surgery, Northwestern Meml Hosp 1977; Plastic Surgery, Northwestern Meml Hosp 1979; **Fellow:** Hand Surgery, UCSF Med Ctr 1979; **Fac Appt:** Assoc Clin Prof S, Northwestern Univ

Hastings II, Hill MD [HS] - **Spec Exp:** Wrist Surgery; Elbow Reconstruction; Fractures & Tendon Transfers; Arthritis; **Hospital:** St Vincent Indianapolis Hosp; **Address:** 8501 Harcourt Rd, Indianapolis, IN 46280-0434; **Phone:** 317-875-9105; **Board Cert:** Orthopaedic Surgery 1982; Hand Surgery 2000; **Med School:** USC Sch Med 1974; **Resid:** Surgery, Univ Colorado Med Ctr 1976; Orthopaedic Surgery, Mass Genl Hosp 1980; **Fellow:** Hand Surgery, St Vincent Hosp 1981; **Fac Appt:** Clin Prof OrS, Indiana Univ

Kleinman, William B MD [HS] - **Spec Exp:** Upper Extremity Surgery-Pediatric; Congenital Hand Deformities; **Hospital:** St Vincent Indianapolis Hosp; **Address:** 8501 Harcourt Rd, Indianapolis, IN 46280; **Phone:** 317-875-9105; **Board Cert:** Orthopaedic Surgery 1979; Hand Surgery 2000; **Med School:** Cornell Univ-Weill Med Coll 1972; **Resid:** Surgery, Univ Colorado 1974; Orthopaedic Surgery, NY Orthopaedic Hosp/Columbia 1977; **Fellow:** Hand Surgery, Columbia-Presby Med Ctr 1978; Microvascular Surgery, Duke Univ 1979; **Fac Appt:** Clin Prof OrS, Indiana Univ

Light, Terry R MD [HS] - **Spec Exp:** Hand-Congenital Anomaly; Hand Injuries-Pediatric; Arthritis; Thumb-Absence; **Hospital:** Loyola Univ Med Ctr, Chicago Shriners Hosp; **Address:** Loyola Univ Med Ctr, Dept Ortho Surg, 2160 S First Ave Maguire Bldg - rm 1700, Maywood, IL 60153-5590; **Phone:** 708-216-4570; **Board Cert:** Orthopaedic Surgery 1979; Hand Surgery 2000; **Med School:** Ros Franklin Univ/Chicago Med Sch 1973; **Resid:** Orthopaedic Surgery, Yale-New Haven Hosp 1977; **Fellow:** Hand Surgery, Hartford Combined Prog 1977; **Fac Appt:** Prof OrS, Loyola Univ-Stritch Sch Med

Hand Surgery

Manske, Paul MD [HS] - **Spec Exp:** Congenital Hand Deformities; Pediatric Hand Surgery; **Hospital:** Barnes-Jewish Hosp; **Address:** Wash Univ Sch Med, Dept Ortho Surg, 4921 Parkview Pl, Ste 6A, St Louis, MO 63110; **Phone:** 314-747-2500; **Board Cert:** Orthopaedic Surgery 1974; Hand Surgery 2000; **Med School:** Washington Univ, St Louis 1964; **Resid:** Surgery, Univ Wash Med Ctr 1966; Orthopaedic Surgery, Barnes Hosp-Wash Univ 1972; **Fellow:** Hand Surgery, Univ Louisville Hosp 1971; **Fac Appt:** Prof OrS, Washington Univ, St Louis

Mass, Daniel MD [HS] - **Spec Exp:** Tendon Surgery; Shoulder Reconstruction; Elbow Reconstruction; Wrist Surgery; **Hospital:** Univ of Chicago Med Ctr; **Address:** 5841 S Maryland Ave, MC 3079, Chicago, IL 60637-1448; **Phone:** 773-834-3531; **Board Cert:** Orthopaedic Surgery 2007; Hand Surgery 2007; **Med School:** Univ Chicago-Pritzker Sch Med 1975; **Resid:** Orthopaedic Surgery, Univ Chicago Hosp 1979; **Fellow:** Hand Surgery, St Francis Hosp 1980; **Fac Appt:** Prof S, Univ Chicago-Pritzker Sch Med

Mih, Alexander D MD [HS] - **Spec Exp:** Microsurgery; Arthritis; Hand Disorders-Pediatric; **Hospital:** Indiana Univ Hosp, St Vincent Indianapolis Hosp; **Address:** Indiana Hand Center, 8501 Harcourt Rd, Indianapolis, IN 46260; **Phone:** 317-471-4318; **Board Cert:** Orthopaedic Surgery 2003; Hand Surgery 2003; **Med School:** Johns Hopkins Univ 1984; **Resid:** Orthopaedic Surgery, Mayo Clinic 1989; **Fellow:** Hand Surgery, Indiana Ctr for Hand Surg 1990; **Fac Appt:** Assoc Prof OrS, Indiana Univ

Nagle, Daniel J MD [HS] - **Spec Exp:** Wrist Surgery; Carpal Tunnel Syndrome; **Hospital:** Northwestern Meml Hosp, Children's Mem Hosp; **Address:** Chicago Hand Surgery, 737 N Michigan Ave, Ste 700, Chicago, IL 60611-7108; **Phone:** 312-337-6960; **Board Cert:** Orthopaedic Surgery 2007; Hand Surgery 2007; **Med School:** Belgium 1978; **Resid:** Orthopaedic Surgery, Northwestern Univ Med Sch 1983; **Fellow:** Hand Surgery, Christine Kleinert 1984; **Fac Appt:** Prof OrS, Northwestern Univ

Putnam, Matthew D MD [HS] - **Spec Exp:** Wrist Surgery; Fracture Deformities/Arm; Arthritis; Nerve Disorders/Surgery; **Hospital:** Univ Minn Med Ctr, Fairview - Univ Campus, Univ Minn Med Ctr, Fairview - Riverside Campus; **Address:** 2450 Riverside Ave S, Ste R200, Minneapolis, MN 55454; **Phone:** 612-273-9400; **Board Cert:** Hand Surgery 2001; **Med School:** Dartmouth Med Sch 1977; **Resid:** Surgery, Roosevelt Hosp 1979; Orthopaedic Surgery, Univ Pittsburgh 1984; **Fellow:** Hand Surgery, NYOH 1985; **Fac Appt:** Prof OrS, Univ Minn

Seitz, William H MD [HS] - **Spec Exp:** Hand & Upper Extremity Surgery; Shoulder Surgery; **Hospital:** Lutheran Med Ctr - Cleveland, Cleveland Clin Fdn (page 56); **Address:** 1730 W 25th St, Ste 2C, Beachwood, OH 44113; **Phone:** 216-363-2331; **Board Cert:** Orthopaedic Surgery 2008; Hand Surgery 2008; **Med School:** Columbia P&S 1979; **Resid:** Surgery, St Vincents Med Ctr 1981; Orthopaedic Surgery, Columbia-Presby Med Ctr 1984; **Fellow:** Hand & Microvascular Surgery, Columbia-Presby Med Ctr 1985; **Fac Appt:** Assoc Clin Prof OrS, Case West Res Univ

Steinmann, Scott P MD [HS] - **Spec Exp:** Shoulder Surgery; Elbow Surgery; Brachial Plexus Palsy; Reconstructive Microvascular Surgery; **Hospital:** Mayo Med Ctr & Clin - Rochester; **Address:** Mayo Clin, Gonda 15, 200 1st St SW, Rochester, MN 55905; **Phone:** 507-284-3399; **Board Cert:** Orthopaedic Surgery 2004; Hand Surgery 2004; **Med School:** Cornell Univ-Weill Med Coll 1988; **Resid:** Orthopaedic Surgery, Hosp Spec Surgery 1992; **Fellow:** Shoulder Surgery, Columbia-Presby Med Ctr 1995; Hand Surgery, Mayo Clin 1998; **Fac Appt:** Prof OrS, Mayo Med Sch

Stern, Peter J MD [HS] - **Spec Exp:** Hand & Wrist Surgery; Microsurgery; **Hospital:** Good Samaritan Hosp - Cincinnati, Univ Hosp - Cincinnati; **Address:** Hand Surg Specialists, 538 Oak St, Ste 200, Cincinnati, OH 45219; **Phone:** 513-961-4263; **Board Cert:** Orthopaedic Surgery 1985; Hand Surgery 2000; **Med School:** Washington Univ, St Louis 1970; **Resid:** Surgery, Beth Israel Hosp 1972; Orthopaedic Surgery, Harvard Combined Prgm 1977; **Fellow:** Hand Surgery, Univ Louisville Hosps 1979; **Fac Appt:** Prof OrS, Univ Cincinnati

Great Plains and Mountains

Idler, Richard S MD [HS] - **Spec Exp:** Upper Extremity Surgery; **Hospital:** Penrose - St Francis Hlth Sys; **Address:** 3010 N Circle Drive, Ste 100, Colorado, CO 80919-1174; **Phone:** 719-632-7669; **Board Cert:** Orthopaedic Surgery 1985; Hand Surgery 2000; **Med School:** Dartmouth Med Sch 1975; **Resid:** Surgery, UCLA Med Ctr 1977; Plastic Surgery, UCLA Med Ctr 1978; **Fellow:** Orthopaedic Surgery, Mass Genl Hosp-Harvard 1981; Hand Surgery, St Vincent Hosp 1982; **Fac Appt:** Asst Clin Prof OrS, Indiana Univ

Southwest

Ezaki, Marybeth MD [HS] - **Spec Exp:** Hand-Congenital Anomaly; Hand Reconstruction-Pediatric; **Hospital:** Texas Scottish Rite Hosp for Chldn; **Address:** 2222 Welborn St, Dallas, TX 75219; **Phone:** 214-559-7842; **Board Cert:** Orthopaedic Surgery 1985; Hand Surgery 2000; **Med School:** Yale Univ 1977; **Resid:** Orthopaedic Surgery, Univ Tex SW Med Ctr 1982; **Fellow:** Hand Surgery, Weyham Pk Hosp 1982; **Fac Appt:** Assoc Prof OrS, Univ Tex SW, Dallas

Moneim, Moheb S MD [HS] - **Hospital:** Univ NM Hlth & Sci Ctr; **Address:** 1 University of New Mexico, Dept Orthopedics, MSC10 5600, Albuquerque, NM 87106; **Phone:** 505-272-4107; **Board Cert:** Orthopaedic Surgery 1998; Hand Surgery 1998; **Med School:** Egypt 1963; **Resid:** Orthopaedic Surgery, Duke Univ Med Ctr 1975; **Fellow:** Hand Surgery, Hosp for Spec Surgery 1976; **Fac Appt:** Prof OrS, Univ New Mexico

Rayan, Ghazi M MD [HS] - **Spec Exp:** Microsurgery; Congenital Limb Deformities; Arthritis; **Hospital:** Integris Baptist Med Ctr - OK, OU Med Ctr; **Address:** 3366 Northwest Expressway, Ste 700, Oklahoma City, OK 73112-4439; **Phone:** 405-945-4888; **Board Cert:** Orthopaedic Surgery 2000; Hand Surgery 2000; **Med School:** Egypt 1973; **Resid:** Surgery, S Baltimore Genl Hosp 1977; Orthopaedic Surgery, Union Meml Hosp 1980; **Fellow:** Hand & Microvascular Surgery, Union Meml Hosp 1980; **Fac Appt:** Clin Prof OrS, Univ Okla Coll Med

West Coast and Pacific

Atkinson, Robert E MD [HS] - **Spec Exp:** Arthritis; Arthroscopic Surgery; Nerve Disorders/Surgery; **Hospital:** Queen's Med Ctr - Honolulu, Kapiolani Med Ctr @ Pali Momi; **Address:** Queen's Physicians' Office Bldg 1, 1380 Lusitana St, Ste 604, Honolulu, HI 96813; **Phone:** 808-521-8128; **Board Cert:** Orthopaedic Surgery 1985; **Med School:** Jefferson Med Coll 1977; **Resid:** Orthopaedic Surgery, Hosp Special Surgery 1982; **Fellow:** Hand Surgery, Mass Genl Hosp 1983; **Fac Appt:** Clin Prof OrS, Univ Hawaii JA Burns Sch Med

Godzik, Cathleen A MD [HS] - **Spec Exp:** Congenital Hand Deformities; Sports Injuries; Dupuytren's Contracture; Arthritis; **Hospital:** Good Samaritan Hosp - LA, California Hosp Med Ctr; **Address:** 1245 Wilshire Blvd, Ste 611, Los Angeles, CA 90017; **Phone:** 213-482-6100; **Board Cert:** Orthopaedic Surgery 2001; Hand Surgery 2001; **Med School:** NY Med Coll 1981; **Resid:** Surgery, Brown Univ Sch Med 1983; Orthopaedic Surgery, Univ Conn Sch Med 1985; **Fellow:** Hand Surgery, Joseph Boyes Hand Fell-USC 1987

Hanel, Douglas P MD [HS] - **Spec Exp:** Reconstructive Microvascular Surgery; Hand-Congenital Anomaly; Elbow Reconstruction; **Hospital:** Harborview Med Ctr, Chldns Hosp and Regl Med Ctr - Seattle; **Address:** Harborview Medical Ctr, 325 9th Ave, Box 359798, Seattle, WA 98104-2420; **Phone:** 206-731-3462; **Board Cert:** Orthopaedic Surgery 2007; Hand Surgery 2007; **Med School:** St Louis Univ 1977; **Resid:** Orthopaedic Surgery, St Louis Univ Hosp 1982; **Fellow:** Hand Surgery, Univ Louisville Hosp 1983; Microsurgery, Univ Louisville Hosp 1983; **Fac Appt:** Prof OrS, Univ Wash

Hand Surgery

Hentz, Vincent R MD [HS] - **Spec Exp:** Hand Plastic Surgery; **Hospital:** Stanford Univ Med Ctr; **Address:** 1000 Welch Rd, Ste 100, Palto Alto, CA 94304; **Phone:** 650-723-5256; **Board Cert:** Plastic Surgery 1977; **Med School:** Univ Fla Coll Med 1968; **Resid:** Plastic Surgery, Stanford Univ Hosp 1974; **Fellow:** Hand Surgery, Roosevelt Hosp 1975; **Fac Appt:** Prof S, Stanford Univ

Meals, Roy A MD [HS] - **Hospital:** UCLA Ronald Reagan Med Ctr; **Address:** 100 UCLA Medical Plaza, Ste 305, Los Angeles, CA 90024; **Phone:** 310-206-6337; **Board Cert:** Orthopaedic Surgery 1980; Hand Surgery 2000; **Med School:** Vanderbilt Univ 1971; **Resid:** Surgery, Johns Hopkins Hosp 1973; Orthopaedic Surgery, Johns Hopkins Hosp 1978; **Fellow:** Hand Surgery, Mass Genl Hosp 1979; **Fac Appt:** Clin Prof S, UCLA

Slutsky, David J MD [HS] - **Spec Exp:** Hand Reconstruction; Wrist Surgery; Peripheral Nerve Surgery; Arthroscopic Surgery; **Hospital:** LAC - Harbor - UCLA Med Ctr, Torrance Memorial Med Ctr; **Address:** The Slutsky Hand & Wrist Inst, 2808 Columbia St, Torrance, CA 90503; **Phone:** 310-618-9922; **Board Cert:** Orthopaedic Surgery 2002; Hand Surgery 2002; **Med School:** Univ Manitoba 1981; **Resid:** Orthopaedic Surgery, Univ Manitoba Med Ctr 1987; **Fellow:** Hand & Microvascular Surgery, Loma Linda Univ Med Ctr 1989; **Fac Appt:** Asst Prof OrS, UCLA

Szabo, Robert M MD [HS] - **Spec Exp:** Peripheral Nerve Surgery; Hand Injuries; Hand & Upper Extremity Tumors; **Hospital:** UC Davis Med Ctr, Mercy General Hosp - Sacramento; **Address:** UC Davis, Dept Orthopaedics, 4860 Y St, Ste 3800, Sacramento, CA 95817-2307; **Phone:** 916-734-3678; **Board Cert:** Orthopaedic Surgery 2009; Hand Surgery 2009; **Med School:** SUNY Buffalo 1977; **Resid:** Surgery, Mt Sinai Hosp 1979; Orthopaedic Surgery, Mt Sinai Hosp 1982; **Fellow:** Hand Surgery, UCSD Med Ctr 1983; Epidemiology, UC Berkeley 1995; **Fac Appt:** Prof OrS, UC Davis

Trumble, Thomas MD [HS] - **Spec Exp:** Nerve Disorders/Surgery; Upper Extremity Trauma; **Hospital:** Univ Wash Med Ctr, Harborview Med Ctr; **Address:** 4245 Roosevelt Way NE, Seattle, WA 98105; **Phone:** 206-598-4288; **Board Cert:** Orthopaedic Surgery 2009; Hand Surgery 2009; **Med School:** Yale Univ 1979; **Resid:** Orthopaedic Surgery, Yale-New Haven Hosp 1984; **Fellow:** Microvascular Surgery, Duke Univ Med Ctr 1984; Hand Surgery, Mass Genl Hosp 1985; **Fac Appt:** Prof S, Univ Wash

Cleveland Clinic

Upper Extremity Center

The Cleveland Clinic Upper Extremity Center, a division of the Department of Orthopaedic Surgery, provides a centralized, comprehensive diagnostic and treatment center for problems affecting the hand, wrist, elbow and shoulder. If you are among the millions of Americans experiencing hand and upper extremity problems each year, finding expert care is all-important. For the past several years, *U.S.News & World Report* has consistently ranked the Department of Orthopaedic Surgery among the nation's top five orthopaedic programs.

Our surgeons treat all disorders of the upper extremity. Following is a list of many of the injuries and disorders we see. We encourage you to ask about our experience with your particular problem.

Shoulder
Fractures and dislocations
Arthritis
Chronic instability
Rotator cuff tears
Brachial plexus injuries

Wrist
Fractures and nonunions
Dislocations
Instability
Carpal tunnel syndrome
Tendinitis
Rheumatoid wrist

Elbow
Fractures and dislocations
Tennis and golfer's elbow
Arthritis
Throwing elbow

Hand
Fractures and dislocations
Trigger finger
Cysts and tumors
Burns

Surgery of the Upper Extremity
Our surgeons are experts in the operative care of a wide array of upper extremity disorders. For some injuries, we offer the newest surgical techniques, such as microsurgery and minimally invasive surgery.

Work-Related Disorders
Acute injuries and chronic problems of the hand and upper extremity can result from occupational activity. Our surgeons are experts in determining whether a disorder is work-related and at determining a treatment course that will help you meet the physical demands of your job.

For more information about the Cleveland Clinic Upper Extremity Center, to schedule a second opinion or to learn about assistance for out-of-town patients, call 800.890.2467 or visit www.clevelandclinic.org/orthotopdocs.

Upper Extremity Center
9500 Euclid Avenue / AC311 | Cleveland OH 44195

NYU Hospital for Joint Diseases
NYU LANGONE MEDICAL CENTER

301 East 17th Street
(at Second Avenue)
New York, NY 10003
212-598-6000 FAX: 212-260-1203
www.nyuhjd.org

HAND SURGERY

About Hand Surgery Services:

The Hospital for Joint Diseases (HJD) at NYU Langone Medical Center provides comprehensive care for patients with hand and wrist disorders including: fractures, congenital anomalies, soft tissue and skeletal trauma, degenerative and rheumatoid arthritis, sports-related injuries, vascular disorders, tumors and occupational disorders. Care is provided by specialists encompassing all aspects of diagnosis and treatment affecting the hand and wrist.

We specialize in the following areas:

ORTHOPAEDIC HAND PROGRAM

Through its Division of Hand Surgery, the Hospital for Joint Diseases at NYU Langone Medical Center provides specific emphasis on fractures of the wrist and distal radius and reconstructive hand surgery. Hand surgery experts specialize in post traumatic injuries, arthritis and congenital, neuromuscular and neoplastic conditions. Offering one of the largest Hand Programs in the United States, NYU Langone Medical Center provides comprehensive care for the many problems that affect the upper extremity including: acute traumatic injuries (fractures, dislocations and tendon, nerve and vascular lacerations), post-traumatic and arthritic deformities, acquired problems (nerve compressions and tumors), congenital deformities and neuromuscular disorders such as cerebral palsy. The board-certified and fellowship-trained orthopaedists perform more than 5,000 operative procedures on adults and children each year.

REHABILITATION

After surgery, the outpatient Hand Therapy Unit at the Rusk Institute of Rehabilitation Medicine at NYU Langone Medical Center helps surgical patients recover full or partial use of their hands, providing comprehensive rehabilitation for a variety of ailments associated with the hand and upper body. The Unit specializes in fractures, traumatic injuries, tendonitis, sports injuries, work-related injuries, repetitive stress injuries, carpal tunnel syndrome, tendon and nerve repairs and arthritis. The Unit is staffed by expert occupational therapists that specialize in treatments of the hand and upper extremities.

RESEARCH

The research focus of the Hospital for Joint Diseases' Hand Service program at NYU Langone Medical Center is on a variety of clinical problems, including wrist fractures, non-unions of the scaphoid (bone between the hand and the forearm), Kienbock's disease (death and fracture of bone tissue due to interruption of blood supply), intercarpal subluxations (incomplete or partial dislocation) and neuropathies (disorders of the nerves) of the upper extremities.

Hematology &
Medical Oncology
a subspecialty of Internal Medicine

Hematology: An internist with additional training who specializes in diseases of the blood, spleen and lymph glands. This specialist treats conditions such as anemia, clotting disorders, sickle cell disease, hemophilia, leukemia and lymphoma.

Medical Oncology: An internist who specializes in the diagnosis and treatment of all types of cancer and other benign and malignant tumors. This specialist decides on and administers chemotherapy for malignancy, as well as consulting with surgeons and radiotherapists on other treatments for cancer.

Training Required: Three years in internal medicine *plus* additional training and examination for certification in hematology or medical oncology.

HEMATOLOGY

New England

Anderson, Kenneth C MD [Hem] - **Spec Exp:** Multiple Myeloma; Hematologic Malignancies; **Hospital:** Dana-Farber Cancer Inst, Brigham & Women's Hosp; **Address:** 44 Binney St Mayer Bldg - rm 557, Dana-Farber Cancer Inst, Div Hematology, Boston, MA 02115; **Phone:** 617-632-2144; **Board Cert:** Internal Medicine 1980; **Med School:** Johns Hopkins Univ 1977; **Resid:** Internal Medicine, Johns Hopkins Hosp 1980; **Fellow:** Hematology & Oncology, Dana Farber Cancer Inst 1983; **Fac Appt:** Prof Med, Harvard Med Sch

Comenzo, Raymond MD [Hem] - **Spec Exp:** Plasma Cell Disorders; **Hospital:** Tufts Med Ctr; **Address:** 800 Washington St, Box 826, Boston, MA 02111; **Phone:** 617-636-6454; **Board Cert:** Internal Medicine 1989; Hematology 2004; Blood Banking Transfusion Medicine 1992; **Med School:** Boston Univ 1986; **Resid:** Internal Medicine, Boston City Hosp 1989; **Fellow:** Hematology & Oncology, New Engl Med Ctr 1991

Dezube, Bruce J MD [Hem] - **Spec Exp:** AIDS Related Cancers; Clinical Trials; **Hospital:** Beth Israel Deaconess Med Ctr - Boston; **Address:** BIDMC-Division of Hematology/Oncology, 330 Brookline Ave, MASCO 414, Boston, MA 02215; **Phone:** 617-632-9258; **Board Cert:** Internal Medicine 1986; Medical Oncology 1989; Hematology 1988; **Med School:** Tufts Univ 1983; **Resid:** Internal Medicine, New England Med Ctr 1986; **Fellow:** Hematology & Oncology, Beth Israel Deaconess Hosp 1989; **Fac Appt:** Assoc Prof Med, Harvard Med Sch

Duffy, Thomas P MD [Hem] - **Spec Exp:** Mast Cell Diseases; Leukemia; Lymphoma; **Hospital:** Yale-New Haven Hosp; **Address:** Yale Univ, Sect Hematology, 333 Cedar St, rm 403-WWW, Box 208021, New Haven, CT 06520-8021; **Phone:** 203-785-4744; **Board Cert:** Internal Medicine 1972; Hematology 1974; **Med School:** Johns Hopkins Univ 1962; **Resid:** Internal Medicine, Johns Hopkins Hosp 1965; **Fellow:** Hematology, Johns Hopkins Hosp 1970; **Fac Appt:** Prof Med, Yale Univ

Ellman, Leonard MD [Hem] - **Spec Exp:** Multiple Myeloma; Leukemia; **Hospital:** Mass Genl Hosp; **Address:** Mass Genl Hosp, 15 Parkman St, rm 516, Boston, MA 02114; **Phone:** 617-726-3448; **Board Cert:** Internal Medicine 1972; Hematology 1974; **Med School:** Harvard Med Sch 1967; **Resid:** Internal Medicine, Mass Genl Hosp 1969; **Fellow:** Hematology, Natl Inst Hlth 1971; **Fac Appt:** Assoc Prof Med, Harvard Med Sch

Forget, Bernard MD [Hem] - **Spec Exp:** Thalassemia; Anemias & Red Cell Disorders; Leukemia; Sickle Cell Anemia; **Hospital:** Yale-New Haven Hosp; **Address:** Yale Univ Sch Med, Div Hematology, PO Box 208021, New Haven, CT 06520-8021; **Phone:** 203-785-4144; **Board Cert:** Internal Medicine 1971; Hematology 1972; **Med School:** McGill Univ 1963; **Resid:** Internal Medicine, Mass Genl Hosp 1965; Clinical Pathology, Mass Genl Hosp 1968; **Fellow:** Hematology, Peter Bent Brigham Hosp 1971; **Fac Appt:** Prof Med, Yale Univ

Meehan, Kenneth MD [Hem] - **Spec Exp:** Bone Marrow Transplant; **Hospital:** Dartmouth - Hitchcock Med Ctr; **Address:** Norris Cotton Cancer Ctr, Dartmouth-Hitchcock Med Ctr, 1 Medical Center Drive, Lebanon, NH 03756; **Phone:** 603-650-4628; **Board Cert:** Internal Medicine 1989; Hematology 2004; **Med School:** Georgetown Univ 1986; **Resid:** Internal Medicine, Georgetown Univ 1989; **Fellow:** Hematology & Oncology, Dartmouth-Hitchcock Med Ctr 1992; **Fac Appt:** Assoc Prof Med, Dartmouth Med Sch

Miller, Kenneth B MD [Hem] - **Spec Exp:** Bone Marrow Transplant; Leukemia; Myelodysplastic Syndromes; **Hospital:** Tufts Med Ctr; **Address:** Dept Medicine, 750 Washington St, Box 245, Boston, MA 02211; **Phone:** 617-636-2600; **Board Cert:** Internal Medicine 1976; Hematology 1980; **Med School:** NY Med Coll 1972; **Resid:** Internal Medicine, NYU Med Ctr/VA Hosp 1976; Internal Medicine, NYU Med Ctr 1976; **Fellow:** Hematology, New England Med Ctr 1979; **Fac Appt:** Prof Med, Tufts Univ

Schiffman, Fred J MD [Hem] - **Spec Exp:** Hematologic Malignancies; Anemia; Coagulation/Bleeding Disorders; **Hospital:** Miriam Hosp; **Address:** Comp Cancer Ctr at Miriam Hospital, 164 Summit Ave Fain Bldg Fl 3, Providence, RI 02906; **Phone:** 401-793-2920; **Board Cert:** Internal Medicine 1979; Hematology 1982; Medical Oncology 1987; **Med School:** NYU Sch Med 1973; **Resid:** Internal Medicine, Yale-New Haven Hosp 1975; Internal Medicine, Yale-New Haven Hosp 1979; **Fellow:** Hematology, Yale-New Haven Hosp 1981; **Fac Appt:** Prof Med, Brown Univ

Spitzer, Thomas R MD [Hem] - **Spec Exp:** Bone Marrow Transplant; Leukemia; **Hospital:** Mass Genl Hosp; **Address:** Mass Genl Hosp-Bone Marrow Tranplant Program, 55 Fruit St, Emerson Pl, Ste 118, Boston, MA 02114; **Phone:** 617-724-1124; **Board Cert:** Internal Medicine 1977; Medical Oncology 1983; Hematology 1984; **Med School:** Univ Rochester 1974; **Resid:** Internal Medicine, NYew York Hosp-Cornell Med Ctr 1977; Internal Medicine, Mem Sloan Kettering Cancer Ctr 1977; **Fellow:** Hematology & Oncology, Case West Res Univ 1983; **Fac Appt:** Prof Med, Harvard Med Sch

Stone, Richard M MD [Hem] - **Spec Exp:** Leukemia; **Hospital:** Dana-Farber Cancer Inst, Brigham & Women's Hosp; **Address:** Dana Farber Cancer Inst, Adult Leukemia Program, 44 Binney St, Ste M1B17, Boston, MA 02115-6084; **Phone:** 617-632-2214; **Board Cert:** Internal Medicine 1984; Medical Oncology 1987; Hematology 1988; **Med School:** Harvard Med Sch 1981; **Resid:** Internal Medicine, Brigham & Womens Hosp 1984; **Fellow:** Medical Oncology, Dana Farber Cancer Inst 1987; **Fac Appt:** Prof Med, Harvard Med Sch

Mid Atlantic

Abrams, Charles S MD [Hem] - **Spec Exp:** Bleeding/Coagulation Disorders; Thrombotic Disorders; **Hospital:** Hosp Univ Penn - UPHS (page 60); **Address:** Univ Penn, Dept Hem/Onc, 421 Curie Blvd, Bio Medical Research Bldg 2/3, Philadelphia, PA 19104-6160; **Phone:** 215-573-3288; **Board Cert:** Internal Medicine 1987; Medical Oncology 1989; Hematology 2005; **Med School:** Yale Univ 1984; **Resid:** Internal Medicine, Hosp Univ Penn 1987; **Fellow:** Hematology & Oncology, Hosp Univ Penn 1988; **Fac Appt:** Assoc Prof Med, Univ Pennsylvania

Baer, Maria R MD [Hem] - **Spec Exp:** Leukemia; Myelodysplastic Syndromes; Myeloproliferative Disorders; **Hospital:** Univ of MD Med Ctr; **Address:** Univ Maryland, Greenebaum Cancer Ctr, 22 S Greene St, rm S9D04, Baltimore, MD 21201; **Phone:** 410-328-7904; **Board Cert:** Internal Medicine 1983; Hematology 1984; **Med School:** Johns Hopkins Univ 1979; **Resid:** Internal Medicine, Vanderbilt Univ Hosp 1982; **Fellow:** Hematology, Vanderbilt Univ Hosp 1984; **Fac Appt:** Prof Med, Univ MD Sch Med

Cheson, Bruce D MD [Hem] - **Spec Exp:** Leukemia; Hematologic Malignancies; **Hospital:** Georgetown Univ Hosp; **Address:** GUMC - Lombardi Cancer Ctr, 3800 Reservoir Rd NW, Podium B, Washington, DC 20007; **Phone:** 202-444-7932; **Board Cert:** Internal Medicine 1974; Hematology 1976; **Med School:** Tufts Univ 1971; **Resid:** Internal Medicine, Univ Virginia Hosp 1974; **Fellow:** Hematology, New England Med Ctr Hosp 1976

Hematology

Coller, Barry MD [Hem] - **Spec Exp:** Glanzmann's Thrombasthenia; Bleeding/Coagulation Disorders; **Hospital:** Rockefeller Univ, Mount Sinai Med Ctr (page 64); **Address:** Rockefeller Univ, 1230 York Ave, New York, NY 10065; **Phone:** 212-327-7490; **Board Cert:** Internal Medicine 1973; Hematology 1975; **Med School:** NYU Sch Med 1970; **Resid:** Internal Medicine, Bellevue Hosp 1972; **Fellow:** Hematology, Natl Inst Hlth Clin Ctr 1974; **Fac Appt:** Clin Prof Med, Mount Sinai Sch Med

Diuguid, David L MD [Hem] - **Spec Exp:** Bleeding/Coagulation Disorders; **Hospital:** NY-Presby Hosp/Columbia (page 66); **Address:** 161 Ft Washington Ave, Irving 10, New York, NY 10032; **Phone:** 212-305-0527; **Board Cert:** Internal Medicine 1982; Hematology 1986; Medical Oncology 1985; **Med School:** Cornell Univ-Weill Med Coll 1979; **Resid:** Internal Medicine, Boston Univ Med Ctr 1983; **Fellow:** Hematology & Oncology, New England Med Ctr 1986; **Fac Appt:** Assoc Prof Med, Columbia P&S

Fruchtman, Steven M MD [Hem] - **Spec Exp:** Myeloproliferative Disorders; Polycythemia Rubra Vera; **Address:** 1111 Park Ave, New York, NY 10128; **Phone:** 212-427-7700; **Board Cert:** Internal Medicine 1980; Hematology 1984; **Med School:** NY Med Coll 1977; **Resid:** Internal Medicine, Univ Hosp 1981; **Fellow:** Hematology, Mount Sinai Med Ctr 1984; Hematology, Meml Sloan Kettering Cancer Ctr 1985; **Fac Appt:** Assoc Prof Med, NY Med Coll

Gewirtz, Alan M MD [Hem] - **Spec Exp:** Leukemia; Gene Therapy; **Hospital:** Hosp Univ Penn - UPHS (page 60); **Address:** Perelman Ctr for Advanced Medicine Fl 2, 3400 Civic Center Blvd, Philadelphia, PA 19104; **Phone:** 215-615-5858; **Board Cert:** Internal Medicine 1979; Medical Oncology 1981; Hematology 1982; **Med School:** SUNY Buffalo 1976; **Resid:** Internal Medicine, Mt Sinai Hosp 1979; **Fellow:** Medical Oncology, Yale-New Haven Hosp 1981; Hematology, Yale-New Haven Hosp 1982; **Fac Appt:** Prof Med, Univ Pennsylvania

Goldberg, Jack MD [Hem] - **Spec Exp:** Leukemia; Lymphoma; Breast Cancer; Bone Marrow Transplant; **Hospital:** Penn Presby Med Ctr - UPHS (page 60), Virtua West Jersey Hosp - Voorhees; **Address:** 409 Route 70 E, Cherry Hill, NJ 08034; **Phone:** 856-429-1519; **Board Cert:** Internal Medicine 1976; Hematology 1980; Medical Oncology 1989; **Med School:** SUNY Upstate Med Univ 1973; **Resid:** Internal Medicine, Boston Univ Hosp 1975; **Fellow:** Hematology & Oncology, SUNY Syracuse Med Ctr 1977; **Fac Appt:** Clin Prof Med, Univ Pennsylvania

Kempin, Sanford J MD [Hem] - **Spec Exp:** Bleeding/Coagulation Disorders; Leukemia; Lymphoma; **Hospital:** St Vincent Cath Med Ctrs - Manhattan; **Address:** St Vincents Cancer Ctr, 325 W 15th St, New York, NY 10011; **Phone:** 212-604-6068; **Board Cert:** Internal Medicine 1976; Medical Oncology 1977; Hematology 1978; **Med School:** Belgium 1971; **Resid:** Internal Medicine, Lemuel Shattuck Hosp 1972; **Fellow:** Hematology, St Jude Chldns Hosp 1975; Medical Oncology, Meml Sloan Kettering Cancer Ctr 1976; **Fac Appt:** Asst Prof Med, NY Med Coll

Kessler, Craig M MD [Hem] - **Spec Exp:** Bleeding/Coagulation Disorders; Hemophilia; Hematologic Malignancies; **Hospital:** Georgetown Univ Hosp; **Address:** GUMC, Lombardi Cancer Ctr, 3800 Reservoir Rd NW, Washington, DC 20007; **Phone:** 202-444-8676; **Board Cert:** Internal Medicine 1976; Hematology 1980; **Med School:** Tulane Univ 1973; **Resid:** Internal Medicine, Ochsner Fdn Hosp 1976; **Fellow:** Hematology, Johns Hopkins Hosp 1978; **Fac Appt:** Prof Med, Georgetown Univ

Kopel, Samuel MD [Hem] - **Spec Exp:** Hematologic Malignancies; Solid Tumors; **Hospital:** Maimonides Med Ctr (page 63); **Address:** MMC Hematology/Oncology, 6300 8th Ave, Brooklyn, NY 11220; **Phone:** 718-765-2600; **Board Cert:** Internal Medicine 1975; Hematology 1978; Medical Oncology 1979; **Med School:** Italy 1972; **Resid:** Internal Medicine, Jewish Hosp 1975; **Fellow:** Hematology & Oncology, Mt Sinai Med Ctr 1978; **Fac Appt:** Asst Prof Med, SUNY Downstate

Mangan, Kenneth F MD [Hem] - **Spec Exp:** Bone Marrow Transplant; **Hospital:** Temple Univ Hosp; **Address:** Temple BMT Program, Friends Hall Physicians Bldg, 7604 Central Ave, Lower Level, Philadelphia, PA 19111-2499; **Phone:** 215-214-3129; **Board Cert:** Internal Medicine 1976; Hematology 1978; **Med School:** Geo Wash Univ 1973; **Resid:** Internal Medicine, G Washington Univ Hosps 1976; **Fellow:** Hematology, Tufts-New England Med Ctr 1977

Marks, Stanley M MD [Hem] - **Spec Exp:** Leukemia; Lymphoma; **Hospital:** UPMC Shadyside; **Address:** 5115 Center Ave Fl 3, Pittsburgh, PA 15232; **Phone:** 412-235-1020; **Board Cert:** Internal Medicine 1976; Hematology 1978; **Med School:** Univ Pittsburgh 1973; **Resid:** Internal Medicine, Presby Univ Hosp 1976; **Fellow:** Hematology & Oncology, Peter Bent Brigham Hosp 1978; **Fac Appt:** Assoc Clin Prof Med, Drexel Univ Coll Med

Mears, John Gregory MD [Hem] - **Spec Exp:** Lymphoma; Leukemia; Multiple Myeloma; Breast Cancer; **Hospital:** NY-Presby Hosp/Columbia (page 66); **Address:** 161 Ft Washington Ave, Ste 923, New York, NY 10032; **Phone:** 212-305-3506; **Board Cert:** Internal Medicine 1976; Hematology 1978; **Med School:** Columbia P&S 1973; **Resid:** Internal Medicine, Boston Univ Med Ctr 1975; **Fellow:** Hematology & Oncology, Columbia-Presby Med Ctr 1978; **Fac Appt:** Clin Prof Med, Columbia P&S

Millenson, Michael M MD [Hem] - **Spec Exp:** Leukemia & Lymphoma; Thromboembolic Disorders; Hematologic Malignancies; **Hospital:** Fox Chase Cancer Ctr (page 58); **Address:** Fox Chase Cancer Center, 7701 Burholme Ave, Ste C307, Philadelphia, PA 19111; **Phone:** 215-728-2600; **Board Cert:** Internal Medicine 1987; Medical Oncology 2000; Hematology 2000; **Med School:** Temple Univ 1984; **Resid:** Internal Medicine, Temple Univ Hosp 1987; **Fellow:** Hematology & Oncology, Beth Israel Hosp 1991

Nimer, Stephen D MD [Hem] - **Spec Exp:** Bone Marrow Transplant; Myelodysplastic Syndromes; Leukemia; Stem Cell Transplant; **Hospital:** Meml Sloan-Kettering Cancer Ctr; **Address:** 1275 York Avenue, New York, NY 10065; **Phone:** 800-525-2225; **Board Cert:** Internal Medicine 1982; Hematology 1986; Medical Oncology 1985; **Med School:** Univ Chicago-Pritzker Sch Med 1979; **Resid:** Internal Medicine, UCLA Med Ctr 1982; **Fellow:** Hematology & Oncology, UCLA Med Ctr 1986; **Fac Appt:** Prof Med, Cornell Univ-Weill Med Coll

Porter, David L MD [Hem] - **Spec Exp:** Leukemia; Bone Marrow Transplant; Lymphoma; **Hospital:** Hosp Univ Penn - UPHS (page 60); **Address:** Perelman Ctr for Advanced Medicine Fl 2, 3400 Civic Center Blvd, Philadelphia, PA 19104; **Phone:** 215-615-5858; **Board Cert:** Hematology 2006; **Med School:** Brown Univ 1987; **Resid:** Internal Medicine, Univ Hosp 1990; **Fellow:** Hematology & Oncology, Brigham & Womens Hosp 1992; **Fac Appt:** Assoc Prof Med, Univ Pennsylvania

Rai, Kanti MD [Hem] - **Spec Exp:** Leukemia; Lymphoma; Multiple Myeloma; **Hospital:** Long Island Jewish Med Ctr; **Address:** 410 Lakeville Rd, Ste 212, New Hyde Park, NY 10042; **Phone:** 718-470-4050; **Board Cert:** Pediatrics 1959; **Med School:** India 1955; **Resid:** Pediatrics, Lincoln Hosp 1958; Pediatrics, North Shore Univ Hosp 1959; **Fellow:** Hematology, LI Jewish Med Ctr 1960; **Fac Appt:** Prof Med, Albert Einstein Coll Med

Rand, Jacob H MD [Hem] - **Spec Exp:** Bleeding/Coagulation Disorders; Pregnancy & Hematologic Abnormalities; Thrombotic Disorders; **Hospital:** Montefiore Med Ctr - Div. Moses; **Address:** Montefiore Medical Ctr, 111 E 210th St, N8 Silverzone, Bronx, NY 10467-2401; **Phone:** 718-920-5991; **Board Cert:** Internal Medicine 1977; Hematology 1978; **Med School:** Albert Einstein Coll Med 1973; **Resid:** Pathology, Montefiore Med Ctr 1974; Internal Medicine, Mount Sinai Hosp 1975; **Fellow:** Hematology, Montefiore Med Ctr 1978; Research, Montefiore Med Ctr 1983; **Fac Appt:** Prof Med, Albert Einstein Coll Med

Hematology

Raphael, Bruce MD [Hem] - **Spec Exp:** Lymphoma; Leukemia; Multiple Myeloma; **Hospital:** NYU Langone Med Ctr (page 67), NY Downtown Hosp; **Address:** 160 E 34th Street Ave Fl 7, NYU Clinical Cancer Ctr, New York, NY 10016-6402; **Phone:** 212-731-5185; **Board Cert:** Internal Medicine 1978; Hematology 1980; Medical Oncology 1981; **Med School:** McGill Univ 1975; **Resid:** Internal Medicine, Jewish Genl Hosp 1977; **Fellow:** Medical Oncology, Meml Sloan Kettering Cancer Ctr 1978; Hematology, NYU Med Ctr 1980; **Fac Appt:** Assoc Prof Med, NYU Sch Med

Roodman, G David MD [Hem] - **Spec Exp:** Multiple Myeloma; **Hospital:** UPMC Shadyside, VA Pittsburgh Hlth Care Sys; **Address:** VA Pittsburgh Healthcare System, R&D 151-U, rm 2E113, University Drive C, Pittsburgh, PA 15240; **Phone:** 412-692-4724; **Board Cert:** Internal Medicine 1978; Hematology 1980; **Med School:** Univ KY Coll Med 1973; **Resid:** Internal Medicine, Univ Minnesota Hosp 1978; **Fellow:** Hematology, Univ Minnesota Hosp 1980; **Fac Appt:** Prof Med, Univ Pittsburgh

Rowley, Scott D MD [Hem] - **Spec Exp:** Stem Cell Transplant; Bone Marrow Transplant; **Hospital:** Hackensack Univ Med Ctr; **Address:** 360 Essex St, Ste 303, Hackensack, NJ 07601; **Phone:** 201-336-8297; **Board Cert:** Internal Medicine 1981; Medical Oncology 1983; Hematology 1984; **Med School:** Univ Mass Sch Med 1978; **Resid:** Internal Medicine, Rhode Island Hosp 1981; **Fellow:** Hematology & Oncology, Rhode Island Hosp 1984; **Fac Appt:** Assoc Prof Med, UMDNJ-NJ Med Sch, Newark

Savage, David G MD [Hem] - **Spec Exp:** Stem Cell Transplant; Multiple Myeloma; Lymphoma; **Hospital:** NY-Presby Hosp/Columbia (page 66); **Address:** 177 Fort Washington Ave, Millstein Bldg Fl 6 - rm 435, New York, NY 10032; **Phone:** 212-305-9783; **Board Cert:** Internal Medicine 1977; Hematology 1982; Medical Oncology 1985; **Med School:** Columbia P&S 1974; **Resid:** Internal Medicine, Harlem Hosp/Columbia Presby Med Ctr 1977; **Fellow:** Hematology & Oncology, Harlem Hosp/Columbia Presby Med Ctr 1979; **Fac Appt:** Assoc Prof Med, Columbia P&S

Schuster, Michael W MD [Hem] - **Spec Exp:** Bone Marrow Transplant; **Hospital:** NY-Presby Hosp/Weill Cornell (page 66); **Address:** NY Weill Cornell Medical Ctr, 525 E 68th St, Starr 341, New York, NY 10021; **Phone:** 212-746-2119; **Board Cert:** Internal Medicine 1984; Hematology 1986; **Med School:** Dartmouth Med Sch 1980; **Resid:** Internal Medicine, New Eng Deaconess Hosp 1983; **Fellow:** Hematology & Oncology, Beth Israel Med Ctr 1987; **Fac Appt:** Assoc Prof Med, Cornell Univ-Weill Med Coll

Slease, Robert B MD [Hem] - **Spec Exp:** Hematologic Malignancies; Hodgkin's Disease; Stem Cell Transplant; Clinical Trials; **Hospital:** Christiana Care Hlth Svs; **Address:** Cristiana Care Hlth Svs, Div Hematology, 4735 Ogletown-Stanton Rd, Ste S-2225, Newark, DE 19713; **Phone:** 302-737-7700; **Board Cert:** Internal Medicine 1975; Hematology 1978; **Med School:** Univ Kans 1972; **Resid:** Internal Medicine, Natl Naval Med Ctr 1975; **Fellow:** Hematology, Natl Naval Med Ctr 1977; **Fac Appt:** Clin Prof Med, Jefferson Med Coll

Spivak, Jerry L MD [Hem] - **Spec Exp:** Myeloproliferative Disorders; Polycythemia Rubra Vera; Leukemia; Anemia; **Hospital:** Johns Hopkins Hosp (page 61); **Address:** 720 Rutland Ave Bldg Ross - Ste 1025, Baltimore, MD 21205; **Phone:** 410-614-0167; **Board Cert:** Internal Medicine 1971; Hematology 1974; **Med School:** Cornell Univ-Weill Med Coll 1964; **Resid:** Internal Medicine, Johns Hopkins Hosp 1966; Internal Medicine, Johns Hopkins Hosp 1972; **Fellow:** Hematology, Natl Cancer Inst 1968; Hematology, Johns Hopkins Hosp 1971; **Fac Appt:** Prof Med, Johns Hopkins Univ

Wisch, Nathaniel MD [Hem] - **Spec Exp:** Lymphoma; Breast Cancer; Leukemia; Anemia-Cancer Related; **Hospital:** Lenox Hill Hosp (page 62), Mount Sinai Med Ctr (page 64); **Address:** 12 E 86th St, New York, NY 10028-0506; **Phone:** 212-861-6660; **Board Cert:** Internal Medicine 1965; Hematology 1972; Medical Oncology 1977; **Med School:** Northwestern Univ 1958; **Resid:** Internal Medicine, VA Hosp 1960; Internal Medicine, Montefiore Hosp 1961; **Fellow:** Hematology, Mount Sinai Hosp 1962; **Fac Appt:** Clin Prof Med, Mount Sinai Sch Med

Zalusky, Ralph MD [Hem] - **Spec Exp:** Anemia; Leukemia; Lymphoma; **Hospital:** Beth Israel Med Ctr - Petrie Division (page 57); **Address:** Beth Israel Med Ctr, First Ave at 16th St, New York, NY 10003; **Phone:** 212-420-4185; **Board Cert:** Internal Medicine 1964; Hematology 1972; **Med School:** Boston Univ 1957; **Resid:** Internal Medicine, Duke Univ Med Ctr 1962; **Fellow:** Hematology, Boston Med Ctr 1961; **Fac Appt:** Prof Med, Albert Einstein Coll Med

Southeast

Adams-Graves, Patricia MD [Hem] - **Spec Exp:** Sickle Cell Disease; **Hospital:** Regional Med Ctr - Memphis; **Address:** Memphis Med Ctr, 880 Madison Ave, Ste 5C01, Memphis, TN 38103-3409; **Phone:** 901-545-8535; **Board Cert:** Internal Medicine 1989; **Med School:** Univ Louisville Sch Med 1986; **Resid:** Internal Medicine, Univ Louisville Affil Hosp 1989; **Fellow:** Hematology & Oncology, Univ Tennessee Hlth Science Ctr 1993; **Fac Appt:** Prof Med, Univ Tenn Coll Med, Memphis

Bigelow, Carolyn L MD [Hem] - **Spec Exp:** Bone Marrow Transplant; Sickle Cell Disease; **Hospital:** Univ Mississippi Med Ctr; **Address:** Univ Mississippi Med Ctr-Div Hematology, 2500 N State St, Jackson, MS 39216; **Phone:** 601-984-5615; **Board Cert:** Internal Medicine 1982; Hematology 1988; **Med School:** Univ Miss 1979; **Resid:** Internal Medicine, Univ Mississippi Med Ctr 1982; **Fellow:** Hematology & Oncology, Univ Washington Med Ctr 1987; **Fac Appt:** Prof Med, Univ Miss

Djulbegovic, Benjamin MD [Hem] - **Spec Exp:** Multiple Myeloma; Lymphoma; Myeloproliferative Disorders; **Hospital:** Univ of S FL - Tampa, H Lee Moffitt Cancer Ctr & Research Inst; **Address:** 12901 Bruce B Downs Blvd, MDC 02, Tampa, FL 33612; **Phone:** 813-396-9178; **Board Cert:** Internal Medicine 2002; Hematology 2004; **Med School:** Bosnia 1976; **Resid:** Internal Medicine, Univ Med Ctr 1983; Internal Medicine, Univ Louisville Med Ctr 1988; **Fellow:** Univ Manchester 1985; Hematology & Oncology, Univ Louisville 1990; **Fac Appt:** Prof Med, Univ S Fla Coll Med

Files, Joe C MD [Hem] - **Spec Exp:** Bone Marrow Transplant; Stem Cell Transplant; Leukemia; **Hospital:** Univ Mississippi Med Ctr; **Address:** Univ Miss Med Ctr-Div Hematology, 2500 N State St, Jackson, MS 39216; **Phone:** 601-984-5615; **Board Cert:** Internal Medicine 1976; Hematology 1980; **Med School:** Univ Miss 1972; **Resid:** Internal Medicine, Univ Miss Med Ctr 1976; **Fellow:** Hematology, Univ Wash Sch Med 1979; **Fac Appt:** Prof Med, Univ Miss

Greer, John P MD [Hem] - **Spec Exp:** Leukemia & Lymphoma; Myelodysplastic Syndromes; Stem Cell Transplant; **Hospital:** Vanderbilt Univ Med Ctr; **Address:** 2665 The Vanderbilt Clinic, 1301 22nd Ave S, Nashville, TN 37232-5505; **Phone:** 615-936-1803; **Board Cert:** Pediatrics 1985; Internal Medicine 1979; Hematology 1984; Medical Oncology 1985; **Med School:** Vanderbilt Univ 1976; **Resid:** Internal Medicine, Tulane Univ Med Ctr 1979; Pediatrics, Med Coll Virginia 1981; **Fellow:** Hematology & Oncology, Vanderbilt Univ Med Ctr 1984; **Fac Appt:** Prof Med, Vanderbilt Univ

Lin, Weei-Chin MD/PhD [Hem] - **Spec Exp:** Hematologic Malignancies; Bleeding/Coagulation Disorders; **Hospital:** Univ of Ala Hosp at Birmingham; **Address:** Univ of Alabama, 1530 3rd Ave S, Ste 520A, Birmingham, AL 35294; **Phone:** 205-934-3980; **Board Cert:** Hematology 1999; Medical Oncology 1999; **Med School:** Taiwan 1986; **Resid:** Internal Medicine, Duke Univ Med Ctr 1996; **Fellow:** Hematology & Oncology, Duke Univ Med Ctr 1999; **Fac Appt:** Assoc Prof Med, Univ Alabama

Hematology

List, Alan F MD [Hem] - **Spec Exp:** Myelodysplastic Syndromes; Leukemia; **Hospital:** H Lee Moffitt Cancer Ctr & Research Inst; **Address:** 12902 Magnolia Drive, MCC-VP, Tampa, FL 33612-9497; **Phone:** 813-745-6086; **Board Cert:** Internal Medicine 1983; Medical Oncology 1985; Hematology 1986; **Med School:** Univ Pennsylvania 1980; **Resid:** Internal Medicine, Good Samaritan Hosp 1983; Oncology, Vanderbilt Univ Med Ctr 1985; **Fellow:** Hematology, Vanderbilt Univ Med Ctr 1986

Ortel, Thomas L MD/PhD [Hem] - **Spec Exp:** Bleeding/Coagulation Disorders; Hemophilia; **Hospital:** Duke Univ Med Ctr; **Address:** Duke Medical Ctr, Box 3422, Durham, NC 27710; **Phone:** 919-668-6688 x22; **Board Cert:** Internal Medicine 1988; Hematology 2002; **Med School:** Indiana Univ 1985; **Resid:** Internal Medicine, Duke Univ Med Ctr 1988; **Fellow:** Hematology & Oncology, Duke Univ Med Ctr 1989; **Fac Appt:** Prof Med, Duke Univ

Powell, Bayard L MD [Hem] - **Spec Exp:** Leukemia; Myelodysplastic Syndromes; **Hospital:** Wake Forest Univ Baptist Med Ctr (page 72); **Address:** Wake Forest Univ Baptist Med Ctr, Med Ctr Blvd-Cancer Center, Winston-Salem, NC 27157-1082; **Phone:** 336-716-7970; **Board Cert:** Internal Medicine 1983; Medical Oncology 1985; **Med School:** Univ NC Sch Med 1980; **Resid:** Internal Medicine, NC Baptist Hosp 1983; **Fellow:** Hematology & Oncology, Wake Forest Univ Sch Med 1986; **Fac Appt:** Prof Med, Wake Forest Univ

Rosenblatt, Joseph D MD [Hem] - **Spec Exp:** Lymphoma; Leukemia; Multiple Myeloma; **Hospital:** Univ of Miami Hosp & Clins/Sylvester Comp Canc Ctr (page 70), Jackson Meml Hosp (page 70); **Address:** Sylvester Comprehensive Cancer Ctr, 1475 NW 12th Ave, D8-4, Ste 3300, Miami, FL 33136; **Phone:** 305-243-4909; **Board Cert:** Internal Medicine 1983; Medical Oncology 1985; **Med School:** UCLA 1980; **Resid:** Internal Medicine, UCLA Med Ctr 1983; **Fellow:** Hematology & Oncology, UCLA Med Ctr 1986; **Fac Appt:** Prof Med, Univ Miami Sch Med

Schwartzberg, Lee S MD [Hem] - **Spec Exp:** Breast Cancer; Lung Cancer; Stem Cell Transplant; **Hospital:** Baptist Memorial Hospital - Memphis; **Address:** The West Clinic, 100 N Humphreys Blvd, Memphis, TN 38120; **Phone:** 901-683-0055; **Board Cert:** Internal Medicine 1983; Hematology 1986; Medical Oncology 1985; **Med School:** NY Med Coll 1980; **Resid:** Internal Medicine, North Shore Univ Hosp 1983; Internal Medicine, Meml Sloan Kettering Cancer Ctr 1985; **Fellow:** Hematology & Oncology, Meml Sloan Kettering Cancer Ctr 1984; Hematology & Oncology, Meml Sloan Kettering Cancer Ctr 1987; **Fac Appt:** Assoc Prof Med, Univ Tenn Coll Med, Memphis

Solberg, Lawrence MD/PhD [Hem] - **Spec Exp:** Bone Marrow Transplant; Myeloproliferative Disorders; Porphyria; **Hospital:** Mayo - Jacksonville, Rochelle Comm Hosp; **Address:** Mayo Clinic-Dept Hem-Onc, 4500 San Pablo Rd Fl 8, Jacksonville, FL 32224; **Phone:** 904-953-7292; **Board Cert:** Internal Medicine 1978; Hematology 1980; **Med School:** St Louis Univ 1975; **Resid:** Internal Medicine, Mayo Clinic 1978; **Fellow:** Hematology, Mayo Clinic 1980; **Fac Appt:** Prof Med, Mayo Med Sch

Telen, Marilyn J MD [Hem] - **Spec Exp:** Transfusion Medicine; Anemias & Red Cell Disorders; Sickle Cell Disease; **Hospital:** Duke Univ Med Ctr; **Address:** Duke Univ Med Ctr, Box 2615, Durham, NC 27710; **Phone:** 919-684-5426; **Board Cert:** Internal Medicine 1980; Hematology 1984; **Med School:** NYU Sch Med 1977; **Resid:** Internal Medicine, Erie Co Med Cr 1980; **Fellow:** Hematology, Duke Univ Med Ctr 1983; **Fac Appt:** Prof Med, Duke Univ

Zuckerman, Kenneth S MD [Hem] - **Spec Exp:** Myeloproliferative Disorders; Leukemia; Lymphoma; Anemia; **Hospital:** H Lee Moffitt Cancer Ctr & Research Inst, Tampa Genl Hosp; **Address:** H Lee Moffitt Cancer Ctr, 12902 Magnolia Drive, FOB3, Tampa, FL 33612-9416; **Phone:** 813-745-8090; **Board Cert:** Internal Medicine 1975; Hematology 1978; **Med School:** Ohio State Univ 1972; **Resid:** Internal Medicine, Ohio State Univ Hosps 1975; **Fellow:** Hematology, Brigham Hosp/Harvard Univ 1978; **Fac Appt:** Prof Med, Univ S Fla Coll Med

Midwest

Baron, Joseph M MD [Hem] - **Spec Exp:** Bleeding/Coagulation Disorders; Lymphoma; Myelo-proliferative Disorders; **Hospital:** Univ of Chicago Med Ctr; **Address:** 5758 S Maryland Ave, MC 9015, Chicago, IL 60637-1463; **Phone:** 773-702-6149; **Board Cert:** Internal Medicine 1969; Hematology 1972; Medical Oncology 1975; **Med School:** Univ Chicago-Pritzker Sch Med 1962; **Resid:** Internal Medicine, Univ Chicago Hosps 1964; Internal Medicine, Univ Chicago Hosps 1968; **Fellow:** Hematology, Univ Chicago Hosps 1968; **Fac Appt:** Assoc Prof Med, Univ Chicago-Pritzker Sch Med

Blinder, Morey MD [Hem] - **Spec Exp:** Bleeding/Coagulation Disorders; Anemia; Sickle Cell Disease; **Hospital:** Barnes-Jewish Hosp; **Address:** Washington Univ School of Medicine, Hematology Division, 660 S Euclid Ave, Box 8125, St Louis, MO 63110; **Phone:** 314-362-8808; **Board Cert:** Internal Medicine 1984; Hematology 1988; Medical Oncology 1987; **Med School:** St Louis Univ 1981; **Resid:** Internal Medicine, Univ Illinois Hosp 1984; **Fellow:** Hematology & Oncology, Univ Wash Med Ctr 1986; **Fac Appt:** Assoc Prof Med, Washington Univ, St Louis

Bockenstedt, Paula MD [Hem] - **Spec Exp:** Bleeding/Coagulation Disorders; Leukemia; Von Willebrand's Disease; **Hospital:** Univ Michigan Hlth Sys; **Address:** Div Hematology, 1500 E Med Ctr Dr, MIB, rm C-344, Ann Arbor, MI 48109-8048; **Phone:** 734-647-8921; **Board Cert:** Internal Medicine 1981; Hematology 1984; **Med School:** Harvard Med Sch 1978; **Resid:** Internal Medicine, Brigham-Womens Hosp 1981; **Fellow:** Hematology, Brigham-Womens Hosp 1984; **Fac Appt:** Assoc Clin Prof Med, Univ Mich Med Sch

Byrd, John C MD [Hem] - **Spec Exp:** Leukemia-Chronic Lymphocytic; **Hospital:** Arthur G James Cancer Hosp & Research Inst; **Address:** Bl02 Starling-Loving Hall, 320 W 10th Ave, Columbus, OH 43210; **Phone:** 614-293-3196; **Board Cert:** Hematology 2007; **Med School:** Univ Ark 1991; **Resid:** Internal Medicine, Walter Reed AMC 1994; **Fellow:** Hematology & Oncology, Walter Reed AMC 1997; **Fac Appt:** Assoc Prof Med, Ohio State Univ

Copelan, Edward A MD [Hem] - **Spec Exp:** Leukemia; Myelodysplastic Syndromes; Bone Marrow Transplant; Multiple Myeloma; **Hospital:** Cleveland Clin Fdn (page 56); **Address:** Cleveland Clinic Fdn, 9500 Euclid Ave, MC R35, Cleveland, OH 44195; **Phone:** 216-445-5647; **Board Cert:** Internal Medicine 1980; Hematology 1982; Medical Oncology 1983; **Med School:** Tufts Univ 1977; **Resid:** Internal Medicine, Ohio State Univ Hosp 1980; **Fellow:** Hematology & Oncology, Ohio State Univ Hosp 1983; Bone Marrow Transplant, UCLA Med Ctr

Di Persio, John MD/PhD [Hem] - **Spec Exp:** Bone Marrow Transplant; Hematologic Malignancies; Leukemia; **Hospital:** Barnes-Jewish Hosp; **Address:** Wash Univ Sch Med, Sect Bone Marrow Transplant & Leukemia, 660 S Euclid Ave, Box 8007, St Louis, MO 63110; **Phone:** 314-454-8306; **Board Cert:** Internal Medicine 1984; Medical Oncology 1987; Hematology 1988; **Med School:** Univ Rochester 1980; **Resid:** Internal Medicine, Parkland Meml Hosp 1984; **Fellow:** Hematology & Oncology, UCLA Med Ctr 1987; **Fac Appt:** Prof Med, Washington Univ, St Louis

Erba, Harry P MD/PhD [Hem] - **Spec Exp:** Leukemia; Myelodysplastic Syndromes; Lymphoma; **Hospital:** Univ Michigan Hlth Sys; **Address:** Univ Michigan Medical Ctr, 1500 E Medical Center Dr, B1-358 Cancer Ctr, Ann Arbor, MI 48109-5848; **Phone:** 734-647-8901; **Board Cert:** Internal Medicine 2004; Hematology 2004; Medical Oncology 2005; **Med School:** Stanford Univ 1988; **Resid:** Internal Medicine, Brigham & Womens Hosp 1990; **Fellow:** Hematology & Oncology, Brigham & Womens Hosp 1993; **Fac Appt:** Assoc Prof Med, Univ Mich Med Sch

Hematology

Farag, Sherif S MD/PhD [Hem] - **Spec Exp:** Multiple Myeloma; Leukemia & Lymphoma; Bone Marrow Transplant; Stem Cell Transplant; **Hospital:** Indiana Univ Hosp; **Address:** 980 W Walnut St, Walther Hall, R3-C400, Indianapolis, IN 46202; **Phone:** 317-274-0843; **Med School:** Australia 1995; **Resid:** Internal Medicine, Univ Melbourne Med Ctr; **Fellow:** Hematology & Oncology, Roswell Park Cancer Inst; **Fac Appt:** Assoc Prof Med, Indiana Univ

Flynn, Patrick MD [Hem] - **Spec Exp:** Hematologic Malignancies; Colon & Rectal Cancer; Clinical Trials; Breast Cancer; **Hospital:** Abbott - Northwestern Hosp, Fairview Southdale Hosp; **Address:** 800 E 28th St, Piper Bldg, Ste 405, Minneapolis, MN 55407; **Phone:** 612-863-8585; **Board Cert:** Internal Medicine 1978; Medical Oncology 1981; Hematology 1982; **Med School:** Univ Minn 1975; **Resid:** Internal Medicine, Hennepin Co Med Ctr 1978; **Fellow:** Hematology & Oncology, Univ Minnesota Hosp 1981

Gaynor, Ellen MD [Hem] - **Spec Exp:** Lymphoma; Genitourinary Cancer; Breast Cancer; **Hospital:** Loyola Univ Med Ctr; **Address:** Loyola Univ Med Ctr, Dept Hematology, 2160 S First Ave Bldg 112 - rm 108, Maywood, IL 60153-3328; **Phone:** 708-327-3214; **Board Cert:** Internal Medicine 1982; Hematology 1986; Medical Oncology 1985; **Med School:** Univ Wisc 1978; **Resid:** Internal Medicine, Loyola Univ Med Ctr 1982; **Fellow:** Medical Oncology, Loyola Univ Med Ctr 1981; Hematology & Oncology, Univ Chicago Hosp 1984; **Fac Appt:** Prof Med, Loyola Univ-Stritch Sch Med

Gertz, Morie MD [Hem] - **Spec Exp:** Multiple Myeloma; Amyloidosis; Waldenstrom's Macroglobulinemia; Plasma Cell Disorders; **Hospital:** Mayo Med Ctr & Clin - Rochester, Rochester Methodist Hosp; **Address:** 200 SW 1st St Fl W10, Rochester, MN 55905; **Phone:** 507-284-2511; **Board Cert:** Internal Medicine 1979; Hematology 1982; Medical Oncology 1983; **Med School:** Loyola Univ-Stritch Sch Med 1975; **Resid:** Internal Medicine, St Lukes Hosp 1979; **Fellow:** Hematology & Oncology, Mayo Clin 1982; **Fac Appt:** Prof Med, Mayo Med Sch

Godwin, John MD [Hem] - **Spec Exp:** Thrombotic Disorders; Leukemia in Elderly; Head & Neck Cancer; Lymphoma; **Hospital:** St John's Hosp - Springfield, Memorial Med Ctr-Springfield; **Address:** SIU School Medicine, Simmons Cooper Cancer Inst, PO Box 19678, Springfield, IL 62794; **Phone:** 217-545-5817; **Board Cert:** Internal Medicine 1981; Hematology 1986; **Med School:** Univ Alabama 1978; **Resid:** Internal Medicine, Baylor Coll Med 1981; Internal Medicine, Baylor Coll Med 1982; **Fellow:** Hematology, Baylor Coll Med 1983; Hematology, North Carolina Meml Hosp 1985; **Fac Appt:** Prof Med, Southern IL Univ

Gordon, Leo I MD [Hem] - **Spec Exp:** Lymphoma, Non-Hodgkin's; Hodgkin's Disease; Bone Marrow Transplant; **Hospital:** Northwestern Meml Hosp; **Address:** 676 N St Clair St, Ste 850, Chicago, IL 60611-3124; **Phone:** 312-695-4546; **Board Cert:** Internal Medicine 1976; Hematology 1978; Medical Oncology 1979; **Med School:** Univ Cincinnati 1973; **Resid:** Internal Medicine, Univ Chicago Hosps 1976; **Fellow:** Hematology, Univ Minnesota Hosps 1978; Hematology & Oncology, Univ Chicago Hosps 1979; **Fac Appt:** Prof Med, Northwestern Univ

Gregory, Stephanie A MD [Hem] - **Spec Exp:** Lymphoma; Leukemia; Plasma Cell Disorders; Multiple Myeloma; **Hospital:** Rush Univ Med Ctr; **Address:** 1725 W Harrison St, Ste 834, Rush Professional Office Bldg, Chicago, IL 60612-3861; **Phone:** 312-942-5982; **Board Cert:** Internal Medicine 1972; Hematology 1972; **Med School:** Med Coll PA Hahnemann 1965; **Resid:** Internal Medicine, Rush/Presby-St Luke's Med Ctr 1969; **Fellow:** Hematology, Rush/Presby-St Luke's Med Ctr 1972; **Fac Appt:** Prof Med, Rush Med Coll

Greipp, Philip R MD [Hem] - **Spec Exp:** Multiple Myeloma; **Hospital:** Mayo Med Ctr & Clin - Rochester; **Address:** Mayo Clinic, Div Hematology, 200 First St SW Mayo Bldg Fl W-10, Rochester, MN 55905-0001; **Phone:** 507-284-3159; **Board Cert:** Internal Medicine 1974; Hematology 1994; **Med School:** Georgetown Univ 1968; **Resid:** Internal Medicine, Mayo Clinic 1973; **Fellow:** Hematology, Mayo Clinic 1975; **Fac Appt:** Prof Med, Mayo Med Sch

Grever, Michael R MD [Hem] - **Spec Exp:** Hematologic Malignancies; Leukemia; Drug Development; Clinical Trials; **Hospital:** Ohio St Univ Med Ctr; **Address:** 215 Means Hall, 1654 Upham Drive, Columbus, OH 43210; **Phone:** 614-293-8724; **Board Cert:** Internal Medicine 1975; Hematology 1988; Medical Oncology 1979; **Med School:** Univ Pittsburgh 1971; **Resid:** Internal Medicine, Univ of Pittsburgh 1974; **Fellow:** Hematology & Oncology, Ohio State Univ 1978; **Fac Appt:** Prof Med, Ohio State Univ

Habermann, Thomas M MD [Hem] - **Spec Exp:** Lymphoma; Hodgkin's Disease; Leukemia; **Hospital:** Mayo Med Ctr & Clin - Rochester; **Address:** Mayo Clinic, 200 1st St SW, Rochester, MN 55905; **Phone:** 507-284-3159; **Board Cert:** Internal Medicine 1982; Hematology 1984; **Med School:** Creighton Univ 1979; **Resid:** Internal Medicine, Mayo Clinic 1982; **Fellow:** Hematology, Mayo Clinic 1985; **Fac Appt:** Prof Med, Mayo Med Sch

Juckett, Mark B MD [Hem] - **Spec Exp:** Bone Marrow Transplant; **Hospital:** Univ WI Hosp & Clins; **Address:** 600 Highland Ave, Ste H4/534, 2817 New Pinery Rd, Portage, WI 53901; **Phone:** 608-745-5660; **Board Cert:** Internal Medicine 2001; Hematology 2004; Medical Oncology 2005; **Med School:** Univ Louisville Sch Med 1987; **Resid:** Internal Medicine, Univ Minnesota 1990; **Fellow:** Hematology & Oncology, Univ Minnesota 1992; **Fac Appt:** Assoc Prof Med, Univ Wisc

Kraut, Eric H MD [Hem] - **Spec Exp:** Hematologic Malignancies; Leukemia; Drug Development; Clinical Trials; **Hospital:** Ohio St Univ Med Ctr; **Address:** B405 Starling Loving Hall, 320 W 10th Ave, Columbus, OH 43210; **Phone:** 614-293-2887; **Board Cert:** Internal Medicine 1975; Hematology 1978; Medical Oncology 1977; **Med School:** Temple Univ 1972; **Resid:** Internal Medicine, Univ Pittsburgh 1975; **Fellow:** Hematology & Oncology, Ohio State Univ Hosp 1977; **Fac Appt:** Prof Med, Ohio State Univ

Kuriakose, Philip MD [Hem] - **Spec Exp:** Leukemia; **Hospital:** Henry Ford Hosp; **Address:** Henry Ford Hosp, Hematology/Oncology, 2799 W Grand Blvd, Detroit, MI 48202; **Phone:** 313-916-1841; **Board Cert:** Internal Medicine 1999; Medical Oncology 2002; Hematology 2002; **Med School:** India 1990; **Resid:** Internal Medicine, Christian Med Coll 1992; Internal Medicine, Henry Ford Hosp 1994; **Fellow:** Hematology & Oncology, Mayo Clinic 1995

Kuzel, Timothy M MD [Hem] - **Spec Exp:** Kidney Cancer; Melanoma; Cutaneous Lymphoma; **Hospital:** Northwestern Meml Hosp; **Address:** Northwestern Meml Hosp, 675 N St Clair, Ste 21-100, Chicago, IL 60611; **Phone:** 312-695-0990; **Board Cert:** Internal Medicine 1987; Hematology 2000; Medical Oncology 1989; **Med School:** Univ Mich Med Sch 1984; **Resid:** Internal Medicine, McGraw MC-Northwestern Univ 1987; **Fellow:** Hematology & Oncology, McGraw MC-Northwestern Univ 1990; **Fac Appt:** Prof Med, Northwestern Univ

Larson, Richard A MD [Hem] - **Spec Exp:** Leukemia & Lymphoma; Bone Marrow Transplant; Myelodysplastic Syndromes; **Hospital:** Univ of Chicago Med Ctr; **Address:** Univ Chicago Hosps, 5841 S Maryland Ave, MC 2115, Chicago, IL 60637; **Phone:** 773-702-6149; **Board Cert:** Internal Medicine 1980; Hematology 1982; Medical Oncology 1983; **Med School:** Stanford Univ 1977; **Resid:** Internal Medicine, Univ Chicago Hosps 1980; **Fellow:** Hematology & Oncology, Univ Chicago Hosps 1983; **Fac Appt:** Prof Med, Univ Chicago-Pritzker Sch Med

Laughlin, Mary J MD [Hem] - **Spec Exp:** Bone Marrow Transplant; **Hospital:** Univ Hosps Case Med Ctr; **Address:** 2103 Cornell Rd, WRB 2-129, Cleveland, OH 44106; **Phone:** 216-844-5182; **Board Cert:** Internal Medicine 2003; Hematology 2004; **Med School:** SUNY Buffalo 1988; **Resid:** Internal Medicine, Duke Univ Med Ctr 1991; **Fellow:** Hematology & Oncology, Duke Univ Med Ctr 1992; Bone Marrow Transplant, Rosewell Park Cancer Inst 1994; **Fac Appt:** Assoc Prof Med, Case West Res Univ

Hematology

Lazarus, Hillard M MD [Hem] - **Spec Exp:** Bone Marrow Transplant; Stem Cell Transplant; Leukemia; **Hospital:** Univ Hosps Case Med Ctr; **Address:** 11100 Euclid Ave, Cleveland, OH 44106-5065; **Phone:** 216-844-3629; **Board Cert:** Internal Medicine 1977; Medical Oncology 1979; Hematology 1980; **Med School:** Univ Rochester 1974; **Resid:** Internal Medicine, Univ Hosps 1977; **Fellow:** Hematology & Oncology, Univ Hosps 1979; **Fac Appt:** Prof Med, Case West Res Univ

Litzow, Mark R MD [Hem] - **Spec Exp:** Bone Marrow Transplant; Leukemia; **Hospital:** Mayo Med Ctr & Clin - Rochester; **Address:** Mayo Clinic, Div Hematology, 200 First St SW, Rochester, MN 55905; **Phone:** 507-284-0923; **Board Cert:** Internal Medicine 1983; Hematology 1988; Medical Oncology 1989; **Med School:** Univ Chicago-Pritzker Sch Med 1980; **Resid:** Internal Medicine, Mayo Clinic 1984; **Fellow:** Medical Oncology, Mayo Clinic 1990; **Fac Appt:** Asst Prof Med, Mayo Med Sch

Maciejewski, Jaroslaw P MD/PhD [Hem] - **Spec Exp:** Anemia-Aplastic; Hematologic Malignancies; Stem Cell Transplant; **Hospital:** Cleveland Clin Fdn (page 56); **Address:** Cleveland Clinic, 9500 Euclid Ave, Desk R40, Cleveland, OH 44195; **Phone:** 216-445-5962; **Board Cert:** Internal Medicine 1999; Hematology 2001; **Med School:** Germany 1990; **Resid:** Internal Medicine, Univ Nevada Med Ctr 1997; **Fellow:** Hematology, Natl Inst Hlth 2000; **Fac Appt:** Prof Med, Case West Res Univ

McGlave, Philip B MD [Hem] - **Spec Exp:** Leukemia; Bone Marrow Transplant; **Hospital:** Univ Minn Med Ctr, Fairview - Univ Campus; **Address:** Univ Minn, Dept Med - Div Hem/Onc, Mayo Mail Code 480, 420 Delaware St SE, Minneapolis, MN 55455; **Phone:** 612-626-2446; **Board Cert:** Internal Medicine 1977; Hematology 1980; **Med School:** Univ IL Coll Med 1974; **Resid:** Internal Medicine, Univ Minnesota Med Ctr 1977; **Fellow:** Hematology & Oncology, Univ Minnesota Med Ctr 1980; **Fac Appt:** Prof Med, Univ Minn

Mosher, Deane F MD [Hem] - **Hospital:** Univ WI Hosp & Clins; **Address:** Dept Hematology, 600 Highland Ave Fl 5, Madison, WI 53792; **Phone:** 608-263-7022; **Board Cert:** Internal Medicine 1973; Hematology 1980; **Med School:** Harvard Med Sch 1968; **Resid:** Internal Medicine, Beth Israel Hosp 1970; **Fellow:** Hematology, Harvard Med Sch 1972; **Fac Appt:** Prof Med, Univ Wisc

Nand, Sucha MD [Hem] - **Spec Exp:** Myelodysplastic Syndromes; Myeloproliferative Disorders; Leukemia; Lymphoma, Non-Hodgkin's; **Hospital:** Loyola Univ Med Ctr; **Address:** Cardinal Bernardin Cancer Ctr, 2160 S First Ave Bldg 112 - rm 342, Maywood, IL 60153-3304; **Phone:** 708-327-3217; **Board Cert:** Internal Medicine 1979; Medical Oncology 1981; Hematology 1982; **Med School:** India 1971; **Resid:** Physical Medicine & Rehabilitation, Northwestern Meml Hosp 1976; Internal Medicine, North Chicago VA Hosp 1978; **Fellow:** Medical Oncology, Northwestern Meml Hosp 1981; **Fac Appt:** Prof Med, Loyola Univ-Stritch Sch Med

Palascak, Joseph E MD [Hem] - **Spec Exp:** Hemophilia; Bleeding/Coagulation Disorders; Thrombotic Disorders; **Hospital:** Univ Hosp - Cincinnati; **Address:** 234 Goodman, ML 501, Cincinnati, OH 45219; **Phone:** 513-584-1937; **Board Cert:** Internal Medicine 1975; Hematology 1978; **Med School:** Jefferson Med Coll 1968; **Resid:** Internal Medicine, Thomas Jefferson Univ Hosp 1971; **Fellow:** Hematology, Thomas Jefferson Univ Hosp 1972; Hematology, Thomas Jefferson Univ Hosp 1976; **Fac Appt:** Prof Med, Univ Cincinnati

Porcu, Pierluigi MD [Hem] - **Spec Exp:** Lymphoma; Lymphoma, Non-Hodgkin's; Immunotherapy; **Hospital:** Ohio St Univ Med Ctr; **Address:** 320 W 10th Ave, B320 Starling Loving Hall, Columbus, OH 43210; **Phone:** 614-293-9273; **Board Cert:** Hematology 1999; Medical Oncology 1999; **Med School:** Italy 1987; **Resid:** Internal Medicine, Indiana Univ Hosp 1996; **Fellow:** Hematology & Oncology, Indiana Univ Hosp 1999; **Fac Appt:** Asst Prof Med, Ohio State Univ

Silverstein, Roy L MD [Hem] - **Spec Exp:** Thrombotic Disorders; Bleeding/Coagulation Disorders; **Hospital:** Cleveland Clin Fdn (page 56); **Address:** Dept Cell Biology, Lerner Rsch Inst, 9500 Euclid Ave, NC10, Cleveland, OH 44195; **Phone:** 216-444-5220; **Board Cert:** Internal Medicine 1982; Hematology 1984; Medical Oncology 1985; **Med School:** Emory Univ 1979; **Resid:** Internal Medicine, NY Hosp-Cornell Med Ctr 1982; Hematology & Oncology, NY Hosp-Cornell Med Ctr 1984; **Fac Appt:** Prof Med, Cleveland Cl Coll Med/Case West Res

Singhal, Seema MD [Hem] - **Spec Exp:** Multiple Myeloma; **Hospital:** Northwestern Meml Hosp; **Address:** 675 N St Claire St, Ste 21-100, Chicago, IL 60611; **Phone:** 312-695-0990; **Board Cert:** Internal Medicine 2005; **Med School:** India 1989; **Resid:** Internal Medicine, King Edward Meml Hosp 1991; Hematology, King Edward Meml Hosp 1991; **Fellow:** Bone Marrow Transplant, Hadassah Univ Hosp 1992; **Fac Appt:** Prof Med, Northwestern Univ

Stiff, Patrick J MD [Hem] - **Spec Exp:** Bone Marrow Transplant; Lymphoma, Non-Hodgkin's; Leukemia; **Hospital:** Loyola Univ Med Ctr; **Address:** Cardinal Bernadin Cancer Ctr, 2160 S First Ave Bldg 112 - rm 255, Maywood, IL 60153; **Phone:** 708-327-3304; **Board Cert:** Internal Medicine 1978; Medical Oncology 1981; Hematology 1982; **Med School:** Loyola Univ-Stritch Sch Med 1975; **Resid:** Internal Medicine, Cleveland Clinic Fdn 1978; **Fellow:** Hematology & Oncology, Meml Sloan Kettering Cancer Ctr 1981; **Fac Appt:** Prof Med, Loyola Univ-Stritch Sch Med

Sweetenham, John MD [Hem] - **Spec Exp:** Leukemia; Lymphoma; **Hospital:** Cleveland Clin Fdn (page 56); **Address:** Cleveland Clinic, Taussig Cancer Inst, 9500 Euclid Ave, MC R35, Cleveland, OH 44195; **Phone:** 216-445-6707; **Med School:** England, UK 1980; **Resid:** Internal Medicine, Royal United Hosp 1984; **Fellow:** Hematology & Oncology, Univ Southampton 1989; **Fac Appt:** Prof Med, Univ Colorado

Tallman, Martin S MD [Hem] - **Spec Exp:** Bone Marrow Transplant; Leukemia; Lymphoma; **Hospital:** Northwestern Meml Hosp; **Address:** 675 N St Clair St, Ste 21-100, Chicago, IL 60611; **Phone:** 312-695-0990; **Board Cert:** Internal Medicine 1983; Medical Oncology 1987; Hematology 1988; **Med School:** Ros Franklin Univ/Chicago Med Sch 1980; **Resid:** Internal Medicine, Evanston Hosp 1983; **Fellow:** Medical Oncology, Fred Hutchinson Cancer Ctr 1987; **Fac Appt:** Prof Med, Northwestern Univ

Uberti, Joseph P MD/PhD [Hem] - **Spec Exp:** Bone Marrow Transplant; Stem Cell Transplant; **Hospital:** Detroit Med Ctr; **Address:** Barbara Ann Karmanos Cancer Inst, 4100 John R St, MC HWO4HO, Detroit, MI 48201; **Phone:** 313-576-8760; **Board Cert:** Internal Medicine 1986; Medical Oncology 1989; **Med School:** Wayne State Univ 1983; **Resid:** Internal Medicine, Detroit Receiving Hosp 1986; **Fellow:** Hematology & Oncology, Wayne State Univ Hosps 1988; **Fac Appt:** Prof Med, Wayne State Univ

van Besien, Koen W MD [Hem] - **Spec Exp:** Lymphoma; Stem Cell Transplant; **Hospital:** Univ of Chicago Med Ctr; **Address:** Stem Cell Transplant Program, 5841 S Maryland Ave, MC 2115, Chicago, IL 60637; **Phone:** 773-702-4400; **Board Cert:** Internal Medicine 2005; Medical Oncology 2005; Hematology 2006; **Med School:** Belgium 1984; **Resid:** Internal Medicine, Univ Leuven Med Ctr 1987; **Fellow:** Hematology & Oncology, Indiana Univ Med Ctr 1990; **Fac Appt:** Prof Med, Univ Chicago-Pritzker Sch Med

Winter, Jane N MD [Hem] - **Spec Exp:** Lymphoma, Non-Hodgkin's; Hodgkin's Disease; Bone Marrow Transplant; **Hospital:** Northwestern Meml Hosp; **Address:** Northwestern Univ - Div Hem/Oncology, 675 N St Clair St, Ste 21-100, Chicago, IL 60611; **Phone:** 312-695-0990; **Board Cert:** Internal Medicine 1980; Hematology 1982; Medical Oncology 1983; **Med School:** Univ Pennsylvania 1977; **Resid:** Internal Medicine, Univ Chicago Hosps 1980; **Fellow:** Hematology & Oncology, Columbia Presby Hosp 1981; Hematology & Oncology, Northwestern Univ 1983; **Fac Appt:** Prof Med, Northwestern Univ

Hematology

Great Plains and Mountains

Vose, Julie M MD [Hem] - **Spec Exp:** Lymphoma; **Hospital:** Nebraska Med Ctr; **Address:** 987680 Nebraska Med Ctr, Emile @ 42nd St, Omaha, NE 68198-7680; **Phone:** 402-559-5600; **Board Cert:** Internal Medicine 1987; Medical Oncology 2000; Hematology 2000; **Med School:** Univ Nebr Coll Med 1984; **Resid:** Internal Medicine, Univ Nebraska Med Ctr 1987; **Fellow:** Hematology & Oncology, Univ Nebraska Med Ctr 1990; **Fac Appt:** Prof Med, Univ Nebr Coll Med

Southwest

Barlogie, Bart MD/PhD [Hem] - **Spec Exp:** Bone Marrow Transplant; Plasma Cell Disorders; Multiple Myeloma; **Hospital:** UAMS Med Ctr; **Address:** UAMS-Myeloma Inst Rsch & Therapy, 4301 West Markham St, Slot 816, Little Rock, AR 72205; **Phone:** 501-526-2873; **Med School:** Germany 1969; **Resid:** Internal Medicine, Univ Muenster Med Sch; **Fellow:** Medical Oncology, MD Anderson Cancer Ctr-Tumor Inst 1976; **Fac Appt:** Prof Med, Univ Ark

Brenner, Malcolm K MD/PhD [Hem] - **Spec Exp:** Gene Therapy; Bone Marrow Transplant; **Hospital:** Methodist Hosp - Houston, Texas Chldns Hosp; **Address:** 6621 Fannin St, rm 3-3320, Houston, TX 77030; **Phone:** 832-824-4671; **Med School:** England, UK 1975; **Resid:** Internal Medicine, Cambridge Univ 1979; **Fellow:** Immunology, Clinical Rsch Ctr 1984; Hematology & Oncology, Royal Free Hosp 1986; **Fac Appt:** Prof Med, Baylor Coll Med

Champlin, Richard E MD [Hem] - **Spec Exp:** Bone Marrow Transplant; Stem Cell Transplant; Leukemia & Lymphoma; **Hospital:** UT MD Anderson Cancer Ctr; **Address:** MD Anderson Cancer Ctr, Stem Cell Transplantation Ctr, 1515 Holcombe Blvd, Box 0423, Houston, TX 77030; **Phone:** 713-792-6100; **Board Cert:** Internal Medicine 1978; Hematology 1980; Medical Oncology 1981; **Med School:** Univ Chicago-Pritzker Sch Med 1975; **Resid:** Internal Medicine, LA Co Harbor/UCLA Med Ctr 1978; **Fellow:** Hematology & Oncology, LA Co Harbor/UCLA Med Ctr 1980; **Fac Appt:** Prof Med, Univ Tex, Houston

Cobos, Everardo MD [Hem] - **Spec Exp:** Bone Marrow Transplant; Bleeding/Coagulation Disorders; **Hospital:** Univ Med Ctr-Lubbock; **Address:** Texas Tech Univ Med Sch, Dept Med, 3601 4th St, MS 9410, Lubbock, TX 79430; **Phone:** 806-775-8600; **Board Cert:** Internal Medicine 1985; Medical Oncology 1987; Hematology 1988; **Med School:** Univ Tex, San Antonio 1981; **Resid:** Internal Medicine, Letterman Army Med Ctr 1985; **Fellow:** Hematology & Oncology, Letterman Army Med Ctr 1988; **Fac Appt:** Prof Med, Texas Tech Univ

Cooper, Barry MD [Hem] - **Spec Exp:** Leukemia; Lymphoma; Bleeding/Coagulation Disorders; **Hospital:** Baylor Univ Medical Ctr; **Address:** 3535 Worth St, Ste 200, Dallas, TX 75246-2096; **Phone:** 214-370-1002; **Board Cert:** Internal Medicine 1974; Medical Oncology 1977; Hematology 1978; **Med School:** Johns Hopkins Univ 1971; **Resid:** Internal Medicine, Johns Hopkins Hosp 1973; **Fellow:** Metabolism, Natl Inst of Health 1975; Hematology, Peter Bent Brigham Hosp 1977; **Fac Appt:** Clin Prof Med, Univ Tex SW, Dallas

Emanuel, Peter D MD [Hem] - **Spec Exp:** Lymphoma; Leukemia; Hodgkin's Disease; Multiple Myeloma; **Hospital:** UAMS Med Ctr; **Address:** 4301 W Markham, Slot 623, Little Rock, AR 72205; **Phone:** 501-526-2272; **Board Cert:** Internal Medicine 1988; **Med School:** Univ Wisc 1985; **Resid:** Internal Medicine, Univ Alabama Hosp 1988; **Fellow:** Hematology & Oncology, Univ Alabama 1991; **Fac Appt:** Prof Med, Univ Ark

Fonseca, Rafael MD [Hem] - **Spec Exp:** Multiple Myeloma; **Hospital:** Mayo Clinic - Scottsdale; **Address:** 13400 E Shea Blvd, MCCRB 3-001, Scottsdale, AZ 85259; **Phone:** 480-301-4280; **Board Cert:** Hematology 1998; **Med School:** Mexico 1991; **Resid:** Internal Medicine, Jackson Meml Hosp 1994; **Fellow:** Hematology & Oncology, Mayo Clinic 1998; **Fac Appt:** Assoc Prof Med, Mayo Med Sch

Kantarjian, Hagop M MD [Hem] - **Spec Exp:** Leukemia; **Hospital:** UT MD Anderson Cancer Ctr; **Address:** 1400 Holcombe Blvd, Unit 428, Houston, TX 77030; **Phone:** 713-792-7026; **Board Cert:** Internal Medicine 1983; Medical Oncology 1985; **Med School:** Amer Univ Beirut 1979; **Resid:** Internal Medicine, Univ Tex MD Anderson Cancer Ctr 1983; **Fellow:** Hematology & Oncology, Univ Tex MD Anderson Cancer Ctr 1983; **Fac Appt:** Prof Med, Univ Tex, Houston

Keating, Michael MD [Hem] - **Spec Exp:** Leukemia; **Hospital:** UT MD Anderson Cancer Ctr; **Address:** MD Anderson Cancer Ctr, 1400 Holcombe Blvd, Unit 428, Houston, TX 77030-4000; **Phone:** 713-745-2376; **Med School:** Australia 1966; **Resid:** Internal Medicine, St Vincents Hosp 1973; **Fellow:** Hematology, MD Anderson Cancer Ctr 1975; **Fac Appt:** Prof Med, Univ Tex, Houston

Lyons, Roger M MD [Hem] - **Spec Exp:** Leukemia & Lymphoma; Multiple Myeloma; Bleeding/Coagulation Disorders; Platelet Disorders; **Hospital:** SW TX Meth Hosp, Methodist Spec & Transpl Hosp; **Address:** 4411 Medical Drive, Ste 100, San Antonio, TX 78229-3325; **Phone:** 210-595-5300; **Board Cert:** Internal Medicine 1981; Hematology 1982; **Med School:** Canada 1967; **Resid:** Internal Medicine, Winnipeg Genl Hosp 1969; Internal Medicine, Barnes-Wohl Hosps 1972; **Fellow:** Hematology, Washington Univ Hosps 1975; **Fac Appt:** Clin Prof Med, Univ Tex, San Antonio

Maddox, Anne Marie MD [Hem] - **Spec Exp:** Hematologic Malignancies; Lung Cancer; Head & Neck Cancer; Clinical Trials; **Hospital:** UAMS Med Ctr; **Address:** Univ Arkansas Med Ctr, 4301 W Markham St, Slot 74-5, Little Rock, AR 72205; **Phone:** 501-686-8530; **Board Cert:** Internal Medicine 1979; Medical Oncology 1985; Hematology 2004; **Med School:** Dalhousie Univ 1975; **Resid:** Internal Medicine, Univ Toronto 1978; **Fellow:** Medical Oncology, TX MD Anderson Cancer Ctr 1982; **Fac Appt:** Prof, Univ Ark

Miro-Quesada, Miguel MD [Hem] - **Hospital:** Meml Hermann Hosp - Texas Med Ctr, St Luke's Episcopal Hosp-Houston; **Address:** 925 Gessner, Ste 600, Houston, TX 77024; **Phone:** 713-827-9525; **Board Cert:** Internal Medicine 1972; Hematology 1974; Medical Oncology 1985; **Med School:** Johns Hopkins Univ 1969; **Resid:** Internal Medicine, Northwestern Univ Hosp 1971; Internal Medicine, Rush-Presby-St Luke's Med Ctr 1972; **Fellow:** Hematology, Montefiore Hosp 1974

Munker, Reinhold MD [Hem] - **Spec Exp:** Leukemia & Lymphoma; Bone Marrow Transplant; Hematologic Malignancies; **Hospital:** Louisiana State Univ Hosp; **Address:** LSUHSC-Shreveport, Feist-Weiller Cancer Ctr, 1501 Kings Hwy, Shreveport, LA 71130; **Phone:** 318-813-1016; **Board Cert:** Internal Medicine 2004; Hematology 2006; **Med School:** Germany 1979; **Resid:** Internal Medicine, Universit%otsklinikum Gro?hadern 1989; **Fellow:** Hematology & Oncology, Universit%otsklinikum Gro?hadern 1993; Blood Banking, Universit%otsklinikum Gro?hadern 1997; **Fac Appt:** Assoc Prof Med, Louisiana State U, Shrevport

Strauss, James F MD [Hem] - **Spec Exp:** Bleeding/Coagulation Disorders; Leukemia; Lymphoma; **Hospital:** Presby Hosp of Dallas; **Address:** Texas Oncology at Presbyterian, 8220 Walnut Hill Ln Bldg 2 - Ste 700, Dallas, TX 75231; **Phone:** 214-739-4175; **Board Cert:** Internal Medicine 1976; Hematology 1978; Medical Oncology 1981; **Med School:** NYU Sch Med 1972; **Resid:** Internal Medicine, Baylor Univ Medical Ctr 1976; **Fellow:** Hematology, Univ Texas SW Medical Ctr 1977

Hematology

Yeager, Andrew M MD [Hem] - **Spec Exp:** Bone Marrow & Stem Cell Transplant; Graft vs Host Disease; Leukemia; **Hospital:** Univ Med Ctr - Tucson; **Address:** Arizona Cancer Ctr, 1515 N Campbell Ave, Ste 2956, Tucson, AZ 85724-0001; **Phone:** 520-626-0662; **Board Cert:** Pediatrics 1979; Pediatric Hematology-Oncology 1980; **Med School:** Johns Hopkins Univ 1975; **Resid:** Pediatrics, Johns Hopkins Hosp 1978; Pediatrics, Johns Hopkins Hosp 1982; **Fellow:** Pediatric Hematology-Oncology, Johns Hopkins Hosp 1980; **Fac Appt:** Prof Med, Univ Ariz Coll Med

West Coast and Pacific

Damon, Lloyd E MD [Hem] - **Spec Exp:** Leukemia; Lymphoma; Stem Cell Transplant; **Hospital:** UCSF Med Ctr; **Address:** UCSF Comprehensive Cancer Ctr, 400 Parnassus Ave, Ste A502, San Francisco, CA 94143; **Phone:** 415-353-2421; **Board Cert:** Internal Medicine 1985; Medical Oncology 1987; Hematology 1988; **Med School:** Univ Mich Med Sch 1982; **Resid:** Internal Medicine, UCSF Med Ctr 1985; **Fellow:** Hematology & Oncology, UCSF Med Ctr 1988; **Fac Appt:** Prof Med, UCSF

Forman, Stephen J MD [Hem] - **Spec Exp:** Lymphoma; Leukemia; Bone Marrow Transplant; **Hospital:** City of Hope Natl Med Ctr & Beckman Rsch; **Address:** City Hope National Medical Ctr, 1500 E Duarte Rd, rm 3002, Duarte, CA 91010-3012; **Phone:** 626-256-4673 x62403; **Board Cert:** Internal Medicine 1977; **Med School:** USC Sch Med 1974; **Resid:** Internal Medicine, LAC-Harbor-UCLA Med Ctr 1976; **Fellow:** Hematology, LAC-USC Med Ctr 1978; Hematology, City of Hope Med Ctr 1979; **Fac Appt:** Clin Prof Med, USC Sch Med

Heinrich, Michael C MD [Hem] - **Spec Exp:** Hematologic Malignancies; Sarcoma; Gastrointestinal Stromal Tumors; **Hospital:** VA Medical Center - Portland, OR Hlth & Sci Univ; **Address:** 3710 SW US Veteran's Hospital Rd, Portland, OR 97239; **Phone:** 503-220-8262 x51169; **Board Cert:** Internal Medicine 1987; Hematology 2000; Medical Oncology 2001; **Med School:** Johns Hopkins Univ 1984; **Resid:** Internal Medicine, Oreg Hlth Scis Univ 1988; **Fellow:** Hematology & Oncology, Oreg Hlth Scis Univ 1991; **Fac Appt:** Prof Med, Oregon Hlth & Sci Univ

Kipps, Thomas J MD/PhD [Hem] - **Spec Exp:** Leukemia; Lymphoma, Non-Hodgkin's; **Hospital:** UCSD Med Ctr; **Address:** Moores UCSD Cancer Ctr, 3855 Health Sciences Drive, La Jolla, CA 92093; **Phone:** 858-822-5635; **Board Cert:** Internal Medicine 1982; Hematology 1984; **Med School:** Harvard Med Sch 1979; **Resid:** Internal Medicine, Stanford Univ Med Ctr 1981; **Fellow:** Hematology & Oncology, Stanford Univ Med Ctr 1984; **Fac Appt:** Prof Med, UCSD

Leung, Lawrence L MD [Hem] - **Spec Exp:** Thrombotic Disorders; **Hospital:** Stanford Univ Med Ctr, VA Hlth Care Sys - Palo Alto; **Address:** Stanford Univ Med Ctr, Hematology Div, 269 Campus Drive CCSR Bldg - rm 1155, Stanford, CA 94305-5156; **Phone:** 650-723-9729; **Board Cert:** Internal Medicine 1978; Hematology 1980; Medical Oncology 1981; **Med School:** Columbia P&S 1975; **Resid:** Internal Medicine, NY Hosp/Cornell Med Ctr 1978; **Fellow:** Hematology & Oncology, NY Hosp/Cornell Med Ctr 1981; **Fac Appt:** Prof Med, Stanford Univ

Levine, Alexandra M MD [Hem] - **Spec Exp:** Lymphoma; AIDS Related Cancers; AIDS/HIV; **Hospital:** City of Hope Natl Med Ctr & Beckman Rsch; **Address:** 1500 E Duarte Rd, Needleman 213, Duarte, CA 91010; **Phone:** 626-471-7213; **Med School:** USC Sch Med 1971; **Resid:** Internal Medicine, LAC-USC Med Ctr 1974; **Fellow:** Hematology & Oncology, Grady Meml Hosp-Emory Univ 1975; Hematology, LAC-USC Med Ctr 1978; **Fac Appt:** Prof Med, USC Sch Med

Lill, Michael MD [Hem] - **Spec Exp:** Lymphoma; Stem Cell Transplant; Hematologic Malignancies; **Hospital:** Cedars-Sinai Med Ctr; **Address:** Cedars-Sinai Med Ctr-Outpt Cancer Ctr, 8700 Beverly Blvd, Ste AC 1070, Los Angeles, CA 90048; **Phone:** 310-423-1160; **Med School:** Australia 1982; **Resid:** Internal Medicine, Sir Charles Gairdner Hospital 1985; **Fellow:** Hematology, Royal Perth Hospital 1988; **Fac Appt:** Prof Med, UCLA

Linenberger, Michael MD [Hem] - **Spec Exp:** Bone Marrow Transplant; Leukemia & Lymphoma; Multiple Myeloma; **Hospital:** Univ Wash Med Ctr; **Address:** 825 Eastlake Ave E, MS G6-800, Seattle, WA 98109; **Phone:** 206-288-1260; **Board Cert:** Internal Medicine 1985; Hematology 1988; **Med School:** Univ Kans 1982; **Resid:** Internal Medicine, Rhode Island Hosp 1985; **Fellow:** Hematology, Univ Wash Med Ctr 1989; **Fac Appt:** Assoc Prof Med, Univ Wash

Linker, Charles A MD [Hem] - **Spec Exp:** Leukemia; Bone Marrow Transplant; Multiple Myeloma; **Hospital:** UCSF Med Ctr, St Francis Memorial Hosp; **Address:** 400 Parnassus Ave, Ste A502, San Francisco, CA 94143; **Phone:** 415-353-2421; **Board Cert:** Internal Medicine 1978; Hematology 1980; Medical Oncology 1981; **Med School:** Stanford Univ 1974; **Resid:** Internal Medicine, Stanford Univ Hosp 1978; **Fellow:** Hematology & Oncology, UCSF Med Ctr 1981; **Fac Appt:** Clin Prof Med, UCSF

Maziarz, Richard MD [Hem] - **Spec Exp:** Leukemia; Immunotherapy; Bone Marrow Transplant; Lymphoma; **Hospital:** OR Hlth & Sci Univ; **Address:** OHSU Ctr Hematologic Malignancies, 3181 SW Sam Jackson Park Rd, UHN 73C, Portland, OR 97239; **Phone:** 503-494-4601; **Board Cert:** Internal Medicine 1982; Hematology 1988; Medical Oncology 1989; **Med School:** Harvard Med Sch 1979; **Resid:** Internal Medicine, Univ Hosp 1982; **Fellow:** Hematology & Oncology, Brigham & Womens Hosp 1988; **Fac Appt:** Prof Med, Oregon Hlth & Sci Univ

Mitchell, Beverly S MD [Hem] - **Spec Exp:** Hematologic Malignancies; Leukemia; Lymphoma; **Hospital:** Stanford Univ Med Ctr; **Address:** Stanford Cancer Center, 800 Welch Rd, Ste 280, MC 5-5796, Stanford, CA 94305-5402; **Phone:** 650-736-7716; **Board Cert:** Internal Medicine 1973; Hematology 1978; **Med School:** Harvard Med Sch 1969; **Resid:** Internal Medicine, Univ Washington Med Ctr 1972; **Fellow:** Metabolism, Univ Zurich 1975; Hematology & Oncology, Univ Michigan 1977; **Fac Appt:** Prof Med, Stanford Univ

Nademanee, Auayporn P MD [Hem] - **Spec Exp:** Lymphoma; Hematologic Malignancies; Clinical Trials; **Hospital:** City of Hope Natl Med Ctr & Beckman Rsch; **Address:** City of Hope Med Ctr-Dept Hematology, 1500 Duarte Rd, Duarte, CA 91010; **Phone:** 626-256-4673 x62691; **Board Cert:** Hematology 1982; Medical Oncology 1983; Internal Medicine 1978; **Med School:** Thailand 1973; **Resid:** Internal Medicine, Touro Infirm-Tulane Univ 1978; **Fellow:** Hematology & Oncology, Sepulveda VA Hosp 1980; Hematology & Oncology, USC Med Ctr 1981; **Fac Appt:** Prof Med, UCLA

Negrin, Robert S MD [Hem] - **Spec Exp:** Bone Marrow Transplant; **Hospital:** Stanford Univ Med Ctr; **Address:** BMT Program, 300 Pasteur Drive, rm H3249, MC 5623, Stanford, CA 94305; **Phone:** 650-723-0822; **Board Cert:** Internal Medicine 1987; Hematology 2007; **Med School:** Harvard Med Sch 1984; **Resid:** Internal Medicine, Stanford Univ Hosp 1987; **Fellow:** Hematology, Stanford Univ Hosp 1990; **Fac Appt:** Prof Med, Stanford Univ

O'Donnell, Margaret R MD [Hem] - **Spec Exp:** Leukemia; Clinical Trials; **Hospital:** City of Hope Natl Med Ctr & Beckman Rsch; **Address:** City of Hope National Med Ctr, 1500 E Duarte Rd, MOB-rm 3001, Duarte, CA 91010; **Phone:** 626-359-8111 x62405; **Board Cert:** Internal Medicine 1978; Hematology 1980; Medical Oncology 1979; **Med School:** Med Coll PA 1974; **Resid:** Internal Medicine, Montreal Genl Hosp 1976; Hematology, Royal Victoria Hosp-Montreal 1977; **Fellow:** Hematology & Oncology, Fred Hutchinson Cancer Ctr 1979

Saven, Alan MD [Hem] - **Spec Exp:** Leukemia; Lymphoma; **Hospital:** Scripps Green Hosp; **Address:** Scripps Green Hosp, 10666 N Torrey Pines Rd, MS 312, La Jolla, CA 92037; **Phone:** 858-554-9489; **Board Cert:** Internal Medicine 1987; Medical Oncology 1989; **Med School:** South Africa 1982; **Resid:** Internal Medicine, Albert Einstein Med Ctr 1986; **Fellow:** Hematology & Oncology, Scripps Clinic 1987

Hematology

Schiller, Gary J MD [Hem] - **Spec Exp:** Leukemia; **Hospital:** UCLA Ronald Reagan Med Ctr; **Address:** 10833 Le Conte Ave, rm 42-121 CHS, Los Angeles, CA 90095; **Phone:** 310-825-5513; **Board Cert:** Internal Medicine 1987; Medical Oncology 1989; Hematology 2000; **Med School:** USC Sch Med 1984; **Resid:** Internal Medicine, UCLA Med Ctr 1987; **Fellow:** Hematology & Oncology, UCLA Med Ctr 1990; **Fac Appt:** Prof Med, UCLA

Snyder, David S MD [Hem] - **Spec Exp:** Leukemia; Bone Marrow Transplant; **Hospital:** City of Hope Natl Med Ctr & Beckman Rsch; **Address:** 1500 E Duarte Rd, rm 003, Duarte, CA 91010-3012; **Phone:** 626-256-4673; **Board Cert:** Internal Medicine 1980; Hematology 1984; **Med School:** Harvard Med Sch 1977; **Resid:** Internal Medicine, Beth Israel Hosp 1980; **Fellow:** Immunology, Harvard Med Sch 1982; Hematology & Oncology, New England Med Ctr 1984

MEDICAL ONCOLOGY

New England

Antin, Joseph H MD [Onc] - **Spec Exp:** Bone Marrow Transplant; Stem Cell Transplant; Leukemia; **Hospital:** Brigham & Women's Hosp, Dana-Farber Cancer Inst; **Address:** 44 Binney St, rm D1B20, Boston, MA 02115-6013; **Phone:** 617-632-3667; **Board Cert:** Internal Medicine 1981; Medical Oncology 1983; Hematology 1984; **Med School:** Cornell Univ-Weill Med Coll 1978; **Resid:** Internal Medicine, Peter Bent Brigham Hosp 1981; **Fellow:** Hematology & Oncology, Brigham & Womens Hosp/Dana Farber 1984; **Fac Appt:** Prof Med, Harvard Med Sch

Atkins, Michael B MD [Onc] - **Spec Exp:** Melanoma; Kidney Cancer; Immunotherapy; **Hospital:** Beth Israel Deaconess Med Ctr - Boston; **Address:** Beth Israel Deaconess Med Ctr, Cancer Clinical Trials 375 Longwood Ave, Masco Bldg Fl 4 - Ste 412, Boston, MA 02215; **Phone:** 617-632-9250; **Board Cert:** Internal Medicine 1983; Medical Oncology 1987; **Med School:** Tufts Univ 1980; **Resid:** Internal Medicine, New England Med Ctr 1983; **Fellow:** Hematology & Oncology, New England Med Ctr 1987; **Fac Appt:** Prof Med, Harvard Med Sch

Bubley, Glenn J MD [Onc] - **Spec Exp:** Prostate Cancer; **Hospital:** Beth Israel Deaconess Med Ctr - Boston; **Address:** Beth Israel Deaconess Med Ctr, 330 Brookline Ave, Shapiro Bldg Fl 9, Boston, MA 02215; **Phone:** 617-735-2062; **Board Cert:** Internal Medicine 1980; Medical Oncology 1983; **Med School:** Mich State Univ 1977; **Resid:** Internal Medicine, St Francis Hosp 1980; **Fellow:** Hematology & Oncology, Beth Israel Deaconess Med Ctr 1983; **Fac Appt:** Assoc Prof Med, Harvard Med Sch

Burstein, Harold J MD [Onc] - **Spec Exp:** Breast Cancer; **Hospital:** Dana-Farber Cancer Inst, Brigham & Women's Hosp; **Address:** Dana Farber Cancer Inst, 44 Binney St, Ste Mayer 2, Boston, MA 02115; **Phone:** 617-632-4587; **Board Cert:** Medical Oncology 2000; **Med School:** Harvard Med Sch 1994; **Resid:** Internal Medicine, Mass Genl Hosp 1996; **Fellow:** Medical Oncology, Dana Farber Cancer Inst 1999; **Fac Appt:** Asst Prof Med, Harvard Med Sch

Canellos, George P MD [Onc] - **Spec Exp:** Lymphoma; Leukemia; Breast Cancer; **Hospital:** Dana-Farber Cancer Inst, Brigham & Women's Hosp; **Address:** 44 Binney St, Boston, MA 02115; **Phone:** 617-632-3470; **Board Cert:** Internal Medicine 1967; Hematology 1972; Medical Oncology 1973; **Med School:** Columbia P&S 1960; **Resid:** Internal Medicine, Mass Genl Hosp 1963; Internal Medicine, Mass Genl Hosp 1966; **Fellow:** Medical Oncology, Natl Cancer Inst 1965; Hematology, Hammersmith Hosp 1967; **Fac Appt:** Prof Med, Harvard Med Sch

America's Top Doctors® 9th Edition

Cannistra, Stephen A MD [Onc] - **Spec Exp:** Gynecologic Cancer; **Hospital:** Beth Israel Deaconess Med Ctr - Boston, Dana-Farber Cancer Inst; **Address:** Beth Israel Deaconess Med Ctr, 330 Brookline Ave, KS 158, Boston, MA 02215; **Phone:** 617-667-1909; **Board Cert:** Internal Medicine 1982; Medical Oncology 1985; **Med School:** Brown Univ 1979; **Resid:** Internal Medicine, Johns Hopkins Hosp 1982; **Fellow:** Medical Oncology, Dana-Farber Cancer Inst 1985; **Fac Appt:** Prof Med, Harvard Med Sch

Chabner, Bruce A MD [Onc] - **Spec Exp:** Colon & Rectal Cancer; Breast Cancer; **Hospital:** Mass Genl Hosp; **Address:** Mass General Hospital, 55 Fruit St, Lawrence House 214, Boston, MA 02114; **Phone:** 617-724-3200; **Board Cert:** Internal Medicine 1971; Medical Oncology 1973; **Med School:** Harvard Med Sch 1965; **Resid:** Internal Medicine, Peter Bent Brigham Hosp 1967; Internal Medicine, Yale-New Haven Hosp 1970; **Fellow:** Medical Oncology, Natl Inst Hlth 1969; **Fac Appt:** Prof Med, Harvard Med Sch

Chu, Edward MD [Onc] - **Spec Exp:** Colon & Rectal Cancer; Gastrointestinal Cancer; Clinical Trials; **Hospital:** Yale-New Haven Hosp, VA Conn Hlthcre Sys; **Address:** Yale Cancer Ctr, 333 Cedar St, Room WWW221, New Haven, CT 06520-8032; **Phone:** 203-785-6879; **Board Cert:** Internal Medicine 1986; Medical Oncology 1989; **Med School:** Brown Univ 1983; **Resid:** Internal Medicine, Roger Williams Hosp 1987; **Fellow:** Hematology & Oncology, Natl Cancer Inst 1990; Internal Medicine, Natl Cancer Inst 1992; **Fac Appt:** Prof Med, Yale Univ

Come, Steven E MD [Onc] - **Spec Exp:** Breast Cancer; Hodgkin's Disease; **Hospital:** Beth Israel Deaconess Med Ctr - Boston, Dana-Farber Cancer Inst; **Address:** Beth Israel Deaconess Hosp, 330 Brookline Ave, Ste CC913, Boston, MA 02215-5400; **Phone:** 617-667-4599; **Board Cert:** Internal Medicine 1975; Medical Oncology 1979; **Med School:** Harvard Med Sch 1972; **Resid:** Internal Medicine, Beth Israel Hosp 1977; **Fellow:** Medical Oncology, Natl Cancer Inst 1976; **Fac Appt:** Assoc Prof Med, Harvard Med Sch

Demetri, George D MD [Onc] - **Spec Exp:** Sarcoma; Bone Tumors; **Hospital:** Dana-Farber Cancer Inst; **Address:** Dana Farber Cancer Inst, 44 Binney St, D1212, Boston, MA 02115; **Phone:** 617-632-3985; **Board Cert:** Internal Medicine 1986; Medical Oncology 1989; **Med School:** Stanford Univ 1983; **Resid:** Internal Medicine, Univ Wash Med Ctr 1986; **Fellow:** Medical Oncology, Dana Farber Cancer Inst 1989; **Fac Appt:** Assoc Prof Med, Harvard Med Sch

DeVita Jr, Vincent T MD [Onc] - **Spec Exp:** Lymphoma Consultation; Hodgkin's Disease Consultation; **Hospital:** Yale-New Haven Hosp; **Address:** Yale Cancer Ctr, 333 Cedar St, rm WWW-211B, New Haven, CT 06520-8028; **Phone:** 203-737-1010; **Board Cert:** Internal Medicine 1974; Hematology 1972; Medical Oncology 1973; **Med School:** Geo Wash Univ 1961; **Resid:** Internal Medicine, Geo Wash Hosp 1963; Internal Medicine, Yale-New Haven Hosp 1966; **Fellow:** Medical Oncology, Natl Cancer Inst 1965; **Fac Appt:** Prof Med, Yale Univ

Erban III, John K MD [Onc] - **Spec Exp:** Breast Cancer; Hematologic Malignancies; Stem Cell Transplant; **Hospital:** Mass Genl Hosp; **Address:** Mass Genl Hosp, Yawkey Center, Ste 9A, 55 Fruit St, Boston, MA 02114; **Phone:** 617-726-6500; **Board Cert:** Internal Medicine 1984; Medical Oncology 1989; Hematology 1999; **Med School:** Tufts Univ 1981; **Resid:** Internal Medicine, Hosp Univ Penn 1984; **Fellow:** Hematology & Oncology, New England Med Ctr 1990; **Fac Appt:** Assoc Prof Med, Harvard Med Sch

Foss, Francine M MD [Onc] - **Spec Exp:** Lymphoma, Cutaneous T Cell (CTCL); Stem Cell Transplantation; Graft vs Host Disease; Multiple Myeloma; **Hospital:** Yale-New Haven Hosp; **Address:** Yale Cancer Ctr, 333 Cedar St, Box 208032, New Haven, CT 06520; **Phone:** 203-737-5312; **Board Cert:** Internal Medicine 1985; Medical Oncology 1987; **Med School:** Univ Mass Sch Med 1982; **Resid:** Internal Medicine, Brigham & Womens Hosp 1985; **Fellow:** Medical Oncology, Natl Cancer Inst 1988; **Fac Appt:** Prof Med, Yale Univ

Medical Oncology

Fuchs, Charles S MD [Onc] - **Spec Exp:** Gastrointestinal Cancer; **Hospital:** Dana-Farber Cancer Inst, Brigham & Women's Hosp; **Address:** 44 Binney St, Dana 1220, Boston, MA 02115; **Phone:** 617-632-5840; **Board Cert:** Internal Medicine 1989; Medical Oncology 2002; **Med School:** Harvard Med Sch 1986; **Resid:** Internal Medicine, Brigham & Womens Hosp 1989; **Fellow:** Hematology & Oncology, Dana Farber Cancer Inst 1992; **Fac Appt:** Assoc Prof Med, Harvard Med Sch

Garber, Judy E MD [Onc] - **Spec Exp:** Breast Cancer; **Hospital:** Dana-Farber Cancer Inst, Brigham & Women's Hosp; **Address:** Dana Farber Cancer Inst, 44 Binney St, Smith 210, Boston, MA 02115; **Phone:** 617-632-5770; **Board Cert:** Internal Medicine 1984; Medical Oncology 1987; Hematology 1988; **Med School:** Yale Univ 1981; **Resid:** Internal Medicine, Brigham & Womens Hosp 1984; **Fellow:** Medical Oncology, Dana Farber Cancer Inst 1988; Epidemiology, Dana Farber Cancer Inst 1990; **Fac Appt:** Assoc Prof Med, Harvard Med Sch

Garnick, Marc B MD [Onc] - **Spec Exp:** Prostate Cancer; Urologic Cancer; **Hospital:** Beth Israel Deaconess Med Ctr - Boston; **Address:** Beth Israel Deaconess Medical Ctr, SCC9, 330 Brookline Ave, Boston, MA 02215; **Phone:** 617-735-2062; **Board Cert:** Internal Medicine 1976; Medical Oncology 1979; **Med School:** Univ Pennsylvania 1972; **Resid:** Internal Medicine, Hosp Univ Penn 1974; **Fellow:** Research, Natl Inst Hlth 1976; Medical Oncology, Dana-Farber Cancer Inst 1978; **Fac Appt:** Clin Prof Med, Harvard Med Sch

Grunberg, Steven M MD [Onc] - **Spec Exp:** Lung Cancer; Head & Neck Cancer; **Hospital:** Fletcher Allen Health Care- Med Ctr Campus; **Address:** FAHC Division of Hematology/Oncology, 89 Beaumont Ave, Given Bldg, E214, Burlington, VT 05405; **Phone:** 802-847-8400; **Board Cert:** Internal Medicine 1978; Medical Oncology 1983; **Med School:** Cornell Univ-Weill Med Coll 1975; **Resid:** Internal Medicine, Mofitt Hosp-U Calif 1978; **Fellow:** Medical Oncology, Sidney Farber Cancer Ctr 1981; **Fac Appt:** Prof Med, Univ VT Coll Med

Hammond, Denis B MD [Onc] - **Spec Exp:** Breast Cancer; Prostate Cancer; **Hospital:** Elliot Hosp, Catholic Med Ctr; **Address:** NH Oncology, 200 Technology Drive, Hooksett, NH 03106; **Phone:** 603-622-6484; **Board Cert:** Internal Medicine 1977; Hematology 1978; **Med School:** Tufts Univ 1973; **Resid:** Internal Medicine, SUNY Buffalo Affil Hosps 1976; **Fellow:** Hematology, Mass Genl Hosp 1977; Medical Oncology, Dartmouth Med Sch 1978

Johnson, Bruce E MD [Onc] - **Spec Exp:** Lung Cancer; Thoracic Cancers; Merkel Cell Carcinoma; **Hospital:** Dana-Farber Cancer Inst, Brigham & Women's Hosp; **Address:** Lowe Ctr Thoracic Oncology, 44 Binney St, Ste D-1234, Boston, MA 02115; **Phone:** 617-632-6875; **Board Cert:** Internal Medicine 1982; Medical Oncology 1985; **Med School:** Univ Minn 1979; **Resid:** Internal Medicine, Univ Chicago Hosps 1982; **Fellow:** Medical Oncology, Natl Cancer Inst 1985; **Fac Appt:** Assoc Prof Med, Harvard Med Sch

Kantoff, Philip W MD [Onc] - **Spec Exp:** Genitourinary Cancer; Prostate Cancer; **Hospital:** Dana-Farber Cancer Inst, Brigham & Women's Hosp; **Address:** 44 Binney St Fl 11, Boston, MA 02115; **Phone:** 617-632-1914; **Board Cert:** Internal Medicine 1982; Medical Oncology 1989; **Med School:** Brown Univ 1979; **Resid:** Internal Medicine, NYU/Bellevue Hosp 1983; **Fellow:** Gene Therapy Research, NIH 1986; **Fac Appt:** Prof Med, Harvard Med Sch

Kaufman, Peter A MD [Onc] - **Spec Exp:** Breast Cancer; Clinical Trials; **Hospital:** Dartmouth - Hitchcock Med Ctr; **Address:** Dept Hematology-Oncology, One Medical Center Drive, Lebanon, NH 03756; **Phone:** 603-653-6181; **Board Cert:** Internal Medicine 1986; Medical Oncology 1989; **Med School:** NYU Sch Med 1983; **Resid:** Internal Medicine, Duke Univ Med Ctr 1986; **Fellow:** Hematology & Oncology, Duke Univ Med Ctr 1989; **Fac Appt:** Assoc Prof Med, Dartmouth Med Sch

Kelly, William K DO [Onc] - **Spec Exp:** Prostate Cancer; Genitourinary Cancer; Solid Tumors; **Hospital:** Yale-New Haven Hosp; **Address:** Yale Physicians Bldg - 2nd FL, 800 Howard Ave, New Haven, CT 06510; **Phone:** 203-785-4191; **Board Cert:** Medical Oncology 2003; **Med School:** Philadelphia Coll Osteo Med 1986; **Resid:** Internal Medicine, Montefiore Med Ctr 1990; **Fellow:** Hematology & Oncology, Meml Sloan Kettering Cancer Ctr 1993; **Fac Appt:** Assoc Prof Med, Yale Univ

Lacy, Jill MD [Onc] - **Spec Exp:** Colon & Rectal Cancer; Brain Tumors; Gastrointestinal Cancer; Pancreatic Cancer; **Hospital:** Yale-New Haven Hosp; **Address:** Yale Univ Sch Med-Div Medical Oncology, 333 Cedar St, PO Box 208032, New Haven, CT 06520-8032; **Phone:** 203-785-4191; **Board Cert:** Internal Medicine 1982; Medical Oncology 2005; **Med School:** Yale Univ 1978; **Resid:** Internal Medicine, Yale-New Haven Hosp 1981; **Fellow:** Medical Oncology, Yale-New Haven Hosp 1985; **Fac Appt:** Assoc Prof Med, Yale Univ

Legare, Robert D MD [Onc] - **Spec Exp:** Breast Cancer; Breast Cancer Risk Assessment; **Hospital:** Women & Infants Hosp of RI; **Address:** Women & Infants Hospital, 101 Dudeley St, Providence, RI 02905; **Phone:** 401-453-7520; **Board Cert:** Internal Medicine 2005; Hematology 2006; Medical Oncology 2008; **Med School:** Tufts Univ 1990; **Resid:** Internal Medicine, Yale-New Haven Hosp 1992; **Fellow:** Hematology & Oncology, Brigham & Women's Hosp 1996; **Fac Appt:** Asst Prof Med, Brown Univ

Lynch, Thomas MD [Onc] - **Spec Exp:** Lung Cancer; Thoracic Cancers; **Hospital:** Yale-New Haven Hosp; **Address:** 333 Cedar St, New Haven, CT 06510; **Phone:** 203-785-4371; **Board Cert:** Internal Medicine 1989; Medical Oncology 2003; **Med School:** Yale Univ 1986; **Resid:** Internal Medicine, Mass Genl Hosp 1989; **Fellow:** Medical Oncology, Dana-Farber Cancer Inst 1991; **Fac Appt:** Assoc Prof Med, Yale Univ

Mathew, Paul MD [Onc] - **Spec Exp:** Prostate Cancer; **Hospital:** Tufts Med Ctr; **Address:** 800 Washington St, Box 245, Boston, MA 02111; **Phone:** 617-636-8483; **Board Cert:** Internal Medicine 2000; Medical Oncology 2003; Hematology 2004; **Med School:** Chile 1985; **Resid:** Internal Medicine, Cook Co Hos 1990; **Fellow:** Hematology & Oncology, Mayo Clinic 1994; **Fac Appt:** Assoc Prof Med, Boston Univ

Matulonis, Ursula A MD [Onc] - **Spec Exp:** Gynecologic Cancer; Ovarian Cancer; Breast Cancer; Drug Development; **Hospital:** Dana-Farber Cancer Inst; **Address:** Gynecologic Oncology Program, Dana Farber Cancer Institute, 44 Binney St, Ste Dana 1210, Boston, MA 02115; **Phone:** 617-632-2334; **Board Cert:** Internal Medicine 2000; Medical Oncology 2000; **Med School:** Albany Med Coll 1987; **Resid:** Internal Medicine, Univ Pittsburgh Hosp 1990; **Fellow:** Medical Oncology, Dana Farber Cancer Inst 1993; **Fac Appt:** Asst Prof Med, Harvard Med Sch

Nadler, Lee M MD [Onc] - **Spec Exp:** Lymphoma; **Hospital:** Dana-Farber Cancer Inst, Brigham & Women's Hosp; **Address:** Dana Farber Cancer Inst, 44 Binney St, SM 339A, Boston, MA 02115; **Phone:** 617-632-3331; **Board Cert:** Internal Medicine 1976; **Med School:** Harvard Med Sch 1973; **Resid:** Internal Medicine, Columbia-Presby Hosp 1975; **Fellow:** Medical Oncology, Natl Cancer Inst 1977; Medical Oncology, Dana-Farber Cancer Inst 1978; **Fac Appt:** Prof Med, Harvard Med Sch

Posner, Marshall R MD [Onc] - **Spec Exp:** Head & Neck Cancer; Skin Cancer-Head & Neck; **Hospital:** Dana-Farber Cancer Inst, Beth Israel Deaconess Med Ctr - Boston; **Address:** Dana-Farber Cancer Inst, Head & Neck Cancer Ctr, 44 Binney St, rm G430, Boston, MA 02115; **Phone:** 617-632-3090; **Board Cert:** Internal Medicine 1978; Medical Oncology 1981; **Med School:** Tufts Univ 1975; **Resid:** Internal Medicine, Boston City Hosp 1978; **Fellow:** Oncology, Dana-Farber Cancer Inst 1981; **Fac Appt:** Assoc Prof Med, Harvard Med Sch

Medical Oncology

Schnipper, Lowell E MD [Onc] - **Spec Exp:** Breast Cancer; Lymphoma; **Hospital:** Beth Israel Deaconess Med Ctr - Boston; **Address:** Beth Israel Deaconess Med Ctr, 330 Brookline Ave, RABB 430, Boston, MA 02215; **Phone:** 617-667-1198; **Board Cert:** Internal Medicine 1973; Medical Oncology 1983; **Med School:** SUNY Downstate 1968; **Resid:** Internal Medicine, Yale-New Haven Hosp 1970; Medical Oncology, Natl Cancer Inst 1973; **Fellow:** Hematology & Oncology, Barnes Jewish Hosp 1974; **Fac Appt:** Prof Med, Harvard Med Sch

Shulman, Lawrence N MD [Onc] - **Spec Exp:** Breast Cancer; **Hospital:** Dana-Farber Cancer Inst; **Address:** Dana-Farber Cancer Inst, 44 Binney St, rm Dana-1608, Boston, MA 02115; **Phone:** 617-632-2277; **Board Cert:** Internal Medicine 1978; Medical Oncology 1981; Hematology 1982; **Med School:** Harvard Med Sch 1975; **Resid:** Internal Medicine, Beth Israel Hosp 1977; **Fellow:** Hematology & Oncology, Beth Israel Hosp 1980; **Fac Appt:** Assoc Prof Med, Harvard Med Sch

Smith, Matthew R MD/PhD [Onc] - **Spec Exp:** Prostate Cancer; **Hospital:** Mass Genl Hosp; **Address:** Mass Genl Hosp, Hematology/Oncology, 55 Fruit St, Yawkey 7E, Boston, MA 02114; **Phone:** 617-724-5257; **Board Cert:** Medical Oncology 1997; **Med School:** Duke Univ 1992; **Resid:** Internal Medicine, Brigham & Women's Hosp 1994; **Fellow:** Medical Oncology, Dana Farber Cancer Inst 1997; **Fac Appt:** Assoc Prof Med, Harvard Med Sch

Soiffer, Robert J MD [Onc] - **Spec Exp:** Stem Cell Transplant; Bone Marrow Transplant; Leukemia; Lymphoma; **Hospital:** Dana-Farber Cancer Inst, Brigham & Women's Hosp; **Address:** Dana-Farber Cancer Inst, 44 Binney St, Dana 1B11, Boston, MA 02115; **Phone:** 617-632-4731; **Board Cert:** Internal Medicine 1986; Medical Oncology 1989; **Med School:** NYU Sch Med 1983; **Resid:** Internal Medicine, Brigham & Women's Hosp 1986; **Fellow:** Medical Oncology, Brigham & Women's Hosp 1989; **Fac Appt:** Clin Prof Med, Harvard Med Sch

Strauss, Gary M MD [Onc] - **Spec Exp:** Melanoma; **Hospital:** Tufts Med Ctr; **Address:** Tufts Medical Ctr, 800 Washington St, Box 245, Boston, MA 02111; **Phone:** 617-636-5627; **Board Cert:** Internal Medicine 1975; Medical Oncology 1979; Hematology 1980; **Med School:** Yale Univ 1972; **Resid:** Internal Medicine, Boston City Hosp 1976; **Fellow:** Medical Oncology, Natl Cancer Inst 1976; Hematology & Oncology, Mass General Hosp 1979

Taplin, Mary-Ellen MD [Onc] - **Spec Exp:** Prostate Cancer; Genitourinary Cancer; **Hospital:** Dana-Farber Cancer Inst, Brigham & Women's Hosp; **Address:** Dana Farber Cancer Inst, 44 Binney St, rm D1230, Boston, MA 02115; **Phone:** 617-632-3237; **Board Cert:** Internal Medicine 1989; Hematology 2006; Medical Oncology 2003; **Med School:** Univ Mass Sch Med 1986; **Resid:** Internal Medicine, Univ Mass Med Ctr 1990; **Fellow:** Hematology & Oncology, Beth Israel Deaconess Hosp 1993; **Fac Appt:** Assoc Prof Med

Treon, Steven P MD/PhD [Onc] - **Spec Exp:** Waldenstrom's Macroglobulinemia; Multiple Myeloma; **Hospital:** Dana-Farber Cancer Inst; **Address:** Dana-Farber Cancer Inst, 44 Binney St, Ste Dana 1B, Boston, MA 02115; **Phone:** 617-632-2681; **Med School:** Boston Univ 1993; **Resid:** Internal Medicine, Boston Univ Med Ctr 1995; **Fellow:** Hematology & Oncology, Mass Genl Hosp 1996; Research, Dana Farber Cancer Inst 1997; **Fac Appt:** Assoc Prof Med, Harvard Med Sch

Weisberg, Tracey MD [Onc] - **Spec Exp:** Breast Cancer; **Hospital:** Maine Med Ctr; **Address:** 100 Campus Drive, Unit 108, Scarborough, ME 04074; **Phone:** 207-885-7600; **Board Cert:** Internal Medicine 1987; Medical Oncology 1989; **Med School:** SUNY Stony Brook 1983; **Resid:** Internal Medicine, Mount Sinai Hosp 1985; Internal Medicine, Hartford Hosp 1986; **Fellow:** Medical Oncology, Yale Univ Hosp 1988

Winer, Eric P MD [Onc] - **Spec Exp:** Breast Cancer; **Hospital:** Dana-Farber Cancer Inst, Brigham & Women's Hosp; **Address:** Dana Farber Cancer Inst, 44 Binney St Fl 9th, Boston, MA 02115; **Phone:** 617-582-7933; **Board Cert:** Internal Medicine 1987; Medical Oncology 1989; **Med School:** Yale Univ 1983; **Resid:** Internal Medicine, Yale-New Haven Hosp 1987; **Fellow:** Hematology & Oncology, Duke Univ 1989; **Fac Appt:** Assoc Prof Med, Harvard Med Sch

Mid Atlantic

Adler, Kenneth R MD [Onc] - **Spec Exp:** Breast Cancer; Myeloproliferative Disorders; Lymphoma; **Hospital:** Morristown Mem Hosp; **Address:** 100 Madison Ave Fl 2, Box 1089, Morristown, NJ 07962; **Phone:** 973-538-5210; **Board Cert:** Internal Medicine 1976; Hematology 1978; **Med School:** Albany Med Coll 1973; **Resid:** Internal Medicine, Albany Med Ctr 1976; **Fellow:** Hematology & Oncology, Albany Med Ctr 1978; **Fac Appt:** Asst Clin Prof Med, UMDNJ-NJ Med Sch, Newark

Ahlgren, James D MD [Onc] - **Spec Exp:** Gastrointestinal Cancer; **Hospital:** G Washington Univ Hosp; **Address:** Geo Wash Univ Med Ctr, Div Hem/Oncology, 2150 Pennsylvania Ave NW, Ste 3-428, Washington, DC 20037-3201; **Phone:** 202-741-2478; **Board Cert:** Internal Medicine 1980; Medical Oncology 1989; **Med School:** Georgetown Univ 1977; **Resid:** Internal Medicine, Georgetown Univ Hosp 1979; **Fellow:** Medical Oncology, Georgetown Univ Hosp 1981; **Fac Appt:** Prof Med, Geo Wash Univ

Aisner, Joseph MD [Onc] - **Spec Exp:** Lung Cancer; Solid Tumors; **Hospital:** Robert Wood Johnson Univ Hosp - New Brunswick; **Address:** Cancer Inst of New Jersey, 195 Little Albany St, rm 2006, New Brunswick, NJ 08903-2681; **Phone:** 732-235-6777; **Board Cert:** Internal Medicine 1973; Medical Oncology 1975; **Med School:** Wayne State Univ 1970; **Resid:** Internal Medicine, Georgetown Univ Hosp 1972; **Fellow:** Medical Oncology, Natl Cancer Inst 1975

Algazy, Kenneth M MD [Onc] - **Spec Exp:** Lung Cancer; Mesothelioma; Hematologic Malignancies; **Hospital:** Hosp Univ Penn - UPHS (page 60), VA Med Ctr; **Address:** Hosp Univ Pennsylvania, 3400 Spruce St, 12 Penn Tower, Philadelphia, PA 19104; **Phone:** 215-614-1858; **Board Cert:** Internal Medicine 1972; Hematology 1974; Medical Oncology 1979; **Med School:** Temple Univ 1969; **Resid:** Internal Medicine, Univ Rochester-Strong Meml Hosp 1972; **Fellow:** Hematology & Oncology, Johns Hopkins Med Ctr 1974; **Fac Appt:** Clin Prof Med, Univ Pennsylvania

Ambinder, Richard F MD/PhD [Onc] - **Spec Exp:** Lymphoma; Hodgkin's Disease; AIDS Related Cancers; **Hospital:** Johns Hopkins Hosp (page 61); **Address:** Cancer Research Bldg, 1650 Orleans St, rm CRB 389, Baltimore, MD 21231; **Phone:** 410-955-8964; **Board Cert:** Internal Medicine 1982; Medical Oncology 1985; **Med School:** Johns Hopkins Univ 1979; **Resid:** Internal Medicine, Johns Hopkins Hosp 1981; **Fellow:** Internal Medicine, Johns Hopkins Hosp 1982; Medical Oncology, Johns Hopkins Hosp 1985; **Fac Appt:** Prof Med, Johns Hopkins Univ

Argiris, Athanassios MD [Onc] - **Spec Exp:** Lung Cancer; Head & Neck Cancer; Clinical Trials; **Hospital:** UPMC Presby, Pittsburgh, UPMC Shadyside; **Address:** UPMC Presbyterian Cancer Ctr, 5115 Centre Ave Fl 2, Pittsburgh, PA 15232; **Phone:** 412-692-4724; **Board Cert:** Internal Medicine 1997; Medical Oncology 2000; **Med School:** Greece 1990; **Resid:** Internal Medicine, Beth Israel Med Ctr 1997; **Fellow:** Medical Oncology, Yale-New Haven Hosp 2000; **Fac Appt:** Assoc Prof Med, Univ Pittsburgh

Medical Oncology

Arlen, Philip M MD [Onc] - **Spec Exp:** Prostate Cancer-Vaccine Therapy; Vaccine Therapy-Clinical Trials Only; Clinical Trials Only; **Hospital:** Natl Inst of Hlth - Clin Ctr, Natl Naval Med Ctr; **Address:** National Cancer Inst, MSC 1750, 10 Center Drive Bldg 10 - rm 5B52, Bethesda, MD 20892-1750; **Phone:** 301-496-0629; **Board Cert:** Medical Oncology 1998; **Med School:** Med Coll GA 1991; **Resid:** Internal Medicine, Georgia Baptist Hlth Care Syst 1994; **Fellow:** Hematology & Oncology, Emory Univ Med Ctr 1994; NCI/NIH 1999

Attas, Lewis MD [Onc] - **Spec Exp:** Breast Cancer; Lymphoma; Bleeding/Coagulation Disorders; **Hospital:** Englewood Hosp & Med Ctr, Holy Name Hosp; **Address:** 25 Rockwood Pl Fl 1, Englewood, NJ 07631-4957; **Phone:** 201-568-5250; **Board Cert:** Internal Medicine 1985; Medical Oncology 1987; Hematology 1988; **Med School:** Mount Sinai Sch Med 1982; **Resid:** Internal Medicine, Montefiore Hosp Med Ctr 1985; **Fellow:** Hematology & Oncology, North Shore Univ Hosp 1988; **Fac Appt:** Assoc Clin Prof Med, Mount Sinai Sch Med

Axelrod, Rita S MD [Onc] - **Spec Exp:** Head & Neck Cancer; Lung Cancer; Complementary Medicine; **Hospital:** Thomas Jefferson Univ Hosp; **Address:** Thomas Jefferson Univ Hosp, 111 S 11th St, Ste 4240, Gibbon Bldg, Philadelphia, PA 19107; **Phone:** 215-955-8874; **Board Cert:** Internal Medicine 1976; Medical Oncology 1977; Hematology 1978; **Med School:** NYU Sch Med 1970; **Resid:** Internal Medicine, Med Coll Georgia Hosps 1973; **Fellow:** Hematology & Oncology, Hosp Univ Penn 1975; **Fac Appt:** Assoc Prof Med, Thomas Jefferson Univ

Bashevkin, Michael MD [Onc] - **Spec Exp:** Solid Tumors; Bleeding/Coagulation Disorders; Hematologic Malignancies; **Hospital:** Maimonides Med Ctr (page 63); **Address:** 1660 E 14st St, Ste 501, Brooklyn, NY 11229; **Phone:** 718-382-8500 x501; **Board Cert:** Internal Medicine 1976; Hematology 1978; Medical Oncology 1979; **Med School:** SUNY Downstate 1973; **Resid:** Internal Medicine, VA Med Ctr 1976; Hematology & Oncology, Maimonides Med Ctr 1979

Belani, Chandra P MD [Onc] - **Spec Exp:** Lung Cancer; Drug Discovery; **Hospital:** Penn State Milton S Hershey Med Ctr; **Address:** Penn State Hershey Cancer Ctr, 500 University Drive, MC H072, Hershey, PA 17033; **Phone:** 717-531-1078; **Board Cert:** Internal Medicine 1986; Medical Oncology 1987; **Med School:** India 1978; **Resid:** Internal Medicine, SMS Med Hosp 1981; Internal Medicine, Good Samaritan/Univ MD Hosps 1984; **Fellow:** Hematology & Oncology, Univ Maryland Hosp 1987; **Fac Appt:** Prof Med, Univ Pittsburgh

Biggs, David D MD [Onc] - **Spec Exp:** Breast Cancer; Kidney Cancer; Melanoma; Skin Cancer; **Hospital:** Christiana Care Hlth Svs; **Address:** Med. Onc. Hem. Consultants, 4701 Ogletown-Stanton Rd, Ste 3400, Newark, DE 19713; **Phone:** 302-366-1200; **Board Cert:** Internal Medicine 1988; Hematology 2002; Medical Oncology 2001; **Med School:** Univ Kans 1984; **Resid:** Internal Medicine, Med Coll Wisconsin 1989; **Fellow:** Hematology & Oncology, Hosp Univ Penn 1991; **Fac Appt:** Asst Clin Prof Med

Bosl, George MD [Onc] - **Spec Exp:** Testicular Cancer; **Hospital:** Meml Sloan-Kettering Cancer Ctr; **Address:** 1275 York Avenue, New York, NY 10065; **Phone:** 800-525-2225; **Board Cert:** Internal Medicine 1976; Medical Oncology 1979; **Med School:** Creighton Univ 1973; **Resid:** Internal Medicine, NY Hosp 1975; Internal Medicine, Meml Sloan-Kettering Cancer Ctr 1977; **Fellow:** Medical Oncology, Univ Minn Hosps 1979; **Fac Appt:** Prof Med, Cornell Univ-Weill Med Coll

Brufsky, Adam M MD/PhD [Onc] - **Spec Exp:** Breast Cancer; **Hospital:** Magee-Womens Hosp - UPMC, UPMC Presby, Pittsburgh; **Address:** Univ Pitt Cancer Inst/Magee-Women's Hosp, 300 Halket St, Ste 4628, Pittsburgh, PA 15213; **Phone:** 412-641-4530; **Board Cert:** Internal Medicine 2004; Medical Oncology 2005; **Med School:** Univ Conn 1990; **Resid:** Internal Medicine, Brigham & Womens Hosp 1992; **Fellow:** Medical Oncology, Dana Farber Cancer Inst 1995; Medical Microbiology, Brigham & Womens Hosp 1995; **Fac Appt:** Asst Prof Med, Univ Pittsburgh

Carabasi, Matthew H MD [Onc] - **Spec Exp:** Bone Marrow Transplant; Stem Cell Transplant; **Hospital:** Thomas Jefferson Univ Hosp; **Address:** Jefferson Univ Hosp, 111 S 11th St, Gibbon Bldg - Ste 4240, Philadelphia, PA 19107; **Phone:** 215-955-8874; **Board Cert:** Internal Medicine 1983; Medical Oncology 1987; **Med School:** Jefferson Med Coll 1980; **Resid:** Internal Medicine, Hahnemann MC Hosp 1984; **Fellow:** Hematology & Oncology, Meml Sloan-Kettering Cancer Ctr 1988; Research, Meml Sloan-Kettering Cancer Ctr 1989; **Fac Appt:** Assoc Prof Med, Jefferson Med Coll

Carducci, Michael A MD [Onc] - **Spec Exp:** Urologic Cancer; Drug Discovery & Development; Vaccine Therapy; Clinical Trials; **Hospital:** Johns Hopkins Hosp (page 61); **Address:** Sidney Kimmel Cancer Ctr, 1650 Orleans St 1M59 BB Bldg, Baltimore, MD 21231; **Phone:** 410-614-3977; **Board Cert:** Internal Medicine 2001; Medical Oncology 2005; **Med School:** Wayne State Univ 1988; **Resid:** Internal Medicine, Univ Colorado Hlth Sci Ctr 1992; **Fellow:** Medical Oncology, Johns Hopkins Hosp 1995; **Fac Appt:** Prof Med, Johns Hopkins Univ

Chachoua, Abraham MD [Onc] - **Spec Exp:** Lung Cancer; **Hospital:** NYU Langone Med Ctr (page 67); **Address:** NYU Clinical Cancer Ctr, 160 E 34th St Fl 8, New York, NY 10016; **Phone:** 212-731-5388; **Med School:** Australia 1978; **Resid:** Internal Medicine, Alfred Hosp 1982; **Fellow:** Hematology & Oncology, Alfred Hosp 1985; Hematology & Oncology, NYU Med Ctr 1988; **Fac Appt:** Asst Prof Med, NYU Sch Med

Chanan-Khan, Asher A MD [Onc] - **Spec Exp:** Multiple Myeloma; Leukemia; **Hospital:** Roswell Park Cancer Inst; **Address:** Roswell Park Cancer Inst, Elm & Carlton Sts, Buffalo, NY 14263; **Phone:** 716-845-3221; **Board Cert:** Medical Oncology 2001; Hematology 2004; **Med School:** Pakistan 1993; **Resid:** Internal Medicine, Harlem Hosp Ctr 1997; **Fellow:** Hematology & Oncology, NYU Med Ctr 1999; **Fac Appt:** Asst Prof Med, SUNY Buffalo

Chapman, Paul B MD [Onc] - **Spec Exp:** Melanoma; Immunotherapy; Vaccine Therapy; **Hospital:** Meml Sloan-Kettering Cancer Ctr; **Address:** 1275 York Avenue, New York, NY 10065; **Phone:** 646-888-2378; **Board Cert:** Internal Medicine 1984; Medical Oncology 1987; **Med School:** Cornell Univ-Weill Med Coll 1981; **Resid:** Internal Medicine, Univ Chicago Hosps 1984; **Fellow:** Medical Oncology, Meml Sloan-Kettering Cancer Ctr 1987; **Fac Appt:** Prof Med, Cornell Univ-Weill Med Coll

Claxton, David F MD [Onc] - **Spec Exp:** Leukemia; Bone Marrow Transplant; Hematologic Malignancies; **Hospital:** Penn State Milton S Hershey Med Ctr; **Address:** MS Hershey Med Ctr, Medical Oncology, 500 University Drive, MC HO46, Hershey, PA 17033; **Phone:** 717-531-8677; **Board Cert:** Internal Medicine 1984; Medical Oncology 2004; **Med School:** McGill Univ 1978; **Resid:** Internal Medicine, Royal Victoria Hosp 1984; **Fellow:** Hematology, Royal Victoria Hosp 1986; Medical Oncology, UTMD Anderson Cancer Ctr 1989; **Fac Appt:** Assoc Prof Med, Penn State Univ-Hershey Med Ctr

Cohen, Philip MD [Onc] - **Spec Exp:** Breast Cancer; **Hospital:** Georgetown Univ Hosp; **Address:** Georgetown Univ Hosp, Lombardi Cancer Ctr, 3800 Reservoir Rd NW, Washington, DC 20007; **Phone:** 202-444-2198; **Board Cert:** Internal Medicine 1973; Medical Oncology 1975; Hematology 1976; **Med School:** Harvard Med Sch 1970; **Resid:** Internal Medicine, Mass Genl Hosp 1972; **Fellow:** Medical Oncology, Natl Cancer Inst 1974; **Fac Appt:** Assoc Prof Med, Geo Wash Univ

Cohen, Roger MD [Onc] - **Spec Exp:** Drug Discovery & Development; Clinical Trials; Thyroid Cancer; Lung Cancer; **Hospital:** Fox Chase Cancer Ctr (page 58); **Address:** Fox Chase Cancer Ctr, 333 Cottman Ave, Ste C307, Philadelphia, PA 19111; **Phone:** 215-728-2570; **Board Cert:** Internal Medicine 1984; Medical Oncology 1993; Hematology 1986; **Med School:** Harvard Med Sch 1980; **Resid:** Internal Medicine, Mt Sinai Hosp 1982; **Fellow:** Research, Sloan Kettering Cancer Inst 1985; Hematology, Mt Sinai Hosp 1986

Medical Oncology

Cohen, Seymour M MD [Onc] - **Spec Exp:** Breast Cancer; Melanoma; Lung Cancer; Merkel Cell Carcinoma; **Hospital:** Mount Sinai Med Ctr (page 64); **Address:** 1150 5th Ave, New York, NY 10128; **Phone:** 212-249-9141; **Board Cert:** Internal Medicine 1971; Medical Oncology 1973; **Med School:** Univ Pittsburgh 1962; **Resid:** Internal Medicine, Montefiore Med Ctr 1964; Internal Medicine, Mount Sinai Med Ctr 1965; **Fellow:** Hematology, Mount Sinai Med Ctr 1966; Hematology & Oncology, LI Jewish Hosp 1969; **Fac Appt:** Assoc Clin Prof Med, Mount Sinai Sch Med

Coleman, Morton MD [Onc] - **Spec Exp:** Leukemia & Lymphoma; Hodgkin's Disease; Multiple Myeloma; Waldenstrom's Macroglobulinemia; **Hospital:** NY-Presby Hosp/Weill Cornell (page 66); **Address:** 407 E 70th St, FL 3, New York, NY 10021-5302; **Phone:** 212-517-5900; **Board Cert:** Internal Medicine 1971; Hematology 1972; Medical Oncology 1973; **Med School:** Med Coll VA 1963; **Resid:** Internal Medicine, Grady Meml Hosp-Emory 1965; Internal Medicine, NY Hosp-Cornell 1968; **Fellow:** Hematology & Oncology, NY Hosp-Cornell 1970; **Fac Appt:** Clin Prof Med, Cornell Univ-Weill Med Coll

Cullen, Kevin MD [Onc] - **Spec Exp:** Head & Neck Cancer; **Hospital:** Univ of MD Med Ctr; **Address:** Univ Md Greenbaum Cancer Ctr, 22 S Greene St, rm N9E22, Baltimore, MD 21201; **Phone:** 410-328-5506; **Board Cert:** Internal Medicine 1986; Medical Oncology 1989; **Med School:** Harvard Med Sch 1983; **Resid:** Internal Medicine, Beth Israel Hosp 1986; Internal Medicine, Hammersmith Hosp 1985; **Fellow:** Medical Oncology, Natl Cancer Inst 1988

Czuczman, Myron S MD [Onc] - **Spec Exp:** Lymphoma; Multiple Myeloma; Leukemia; **Hospital:** Roswell Park Cancer Inst, Buffalo General Hosp; **Address:** Roswell Park Cancer Inst, Elm & Carlton Sts, Buffalo, NY 14263; **Phone:** 716-845-7695; **Board Cert:** Internal Medicine 1988; **Med School:** Penn State Univ-Hershey Med Ctr 1985; **Resid:** Internal Medicine, North Shore Univ Hosp 1988; **Fellow:** Hematology & Oncology, Meml Sloan-Kettering Cancer Ctr 1992; **Fac Appt:** Assoc Prof Med, SUNY Buffalo

Daly, Mary B MD/PhD [Onc] - **Spec Exp:** Breast Cancer; Breast Cancer Risk Assessment; Cancer Prevention; Ovarian Cancer Risk Assessment; **Hospital:** Fox Chase Cancer Ctr (page 58); **Address:** Fox Chase Cancer Ctr, 333 Cottman Ave, P1054, Philadelphia, PA 19111; **Phone:** 215-728-2791; **Board Cert:** Internal Medicine 1981; Medical Oncology 1983; **Med School:** Univ NC Sch Med 1978; **Resid:** Internal Medicine, Univ Texas Hlth Sci Ctr 1981; **Fellow:** Medical Oncology, Univ Texas Hlth Sci Ctr 1983; **Fac Appt:** Clin Prof Med, Temple Univ

Davidson, Nancy E MD [Onc] - **Spec Exp:** Breast Cancer; **Hospital:** UPMC Shadyside, Magee-Womens Hosp - UPMC; **Address:** Univ Pittsburgh Cancer Inst, 5150 Centre Ave, Ste 500, Pittsburgh, PA 15232; **Phone:** 412-623-3205; **Board Cert:** Internal Medicine 1982; Medical Oncology 1985; **Med School:** Harvard Med Sch 1979; **Resid:** Internal Medicine, Johns Hopkins Hosp 1982; **Fellow:** Medical Oncology, Natl Cancer Inst 1986; **Fac Appt:** Prof Med, Univ Pittsburgh

Dawson, Nancy MD [Onc] - **Spec Exp:** Prostate Cancer; Kidney Cancer; Bladder Cancer; **Hospital:** Georgetown Univ Hosp; **Address:** Lombardi Cancer Ctr, Georgetown Univ Hosp, 3800 Reservoir Rd NW, Washington, DC 20007; **Phone:** 202-444-9094; **Board Cert:** Internal Medicine 1982; Hematology 1984; Medical Oncology 1985; **Med School:** Georgetown Univ 1979; **Resid:** Internal Medicine, Walter Reed AMC 1982; **Fellow:** Hematology & Oncology, Walter Reed AMC 1985; **Fac Appt:** Prof Med, Georgetown Univ

Dickler, Maura MD [Onc] - **Spec Exp:** Breast Cancer; **Hospital:** Meml Sloan-Kettering Cancer Ctr; **Address:** 1275 York Avenue, New York, NY 10065; **Phone:** 800-525-2225; **Board Cert:** Medical Oncology 1998; **Med School:** Univ Chicago-Pritzker Sch Med 1991; **Resid:** Internal Medicine, Univ Chicago Hosps 1994; **Fellow:** Medical Oncology, Meml Sloan Kettering Cancer Ctr 1998; **Fac Appt:** Asst Prof Med, Cornell Univ-Weill Med Coll

Donehower, Ross Carl MD [Onc] - **Spec Exp:** Pancreatic Cancer; Colon Cancer; Prostate Cancer; **Hospital:** Johns Hopkins Hosp (page 61); **Address:** Hopkins Kimmel Cancer Ctr, 1650 Orleans St, CRB-I, rm 187, Baltimore, MD 21231-1000; **Phone:** 410-955-8964; **Board Cert:** Internal Medicine 1977; Medical Oncology 1979; **Med School:** Univ Minn 1974; **Resid:** Internal Medicine, Johns Hopkins Hosp 1976; **Fellow:** Medical Oncology, Natl Inst Hlth 1980; **Fac Appt:** Prof Med, Johns Hopkins Univ

Doroshow, James H MD [Onc] - **Spec Exp:** Drug Discovery & Development; Colon Cancer; Breast Cancer; **Hospital:** Natl Inst of Hlth - Clin Ctr; **Address:** National Cancer Institute, Div Cancer Treatment & Diagnosis, 31 Center, Bldg 31-rm 3A44, Bethesda, MD 20892-2440; **Phone:** 301-496-4291; **Board Cert:** Internal Medicine 1976; Medical Oncology 1977; **Med School:** Harvard Med Sch 1973; **Resid:** Internal Medicine, Mass Genl Hosp 1975; **Fellow:** Medical Oncology, Natl Cancer Inst 1978

Edelman, Martin J MD [Onc] - **Spec Exp:** Thoracic Cancers; Lung Cancer; Drug Discovery & Development; **Hospital:** Univ of MD Med Ctr; **Address:** Greenebaum Cancer Ctr-Univ MD, 22 S Greene St, rm N9808, Baltimore, MD 21201; **Phone:** 410-328-2703; **Board Cert:** Internal Medicine 1986; Medical Oncology 1989; **Med School:** Albany Med Coll 1982; **Resid:** Internal Medicine, Naval Hosp 1986; **Fellow:** Hematology & Oncology, Naval Hosp 1990; **Fac Appt:** Prof Med, Univ MD Sch Med

Eisenberger, Mario MD [Onc] - **Spec Exp:** Prostate Cancer; **Hospital:** Johns Hopkins Hosp (page 61); **Address:** 1650 Orleans St, rm 1M51, Baltimore, MD 21231; **Phone:** 410-614-3511; **Board Cert:** Internal Medicine 1976; Medical Oncology 1979; **Med School:** Brazil 1972; **Resid:** Internal Medicine, Michael Reese Hosp 1975; **Fellow:** Hematology, Michael Reese Hosp 1976; Medical Oncology, Jackson Meml Hosp/Univ Miami 1979; **Fac Appt:** Prof Med, Johns Hopkins Univ

Engstrom, Paul F MD [Onc] - **Spec Exp:** Colon & Rectal Cancer; Gastrointestinal Cancer; Neuroendocrine Cancer; Chemoprevention; **Hospital:** Fox Chase Cancer Ctr (page 58); **Address:** Fox Chase Cancer Ctr, Dept Medical Oncology, 333 Cottman Ave, Philadelphia, PA 19111; **Phone:** 215-728-2986; **Board Cert:** Internal Medicine 1969; Medical Oncology 1973; **Med School:** Univ Minn 1962; **Resid:** Internal Medicine, Univ Minn Hosp 1965; **Fac Appt:** Prof Med, Temple Univ

Ettinger, David S MD [Onc] - **Spec Exp:** Lung Cancer; Sarcoma; Clinical Trials; **Hospital:** Johns Hopkins Hosp (page 61); **Address:** Bunting Blaustein Cancer Rsrch Bldg, 1650 Orleans St, rm G88, Baltimore, MD 21231-1000; **Phone:** 410-955-8847; **Board Cert:** Internal Medicine 1976; Medical Oncology 1977; **Med School:** Univ Louisville Sch Med 1967; **Resid:** Internal Medicine, Mayo Grad Schl 1971; **Fellow:** Medical Oncology, Johns Hopkins Hosp 1975; **Fac Appt:** Prof Med, Johns Hopkins Univ

Fanucchi, Michael P MD [Onc] - **Spec Exp:** Sarcoma; Aerodigestive Tract Cancer; Lung Cancer; **Hospital:** St Vincent Cath Med Ctrs - Manhattan; **Address:** 325 W 15th St, New York, NY 10011; **Phone:** 212-604-6011; **Board Cert:** Internal Medicine 1980; Medical Oncology 1985; **Med School:** Columbia P&S 1977; **Resid:** Internal Medicine, Bronx Muni Hosp Ctr 1981; **Fellow:** Medical Oncology, Meml Sloan-Kettering Cancer Ctr 1984; **Fac Appt:** Assoc Prof Med, Emory Univ

Fine, Howard Alan MD [Onc] - **Spec Exp:** Brain Tumors; **Hospital:** Natl Inst of Hlth - Clin Ctr; **Address:** NIH/NCI/NOB, Bloch Building 82, Rm 225 MSC 8202, 9030 Old Georgetown Rd, Bethesda, MD 20892-0001; **Phone:** 301-402-6298; **Board Cert:** Internal Medicine 1987; Medical Oncology 1989; **Med School:** Mount Sinai Sch Med 1984; **Resid:** Internal Medicine, Hosp Univ Penn 1987; **Fellow:** Medical Oncology, Dana Farber Cancer Ctr 1990

Medical Oncology

Fine, Robert MD [Onc] - **Spec Exp:** Pancreatic Cancer; Drug Development; Brain Tumors; Clinical Trials; **Hospital:** NY-Presby Hosp/Columbia (page 66); **Address:** Columbia Univ Comprehensive Cancer Ctr, 650 W 168th St, rm BB 20-05, New York, NY 10032; **Phone:** 212-305-1168; **Board Cert:** Internal Medicine 1983; Medical Oncology 1985; **Med School:** Univ Chicago-Pritzker Sch Med 1979; **Resid:** Internal Medicine, Stanford Univ Med Ctr 1982; **Fellow:** Medical Oncology, National Cancer Inst 1988; **Fac Appt:** Assoc Prof Med, Columbia P&S

Fisher, Richard I MD [Onc] - **Spec Exp:** Lymphoma; Hodgkin's Disease; **Hospital:** Univ of Rochester Strong Meml Hosp; **Address:** James P Wilmot Cancer Ctr, 601 Elmwood Ave, Box 704, Rochester, NY 14642; **Phone:** 585-275-5823; **Board Cert:** Internal Medicine 1973; Medical Oncology 1977; **Med School:** Harvard Med Sch 1970; **Resid:** Internal Medicine, Mass Genl Hosp 1972; **Fac Appt:** Prof Med, Univ Rochester

Flomenberg, Neal MD [Onc] - **Spec Exp:** Bone Marrow Transplant; Stem Cell Transplant; Leukemia & Lymphoma; **Hospital:** Thomas Jefferson Univ Hosp; **Address:** Thomas Jefferson Univ Hosp, 125 S 9th St, Ste 801, Philadelphia, PA 19107; **Phone:** 215-955-0356; **Board Cert:** Internal Medicine 1979; Medical Oncology 1981; Hematology 1982; **Med School:** Jefferson Med Coll 1976; **Resid:** Internal Medicine, Montefiore Med Ctr 1979; **Fellow:** Hematology & Oncology, Meml Sloan Kettering Cancer Ctr 1982; **Fac Appt:** Clin Prof Med, Thomas Jefferson Univ

Forastiere, Arlene A MD [Onc] - **Spec Exp:** Esophageal Cancer; Head & Neck Cancer; **Hospital:** Johns Hopkins Hosp (page 61); **Address:** Bunting Blaustein Cancer Research Bldg, 1650 Orleans St, rm G90, Baltimore, MD 21231; **Phone:** 410-955-8964; **Board Cert:** Internal Medicine 1978; Medical Oncology 1981; **Med School:** NY Med Coll 1975; **Resid:** Internal Medicine, Albert Einstein Med Ctr 1977; Internal Medicine, Univ Conn Health Ctr 1978; **Fellow:** Medical Oncology, Meml Sloan Kettering Cancer Ctr 1980; **Fac Appt:** Prof Med, NY Med Coll

Fox, Kevin R MD [Onc] - **Spec Exp:** Breast Cancer; **Hospital:** Hosp Univ Penn - UPHS (page 60); **Address:** 3400 Spruce St, 14 Penn Tower, Philadelphia, PA 19104; **Phone:** 215-662-7469; **Board Cert:** Internal Medicine 1985; Medical Oncology 1987; **Med School:** Johns Hopkins Univ 1981; **Resid:** Internal Medicine, Johns Hopkins Hosp 1984; **Fellow:** Hematology & Oncology, Hosp Univ Penn 1987; **Fac Appt:** Prof Med, Univ Pennsylvania

Friedberg, Jonathan MD [Onc] - **Spec Exp:** Lymphoma; Hodgkin's Disease; **Hospital:** Univ of Rochester Strong Meml Hosp; **Address:** James P Wilmot Cancer Ctr, 601 Elmwood Ave, Box 704, Rochester, NY 14642-8704; **Phone:** 585-275-4911; **Board Cert:** Internal Medicine 1997; Hematology 2000; Medical Oncology 2000; **Med School:** Harvard Med Sch 1994; **Resid:** Internal Medicine, Mass Genl Hosp 1997; Hematology & Oncology, Dana-Farber/Partners Cancer Ctr 1999; **Fac Appt:** Asst Prof Med, Univ Rochester

Gabrilove, Janice MD [Onc] - **Spec Exp:** Myelodysplastic Syndromes; Leukemia; Hematologic Malignancies; Myeloproliferative Disorders; **Hospital:** Mount Sinai Med Ctr (page 64); **Address:** Mount Sinai Med Ctr, One Gustave L Levy Pl, Box 1079, Dept Hem Onc, New York, NY 10029-6574; **Phone:** 212-241-9650; **Board Cert:** Internal Medicine 1980; Medical Oncology 1983; **Med School:** Mount Sinai Sch Med 1977; **Resid:** Internal Medicine, Columbia-Presby Med Ctr 1980; **Fellow:** Hematology & Oncology, Meml Sloan-Kettering Cancer Ctr 1983; **Fac Appt:** Prof Med, Mount Sinai Sch Med

Gelmann, Edward P MD [Onc] - **Spec Exp:** Prostate Cancer; Testicular Cancer; **Hospital:** NY-Presby Hosp/Columbia (page 66); **Address:** Columbia Univ Med Ctr, Milstein Hosp Bldg 6-435, 177 Fort Washington Ave, New York, NY 10032; **Phone:** 212-305-8602; **Board Cert:** Internal Medicine 1979; Medical Oncology 1981; **Med School:** Stanford Univ 1976; **Resid:** Internal Medicine, Univ Chicago Hosps 1978; **Fellow:** Medical Oncology, National Cancer Inst 1981; **Fac Appt:** Prof Med, Columbia P&S

Geyer Jr, Charles E MD [Onc] - **Spec Exp:** Breast Cancer; **Hospital:** Allegheny General Hosp; **Address:** Allegheny Cancer Ctr, 320 E North Ave Fl 3, Pittsburgh, PA 15212; **Phone:** 412-359-6147; **Board Cert:** Internal Medicine 1983; Medical Oncology 1987; **Med School:** Texas Tech Univ 1980; **Resid:** Internal Medicine, Baylor Affil Hosps 1983; **Fellow:** Medical Oncology, Baylor Affil Hosps 1985

Glick, John H MD [Onc] - **Spec Exp:** Breast Cancer; Hodgkin's Disease; Lymphoma, Non-Hodgkin's; **Hospital:** Hosp Univ Penn - UPHS (page 60); **Address:** Abramson Cancer Ctr of Univ Penn, 3400 Spruce St, 1218 Penn Tower, Philadelphia, PA 19104; **Phone:** 215-662-6065; **Board Cert:** Internal Medicine 1973; Medical Oncology 1975; **Med School:** Columbia P&S 1969; **Resid:** Internal Medicine, Presbyterian Hosp 1971; **Fellow:** Medical Oncology, Natl Cancer Inst 1973; Medical Oncology, Stanford Univ 1974; **Fac Appt:** Prof Med, Univ Pennsylvania

Goldstein, Lori J MD [Onc] - **Spec Exp:** Breast Cancer; **Hospital:** Fox Chase Cancer Ctr (page 58); **Address:** Fox Chase Cancer Ctr, Dept Med Oncology, 333 Cottman Ave, Philadelphia, PA 19111; **Phone:** 215-728-2689; **Board Cert:** Internal Medicine 1985; Medical Oncology 2002; **Med School:** SUNY Upstate Med Univ 1982; **Resid:** Internal Medicine, Presby Univ Hosp 1985; **Fellow:** Medical Oncology, Natl Cancer Inst/NIH 1990

Goy, Andre MD [Onc] - **Spec Exp:** Lymphoma; Hodgkin's Disease; **Hospital:** Hackensack Univ Med Ctr; **Address:** 20 Prospect Ave, Ste 400, Hackensack, NJ 07601; **Phone:** 201-996-5900; **Med School:** France 1988; **Resid:** Internal Medicine, Grenoble Univ Med Ctr 1992; **Fellow:** Hematology & Oncology, Grenoble Univ Med Ctr 1993

Grana, Generosa MD [Onc] - **Spec Exp:** Breast Cancer; Cancer Genetics; Cancer Prevention; **Hospital:** Cooper Univ Hosp, Virtua West Jersey Hosp - Voorhees; **Address:** 900 Centennial Blvd, Ste M, Voorhees, NJ 08043; **Phone:** 856-325-6740; **Board Cert:** Internal Medicine 1988; Medical Oncology 2001; **Med School:** Northwestern Univ 1985; **Resid:** Internal Medicine, Temple Univ Hosp 1988; **Fellow:** Hematology & Oncology, Fox Chase Cancer Ctr 1992; **Fac Appt:** Assoc Prof Med, UMDNJ-RW Johnson Med Sch

Grossbard, Michael L MD [Onc] - **Spec Exp:** Lymphoma; Breast Cancer; Gastrointestinal Cancer; **Hospital:** St Luke's - Roosevelt Hosp Ctr - Roosevelt Div (page 57), Beth Israel Med Ctr - Petrie Division (page 57); **Address:** 1000 10th Ave Fl 11 - Ste C02, New York, NY 10019; **Phone:** 212-523-5419; **Board Cert:** Internal Medicine 1989; Medical Oncology 2001; **Med School:** Yale Univ 1986; **Resid:** Internal Medicine, Mass Genl Hosp 1989; **Fellow:** Medical Oncology, Dana Farber Cancer Inst 1991; **Fac Appt:** Clin Prof Med, Columbia P&S

Grossman, Stuart MD [Onc] - **Spec Exp:** Brain Tumors; Neuro-Oncology; Pain-Cancer; **Hospital:** Johns Hopkins Hosp (page 61); **Address:** Cancer Research Bldg 2, rm 1M16, 1551 Orleans St, Baltimore, MD 21231; **Phone:** 410-955-8837; **Board Cert:** Internal Medicine 1976; Medical Oncology 1983; **Med School:** Univ Rochester 1973; **Resid:** Internal Medicine, Strong Meml Hosp 1976; **Fellow:** Medical Oncology, Johns Hopkins Hosp 1981; **Fac Appt:** Prof Med, Johns Hopkins Univ

Gulley, James L MD/PhD [Onc] - **Spec Exp:** Prostate Cancer-Vaccine Therapy; Vaccine Therapy-Clinical Trials Only; Clinical Trials Only; **Hospital:** Natl Inst of Hlth - Clin Ctr; **Address:** NIH Cancer Research Ctr, MSC 1750, 10 Center Drive Bldg 10 - rm 5B52, Bethesda, MD 20892; **Phone:** 301-435-2956; **Board Cert:** Internal Medicine 1999; Medical Oncology 2000; **Med School:** Loma Linda Univ 1995; **Resid:** Internal Medicine, Emory Univ Med Ctr 1998; **Fellow:** Medical Oncology, Natl Cancer Inst 2000

Medical Oncology

Haas, Naomi S Balzer MD [Onc] - **Spec Exp:** Genitourinary Cancer; Kidney Cancer; Clinical Trials; **Hospital:** Hosp Univ Penn - UPHS (page 60); **Address:** Abramson Cancer Ctr, 12 Penn Tower, 3400 Spruce St, Philadelphia, PA 19104; **Phone:** 215-615-5121; **Board Cert:** Internal Medicine 1988; Medical Oncology 2005; **Med School:** NE Ohio Univ 1985; **Resid:** Internal Medicine, Abington Meml Hosp 1988; **Fellow:** Hematology & Oncology, Fox Chase Cancer Ctr 1989

Haller, Daniel G MD [Onc] - **Spec Exp:** Gastrointestinal Cancer; Colon & Rectal Cancer; Cancer Prevention; **Hospital:** Hosp Univ Penn - UPHS (page 60); **Address:** Hosp Univ Penn, Div Hematology/Oncology, 3400 Spruce St, 12 Penn Tower, Philadelphia, PA 19104; **Phone:** 215-662-6318; **Board Cert:** Internal Medicine 1976; Medical Oncology 1979; **Med School:** Univ Pittsburgh 1973; **Resid:** Internal Medicine, Georgetown Univ Hosp 1976; **Fellow:** Medical Oncology, Georgetown Univ Hosp 1978; **Fac Appt:** Prof Med, Univ Pennsylvania

Himelstein, Andrew L MD [Onc] - **Spec Exp:** Leukemia & Lymphoma; Palliative Care; **Hospital:** Christiana Hospital; **Address:** Med. Onc. Hem. Consultants, PA, 4701 Ogletown-Stanton Rd, Ste 3400, Newark, DE 19713; **Phone:** 302-366-1200; **Board Cert:** Internal Medicine 1988; Medical Oncology 2000; Hematology 2000; **Med School:** Washington Univ, St Louis 1985; **Resid:** Internal Medicine, Mt Sinai Hosp 1988; **Fellow:** Hematology & Oncology, Colum-Presby Univ Hosp 1991

Hochster, Howard S MD [Onc] - **Spec Exp:** Gastrointestinal Cancer; Gynecologic Cancer; Colon & Rectal Cancer; **Hospital:** NYU Langone Med Ctr (page 67); **Address:** NYU Cancer Institute, 160 E 34 St Fl 9, New York, NY 10016; **Phone:** 212-731-5100; **Board Cert:** Internal Medicine 1983; Medical Oncology 1985; Hematology 1986; **Med School:** Yale Univ 1980; **Resid:** Internal Medicine, NYU Med Ctr 1983; **Fellow:** Hematology & Oncology, NYU Med Ctr 1985; Medical Oncology, Jules Bordet Inst 1986; **Fac Appt:** Prof Med, NYU Sch Med

Hogan, Thomas F MD [Onc] - **Spec Exp:** Genitourinary Cancer; Kidney Cancer; Urologic Cancer; **Hospital:** WV Univ Hosp - Ruby Memorial; **Address:** WVU HSC-Dept Med-Hem/Onc, 1 Med Ctr Drive, P.O. Box 9162, Morgantown, WV 26506; **Phone:** 304-293-4500; **Board Cert:** Anatomic Pathology 1997; Internal Medicine 1975; Medical Oncology 1977; **Med School:** Med Coll VA 1972; **Resid:** Internal Medicine, Jefferson Hosp 1975; **Fellow:** Medical Oncology, Univ Wisconsin 1977; **Fac Appt:** Prof Med, W VA Univ

Holland, James F MD [Onc] - **Spec Exp:** Breast Cancer; Colon Cancer; Lung Cancer; Pancreatic Cancer; **Hospital:** Mount Sinai Med Ctr (page 64); **Address:** Ruttenberg Cancer Ctr, Div Med Oncology, 1 Gustave L Levy Pl, Box 1129, New York, NY 10029-6500; **Phone:** 212-241-4495; **Board Cert:** Internal Medicine 1955; **Med School:** Columbia P&S 1947; **Resid:** Internal Medicine, Columbia-Presby Hosp 1949; **Fellow:** Medical Oncology, Francis Delafield Hosp 1953; **Fac Appt:** Prof Med, Mount Sinai Sch Med

Horwitz, Steven MD [Onc] - **Spec Exp:** Lymphoma, Cutaneous T Cell (CTCL); **Hospital:** Meml Sloan-Kettering Cancer Ctr; **Address:** Meml Sloan-Kettering Cancer Ctr, 1275 York Ave, New York, NY 10021; **Phone:** 212-639-3045; **Board Cert:** Medical Oncology 2001; **Med School:** Case West Res Univ 1993; **Resid:** Internal Medicine, Strong Memorial Hosp 1996; **Fellow:** Medical Oncology, Stanford Univ Med Ctr 1999

Hudes, Gary R MD [Onc] - **Spec Exp:** Prostate Cancer; Genitourinary Cancer; Kidney Cancer; **Hospital:** Fox Chase Cancer Ctr (page 58); **Address:** 333 Cottman Ave, rm C307, Philadelphia, PA 19111; **Phone:** 215-728-3889; **Board Cert:** Internal Medicine 1982; Hematology 1984; Medical Oncology 1985; **Med School:** SUNY Downstate 1979; **Resid:** Internal Medicine, Graduate Hosp 1982; **Fellow:** Hematology & Oncology, Presby-Univ Penn Med Ctr 1985

Hudis, Clifford A MD [Onc] - **Spec Exp:** Breast Cancer; **Hospital:** Meml Sloan-Kettering Cancer Ctr; **Address:** 1275 York Avenue, New York, NY 10065; **Phone:** 800-525-2225; **Board Cert:** Internal Medicine 1986; Medical Oncology 2001; **Med School:** Med Coll PA Hahnemann 1983; **Resid:** Internal Medicine, Hosp Med Coll Penn 1986; **Fellow:** Medical Oncology, Meml Sloan Kettering Cancer Ctr 1991; **Fac Appt:** Prof Med, Cornell Univ-Weill Med Coll

Ilson, David H MD [Onc] - **Spec Exp:** Esophageal Cancer; Colon & Rectal Cancer; Mesothelioma; Unknown Primary Cancer; **Hospital:** Meml Sloan-Kettering Cancer Ctr; **Address:** 1275 York Avenue, New York, NY 10065; **Phone:** 800-525-2225; **Board Cert:** Internal Medicine 1989; Medical Oncology 2002; **Med School:** NYU Sch Med 1986; **Resid:** Internal Medicine, Bellevue-NYU Sch Med 1989; **Fellow:** Medical Oncology, Meml Sloan Kettering Hosp 1992; **Fac Appt:** Assoc Prof Med, Cornell Univ-Weill Med Coll

Isaacs, Claudine J MD [Onc] - **Spec Exp:** Breast Cancer; Breast Cancer Risk Assessment; **Hospital:** Georgetown Univ Hosp; **Address:** Lombardi Cancer Ctr, Podium B, 3800 Reservoir Rd NW, Washington, DC 20007; **Phone:** 202-444-3677; **Board Cert:** Internal Medicine 2002; Medical Oncology 2003; **Med School:** McGill Univ 1987; **Resid:** Internal Medicine, Montreal Genl Hosp 1990; Hematology & Oncology, McGill Univ Hosp 1992; **Fellow:** Medical Oncology, Georgetown Univ Med Ctr 1993; **Fac Appt:** Assoc Prof Med, Georgetown Univ

Jurcic, Joseph G MD [Onc] - **Spec Exp:** Leukemia; Myelodysplastic Syndromes; Clinical Trials; **Hospital:** Meml Sloan-Kettering Cancer Ctr; **Address:** 1275 York Avenue, New York, NY 10065; **Phone:** 800-525-2225; **Board Cert:** Internal Medicine 2001; Medical Oncology 2005; Hematology 1998; **Med School:** Univ Pennsylvania 1988; **Resid:** Internal Medicine, Barnes Hosp 1991; **Fellow:** Hematology & Oncology, Meml Sloan Kettering Cancer Ctr 1994; **Fac Appt:** Assoc Prof Med, Cornell Univ-Weill Med Coll

Karp, Judith MD [Onc] - **Spec Exp:** Leukemia; Clinical Trials; Myelodysplastic Syndromes; **Hospital:** Johns Hopkins Hosp (page 61); **Address:** 1650 Orleans St, CRB1 Bldg - rm 289, Baltimore, MD 21287; **Phone:** 410-502-7726; **Board Cert:** Internal Medicine 1976; **Med School:** Stanford Univ 1971; **Resid:** Internal Medicine, John Hopkins Hosp 1974; **Fellow:** Medical Oncology, John Hopkins Hosp 1977; **Fac Appt:** Prof Med, Johns Hopkins Univ

Kelsen, David MD [Onc] - **Spec Exp:** Gastrointestinal Cancer; Neuroendocrine Tumors; Unknown Primary Cancer; Merkel Cell Carcinoma; **Hospital:** Meml Sloan-Kettering Cancer Ctr; **Address:** 1275 York Avenue, New York, NY 10065; **Phone:** 212-639-8470; **Board Cert:** Internal Medicine 1976; Medical Oncology 1979; **Med School:** Hahnemann Univ 1972; **Resid:** Internal Medicine, Temple Univ Hosp 1976; **Fellow:** Medical Oncology, Meml Sloan Kettering Cancer Ctr 1978; **Fac Appt:** Prof Med, Cornell Univ-Weill Med Coll

Kemeny, Nancy MD [Onc] - **Spec Exp:** Colon Cancer; Rectal Cancer; Liver Cancer; **Hospital:** Meml Sloan-Kettering Cancer Ctr; **Address:** 1275 York Avenue, New York, NY 10065; **Phone:** 800-525-2225; **Board Cert:** Internal Medicine 1974; Medical Oncology 1981; **Med School:** UMDNJ-NJ Med Sch, Newark 1971; **Resid:** Internal Medicine, St Luke's Hosp 1974; **Fellow:** Medical Oncology, Mem Sloan Kettering Cancer Ctr 1976; **Fac Appt:** Prof Med, Cornell Univ-Weill Med Coll

Kirkwood, John M MD [Onc] - **Spec Exp:** Melanoma; Immunotherapy; **Hospital:** UPMC Presby, Pittsburgh, UPMC Shadyside; **Address:** Hillman Cancer Research Pavilion, 5117 Centre Ave, Ste 1.32, Pittsburgh, PA 15213-1862; **Phone:** 412-623-7707; **Board Cert:** Internal Medicine 1976; Medical Oncology 1981; **Med School:** Yale Univ 1973; **Resid:** Internal Medicine, Yale-New Haven Hosp 1976; **Fellow:** Medical Oncology, Dana Farber Cancer Inst 1979; **Fac Appt:** Prof Med, Univ Pittsburgh

Medical Oncology

Kris, Mark G MD [Onc] - **Spec Exp:** Lung Cancer; Mediastinal Tumors; Thymoma; Thoracic Cancers; **Hospital:** Meml Sloan-Kettering Cancer Ctr; **Address:** 1275 York Avenue, New York, NY 10065; **Phone:** 212-639-7590; **Board Cert:** Internal Medicine 1980; Medical Oncology 1983; **Med School:** Cornell Univ-Weill Med Coll 1977; **Resid:** Internal Medicine, New York Hosp 1980; **Fellow:** Medical Oncology, Meml Sloan Kettering Cancer Ctr 1983; **Fac Appt:** Prof Med, Cornell Univ-Weill Med Coll

Langer, Corey J MD [Onc] - **Spec Exp:** Lung Cancer; Head & Neck Cancer; Mesothelioma; Thoracic Cancers; **Hospital:** Hosp Univ Penn - UPHS (page 60); **Address:** Hospital U Penn, Abramson Cancer Ctr, Div Hem/Oncology, 16 Penn Tower, 3400 Spruce St, Philadelphia, PA 19104; **Phone:** 215-615-5121; **Board Cert:** Internal Medicine 1984; Hematology 1986; Medical Oncology 1987; **Med School:** Boston Univ 1981; **Resid:** Internal Medicine, Graduate Hosp 1984; Hematology & Oncology, Presby Hosp 1986; **Fellow:** Medical Oncology, Fox Chase Cancer Ctr 1987; **Fac Appt:** Prof Med, Univ Pennsylvania

Levine, Ellis G MD [Onc] - **Spec Exp:** Breast Cancer; Testicular Cancer; Bladder Cancer; Prostate Cancer; **Hospital:** Roswell Park Cancer Inst; **Address:** Roswell Park Cancer Inst, Elm & Carlton St, Buffalo, NY 14263-0001; **Phone:** 716-845-8547; **Board Cert:** Internal Medicine 1982; Medical Oncology 1985; **Med School:** Univ Pittsburgh 1979; **Resid:** Internal Medicine, Univ Minn Hosps 1982; **Fellow:** Medical Oncology, Univ Minn Hosps 1984; **Fac Appt:** Assoc Prof Med, SUNY Buffalo

Levy, Michael H MD/PhD [Onc] - **Spec Exp:** Pain Management; Palliative Care; Pain-Cancer; Ethics; **Hospital:** Fox Chase Cancer Ctr (page 58); **Address:** Fox Chase Cancer Ctr, Div Med Oncology, 333 Cottman Ave, Ste C307, Philadelphia, PA 19111; **Phone:** 215-728-3637; **Board Cert:** Internal Medicine 1979; Medical Oncology 1981; **Med School:** Jefferson Med Coll 1976; **Resid:** Internal Medicine, Mt Sinai Med Ctr 1978; Internal Medicine, Hosp Univ Penn 1979; **Fellow:** Hematology & Oncology, Hosp Univ Penn 1981

Livingston, Philip O MD [Onc] - **Spec Exp:** Melanoma; Vaccine Therapy; Immunotherapy; **Hospital:** Meml Sloan-Kettering Cancer Ctr; **Address:** 1275 York Avenue, New York, NY 10065; **Phone:** 800-525-2225; **Board Cert:** Internal Medicine 1980; Allergy & Immunology 1974; Rheumatology 1974; Medical Oncology 1981; **Med School:** Harvard Med Sch 1969; **Resid:** Internal Medicine, North Shore Hosp-Cornell 1971; **Fellow:** Immunology, NYU Med Ctr 1973; Medical Oncology, Meml Sloan Kettering Cancer Inst 1977; **Fac Appt:** Prof Med, Cornell Univ-Weill Med Coll

Marshall, John L MD [Onc] - **Spec Exp:** Gastrointestinal Cancer; Drug Development; **Hospital:** Georgetown Univ Hosp; **Address:** Lombardi Cancer Ctr, Podium A, 3800 Reservoir Rd NW, Washington, DC 20007; **Phone:** 202-444-7064; **Board Cert:** Internal Medicine 2001; Medical Oncology 2003; **Med School:** Univ Louisville Sch Med 1988; **Resid:** Internal Medicine, Georgetown Univ Hosp 1991; **Fellow:** Medical Oncology, Georgetown Univ Hosp 1993; **Fac Appt:** Assoc Prof Med, Georgetown Univ

Maslak, Peter G MD [Onc] - **Spec Exp:** Leukemia; Stem Cell Transplant; Myelodysplastic Syndromes; Clinical Trials; **Hospital:** Meml Sloan-Kettering Cancer Ctr; **Address:** 1275 York Avenue, New York, NY 10065; **Phone:** 800-525-2225; **Board Cert:** Internal Medicine 1987; Hematology 2000; Medical Oncology 1989; **Med School:** Mount Sinai Sch Med 1984; **Resid:** Internal Medicine, Univ Michigan Med Ctr 1987; **Fellow:** Hematology & Oncology, Meml Sloan Kettering Cancer Ctr 1990

Masters, Gregory A MD [Onc] - **Spec Exp:** Lung Cancer; Esophageal Cancer; Thoracic Cancers; **Hospital:** Christiana Hospital; **Address:** Medical Oncology-Hematology Consultants, Graham Cancer Ctr, 4701 Ogletown-Stanton Rd, Ste 2200, Newark, DE 19713; **Phone:** 302-366-1200; **Board Cert:** Internal Medicine 2003; Medical Oncology 2005; **Med School:** Northwestern Univ 1990; **Resid:** Internal Medicine, Hosp Univ Penn 1993; **Fellow:** Medical Oncology, Univ Chicago Hosps 1995; **Fac Appt:** Assoc Prof Med, Thomas Jefferson Univ

McGuire III, William P MD [Onc] - **Spec Exp:** Gynecologic Cancer; Ovarian Cancer; Breast Cancer; **Hospital:** Franklin Square Hosp; **Address:** Harry & Jeanette Weinberg Cancer Inst, 9103 Franklin Square Drive, Ste 2200, Baltimore, MD 21287; **Phone:** 443-777-7826; **Board Cert:** Internal Medicine 1974; Medical Oncology 1981; **Med School:** Baylor Coll Med 1971; **Resid:** Internal Medicine, Yale-New Haven Hosp 1973; **Fac Appt:** Clin Prof Med, Univ MD Sch Med

Miller, Vincent A MD [Onc] - **Spec Exp:** Lung Cancer; Drug Development; **Hospital:** Meml Sloan-Kettering Cancer Ctr; **Address:** Memorial Sloan-Kettering Cancer Ctr, 1275 York Ave, New York, NY 10065; **Phone:** 800-525-2225; **Board Cert:** Internal Medicine 2002; Medical Oncology 2005; **Med School:** UMDNJ-NJ Med Sch, Newark 1987; **Resid:** Internal Medicine, Thos Jefferson Univ Hosp 1991; **Fellow:** Medical Oncology, Meml Sloan Kettering Cancer Ctr 1994; **Fac Appt:** Assoc Prof Med, Cornell Univ-Weill Med Coll

Mintzer, David M MD [Onc] - **Spec Exp:** Breast Cancer; Gastrointestinal Cancer; Head & Neck Cancer; **Hospital:** Pennsylvania Hosp (page 60); **Address:** 230 W Washington Square Fl 2, Philadelphia, PA 19106; **Phone:** 215-829-6088; **Board Cert:** Internal Medicine 1980; Hematology 1982; Medical Oncology 1983; **Med School:** Jefferson Med Coll 1977; **Resid:** Internal Medicine, Pennsylvania Hosp 1980; **Fellow:** Hematology, Jefferson Med Coll 1982; Medical Oncology, Meml Sloan Kettering Cancer Ctr 1984; **Fac Appt:** Assoc Clin Prof Med, Univ Pennsylvania

Moore, Anne MD [Onc] - **Spec Exp:** Breast Cancer; **Hospital:** NY-Presby Hosp/Weill Cornell (page 66); **Address:** Weill Cornell Breast Ctr, 425 E 61st St Fl 8, New York, NY 10065; **Phone:** 212-821-0654; **Board Cert:** Internal Medicine 1973; Hematology 1976; Medical Oncology 2008; **Med School:** Columbia P&S 1969; **Resid:** Internal Medicine, Cornell Univ Med Ctr 1973; **Fellow:** Medical Oncology, Rockefeller Univ 1973; **Fac Appt:** Prof Med, Cornell Univ-Weill Med Coll

Motzer, Robert J MD [Onc] - **Spec Exp:** Kidney Cancer; Testicular Cancer; Prostate Cancer; **Hospital:** Meml Sloan-Kettering Cancer Ctr; **Address:** 1275 York Avenue, New York, NY 10065; **Phone:** 800-525-2225; **Board Cert:** Internal Medicine 1984; Medical Oncology 1987; **Med School:** Univ Mich Med Sch 1981; **Resid:** Internal Medicine, Meml Sloan Kettering Cancer Ctr 1984; **Fellow:** Medical Oncology, Meml Sloan Kettering Cancer Ctr 1987; **Fac Appt:** Assoc Prof Med, Cornell Univ-Weill Med Coll

Muggia, Franco MD [Onc] - **Spec Exp:** Gynecologic Cancer; **Hospital:** NYU Langone Med Ctr (page 67); **Address:** NYU Clinical Cancer Ctr, 160 E 34th St Fl 8, New York, NY 10016; **Phone:** 212-731-5433; **Board Cert:** Internal Medicine 1968; Medical Oncology 1973; Hematology 1974; **Med School:** Cornell Univ-Weill Med Coll 1961; **Resid:** Internal Medicine, Hartford Hosp 1964; Internal Medicine, Francis A Delafield Hosp 1966; **Fac Appt:** Prof Med, NYU Sch Med

Nissenblatt, Michael MD [Onc] - **Spec Exp:** Breast Cancer; Colon Cancer; Hereditary Cancer; Lymphoma; **Hospital:** Robert Wood Johnson Univ Hosp - New Brunswick, St Peter's Univ Hosp; **Address:** 205 Easton Ave, New Brunswick, NJ 08901-1722; **Phone:** 732-828-9570; **Board Cert:** Internal Medicine 1976; Medical Oncology 1979; **Med School:** Columbia P&S 1973; **Resid:** Internal Medicine, Johns Hopkins Hosp 1976; **Fellow:** Medical Oncology, Johns Hopkins Hosp 1978; **Fac Appt:** Clin Prof Med, Robert W Johnson Med Sch

Medical Oncology

Norton, Larry MD [Onc] - **Spec Exp:** Breast Cancer; **Hospital:** Meml Sloan-Kettering Cancer Ctr; **Address:** 1275 York Avenue, New York, NY 10065; **Phone:** 800-525-2225; **Board Cert:** Internal Medicine 1975; Medical Oncology 1977; **Med School:** Columbia P&S 1972; **Resid:** Internal Medicine, Bronx Muni Hosp 1974; **Fellow:** Medical Oncology, Natl Cancer Inst 1977; **Fac Appt:** Prof Med, Cornell Univ-Weill Med Coll

O'Reilly, Eileen M MD [Onc] - **Spec Exp:** Pancreatic Cancer; Liver Cancer; Biliary Cancer; Neuroendocrine Tumors; **Hospital:** Meml Sloan-Kettering Cancer Ctr, NY-Presby Hosp/Weill Cornell (page 66); **Address:** 1275 York Avenue, Meml Sloan-Kettering Cancer Ctr, New York, NY 10065; **Phone:** 212-639-6672; **Med School:** Ireland 1990; **Resid:** Internal Medicine, St Vincent's Hosp 1994; **Fellow:** Hematology, St Vincent's Hosp 1995; Medical Oncology, Memorial-Sloan Kettering Cancer Ctr 1997; **Fac Appt:** Assoc Prof Med, Cornell Univ-Weill Med Coll

Offit, Kenneth MD [Onc] - **Spec Exp:** Cancer Genetics; Breast Cancer; Lymphoma; **Hospital:** Meml Sloan-Kettering Cancer Ctr; **Address:** 1275 York Avenue, New York, NY 10065; **Phone:** 800-525-2225; **Board Cert:** Internal Medicine 1985; Medical Oncology 1987; **Med School:** Harvard Med Sch 1982; **Resid:** Internal Medicine, Lenox Hill Hosp 1985; **Fellow:** Hematology & Oncology, Meml Sloan Kettering Cancer Ctr 1988; **Fac Appt:** Prof Med, Cornell Univ-Weill Med Coll

Oh, William K MD [Onc] - **Spec Exp:** Genitourinary Cancer; Prostate Cancer; Testicular Cancer; **Hospital:** Mount Sinai Med Ctr (page 64); **Address:** Mount Sinai Medical Ctr, Gustave Levy Pl, Box 1079, New York, NY 10029; **Phone:** 212-241-5293; **Board Cert:** Medical Oncology 1998; **Med School:** NYU Sch Med 1992; **Resid:** Internal Medicine, Brigham & Womens Hosp 1995; **Fellow:** Medical Oncology, Dana-Farber Cancer Inst 1997; **Fac Appt:** Prof Med, Mount Sinai Sch Med

Oratz, Ruth MD [Onc] - **Spec Exp:** Breast Cancer; Ovarian Cancer; **Hospital:** NYU Langone Med Ctr (page 67); **Address:** 345 E 37th St, Ste 202, New York, NY 10016; **Phone:** 212-400-4904; **Board Cert:** Internal Medicine 1985; Medical Oncology 1989; **Med School:** Albert Einstein Coll Med 1982; **Resid:** Internal Medicine, NYU Med Ctr 1982; **Fellow:** Medical Oncology, NYU Med Ctr 1985; **Fac Appt:** Assoc Clin Prof Med, NYU Sch Med

Oster, Martin W MD [Onc] - **Spec Exp:** Breast Cancer; Gastrointestinal Cancer; Head & Neck Cancer; **Hospital:** NY-Presby Hosp/Columbia (page 66); **Address:** NY Presby Hosp-Columbia Presby Med Ctr, 161 Fort Washington Ave, New York, NY 10032-3713; **Phone:** 212-305-8231; **Board Cert:** Internal Medicine 1974; Medical Oncology 1975; **Med School:** Columbia P&S 1971; **Resid:** Internal Medicine, Mass Genl Hosp 1973; **Fellow:** Medical Oncology, Natl Cancer Inst/NIH 1976; **Fac Appt:** Assoc Clin Prof Med, Columbia P&S

Pasmantier, Mark W MD [Onc] - **Spec Exp:** Lung Cancer; Ovarian Cancer; Breast Cancer; Lymphoma; **Hospital:** NY-Presby Hosp/Weill Cornell (page 66); **Address:** 407 E 70th St Fl 3, New York, NY 10021-5302; **Phone:** 212-517-5900; **Board Cert:** Internal Medicine 1972; Hematology 1974; Medical Oncology 1975; **Med School:** NYU Sch Med 1966; **Resid:** Internal Medicine, Harlem Hosp 1970; **Fellow:** Hematology, Montefiore Med Ctr 1971; Medical Oncology, NY Hosp 1972; **Fac Appt:** Clin Prof Med, Cornell Univ-Weill Med Coll

Pecora, Andrew L MD [Onc] - **Spec Exp:** Stem Cell Transplant; Myelodysplastic Syndromes; Melanoma; Immunotherapy; **Hospital:** Hackensack Univ Med Ctr; **Address:** The Cancer Ctr-Hackensack Univ Med Ctr, 20 Prospect Ave, Ste 400, Hackensack, NJ 07601; **Phone:** 201-996-5900; **Board Cert:** Internal Medicine 1986; Hematology 1988; Medical Oncology 1989; **Med School:** UMDNJ-NJ Med Sch, Newark 1983; **Resid:** Internal Medicine, New York Hosp 1986; **Fellow:** Hematology & Oncology, Meml Sloan Kettering Cancer Ctr 1988; **Fac Appt:** Prof Med, UMDNJ-NJ Med Sch, Newark

Perry, David J MD [Onc] - **Spec Exp:** Gastrointestinal Cancer; Lung Cancer; Genitourinary Cancer; Clinical Trials; **Hospital:** Washington Hosp Ctr; **Address:** Washington Hosp Ctr-Dept Med Oncology, 110 Irving St NW Fl 2nd - rm CI-2151, Washington, DC 20010; **Phone:** 202-877-2843; **Board Cert:** Internal Medicine 1979; Hematology 1982; Medical Oncology 1981; **Med School:** Univ Pennsylvania 1974; **Resid:** Internal Medicine, Walter Reed AMC 1979; **Fellow:** Hematology & Oncology, Walter Reed AMC 1979; **Fac Appt:** Assoc Prof Med, Eastern VA Med Sch

Petrylak, Daniel P MD [Onc] - **Spec Exp:** Genitourinary Cancer; Prostate Cancer; Bladder Cancer; Kidney Cancer; **Hospital:** NY-Presby Hosp/Columbia (page 66); **Address:** 161 Fort Washington Ave, New York, NY 10032-3729; **Phone:** 212-305-1731; **Board Cert:** Internal Medicine 2001; Medical Oncology 2003; **Med School:** Case West Res Univ 1985; **Resid:** Internal Medicine, Jacobi Med Ctr 1988; **Fellow:** Oncology, Meml-Sloan Kettering Cancer Ctr 1991; **Fac Appt:** Assoc Prof Med, Columbia P&S

Pfister, David G MD [Onc] - **Spec Exp:** Head & Neck Cancer; Laryngeal Cancer; Thyroid Cancer; Skin Cancer; **Hospital:** Meml Sloan-Kettering Cancer Ctr; **Address:** 1275 York Avenue, New York, NY 10065; **Phone:** 800-525-2225; **Board Cert:** Internal Medicine 1985; Medical Oncology 1989; **Med School:** Univ Pennsylvania 1982; **Resid:** Internal Medicine, Hosp Univ Penn 1985; **Fellow:** Epidemiology, Yale-New Haven Hosp 1987; Hematology & Oncology, Meml Sloan Kettering Cancer Ctr 1989; **Fac Appt:** Prof Med, Cornell Univ-Weill Med Coll

Raptis, George MD [Onc] - **Spec Exp:** Breast Cancer; **Hospital:** Mount Sinai Med Ctr (page 64); **Address:** 1190 5th Ave, Box 1132, New York, NY 10029; **Phone:** 212-241-6756; **Board Cert:** Medical Oncology 2003; **Med School:** Mount Sinai Sch Med 1987; **Resid:** Internal Medicine, Mt Sinai Med Ctr 1990; **Fellow:** Hematology & Oncology, Meml Sloan-Kettering Canc Ctr 1993; **Fac Appt:** Assoc Prof Med, Mount Sinai Sch Med

Remick, Scot C MD [Onc] - **Spec Exp:** AIDS Related Cancers; Clinical Trials; Drug Development; Thyroid Cancer; **Hospital:** WV Univ Hosp - Ruby Memorial; **Address:** WVU Mary Babb Randolph Cancer Ctr, Box 9300, Morgantown, WV 26506-9300; **Phone:** 304-598-4552; **Board Cert:** Internal Medicine 1985; Medical Oncology 1988; **Med School:** NY Med Coll 1982; **Resid:** Internal Medicine, Johns Hopkins Hosp 1985; **Fellow:** Medical Oncology, Univ Wisconsin Clin Cancer Ctr 1988; **Fac Appt:** Prof Med, W VA Univ

Ruggiero, Joseph T MD [Onc] - **Spec Exp:** Colon Cancer; Breast Cancer; **Hospital:** NY-Presby Hosp/Weill Cornell (page 66); **Address:** 428 E 72nd St, Ste 300, New York, NY 10021-4635; **Phone:** 212-746-2083; **Board Cert:** Internal Medicine 1980; Hematology 1982; Medical Oncology 1983; **Med School:** NYU Sch Med 1977; **Resid:** Internal Medicine, New York Hosp 1980; **Fellow:** Hematology & Oncology, New York Hosp/Cornell 1983; **Fac Appt:** Assoc Clin Prof Med, Cornell Univ-Weill Med Coll

Saltz, Leonard B MD [Onc] - **Spec Exp:** Colon & Rectal Cancer; Gastrointestinal Cancer & Rare Tumors; Liver Cancer; Neuroendocrine Tumors; **Hospital:** Meml Sloan-Kettering Cancer Ctr; **Address:** 1275 York Avenue, New York, NY 10065; **Phone:** 646-497-9053; **Board Cert:** Internal Medicine 1986; Hematology 1988; Medical Oncology 1989; **Med School:** Yale Univ 1983; **Resid:** Internal Medicine, New Yor Hosp 1986; **Fellow:** Hematology & Oncology, New York Hosp-Cornell/Rockefeller Univ 1987; **Fac Appt:** Prof Med, Cornell Univ-Weill Med Coll

Scheinberg, David MD/PhD [Onc] - **Spec Exp:** Leukemia; Immunotherapy; Vaccine Therapy; **Hospital:** Meml Sloan-Kettering Cancer Ctr; **Address:** 1275 York Avenue, New York, NY 10065; **Phone:** 800-525-2225; **Board Cert:** Internal Medicine 1986; Medical Oncology 2005; **Med School:** Johns Hopkins Univ 1983; **Resid:** Internal Medicine, NY Hosp-Cornell Med Ctr 1985; **Fellow:** Medical Oncology, Meml Sloan Kettering Cancer Ctr 1987; **Fac Appt:** Prof Med, Cornell Univ-Weill Med Coll

Scher, Howard MD [Onc] - **Spec Exp:** Genitourinary Cancer; Prostate Cancer; Bladder Cancer; **Hospital:** Meml Sloan-Kettering Cancer Ctr; **Address:** 1275 York Avenue, New York, NY 10065; **Phone:** 800-525-2225; **Board Cert:** Internal Medicine 1979; Medical Oncology 1985; **Med School:** NYU Sch Med 1976; **Resid:** Internal Medicine, Bellevue Hosp 1980; **Fellow:** Medical Oncology, Meml Sloan Kettering Cancer Ctr 1983; **Fac Appt:** Prof Med, Cornell Univ-Weill Med Coll

Schilder, Russell J MD [Onc] - **Spec Exp:** Gynecologic Cancer; Hematologic Malignancies; Drug Development; Clinical Trials; **Hospital:** Fox Chase Cancer Ctr (page 58); **Address:** Fox Chase Cancer Center, 333 Cottman Ave, Philadelphia, PA 19111; **Phone:** 215-728-4300; **Board Cert:** Internal Medicine 1986; Hematology 1988; Medical Oncology 1989; **Med School:** Univ Miami Sch Med 1983; **Resid:** Internal Medicine, Temple Univ Hosp 1986; **Fellow:** Hematology & Oncology, Fox Chase Cancer Ctr 1989; **Fac Appt:** Prof Med, Temple Univ

Schuchter, Lynn M MD [Onc] - **Spec Exp:** Melanoma; Breast Cancer; Clinical Trials; **Hospital:** Hosp Univ Penn - UPHS (page 60); **Address:** Univ Penn/Abramson Cancer Ctr, 3400 Spruce St, 16 Penn Tower, Philadelphia, PA 19104-4206; **Phone:** 215-662-7907; **Board Cert:** Internal Medicine 1985; Medical Oncology 1989; **Med School:** Ros Franklin Univ/Chicago Med Sch 1982; **Resid:** Internal Medicine, Michael Reese Hosp 1985; **Fellow:** Medical Oncology, Johns Hopkins Hosp 1989; **Fac Appt:** Prof Med, Univ Pennsylvania

Selvaggi, Kathy J MD [Onc] - **Spec Exp:** Palliative Care; Pain-Cancer; **Hospital:** Allegheny General Hosp; **Address:** West Penn Allegheny Health System, 4815 Liberty Ave, Ste 435, Pittsburgh, PA 15224; **Phone:** 412-578-1112; **Board Cert:** Internal Medicine 1989; Medical Oncology 2005; **Med School:** Penn State Univ-Hershey Med Ctr 1985; **Resid:** Internal Medicine, UPMC Shadyside Hosp 1989; **Fellow:** Medical Oncology, UPMC Shadyside Hosp 1992

Shields, Peter G MD [Onc] - **Spec Exp:** Hematologic Malignancies; **Hospital:** Georgetown Univ Hosp; **Address:** Lombardi Cancer Ctr, 3800 Reservoir Rd NW, First Floor, Washington, DC 20007; **Phone:** 202-444-9495; **Board Cert:** Internal Medicine 1986; Medical Oncology 1989; **Med School:** Mount Sinai Sch Med 1983; **Resid:** Internal Medicine, George Washington Univ Hosp 1986; **Fellow:** Hematology & Oncology, George Washington Univ Hosp 1990; **Fac Appt:** Prof Med, Georgetown Univ

Silverman, Lewis R MD [Onc] - **Spec Exp:** Myelodysplastic Syndromes; Leukemia & Lymphoma; Multiple Myeloma; **Hospital:** Mount Sinai Med Ctr (page 64); **Address:** 1190 5th Ave, Ruttenberg Treatment Ctr, New York, NY 10029; **Phone:** 212-241-6756; **Board Cert:** Internal Medicine 1981; Medical Oncology 1987; **Med School:** Belgium 1978; **Resid:** Internal Medicine, Metro Hospital 1980; Internal Medicine, Montefiore Med Ctr 1981; **Fellow:** Hematology, Montefiore Med Ctr 1982; Neoplastic Diseases, Mt Sinai Med Ctr 1984; **Fac Appt:** Assoc Prof Med, Mount Sinai Sch Med

Simon, George R MD [Onc] - **Spec Exp:** Mesothelioma; Lung Cancer; **Hospital:** Fox Chase Cancer Ctr (page 58); **Address:** Fox Chase Cancer Ctr, 333 Cottman Ave, Philadelphia, PA 19111; **Phone:** 215-728-2570; **Board Cert:** Internal Medicine 2007; Medical Oncology 2007; Hematology 1999; **Med School:** India 1986; **Resid:** Internal Medicine, St Joseph's Hosp 1995; **Fellow:** Hematology & Oncology, Univ Colorado Hlth Sciences Ctr 1997

Smith, Mitchell R MD/PhD [Onc] - **Spec Exp:** Lymphoma; Leukemia; Hodgkin's Disease; Multiple Myeloma; **Hospital:** Fox Chase Cancer Ctr (page 58); **Address:** Fox Chase Cancer Center, 333 Cottman Ave, Ste C307, Philadelphia, PA 19111; **Phone:** 215-728-2570; **Board Cert:** Internal Medicine 1985; Medical Oncology 1987; Hematology 1988; **Med School:** Case West Res Univ 1979; **Resid:** Pathology, Barnes Jewish Hosp 1983; Internal Medicine, Barnes Jewish Hosp 1984; **Fellow:** Medical Oncology, Meml Sloan-Ketter Cancer Ctr 1988

Speyer, James MD [Onc] - **Spec Exp:** Ovarian Cancer; Breast Cancer; Cardiac Toxicity in Cancer Therapy; **Hospital:** NYU Langone Med Ctr (page 67); **Address:** NYU Clinical Cancer Center, 160 E 34th St Fl 8, New York, NY 10016-4750; **Phone:** 212-731-5432; **Board Cert:** Internal Medicine 1977; Hematology 1978; Medical Oncology 1979; **Med School:** Johns Hopkins Univ 1974; **Resid:** Internal Medicine, Columbia-Presby Med Ctr 1976; Hematology, Columbia-Presby Med Ctr 1977; **Fellow:** Medical Oncology, Natl Cancer Inst 1979; **Fac Appt:** Prof Med, NYU Sch Med

Spriggs, David R MD [Onc] - **Spec Exp:** Ovarian Cancer; Drug Development; Uterine Cancer; **Hospital:** Meml Sloan-Kettering Cancer Ctr; **Address:** 1275 York Avenue, New York, NY 10065; **Phone:** 800-525-2225; **Board Cert:** Internal Medicine 1981; Medical Oncology 2006; **Med School:** Univ Wisc 1977; **Resid:** Internal Medicine, Columbia-Presby Hosp 1981; **Fellow:** Medical Oncology, Dana-Farber Cancer Inst 1985; **Fac Appt:** Prof Med, Cornell Univ-Weill Med Coll

Stadtmauer, Edward A MD [Onc] - **Spec Exp:** Bone Marrow & Stem Cell Transplant; Leukemia; Multiple Myeloma; **Hospital:** Hosp Univ Penn - UPHS (page 60); **Address:** Abramson Cancer Ctr, Univ of Penn, 2 PCAM, 34th & Cancer Ctr Blvd, Philadelphia, PA 19104; **Phone:** 215-662-7910; **Board Cert:** Internal Medicine 1986; Hematology 1988; Medical Oncology 1989; **Med School:** Univ Pennsylvania 1983; **Resid:** Internal Medicine, Bronx Muni Hosp 1986; **Fellow:** Hematology & Oncology, Hosp Univ Penn 1989; **Fac Appt:** Assoc Prof Med, Univ Pennsylvania

Stoopler, Mark MD [Onc] - **Spec Exp:** Lung Cancer; Esophageal Cancer; Unknown Primary Cancer; **Hospital:** NY-Presby Hosp/Columbia (page 66); **Address:** 161 Fort Washington Ave, Ste 936, New York, NY 10032-3713; **Phone:** 212-305-8230; **Board Cert:** Internal Medicine 1978; Medical Oncology 1981; **Med School:** Cornell Univ-Weill Med Coll 1975; **Resid:** Internal Medicine, North Shore Univ Hosp 1978; Internal Medicine, Meml Hosp 1978; **Fellow:** Medical Oncology, Meml-Sloan Kettering Cancer Ctr 1980; **Fac Appt:** Assoc Clin Prof Med, Columbia P&S

Straus, David J MD [Onc] - **Spec Exp:** Lymphoma; Multiple Myeloma; **Hospital:** Meml Sloan-Kettering Cancer Ctr; **Address:** 1275 York Avenue, New York, NY 10065; **Phone:** 212-639-8365; **Board Cert:** Internal Medicine 1972; Hematology 1976; Medical Oncology 1977; **Med School:** Marquette Sch Med 1969; **Resid:** Internal Medicine, Montefiore Med Ctr 1972; Medical Oncology, Meml Sloan Kettering Cancer Ctr 1977; **Fellow:** Hematology, Beth Israel Hosp 1973; **Fac Appt:** Prof Med, Cornell Univ-Weill Med Coll

Sun, Weijing MD [Onc] - **Spec Exp:** Gastrointestinal Cancer; Pancreatic Cancer; **Hospital:** Hosp Univ Penn - UPHS (page 60); **Address:** Hosp of the Univ of Pennsylvania, Division of Hematology-Oncology, 3400 Spruce St, 15 Penn Tower, Philadelphia, PA 19104; **Phone:** 215-662-6319; **Board Cert:** Internal Medicine 1998; Medical Oncology 2001; **Med School:** China 1982; **Resid:** Internal Medicine, Loyola U Med Ctr 1998; **Fellow:** Hematology & Oncology, Hosp Univ Penn 2001; **Fac Appt:** Assoc Prof Med, Univ Pennsylvania

Swain, Sandra MD [Onc] - **Spec Exp:** Breast Cancer; **Hospital:** Washington Hosp Ctr; **Address:** Washington Cancer Inst, 110 Irving St NW, Washington, DC 20010; **Phone:** 202-877-8112; **Board Cert:** Internal Medicine 1983; Medical Oncology 1985; **Med School:** Univ Fla Coll Med 1980; **Resid:** Internal Medicine, Vanderbilt Univ Affil Hosp 1980; **Fellow:** Medical Oncology, NIH-Natl Cancer Inst 1986; **Fac Appt:** Assoc Prof Med, Georgetown Univ

Tepler, Jeffrey MD [Onc] - **Spec Exp:** Breast Cancer; Leukemia & Lymphoma; Multiple Myeloma; Bleeding/Coagulation Disorders; **Hospital:** NY-Presby Hosp/Weill Cornell (page 66); **Address:** 310 E 72nd St, New York, NY 10021; **Phone:** 212-650-1780; **Board Cert:** Internal Medicine 1985; Medical Oncology 1987; Hematology 1988; **Med School:** Yale Univ 1982; **Resid:** Internal Medicine, NY Hosp 1985; **Fellow:** Hematology & Oncology, NY Hosp 1988; **Fac Appt:** Asst Clin Prof Med, Cornell Univ-Weill Med Coll

Medical Oncology

Tkaczuk, Katherine H MD [Onc] - **Spec Exp:** Breast Cancer; **Hospital:** Univ of MD Med Ctr; **Address:** Univ MD Cancer Ctr, 22 S Greene St, rm S9D12, Baltimore, MD 21201; **Phone:** 410-328-7904; **Board Cert:** Internal Medicine 1989; Medical Oncology 2001; **Med School:** Poland 1984; **Resid:** Internal Medicine, St Agnes Hosp 1989; **Fellow:** Hematology & Oncology, Univ Maryland Cancer Ctr 1992; **Fac Appt:** Assoc Prof Med, Univ MD Sch Med

Trump, Donald L MD [Onc] - **Spec Exp:** Prostate Cancer; Genitourinary Cancer; Drug Discovery & Development; **Hospital:** Roswell Park Cancer Inst; **Address:** Elm & Carlton St, Buffalo, NY 14263; **Phone:** 716-845-3499; **Board Cert:** Internal Medicine 1973; Medical Oncology 1977; **Med School:** Johns Hopkins Univ 1970; **Resid:** Internal Medicine, Johns Hopkins Hosp 1975; **Fellow:** Medical Oncology, Johns Hopkins Hosp 1974; **Fac Appt:** Prof Med, SUNY Buffalo

Vaughn, David J MD [Onc] - **Spec Exp:** Testicular Cancer; Bladder Cancer; Prostate Cancer; Genitourinary Cancer; **Hospital:** Hosp Univ Penn - UPHS (page 60), Penn Presby Med Ctr - UPHS (page 60); **Address:** Hosp Univ of Pennsylvania-16 Penn Tower, 3400 Spruce St, Philadelphia, PA 19104; **Phone:** 215-349-8140; **Board Cert:** Medical Oncology 2003; **Med School:** Harvard Med Sch 1987; **Resid:** Internal Medicine, NY Hosp-Cornell Med Ctr 1990; **Fellow:** Hematology & Oncology, Hosp U Penn 1993; **Fac Appt:** Assoc Prof Med, Univ Pennsylvania

von Mehren, Margaret MD [Onc] - **Spec Exp:** Sarcoma; Melanoma; Immunotherapy; Gastrointestinal Stromal Tumors; **Hospital:** Fox Chase Cancer Ctr (page 58); **Address:** Fox Chase Cancer Ctr, Dept Med Oncology, 333 Cottman Ave, Philadelphia, PA 19111-2434; **Phone:** 215-728-2570; **Board Cert:** Medical Oncology 2007; **Med School:** Albany Med Coll 1989; **Resid:** Internal Medicine, NYU Med Ctr 1993; **Fellow:** Hematology & Oncology, Fox Chase Cancer Ctr 1996; **Fac Appt:** Assoc Prof Med, Temple Univ

Waintraub, Stanley MD [Onc] - **Spec Exp:** Breast Cancer; Gynecologic Cancer; Bleeding/Coagulation Disorders; **Hospital:** Hackensack Univ Med Ctr, Holy Name Hosp; **Address:** Northern NJ Cancer Associates, 20 Prospect Ave, Fl 4, Hackensack, NJ 07601-1997; **Phone:** 201-996-5900; **Board Cert:** Internal Medicine 1980; Hematology 1982; Medical Oncology 1983; **Med School:** NY Med Coll 1977; **Resid:** Internal Medicine, Metropolitan Hosp Ctr 1980; **Fellow:** Hematology, Montefiore Hosp Med Ctr 1982; Medical Oncology, Meml Sloan Kettering Cancer Ctr 1983; **Fac Appt:** Asst Clin Prof Med, UMDNJ-NJ Med Sch, Newark

Weiner, Louis M MD [Onc] - **Spec Exp:** Gastrointestinal Cancer; Immunotherapy; Liver Cancer; **Hospital:** Georgetown Univ Hosp; **Address:** Lombardi Cancer Ctr, Georgetown Univ, Research Bldg - rm E501, 3970 Reservoir Rd NW, Washington, DC 20057; **Phone:** 202-687-2110; **Board Cert:** Internal Medicine 1980; Medical Oncology 1985; **Med School:** Mount Sinai Sch Med 1977; **Resid:** Internal Medicine, Med Ctr Hosp Vermont 1981; **Fellow:** Hematology & Oncology, New England Med Ctr 1984; **Fac Appt:** Prof Med, Georgetown Univ

Wetzler, Meir MD [Onc] - **Spec Exp:** Leukemia; **Hospital:** Roswell Park Cancer Inst; **Address:** Roswell Park Cancer Inst, Elm and Carlton Streets, Buffalo, NY 14263; **Phone:** 716-845-8447; **Board Cert:** Internal Medicine 2001; Medical Oncology 2003; **Med School:** Israel 1980; **Resid:** Internal Medicine, Kaplan Hosp 1986; **Fellow:** Medical Oncology, MD Anderson Cancer Ctr 1992; Clinical Immunology, MD Anderson Cancer Ctr 1992; **Fac Appt:** Prof Med, SUNY Buffalo

Wilson, Wyndham MD [Onc] - **Spec Exp:** Lymphoma; **Hospital:** Natl Inst of Hlth - Clin Ctr; **Address:** National Cancer Inst, Bldg 10 - rm 12N-226, 9000 Rockville Pike, Bethesda, MD 20892; **Phone:** 301-435-2415; **Board Cert:** Internal Medicine 1985; Medical Oncology 1987; **Med School:** Stanford Univ 1981; **Resid:** Internal Medicine, Stanford Univ 1984; **Fellow:** Oncology, NCI-NIH 1987

Wolff, Antonio C MD [Onc] - **Spec Exp:** Breast Cancer; Drug Development; **Hospital:** Johns Hopkins Hosp (page 61); **Address:** 1650 Orleans St, rm 189, crb-1 Bldg, Baltimore, MD 21231; **Phone:** 410-614-4192; **Board Cert:** Internal Medicine 2000; Medical Oncology 2000; **Med School:** Brazil 1986; **Resid:** Internal Medicine, Mt Sinai Med Ctr 1991; **Fellow:** Hematology & Oncology, Washington Univ Med Ctr 1992; Medical Oncology, Johns Hopkins Hosp 1995; **Fac Appt:** Assoc Prof Med, Johns Hopkins Univ

Zelenetz, Andrew D MD/PhD [Onc] - **Spec Exp:** Lymphoma; **Hospital:** Meml Sloan-Kettering Cancer Ctr; **Address:** 1275 York Avenue, New York, NY 10065; **Phone:** 800-525-2225; **Med School:** Harvard Med Sch 1984; **Resid:** Internal Medicine, Stanford Univ Med Ctr 1986; **Fellow:** Medical Oncology, Stanford Univ Med Ctr 1991; **Fac Appt:** Asst Prof Med, Cornell Univ-Weill Med Coll

Southeast

Antonia, Scott J MD/PhD [Onc] - **Spec Exp:** Kidney Cancer; Lung Cancer; **Hospital:** H Lee Moffitt Cancer Ctr & Research Inst; **Address:** H Lee Moffitt Cancer Ctr, 12902 Magnolia Drive, Tampa, FL 33612; **Phone:** 813-979-3883; **Board Cert:** Internal Medicine 2002; Medical Oncology 2006; **Med School:** Univ Conn 1989; **Resid:** Internal Medicine, Yale-New Haven Hosp 1991; **Fellow:** Medical Oncology, Yale-New Haven Hosp 1994; **Fac Appt:** Assoc Prof Med, Univ S Fla Coll Med

Arteaga, Carlos L MD [Onc] - **Spec Exp:** Breast Cancer; **Hospital:** Vanderbilt Univ Med Ctr, VA Med Ctr - Nashville; **Address:** Vanderbilt-Ingram Cancer Ctr, 2220 Pierce Ave, 777-PRB, Nashville, TN 37232-6838; **Phone:** 615-936-3524; **Board Cert:** Internal Medicine 1984; Medical Oncology 1989; **Med School:** Ecuador 1980; **Resid:** Internal Medicine, Grady Meml Hosp 1984; **Fellow:** Hematology & Oncology, Univ Texas Hlth Sci Ctr 1987; **Fac Appt:** Prof Med, Vanderbilt Univ

Balducci, Lodovico MD [Onc] - **Spec Exp:** Genitourinary Cancer; Breast Cancer; **Hospital:** H Lee Moffitt Cancer Ctr & Research Inst, Tampa Genl Hosp; **Address:** H Lee Moffitt Cancer Ctr, 12902 Magnolia Drive, Tampa, FL 33612; **Phone:** 813-745-8658; **Board Cert:** Internal Medicine 1987; Hematology 1978; Medical Oncology 1979; **Med School:** Italy 1968; **Resid:** Internal Medicine, Univ Miss Med Ctr 1976; Hematology & Oncology, Univ Miss Med Ctr 1979; **Fellow:** Internal Medicine, A Gemelli Genl Hosp 1970; **Fac Appt:** Prof Med, Univ S Fla Coll Med

Benedetto, Pasquale W MD [Onc] - **Spec Exp:** Genitourinary Cancer; Bladder Cancer; Kidney Cancer; Pancreatic Cancer; **Hospital:** Univ of Miami Hosp & Clins/Sylvester Comp Canc Ctr (page 70), Jackson Meml Hosp (page 70); **Address:** Sylvester Comp Cancer Ctr, Med Oncology, 1475 NW 12th Ave, Ste 3310, Locator D8-4, Miami, FL 33136; **Phone:** 305-243-4909; **Board Cert:** Internal Medicine 1979; Medical Oncology 1981; Hematology 1982; **Med School:** Cornell Univ-Weill Med Coll 1976; **Resid:** Internal Medicine, Johns Hopkins Hosp 1979; **Fellow:** Medical Oncology, Meml Sloan Kettering Cancer Ctr 1981; **Fac Appt:** Prof Med, Univ Miami Sch Med

Berlin, Jordan D MD [Onc] - **Spec Exp:** Gastrointestinal Cancer; Pancreatic Cancer; Liver Cancer; **Hospital:** Vanderbilt Univ Med Ctr; **Address:** 777 Preston Research Building, Nashville, TN 37232-0001; **Phone:** 615-322-6053; **Board Cert:** Internal Medicine 2002; Medical Oncology 2005; **Med School:** Univ IL Coll Med 1989; **Resid:** Internal Medicine, Univ Cincinnati 1992; **Fellow:** Medical Oncology, Univ Wisconsin 1995; **Fac Appt:** Assoc Prof Med, Vanderbilt Univ

Medical Oncology

Bernard, Stephen MD [Onc] - **Spec Exp:** Gastrointestinal Cancer; Palliative Care; Clinical Trials; **Hospital:** Univ NC Hosps; **Address:** Univ North Carolina Sch Med, 170 Manning Drive, CB 7305, Chapel Hill, NC 27599; **Phone:** 919-966-0000; **Board Cert:** Internal Medicine 1987; Medical Oncology 1979; Hospice & Palliative Medicine 2004; **Med School:** Univ NC Sch Med 1973; **Resid:** Internal Medicine, Columbia-Presby Med Ctr 1976; **Fellow:** Hematology & Oncology, Wash Univ Hosps 1978; **Fac Appt:** Prof Med, Univ NC Sch Med

Bolger, Graeme B MD [Onc] - **Spec Exp:** Prostate Cancer; Testicular Cancer; **Hospital:** Univ of Ala Hosp at Birmingham; **Address:** 1530 3rd Ave S, Ste FOT-1105, Birmingham, AL 35294; **Phone:** 205-934-2992; **Board Cert:** Internal Medicine 1984; Medical Oncology 2000; **Med School:** McGill Univ 1981; **Resid:** Internal Medicine, Johns Hopkins Hosp 1984; **Fellow:** Medical Oncology, Fred Hutchinson Cancer Rsch 1985; Oncology, Meml Sloan-Kettering Cancer Ctr 1992; **Fac Appt:** Assoc Prof Med, Univ Alabama

Boston, Barry MD [Onc] - **Spec Exp:** Gastrointestinal Cancer; Genitourinary Cancer; Prostate Cancer; **Hospital:** St Francis Hosp - Memphis, Methodist Univ Hosp - Memphis; **Address:** Univ of Tennessee Cancer Inst, 7945 Wolf River Blvd, Ste 300, Germantown, TN 38138; **Phone:** 901-752-6131; **Board Cert:** Internal Medicine 1974; Medical Oncology 1977; **Med School:** Louisiana State U, New Orleans 1971; **Resid:** Internal Medicine, Univ Tenn Hosp-VA Hosp 1973; Hematology, Univ Tenn Hosp-VA Hosp 1973; **Fellow:** Medical Oncology, Yale-New Haven Hosp 1975; **Fac Appt:** Assoc Prof Med, Univ Tenn Coll Med, Memphis

Brescia, Frank J MD [Onc] - **Spec Exp:** Palliative Care; Breast Cancer; Gastrointestinal Cancer; Ethics; **Hospital:** Roper Hosp, MUSC Med Ctr; **Address:** Low Country Hematology & Oncology, 900 Bowman Drive, Mount Pleasant, SC 29464; **Phone:** 843-881-5844; **Board Cert:** Internal Medicine 1974; Medical Oncology 1975; **Med School:** UMDNJ-NJ Med Sch, Newark 1968; **Resid:** Internal Medicine, North Shore Univ Hosp 1970; **Fellow:** Medical Oncology, Meml Sloan Kettering Cancer Ctr 1974; **Fac Appt:** Prof Med, Med Univ SC

Burris III, Howard A MD [Onc] - **Spec Exp:** Drug Development; Drug Discovery; Breast Cancer; **Hospital:** Centennial Med Ctr, Baptist Hosp - Nashville; **Address:** 250 25th Ave N Atrium Bldg - Ste 100, Nashville, TN 37203; **Phone:** 615-329-7276; **Board Cert:** Internal Medicine 1988; Medical Oncology 2001; **Med School:** Univ S Ala Coll Med 1985; **Resid:** Internal Medicine, Brooke Army Med Ctr 1988; **Fellow:** Medical Oncology, Brooke Army Med Ctr 1991

Butler, William M MD [Onc] - **Spec Exp:** Breast Cancer; Prostate Cancer; Lung Cancer; Clinical Trials; **Hospital:** Palmetto Richland Mem Hosp; **Address:** SC Oncology Associates, 166 Stoneridge St, Columbia, SC 29210; **Phone:** 803-461-3000; **Board Cert:** Internal Medicine 1975; Hematology 1980; Medical Oncology 1979; **Med School:** Tulane Univ 1972; **Resid:** Internal Medicine, Charity Hosp 1975; **Fellow:** Hematology & Oncology, Walter Reed AMC 1980; **Fac Appt:** Clin Prof Med, Univ SC Sch Med

Carbone, David MD/PhD [Onc] - **Spec Exp:** Lung Cancer; **Hospital:** Vanderbilt Univ Med Ctr; **Address:** Vanderbilt-Ingram Cancer Ctr, 685 Preston Rsch Bldg, 2200 Pierce Ave, Nashville, TN 37232-6838; **Phone:** 615-936-1279; **Board Cert:** Internal Medicine 1988; Medical Oncology 2001; **Med School:** Johns Hopkins Univ 1985; **Resid:** Internal Medicine, Johns Hopkins Hosp 1988; **Fellow:** Oncology, Natl Cancer Inst 1991; **Fac Appt:** Prof Med, Vanderbilt Univ

Carey, Lisa A MD [Onc] - **Spec Exp:** Breast Cancer; **Hospital:** Univ NC Hosps; **Address:** Univ North Carolina-Div Hem/Onc, Campus Box 7305, 3009 Old Clinic Bldg, Chapel Hill, NC 27599; **Phone:** 919-966-4431; **Board Cert:** Internal Medicine 2003; Medical Oncology 2007; **Med School:** Johns Hopkins Univ 1990; **Resid:** Internal Medicine, Johns Hopkins Hosp 1993; **Fellow:** Oncology, Johns Hopkins Hosp 1996; **Fac Appt:** Asst Prof Med, Univ NC Sch Med

Carpenter Jr, John T MD [Onc] - **Spec Exp:** Breast Cancer; **Hospital:** Univ of Ala Hosp at Birmingham; **Address:** Univ Alabama Birmingham, 1530 3rd Ave S, Birmingham, AL 35294-3300; **Phone:** 205-934-2084; **Board Cert:** Internal Medicine 1972; Hematology 1981; Medical Oncology 1975; **Med School:** Tulane Univ 1968; **Resid:** Internal Medicine, Grady Meml Hosp 1971; **Fellow:** Hematology & Oncology, Emory Univ 1973; **Fac Appt:** Prof Med, Univ Alabama

Chao, Nelson Jen An MD [Onc] - **Spec Exp:** Bone Marrow Transplant; Lymphoma; Leukemia; **Hospital:** Duke Univ Med Ctr; **Address:** Duke Univ Med Ctr, Box 3961, Durham, NC 27710; **Phone:** 919-668-1002; **Board Cert:** Internal Medicine 1984; Medical Oncology 1987; **Med School:** Yale Univ 1981; **Resid:** Internal Medicine, Stanford Univ Med Ctr 1984; **Fellow:** Oncology, Stanford Univ Med Ctr 1987; **Fac Appt:** Prof Med, Duke Univ

Colon-Otero, Gerardo MD [Onc] - **Spec Exp:** Ovarian Cancer; Breast Cancer; Hematologic Malignancies; **Hospital:** Mayo - Jacksonville, St Luke's Hosp - Jacksonville; **Address:** Mayo Clinic Jacksonville, 4500 San Pablo Rd S, Jacksonville, FL 32224-1865; **Phone:** 904-953-2000; **Board Cert:** Internal Medicine 1982; Hematology 1984; Medical Oncology 1985; **Med School:** Puerto Rico 1979; **Resid:** Internal Medicine, Mayo Clinic 1982; **Fellow:** Hematology, Mayo Clinic 1984; Medical Oncology, Univ Va Med Ctr 1986; **Fac Appt:** Assoc Prof Med, Mayo Med Sch

Conry, Robert M MD [Onc] - **Spec Exp:** Melanoma; Lung Cancer; Colon & Rectal Cancer; Sarcoma; **Hospital:** Univ of Ala Hosp at Birmingham; **Address:** The Kirklin Clinic At Acton Rd, 2145 Bonner Way, Birmingham, AL 35243; **Phone:** 205-978-0250; **Board Cert:** Hematology 2001; **Med School:** Univ Alabama 1987; **Resid:** Internal Medicine, Univ Alabama Hosp 1990; **Fellow:** Medical Oncology, Univ Alabama Hosp 1993; **Fac Appt:** Assoc Prof Med, Univ Alabama

Crawford, Jeffrey MD [Onc] - **Spec Exp:** Lung Cancer; **Hospital:** Duke Univ Med Ctr; **Address:** Duke Univ Med Ctr, Box 3476, Durham, NC 27710-0001; **Phone:** 919-668-6688; **Board Cert:** Internal Medicine 1977; Hematology 1980; Medical Oncology 1981; **Med School:** Ohio State Univ 1974; **Resid:** Internal Medicine, Duke Univ Med Ctr 1977; **Fellow:** Hematology & Oncology, Duke Univ Med Ctr 1981; **Fac Appt:** Prof Med, Duke Univ

De Simone, Philip MD [Onc] - **Spec Exp:** Colon Cancer; Pancreatic Cancer; **Hospital:** Univ of Kentucky Chandler Hosp; **Address:** UKMC Markey Cancer Ctr, 800 Rose St, rm 134, Whitney-Hendrickson bldg, Lexington, KY 40536; **Phone:** 859-323-8043; **Board Cert:** Internal Medicine 1972; Hematology 1974; **Med School:** Univ VT Coll Med 1967; **Resid:** Internal Medicine, Univ Kentucky Hosp 1972; **Fellow:** Hematology & Oncology, Univ Kentucky Hosp 1974; **Fac Appt:** Prof Med, Univ KY Coll Med

Dunphy, Frank R MD [Onc] - **Spec Exp:** Lung Cancer; Head & Neck Cancer; **Hospital:** Duke Univ Med Ctr; **Address:** Duke Univ Med Ctr, Box 3685, Durham, NC 27710; **Phone:** 919-668-6688; **Board Cert:** Internal Medicine 1984; Hematology 1986; Medical Oncology 1989; **Med School:** Louisiana State U, New Orleans 1979; **Resid:** Internal Medicine, Lousiana St Univ Hosp 1983; **Fellow:** Hematology & Oncology, Louisiana St Univ Hosp 1985; **Fac Appt:** Assoc Prof Med, Duke Univ

Flinn, Ian W MD/PhD [Onc] - **Spec Exp:** Hematologic Malignancies; Lymphoma; Bone Marrow Transplant; Clinical Trials; **Hospital:** Centennial Med Ctr; **Address:** Tennessee Oncology, 250 25th Ave N, Ste 412, Nashville, TN 37203; **Phone:** 615-986-7600; **Board Cert:** Hematology 2007; Medical Oncology 2008; **Med School:** Johns Hopkins Univ 1990; **Resid:** Internal Medicine, Univ Michigan Med Ctr 1993; **Fellow:** Hematology & Oncology, Johns Hopkins Univ Hosps 1993

Forero, Andres MD [Onc] - **Spec Exp:** Lymphoma; **Hospital:** Univ of Ala Hosp at Birmingham; **Address:** 615 18th St S, Birmingham, AL 35233; **Phone:** 205-934-9999; **Med School:** Colombia 1982; **Resid:** Internal Medicine, Javeriana Univ 1987; **Fellow:** Medical Oncology, Javeriana Univ 1991; **Fac Appt:** Assoc Prof Med, Univ Alabama

Medical Oncology

Fracasso, Paula M MD/PhD [Onc] - **Spec Exp:** Gynecologic Cancer; Breast Cancer; **Hospital:** Univ Virginia Med Ctr; **Address:** Dept Medicine, Div Hem/Onc, PO Box 800716, Charlottesville, VA 22908; **Phone:** 434-243-6143; **Board Cert:** Internal Medicine 1987; Medical Oncology 2003; **Med School:** Yale Univ 1984; **Resid:** Internal Medicine, Beth Israel Hosp 1987; **Fellow:** Cancer Research, Mass Inst Tech 1989; Hematology & Oncology, Tufts-New England Med Ctr 1991; **Fac Appt:** Prof Med, Univ VA Sch Med

Garst, Jennifer L MD [Onc] - **Spec Exp:** Lung Cancer; Thoracic Cancers; Cancer Survivors-Late Effects of Therapy; **Hospital:** Duke Univ Med Ctr; **Address:** Reg Cancer Care Ctr, 4411 Ben Franklin Blvd, Durham, NC 27704; **Phone:** 919-477-0047; **Board Cert:** Internal Medicine 2008; **Med School:** Med Coll GA 1990; **Resid:** Internal Medicine, Univ SW Texas Hosp 1993; **Fellow:** Hematology & Oncology, Duke Univ Med Ctr 1996; **Fac Appt:** Assoc Prof Med, Duke Univ

Gockerman, Jon Paul MD [Onc] - **Spec Exp:** Leukemia; Lymphoma; **Hospital:** Duke Univ Med Ctr; **Address:** Duke Univ Med Ctr, 1 Trent Drive, rm 25153, Box 3872, Morris Bldg, Durham, NC 27710; **Phone:** 919-684-8964; **Board Cert:** Internal Medicine 1972; Hematology 1974; Medical Oncology 1973; **Med School:** Univ Chicago-Pritzker Sch Med 1967; **Resid:** Internal Medicine, Duke Univ Med Ctr 1969; **Fellow:** Hematology & Oncology, Duke Univ Med Ctr 1971

Godley, Paul A MD/PhD [Onc] - **Spec Exp:** Prostate Cancer (advanced); Testicular Cancer; Penile Cancer; Bladder Cancer; **Hospital:** Univ NC Hosps; **Address:** UNC Hematology/Oncology, 3009 Old Clinic Bldg, rm 7305, Chapel Hill, NC 27599; **Phone:** 919-966-4431; **Board Cert:** Internal Medicine 1987; Medical Oncology 2002; **Med School:** Harvard Med Sch 1984; **Resid:** Internal Medicine, Univ Hosps 1987; **Fellow:** Epidemiology, Univ NC Sch of Public Hlth 1989; Hematology & Oncology, Univ NC Hosps 1991; **Fac Appt:** Assoc Prof Med, Univ NC Sch Med

Goldberg, Richard M MD [Onc] - **Spec Exp:** Stomach Cancer; Esophageal Cancer; Pancreatic Cancer; Neuroendocrine Tumors; **Hospital:** Univ NC Hosps; **Address:** Division of Hematology/Oncology, CB 7305, 3009 Old Clinic Bldg SW, Chapel Hill, NC 27599-0001; **Phone:** 919-843-7711; **Board Cert:** Internal Medicine 1982; Medical Oncology 1985; **Med School:** SUNY Upstate Med Univ 1979; **Resid:** Internal Medicine, Emory Univ Med Ctr 1982; **Fellow:** Medical Oncology, Georgetown Univ Med Ctr 1984; **Fac Appt:** Prof Med, Univ NC Sch Med

Graham II, Mark L MD [Onc] - **Spec Exp:** Breast Cancer; Breast Cancer Genetics; **Hospital:** WakeMed Cary; **Address:** Waverly Hematology/Oncology, 300 Ashville Ave, Ste 310, Cary, NC 27518; **Phone:** 919-233-8585; **Board Cert:** Internal Medicine 1989; **Med School:** Mayo Med Sch 1982; **Resid:** Internal Medicine, Duke Univ Med Ctr 1985; **Fellow:** Medical Oncology, Univ CO Hlth Sci Ctr 1990; Medical Oncology, Mayo Clinic 1991; **Fac Appt:** Assoc Clin Prof Med, Univ NC Sch Med

Greco, F Anthony MD [Onc] - **Spec Exp:** Lung Cancer; Unknown Primary Cancer; **Hospital:** Centennial Med Ctr; **Address:** Sarah Cannon Research Inst, 250 25th Ave N Atrium Bldg - Ste 100, Nashville, TN 37203; **Phone:** 615-320-5090; **Board Cert:** Internal Medicine 1975; Medical Oncology 1977; **Med School:** W VA Univ 1972; **Resid:** Internal Medicine, Univ West Virginia Hosp 1974; **Fellow:** Medical Oncology, Natl Cancer Inst 1976

Grosh, William W MD [Onc] - **Spec Exp:** Melanoma; Sarcoma; Neuroendocrine Tumors; **Hospital:** Univ Virginia Med Ctr; **Address:** UVA Health System, Div Hem/Oncology, PO Box 800716, Charlottesville, VA 22908; **Phone:** 434-924-1904; **Board Cert:** Internal Medicine 1978; Medical Oncology 1985; **Med School:** Columbia P&S 1974; **Resid:** Internal Medicine, Vanderbilt Univ Med Ctr 1977; **Fellow:** Medical Oncology, Vanderbilt Univ Med Ctr 1983; **Fac Appt:** Assoc Prof Med, Univ VA Sch Med

Hande, Kenneth R MD [Onc] - **Spec Exp:** Drug Discovery; Sarcoma; Carcinoid Tumors; **Hospital:** Vanderbilt Univ Med Ctr, VA Med Ctr - Nashville; **Address:** Vanderbilt Univ Med Ctr, 777 Preston Research Building, Nashville, TN 37232-6307; **Phone:** 615-322-4967; **Board Cert:** Internal Medicine 1975; Medical Oncology 1977; **Med School:** Johns Hopkins Univ 1972; **Resid:** Internal Medicine, Barnes Hosp 1974; **Fellow:** Medical Oncology, Natl Cancer Inst 1977; **Fac Appt:** Prof Med, Vanderbilt Univ

Hurd, David MD [Onc] - **Spec Exp:** Lymphoma; Leukemia; Bone Marrow Transplant; **Hospital:** Wake Forest Univ Baptist Med Ctr (page 72); **Address:** Wake Forest Sch Med, Comp Cancer Ctr, Medical Center Boulevard, Winston-Salem, NC 27157-1082; **Phone:** 336-713-5440; **Board Cert:** Internal Medicine 1977; Medical Oncology 1981; **Med School:** Univ IL Coll Med 1974; **Resid:** Internal Medicine, Univ Minn Hosp 1977; **Fellow:** Medical Oncology, Univ Minn Hosp 1979; **Fac Appt:** Prof Med, Wake Forest Univ

Jahanzeb, Mohammad MD [Onc] - **Spec Exp:** Breast Cancer; Lung Cancer; **Hospital:** Boca Raton Comm Hosp; **Address:** 21020 State Rd 7, Boca Raton, FL 33428; **Phone:** 561-883-7600; **Board Cert:** Medical Oncology 2003; Hematology 2005; **Med School:** Pakistan 1986; **Resid:** Internal Medicine, New Britain Genl Hosp 1990; **Fellow:** Hematology & Oncology, Washington Univ 1993

Jillella, Anand MD [Onc] - **Spec Exp:** Bone Marrow Transplant; Leukemia; Lymphoma; Multiple Myeloma; **Hospital:** Med Coll of GA Hosp and Clin (MCG Health Inc); **Address:** Med Coll Ga - BMT Program, 1120 15th St, BAA 5407, Augusta, GA 30912-3125; **Phone:** 706-721-2505; **Board Cert:** Medical Oncology 1997; **Med School:** India 1985; **Resid:** Internal Medicine, Med Coll Georgia 1992; **Fellow:** Medical Oncology, Yale-New Haven Hosp 1996; **Fac Appt:** Prof Med, Med Coll GA

Johnson, David H MD [Onc] - **Spec Exp:** Lung Cancer; Breast Cancer; Drug Development; **Hospital:** Vanderbilt Univ Med Ctr; **Address:** Vanderbilt Univ Med Ctr, Div Med Onc, 2220 Pierce Ave, 777 PRB, Nashville, TN 37232-0021; **Phone:** 615-322-6053; **Board Cert:** Internal Medicine 1979; Medical Oncology 2008; **Med School:** Med Coll GA 1976; **Resid:** Internal Medicine, Univ South Alabama Med Ctr 1979; Internal Medicine, Med Coll Georgia Hosps 1980; **Fellow:** Medical Oncology, Vanderbilt Univ Med Ctr 1983; **Fac Appt:** Prof Med, Vanderbilt Univ

Khuri, Fadlo MD [Onc] - **Spec Exp:** Lung Cancer; Head & Neck Cancer; **Hospital:** Emory Univ Hosp, Grady Hlth Sys; **Address:** Winship Cancer Institute, 1365 Clifton Rd NE, C Bldg Fl 2, Atlanta, GA 30322; **Phone:** 404-778-1900; **Board Cert:** Medical Oncology 2008; **Med School:** Columbia P&S 1989; **Resid:** Internal Medicine, Boston City Hosp 1992; **Fellow:** Medical Oncology, New England Med Ctr-Tufts 1995; **Fac Appt:** Prof Hem & Onc, Emory Univ

Kraft, Andrew S MD [Onc] - **Spec Exp:** Prostate Cancer; Sarcoma; Drug Development; Clinical Trials; **Hospital:** MUSC Med Ctr; **Address:** 86 Jonathan Lucas St, PO BOX 250955, Charleston, SC 29425; **Phone:** 843-792-8284; **Board Cert:** Internal Medicine 1980; Medical Oncology 1985; **Med School:** Univ Pennsylvania 1975; **Resid:** Internal Medicine, Mt Sinai Hosp 1979; **Fellow:** Medical Oncology, Natl Cancer Inst 1983; **Fac Appt:** Prof Med, Med Univ SC

Kucuk, Omer MD [Onc] - **Spec Exp:** Genitourinary Cancer; Nutrition in Cancer Therapy; Prostate Cancer; Nutrition & Cancer Prevention/Control; **Hospital:** Emory Univ Hosp; **Address:** Winship Cancer Inst, 1365C Clifton Rd, Ste 2110, Atlanta, GA 30322; **Phone:** 404-778-1900; **Board Cert:** Internal Medicine 1978; Hematology 1984; Medical Oncology 1989; **Med School:** Turkey 1975; **Resid:** Internal Medicine, St Francis Hosp 1978; **Fellow:** Hematology & Oncology, Northwestern Univ 1981; **Fac Appt:** Prof Hem & Onc, Emory Univ

Medical Oncology

Kvols, Larry K MD [Onc] - **Spec Exp:** Gastrointestinal Cancer; Carcinoid Tumors; Neuroendocrine Tumors; **Hospital:** H Lee Moffitt Cancer Ctr & Research Inst; **Address:** H Lee Moffitt Cancer Ctr & Research Inst, 12902 Magnolia Drive, WCB-GI Program, Tampa, FL 33612-9497; **Phone:** 813-745-7257; **Board Cert:** Internal Medicine 1976; Medical Oncology 1977; **Med School:** Baylor Coll Med 1970; **Resid:** Internal Medicine, Johns Hopkins Hosp 1972; **Fellow:** Hematology & Oncology, Johns Hopkins Hosp 1973; **Fac Appt:** Prof Med, Mayo Med Sch

Lawson, David H MD [Onc] - **Spec Exp:** Melanoma; **Hospital:** Emory Univ Hosp; **Address:** Winship Cancer Institute, 1365 Clifton Rd NE C Bldg, Atlanta, GA 30322; **Phone:** 404-778-1900; **Board Cert:** Internal Medicine 1977; Medical Oncology 1979; **Med School:** Emory Univ 1974; **Resid:** Internal Medicine, Emory Univ Hosps 1977; **Fellow:** Medical Oncology, Emory Univ Hosps 1979; **Fac Appt:** Assoc Prof Med, Emory Univ

Lesser, Glenn J MD [Onc] - **Spec Exp:** Neuro-Oncology; Brain Tumors; **Hospital:** Wake Forest Univ Baptist Med Ctr (page 72); **Address:** Wake Forest Univ-Div Hematolgy/Oncology, Medical Center Blvd, Winston-Salem, NC 27157-1082; **Phone:** 336-716-9527; **Board Cert:** Medical Oncology 2007; **Med School:** Penn State Univ-Hershey Med Ctr 1987; **Resid:** Internal Medicine, NC Baptist Hosp/Bowman Gray Sch Med 1991; **Fellow:** Medical Oncology, Johns Hopkins Hosp 1994; **Fac Appt:** Assoc Prof Med, Wake Forest Univ

Lilenbaum, Rogerio MD [Onc] - **Spec Exp:** Lung Cancer; **Hospital:** Mount Sinai Med Ctr - Miami; **Address:** Mount Sinai Cancer Ctr, 4306 Alton Rd, Ste 3, Miami, FL 33140-2840; **Phone:** 305-535-3310; **Board Cert:** Internal Medicine 2005; Hematology 1998; Medical Oncology 2007; **Med School:** Brazil 1986; **Resid:** Internal Medicine, Univ Hosp-Rio de Janeiro 1989; **Fellow:** Hematology & Oncology, Washington Univ Sch Med 1992; Oncology, UCSD 1994; **Fac Appt:** Assoc Clin Prof Med, Univ Miami Sch Med

Limentani, Steven A MD [Onc] - **Spec Exp:** Breast Cancer; Multiple Myeloma; Clinical Trials; **Hospital:** Carolinas Med Ctr; **Address:** 1100 S Tryon St, Ste 400, Charlotte, NC 28203; **Phone:** 704-446-9046; **Board Cert:** Internal Medicine 1989; Medical Oncology 2001; Hematology 2002; **Med School:** Tufts Univ 1986; **Resid:** Internal Medicine, New England Deaconess Hosp 1989; **Fellow:** Hematology & Oncology, New England Med Ctr 1992; **Fac Appt:** Clin Prof Med, Univ NC Sch Med

Lippman, Marc E MD [Onc] - **Spec Exp:** Breast Cancer; **Hospital:** Univ of Miami Hosp & Clins/Sylvester Comp Canc Ctr (page 70); **Address:** Leonard M Miller Sch Med, Dept Med, 1430 NW 11th Ave, MTSL, Ste 1001, Miami, FL 33136; **Phone:** 305-243-9120; **Board Cert:** Internal Medicine 1987; Endocrinology 1975; Medical Oncology 1977; **Med School:** Yale Univ 1968; **Resid:** Internal Medicine, Johns Hopkins Hosp 1970; **Fellow:** Medical Oncology, Natl Cancer Inst 1973; Endocrinology, Yale-New Haven Hosp 1974; **Fac Appt:** Prof Med, Univ Mich Med Sch

Lossos, Izidore MD [Onc] - **Spec Exp:** Lymphoma; Hodgkin's Disease; Leukemia; **Hospital:** Univ of Miami Hosp & Clins/Sylvester Comp Canc Ctr (page 70), Jackson Meml Hosp (page 70); **Address:** Univ Miami - Sylvester Comp Cancer Ctr, 1475 NW 12th Ave, D8-4, Miami, FL 33136; **Phone:** 305-243-4785; **Med School:** Israel 1987; **Resid:** Internal Medicine, Hadassah Univ Hosp 1995; **Fellow:** Hematology & Oncology, Hadassah Univ Hosp 1997; Medical Oncology, Stanford Univ 2001; **Fac Appt:** Prof Med, Univ Miami Sch Med

Lyckholm, Laurel J MD [Onc] - **Spec Exp:** Neuro-Oncology; **Hospital:** Med Coll of VA Hosp; **Address:** Med Coll of VA, Div Hem/Onc, PO Box 980230, Richmond, VA 23298; **Phone:** 804-828-9723; **Board Cert:** Internal Medicine 1989; Medical Oncology 2003; Hematology 2004; **Med School:** Creighton Univ 1985; **Resid:** Internal Medicine, Creighton Univ 1989; **Fellow:** Hematology & Oncology, Univ IA Coll Med 1992; **Fac Appt:** Assoc Prof Med, Med Coll VA

Lyman, Gary H MD [Onc] - **Spec Exp:** Breast Cancer; **Hospital:** Duke Univ Med Ctr; **Address:** Duke Comprehensive Cancer Center, Hock Plaza, 2424 Erwin Rd, Ste 602 - rm 6038, Box 3645, Durham, NC 27710; **Phone:** 919-681-1736; **Board Cert:** Internal Medicine 1987; Medical Oncology 1977; Hematology 1978; **Med School:** SUNY Buffalo 1972; **Resid:** Internal Medicine, Univ North Carolina Hosp 1974; **Fellow:** Medical Oncology, Roswell Park Meml Inst 1976; Biostatistics, Harvard Med Sch 1982; **Fac Appt:** Prof Med, Duke Univ

Lynch Jr, James W MD [Onc] - **Spec Exp:** Lymphoma; Immunotherapy; Lung Cancer; **Hospital:** Shands at Univ of FL; **Address:** Shands Hlthcare, Div Hematology/Oncology, PO Box 100383, Gainesville, FL 32610-0383; **Phone:** 352-265-0725; **Board Cert:** Internal Medicine 1987; Medical Oncology 2001; **Med School:** Eastern VA Med Sch 1984; **Resid:** Internal Medicine, Univ Florida 1987; **Fellow:** Medical Oncology, Natl Cancer Inst 1991; **Fac Appt:** Prof Med, Univ Fla Coll Med

Marcom, Paul K MD [Onc] - **Spec Exp:** Breast Cancer; Clinical Trials; Cancer Genetics; **Hospital:** Duke Univ Med Ctr; **Address:** Duke Univ Med Ctr, Box 3147, Seeley G Mudd Bldg, Ste 461, Durham, NC 27710; **Phone:** 919-684-3877; **Board Cert:** Internal Medicine 2003; Medical Oncology 2005; **Med School:** Baylor Coll Med 1989; **Resid:** Internal Medicine, Duke Univ Med Ctr 1992; Hematology & Oncology, Duke Univ Med Ctr 1995; **Fac Appt:** Assoc Prof Med, Duke Univ

Miller, Antonius A MD [Onc] - **Spec Exp:** Lung Cancer; **Hospital:** Wake Forest Univ Baptist Med Ctr (page 72); **Address:** Wake Forest Baptist Med Ctr, Comp Cancer Ctr, 3rd Fl (Hem/Onc), Medical Center Boulevard, Winston-Salem, NC 27157; **Phone:** 336-713-4392; **Med School:** Germany 1977; **Resid:** Internal Medicine, Univ Essen Med Sch 1979; **Fellow:** Hematology & Oncology, UT MD Anderson Cancer Ctr 1981; **Fac Appt:** Prof Med, Wake Forest Univ

Miller, Donald M MD/PhD [Onc] - **Spec Exp:** Melanoma; Lung Cancer; **Hospital:** Univ of Louisville Hosp; **Address:** 529 S Jackson St, Louisville, KY 40202; **Phone:** 502-562-4790; **Board Cert:** Internal Medicine 1979; **Med School:** Duke Univ 1973; **Resid:** Internal Medicine, Peter Bent Brigham Hosp 1975; **Fellow:** Internal Medicine, Peter Bent Brigham Hosp 1978; Medical Oncology, Natl Cancer Inst 1979; **Fac Appt:** Prof Med, Univ Louisville Sch Med

Moore, Joseph O MD [Onc] - **Spec Exp:** Leukemia; Hodgkin's Disease; Lymphoma, Non-Hodgkin's; Neuroendocrine Tumors; **Hospital:** Duke Univ Med Ctr; **Address:** Duke Univ Med Ctr, Box 3872, Durham, NC 27710; **Phone:** 919-684-8964; **Board Cert:** Internal Medicine 1975; Medical Oncology 1977; **Med School:** Johns Hopkins Univ 1970; **Resid:** Internal Medicine, Johns Hopkins Hosp 1975; **Fellow:** Hematology & Oncology, Duke Univ 1977; **Fac Appt:** Prof Med, Duke Univ

Muss, Hyman B MD [Onc] - **Spec Exp:** Breast Cancer; **Hospital:** Univ NC Hosps; **Address:** Div of Hem/Onc, Physicians Office Bldg, 170 Manning Drive Fl 3 - rm 3120, Box 7305, Chapel Hill, NC 27599-7305; **Phone:** 919-966-0840; **Board Cert:** Internal Medicine 1973; Hematology 1974; Medical Oncology 1975; **Med School:** SUNY Downstate 1968; **Resid:** Internal Medicine, Peter Bent Brigham Hosp 1971; **Fellow:** Hematology & Oncology, Peter Bent Brigham Hosp 1974

Nabell, Lisle M MD [Onc] - **Spec Exp:** Breast Cancer; Head & Neck Cancer; **Hospital:** Univ of Ala Hosp at Birmingham; **Address:** Univ of Alabama, 1530 3rd Ave S, Ste WTI237, Birmingham, AL 35294; **Phone:** 205-934-3061; **Board Cert:** Internal Medicine 2000; Medical Oncology 2000; **Med School:** Univ NC Sch Med 1987; **Resid:** Internal Medicine, Univ Alabama Hosp 1990; **Fellow:** Hematology & Oncology, Univ Alabama Hosp 1992; **Fac Appt:** Assoc Prof Med, Univ Alabama

O'Regan, Ruth M MD [Onc] - **Spec Exp:** Breast Cancer; Breast Cancer Risk Assessment; Cancer Prevention; Clinical Trials; **Hospital:** Emory Univ Hosp; **Address:** Emory Univ Winship Cancer Inst, 1365C Clifton Rd, Ste 4005, Atlanta, GA 30322; **Phone:** 404-778-1900; **Board Cert:** Internal Medicine 1999; Medical Oncology 2000; **Med School:** Ireland 1988; **Resid:** Internal Medicine, Med Coll Wisconsin 1995; Medical Oncology, Northwestern Univ Hosp 1999; **Fellow:** Medical Oncology, Northwestern Univ Hosp 1998; **Fac Appt:** Assoc Prof Med, Emory Univ

Pasche, Boris C MD/PhD [Onc] - **Spec Exp:** Cancer Genetics; Gastrointestinal Cancer; **Hospital:** Univ of Ala Hosp at Birmingham; **Address:** 2000 Morris Ave, Ste 1610, Birmingham, AL 35203; **Phone:** 205-934-9591; **Board Cert:** Medical Oncology 2008; Hematology 1999; **Med School:** Sweden 1986; **Resid:** Internal Medicine, NY Hosp/Cornell Med Ctr 1994; **Fellow:** Hematology & Oncology, Meml Sloan Kettering Cancer Ctr 1996; **Fac Appt:** Assoc Prof Med, Northwestern Univ

Perez, Edith A MD [Onc] - **Spec Exp:** Breast Cancer; Breast Cancer Risk Assessment; Clinical Trials; **Hospital:** Mayo - Jacksonville; **Address:** Mayo Clinic-Jacksonville, 4500 San Pablo Rd Davis Bldg Fl 8, Jacksonville, FL 32224; **Phone:** 904-953-7283; **Board Cert:** Internal Medicine 1983; Hematology 1986; Medical Oncology 1987; **Med School:** Univ Puerto Rico 1979; **Resid:** Internal Medicine, Loma Linda Univ Med Ctr 1982; **Fellow:** Hematology & Oncology, Martinez VA Hosp/UC Davis 1987; **Fac Appt:** Prof Med, Mayo Med Sch

Posey III, James A MD [Onc] - **Spec Exp:** Gastrointestinal Cancer; Colon Cancer; Liver Cancer; Biliary Cancer; **Hospital:** Univ of Ala Hosp at Birmingham; **Address:** 1806 6th Ave S, NP-2540U, Birmingham, AL 35294-3300; **Phone:** 205-934-0916; **Board Cert:** Medical Oncology 1997; **Med School:** Howard Univ 1991; **Resid:** Internal Medicine, Georgetown Univ Med Ctr 1994; **Fellow:** Hematology & Oncology, Georgetown Univ Med Ctr 1997; **Fac Appt:** Assoc Prof Med, Univ Alabama

Ready, Neal E MD/PhD [Onc] - **Spec Exp:** Lung Cancer; Head & Neck Cancer; Clinical Trials; **Hospital:** Duke Univ Med Ctr; **Address:** Duke Univ Medical Ctr, DUMC, Box 3198, Durham, NC 27710; **Phone:** 919-681-6932; **Board Cert:** Internal Medicine 1989; Hematology 2005; Medical Oncology 2005; **Med School:** Vanderbilt Univ 1986; **Resid:** Internal Medicine, Rhode Island Hosp 1989; **Fellow:** Hematology, Rhode Island Hosp 1992; Medical Oncology, New England Med Ctr 1994

Robert, Nicholas J MD [Onc] - **Spec Exp:** Breast Cancer; **Hospital:** Inova Fairfax Hosp; **Address:** 8503 Arlington Blvd, Ste 400, Fairfax, VA 22031; **Phone:** 703-280-5390; **Board Cert:** Internal Medicine 1978; Anatomic Pathology 1979; Medical Oncology 1981; Hematology 1984; **Med School:** McGill Univ 1974; **Resid:** Internal Medicine, Royal Victoria Hosp 1976; Pathology, Mass Genl Hosp 1979; **Fellow:** Hematology, Peter Bent Brigham Hosp 1980; Medical Oncology, Dana Farber Cancer Inst 1981

Robert-Vizcarrondo, Francisco MD [Onc] - **Spec Exp:** Lung Cancer; Mesothelioma; Drug Development; Clinical Trials; **Hospital:** Univ of Ala Hosp at Birmingham; **Address:** 1802 6th Ave S, rm NP-2555D, Birmingham, AL 35294-0001; **Phone:** 205-934-5077; **Board Cert:** Internal Medicine 1973; Medical Oncology 1975; Hematology 1976; **Med School:** Puerto Rico 1969; **Resid:** Internal Medicine, Univ PR Hosp 1972; Hematology, Univ PR Hosp 1974; **Fellow:** Medical Oncology, Univ AL Hosp at Birmingham 1976; **Fac Appt:** Prof Med, Univ Alabama

Romond, Edward H MD [Onc] - **Spec Exp:** Breast Cancer; Hemophilia; **Hospital:** Univ of Kentucky Chandler Hosp; **Address:** Univ Kentucky Med Ctr, Div Hematology/Oncology, CC413 Markey Cancer Center, Lexington, KY 40536-0093; **Phone:** 859-323-8043; **Board Cert:** Internal Medicine 1980; Hematology 1984; Medical Oncology 1983; **Med School:** Univ KY Coll Med 1977; **Resid:** Internal Medicine, Michigan State Univ Hosps 1980; **Fellow:** Hematology & Oncology, Michigan State Univ 1983; **Fac Appt:** Prof Med, Univ KY Coll Med

Roth, Bruce J MD [Onc] - **Spec Exp:** Prostate Cancer; Bladder Cancer; Testicular Cancer; **Hospital:** Vanderbilt Univ Med Ctr; **Address:** Vanderbilt Ingram Cancer Center, 777 Preston Research Bldg, Nashville, TN 37232-6307; **Phone:** 615-343-4070; **Board Cert:** Internal Medicine 1983; Medical Oncology 1985; **Med School:** St Louis Univ 1980; **Resid:** Internal Medicine, Indiana Univ Med Ctr 1983; **Fellow:** Hematology & Oncology, Indiana Univ Med Ctr 1986; **Fac Appt:** Prof Med, Vanderbilt Univ

Schwartz, Michael A MD [Onc] - **Spec Exp:** Breast Cancer; Lymphoma; Colon Cancer; **Hospital:** Mount Sinai Med Ctr - Miami, Miami Heart Inst; **Address:** 4306 Alton Rd Fl 3, Miami Beach, FL 33140; **Phone:** 305-535-3310; **Board Cert:** Internal Medicine 1989; Medical Oncology 2004; Hematology 2004; **Med School:** UMDNJ-RW Johnson Med Sch 1986; **Resid:** Internal Medicine, Mt Sinai Medical Ctr 1989; **Fellow:** Hematology & Oncology, Meml Sloan Kettering Cancer Ctr 1992; **Fac Appt:** Asst Clin Prof Med, Univ Miami Sch Med

Serody, Jonathan S MD [Onc] - **Spec Exp:** Breast Cancer Vaccine Therapy; Clinical Trials; Lymphoma; **Hospital:** Univ NC Hosps; **Address:** Lineberger Comprehensive Cancer Ctr, 450 West Drive, CB 7295, Chapel Hill, NC 27599-7295; **Phone:** 919-966-8644; **Board Cert:** Internal Medicine 1989; Hematology 2007; **Med School:** Univ VA Sch Med 1986; **Resid:** Internal Medicine, Univ NC Med Ctr 1989; **Fellow:** Hematology, Univ NC Med Ctr 1992; Bone Marrow Transplant, Fred Hutchinson Transplant Program 1993; **Fac Appt:** Assoc Prof Med, Univ NC Sch Med

Shea, Thomas MD [Onc] - **Spec Exp:** Bone Marrow Transplant; Lymphoma; Leukemia; **Hospital:** Univ NC Hosps; **Address:** Univ N Carolina, Dept Medicine, 170 Manning Drive, CB 7305, Chapel Hill, NC 27599; **Phone:** 919-966-7746; **Board Cert:** Internal Medicine 1982; Hematology 1984; Medical Oncology 1985; **Med School:** Univ NC Sch Med 1978; **Resid:** Internal Medicine, Beth Israel Deaconess Med Ctr 1982; **Fellow:** Hematology & Oncology, Beth Israel Deaconess Med Ctr 1985; Bone Marrow Transplant, Dana Farber Cancer Inst 1988; **Fac Appt:** Prof Med, Univ NC Sch Med

Sherman, Carol A MD [Onc] - **Spec Exp:** Lung Cancer; Thoracic Cancers; **Hospital:** MUSC Med Ctr; **Address:** 96 Jonathan Lucas St, Ste CSB-903, Charleston, SC 29425; **Phone:** 843-792-9621; **Board Cert:** Internal Medicine 1987; Medical Oncology 1989; **Med School:** Univ Mass Sch Med 1984; **Resid:** Internal Medicine, Univ Mass Med Ctr 1987; **Fellow:** Hematology & Oncology, Univ Mass Med Ctr 1989; **Fac Appt:** Assoc Prof Med, Med Univ SC

Shin, Dong Moon MD [Onc] - **Spec Exp:** Head & Neck Cancer; Cancer Prevention; Mesothelioma; Thymoma; **Hospital:** Emory Univ Hosp; **Address:** Emory Winship Cancer Inst, 1365 C Clifton Rd NE, Ste 3090, Atlanta, GA 30322; **Phone:** 404-778-5990; **Board Cert:** Internal Medicine 1985; Medical Oncology 1989; **Med School:** South Korea 1975; **Resid:** Internal Medicine, Cook Co Hosp 1985; **Fellow:** Medical Oncology, Univ Texas MD Anderson Cancer Ctr 1986; **Fac Appt:** Prof Med, Emory Univ

Smith, Thomas Joseph MD [Onc] - **Spec Exp:** Breast Cancer; Palliative Care; **Hospital:** Med Coll of VA Hosp; **Address:** Med Coll Va, Div Hem/Onc, PO Box 980230, Richmond, VA 23298-0230; **Phone:** 804-828-9992; **Board Cert:** Internal Medicine 1982; Medical Oncology 1987; Hospice & Palliative Medicine 2003; **Med School:** Yale Univ 1979; **Resid:** Internal Medicine, Hosp Univ Penn 1982; **Fellow:** Medical Oncology, Med Coll Virginia 1987; **Fac Appt:** Prof Med, Med Coll VA

Socinski, Mark A MD [Onc] - **Spec Exp:** Lung Cancer; **Hospital:** Univ NC Hosps; **Address:** UNC Chapel Hill, Div Hem/Onc, 170 Manning Drive, CB 7305, Chapel Hill, NC 27599-7305; **Phone:** 919-966-0000; **Board Cert:** Internal Medicine 1988; Medical Oncology 2002; **Med School:** Univ VT Coll Med 1984; **Resid:** Internal Medicine, Beth Israel Hosp 1986; **Fellow:** Medical Oncology, Dana-Farber Cancer Inst 1989; **Fac Appt:** Assoc Prof Med, Univ NC Sch Med

Medical Oncology

Sosman, Jeffrey MD [Onc] - **Spec Exp:** Kidney Cancer; Melanoma; Drug Discovery; **Hospital:** Vanderbilt Univ Med Ctr; **Address:** Vanderbilt Ingram Cancer Ctr, 777 Preston Research Bldg, Nashville, TN 37232-6307; **Phone:** 615-322-4967; **Board Cert:** Anatomic Pathology 1985; Internal Medicine 1987; Medical Oncology 1989; **Med School:** Albert Einstein Coll Med 1981; **Resid:** Anatomic Pathology, Univ Chicago Hosps 1985; Internal Medicine, Univ Wisconsin Hosp 1986; **Fellow:** Medical Oncology, Univ Wisconsin 1989; **Fac Appt:** Clin Prof Med, Vanderbilt Univ

Sotomayor, Eduardo M MD [Onc] - **Spec Exp:** Lymphoma; Gene Therapy; Vaccine Therapy; Clinical Trials; **Hospital:** H Lee Moffitt Cancer Ctr & Research Inst; **Address:** H Lee Moffitt Cancer Inst, 12902 Magnolia Drive, MRC 3 East, Ste 3056D, Tampa, FL 33612; **Phone:** 813-745-1387; **Med School:** Peru 1988; **Resid:** Internal Medicine, Univ Miami Sch Med 1995; **Fellow:** Immunology, Univ Mlami Sch Med 1989; Oncology, Johns Hopkins Hosp 1998; **Fac Appt:** Assoc Prof Med, Univ S Fla Coll Med

Stone, Joel MD [Onc] - **Spec Exp:** Lung Cancer; Breast Cancer; **Hospital:** St Vincent's Med Ctr - Jacksonville; **Address:** St Vincent's Med Ctr, 2 Shircliff Way, Ste 800, Jacksonville, FL 32204; **Phone:** 904-388-2619; **Board Cert:** Internal Medicine 1977; Medical Oncology 1979; **Med School:** Univ VA Sch Med 1974; **Resid:** Internal Medicine, Univ KY Med Ctr 1977; **Fellow:** Hematology & Oncology, Emory Univ 1979

Sutton, Linda Marie MD [Onc] - **Spec Exp:** Breast Cancer; Palliative Care; **Hospital:** Duke Univ Med Ctr; **Address:** University Tower, 3100 Tower Blvd, Ste 600, Durham, NC 27707; **Phone:** 919-419-5005; **Board Cert:** Internal Medicine 2002; Medical Oncology 2003; **Med School:** Univ Mass Sch Med 1987; **Resid:** Internal Medicine, Montefiore Med Ctr 1990; **Fellow:** Hematology & Oncology, Duke Univ Med Ctr 1993

Thigpen, James T MD [Onc] - **Spec Exp:** Gynecologic Cancer; Breast Cancer; Lung Cancer; **Hospital:** Univ Mississippi Med Ctr; **Address:** Univ Mississippi Med Ctr, Div Med Onc, 2500 N State St, Jackson, MS 39216; **Phone:** 601-984-5590; **Board Cert:** Internal Medicine 1972; Hematology 1974; Medical Oncology 1975; **Med School:** Univ Miss 1969; **Resid:** Internal Medicine, Univ Miss Med Ctr 1971; **Fellow:** Hematology & Oncology, Univ Miss Med Ctr 1973; **Fac Appt:** Prof Med, Univ Miss

Torti, Frank M MD [Onc] - **Spec Exp:** Prostate Cancer; Urologic Cancer; **Hospital:** Wake Forest Univ Baptist Med Ctr (page 72); **Address:** Wake Forest Med Ctr-Comp Cancer Ctr, Medical Center Blvd, Winston-Salem, NC 27157-1082; **Phone:** 336-716-7971; **Board Cert:** Internal Medicine 1978; Medical Oncology 1979; **Med School:** Harvard Med Sch 1974; **Resid:** Internal Medicine, Beth Israel Hosp 1976; **Fellow:** Medical Oncology, Stanford Univ Med Ctr 1979; **Fac Appt:** Prof Med, Wake Forest Univ

Troner, Michael MD [Onc] - **Spec Exp:** Head & Neck Cancer; Urologic Cancer; **Hospital:** Baptist Hosp of Miami; **Address:** 8940 N Kendall Drive, Ste 300, East Tower, Miami, FL 33176-2132; **Phone:** 305-595-2141; **Board Cert:** Internal Medicine 1972; Medical Oncology 1973; **Med School:** SUNY Downstate 1968; **Resid:** Internal Medicine, Univ Maryland Hosp 1971; **Fellow:** Medical Oncology, Univ Miami Med Ctr 1973; **Fac Appt:** Assoc Clin Prof Med, Univ Miami Sch Med

Vance, Ralph MD [Onc] - **Spec Exp:** Lung Cancer; **Hospital:** Univ Mississippi Med Ctr; **Address:** Univ Mississippi Med Ctr, Div Med Onc, 2500 N State St, Jackson, MS 39216; **Phone:** 601-984-5590; **Med School:** Univ Miss 1972; **Resid:** Internal Medicine, Univ Hosp; **Fellow:** Hematology & Oncology, Univ Hosp; **Fac Appt:** Prof Med, Univ Miss

Vaughan, William P MD [Onc] - **Spec Exp:** Bone Marrow Transplant; Breast Cancer; **Hospital:** Univ of Ala Hosp at Birmingham; **Address:** 1900 University Blvd, rm 541, Tinsley Harrison Twr, Birmingham, AL 35294; **Phone:** 205-934-1908; **Board Cert:** Internal Medicine 1975; Medical Oncology 1979; **Med School:** Univ Conn 1972; **Resid:** Internal Medicine, Univ Chicago Hosps 1975; **Fellow:** Oncology, Johns Hopkins Hosp 1977; **Fac Appt:** Prof Med, Univ Alabama

Weber, Jeffrey S MD/PhD [Onc] - **Spec Exp:** Melanoma; **Hospital:** H Lee Moffitt Cancer Ctr & Research Inst; **Address:** H Lee Moffitt Cancer Ctr, 12902 Magnolia Ave, MS SRB-2, Tampa, FL 33612; **Phone:** 813-745-2691; **Board Cert:** Internal Medicine 1983; Medical Oncology 1987; **Med School:** NYU Sch Med 1980; **Resid:** Internal Medicine, UCSD Med Ctr 1983; **Fellow:** Medical Oncology, Natl Cancer Inst 1990; **Fac Appt:** Assoc Prof Med, USC Sch Med

Weiss, Geoffrey R MD [Onc] - **Spec Exp:** Gastrointestinal Cancer; Genitourinary Cancer; Melanoma; **Hospital:** Univ Virginia Med Ctr; **Address:** Univ Virginia Hlth System, Div Hem/Onc, PO Box 800716, Charlottesville, VA 22908-0716; **Phone:** 434-243-0066; **Board Cert:** Internal Medicine 1977; Medical Oncology 1981; **Med School:** St Louis Univ 1974; **Resid:** Internal Medicine, Temple Univ Hosp 1978; **Fellow:** Medical Oncology, Dana Farber Cancer Inst 1982; **Fac Appt:** Prof Med, Univ VA Sch Med

Williams, Michael E MD [Onc] - **Spec Exp:** Lymphoma; Multiple Myeloma; Leukemia; **Hospital:** Univ Virginia Med Ctr; **Address:** UVA Hlth System, Div Hem/Oncology, PO Box 800716, Charlottesville, VA 22908-0716; **Phone:** 434-924-9637; **Board Cert:** Internal Medicine 1982; Medical Oncology 1987; Hematology 1988; **Med School:** Univ Cincinnati 1979; **Resid:** Internal Medicine, Univ Virginia Med Ctr 1983; **Fellow:** Hematology & Oncology, Univ Virginia Med Ctr 1986; **Fac Appt:** Prof Med, Univ VA Sch Med

Wingard, John R MD [Onc] - **Spec Exp:** Bone Marrow Transplant; Leukemia; Multiple Myeloma; Lymphoma; **Hospital:** Shands at Univ of FL; **Address:** 1376 Mowry Rd, rm 458, Box 103633, Gainesville, FL 32610; **Phone:** 352-265-0062; **Board Cert:** Internal Medicine 1977; Medical Oncology 1983; **Med School:** Johns Hopkins Univ 1973; **Resid:** Internal Medicine, Memphis City Hosps 1976; Internal Medicine, VA Hosp 1977; **Fellow:** Medical Oncology, Johns Hopkins Hosp 1979; **Fac Appt:** Prof Med, Univ Fla Coll Med

Yunus, Furhan MD [Onc] - **Spec Exp:** Multiple Myeloma; Lymphoma; **Hospital:** Methodist Univ Hosp - Memphis, Regional Med Ctr - Memphis; **Address:** Univ TN Cancer Inst, 1331 Union Ave, Ste 800, Memphis, TN 38104; **Phone:** 901-725-1785; **Board Cert:** Medical Oncology 2008; **Med School:** Pakistan 1986; **Resid:** Internal Medicine, Methodist Hosp 1993; **Fellow:** Hematology & Oncology, Univ Ariz Coll Med Affil Hosp 1995; **Fac Appt:** Asst Prof Med, Univ Tenn Coll Med, Memphis

Midwest

Adelstein, David J MD [Onc] - **Spec Exp:** Head & Neck Cancer; Esophageal Cancer; Lung Cancer; **Hospital:** Cleveland Clin Fdn (page 56); **Address:** Cleveland Clinic Fdn, Taussig Cancer Ctr, 9500 Euclid Ave, R35, Cleveland, OH 44195; **Phone:** 216-444-9310; **Board Cert:** Internal Medicine 1978; Medical Oncology 1981; Hematology 1982; **Med School:** NYU Sch Med 1975; **Resid:** Internal Medicine, Univ Hosps Cleveland 1978; **Fellow:** Hematology & Oncology, Univ Hosps Cleveland 1981; **Fac Appt:** Prof Med, Cleveland Cl Coll Med/Case West Res

Medical Oncology

Albain, Kathy S MD [Onc] - **Spec Exp:** Breast Cancer; Lung Cancer; Cancer Survivors-Late Effects of Therapy; **Hospital:** Loyola Univ Med Ctr; **Address:** Loyola Univ Med Ctr, 2160 S First Ave, Bldg 112 - Ste 109, Maywood, IL 60153-5590; **Phone:** 708-327-3102; **Board Cert:** Internal Medicine 1981; Medical Oncology 1983; **Med School:** Univ Mich Med Sch 1978; **Resid:** Internal Medicine, Univ Illinois Med Ctr 1981; **Fellow:** Hematology & Oncology, Univ Chicago Hosps 1984; **Fac Appt:** Prof Med, Loyola Univ-Stritch Sch Med

Albertini, Mark R MD [Onc] - **Spec Exp:** Melanoma; Melanoma-Metastatic; **Hospital:** Univ WI Hosp & Clins; **Address:** Univ Wisconsin Medical Oncology, 600 Highland Ave, K6-930 CSC, Madison, WI 53792; **Phone:** 608-265-1700; **Board Cert:** Internal Medicine 1987; Medical Oncology 2002; **Med School:** Univ VT Coll Med 1984; **Resid:** Internal Medicine, Univ Wisc Hosps Clins 1987; **Fellow:** Medical Oncology, Univ Wisconsin 1991; **Fac Appt:** Assoc Prof Med, Univ Wisc

Anderson, Joseph M MD [Onc] - **Spec Exp:** Breast Cancer; Palliative Care; Neuro-Oncology; **Hospital:** Henry Ford Hosp; **Address:** 2799 W Grand Blvd, Ste K13, Detroit, MI 48202; **Phone:** 313-916-1854; **Board Cert:** Internal Medicine 1985; Medical Oncology 1989; **Med School:** Univ Mich Med Sch 1982; **Resid:** Internal Medicine, Henry Ford Hosp 1986; **Fellow:** Medical Oncology, Henry Ford Hosp 1988

Benson III, Al B MD [Onc] - **Spec Exp:** Colon Cancer; Carcinoid Tumors; Pancreatic Cancer; **Hospital:** Northwestern Meml Hosp, Jesse A Brown VA Med Ctr; **Address:** 675 N St Clair St, Ste 21-100, Chicago, IL 60611; **Phone:** 312-695-0990; **Board Cert:** Internal Medicine 1979; Medical Oncology 1983; **Med School:** SUNY Buffalo 1976; **Resid:** Internal Medicine, Univ Wisc Hosps 1979; **Fellow:** Medical Oncology, Univ Wisc Hosps 1984; **Fac Appt:** Prof Med, Northwestern Univ

Bitran, Jacob D MD [Onc] - **Spec Exp:** Breast Cancer; Bone Marrow Transplant; Lung Cancer; **Hospital:** Adv Luth Genl Hosp, Skokie/North Shore Univ Htlh Syst; **Address:** Lutheran Genl Cancer Care Specialists, 1700 Luther Lane, Park Ridge, IL 60068-1270; **Phone:** 866-611-1991; **Board Cert:** Internal Medicine 1974; Hematology 1986; Medical Oncology 1977; **Med School:** Univ IL Coll Med 1971; **Resid:** Pathology, Rush Presby St Lukes Hosp 1973; Internal Medicine, Michael Reese Hosp 1975; **Fellow:** Hematology & Oncology, Univ Chicago Hosps 1977; **Fac Appt:** Prof Med, Ros Franklin Univ/Chicago Med Sch

Bolwell, Brian J MD [Onc] - **Spec Exp:** Bone Marrow Transplant; Hematologic Malignancies; **Hospital:** Cleveland Clin Fdn (page 56); **Address:** 9500 Euclid Ave, Desk R32, Cleveland, OH 44195; **Phone:** 216-444-6922; **Board Cert:** Internal Medicine 1985; Medical Oncology 1987; **Med School:** Case West Res Univ 1981; **Resid:** Internal Medicine, Univ Hosp 1984; **Fellow:** Hematology & Oncology, Hosp Univ Penn 1987; **Fac Appt:** Prof Med, Cleveland Cl Coll Med/Case West Res

Bonomi, Philip D MD [Onc] - **Spec Exp:** Lung Cancer; Thymoma; Mesothelioma; **Hospital:** Rush Univ Med Ctr; **Address:** 1725 W Harrison St, Ste 821, Chicago, IL 60612; **Phone:** 312-942-3312; **Board Cert:** Internal Medicine 1975; Medical Oncology 1977; **Med School:** Univ IL Coll Med 1970; **Resid:** Internal Medicine, Geisinger Med Ctr 1972; Internal Medicine, Geisinger Med Ctr 1975; **Fellow:** Medical Oncology, Rush Presby-St Luke's Med Ctr 1977; **Fac Appt:** Prof Med, Rush Med Coll

Borden, Ernest C MD [Onc] - **Spec Exp:** Melanoma; Immunotherapy; Sarcoma; Vaccine Therapy; **Hospital:** Cleveland Clin Fdn (page 56); **Address:** 9500 Euclid Ave, Desk R40, Cleveland, OH 44195; **Phone:** 216-444-8183; **Board Cert:** Internal Medicine 1973; Medical Oncology 1975; **Med School:** Duke Univ 1966; **Resid:** Internal Medicine, Hosp Univ Penn 1968; **Fellow:** Medical Oncology, Johns Hopkins Hosp 1973; **Fac Appt:** Prof Med, Cleveland Cl Coll Med/Case West Res

Bricker, Leslie J MD [Onc] - **Spec Exp:** Palliative Care; **Hospital:** Henry Ford Hosp; **Address:** Henry Ford Hospital, 2799 W Grand Blvd, CFP 5, Detroit, MI 48202; **Phone:** 313-916-1859; **Board Cert:** Internal Medicine 1980; Hematology 1982; Medical Oncology 1983; Hospice & Palliative Medicine 2008; **Med School:** Wayne State Univ 1977; **Resid:** Internal Medicine, Sinai Hosp 1980; **Fellow:** Hematology & Oncology, Univ Mich Hosp 1983; **Fac Appt:** Assoc Prof Med, Wayne State Univ

Brockstein, Bruce E MD [Onc] - **Spec Exp:** Head & Neck Cancer; Sarcoma; Melanoma; **Hospital:** Evanston/Northshore Univ Hlth Syst, Highland Park/North Shore Univ Hlth Syst; **Address:** Evanston Northwestern Healthcare, Div Hematology/Oncology, 2650 Ridge Ave, rm 5134, Evanston, IL 60201; **Phone:** 847-570-2515; **Board Cert:** Internal Medicine 2003; Medical Oncology 2005; **Med School:** Univ Chicago-Pritzker Sch Med 1990; **Resid:** Internal Medicine, Hosp Univ Penn 1993; **Fellow:** Hematology & Oncology, Univ Chicago Hosps 1996; **Fac Appt:** Assoc Prof Med, Northwestern Univ

Buckner, Jan Craig MD [Onc] - **Spec Exp:** Brain Tumors; Neuro-Oncology; **Hospital:** Mayo Med Ctr & Clin - Rochester; **Address:** Mayo Clinic, 200 First St SW, Rochester, MN 55905; **Phone:** 507-284-4320; **Board Cert:** Internal Medicine 1983; Medical Oncology 1985; **Med School:** Univ NC Sch Med 1980; **Resid:** Internal Medicine, Butterworth Hosp 1983; **Fellow:** Medical Oncology, Mayo Clinic 1985; **Fac Appt:** Prof Med, Mayo Med Sch

Budd, George T MD [Onc] - **Spec Exp:** Breast Cancer; **Hospital:** Cleveland Clin Fdn (page 56); **Address:** Cleveland Clinic, Taussig Cancer Ctr, 9500 Euclid Ave, Desk R35, Cleveland, OH 44195; **Phone:** 216-444-6480; **Board Cert:** Internal Medicine 1980; Medical Oncology 1983; **Med School:** Univ Kans 1976; **Resid:** Internal Medicine, Cleveland Clinic 1980; **Fellow:** Hematology & Oncology, Cleveland Clinic 1982

Burt, Richard K MD [Onc] - **Spec Exp:** Stem Cell Transplant in Lupus/Crohn's; Stem Cell Transplant in MS; Autoimmune Disease; **Hospital:** Northwestern Meml Hosp; **Address:** Div Immunotherapy, 750 N Lakeshore Drive, rm 649, Chicago, IL 60611; **Phone:** 312-908-0059; **Board Cert:** Internal Medicine 1989; **Med School:** St Louis Univ 1984; **Resid:** Internal Medicine, Baylor Coll Med 1988; **Fellow:** Medical Oncology, Natl Inst Hlth Clin Ctr 1991; Hematology, Nat Inst Hlth Clin Ctr 1993; **Fac Appt:** Assoc Prof Med, Northwestern Univ

Chapman, Robert A MD [Onc] - **Spec Exp:** Lung Cancer; **Hospital:** Henry Ford Hosp; **Address:** 2799 W Grand Blvd, Fl K13, Detroit, MI 48202; **Phone:** 313-916-1841; **Board Cert:** Internal Medicine 1985; Medical Oncology 1989; **Med School:** Cornell Univ-Weill Med Coll 1976; **Resid:** Internal Medicine, Henry Ford Hosp 1979; **Fellow:** Medical Oncology, Meml Sloan Kettering Cancer Ctr 1981

Chitambar, Christopher R MD [Onc] - **Spec Exp:** Lymphoma; Leukemia; Breast Cancer; **Hospital:** Froedtert Meml Lutheran Hosp; **Address:** Div Neoplastic Disease, 9200 W Wisconsin Ave, Milwaukee, WI 53226-3522; **Phone:** 414-805-4600; **Board Cert:** Internal Medicine 1980; Hematology 1982; Medical Oncology 1983; **Med School:** India 1977; **Resid:** Internal Medicine, Brackenridge Hosp 1980; **Fellow:** Hematology & Oncology, Univ CO Hlth Sci Ctr 1983; **Fac Appt:** Prof Med, Med Coll Wisc

Clamon, Gerald H MD [Onc] - **Spec Exp:** Lung Cancer; Drug Development; **Hospital:** Univ Iowa Hosp & Clinics; **Address:** Univ Iowa Hosps & Clins, Dept Internal Med, 200 Hawkins Drive, rm 5970 JPP, Iowa City, IA 52242; **Phone:** 319-356-1932; **Board Cert:** Internal Medicine 1976; Medical Oncology 1979; **Med School:** Washington Univ, St Louis 1971; **Resid:** Internal Medicine, Barnes Hosp 1976; **Fellow:** Natl Cancer Inst 1974; Medical Oncology, Univ Iowa Hosp & Clinics 1977; **Fac Appt:** Prof Med, Univ Iowa Coll Med

Medical Oncology

Clark, Joseph I MD [Onc] - **Spec Exp:** Kidney Cancer; Melanoma; Head & Neck Cancer; **Hospital:** Loyola Univ Med Ctr, Hines VA Hosp; **Address:** Cardinal Bernardin Cancer Ctr, Loyola Univ Med Ctr, 2160 S 1st Ave, rm 346, Maywood, IL 60153-5500; **Phone:** 708-327-3236; **Board Cert:** Internal Medicine 2002; Medical Oncology 2006; **Med School:** Loyola Univ-Stritch Sch Med 1989; **Resid:** Internal Medicine, Loyola Univ Med Ctr/Hines VA Hosp 1992; **Fellow:** Hematology & Oncology, Fox Chase Cancer Ctr/Temple Univ Hosp 1995; **Fac Appt:** Prof Med, Loyola Univ-Stritch Sch Med

Cleary, James F MD [Onc] - **Spec Exp:** Palliative Care; Head & Neck Cancer; **Hospital:** Univ WI Hosp & Clins; **Address:** K6546 CSC, 600 Highland Ave, Madison, WI 53792; **Phone:** 608-263-8090; **Med School:** Australia 1984; **Resid:** Internal Medicine, Royal Adelaide Hosp 1987; **Fellow:** Medical Oncology, Royal Adelaide Hosp 1990; **Fac Appt:** Assoc Prof Med, Univ Wisc

Clinton, Steven K MD/PhD [Onc] - **Spec Exp:** Genitourinary Cancer; Prostate Cancer; Nutrition & Cancer Prevention/Control; **Hospital:** Ohio St Univ Med Ctr; **Address:** A434 Starling Loving Hall, 320 W 10th Ave, Columbus, OH 43210; **Phone:** 614-293-7560; **Board Cert:** Internal Medicine 1987; **Med School:** Univ IL Coll Med 1984; **Resid:** Internal Medicine, Univ Chicago Hosps 1987; **Fellow:** Medical Oncology, Dana Farber Cancer Inst/Harvard 1991; **Fac Appt:** Assoc Prof Med, Ohio State Univ

Cobleigh, Melody A MD [Onc] - **Spec Exp:** Breast Cancer; **Hospital:** Rush Univ Med Ctr; **Address:** Rush Univ Med Ctr, 1725 W Harrison St, Ste 821, Chicago, IL 60612-3828; **Phone:** 312-942-5904; **Board Cert:** Internal Medicine 1979; Medical Oncology 1981; **Med School:** Rush Med Coll 1976; **Resid:** Internal Medicine, Rush Presby-St Lukes Med Ctr 1979; **Fellow:** Medical Oncology, Indiana Univ 1981; **Fac Appt:** Prof Med, Rush Med Coll

Daugherty, Christopher K MD [Onc] - **Spec Exp:** Leukemia & Lymphoma; Stem Cell Transplant; **Hospital:** Univ of Chicago Med Ctr; **Address:** Univ Chicago Hosps, 5758 S Maryland Ave, MC 2115, Chicago, IL 60637; **Phone:** 773-702-6149; **Med School:** Indiana Univ 1989; **Resid:** Internal Medicine, Indiana Univ 1993; **Fellow:** Hematology & Oncology, Univ Chicago Hosps 1997; Medical Ethics, Univ Chicago Hosps

Davis, Mellar P MD [Onc] - **Spec Exp:** Palliative Care; Lung Cancer (advanced); **Hospital:** Cleveland Clin Fdn (page 56); **Address:** Cleveland Clin Fdn, 9500 Euclid Ave, Desk R35, Cleveland, OH 44195-0002; **Phone:** 216-445-4622; **Board Cert:** Internal Medicine 1980; Hematology 1982; Medical Oncology 1983; Hospice & Palliative Medicine 2004; **Med School:** Ohio State Univ 1977; **Resid:** Internal Medicine, Riverside Methodist Hosp 1979; **Fellow:** Hematology, Mayo Clinic 1981; Medical Oncology, Mayo Clinic 1982

Dreicer, Robert MD [Onc] - **Spec Exp:** Prostate Cancer; Kidney Cancer; Bladder Cancer; Testicular Cancer; **Hospital:** Cleveland Clin Fdn (page 56); **Address:** Cleveland Clinic, Taussig Cancer Ctr, 9500 Euclid Ave, Desk R35, Cleveland, OH 44195; **Phone:** 216-445-4623; **Board Cert:** Internal Medicine 1986; Medical Oncology 1989; **Med School:** Univ Tex, Houston 1983; **Resid:** Internal Medicine, Ind Univ Med Ctr 1986; **Fellow:** Medical Oncology, Univ Wisconsin Hosp 1989; **Fac Appt:** Prof Med, Cleveland Cl Coll Med/Case West Res

Einhorn, Lawrence H MD [Onc] - **Spec Exp:** Testicular Cancer; Lung Cancer; Urologic Cancer; **Hospital:** Indiana Univ Hosp; **Address:** 535 Barnhill Drive, rm 473, Indianapolis, IN 46202; **Phone:** 317-278-0054; **Board Cert:** Internal Medicine 1972; Medical Oncology 1975; **Med School:** UCLA 1967; **Resid:** Internal Medicine, Indiana Univ Hosp 1969; **Fellow:** Medical Oncology, Indiana Univ Hosp 1972; **Fac Appt:** Prof Med, Indiana Univ

America's Top Doctors® 9th Edition

Ellis, Matthew J MD/PhD [Onc] - **Spec Exp:** Breast Cancer; **Hospital:** Barnes-Jewish Hosp; **Address:** Washington University, 660 S Euclid Ave, Box 8056, St Louis, MO 63110; **Phone:** 314-747-1171; **Board Cert:** Internal Medicine 2004; Medical Oncology 2005; **Med School:** England, UK 1984; **Fellow:** Research, Georgetown Univ Med Ctr 1992; Medical Oncology, Georgetwon Univ Med Ctr 1994; **Fac Appt:** Prof Med, Washington Univ, St Louis

Eng, Charis MD [Onc] - **Spec Exp:** Breast Cancer; Ovarian Cancer; Cancer Genetics; **Hospital:** Cleveland Clin Fdn (page 56); **Address:** Cleveland Clinic Foundation, 9500 Euclid Ave, MC NE50, Cleveland, OH 44195; **Phone:** 216-444-3440; **Board Cert:** Internal Medicine 1991; Medical Oncology 1997; **Med School:** Univ Chicago-Pritzker Sch Med 1988; **Resid:** Internal Medicine, Beth Israel Hosp 1991; **Fellow:** Medical Oncology, Dana-Farber Cancer Inst 1995

Ensminger, William D MD/PhD [Onc] - **Spec Exp:** Gastrointestinal Cancer; Liver Cancer; Clinical Trials; **Hospital:** Univ Michigan Hlth Sys; **Address:** 1150 W Med Ctr Drive, Med Sci II Rm #4742, Ann Arbor, MI 48109-5633; **Phone:** 734-764-5468; **Board Cert:** Internal Medicine 1976; Medical Oncology 1979; **Med School:** Harvard Med Sch 1973; **Resid:** Internal Medicine, Beth Israel Hosp 1975; **Fellow:** Medical Oncology, Dana Farber Cancer Inst 1977; **Fac Appt:** Prof Med, Univ Mich Med Sch

Fleming, Gini F MD [Onc] - **Spec Exp:** Breast Cancer-Novel Therapies; Gynecologic Cancer; Ovarian Cancer; **Hospital:** Univ of Chicago Med Ctr; **Address:** Univ Chicago Hosps, 5841 S Maryland MC2115, Chicago, IL 60637-1470; **Phone:** 773-702-6149; **Board Cert:** Internal Medicine 1988; Medical Oncology 2001; Hematology 2002; **Med School:** Univ IL Coll Med 1985; **Resid:** Internal Medicine, Univ Chicago Hosps 1988; **Fellow:** Hematology & Oncology, Univ Chicago Hosps 1992; **Fac Appt:** Prof Med, Univ Chicago-Pritzker Sch Med

Gerson, Stanton MD [Onc] - **Spec Exp:** Leukemia; Lymphoma, Non-Hodgkin's; Stem Cell Transplant; **Hospital:** Univ Hosps Case Med Ctr; **Address:** Ireland Cancer Ctr, 11000 Euclid Ave, 1 WEARN 151, Cleveland, OH 44106-5065; **Phone:** 216-844-1232; **Board Cert:** Internal Medicine 1980; Medical Oncology 1983; Hematology 1982; **Med School:** Harvard Med Sch 1977; **Resid:** Internal Medicine, Hosp Univ Penn 1980; **Fellow:** Hematology & Oncology, Hosp Univ Penn 1983; **Fac Appt:** Prof Med, Case West Res Univ

Golomb, Harvey M MD [Onc] - **Spec Exp:** Lung Cancer; Leukemia; Lymphoma; **Hospital:** Univ of Chicago Med Ctr; **Address:** Univ Chicago Hosp, 5758 S Maryland Ave, MC 9015, Chicago, IL 60637-1463; **Phone:** 773-702-6115; **Board Cert:** Internal Medicine 1975; Medical Oncology 1979; **Med School:** Univ Pittsburgh 1968; **Resid:** Internal Medicine, Johns Hopkins Hosp 1972; Clinical Genetics, Johns Hopkins Hosp 1973; **Fellow:** Hematology & Oncology, Univ Chicago Hosps 1975; **Fac Appt:** Prof Med, Univ Chicago-Pritzker Sch Med

Gradishar, William J MD [Onc] - **Spec Exp:** Breast Cancer; **Hospital:** Northwestern Meml Hosp; **Address:** 676 N St Claire St, Ste 21-100, Chicago, IL 60611; **Phone:** 312-695-0990; **Board Cert:** Internal Medicine 1985; Medical Oncology 1989; **Med School:** Univ IL Coll Med 1982; **Resid:** Internal Medicine, Michael Reese Hosp 1985; **Fellow:** Hematology & Oncology, Univ Chicago Hosps 1990; **Fac Appt:** Prof Med, Northwestern Univ

Gruber, Stephen B MD/PhD [Onc] - **Spec Exp:** Cancer Genetics; Colon & Rectal Cancer; Melanoma; **Hospital:** Univ Michigan Hlth Sys; **Address:** 109 Zina Pitcher Pl, Ann Arbor, MI 48109-2200; **Phone:** 734-615-9712; **Board Cert:** Internal Medicine 1995; Medical Oncology 1998; **Med School:** Univ Pennsylvania 1992; **Resid:** Internal Medicine, Hosp Univ Penn 1994; **Fellow:** Medical Oncology, Johns Hopkins Hosp 1997; Clinical Genetics, Univ Michigan Hlth Sys 1999; **Fac Appt:** Assoc Prof Med, Univ Mich Med Sch

Medical Oncology

Hartmann, Lynn Carol MD [Onc] - **Spec Exp:** Ovarian Cancer; **Hospital:** Mayo Med Ctr & Clin - Rochester; **Address:** Mayo Clinic Gonda 10 South, 200 First St SW, Rochester, MN 55905; **Phone:** 507-284-3903; **Board Cert:** Internal Medicine 1986; Medical Oncology 1989; **Med School:** Northwestern Univ 1983; **Resid:** Internal Medicine, Univ Ia Hosps/Clinics 1986; **Fellow:** Medical Oncology, Mayo Clinic 1989; **Fac Appt:** Prof Med, Mayo Med Sch

Hayes, Daniel F MD [Onc] - **Spec Exp:** Breast Cancer; **Hospital:** Univ Michigan Hlth Sys; **Address:** Univ Michigan Comprehensive Cancer Ctr, 6312 CCC SPC, 5942, Ann Arbor, MI 48109-5942; **Phone:** 734-615-6725; **Board Cert:** Internal Medicine 1982; Medical Oncology 1985; **Med School:** Indiana Univ 1979; **Resid:** Internal Medicine, Parkland Meml Hosp 1982; **Fellow:** Medical Oncology, Dana Farber Cancer Inst 1985; **Fac Appt:** Prof Med, Univ Mich Med Sch

Hoffman, Philip C MD [Onc] - **Spec Exp:** Lung Cancer; Breast Cancer; Esophageal Cancer; **Hospital:** Univ of Chicago Med Ctr, Little Company of Mary Hosp & Hlth Care Ctrs; **Address:** 5841 S Maryland Ave, MC 2115, Chicago, IL 60637-1447; **Phone:** 773-834-7424; **Board Cert:** Internal Medicine 1975; Hematology 1980; Medical Oncology 1981; **Med School:** Jefferson Med Coll 1972; **Resid:** Internal Medicine, Hosp Univ Penn 1975; **Fellow:** Hematology & Oncology, Univ Chicago Hosps 1980; **Fac Appt:** Prof Med, Univ Chicago-Pritzker Sch Med

Hussain, Maha H MD [Onc] - **Spec Exp:** Prostate Cancer; Bladder Cancer; Testicular Cancer; Genitourinary Cancer; **Hospital:** Univ Michigan Hlth Sys; **Address:** Univ Michigan Cancer Ctr, 1500 E Medical Ctr Drive, rm 7310, Ann Arbor, MI 48109; **Phone:** 734-936-8906; **Board Cert:** Internal Medicine 1986; Medical Oncology 1989; **Med School:** Iraq 1980; **Resid:** Internal Medicine, Wayne State Univ Affil Hosps 1986; **Fellow:** Medical Oncology, Wayne State Univ Affil Hosps 1989; **Fac Appt:** Prof Med, Univ Mich Med Sch

Ingle, James N MD [Onc] - **Spec Exp:** Breast Cancer; **Hospital:** Rochester Methodist Hosp, Mayo Med Ctr & Clin - Rochester; **Address:** Mayo Clinic, 200 First St SW, Gonda Bldg Fl 10, Rochester, MN 55905-0001; **Phone:** 507-284-8432; **Board Cert:** Internal Medicine 1974; Medical Oncology 1975; **Med School:** Johns Hopkins Univ 1971; **Resid:** Internal Medicine, Johns Hopkins Hosp 1976; Medical Oncology, Natl Cancer Inst 1975; **Fac Appt:** Prof Med, Mayo Med Sch

Kalaycio, Matt E MD [Onc] - **Spec Exp:** Leukemia; Bone Marrow Transplant; **Hospital:** Cleveland Clin Fdn (page 56); **Address:** Taussig Cancer Ctr, 9500 Euclid Ave, Desk R35, Cleveland, OH 44195; **Phone:** 216-444-3705; **Board Cert:** Internal Medicine 2002; Hematology 2004; Medical Oncology 2005; **Med School:** W VA Univ 1988; **Resid:** Internal Medicine, Mercy Hosp 1991; **Fellow:** Hematology & Oncology, Cleveland Clinic 1994; **Fac Appt:** Prof Med, Cleveland Cl Coll Med/Case West Res

Kalemkerian, Gregory MD [Onc] - **Spec Exp:** Lung Cancer; Mesothelioma; Thymoma; **Hospital:** Univ Michigan Hlth Sys; **Address:** 1500 E Medical Center Dr, C350MIB, Ann Arbor, MI 48109-0848; **Phone:** 734-232-6046; **Board Cert:** Internal Medicine 1988; Medical Oncology 2001; **Med School:** Northwestern Univ 1985; **Resid:** Internal Medicine, Northwestern Meml Hosp 1988; **Fac Appt:** Prof Med, Univ Mich Med Sch

Kaminski, Mark S MD [Onc] - **Spec Exp:** Lymphoma; Bone Marrow Transplant; Drug Development; Clinical Trials; **Hospital:** Univ Michigan Hlth Sys; **Address:** Univ Michigan Cancer Ctr, 1500 E Medical Ctr Drive, rm 4316, Ann Arbor, MI 48109-0936; **Phone:** 734-936-5310; **Board Cert:** Internal Medicine 1981; Medical Oncology 1983; **Med School:** Stanford Univ 1978; **Resid:** Internal Medicine, Barnes Hosp 1981; **Fellow:** Medical Oncology, Stanford Univ Med Ctr 1985; **Fac Appt:** Prof Med, Univ Mich Med Sch

Kindler, Hedy Lee MD [Onc] - **Spec Exp:** Mesothelioma; Pancreatic Cancer; Colon & Rectal Cancer; **Hospital:** Univ of Chicago Med Ctr; **Address:** Univ of Chicago Hospital, 5841 S Maryland Ave, MC 2115, Chicago, IL 60637-1470; **Phone:** 773-834-7424; **Board Cert:** Internal Medicine 2002; Medical Oncology 2005; **Med School:** SUNY Buffalo 1985; **Resid:** Internal Medicine, UCLA Med Ctr 1992; **Fellow:** Medical Oncology, Meml Sloan Kettering Cancer Ctr 1995; **Fac Appt:** Assoc Prof Med, Univ Chicago-Pritzker Sch Med

Loehrer, Patrick J MD [Onc] - **Spec Exp:** Gastrointestinal Cancer; Thymoma; Genitourinary Cancer; **Hospital:** Indiana Univ Hosp; **Address:** Indiana Cancer Pavilion, 535 Barnhill Drive, rm 473, Indianapolis, IN 46202-5112; **Phone:** 317-278-7418; **Board Cert:** Internal Medicine 1981; Medical Oncology 2006; **Med School:** Rush Med Coll 1978; **Resid:** Internal Medicine, Rush-Presby-St Lukes Hosp 1981; **Fellow:** Medical Oncology, Indiana Univ 1983; **Fac Appt:** Prof Med, Indiana Univ

Loprinzi, Charles L MD [Onc] - **Spec Exp:** Breast Cancer; **Hospital:** Mayo Med Ctr & Clin - Rochester; **Address:** Mayo Clinic, Dept Med Oncology, 200 First St SW, Rochester, MN 55905-0001; **Phone:** 507-284-4137; **Board Cert:** Internal Medicine 1982; Medical Oncology 1985; **Med School:** Oregon Hlth & Sci Univ 1979; **Resid:** Internal Medicine, Maricopa Co Hosp 1982; **Fellow:** Medical Oncology, Univ Wisconsin Med Ctr 1984; **Fac Appt:** Prof Med, Mayo Med Sch

Markowitz, Sanford D MD [Onc] - **Spec Exp:** Colon & Rectal Cancer; Hereditary Cancer; **Hospital:** Univ Hosps Case Med Ctr; **Address:** Ireland Cancer Ctr, 11100 Euclid Ave Fl 6, Cleveland, OH 44106; **Phone:** 216-844-6966; **Board Cert:** Internal Medicine 1984; Medical Oncology 1987; **Med School:** Yale Univ 1980; **Resid:** Internal Medicine, Univ Chicago Hosp 1984; **Fellow:** Medical Oncology, Natl Cancer Inst 1986; **Fac Appt:** Prof Med, Case West Res Univ

Olopade, Olufunmilayo I F MD [Onc] - **Spec Exp:** Breast Cancer; Hereditary Cancer; Breast Cancer Genetics; **Hospital:** Univ of Chicago Med Ctr; **Address:** Univ Chicago Hospital, 5841 S Maryland Ave, MC 2115, Section, Hematology-Oncology, Chicago, IL 60637-1470; **Phone:** 773-702-6149; **Board Cert:** Internal Medicine 1986; Hematology 2001; Medical Oncology 1989; **Med School:** Nigeria 1980; **Resid:** Internal Medicine, Cook Co Hosp 1986; **Fellow:** Hematology & Oncology, Univ Chicago Hosps 1991; **Fac Appt:** Prof Med, Univ Chicago-Pritzker Sch Med

Peereboom, David M MD [Onc] - **Spec Exp:** Neuro-Oncology; Brain Tumors; Drug Development; **Hospital:** Cleveland Clin Fdn (page 56); **Address:** Cleveland Clinic Taussig Cancer Ctr, 9500 Euclid Ave, MC R35, Cleveland, OH 44195; **Phone:** 216-445-6068; **Board Cert:** Internal Medicine 1989; Medical Oncology 2004; **Med School:** Med Coll VA 1986; **Resid:** Internal Medicine, Univ Hosp of Cleveland 1990; **Fellow:** Medical Oncology, Johns Hopkins Hosp 1993

Perry, Michael C MD [Onc] - **Spec Exp:** Lung Cancer; Breast Cancer; **Hospital:** Univ of Missouri Hosp & Clins; **Address:** Ellis Fischel Cancer Ctr, 115 Business Loop 70 W, DC 116.71, rm 524, Columbia, MO 65203-3299; **Phone:** 573-882-4979; **Board Cert:** Internal Medicine 1987; Hematology 1974; Medical Oncology 1975; **Med School:** Wayne State Univ 1970; **Resid:** Internal Medicine, Mayo Grad Sch 1972; **Fellow:** Hematology, Mayo Grad Sch 1974; Medical Oncology, Mayo Grad Sch 1975; **Fac Appt:** Prof Med, Univ MO-Columbia Sch Med

Peterson, Bruce MD [Onc] - **Spec Exp:** Lymphoma; Leukemia; **Hospital:** Univ Minn Med Ctr, Fairview - Univ Campus; **Address:** Univ of Minnesota, MMC 480, 420 Delaware St SE, Minneapolis, MN 55455; **Phone:** 612-625-5411; **Board Cert:** Internal Medicine 1974; Medical Oncology 1977; **Med School:** Univ Minn 1971; **Resid:** Internal Medicine, Fletcher Allen Hlthcare 1973; Internal Medicine, Fairview-Univ Med Ctr 1974; **Fellow:** Medical Oncology, Fairview-Univ Med Ctr 1977; **Fac Appt:** Prof Med, Univ Minn

Medical Oncology

Picus, Joel MD [Onc] - **Spec Exp:** Pancreatic Cancer; Prostate Cancer; Colon Cancer; Bladder Cancer; **Hospital:** Barnes-Jewish Hosp; **Address:** Washington University School of Medicine, Dept Medicine, 660 S Euclid Ave Campus Box 8056, St Louis, MO 63110; **Phone:** 314-362-5737; **Board Cert:** Internal Medicine 1987; Medical Oncology 1989; **Med School:** Harvard Med Sch 1984; **Resid:** Internal Medicine, Duke Univ Med Ctr 1987; **Fellow:** Hematology & Oncology, UCSF Med Ctr 1991; **Fac Appt:** Assoc Prof Med, Washington Univ, St Louis

Pienta, Kenneth J MD [Onc] - **Spec Exp:** Prostate Cancer; **Hospital:** Univ Michigan Hlth Sys; **Address:** Cancer Center/Geriatrics Center, 1500 E Medical Center Drive, rm 7303 CCC, Ann Arbor, MI 48109-5946; **Phone:** 734-647-3421; **Board Cert:** Internal Medicine 2001; Medical Oncology 2001; **Med School:** Johns Hopkins Univ 1986; **Resid:** Internal Medicine, Univ Chicago Hosps 1988; **Fellow:** Medical Oncology, Johns Hopkins Hosp 1991; **Fac Appt:** Prof Med, Univ Mich Med Sch

Pohlman, Brad L MD [Onc] - **Spec Exp:** Lymphoma; Lymphoma, Non-Hodgkin's; Bone Marrow Transplant; **Hospital:** Cleveland Clin Fdn (page 56); **Address:** Cleveland Clinic Fdn, 9500 Euclid Ave R35, Cleveland, OH 44195; **Phone:** 216-445-6070; **Board Cert:** Internal Medicine 1988; **Med School:** Indiana Univ 1985; **Resid:** Internal Medicine, Univ Wisconsin Hosp 1988; **Fellow:** Hematology, Univ Minnesota Hosp 1992

Raghavan, Derek MD/PhD [Onc] - **Spec Exp:** Prostate Cancer; Testicular Cancer; Bladder Cancer; Genitourinary Cancer; **Hospital:** Cleveland Clin Fdn (page 56); **Address:** Cleveland Clinic Taussig Cancer Inst, 9500 Euclid Ave, MC R35, Cleveland, OH 44195; **Phone:** 216-445-6888; **Med School:** Australia 1974; **Resid:** Internal Medicine, Royal Prince Alfred Hosp 1977; **Fellow:** Medical Oncology, Royal Prince Alfred Hosp 1979; Medical Oncology, Royal Marsden Hosp 1980; **Fac Appt:** Prof Med, Cleveland Cl Coll Med/Case West Res

Ratain, Mark J MD [Onc] - **Spec Exp:** Solid Tumors; Drug Discovery & Development; **Hospital:** Univ of Chicago Med Ctr; **Address:** Univ Chicago Med Ctr, 5841 S Maryland Ave, MC 211, Chicago, IL 60637; **Phone:** 773-702-6149; **Board Cert:** Internal Medicine 1983; Hematology 1986; Medical Oncology 1985; **Med School:** Yale Univ 1980; **Resid:** Internal Medicine, Johns Hopkins Hosp 1983; **Fellow:** Hematology & Oncology, Univ Chicago 1986; **Fac Appt:** Prof Med, Univ Chicago-Pritzker Sch Med

Richards, Jon M MD/PhD [Onc] - **Spec Exp:** Testicular Cancer; Prostate Cancer; Melanoma; **Hospital:** Adv Luth Genl Hosp, Skokie/North Shore Univ Htlh Syst; **Address:** Center for Advanced Care, 1700 Luther Ln Fl 2, Park Ridge, IL 60068; **Phone:** 847-268-8200; **Board Cert:** Internal Medicine 1998; Medical Oncology 2007; **Med School:** Cornell Univ-Weill Med Coll 1983; **Resid:** Internal Medicine, Univ Chicago Hosp 1985; **Fellow:** Hematology & Oncology, Univ Chicago Hosp 1988; **Fac Appt:** Asst Prof Med, Univ IL Coll Med

Rosen, Steven T MD [Onc] - **Spec Exp:** Hematologic Malignancies; Breast Cancer; Lymphoma; **Hospital:** Northwestern Meml Hosp; **Address:** Northwestern Univ, 303 E Chicago Ave, Lurie 3-125, Chicago, IL 60611-3013; **Phone:** 312-695-0990; **Board Cert:** Internal Medicine 1979; Medical Oncology 1981; Hematology 1984; **Med School:** Northwestern Univ 1976; **Resid:** Internal Medicine, Northwestern Univ Hosp 1979; **Fellow:** Medical Oncology, Natl Cancer Inst 1981; **Fac Appt:** Prof Med, Northwestern Univ

Ruckdeschel, John C MD [Onc] - **Spec Exp:** Lung Cancer; Mesothelioma; **Hospital:** Karmanos Cancer Inst; **Address:** Barbara Ann Karmanos Cancer Inst, 4100 John R, Detoit, MI 48201; **Phone:** 313-576-8670; **Board Cert:** Internal Medicine 1976; Medical Oncology 1977; **Med School:** Albany Med Coll 1971; **Resid:** Internal Medicine, Johns Hopkins Hosp 1972; Internal Medicine, Beth Israel Hosp 1976; **Fellow:** Medical Oncology, Natl Cancer Inst 1975

Salgia, Ravi MD/PhD [Onc] - **Spec Exp:** Lung Cancer; Mesothelioma; Thoracic Cancers; **Hospital:** Univ of Chicago Med Ctr; **Address:** Univ Chicago Hosps, 5841 S Maryland Ave, MC 2115, Chicago, IL 60637; **Phone:** 773-702-4400; **Board Cert:** Medical Oncology 2006; **Med School:** Loyola Univ-Stritch Sch Med 1987; **Resid:** Internal Medicine, Johns Hopkins Hosp 1990; **Fellow:** Medical Oncology, Dana-Farber Cancer Inst 1993; **Fac Appt:** Assoc Prof Med, Univ IL Coll Med

Schiffer, Charles A MD [Onc] - **Spec Exp:** Leukemia; Lymphoma; Multiple Myeloma; **Hospital:** Karmanos Cancer Inst, Harper Univ Hosp; **Address:** Karmanos Cancer Inst, Cancer Research Ctr, 4100 John R, 4 CRC-Hudson Webber, Detroit, MI 48201; **Phone:** 313-576-8737; **Board Cert:** Internal Medicine 1972; Medical Oncology 1973; **Med School:** NYU Sch Med 1968; **Resid:** Internal Medicine, Bellevue-NY VA Hosp-NYU 1972; **Fellow:** Medical Oncology, Natl Cancer Inst 1974; **Fac Appt:** Prof Med, Wayne State Univ

Schilsky, Richard MD [Onc] - **Spec Exp:** Gastrointestinal Cancer; Pancreatic Cancer; Drug Development; **Hospital:** Univ of Chicago Med Ctr; **Address:** Univ Chicago- Bio Sciences Div, 5841 S Maryland Ave, MC 2115, Chicago, IL 60637; **Phone:** 773-834-3914; **Board Cert:** Internal Medicine 1978; Medical Oncology 1979; **Med School:** Univ Chicago-Pritzker Sch Med 1975; **Resid:** Internal Medicine, Univ Texas 1977; **Fellow:** Medical Oncology, Natl Cancer Inst 1980; **Fac Appt:** Prof Med, Univ Chicago-Pritzker Sch Med

Schwartz, Burton S MD [Onc] - **Spec Exp:** Lymphoma; Breast Cancer; **Hospital:** Abbott - Northwestern Hosp; **Address:** 800 E 28th St, Piper Bldg, Ste 405, Minneapolis, MN 55407; **Phone:** 612-863-8585; **Board Cert:** Internal Medicine 1980; Hematology 1976; Medical Oncology 1977; **Med School:** Meharry Med Coll 1968; **Resid:** Internal Medicine, Michael Reese Hosp 1971; **Fellow:** Hematology, Univ Minn Hosp 1976; **Fac Appt:** Clin Prof Med, Univ Minn

Shapiro, Charles L MD [Onc] - **Spec Exp:** Breast Cancer; **Hospital:** Arthur G James Cancer Hosp & Research Inst; **Address:** Starling Loving Hall, rm B420, 320 W 10th Ave, Columbus, OH 43210; **Phone:** 614-293-6401; **Board Cert:** Internal Medicine 1987; Medical Oncology 2005; **Med School:** SUNY Buffalo 1984; **Resid:** Internal Medicine, Temple Univ Hosp 1987; **Fellow:** Medical Oncology, Dana Farber Cancer Inst 1991; **Fac Appt:** Assoc Prof Med, Ohio State Univ

Silver, Samuel M MD [Onc] - **Spec Exp:** Hematologic Malignancies; Bleeding/Coagulation Disorders; Myelodyplastic Syndromes; Myeloproliferative Disorders; **Hospital:** Univ Michigan Hlth Sys; **Address:** Univ Michigan Med Ctr / Cancer Ctr, 1500 E Med Ctr Drive, C-412MIB, SPC5843, Ann Arbor, MI 48109; **Phone:** 734-936-4991; **Board Cert:** Internal Medicine 1982; Medical Oncology 1985; Hematology 1984; **Med School:** Cornell Univ-Weill Med Coll 1978; **Resid:** Internal Medicine, UCSF-Moffit Hosp 1982; **Fellow:** Hematology & Oncology, Univ Penn 1985; **Fac Appt:** Clin Prof Med, Univ Mich Med Sch

Silverman, Paula MD [Onc] - **Spec Exp:** Breast Cancer; **Hospital:** Univ Hosps Case Med Ctr; **Address:** Univ Hosp Cleveland, Ireland Cancer Ctr, 11100 Euclid Ave Bolwell Bldg Fl 6, Cleveland, OH 44106; **Phone:** 216-844-8510; **Board Cert:** Internal Medicine 1984; Medical Oncology 1989; **Med School:** Case West Res Univ 1981; **Resid:** Internal Medicine, Univ Hosps 1984; **Fellow:** Hematology & Oncology, Case Western Reserve Univ 1987; **Fac Appt:** Assoc Prof Med, Case West Res Univ

Sledge Jr, George W MD [Onc] - **Spec Exp:** Breast Cancer; **Hospital:** Indiana Univ Hosp; **Address:** 535 Barnhill Drive, rm 473, Indianapolis, IN 46202; **Phone:** 317-274-0920; **Board Cert:** Internal Medicine 1980; Medical Oncology 1983; **Med School:** Tulane Univ 1977; **Resid:** Internal Medicine, St Louis Univ 1980; **Fellow:** Medical Oncology, Univ Texas 1983; **Fac Appt:** Prof Med, Indiana Univ

Medical Oncology

Stadler, Walter M MD [Onc] - **Spec Exp:** Kidney Cancer; Bladder Cancer; Prostate Cancer; Testicular Cancer; **Hospital:** Univ of Chicago Med Ctr; **Address:** Div Hem/Onc, 5841 S Maryland Ave, MC 2115, Chicago, IL 60637; **Phone:** 773-834-7424; **Board Cert:** Internal Medicine 2002; Medical Oncology 2003; **Med School:** Yale Univ 1988; **Resid:** Internal Medicine, Michael Reese Hosp 1991; **Fellow:** Medical Oncology, Univ Chicago Hosps 1994; **Fac Appt:** Prof Med, Univ Chicago-Pritzker Sch Med

Triozzi, Pierre L MD [Onc] - **Spec Exp:** Melanoma; Vaccine Therapy; Clinical Trials; **Hospital:** Cleveland Clin Fdn (page 56); **Address:** Cleveland Clinic Fdn, 9500 Euclid Ave, MC R40, Cleveland, OH 44195; **Phone:** 216-445-5141; **Board Cert:** Internal Medicine 1983; Medical Oncology 1987; Hematology 1988; **Med School:** Ohio State Univ 1980; **Resid:** Internal Medicine, Duke Univ Med Ctr 1983; **Fellow:** Hematology & Oncology, Duke Univ Med Ctr 1987; **Fac Appt:** Prof Med, Case West Res Univ

Urba, Susan G MD [Onc] - **Spec Exp:** Head & Neck Cancer; **Hospital:** Univ Michigan Hlth Sys; **Address:** Comp Cancer Ctr & Geriatrics Ctr, 1500 E Med Ctr Drive, rm 4214, Ann Arbor, MI 48109-0922; **Phone:** 734-647-8902; **Board Cert:** Internal Medicine 1986; Medical Oncology 2002; **Med School:** Univ Mich Med Sch 1983; **Resid:** Internal Medicine, Univ Mich Med Ctr 1986; **Fellow:** Hematology & Oncology, Univ Mich Med Ctr 1988; **Fac Appt:** Assoc Prof Med, Univ Mich Med Sch

Von Roenn, Jamie H MD [Onc] - **Spec Exp:** Palliative Care; AIDS Related Cancers; Breast Cancer; **Hospital:** Northwestern Meml Hosp; **Address:** 675 N St Clair, Ste 21-100, Chicago, IL 60611; **Phone:** 312-695-6180; **Board Cert:** Internal Medicine 1983; Medical Oncology 1985; Hospice & Palliative Medicine 2003; **Med School:** Rush Med Coll 1980; **Resid:** Internal Medicine, Rush-Presby-St Lukes Hosp 1983; **Fellow:** Medical Oncology, Rush-Presby-St Lukes Hosp 1985; **Fac Appt:** Prof Med, Northwestern Univ

Wade, James C MD [Onc] - **Spec Exp:** Infections in Cancer Patients; Bone Marrow Transplant; Leukemia; **Hospital:** Froedtert Meml Lutheran Hosp; **Address:** 9200 W Wisconsin Ave, CLCC4193, Milwaukee, WI 53226-3522; **Phone:** 414-805-4693; **Board Cert:** Internal Medicine 1977; Infectious Disease 1982; Medical Oncology 1981; **Med School:** Univ Utah 1974; **Resid:** Internal Medicine, Johns Hopkins Hosp 1977; **Fellow:** Medical Oncology, Natl Cancer Inst/NIH 1979; Infectious Disease, Univ Wash/Fred Hutchinson Cancer Rsch Ctr 1982; **Fac Appt:** Prof Med, Med Coll Wisc

Weiner, George J MD [Onc] - **Spec Exp:** Lymphoma; Leukemia; Immunotherapy; **Hospital:** Univ Iowa Hosp & Clinics; **Address:** Holden Comprehensive Cancer Center, 200 Hawkins Drive Bldg 5970JPP, Iowa City, IA 52242; **Phone:** 319-356-1932; **Board Cert:** Internal Medicine 1985; Hematology 1988; Medical Oncology 1987; **Med School:** Ohio State Univ 1981; **Resid:** Medical Oncology, Med Coll Ohio 1984; **Fellow:** Hematology & Oncology, Univ Mich Med Ctr 1987; **Fac Appt:** Prof Med, Univ Iowa Coll Med

Weissman, David E MD [Onc] - **Spec Exp:** Palliative Care; Pain-Cancer; **Hospital:** Froedtert Meml Lutheran Hosp; **Address:** Med Coll Wisc, Dept Hem/Onc, 9200 W Wisconsin Ave, Milwaukee, WI 53226-3596; **Phone:** 414-805-6800; **Board Cert:** Internal Medicine 1983; Medical Oncology 1985; **Med School:** UCSD 1980; **Resid:** Internal Medicine, UCSD Univ Hosp 1983; **Fellow:** Medical Oncology, Johns Hopkins Hosp 1985; **Fac Appt:** Prof Med, Univ Wisc

Wicha, Max S MD [Onc] - **Spec Exp:** Breast Cancer; Stem Cell Transplant; **Hospital:** Univ Michigan Hlth Sys; **Address:** Comp Cancer Ctr & Geriatrics Ctr, 1500 E Med Ctr Dr, rm 6302 CC, Ann Arbor, MI 48109-5942; **Phone:** 734-936-1831; **Board Cert:** Internal Medicine 1977; Medical Oncology 1983; **Med School:** Stanford Univ 1974; **Resid:** Internal Medicine, Univ Chicago Hosp 1977; **Fellow:** Medical Oncology, Natl Inst Hlth 1980; **Fac Appt:** Prof Med, Univ Mich Med Sch

Wilding, George MD [Onc] - **Spec Exp:** Prostate Cancer; Kidney Cancer; Genitourinary Cancer; Drug Discovery & Development; **Hospital:** Univ WI Hosp & Clins; **Address:** 1111 Highland Ave, Ste 7057WIMR, Madison, WI 53705; **Phone:** 608-263-8610; **Board Cert:** Internal Medicine 1983; Medical Oncology 1985; **Med School:** Univ Mass Sch Med 1980; **Resid:** Internal Medicine, Univ Mass Med Ctr 1983; **Fellow:** Medical Oncology, Natl Cancer Inst 1985; **Fac Appt:** Prof Med, Univ Wisc

Worden, Francis P MD [Onc] - **Spec Exp:** Head & Neck Cancer; Palliative Care; Clinical Trials; **Hospital:** Univ Michigan Hlth Sys; **Address:** Cancer Center & Geriatric Center, 1500 E Medical Center Drive, rm 4214, Ann Arbor, MI 48109; **Phone:** 734-647-8902; **Board Cert:** Medical Oncology 2000; **Med School:** Indiana Univ 1993; **Resid:** Internal Medicine & Pediatrics, Detroit Med Ctr 1997; **Fellow:** Medical Oncology, Detroit Med Ctr 1920; **Fac Appt:** Asst Clin Prof Med, Univ Mich Med Sch

Yee, Douglas MD [Onc] - **Spec Exp:** Breast Cancer; **Hospital:** Univ Minn Med Ctr, Fairview - Univ Campus; **Address:** Univ Minnesota Cancer Ctr, 420 Delaware St SE, MMC 806, Minneapolis, MN 55455; **Phone:** 612-625-5411; **Board Cert:** Internal Medicine 1984; Medical Oncology 1987; **Med School:** Univ Chicago-Pritzker Sch Med 1981; **Resid:** Internal Medicine, Univ NC Med Ctr 1984; **Fellow:** Medical Oncology, NIH-Clin Ctr 1987; **Fac Appt:** Prof Med, Univ Minn

Great Plains and Mountains

Akerley, Wallace MD [Onc] - **Spec Exp:** Lung Cancer; Clinical Trials; **Hospital:** Univ Utah Hosps and Clins; **Address:** Huntsman Cancer Inst, 2000 Circle of Hope, rm 2165, Salt Lake City, UT 84112; **Phone:** 801-585-0100; **Board Cert:** Internal Medicine 1984; Medical Oncology 1987; Hematology 1988; **Med School:** Brown Univ 1981; **Resid:** Internal Medicine, USC Medical Ctr 1985; **Fellow:** Medical Oncology, USC Medical Ctr 1986; Hematology, Norris Cotton Cancer Ctr/Dartmouth 1988; **Fac Appt:** Prof Med, Univ Utah

Armitage, James MD [Onc] - **Spec Exp:** Lymphoma; Bone Marrow Transplant; **Hospital:** Nebraska Med Ctr; **Address:** 987680 Nebraska Medical Center, Omaha, NE 68198-7680; **Phone:** 402-559-7290; **Board Cert:** Internal Medicine 1976; Medical Oncology 1977; Hematology 1984; **Med School:** Univ Nebr Coll Med 1973; **Resid:** Internal Medicine, Univ Nebraska Med Ctr 1975; **Fellow:** Hematology & Oncology, Univ Iowa Hosp 1977; **Fac Appt:** Prof Med, Univ Nebr Coll Med

Beatty, Patrick G MD [Onc] - **Spec Exp:** Hematologic Malignancies; Lymphoma; **Hospital:** St Patrick Hospital - Missoula; **Address:** PO Box 7877, Missoula, MT 59807; **Phone:** 406-728-2539; **Board Cert:** Internal Medicine 1980; Medical Oncology 1985; **Resid:** Internal Medicine, Vanderbilt Univ Med Ctr 1979; **Fellow:** Oncology, Univ Washington Hosps 1982

Bierman, Philip J MD [Onc] - **Spec Exp:** Lymphoma; Bone Marrow Transplant; **Hospital:** Nebraska Med Ctr; **Address:** Nebraska Medical Ctr, Dept Hem/Oncology, 987680 Nebraska Medical Ctr, Omaha, NE 68198-7680; **Phone:** 402-559-5520; **Board Cert:** Internal Medicine 1982; Medical Oncology 1985; Hematology 1986; **Med School:** Univ MO-Kansas City 1979; **Resid:** Internal Medicine, Univ Nebraska Med Ctr 1983; **Fellow:** Medical Oncology, Univ Nebraska Med Ctr 1985; Hematology, City of Hope Natl Med Ctr 1986; **Fac Appt:** Assoc Prof Med, Univ Nebr Coll Med

Bunn Jr, Paul A MD [Onc] - **Spec Exp:** Lung Cancer; Clinical Trials; **Hospital:** Univ Colorado Hosp, Vail Valley Med Ctr; **Address:** Univ Colorado Hosp Cancer Ctr, 1665 Aurora Ct, Ste MS F-704, 1665 Aurora Court, Aurora, CO 80045-0510; **Phone:** 303-724-4499; **Board Cert:** Internal Medicine 1974; Medical Oncology 1975; **Med School:** Cornell Univ-Weill Med Coll 1971; **Resid:** Internal Medicine, Moffitt Hosp/ UCSF Med Ctr 1973; **Fellow:** Medical Oncology, Natl Cancer Inst 1976; **Fac Appt:** Prof Med, Univ Colorado

Medical Oncology

Buys, Saundra S MD [Onc] - **Spec Exp:** Breast Cancer; Breast Cancer Risk Assessment; Breast Cancer Genetics; **Hospital:** Univ Utah Hosps and Clins; **Address:** Huntsman Cancer Institute, 2000 Circle of Hope, Ste 210, Salt Lake City, UT 84112; **Phone:** 801-585-3525; **Board Cert:** Internal Medicine 1982; Medical Oncology 1985; Hematology 1984; **Med School:** Tufts Univ 1979; **Resid:** Internal Medicine, Univ Utah Hosps 1982; **Fellow:** Hematology & Oncology, Univ Utah Hosps 1985; **Fac Appt:** Prof Med, Univ Utah

Cowan, Kenneth H MD/PhD [Onc] - **Spec Exp:** Breast Cancer; **Hospital:** Nebraska Med Ctr; **Address:** Eppley Cancer Center, 986805 Nebraska Medical Ctr, Omaha, NE 68198-6805; **Phone:** 402-559-4238; **Board Cert:** Internal Medicine 1978; Medical Oncology 1981; **Med School:** Case West Res Univ 1974; **Resid:** Internal Medicine, Parkland Meml Hosp 1977

Dakhil, Shaker MD [Onc] - **Spec Exp:** Leukemia; Mesothelioma; Lymphoma; **Hospital:** Univ of Kansas Hosp; **Address:** Cancer Center Kansas, 818 N Emporia, Ste 403, Wichita, KS 67214; **Phone:** 316-262-4467; **Board Cert:** Internal Medicine 1978; Medical Oncology 1981; **Med School:** Lebanon 1976; **Resid:** Internal Medicine, Wayne State Univ Hosp 1978; **Fellow:** Hematology & Oncology, Univ Michigan Sch Med 1981; **Fac Appt:** Assoc Clin Prof Med, Univ Kans

Eckhardt, S Gail MD [Onc] - **Spec Exp:** Gastrointestinal Cancer; Drug Development; **Hospital:** Univ Colorado Hosp; **Address:** Univ Colorado Hosp Cancer Ctr, PO Box 6510, MS F-704, 1665 Aurora Court, Aurora, CO 80045-0510; **Phone:** 720-848-0300; **Board Cert:** Internal Medicine 1988; Medical Oncology 2006; **Med School:** Univ Tex Med Br, Galveston 1985; **Resid:** Internal Medicine, Univ Virginia Med Ctr 1988; **Fellow:** Research, Scripps Clinic 1989; Medical Oncology, UCSD Med Ctr 1992; **Fac Appt:** Prof Med, Univ Colorado

Elias, Anthony D MD [Onc] - **Spec Exp:** Breast Cancer; **Hospital:** Univ Colorado Hosp; **Address:** UCH Breast Ctr, Anschutz OPD Pavillion, 1635 Aurora Ct, MS F724, Aurora, CO 80045; **Phone:** 720-848-1030; **Board Cert:** Internal Medicine 1983; Medical Oncology 1985; **Med School:** NYU Sch Med 1980; **Resid:** Internal Medicine, Johns Hopkins Hsop 1983; **Fellow:** Medical Oncology, Dana-Farber Cancer Inst 1983; **Fac Appt:** Assoc Prof Med, Univ Colorado

Fabian, Carol J MD [Onc] - **Spec Exp:** Breast Cancer; Breast Cancer Risk Assessment; **Hospital:** Univ of Kansas Hosp; **Address:** Univ Kansas Med Ctr, Div Clinical Onc, 2330 Shawnee Mission Pkwy, Ste 1102, MS 5015, Kansas City, KS 66160-7418; **Phone:** 913-588-7791; **Board Cert:** Internal Medicine 1976; Medical Oncology 1977; **Med School:** Univ Kans 1972; **Resid:** Internal Medicine, Wesley Med Ctr 1975; **Fellow:** Medical Oncology, Univ Kansas Med Ctr 1977; **Fac Appt:** Prof Med, Univ Kans

Glode, L Michael MD [Onc] - **Spec Exp:** Prostate Cancer; Genitourinary Cancer; **Hospital:** Univ Colorado Hosp; **Address:** U Colo Hlth Scis Ctr, Div Med Oncology, PO Box 6510, MS F710, Aurora, CO 80045-0510; **Phone:** 720-848-0170; **Board Cert:** Internal Medicine 1975; Medical Oncology 1981; **Med School:** Washington Univ, St Louis 1972; **Resid:** Internal Medicine, Univ Texas SW Med Sch 1973; Immunology, Natl Inst Hlth 1976; **Fellow:** Medical Oncology, Dana Farber Cancer Inst 1978; **Fac Appt:** Prof Med, Univ Colorado

Grem, Jean L MD [Onc] - **Spec Exp:** Colon & Rectal Cancer; Pancreatic Cancer; Stomach Cancer; Esophageal Cancer; **Hospital:** Nebraska Med Ctr; **Address:** 987680 Nebraska Medical Ctr, Omaha, NE 68198-7680; **Phone:** 402-559-6210; **Board Cert:** Internal Medicine 1983; Medical Oncology 1985; **Med School:** Jefferson Med Coll 1980; **Resid:** Internal Medicine, Univ Iowa Hosps & Clinics 1983; **Fellow:** Medical Oncology, Univ Wisc Clin Cancer Ctr 1986; **Fac Appt:** Prof Med, Univ Nebr Coll Med

Hauke, Ralph J MD [Onc] - **Spec Exp:** Urologic Cancer; Clinical Trials; Testicular Cancer; Prostate Cancer; **Hospital:** Methodist Hosp - Omaha, Alegent Hlth - Bergan Mercy Med Ctr; **Address:** 8303 Dodge St, Ste 250, Omaha, NE 68114; **Phone:** 402-354-8124; **Board Cert:** Medical Oncology 2001; **Med School:** Panama 1990; **Resid:** Internal Medicine, Univ Nebraska Med Ctr 1996; **Fellow:** Medical Oncology, Univ Nebraska Med Ctr 2001; **Fac Appt:** Assoc Prof Med, Univ Nebr Coll Med

Kane, Madeleine A MD/PhD [Onc] - **Spec Exp:** Head & Neck Cancer; Gastrointestinal Cancer; Neuroendocrine Tumors; **Hospital:** Univ Colorado Hosp, VA Med Ctr; **Address:** Univ Colorado Hosp Cancer Ctr, PO Box 6510, MS F-704, 1665 Aurora Court, Aurora, CO 80045; **Phone:** 720-848-0300; **Board Cert:** Internal Medicine 1981; Medical Oncology 1983; Hematology 1986; **Med School:** Univ Miami Sch Med 1978; **Resid:** Internal Medicine, Stanford Univ Med Ctr 1981; **Fellow:** Hematology & Oncology, Univ Colo Hlth Sci Ctr 1984; **Fac Appt:** Prof Med, Univ Colorado

Kelly, Karen Lee MD [Onc] - **Spec Exp:** Lung Cancer; **Hospital:** Univ of Kansas Hosp; **Address:** Univ Kansas Cancer Ctr, 4030 Robinson, MS #1027, 3901 Rainbow Blvd, Kansas City, KS 66160; **Phone:** 913-588-4761; **Board Cert:** Internal Medicine 1987; Medical Oncology 2003; **Med School:** Univ Kans 1984; **Resid:** Internal Medicine, Univ Colo Hlth Sci Ctr 1987; **Fellow:** Medical Oncology, Univ Colo Hlth Sci Ctr 1990; **Fac Appt:** Assoc Prof Med, Univ Colorado

Samuels, Brian L MD [Onc] - **Spec Exp:** Sarcoma; **Hospital:** Kootenai Med Ctr; **Address:** North Idaho Cancer Center, 700 W Ironwood Drive, Ste 103, Coeur D'Alene, ID 83814; **Phone:** 208-666-3800; **Board Cert:** Internal Medicine 1984; Medical Oncology 1987; **Med School:** Zimbabwe 1976; **Resid:** Internal Medicine, Albert Einstein Med Ctr 1981; Internal Medicine, Albert Einstein Med Ctr 1984; **Fellow:** Hematology & Oncology, Univ Chicago Hosps 1988

Ward, John H MD [Onc] - **Spec Exp:** Breast Cancer; Gastrointestinal Cancer; **Hospital:** Univ Utah Hosps and Clins; **Address:** Huntsman Cancer Inst, 2000 Circle of Hope, Ste 2100, Salt Lake City, UT 84112-5550; **Phone:** 801-585-0255; **Board Cert:** Internal Medicine 1979; Medical Oncology 1981; Hematology 1982; **Med School:** Univ Utah 1976; **Resid:** Internal Medicine, Duke Univ Med Ctr 1979; **Fellow:** Hematology & Oncology, Univ Utah 1982; **Fac Appt:** Prof Med, Univ Utah

Southwest

Abbruzzese, James L MD [Onc] - **Spec Exp:** Gastrointestinal Cancer; Pancreatic Cancer; Clinical Trials; **Hospital:** UT MD Anderson Cancer Ctr; **Address:** Univ Tex MD Anderson Cancer Ctr, 1515 Holcombe Blvd, Unit 426, Houston, TX 77030; **Phone:** 713-792-2828; **Board Cert:** Internal Medicine 1981; Medical Oncology 1983; **Med School:** Univ Chicago-Pritzker Sch Med 1978; **Resid:** Internal Medicine, Johns Hopkins Hosp 1981; **Fellow:** Medical Oncology, Dana-Farber Cancer Inst 1983; **Fac Appt:** Prof Med, Univ Tex, Houston

Ahmann, Frederick R MD [Onc] - **Spec Exp:** Prostate Cancer; Testicular Cancer; Bladder Cancer; **Hospital:** Univ Med Ctr - Tucson; **Address:** Arizona Cancer Ctr, 1515 N Campbell Ave, Box 245024, Tucson, AZ 85724; **Phone:** 520-694-2873; **Board Cert:** Internal Medicine 1977; Medical Oncology 1981; **Med School:** Univ MO-Columbia Sch Med 1974; **Resid:** Internal Medicine, Georgetown Univ Med Ctr 1977; **Fellow:** Medical Oncology, Univ Med Ctr 1980; **Fac Appt:** Prof Med, Univ Ariz Coll Med

Medical Oncology

Ajani, Jaffer A MD [Onc] - **Spec Exp:** Gastrointestinal Cancer; Esophageal Cancer; Stomach Cancer; Neuroendocrine Tumors; **Hospital:** UT MD Anderson Cancer Ctr; **Address:** Univ Tex MD Anderson Cancer Ctr, Faculty Ctr Unit 426, Houston, TX 77230; **Phone:** 713-792-2828; **Board Cert:** Internal Medicine 1979; Medical Oncology 1983; **Med School:** India 1971; **Resid:** Family Medicine, Penn Stae Univ-Altoona 1977; Internal Medicine, Tulane Univ Sch Med 1980; **Fellow:** Medical Oncology, MD Anderson Cancer Ctr 1983; **Fac Appt:** Prof Med, Univ Tex, Houston

Alberts, David S MD [Onc] - **Spec Exp:** Cancer Prevention; Ovarian Cancer; **Hospital:** Univ Med Ctr - Tucson; **Address:** Arizona Cancer Center, 1515N Campbell Ave, PO Box 245024, Tucson, AZ 85724; **Phone:** 520-626-7685; **Board Cert:** Internal Medicine 1973; Medical Oncology 1973; **Med School:** Univ VA Sch Med 1966; **Resid:** Medical Oncology, Natl Cancer Inst-NIH 1969; Internal Medicine, Univ Minn Hosps 1971; **Fellow:** Clinical Pharmacology, UC San Francisco 1974; **Fac Appt:** Prof Med, Univ Ariz Coll Med

Anthony, Lowell B MD [Onc] - **Spec Exp:** Gastrointestinal Cancer; Carcinoid Tumors; Neuroendocrine Tumors; **Hospital:** LSU Interim Public Hosp; **Address:** 200 W Esplanade, Ste 200, Kenner, LA 70065; **Phone:** 504-464-8500; **Board Cert:** Internal Medicine 1983; Medical Oncology 1989; **Med School:** Vanderbilt Univ 1979; **Resid:** Internal Medicine, Vanderbilt Univ Med Ctr 1982; **Fellow:** Medical Oncology, Vanderbilt Univ Med Ctr 1985; **Fac Appt:** Assoc Prof Med, Louisiana State U, New Orleans

Arun, Banu K MD [Onc] - **Spec Exp:** Breast Cancer; Cancer Prevention; Clinical Trials; **Hospital:** UT MD Anderson Cancer Ctr; **Address:** 1515 Holcombe Blvd, Unit 1354, Houston, TX 77030; **Phone:** 713-792-2817; **Med School:** Turkey 1990; **Resid:** Internal Medicine, Univ Istanbul 1994; **Fellow:** Hematology & Oncology, Lombardi Cancer Ctr-Georgetown Univ 1997; **Fac Appt:** Assoc Prof Med, Univ Tex, Houston

Benjamin, Robert S MD [Onc] - **Spec Exp:** Sarcoma; **Hospital:** UT MD Anderson Cancer Ctr; **Address:** UT MD Anderson Cancer Ctr, 1515 Holcombe Blvd, Unit 450, Houston, TX 77030; **Phone:** 713-792-3626; **Board Cert:** Internal Medicine 1973; Medical Oncology 1973; **Med School:** NYU Sch Med 1968; **Resid:** Internal Medicine, Bellevue Hosp Ctr-NYU 1970; **Fellow:** Medical Oncology, Baltimore Cancer Rsch Ctr 1972; **Fac Appt:** Prof Med, Univ Tex, Houston

Bergsagel, Peter Leif MD [Onc] - **Spec Exp:** Multiple Myeloma; Hematologic Malignancies; **Hospital:** Mayo Clinic - Scottsdale; **Address:** 13400 E Shea Blvd, Scottsdale, AZ 85259; **Phone:** 480-301-8335; **Board Cert:** Internal Medicine 1987; Medical Oncology 1989; **Med School:** Univ Toronto 1984; **Resid:** Internal Medicine, Stanford Univ Med Ctr 1986; Internal Medicine, Sunnybrook Med Ctr 1987; **Fellow:** Medical Oncology, NIH Natl Cancer Inst 1990; **Fac Appt:** Prof Med, Mayo Med Sch

Bruera, Eduardo MD [Onc] - **Spec Exp:** Palliative Care; **Hospital:** UT MD Anderson Cancer Ctr; **Address:** 1515 Holcombe Blvd, Unit 8, Houston, TX 77030; **Phone:** 713-792-6085; **Med School:** Argentina 1979; **Resid:** Internal Medicine, Hospital Privado; **Fellow:** Medical Oncology, Cross Cancer Inst; **Fac Appt:** Prof Med, Univ Tex, Houston

Buzdar, Aman U MD [Onc] - **Spec Exp:** Breast Cancer; **Hospital:** UT MD Anderson Cancer Ctr; **Address:** UT MD Anderson Canc Ctr, Dept Breast Oncology, PO Box 301429, Unit 1354, Houston, TX 77030; **Phone:** 713-792-2817; **Board Cert:** Internal Medicine 1975; Medical Oncology 1979; **Med School:** Pakistan 1967; **Resid:** Internal Medicine, Norwalk Hosp 1973; Internal Medicine, Lakewood Hosp 1971; **Fellow:** Hematology, Norwalk Hosp 1974; Oncology, MD Anderson Cancer Ctr 1975; **Fac Appt:** Prof Med, Univ Tex, Houston

Camoriano, John MD [Onc] - **Spec Exp:** Lymphoma; Breast Cancer; Bone Marrow Transplant; Castleman's Disease; **Hospital:** Mayo Clinic - Scottsdale; **Address:** Mayo Clinic - Scottsdale, 13400 E Shea Blvd Fl 3, Scottsdale, AZ 85259; **Phone:** 480-301-8335; **Board Cert:** Internal Medicine 1985; Hematology 1988; Medical Oncology 1989; **Med School:** Univ Nebr Coll Med 1982; **Resid:** Internal Medicine, Univ OK 1985; **Fellow:** Hematology & Oncology, Mayo Grad Sch Med 1989; **Fac Appt:** Asst Prof Med, Mayo Med Sch

Chang, Jenny C N MD [Onc] - **Spec Exp:** Breast Cancer; Clinical Trials; **Hospital:** Methodist Hosp - Houston; **Address:** One Baylor Plaza, MS BCM600, Houston, TX 77030; **Phone:** 713-798-1034; **Board Cert:** Internal Medicine 2004; **Med School:** England, UK 1989; **Resid:** Internal Medicine 1993; **Fellow:** Medical Oncology, Royal Marsden Hosp 1997; **Fac Appt:** Assoc Prof Med, Baylor Coll Med

Fay, Joseph W MD [Onc] - **Spec Exp:** Bone Marrow Transplant; Melanoma; Leukemia & Lymphoma; **Hospital:** Baylor Univ Medical Ctr; **Address:** 3535 Worth St, Sammons Tower, Suite 500, Dallas, TX 75246; **Phone:** 214-370-1500; **Board Cert:** Internal Medicine 1975; Medical Oncology 1977; Hematology 1978; **Med School:** Ohio State Univ 1972; **Resid:** Internal Medicine, Duke Med Ctr 1974; Oncology, Natl Cancer Institute 1976; **Fellow:** Hematology, Duke Med Ctr 1977; **Fac Appt:** Clin Prof Med, Univ Tex SW, Dallas

Fitch, Tom R MD [Onc] - **Spec Exp:** Breast Cancer; Sarcoma; Cancer Prevention; Palliative Care; **Hospital:** Mayo Clinic - Scottsdale; **Address:** Mayo Clinic - Scottsdale, 13400 E Shea Blvd Fl 3, Scottsdale, AZ 85259; **Phone:** 480-301-8335; **Board Cert:** Internal Medicine 1985; Medical Oncology 1987; Hematology 1988; **Med School:** Univ Kans 1982; **Resid:** Internal Medicine, Univ Michigan Med Ctr 1985; **Fellow:** Hematology & Oncology, Mayo Clinic 1988; **Fac Appt:** Asst Prof Med, Mayo Med Sch

Fossella, Frank V MD [Onc] - **Spec Exp:** Lung Cancer; **Hospital:** UT MD Anderson Cancer Ctr; **Address:** Dept Thoracic Head/Neck Med Oncol, Unit 432, 1400 Holcombe Blvd, Houston, TX 77030; **Phone:** 713-792-6363; **Board Cert:** Internal Medicine 1985; Medical Oncology 1987; **Med School:** Baylor Coll Med 1982; **Resid:** Internal Medicine, Baylor Coll Med 1985; **Fellow:** Medical Oncology, Baylor Coll Med 1987; **Fac Appt:** Prof Med, Univ Tex, Houston

Glisson, Bonnie S MD [Onc] - **Spec Exp:** Head & Neck Cancer; Lung Cancer; **Hospital:** UT MD Anderson Cancer Ctr; **Address:** 1515 Holcombe Blvd, Unit 432, Houston, TX 77030; **Phone:** 713-792-6363; **Board Cert:** Internal Medicine 1982; Medical Oncology 1985; **Med School:** Ohio State Univ 1979; **Resid:** Internal Medicine, Univ Va Med Ctr 1982; **Fellow:** Medical Oncology, Univ Fla Health Sci Ctr 1985; **Fac Appt:** Prof Med, Univ Tex, Houston

Haley, Barbara MD [Onc] - **Spec Exp:** Breast Cancer; **Hospital:** UT Southwestern Med Ctr at Dallas; **Address:** 5323 Harry Hines Blvd, Dallas, TX 75390-8852; **Phone:** 214-648-4180; **Board Cert:** Internal Medicine 1979; Hematology 1984; **Med School:** Univ Tex SW, Dallas 1976; **Resid:** Internal Medicine, Parkland Meml Hosp 1979; **Fellow:** Hematology & Oncology, Parkland Meml Hosp 1981; **Fac Appt:** Prof Med, Univ Tex SW, Dallas

Herbst, Roy S MD/PhD [Onc] - **Spec Exp:** Lung Cancer; Head & Neck Cancer; Breast Cancer; Drug Development; **Hospital:** UT MD Anderson Cancer Ctr; **Address:** Thoracic/Head & Neck Med Onc - Unit 432, UT MD Anderson Cancer Ctr, PO Box 301402, Houston, TX 77230-1402; **Phone:** 713-792-6363; **Board Cert:** Medical Oncology 2007; **Med School:** Cornell Univ-Weill Med Coll 1991; **Resid:** Internal Medicine, Brigham & Women's Hosp 1994; **Fellow:** Medical Oncology, Dana Farber Cancer Inst 1996; **Fac Appt:** Assoc Prof Med, Univ Tex, Houston

Medical Oncology

Hong, Waun Ki MD [Onc] - **Spec Exp:** Lung Cancer; Head & Neck Cancer; Thoracic Cancers; **Hospital:** UT MD Anderson Cancer Ctr; **Address:** Dept Thoracic Head/Neck, Unit 432, 1400 Holcombe Blvd, Houston, TX 77030; **Phone:** 713-792-6363; **Board Cert:** Internal Medicine 1976; Medical Oncology 1979; **Med School:** South Korea 1967; **Resid:** Internal Medicine, Boston VA Hosp 1973; **Fellow:** Medical Oncology, Meml Sloan-Kettering Cancer Ctr 1975; **Fac Appt:** Prof Med, Univ Tex, Houston

Hortobagyi, Gabriel N MD [Onc] - **Spec Exp:** Breast Cancer; Clinical Trials; Gene Therapy; **Hospital:** UT MD Anderson Cancer Ctr; **Address:** UT MD Anderson Cancer Ctr, Dept Breast Oncology, PO Box 301429, Unit 1354, Houston, TX 77030-1439; **Phone:** 713-792-2817; **Board Cert:** Internal Medicine 1975; Medical Oncology 1977; **Med School:** Colombia 1970; **Resid:** Internal Medicine, St Lukes Hosp 1974; **Fellow:** Medical Oncology, MD Anderson Cancer Ctr 1976; **Fac Appt:** Prof Med

Hutchins, Laura F MD [Onc] - **Spec Exp:** Breast Cancer; Melanoma; **Hospital:** UAMS Med Ctr; **Address:** Univ Arkansas Med Scis, Dept Hem/Onc, 4301 W Markham St, MS 721-5, Little Rock, AR 72205-7101; **Phone:** 501-686-8511; **Board Cert:** Internal Medicine 1980; Hematology 1984; Medical Oncology 1987; **Med School:** Univ Ark 1977; **Resid:** Internal Medicine, Univ Ark Affil Hosp 1980; **Fellow:** Hematology & Oncology, Univ Arkansas 1983; **Fac Appt:** Prof Med, Univ Ark

Karp, Daniel D MD [Onc] - **Spec Exp:** Lung Cancer; **Hospital:** UT MD Anderson Cancer Ctr; **Address:** 1515 Holcombe Blvd, Unit 432, Houston, TX 77030-4009; **Phone:** 713-792-6363; **Board Cert:** Internal Medicine 1976; Hematology 1980; Medical Oncology 1981; **Med School:** Duke Univ 1973; **Resid:** Internal Medicine, Dartmouth-Hitchcock Med Ctr 1976; **Fellow:** Hematology, Dartmouth-Hitchcock Med Ctr 1978; Medical Oncology, Dana Farber Cancer Inst 1979; **Fac Appt:** Prof Med, Univ Tex, Houston

Kies, Merrill S MD [Onc] - **Spec Exp:** Head & Neck Cancer; Lung Cancer; **Hospital:** UT MD Anderson Cancer Ctr; **Address:** Dept Thoracic, Head & Neck Oncology, 1515 Holcombe Blvd, Unit 432, Houston, TX 77030; **Phone:** 713-792-6363; **Board Cert:** Internal Medicine 1976; Medical Oncology 1979; **Med School:** Loyola Univ-Stritch Sch Med 1973; **Resid:** Internal Medicine, Walter Reed AMC 1976; **Fellow:** Medical Oncology, Brooke AMC 1978; **Fac Appt:** Prof Med, Univ Tex, Houston

Kwak, Larry W MD/PhD [Onc] - **Spec Exp:** Lymphoma; Multiple Myeloma; Vaccine Therapy; Immunotherapy; **Hospital:** UT MD Anderson Cancer Ctr; **Address:** MD Anderson Cancer Ctr, Dept Lymphoma/Myeloma, 1515 Holcombe Blvd, Unit 429, Houston, TX 77030; **Phone:** 713-745-4244; **Board Cert:** Internal Medicine 1987; Medical Oncology 1989; **Med School:** Northwestern Univ 1982; **Resid:** Internal Medicine, Stanford Univ Hosp 1987; **Fellow:** Oncology, Stanford Univ Hosp 1989

Lippman, Scott M MD [Onc] - **Spec Exp:** Cancer Prevention; Lung Cancer; Head & Neck Cancer; **Hospital:** UT MD Anderson Cancer Ctr; **Address:** UT MD Anderson Cancer Ctr, 1515 Holcombe Blvd, Box 432, Houston, TX 77030-1439; **Phone:** 713-745-5439; **Board Cert:** Internal Medicine 1987; Hematology 1988; Medical Oncology 1989; **Med School:** Johns Hopkins Univ 1981; **Resid:** Internal Medicine, Harbor-UCLA Med Ctr 1983; **Fellow:** Hematology, Stanford Univ Med Ctr 1985; Hematology & Oncology, Univ Ariz Hlth Scis Ctr 1987; **Fac Appt:** Prof Med, Univ Tex, Houston

Livingston, Robert B MD [Onc] - **Spec Exp:** Bone Marrow Transplant; Breast Cancer; Lung Cancer; **Hospital:** Univ Med Ctr - Tucson; **Address:** University Medical Center, 3838 N Campbell Ave, Tucson, AZ 85719; **Phone:** 520-694-2873; **Board Cert:** Internal Medicine 1972; Medical Oncology 1973; **Med School:** Univ Okla Coll Med 1965; **Resid:** Internal Medicine, Univ Oklahoma Med Ctr 1971; **Fellow:** Medical Oncology, Univ Texas Cancer Ctr 1973; **Fac Appt:** Prof Med, Univ Wash

Logothetis, Christopher J MD [Onc] - **Spec Exp:** Prostate Cancer; Bladder Cancer; **Hospital:** UT MD Anderson Cancer Ctr; **Address:** UT MD Anderson Cancer Ctr, Dept GU Onc, Unit 1374, Box 301439, Houston, TX 77230-1439; **Phone:** 713-745-7020; **Board Cert:** Internal Medicine 1978; Medical Oncology 1981; **Med School:** Greece 1974; **Resid:** Internal Medicine, Univ Texas 1979; **Fellow:** Hematology & Oncology, Univ Tex-MD Anderson Cancer Ctr 1981; **Fac Appt:** Prof Med, Univ Tex, Houston

Markman, Maurie MD [Onc] - **Spec Exp:** Ovarian Cancer; Gynecologic Cancer; Drug Development; Palliative Care; **Hospital:** UT MD Anderson Cancer Ctr; **Address:** Univ Texas MD Anderson Cancer Ctr, 1515 Holcombe Blvd, Box 1435, Houston, TX 77030-4009; **Phone:** 713-745-7140; **Board Cert:** Internal Medicine 1977; Hematology 1982; Medical Oncology 1981; **Med School:** NYU Sch Med 1974; **Resid:** Internal Medicine, Bellevue Hosp Ctr 1978; **Fellow:** Medical Oncology, Johns Hopkins Hosp 1980; **Fac Appt:** Prof Med, Univ Tex, Houston

Miller, Thomas P MD [Onc] - **Spec Exp:** Lymphoma; **Hospital:** Univ Med Ctr - Tucson; **Address:** Arizona Cancer Ctr, 1515 N Campbell Ave, PO Box 245024, Tucson, AZ 85724; **Phone:** 520-626-2667; **Board Cert:** Internal Medicine 1977; Medical Oncology 1981; **Med School:** Univ IL Coll Med 1972; **Resid:** Internal Medicine, Univ Illinois Hosps 1977; **Fellow:** Hematology & Oncology, Univ Med Ctr 1980; **Fac Appt:** Prof Med, Univ Ariz Coll Med

Nemunaitis, John G MD [Onc] - **Spec Exp:** Cancer Genetics; Vaccine Therapy; Lung Cancer; **Hospital:** Baylor Univ Medical Ctr; **Address:** Mary Crowley Med Rsch Ctr, 3535 Worth St, Ste 302, Dallas, TX 75246; **Phone:** 214-370-1870; **Board Cert:** Internal Medicine 1987; **Med School:** Case West Res Univ 1982; **Resid:** Internal Medicine, Boston City Hosp 1985; **Fellow:** Hematology & Oncology, Fred Hutchinson Cancer Rsch Ctr 1989

Northfelt, Donald W MD [Onc] - **Spec Exp:** Breast Cancer; Colon & Rectal Cancer; Lung Cancer; **Hospital:** Mayo Clinic - Scottsdale; **Address:** Mayo Clinic Scottsdale, 13400 E Shea Blvd Fl 3, Scottsdale, AZ 85259; **Phone:** 480-301-8335; **Board Cert:** Internal Medicine 1988; Medical Oncology 2001; **Med School:** Univ Minn 1985; **Resid:** Internal Medicine, UCLA Med Ctr 1988; **Fellow:** Hematology & Oncology, UCSF Med Ctr 1991; **Fac Appt:** Assoc Prof Med, Mayo Med Sch

O'Brien, Susan M MD [Onc] - **Spec Exp:** Leukemia; Lymphoma; **Hospital:** UT MD Anderson Cancer Ctr; **Address:** Univ Texas MD Anderson Cancer Ctr, Dept Leukemia, Unit 428, Box 301439, Houston, TX 77230; **Phone:** 713-792-7305; **Board Cert:** Internal Medicine 1983; Medical Oncology 1987; **Med School:** UMDNJ-NJ Med Sch, Newark 1980; **Resid:** Internal Medicine, UMDNJ Med Ctr 1983; **Fellow:** Medical Oncology, Univ TX MD Anderson Med Ctr 1987; **Fac Appt:** Prof Med, Univ Tex, Houston

O'Shaughnessy, Joyce A MD [Onc] - **Spec Exp:** Breast Cancer; **Hospital:** Baylor Univ Medical Ctr; **Address:** US Oncology, 3535 Worth St, Ste 600, Dallas, TX 75246; **Phone:** 214-370-1000; **Board Cert:** Internal Medicine 1985; Medical Oncology 1987; **Med School:** Yale Univ 1982; **Resid:** Internal Medicine, Mass Genl Hosp 1985; **Fellow:** Medical Oncology, National Cancer Inst 1988

Orlowski, Robert Z MD/PhD [Onc] - **Spec Exp:** Multiple Myeloma; Lymphoma, Non-Hodgkin's; Leukemia; Clinical Trials; **Hospital:** UT MD Anderson Cancer Ctr; **Address:** MD Anderson Cancer Ctr, Lymphoma & Myeloma Clinic, 1515 Holcombe Blvd, Box 429, Houston, TX 77030; **Phone:** 713-792-3510; **Med School:** Yale Univ 1991; **Resid:** Internal Medicine, Barnes Hosp/Wash Univ 1994; **Fellow:** Hematology & Oncology, Johns Hopkins Hosp 1998

Medical Oncology

Osborne, Charles K MD [Onc] - **Spec Exp:** Breast Cancer; **Hospital:** Methodist Hosp - Houston; **Address:** 1 Baylor Plaza, MS BCM600, Houston, TX 77030; **Phone:** 713-798-1641; **Board Cert:** Internal Medicine 1975; Medical Oncology 1977; **Med School:** Univ MO-Columbia Sch Med 1972; **Resid:** Internal Medicine, Johns Hopkins Hosp 1974; **Fellow:** Medical Oncology, Natl Cancer Inst 1977; **Fac Appt:** Prof Med, Baylor Coll Med

Papadopoulos, Nicholas E MD [Onc] - **Spec Exp:** Melanoma; **Hospital:** UT MD Anderson Cancer Ctr; **Address:** 1515 Holcombe Blvd, Unit 430, Houston, TX 77030; **Phone:** 713-792-2828; **Med School:** Greece 1966; **Resid:** Internal Medicine, Baylor Coll Med 1976; **Fellow:** Medical Oncology, MD Anderson Cancer Ctr 1978; **Fac Appt:** Assoc Prof Med, Univ Tex, Houston

Patel, Shreyaskumar MD [Onc] - **Spec Exp:** Sarcoma; **Hospital:** UT MD Anderson Cancer Ctr; **Address:** 1515 Holcombe Blvd, Box 0450, Houston, TX 77030; **Phone:** 713-792-3626; **Board Cert:** Internal Medicine 1987; Medical Oncology 2000; **Med School:** India 1983; **Resid:** Internal Medicine, Wayne State Univ 1987; **Fellow:** Medical Oncology, Mayo Clinic 1990

Patt, Yehuda Z MD [Onc] - **Spec Exp:** Liver Cancer; Biliary Cancer; Colon & Rectal Cancer; Gastrointestinal Cancer; **Hospital:** Univ NM Hlth & Sci Ctr; **Address:** Univ New Mexico CRTC, Div Hem/Onc, 900 Camino de Salud NE, MSC 084630, Albuquerque, NM 87131-0001; **Phone:** 505-272-5837; **Board Cert:** Internal Medicine 1982; Medical Oncology 1987; **Med School:** Israel 1967; **Resid:** Internal Medicine, Tel Aviv-Sheba Med Ctr 1974; **Fellow:** Medical Oncology, UT MD Anderson Cancer Ctr 1977; **Fac Appt:** Prof Med, Univ New Mexico

Pisters, Katherine M W MD [Onc] - **Spec Exp:** Lung Cancer; **Hospital:** UT MD Anderson Cancer Ctr; **Address:** UT MD Anderson Cancer Ctr, 1414 Holcombe Blvd, Houston, TX 77030; **Phone:** 713-792-6110; **Board Cert:** Internal Medicine 1988; Medical Oncology 2002; **Med School:** Univ Western Ontario 1985; **Resid:** Internal Medicine, N Shore Univ Hosp 1988; **Fellow:** Medical Oncology, Meml Sloan Kettering Cancer Ctr 1991; **Fac Appt:** Prof Med, Univ Tex, Houston

Romaguera, Jorge MD [Onc] - **Spec Exp:** Lymphoma; **Hospital:** UT MD Anderson Cancer Ctr; **Address:** 1515 Holcombe Blvd, Box 0429, Houston, TX 77030; **Phone:** 713-745-4246; **Board Cert:** Internal Medicine 1988; Medical Oncology 1989; **Med School:** Univ Puerto Rico 1982; **Resid:** Internal Medicine, Univ Hosp 1985; **Fellow:** Hematology & Oncology, Univ Hosp 1987

Ross, Helen J MD [Onc] - **Spec Exp:** Lung Cancer; Mesothelioma; Esophageal Cancer; **Hospital:** Mayo Clinic - Scottsdale; **Address:** Mayo Clinic, 13400 E Shea Blvd, Scottsdale, AZ 85259; **Phone:** 480-301-8335; **Board Cert:** Internal Medicine 1987; Medical Oncology 1989; **Med School:** UCLA 1984; **Resid:** Internal Medicine, Cedars Sinai Med Ctr 1987; **Fellow:** Medical Oncology, UCLA Med Ctr 1989; **Fac Appt:** Assoc Prof Med, Mayo Med Sch

Saiki, John H MD [Onc] - **Hospital:** Univ NM Hlth & Sci Ctr; **Address:** Univ of New Mexico Cancer Ctr, 900 Camino de Salud NE, MSC 084630, Albuquerque, NM 87131-0001; **Phone:** 505-272-8740; **Board Cert:** Internal Medicine 1970; Medical Oncology 1973; **Med School:** McGill Univ 1961; **Resid:** Internal Medicine, Univ New Mexico 1968; Hematology, Univ New Mexico 1969; **Fellow:** Medical Oncology, MD Anderson Hosp 1970; **Fac Appt:** Prof Emeritus Med, Univ New Mexico

Schiller, Joan H MD [Onc] - **Spec Exp:** Lung Cancer; **Hospital:** UT Southwestern Med Ctr at Dallas; **Address:** Univ Texas SW, 5323 Harry Hines Blvd, Dallas, TX 75390-8852; **Phone:** 214-648-4180; **Board Cert:** Internal Medicine 1983; Medical Oncology 1987; **Med School:** Univ IL Coll Med 1980; **Resid:** Internal Medicine, Northwestern Meml Hosp 1983; **Fellow:** Medical Oncology, Univ Wisconsin Hosp 1986; **Fac Appt:** Prof Med, Univ Wisc

Stopeck, Alison T MD [Onc] - **Spec Exp:** Breast Cancer; Breast Cancer Risk Assessment; **Hospital:** Univ Med Ctr - Tucson; **Address:** 1515 N Campbell Ave, PO Box 245024, Tucson, AZ 85724; **Phone:** 520-626-2816; **Board Cert:** Internal Medicine 1988; Medical Oncology 2002; Hematology 2002; **Med School:** Columbia P&S 1985; **Resid:** Internal Medicine, Columbia-Presby Med Ctr 1988; **Fellow:** Hematology & Oncology, New York Hosp 1991; **Fac Appt:** Assoc Prof Med, Univ Ariz Coll Med

Valero, Vicente MD [Onc] - **Spec Exp:** Breast Cancer; **Hospital:** UT MD Anderson Cancer Ctr, LBJ General Hosp; **Address:** Univ Texas MD Anderson Cancer Ctr, 1515 Holcombe Blvd, Unit 1354, Houston, TX 77030; **Phone:** 713-792-2817; **Board Cert:** Internal Medicine 1985; Medical Oncology 1987; Hematology 1988; **Med School:** Mexico 1980; **Resid:** Internal Medicine, Univ Cincinnati Med Ctr 1985; Hematology & Oncology, Univ Cincinnati Med Ctr 1987; **Fellow:** Hematology & Oncology, Univ Texas Med Br 1988; **Fac Appt:** Prof Med, Univ Tex, Houston

Varadhachary, Gauri MD [Onc] - **Spec Exp:** Unknown Primary Cancer; Pancreatic Cancer; **Hospital:** UT MD Anderson Cancer Ctr; **Address:** 1515 Holcombe Blvd, Box 426, Houston, TX 77030; **Phone:** 713-792-2828; **Board Cert:** Internal Medicine 2004; Hematology 1998; Medical Oncology 2008; **Med School:** India 1991; **Resid:** Internal Medicine, Greater Baltimore Med Ctr 1995; **Fellow:** Hematology & Oncology, Baylor Univ 1998

Verschraegen, Claire F MD [Onc] - **Spec Exp:** Ovarian Cancer; Drug Discovery; Mesothelioma; **Hospital:** Univ NM Hlth & Sci Ctr; **Address:** UNM Cancer Research & Treatment Ctr, 900 Camino de Salud NE, rm MS C084630, Albuquerque, NM 87131-0001; **Phone:** 505-272-6760; **Board Cert:** Internal Medicine 2000; Medical Oncology 2000; **Med School:** Belgium 1982; **Resid:** Internal Medicine, Bordet 1985; Internal Medicine, Univ Texas 1991; **Fellow:** Cancer Research, Stehlin Fdn for Cancer Research 1988; Oncology, MD Anderson Cancer Ctr 1994; **Fac Appt:** Prof Med, Univ New Mexico

Von Burton, Gary MD [Onc] - **Spec Exp:** Breast Cancer; Sarcoma; Brain Tumors; **Hospital:** Louisiana State Univ Hosp; **Address:** LSUHSC-Shreveport, Feist-Weiller Cancer Ctr, 1501 Kings Hwy, PO Box 33932, Shreveport, LA 71130; **Phone:** 318-675-5972; **Board Cert:** Internal Medicine 1981; Medical Oncology 1983; **Med School:** Univ Utah 1978; **Resid:** Internal Medicine, Duke Univ Med Ctr 1981; **Fellow:** Hematology & Oncology, Duke Univ Med Ctr 1983; **Fac Appt:** Prof Med, Louisiana State U, Shrevport

Von Hoff, Daniel D MD [Onc] - **Spec Exp:** Pancreatic Cancer; Breast Cancer; Drug Discovery; **Hospital:** Scottsdale Hlthcare - Shea; **Address:** Translational Genomics Research Inst, 445 N 5th St, Ste 600, Phoenix, AZ 85004; **Phone:** 602-343-8492; **Board Cert:** Internal Medicine 1976; Medical Oncology 1979; **Med School:** Columbia P&S 1973; **Resid:** Internal Medicine, UCSF Med Ctr 1975; **Fac Appt:** Prof Med, Univ Ariz Coll Med

Willson, James KV MD [Onc] - **Spec Exp:** Gastrointestinal Cancer; Colon Cancer; Pancreatic Cancer; **Hospital:** UT Southwestern Med Ctr at Dallas; **Address:** 5323 Harry Hines Blvd, Dallas, TX 75390-8590; **Phone:** 214-645-4673; **Board Cert:** Internal Medicine 1980; Medical Oncology 1981; **Med School:** Univ Alabama 1976; **Resid:** Internal Medicine, Johns Hopkins Hosp 1978; **Fellow:** Medical Oncology, Natl Cancer Inst-NIH 1980; **Fac Appt:** Prof Med, Univ Tex SW, Dallas

Medical Oncology

West Coast and Pacific

Abrams, Donald I MD [Onc] - **Spec Exp:** AIDS Related Cancers; Complementary Medicine; **Hospital:** San Francisco Genl Hosp; **Address:** Positive Hlth Program-SF Genl Hosp, 995 Potrero Ave, Bldg 80, Ward 84, San Francisco, CA 94110; **Phone:** 415-476-4082 x444; **Board Cert:** Internal Medicine 1980; Medical Oncology 1983; **Med School:** Stanford Univ 1977; **Resid:** Internal Medicine, Kaiser Fdn Hosp 1980; **Fellow:** Medical Oncology, UCSF Cancer Rsch 1982; **Fac Appt:** Clin Prof Med, UCSF

Appelbaum, Frederick R MD [Onc] - **Spec Exp:** Bone Marrow Transplant; Leukemia; **Hospital:** Univ Wash Med Ctr; **Address:** 1100 Fairview Ave N, rm D5-310, PO Box 19024, Seattle, WA 98109; **Phone:** 206-288-1024; **Board Cert:** Internal Medicine 1975; Medical Oncology 1977; **Med School:** Tufts Univ 1972; **Resid:** Internal Medicine, Univ Michigan Med Ctr 1974; **Fellow:** Medical Oncology, Natl Cancer Inst 1976; **Fac Appt:** Prof Med, Univ Wash

Back, Anthony MD [Onc] - **Spec Exp:** Palliative Care; Gastrointestinal Cancer; **Hospital:** Univ Wash Med Ctr; **Address:** Seattle Cancer Care Alliance, 825 Eastlake Ave E, Seattle, WA 98109; **Phone:** 206-288-6478; **Board Cert:** Internal Medicine 1987; Medical Oncology 2001; **Med School:** Harvard Med Sch 1984; **Resid:** Internal Medicine, Univ Washington Med Ctr 1988; **Fellow:** Oncology, Univ Washington Med Ctr 1991; **Fac Appt:** Prof Med, Univ Wash

Ball, Edward D MD [Onc] - **Spec Exp:** Bone Marrow & Stem Cell Transplant; Leukemia & Lymphoma; Multiple Myeloma; Immunotherapy; **Hospital:** UCSD Med Ctr; **Address:** 3855 Health Sciences Dr, #0960, La Jolla, CA 92093; **Phone:** 858-822-6600; **Board Cert:** Internal Medicine 1979; Medical Oncology 1983; Hematology 2000; **Med School:** Case West Res Univ 1976; **Resid:** Internal Medicine, Hartford Hosp 1979; **Fellow:** Hematology & Oncology, Univ Hosps Cleveland 1981; Hematology & Oncology, Dartmouth-Hitchcock Hosp 1982; **Fac Appt:** Prof Med, UCSD

Beer, Tomasz M MD [Onc] - **Spec Exp:** Prostate Cancer; **Hospital:** OR Hlth & Sci Univ; **Address:** 3303 SW Bond Ave, CH14R, Portland, OR 97239; **Phone:** 503-494-6594; **Board Cert:** Medical Oncology 2000; **Med School:** Johns Hopkins Univ 1991; **Resid:** Internal Medicine, Oreg Hlth Scis Univ 1994; Internal Medicine, Oreg Hlth Scis Univ 1996; **Fellow:** Hematology & Oncology, Oreg Hlth Scis Univ 1999; **Fac Appt:** Assoc Prof Med, Oregon Hlth & Sci Univ

Bensinger, William I MD [Onc] - **Spec Exp:** Multiple Myeloma; Stem Cell Transplant; **Hospital:** Univ Wash Med Ctr; **Address:** Fred Hutchinson Cancer Research Ctr, 1100 Fairview Ave N, MS DS-390, Seattle, WA 98109-1024; **Phone:** 206-288-1024; **Board Cert:** Internal Medicine 1978; Medical Oncology 1979; **Med School:** Northwestern Univ 1973; **Resid:** Internal Medicine, Univ Wash Hosps 1978; **Fellow:** Medical Oncology, Univ Wash Hosps 1979; **Fac Appt:** Assoc Prof Med, Univ Wash

Carlson, Robert W MD [Onc] - **Spec Exp:** Breast Cancer; **Hospital:** Stanford Univ Med Ctr; **Address:** Stanford Comprehensive Cancer Ctr, 875 Blake Wilbur Drive, MC 5826, Stanford, CA 94305; **Phone:** 650-498-6000; **Board Cert:** Internal Medicine 1981; Medical Oncology 1983; **Med School:** Stanford Univ 1978; **Resid:** Internal Medicine, Barnes Hosp 1980; Internal Medicine, Stanford Univ Hosp 1981; **Fellow:** Medical Oncology, Stanford Univ Hosp 1983; **Fac Appt:** Prof Med, Stanford Univ

Chap, Linnea MD [Onc] - **Spec Exp:** Breast Cancer; **Hospital:** St John's Hlth Ctr, Santa Monica; **Address:** Premier Oncology, 2020 Santa Monica Blvd, Ste 600, Santa Monica, CA 90404-2023; **Phone:** 310-633-8400; **Board Cert:** Medical Oncology 2005; **Med School:** Univ Chicago-Pritzker Sch Med 1988; **Resid:** Internal Medicine, Northwestern Meml Hosp 1991; **Fellow:** Hematology & Oncology, UCLA Med Ctr 1992

Chlebowski, Rowan T MD/PhD [Onc] - **Spec Exp:** Breast Cancer; Women's Health; **Hospital:** LAC - Harbor - UCLA Med Ctr; **Address:** 1124 W Carson St J3 Bldg, Torrance, CA 90502; **Phone:** 310-222-2218; **Board Cert:** Internal Medicine 1980; Medical Oncology 1981; **Med School:** Case West Res Univ 1974; **Resid:** Internal Medicine, MetroHealth Med Ctr 1976; Medical Oncology, LAC-USC Med Ctr 1979; **Fac Appt:** Prof Med, UCLA

Chow, Warren A MD [Onc] - **Spec Exp:** Sarcoma-Soft Tissue; Sarcoma; **Hospital:** City of Hope Natl Med Ctr & Beckman Rsch; **Address:** 1500 E Duarte Rd, Duarte, CA 91010; **Phone:** 626-359-8111; **Board Cert:** Internal Medicine 1989; Medical Oncology 2003; Hematology 2004; **Med School:** Ros Franklin Univ/Chicago Med Sch 1986; **Resid:** Internal Medicine, Cedars-Sinai Med Ctr 1990; **Fellow:** Hematology & Oncology, City of Hope Med Ctr 1992; Molecular Genetics, City of Hope Med Ctr 1994; **Fac Appt:** Assoc Prof Med

Crocenzi, Todd MD [Onc] - **Spec Exp:** Gastrointestinal Cancer; **Hospital:** Providence Portland Med Ctr; **Address:** 4805 NE Glisan, Ste 6N40, Portland, OR 97213; **Phone:** 503-215-5696; **Board Cert:** Medical Oncology 2004; **Med School:** Jefferson Med Coll 1994; **Resid:** Internal Medicine, Univ MD Med Ctr 1997; **Fellow:** Hematology & Oncology, Dartmouth Hitchcock Med Ctr 2004; Immunology, Dartmouth Hitchcock Med Ctr 2005

Daud, Adil I MD [Onc] - **Spec Exp:** Melanoma; Skin Cancer; Drug Development; **Hospital:** UCSF Med Ctr; **Address:** 1600 Divisadero St, Box 1706, San Francisco, CA 94115; **Phone:** 415-353-9900; **Board Cert:** Hematology 2000; Medical Oncology 2000; **Med School:** India 1987; **Resid:** Internal Medicine, Indiana Univ; **Fellow:** Hematology & Oncology, Meml Sloan Kettering Cancer Ctr

Deeg, H. Joachim MD [Onc] - **Spec Exp:** Bone Marrow Failure Disorders; Hematologic Malignancies; **Hospital:** Univ Wash Med Ctr; **Address:** Fred Hutchinson Cancer Research Center, 1100 Fairview Avenue N, D1-100, Box 19024, Seattle, WA 98109-1024; **Phone:** 206-667-5985; **Board Cert:** Internal Medicine 1976; Medical Oncology 1979; **Med School:** Germany 1972; **Fac Appt:** Prof Med, Univ Wash

Disis, Mary Lenora MD [Onc] - **Spec Exp:** Breast Cancer; Ovarian Cancer; Clinical Trials; **Hospital:** Univ Wash Med Ctr; **Address:** Univ Washington, Tumor Vaccine Group, 815 Mercer St, Seattle, WA 98109; **Phone:** 206-543-8557; **Board Cert:** Internal Medicine 1989; Medical Oncology 2008; **Med School:** Univ Nebr Coll Med 1986; **Resid:** Internal Medicine, Univ Illinois Med Ctr 1990; **Fellow:** Medical Oncology, Fred Hutchinson Cancer Ctr 1993; **Fac Appt:** Assoc Prof Med, Univ Wash

Druker, Brian J MD [Onc] - **Spec Exp:** Leukemia; **Hospital:** OR Hlth & Sci Univ; **Address:** 3181 SW Sam Jackson Park Rd, MC L592, Portland, OR 97239-3098; **Phone:** 503-494-5058; **Board Cert:** Internal Medicine 1984; Medical Oncology 1987; **Med School:** UCSD 1981; **Resid:** Internal Medicine, Barnes Jewish Hosp 1984; **Fellow:** Medical Oncology, Dana-Farber Cancer Inst 1987; **Fac Appt:** Prof Med, Oregon Hlth & Sci Univ

Ellis, Georgiana K MD [Onc] - **Spec Exp:** Breast Cancer; Clinical Trials; **Hospital:** Univ Wash Med Ctr; **Address:** Univ Washington Sch Med, Div Oncology, SCCA 825 Eastlake Ave E, Box 358081, MS G3-630, Seattle, WA 98109-1023; **Phone:** 206-288-6989; **Board Cert:** Internal Medicine 1985; Medical Oncology 1987; **Med School:** Univ Wash 1982; **Resid:** Internal Medicine, Univ Washington Med Ctr 1985; **Fellow:** Medical Oncology, Univ Washington Med Ctr 1988; **Fac Appt:** Assoc Prof Med, Univ Wash

Medical Oncology

Estey, Elihu H MD [Onc] - **Spec Exp:** Leukemia; Myelodysplastic Syndromes; Clinical Trials; **Hospital:** Univ Wash Med Ctr; **Address:** Seattle Cancer Care Alliance, 825 Eastlake Ave E, UW Box 3587710, Seattle, WA 98109; **Phone:** 206-288-7176; **Board Cert:** Internal Medicine 1975; Medical Oncology 1981; **Med School:** Johns Hopkins Univ 1972; **Resid:** Internal Medicine, Bellevue Hosp Ctr 1975; **Fellow:** Medical Oncology, MD Anderson Cancer Ctr 1978

Figlin, Robert A MD [Onc] - **Spec Exp:** Urologic Cancer; Kidney Cancer; Immunotherapy; **Hospital:** City of Hope Natl Med Ctr & Beckman Rsch; **Address:** Med Oncology & Therapeutics Research, 1500 E Duarte Rd, Duarte, CA 91010; **Phone:** 626-256-4673; **Board Cert:** Internal Medicine 1979; Medical Oncology 1983; **Med School:** Med Coll PA Hahnemann 1976; **Resid:** Internal Medicine, Cedars Sinai Med Ctr 1980; **Fellow:** Hematology & Oncology, UCLA Ctr Hlth Sci 1982; **Fac Appt:** Prof Med, UCLA

Fisher Jr, George A MD/PhD [Onc] - **Spec Exp:** Gastrointestinal Cancer; Pancreatic Cancer; **Hospital:** Stanford Univ Med Ctr; **Address:** Stanford Comp Cancer Ctr, GI Onc, 875 Blake Wilbur Drive, MC 5826, Stanford, CA 94305; **Phone:** 650-723-7621; **Board Cert:** Medical Oncology 1997; **Med School:** Stanford Univ 1987; **Resid:** Internal Medicine, Stanford Univ Med Ctr 1991; **Fellow:** Medical Oncology, Stanford Univ Med Ctr 1993; **Fac Appt:** Assoc Prof Med, Stanford Univ

Ford, James M MD [Onc] - **Spec Exp:** Gastrointestinal Cancer; Colon & Rectal Cancer; Cancer Genetics; **Hospital:** Stanford Univ Med Ctr; **Address:** Stanford Comp Cancer Ctr, 875 Blake Wilbur Drive, Ste Clinic B, Stanford, CA 94305-5820; **Phone:** 650-723-7621; **Board Cert:** Medical Oncology 2005; **Med School:** Yale Univ 1989; **Resid:** Internal Medicine, Stanford Univ Med Ctr 1991; **Fellow:** Medical Oncology, Stanford Univ Med Ctr 1994; **Fac Appt:** Assoc Prof Med, Stanford Univ

Forscher, Charles A MD [Onc] - **Spec Exp:** Bone Tumors; Sarcoma-Soft Tissue; **Hospital:** Cedars-Sinai Med Ctr, UCLA Ronald Reagan Med Ctr; **Address:** Outpatient Cancer Ctr, Lower Level, 8700 Beverly Blvd, rm AC1042D, Los Angeles, CA 90048; **Phone:** 310-423-8045; **Board Cert:** Internal Medicine 1981; Hematology 1986; Medical Oncology 1987; **Med School:** Albert Einstein Coll Med 1978; **Resid:** Internal Medicine, Montefiore Med Ctr 1981; **Fellow:** Hematology, Montefiore Med Ctr 1983; Neoplastic Diseases, Mt Sinai Med Ctr 1985; **Fac Appt:** Clin Prof Med, UCLA

Gandara, David R MD [Onc] - **Spec Exp:** Lung Cancer; **Hospital:** UC Davis Med Ctr; **Address:** UC Davis Cancer Ctr, 4501 X St, Sacramento, CA 95817; **Phone:** 916-734-5959; **Board Cert:** Internal Medicine 1976; Medical Oncology 1979; **Med School:** Univ Tex Med Br, Galveston 1973; **Resid:** Internal Medicine, Madigan Med Ctr 1976; **Fellow:** Hematology & Oncology, Letterman AMC 1978; **Fac Appt:** Asst Prof Med, UC Davis

Ganz, Patricia A MD [Onc] - **Spec Exp:** Breast Cancer; Cancer Survivors-Late Effects of Therapy; **Hospital:** UCLA Ronald Reagan Med Ctr; **Address:** UCLA, Cancer Prev/Control Rsch, A2-125 CHS, 650 Charles Young Drive S, Box 956900, Los Angeles, CA 90095-6900; **Phone:** 310-206-1404; **Board Cert:** Internal Medicine 1976; Medical Oncology 1979; **Med School:** UCLA 1973; **Resid:** Internal Medicine, UCLA Med Ctr 1976; **Fellow:** Hematology, UCLA Med Ctr 1978; **Fac Appt:** Prof Med, UCLA

Glaspy, John A MD [Onc] - **Spec Exp:** Breast Cancer; Melanoma; Lymphoma; **Hospital:** UCLA Ronald Reagan Med Ctr; **Address:** 100 UCLA Medical Plaza, Ste 550, Los Angeles, CA 90095; **Phone:** 310-794-4955; **Board Cert:** Internal Medicine 1982; Medical Oncology 1985; Hematology 1986; **Med School:** UCLA 1979; **Resid:** Internal Medicine, UCLA Med Ctr 1982; **Fellow:** Hematology & Oncology, UCLA Med Ctr 1984; **Fac Appt:** Prof Med, UCLA

Gold, Philip J MD [Onc] - **Spec Exp:** Gastrointestinal Cancer; **Hospital:** Swedish Med Ctr - Seattle; **Address:** Swedish Cancer Inst, 1221 Madison St Fl 2, Seattle, WA 98104; **Phone:** 206-386-2121; **Board Cert:** Internal Medicine 2005; Medical Oncology 2007; **Med School:** Univ Miami Sch Med 1991; **Resid:** Internal Medicine, Univ of Washington Med Ctr 1994; **Fellow:** Medical Oncology, Fred Hutchinson Cancer Rsch Ctr 1997

Gralow, Julie MD [Onc] - **Spec Exp:** Breast Cancer; **Hospital:** Univ Wash Med Ctr; **Address:** Seattle Cancer Care Alliance, 825 Eastlake Ave E, MS G3-630, Seattle, WA 98109; **Phone:** 206-288-7222; **Board Cert:** Medical Oncology 2005; **Med School:** USC Sch Med 1988; **Resid:** Internal Medicine, Brigham & Women's Hosp 1991; **Fellow:** Oncology, Univ Wash Med Ctr 1994; **Fac Appt:** Assoc Prof Med, Univ Wash

Higano, Celestia MD [Onc] - **Spec Exp:** Genitourinary Cancer; Prostate Cancer; Bladder Cancer; Testicular Cancer; **Hospital:** Univ Wash Med Ctr; **Address:** Seattle Cancer Care Alliance, 825 Eastlake Ave E, PO Box 19024, Seattle, WA 98109; **Phone:** 206-288-7222; **Board Cert:** Internal Medicine 1982; Medical Oncology 1985; **Med School:** Univ Mass Sch Med 1979; **Resid:** Internal Medicine, Mayo Clinic 1982; **Fellow:** Oncology, Univ Washington 1985; **Fac Appt:** Assoc Prof Med, Univ Wash

Horning, Sandra J MD [Onc] - **Spec Exp:** Hodgkin's Disease; Bone Marrow & Stem Cell Transplant; Lymphoma; **Hospital:** Stanford Univ Med Ctr; **Address:** Stanford Cancer Center, 875 Blake Wilbur Drive, Clinic C, Palo Alto, CA 94305; **Phone:** 650-723-7621; **Board Cert:** Internal Medicine 1978; Medical Oncology 1981; **Med School:** Univ Iowa Coll Med 1975; **Resid:** Internal Medicine, Strong Meml Hosp 1978; **Fellow:** Medical Oncology, Stanford Univ 1980; **Fac Appt:** Prof Med, Stanford Univ

Jacobs, Charlotte D MD [Onc] - **Spec Exp:** Sarcoma; Unknown Primary Cancer; **Hospital:** Stanford Univ Med Ctr; **Address:** 875 Blake Wilbur Drive, Stanford, CA 94305; **Phone:** 650-498-6000; **Board Cert:** Internal Medicine 1975; Medical Oncology 1977; **Med School:** Washington Univ, St Louis 1972; **Resid:** Internal Medicine, Barnes Hosp 1974; Internal Medicine, UCSF Med Ctr 1975; **Fellow:** Medical Oncology, Stanford Univ 1977; **Fac Appt:** Prof Med, Stanford Univ

Kaplan, Lawrence D MD [Onc] - **Spec Exp:** AIDS Related Cancers; Lymphoma; **Hospital:** UCSF Med Ctr; **Address:** UCSF Medical Center, 400 Parnassus Ave, rm 502, Box 0324, San Francisco, CA 94143-0324; **Phone:** 415-353-2421; **Board Cert:** Internal Medicine 1983; Medical Oncology 1985; **Med School:** UCLA 1980; **Resid:** Internal Medicine, Boston City Hosp 1983; **Fellow:** Hematology & Oncology, UCSF Med Ctr 1985; **Fac Appt:** Clin Prof Med, UCSF

Koczywas, Marianna MD [Onc] - **Spec Exp:** Lung Cancer; **Hospital:** City of Hope Natl Med Ctr & Beckman Rsch; **Address:** City of Hope National Medical Center, 1500 E Duarte Rd, Duarte, CA 91010; **Phone:** 626-359-8111 x62307; **Board Cert:** Hematology 2000; Medical Oncology 2001; **Med School:** Poland 1984; **Resid:** Internal Medicine, Troczewski City Hosp 1988; Internal Medicine, St Francis Med Ctr 1997; **Fellow:** Hematology & Oncology, City of Hope Natl Med Ctr 2000

Lim, Dean Wee MD [Onc] - **Hospital:** City of Hope Natl Med Ctr & Beckman Rsch; **Address:** City of Hope-Medical Oncology Dept, 1500 E Duarte Rd, Duarte, CA 91010; **Phone:** 626-256-4673 x69200; **Board Cert:** Internal Medicine 1985; Medical Oncology 1989; **Med School:** Philippines 1980; **Resid:** Internal Medicine, Cabrini Med Ctr 1985; **Fellow:** Hematology & Oncology, St Lukes Roosevelt Hosp 1987; **Fac Appt:** Asst Clin Prof Med, USC-Keck School of Medicine

Medical Oncology

Maloney, David G MD/PhD [Onc] - **Spec Exp:** Lymphoma; Bone Marrow & Stem Cell Transplant; Vaccine Therapy; **Hospital:** Univ Wash Med Ctr; **Address:** Fred Hutchinson Cancer, Research Ctr Ave, MS D1-100, 1100 Fairview Ave N, Box 19024, Seattle, WA 98109-1024; **Phone:** 206-667-5616; **Board Cert:** Internal Medicine 1988; Medical Oncology 2005; **Med School:** Stanford Univ 1985; **Resid:** Internal Medicine, Brigham & Women's Hosp 1988; **Fellow:** Medical Oncology, Stanford Univ Med Ctr 1994; **Fac Appt:** Prof Med, Univ Wash

Margolin, Kim Allyson MD [Onc] - **Spec Exp:** Melanoma; Kidney Cancer; Germ Cell Tumors; **Hospital:** Univ Wash Med Ctr; **Address:** 825 Eastlake Ave E, PO Box 19024, Seattle, WA 98109; **Phone:** 206-288-7222; **Board Cert:** Internal Medicine 1982; Hematology 1986; Medical Oncology 2006; **Med School:** Stanford Univ 1979; **Resid:** Internal Medicine, Yale-New Haven Hosp 1982; **Fellow:** Hematology & Oncology, UC San Diego Med Ctr 1983; Hematology & Oncology, City of Hope Med Ctr 1985; **Fac Appt:** Prof Med, Univ Wash

Martins, Renato G MD [Onc] - **Spec Exp:** Head & Neck Cancer; Lung Cancer; Mesothelioma; Salivary Gland Tumors; **Hospital:** Univ Wash Med Ctr; **Address:** Seattle Cancer Care Alliance, 825 Eastlake Ave E, MS G4-940, Seattle, WA 98109; **Phone:** 206-288-2048; **Board Cert:** Internal Medicine 2005; Medical Oncology 1998; **Med School:** Brazil 1992; **Resid:** Internal Medicine, Gunderson Clinic 1995; **Fellow:** Medical Oncology, Mass Genl Hosp 1998

Meyskens, Frank MD [Onc] - **Spec Exp:** Cancer Prevention; Melanoma; Sarcoma; **Hospital:** UC Irvine Med Ctr; **Address:** UC Irvine Cancer Ctr, 101 The City Drive Bldg 56 - rm 215, Orange, CA 92868; **Phone:** 714-456-6310; **Board Cert:** Internal Medicine 1975; Medical Oncology 1981; **Med School:** UCSF 1972; **Resid:** Internal Medicine, Moffit-Calif Hosps 1974; **Fellow:** Hematology & Oncology, Natl Cancer Inst 1977; **Fac Appt:** Prof Med, UC Irvine

Mitsuyasu, Ronald T MD [Onc] - **Spec Exp:** AIDS Related Cancers; **Hospital:** UCLA Ronald Reagan Med Ctr; **Address:** 1399 S Roxbury Drive, Ste 100, Los Angeles, CA 90035; **Phone:** 310-557-2273; **Board Cert:** Internal Medicine 1981; **Med School:** UCLA 1978; **Resid:** Internal Medicine, Rush Presby St Lukes Hosp 1981; **Fellow:** Hematology & Oncology, UCLA Med Ctr 1984

Mortimer, Joanne MD [Onc] - **Spec Exp:** Breast Cancer; Clinical Trials; Head & Neck Cancer; **Hospital:** City of Hope Natl Med Ctr & Beckman Rsch; **Address:** 1500 E Duarte Rd, Duarte, CA 91010; **Phone:** 626-471-9200; **Board Cert:** Internal Medicine 1980; Medical Oncology 1983; **Med School:** Loyola Univ-Stritch Sch Med 1977; **Resid:** Internal Medicine, Cleveland Clinic 1980; **Fellow:** Medical Oncology, Cleveland Clinic 1982

Natale, Ronald B MD [Onc] - **Spec Exp:** Lung Cancer; **Hospital:** Cedars-Sinai Med Ctr; **Address:** Cedars-Sinai Outpatient Comp Cancer Ctr, 8700 Beverly Blvd, Ste AC1042B, Los Angeles, CA 90048; **Phone:** 310-423-1101; **Board Cert:** Internal Medicine 1977; Medical Oncology 1979; **Med School:** Wayne State Univ 1974; **Resid:** Internal Medicine, Wayne State Univ 1977; **Fellow:** Hematology & Oncology, Meml Sloan Kettering 1980; **Fac Appt:** Prof Med, Univ Mich Med Sch

Nichols, Craig R MD [Onc] - **Spec Exp:** Testicular Cancer; Hodgkin's Disease; Lymphoma; **Hospital:** Providence Portland Med Ctr; **Address:** Providence Cancer Ctr, Oregon Clinic, 4805 NE Glisan St, Ste 6N40, Portland, OR 97213; **Phone:** 503-215-5696; **Board Cert:** Internal Medicine 1981; Medical Oncology 1985; **Med School:** Oregon Hlth & Sci Univ 1978; **Resid:** Internal Medicine, Oschner Fdn Hosp 1981; **Fellow:** Medical Oncology, Indiana Univ 1985; **Fac Appt:** Prof Med, Oregon Hlth & Sci Univ

O'Day, Steven J MD [Onc] - **Spec Exp:** Melanoma; Melanoma-Advanced; **Hospital:** St John's Hlth Ctr, Santa Monica; **Address:** 11818 Wilshire Blvd, Ste 200, Los Angeles, CA 90025; **Phone:** 310-231-2121; **Med School:** Johns Hopkins Univ 1988; **Resid:** Internal Medicine, Johns Hopkins Hosp 1991; **Fellow:** Medical Oncology, Dana Farber Cancer Inst 1992; **Fac Appt:** Assoc Clin Prof Med, USC-Keck School of Medicine

Parker, Barbara A MD [Onc] - **Spec Exp:** Breast Cancer; Nutrition; **Hospital:** UCSD Med Ctr; **Address:** Moores UCSD Cancer Ctr, Hem/Onc Dept, 3855 Health Sciences Drive, MC 0987, La Jolla, CA 92093; **Phone:** 858-822-6195; **Board Cert:** Internal Medicine 1984; Medical Oncology 1987; **Med School:** Stanford Univ 1981; **Resid:** Internal Medicine, UCSD Med Ctr 1985; **Fellow:** Medical Oncology, UCSD Med Ctr 1987; **Fac Appt:** Prof Med, UCSD

Petersdorf, Stephen MD [Onc] - **Spec Exp:** Lymphoma; Myelodysplastic Syndromes; Leukemia; **Hospital:** Univ Wash Med Ctr; **Address:** Seattle Cancer Care Alliance, 825 Eastlake Ave E, MS G3200, Seattle, WA 98109-1023; **Phone:** 206-288-6202; **Board Cert:** Internal Medicine 1986; Hematology 2001; Medical Oncology 2001; **Med School:** Brown Univ 1983; **Resid:** Internal Medicine, Univ Washington Med Ctr 1986; **Fellow:** Hematology & Oncology, Univ Washington Med Ctr 1989; **Fac Appt:** Assoc Prof Med, Univ Wash

Picozzi Jr, Vincent J MD [Onc] - **Spec Exp:** Pancreatic Cancer; **Hospital:** Virginia Mason Med Ctr; **Address:** Virginia Mason Med Ctr, Div Hem/Onc, MS C2-Hem, Seattle, WA 98111; **Phone:** 206-223-6193; **Board Cert:** Internal Medicine 1981; Hematology 1986; Medical Oncology 1987; **Med School:** Stanford Univ 1978; **Resid:** Internal Medicine, Peter Bent Brigham Med Ctr 1981; **Fellow:** Hematology, Stanford Univ Med Ctr 1983; Medical Oncology, Stanford Univ MEd Ctr 1983; **Fac Appt:** Clin Prof Med, Univ Wash

Pinto, Harlan A MD [Onc] - **Spec Exp:** Head & Neck Cancer; Clinical Trials; **Hospital:** Stanford Univ Med Ctr, VA Hlth Care Sys - Palo Alto; **Address:** Stanford Med Ctr Oncology Div, 875 Blake Wilbur Drive, Stanford, CA 94305; **Phone:** 650-723-7621; **Board Cert:** Internal Medicine 1986; Medical Oncology 2002; **Med School:** Yale Univ 1983; **Resid:** Internal Medicine, Mass Genl Hosp 1986; **Fellow:** Medical Oncology, Stanford Univ Med Sch 1991; **Fac Appt:** Assoc Prof Med, Stanford Univ

Prados, Michael MD [Onc] - **Spec Exp:** Neuro-Oncology; Brain Tumors; **Hospital:** UCSF Med Ctr; **Address:** UCSF Med Ctr, Div Neuro-Oncology, 400 Parnassus Ave, rm A-808, San Francisco, CA 94143; **Phone:** 415-353-2966; **Board Cert:** Internal Medicine 1977; **Med School:** Louisiana State U, New Orleans 1974; **Resid:** Internal Medicine, Earl K Long Hosp 1977; **Fac Appt:** Prof NS, UCSF

Press, Oliver W MD/PhD [Onc] - **Spec Exp:** Lymphoma; Bone Marrow Transplant; **Hospital:** Univ Wash Med Ctr; **Address:** 1100 Fairview Ave N, MS D3-19, Seattle, WA 98109; **Phone:** 206-667-1864; **Board Cert:** Internal Medicine 1982; Medical Oncology 1985; **Med School:** Univ Wash 1979; **Resid:** Internal Medicine, Mass Genl Hosp 1982; Internal Medicine, Univ Hosp 1983; **Fellow:** Medical Oncology, Univ Washington 1985; **Fac Appt:** Prof Med, Univ Wash

Quinn, David MD/PhD [Onc] - **Spec Exp:** Testicular Cancer; Prostate Cancer; Kidney Cancer; **Hospital:** USC Norris Cancer Hosp; **Address:** 1441 Eastlake Ave, Ste 3440, Los Angeles, CA 90033; **Phone:** 323-865-3956; **Med School:** Australia 1987; **Resid:** Internal Medicine, St Vincents Hosp 1992; **Fellow:** Medical Oncology, St Vincents Hosp 1995; **Fac Appt:** Asst Prof Med, USC Sch Med

Reid, Tony R MD/PhD [Onc] - **Spec Exp:** Gastrointestinal Cancer; Pancreatic Cancer; Esophageal Cancer; Liver Cancer; **Hospital:** UCSD Med Ctr; **Address:** 3855 Health Sciences Drive, La Jolla, CA 92093; **Phone:** 858-822-6100; **Board Cert:** Medical Oncology 1999; **Med School:** Stanford Univ 1991; **Resid:** Internal Medicine, Stanford Univ Med Ctr 1997; **Fellow:** Oncology, Stanford Univ Med Ctr 1999; Cancer Research, Stanford Univ Med Ctr 2000; **Fac Appt:** Assoc Prof Med, UCSD

Medical Oncology

Rugo, Hope S MD [Onc] - **Spec Exp:** Breast Cancer; Complementary Medicine; Breast Cancer-Novel Therapies; **Hospital:** UCSF Med Ctr; **Address:** UCSF Comp Cancer Ctr-Breast Care Ctr, 1600 Divisadero St Fl 2, San Francisco, CA 94115; **Phone:** 415-353-7070; **Board Cert:** Internal Medicine 1987; Medical Oncology 1989; **Med School:** Univ Pennsylvania 1984; **Resid:** Internal Medicine, UCSF Med Ctr 1987; **Fellow:** Hematology & Oncology, UCSF Med Ctr 1989; **Fac Appt:** Clin Prof Med, UCSF

Russell, Christy A MD [Onc] - **Spec Exp:** Breast Cancer; **Hospital:** USC Univ Hosp; **Address:** Norris Cancer Ctr, The Breast Ctr, 1441 Eastlake Ave, Los Angeles, CA 90033; **Phone:** 323-865-3371; **Board Cert:** Internal Medicine 1983; Medical Oncology 1985; **Med School:** Med Coll PA Hahnemann 1980; **Resid:** Internal Medicine, Good Sam Med Ctr 1983; **Fellow:** Hematology & Oncology, LAC-USC Med Ctr 1986; **Fac Appt:** Assoc Prof Med, USC Sch Med

Samlowski, Wolfram E MD [Onc] - **Spec Exp:** Kidney Cancer; Melanoma; Immunotherapy; **Address:** Nevada Cancer Institute, One Breakthrough Way, Las Vegas, NV 89135; **Phone:** 702-822-5433; **Board Cert:** Internal Medicine 1981; Medical Oncology 1985; **Med School:** Ohio State Univ 1978; **Resid:** Internal Medicine, Wayne State Univ Affil Hosp 1981; **Fellow:** Hematology & Oncology, Univ Utah Affil Hosp 1984; **Fac Appt:** Prof Hem & Onc, Univ Nevada

Sandler, Alan MD [Onc] - **Spec Exp:** Lung Cancer; Sarcoma; **Hospital:** OR Hlth & Sci Univ; **Address:** 3181 SW Sam Jackson Park Rd, MC L586, Portland, OR 97239; **Phone:** 503-494-5586; **Board Cert:** Medical Oncology 2006; **Med School:** Rush Med Coll 1987; **Resid:** Internal Medicine, Yale-New Haven Hosp 1990; **Fellow:** Medical Oncology, Yale Univ 1993; **Fac Appt:** Prof Med, Oregon Hlth & Sci Univ

Shibata, Stephen I MD [Onc] - **Spec Exp:** Gastrointestinal Cancer; Clinical Trials; **Hospital:** City of Hope Natl Med Ctr & Beckman Rsch; **Address:** City of Hope Cancer Ctr, 1500 E Duarte Rd, Duarte, CA 91010; **Phone:** 626-359-8111 x62307; **Board Cert:** Internal Medicine 1988; Medical Oncology 1991; **Med School:** UC Irvine 1985; **Resid:** Internal Medicine, St Mary Med Ctr 1988; **Fellow:** Medical Oncology, City of Hope Cancer Ctr 1990; Bone Marrow Transplant, City of Hope Cancer Ctr 1991; **Fac Appt:** Assoc Prof Med

Sikic, Branimir I MD [Onc] - **Spec Exp:** Unknown Primary Cancer; Clinical Trials; **Hospital:** Stanford Univ Med Ctr; **Address:** Stanford Comp Cancer Ctr, 875 Blake Wilbur Drive, Clinic C, Palo Alto, CA 94305; **Phone:** 650-723-7621; **Board Cert:** Internal Medicine 1975; Medical Oncology 1979; **Med School:** Ros Franklin Univ/Chicago Med Sch 1972; **Resid:** Internal Medicine, Georgetown Univ Hosp 1975; **Fellow:** Medical Oncology, Natl Cancer Inst 1978; Medical Oncology, Georgetown Univ Hosp 1979; **Fac Appt:** Prof Med, Stanford Univ

Small, Eric J MD [Onc] - **Spec Exp:** Prostate Cancer; Vaccine Therapy; Genitourinary Cancer; **Hospital:** UCSF Med Ctr; **Address:** UCSF Urologic Oncology Practice, 1600 Divisadero St Fl 3, San Francisco, CA 94115-1711; **Phone:** 415-353-7171; **Board Cert:** Internal Medicine 1988; Medical Oncology 2001; **Med School:** Case West Res Univ 1985; **Resid:** Internal Medicine, Beth Israel Hosp 1988; **Fellow:** Hematology & Oncology, Cancer Research Inst/UCSF 1991; **Fac Appt:** Prof Med, UCSF

Stewart, Forrest M MD [Onc] - **Spec Exp:** Unknown Primary Cancer; Sarcoma; **Hospital:** Univ Wash Med Ctr; **Address:** Seattle Cancer Care Alliance, 825 Eastlake Ave E, Box 19023, Seattle, WA 98109; **Phone:** 206-288-7222; **Board Cert:** Internal Medicine 1980; Hematology 1982; Medical Oncology 1985; **Med School:** Indiana Univ 1977; **Resid:** Internal Medicine, Indiana Univ Med Ctr 1980; Medical Oncology, Indiana Univ Med Ctr 1981; **Fellow:** Hematology, Univ Virginia Med Ctr 1983; **Fac Appt:** Prof Med, Univ Wash

Stockdale, Frank E MD/PhD [Onc] - **Spec Exp:** Breast Cancer; **Hospital:** Stanford Univ Med Ctr; **Address:** Stanford Univ Medical Ctr, 875 Blake Wilbur Drive, Stanford, CA 94305-5826; **Phone:** 650-723-6449; **Med School:** Univ Pennsylvania 1963; **Resid:** Internal Medicine, Stanford Univ Med Ctr 1967; Hematology & Oncology, Stanford Univ Med Ctr; **Fac Appt:** Prof Emeritus Med, Stanford Univ

Tempero, Margaret MD [Onc] - **Spec Exp:** Pancreatic Cancer; Gastrointestinal Cancer; **Hospital:** UCSF Med Ctr; **Address:** UCSF, Multi-Disciplinary Practice, 1600 Divisadero St Fl 4 - rm 4202, San Francisco, CA 94115; **Phone:** 415-353-9888; **Board Cert:** Internal Medicine 1980; Medical Oncology 1983; Hematology 1984; **Med School:** Univ Nebr Coll Med 1977; **Resid:** Internal Medicine, Univ Nebraska Hosp 1980; **Fellow:** Medical Oncology, Univ Nebraska 1982

Thompson, John A MD [Onc] - **Spec Exp:** Melanoma; **Hospital:** Univ Wash Med Ctr; **Address:** Seattle Cancer Care Alliance, 825 Eastlake Ave E, MS G4-200, Seattle, WA 98109-1023; **Phone:** 206-288-2015; **Board Cert:** Internal Medicine 1982; Medical Oncology 1985; **Med School:** Univ Alabama 1979; **Resid:** Internal Medicine, Univ Wash Med Ctr 1982; **Fellow:** Medical Oncology, Univ Washington 1985

Tripathy, Debasish MD [Onc] - **Spec Exp:** Breast Cancer; Clinical Trials; **Hospital:** USC Norris Cancer Hosp; **Address:** USC Norris Cancer Ctr, 1441 Eastlake Ave, Ste 3447, Los Angeles, CA 90033; **Phone:** 323-865-3105; **Board Cert:** Internal Medicine 1988; Medical Oncology 2001; **Med School:** Duke Univ 1985; **Resid:** Internal Medicine, Duke Univ Med Ctr 1988; **Fellow:** Hematology & Oncology, USCF Med Ctr 1991; **Fac Appt:** Prof Med, Univ SC Sch Med

Twardowski, Przemyslaw MD [Onc] - **Spec Exp:** Genitourinary Cancer; **Hospital:** City of Hope Natl Med Ctr & Beckman Rsch; **Address:** 1500 E Duarte Rd, Duarte, CA 91010; **Phone:** 626-256-4673; **Board Cert:** Medical Oncology 1998; Hematology 1998; **Med School:** Univ MO-Columbia Sch Med 1990; **Resid:** Internal Medicine, Northwestern Meml Hosp 1994; **Fellow:** Hematology & Oncology, Northwestern Meml Hosp 1996; **Fac Appt:** Asst Prof Med, UCLA

Urba, Walter J MD/PhD [Onc] - **Spec Exp:** Breast Cancer; **Hospital:** Providence Portland Med Ctr; **Address:** Providence Oncology, 4805 NE Glisan Rd, Ste 6N40, Portland, OR 97213; **Phone:** 503-215-5696; **Board Cert:** Internal Medicine 1985; Medical Oncology 1987; **Med School:** Univ Miami Sch Med 1981; **Resid:** Internal Medicine, Morristown Meml Hosp 1983; **Fellow:** Medical Oncology, Natl Cancer Inst 1986; **Fac Appt:** Assoc Clin Prof Med, Oregon Hlth & Sci Univ

Venook, Alan P MD [Onc] - **Spec Exp:** Gastrointestinal Cancer; Colon & Rectal Cancer; Liver Cancer; **Hospital:** UCSF Med Ctr; **Address:** UCSF Comprehensive Cancer Ctr, Multi Disciplinary Practice, 1600 Divisadero St Fl 4 - rm 4202, San Francisco, CA 94115; **Phone:** 415-353-9888; **Board Cert:** Internal Medicine 1985; Medical Oncology 1987; Hematology 1988; **Med School:** UCSF 1980; **Resid:** Internal Medicine, UC Davis Med Ctr 1985; **Fellow:** Hematology & Oncology, UCSF Med Ctr 1987; **Fac Appt:** Prof Med

Vescio, Robert A MD [Onc] - **Spec Exp:** Multiple Myeloma; Amyloidosis; **Hospital:** Cedars-Sinai Med Ctr; **Address:** Cedars Sinai Med Ctr, Dept Hem/Oncology, 8700 Beverly Blvd, Los Angeles, CA 90048; **Phone:** 310-423-1825; **Board Cert:** Internal Medicine 1989; Hematology 2004; Medical Oncology 2003; **Med School:** UCSD 1986; **Resid:** Internal Medicine, UCSD Med Ctr 1989; **Fellow:** Hematology & Oncology, UCLA Med Ctr 1993; **Fac Appt:** Assoc Prof Med, UCLA

Medical Oncology

Vogelzang, Nicholas J MD [Onc] - **Spec Exp:** Prostate Cancer; Mesothelioma; Kidney Cancer; **Hospital:** Univ Med Ctr - Las Vegas, Summerlin Hosp Med Ctr; **Address:** Nevada Cancer Institute, One Breakthrough Way, Las Vegas, NV 89135; **Phone:** 702-822-5100; **Board Cert:** Internal Medicine 1977; Medical Oncology 1981; **Med School:** Univ IL Coll Med 1974; **Resid:** Internal Medicine, Rush-Presby St Luke's Med Ctr 1977; **Fellow:** Medical Oncology, Univ Minn Med Ctr 1980; **Fac Appt:** Prof Med, Univ Nevada

Volberding, Paul Arthur MD [Onc] - **Spec Exp:** AIDS Related Cancers; **Hospital:** UCSF Med Ctr, VA Med Ctr - San Francisco; **Address:** 4150 Clement St, VAMC 111, San Francisco, CA 94121; **Phone:** 415-750-2203; **Board Cert:** Internal Medicine 1978; Medical Oncology 1981; **Med School:** Univ Minn 1975; **Resid:** Internal Medicine, Univ Utah Med Ctr 1978; **Fellow:** Medical Oncology, UCSF Med Ctr 1981; **Fac Appt:** Prof Med, UCSF

von Gunten, Charles MD/PhD [Onc] - **Spec Exp:** Palliative Care; **Hospital:** San Diego Hospice; **Address:** San Diego Hospice, 4311 Third Ave, San Diego, CA 92103; **Phone:** 619-688-1600; **Board Cert:** Internal Medicine 2002; Medical Oncology 2003; Hospice & Palliative Medicine 2001; **Med School:** Univ Colorado 1988; **Resid:** Internal Medicine, Northwestern Univ 1991; **Fellow:** Medical Oncology, Northwestern Univ 1993; **Fac Appt:** Assoc Clin Prof Med, UCSD

Wierman, Ann MD [Onc] - **Spec Exp:** Breast Cancer; Lymphoma; Lung Cancer; **Hospital:** Univ Med Ctr - Las Vegas; **Address:** 2851 N Tenaya Way, Ste 101, Las Vegas, NV 89128; **Phone:** 702-735-7154; **Board Cert:** Internal Medicine 2002; Medical Oncology 2007; Hematology 1998; **Med School:** Baylor Coll Med 1989; **Resid:** Internal Medicine, Baylor Hosps 1992; Internal Medicine, Ben Taub Genl Hosp 1993; **Fellow:** Hematology & Oncology, Univ CO Hlth Sci Ctr 1996; **Fac Appt:** Assoc Clin Prof Med, Univ Nevada

Yen, Yun MD/PhD [Onc] - **Spec Exp:** Liver Cancer; Biliary Cancer; **Hospital:** City of Hope Natl Med Ctr & Beckman Rsch; **Address:** City of Hope Comprehensive Cancer Ctr, 1500 E Duarte Rd, Duarte, CA 91010; **Phone:** 626-359-8111 x62307; **Board Cert:** Medical Oncology 2003; **Med School:** Taiwan 1982; **Resid:** Internal Medicine, St Luke's Hosp 1990; **Fellow:** Hematology & Oncology, Yale-New Haven Hosp 1993; **Fac Appt:** Prof Med, USC Sch Med

Cleveland Clinic

Innovative Research and Outstanding Outcomes

At Cleveland Clinic Taussig Cancer Institute, more than 250 cancer specialists, researchers, nurses and technicians are dedicated to developing and applying the latest and most effective medical techniques to achieve the long-term survival and improve the quality of life for 7,500 new cancer patients every year. Because of our innovative research, 350 clinical trials and state-of-the-art medical technologies, *U.S.News & World Report* has ranked Taussig Cancer Institute one of the top cancer centers in the nation.

The Taussig Cancer Institute has more than 200,000 annual cancer patient visits at its main campus in Cleveland and at 10 locations throughout Northeast Ohio. Our areas of expertise include prostate and other urologic cancers, melanoma, blood and bone marrow cancers, multiple myeloma, colorectal cancer, lung cancer, breast cancer and brain and spinal cord tumors.

Because of Taussig Cancer Institute's extensive cancer care system, the Leukemia & Lymphoma Society forged a groundbreaking partnership with Taussig Cancer Institute to make blood cancer clinical trials available to patients in their communities. This enables patients to stay with their primary doctors and participate in clinical trials near their hometown.

Clinical Trials Now Online

Cleveland Clinic offers a new online tool for patients, caregivers and physicians to search for open clinical trials. The site lists more than 100 trials being managed by oncologists in the Taussig Cancer Institute that are accepting patients at all Cleveland Clinic campuses, including main campus and our regional hospitals.

Patients, family members and physicians who have questions about a specific trial or who are interested in enrolling in an open study can call the Cancer Answer Line at 866.223.8100 for more information.

Outstanding Outcomes: One example is our Bone Marrow Transplant outcomes, which are unsurpassed by any program in the world. We have one of the most experienced teams in the nation, having performed more than 2,900 bone marrow transplant procedures since 1977.

Innovative Research: Taussig Cancer Institute is at the forefront of cancer research. Our world-renowned scientists are dedicated to developing novel, effective therapeutic options for cancer patients. Through understanding cellular abnormalities that lead to cancer, our researchers target specific genes with drugs or combinations of drugs to improve outcomes.

Cancer Genetics at the Center for Personalized Genetic Healthcare: Because some families are prone to developing cancer, advances in genetic research help us identify some of the risk factors. Cleveland Clinic's Center for Personalized Genetic Healthcare aims to prevent cancer by identifying high risk individuals and offers personalized medical management to them and their family members.

In our multidisciplinary clinics, medical, radiation and surgical oncologists work closely with pathologists, radiologists, oncology nurses and social workers to optimize the options for individual patients with complex problems.

For more information about the Cleveland Clinic Taussig Cancer Institute, to schedule a second opinion or to learn about assistance for out-of-town patients, call 800.890.2467 or visit www.clevelandclinic.org/cancertopdocs.
Cleveland Clinic Taussig Cancer Institute
9500 Euclid Avenue / AC311 | Cleveland OH 44195

Continuum Cancer Centers of New York

(212) 844-6027

The hospitals of Continuum – Beth Israel Medical Center, St. Luke's and Roosevelt Hospitals, Long Island College Hospital of Brooklyn and the New York Eye and Ear Infirmary – are leading providers of cancer care through Continuum Cancer Centers of New York. Our integrated system allows us to build on the clinical strengths found at each of our partner hospitals.

The goal – and result – is delivery of care in ways that are more efficient, more attractive and more convenient for patients. Specifically, it means that cancer patients at any Continuum hospital can benefit from system-wide cancer expertise, facilities and resources. Continuum Cancer Centers feature world-renowned cancer specialists, including top-rated surgeons, medical oncologists, radiation oncologists, radiologists, pathologists, and oncology nurses.

Comprehensive diagnostic and treatment services are available for breast cancer, prostate cancer, head and neck and thyroid cancers, skin cancer, lung cancer, colorectal and other gastrointestinal cancers, lymphoma/Hodgkin's Disease, gynecological cancers, and cancers of the brain and central nervous system. Delivered efficiently in a friendly and supportive environment, our services include prevention programs – such as community education, screenings and early detection – expert diagnosis, outpatient treatment, inpatient services and home care. In addition, our Research Program offers patients access to investigational protocols through a wide number of clinical trials. Our physicians are leaders in both non-invasive and minimally invasive cancer treatments that focus on maximizing both the cure rate and the quality of life.

Support Services play an important role at Continuum Cancer Centers.

Nurses, social workers, psychiatrists, chaplains, pharmacists, rehabilitation therapists and nutritionists all have specialized knowledge and expertise in the field of oncology.

In February 2007, Continuum Cancer Centers of New York received a full three-year accreditation with commendations from the American College of Surgeons, Commission on Cancer (CoC). Continuum is the first hospital system in New York State to earn this network accreditation; fewer than 25 networks in the entire United States are so accredited by the Commission.

For help finding the services and care you need, please call us at (212) 844 – 6027.

Beth Israel   Roosevelt Hospital   St. Luke's Hospital   Long Island College Hospital   NY Eye & Ear Infirmary

www.chpnyc.org

Advancing Cancer Care

Penn Medicine is known for its innovative approach to the prevention, diagnosis and treatment of cancer. Through clinical excellence, advanced research and supportive care services, patients and their families are provided with outstanding comprehensive cancer care.

Abramson Cancer Center of the University of Pennsylvania

The Abramson Cancer Center is one of a select group of cancer centers in the country awarded the prestigious designation of *Comprehensive Cancer Center* by the National Cancer Institute (NCI).

The Cancer Center has established a variety of interdisciplinary centers dedicated to specific cancers. Each center offers patients a complete evaluation and treatment options by a team of doctors with recognized expertise in that type of cancer.

What Sets Abramson Apart?

- More than 400 full-time Penn faculty are actively involved in the diagnosis and treatment of patients with cancer.
- Clinical programs offering cutting-edge treatments such as robotic surgery for prostate, gynecologic cancer, and Transoral Robotic Surgery (TORS) for head and neck cancer.
- Emphasis on patient education to empower our patients to be active participants in their care.
- One of the first cancer risk evaluation programs in the country for women concerned about their risk for breast and ovarian cancer.
- One of the foremost cancer research centers in the country and a leader in translational research, in which scientists translate discoveries from research laboratories into new treatments that benefit cancer patients.
- Comprehensive medical care for patients with other medical conditions such diabetes, pregnancy or heart disease.
- Penn's cancer specialists work closely with a patient's personal physician.
- Designated as a LIVE**STRONG** Center of Excellence™.
- Full range of support services to complement medical care including nutritional counseling, support groups, cancer rehabilitation, complementary and alternative therapies and pain and symptom management.

Joan Karnell Cancer Center at Pennsylvania Hospital

For patients and families facing cancer or blood-related illnesses, the Joan Karnell Cancer Center at Pennsylvania Hospital provides progressive, comprehensive and supportive cancer care through a wide range of services.
- A leader in the treatment of sarcoma and bloodless medicine.
- Committed to providing excellent cancer care in a supportive setting offering an interdisciplinary approach to diagnosis, treatment, research and education to help patients and their families achieve the best quality of life.

The Ruth and Raymond Perelman Center for Advanced Medicine

The Perelman Center is the home of the Abramson Cancer Center, which brings together outstanding cancer specialists with state-of-the-art technology to offer the most advanced cancer treatment options available.

The Roberts Proton Therapy Center

The Center, which is adjacent to the Perelman Center for Advanced Medicine, is the largest proton therapy treatment facility in the world and the first to be located on the campus of an academic medical center, facilitating scientific research to measure and improve this innovative therapy.

Additional Locations

Penn cancer services are also available at:

- Abramson Cancer Center at Penn Presbyterian Medical Center
- Hospital of the University of Pennsylvania
- Penn Medicine at Radnor
- Penn Medicine at Cherry Hill

For more information to schedule an appointment, call 800.789.PENN (7366) or visit PennMedicine.org/cancer.

Maimonides
Medical Center

Maimonides Cancer Center offers a fully integrated, multi-modal approach to cancer care that includes prevention, education, screening, diagnostics, treatment, palliative care and clinical research – all in one location. This free-standing, 50,000 square foot facility contains the following specialty divisions:

Radiation Oncology: equipped with state-of-the art imaging and treatment delivery technologies; offers patients the most precise treatments available, yet does so in an airy, life-affirming environment.

Medical Oncology: provides comprehensive diagnosis, oral drug therapies, intravenous chemotherapy infusions, and biological and hormonal therapies.

Pediatric Oncology: treats children with cancer and diseases of the blood in a child-friendly environment, and features special areas set aside for parent conferences.

Surgical Oncology: provides a convenient location for minor surgical procedures, as well as innovative surgical techniques such as sentinel node mapping and biopsy, skin/tissue-sparing mastectomy, and nerve-sparing prostatectomy.

Brooklyn Breast Cancer Program: provides digital mammography, sonography, computerized interpretation, digital stereotactic biopsies, breast-specific Gamma Imaging, and treatment plans tailored to each patient.

Research Center: conducts clinical trials that not only help advance science but also offer appropriately screened patients, who wish to volunteer, new therapies and medications.

Resource Center: offers access to integrative (complementary) oncology services, a library with Internet resources, social services, and dietary advice.

Physicians at Maimonides are among the small percentage in the US who use computers to enter patient orders, thereby reducing the risk of errors, increasing efficiency and speeding the healing process. Maimonides has appeared on the American Hospital Association's "Most Wired" and "Most Wireless" lists more often than any other health care institution in the metropolitan area. Advanced technology allows our doctors to focus more on caring for their patients.

Maimonides Medical Center
Passionate about medicine.
Compassionate about people.
www.maimonidesmed.org/cancer

MOUNT SINAI
SCHOOL OF
MEDICINE

THE TISCH CANCER INSTITUTE
AT THE MOUNT SINAI MEDICAL CENTER
One Gustave L. Levy Place
Fifth Avenue and 100th Street
New York, NY 10029-6574
Physician Referral: 1-800-MD-SINAI (637-4624)
www.tischcancerinstitute.org

THE TISCH CANCER INSTITUTE, part of The Mount Sinai Medical Center, is located on the Upper East Side of Manhattan. The Mount Sinai Medical Center was founded in 1852 and encompasses one of the oldest teaching hospitals in the country. In an atmosphere of learning, cutting-edge basic and clinical research, and superb patient care, The Tisch Cancer Institute coordinates a full-service diagnostic and treatment program for cancer patients. Because new treatments are developed at the Institute, patients often have access to these therapies before they are available anywhere else in the world.

A Heritage of Breakthroughs – Teams of physicians and scientists at The Tisch Cancer Institute at Mount Sinai work together to rapidly translate laboratory research into new patient treatments. Among the advances pioneered at Mount Sinai are the first successful treatment of tumors of the bladder by transurethral electrocoagulation, the first demonstration of how asbestos can cause cancerous changes in the DNA of cells, and the first development of an ultrasound-guided technique to insert radioactive seeds into the prostate to treat prostate cancer.

Services and Programs – The Tisch Cancer Institute employs a multidisciplinary treatment approach, providing access to clinical breakthroughs, innovative techniques, leading-edge technologies, and a wide range of diagnostic, therapeutic, and support services for all types of cancer. The Institute treats: head and neck cancer; thoracic cancer (including lung and esophagus); gynecologic cancer; hematological malignancies (including myelodysplastic syndrome and myeloproliferative disorders); brain tumors; and prostate, bladder, kidney, and liver cancer. In addition to surgical treatment, the Institute provides radiation and medical oncology therapies as well as bone marrow transplantation.

The Institute's multidisciplinary treatment approach involves collaboration with colleagues across the Medical Center, drawing upon the knowledge of a vast network of specialists who are outstanding in their fields. These experts consist of award-winning physicians and surgeons specializing in cardiac care, neurology, urology, pediatrics, digestive diseases, obstetrics and gynecology, and other therapeutic areas. Furthermore, Mount Sinai's nursing staff is an important part of the Medical Center's focus on delivering exceptional patient care, and it has received the prestigious Magnet Award for nursing excellence.

Mount Sinai is renowned for its palliative care program, which provides the highest level of care, focusing on the relief of pain, symptoms, and stress in cancer patients in both an inpatient and outpatient setting.

THE RUTTENBERG TREATMENT CENTER
The mission of the Ruttenberg Treatment Center at The Mount Sinai Medical Center is to reduce the burden of human cancer through its outstanding interdisciplinary programs in patient care and research, including cancer prevention, treatment, early detection, and education. Oncologists, surgeons, and specialists from across the medical spectrum work together to provide the highest quality care to all cancer patients. The members of the Center—scientists and physicians—are developing cancer therapies and prevention strategies to improve cancer care, and patients at the Center are the first to benefit from these treatments.

NewYork-Presbyterian

The University Hospital of Columbia and Cornell

NewYork-Presbyterian Cancer Centers

Affiliated with Columbia University College of Physicians and Surgeons and Weill Medical College of Cornell University

Herbert Irving Comprehensive Cancer Center
At NewYork-Presbyterian Hospital
Columbia University Medical Center
161 Fort Washington Avenue
New York, NY 10032

Weill Cornell Cancer Center
At NewYork-Presbyterian Hospital
Weill Cornell Medical Center
525 East 68th Street
New York, NY 10021

OVERVIEW:

NewYork-Presbyterian Cancer Centers are dedicated to reducing cancer morbidity and mortality by providing

- a full continuum of multidisciplinary, state-of-the-art screening, diagnostic, treatment and support services for all phases of the disease process;
- cutting-edge basic, clinical, and public health research;
- full range of cancer-related educational programs and resources to clinicians, scientists, patients and survivors, families, and the cancer prevention community.

The Cancer Centers, which treat over 6,000 new patients annually, draw on the innovation and excellence of the NCI- designated Herbert Irving Comprehensive Cancer Center at NewYork-Presbyterian Hospital/Columbia University Medical Center and oncology services at NewYork-Presbyterian Hospital/Weill Cornell Medical Center. Programs include:

- AIDS-related Malignancies
- Bone Marrow Transplant
- Breast Cancer
- Dermatologic/Skin Cancer
- Gastrointestinal Cancers
- Genitourinary Cancers
- Gynecologic Cancers
- Head and Neck Cancers
- Hematologic Malignancies, such as lymphoma, myeloma and leukemias
- Lung Cancer
- Neurologic Cancer
- Ophthalmic Cancer
- Pediatric Hematology/Oncology
- Urologic Cancers, including bladder, kidney and prostate cancer
- Sarcomas and Mesotheiliomas

The Centers are frequent recipients of major grants and gifts to support research programs. Recent highlights include:

- Avon Products Foundation $10 million award to NewYork-Presbyterian Hospital/Columbia University Medical Center and Columbia University for establishment of the Avon Products Breast Center to support basic, clinical and public health research in breast cancer;
- The Leukemia and Lymphoma Society five-year $7.5 million grant to NewYork-Presbyterian Hospital/Weill Cornell Medical Center to study fundamental causes of multiple myeloma

Physician Referral: For a physician referral call toll free **1-877-NYP-WELL** (1-877-697-9355) to learn more about our Cancer Centers visit our website at **www.nypcancer.org**

COMPREHENSIVE SERVICES INCLUDE:

- Access to over 400 clinical trials supported by the National Institutes of Health and many prominent pharmaceutical companies.

- Bone marrow and blood stem cell transplant, including New York State approval to perform transplants using unrelated donors for patients with hematologic malignances

- CT screening for early lung cancer detection

- Sentinel node biopsy to assess spread of breast cancer

- Skin-sparing mastectomy and reconstruction

- Laparoscopic surgery for colon cancer

- Intraoperative brachytherapy for GI, prostate and other cancers

- Stereotactic biopsies for breast cancer and brain cancer

- Stereotactic gamma radiation for brain tumors

NYU Clinical Cancer Institute
160 East 34th Street
New York, NY 10016
www.nyuci.org/atcd

NYU Langone Medical Center
505 First Avenue (at 31st Street)
New York, NY 10016
www.med.nyu.edu

Stephen D. Hassenfeld
Children's CenterFor Cancer and Blood Disorders
160 East 32nd Street, New York, NY 10016
www.nyumc.org/hassenfeld

NYU CANCER INSTITUTE

About the Cancer Institute:

The NYU Cancer Institute is an NCI-designated cancer center and provides personalized patient care that is both compassionate and state of the art. The doctors and researchers work together to develop innovative therapies for patients. The Institute is world-renowned for excellence in cancer-focused research, personalized care, education and community outreach. Its mission is to discover the origins of human cancer and to use that knowledge to eradicate the personal and societal burden of cancer in our community, the nation and the world. The center and its multidisciplinary team of experts provide access to the latest treatment options and clinical trials along with a variety of programs in cancer prevention, screening, diagnostics, genetic counseling and supportive services.

We specialize in the following areas:

PATIENT-FOCUSED SETTING

The NYU Clinical Cancer Center is the principal outpatient facility of The Cancer Institute and serves as home to our patients and their caregivers. The center and its multidisciplinary team of experts provide access to the latest treatment options and clinical trials along with a variety of programs in cancer prevention, screening, diagnostics, genetic counseling and supportive services. In addition the NYUCI emphasizes the importance of a holistic approach to management services in complementary medicine, psychosocial support, survivorship and palliative care.

RENOWNED EXPERTISE

The NYU Cancer Institute brings together experts from a variety of disciplines to create collaborative research endeavors and clinical care teams. The Institute offers a full continuum of personalized care, from prevention through diagnosis, treatment and post-treatment support. The compassion and expertise of our team members helps patients better manage the symptoms of their diseases as well as meet their special needs. Additionally, we have created special emphasis programs in diseases such as breast cancer, melanoma, GI cancer, prostate cancer, hematologic malignancies and lung cancer among others, as well as, translational programs in cancer healthcare disparities, molecularly-targeted therapy, and the cell signaling pathways involved in cancer.

A TRANSLATIONAL APPROACH

NYU Langone Medical Center scientists and other researchers excel in uncovering how cancer develops at the molecular level, and how we can harness that knowledge to reduce the risk of cancer and treat the disease. The Medical Center constantly seeks to create new opportunities for collaboration between investigators within our own institution, those located elsewhere in the NYU network of campuses, and researchers at other institutions.

THE STEPHEN D. HASSENFELD CHILDREN'S CENTER FOR CANCER AND BLOOD DISORDERS

The center is a leading pediatric outpatient facility for the treatment of childhood cancers and blood diseases. Its unique interdisciplinary and family-centered approach combines the most advanced medical treatments with psychosocial and emotional support services for young patients and their families.

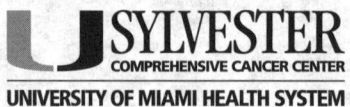

Wake Forest University Baptist
MEDICAL CENTER ®
Comprehensive Cancer Center

Medical Center Boulevard • Winston-Salem, NC 27157 • 336-716-2011
Health On-Call® (Patient Access) 1-800-446-2255
Physician-To-Physician Calls (PAL®) 1-800-277-7654
wfubmc.edu/cancer

TOP RANKINGS

The Comprehensive Cancer Center of Wake Forest University Baptist Medical Center is among an elite group of only 40 U.S. cancer centers designated by the National Cancer Institute as comprehensive, indicating excellence in research, patient care and education. The comprehensive designation was renewed for an additional five years in late 2006.

RESEARCH ADVANTAGES

Wake Forest Baptist offers more cancer-related clinical trials than any other hospital in western N.C. From gene therapy to vitamin and nutrition studies to new surgical and radiological treatments, patients benefit from the leading edge of cancer knowledge and care. Innovative basic science, public health and clinical research promote new discovery about prevention, detection and treatment of cancers. Wake Forest scientists were first in the world to discover cancer resistant cells in mice.

TECHNOLOGY AND TREATMENT STRENGTHS

Wake Forest University Baptist Medical Center is home to North Carolina's first Gamma Knife, a non-invasive, stereotactic radiosurgical tool used to treat malignant and benign brain tumors once considered inoperable. Operated by one of the nation's most experienced treatment teams, the Gamma Knife painlessly bombards tumors with precisely focused beams of gamma energy—sparing normal tissue—and is performed on an outpatient basis. Extracranial body stereotactic radiosurgery offers new options for cancers in the torso.

Wake Forest Baptist offers an integrated brachytherapy unit (IBU) and highly targeted Intensity Modulated Radiation Therapy (IMRT) for treatment of prostate, brain, lung, head and neck, and gynecological cancers. Other treatment innovations include IPHC (intraperitoneal hyperthermic chemotherapy) for abdominal cavity cancers and radiofrequency ablation for liver malignancies.

MULTIDISCIPLINARY EXPERTISE

Expert, subspecialized oncology teams provide patients a consensus opinion on treatment. Multidisciplinary centers include the Breast Care Center, the Brain Tumor Clinic, and the Head and Neck Cancers Multidisciplinary Clinic.

**To make an appointment or find a specialist, call Health On-Call®
at 1-800-446-2255.**

HIGHLIGHTS OF EXCELLENCE

- Western North Carolina's only NCI-designated Comprehensive Cancer Center offers the convenience and comfort of a state-of-the-art Outpatient Cancer Center. The nation's first Cancer Patient Support Group was developed here.

- Wake Forest Baptist is ranked among the nation's best hospitals for cancer care by U.S.News & World Report (2009).

- The Hereditary Cancer Program helps patients understand their risk profile for colorectal, breast, ovarian and melanoma cancers.

- Minimally invasive treatments include high dose rate (HDR) brachytherapy for prostate cancer. Lymph node mapping increases chance for lymph-sparing breast surgery.

- Clinical trials testing new methods of drug delivery offer patients with brain tumors potentially more effective treatment while minimizing effects on healthy tissue.

KNOWLEDGE MAKES ALL THE DIFFERENCE.

Infectious Disease

a subspecialty of Internal Medicine

An internist who deals with infectious diseases of all types and in all organs. Conditions requiring selective use of antibiotics call for this special skill. This physician often diagnoses and treats AIDS patients and patients with fevers which have not been explained. Infectious disease specialists may also have expertise in preventive medicine and conditions associated with travel.

Training Required: Three years in internal medicine *plus* additional training and examination for certification in infectious disease.

INFECTIOUS DISEASE

New England

Craven, Donald Edward MD [Inf] - **Spec Exp:** AIDS/HIV; Hepatitis C; Hospital Acquired Infections; Pneumonia; **Hospital:** Lahey Clin; **Address:** Lahey Clin Med Ctr, Infectious Diseases, 41 Mall Rd, Burlington, MA 01805; **Phone:** 781-744-8608; **Board Cert:** Internal Medicine 1973; Infectious Disease 1982; **Med School:** Albany Med Coll 1970; **Resid:** Internal Medicine, Royal Victoria Hosp-McGill 1973; Internal Medicine, Royal Victoria Hosp 1974; **Fellow:** Infectious Disease, Boston Univ Hosp 1976; NIH/Bureau of Biologics 1979; **Fac Appt:** Prof Med, Tufts Univ

Flanigan, Timothy P MD [Inf] - **Spec Exp:** AIDS/HIV; **Hospital:** Miriam Hosp, Rhode Island Hosp; **Address:** 164 Summit Ave Fain Bldg - Ste E, Providence, RI 02906; **Phone:** 401-793-2928; **Board Cert:** Internal Medicine 1986; Infectious Disease 1988; **Med School:** Cornell Univ-Weill Med Coll 1983; **Resid:** Internal Medicine, Hosp Univ Penn 1986; **Fellow:** Infectious Disease, Case West Res Univ 1987; **Fac Appt:** Prof Med, Brown Univ

Longworth, David L MD [Inf] - **Hospital:** Baystate Med Ctr; **Address:** Baystate Medical Ctr, 759 Chestnut St, Springfield, MA 01199; **Phone:** 413-794-4319; **Board Cert:** Internal Medicine 1981; Infectious Disease 1984; **Med School:** Cornell Univ-Weill Med Coll 1978; **Resid:** Internal Medicine, UCSF-HC Moffitt Hosp 1981; **Fellow:** Infectious Disease, Brigham & Womens Hosp 1983; Research, Harvard Med School 1985; **Fac Appt:** Prof Med, Tufts Univ

Quagliarello, Vincent MD [Inf] - **Spec Exp:** Meningitis; Pneumonia; Endocarditis; **Hospital:** Yale-New Haven Hosp; **Address:** Yale Univ Sch Med, TAC S169A, 300 Cedar St, New Haven, CT 06520-8022; **Phone:** 203-785-3561; **Board Cert:** Internal Medicine 1984; Infectious Disease 1988; **Med School:** Washington Univ, St Louis 1980; **Resid:** Internal Medicine, Yale-New Haven Hosp 1984; **Fellow:** Infectious Disease, Univ VA Hlth Sci Ctr 1987; **Fac Appt:** Prof Med, Yale Univ

Rubin, Robert H MD [Inf] - **Spec Exp:** Infections-Transplant; **Hospital:** Brigham & Women's Hosp; **Address:** Brigham & Women's Hospital, Div Infectious Disease, 15 Francis St, Boston, MA 02115; **Phone:** 617-525-7491; **Board Cert:** Internal Medicine 1972; Infectious Disease 1974; **Med School:** Harvard Med Sch 1966; **Resid:** Internal Medicine, Peter Bent Brigham Hosp 1970; **Fellow:** Infectious Disease, Mass Genl Hosp 1972; **Fac Appt:** Prof Med, Harvard Med Sch

Sax, Paul E MD [Inf] - **Spec Exp:** AIDS/HIV; **Hospital:** Brigham & Women's Hosp; **Address:** Brigham & Women's Hospital, Div Infectious Disease, 15 Francis St Fl 4, Boston, MA 02115; **Phone:** 617-732-8881; **Board Cert:** Internal Medicine 2000; Infectious Disease 2000; **Med School:** Harvard Med Sch 1987; **Resid:** Internal Medicine, Brigham & Womens Hosp 1990; **Fellow:** Infectious Disease, Mass Genl Hosp 1992

Mid Atlantic

Auwaerter, Paul MD [Inf] - **Spec Exp:** Lyme Disease; Ehrlichiosis; Tick-borne Diseases; Fevers of Unknown Origin; **Hospital:** Johns Hopkins Hosp (page 61); **Address:** 10751 Falls Rd, Ste 412, Lutherville, MD 21093; **Phone:** 410-583-2900; **Board Cert:** Internal Medicine 2002; Infectious Disease 2004; **Med School:** Columbia P&S 1988; **Resid:** Internal Medicine, Johns Hopkins Med Ctr 1992; **Fellow:** Infectious Disease, Johns Hopkins Med Ctr 1996; **Fac Appt:** Assoc Prof Med, Johns Hopkins Univ

Bartlett, John G MD [Inf] - **Spec Exp:** AIDS/HIV; Fevers of Unknown Origin; Pseudomembranous Colitis; **Hospital:** Johns Hopkins Hosp (page 61); **Address:** 1830 E Monument St, Ste 439, Baltimore, MD 21205; **Phone:** 410-955-7634; **Board Cert:** Internal Medicine 1972; **Med School:** SUNY Upstate Med Univ 1963; **Resid:** Internal Medicine, Peter Bent Brigham Hosp 1965; Internal Medicine, Univ Hosp Birmingham 1968; **Fellow:** Infectious Disease, Wadsworth VA Hosp 1970

Berkowitz, Leonard B MD [Inf] - **Spec Exp:** AIDS/HIV; **Hospital:** Brooklyn Hosp Ctr-Downtown; **Address:** 121 DeKalb Ave, rm 5H, Brooklyn, NY 11201-5425; **Phone:** 718-250-6922; **Board Cert:** Internal Medicine 1980; Infectious Disease 1984; **Med School:** SUNY Downstate 1977; **Resid:** Internal Medicine, Kings Co Med Ctr 1981; **Fellow:** Infectious Disease, Kings Co Med Ctr 1983; **Fac Appt:** Asst Clin Prof Med, SUNY Hlth Sci Ctr

Brause, Barry MD [Inf] - **Spec Exp:** Bone/Joint Infections; Skin/Soft Tissue Infections; Infections in Prosthetic Devices; **Hospital:** Hosp For Special Surgery (page 59), NY-Presby Hosp/Weill Cornell (page 66); **Address:** 535 E 70th St, New York, NY 10021-5718; **Phone:** 212-774-7411; **Board Cert:** Internal Medicine 1973; Infectious Disease 1976; **Med School:** Univ Pittsburgh 1970; **Resid:** Internal Medicine, NY Hosp 1973; **Fellow:** Infectious Disease, NY Hosp 1975; **Fac Appt:** Clin Prof Med, Cornell Univ-Weill Med Coll

Chaisson, Richard E MD [Inf] - **Spec Exp:** AIDS/HIV; Tuberculosis; **Hospital:** Johns Hopkins Hosp (page 61); **Address:** 1515 Orleans St, IM-08, Baltimore, MD 21231; **Phone:** 410-955-1755; **Board Cert:** Internal Medicine 1985; **Med School:** Univ Mass Sch Med 1982; **Resid:** Internal Medicine, UCSF Med Ctr 1985; **Fellow:** Infectious Disease, UCSF Med Ctr 1987; **Fac Appt:** Prof Med, Johns Hopkins Univ

Cunha, Burke A MD [Inf] - **Spec Exp:** Infections in Immunocompromised Patients; Fevers of Unknown Origin; Pneumonia; Chronic Fatigue Syndrome; **Hospital:** Winthrop - Univ Hosp; **Address:** 222 Station Plz N, Ste 432, Mineola, NY 11501; **Phone:** 516-663-2507; **Board Cert:** Internal Medicine 1977; Infectious Disease 1978; **Med School:** Penn State Univ-Hershey Med Ctr 1972; **Resid:** Internal Medicine, Hartford Hosp 1975; **Fellow:** Infectious Disease, Hartford Hosp 1977; **Fac Appt:** Prof Med, SUNY Stony Brook

Fauci, Anthony S MD [Inf] - **Spec Exp:** AIDS/HIV; Immunotherapy; **Hospital:** Natl Inst of Hlth - Clin Ctr; **Address:** NIAID Bldg 31 - rm 7A03, 31 Center Drive, MSC 2520, Bethesda, MD 20892-2520; **Phone:** 301-496-2263; **Board Cert:** Internal Medicine 1972; Allergy & Immunology 1974; Infectious Disease 1974; **Med School:** Cornell Univ-Weill Med Coll 1966; **Resid:** Internal Medicine, New York Hosp Cornell Med Ctr 1972; **Fellow:** Infectious Disease, Natl Inst Infectious Disease NIH 1971

Frank, Ian MD [Inf] - **Spec Exp:** AIDS/HIV; **Hospital:** Hosp Univ Penn - UPHS (page 60); **Address:** Div Infectious Disease, 3400 Spruce St, Sliverstein Bldg, Fl 3 - Ste D, Philadelphia, PA 19104; **Phone:** 215-662-6932; **Board Cert:** Internal Medicine 1983; Infectious Disease 2006; **Med School:** Dartmouth Med Sch 1980; **Resid:** Internal Medicine, Graduate Hosp 1983; **Fellow:** Infectious Disease, Hosp Univ Penn 1984; **Fac Appt:** Assoc Prof Med, Univ Pennsylvania

Gumprecht, Jeffrey Paul MD [Inf] - **Spec Exp:** AIDS/HIV; Travel Medicine; Infections-Surgical; **Hospital:** Mount Sinai Med Ctr (page 64); **Address:** 1100 Park Ave, New York, NY 10128; **Phone:** 212-427-9550; **Board Cert:** Internal Medicine 1987; Infectious Disease 2003; **Med School:** Albany Med Coll 1983; **Resid:** Internal Medicine, Mt Sinai Hosp 1987; **Fellow:** Infectious Disease, Montefiore Med Ctr 1990; **Fac Appt:** Asst Clin Prof Med, Mount Sinai Sch Med

Infectious Disease

Hammer, Glenn MD [Inf] - **Spec Exp:** AIDS/HIV; Hospital Acquired Infections; Infections-Surgical; **Hospital:** Mount Sinai Med Ctr (page 64); **Address:** 1100 Park Ave, New York, NY 10128-1202; **Phone:** 212-427-9550; **Board Cert:** Infectious Disease 1974; Internal Medicine 1973; **Med School:** NYU Sch Med 1969; **Resid:** Internal Medicine, Mount Sinai Hosp 1972; **Fellow:** Infectious Disease, Mount Sinai Hosp 1974; **Fac Appt:** Asst Clin Prof Med, Mount Sinai Sch Med

Hammer, Scott M MD [Inf] - **Spec Exp:** AIDS/HIV; **Hospital:** NY-Presby Hosp/Columbia (page 66); **Address:** 630 W 168th St, P&S Box 82, New York, NY 10032; **Phone:** 212-305-8039; **Board Cert:** Internal Medicine 1975; Infectious Disease 1980; **Med School:** Columbia P&S 1972; **Resid:** Internal Medicine, Columbia-Presby Hosp 1975; Internal Medicine, Stanford Univ Hosp 1975; **Fellow:** Infectious Disease, Mass Genl Hosp 1981; **Fac Appt:** Prof Med, Columbia P&S

Hartman, Barry Jay MD [Inf] - **Spec Exp:** Endocarditis; Infections-Surgical; Parasitic Infections; **Hospital:** NY-Presby Hosp/Weill Cornell (page 66); **Address:** 407 E 70th St, Fl 4, New York, NY 10021-5302; **Phone:** 212-744-4882; **Board Cert:** Internal Medicine 1976; Infectious Disease 1980; **Med School:** Penn State Univ-Hershey Med Ctr 1973; **Resid:** Internal Medicine, NY Hosp/Cornell Med Ctr 1976; **Fellow:** Infectious Disease, NY Hosp/Cornell Med Ctr 1981; **Fac Appt:** Clin Prof Med, Cornell Univ-Weill Med Coll

Lorber, Bennett MD [Inf] - **Spec Exp:** Foodborne illnesses; **Hospital:** Temple Univ Hosp, Fox Chase Cancer Ctr (page 58); **Address:** Temple Univ Hosp - Inf Diseases, 3401 N Broad St, Parkinson Pavilion, Ste 500, Philadelphia, PA 19140; **Phone:** 215-707-3807; **Board Cert:** Internal Medicine 1974; Infectious Disease 1976; **Med School:** Univ Pennsylvania 1968; **Resid:** Internal Medicine, Temple Univ Hosp 1971; **Fellow:** Infectious Disease, Temple Univ Hosp 1973; **Fac Appt:** Prof Med, Temple Univ

Louie, Eddie MD [Inf] - **Spec Exp:** Lyme Disease; AIDS/HIV; Hospital Acquired Infections; **Hospital:** NYU Langone Med Ctr (page 67); **Address:** 345 E 37th St, New York, NY 10016-3256; **Phone:** 212-682-9202; **Board Cert:** Internal Medicine 1982; Infectious Disease 1986; **Med School:** NYU Sch Med 1979; **Resid:** Internal Medicine, Kings County Hosp 1983; **Fellow:** Infectious Disease, NYU Med Ctr 1985; **Fac Appt:** Assoc Clin Prof Med, NYU Sch Med

Masur, Henry MD [Inf] - **Spec Exp:** Critical Care; AIDS/HIV; **Hospital:** Natl Inst of Hlth - Clin Ctr; **Address:** National Institutes of Health, 10 Center Drive, Clinical Ctr 7D43, Bethesda, MD 20892; **Phone:** 301-496-9320; **Board Cert:** Internal Medicine 1975; Infectious Disease 1978; **Med School:** Cornell Univ-Weill Med Coll 1972; **Resid:** Internal Medicine, New York Hosp 1974; Internal Medicine, Johns Hopkins Hosp 1975; **Fellow:** Infectious Disease, New York Hosp-Cornell 1977

McGowan, Joseph MD [Inf] - **Spec Exp:** AIDS/HIV; HIV in Pregnancy; HIV/Hepatitis Co-Infection; AIDS/HIV in Elderly; **Hospital:** NS-LIJ Hlth Sys; **Address:** 400 Community Drive, Manhasset, NY 11030; **Phone:** 516-562-4280; **Board Cert:** Internal Medicine 2002; Infectious Disease 2002; **Med School:** Mount Sinai Sch Med 1987; **Resid:** Internal Medicine, Montefiore Med Ctr 1990; **Fellow:** Infectious Disease, Montefiore Med Ctr 1993

Mildvan, Donna MD [Inf] - **Spec Exp:** AIDS/HIV; Clinical Trials; **Hospital:** Beth Israel Med Ctr - Petrie Division (page 57); **Address:** Beth Israel Med Ctr, Div Infectious Dis, 1st Ave at 16th St, 19BH17, New York, NY 10003; **Phone:** 212-420-4005; **Board Cert:** Internal Medicine 1972; Infectious Disease 1972; **Med School:** Johns Hopkins Univ 1967; **Resid:** Internal Medicine, Mt Sinai Hosp 1970; **Fellow:** Infectious Disease, Mt Sinai Hosp 1972; **Fac Appt:** Prof Med, Albert Einstein Coll Med

Nahass, Ronald MD [Inf] - **Spec Exp:** Hepatitis B & C; Lyme Disease; Wound Healing/Care; Bone Infections; **Hospital:** Robert Wood Johnson Univ Hosp - New Brunswick, Univ Med Ctr - Princeton; **Address:** 105 Raider Rd, Hillsborough, NJ 08844; **Phone:** 908-281-0221; **Board Cert:** Internal Medicine 1985; Infectious Disease 1988; **Med School:** UMDNJ-RW Johnson Med Sch 1982; **Resid:** Internal Medicine, RWJ Univ Hosp 1986; **Fellow:** Infectious Disease, RWJ Univ Hosp 1988; **Fac Appt:** Clin Prof Med, UMDNJ-RW Johnson Med Sch

Perlman, David MD [Inf] - **Spec Exp:** AIDS/HIV; Lyme Disease; Travel Medicine; Tuberculosis; **Hospital:** Beth Israel Med Ctr - Petrie Division (page 57), Lenox Hill Hosp (page 62); **Address:** Beth Israel Med Ctr, 1st Ave at 16th St, New York, NY 10003; **Phone:** 212-420-4470; **Board Cert:** Internal Medicine 1986; Infectious Disease 1988; **Med School:** Albert Einstein Coll Med 1983; **Resid:** Internal Medicine, New York Hosp/Meml Sloan Kettering 1986; **Fellow:** Infectious Disease, Montefiore Hosp 1988; **Fac Appt:** Prof Med, Albert Einstein Coll Med

Polsky, Bruce W MD [Inf] - **Spec Exp:** AIDS/HIV; Viral Infections; Infections in Cancer Patients; AIDS Related Cancers; **Hospital:** St Luke's - Roosevelt Hosp Ctr - Roosevelt Div (page 57); **Address:** 1111 Amsterdam Ave, New York, NY 10025; **Phone:** 212-523-2525; **Board Cert:** Internal Medicine 1983; Infectious Disease 1986; **Med School:** Wayne State Univ 1980; **Resid:** Internal Medicine, Montefiore Hosp 1983; **Fellow:** Infectious Disease, Meml Sloan Kettering Cancer Ctr 1986; **Fac Appt:** Prof Med, Columbia P&S

Rahal, James MD [Inf] - **Spec Exp:** West Nile Virus; Antibiotic Resistance; Hospital Acquired Infections; **Hospital:** NY Hosp Queens; **Address:** NY Hosp Queens, Div Infectious Disease, 56-45 Main St, Flushing, NY 11355-5095; **Phone:** 718-670-1525; **Board Cert:** Internal Medicine 1967; Infectious Disease 1972; **Med School:** Tufts Univ 1959; **Resid:** Internal Medicine, Bellevue Hosp Ctr 1961; Internal Medicine, New England Ctr Hosp 1964; **Fellow:** Infectious Disease, New England Ctr Hosp 1965; **Fac Appt:** Prof Med, Cornell Univ-Weill Med Coll

Rao, Nalini G MD [Inf] - **Spec Exp:** Bone/Joint Infections; Tropical Diseases; Travel Medicine; **Hospital:** UPMC Presby, Pittsburgh, UPMC Shadyside; **Address:** Centre Commons, Suite 510, 5750 Centre Ave, Pittsburgh, PA 15206-3721; **Phone:** 412-661-1633; **Board Cert:** Internal Medicine 1975; Infectious Disease 1980; **Med School:** India 1970; **Resid:** Internal Medicine, Geo Wash Univ Hosp 1974; **Fellow:** Infectious Disease, Baylor Coll Med 1975; Infectious Disease, Univ Pittsburgh Sch Med 1977; **Fac Appt:** Clin Prof Med, Univ Pittsburgh

Romagnoli, Mario MD [Inf] - **Spec Exp:** AIDS/HIV; Bone/Joint Infections; **Hospital:** Lenox Hill Hosp (page 62); **Address:** 903 Park Ave, New York, NY 10021; **Phone:** 212-396-3390; **Board Cert:** Internal Medicine 1979; Infectious Disease 1982; **Med School:** Columbia P&S 1976; **Resid:** Internal Medicine, Columbia-Presby Med Ctr 1979; **Fellow:** Infectious Disease, Beth Israel Med Ctr 1981; **Fac Appt:** Assoc Prof Med, Columbia P&S

Segal, Brahm H MD [Inf] - **Spec Exp:** Infections in Cancer Patients; Immune Deficiencies-Primary; **Hospital:** Roswell Park Cancer Inst; **Address:** Elm and Carlton Streets, Buffalo, NY 14263; **Phone:** 716-845-5721; **Board Cert:** Infectious Disease 1997; **Med School:** Albert Einstein Coll Med 1992; **Resid:** Internal Medicine, New England Med Ctr 1995; **Fellow:** Infectious Disease, Natl Inst Allergy/Inf Dis 1997; **Fac Appt:** Assoc Prof Med, SUNY Buffalo

Sepkowitz, Kent MD [Inf] - **Spec Exp:** Tuberculosis; Infections in Cancer Patients; Fungal Infections; **Hospital:** Meml Sloan-Kettering Cancer Ctr; **Address:** 1275 York Avenue, New York, NY 10065; **Phone:** 800-525-2225; **Board Cert:** Internal Medicine 1983; Infectious Disease 2000; **Med School:** Univ Okla Coll Med 1980; **Resid:** Internal Medicine, Roosevelt Hosp 1984; **Fellow:** Infectious Disease, Meml Sloan Kettering Cancer Ctr 1991; **Fac Appt:** Prof Med, Cornell Univ-Weill Med Coll

Infectious Disease

Wallach, Frances MD [Inf] - **Spec Exp:** AIDS/HIV; HIV & Blood Transfusions; **Hospital:** Mount Sinai Med Ctr (page 64); **Address:** One Gustave L Levy Pl, Box 1090, New York, NY 10029; **Phone:** 212-241-6492; **Board Cert:** Internal Medicine 1989; Infectious Disease 2002; **Med School:** Albany Med Coll 1985; **Resid:** Internal Medicine, Montefiore Med Ctr 1989; **Fellow:** Nuclear Medicine, Montefiore Med Ctr 1990; Infectious Disease, NY Hosp-Cornell Med Ctr 1992; **Fac Appt:** Asst Prof Med, Mount Sinai Sch Med

Welch, Peter MD [Inf] - **Spec Exp:** Lyme Disease; Tick-borne Diseases; **Hospital:** Northern Westchester Hosp; **Address:** 16 Orchard Drive, Armonk, NY 10504; **Phone:** 914-273-3404; **Board Cert:** Internal Medicine 1977; Infectious Disease 1980; **Med School:** SUNY Buffalo 1974; **Resid:** Internal Medicine, New York Hosp 1977; **Fellow:** Infectious Disease, New York Hosp 1979

Wormser, Gary P MD [Inf] - **Spec Exp:** Lyme Disease; AIDS/HIV; Diagnostic Problems; **Hospital:** Westchester Med Ctr; **Address:** New York Medical College, Munger Pavilion, rm 245, Valhalla, NY 10595; **Phone:** 914-493-8865; **Board Cert:** Internal Medicine 1978; Infectious Disease 1982; **Med School:** Johns Hopkins Univ 1972; **Resid:** Internal Medicine, Mt Sinai Hosp 1975; **Fellow:** Infectious Disease, Mt Sinai Hosp 1977; **Fac Appt:** Prof Med, NY Med Coll

Yancovitz, Stanley MD [Inf] - **Spec Exp:** Lyme Disease; AIDS/HIV; **Hospital:** Beth Israel Med Ctr - Petrie Division (page 57); **Address:** 1st Ave at 16th St, Ste 17 BH10, New York, NY 10003; **Phone:** 212-420-2600; **Board Cert:** Internal Medicine 1973; Infectious Disease 1976; **Med School:** SUNY Downstate 1967; **Resid:** Internal Medicine, Metropolitan Hosp 1969; Internal Medicine, Beth Israel Med Ctr 1972; **Fellow:** Infectious Disease, Mt Sinai Hosp 1975; **Fac Appt:** Clin Prof Med, Albert Einstein Coll Med

Yu, Victor L MD [Inf] - **Spec Exp:** Legionnaire's Disease; Pneumonia; Staphylococcal Infections; **Hospital:** UPMC Presby, Pittsburgh; **Address:** University of Pittsburgh, 1401 Forbes Ave, Ste 209, Pittsburgh, PA 15219; **Phone:** 412-901-7707; **Board Cert:** Internal Medicine 1978; Infectious Disease 1982; **Med School:** Univ Minn 1970; **Resid:** Internal Medicine, Univ Colo Med Ctr 1972; Internal Medicine, Stanford Univ Med Ctr 1975; **Fellow:** Infectious Disease, Stanford Univ Med Ctr 1977; **Fac Appt:** Prof Med, Univ Pittsburgh

Southeast

Alvarez-Elcoro, Salvador MD [Inf] - **Spec Exp:** Tuberculosis; Travel Medicine; Infections-Transplant; **Hospital:** Mayo - Jacksonville; **Address:** Mayo Clinic, Div Infectious Disease, 4500 San Pablo Rd, Jacksonville, FL 32224; **Phone:** 904-953-2419; **Board Cert:** Internal Medicine 1977; Infectious Disease 1982; **Med School:** Mexico 1972; **Resid:** Internal Medicine, Charity Hosp 1977; **Fellow:** Infectious Disease, Boston City Hosp 1979; **Fac Appt:** Prof Med, Univ Fla Coll Med

Blumberg, Henry MD [Inf] - **Spec Exp:** Tuberculosis; **Hospital:** Grady Hlth Sys, Emory Univ Hosp; **Address:** Emory Univ, Div Infectious Diseases, 49 Jesse Hill Jr Drive, Atlanta, GA 30303; **Phone:** 404-616-6145; **Board Cert:** Internal Medicine 1986; Infectious Disease 2000; **Med School:** Vanderbilt Univ 1983; **Resid:** Internal Medicine, Emory Univ Affil Hosps 1986; Internal Medicine, Crawford-Long Hosp 1988; **Fellow:** Infectious Disease, Emory Univ Affil Hosps 1992; **Fac Appt:** Prof Med, Emory Univ

Cancio, Margarita MD [Inf] - **Spec Exp:** AIDS/HIV; **Hospital:** Tampa Genl Hosp; **Address:** 4729 N Habana Ave, Tampa, FL 33614; **Phone:** 813-251-8444; **Board Cert:** Internal Medicine 1985; Infectious Disease 1988; **Med School:** Univ S Fla Coll Med 1982; **Resid:** Internal Medicine, Univ S Florida Affil Hosps 1985; **Fellow:** Infectious Disease, Univ S Florida Affil Hosps 1988; **Fac Appt:** Assoc Prof Med, Univ S Fla Coll Med

Cohen, Myron S MD [Inf] - **Spec Exp:** Infections in Immunocompromised Patients; **Hospital:** Univ NC Hosps; **Address:** UNC-Chapel Hill, Div Infectious Disease, 130 Mason Farm Rd, Ste 2115, Box CB 7030, Chapel Hill, NC 27599-7030; **Phone:** 919-966-7199; **Board Cert:** Internal Medicine 1977; Infectious Disease 1982; **Med School:** Rush Med Coll 1974; **Resid:** Internal Medicine, Univ Michigan Hlth Ctr 1977; **Fellow:** Infectious Disease, Yale-New Haven Hosp 1979; **Fac Appt:** Prof Med, Univ NC Sch Med

Corey, G Ralph MD [Inf] - **Spec Exp:** Tropical Diseases; Travel Medicine; **Hospital:** Duke Univ Med Ctr; **Address:** Duke Univ Med Ctr, Box 3850, Durham, NC 27710; **Phone:** 919-668-7174; **Board Cert:** Internal Medicine 1977; Infectious Disease 1980; **Med School:** Baylor Coll Med 1973; **Resid:** Internal Medicine, Duke Univ Med Ctr 1978; **Fellow:** Infectious Disease, Duke Univ Med Ctr 1980; **Fac Appt:** Prof Med, Duke Univ

Edmond, Michael B MD [Inf] - **Spec Exp:** Bone/Joint Infections; Skin/Soft Tissue Infections; Antibiotic Resistance; Hospital Acquired Infections; **Hospital:** Med Coll of VA Hosp; **Address:** VCU/Med College Virginia, Box 980019, Richmond, VA 23298-0019; **Phone:** 804-828-2121; **Board Cert:** Internal Medicine 1989; Infectious Disease 2002; **Med School:** W VA Univ 1986; **Resid:** Internal Medicine, W Virginia Univ Hosps 1989; **Fellow:** Infectious Disease, Univ Pittsburgh 1992; Epidemiology, Univ Iowa; **Fac Appt:** Prof Med, Med Coll VA

Gorensek, Margaret J MD [Inf] - **Spec Exp:** AIDS/HIV; Infections-Transplant; Chronic Fatigue Syndrome; Pediatric Infectious Disease; **Hospital:** Holy Cross Hosp - Fort Lauderdale, Broward General Med Ctr; **Address:** Holy Cross Medical Group, 1930 NE 47th St, Ste 104, Fort Lauderdale, FL 33308; **Phone:** 954-493-9752; **Board Cert:** Internal Medicine 1985; Pediatrics 1986; Infectious Disease 1988; Pediatric Infectious Disease 2002; **Med School:** Case West Res Univ 1981; **Resid:** Internal Medicine & Pediatrics, Cleveland Clinic Fdn 1985; **Fellow:** Infectious Disease, Cleveland Clinic Fdn 1987; Pediatric Infectious Disease, Chldns Med Ctr 1988; **Fac Appt:** Asst Clin Prof Med, Univ Miami Sch Med

Guerrant, Richard MD [Inf] - **Spec Exp:** Tropical Diseases; Infectious Diarrhea; Travel Medicine; **Hospital:** Univ Virginia Med Ctr; **Address:** Ctr Global Hlth, PO Box 801379, Charlottesville, VA 22908-1379; **Phone:** 434-924-5242; **Board Cert:** Infectious Disease 1976; Internal Medicine 1973; **Med School:** Univ VA Sch Med 1968; **Resid:** Internal Medicine, Boston City Hosp 1970; Internal Medicine, Univ Virginia Hosp 1973; **Fellow:** Infectious Disease, Johns Hopkins 1972; Infectious Disease, Univ Virginia Hosp 1974; **Fac Appt:** Prof Med, Univ VA Sch Med

Katner, Harold P MD [Inf] - **Spec Exp:** AIDS/HIV; **Hospital:** Med Ctr of Central GA; **Address:** Mercer Univ Sch Med, Dept Internal Med, 707 Pine St, Macon, GA 31201; **Phone:** 478-301-5809; **Board Cert:** Internal Medicine 1983; Infectious Disease 1986; **Med School:** Louisiana State U, New Orleans 1980; **Resid:** Internal Medicine, Univ Med Ctr 1983; **Fellow:** Infectious Disease, Ochsner Fdn Hosp 1986; **Fac Appt:** Prof Med, Mercer Univ Sch Med

Pearson, Richard D MD [Inf] - **Spec Exp:** Tropical Diseases; Travel Medicine; Infectious Disease; **Hospital:** Univ Virginia Med Ctr; **Address:** Univ VA Sch Med, Dept Internal Med, McKin Hall, Box 800739, Charlottesville, VA 22908-0001; **Phone:** 434-924-5579; **Board Cert:** Internal Medicine 1976; Infectious Disease 1980; **Med School:** Univ Mich Med Sch 1973; **Resid:** Internal Medicine, Strong Meml Hosp 1976; **Fellow:** Infectious Disease, Strong Meml Hosp 1979; **Fac Appt:** Prof Med, Univ VA Sch Med

Pegram, P Samuel MD [Inf] - **Spec Exp:** AIDS/HIV; **Hospital:** Wake Forest Univ Baptist Med Ctr (page 72); **Address:** Wake Forest Univ School of Med, Medical Ctr Blvd, ID Dept, Winston-Salem, NC 27157-1042; **Phone:** 336-716-2700; **Board Cert:** Infectious Disease 1978; Internal Medicine 1976; **Med School:** Wake Forest Univ 1970; **Resid:** Internal Medicine, NC Baptist Hosp 1975; **Fellow:** Infectious Disease, NC Baptist Hosp 1978; **Fac Appt:** Prof Med, Wake Forest Univ

Infectious Disease

Ratzan, Kenneth MD [Inf] - **Spec Exp:** AIDS/HIV; **Hospital:** Mount Sinai Med Ctr - Miami, Miami Heart Inst; **Address:** Mount Sinai Medical Ctr, 4300 Alton Rd, Ste 450, Miami Beach, FL 33140-2800; **Phone:** 305-673-5490; **Board Cert:** Internal Medicine 1977; Infectious Disease 1974; **Med School:** Harvard Med Sch 1965; **Resid:** Internal Medicine, Columbia Presby Med Ctr 1967; Infectious Disease, Tufts New England Med Ctr 1972; **Fellow:** Infectious Disease, Tufts New England Med Ctr 1971; **Fac Appt:** Prof Med, Univ Miami Sch Med

Saag, Michael S MD [Inf] - **Spec Exp:** AIDS/HIV; **Hospital:** Univ of Ala Hosp at Birmingham; **Address:** UAB Div Infectious Diseases, 908 20 St S, Birmingham, AL 35294; **Phone:** 205-934-1917; **Board Cert:** Internal Medicine 1985; Infectious Disease 1988; **Med School:** Univ Louisville Sch Med 1981; **Resid:** Internal Medicine, Univ Ala Hosp 1984; **Fellow:** Infectious Disease, Univ Ala Hosp 1987

Scheld, W Michael MD [Inf] - **Spec Exp:** Meningitis; Septic Shock; AIDS/HIV; Antibiotic Resistance; **Hospital:** Univ Virginia Med Ctr; **Address:** Univ VA Hlth Sci Ctr, PO Box 801342, Charlottesville, VA 22908; **Phone:** 434-924-5991; **Board Cert:** Internal Medicine 1976; Infectious Disease 1978; **Med School:** Cornell Univ-Weill Med Coll 1973; **Resid:** Internal Medicine, Univ VA Med Ctr 1976; **Fellow:** Infectious Disease, Univ VA Med Ctr 1979; **Fac Appt:** Prof Med, Univ VA Sch Med

van der Horst, Charles M MD [Inf] - **Spec Exp:** AIDS/HIV; Fungal Infections; Viral Infections; **Hospital:** Univ NC Hosps; **Address:** Univ NC-Dept Med, Box CB3368, Chapel Hill, NC 27599-3368; **Phone:** 919-843-7199; **Board Cert:** Internal Medicine 1982; Infectious Disease 1986; **Med School:** Harvard Med Sch 1979; **Resid:** Internal Medicine, Montefiore Med Ctr 1982; **Fellow:** Infectious Disease, NC Meml Hosp 1985; **Fac Appt:** Prof Med, Univ NC Sch Med

Wallace, Mark R MD [Inf] - **Spec Exp:** Fever in Returning Travelers; Travel Medicine; Valley Fever; **Hospital:** Orlando Regl Med Ctr; **Address:** 77 W Underwood, Ste 4B, Orlando, FL 32806; **Phone:** 321-841-7750; **Board Cert:** Internal Medicine 1984; Infectious Disease 2000; **Med School:** St Louis Univ 1981; **Resid:** Internal Medicine, Univ Washington Hosp 1984; **Fellow:** Infectious Disease, Naval Hosp 1989; **Fac Appt:** Prof Med, Uniformed Srvs Univ, Bethesda

Midwest

Bakken, Johan S MD/PhD [Inf] - **Spec Exp:** Human Granulocytic Anaplasmosis; Tick-borne Diseases; Diarrheal Diseases; Ehrlichiosis; **Hospital:** St Luke's Hosp - Duluth, St Mary's Med Ctr - Duluth; **Address:** 1001 E Superior St, Ste L201, Duluth, MN 55802; **Phone:** 218-249-7990; **Board Cert:** Internal Medicine 1999; **Med School:** Univ Wash 1972; **Resid:** Internal Medicine, Univ Wash Hosps 1978; Internal Medicine, Lillehammer Fylkessykehus 1981; **Fellow:** Infectious Disease, Ulleval Hosp 1985; Microbiology, Creighton Univ 1987; **Fac Appt:** Assoc Clin Prof FMed, Univ Minn

Campbell, J William MD [Inf] - **Spec Exp:** AIDS/HIV; **Hospital:** St Luke's Hosp - Chesterfield, MO, Barnes-Jewish Hosp; **Address:** 222 S Woods Mill Rd, Ste 750N, Chesterfield, MO 63017; **Phone:** 314-205-6600; **Board Cert:** Internal Medicine 1980; Infectious Disease 1982; **Med School:** Washington Univ, St Louis 1977; **Resid:** Internal Medicine, Barnes Hosp-Wash Univ 1980; **Fellow:** Infectious Disease, Univ Tex Hlth Sci Ctr 1981; Infectious Disease, Wash Univ 1982; **Fac Appt:** Clin Prof Med, Washington Univ, St Louis

Flaherty, John P MD [Inf] - **Spec Exp:** AIDS/HIV; Travel Medicine; Orthopaedic Infectious Disease; **Hospital:** Northwestern Meml Hosp; **Address:** 676 St Clair St, Ste 205, Chicago, IL 60611; **Phone:** 312-926-8358; **Board Cert:** Internal Medicine 1986; Infectious Disease 1988; **Med School:** Univ IL Coll Med 1983; **Resid:** Internal Medicine, Univ Iowa Hosp 1986; **Fellow:** Infectious Disease, Univ Chicago Hosps 1988; **Fac Appt:** Prof Med, Northwestern Univ

Kazanjian Jr, Powel H MD [Inf] - **Spec Exp:** AIDS/HIV; **Hospital:** Univ Michigan Hlth Sys; **Address:** Infectious Disease Clin, TC Level 3, Reception D, 1500 E Med Ctr Drive, Ann Arbor, MI 48109-0999; **Phone:** 734-647-5899; **Board Cert:** Internal Medicine 1982; Infectious Disease 1986; **Med School:** Tufts Univ 1979; **Resid:** Internal Medicine, Univ Chicago Hosp 1982; **Fellow:** Infectious Disease, Brigham & Womens Hosp 1984; **Fac Appt:** Assoc Prof Med, Univ Mich Med Sch

Maki, Dennis G MD [Inf] - **Spec Exp:** Urinary Tract Infections; Critical Care; **Hospital:** Univ WI Hosp & Clins; **Address:** 600 Highland Ave, MC 2442, Madison, WI 53792-5158; **Phone:** 608-263-0946; **Board Cert:** Internal Medicine 1972; Infectious Disease 1974; **Med School:** Univ Wisc 1967; **Resid:** Infectious Disease, Mass Genl Hosp 1972; Internal Medicine, Harvard-Boston City Hosp 1973; **Fellow:** Infectious Disease, Mass Genl Hosp 1974; **Fac Appt:** Prof Med, Univ Wisc

O'Keefe, J Paul MD [Inf] - **Spec Exp:** AIDS/HIV; Fungal Infections; Infections-Surgical; Travel Medicine; **Hospital:** Loyola Univ Med Ctr; **Address:** 2160 S 1st Ave, Maywood, IL 60153-3304; **Phone:** 708-216-8563; **Board Cert:** Internal Medicine 1974; Infectious Disease 1978; **Med School:** Loyola Univ-Stritch Sch Med 1971; **Resid:** Internal Medicine, Loyola Univ Med Ctr 1974; **Fellow:** Infectious Disease, VA Hosp 1975; Infectious Disease, Tufts New England Med Ctr 1977; **Fac Appt:** Prof Med, Loyola Univ-Stritch Sch Med

Sha, Beverly MD [Inf] - **Spec Exp:** AIDS/HIV in Women; **Hospital:** Rush Univ Med Ctr; **Address:** 600 S Paulina St, Ste 140, Chicago, IL 60612-3806; **Phone:** 312-942-5865; **Board Cert:** Internal Medicine 1989; Infectious Disease 2002; **Med School:** Johns Hopkins Univ 1986; **Resid:** Internal Medicine, Rush-Presby St Lukes Med Ctr 1989; **Fellow:** Infectious Disease, Rush-Presby St Lukes Med Ctr 1991; **Fac Appt:** Assoc Prof Med, Rush Med Coll

Slama, Thomas G MD [Inf] - **Spec Exp:** Fungal Infections; Bone Infections; Infective Endocarditis; **Hospital:** St Vincent Indianapolis Hosp; **Address:** 8240 Naab Rd, Ste 300, Indianapolis, IN 46260; **Phone:** 317-870-1970; **Board Cert:** Internal Medicine 1976; Infectious Disease 1978; **Med School:** Indiana Univ 1973; **Resid:** Internal Medicine, Indianapolis Meth Hosp 1976; **Fellow:** Infectious Disease, Ohio State Univ Hosps 1978; **Fac Appt:** Clin Prof Med, Indiana Univ

Sobel, Jack MD [Inf] - **Spec Exp:** Vaginitis; Fungal Infections; Urinary Tract Infections; **Hospital:** Harper Univ Hosp, Detroit Receiving Hospital; **Address:** 3750 Woodward Ave, Ste 200, Detroit, MI 48201; **Phone:** 313-745-9035; **Board Cert:** Internal Medicine 1978; Infectious Disease 1982; **Med School:** South Africa 1965; **Resid:** Internal Medicine 1970; **Fellow:** Infectious Disease, Univ Penn Hosps 1977; Research, Natl Inst Hlth 1978; **Fac Appt:** Prof Med, Wayne State Univ

Tomford, John Walton MD [Inf] - **Hospital:** Cleveland Clin Fdn (page 56); **Address:** Cleveland Clinic, 9500 Euclid Ave, Desk S32, Cleveland, OH 44195; **Phone:** 216-444-2764; **Board Cert:** Internal Medicine 1978; Infectious Disease 1980; **Med School:** Johns Hopkins Univ 1975; **Resid:** Internal Medicine, Johns Hopkins Hosp 1978; **Fellow:** Infectious Disease, Cleveland Univ Hosp 1980; **Fac Appt:** Assoc Prof Med, Cleveland Cl Coll Med/Case West Res

Trenholme, Gordon M MD [Inf] - **Spec Exp:** Fevers of Unknown Origin; Malaria; Tropical Diseases; **Hospital:** Rush Univ Med Ctr; **Address:** Rush Univ Med Ctr, Infectious Disease, 600 S Paulina St, Ste 143AAC, Chicago, IL 60612-3809; **Phone:** 312-942-3665; **Board Cert:** Internal Medicine 1972; Infectious Disease 1976; **Med School:** Med Coll Wisc 1970; **Resid:** Internal Medicine, Univ Chicago Hosp 1973; **Fellow:** Infectious Disease, Rush/Presby-St Luke's Med Ctr 1975; **Fac Appt:** Prof Med, Rush Med Coll

Infectious Disease

Wilson, Walter Ray MD [Inf] - **Spec Exp:** Musculoskeletal Infections; **Hospital:** Mayo Med Ctr & Clin - Rochester; **Address:** Mayo Clin, Div Infectious Disease, 200 First St SW, Rochester, MN 55905; **Phone:** 507-255-7761; **Board Cert:** Internal Medicine 1973; Infectious Disease 1974; Medical Microbiology 1975; **Med School:** Baylor Coll Med 1967; **Resid:** Internal Medicine, Methodist Hosp 1968; Internal Medicine, Mayo Clin 1973; **Fellow:** Infectious Disease, Mayo Clin 1974; Microbiology, Mayo Clin 1975; **Fac Appt:** Prof Med, Mayo Med Sch

Great Plains and Mountains

Cohn, David L MD [Inf] - **Spec Exp:** Tuberculosis; AIDS/HIV; **Hospital:** Denver Health Med Ctr; **Address:** Denver Public Hlth, 605 Bannock Street, Denver, CO 80204-4507; **Phone:** 303-602-8763; **Board Cert:** Internal Medicine 1986; Infectious Disease 1982; **Med School:** Univ IL Coll Med 1975; **Resid:** Internal Medicine, Univ Wisconsin Hosp 1978; **Fellow:** Infectious Disease, Univ Colorado Hosp 1981; **Fac Appt:** Prof Med, Univ Colorado

Huitt, Gwen A MD [Inf] - **Spec Exp:** Tuberculosis; Cystic Fibrosis Infection; Mycobacterial Infections; **Hospital:** Natl Jewish Med & Rsch Ctr; **Address:** Natl Jewish Med & Research Ctr, 1400 Jackson St, rm J222, Denver, CO 80206; **Phone:** 303-398-1667; **Board Cert:** Internal Medicine 2003; Infectious Disease 2004; **Med School:** Univ Colorado 1988; **Resid:** Internal Medicine, Univ Colorado Hlth Sci Ctr 1991; **Fellow:** Infectious Disease, Univ Colorado Hlth Sci Ctr 1993; **Fac Appt:** Assoc Prof Med, Univ Colorado

Southwest

Atmar, Robert MD [Inf] - **Spec Exp:** Infectious Disease-Lung; Infections-Respiratory; Viral Infections; **Hospital:** Ben Taub Genl Hosp; **Address:** 1 Baylor Plaza, Ste 221D, MS BCM 280, Houston, TX 77030; **Phone:** 713-798-4469; **Board Cert:** Internal Medicine 1986; Infectious Disease 2007; **Med School:** Baylor Coll Med 1981; **Resid:** Internal Medicine, Baylor Coll of Med Affil Hosp 1986; **Fellow:** Infectious Disease, Baylor Coll of Med Affil Hosp 1990; **Fac Appt:** Prof Med, Baylor Coll Med

DuPont, Herbert L MD [Inf] - **Spec Exp:** Tropical Diseases; Diarrheal Diseases; Travel Medicine; **Hospital:** St Luke's Episcopal Hosp-Houston; **Address:** 6720 Bertner Ave, MC 1-164, Houston, TX 77030-1602; **Phone:** 832-355-4122; **Board Cert:** Internal Medicine 1972; **Med School:** Emory Univ 1965; **Resid:** Internal Medicine, Univ Minn Hosps 1967; **Fellow:** Infectious Disease, Univ Maryland Hosp 1969; **Fac Appt:** Prof Med, Baylor Coll Med

Keiser, Philip MD [Inf] - **Spec Exp:** AIDS/HIV; **Hospital:** UT Southwestern Med Ctr at Dallas; **Address:** 1936 Amelia Ct, Dallas, TX 75235-9173; **Phone:** 214-590-5647; **Board Cert:** Internal Medicine 1989; **Med School:** Univ MD Sch Med 1986; **Resid:** Internal Medicine, Francis Scott Key Med Ctr 1989; **Fellow:** Infectious Disease, Univ Md 1989; **Fac Appt:** Assoc Prof Med, Univ Tex SW, Dallas

Luby, James P MD [Inf] - **Spec Exp:** Viral Infections; **Hospital:** Parkland Hlth & Hosp Sys, UT Southwestern Med Ctr at Dallas; **Address:** Univ Tex SW Med Ctr, Div Inf Dis, 5303 Harry Hines Blvd, Fl 8th - Ste 400, Dallas, TX 75390-9113; **Phone:** 214-648-3480; **Board Cert:** Internal Medicine 1968; Infectious Disease 1972; **Med School:** Northwestern Univ 1961; **Resid:** Internal Medicine, Northwestern Univ 1964; **Fac Appt:** Prof Med, Univ Tex SW, Dallas

Patterson, Jan E Evans MD [Inf] - **Spec Exp:** Hospital Acquired Infections; Antibiotic Resistance; **Hospital:** Univ Hlth Syst-San Antonio; **Address:** 7400 Merton Minter Blvd, MC 111, San Antonio, TX 78229-3900; **Phone:** 210-617-5120; **Board Cert:** Internal Medicine 1985; Infectious Disease 1988; **Med School:** Univ Tex, Houston 1982; **Resid:** Internal Medicine, Vanderbilt Univ Hosp 1985; **Fellow:** Infectious Disease, Yale-New Haven Hosp 1988; **Fac Appt:** Prof Med, Univ Tex, San Antonio

Patterson, Thomas F MD [Inf] - **Spec Exp:** Fungal Infections; **Hospital:** Univ Hlth Syst-San Antonio; **Address:** Univ Texas HSC, Dept Medicine, Div Infectious Dis, 7703 Floyd Curl Drive, MC 7881, San Antonio, TX 78229-3900; **Phone:** 210-567-4823; **Board Cert:** Internal Medicine 1986; Infectious Disease 1988; **Med School:** Univ Tex, Houston 1983; **Resid:** Internal Medicine, Vanderbilt Univ Hosp 1985; Internal Medicine, Yale-New Haven Hosp 1986; **Fellow:** Infectious Disease, Yale-New Haven Hosp 1989; **Fac Appt:** Prof Med, Univ Tex, San Antonio

Wallace Jr, Richard James MD [Inf] - **Spec Exp:** Non Tuberculous Mycobacteria; Nocardia Infection; **Hospital:** UT Hlth Ctr at Tyler; **Address:** 11937 US Hwy 271, Tyler, TX 75708; **Phone:** 903-877-5122; **Board Cert:** Internal Medicine 1975; Infectious Disease 1976; **Med School:** Baylor Coll Med 1972; **Resid:** Internal Medicine, Boston City Hosp 1974; **Fellow:** Infectious Disease, Boston City Hosp 1975; Infectious Disease, Baylor Coll Med 1977

West Coast and Pacific

Ballon-Landa, Gonzalo MD [Inf] - **Spec Exp:** Hospital Acquired Infections; AIDS/HIV; Travel Medicine; **Hospital:** Scripps Mercy Hosp & Med Ctr; **Address:** 4136 Bachman Pl, San Diego, CA 92103; **Phone:** 619-298-1443; **Board Cert:** Internal Medicine 1980; Infectious Disease 1984; **Med School:** Northwestern Univ 1977; **Resid:** Internal Medicine, Evanston Hosp 1981; **Fellow:** Infectious Disease, UCSD Med Ctr 1983

Bayer, Arnold MD [Inf] - **Spec Exp:** Infective Endocarditis; Arthritis-Septic; Coccidioidomycosis; **Hospital:** LAC - Harbor - UCLA Med Ctr, UCLA Ronald Reagan Med Ctr; **Address:** 1124 W Carson St, RB2 Fl 2, Torrance, CA 90502; **Phone:** 310-222-3813; **Board Cert:** Internal Medicine 1973; Infectious Disease 1978; **Med School:** Temple Univ 1970; **Resid:** Internal Medicine, Thomas Jefferson Univ Hosp 1972; Internal Medicine, LAC-Harbor UCLA Med Ctr 1974; **Fellow:** Infectious Disease, VA Med Ctr 1976; Infectious Disease, LAC-Harbor UCLA Med Ctr 1977; **Fac Appt:** Prof Med, UCLA

Corey, Lawrence MD [Inf] - **Spec Exp:** Viral Infections; AIDS/HIV; **Hospital:** Univ Wash Med Ctr; **Address:** Fred Hutchinson Cancer Ctr, 1100 Fairview Ave N, Ste LE-500, Seattle, WA 98109; **Phone:** 206-667-6702; **Board Cert:** Internal Medicine 1974; **Med School:** Univ Mich Med Sch 1971; **Resid:** Internal Medicine, Univ Mich Med Ctr 1973; **Fellow:** Infectious Disease, Univ Wash Hosp 1977; **Fac Appt:** Prof Med, Univ Wash

Daar, Eric S MD [Inf] - **Spec Exp:** AIDS/HIV; Infectious Disease; **Hospital:** LAC - Harbor - UCLA Med Ctr; **Address:** 1000 W Carson St, Box 449, Torrance, CA 90502; **Phone:** 310-222-2467; **Board Cert:** Internal Medicine 1988; **Med School:** Georgetown Univ 1985; **Resid:** Internal Medicine, Cedars-Sinai Med Ctr 1988; **Fellow:** Infectious Disease, Cedars-Sinai Med Ctr 1991

Edwards Jr, John Ellis MD [Inf] - **Spec Exp:** Fungal Infections; Infections in Immunocompromised Patients; **Hospital:** LAC - Harbor - UCLA Med Ctr; **Address:** 1124 W Carson St, RB2 Fl 2, Torrance, CA 90502; **Phone:** 310-222-3813; **Board Cert:** Internal Medicine 1980; Infectious Disease 1974; **Med School:** UC Irvine 1968; **Resid:** Internal Medicine, Harbor-UCLA Med Ctr 1971; **Fellow:** Infectious Disease, Harbor-UCLA Med Ctr 1973; **Fac Appt:** Prof Med, UCLA

Infectious Disease

Palefsky, Joel M MD [Inf] - **Spec Exp:** AIDS Related Cancers; **Hospital:** UCSF - Mt Zion Med Ctr; **Address:** UCSF Med Ctr, Div Infectious Disease, 505 Parnassus Ave, Box 0162, San Francisco, CA 94143-0126; **Phone:** 415-476-1574; **Board Cert:** Internal Medicine 1984; Infectious Disease 1988; **Med School:** McGill Univ 1980; **Resid:** Internal Medicine, Royal Victoria Hosp 1984; **Fellow:** Infectious Disease, Stanford Univ 1989

Richman, Douglas D MD [Inf] - **Spec Exp:** AIDS/HIV; **Hospital:** VA San Diego Hlthcre Sys, UCSD Med Ctr; **Address:** UCSD-Stein Clin Rsch Bldg, 9500 Gilman, MC 0679, La Jolla, CA 92093-0679; **Phone:** 858-552-7439; **Board Cert:** Internal Medicine 1973; Infectious Disease 1976; **Med School:** Stanford Univ 1970; **Resid:** Internal Medicine, Stanford Univ Hosp 1972; **Fellow:** Infectious Disease, NIAID/NIH 1975; Infectious Disease, Beth Israel/Chldns Hosp-Harvard 1976; **Fac Appt:** Prof Med, UCSD

Schooley, Robert T MD [Inf] - **Spec Exp:** AIDS/HIV; Infectious Disease; **Hospital:** UCSD Med Ctr; **Address:** UCSD - Stein Rsch Bldg, rm 401, MC 071, 9500 Gilman Drive, La Jolla, CA 92023-0665; **Phone:** 858-822-0216; **Board Cert:** Internal Medicine 1977; **Med School:** Johns Hopkins Univ 1974; **Resid:** Internal Medicine, Johns Hopkins Hosp 1976; **Fellow:** Infectious Disease, Natl Inst Hlth 1979; Infectious Disease, Mass Genl Hosp 1981; **Fac Appt:** Prof Med, UCSD

Wiviott, Lory David MD [Inf] - **Spec Exp:** AIDS/HIV; **Hospital:** CA Pacific Med Ctr - Pacific Campus, CA Pacific Med Ctr - Davies Campus; **Address:** 2100 Webster St, Ste 400, San Francisco, CA 94115; **Phone:** 415-923-3883; **Board Cert:** Internal Medicine 1986; Infectious Disease 2000; **Med School:** Albert Einstein Coll Med 1982; **Resid:** Internal Medicine, Columbia Presby Med Ctr 1985; **Fellow:** Infectious Disease, UCSF Med Ctr 1989; **Fac Appt:** Asst Clin Prof Med, UCSF

Yoshikawa, Thomas T MD [Inf] - **Spec Exp:** Infections in the Elderly; **Hospital:** VA Med Ctr - W Los Angeles; **Address:** 11301 Wilshire Blvd, Bldg 220-Rm# 309, Los Angeles, CA 90073; **Phone:** 310-478-3711; **Board Cert:** Internal Medicine 1971; Infectious Disease 1974; **Med School:** Univ Mich Med Sch 1966; **Resid:** Internal Medicine, Harbor Genl Hosp 1970; **Fellow:** Infectious Disease, Harbor Genl Hosp 1972; **Fac Appt:** Prof Med, Charles Drew Univ Med & Sci

Cleveland Clinic

Infectious Disease

The mission of the Cleveland Clinic Department of Infectious Disease in the Medicine Institute is to provide all patients with the most technologically advanced, compassionate medical care available anywhere. We diagnose and treat patients with a wide range of both opportunistic and acquired infections. The department is an integral part of Cleveland Clinic, a not-for-profit multispecialty academic medical center ranked by *U.S.News & World Report* as one of the nation's best hospitals.

We provide around-the-clock inpatient care, including three general infectious disease consultation services as well as dedicated solid organ transplant, bone marrow transplant, cardiothoracic intensive care and medical/surgical intensive infectious disease services. The department also operates several specialty outpatient clinics. Both services are designed to provide patients with optimal care, while supporting research and education initiatives. The department's outpatient subspecialty clinics include:

Granuloma Clinic: Granulomas are tumor-like masses often caused by tissue infections. One of the most common types of infections that cause granulomatous disease in Northeast Ohio is histoplasmosis. Granulomas are non-cancerous, but many types require special care because they can spread from person to person. Tuberculosis is an example of a contagious and potentially fatal granuloma. Other conditions treated by Cleveland Clinic's Granuloma Clinic include coccidoidmycosis, cyptococcosis and mycobacterial avium-intracellulare complex.

Endocarditis Clinic: Endocarditis is an inflammation of the endocardium, or the inner lining of the heart and the heart valves. The disease is most commonly caused by a bacterial pathogen but can be due to fungal pathogens as well. Major symptoms of bacterial endocarditis include fever, fatigue, heart murmur, enlarged spleen and areas of tissue death. In addition to bacterial endocarditis, Cleveland Clinic's Endocarditis Clinic also treats infections of the endocardium caused by cardiac devices, grafts or implants.

HIV/AIDS Clinic: This specialty clinic provides care and support for patients infected with the human immunodeficiency virus, or HIV. This virus attacks the immune system, weakening a person's ability to fight infections and cancer.

International Traveler's Health Clinic: This specialty clinic provides pre-travel health and safety advice to anyone planning to journey abroad. All vaccinations and prescription medications necessary to facilitate safe travel are administered or prescribed. The International Traveler's Health Clinic also provides a comprehensive itinerary review, developing individualized packets of information for every client. Post-travel evaluation is available as needed.

Outpatient Parenteral Antimicrobial Therapy Program: This program works with patients receiving intravenous treatments for serious infections while living at home or outside a hospital setting. We play an integral role in the managing this program, which has one of the highest volumes of any center in the United States.

The Bone and Joint Infection Program: This service at Cleveland Clinic employs a multi-disciplinary team approach in the inpatient and outpatient settings for diagnosis, management, and prevention of infections of the musculoskeletal system. Infectious Disease specialists and orthopaedic surgeons work hand in hand with colleagues in microbiology, pathology, pharmacy, and infection control to treat complex infections such as prosthetic joint infections and osteomyelitis.

For more information about the Cleveland Clinic Medicine Institute's Department of Infectious Disease, to schedule a second opinion or to learn about assistance for out-of-town patients, call 800.890.2467 or visit www.clevelandclinic.org/infectioustopdocs.

Department of Infectious Disease | 9500 Euclid Avenue / AC311 | Cleveland OH 44195

NYU **Langone Medical Center**

550 First Avenue (at 31St Street)
New York, NY 10016
Physician Referral:
(888)7-NYU-MED (888-769-8633)
www.med.nyu.edu

INFECTIOUS DISEASES

About the Division of Infectious Diseases and Immunology:

Developing effective treatment for infectious diseases is among the miracles of the last century's science, but today we are faced with deadly new infections and old ones that were never tamed. These and the rapidly emerging problem of resistance to antibiotics place the study and treatment of infectious diseases at the forefront of modern medicine. NYU Langone Medical Center faculty and fellows within the Division of Infectious Diseases and Immunology have expertise in the diagnosis, treatment and prevention of rare and common acute and chronic infectious diseases. Physicians within the Division are actively involved in the management of complicated bone and joint infections, prevention of infection in cancer and transplant patients and developing strategies for managing hepatitis B and C. The Division also offers the opportunity for patients with HIV to enroll in clinical trials of new drugs that are not yet widely available.

We specialize in the following areas:

MEDICAL AND MOLECULAR PARASITOLOGY
The NYU Division of Infectious Diseases and Immunology works alongside NYU Langone Medical Center's Department of Medical Parasitology to bring malaria and other parasitic diseases under control.

AIDS CLINICAL TRIALS
The NYU AIDS Clinical Trials Unit is one of 35 such units designated and supported by the National Institute of Allergy and Infectious Diseases and is a dedicated resource for healthcare providers, researchers and scientists working in the field of HIV/AIDS research. It is one of the most productive units in the nation and enrolls adult and pediatric patients in clinical trials supported by the NIH. The data produced by the unit has supported the licensing of several drugs and plays an essential role in defining optimal therapies and preventing complications.

HIV PREVENTION
The NYU Division of Infectious Diseases and Immunology has developed a uniquely effective program in HIV prevention that has gained wide recognition and has extended the hospital's expertise from New York City to West and East Africa.

POPULATION BIOLOGY OF INFECTIOUS DISEASES
This novel program combines laboratory and clinical studies with epidemiology (examines factors affecting the health and illness of populations) and genetics to reach maximum results.

RESEARCH
Doctors in the Division of Infectious Diseases and Immunology are extensively involved in local and international research into the early diagnosis, treatment and prevention of chronic infections such as tuberculosis and Helicobacter (bacteria associated with stomach ulcers).

Internal Medicine

A personal physician who provides long-term, comprehensive care in the office and the hospital, managing both common and complex illness of adolescents, adults and the elderly. Internists are trained in the diagnosis and treatment of cancer, infections and diseases affecting the heart, blood, kidneys, joints and digestive, respiratory and vascular systems. They are also trained in the essentials of primary care internal medicine which incorporates an understanding of disease prevention, wellness, substance abuse, mental health and effective treatment of common problems of the eyes, ears, skin, nervous system and reproductive organs.

Note: *Internal Medicine normally includes many primary care physicians. However, for purposes of this directory, no primary care physicians are included.*

Training Required: Three years

INTERNAL MEDICINE

New England

Gillman, Matthew MD [IM] - **Spec Exp:** Obesity; Nutrition & Disease Prevention/Control; Diabetes in Pregnancy; Clinical Trials Only; **Hospital:** Children's Hospital - Boston, Brigham & Women's Hosp; **Address:** Harvard Med School, Dept of Population Medicine, 133 Brookline Ave Fl 6, Boston, MA 02215; **Phone:** 617-509-9968; **Board Cert:** Internal Medicine 1985; Pediatrics 1986; **Med School:** Duke Univ 1981; **Resid:** Internal Medicine, N Carolina Meml Hosp 1984; Pediatrics, N Carolina Meml Hosp 1985; **Fellow:** Research, Harvard Univ 1990; **Fac Appt:** Prof Med, Harvard Med Sch

Jackson, Vicki MD [IM] - **Spec Exp:** Palliative Care; **Hospital:** Mass Genl Hosp; **Address:** Palliative Care Svc, 55 Fruit St, FND 600, Boston, MA 02114; **Phone:** 617-724-9197; **Board Cert:** Internal Medicine 1998; Hospice & Palliative Medicine 2002; **Med School:** Univ Wisc 1995; **Resid:** Internal Medicine, Cambridge Hlth Alliance 1998

Mid Atlantic

Arnold, Robert M MD [IM] - **Spec Exp:** Palliative Care; Ethics; Pain-HIV patients; **Hospital:** UPMC Montefiore, UPMC Presby, Pittsburgh; **Address:** UPMC Montefiore, Div Internal Medicine, Section of Palliative Care & Ethics, 3459 Fifth Ave, Ste 932W, Pittsburgh, PA 15213; **Phone:** 412-692-4834; **Board Cert:** Internal Medicine 1986; **Med School:** Univ MO-Kansas City 1983; **Resid:** Internal Medicine, Rhode Island Hosp 1986; Internal Medicine, Hosp Univ Penn 1988; **Fellow:** Public Health, Robert Wood Johnson Univ Affil Hosp 1998; **Fac Appt:** Prof Med, Univ Pittsburgh

Braunstein, Seth N MD/PhD [IM] - **Spec Exp:** Diabetes; **Hospital:** Hosp Univ Penn - UPHS (page 60); **Address:** Hosp of Univ Penn, Diabetes Ctr, 3400 Spruce St, 4 Penn Tower, Philadelphia, PA 19104-4219; **Phone:** 215-662-2468; **Board Cert:** Internal Medicine 1975; **Med School:** NYU Sch Med 1972; **Resid:** Internal Medicine, Hosp U Penn 1975; **Fac Appt:** Assoc Prof Med, Univ Pennsylvania

Cirigliano, Michael D MD [IM] - **Spec Exp:** Complementary Medicine; Women's Health; **Hospital:** Hosp Univ Penn - UPHS (page 60); **Address:** Penn Internal Med Practice, UPHS, 3701 Market St Fl 3, Philadelphia, PA 19104; **Phone:** 215-615-0878; **Board Cert:** Internal Medicine 2005; **Med School:** Univ Pennsylvania 1990; **Resid:** Internal Medicine, Hosp U Penn 1993; **Fac Appt:** Assoc Prof Med, Univ Pennsylvania

Galland, Leo MD [IM] - **Spec Exp:** Nutrition; Chronic Illness; Complementary Medicine; **Address:** 156 5th Ave, Ste 820, New York, NY 10010; **Phone:** 212-989-6733; **Board Cert:** Internal Medicine 1972; **Med School:** NYU Sch Med 1968; **Resid:** Internal Medicine, Bellevue Hosp 1972; **Fellow:** Behavioral Medicine, Univ Conn Hlth Ctr 1981

Legato, Marianne J MD [IM] - **Spec Exp:** Cardiovascular Disease; Women's Health; Gender Specific Medicine; **Hospital:** NY-Presby Hosp/Columbia (page 66), St Luke's - Roosevelt Hosp Ctr - Roosevelt Div (page 57); **Address:** 962 Park Ave, New York, NY 10028-2433; **Phone:** 212-737-5663; **Board Cert:** Internal Medicine 2003; **Med School:** NYU Sch Med 1962; **Resid:** Internal Medicine, Columbia-Presby Med Ctr 1965; **Fellow:** Cardiovascular Disease, Columbia-Presby Med Ctr 1968; **Fac Appt:** Prof Emeritus Med, Columbia P&S

Lewin, Neal A MD [IM] - **Spec Exp:** Preventive Medicine; Toxicology; Headache; **Hospital:** NYU Langone Med Ctr (page 67); **Address:** 120 E 36th St, Ste 1B, New York, NY 10016-3426; **Phone:** 212-889-2813; **Board Cert:** Internal Medicine 1977; Emergency Medicine 2002; Medical Toxicology 1983; **Med School:** SUNY Downstate 1974; **Resid:** Internal Medicine, NYU-Bellevue Hosp 1977; **Fac Appt:** Prof Med, NYU Sch Med

Quill, Timothy E MD [IM] - **Spec Exp:** Palliative Care; **Hospital:** Univ of Rochester Strong Meml Hosp; **Address:** University of Rochester Medical Ctr, 601 Elmwood Ave, Box 687, Rochester, NY 14642; **Phone:** 585-273-1154; **Board Cert:** Internal Medicine 1979; Hospice & Palliative Medicine 1990; **Med School:** Univ Rochester 1976; **Resid:** Internal Medicine, U Rochester/Strong Meml Hosp 1979; **Fellow:** Liaison Psychiatry, U Rochester Med Psych Liason Program 1980; **Fac Appt:** Prof Med, Univ Rochester

Rader, Daniel J MD [IM] - **Spec Exp:** Cholesterol/Lipid Disorders; Preventive Cardiology; Metabolic Disorders; **Hospital:** Hosp Univ Penn - UPHS (page 60), Penn Presby Med Ctr - UPHS (page 60); **Address:** Univ Penn-UPHS, 52 N 39th St, PHI Bldg - Ste 2A, Philadelphia, PA 19104; **Phone:** 215-662-9993; **Board Cert:** Internal Medicine 1987; **Med School:** Med Coll PA Hahnemann 1984; **Resid:** Internal Medicine, Yale-New Haven Hosp 1987; **Fellow:** Research, Natl Inst Hlth 1992; **Fac Appt:** Prof Med, Univ Pennsylvania

Rivlin, Richard S MD [IM] - **Spec Exp:** Nutrition & Cancer Prevention/Control; Breast Cancer; Prostate Cancer; Colon Cancer; **Hospital:** NY-Presby Hosp/Weill Cornell (page 66); **Address:** 428 E 72nd St, Ste 600, New York, NY 10021; **Phone:** 646-898-2749; **Board Cert:** Internal Medicine 1969; **Med School:** Harvard Med Sch 1959; **Resid:** Internal Medicine, Johns Hopkins Hosp 1961; Internal Medicine, Johns Hopkins Hosp 1964; **Fellow:** Endocrinology, Diabetes & Metabolism, Natl Inst Hlth 1963; Biochemistry, Johns Hopkins Hosp 1966; **Fac Appt:** Prof Med, Cornell Univ-Weill Med Coll

Selwyn, Peter MD [IM] - **Spec Exp:** AIDS/HIV; Palliative Care; Addiction/Substance Abuse; **Hospital:** Montefiore Med Ctr - Div. Moses; **Address:** Montfiore Med Ctr, 3544 Jerome Ave, Bronx, NY 10467; **Phone:** 718-920-4678; **Board Cert:** Family Medicine 2005; **Med School:** Harvard Med Sch 1981; **Resid:** Family Medicine, Montefiore Med Ctr 1984; **Fac Appt:** Prof Med, Albert Einstein Coll Med

Yaffe, Bruce MD [IM] - **Spec Exp:** Gastroscopy; Colonoscopy; **Hospital:** Lenox Hill Hosp (page 62); **Address:** 201 E 65th St, New York, NY 10021-6701; **Phone:** 212-879-4700; **Board Cert:** Internal Medicine 1979; Gastroenterology 1981; **Med School:** Geo Wash Univ 1976; **Resid:** Internal Medicine, Mount Sinai Hosp 1979; Hepatology, Mount Sinai Hosp 1980; **Fellow:** Gastroenterology, Lenox Hill Hosp 1982

Southeast

Cushman, William C MD [IM] - **Spec Exp:** Hypertension; Preventive Cardiology; Cholesterol/Lipid Disorders; **Hospital:** VA Med Ctr - Memphis; **Address:** VA Medical Ctr, 1030 Jefferson Ave, MC 111Q, Memphis, TN 38104-2127; **Phone:** 901-523-8990 x6605; **Board Cert:** Internal Medicine 1977; **Med School:** Univ Miss 1974; **Resid:** Internal Medicine, Univ Mississippi Med Ctr 1977; **Fac Appt:** Prof Med, Univ Tenn Coll Med, Memphis

Heimburger, Douglas C MD [IM] - **Spec Exp:** Nutrition & Disease Prevention/Control; Nutrition & Cancer Prevention; **Hospital:** Univ of Ala Hosp at Birmingham, VA Med Ctr; **Address:** UAB, Dept Nutrition Sci & Med, 1675 University Blvd Webb Bldg - rm 439, Birmingham, AL 35294-3360; **Phone:** 205-996-5400; **Board Cert:** Internal Medicine 1981; **Med School:** Vanderbilt Univ 1978; **Resid:** Internal Medicine, Washington Univ Hosps 1981; **Fellow:** Nutrition, Univ Alabama Med Ctr 1982

Internal Medicine

Tucker, Rodney O MD [IM] - **Spec Exp:** Palliative Care; **Hospital:** Univ of Ala Hosp at Birmingham; **Address:** UAB Center for Palliative Care, CH19 219U, 1530 3rd Ave S, Birmingham, AL 35294-2041; **Phone:** 205-975-8197; **Board Cert:** Internal Medicine 2002; **Med School:** Univ Alabama 1989; **Resid:** Internal Medicine, Carraway Methodist Med Ctr 1993; **Fac Appt:** Asst Prof Med, Univ Alabama

Tulsky, James A MD [IM] - **Spec Exp:** Palliative Care; **Hospital:** Duke Univ Med Ctr; **Address:** Ctr for Palliative Care, Hock Plaza, 2424 Erwin Rd, Ste 1105, Durham, NC 27705; **Phone:** 919-668-7215; **Board Cert:** Internal Medicine 2000; Hospice & Palliative Medicine 2006; **Med School:** Univ IL Coll Med 1987; **Resid:** Internal Medicine, UCSF Med Ctr 1990; **Fellow:** Pain & Palliative Care, UCSF Med Ctr 1993; **Fac Appt:** Prof Med, Duke Univ

Midwest

Santa-Emma, Philip H MD [IM] - **Spec Exp:** Palliative Care; **Hospital:** Mt Carmel W Hosp; **Address:** 1144 Dublin Rd, Columbus, OH 43215; **Phone:** 614-234-5000; **Board Cert:** Family Medicine 2003; Hospice & Palliative Medicine 2003; **Med School:** Ohio State Univ 1988; **Resid:** Family Medicine, Mt Carmel Med Ctr 1991

Weder, Alan B MD [IM] - **Spec Exp:** Hypertension; Renovascular Disease; Peripheral Vascular Disease; Carotid Artery Disease; **Hospital:** Univ Michigan Hlth Sys; **Address:** Univ Mich, Div Cardiovascular Med, 1500 E Med Ctr Drive, Floor 3 Reception: B, Ann Arbor, MI 48109; **Phone:** 734-647-7321; **Board Cert:** Internal Medicine 1978; **Med School:** Hahnemann Univ 1975; **Resid:** Internal Medicine, Univ Chicago Hosps 1978; **Fac Appt:** Prof Med, Univ Mich Med Sch

Wright Jr, Jackson T MD/PhD [IM] - **Spec Exp:** Hypertension; **Hospital:** Univ Hosps Case Med Ctr; **Address:** CWRU Div Hypertension, 11100 Euclid Ave, Bolwell Bldg - rm 2200, Cleveland, OH 44106; **Phone:** 216-844-5174; **Board Cert:** Internal Medicine 1980; **Med School:** Univ Pittsburgh 1976; **Resid:** Internal Medicine, Univ Michigan Hosps 1987; **Fellow:** Pharmacology, Univ Health Ctr 1980; **Fac Appt:** Prof Med, Case West Res Univ

Great Plains and Mountains

Mehler, Philip S MD [IM] - **Spec Exp:** Eating Disorders; Substance Abuse; Hypertension; **Hospital:** Denver Health Med Ctr; **Address:** Denver Health Med Ctr, 777 Bannock St, MC 0278, Denver, CO 80204; **Phone:** 303-436-3234; **Board Cert:** Internal Medicine 1989; **Med School:** Univ Colorado 1983; **Resid:** Internal Medicine, Univ Colorado Affil Hosp 1987; **Fac Appt:** Prof Med, Univ Colorado

Southwest

Fine, Robert L MD [IM] - **Spec Exp:** Palliative Care; **Hospital:** Baylor Univ Medical Ctr; **Address:** 3434 Swiss Ave, Dallas, TX 75204; **Phone:** 214-828-5090; **Board Cert:** Internal Medicine 1981; Hospice & Palliative Medicine 1993; **Med School:** Univ Tex SW, Dallas 1978; **Resid:** Internal Medicine, Baylor Univ Med Ctr 1981

Wolff, Robert A MD [IM] - **Spec Exp:** Gastrointestinal Cancer; Pancreatic Cancer; Colon & Rectal Cancer; Clinical Trials; **Hospital:** UT MD Anderson Cancer Ctr; **Address:** 1515 Holcombe Blvd, Unit 421, Houston, TX 77030; **Phone:** 713-745-5476; **Board Cert:** Internal Medicine 1989; **Med School:** Albany Med Coll 1986; **Resid:** Internal Medicine, Duke Univ Med Ctr 1989; **Fellow:** Hematology & Oncology, Duke Univ Med Ctr 1992

West Coast and Pacific

Bissell Jr, Dwight M MD [IM] - **Spec Exp:** Porphyria; **Hospital:** UCSF Med Ctr; **Address:** UCSF Med Ctr, Dept Gastroenterology, 350 Parnassus Ave, rm 410, San Francisco, CA 94117; **Phone:** 415-353-2318; **Board Cert:** Internal Medicine 1974; **Med School:** Harvard Med Sch 1967; **Resid:** Internal Medicine, Boston City Hosp-Harvard 1970; **Fellow:** Gastroenterology, UCSF Med Ctr 1973; **Fac Appt:** Prof Med, UCSF

Ferris, Frank D MD [IM] - **Spec Exp:** Palliative Care; **Hospital:** San Diego Hospice; **Address:** 4311 3rd Ave, San Diego, CA 92103-1407; **Phone:** 619-688-1600; **Board Cert:** Hospice & Palliative Medicine 1998; **Med School:** Canada 1981; **Resid:** Internal Medicine, Univ Toronto; Radiation Oncology, Univ Toronto; **Fellow:** Pain Management, Toronto-Sunnybrook Reg Cancer Ctr

Pantilat, Steven MD [IM] - **Spec Exp:** Palliative Care; **Hospital:** UCSF Med Ctr; **Address:** 521 Parnassus Ave, Box 0903, San Francisco, CA 94143-0903; **Phone:** 415-502-1414; **Board Cert:** Internal Medicine 2003; Hospice & Palliative Medicine 2001; **Med School:** UCSF 1989; **Resid:** Internal Medicine, UCSF Med Ctr 1992; **Fac Appt:** Asst Clin Prof Med, UCSF

Rabow, Michael W MD [IM] - **Spec Exp:** Palliative Care; **Hospital:** UCSF - Mt Zion Med Ctr; **Address:** 1701 Divisadero St, Ste 500, UCSF, San Francisco, CA 94143; **Phone:** 415-353-7300; **Board Cert:** Internal Medicine 1996; Hospice & Palliative Medicine 2002; **Med School:** UCSF 1993; **Resid:** Internal Medicine, UCSF Med Ctr 1996; **Fellow:** Gastroenterology, UCSF Med Ctr 1997; **Fac Appt:** Assoc Clin Prof Med, UCSF

White, Jocelyn C MD [IM] - **Spec Exp:** Palliative Care; **Hospital:** Legacy Good Samaritan Hosp and Med Ctr; **Address:** 1015 NW 22nd Ave, Portland, OR 97210; **Phone:** 503-413-8423; **Board Cert:** Internal Medicine 2000; Hospice & Palliative Medicine 2001; **Med School:** NYU Sch Med 1987; **Resid:** Internal Medicine, Good Samaritan Hosp 1991

NYU **Langone Medical Center**

550 First Avenue (at 31St Street)
New York, NY 10016
Physician Referral:
(888)7-NYU-MED (888-769-8633)
www.med.nyu.edu

INTERNAL MEDICINE

About the Division of General Internal Medicine, Department of Medicine:

Famous equally for cutting-edge research and for nurturing lifelong physician-patient relationships, the internal medicine physicians of NYU Langone Medical Center are dedicated to treating the whole patient. Internists at the Medical Center meet the highest standards of the medical profession, addressing physical and psychological aspects of health and disease through clear communication and integration of diverse elements of care. The Division of General Medicine at NYU Langone Medical Center attracts internists whose passion is the care of patients with multiple problems and who specialize in keeping people healthy.

We specialize in the following areas:

PRIMARY AND SPECIALIZED HEALTHCARE

The Division of General Internal Medicine offers physical examinations as well as specialized care in illnesses involving the heart, lungs, gastrointestinal tract, joints, bones, muscles, endocrine organs and kidneys. Division faculty believe in integrating the care of multiple conditions, and place a premium on coordinating care that is often spread across a wide variety of doctor's offices. A wide range of laboratory, imaging and advanced diagnostic testing, ranging from throat cultures to the complex mapping of the electrical surface of the heart, are also available on-site or by referral. The Division also provides comprehensive women's healthcare, including cancer screening and osteoporosis prevention and treatment.

GERIATRICS

The Division of Geriatrics at NYU Langone Medical Center provides comprehensive and multidisciplinary care, consultation and follow-up for elderly patients ranging across the full spectrum from prevention and healthy aging to the treatment and care of chronic conditions including dementia, functional impairment and degenerative disorders.

CENTER FOR HEALTHFUL BEHAVIOR CHANGE (CHBC)

The Center for Healthful Behavior Change (CHBC) focuses on developing evidence-based behavioral interventions aimed at improving patient health by altering unhealthy behaviors. The CHBC originates, tests and spreads innovative evidence-based behavioral interventions into everyday clinical practice and community settings for patients with high blood pressure and other conditions associated with cardiovascular risk including obesity and high cholesterol.

Maternal & Fetal Medicine
a subspecialty of Obstetrics & Gynecology

An obstetrician/gynecologist possesses special knowledge, skills and professional capability in the medical and surgical care of the female reproductive system and associated disorders. This physician serves as a consultant to other physicians and as a primary physician for women.

Training Required: Four years *plus* two years in clinical practice before certification in obstetrics and gynecology is complete *plus* additional training and examination in maternal-fetal medicine.

MATERNAL & FETAL MEDICINE

New England

Acker, David B MD [MF] - **Spec Exp:** Multiple Gestation; Pregnancy-High Risk; **Hospital:** Brigham & Women's Hosp; **Address:** Brigham & Womens Hosp, Dept Ob/Gyn, 75 Francis St, ASB1-3, Boston, MA 02115-6110; **Phone:** 617-732-5445; **Board Cert:** Obstetrics & Gynecology 2007; Maternal & Fetal Medicine 2007; **Med School:** NYU Sch Med 1968; **Resid:** Obstetrics & Gynecology, Einstein Affil Hosp 1971; Obstetrics & Gynecology, Vanderbilt Univ Affil Hosp 1974; **Fellow:** Maternal & Fetal Medicine, Boston Lying-In Hosp 1979; **Fac Appt:** Assoc Prof ObG, Harvard Med Sch

Baker, Emily MD [MF] - **Spec Exp:** Ultrasound; **Hospital:** Dartmouth - Hitchcock Med Ctr; **Address:** Dartmouth-Hitchcock Med Ctr, Dept Ob/Gyn, One Medical Center Drive, Lebanon, NH 03756; **Phone:** 603-653-9306; **Board Cert:** Obstetrics & Gynecology 2007; Maternal & Fetal Medicine 2007; **Med School:** Stanford Univ 1986; **Resid:** Obstetrics & Gynecology, Univ Chicago Hosps 1990; Maternal & Fetal Medicine, Univ Washington Med Ctr 1991; **Fellow:** Maternal & Fetal Medicine, St Margaret's Hosp-Tufts Univ 1992; **Fac Appt:** Assoc Prof ObG, Dartmouth Med Sch

Carr, Stephen R MD [MF] - **Spec Exp:** Twin to Twin Transfusion Syndrome (TTTS); Multiple Gestation; Fetal Surgery; **Hospital:** Women & Infants Hosp of RI; **Address:** Women & Infants Hosp, Div Mat-Fet Med, 101 Dudley St, Providence, RI 02903; **Phone:** 401-274-1122; **Board Cert:** Obstetrics & Gynecology 2000; Maternal & Fetal Medicine 1998; **Med School:** Univ Hawaii JA Burns Sch Med 1982; **Resid:** Obstetrics & Gynecology, Univ Illinois Med Ctr 1986; **Fellow:** Maternal & Fetal Medicine, Brown Univ 1988; **Fac Appt:** Assoc Prof ObG, Brown Univ

Copel, Joshua A MD [MF] - **Spec Exp:** Prenatal Diagnosis; Fetal Echocardiography; Pregnancy-High Risk; Fetal Diagnosis & Therapy; **Hospital:** Yale-New Haven Hosp; **Address:** Yale Univ Sch Med, Dept OB/GYN, 333 Cedar St, Box 208063, New Haven, CT 06520-3206; **Phone:** 203-785-5682; **Board Cert:** Obstetrics & Gynecology 2007; Maternal & Fetal Medicine 2007; **Med School:** Tufts Univ 1979; **Resid:** Obstetrics & Gynecology, Pennsylvania Hosp 1983; **Fellow:** Maternal & Fetal Medicine, Yale-New Haven Hosp 1985; **Fac Appt:** Prof ObG, Yale Univ

Greene, Michael F MD [MF] - **Spec Exp:** Pregnancy-High Risk; Multiple Gestation; Seizure Disorders & Pregnancy; **Hospital:** Mass Genl Hosp; **Address:** Mass Genl Hosp, Dept Ob/Gyn, 32 Fruit St Yawkey Bldg - rm 4F, Boston, MA 02114; **Phone:** 617-724-2229; **Board Cert:** Obstetrics & Gynecology 2007; Maternal & Fetal Medicine 2007; **Med School:** SUNY Downstate 1976; **Resid:** Obstetrics & Gynecology, Boston Hosp Women 1980; **Fellow:** Maternal & Fetal Medicine, Brigham Hosp Women 1982; **Fac Appt:** Prof ObG, Harvard Med Sch

Heffner, Linda MD/PhD [MF] - **Spec Exp:** Pregnancy-Advanced Maternal Age; Pregnancy-High Risk; **Hospital:** Boston Med Ctr; **Address:** 85 E Concord St Fl 6, Boston, MA 02118; **Phone:** 617-414-5175; **Board Cert:** Obstetrics & Gynecology 1998; Maternal & Fetal Medicine 1998; **Med School:** Johns Hopkins Univ 1977; **Resid:** Obstetrics & Gynecology, Hosp Univ Penn 1983; **Fellow:** Maternal & Fetal Medicine, Brigham-Womens Hosp 1987; **Fac Appt:** Prof ObG, Boston Univ

Lockwood, Charles MD [MF] - **Spec Exp:** Prematurity Prevention; Miscarriage-Recurrent; Multiple Gestation; **Hospital:** Yale-New Haven Hosp; **Address:** Yale Univ Sch Med, Dept Ob-Gyn, 333 Cedar St, rm FMB 302, New Haven, CT 06520-8063; **Phone:** 203-737-2970; **Board Cert:** Obstetrics & Gynecology 2007; Maternal & Fetal Medicine 2007; **Med School:** Univ Pennsylvania 1981; **Resid:** Obstetrics & Gynecology, Penn Hosp 1985; **Fellow:** Maternal & Fetal Medicine, Yale-New Haven Hosp 1987; Thrombosis, Mt Sinai Med Ctr 1991; **Fac Appt:** Prof ObG, Yale Univ

Paidas, Michael J MD [MF] - **Spec Exp:** Pregnancy-High Risk; Clotting Disorders in Pregnancy; Miscarriage-Recurrent; **Hospital:** Yale-New Haven Hosp; **Address:** Dept Ob/Gyn & Reproductive Scis, Yale-New Haven Hosp, 333 Cedar St, FMB 308, New Haven, CT 06520-8063; **Phone:** 203-785-5682; **Board Cert:** Obstetrics & Gynecology 2007; Maternal & Fetal Medicine 2007; **Med School:** Tufts Univ 1987; **Resid:** Obstetrics & Gynecology, Pennsylvania Hosp 1991; **Fellow:** Maternal & Fetal Medicine, Mount Sinai Med Ctr 1993; **Fac Appt:** Assoc Prof ObG, Yale Univ

Riley, Laura E MD [MF] - **Spec Exp:** AIDS/HIV in Pregnancy; Infectious Disease in Pregnancy; Pregnancy-High Risk; **Hospital:** Mass Genl Hosp; **Address:** Mass Genl Hosp, Yawkey Bldg, 32 Fruit St, Ste 4200, Boston, MA 02114; **Phone:** 617-724-2229; **Board Cert:** Obstetrics & Gynecology 2007; Maternal & Fetal Medicine 2007; **Med School:** Univ Pittsburgh 1985; **Resid:** Obstetrics & Gynecology, Univ Pittsburgh Med Ctr 1988; **Fellow:** Maternal & Fetal Medicine, Brigham & Womens Hosp 1990; **Fac Appt:** Assoc Prof ObG, Harvard Med Sch

Robinson, Julian N MD [MF] - **Spec Exp:** Prenatal Diagnosis; Fetal Echocardiography; Amniocentesis; Ultrasound; **Hospital:** Newton - Wellesley Hosp; **Address:** Newton-Wellesley Hospital, 2014 Washington St, Newton, MA 02462; **Phone:** 617-243-5909; **Board Cert:** Obstetrics & Gynecology 2008; Maternal & Fetal Medicine 2008; **Med School:** England, UK 1986; **Resid:** Obstetrics & Gynecology, Eastern VA Med Sch 1997; **Fellow:** Maternal & Fetal Medicine, Brigham & Women's Hosp 1998

Mid Atlantic

Berkowitz, Richard MD [MF] - **Spec Exp:** Fetal Therapy; Multiple Gestation; Pregnancy & Hematologic Abnormalities; **Hospital:** NY-Presby Hosp/Columbia (page 66); **Address:** 16 E 60th St Fl 4, New York, NY 10022; **Phone:** 212-326-8951; **Board Cert:** Obstetrics & Gynecology 2005; Maternal & Fetal Medicine 2005; **Med School:** NYU Sch Med 1965; **Resid:** Obstetrics & Gynecology, NY Hosp-Cornell Univ 1972; **Fac Appt:** Prof ObG, Columbia P&S

Caritis, Steve N MD [MF] - **Hospital:** Magee-Womens Hosp - UPMC; **Address:** Dept Maternal/Fetal Medicine, 300 Halket St, Ste 0610, Pittsburgh, PA 15213-3180; **Phone:** 412-641-6361; **Board Cert:** Obstetrics & Gynecology 1999; Maternal & Fetal Medicine 1999; **Med School:** W VA Univ 1969; **Resid:** Obstetrics & Gynecology, Univ Pittsburgh Med Ctr 1973; **Fellow:** Maternal & Fetal Medicine, Columbia-Presby Med Ctr 1975; **Fac Appt:** Prof ObG, Univ Pittsburgh

Chervenak, Francis A MD [MF] - **Spec Exp:** Ultrasound; Pregnancy-High Risk; Ethics; **Hospital:** NY-Presby Hosp/Weill Cornell (page 66); **Address:** 525 E 68th St, Ste J-130, New York, NY 10021-4870; **Phone:** 212-746-3184; **Board Cert:** Obstetrics & Gynecology 1984; Maternal & Fetal Medicine 1985; **Med School:** Jefferson Med Coll 1976; **Resid:** Obstetrics & Gynecology, NY Med Coll-Flower Fifth Ave Hosp 1979; Obstetrics & Gynecology, St Lukes Hosp 1981; **Fellow:** Maternal & Fetal Medicine, Yale-New Haven Hosp 1983; **Fac Appt:** Prof ObG, Cornell Univ-Weill Med Coll

Collea, Joseph Vincent MD [MF] - **Spec Exp:** Multiple Gestation; Obstetric Ultrasound; **Hospital:** Georgetown Univ Hosp, Sibley Mem Hosp; **Address:** GUMC PHC Bldg Fl 3, 3800 Reservoir Rd NW, Washington, DC 20007-2194; **Phone:** 202-444-8531; **Board Cert:** Obstetrics & Gynecology 1974; Maternal & Fetal Medicine 1981; **Med School:** SUNY Upstate Med Univ 1966; **Resid:** Obstetrics & Gynecology, Johns Hopkins Hosp 1972; **Fellow:** Perinatal Medicine, LAC-USC Med Ctr 1976; **Fac Appt:** Prof ObG, Georgetown Univ

Maternal & Fetal Medicine

D'Alton, Mary Elizabeth MD [MF] - **Spec Exp:** Pregnancy-High Risk; Multiple Gestation; Prenatal Diagnosis; **Hospital:** NY-Presby Hosp/Columbia (page 66); **Address:** 16 E 60th St, Ste 480, New York, NY 10022; **Phone:** 212-326-8951; **Board Cert:** Obstetrics & Gynecology 2001; Maternal & Fetal Medicine 2001; **Med School:** Ireland 1976; **Resid:** Obstetrics & Gynecology, Ottawa Genl Hosp 1982; **Fellow:** Maternal & Fetal Medicine, Tufts-New Eng Med Ctr 1984; **Fac Appt:** Clin Prof ObG, Columbia P&S

Fox, Harold E MD [MF] - **Spec Exp:** Pregnancy-High Risk; Prematurity Prevention; Multiple Gestation; **Hospital:** Johns Hopkins Hosp (page 61); **Address:** 600 N Wolfe St Phipps Bldg - rm 264, Baltimore, MD 21287; **Phone:** 410-614-0178; **Board Cert:** Obstetrics & Gynecology 2007; Maternal & Fetal Medicine 2007; **Med School:** Univ Rochester 1972; **Resid:** Obstetrics & Gynecology, Strong Meml Hosp 1975; **Fellow:** Maternal & Fetal Medicine, Univ Rochester Hosps 1977; **Fac Appt:** Prof ObG, Johns Hopkins Univ

Landy, Helain J MD [MF] - **Spec Exp:** Pregnancy-High Risk; Miscarriage-Recurrent; Multiple Gestation; Diabetes in Pregnancy; **Hospital:** Georgetown Univ Hosp, Sibley Mem Hosp; **Address:** Georgetown Univ Dept Ob/Gyn, 3800 Reservoir Rd NW, 3PHC, Washington, DC 20007-2113; **Phone:** 202-444-8531; **Board Cert:** Obstetrics & Gynecology 1998; Maternal & Fetal Medicine 1998; **Med School:** Northwestern Univ 1982; **Resid:** Obstetrics & Gynecology, Penn Hosp 1986; **Fellow:** Maternal & Fetal Medicine, Geo Washington Univ Med Ctr 1988; **Fac Appt:** Prof ObG, Georgetown Univ

Parry, Samuel I MD [MF] - **Hospital:** Hosp Univ Penn - UPHS (page 60); **Address:** Dept Maternal & Fetal Medicine, 3400 Spruce St, 2000 Courtyard Bldg, Philadephia, PA 19104; **Phone:** 215-662-6913; **Board Cert:** Obstetrics & Gynecology 2007; Maternal & Fetal Medicine 2007; **Med School:** Cornell Univ-Weill Med Coll 1990; **Resid:** Obstetrics & Gynecology, SUNY Buffalo Med Ctr 1994; **Fellow:** Maternal & Fetal Medicine, Hosp Univ Penn 1996; **Fac Appt:** Assoc Prof ObG, Univ Pennsylvania

Pinckert, Thomas L MD [MF] - **Spec Exp:** Pregnancy-High Risk; **Hospital:** Shady Grove Adven Hosp, Holy Cross Hospital - Silver Spring; **Address:** Greater Washington Maternal-Fetal Medicine, 9707 Medical Ctr Drive, Ste 230, Rockville, MD 20850; **Phone:** 301-279-6060; **Board Cert:** Obstetrics & Gynecology 2007; Clinical Genetics 1990; Maternal & Fetal Medicine 2007; **Med School:** Oregon Hlth & Sci Univ 1979; **Resid:** Obstetrics & Gynecology, David Grant Med Ctr 1983; **Fellow:** Maternal & Fetal Medicine, UCSF Med Ctr 1989; Clinical Genetics, UCSF Med Ctr 1990

Repke, John T MD [MF] - **Spec Exp:** Pregnancy-High Risk; Hypertension in Pregnancy; Women's Health; **Hospital:** Penn State Milton S Hershey Med Ctr; **Address:** MS Hershey Med Ctr Maternal Fetal Med, 500 University Drive, MC H103, Hershey, PA 17033; **Phone:** 717-531-3503 x4; **Board Cert:** Obstetrics & Gynecology 2007; Maternal & Fetal Medicine 2007; **Med School:** NY Med Coll 1978; **Resid:** Obstetrics & Gynecology, Johns Hopkins Hosp 1982; **Fellow:** Maternal & Fetal Medicine, Johns Hopkins Hosp 1984; **Fac Appt:** Prof ObG, Penn State Univ-Hershey Med Ctr

Wapner, Ronald J MD [MF] - **Spec Exp:** Perinatal Medicine; Genetic Disorders; Multiple Gestation; Vomiting-Cyclic; **Hospital:** NY-Presby Hosp/Columbia (page 66); **Address:** Div Maternal/Fetal Medicine, 16 E 60th St, rm 480, New York, NY 10022; **Phone:** 212-326-8951; **Board Cert:** Obstetrics & Gynecology 2000; Maternal & Fetal Medicine 2000; Clinical Genetics 2006; **Med School:** Jefferson Med Coll 1972; **Resid:** Obstetrics & Gynecology, Jefferson Univ Hosp 1976; **Fellow:** Maternal & Fetal Medicine, Jefferson Med Coll 1978; **Fac Appt:** Prof ObG, Columbia P&S

Southeast

Abuhamad, Alfred Z MD [MF] - **Spec Exp:** Twin to Twin Transfusion Syndrome (TTTS); Prenatal Diagnosis; Prenatal Ultrasound; Multiple Gestation; **Hospital:** Sentara Norfolk Genl Hosp; **Address:** E VA Med Sch, Div Mat Fetal Med, 825 Fairfax Ave, Ste 310, Norfolk, VA 23507; **Phone:** 757-446-7900; **Board Cert:** Obstetrics & Gynecology 2007; Maternal & Fetal Medicine 2007; **Med School:** Amer Univ Beirut 1985; **Resid:** Obstetrics & Gynecology, Jackson Meml Hosp 1989; **Fellow:** Maternal & Fetal Medicine, Jackson Meml Hosp-Univ Miami 1991; Ultrasound, Yale Univ 1991; **Fac Appt:** Prof ObG, Eastern VA Med Sch

Duff, W Patrick MD [MF] - **Spec Exp:** Pregnancy-High Risk; Infections in Pregnancy; **Hospital:** Shands at Univ of FL; **Address:** Women's Health Magnolia Parke, 3951 NW 48th Terr, Ste 101, Gainesville, FL 32606; **Phone:** 352-265-6200; **Board Cert:** Obstetrics & Gynecology 2003; Maternal & Fetal Medicine 2003; **Med School:** Georgetown Univ 1974; **Resid:** Obstetrics & Gynecology, Walter Reed Med Ctr 1978; **Fellow:** Maternal & Fetal Medicine, UT - San Antonio 1983; **Fac Appt:** Prof ObG, Univ S Fla Coll Med

Ferguson II, James E MD [MF] - **Spec Exp:** Pregnancy-High Risk; Ultrasound; **Hospital:** Univ Virginia Med Ctr; **Address:** Dept Ob/Gyn, Univ Virginia Sch Med, P.O. Box 800712, Charlottesville, VA 22908-0712; **Phone:** 434-924-9937; **Board Cert:** Obstetrics & Gynecology 2007; Maternal & Fetal Medicine 2007; **Med School:** Wake Forest Univ 1977; **Resid:** Obstetrics & Gynecology, Stanford Univ Med Ctr 1980; **Fellow:** Maternal & Fetal Medicine, Stanford Univ Med Ctr 1984; **Fac Appt:** Prof ObG, Univ KY Coll Med

McLaren, Rodney A MD [MF] - **Spec Exp:** Prenatal Diagnosis; Amniocentesis; Pregnancy-High Risk; **Hospital:** Virginia Hosp Ctr - Arlington, Georgetown Univ Hosp; **Address:** Dept Maternal & Fetal Med, 1635 N George Mason Drive, Ste 190, Arlington, VA 22205-3698; **Phone:** 703-558-6077; **Board Cert:** Obstetrics & Gynecology 2003; Maternal & Fetal Medicine 2003; **Med School:** Tufts Univ 1983; **Resid:** Obstetrics & Gynecology, LI Coll Hosp 1987; **Fellow:** Maternal & Fetal Medicine, Georgetown Univ 1989; **Fac Appt:** Assoc Prof ObG, Georgetown Univ

Miller, Franklin C MD [MF] - **Spec Exp:** Pregnancy-High Risk; Fetal Assessment; **Hospital:** Univ of Kentucky Chandler Hosp; **Address:** Univ Kentucky Med Ctr, Div High Risk Obstetrics, 800 Rose St, Ste C358, Lexington, KY 40536-0084; **Phone:** 859-257-5158; **Board Cert:** Obstetrics & Gynecology 1999; Maternal & Fetal Medicine 1999; **Med School:** Univ Louisville Sch Med 1962; **Resid:** Obstetrics & Gynecology, Tripler Genl Hosp 1969; **Fellow:** Maternal & Fetal Medicine, USC Med Ctr 1974; **Fac Appt:** Prof ObG, Univ KY Coll Med

Thorp Jr, John M MD [MF] - **Spec Exp:** Multiple Gestation; Premature Labor; **Hospital:** Univ NC Hosps; **Address:** UNC-Chapel Hill, 101 Manning Drive, Box 7600, Chapel Hill, NC 27599; **Phone:** 919-966-2496; **Board Cert:** Obstetrics & Gynecology 2007; Maternal & Fetal Medicine 2007; **Med School:** E Carolina Univ 1983; **Resid:** Obstetrics & Gynecology, Univ NC Hosp 1987; **Fellow:** Maternal & Fetal Medicine, Univ NC Hosp 1989; **Fac Appt:** Prof ObG, Univ NC Sch Med

Van Dorsten, J Peter MD [MF] - **Spec Exp:** Pregnancy-High Risk; **Hospital:** MUSC Med Ctr; **Address:** MUSC Med Ctr, Dept ObGyn, 96 Jonathan Lucas St, Charleston, SC 29425; **Phone:** 843-792-4509; **Board Cert:** Obstetrics & Gynecology 2008; Maternal & Fetal Medicine 2008; **Med School:** Univ NC Sch Med 1971; **Resid:** Obstetrics & Gynecology, Med Univ SC Hosp 1976; **Fellow:** Maternal & Fetal Medicine, USC-LAC Hosp 1981; **Fac Appt:** Prof ObG, Med Univ SC

Maternal & Fetal Medicine

Wenstrom, Katharine D MD [MF] - **Spec Exp:** Reproductive Genetics; Pregnancy-High Risk; **Hospital:** Vanderbilt Univ Med Ctr; **Address:** Vanderbilt Med Ctr, Dept OB/GYN, 1161 21st Ave S, Ste B1100, Nashville, TN 37232; **Phone:** 615-343-4673; **Board Cert:** Obstetrics & Gynecology 2006; Maternal & Fetal Medicine 2006; Clinical Genetics 1990; **Med School:** Case West Res Univ 1983; **Resid:** Obstetrics & Gynecology, Univ Illinois Hosp 1987; **Fellow:** Maternal & Fetal Medicine, Univ Illinois Hosp 1989; Clinical Genetics, Univ Iowa Med Ctr 1990; **Fac Appt:** Prof ObG, Vanderbilt Univ

Midwest

Bahado-Singh, Ray O MD [MF] - **Spec Exp:** Pregnancy-High Risk; Genetic Disorders; Obstetric Ultrasound; Twin to Twin Transfusion Syndrome (TTTS); **Hospital:** Hutzel Hosp - Detroit; **Address:** 3990 John R, 4 Webber N, Detroit, MI 48201; **Phone:** 313-745-7619; **Board Cert:** Obstetrics & Gynecology 2007; Maternal & Fetal Medicine 2007; Clinical Genetics 2006; **Med School:** Jamaica 1979; **Resid:** Obstetrics & Gynecology, Metropolitan Hosp 1985; **Fellow:** Perinatal Medicine, UC-Irvine 1987; Clinical Genetics, Yale Univ 1993

Bartelsmeyer, James MD [MF] - **Spec Exp:** Pregnancy-High Risk; Multiple Gestation; **Hospital:** St John's Mercy Med Ctr - St Louis; **Address:** 621 S New Ballas Rd, Ste 2007B, St Louis, MO 63141; **Phone:** 314-991-5000; **Board Cert:** Obstetrics & Gynecology 2007; Maternal & Fetal Medicine 2007; **Med School:** Univ IL Coll Med 1985; **Resid:** Obstetrics & Gynecology, Univ Ill Coll Med Hosps 1989; **Fellow:** Maternal & Fetal Medicine, Barnes Hosp-Univ Wash 1991; **Fac Appt:** Assoc Prof ObG, Washington Univ, St Louis

Besinger, Richard MD [MF] - **Spec Exp:** Prenatal Diagnosis; Premature Labor; Critical Care; **Hospital:** Loyola Univ Med Ctr; **Address:** Loyola Univ Med Ctr, Bldg 103, 2160 S First Ave, Ste 1013, Outpatient Ctr, Maywood, IL 60153-5590; **Phone:** 708-216-6444; **Board Cert:** Obstetrics & Gynecology 1998; Maternal & Fetal Medicine 1998; **Med School:** Loyola Univ-Stritch Sch Med 1982; **Resid:** Obstetrics & Gynecology, Univ Mich Med Ctr 1986; **Fellow:** Maternal & Fetal Medicine, Johns Hopkins Hosp 1988; **Fac Appt:** Prof ObG, Loyola Univ-Stritch Sch Med

Dooley, Sharon L MD [MF] - **Spec Exp:** Fetal Abnormalities; Pregnancy-High Risk; Multiple Gestation; **Hospital:** Northwestern Meml Hosp; **Address:** 675 N St Clair Fl 14 - Ste 200, Chicago, IL 60611; **Phone:** 312-695-7542; **Board Cert:** Obstetrics & Gynecology 2005; Maternal & Fetal Medicine 2005; **Med School:** Univ VA Sch Med 1973; **Resid:** Obstetrics & Gynecology, Northwestern Meml Hosp 1977; **Fac Appt:** Prof ObG, Northwestern Univ

Gianopoulos, John MD [MF] - **Spec Exp:** Perinatal Medicine; Premature Labor; Critical Care; **Hospital:** Loyola Univ Med Ctr; **Address:** Loyola Univ Med Ctr, 2160 S 1st Ave, Bldg 103 - Ste 1019, Maywood, IL 60153; **Phone:** 708-216-5423; **Board Cert:** Obstetrics & Gynecology 2007; Maternal & Fetal Medicine 2007; **Med School:** Loyola Univ-Stritch Sch Med 1977; **Resid:** Obstetrics & Gynecology, Loyola Univ Med Ctr 1981; **Fellow:** Maternal & Fetal Medicine, Loyola Univ Med Ctr 1983; **Fac Appt:** Prof ObG, Loyola Univ-Stritch Sch Med

Hibbard, Judith MD [MF] - **Spec Exp:** Pregnancy-High Risk; Heart Disease in Pregnancy; Prenatal Diagnosis; Ultrasound; **Hospital:** Univ of IL Med Ctr at Chicago; **Address:** Univ Illinois at Chicago, Dept OB-GYN, 1801 W Taylor St, MS 808, Chicago, IL 60612; **Phone:** 312-413-7500; **Board Cert:** Obstetrics & Gynecology 1999; Maternal & Fetal Medicine 1999; **Med School:** Loyola Univ-Stritch Sch Med 1982; **Resid:** Obstetrics & Gynecology, Univ Chicago Hosps 1986; **Fellow:** Maternal & Fetal Medicine, Univ Chicago Hosps 1988; **Fac Appt:** Prof ObG, Univ IL Coll Med

Hussey, Michael J MD [MF] - **Spec Exp:** Perinatal Medicine; Congenital Anomalies; Multiple Gestation; **Hospital:** Rush Univ Med Ctr; **Address:** 1725 W Harrison St, Ste 408, Chicago, IL 60612; **Phone:** 312-997-2229; **Board Cert:** Obstetrics & Gynecology 2007; Maternal & Fetal Medicine 2007; **Med School:** Univ IL Coll Med 1986; **Resid:** Obstetrics & Gynecology, Loyola Univ Med Ctr 1993; **Fellow:** Maternal & Fetal Medicine, Rush-Presby-St Lukes Hosp 1995; Ultrasound, Univ Col Hlth Sci Ctr 1996; **Fac Appt:** Asst Prof ObG, Rush Med Coll

Ismail, Mahmoud A MD [MF] - **Spec Exp:** Pregnancy-High Risk; Perinatal Medicine; Infections-Neonatal; Infections in Pregnancy; **Hospital:** Univ of Chicago Med Ctr; **Address:** Dept Ob/Gyn, 5841 S Maryland Ave, MC 2050, Chicago, IL 60637-1463; **Phone:** 773-702-5200; **Board Cert:** Obstetrics & Gynecology 2005; Maternal & Fetal Medicine 2005; **Med School:** Egypt 1970; **Resid:** Obstetrics & Gynecology, Wayne St Univ Affil Hosps 1977; **Fellow:** Maternal & Fetal Medicine, Univ Chicago Hosps 1982; **Fac Appt:** Prof ObG, Univ Chicago-Pritzker Sch Med

Johnson, Timothy R B MD [MF] - **Spec Exp:** Fetal Assessment; Prenatal Diagnosis; **Hospital:** Univ Michigan Hlth Sys; **Address:** Univ Mich, Dept Ob/Gyn, 1500 E Med Ctr, rm L4000, Box 5276, Ann Arbor, MI 48109; **Phone:** 734-764-8123; **Board Cert:** Obstetrics & Gynecology 2001; Maternal & Fetal Medicine 2001; **Med School:** Univ VA Sch Med 1975; **Resid:** Obstetrics & Gynecology, Univ Michigan Med Ctr 1979; **Fellow:** Maternal & Fetal Medicine, Johns Hopkins Hosp 1981; **Fac Appt:** Prof ObG, Univ Mich Med Sch

Landers, Daniel V MD [MF] - **Spec Exp:** Infectious Disease; **Hospital:** Univ Minn Med Ctr, Fairview - Riverside Campus; **Address:** 606 S 24th Ave S, Professional Bldg Fl 4, Minneapolis, MN 55454; **Phone:** 612-273-2223; **Board Cert:** Obstetrics & Gynecology 1998; Maternal & Fetal Medicine 1998; **Med School:** UCSF 1980; **Resid:** Obstetrics & Gynecology, UCSF Med Ctr 1984; **Fellow:** Maternal & Fetal Medicine, UCSF Med Ctr 1986; Infectious Disease, UCSF Med Ctr 1988; **Fac Appt:** Prof ObG, Univ Minn

Leslie, Kimberly K MD [MF] - **Spec Exp:** Uterine Cancer; **Hospital:** Univ Iowa Hosp & Clinics; **Address:** 200 Hawkins Drive, Iowa City, IA 52242; **Phone:** 319-356-1976; **Board Cert:** Obstetrics & Gynecology 2007; Maternal & Fetal Medicine 2007; **Med School:** Univ Tex SW, Dallas 1981; **Resid:** Obstetrics & Gynecology, Georgetown Univ 1983; **Fellow:** Maternal & Fetal Medicine, Georgetown Univ 1987; **Fac Appt:** Prof ObG, Univ Iowa Coll Med

Macones, George A MD [MF] - **Spec Exp:** Pregnancy-High Risk; Premature Labor; **Hospital:** Barnes-Jewish Hosp, St Louis Chldns Hosp; **Address:** Washington Univ Dept Ob/Gyn, 660 S Euclid Ave, Box 8064, St Louis, MO 63110; **Phone:** 314-996-6056; **Board Cert:** Obstetrics & Gynecology 2007; Maternal & Fetal Medicine 2007; **Med School:** Jefferson Med Coll 1988; **Resid:** Obstetrics & Gynecology, Pennsylvania Hosp 1992; **Fellow:** Maternal & Fetal Medicine, Jefferson Univ Hosp 1994; **Fac Appt:** Prof ObG, Washington Univ, St Louis

Philipson, Elliot MD [MF] - **Spec Exp:** Pregnancy-High Risk; Amniocentesis; **Hospital:** Hillcrest Hosp-Mayfield Hts, Cleveland Clin Fdn (page 56); **Address:** Hillcrest Hosp, Dept OB/Gyn, 6770 Mayfield Rd, Ste 336, Mayfield Heights, OH 44124; **Phone:** 440-312-7774; **Board Cert:** Obstetrics & Gynecology 2007; Maternal & Fetal Medicine 2007; **Med School:** Italy 1975; **Resid:** Obstetrics & Gynecology, Albany Med Ctr 1980; **Fellow:** Maternal & Fetal Medicine, Metro Genl Hosp 1982; **Fac Appt:** Assoc Prof ObG, Cleveland Cl Coll Med/Case West Res

Socol, Michael MD [MF] - **Spec Exp:** Diabetes in Pregnancy; Multiple Gestation; Premature Labor; **Hospital:** Northwestern Meml Hosp; **Address:** Prentice Womens Hosp, 250 E Superior St, Ste 3-2307, Chicago, IL 60611-3056; **Phone:** 312-472-3970; **Board Cert:** Obstetrics & Gynecology 1989; Maternal & Fetal Medicine 1981; **Med School:** Univ IL Coll Med 1974; **Resid:** Obstetrics & Gynecology, Univ Illinois Med Ctr 1977; **Fellow:** Maternal & Fetal Medicine, USC Med Ctr 1979; **Fac Appt:** Prof ObG, Northwestern Univ

Maternal & Fetal Medicine

Strassner, Howard T MD [MF] - **Spec Exp:** Pregnancy-High Risk; Amniocentesis; Obstetric Ultrasound; **Hospital:** Rush Univ Med Ctr, Resurrection Hlth Care St Joseph Hosp; **Address:** Women's Hlth Consultants, 1725 W Harrison St, Ste 408, Chicago, IL 60612; **Phone:** 312-997-2229; **Board Cert:** Obstetrics & Gynecology 2007; Maternal & Fetal Medicine 2007; **Med School:** Univ Chicago-Pritzker Sch Med 1974; **Resid:** Obstetrics & Gynecology, Columbia Presby Med Ctr 1978; **Fellow:** Maternal & Fetal Medicine, LA Co-USC Med Ctr 1980; **Fac Appt:** Prof ObG, Rush Med Coll

Treadwell, Marjorie C MD [MF] - **Spec Exp:** Ultrasound; Pregnancy-High Risk; Fetal Diagnosis & Therapy; **Hospital:** Univ Michigan Hlth Sys; **Address:** 1500 E Med Ctr Drive, F4835 MOTT Bldg, Ann Arbor, MI 48109-0264; **Phone:** 734-763-4264; **Board Cert:** Obstetrics & Gynecology 2000; Maternal & Fetal Medicine 2000; **Med School:** Univ Mich Med Sch 1984; **Resid:** Obstetrics & Gynecology, Wayne State Univ 1988; **Fellow:** Maternal & Fetal Medicine, Wayne State Univ 1990; **Fac Appt:** Prof ObG, Univ Mich Med Sch

Wilkins, Isabelle MD [MF] - **Spec Exp:** Multiple Gestation; Prenatal Ultrasound; Premature Labor; Prematurity/Low Birth Weight Infants; **Hospital:** Univ of IL Med Ctr at Chicago; **Address:** Univ Illinois Med Ctr at Chicago, Center for Womens Health, 1801 W Taylor, MS 650, Chicago, IL 60612; **Phone:** 312-413-7500; **Board Cert:** Obstetrics & Gynecology 2008; Maternal & Fetal Medicine 2008; **Med School:** Duke Univ 1980; **Resid:** Obstetrics & Gynecology, Mt Sinai Med Ctr 1984; **Fellow:** Maternal & Fetal Medicine, Mt Sinai Med Ctr 1986; **Fac Appt:** Prof ObG, Univ IL Coll Med

Winn, Hung MD [MF] - **Spec Exp:** Multiple Gestation; Pregnancy-High Risk; **Hospital:** Univ of Missouri Hosp & Clins; **Address:** 500 N Keene St, Ste 405-5, Columbia, MO 65201; **Phone:** 573-882-6361; **Board Cert:** Obstetrics & Gynecology 2000; Maternal & Fetal Medicine 2000; **Med School:** Univ IL Coll Med 1982; **Resid:** Obstetrics & Gynecology, Univ Ill Hosp 1986; **Fellow:** Maternal & Fetal Medicine, Yale-New Haven Hosp 1988; **Fac Appt:** Prof ObG, Univ MO-Columbia Sch Med

Great Plains and Mountains

Dugoff, Lorraine MD [MF] - **Spec Exp:** Pregnancy-High Risk; Prenatal Diagnosis; Ultrasound; **Hospital:** Univ Colorado Hosp; **Address:** 1635 Aurora Ct, rm F711, Aurora, CO 80045; **Phone:** 720-848-1060; **Board Cert:** Clinical Genetics 2009; **Med School:** Georgetown Univ 1989; **Resid:** Obstetrics & Gynecology, Philadelphia Hosp 1990; Obstetrics & Gynecology, Univ Colorado Hlth Sci Ctr 1993; **Fellow:** Maternal & Fetal Medicine, Univ Colorado Hlth Sci Ctr 1995; Clinical Genetics, Univ Colorado Hlth Sci Ctr 1996; **Fac Appt:** Assoc Prof ObG, Univ Colorado

Gibbs, Ronald S MD [MF] - **Spec Exp:** Infectious Disease; **Hospital:** Univ Colorado Hosp; **Address:** Dept of Ob/Gyn, MS B198-1, PO Box 6511, Aurora, CO 80045; **Phone:** 720-848-1060; **Board Cert:** Obstetrics & Gynecology 1989; Maternal & Fetal Medicine 1981; **Med School:** Univ Pennsylvania 1969; **Resid:** Obstetrics & Gynecology, Hosp Univ Penn 1974; **Fellow:** Maternal & Fetal Medicine, Univ Tex Hlth Sci Ctr 1978; **Fac Appt:** Prof ObG, Univ Colorado

Tomich, Paul MD [MF] - **Spec Exp:** Pregnancy-High Risk; Prenatal Ultrasound; **Hospital:** Nebraska Med Ctr; **Address:** 983255 Nebraska Med Ctr, Omaha, NE 68198-3255; **Phone:** 402-559-6150; **Board Cert:** Obstetrics & Gynecology 2007; Maternal & Fetal Medicine 2007; **Med School:** Loyola Univ-Stritch Sch Med 1973; **Resid:** Obstetrics & Gynecology, Mayo Clinic 1978; **Fellow:** Maternal & Fetal Medicine, Barnes Hosp-Wash Univ 1980; **Fac Appt:** Prof ObG, Univ Nebr Coll Med

Southwest

Elliott, John P MD [MF] - **Spec Exp:** Twin to Twin Transfusion Syndrome (TTTS); Multiple Gestation; Premature Labor; **Hospital:** Banner Good Samaritan Regl Med Ctr - Phoenix, Banner Desert Med Ctr; **Address:** 6320 W Union Hills Drive, Ste B1400, Glendale, AZ 85308; **Phone:** 623-561-0043; **Board Cert:** Obstetrics & Gynecology 1980; Maternal & Fetal Medicine 1982; **Med School:** Univ Colorado 1972; **Resid:** Obstetrics & Gynecology, Fitzsimmons Army Med Ctr 1976; **Fellow:** Maternal & Fetal Medicine, Long Beach Meml Hosp/UC Irvine 1980; **Fac Appt:** Clin Prof ObG, Univ Ariz Coll Med

Hankins, Gary D V MD [MF] - **Spec Exp:** Pregnancy-High Risk; Hypertension in Pregnancy; **Hospital:** UT Med Br Hosp at Galveston; **Address:** 301 University Blvd, 3.400 JSA, Galveston, TX 77555-0587; **Phone:** 409-772-1957; **Board Cert:** Obstetrics & Gynecology 2000; Maternal & Fetal Medicine 2000; **Med School:** Med Coll VA 1977; **Resid:** Obstetrics & Gynecology, Wilford Hall Med Ctr 1981; **Fellow:** Critical Care Medicine, Wilford Hall Med Ctr 1982; Maternal & Fetal Medicine, Parkland Hosp 1984; **Fac Appt:** Prof ObG, Univ Tex Med Br, Galveston

Horsager, Robyn Boehrer MD [MF] - **Hospital:** UT Southwestern Med Ctr at Dallas; **Address:** 5939 Harry Hines Blvd, Ste 300, MC 9102, Dallas, TX 75390-9102; **Phone:** 214-645-3837; **Board Cert:** Obstetrics & Gynecology 2007; Maternal & Fetal Medicine 2007; **Med School:** Univ IL Coll Med 1987; **Resid:** Obstetrics & Gynecology, Parkland Meml Hosp 1991; **Fellow:** Maternal & Fetal Medicine, Univ Texas SW Med Ctr 1993; **Fac Appt:** Assoc Prof ObG, Univ Tex SW, Dallas

Pridjian, Gabriella C MD [MF] - **Spec Exp:** Pregnancy-High Risk; Prenatal Diagnosis; Genetic Disorders; Prenatal Ultrasound; **Hospital:** Tulane-Lakeside Hosp; **Address:** 4720 S I-10 Service Rd, Ste 300, Metairie, LA 70001; **Phone:** 504-988-8070; **Board Cert:** Obstetrics & Gynecology 2007; Clinical Genetics 2007; Maternal & Fetal Medicine 2007; **Med School:** Med Coll Wisc 1982; **Resid:** Obstetrics & Gynecology, Univ Chicago Affil Hosp 1986; **Fellow:** Maternal & Fetal Medicine, Univ Chicago Affil Hosp 1989; Clinical Genetics, Hayward Gentics Ctr/Tulane Univ 1994; **Fac Appt:** Prof ObG, Tulane Univ

Reed, Kathryn L MD [MF] - **Spec Exp:** Prenatal Diagnosis; Ultrasound; Fetal Echocardiography; **Hospital:** Univ Med Ctr - Tucson; **Address:** University Medical Ctr, Womens Resource Ctr, 1501 N Campbell Ave Fl 8, Tucson, AZ 85724; **Phone:** 520-694-6010; **Board Cert:** Obstetrics & Gynecology 1994; Maternal & Fetal Medicine 1987; **Med School:** Univ Ariz Coll Med 1977; **Resid:** Obstetrics & Gynecology, Ariz Hlth Scis Ctr 1981; Maternal & Fetal Medicine, Ariz Hlth Scis Ctr 1983; **Fac Appt:** Prof ObG, Univ Ariz Coll Med

West Coast and Pacific

Benedetti, Thomas J MD [MF] - **Spec Exp:** Prematurity Prevention; Fetal Macrosomia; **Hospital:** Univ Wash Med Ctr, Yakima Valley Mem Hosp; **Address:** 1959 NE Pacific St, Box 356460, Seattle, WA 98195; **Phone:** 206-543-3729; **Board Cert:** Obstetrics & Gynecology 1980; Maternal & Fetal Medicine 1981; **Med School:** Univ Wash 1973; **Resid:** Obstetrics & Gynecology, LAC-USC Med Ctr 1977; **Fellow:** Maternal & Fetal Medicine, LAC-USC Med Ctr 1979; **Fac Appt:** Prof ObG, Univ Wash

Chmait, Ramen H MD [MF] - **Spec Exp:** Fetal Surgery; Twin to Twin Transfusion Syndrome (TTTS); **Hospital:** Hollywood Presby Med Ctr; **Address:** Hollywood Presbyterian Med Ctr, 1300 N Vermont Ave, Ste 706, Los Angles, CA 90027; **Phone:** 323-361-6074; **Board Cert:** Obstetrics & Gynecology 2007; Maternal & Fetal Medicine 2007; **Med School:** UCLA 1996; **Resid:** Obstetrics & Gynecology, LAC/USC Med Ctr 2001; **Fellow:** Maternal & Fetal Medicine, UCSD Med Ctr 2003

Maternal & Fetal Medicine

Druzin, Maurice L MD [MF] - **Spec Exp:** Lupus/SLE in Pregnancy; Fetal Electronic Monitors; Miscarriage-Recurrent; **Hospital:** Lucile Packard Chldn's Hosp; **Address:** Stanford Univ, Dept Ob/Gyn, 300 Pasteur Drive, rm HH333, MC 5317, Stanford, CA 94305-5317; **Phone:** 650-498-4069; **Board Cert:** Obstetrics & Gynecology 2008; Maternal & Fetal Medicine 2008; **Med School:** South Africa 1970; **Resid:** Obstetrics & Gynecology, Rose Med Ctr-Univ Colo 1977; **Fellow:** Maternal & Fetal Medicine, LAC-USC Med Ctr 1979; **Fac Appt:** Prof ObG, Stanford Univ

Goldberg, James D MD [MF] - **Spec Exp:** Prenatal Diagnosis; Fetal Diagnosis & Therapy; **Hospital:** CA Pacific Med Ctr - Pacific Campus; **Address:** San Francisco Perinatal Assoc, One Daniel Burnham Ct, Ste 230C, San Francisco, CA 94109; **Phone:** 415-202-1200; **Board Cert:** Obstetrics & Gynecology 2009; Clinical Genetics 1987; Maternal & Fetal Medicine 2009; **Med School:** Univ Minn 1979; **Resid:** Obstetrics & Gynecology, UCSF Med Ctr 1983; **Fellow:** Maternal & Fetal Medicine, Mt Sinai Hosp 1985; Clinical Genetics, Mt Sinai Hosp 1985

Gravett, Michael G MD [MF] - **Spec Exp:** Infectious Disease-Perinatal; **Hospital:** Univ Wash Med Ctr; **Address:** Univ Washington, Dept OB/GYN, 1959 NE Pacific St, Box 356460, Seattle, WA 98195-6460; **Phone:** 206-598-4070; **Board Cert:** Obstetrics & Gynecology 1985; Maternal & Fetal Medicine 1987; **Med School:** UCLA 1977; **Resid:** Obstetrics & Gynecology, Univ Wash Med Ctr 1981; **Fellow:** Maternal & Fetal Medicine, Univ Wash Med Ctr 1983; **Fac Appt:** Prof ObG, Univ Wash

Kelly, Thomas F MD [MF] - **Spec Exp:** Pregnancy-High Risk; **Hospital:** UCSD Med Ctr; **Address:** UCSD Med Ctr, Dept Reproductive Med, 200 W Arbor Drive, San Diego, CA 92103; **Phone:** 619-543-2284; **Board Cert:** Obstetrics & Gynecology 2008; Maternal & Fetal Medicine 2008; **Med School:** Univ Nevada 1986; **Resid:** Obstetrics & Gynecology, USCD Med Ctr 1990; **Fellow:** Maternal & Fetal Medicine, USCD Med Ctr 1992; **Fac Appt:** Prof ObG, UCSD

Koos, Brian J MD [MF] - **Spec Exp:** Pregnancy-High Risk; Fetal Diagnosis & Therapy; Heart Disease in Pregnancy; **Hospital:** UCLA Ronald Reagan Med Ctr; **Address:** UCLA Medical Ctr, 10833 Le Conte Ave, MC 3075, Los Angeles, CA 90095-3075; **Phone:** 310-794-7852; **Board Cert:** Obstetrics & Gynecology 1999; Maternal & Fetal Medicine 1999; **Med School:** Loma Linda Univ 1974; **Resid:** Obstetrics & Gynecology, Brigham & Womens Hosp 1979; **Fellow:** Maternal & Fetal Medicine, Womens Hosp 1983; **Fac Appt:** Prof ObG, UCLA

Moore, Thomas R MD [MF] - **Spec Exp:** Diabetes in Pregnancy; Fetal Diagnosis & Therapy; **Hospital:** UCSD Med Ctr, Scripps Meml Hosp - La Jolla; **Address:** 200 W Arbor Drive, MC 8433, San Diego, CA 92103; **Phone:** 619-543-7900; **Board Cert:** Obstetrics & Gynecology 2006; Maternal & Fetal Medicine 2006; **Med School:** Yale Univ 1979; **Resid:** Obstetrics & Gynecology, Naval Hosp 1983; **Fellow:** Maternal & Fetal Medicine, UCSD 1985; **Fac Appt:** Prof ObG, UCSD

Platt, Lawrence D MD [MF] - **Spec Exp:** Ultrasound; Prenatal Diagnosis; **Hospital:** Cedars-Sinai Med Ctr, St John's Hlth Ctr, Santa Monica; **Address:** 6310 W San Vincente Blvd, Ste 520, Los Angeles, CA 90048; **Phone:** 323-857-1952; **Board Cert:** Obstetrics & Gynecology 1979; Maternal & Fetal Medicine 1981; **Med School:** Wayne State Univ 1972; **Resid:** Obstetrics & Gynecology, Sinai Hosp 1976; **Fellow:** Maternal & Fetal Medicine, USC Med Ctr 1978; **Fac Appt:** Prof ObG, UCLA

Tabsh, Khalil M A MD [MF] - **Spec Exp:** Pregnancy-High Risk; **Hospital:** UCLA Ronald Reagan Med Ctr, Santa Monica - UCLA Med Ctr & Ortho Hosp; **Address:** 200 Medical Plaza, Ste 430, Los Angeles, CA 90095; **Phone:** 310-208-4492; **Board Cert:** Obstetrics & Gynecology 1981; Maternal & Fetal Medicine 1982; **Med School:** Lebanon 1974; **Resid:** Obstetrics & Gynecology, American Univ Beirut Med Ctr 1976; Obstetrics & Gynecology, Yale-New Haven Hosp 1978; **Fellow:** Maternal & Fetal Medicine, UCLA Med Ctr 1979; **Fac Appt:** Clin Prof ObG, UCLA-David Geffen Sch Med

WOMEN'S HEALTH
OBSTETRICS AND GYNECOLOGY

About the Department of Obstetrics and Gynecology:

NYU Langone Medical Center provides a comprehensive group of programs and services designed specifically for women's medical needs. Services range from primary care to the most specialized programs. Supported by sophisticated research and advanced training, the Department of Obstetrics and Gynecology at NYU Langone Medical Center offers high-quality therapies and regiments.

We specialize in the following areas:

FERTILITY-RELATED SERVICES
The Fertility Center at NYU Langone Medical Center offers state-of-the-art programs in egg donation, egg freezing and wellness (acupuncture, mind/body, psychology and yoga). Diagnosis and treatment includes ovulation induction, assisted reproductive technologies and surgical options that incorporate the latest endoscopic techniques. The Center also tests for genetic abnormalities, as well as immunity and infectious diseases.

GYNECOLOGIC ONCOLOGY
The National Ovarian Cancer Early Detection Program at NYU Langone Medical Center provides focused, high-quality, innovative care and services for asymptomatic women at increased risk of developing ovarian cancer. Additionally, the Women's Cancer program at NYU Langone Medical Center specializes in the treatment of all forms of gynecologic cancer, including cervical cancer, endometrial cancer, ovarian cancer, uterine cancer, vaginal cancer and vulvar cancer. The Program also provides treatment for uterine sarcoma, molar pregnancy and all types of gestational trophoblastic disease.

MATERNAL FETAL MEDICINE
The Division of Maternal-Fetal Medicine at NYU Langone Medical Center offers prenatal care for high-risk pregnancies as well as detailed consultations before, during and after pregnancy. Special attention is given to multifetal pregnancies and to women who have other medical conditions that may complicate a pregnancy such as diabetes, heart problems, high blood pressure and lupus.

OBSTETRICS
The Obstetrics Program offers a broad range of services including: prenatal care that gives equal emphasis to the well-being of the mother and of the fetus; fetal monitoring through ultrasound and other techniques; childbirth preparedness and breastfeeding classes; and consultation for high-risk pregnancies, including treatment for women who experience recurrent pregnancy loss.

SPECIALTY SERVICES
In addition to routine gynecological care, many other services are offered in Women's Health including: pelvic ultrasound; aspiration of breast cysts; evaluation of infertility (including the special needs of same-sex couples); colposcopy (a diagnostic evaluation of abnormal pap smears); LEEP (a loop electrosurgical procedure used to diagnose and treat cervical cancer); cryotherapy for vaginal warts; and bone density testing for osteoporosis prevention and treatment.

UROGYNECOLOGY AND RECONSTRUCTIVE PELVIC SURGERY
The Division of Urogynecology and Reconstructive Plastic Surgery at NYU Langone Medical Center focuses on using state-of-the-art diagnostic modalities for all forms of incontinence and pelvic disorders, as well as correcting malformations of the reproductive tract found at birth, during childhood or in young adults. The Division's urogynecologists are experts in providing comprehensive care for women with a wide range of conditions such as overactive bladder, urinary and/or fecal incontinence and pelvic organ prolapse.

Neonatal-Perinatal Medicine
a subspecialty of Pediatrics

A subspecialist in neonatal-perinatal medicine is a pediatrician who is the principal care provider for sick newborn infants. Clinical expertise is used for direct patient care and for consulting with obstetrical colleagues to plan for the care of mothers who have high-risk pregnancies.

Training Required: Three years in pediatrics *plus* additional training and examination.

NEONATAL-PERINATAL MEDICINE

New England

Cloherty, John MD [NP] - **Spec Exp:** Neonatology; **Hospital:** Children's Hospital - Boston, Brigham & Women's Hosp; **Address:** 319 Longwood Ave, Fl 4, Boston, MA 02115; **Phone:** 617-277-7320; **Board Cert:** Pediatrics 1986; Neonatal-Perinatal Medicine 1986; **Med School:** Boston Univ 1962; **Resid:** Pediatrics, Mass Genl Hosp 1969; **Fellow:** Neonatal-Perinatal Medicine, Chldns Hosp; **Fac Appt:** Assoc Clin Prof Ped, Harvard Med Sch

Davis, Jonathan M MD [NP] - **Spec Exp:** Lung Disease in Newborns; Brain Injury; Infections-Neonatal; **Hospital:** Tufts Med Ctr; **Address:** Tufts-New England Med Ctr, 750 Washington St, Box 44, Boston, MA 02111; **Phone:** 617-636-5322; **Board Cert:** Pediatrics 1985; Neonatal-Perinatal Medicine 1987; **Med School:** McGill Univ 1981; **Resid:** Pediatrics, Chldns Hosp 1984; **Fellow:** Neonatal-Perinatal Medicine, Chldns Hosp 1986; **Fac Appt:** Prof Ped, Tufts Univ

Ehrenkranz, Richard MD [NP] - **Spec Exp:** Nutrition; Chronic Obstructive Lung Disease (COPD); **Hospital:** Yale-New Haven Hosp; **Address:** Yale Univ-Dept Ped, PO Box 208064, New Haven, CT 06520-8064; **Phone:** 203-688-2320; **Board Cert:** Pediatrics 1977; Neonatal-Perinatal Medicine 1979; **Med School:** SUNY Downstate 1972; **Resid:** Pediatrics, Yale-New Haven Hosp 1974; **Fellow:** Neonatal-Perinatal Medicine, Yale-New Haven Hosp 1978; **Fac Appt:** Prof Ped, Yale Univ

Gross, Ian MD [NP] - **Spec Exp:** Breathing Disorders; Critical Care; **Hospital:** Yale-New Haven Hosp; **Address:** Yale Sch Med, Dept Peds, 333 Cedar St, PO Box 208064, New Haven, CT 06520-8064; **Phone:** 203-688-2320; **Board Cert:** Pediatrics 1974; Neonatal-Perinatal Medicine 1977; **Med School:** South Africa 1967; **Resid:** Pediatrics, Univ Witwatersrand Affil Hosps 1971; Pediatrics, Chldns Hosp Med Ctr 1973; **Fellow:** Neonatal-Perinatal Medicine, Yale-New Haven Hosp 1974; **Fac Appt:** Prof Ped, Yale Univ

Horbar, Jeffrey D MD [NP] - **Hospital:** Fletcher Allen Health Care- Med Ctr Campus; **Address:** Vermont Oxford Network, 33 Kilburn St, Burlington, VT 05401; **Phone:** 802-865-4814; **Board Cert:** Pediatrics 1982; Neonatal-Perinatal Medicine 1983; **Med School:** SUNY Downstate 1977; **Resid:** Pediatrics, Med Ctr Hosp Vermont 1979; **Fellow:** Obstetrics & Gynecology, Med Ctr Hosp Vermont 1981; **Fac Appt:** Assoc Prof Ped, Univ VT Coll Med

Van Marter, Linda J MD [NP] - **Spec Exp:** Neonatal Chronic Lung Disease (CLD); Lung Disease in Newborns; Pulmonary Hypertension of Newborn (PPHN); **Hospital:** Brigham & Women's Hosp, Children's Hospital - Boston; **Address:** 300 Longwood Ave, Hunnewell 430 - Newborn Med, Boston, MA 02115; **Phone:** 617-355-6027; **Board Cert:** Pediatrics 1985; Neonatal-Perinatal Medicine 1985; **Med School:** Univ Pittsburgh 1980; **Resid:** Pediatrics, Childrens Hosp Med Ctr 1983; **Fellow:** Neonatology, Harvard Med Sch 1986; **Fac Appt:** Assoc Prof Ped, Harvard Med Sch

Mid Atlantic

Davidson, Dennis MD [NP] - **Spec Exp:** Lung Disease in Newborns; **Hospital:** Schneider Chldn's Hosp; **Address:** Schneider Chldns Hosp, Neonatal Div, 269-01 76th Ave, Ste 344, New Hyde Park, NY 11040; **Phone:** 718-470-3440; **Board Cert:** Pediatrics 1980; Neonatal-Perinatal Medicine 1981; **Med School:** Loyola Univ-Stritch Sch Med 1974; **Resid:** Pediatrics, Babies Hosp-Columbia Univ 1978; **Fellow:** Neonatal-Perinatal Medicine, Babies Hosp-Columbia Univ 1981; **Fac Appt:** Assoc Prof Ped, Albert Einstein Coll Med

Delivoria-Papadopoulos, Maria MD [NP] - **Spec Exp:** Neonatology; Prematurity/Low Birth Weight Infants; Breathing Disorders; Brain Injury; **Hospital:** St Christopher's Hosp for Chldn, Hahnemann Univ Hosp; **Address:** St Christopher's Hosp for Children, Erie Ave at Front St, Ste 2212, Neonatology, Philadelphia, PA 19134; **Phone:** 215-427-5202; **Board Cert:** Pediatrics 1971; Neonatal-Perinatal Medicine 1975; **Med School:** Greece 1957; **Resid:** Pediatrics, Chldns Hosp 1959; Psychiatry, Colo State Hosp 1962; **Fellow:** Neonatology, Hosp Sick Chldn 1964; **Fac Appt:** Prof Ped

Hendricks-Munoz, Karen MD [NP] - **Spec Exp:** Breathing Disorders; Neonatal Neurology; Retinopathy of Prematurity; **Hospital:** NYU Langone Med Ctr (page 67), Bellevue Hosp Ctr; **Address:** NYU Med Ctr, Dept Neonatology, 530 1st Ave, Ste HCC-7A, New York, NY 10016-6402; **Phone:** 212-263-7477; **Board Cert:** Pediatrics 1985; Neonatal-Perinatal Medicine 1987; **Med School:** Yale Univ 1978; **Resid:** Pediatrics, Yale-New Haven Hosp 1981; **Fellow:** Neonatology, Strong Meml Hosp 1984; **Fac Appt:** Assoc Prof Ped, NYU Sch Med

Holzman, Ian R MD [NP] - **Spec Exp:** Neonatal Nutrition; Necrotizing Enterocolitis; Ethics; Prematurity/Low Birth Weight Infants; **Hospital:** Mount Sinai Med Ctr (page 64), Elmhurst Hosp Ctr; **Address:** Newborn Assocs, 1 Gustave L Levy Pl, Box 1508, New York, NY 10029-6500; **Phone:** 212-241-5446; **Board Cert:** Pediatrics 1975; Neonatal-Perinatal Medicine 1977; **Med School:** Univ Pittsburgh 1971; **Resid:** Pediatrics, Chldns Hosp 1975; **Fellow:** Neonatal-Perinatal Medicine, Univ Colorado Hosp 1977; **Fac Appt:** Prof Ped, Mount Sinai Sch Med

Hurt, Hallam MD [NP] - **Spec Exp:** Neonatology; **Hospital:** Chldns Hosp of Philadelphia, The, Hosp Univ Penn - UPHS (page 60); **Address:** Chldns Hosp of Philadelphia, 3535 Market St, rm 1509, Philadelphia, PA 19104; **Phone:** 215-590-0560; **Board Cert:** Pediatrics 1976; Neonatal-Perinatal Medicine 2002; **Med School:** Univ VA Sch Med 1971; **Resid:** Pediatrics, Univ Virginia Hosp 1974; **Fellow:** Neonatal-Perinatal Medicine, Univ Virginia Hosp 1976; **Fac Appt:** Prof Ped, Temple Univ

La Gamma, Edmund F MD [NP] - **Spec Exp:** Neonatal Infections; Prematurity/Low Birth Weight Infants; Necrotizing Enterocolitis; **Hospital:** Westchester Med Ctr; **Address:** Maria Fareri Chldns Hosp, Grasslands Rd Fl 2, Valhalla, NY 10595-0001; **Phone:** 914-493-8558; **Board Cert:** Pediatrics 1981; Neonatal-Perinatal Medicine 1981; **Med School:** NY Med Coll 1976; **Resid:** Pediatrics, NY Hosp-Cornell Med Ctr 1978; **Fellow:** Neonatal-Perinatal Medicine, NY Hosp-Cornell Med Ctr 1980; Cardiovascular Disease, UCSF Med Ctr 1981; **Fac Appt:** Prof Ped, NY Med Coll

Lawson, Edward E MD [NP] - **Spec Exp:** Prematurity/Low Birth Weight Infants; Respiratory Distress Syndrome (RDS); Neonatal Critical Care; Breathing Disorders; **Hospital:** Johns Hopkins Hosp (page 61), Johns Hopkins Bayview Med Ctr (page 61); **Address:** Johns Hopkins Chldns Ctr, 600 N Wolfe St, Nelson 2-133, Baltimore, MD 21287; **Phone:** 410-955-5259; **Board Cert:** Pediatrics 1990; Neonatal-Perinatal Medicine 1997; **Med School:** Northwestern Univ 1972; **Resid:** Pediatrics, Chldns Hosp Med Ctr 1975; **Fellow:** Neonatal-Perinatal Medicine, Harvard Med Sch 1977; **Fac Appt:** Prof Ped, Johns Hopkins Univ

Nogee, Lawrence M MD [NP] - **Spec Exp:** Lung Disease in Newborns-Genetic; **Hospital:** Johns Hopkins Hosp (page 61); **Address:** Johns Hopkins Hosp, Div Neonatolgy, 600 N Wolfe St, CMSC 6-104, Baltimore, MD 21287-3200; **Phone:** 410-502-6794; **Board Cert:** Pediatrics 1986; Neonatal-Perinatal Medicine 1987; **Med School:** Johns Hopkins Univ 1981; **Resid:** Pediatrics, Johns Hopkins Hosp 1984; **Fellow:** Neonatal-Perinatal Medicine, Chldns Hosp Med Ctr 1986; **Fac Appt:** Assoc Prof Ped, Johns Hopkins Univ

Neonatal-Perinatal Medicine

Perlman, Jeffrey M MD [NP] - **Spec Exp:** Neonatal Critical Care; Prematurity/Low Birth Weight Infants; Neonatal Neurology; Lung Disease in Newborns; **Hospital:** NY-Presby Hosp/Weill Cornell (page 66); **Address:** 525 E 68th St, Ste N 506, New York, NY 10065; **Phone:** 212-746-3530; **Board Cert:** Pediatrics 1983; Neonatal-Perinatal Medicine 1983; **Med School:** South Africa 1974; **Resid:** Pediatrics, Johannesburg Chldns Hosp 1979; Pediatrics, St Louis Chldns Hosp 1981; **Fellow:** Neonatology, St Louis Chldns Hosp 1983; **Fac Appt:** Prof Ped, Cornell Univ-Weill Med Coll

Polin, Richard MD [NP] - **Spec Exp:** Neonatal Infections; **Hospital:** NYPresby-Morgan Stanley Children's Hosp (page 66); **Address:** Morgan Stanley Chlds Hosp, 3959 Broadway, CHC 115, New York, NY 10032; **Phone:** 212-305-5827; **Board Cert:** Pediatrics 1975; Neonatal-Perinatal Medicine 1977; **Med School:** Temple Univ 1970; **Resid:** Pediatrics, Chldns Meml Hosp 1972; Pediatrics, Babies Hosp 1975; **Fellow:** Neonatal-Perinatal Medicine, Babies Hosp-Columbia 1974; **Fac Appt:** Prof Ped, Columbia P&S

Short, Billie Lou MD [NP] - **Hospital:** Chldns Natl Med Ctr; **Address:** Div Neonatology, 111 Michigan Ave NW, Washington, DC 20010; **Phone:** 202-476-3314; **Board Cert:** Pediatrics 1979; Neonatal-Perinatal Medicine 1979; **Med School:** Univ Okla Coll Med 1974; **Resid:** Pediatrics, Chldn's Hosp-Oklahoma 1977; **Fellow:** Neonatal-Perinatal Medicine, Chldn's Hosp Med Ctr 1979; **Fac Appt:** Prof Ped, Geo Wash Univ

Silverman, Gary A MD/PhD [NP] - **Hospital:** Children's Inst - Pittsburgh, Magee-Womens Hosp - UPMC; **Address:** Div Neonatology & Developmental Biology, 300 Halket St, Pittsburgh, PA 15213; **Phone:** 412-641-4111; **Board Cert:** Neonatal-Perinatal Medicine 2004; **Med School:** Univ Chicago-Pritzker Sch Med 1984; **Resid:** Pediatrics, Children's Hosp 1087; **Fellow:** Neonatology, St Louis Chldns Hosp 1989; Research, Washington U Sch Med 1991; **Fac Appt:** Prof Ped, Univ Pittsburgh

Sison, Joseph S MD [NP] - **Spec Exp:** Neonatology; **Hospital:** Englewood Hosp & Med Ctr, Mount Sinai Med Ctr (page 64); **Address:** 350 Engle St, Englewood, NJ 07631-1808; **Phone:** 201-894-3321; **Board Cert:** Pediatrics 2007; Neonatal-Perinatal Medicine 2005; **Med School:** Philippines 1984; **Resid:** Pediatrics, Jersey Shore Med Ctr 1992; Neonatal-Perinatal Medicine, Vanderbilt Univ Hosp 1993; **Fellow:** Neonatal-Perinatal Medicine, New York Hosp 1995; **Fac Appt:** Clin Prof Ped, Mount Sinai Sch Med

Watchko, Jon F MD [NP] - **Hospital:** Magee-Womens Hosp - UPMC; **Address:** Div Neonatology & Developmental Biology, 300 Halket St, Pittsburg, PA 15213; **Phone:** 412-641-1834; **Board Cert:** Pediatrics 1985; Neonatal-Perinatal Medicine 1985; **Med School:** Univ Pittsburgh 1980; **Resid:** Pediatrics, Upstate Med Ctr 1983; **Fellow:** Neonatology, Univ Washington Med Ctr 1986; **Fac Appt:** Prof Ped, Univ Pittsburgh

Zubrow, Alan B MD [NP] - **Spec Exp:** Neonatology; **Hospital:** St Christopher's Hosp for Chldn, Hahnemann Univ Hosp; **Address:** St Christopher's Hosp for Chldn, Erie Ave at Front St, Ste 2212, Philadelphia, PA 19134; **Phone:** 215-427-5202; **Board Cert:** Pediatrics 1980; Neonatal-Perinatal Medicine 1981; **Med School:** Univ Pennsylvania 1976; **Resid:** Pediatrics, Chldns Hosp 1979; **Fellow:** Neonatology, Columbia-Presby Med Ctr 1981; **Fac Appt:** Prof Ped, Drexel Univ Coll Med

Southeast

Bancalari, Eduardo MD [NP] - **Spec Exp:** Neonatology; **Hospital:** Jackson Meml Hosp (page 70); **Address:** Dept Pediatrics (R-131), PO Box 016960, Miami, FL 33101; **Phone:** 305-585-2328; **Board Cert:** Neonatal-Perinatal Medicine 1993; Pediatrics 1993; **Med School:** Chile 1966; **Resid:** Pediatrics, Hosp Luis Calvo Mackenna 1969; **Fellow:** Pediatric Cardiology, Univ Miami Med Ctr; **Fac Appt:** Prof Ped, Univ Miami Sch Med

Boyle, Robert J MD [NP] - **Spec Exp:** Neonatology; Ethics; **Hospital:** Univ Virginia Med Ctr; **Address:** UVA Hlth Sci Ctr, Dept Peds, PO Box 800386, Charlottesville, VA 22908; **Phone:** 434-924-5429; **Board Cert:** Pediatrics 1978; Neonatal-Perinatal Medicine 1979; **Med School:** Johns Hopkins Univ 1973; **Resid:** Pediatrics, Rainbow Babies Chldns Hosp 1976; **Fellow:** Neonatal-Perinatal Medicine, Women & Infants Hosp 1978; **Fac Appt:** Prof Ped, Univ VA Sch Med

Bucciarelli, Richard L MD [NP] - **Spec Exp:** Neonatal Cardiology; **Hospital:** Shands at Univ of FL; **Address:** Shands Healthcare, 1600 SW Archer Rd, rm R1-118, Gainesville, FL 32610; **Phone:** 352-392-3337; **Board Cert:** Pediatrics 1977; Neonatal-Perinatal Medicine 1977; Pediatric Cardiology 1977; **Med School:** Univ Mich Med Sch 1972; **Resid:** Pediatrics, Shands Hosp-Univ Fla 1975; **Fellow:** Neonatal-Perinatal Medicine, Shands Hosp-Univ Fla 1977; **Fac Appt:** Prof Ped, Univ Fla Coll Med

Dhanireddy, Ramasubbareddy MD [NP] - **Spec Exp:** Neonatology; Prematurity/Low Birth Weight Infants; **Hospital:** Regional Med Ctr - Memphis, Le Bonheur Chldns Med Ctr; **Address:** Memphis Med Ctr, 853 Jefferson Ave, rm 201, Memphis, TN 38163; **Phone:** 901-448-5950; **Board Cert:** Pediatrics 1980; Neonatal-Perinatal Medicine 1997; **Med School:** India 1974; **Resid:** Pediatrics, Lousiana State Univ Med Ctr 1978; **Fellow:** Neonatology, Georgetown Univ Med Ctr 1980; **Fac Appt:** Prof Ped, Univ Tenn Coll Med, Memphis

Holtzman, Ronald B MD [NP] - **Spec Exp:** Neonatology; Lung Disease in Newborns; **Hospital:** Gaston Meml Hosp; **Address:** Gaston Meml Hosp, NICU Office, 2525 Court Drive, Gastonia, NC 28053; **Phone:** 704-834-3390; **Board Cert:** Pediatrics 1987; Neonatal-Perinatal Medicine 2004; **Med School:** Rush Med Coll 1983; **Resid:** Pediatrics, Chldns Meml/Northwestern Univ 1986; **Fellow:** Neonatal-Perinatal Medicine, Chldns Meml/Northwestern Univ 1986

Kattwinkel, John MD [NP] - **Spec Exp:** Lung Disease in Newborns; Sudden Infant Death Syndrome (SIDS); **Hospital:** Univ Virginia Med Ctr; **Address:** Univ Va Hosp, Div Neonatology, Dept Peds, PO Box 800386, Charlottesville, VA 22908-0386; **Phone:** 434-924-5428; **Board Cert:** Pediatrics 1986; Neonatal-Perinatal Medicine 1986; **Med School:** Harvard Med Sch 1968; **Resid:** Pediatrics, Duke Univ Med Ctr 1970; **Fellow:** Neonatology, Case-West Res Univ 1974; **Fac Appt:** Prof Ped, Univ VA Sch Med

Neu, Josef MD [NP] - **Spec Exp:** Neonatal Nutrition; Neonatal Gastroenterology; **Hospital:** Shands at Univ of FL; **Address:** Shands Healthcare-Univ Fla, 1600 SW Archer Rd, rm HD513, Gainesville, FL 32610; **Phone:** 352-392-8179; **Board Cert:** Pediatrics 1980; Neonatal-Perinatal Medicine 1981; **Med School:** Univ Wisc 1975; **Resid:** Pediatrics, Johns Hopkins Hosp 1978; **Fellow:** Neonatal-Perinatal Medicine, Stanford Univ 1980; **Fac Appt:** Prof Ped, Univ Fla Coll Med

Stiles, Alan D MD [NP] - **Spec Exp:** Neonatology; **Hospital:** Univ NC Hosps; **Address:** Dept of Pediatrics CB # 7220, Chapel Hill, NC 27599-7220; **Phone:** 919-966-4427; **Board Cert:** Pediatrics 1984; Neonatal-Perinatal Medicine 1985; **Med School:** Univ NC Sch Med 1977; **Resid:** Pediatrics, North Carolina Meml Hosp 1982; **Fellow:** Neonatal-Perinatal Medicine, Chldns Hosp/Brigham Hosp 1985; **Fac Appt:** Prof Ped, Univ NC Sch Med

Midwest

Bell, Edward F MD [NP] - **Spec Exp:** Neonatal Critical Care; Prematurity/Low Birth Weight Infants; **Hospital:** Univ Iowa Hosp & Clinics, Genesis Med Ctr; **Address:** Univ Iowa Hosps, Dept Pediatrics, 200 Hawkins Drive, rm 8811 JPP, Iowa City, IA 52242; **Phone:** 319-356-4006; **Board Cert:** Pediatrics 1978; Neonatal-Perinatal Medicine 1995; **Med School:** Columbia P&S 1973; **Resid:** Pediatrics, Babies Hosp-Columbia Presby 1976; **Fellow:** Neonatology, McMaster Univ Med Ctr 1977; Neonatology, Women & Infants Hosp-Brown Univ 1979; **Fac Appt:** Prof Ped, Univ Iowa Coll Med

Neonatal-Perinatal Medicine

Cole, Francis Sessions MD [NP] - **Spec Exp:** Neonatal Chronic Lung Disease (CLD); Respiratory Distress Syndrome (RDS); Surfactant Biology; Prematurity/Low Birth Weight Infants; **Hospital:** St Louis Chldns Hosp, Barnes-Jewish Hosp; **Address:** St Louis Chldns Hosp, 1 Children's Pl, Box 8116/NWT, St Louis, MO 63110; **Phone:** 314-454-6148; **Board Cert:** Pediatrics 1980; Neonatal-Perinatal Medicine 1983; **Med School:** Yale Univ 1973; **Resid:** Pediatrics, Chldns Hosp Med Ctr 1978; **Fellow:** Neonatology, Brigham & Womens Hosp 1981; **Fac Appt:** Prof Ped, Washington Univ, St Louis

Donn, Steven M MD [NP] - **Spec Exp:** Breathing Disorders; Respiratory Distress Syndrome (RDS); Pulmonary Hypertension of Newborn (PPHN); Surfactant Biology; **Hospital:** Mott Chldns Hosp, Univ Michigan Hlth Sys; **Address:** F5790 Mott Hosp/ 0254, 1500 E Med Ctr Drive, Ann Arbor, MI 48109-0254; **Phone:** 734-763-4109; **Board Cert:** Pediatrics 1981; Neonatal-Perinatal Medicine 1981; **Med School:** Tulane Univ 1974; **Resid:** Pediatrics, Univ Vermont Med Ctr 1978; **Fellow:** Neonatology, Univ Michigan 1980; **Fac Appt:** Prof Ped, Univ Mich Med Sch

Gewolb, Ira MD [NP] - **Spec Exp:** Breathing Disorders; Gastroesophageal Reflux Disease (GERD); **Hospital:** Mich State Univ-Sparrow Hos; **Address:** Sparrow Hosp, Div Neonatology Michigan State Univ., 1215 E Michigan Ave Fl 3, Lansing, MI 48912; **Phone:** 517-364-2670; **Board Cert:** Pediatrics 1980; Neonatal-Perinatal Medicine 1981; **Med School:** Yale Univ 1976; **Resid:** Pediatrics, Childrens Hosp Med Ctr 1979; **Fellow:** Neonatology, Yale Univ 1981; **Fac Appt:** Prof Ped, Mich State Univ

Hamvas, Aaron MD [NP] - **Spec Exp:** Lung Disease in Newborns-Genetic; **Hospital:** St Louis Chldns Hosp, Barnes-Jewish Hosp; **Address:** Wash Univ-Div Newborn Med, 660 S Euclid Ave, Box 8116, St Louis, MO 63110; **Phone:** 314-454-6148; **Board Cert:** Pediatrics 1989; Neonatal-Perinatal Medicine 2006; **Med School:** Washington Univ, St Louis 1981; **Resid:** Pediatrics, St Louis Chldns Hosp 1984; **Fellow:** Neonatology, St Louis Chldns Hosp 1990; **Fac Appt:** Prof Ped, Washington Univ, St Louis

Lemons, James A MD [NP] - **Spec Exp:** Nutrition; Ethics; **Hospital:** Riley Hosp for Children, Indiana Univ Hosp; **Address:** 699 West Drive, RR-208, Indianapolis, IN 46202-5119; **Phone:** 317-274-4716; **Board Cert:** Pediatrics 1993; Neonatal-Perinatal Medicine 1993; **Med School:** Northwestern Univ 1969; **Resid:** Pediatrics, Univ Mich Med Sch 1972; **Fellow:** Neonatal-Perinatal Medicine, Univ Colo Med Ctr 1975; **Fac Appt:** Prof Ped, Indiana Univ

Martin, Richard J MD [NP] - **Spec Exp:** Breathing Disorders; **Hospital:** Rainbow Babies & Chldns Hosp; **Address:** 11100 Euclid Ave, Div Neonatology, Cleveland, OH 44106-6010; **Phone:** 216-844-3387; **Board Cert:** Pediatrics 1976; Neonatal-Perinatal Medicine 2005; **Med School:** Australia 1970; **Resid:** Pediatrics, Univ Missouri 1973; **Fellow:** Neonatal-Perinatal Medicine, Case West Res Univ 1975; **Fac Appt:** Prof Ped, Case West Res Univ

Meadow, William Lee MD/PhD [NP] - **Spec Exp:** Infections-Neonatal; Ethics; **Hospital:** Univ of Chicago Med Ctr; **Address:** 5841 S Maryland Ave, MC-6060, Chicago, IL 60637; **Phone:** 773-702-6210; **Board Cert:** Pediatrics 1979; Neonatal-Perinatal Medicine 1981; **Med School:** Univ Pennsylvania 1974; **Resid:** Pediatrics, Chldns Meml Hosp 1978; **Fellow:** Neonatology, Wyler Chldns Hosp 1981; Infectious Disease, Wyler Chldns Hosp 1981; **Fac Appt:** Prof Ped, Univ Chicago-Pritzker Sch Med

Muraskas, Jonathan MD [NP] - **Spec Exp:** Prematurity/Low Birth Weight Infants; Multiple Gestation; Conjoined Twins; Ethics; **Hospital:** Loyola Univ Med Ctr; **Address:** Loyola University Medical Ctr, Bldg 107, 2160 S First Ave Fl 5 - rm 5810, Maywood, IL 60153-5500; **Phone:** 708-216-1067; **Board Cert:** Pediatrics 1987; Neonatal-Perinatal Medicine 1987; **Med School:** Loyola Univ-Stritch Sch Med 1982; **Resid:** Pediatrics, Loyola Univ Med Ctr 1985; **Fellow:** Neonatal-Perinatal Medicine, Loyola Univ Med Ctr 1987; **Fac Appt:** Prof Ped, Loyola Univ-Stritch Sch Med

Steinhorn, Robin H MD [NP] - **Spec Exp:** Pulmonary Hypertension; **Hospital:** Children's Mem Hosp, Northwestern Meml Hosp; **Address:** 2300 Children's Plaza, Box 45, Chicago, IL 60614; **Phone:** 773-880-4142; **Board Cert:** Neonatal-Perinatal Medicine 2004; **Med School:** Washington Univ, St Louis 1980; **Resid:** Obstetrics & Gynecology, Barnes Hosp 1983; Pediatrics, Univ Minn Affil Hosp 1986; **Fellow:** Neonatal-Perinatal Medicine, Univ Minn Affil Hosp 1988; **Fac Appt:** Prof Ped, Northwestern Univ

Whitsett, Jeffrey A MD [NP] - **Spec Exp:** Lung Disease in Newborns-Genetic; **Hospital:** Cincinnati Chldns Hosp Med Ctr, Good Samaritan Hosp - Cincinnati; **Address:** Cincinnati Chldns Hosp, Div Neonatalogy, 3333 Burnet Ave, Cincinnati, OH 45229-3039; **Phone:** 513-636-4830; **Board Cert:** Pediatrics 1979; Neonatal-Perinatal Medicine 1979; **Med School:** Columbia P&S 1973; **Resid:** Pediatrics, Mt Sinai Hosp 1976; **Fellow:** Neonatology, Chldns Hosp Med Ctr 1977; **Fac Appt:** Prof Ped, Univ Cincinnati

Great Plains and Mountains

Milley, J Ross MD/PhD [NP] - **Spec Exp:** Nutrition; **Hospital:** Primary Children's Med Ctr, Univ Utah Hosps and Clins; **Address:** Univ Utah - Dept Pediatrics/Neonatology, Williams Bldg, PO Box 581289, Salt Lake City, UT 84158; **Phone:** 801-581-7085; **Board Cert:** Pediatrics 1980; Neonatal-Perinatal Medicine 1981; **Med School:** Univ Chicago-Pritzker Sch Med 1975; **Resid:** Pediatrics, Johns Hopkins Hosp 1978; **Fellow:** Neonatology, Johns Hopkins Hosp 1980; **Fac Appt:** Prof Ped, Univ Utah

Zach, Terence MD [NP] - **Spec Exp:** Neonatal Critical Care; **Hospital:** Creighton Univ Med Ctr; **Address:** 600 S 42nd St, Omaha, NE 68198; **Phone:** 402-559-6750; **Board Cert:** Pediatrics 1987; Neonatal-Perinatal Medicine 2004; **Med School:** Univ Nebr Coll Med 1983; **Resid:** Pediatrics, Univ Nebr Med Ctr 1986; **Fellow:** Neonatology, Univ Minnesota 1986; **Fac Appt:** Prof Ped, Creighton Univ

Southwest

Adams, James M MD [NP] - **Spec Exp:** Lung Disease in Newborns; **Hospital:** Texas Chldns Hosp; **Address:** 6621 Fannin St, MC WT-6104, Houston, TX 77030; **Phone:** 832-826-1380; **Board Cert:** Pediatrics 1975; Neonatal-Perinatal Medicine 1975; **Med School:** Baylor Coll Med 1970; **Resid:** Pediatrics, Baylor Affil Hosps 1973; **Fellow:** Neonatal-Perinatal Medicine, Baylor Affil Hosps 1975; **Fac Appt:** Prof Ped, Baylor Coll Med

Denson, Susan E MD [NP] - **Spec Exp:** Neonatology; **Hospital:** Meml Hermann Hosp - Texas Med Ctr, LBJ General Hosp; **Address:** Univ Tex Houston Med Sch, Dept Peds, 6431 Fannin, Ste 2.106, Houston, TX 77030; **Phone:** 713-500-5727; **Board Cert:** Pediatrics 1978; Neonatal-Perinatal Medicine 1979; **Med School:** Univ Tex SW, Dallas 1972; **Resid:** Pediatrics, Univ Ariz 1974; **Fellow:** Neonatal-Perinatal Medicine, Univ Ariz 1975; Neonatal-Perinatal Medicine, Univ Tex Med Sch 1976; **Fac Appt:** Prof Ped, Univ Tex, Houston

Escobedo, Marilyn B MD [NP] - **Spec Exp:** Neonatology; Nutrition; **Hospital:** Chldns Hosp OU Med Ctr; **Address:** 1200 Everett Dr, 7th Fl, North Pavilion, Oklahoma City, OK 73104; **Phone:** 405-271-5215; **Board Cert:** Pediatrics 1986; Neonatal-Perinatal Medicine 2004; **Med School:** Washington Univ, St Louis 1970; **Resid:** Pediatrics, Chldns Hosp 1972; Neonatal-Perinatal Medicine, Chldns Hosp 1973; **Fellow:** Neonatal-Perinatal Medicine, Vanderbilt Univ 1976; **Fac Appt:** Prof Ped, Univ Okla Coll Med

Neonatal-Perinatal Medicine

Garcia-Prats, Joseph MD [NP] - **Spec Exp:** Lung Disease in Newborns; Neonatology; **Hospital:** Texas Chldns Hosp, Ben Taub Genl Hosp; **Address:** 6621 Fannin St, MC WT-6104, Houston, TX 77030-1608; **Phone:** 832-826-1380; **Board Cert:** Pediatrics 1977; Neonatal-Perinatal Medicine 1977; **Med School:** Tulane Univ 1972; **Resid:** Pediatrics, Baylor Affil Hosp 1975; **Fellow:** Neonatal-Perinatal Medicine, Baylor Affil Hosp 1977; **Fac Appt:** Prof Ped, Baylor Coll Med

Odom, Michael W MD [NP] - **Spec Exp:** Neonatology; **Hospital:** Univ Hlth Syst-San Antonio; **Address:** Dept Peds, 7703 Floyd Curl Drive, MC 7812, San Antonio, TX 78229-3900; **Phone:** 210-567-5225; **Board Cert:** Pediatrics 1987; Neonatal-Perinatal Medicine 2004; **Med School:** Univ Tex SW, Dallas 1983; **Resid:** Pediatrics, Vanderbilt Univ Affil Hosps 1986; **Fellow:** Neonatal-Perinatal Medicine, Mt Zion Med Ctr-UCSF 1989; **Fac Appt:** Assoc Prof Ped, Univ Tex, San Antonio

Seidner, Steven R MD [NP] - **Spec Exp:** Neonatal Chronic Lung Disease (CLD); Respiratory Distress Syndrome (RDS); Pulmonary Hypertension of Newborn (PPHN); **Hospital:** Univ Hlth Syst-San Antonio; **Address:** Dept Peds, 7703 Floyd Curl Drive, MC 7812, San Antonio, TX 78229-3901; **Phone:** 210-567-5225; **Board Cert:** Pediatrics 1987; Neonatal-Perinatal Medicine 1987; **Med School:** Univ Ariz Coll Med 1982; **Resid:** Pediatrics, Harbor-UCLA Med Ctr 1985; **Fellow:** Neonatal-Perinatal Medicine, Harbor-UCLA Med Ctr 1988; **Fac Appt:** Prof Ped, Univ Tex, San Antonio

Tyson, Jon E MD [NP] - **Spec Exp:** Neonatology; Epidemiology; **Hospital:** Meml Hermann Hosp - Texas Med Ctr; **Address:** Univ Tex, Ctr Clin Rsch, 6431 Fannin St, Ste 2.106, Houston, TX 77030; **Phone:** 713-500-5651; **Board Cert:** Pediatrics 1973; Neonatal-Perinatal Medicine 1975; **Med School:** Tulane Univ 1968; **Resid:** Pediatrics, Univ Tenn/Memphis Hosp 1971; **Fellow:** Neonatology, McMaster Univ 1975; **Fac Appt:** Prof Ped, Univ Tex, Houston

West Coast and Pacific

Ariagno, Ronald L MD [NP] - **Spec Exp:** Prematurity/Low Birth Weight Infants; Neonatal Critical Care; Sudden Infant Death Syndrome (SIDS); **Hospital:** Stanford Univ Med Ctr; **Address:** Stanford Univ, Div Neonatology, 750 Welch Rd, Ste 315, Palo Alto, CA 94304; **Phone:** 650-723-5711; **Board Cert:** Pediatrics 1973; Neonatal-Perinatal Medicine 1975; **Med School:** Univ IL Coll Med 1968; **Resid:** Pediatrics, Presby-St Lukes Hosp 1971; **Fellow:** Neonatology, Chldns Hosp, UCSF 1975; **Fac Appt:** Prof Ped, Stanford Univ

Stevenson, David K MD [NP] - **Spec Exp:** Neonatology; **Hospital:** Lucile Packard Chldn's Hosp; **Address:** 750 Welch Rd, Ste 315, Palo Alto, CA 94304-1510; **Phone:** 650-723-5711; **Board Cert:** Pediatrics 1979; Neonatal-Perinatal Medicine 2004; **Med School:** Univ Wash 1975; **Resid:** Pediatrics, Univ Washington 1977; **Fellow:** Neonatal-Perinatal Medicine, Stanford Univ 1979; **Fac Appt:** Prof Ped, Stanford Univ

NYU **Langone Medical Center**

550 First Avenue (at 31St Street)
New York, NY 10016
Physician Referral:
(888)7-NYU-MED (888-769-8633)
www.med.nyu.edu

NEONATAL PERINATAL MEDICINE

About the Neonatology Program, Department of Pediatrics:

The Neonatology Program at NYU Langone Medical Center understands that infants have different and unique emotional and developmental needs from those of adults. The Program combines family-centered care and state-of-the art technology to offer positive early experiences and simultaneously, enhance the quality of medical care for newborns and infants.

We specialize in the following areas:

CONTINUING CARE

Because many premature babies may be at an increased risk for problems in growth and development, the Neonatal Comprehensive Continuing Care Program (NCCCP) follows these infants from birth through pre-school, providing evaluation and assessment of problems as soon as they arise.

HYPOTHERMIA PROGRAM

The Hypothermia Program at NYU Langone Medical Center is a full multidisciplinary service with neonatal transport and inpatient and outpatient follow-up services. The Program provides rapid assessment and treatment implementation for those infants affected.

INFANT APNEA AND SIDS

The Infant Apnea and SIDS Program at the Bellevue Hospital Center, an affiliate of NYU Langone Medical Center, provides treatment to critically ill infants from the Neonatal Intensive Care Unit and other children at risk for apnea, sudden infant death syndrome (SIDS) and other acute life-threatening events. The Program offers parent CPR education and support for as long as the infant requires monitored care.

NEONATAL INTENSIVE CARE

The Neonatal Intensive Care Unit (NICU) at Tisch Hospital at NYU Langone Medical Center provides the most advanced care in New York City, including general and cardiac surgery, neurosurgery and craniofacial surgery. In addition to providing maternal-fetal medicine services and a NICU, the Program offers early intervention evaluation services and comprehensive family support and education. The relaxed setting includes covered incubators, drawn shades and parents holding pre-term infants skin-to-skin. Studies from NYU Langone Medical Center show that this approach has decreased the need for ventilator support and the risk of chronic lung disease. It has also enhanced weight gain and improved overall neurological development.

Nephrology

a subspecialty of Internal Medicine

An internist who treats disorders of the kidney, high blood pressure, fluid and mineral balance and dialysis of body wastes when the kidneys do not function. This specialist consults with surgeons about kidney transplantation.

Training Required: Three years in internal medicine *plus* additional training and examination for certification in nephrology.

NEPHROLOGY

New England

Aronson, Peter S MD [Nep] - **Spec Exp:** Electrolyte Disorders; Kidney Stones; **Hospital:** Yale-New Haven Hosp, VA Conn Hlthcre Sys; **Address:** Yale Sch Med, Dept Medicine, PO Box 208029, New Haven, CT 06520-8029; **Phone:** 203-785-4186; **Board Cert:** Internal Medicine 1973; Nephrology 1976; **Med School:** NYU Sch Med 1970; **Resid:** Internal Medicine, NC Meml Hosp 1972; **Fellow:** Nephrology, Yale-New Haven Hosp 1977; **Fac Appt:** Prof Med, Yale Univ

Bazari, Hasan MD [Nep] - **Spec Exp:** Kidney Failure-Acute; Nephrotic Syndrome; Hypertension; **Hospital:** Mass Genl Hosp; **Address:** Renal Assocs, Mass Genl Hosp, 55 Fruit St Gray Bldg - Ste 1003, Boston, MA 02114; **Phone:** 617-726-5050; **Board Cert:** Internal Medicine 1986; Nephrology 1988; **Med School:** Albert Einstein Coll Med 1983; **Resid:** Internal Medicine, Mass Genl Hosp 1986; **Fellow:** Nephrology, Mass Genl Hosp 1988

Brenner, Barry M MD [Nep] - **Spec Exp:** Hypertension; Diabetic Kidney Disease; Kidney Failure-Acute; Kidney Failure-Chronic; **Hospital:** Brigham & Women's Hosp; **Address:** Brigham & Women's Hosp, Renal Div, 75 Francis St, Boston, MA 02115; **Phone:** 617-732-5850; **Med School:** Univ Pittsburgh 1962; **Resid:** Internal Medicine, Albert Einstein Coll Med 1966; **Fellow:** Nephrology, Nat Inst Health 1969; **Fac Appt:** Prof Med, Harvard Med Sch

Coggins, Cecil MD [Nep] - **Spec Exp:** Kidney Disease; Hypertension; **Hospital:** Mass Genl Hosp; **Address:** 165 Cambridge St, Ste 501, Boston, MA 02114-2712; **Phone:** 617-726-4900; **Board Cert:** Internal Medicine 1965; Nephrology 1974; **Med School:** Harvard Med Sch 1958; **Resid:** Internal Medicine, Stanford Univ Med Ctr 1965; Internal Medicine; **Fellow:** Nephrology, Stanford Univ Med Ctr 1963; Nephrology, Mass Genl Hosp 1967; **Fac Appt:** Assoc Prof Med, Harvard Med Sch

Kliger, Alan MD [Nep] - **Spec Exp:** Kidney Disease; Kidney Disease-Metabolic; **Hospital:** Hosp of St Raphael; **Address:** 136 Sherman Ave, New Haven, CT 06511-5238; **Phone:** 203-787-0117 x307; **Board Cert:** Internal Medicine 1973; Nephrology 1976; **Med School:** SUNY Upstate Med Univ 1970; **Resid:** Internal Medicine, SUNY Upstate Med Ctr 1973; **Fellow:** Nephrology, Georgetown Univ Hosp 1975; **Fac Appt:** Clin Prof Med, Yale Univ

Perrone, Ronald MD [Nep] - **Spec Exp:** Kidney Disease-Chronic; Kidney Failure-Acute; Polycystic Kidney Disease; **Hospital:** Tufts Med Ctr; **Address:** Tufts-New Eng Med Ctr, Div Nephrology, 750 Washington St, Box 391, Boston, MA 02111; **Phone:** 617-636-5866; **Board Cert:** Internal Medicine 1979; Nephrology 1982; **Med School:** Hahnemann Univ 1975; **Resid:** Internal Medicine, Grady Meml Hosp 1978; **Fellow:** Nephrology, Boston Med Ctr 1982; **Fac Appt:** Prof Med, Tufts Univ

Salant, David MD [Nep] - **Spec Exp:** Kidney Disease-Glomerular; Kidney Disease-Autoimmune; Lupus Nephritis; **Hospital:** Boston Med Ctr; **Address:** 720 Harrison Ave, Boston, MA 02118-2371; **Phone:** 617-638-7480; **Board Cert:** Internal Medicine 1978; Nephrology 1980; **Med School:** South Africa 1969; **Resid:** Internal Medicine, Johannesburg Genl Hosp 1973; **Fellow:** Nephrology, Boston Univ Med Ctr 1978; **Fac Appt:** Prof Med, Boston Univ

Seifter, Julian L MD [Nep] - **Spec Exp:** Diabetic Kidney Disease; Kidney Failure-Chronic; Kidney Stones; **Hospital:** Brigham & Women's Hosp; **Address:** Brigham & Women's Hosp, Div Renal Med, 45 Francis St, Boston, MA 02115; **Phone:** 617-732-6383; **Board Cert:** Internal Medicine 1978; Nephrology 1980; **Med School:** Albert Einstein Coll Med 1975; **Resid:** Internal Medicine, Bronx Muni Hosp Ctr 1981; **Fellow:** Nephrology, Yale-New Haven Hosp 1982; **Fac Appt:** Assoc Prof Med, Harvard Med Sch

Tolkoff-Rubin, Nina MD [Nep] - **Spec Exp:** Transplant Medicine-Kidney; Hypertension; Kidney Failure-Acute; **Hospital:** Mass Genl Hosp; **Address:** 55 Fruit St, GRB 103J, Boston, MA 02114; **Phone:** 617-726-3706; **Board Cert:** Nephrology 1974; Internal Medicine 1972; **Med School:** Harvard Med Sch 1968; **Resid:** Internal Medicine, Mass Genl Hosp 1970; Internal Medicine, Mass Genl Hosp 1972; **Fellow:** Nephrology, Mass Genl Hosp 1971; **Fac Appt:** Assoc Prof Med, Harvard Med Sch

Mid Atlantic

Appel, Gerald MD [Nep] - **Spec Exp:** Glomerulonephritis; Lupus Nephritis; Nephrotic Syndrome; **Hospital:** NY-Presby Hosp/Columbia (page 66); **Address:** 622 W 168th St, Ste PH4-124, New York, NY 10032-3720; **Phone:** 212-305-0320; **Board Cert:** Internal Medicine 1975; Nephrology 1978; **Med School:** Albert Einstein Coll Med 1972; **Resid:** Internal Medicine, Columbia Presby Hosp 1975; **Fellow:** Nephrology, Columbia Presby Hosp 1976; Nephrology, Yale-New Haven Hosp 1978; **Fac Appt:** Clin Prof Med, Columbia P&S

August, Phyllis MD [Nep] - **Spec Exp:** Hypertension; Hypertension in Pregnancy; **Hospital:** NY-Presby Hosp/Weill Cornell (page 66); **Address:** 525 E 68th St, Ste L-1, Hypertension Center, New York, NY 10021-4870; **Phone:** 212-746-2210; **Board Cert:** Internal Medicine 1980; Nephrology 1982; **Med School:** Yale Univ 1977; **Resid:** Internal Medicine, NY Hosp-Cornell Med Ctr 1980; **Fellow:** Nephrology, NY Hosp-Cornell Med Ctr 1983; **Fac Appt:** Prof Med, Cornell Univ-Weill Med Coll

Blumenfeld, Jon D MD [Nep] - **Spec Exp:** Hypertension; Polycystic Kidney Disease; Adrenal Disorders; **Hospital:** NY-Presby Hosp/Weill Cornell (page 66), Rockefeller Univ; **Address:** The Rogosin Institute, 505 E 70th St, rm HT230, New York, NY 10021; **Phone:** 212-746-1495; **Board Cert:** Internal Medicine 1984; Nephrology 1986; **Med School:** Yale Univ 1981; **Resid:** Internal Medicine, New York Hosp 1984; **Fellow:** Nephrology, Brigham & Womens Hosp 1988; **Fac Appt:** Prof Med, Cornell Univ-Weill Med Coll

Cohen, David J MD [Nep] - **Spec Exp:** Transplant Medicine-Kidney; Glomerulonephritis; **Hospital:** NY-Presby Hosp/Columbia (page 66); **Address:** Columbia Univ Med Ctr, 622 W 168th St, rm PH 4-124, New York, NY 10032-3720; **Phone:** 212-305-0320; **Board Cert:** Internal Medicine 1980; Nephrology 1984; **Med School:** Albert Einstein Coll Med 1977; **Resid:** Internal Medicine, Mount Sinai Hosp 1980; **Fellow:** Nephrology, Columbia-Presby Hosp 1981; Transplant Immunobiology, Brigham & Womens Hosp 1983; **Fac Appt:** Clin Prof Med, Columbia P&S

Johnston, James R MD [Nep] - **Spec Exp:** Diabetic Kidney Disease; Hypertension; **Hospital:** UPMC Presby, Pittsburgh; **Address:** Univ Pittsburgh Physicians, Renal Div, 3550 Terrace St, Scaife Hall, rm A915, Pittsburgh, PA 15261; **Phone:** 412-802-3043; **Board Cert:** Internal Medicine 1982; Nephrology 1984; **Med School:** Univ Pittsburgh 1979; **Resid:** Internal Medicine, Montefiore Hosp 1982; **Fellow:** Nephrology, Univ Pittsburgh Med Ctr 1983; Nephrology, Brigham & Women's Hosp 1986; **Fac Appt:** Prof Med, Univ Pittsburgh

Nephrology

Kelepouris, Ellie MD [Nep] - **Spec Exp:** Kidney Stones; Hypertension; **Hospital:** Temple Univ Hosp; **Address:** 3322 N Broad St, Medical Office Bldg, Ste 201, Philadelphia, PA 19140; **Phone:** 215-707-7944; **Board Cert:** Nephrology 2008; **Med School:** Greece 1976; **Resid:** Internal Medicine, Mercy Cath Med Ctr 1979; **Fellow:** Nephrology, Hosp U Penn 1982; **Fac Appt:** Prof Med, Temple Univ

Kobrin, Sidney M MD [Nep] - **Spec Exp:** Diabetic Kidney Disease; Kidney Failure; Hypertension; **Hospital:** Hosp Univ Penn - UPHS (page 60); **Address:** Div Nephrology, 3400 Civic Center Blvd, Fl 1 - Ste 300 South, Philadelphia, PA 19104; **Phone:** 215-662-2638; **Board Cert:** Nephrology 2002; **Med School:** South Africa 1978; **Resid:** Internal Medicine, Johannesburg Tchg Hosp 1984; **Fellow:** Nephrology, Einstein Med Ctr 1988; **Fac Appt:** Assoc Prof Med, Univ Pennsylvania

Piraino, Beth Marie MD [Nep] - **Spec Exp:** Kidney Failure; Hypertension; **Hospital:** UPMC Presby, Pittsburgh; **Address:** 3504 Fifth Ave, Ste 200, Pittsburgh, PA 15213; **Phone:** 412-383-4899; **Board Cert:** Internal Medicine 1980; Nephrology 1982; **Med School:** Med Coll PA Hahnemann 1977; **Resid:** Internal Medicine, Presby Univ Hosp 1980; **Fellow:** Nephrology, Presby Univ Hosp 1982; **Fac Appt:** Prof Med, Univ Pittsburgh

Rudnick, Michael R MD [Nep] - **Spec Exp:** Hypertension; Kidney Disease; **Hospital:** Penn Presby Med Ctr - UPHS (page 60); **Address:** Presbyterian Medical Ctr, Medical Office Bldg, 39th and Market Sts, Ste 240, Philadelphia, PA 19104; **Phone:** 215-662-8730; **Board Cert:** Internal Medicine 1975; Nephrology 1976; **Med School:** Hahnemann Univ 1972; **Resid:** Internal Medicine, Hahnemann U Med Ctr 1974; **Fellow:** Nephrology, Hosp U Penn 1976; **Fac Appt:** Assoc Prof Med, Univ Pennsylvania

Scheinman, Steven J MD [Nep] - **Spec Exp:** Kidney Stones; Bartter's Syndrome; Gitelman's Syndrome; **Hospital:** Univ Hosp - SUNY Upstate, Crouse Hosp; **Address:** SUNY Upstate Med Univ, Office of the Dean, 750 E Adams St, Syracuse, NY 13210; **Phone:** 315-464-3834; **Board Cert:** Internal Medicine 1980; Nephrology 1984; **Med School:** Yale Univ 1977; **Resid:** Internal Medicine, Yale New Haven Hosp 1990; Internal Medicine, Upstate Med Ctr 1981; **Fellow:** Nephrology, Upstate Med Ctr 1983; Nephrology, Yale New Haven Hosp 1984; **Fac Appt:** Prof Med, SUNY Upstate Med Univ

Townsend, Raymond R MD [Nep] - **Spec Exp:** Hypertension-Complex; Renal Artery Stenosis; **Hospital:** Hosp Univ Penn - UPHS (page 60); **Address:** Div Nephrology, 3400 Civic Center Blvd, Fl 1 - Ste 300 South, Philadelphia, PA 19104; **Phone:** 215-662-2638; **Board Cert:** Internal Medicine 1982; Nephrology 1984; **Med School:** Hahnemann Univ 1979; **Resid:** Internal Medicine, Allegheny Genl Hosp 1982; **Fellow:** Nephrology, Temple Univ Hosp 1984; **Fac Appt:** Assoc Prof Med, Univ Pennsylvania

Wilcox, Christopher S MD [Nep] - **Spec Exp:** Hypertension-Renovascular; Hypertension-Drug Resistent; **Hospital:** Georgetown Univ Hosp; **Address:** Georgetown Univ Med Ctr, 3800 Reservoir Rd NW, PHC Fl 6th, Washington, DC 20007-2113; **Phone:** 202-444-9183; **Board Cert:** Internal Medicine 1983; Nephrology 1986; **Med School:** England, UK 1968; **Resid:** Internal Medicine, Middlesex Hosp 1971; Nephrology, Middlesex Hosp 1972; **Fellow:** Nephrology, Middlesex Hosp 1975; **Fac Appt:** Prof Med, Georgetown Univ

Southeast

Allon, Michael MD [Nep] - **Spec Exp:** Dialysis Care; **Hospital:** Univ of Ala Hosp at Birmingham; **Address:** 1530 3rd Ave S, PB226, Birmingham, AL 35294; **Phone:** 205-975-9676; **Board Cert:** Internal Medicine 1985; Nephrology 1988; **Med School:** Univ Mich Med Sch 1982; **Resid:** Internal Medicine, Emory Univ Hosp 1985; **Fellow:** Nephrology, Emory Univ Hosp 1987; **Fac Appt:** Prof Med, Univ Alabama

Bolton, W Kline MD [Nep] - **Spec Exp:** Kidney Disease-Glomerular; Kidney Disease-Chronic; **Hospital:** Univ Virginia Med Ctr; **Address:** Univ VA Hlth Scis Ctr, Box 800 133, Charlottesville, VA 22908-0001; **Phone:** 434-924-5125; **Board Cert:** Internal Medicine 1972; Nephrology 1974; **Med School:** Univ VA Sch Med 1969; **Resid:** Internal Medicine, Boston City Hosp 1971; **Fellow:** Nephrology, Univ Chicago 1973; **Fac Appt:** Prof Med, Univ VA Sch Med

Coffman, Thomas M MD [Nep] - **Spec Exp:** Transplant Medicine-Kidney; Hypertension; **Hospital:** VA Med Ctr - Durham, Duke Univ Med Ctr; **Address:** Duke Univ Med Center, Box 103015, Durham, NC 27710; **Phone:** 919-684-9788; **Board Cert:** Internal Medicine 1983; Nephrology 1988; **Med School:** Ohio State Univ 1980; **Resid:** Internal Medicine, Duke Univ Med Ctr 1983; **Fellow:** Nephrology, Duke Univ Med Ctr 1985; **Fac Appt:** Prof Med, Duke Univ

Falk, Ronald J MD [Nep] - **Spec Exp:** Glomerulonephritis; Lupus Nephritis; Wegener's Granu-lomatosis; Vasculitis; **Hospital:** Univ NC Hosps; **Address:** Univ North Carolina Kidney Ctr, 7024 Burnett Womack Bldg CB #7155, Chapel Hill, NC 27599-7155; **Phone:** 919-966-2561; **Board Cert:** Internal Medicine 1980; Nephrology 1982; **Med School:** Univ NC Sch Med 1977; **Resid:** Internal Medicine, Univ North Carolina Hosps 1980; Nephrology, Univ NC 1981; **Fellow:** Research, Univ Minn 1983; **Fac Appt:** Prof Med, Univ NC Sch Med

Freedman, Barry MD [Nep] - **Spec Exp:** Hypertension; Inherited Metabolic Disorders; Dia-betes; Kidney Failure; **Hospital:** Wake Forest Univ Baptist Med Ctr (page 72); **Address:** Wake Forest Univ, Nephrology Dept, Medical Ctr Blvd, Winston-Salem, NC 27157; **Phone:** 336-716-8817; **Board Cert:** Internal Medicine 1987; Nephrology 1999; **Med School:** SUNY Downstate 1984; **Resid:** Internal Medicine, E Virgina Univ Affil Hosp 1987; **Fellow:** Nephrology, NC Baptist Hosp 1989; **Fac Appt:** Prof Med, Wake Forest Univ

Helderman, J Harold MD [Nep] - **Spec Exp:** Transplant Medicine-Kidney; Kidney Disease; **Hospital:** Vanderbilt Univ Med Ctr; **Address:** Vanderbilt-Div Nephrology & Hypertension, 1161 21st Ave S, S-3223 MCN, Nashville, TN 37232-2372; **Phone:** 615-343-7592; **Board Cert:** Internal Medicine 1974; **Med School:** SUNY Downstate 1971; **Resid:** Internal Medicine, Johns Hopkins Hosp 1973; **Fellow:** Nephrology, Brigham & Womens Hosp-Harvard 1976; **Fac Appt:** Prof Med, Vanderbilt Univ

Lea, Janice I MD [Nep] - **Spec Exp:** Hypertension-Complex; Kidney Disease-Chronic; **Hospi-tal:** Emory Univ Hosp Midtown; **Address:** Emory Midtown-Div Nephrology, 550 Peachtree St Fl 8, At-lanta, GA 30308; **Phone:** 404-686-5038; **Board Cert:** Nephrology 2005; **Med School:** Univ Tex Med Br, Galveston 1988; **Resid:** Internal Medicine, Emory Univ Affil Hosps 1991; **Fellow:** Nephrol-ogy, Emory Univ Affil Hosps 1994; **Fac Appt:** Assoc Prof Med, Emory Univ

Okusa, Mark D MD [Nep] - **Spec Exp:** Kidney Failure-Chronic; Nephrotic Syndrome; Kidney Failure-Acute; **Hospital:** Univ Virginia Med Ctr; **Address:** Univ VA Hlth Sci Ctr, Div Nephrology, Lee St, Box 800-133, Charlottesville, VA 22908-0001; **Phone:** 434-924-5125; **Board Cert:** Internal Medicine 1985; Nephrology 1988; **Med School:** Med Coll VA 1982; **Resid:** Internal Medicine, Med Coll Virginia 1985; **Fellow:** Nephrology, Yale Univ Sch Med 1988; **Fac Appt:** Prof Med, Univ VA Sch Med

Rakowski, Thomas A MD [Nep] - **Spec Exp:** Polycystic Kidney Disease; Kidney Disease-Glomerular; **Hospital:** Virginia Hosp Ctr - Arlington, Inova Fairfax Hosp; **Address:** Virginia Nephrol-ogy Group, 1635 N George Mason Drive, Ste 215, Arlington, VA 22205; **Phone:** 703-841-0707; **Board Cert:** Internal Medicine 1972; Nephrology 1974; **Med School:** Hahnemann Univ 1969; **Resid:** Internal Medicine, Georgetown Univ 1971; **Fellow:** Nephrology, Georgetown Univ 1973; **Fac Appt:** Assoc Prof Med, Georgetown Univ

Nephrology

Roth, David MD [Nep] - **Spec Exp:** Transplant Medicine-Kidney; Kidney Failure-Chronic; **Hospital:** Jackson Meml Hosp (page 70), Univ of Miami Hosp & Clins/Sylvester Comp Canc Ctr (page 70); **Address:** Univ Miami Div Nephrology, PO Box 016960 (R-126), Miami, FL 33101; **Phone:** 305-243-6251; **Board Cert:** Internal Medicine 1980; Nephrology 1982; **Med School:** SUNY Downstate 1977; **Resid:** Internal Medicine, Jackson Meml Hosp 1980; **Fellow:** Nephrology, Jackson Meml Hosp 1982; **Fac Appt:** Prof Med, Univ Miami Sch Med

Vachharajani, Tushar J MD [Nep] - **Spec Exp:** Interventional Nephrology; Dialysis Care; Hypertension; **Hospital:** Wake Forest Univ Baptist Med Ctr (page 72); **Address:** Wake Forrest Univ School of Medicine, Wattington Hall, Medical Center Blvd, Winston Salem, NC 27127; **Phone:** 336-716-8341; **Board Cert:** Internal Medicine 2001; Nephrology 2002; **Med School:** India 1986; **Resid:** Nephrology, Bombay Hosp, Mumbai & St Batholomew's Hosp, London 1996; Internal Medicine, LSU Med Hlth Sci Ctr 1999; **Fellow:** Nephrology, LSU Med Hlth Sci Ctr 2000; Interventional Nephrology, LSU Med Hlth Sci Ctr 2001; **Fac Appt:** Assoc Prof Med, Wake Forest Univ

Warnock, David G MD [Nep] - **Spec Exp:** Liddle's Syndrome; Kidney Stones; Nephrotic Syndrome; **Hospital:** Univ of Ala Hosp at Birmingham; **Address:** UAB Dept Medicine, 1530 3rd Ave S, ZRB 614, Birmingham, AL 35294-0006; **Phone:** 205-934-9349509; **Board Cert:** Internal Medicine 1973; Nephrology 2000; **Med School:** UCSF 1970; **Resid:** Internal Medicine, UCSF Med Ctr 1973; **Fellow:** Nephrology, Natl Inst Hlth 1975; **Fac Appt:** Prof Med, Univ Alabama

Weiner, I David MD [Nep] - **Spec Exp:** Kidney Disease; Fluid/Electrolyte Balance; Kidney Stones; Hypertension; **Hospital:** Shands at Univ of FL; **Address:** Shands at Univ Florida, Dept Nephrology, PO Box 100224, Gainesville, FL 32610-0224; **Phone:** 352-273-8821; **Board Cert:** Internal Medicine 1987; Nephrology 2000; **Med School:** Vanderbilt Univ 1984; **Resid:** Internal Medicine, Univ Texas Hlth Sci Ctr 1987; **Fellow:** Nephrology, Wash Univ 1990; **Fac Appt:** Assoc Prof Med, Univ Fla Coll Med

Midwest

Brennan, Daniel C MD [Nep] - **Spec Exp:** Transplant Medicine-Kidney; **Hospital:** Barnes-Jewish Hosp; **Address:** Wash Univ School Med, Div Renal Diseases, 660 S Euclid Ave, Box 8126, St Louis, MO 63110; **Phone:** 314-362-8351; **Board Cert:** Internal Medicine 1988; Nephrology 2002; **Med School:** Univ Iowa Coll Med 1985; **Resid:** Internal Medicine, U Iowa Hosps 1988; **Fellow:** Nephrology, Brigham & Womens Hosp 1992; **Fac Appt:** Assoc Prof Med, Washington Univ, St Louis

Coe, Fredric MD [Nep] - **Spec Exp:** Kidney Stones; Fluid/Electrolyte Balance; **Hospital:** Univ of Chicago Med Ctr; **Address:** 5841 S Maryland Ave, MC 5100, Chicago, IL 60637-1463; **Phone:** 773-702-1475; **Board Cert:** Internal Medicine 1968; **Med School:** Univ Chicago-Pritzker Sch Med 1961; **Resid:** Internal Medicine, Michael Reese Hosp 1965; **Fellow:** Renal Disease, Univ Texas SW 1969; **Fac Appt:** Prof Med, Univ Chicago-Pritzker Sch Med

Delmez, James MD [Nep] - **Spec Exp:** Kidney Disease; **Hospital:** Barnes-Jewish Hosp, Washington Univ Med Ctr; **Address:** Wash Univ Sch Med, Div Renal Disease, 4921 Parkview Pl, St Louis, MO 63110; **Phone:** 314-362-7603; **Board Cert:** Internal Medicine 1976; Nephrology 1982; **Med School:** Univ Rochester 1973; **Resid:** Internal Medicine, Barnes Hosp 1976; **Fellow:** Nephrology, Barnes Hosp 1978; **Fac Appt:** Prof Med, Washington Univ, St Louis

America's Top Doctors® 9th Edition

Hruska, Keith MD [Nep] - **Spec Exp:** Kidney Disease-Pediatric & Adult; Kidney Stones; Bone Disorders; **Hospital:** St Louis Chldns Hosp, Barnes-Jewish Hosp; **Address:** St Louis Chldn's Hospital, Dept Peds, 660 S Euclid Ave Fl 5MPRB, Box 8208, St Louis, MO 63110-1010; **Phone:** 314-286-2772; **Board Cert:** Internal Medicine 1972; Nephrology 1976; **Med School:** Creighton Univ 1969; **Resid:** Internal Medicine, New York Hosp-Cornell 1971; Internal Medicine, Barnes Hosp-Wash Univ 1972; **Fellow:** Nephrology, Barnes Hosp-Wash Univ 1974; **Fac Appt:** Prof Ped, Washington Univ, St Louis

Josephson, Michelle A MD [Nep] - **Spec Exp:** Transplant Medicine-Kidney; Hypertension; **Hospital:** Univ of Chicago Med Ctr; **Address:** Div Nephrology, 5841 S Maryland Ave, MC 5100, Chicago, IL 60637; **Phone:** 773-702-6134; **Board Cert:** Internal Medicine 1986; Nephrology 2000; **Med School:** Univ Pennsylvania 1983; **Resid:** Internal Medicine, Univ Chicago Hosps 1986; **Fellow:** Nephrology, Univ Chicago Hosps 1991; **Fac Appt:** Assoc Clin Prof Med, Univ Chicago-Pritzker Sch Med

Kasiske, Bertram MD [Nep] - **Spec Exp:** Transplant Medicine-Kidney; Kidney Disease-Geriatric; **Hospital:** Hennepin Cnty Med Ctr; **Address:** Div Nephrology, Hennepin Co Med Ctr, 701 Park Ave, Minneapolis, MN 55415; **Phone:** 612-347-6088; **Board Cert:** Internal Medicine 1980; Nephrology 1982; **Med School:** Univ Iowa Coll Med 1976; **Resid:** Internal Medicine, Hennepin Co Med Ctr 1980; **Fellow:** Nephrology, Hennepin Co Med Ctr 1983; **Fac Appt:** Prof Med, Univ Minn

Kraus, Michael A MD [Nep] - **Spec Exp:** Dialysis Care; Kidney Failure-Acute; **Hospital:** Indiana Univ Hosp, Wishard Hlth Srvs; **Address:** Indiana University Hosp, 550 N University Blvd, Ste 1115, Indianapolis, IN 46202; **Phone:** 317-274-5292; **Board Cert:** Internal Medicine 1988; Nephrology 2002; **Med School:** Indiana Univ 1985; **Resid:** Internal Medicine, Indiana Univ Med Ctr 1988; **Fellow:** Nephrology, Univ Iowa Hosps & Clins 1991; **Fac Appt:** Clin Prof Med, Indiana Univ

Pohl, Marc MD [Nep] - **Spec Exp:** Hypertension; Kidney Disease; Diabetes; **Hospital:** Cleveland Clin Fdn (page 56); **Address:** Dept Nephrology & Hypertension, 9500 Euclid Ave, Desk Q7, Cleveland, OH 44195; **Phone:** 216-444-6776; **Board Cert:** Internal Medicine 1972; Nephrology 1978; **Med School:** Case West Res Univ 1966; **Resid:** Internal Medicine, Univ Hosps 1968; Internal Medicine, Mass Genl Hosp 1971; **Fellow:** Nephrology, Boston City Hosp-Boston Univ 1972; Nephrology, Mass Genl Hosp 1973

Rodby, Roger A MD [Nep] - **Spec Exp:** Diabetic Kidney Disease; Glomerulonephritis; Lupus Nephritis; **Hospital:** Rush Univ Med Ctr; **Address:** 1426 W Washington Blvd, Chicago, IL 60612-3809; **Phone:** 312-850-8434; **Board Cert:** Internal Medicine 1985; Nephrology 1988; **Med School:** Univ IL Coll Med 1982; **Resid:** Internal Medicine, UMDNJ-Rutgers 1985; **Fellow:** Nephrology, Rush/Presby-St Lukes 1987; **Fac Appt:** Assoc Prof Med, Rush Med Coll

Schwartz, Gary Lee MD [Nep] - **Spec Exp:** Hypertension; Hypotension; Diabetic Kidney Disease; **Hospital:** St Mary's Hosp - Rochester, Rochester Methodist Hosp; **Address:** Mayo Clinic, 200 1st St SW, Rochester, MN 55905-0002; **Phone:** 507-284-4083; **Board Cert:** Internal Medicine 1980; Nephrology 1982; **Med School:** Univ Wisc 1977; **Resid:** Internal Medicine, Mayo Clinic 1980; **Fellow:** Nephrology, Mayo Clinic 1982; **Fac Appt:** Assoc Clin Prof Med, Mayo Med Sch

Somerville, James H MD [Nep] - **Hospital:** Fairview Southdale Hosp, Fairview Ridges Hosp; **Address:** 6363 France Ave S, Ste 400, Edina, MN 55435; **Phone:** 952-920-2070; **Board Cert:** Internal Medicine 1978; Nephrology 1982; **Med School:** Univ MD Sch Med 1975; **Resid:** Internal Medicine, Hennepin Co Med Ctr 1978; **Fellow:** Nephrology, Hennepin Co Med Ctr 1980

Nephrology

Swartz, Richard D MD [Nep] - **Spec Exp:** Kidney Failure; Dialysis Care; **Hospital:** Univ Michigan Hlth Sys; **Address:** Univ Mich, Div Nephrology, 1500 E Med Ctr Drive, 3914 Taubman Ctr, Ann Arbor, MI 48109-0364; **Phone:** 734-647-9342; **Board Cert:** Internal Medicine 1975; Nephrology 1978; **Med School:** Univ Mich Med Sch 1970; **Resid:** Internal Medicine, Boston City Hosp 1975; Nephrology, Beth Israel Hosp-Harvard 1977; **Fac Appt:** Prof Med, Univ Mich Med Sch

Textor, Stephen C MD [Nep] - **Spec Exp:** Transplant Medicine-Kidney; Hypertension; Renal Artery Stenosis; **Hospital:** Mayo Med Ctr & Clin - Rochester; **Address:** Mayo Clinic, Div Nephrology/Hypertension Fl W19A, 200 First St SW, Rochester, MN 55905; **Phone:** 507-284-4083; **Board Cert:** Internal Medicine 1977; Nephrology 1980; **Med School:** UCLA 1973; **Resid:** Internal Medicine, Boston City Hosp 1977; **Fellow:** Nephrology, Boston Univ 1978; Hypertension, Fogarty Inst 1980; **Fac Appt:** Prof Med, Mayo Med Sch

Torres, Vicente Esbarranch MD [Nep] - **Spec Exp:** Polycystic Kidney Disease; **Hospital:** Mayo Med Ctr & Clin - Rochester; **Address:** Mayo Clin, Eisenberg Bldg-Rm SL 24, 200 First St SW, Rochester, MN 55905; **Phone:** 507-266-7093; **Board Cert:** Internal Medicine 1977; Nephrology 1980; **Med School:** Spain 1969; **Resid:** Internal Medicine, Mayo Grad Sch Med 1977; **Fellow:** Nephrology, Mayo Grad Sch Med 1979; **Fac Appt:** Prof Med, Mayo Med Sch

Venkat, K K MD [Nep] - **Spec Exp:** Transplant Medicine-Kidney; Kidney Disease; **Hospital:** Henry Ford Hosp; **Address:** Henry Ford Hosp, Div Nephrology, 2799 W Grand Blvd, rm CFP5, Detroit, MI 48202-2689; **Phone:** 313-916-2702; **Board Cert:** Internal Medicine 1977; Nephrology 1978; **Med School:** India 1970; **Resid:** Internal Medicine, Henry Ford Hosp 1976; **Fellow:** Nephrology, Henry Ford Hosp 1978

Great Plains and Mountains

Berl, Tomas MD [Nep] - **Spec Exp:** Fluid/Electrolyte Balance; Kidney Failure-Chronic; **Hospital:** Univ Colorado Hosp; **Address:** Univ Colorado-Denver, 1635 Aurora Court, MS F747, Aurora, CO 80045; **Phone:** 720-848-0749; **Board Cert:** Internal Medicine 1972; Nephrology 1976; **Med School:** NYU Sch Med 1968; **Resid:** Internal Medicine, Bronx Municipal Hosp 1970; **Fellow:** Renal Disease, Moffit Hosp-UCSF 1971

Schrier, Robert W MD [Nep] - **Spec Exp:** Hypertension; Polycystic Kidney Disease; **Hospital:** Univ Colorado Hosp; **Address:** Univ Colorado Denver, 12700 E 19th Ave, Box 6511, Box C281, Aurora, CO 80045; **Phone:** 303-315-7297; **Board Cert:** Internal Medicine 1969; **Med School:** Indiana Univ 1962; **Resid:** Internal Medicine, Univ Wash Hosp 1965; **Fellow:** Research, PB Brigham Hosp/Harvard 1966; **Fac Appt:** Prof Med, Univ Colorado

Southwest

Brennan, Stephen T MD [Nep] - **Spec Exp:** Transplant Medicine-Kidney; Kidney Stones; Kidney Failure-Chronic; **Hospital:** Methodist Hosp - Houston, St Luke's Episcopal Hosp-Houston; **Address:** 1415 La Concha Ln, Houston, TX 77054; **Phone:** 713-790-9080; **Board Cert:** Internal Medicine 1983; Nephrology 1988; **Med School:** Loyola Univ-Stritch Sch Med 1979; **Resid:** Internal Medicine, Loyola Univ Med Ctr 1983; **Fellow:** Nephrology, Univ Wash-Barnes Hosp 1986; **Fac Appt:** Assoc Clin Prof Med, Baylor Coll Med

Fadem, Stephen Z MD [Nep] - **Spec Exp:** Kidney Disease-Chronic; Kidney Failure; Hypertension; **Hospital:** Methodist Hosp - Houston, St Luke's Episcopal Hosp-Houston; **Address:** Kidney Associates, 6624 Fannin St, Ste 1400, Houston, TX 77030; **Phone:** 713-795-5511; **Board Cert:** Internal Medicine 1976; Nephrology 1978; **Med School:** Univ Okla Coll Med 1973; **Resid:** Internal Medicine, Univ Texas/ Affil MD Anderson Hosp 1976; **Fellow:** Renal Disease, Univ Texas Hlth Sci Ctr 1978; **Fac Appt:** Clin Prof Med, Baylor Coll Med

Hura, Claudia E MD [Nep] - **Spec Exp:** Transplant Medicine-Kidney; Glomerulonephritis; Lupus Nephritis; **Hospital:** Methodist Spec & Transpl Hosp, SW TX Meth Hosp; **Address:** 8042 Wurzbach St, Physician Plaza 2, Ste 500, San Antonio, TX 78229; **Phone:** 210-692-7228; **Board Cert:** Internal Medicine 1982; Nephrology 1986; **Med School:** Ohio State Univ 1979; **Resid:** Internal Medicine, Indiana Univ Med Ctr 1983; **Fellow:** Nephrology, Univ Tex Hlth Sci Ctr 1986; **Fac Appt:** Assoc Clin Prof Med, Univ Tex, San Antonio

Kasinath, Balakuntalam S MD [Nep] - **Spec Exp:** Glomerulonephritis; Diabetic Kidney Disease; **Hospital:** Univ Hlth Syst-San Antonio, Audie L Murphy Meml Vets Hosp; **Address:** Univ Tex Hlth Sci Ctr, Dept Med/Div Neph, 7703 Floyd Curl Drive, MC 7882, San Antonio, TX 78229-3901; **Phone:** 210-567-4707; **Board Cert:** Internal Medicine 1980; Nephrology 1982; **Med School:** India 1975; **Resid:** Internal Medicine, Ill Masonic Med Ctr 1980; **Fellow:** Nephrology, Univ Chicago Hosp 1983; **Fac Appt:** Prof Med, Univ Tex, San Antonio

Mitch, William MD [Nep] - **Spec Exp:** Nutrition; Hypertension; Kidney Failure; **Hospital:** Baylor Univ Medical Ctr, Ben Taub Genl Hosp; **Address:** Baylor Clin, 6620 Main St, Ste 1375, Houston, TX 77030; **Phone:** 713-798-2500; **Board Cert:** Internal Medicine 1972; Nephrology 1978; **Med School:** Harvard Med Sch 1967; **Resid:** Internal Medicine, Brigham & Women's Hosp 1974; Nat Cancer Inst-NIH 1972; **Fellow:** Nephrology, Johns Hopkins Hosp 1973; **Fac Appt:** Prof Med, Baylor Coll Med

Olivero, Juan J MD [Nep] - **Spec Exp:** Kidney Failure-Acute; Kidney Failure-Chronic; Fluid/Electrolyte Balance; Hypertension; **Hospital:** Methodist Hosp - Houston, St Luke's Episcopal Hosp-Houston; **Address:** 6560 Fannin St, Scurlock Twr, Ste 2206, Houston, TX 77030; **Phone:** 713-790-4615; **Board Cert:** Internal Medicine 1974; Nephrology 1976; **Med School:** Guatemala 1970; **Resid:** Internal Medicine, Baylor Affil Hosps 1973; Internal Medicine, Ben Taub Genl Hosp 1974; **Fellow:** Nephrology, Baylor Affil Hosps 1975; **Fac Appt:** Clin Prof Med, Baylor Coll Med

Suki, Wadi N MD [Nep] - **Spec Exp:** Transplant Medicine-Kidney; Hypertension; Lupus Nephritis; **Hospital:** Methodist Hosp - Houston, St Luke's Episcopal Hosp-Houston; **Address:** 1415 La Concha Ln, Houston, TX 77054; **Phone:** 713-790-9080; **Board Cert:** Internal Medicine 1967; Nephrology 1972; **Med School:** Sudan 1959; **Resid:** Internal Medicine, Parkland Meml Hosp 1963; **Fellow:** Nephrology, Univ Tex SW Med Ctr 1961; Nephrology, Univ Tex SW Med Ctr 1965; **Fac Appt:** Clin Prof Med, Baylor Coll Med

Toto, Robert D MD [Nep] - **Spec Exp:** Hypertension/Kidney Disease; Dialysis Care; Diabetic Kidney Disease; Kidney Failure-Acute; **Hospital:** UT Southwestern Med Ctr at Dallas; **Address:** 5323 Harry Hines Blvd, Dallas, TX 75390-8523; **Phone:** 214-648-3442; **Board Cert:** Internal Medicine 1980; Nephrology 1982; **Med School:** Univ IL Coll Med 1977; **Resid:** Internal Medicine, Univ Michigan Med Ctr 1979; Internal Medicine, Baylor Univ Med Ctr 1980; **Fellow:** Nephrology, US Public Health Service Hosp 1981; Nephrology, UTSW Med Ctr 1983; **Fac Appt:** Prof Med, Univ Tex SW, Dallas

Nephrology

West Coast and Pacific

Ahmad, Suhail MD [Nep] - **Spec Exp:** Hypertension; Kidney Failure-Chronic; Kidney Stones; **Hospital:** Univ Wash Med Ctr; **Address:** 2150 N 107th St, Ste 160, Seattle, WA 98133; **Phone:** 206-363-5090; **Med School:** India 1968; **Resid:** Internal Medicine, Univ Allahabad 1971; **Fellow:** Nephrology, Univ Washington 1978; **Fac Appt:** Assoc Prof Med, Univ Wash

Bennett, William M MD [Nep] - **Spec Exp:** Polycystic Kidney Disease; Transplant Medicine-Kidney; Drug Toxicity-Kidneys; **Hospital:** Legacy Good Samaritan Hosp and Med Ctr, Legacy Emanuel Hospitals; **Address:** Legacy Good Samaritan Hosp, Transplant Svcs, 1040 NW 22nd, Ste 480, Portland, OR 97210; **Phone:** 503-413-6555; **Board Cert:** Internal Medicine 2003; Nephrology 2003; **Med School:** Northwestern Univ 1963; **Resid:** Internal Medicine, Northwestern Univ 1965; Internal Medicine, Ore Hlth Sci Univ 1966; **Fellow:** Nephrology, Mass Genl Hosp 1970

Ellison, David H MD [Nep] - **Spec Exp:** Bartter's Syndrome; Gitelman's Syndrome; Hypertension; **Hospital:** OR Hlth & Sci Univ, VA Medical Center - Portland; **Address:** OHSU-Div Nephrology, 3314 SW US Veteran's Hospital Rd, MC PP262, Portland, OR 97239-3098; **Phone:** 503-494-8490; **Board Cert:** Internal Medicine 1981; Nephrology 1986; **Med School:** Rush Med Coll 1978; **Resid:** Internal Medicine, Oregon Hlth Scis Univ 1981; **Fellow:** Research, Oregon Hlth Scis Univ 1982; Nephrology, Yale Univ 1985; **Fac Appt:** Prof Med, Oregon Hlth & Sci Univ

Gluck, Stephen L MD [Nep] - **Spec Exp:** Kidney Disease; Fluid/Electrolyte Balance; Hypertension; Kidney Stones; **Hospital:** UCSF Med Ctr; **Address:** UCSF, Div Nephrology, C442, 521 Parnassus Ave, rm C443, Box 0532, San Francisco, CA 94143-0532; **Phone:** 415-476-2173; **Board Cert:** Internal Medicine 1980; Nephrology 1984; **Med School:** UCLA 1977; **Resid:** Internal Medicine, Columbia Presby Med Ctr 1980; **Fellow:** Nephrology, Columbia Presby Med Ctr 1983; **Fac Appt:** Prof Med, UCSF

Kaysen, George Alan MD/PhD [Nep] - **Spec Exp:** Kidney Disease-Metabolic; Kidney Failure-Chronic; **Hospital:** UC Davis Med Ctr; **Address:** UC Davis Med Ctr, Div Nephr, One Shields Ave, GBSF 6310, Davis, CA 95616; **Phone:** 530-752-4010; **Board Cert:** Internal Medicine 1975; Nephrology 1980; **Med School:** Albert Einstein Coll Med 1972; **Resid:** Internal Medicine, Bronx Muni Hosp 1975; **Fellow:** Renal Disease, Bronx Muni Hosp 1977; **Fac Appt:** Prof Med, UC Davis

King, Andrew J MD [Nep] - **Spec Exp:** Kidney Disease-Chronic; Hypertension; Dialysis Care; **Hospital:** Scripps Green Hosp; **Address:** Scripps Green Hospital, 10666 N Torrey Pines Rd, MC N239, La Jolla, CA 92037-1027; **Phone:** 858-554-9765; **Board Cert:** Internal Medicine 1986; Nephrology 1988; **Med School:** Northwestern Univ 1983; **Resid:** Internal Medicine, Northwestern Meml Hosp 1986; **Fellow:** Nephrology, Brigham & Women's Hosp 1990; **Fac Appt:** Clin Prof Med, UCSD

Ott, Susan M MD [Nep] - **Spec Exp:** Bone Disorders-Metabolic; Osteoporosis; **Hospital:** Univ Wash Med Ctr; **Address:** Bone & Joint Center, UWMC- Roosevelt, 4245 Roosevelt Way NE, Box 354740, Seattle, WA 98105-6920; **Phone:** 206-598-4288; **Board Cert:** Internal Medicine 1978; Nephrology 1982; **Med School:** Univ Wash 1974; **Resid:** Family Medicine, UC Davis Med Ctr 1978; **Fellow:** Nephrology, Univ Wash Med Ctr 1982; **Fac Appt:** Assoc Prof Med, Univ Wash

Riordan, John W MD [Nep] - **Hospital:** CA Pacific Med Ctr - Pacific Campus; **Address:** 2100 Webster St, Ste 412, San Francisco, CA 94115; **Phone:** 415-923-3815; **Board Cert:** Nephrology 2005; **Med School:** Univ Tex Med Br, Galveston 1987; **Resid:** Internal Medicine, Univ Texas Hlth Sci Ctr 1990; **Fellow:** Nephrology, UCSF Med Ctr 1995

Scandling Jr, John David MD [Nep] - **Spec Exp:** Transplant Medicine-Kidney; **Hospital:** Stanford Univ Med Ctr; **Address:** 750 Welch Rd, Ste 200, Palo Alto, CA 94304-1509; **Phone:** 650-725-9891; **Board Cert:** Internal Medicine 1981; Nephrology 1984; **Med School:** Med Coll VA 1978; **Resid:** Internal Medicine, West Virginia Univ Hosp 1981; **Fellow:** Nephrology, Univ Rochester 1983; **Fac Appt:** Prof Med, Stanford Univ

Cleveland Clinic

Nephrology and Hypertension

The Glickman Urological and Kidney Institute's Department of Nephrology and Hypertension provides comprehensive diagnostic and therapeutic services for patients with kidney disease and hypertension. The department participates in an active kidney transplant program, all modalities of dialysis care, and clinical research studies of diabetic and other glomerular disease. In addition to unique diagnostic capabilities, the department is renowned for its expertise in the areas of renovascular hypertension, primary aldosteronism and pheochromocytoma.

Intensive Care Nephrology Services

The Department of Nephrology and Hypertension is a major participant in the intensive care setting. Institute nephrologists are leaders in research into the risk factors for acute renal failure after surgeries and in evaluations of different techniques for treatment of acute renal failure such as slow continuous ultrafiltration, continuous arteriovenous hemofiltration and venovenous hemofiltration.

Research and Clinical Trials

The Department of Nephrology and Hypertension is actively involved in clinical and basic research. Its legacy of excellence in hypertension research began in 1945.

For more than 30 years, the Clinic has received support from the National Institutes of Health (NIH) for its research into the causes of hypertension.

Kidney/Kidney-Pancreas Transplant

Cleveland Clinic's kidney transplant program dates to January 1963. Since then, more than 3,000 kidney transplants have been performed here. Each year, between 75 and 100 kidney transplants are performed.

For more information about Glickman Urological and Kidney Institute's Department of Nephrology and Hypertension, to schedule a second opinion or learn about assistance for out-of-state patients, call 800.890.2467 or visit www.clevelandclinic.org/nephrologytopdocs.

Glickman Urological & Kidney Institute
Department of Nephrology and Hypertension
Cleveland Clinic | 9500 Euclid Avenue / AC311 | Cleveland OH 44195

Neurological Surgery

A neurological surgeon provides the operative and non-operative management (i.e., prevention, diagnosis, evaluation, treatment, critical care and rehabilitation) of disorders of the central, peripheral and autonomic nervous systems, including their supporting structures and vascular supply; the evaluation and treatment of pathological processes which modify function or activity of the nervous system; and the operative and non-operative management of pain. A neurological surgeon treats patients with disorders of the nervous system; disorders of the brain, meninges, skull and their blood supply, including the extracranial carotid and vertebral arteries; disorders of the pituitary gland; disorders of the spinal cord, meninges and vertebral column, including those which may require treatment by spinal fusion or instrumentation; and disorders of the cranial and spinal nerves throughout their distribution.

Training Required: Seven years (including general surgery)

The American Board of Pediatric Neurological Surgery (ABPNS) is not a recognized ABMS subspecialty. However, this designation has been included because the certification process is meaningful and rigorous. It is awarded to those doctors who hold a current ABMS certification in Neurological Surgery, have completed a fully accredited one year, post-graduate fellowship in pediatric neurological surgery, and have submitted surgical logs indicating a practice of pediatric neurological surgery for one year, followed by a written examination.

NEUROLOGICAL SURGERY

New England

Black, Peter MD/PhD [NS] - **Spec Exp:** Brain Tumors; Pituitary Tumors; Seizure Disorders; **Hospital:** Brigham & Women's Hosp, Children's Hospital - Boston; **Address:** Brigham & Women's Hosp, Dept Neurosurg, 75 Francis St, Boston, MA 02115-6106; **Phone:** 617-732-6600; **Board Cert:** Neurological Surgery 1984; **Med School:** McGill Univ 1970; **Resid:** Surgery, Mass Genl Hosp 1972; Neurological Surgery, Mass Genl Hosp 1980; **Fellow:** Neurosurgical Oncology, Mass Genl Hosp 1976; **Fac Appt:** Prof NS, Harvard Med Sch

Borges, Lawrence F MD [NS] - **Spec Exp:** Spinal Surgery; Spinal Tumors; **Hospital:** Mass Genl Hosp; **Address:** Mass Genl Hosp, Div Neurosurg Svcs, 55 Fruit St, Ste 1205, Boston, MA 02114-2696; **Phone:** 617-726-6156; **Board Cert:** Neurological Surgery 1986; **Med School:** Johns Hopkins Univ 1977; **Resid:** Neurological Surgery, Mass Genl Hosp 1983; **Fac Appt:** Assoc Prof S, Harvard Med Sch

Cosgrove, G Rees MD [NS] - **Spec Exp:** Epilepsy/Seizure Disorders; Brain Tumors; **Hospital:** Lahey Clin, Emerson Hosp; **Address:** Lahey Clinic, 41 Mall Rd, Burlington, MA 01805; **Phone:** 781-744-1990; **Board Cert:** Neurological Surgery 1989; **Med School:** Queens Univ 1980; **Resid:** Neurological Surgery, Montreal Neur Inst 1986; **Fac Appt:** Prof NS, Tufts Univ

David, Carlos MD [NS] - **Spec Exp:** Cerebrovascular Surgery; Skull Base Tumors & Surgery; **Hospital:** Lahey Clin, Emerson Hosp; **Address:** Lahey Clinic, Dept Neurosurgery, 41 Mall Rd, Burlington, MA 01805; **Phone:** 781-744-8643; **Board Cert:** Neurological Surgery 2001; **Med School:** Univ Miami Sch Med 1990; **Resid:** Neurological Surgery, Jackson Memorial Hosp 1995; **Fellow:** Cerebrovascular & Skull Base Surgery, Barrow Neuro Inst 1997; **Fac Appt:** Assoc Clin Prof NS, Tufts Univ

Day, Arthur L MD [NS] - **Spec Exp:** Cerebrovascular Surgery; Orbital Tumors/Cancer; Carotid Artery Surgery; Skull Base Tumors; **Hospital:** Brigham & Women's Hosp, Children's Hospital - Boston; **Address:** Brigham & Womens Hosp, Dept Neurosurgery, 75 Francis St, Boston, MA 02115; **Phone:** 617-732-6600; **Board Cert:** Neurological Surgery 1980; **Med School:** Louisiana State U, New Orleans 1972; **Resid:** Neurological Surgery, Shands-Univ Florida Hosp 1977; **Fellow:** Neurological Pathology, Shands-Univ Florida Hosp 1978; **Fac Appt:** Prof NS, Harvard Med Sch

Duhaime, Ann Christine MD [NS] - **Spec Exp:** Pediatric Neurosurgery; Brain Tumors; Epilepsy; Craniofacial Surgery; **Hospital:** Dartmouth - Hitchcock Med Ctr; **Address:** Chldns Hosp at Dartmouth-Hitchcock Med Ctr, One Medical Center Drive, Lebanon, NH 03756; **Phone:** 603-653-9880; **Board Cert:** Neurological Surgery 1990; Pediatric Neurological Surgery 2005; **Med School:** Univ Pennsylvania 1981; **Resid:** Neurological Surgery, Hosp Univ Penn 1987; **Fellow:** Pediatric Neurological Surgery, Chldns Hosp 1987; **Fac Appt:** Prof S, Dartmouth Med Sch

Goumnerova, Liliana MD [NS] - **Spec Exp:** Pediatric Neurosurgery; Brain Tumors; Endoscopic Surgery/Ventriculoscopy; **Hospital:** Children's Hospital - Boston, Dana-Farber Cancer Inst; **Address:** Chldns Hosp, 300 Longwood Ave, Hunnewell 2, Boston, MA 02115; **Phone:** 617-355-6364; **Board Cert:** Neurological Surgery 1992; Pediatric Neurological Surgery 2006; **Med School:** Canada 1980; **Resid:** Neurological Surgery, Univ Ottawa 1986; **Fellow:** Pediatric Neurological Surgery, Hosp for Sick Chldn 1988; Neurological Science, Univ Penn 1990; **Fac Appt:** Assoc Prof S, Harvard Med Sch

Heilman, Carl B MD [NS] - **Spec Exp:** Skull Base Surgery; Pediatric Neurosurgery; **Hospital:** Tufts Med Ctr; **Address:** Tufts-NE Med Ctr, Dept Neurosurgery, 800 Washington St, Box 178, Bsoton, MA 02111; **Phone:** 617-636-5858; **Board Cert:** Neurological Surgery 1996; **Med School:** Univ Pennsylvania 1986; **Resid:** Neurological Surgery, Tufts New England Med Ctr 1993; **Fellow:** Skull Base Surgery, Baptist Meml Hosp 1993; **Fac Appt:** Assoc Prof NS, Tufts Univ

Madsen, Joseph MD [NS] - **Spec Exp:** Pediatric Neurosurgery; Epilepsy/Seizure Disorders; **Hospital:** Children's Hospital - Boston; **Address:** 300 Longwood Ave, Bader 3, Boston, MA 02115; **Phone:** 617-355-6005; **Board Cert:** Neurological Surgery 1994; Pediatric Neurological Surgery 1997; **Med School:** Harvard Med Sch 1981; **Resid:** Neurological Surgery, Mass Genl Hosp 1989; **Fellow:** Research, Beth Israel Hosp 1983; **Fac Appt:** Assoc Prof NS, Harvard Med Sch

Martuza, Robert L MD [NS] - **Spec Exp:** Brain Tumors; Acoustic Neuroma; Skull Base Surgery; **Hospital:** Mass Genl Hosp; **Address:** Mass General Hosp, 55 Fruit St, MGH-White 502, Boston, MA 02114; **Phone:** 617-726-8581; **Board Cert:** Neurological Surgery 1983; **Med School:** Harvard Med Sch 1973; **Resid:** Neurological Surgery, Mass Genl Hosp 1980; **Fac Appt:** Prof NS, Harvard Med Sch

Penar, Paul L MD [NS] - **Spec Exp:** Brain & Spinal Tumors; Epilepsy/Seizure Disorders; Movement Disorders; Stereotactic Radiosurgery; **Hospital:** Fletcher Allen Health Care- Med Ctr Campus; **Address:** Fletcher Allen Health Care, 111 Colchester Ave, Burlington, VT 05401; **Phone:** 802-847-4590; **Board Cert:** Neurological Surgery 1989; **Med School:** Univ Mich Med Sch 1981; **Resid:** Neurological Surgery, Yale-New Haven Hosp 1987

Piepmeier, Joseph MD [NS] - **Spec Exp:** Neuro-Oncology; Brain & Spinal Cord Tumors; **Hospital:** Yale-New Haven Hosp; **Address:** Yale Sch Med, Dept Neurosurgery, 333 Cedar St Fl TMP-410, New Haven, CT 06520; **Phone:** 203-785-2791; **Board Cert:** Neurological Surgery 1984; **Med School:** Univ Tenn Coll Med, Memphis 1975; **Resid:** Neurological Surgery, Yale-New Haven Hosp 1982; **Fac Appt:** Prof NS, Yale Univ

Spencer, Dennis D MD [NS] - **Spec Exp:** Epilepsy/Seizure Disorders; Brain Tumors; **Hospital:** Yale-New Haven Hosp; **Address:** Yale Univ Sch Med, Dept Neurosurgery, 333 Cedar St, TMP-4, New Haven, CT 06520; **Phone:** 203-785-4891; **Board Cert:** Neurological Surgery 1980; **Med School:** Washington Univ, St Louis 1971; **Resid:** Surgery, Barnes Hosp 1972; Neurological Surgery, Yale-New Haven Hosp 1976; **Fac Appt:** Prof NS, Yale Univ

Mid Atlantic

Andrews, David MD [NS] - **Spec Exp:** Brain Tumors; Stereotactic Radiosurgery; **Hospital:** Thomas Jefferson Univ Hosp; **Address:** Thom Jefferson Univ Hosp, Dept Neurosurg, 909 Walnut St Fl 2, Philadelphia, PA 19107-5109; **Phone:** 215-503-7005; **Board Cert:** Neurological Surgery 1992; **Med School:** Univ Colorado 1983; **Resid:** Neurological Surgery, NY Presby Hos-Cornell Med Ctr 1989; **Fellow:** Neuro-Oncology, Meml Sloan Kettering Cancer Ctr 1987; **Fac Appt:** Prof NS, Thomas Jefferson Univ

Baltuch, Gordon MD/PhD [NS] - **Spec Exp:** Movement Disorders; Parkinson's Disease; Epilepsy/Seizure Disorders; **Hospital:** Hosp Univ Penn - UPHS (page 60), Pennsylvania Hosp (page 60); **Address:** Penn Neurological Institute, 3400 Spruce St, Silverstein Bldg Fl 3, Philadelphia, PA 19104; **Phone:** 215-662-7788; **Board Cert:** Neurological Surgery 1998; **Med School:** McGill Univ 1986; **Resid:** Surgery, Montreal Genl Hosp 1988; Neurological Surgery, Montreal Neuro Inst 1994; **Fellow:** Neurological Surgery, Centre Hospitalier Univ Vaudois 1995; **Fac Appt:** Assoc Prof NS, Univ Pennsylvania

Neurological Surgery

Bederson, Joshua B MD [NS] - **Spec Exp:** Brain & Spinal Cord Tumors; Aneurysm-Cerebral; Meningioma; Pituitary Tumors; **Hospital:** Mount Sinai Med Ctr (page 64); **Address:** Mount Sinai Med Ctr, 1 Gustave Levy Pl, Box 1136, New York, NY 10029; **Phone:** 212-241-2377; **Board Cert:** Neurological Surgery 1993; **Med School:** UCSF 1984; **Resid:** Neurological Surgery, UCSF Med Ctr 1990; **Fellow:** Neurological Vascular Surgery, Barrow Neur Inst 1990; Neurological Vascular Surgery, Univ Hosp Zurich 1990; **Fac Appt:** Prof NS, Mount Sinai Sch Med

Belzberg, Allan J MD [NS] - **Spec Exp:** Peripheral Nerve Disorders; Nerve Surgery & Transplantation; Nerve Tumors; Pediatric Neurosurgery; **Hospital:** Johns Hopkins Hosp (page 61); **Address:** Johns Hopkins Dept Neurosurgery, 600 N Wolfe St, Meyer 5-109, Baltimore, MD 21287; **Phone:** 410-955-5810; **Board Cert:** Neurological Surgery 1997; **Med School:** Univ Calgary 1982; **Resid:** Neurological Surgery, Univ Calgary Affil Hosps 1990; **Fellow:** Neurological Surgery, Johns Hopkins Univ 1992; **Fac Appt:** Assoc Prof NS, Johns Hopkins Univ

Bilsky, Mark H MD [NS] - **Spec Exp:** Spinal Tumors; Skull Base Tumors; Brain Tumors; Spinal Reconstructive Surgery; **Hospital:** Meml Sloan-Kettering Cancer Ctr, NY-Presby Hosp/Weill Cornell (page 66); **Address:** 1275 York Avenue, New York, NY 10065; **Phone:** 800-525-2225; **Board Cert:** Neurological Surgery 1999; **Med School:** Emory Univ 1988; **Resid:** Neurological Surgery, NY Hosp-Cornell Med Ctr 1994; **Fellow:** Neuro-Oncology, Louisville Univ Med Ctr 1995; **Fac Appt:** Assoc Prof NS, Cornell Univ-Weill Med Coll

Brem, Henry MD [NS] - **Spec Exp:** Brain & Spinal Cord Tumors; Skull Base Tumors; Pituitary Tumors; **Hospital:** Johns Hopkins Hosp (page 61), Johns Hopkins Bayview Med Ctr (page 61); **Address:** Johns Hopkins Med Ctr-Dept Neuro Surgery, 600 N Wolfe St Meyer 7 Bldg - rm 113, Baltimore, MD 21287; **Phone:** 410-955-2248; **Board Cert:** Neurological Surgery 1986; **Med School:** Harvard Med Sch 1978; **Resid:** Neurological Surgery, Columbia-Presby Med Ctr 1984; **Fellow:** Neurological Surgery, Johns Hopkins Hosp 1980; **Fac Appt:** Prof NS, Johns Hopkins Univ

Bruce, Jeffrey MD [NS] - **Spec Exp:** Brain Tumors; Pituitary Tumors; Skull Base Surgery; Pineal Tumors; **Hospital:** NY-Presby Hosp/Columbia (page 66); **Address:** NY Presby Hosp, Dept Neurosurgery, 710 W 168th St N1 Bldg Fl 4 - rm 434, New York, NY 10032-3726; **Phone:** 212-305-7346; **Board Cert:** Neurological Surgery 1993; **Med School:** UMDNJ-RW Johnson Med Sch 1983; **Resid:** Neurological Surgery, Columbia-Presby Med Ctr 1990; **Fellow:** Neurological Surgery, Nat Inst Health 1985; **Fac Appt:** Prof NS, Columbia P&S

Caputy, Anthony J MD [NS] - **Spec Exp:** Epilepsy/Seizure Disorders; Spinal Surgery; Brain & Spinal Tumors; Minimally Invasive Surgery; **Hospital:** G Washington Univ Hosp, Suburban Hosp; **Address:** Geo Wash Univ, Dept Neurosurgery, 2150 Pennsylvania Ave NW, Ste 7-420, Washington, DC 20037; **Phone:** 202-741-2735; **Board Cert:** Neurological Surgery 1989; **Med School:** Univ VA Sch Med 1980; **Resid:** Neurological Surgery, Georgetown Univ Hosp 1986; **Fac Appt:** Prof NS, Geo Wash Univ

Carson, Benjamin S MD [NS] - **Spec Exp:** Brain Injury; Brain & Spinal Cord Tumors; Pediatric Neurosurgery; Rasmussen's Syndrome; **Hospital:** Johns Hopkins Hosp (page 61); **Address:** 600 N Wolfe St, Harvey 811, Baltimore, MD 21287-8811; **Phone:** 410-955-7888; **Board Cert:** Neurological Surgery 1988; Pediatric Neurological Surgery 1997; **Med School:** Univ Mich Med Sch 1977; **Resid:** Neurological Surgery, Johns Hopkins Hosp 1983; **Fellow:** Pediatric Neurological Surgery, Queen Elizabeth II Med Ctr 1984; **Fac Appt:** Assoc Prof NS, Johns Hopkins Univ

Chen, Chun Siang MD [NS] - **Spec Exp:** Skull Base Tumors; Skull Base Surgery; Microsurgery; Brain & Spinal Surgery; **Hospital:** Mount Sinai Med Ctr (page 64); **Address:** Mount Sinai Med Ctr, Annenberg Bldg, One Gustave L Levy Pl Fl 8 - rm 10, New York, NY 10029; **Phone:** 212-241-8480; **Med School:** Brazil 1978; **Resid:** Neurological Surgery, Santa Casa de Misericordia of Sao Paulo Med Sch 1983; Neurological Surgery, Mt Sinai Med Ctr 2005; **Fellow:** Skull Base Surgery, St Lukes Roosevelt Hosp 2006; **Fac Appt:** Asst Prof NS, Mount Sinai Sch Med

Di Giacinto, George V MD [NS] - **Spec Exp:** Spinal Surgery; Pain Management; **Hospital:** St Luke's - Roosevelt Hosp Ctr - Roosevelt Div (page 57); **Address:** 425 W 59th St, Ste 4E, New York, NY 10019; **Phone:** 212-523-8500; **Board Cert:** Neurological Surgery 1981; **Med School:** Harvard Med Sch 1970; **Resid:** Neurological Surgery, Columbia-Presby Hosp 1978

Dias, Mark S MD [NS] - **Spec Exp:** Pediatric Neurosurgery; Spina Bifida; Hydrocephalus; Craniosynostosis; **Hospital:** Penn State Milton S Hershey Med Ctr; **Address:** Penn State-Hersey Med Ctr, Dept Neurosurg, EC110 30 Hope Drive, Hersey, PA 17033; **Phone:** 717-531-8807; **Board Cert:** Neurological Surgery 1995; Pediatric Neurological Surgery 2006; **Med School:** Johns Hopkins Univ 1982; **Resid:** Neurological Surgery, Univ Pittsburgh Med Ctr 1989; **Fellow:** Pediatric Neurological Surgery, Univ Utah-Primary Chldns Hosp 1991; **Fac Appt:** Prof NS, Penn State Univ Coll Med

Eisenberg, Howard M MD [NS] - **Spec Exp:** Acoustic Neuroma; Skull Base Surgery; Deep Brain Stimulation; Epilepsy/Seizure Disorders; **Hospital:** Univ of MD Med Ctr, Greater Baltimore Med Ctr; **Address:** Univ MD Sch Med, Dept Neurosurg, 22 S Greene St, Ste S-12-D, Baltimore, MD 21201-1544; **Phone:** 410-328-3514; **Board Cert:** Neurological Surgery 1973; **Med School:** SUNY Downstate 1964; **Resid:** Surgery, New York Hosp 1966; Neurological Surgery, Peter Bent Brigham Hosp/Chldns Hosp 1970; **Fellow:** Harvard Univ 1970; **Fac Appt:** Prof NS, Univ MD Sch Med

Feldstein, Neil A MD [NS] - **Spec Exp:** Pediatric Neurosurgery; Chiari's Deformity; Brain Tumors-Pediatric; Spinal Cord Surgery-Pediatric; **Hospital:** NY-Presby Hosp/Columbia (page 66); **Address:** Neurological Inst, 710 W 168th St Fl 2 - rm 213, New York, NY 10032; **Phone:** 212-305-1396; **Board Cert:** Neurological Surgery 1995; Pediatric Neurological Surgery 2007; **Med School:** NYU Sch Med 1984; **Resid:** Neurological Surgery, Baylor Coll Med 1989; **Fellow:** Pediatric Neurological Surgery, NYU Med Ctr 1991; **Fac Appt:** Assoc Prof NS, Columbia P&S

Gokaslan, Ziya L MD [NS] - **Spec Exp:** Spinal Tumors; Spinal Surgery-Complex; Spinal Reconstructive Surgery; **Hospital:** Johns Hopkins Hosp (page 61), Johns Hopkins Bayview Med Ctr (page 61); **Address:** Johns Hopkins Hosp, Dept Neurosurg, 600 N Wolfe St, Meyer 7-109, Baltimore, MD 21287; **Phone:** 410-955-4424; **Board Cert:** Neurological Surgery 1997; **Med School:** Turkey 1983; **Resid:** Neurological Surgery, Baylor Coll Med 1993; **Fellow:** Neurological Trauma, Baylor Coll Med 1988; Spinal Surgery, NYU Med Ctr 1994; **Fac Appt:** Prof NS, Johns Hopkins Univ

Golfinos, John G MD [NS] - **Spec Exp:** Brain Tumors; Acoustic Neuroma; Stereotactic Radiosurgery; Skull Base Surgery; **Hospital:** NYU Langone Med Ctr (page 67), Lenox Hill Hosp (page 62); **Address:** NYU Med Ctr, Dept Neurosurgery, 530 1st Ave, Ste 8R, New York, NY 10016-6402; **Phone:** 212-263-2950; **Board Cert:** Neurological Surgery 1998; **Med School:** Columbia P&S 1988; **Resid:** Neurological Surgery, Barrow Neuro Inst 1995; **Fac Appt:** Assoc Prof NS, NYU Sch Med

Goodman, Robert R MD/PhD [NS] - **Spec Exp:** Parkinson's Disease/Movement Disorders; Epilepsy; Trigeminal Neuralgia; Hydrocephalus-Adult; **Hospital:** NY-Presby Hosp/Columbia (page 66); **Address:** 710 W 168th St, rm 426, New York, NY 10032-2603; **Phone:** 212-305-3774; **Board Cert:** Neurological Surgery 1993; **Med School:** Johns Hopkins Univ 1982; **Resid:** Neurological Surgery, Columbia-Presby Med Ctr 1989; **Fac Appt:** Assoc Prof NS, Columbia P&S

Goodrich, James T MD [NS] - **Spec Exp:** Craniofacial Surgery/Reconstruction; Spina Bifida; Brain Tumors-Pediatric; Pediatric Neurosurgery; **Hospital:** Montefiore Med Ctr - Div. Moses, Jacobi Med Ctr; **Address:** Montefiore Med Ctr, Dept Ped Neurosurgery, 111 E 210th St, Bronx, NY 10467-2401; **Phone:** 718-920-4197; **Board Cert:** Neurological Surgery 1989; Pediatric Neurological Surgery 2007; **Med School:** Columbia P&S 1980; **Resid:** Neurological Surgery, NY Neurological Inst 1986; **Fac Appt:** Prof NS, Albert Einstein Coll Med

Neurological Surgery

Grady, M Sean MD [NS] - **Spec Exp:** Cerebrovascular Surgery; Aneurysm-Cerebral; Arteriovenous Malformations; **Hospital:** Hosp Univ Penn - UPHS (page 60), Pennsylvania Hosp (page 60); **Address:** Dept Neurosurgery, 3400 Spruce St, Silverstein Bldg Fl 3, Philadelphia, PA 19104; **Phone:** 215-662-3483; **Board Cert:** Neurological Surgery 1990; **Med School:** Georgetown Univ 1981; **Resid:** Neurological Surgery, Univ Virginia Hosp 1987; **Fac Appt:** Prof NS, Univ Pennsylvania

Gutin, Philip MD [NS] - **Spec Exp:** Brain Tumors; Meningioma; Acoustic Neuroma; **Hospital:** Meml Sloan-Kettering Cancer Ctr, NY-Presby Hosp/Weill Cornell (page 66); **Address:** 1275 York Avenue, New York, NY 10065; **Phone:** 800-525-2225; **Board Cert:** Neurological Surgery 1981; **Med School:** Univ Pennsylvania 1971; **Resid:** Neurological Surgery, UCSF Med Ctr 1979; **Fellow:** Natl Cancer Inst 1976; **Fac Appt:** Prof NS, Cornell Univ-Weill Med Coll

Harbaugh, Robert E MD [NS] - **Spec Exp:** Carotid Artery Surgery; Aneurysm-Cerebral; Arteriovenous Malformations; **Hospital:** Penn State Milton S Hershey Med Ctr; **Address:** Penn State-Hershey Med Ctr, Dept of Neurosurgery, 30 Hope Drive, Hershey, PA 17033-0850; **Phone:** 717-531-8807; **Board Cert:** Neurological Surgery 1989; **Med School:** Penn State Univ-Hershey Med Ctr 1978; **Resid:** Surgery, Dartmouth-Hitchcock Med Ctr 1980; Neurological Surgery, Dartmouth-Hitchcock Med Ctr 1985; **Fac Appt:** Prof NS, Penn State Univ-Hershey Med Ctr

Hartl, Roger MD [NS] - **Spec Exp:** Spinal Surgery-Complex; Minimally Invasive Spinal Surgery; Spinal Disc Replacement; **Hospital:** NY-Presby Hosp/Weill Cornell (page 66); **Address:** Cornell Neurosurgery, 525 E 68th St, Starr 651, New York, NY 10065; **Phone:** 212-746-2152; **Board Cert:** Neurological Surgery 2008; **Med School:** Germany 1993; **Resid:** Neurological Surgery, NY Presby-Cornell Med Ctr 2003; **Fellow:** Spinal Surgery, Barrow Neurological Inst

Hopkins, L Nelson MD [NS] - **Spec Exp:** Cerebrovascular Disease; Endovascular Surgery; **Hospital:** Millard Fillmore Gates Cir Hosp; **Address:** Univ Buffalo Neurosurgery, 3 Gates Circle, Buffalo, NY 14209; **Phone:** 716-887-5200; **Board Cert:** Neurological Surgery 1977; **Med School:** Albany Med Coll 1969; **Resid:** Neurological Surgery, SUNY Buffalo Med Ctr 1975; **Fac Appt:** Prof NS, SUNY Buffalo

Jallo, George I MD [NS] - **Spec Exp:** Pediatric Neurosurgery; Chiari's Deformity; Brain & Spinal Cord Tumors; Epilepsy; **Hospital:** Johns Hopkins Hosp (page 61), Johns Hopkins Bayview Med Ctr (page 61); **Address:** Johns Hopkins Hosp, Dept of Neurosurgery, 600 N Wolfe St, Ste Harvey 811, Baltimore, MD 21287; **Phone:** 410-955-7851; **Board Cert:** Neurological Surgery 2002; Pediatric Neurological Surgery 2004; **Med School:** Univ VA Sch Med 1991; **Resid:** Neurological Surgery, NYU Med Ctr 1998; **Fellow:** Pediatric Neurological Surgery, Beth Israel Med Ctr 1999; **Fac Appt:** Assoc Prof NS, Johns Hopkins Univ

Jho, Hae-Dong MD/PhD [NS] - **Spec Exp:** Minimally Invasive Surgery; **Hospital:** Allegheny General Hosp; **Address:** Jho Inst for Min Invasive Neurosurgery, 320 E North Ave, Snyder Pavilion, Fl 7, Pittsburgh, PA 15212-4746; **Phone:** 412-359-6110; **Board Cert:** Neurological Surgery 1991; **Med School:** Korea 1971; **Resid:** Neurological Surgery, Hanyang Univ Hosp 1979; Neurological Surgery, Univ Pittsburgh 1989; **Fellow:** Microsurgery, Univ Pittsburgh 1983; **Fac Appt:** Prof NS, Drexel Univ Coll Med

Judy, Kevin MD [NS] - **Spec Exp:** Brain Tumors; **Hospital:** Hosp Univ Penn - UPHS (page 60), Pennsylvania Hosp (page 60); **Address:** Hosp Univ Penn-Dept Neurosurg, 3400 Spruce St, 3 Silverstein, Philadelphia, PA 19104; **Phone:** 215-662-7854; **Board Cert:** Neurological Surgery 1997; **Med School:** Univ Pittsburgh 1984; **Resid:** Surgery, Mercy Hosp 1986; Neurological Surgery, Johns Hopkins Hosp 1992; **Fellow:** Neurological Surgery, Johns Hopkins Hosp 1991; **Fac Appt:** Assoc Prof NS, Univ Pennsylvania

Kaplitt, Michael G MD/PhD [NS] - **Spec Exp:** Parkinson's Disease/Movement Disorders; Gene Therapy; Stereotactic Radiosurgery; Trigeminal Neuralgia; **Hospital:** NY-Presby Hosp/Weill Cornell (page 66); **Address:** 525 E 68th St, Box 99, New York, NY 10065; **Phone:** 212-746-4966; **Board Cert:** Neurological Surgery 2005; **Med School:** Cornell Univ-Weill Med Coll 1995; **Resid:** Neurological Surgery, New York Hosp 2000; **Fellow:** Stereo Neurological Surgery, Toronto Western Hosp 2001; **Fac Appt:** Assoc Prof NS, Cornell Univ-Weill Med Coll

Kassam, Amin MD [NS] - **Spec Exp:** Skull Base Tumors & Surgery; Cranial Nerve Disorders; Cerebrovascular Surgery; Endoscopic Surgery; **Hospital:** UPMC Presby, Pittsburgh, UPMC Mercy, Pittsburgh; **Address:** Univ Pittsburgh Med Ctr, Dept Neurosurgery, 200 Lothrop St, Ste B400, Pittburgh, PA 15213; **Phone:** 412-647-6778; **Med School:** Univ Toronto 1991; **Resid:** Neurological Surgery, Univ Ottawa Med Ctr 1997; **Fac Appt:** Assoc Prof NS, Univ Pittsburgh

Khan, Agha S MD [NS] - **Spec Exp:** Skull Base Surgery; Spinal Surgery; **Hospital:** Sinai Hosp - Baltimore, Maryland Genl Hosp; **Address:** 2411 W Belvedere Ave, Ste 402, Baltimore, MD 21215; **Phone:** 410-601-8314; **Board Cert:** Neurological Surgery 1995; **Med School:** Pakistan 1979; **Resid:** Neurological Surgery, Univ Wisconsin Hosp 1990; **Fellow:** Surgical Oncology, Roswell Park Meml Inst 1982; Neurological Surgery, Allegheny Genl Hosp 1991

Kobrine, Arthur MD/PhD [NS] - **Spec Exp:** Spinal Cord Surgery; Brain & Spinal Cord Tumors; **Hospital:** Sibley Mem Hosp, Georgetown Univ Hosp; **Address:** 2440 M St NW, Ste 315, Washington, DC 20037-1404; **Phone:** 202-293-7136; **Board Cert:** Neurological Surgery 1976; **Med School:** Northwestern Univ 1968; **Resid:** Neurological Surgery, Northwestern Univ Hosp 1970; Neurological Surgery, Walter Reed Army Hosp 1973; **Fellow:** Physiology, Geo Wash Univ 1979; **Fac Appt:** Clin Prof NS, Georgetown Univ

Kondziolka, Douglas MD [NS] - **Spec Exp:** Brain Tumors-Adult & Pediatric; Brain Tumors-Metastatic; Stereotactic Radiosurgery; Movement Disorders; **Hospital:** UPMC Presby, Pittsburgh, Chldns Hosp of Pittsburgh - UPMC; **Address:** Univ Pittsburgh Med Ctr, Dept Neurological Surgery, 200 Lothrop St, Ste B400, Pittsburgh, PA 15213; **Phone:** 412-647-9990; **Board Cert:** Neurological Surgery 1994; **Med School:** Univ Toronto 1985; **Resid:** Neurological Surgery, Univ Toronto 1991; **Fellow:** Stereo Neurological Surgery, UPMC Presby Med Ctr 1991; **Fac Appt:** Prof NS, Univ Pittsburgh

Kotapka, Mark J MD [NS] - **Spec Exp:** Pituitary Tumors; Skull Base Surgery; Spinal Surgery; **Hospital:** Albert Einstein Med Ctr; **Address:** Albert Einstein Medical Ctr, Klein Bldg - Ste 501, 5401 Old York Rd, Philadelphia, PA 19141; **Phone:** 215-456-6127; **Board Cert:** Neurological Surgery 1997; **Med School:** Univ MD Sch Med 1985; **Resid:** Neurological Surgery, Hosp Univ Penn 1991; **Fellow:** Pediatric Neurological Surgery, Children's Hosp Philadelphia 1992; Skull Base Surgery, Univ Pittsburgh Med Ctr 1992; **Fac Appt:** Prof NS, Albert Einstein Coll Med

Laske, Douglas W MD [NS] - **Spec Exp:** Brain & Spinal Cord Tumors; Stereotactic Radiosurgery; Brain Tumors-Metastatic; **Hospital:** Temple Univ Hosp, Fox Chase Cancer Ctr (page 58); **Address:** Temple Univ Hosp-Dept Neuro-Surgery, 3509 N Broad St, Boyer Pavillio-5th flr, Phildelphia, PA 19140; **Phone:** 215-707-7200; **Board Cert:** Neurological Surgery 1996; **Med School:** Columbia P&S 1985; **Resid:** Neurology, Med Coll Virginia 1991; **Fellow:** Neurosurgical Oncology, Natl Inst Hlth 1995; **Fac Appt:** Assoc Prof NS, Temple Univ

Lavyne, Michael H MD [NS] - **Spec Exp:** Spinal Surgery; Spinal Tumors; Spinal Disorders; **Hospital:** NY-Presby Hosp/Weill Cornell (page 66), Hosp For Special Surgery (page 59); **Address:** 110 E 55th St Fl 9, New York, NY 10022; **Phone:** 212-486-9100; **Board Cert:** Neurological Surgery 1982; **Med School:** Cornell Univ-Weill Med Coll 1972; **Resid:** Neurological Surgery, Mass Genl Hosp 1979; **Fellow:** Neurology, Beth Israel Hosp 1974; **Fac Appt:** Clin Prof NS, Cornell Univ-Weill Med Coll

Neurological Surgery

Loftus, Christopher M MD [NS] - **Spec Exp:** Carotid Artery Surgery; Aneurysm-Cerebral; Arteriovenous Malformations; Cerebrovascular Surgery; **Hospital:** Temple Univ Hosp; **Address:** Temple Univ School Med, 3401 N Broad St, Parkinson Pavilion 540, Philadelphia, PA 19140; **Phone:** 215-707-4109; **Board Cert:** Neurological Surgery 1987; **Med School:** SUNY Downstate 1979; **Resid:** Neurological Surgery, Columbia-Presby Med Ctr 1985; **Fac Appt:** Prof NS, Temple Univ

Lunsford, L Dade MD [NS] - **Spec Exp:** Brain Tumors; Stereotactic Radiosurgery; Movement Disorders; Vascular Malformations; **Hospital:** UPMC Presby, Pittsburgh, Chldns Hosp of Pittsburgh - UPMC; **Address:** UPMC Presbyterian Hosp, 200 Lothrop St, Ste B400, Pittsburgh, PA 15213-2536; **Phone:** 412-647-0953; **Board Cert:** Neurological Surgery 1983; **Med School:** Columbia P&S 1974; **Resid:** Neurological Surgery, Univ Pittsburgh Med Ctr 1980; **Fellow:** Stereo Neurological Surgery, Karolinska Hospital 1981; **Fac Appt:** Prof NS, Univ Pittsburgh

Maroon, Joseph C MD [NS] - **Spec Exp:** Minimally Invasive Surgery; Microdiscectomy; Brain Injury-Traumatic; **Hospital:** UPMC Presby, Pittsburgh, UPMC Passavant; **Address:** UPMC Presbyterian, Dept Neuro Surg, 200 Lothrop St, Ste 5-C, Pittsburgh, PA 15213; **Phone:** 412-647-3604; **Board Cert:** Neurological Surgery 1973; **Med School:** Indiana Univ 1965; **Resid:** Surgery, Georgetown Univ Hosp 1967; Neurological Surgery, Indiana Univ Med Ctr 1971; **Fellow:** Neurological Surgery, Radcliffe Infirmary 1969; Microsurgery, Univ Vermont Affil Hosp 1972; **Fac Appt:** Prof NS, Univ Pittsburgh

McCormick, Paul C MD [NS] - **Spec Exp:** Spinal Surgery; Spinal Tumors; **Hospital:** NY-Presby Hosp/Columbia (page 66), Valley Hosp; **Address:** 710 W 168th St, Ste 506, New York, NY 10032-2603; **Phone:** 212-305-7976; **Board Cert:** Neurological Surgery 1993; **Med School:** Columbia P&S 1982; **Resid:** Neurological Surgery, Columbia Presby Med Ctr 1989; **Fellow:** Neurological Surgery, Natl Inst Hlth 1984; Spinal Surgery, Med Coll Wisconsin 1990; **Fac Appt:** Prof NS, Columbia P&S

Murali, Raj MD [NS] - **Spec Exp:** Trigeminal Neuralgia; Skull Base Surgery; Aneurysm-Cerebral; Pituitary Tumors; **Hospital:** Westchester Med Ctr, St Vincent Cath Med Ctrs - Manhattan; **Address:** Westchester Med Ctr, Dept Neurosurgery, Munger Pavilion, Ste 329, Valhalla, NY 10595; **Phone:** 914-493-8392; **Board Cert:** Neurological Surgery 1982; **Med School:** India 1968; **Resid:** Neurological Surgery, Royal Infirm-Univ Edinburgh 1974; Neurological Surgery, NYU Med Ctr 1979; **Fac Appt:** Prof NS, NY Med Coll

O'Rourke, Donald MD [NS] - **Spec Exp:** Neuro-Oncology; Brain Tumors; Spinal Surgery-Cervical; **Hospital:** Hosp Univ Penn - UPHS (page 60); **Address:** Hosp Univ Penn - Dept Neurosurg, 3400 Spruce St, 3 Silverstein, Philadelphia, PA 19104; **Phone:** 215-662-3490; **Board Cert:** Neurological Surgery 1998; **Med School:** Univ Pennsylvania 1987; **Resid:** Neurological Surgery, Hosp Univ Penn 1994; **Fac Appt:** Assoc Prof NS, Univ Pennsylvania

Piatt, Joseph H MD [NS] - **Spec Exp:** Brachial Plexus Palsy-Pediatric; Spasticity & Movement Disorders; Chiari's Deformity; Syringomyelia & Spinal Cord Diseases; **Hospital:** St Christopher's Hosp for Chldn; **Address:** St Christopher's Hosp-Div Neurosurg, Erie Ave & Front St, Ste 2202, Philadelphia, PA 19134; **Phone:** 215-427-5196; **Board Cert:** Neurological Surgery 1989; Pediatric Neurological Surgery 2006; **Med School:** Univ Pennsylvania 1979; **Resid:** Neurological Surgery, Duke Univ Med Ctr 1986; **Fellow:** Pediatric Neurological Surgery, Hosp Sick Chldn 1987; **Fac Appt:** Prof NS, Drexel Univ Coll Med

Pollack, Ian F MD [NS] - **Spec Exp:** Pediatric Neurosurgery; Brain Tumors; Craniofacial Surgery; Neuro-Oncology; **Hospital:** Chldns Hosp of Pittsburgh - UPMC, UPMC Presby, Pittsburgh; **Address:** Chldns Hosp Pittsburgh, Div Neurosurgery, 3705 Fifth Ave, Ste 3670A, Pittsburgh, PA 15213-2524; **Phone:** 412-692-5881; **Board Cert:** Neurological Surgery 1996; Pediatric Neurological Surgery 2006; **Med School:** Johns Hopkins Univ 1984; **Resid:** Neurological Surgery, Univ Pittsburgh Med Ctr 1991; **Fellow:** Pediatric Neurological Surgery, Hosp Sick Chldn 1992; **Fac Appt:** Prof NS, Univ Pittsburgh

Rigamonti, Daniele MD [NS] - **Spec Exp:** Hydrocephalus-Adult; Brain Tumors; Spinal Disorders; Vascular Neurosurgery; **Hospital:** Johns Hopkins Hosp (page 61); **Address:** Johns Hopkins Hosp, Dept Neurosurgery, 600 N Wolfe St, Phipps 126, Baltimore, MD 21287; **Phone:** 410-955-2259; **Board Cert:** Neurological Surgery 1988; **Med School:** Italy 1976; **Resid:** Neurological Surgery, Mt Sinai Hosp Med Ctr 1984; **Fellow:** Neurological Vascular Surgery, Barrow Neuro Inst 1987; **Fac Appt:** Prof NS, Johns Hopkins Univ

Riina, Howard A MD [NS] - **Spec Exp:** Neuroradiology; Cerebrovascular Disease; Cerebrovascular Malformations; Stroke; **Hospital:** NY-Presby Hosp/Weill Cornell (page 66); **Address:** 525 E 68th St, Starr 651, Nwe York, NY 10021; **Phone:** 212-746-5149; **Board Cert:** Neurological Surgery 2004; **Med School:** Temple Univ 1993; **Resid:** Neurological Surgery, Hosp Univ Penn 2000; **Fellow:** Skull Base Surgery, Barrow Neuro Inst 2001; **Fac Appt:** Assoc Prof NS, Cornell Univ-Weill Med Coll

Rosenwasser, Robert H MD [NS] - **Spec Exp:** Aneurysm-Cerebral; Cerebrovascular Surgery; Arteriovenous Malformations; **Hospital:** Thomas Jefferson Univ Hosp; **Address:** Thomas Jefferson University Hospital, 909 Walnut St Fl 2, Philadelphia, PA 19107; **Phone:** 215-955-7000; **Board Cert:** Neurological Surgery 1987; **Med School:** Louisiana State U, New Orleans 1979; **Resid:** Neurological Surgery, Temple Univ Hosp 1984; **Fellow:** Neurological Vascular Surgery, Univ West Ontarion 1985; Interventional Neuroradiology, NYU Med Ctr 1993; **Fac Appt:** Prof NS, Thomas Jefferson Univ

Sen, Chandranath MD [NS] - **Spec Exp:** Brain Tumors; Skull Base Tumors; Skull Base Surgery; **Hospital:** St Luke's - Roosevelt Hosp Ctr - Roosevelt Div (page 57); **Address:** St Lukes Roosevelt Hosp Ctr, Dept Neurosurgery, 1000 10th Ave, Ste 5G-80, New York, NY 10019; **Phone:** 212-523-6720; **Board Cert:** Neurological Surgery 1989; **Med School:** India 1976; **Resid:** Surgery, Univ Wisconsin Hosps 1980; Neurological Surgery, Univ Wisconsin Hosps 1985; **Fellow:** Microsurgery, Univ Pittsburgh Med Ctr 1986

Sisti, Michael B MD [NS] - **Spec Exp:** Acoustic Neuroma; Brain Tumors; Stereotactic Radiosurgery; Meningioma; **Hospital:** NY-Presby Hosp/Columbia (page 66); **Address:** 710 W 168th St, New York, NY 10032-2603; **Phone:** 212-305-1728; **Board Cert:** Neurological Surgery 1991; **Med School:** Columbia P&S 1981; **Resid:** Neurological Surgery, Neuro Inst-Columbia-Presby Med Ctr 1988; **Fellow:** Neurological Surgery, Natl Inst Hlth 1983; **Fac Appt:** Asst Prof NS, Columbia P&S

Solomon, Robert A MD [NS] - **Spec Exp:** Aneurysm-Cerebral; Arteriovenous Malformations; **Hospital:** NY-Presby Hosp/Columbia (page 66); **Address:** 710 W 168th St, Ste 439, New York, NY 10032; **Phone:** 212-305-4118; **Board Cert:** Neurological Surgery 1988; **Med School:** Johns Hopkins Univ 1980; **Resid:** Neurological Surgery, Neuro Inst-Columbia 1986; **Fac Appt:** Prof NS, Columbia P&S

Neurological Surgery

Stieg, Philip E MD/PhD [NS] - **Spec Exp:** Cerebrovascular Surgery; Acoustic Neuroma; Skull Base Surgery; Meningioma; **Hospital:** NY-Presby Hosp/Weill Cornell (page 66); **Address:** 525 E 68th St, STARR 651, New York, NY 10021-9800; **Phone:** 212-746-4684; **Board Cert:** Neurological Surgery 1992; **Med School:** Med Coll Wisc 1983; **Resid:** Neurological Surgery, Dallas Chldns Hosp/Parkland Meml Hosp 1988; **Fellow:** Neurological Biology, Karolinska Inst 1988; **Fac Appt:** Prof NS, Cornell Univ-Weill Med Coll

Sutton, Leslie N MD [NS] - **Spec Exp:** Brain Tumors-Pediatric; Fetal Neurosurgery; Hydrocephalus; **Hospital:** Chldns Hosp of Philadelphia, The; **Address:** Childrens Hosp of Phila -Div Neurosurgery, 34th St & Civic Ctr Blvd Wood 6 Bldg, Philadelphia, PA 19104; **Phone:** 215-590-2780; **Board Cert:** Neurological Surgery 1984; Pediatric Neurological Surgery 1996; **Med School:** Univ Pennsylvania 1975; **Resid:** Neurological Surgery, Hosp Univ Penn 1981; **Fac Appt:** Prof NS, Univ Pennsylvania

Tamargo, Rafael J MD [NS] - **Spec Exp:** Vascular Neurosurgery; Skull Base Surgery; **Hospital:** Johns Hopkins Hosp (page 61); **Address:** Johns Hopkins Hosp, Dept Neurosurgery, 600 N Wolfe St, Meyer 8-181, Baltimore, MD 21287; **Phone:** 410-614-1533; **Board Cert:** Neurological Surgery 1995; **Med School:** Columbia P&S 1984; **Resid:** Neurological Surgery, Johns Hopkins Hosps 1992; **Fac Appt:** Prof NS, Johns Hopkins Univ

Turtz, Alan R MD [NS] - **Spec Exp:** Brain Tumors; Pituitary Tumors; Spinal Surgery; Neuro-Endoscopy; **Hospital:** Cooper Univ Hosp; **Address:** 3 Cooper Plaza, Ste 104, Camden, NJ 08103; **Phone:** 856-968-7965; **Board Cert:** Neurological Surgery 1995; **Med School:** Med Coll PA 1986; **Resid:** Neurological Surgery, Med Coll Penn 1992; **Fac Appt:** Assoc Prof NS, UMDNJ-RW Johnson Med Sch

Weiner, Howard L MD [NS] - **Spec Exp:** Pediatric Neurosurgery; Epilepsy; Brain Tumors; Tuberous Sclerosis; **Hospital:** NYU Langone Med Ctr (page 67); **Address:** NYU Med Ctr, Div Pediatric Neurosurgery, 317 E 34th St, Ste 1002, New York, NY 10016; **Phone:** 212-263-6419; **Board Cert:** Neurological Surgery 2001; **Med School:** Cornell Univ 1989; **Resid:** Neurological Surgery, NYU Med Ctr 1996; **Fellow:** Pediatric Neurological Surgery, NYU Med Ctr 1997; **Fac Appt:** Assoc Prof NS, NYU Sch Med

Welch, William C MD [NS] - **Spec Exp:** Spinal Surgery; **Hospital:** Pennsylvania Hosp (page 60); **Address:** Pennsylvania Hospital, Garfield-Duncan Bldg, 301 S 8th St, Ste 4B, Philadelphia, PA 19106; **Phone:** 215-829-6700; **Board Cert:** Neurological Surgery 1995; **Med School:** SUNY Downstate 1985; **Resid:** Neurological Surgery, Univ Rochester/Strong Meml Hosp 1991; **Fellow:** Neuro-Oncology, Montefiore Med Ctr 1992; Spinal Surgery, Montefiore Med Ctr/Albert Einstein 1993; **Fac Appt:** Prof NS, Univ Pennsylvania

Whiting, Donald M MD [NS] - **Spec Exp:** Movement Disorders; Pain & Spasticity; Spinal Disorders; **Hospital:** Allegheny General Hosp, Washington Hosp, The; **Address:** 380 West Chestnut St, Washington, PA 15301-4657; **Phone:** 724-228-1414; **Board Cert:** Neurological Surgery 1995; **Med School:** Jefferson Med Coll 1985; **Resid:** Surgery, Geisinger Med Ctr 1986; Neurological Surgery, Cleveland Clinic 1991; **Fellow:** Neurological Trauma, Allegheny Genl Hosp 1990; **Fac Appt:** Assoc Prof NS, Drexel Univ Coll Med

Wisoff, Jeffrey H MD [NS] - **Spec Exp:** Pediatric Neurosurgery; Brain Tumors-Pediatric; Hydrocephalus; Chiari's Deformity; **Hospital:** NYU Langone Med Ctr (page 67), Maimonides Med Ctr (page 63); **Address:** 317 E 34th St, Ste 1002, New York, NY 10016-4974; **Phone:** 212-263-6419; **Board Cert:** Neurological Surgery 1990; Pediatric Neurological Surgery 2008; **Med School:** Geo Wash Univ 1978; **Resid:** Neurological Surgery, NYU/Bellevue Hosp 1984; **Fellow:** Pediatric Neurological Surgery, NYU Med Ctr 1985; **Fac Appt:** Assoc Prof NS, NYU Sch Med

Zager, Eric L MD [NS] - **Spec Exp:** Peripheral Nerve Disorders; Carpal Tunnel Syndrome; Pediatric Neurosurgery; **Hospital:** Hosp Univ Penn - UPHS (page 60), Chldns Hosp of Philadelphia, The; **Address:** Hospital Univ Penn, Neurosurgery, 3400 Spruce St, 3 Silverstein, Philadelphia, PA 19104; **Phone:** 215-662-3497; **Board Cert:** Neurological Surgery 1992; **Med School:** Stanford Univ 1982; **Resid:** Neurological Surgery, Mass Genl Hosp 1988; **Fellow:** Peripheral Nerve Surgery, Univ Toronto 1989; Peripheral Nerve Surgery, LSU Med Ctr 1989; **Fac Appt:** Prof NS, Univ Pennsylvania

Southeast

Asher, Anthony MD [NS] - **Spec Exp:** Brain Tumors; Stereotactic Radiosurgery; Epilepsy; **Hospital:** Carolinas Med Ctr, Presby Hosp - Charlotte; **Address:** 225 Baldwin Ave, Charlotte, NC 28204; **Phone:** 704-376-1605; **Board Cert:** Neurological Surgery 1998; **Med School:** Wayne State Univ 1987; **Resid:** Neurological Surgery, Univ Mich Med Ctr 1995; **Fellow:** Surgical Oncology, Natl Cancer Inst 1991

Barrow, Daniel L MD [NS] - **Spec Exp:** Cerebrovascular Disease; Stroke; Aneurysm-Cerebral; Microsurgery; **Hospital:** Emory Univ Hosp; **Address:** Emory Clinic-Dept Neurosurgery, 1365B Clifton Rd NE, Ste 2200, Atlanta, GA 30322; **Phone:** 404-778-5770; **Board Cert:** Neurological Surgery 1988; **Med School:** Southern IL Univ 1979; **Resid:** Neurological Surgery, Emory Univ Hosps 1985; **Fellow:** Mayo Clinic 1986; **Fac Appt:** Prof NS, Emory Univ

Boop, Frederick A MD [NS] - **Spec Exp:** Pediatric Neurosurgery; Epilepsy; Brain Tumors; **Hospital:** Le Bonheur Chldns Med Ctr, Methodist Univ Hosp - Memphis; **Address:** Semmes Murphy Clinic, 1211 Union Ave, Ste 200, Memphis, TN 38104; **Phone:** 901-259-5340; **Board Cert:** Neurological Surgery 1993; Pediatric Neurological Surgery 2005; **Med School:** Univ Ark 1983; **Resid:** Neurological Surgery, Univ Tex Hlth Sci Ctr 1989; Neurological Surgery, Inst Neur/Hosp Sick Chldn 1987; **Fellow:** Epilepsy, Univ Minn 1989; Pediatric Neurological Surgery, Ark Chldns Hosp 1990; **Fac Appt:** Assoc Prof NS, Univ Tenn Coll Med, Memphis

Branch Jr, Charles L MD [NS] - **Spec Exp:** Spinal Reconstructive Surgery; Minimally Invasive Spinal Surgery; Stereotactic Radiosurgery; **Hospital:** Wake Forest Univ Baptist Med Ctr (page 72), Forsyth Med Ctr; **Address:** WFU Baptist Med Ctr, Medical Center Blvd, Winston-Salem, NC 27157-1029; **Phone:** 336-716-4083; **Board Cert:** Neurological Surgery 1991; **Med School:** Univ Tex SW, Dallas 1981; **Resid:** Neurological Surgery, NC Baptist Hosp 1987; **Fac Appt:** Prof NS, Wake Forest Univ

Brem, Steven MD [NS] - **Spec Exp:** Brain Tumors; Pituitary Tumors; Clinical Trials; Neuro-Oncology; **Hospital:** H Lee Moffitt Cancer Ctr & Research Inst; **Address:** H Lee Moffitt Cancer Ctr/Neurosurgery, 12902 Magnolia Drive, Neuro Program, Tampa, FL 33612-9497; **Phone:** 813-745-3056; **Board Cert:** Neurological Surgery 1983; **Med School:** Harvard Med Sch 1972; **Resid:** Neurological Surgery, Massachusetts Genl Hosp 1981; **Fellow:** Oncology, Natl Cancer Inst 1976; **Fac Appt:** Prof NS, Univ S Fla Coll Med

Ewend, Matthew MD [NS] - **Spec Exp:** Brain Tumors; Pituitary Tumors; Pediatric Neurosurgery; Epilepsy; **Hospital:** Univ NC Hosps; **Address:** Univ North Carolina Neurosurgery, 3015 Burnett Womack Bldg, CB# 7060, Chapel Hill, NC 27599; **Phone:** 919-966-1374; **Board Cert:** Neurological Surgery 2001; **Med School:** Johns Hopkins Univ 1990; **Resid:** Neurological Surgery, Johns Hopkins Hospital 1994; **Fellow:** Neuro-Oncology, National Institutes of Health 1996; **Fac Appt:** Asst Prof NS, Univ NC Sch Med

Neurological Surgery

Foley, Kevin MD [NS] - **Spec Exp:** Spinal Surgery; Minimally Invasive Spinal Surgery; **Hospital:** Methodist Univ Hosp - Memphis, Baptist Memorial Hospital - Memphis; **Address:** Semmes-Murphy Clin, 1211 Union Ave, Ste 200, Memphis, TN 38104; **Phone:** 901-259-5340; **Board Cert:** Neurological Surgery 1987; **Med School:** UCLA 1979; **Resid:** Neurological Surgery, UCLA Med Ctr 1985; **Fac Appt:** Prof NS, Univ Tenn Coll Med, Memphis

Freeman, Thomas B MD [NS] - **Spec Exp:** Parkinson's Disease; Nerve Surgery & Transplantation; Spinal Surgery; **Hospital:** Tampa Genl Hosp; **Address:** 2 Tampa Genl Circle Drive Fl 7th, Tampa, FL 33606; **Phone:** 813-259-0889; **Board Cert:** Neurological Surgery 1993; **Med School:** Johns Hopkins Univ 1981; **Resid:** Neurological Surgery, NYU Med Ctr 1988; **Fac Appt:** Prof NS, Univ S Fla Coll Med

Friedman, Allan H MD [NS] - **Spec Exp:** Brain Tumors; Skull Base Tumors; Cerebrovascular Surgery; **Hospital:** Duke Univ Med Ctr; **Address:** Duke Univ Med Ctr, DUMC 3807, Durham, NC 27710; **Phone:** 919-681-6421; **Board Cert:** Neurological Surgery 1983; **Med School:** Univ IL Coll Med 1974; **Resid:** Neurological Surgery, Duke Univ Med Ctr 1980; **Fellow:** Vascular Surgery, Univ Western Ontario 1981; **Fac Appt:** Prof S, Duke Univ

Green, Barth A MD [NS] - **Spec Exp:** Spinal Surgery; **Hospital:** Jackson Meml Hosp (page 70), Univ of Miami Hosp & Clins/Sylvester Comp Canc Ctr (page 70); **Address:** Univ Miami Dept Neurosurgery, 1095 NW 14th Terrace Fl 2, Miami, FL 33136; **Phone:** 305-243-6946; **Board Cert:** Neurological Surgery 1978; **Med School:** Indiana Univ 1969; **Resid:** Neurological Surgery, Northwestern Univ Hosp 1975; **Fac Appt:** Prof NS, Univ Miami Sch Med

Guthrie, Barton L MD [NS] - **Spec Exp:** Brain Tumors; Stereotactic Radiosurgery; Parkinson's Disease/Movement Disorders; **Hospital:** Univ of Ala Hosp at Birmingham; **Address:** Univ Alabama, Div Neurosurg, 510 20th St S, FOT 1038, Birmingham, AL 35294-3410; **Phone:** 205-934-8136; **Board Cert:** Neurological Surgery 1992; **Med School:** Univ Alabama 1980; **Resid:** Neurological Surgery, Mayo Clinic 1988; **Fellow:** Neurological Surgery, Stanford Univ Med Ctr 1988; **Fac Appt:** Assoc Prof NS, Univ Alabama

Hadley, Mark N MD [NS] - **Spec Exp:** Spinal Surgery-Complex; Spinal Disorders-Degenerative; **Hospital:** Univ of Ala Hosp at Birmingham; **Address:** UAB Sch Med, Div Neurosurgery, 510 20th St S, Ste FOT 1030, Birmingham, AL 35294-3410; **Phone:** 205-934-1439; **Board Cert:** Neurological Surgery 1992; **Med School:** Albany Med Coll 1982; **Resid:** Neurological Surgery, St Josephs Hosp Med Ctr 1988; **Fac Appt:** Prof NS, Univ Alabama

Haid Jr, Regis W MD [NS] - **Spec Exp:** Spinal Surgery; Minimally Invasive Spinal Surgery; Spinal Disc Replacement; Microdiscectomy; **Hospital:** Piedmont Hosp; **Address:** Atlanta Brain & Spine Care, 2001 Peachtree Rd NE, Ste 645, Atlanta, GA 30309; **Phone:** 404-350-0106; **Board Cert:** Neurological Surgery 2000; **Med School:** W VA Univ 1982; **Resid:** Surgery, W Va Univ Hosps 1983; Neurological Surgery, W Va Univ Hosps 1988; **Fellow:** Spinal Surgery, Univ Fl Affil Hosps 1989; **Fac Appt:** Assoc Prof NS, Emory Univ

Heros, Roberto MD [NS] - **Spec Exp:** Cerebrovascular Surgery; Skull Base Surgery; Brain Tumors; **Hospital:** Jackson Meml Hosp (page 70), Univ of Miami Hosp & Clins/Sylvester Comp Canc Ctr (page 70); **Address:** Univ Miami, Dept Neurosurgery, 1095 NW 14th Terrace, Miami, FL 33136; **Phone:** 305-243-4572; **Board Cert:** Neurological Surgery 1979; **Med School:** Univ Tenn Coll Med, Memphis 1968; **Resid:** Surgery, Mass Genl Hosp 1970; Neurological Surgery, Mass Genl Hosp 1976; **Fac Appt:** Prof NS, Univ Miami Sch Med

Landy, Howard J MD [NS] - **Spec Exp:** Stereotactic Radiosurgery; **Hospital:** Jackson Meml Hosp (page 70); **Address:** University of Miami, Neurosurgery, 1095 NW 14th Terrace Fl 2, Miami, FL 33136; **Phone:** 305-243-4675; **Board Cert:** Neurological Surgery 1991; **Med School:** Univ Miami Sch Med 1980; **Resid:** Neurological Surgery, Jackson Meml Hosp 1987; **Fac Appt:** Prof NS, Univ Miami Sch Med

Markert Jr, James M MD [NS] - **Spec Exp:** Brain Tumors; Stereotactic Radiosurgery; Clinical Trials; **Hospital:** Univ of Ala Hosp at Birmingham; **Address:** Univ Alabama, Div Neurosurgery, 510 20th St S, FOT, rm 1060, Birmingham, AL 35294; **Phone:** 205-975-6985; **Board Cert:** Neurological Surgery 1999; **Med School:** Columbia P&S 1988; **Resid:** Neurological Surgery, Univ Mich Med Ctr 1995; **Fellow:** Neuro-Oncology, Mass Genl Hosp; **Fac Appt:** Prof NS, Univ Alabama

Morrison, Glenn MD [NS] - **Spec Exp:** Pediatric Neurosurgery; Epilepsy; Craniofacial Surgery; Spinal Cord Tumors; **Hospital:** Miami Children's Hosp, Jackson Meml Hosp (page 70); **Address:** Ambulatory Care Bldg, 3215 SW 62nd Ave, Ste 3109, Miami, FL 33155; **Phone:** 305-662-8386; **Board Cert:** Neurological Surgery 1976; Pediatric Neurological Surgery 1996; **Med School:** Case West Res Univ 1967; **Resid:** Neurological Surgery, Case Western Univ Hosp 1974; **Fac Appt:** Prof NS, Univ Miami Sch Med

Myseros, John S MD [NS] - **Spec Exp:** Pediatric Neurosurgery; Brain Tumors; Congenital Nervous System Malformations; **Hospital:** Inova Fairfax Hosp for Chldn; **Address:** 8501 Arlington Blvd, Ste 450, Fairfax, VA 22031; **Phone:** 571-226-8330; **Board Cert:** Neurological Surgery 2000; **Med School:** Johns Hopkins Univ 1990; **Resid:** Neurological Surgery, Med Coll Virginia 1996; **Fellow:** Pediatric Neurological Surgery, Hosp for Sick Children 1997; **Fac Appt:** Assoc Prof NS, Geo Wash Univ

Oakes, W Jerry MD [NS] - **Spec Exp:** Pediatric Neurosurgery; Chiari's Deformity; Occult Spinal Dysraphism (OSD); **Hospital:** Children's Hospital - Birmingham; **Address:** Children's Hosp Alabama, 1600 7th Ave S ACC 400 Bldg, Birmingham, AL 35233; **Phone:** 205-939-9653; **Board Cert:** Neurological Surgery 1981; Pediatric Neurological Surgery 2005; **Med School:** Duke Univ 1972; **Resid:** Neurological Surgery, Duke Univ Hosp 1978; **Fellow:** Neurological Surgery, Hosp for Sick Chldn 1975; Neurological Surgery, Great Ormond St Hosp 1979; **Fac Appt:** Prof NS, Univ Alabama

Olson, Jeffrey J MD [NS] - **Spec Exp:** Neuro-Oncology; Brain Tumors; Stereotactic Radiosurgery; **Hospital:** Emory Univ Hosp, Emory Univ Hosp Midtown; **Address:** Emory Univ, Dept Neurosurgery, 1365B Clifton Rd NE, Ste 2200, Atlanta, GA 30322; **Phone:** 404-778-5770; **Board Cert:** Neurological Surgery 1989; **Med School:** Univ Minn 1981; **Resid:** Neurological Surgery, Univ Iowa Hosps & Clinics 1987; **Fellow:** Neurological Surgery, Natl Inst Hlth 1990; **Fac Appt:** Prof NS, Emory Univ

Parent, Andrew D MD [NS] - **Spec Exp:** Pediatric Neurosurgery; Neuroendocrine Tumors; Pituitary Tumors; **Hospital:** Univ Mississippi Med Ctr; **Address:** Univ Miss Med Ctr- Dept Neurosurgery, 2500 N State St, Jackson, MS 39216-4500; **Phone:** 601-984-5702; **Board Cert:** Neurological Surgery 1981; Pediatric Neurological Surgery 2005; **Med School:** Univ VT Coll Med 1970; **Resid:** Neurological Surgery, Emory Univ 1978; **Fellow:** Neurological Surgery, Univ Tex Med Br 1974; **Fac Appt:** Prof NS, Univ Miss

Patel, Sunil J MD [NS] - **Spec Exp:** Brain Tumors; Skull Base Surgery; Pain-Facial; Trigeminal Neuralgia; **Hospital:** MUSC Med Ctr, R H Johnson VA Med Ctr; **Address:** MUSC-Adult Neurological Surgery, CSB, Ste 428, Charleston, SC 29425; **Phone:** 843-792-7700; **Board Cert:** Neurological Surgery 1996; **Med School:** Med Univ SC 1985; **Resid:** Neurological Surgery, Univ South Carolina 1991; **Fellow:** Neurological Surgery, Nagoya Univ Med School 1991; Skull Base Surgery, Univ Pittsburgh 1993; **Fac Appt:** Prof NS, Med Univ SC

Neurological Surgery

Reid, William S MD [NS] - **Spec Exp:** Spinal Surgery; Spinal Cord Surgery; Brain & Spinal Cord Tumors; **Hospital:** Univ of Tennesee Mem Hosp; **Address:** 1932 Alcoa Hwy, Bldg C, Ste 280, Knoxville, TN 37920; **Phone:** 865-329-4003; **Board Cert:** Neurological Surgery 1980; **Med School:** Univ Ariz Coll Med 1971; **Resid:** Neurological Surgery, Univ Texas Hlth Sci Ctr 1975; **Fac Appt:** Assoc Clin Prof NS, Univ Tex SW, Dallas

Rodts Jr, Gerald E MD [NS] - **Spec Exp:** Spinal Surgery; **Hospital:** Emory Univ Hosp Midtown, Emory Univ Hosp; **Address:** Emory Spine Center, 59 Executive Park South, Ste 3000, Atlanta, GA 30329; **Phone:** 404-778-6227; **Board Cert:** Neurological Surgery 1998; **Med School:** Columbia P&S 1987; **Resid:** Neurological Surgery, UCLA Med Ctr 1994; **Fellow:** Spinal Surgery, Emory Univ Hosp 1995; **Fac Appt:** Prof NS, Emory Univ

Sampson, John H MD/PhD [NS] - **Spec Exp:** Brain Tumors; Clinical Trials; **Hospital:** Duke Univ Med Ctr; **Address:** Duke Univ Med Ctr, Box 3050, Durham, NC 27710; **Phone:** 919-684-9041; **Board Cert:** Neurological Surgery 2002; **Med School:** Univ Manitoba 1990; **Resid:** Neurological Surgery, Duke Univ Med Ctr 1998; **Fellow:** Neurological Intensive Care, Duke Univ Med Ctr 1999; **Fac Appt:** Assoc Prof S, Duke Univ

Sanford, Robert A MD [NS] - **Spec Exp:** Pediatric Neurosurgery; Brain Tumors-Pediatric; **Hospital:** Le Bonheur Chldns Med Ctr, St Jude Children's Research Hosp; **Address:** 6325 Humphreys Blvd, Memphis, TN 38120; **Phone:** 901-522-7762; **Board Cert:** Neurological Surgery 1976; Pediatric Neurological Surgery 2005; **Med School:** Univ Ark 1967; **Resid:** Neurological Surgery, Univ Minneapolis Med Ctr 1973; **Fac Appt:** Prof NS, Univ Tenn Coll Med, Memphis

Shaffrey, Christopher I MD [NS] - **Spec Exp:** Spinal Surgery; Spinal Surgery-Pediatric; **Hospital:** Univ Virginia Med Ctr; **Address:** Univ Virg, Dept Neurosurg, Hosp Drive, Private Clinic 3rd Fl, Rm 3508, Charlottesville, VA 22908; **Phone:** 434-243-7026; **Board Cert:** Neurological Surgery 1997; Orthopaedic Surgery 2008; **Med School:** Univ VA Sch Med 1986; **Resid:** Neurological Surgery, Univ Virginia Med Ctr 1992; Orthopaedic Surgery, Univ Virginia Med Ctr 1995; **Fellow:** Spinal Surgery, Univ Virginia Med Ctr 1996; **Fac Appt:** Prof NS, Univ VA Sch Med

Shaffrey, Mark E MD [NS] - **Spec Exp:** Brain Tumors; Clinical Trials; Spinal Cord Tumors; Spinal Tumors; **Hospital:** Univ Virginia Med Ctr; **Address:** UVA Health System, Dept Neurosurgery, PO Box 800212, Charlottesville, VA 22908; **Phone:** 434-924-1843; **Board Cert:** Neurological Surgery 2000; **Med School:** Univ VA Sch Med 1987; **Resid:** Neurological Surgery, Univ Virginia Med Ctr 1991; **Fellow:** Microvascular Physiology, NIH 1992; Neurological Pathology, Univ Virginia Med Ctr 1993; **Fac Appt:** Prof NS, Univ VA Sch Med

Sills Jr, Allen MD [NS] - **Spec Exp:** Brain & Spinal Tumors; Stereotactic Radiosurgery; Cerebrovascular Disease; **Hospital:** Methodist Univ Hosp - Memphis; **Address:** Semmes-Murphey Clinic, 1211 Union Ave, Ste 200, Memphis, TN 38104; **Phone:** 901-259-5340; **Board Cert:** Neurological Surgery 2002; **Med School:** Johns Hopkins Univ 1990; **Resid:** Neurological Surgery, Johns Hopkins Hosp 1994; **Fellow:** Neuro-Oncology, Hunterian Neurosurg Lab/Johns Hopkins 1996; **Fac Appt:** Prof NS, Univ Tenn Coll Med, Memphis

Swaid, Swaid N MD [NS] - **Spec Exp:** Stereotactic Radiosurgery; **Hospital:** UAB Highlands Hosp; **Address:** 513 Brookwood Blvd, Ste 372, Birmingham, AL 35209; **Phone:** 205-802-6844; **Board Cert:** Neurological Surgery 1983; **Med School:** Univ Alabama 1976; **Resid:** Neurological Surgery, UAB Med Ctr 1981; **Fac Appt:** Assoc Prof NS, Univ Alabama

Tatter, Stephen MD/PhD [NS] - **Spec Exp:** Brain Tumors; Pituitary Tumors; Stereotactic Radiosurgery; **Hospital:** Wake Forest Univ Baptist Med Ctr (page 72); **Address:** Wake Forest Univ Sch Med, Dept Neurosurg, Medical Center Blvd, Winston-Salem, NC 27157-1029; **Phone:** 336-716-4047; **Board Cert:** Neurological Surgery 2004; **Med School:** Cornell Univ-Weill Med Coll 1990; **Resid:** Neurological Surgery, Mass Genl Hosp 1996; **Fellow:** Neurological Surgery, Mass Genl Hosp 1997; **Fac Appt:** Assoc Prof NS, Wake Forest Univ

Thompson, Reid C MD [NS] - **Spec Exp:** Neuro-Oncology; Brain & Spinal Cord Tumors; Neurovascular Surgery; Skull Base Tumors; **Hospital:** Vanderbilt Univ Med Ctr; **Address:** Vanderbilt Univ Med Ctr, Dept Neurosurg, 1500 21st Ave S, Ste 1506, Nashville, TN 37212; **Phone:** 615-322-7417; **Board Cert:** Neurological Surgery 2001; **Med School:** Johns Hopkins Univ 1989; **Resid:** Neurological Surgery, Johns Hopkins Hosp 1995; **Fellow:** Neuro-Oncology, Rsch-Johns Hopkins Hosp 1996; Cerebrovascular Neurosurgery, Stanford Univ Med Ctr 1997; **Fac Appt:** Assoc Prof NS, Vanderbilt Univ

Tiel, Robert L MD [NS] - **Hospital:** Univ Mississippi Med Ctr; **Address:** Univ Mississippi Med Ctr, 2500 N State St, Jackson, MS 39216-4505; **Phone:** 601-984-6445; **Board Cert:** Neurological Surgery 1991; **Med School:** Univ Minn 1980; **Resid:** Neurological Surgery, Henry Ford Hosp 1986; **Fac Appt:** Prof NS, Univ Miss

Van Loveren, Harry R MD [NS] - **Spec Exp:** Trigeminal Neuralgia; Skull Base Surgery; **Hospital:** Tampa Genl Hosp; **Address:** Harbourside Medical Tower, 2 Tampa Genl Cir, Tampa, FL 33606; **Phone:** 813-259-0929; **Board Cert:** Neurological Surgery 1988; **Med School:** Univ Cincinnati 1979; **Resid:** Neurological Surgery, Good Samaritan Hosp 1984; **Fellow:** Neurological Surgery, Universitatspital 1985; **Fac Appt:** Prof NS, Univ S Fla Coll Med

Wharen Jr, Robert E MD [NS] - **Spec Exp:** Parkinson's Disease; Brain Tumors; Epilepsy; **Hospital:** Mayo - Jacksonville; **Address:** Mayo Clinic, Dept Neurosurgery, 4500 San Pablo Rd, Jacksonville, FL 32224-1865; **Phone:** 904-953-2103; **Board Cert:** Neurological Surgery 1988; **Med School:** Penn State Univ-Hershey Med Ctr 1979; **Resid:** Neurological Surgery, Mayo Clinic 1985; **Fac Appt:** Prof NS, Mayo Med Sch

Wilson, John A MD [NS] - **Spec Exp:** Cerebrovascular Surgery; Skull Base Surgery; Spinal Surgery; **Hospital:** Wake Forest Univ Baptist Med Ctr (page 72); **Address:** Wake Forest Univ Medical Ctr, Medical Center Blvd, Box 1029, Winston-Salem, NC 27157-1029; **Phone:** 336-716-4020; **Board Cert:** Neurological Surgery 1996; **Med School:** Jefferson Med Coll 1982; **Resid:** Surgery, Allegheny Gen Hosp 1985; Neurological Surgery, NYU Med Ctr 1986; **Fellow:** Neurological Surgery, New England Med Ctr 1990; **Fac Appt:** Assoc Prof NS, Wake Forest Univ

Young, Byron MD [NS] - **Spec Exp:** Brain Tumors; Stereotactic Radiosurgery; Parkinson's Disease; Trigeminal Neuralgia; **Hospital:** Univ of Kentucky Chandler Hosp; **Address:** Div Neurosurgery, MS 101, 800 Rose St, Lexington, KY 40536-0298; **Phone:** 859-323-5861; **Board Cert:** Neurological Surgery 1974; **Med School:** Univ KY Coll Med 1965; **Resid:** Surgery, Vanderbilt Univ Hosp 1967; Neurological Surgery, Vanderbilt Univ Hosp 1971; **Fac Appt:** Prof NS, Univ KY Coll Med

Midwest

Albright, A Leland MD [NS] - **Spec Exp:** Pediatric Neurosurgery; Spasticity & Movement Disorders; Brain Tumors; **Hospital:** Univ WI Hosp & Clins; **Address:** Dept Neurosurgery, 600 Highland Ave, rm K4/836, Madison, WI 53792; **Phone:** 608-263-9651; **Board Cert:** Neurological Surgery 1981; Pediatric Neurological Surgery 2005; **Med School:** Louisiana State U, New Orleans 1969; **Resid:** Surgery, Wash Hosps 1971; Neurological Surgery, Univ Pittsburgh Med Ctr 1978; **Fellow:** Neurological Surgery, Natl Inst Hlth 1974; Immunopathology, Univ Pittsburgh Med Ctr 1978; **Fac Appt:** Prof NS, Univ Wisc

Atkinson, John L MD [NS] - **Spec Exp:** Pituitary Surgery; Stroke; Cerebrovascular Disease; **Hospital:** Mayo Med Ctr & Clin - Rochester; **Address:** Mayo Clin, Dept Neurosurgery, 200 First St SW, Rochester, MN 55905; **Phone:** 507-284-2376; **Board Cert:** Neurological Surgery 1992; **Med School:** Univ Alabama 1984; **Resid:** Neurological Surgery, Mayo Clin 1990; **Fac Appt:** Assoc Prof NS, Mayo Med Sch

Bakay, Roy AE MD [NS] - **Spec Exp:** Parkinson's Disease/Movement Disorders; Epilepsy; Brain Tumors; **Hospital:** Rush Univ Med Ctr; **Address:** Rush Univ Med Ctr, 1725 W Harrison St, Ste 970, Chicago, IL 60612; **Phone:** 312-942-6644; **Board Cert:** Neurological Surgery 1985; **Med School:** Northwestern Univ 1975; **Resid:** Neurological Surgery, Univ Washington Med Ctr 1981; **Fellow:** Neuronal Plasticity, Natl Inst Hlth 1982; **Fac Appt:** Prof NS, Rush Med Coll

Barnett, Gene H MD [NS] - **Spec Exp:** Brain Tumors; Stereotactic Radiosurgery; **Hospital:** Cleveland Clin Fdn (page 56); **Address:** Cleveland Clinic Brain Tumor Inst, 9500 Euclid Ave, Desk R20, Cleveland, OH 44195; **Phone:** 216-444-5381; **Board Cert:** Neurological Surgery 1990; **Med School:** Case West Res Univ 1980; **Resid:** Neurological Surgery, Cleveland Clinic 1986; **Fellow:** Neurology, Cleveland Clinic 1982; Research, Mass Genl Hosp-Harvard 1987; **Fac Appt:** Prof NS, Cleveland Cl Coll Med/Case West Res

Batjer, Hunt Henry MD [NS] - **Spec Exp:** Aneurysm-Cerebral; Arteriovenous Malformations; Stroke; **Hospital:** Northwestern Meml Hosp, Evanston/Northshore Univ Hlth Syst; **Address:** 675 N St Clair, Galter Bldg Fl 20 - Ste 250, Chicago, IL 60611; **Phone:** 312-695-8143; **Board Cert:** Neurological Surgery 1986; **Med School:** Univ Tex SW, Dallas 1977; **Resid:** Neurological Surgery, Parkland Meml Hosp 1981; **Fellow:** Neurological Surgery, Univ W Ontario Med Ctr 1982; **Fac Appt:** Prof NS, Northwestern Univ

Bauer, Jerry MD [NS] - **Spec Exp:** Pain-Back; Minimally Invasive Surgery; Spinal Surgery; **Hospital:** Adv Luth Genl Hosp; **Address:** Ctr Brain & Spine Surg-Parkside Ctr, 1875 Dempster St, Ste 605, Park Ridge, IL 60068-1168; **Phone:** 847-698-1088; **Board Cert:** Neurological Surgery 1982; **Med School:** Univ IL Coll Med 1974; **Resid:** Neurological Surgery, Univ Illinois Med Ctr 1979; **Fac Appt:** Asst Clin Prof NS, Univ IL Coll Med

Benzel, Edward C MD [NS] - **Spec Exp:** Spinal Surgery; **Hospital:** Cleveland Clin Fdn (page 56); **Address:** 9500 Euclid Ave, Desk S80, Cleveland, OH 44195; **Phone:** 216-445-5514; **Board Cert:** Neurological Surgery 1986; **Med School:** Univ Wisc 1975; **Resid:** Neurological Surgery, Med Coll Wisc Clins 1980; **Fellow:** Spinal Cord Injury Medicine, Wood VA Med Ctr 1981; **Fac Appt:** Prof NS, Case West Res Univ

Bierbrauer, Karin S MD [NS] - **Spec Exp:** Pediatric Neurosurgery; Spina Bifida; Craniosynostosis; Hydrocephalus; **Hospital:** Cincinnati Chldns Hosp Med Ctr; **Address:** Cincinnati Childrens Hospital, 3333 Burnet Ave, MC 2016, Cincinnati, OH 45229; **Phone:** 513-636-7124; **Board Cert:** Neurological Surgery 1994; Pediatric Neurological Surgery 1995; **Med School:** Med Univ SC 1984; **Resid:** Neurological Surgery, Emory Univ Hosp 1990; **Fellow:** Pediatric Neurological Surgery, Chldns Meml Hosp 1991; **Fac Appt:** Assoc Clin Prof NS, Ohio State Univ

Brown, Frederick D MD [NS] - **Spec Exp:** Minimally Invasive Spinal Surgery; Spinal Surgery; Pain-Chronic; **Hospital:** Univ of Chicago Med Ctr; **Address:** Univ Chicago Hosp, Dept Neurosurgery, 5841 S Maryland Ave, MC 3026, Chicago, IL 60617; **Phone:** 773-702-2123; **Board Cert:** Neurological Surgery 1982; **Med School:** Ohio State Univ 1972; **Resid:** Neurological Surgery, Univ Chicago Hosps 1978; **Fac Appt:** Assoc Prof NS, Univ Chicago-Pritzker Sch Med

Chandler, James P MD [NS] - **Spec Exp:** Skull Base Surgery; Neuro-Oncology; Brain Tumors; Spinal Disorders; **Hospital:** Northwestern Meml Hosp; **Address:** 675 N St Clair St, Galter Pavilion, Ste 20-250, Chicago, IL 60611; **Phone:** 312-695-8143; **Board Cert:** Neurological Surgery 2002; **Med School:** Univ MD Sch Med 1990; **Resid:** Neurological Surgery, Northwestern Meml Hosp 1996; **Fellow:** Microvascular Surgery, Inst Neurologico De S„o Paulo 1996; Cranial Base Surgery, George Washington Univ Hosp 1997; **Fac Appt:** Asst Prof NS, Northwestern Univ

Chandler, William F MD [NS] - **Spec Exp:** Pituitary Surgery; Brain Tumors; **Hospital:** Univ Michigan Hlth Sys; **Address:** 1500 E Med Center Drive, Ste 3470, Tauban Center, Ann Arbor, MI 48109; **Phone:** 734-936-5020; **Board Cert:** Neurological Surgery 1980; **Med School:** Univ Mich Med Sch 1971; **Resid:** Neurological Surgery, Michigan Hosp 1977; **Fac Appt:** Prof NS, Univ Mich Med Sch

Chiocca, E Antonio MD [NS] - **Spec Exp:** Brain Tumors; Spinal Cord Tumors; **Hospital:** Arthur G James Cancer Hosp & Research Inst, Ohio St Univ Med Ctr; **Address:** OSU Med Ctr, Dept Neurosurgery, 410 W 10th Ave, 1021-N Doan Hall, Columbus, OH 43210; **Phone:** 614-293-9312; **Board Cert:** Neurological Surgery 2000; **Med School:** Univ Tex, Houston 1988; **Resid:** Neurological Surgery, Mass Genl Hosp 1995; **Fac Appt:** Prof NS, Ohio State Univ

Cohen, Alan R MD [NS] - **Spec Exp:** Pediatric Neurosurgery; Brain & Spinal Tumors-Pediatric; Minimally Invasive Surgery; **Hospital:** Rainbow Babies & Chldns Hosp, Univ Hosps Case Med Ctr; **Address:** 11100 Euclid Ave, Ste B501, Cleveland, OH 44106; **Phone:** 216-844-5741; **Board Cert:** Neurological Surgery 1991; Pediatric Neurological Surgery 2007; **Med School:** Cornell Univ-Weill Med Coll 1978; **Resid:** Surgery, NYU Medical Ctr 1980; Neurological Surgery, NYU Medical Ctr 1987; **Fellow:** Neurology, Natl Hosp Queen's Square 1982; **Fac Appt:** Prof NS, Case West Res Univ

Dacey Jr, Ralph G MD [NS] - **Spec Exp:** Cerebrovascular Surgery; Aneurysm-Cerebral; Brain Tumors; **Hospital:** Barnes-Jewish Hosp, Barnes-Jewish West County Hosp; **Address:** Wash Univ Dept Neurosurgery, 660 S Euclid Ave, Box 8057, St Louis, MO 63110; **Phone:** 314-362-3577; **Board Cert:** Internal Medicine 1978; Neurological Surgery 1985; **Med School:** Univ VA Sch Med 1974; **Resid:** Internal Medicine, Strong Meml Hosp 1977; Neurological Surgery, Univ Virginia Med Ctr 1983; **Fac Appt:** Prof NS, Washington Univ, St Louis

Dempsey, Robert J MD [NS] - **Spec Exp:** Vascular Neurosurgery; Aneurysm-Cerebral; Stroke; **Hospital:** Univ WI Hosp & Clins; **Address:** Dept Neurosurgery, 600 Highland Ave, rm K4-822, Madison, WI 53792; **Phone:** 608-265-5967; **Board Cert:** Neurological Surgery 1985; **Med School:** Univ Chicago-Pritzker Sch Med 1977; **Resid:** Neurological Surgery, Univ Mich Hosps 1983; **Fac Appt:** Prof NS, Univ Wisc

Diaz, Fernando G MD/PhD [NS] - **Spec Exp:** Arteriovenous Malformations; Spinal Surgery; **Hospital:** Providence Hosp - Southfield, William Beaumont Hosp; **Address:** Michigan Head & Spine Institute, 29275 Northwestern Hwy, Ste 100, Southfield, MI 48034; **Phone:** 877-784-3667; **Board Cert:** Neurological Surgery 1980; **Med School:** Mexico 1968; **Resid:** Surgery, Univ Kansas Med Ctr 1973; Neurological Surgery, Univ Minn Med Ctr 1978; **Fellow:** Cerebrovascular Disease, Univ Minn Med Ctr 1979; **Fac Appt:** Prof NS, Wayne State Univ

Fessler, Richard G MD/PhD [NS] - **Spec Exp:** Skull Base Surgery; Spinal Surgery; Minimally Invasive Spinal Surgery; **Hospital:** Northwestern Meml Hosp; **Address:** 676 N St Clair, Ste 2210, Galter Bldg Fl 20, Chicago, IL 60611; **Phone:** 312-695-8143; **Board Cert:** Neurological Surgery 1992; **Med School:** Univ Chicago-Pritzker Sch Med 1983; **Resid:** Neurological Surgery, Univ Chicago Hosp 1989; **Fac Appt:** Prof NS, Northwestern Univ

Neurological Surgery

Frim, David M MD/PhD [NS] - **Spec Exp:** Pediatric Neurosurgery; Hydrocephalus; Brain & Spinal Tumors; Brain & Spinal Malformations; **Hospital:** Univ of Chicago Med Ctr; **Address:** Univ of Chicago Hosps, Pediatric Neurosurgery, 5841 S Maryland Ave, MC 3026, Chicago, IL 60637-1463; **Phone:** 773-702-2475; **Board Cert:** Neurological Surgery 1998; Pediatric Neurological Surgery 1998; **Med School:** Harvard Med Sch 1988; **Resid:** Neurological Surgery, Mass Genl Hosp 1995; **Fellow:** Pediatric Neurological Surgery, Chldns Hosp 1996; **Fac Appt:** Assoc Prof S, Univ Chicago-Pritzker Sch Med

Greene Jr, Clarence S MD [NS] - **Spec Exp:** Pediatric Neurosurgery; Congenital Nervous System Malformations; Brain Tumors; **Hospital:** Chldns Mercy Hosps & Clinics; **Address:** 2401 Gillham Rd, Kansas City, MO 64108; **Phone:** 816-234-3000; **Board Cert:** Neurological Surgery 1984; Pediatric Neurological Surgery 2007; **Med School:** Howard Univ 1974; **Resid:** Neurological Surgery, Chldns Hosp 1981; Neurological Surgery, Peter Bent Brigham Hosp 1981; **Fellow:** Pediatric Neurological Surgery, Chldns Hosp 1985; **Fac Appt:** Assoc Clin Prof NS, UC Irvine

Grubb Jr, Robert L MD [NS] - **Spec Exp:** Brain Tumors; Acoustic Neuroma; Trigeminal Neuralgia; Skull Base Tumors; **Hospital:** Barnes-Jewish Hosp, St Louis Chldns Hosp; **Address:** Wash Univ Sch Med, Dept Neurosurgery, 660 S Euclid Ave, Box 8057, St Louis, MO 63110; **Phone:** 314-362-3567; **Board Cert:** Neurological Surgery 1976; **Med School:** Univ NC Sch Med 1965; **Resid:** Surgery, Barnes Jewish Hosp 1967; Neurological Surgery, Barnes Jewish Hosp 1973; **Fellow:** Neurological Surgery, National Inst Health 1969; **Fac Appt:** Prof NS, Washington Univ, St Louis

Guthikonda, Murali MD [NS] - **Spec Exp:** Skull Base Tumors; Pituitary Tumors; Aneurysm-Cerebral; Spinal Tumors; **Hospital:** Detroit Med Ctr, Harper Univ Hosp; **Address:** Wayne St U Physicians Grp-Neurosurgery, 4160 John R, Ste 930, Detroit, MI 48201; **Phone:** 313-831-0777; **Board Cert:** Neurological Surgery 1982; **Med School:** India 1971; **Resid:** Surgery, St Elizabeth Hosp 1976; Neurological Surgery, Med Ctr Hosp VT 1980; **Fellow:** Skull Base Surgery, Univ Cincinnati 1993; **Fac Appt:** Assoc Prof NS, Wayne State Univ

Gutierrez, Francisco A MD [NS] - **Spec Exp:** Brain Tumors; Cerebrovascular Surgery; Spinal Surgery; **Hospital:** Northwestern Meml Hosp, Resurrection Med Ctr; **Address:** 7447 W Talcott, Ste 340, Galter Pavilion, Chicago, IL 60631; **Phone:** 773-594-0200; **Board Cert:** Neurological Surgery 1976; **Med School:** Colombia 1965; **Resid:** Neurological Surgery, San Juan de Dios Hosp 1967; Neurological Surgery, Northwestern Meml Hosp 1973; **Fac Appt:** Assoc Prof NS, Northwestern Univ

Kaufman, Bruce A MD [NS] - **Spec Exp:** Pediatric Neurosurgery; Brain & Spinal Cord Tumors; Spasticity & Movement Disorders; **Hospital:** Chldns Hosp - Wisconsin; **Address:** Chldns Hosp, Dept Neurosurg, 999 N 92nd St, Ste 310, Milwaukee, WI 53226; **Phone:** 414-266-6435; **Board Cert:** Neurological Surgery 1992; Pediatric Neurological Surgery 2006; **Med School:** Case West Res Univ 1982; **Resid:** Neurological Surgery, Univ Hosp Cleveland/Case West Res 1988; **Fellow:** Pediatric Neurological Surgery, Chldns Meml Hosp/Northwestern Univ 1989; **Fac Appt:** Prof NS, Med Coll Wisc

Levy, Robert M MD/PhD [NS] - **Spec Exp:** Stereotactic Radiosurgery; Brain Tumors; Pain-Chronic; **Hospital:** Northwestern Meml Hosp; **Address:** 675 N Saint Clair St, Ste 2210, Galter Bldg Fl 20, Chicago, IL 60611-2922; **Phone:** 312-695-8143; **Board Cert:** Neurological Surgery 1991; **Med School:** Stanford Univ 1981; **Resid:** Neurological Surgery, UCSF Med Ctr 1987; **Fellow:** Neurological Surgery, UCSF Med Ctr 1986; **Fac Appt:** Prof NS, Northwestern Univ

Link, Michael J MD [NS] - **Spec Exp:** Skull Base Tumors; Brain Tumors; Cerebrovascular Surgery; **Hospital:** Mayo Med Ctr & Clin - Rochester; **Address:** Mayo Clinic, Dept Neurosurgery, 200 First St SW, Rochester, MN 55905; **Phone:** 507-284-8008; **Board Cert:** Neurological Surgery 2000; **Med School:** Mayo Med Sch 1990; **Resid:** Neurological Surgery, Mayo Clinic 1996; **Fellow:** Cerebrovascular & Skull Base Surgery, Univ Cincinnati/Mayfield Clinic 1998; **Fac Appt:** Assoc Prof NS, Mayo Med Sch

Luken, Martin MD [NS] - **Spec Exp:** Brain Tumors; Spinal Surgery; Chiari's Deformity; **Hospital:** Ingalls Meml Hosp, Neuro & Ortho Hosp of Chicago; **Address:** 71 W 156 St, Ste 208, Chicago, IL 60426; **Phone:** 773-331-6669; **Board Cert:** Neurological Surgery 1983; **Med School:** Columbia P&S 1973; **Resid:** Surgery, Univ Illinois Med Ctr 1976; Neurological Surgery, Neurological Inst-Columbia Presby 1980; **Fac Appt:** Asst Prof NS, Rush Med Coll

Malik, Ghaus MD [NS] - **Spec Exp:** Trigeminal Neuralgia; Cerebrovascular Surgery; Brain & Spinal Cord Tumors; **Hospital:** Henry Ford Hosp, William Beaumont Hosp; **Address:** Henry Ford Hosp, Dept Neurosurg, 2799 W Grand Blvd, Detroit, MI 48202; **Phone:** 313-916-1093; **Board Cert:** Neurological Surgery 1978; **Med School:** Pakistan 1968; **Resid:** Surgery, Henry Ford Hosp 1971; Neurological Surgery, Henry Ford Hosp 1975

Menezes, Arnold MD [NS] - **Spec Exp:** Pediatric Neurosurgery; Craniocervical Disorders; Spinal Surgery-Pediatric; **Hospital:** Univ Iowa Hosp & Clinics; **Address:** Univ Iowa Hosp, Dept Neurosurgery, 200 Hawkins Drive, rm 1824JPP, Iowa City, IA 52242; **Phone:** 319-356-2768; **Board Cert:** Neurological Surgery 1976; Pediatric Neurological Surgery 1997; **Med School:** India 1967; **Resid:** Surgery, Univ Iowa Hosps 1970; Neurological Surgery, Univ Iowa Hosps 1974; **Fellow:** Child Neurology, Univ Iowa Hosps; **Fac Appt:** Prof NS, Univ Iowa Coll Med

Meyer, Fredric B MD [NS] - **Spec Exp:** Cerebrovascular Disease; Brain Tumors; Epilepsy; Pituitary Tumors; **Hospital:** Mayo Med Ctr & Clin - Rochester; **Address:** Mayo Clinic Dept Neurosurgery, 200 First St SW, Rochester, MN 55905; **Phone:** 507-284-5317; **Board Cert:** Neurological Surgery 1990; **Med School:** Boston Univ 1981; **Resid:** Neurological Surgery, Mayo Clin 1987; **Fellow:** Neurological Surgery, Mayo Clin 1988; **Fac Appt:** Prof NS, Mayo Med Sch

Nagib, Mahmoud MD [NS] - **Spec Exp:** Pediatric Neurosurgery; Skull Base Surgery; **Hospital:** Chldns Hosp and Clinics - Minneapolis, Abbott - Northwestern Hosp; **Address:** 800 E 28th St Piper Bldg - Ste 305, Minneapolis, MN 55407-3723; **Phone:** 612-871-7278; **Board Cert:** Neurological Surgery 1985; **Med School:** Egypt 1973; **Resid:** Neurological Surgery, Univ Minn Hosps 1982; **Fellow:** Neurological Physiology, Univ Oslo 1976; **Fac Appt:** Clin Prof NS, Univ Minn

Origitano, Thomas MD/PhD [NS] - **Spec Exp:** Skull Base Tumors & Surgery; Cerebrovascular Surgery; Brain Tumors; Hydrocephalus-Adult; **Hospital:** Loyola Univ Med Ctr; **Address:** Loyola Univ Med Ctr, Dept Neurosurgery, 2160 S First Ave Bldg 105 - rm 1900, Maywood, IL 60153-3304; **Phone:** 708-216-8920; **Board Cert:** Neurological Surgery 1995; **Med School:** Loyola Univ-Stritch Sch Med 1984; **Resid:** Neurological Surgery, Loyola Univ Med Ctr 1990; **Fac Appt:** Prof NS, Loyola Univ-Stritch Sch Med

Park, Tae Sung MD [NS] - **Spec Exp:** Pediatric Neurosurgery; Cerebral Palsy-Select Dorsal Rhizotomy; Brachial Plexus Palsy-Pediatric; Neuro-Oncology; **Hospital:** St Louis Chldns Hosp; **Address:** St Louis Children's Hospital, 1 Children's Place, Ste 4-S20, St Louis, MO 63110; **Phone:** 314-454-4629; **Board Cert:** Neurological Surgery 1985; Pediatric Neurological Surgery 2006; **Med School:** Korea 1971; **Resid:** Neurological Surgery, Univ Virginia Hosp 1981; **Fellow:** Pediatric Neurological Surgery, Hosp for Sick Chldn 1983; **Fac Appt:** Prof NS, Washington Univ, St Louis

Neurological Surgery

Piepgras, David MD [NS] - **Spec Exp:** Vascular Neurosurgery; Minimally Invasive Spinal Surgery; Pain-Facial; **Hospital:** Mayo Med Ctr & Clin - Rochester, St Mary's Hosp - Rochester; **Address:** Mayo Clin, Dept Neuro Surg, 200 First St SW, Rochester, MN 55905; **Phone:** 507-284-3331; **Board Cert:** Neurological Surgery 1977; **Med School:** Univ Minn 1965; **Resid:** Surgery, Hennipin Co Genl Hosp 1970; Neurological Surgery, Mayo Clin 1974; **Fac Appt:** Prof NS, Mayo Med Sch

Raffel, Corey MD/PhD [NS] - **Spec Exp:** Pediatric Neurosurgery; Brain Tumors; Medulloblastoma; **Hospital:** Nationwide Chldn's Hosp; **Address:** Nationwide Chldn's Hosp, Dept Neurosurgery, 700 Children's Drive, Columbus, OH 43205; **Phone:** 614-722-2014; **Board Cert:** Neurological Surgery 1990; Pediatric Neurological Surgery 1996; **Med School:** UCSD 1980; **Resid:** Neurological Surgery, UCSF Med Ctr 1986; **Fellow:** Pediatric Neurological Surgery, Hosp Sick Chldn 1988

Rezai, Ali R MD [NS] - **Spec Exp:** Parkinson's Disease; Pain-Chronic; Deep Brain Stimulation; Alzheimer's Disease; **Hospital:** Cleveland Clin Fdn (page 56); **Address:** 9500 Euclid Ave, MC S31, Cleveland, OH 44195; **Phone:** 216-444-8001; **Board Cert:** Neurological Surgery 2003; **Med School:** USC Sch Med 1990; **Resid:** Neurological Surgery, NYU Med Ctr 1997; **Fellow:** Stereo Neurological Surgery, Univ Toronto Med Ctr 1998; Neurological Surgery, Karolinska Inst; **Fac Appt:** Assoc Prof NS, Cleveland Cl Coll Med/Case West Res

Rich, Keith M MD [NS] - **Spec Exp:** Brain Tumors; Neurovascular Surgery; Stereotactic Radiosurgery; **Hospital:** Barnes-Jewish Hosp; **Address:** Wash Univ Dept Neurosurgery, 660 S Euclid Ave, Box 8057, St Louis, MO 63110; **Phone:** 314-362-3577; **Board Cert:** Neurological Surgery 1987; **Med School:** Indiana Univ 1977; **Resid:** Neurological Surgery, Barnes Jewish Hosp 1982; **Fellow:** Neurological Pharmacology, Barnes Jewish Hosp 1984; **Fac Appt:** Assoc Prof NS, Washington Univ, St Louis

Rock, Jack P MD [NS] - **Spec Exp:** Neuro-Oncology; Pituitary Surgery; Skull Base Surgery; Brain Tumors; **Hospital:** Henry Ford Hosp; **Address:** Henry Ford Hosp, Dept Neurosurg, 2799 W Grand Blvd, Detroit, MI 48202; **Phone:** 313-916-2241; **Board Cert:** Neurological Surgery 1989; **Med School:** Univ Miami Sch Med 1979; **Resid:** Neurological Surgery, New York Hosp-Cornell 1985; **Fellow:** Univ Maryland 1986

Rosenblum, Mark L MD [NS] - **Spec Exp:** Brain Tumors; Spinal Surgery; Infections-Neurologic; Neuro-Oncology; **Hospital:** Henry Ford Hosp; **Address:** Henry Ford Hospital, K11, 2799 W Grand Blvd, Detroit, MI 48202; **Phone:** 313-916-1340; **Board Cert:** Neurological Surgery 1982; **Med School:** NY Med Coll 1969; **Resid:** Surgery, UCLA Med Ctr 1973; Neurological Surgery, UCSF Med Ctr 1979; **Fellow:** Neuro-Oncology, NIH/Natl Cancer Inst 1972

Ruge, John MD [NS] - **Spec Exp:** Pediatric Neurosurgery; Brain Tumors; Hydrocephalus; **Hospital:** Adv Luth Genl Hosp; **Address:** Ctr Brain & Spine Surg-Parkside Ctr, 1875 Dempster St, Ste 605, Park Ridge, IL 60068; **Phone:** 847-698-1088; **Board Cert:** Neurological Surgery 1993; **Med School:** Northwestern Univ 1983; **Resid:** Neurological Surgery, Northwestern Meml Hosp 1989; **Fellow:** Pediatric Neurological Surgery, Childrens Hosp 1990; **Fac Appt:** Asst Prof S, Rush Med Coll

Ryken, Timothy C MD [NS] - **Spec Exp:** Brain Tumors; Spinal Surgery; **Hospital:** Covenant Med Ctr; **Address:** Iowa Spine & Brain Institute, 2710 St Francis Drive, Ste 110, Waterloo, IA 50702; **Phone:** 319-272-6700; **Board Cert:** Neurological Surgery 1998; **Med School:** Univ Iowa Coll Med 1988; **Resid:** Neurological Surgery, Univ Iowa 1995; **Fellow:** Cambridge Univ 1996; **Fac Appt:** Assoc Prof NS, Univ Iowa Coll Med

Selman, Warren R MD [NS] - **Spec Exp:** Stroke; Pituitary Surgery; Aneurysm-Cerebral; Microsurgery; **Hospital:** Univ Hosps Case Med Ctr; **Address:** Dept Neurosurgery, 11100 Euclid Ave, 5th Fl Hanna House, Cleveland, OH 44106; **Phone:** 216-844-5745; **Board Cert:** Neurological Surgery 1986; **Med School:** Case West Res Univ 1977; **Resid:** Neurological Surgery, Univ Hosps 1984; **Fellow:** Research, Univ Hosps 1980; Neurological Surgery, Mayo Clinic 1984; **Fac Appt:** Prof NS, Case West Res Univ

Shapiro, Scott A MD [NS] - **Spec Exp:** Brain Tumors; Aneurysm-Cerebral; Spinal Cord Injury; Pituitary Tumors; **Hospital:** Indiana Univ Hosp; **Address:** Inidiana Univ, Wishard Memorial Hosp, 1001 W 10th St, Ste EOP323, Indianapolis, IN 46202; **Phone:** 317-630-7625; **Board Cert:** Neurological Surgery 1990; **Med School:** Indiana Univ 1981; **Resid:** Neurological Surgery, Indiana Univ Med Ctr 1987; **Fac Appt:** Prof NS, Indiana Univ

Thompson, B Gregory MD [NS] - **Spec Exp:** Acoustic Neuroma; Neurovascular Surgery; Skull Base Tumors & Surgery; Aneurysm-Cerebral; **Hospital:** Univ Michigan Hlth Sys; **Address:** Dept Neurosurgery, 3552 Taubman, 1500 E Medical Center Drive, Ann Arbor, MI 48109; **Phone:** 734-936-7493; **Board Cert:** Neurological Surgery 1998; **Med School:** Univ Kans 1986; **Resid:** Neurological Surgery, Univ Pittsburgh 1993; Research, Natl Inst Hlth 1992; **Fellow:** Neurological Surgery, Barrow Neuro Inst 1994; Interventional Radiology, Thomas Jefferson Univ 2005

Tomita, Tadanori MD [NS] - **Spec Exp:** Pediatric Neurosurgery; Brain Tumors-Pediatric; Hydrocephalus; **Hospital:** Children's Mem Hosp, Northwestern Meml Hosp; **Address:** Chldns Meml Hosp, Div Ped Neurosurg, 2300 Children's Plaza, Box 28, Chicago, IL 60614-3363; **Phone:** 773-880-4373; **Board Cert:** Neurological Surgery 1984; Pediatric Neurological Surgery 1996; **Med School:** Japan 1970; **Resid:** Neurological Surgery, Kobe Univ 1974; Neurological Surgery, Northwestern Meml Hosp 1980; **Fellow:** Surgery, Meml Sloan Kettering Canc Ctr 1981; **Fac Appt:** Prof NS, Northwestern Univ

Traynelis, Vincent C MD [NS] - **Spec Exp:** Spinal Surgery; **Hospital:** Rush Univ Med Ctr; **Address:** Rush Univ Med Ctr, Dept Neurosurgery, 1725 W Harrison St, Chicago, IL 60612; **Phone:** 312-942-6628; **Board Cert:** Neurological Surgery 1992; **Med School:** W VA Univ 1983; **Resid:** Neurological Surgery, Univ West Virginia Med Ctr 1989; **Fac Appt:** Prof NS, Rush Med Coll

Warnick, Ronald E MD [NS] - **Spec Exp:** Neuro-Oncology; Brain Tumors; **Hospital:** Univ Hosp - Cincinnati, Good Samaritan Hosp - Cincinnati; **Address:** 222 Piedmont Ave, Ste 3100, Cincinnati, OH 45219; **Phone:** 513-475-8629; **Board Cert:** Neurological Surgery 1995; **Med School:** Univ Rochester 1982; **Resid:** Neurological Surgery, NYU Med Ctr 1989; **Fellow:** Neuro-Oncology, UCSF Med Ctr 1991; **Fac Appt:** Prof NS, Univ Cincinnati

Great Plains and Mountains

Apfelbaum, Ronald I MD [NS] - **Spec Exp:** Spinal Surgery; **Hospital:** Univ Utah Hosps and Clins; **Address:** Clinical Neurosciences Ctr North, 175 N Medical Drive Bldg 550 Fl 4, Salt Lake City, UT 84132-2303; **Phone:** 801-585-7575; **Board Cert:** Neurological Surgery 1976; **Med School:** Hahnemann Univ 1965; **Resid:** Surgery, Montefiore Med Ctr 1969; Neurological Surgery, Montefiore Med Ctr 1974; **Fac Appt:** Prof NS, Univ Utah

Cherny, W Bruce MD [NS] - **Spec Exp:** Pediatric Neurosurgery; Brain Tumors; Spina Bifida; **Hospital:** St. Luke's Reg Med Ctr - Boise; **Address:** 100 E Idaho St, Ste 202, Boise, ID 83712; **Phone:** 208-381-7360; **Board Cert:** Neurological Surgery 2000; **Med School:** Univ Ariz Coll Med 1987; **Resid:** Neurological Surgery, Barrow Neuro Inst/St Joseph's Med Ctr 1994; **Fellow:** Pediatric Neurological Surgery, Primary Chldns Hosp 1995

Neurological Surgery

Couldwell, William MD/PhD [NS] - **Spec Exp:** Brain Tumors; Epilepsy/Movement Disorders; Parkinson's Disease; Pituitary Tumors; **Hospital:** Univ Utah Hosps and Clins; **Address:** Univ Utah, Dept Neurological Surgery, 175 N Medical Drive E, Salt Lake City, UT 84132-2303; **Phone:** 801-581-6908; **Board Cert:** Neurological Surgery 1994; **Med School:** McGill Univ 1984; **Resid:** Neurological Surgery, LAC/USC Med Ctr 1989; **Fellow:** Neurological Immunology, Montreal Neur Inst/McGill Univ 1991; Neurological Surgery, CHUV; **Fac Appt:** Prof NS, Univ Utah

Johnson, Stephen D MD [NS] - **Spec Exp:** Skull Base Tumors & Surgery; **Hospital:** Presby - St Luke's Med Ctr; **Address:** Western Neurological Group, 1601 E 19th Ave, Ste 4400, Denver, CO 80218; **Phone:** 303-861-2266; **Board Cert:** Neurological Surgery 1988; **Med School:** Univ Tenn Coll Med, Memphis 1974; **Resid:** Neurological Surgery, Virginia Mason Med Ctr; Neurological Surgery, New York Hosp; **Fellow:** Neurological Surgery, Univ Tennessee; **Fac Appt:** Assoc Prof NS, Univ Colorado

Kestle, John RW MD [NS] - **Spec Exp:** Pediatric Neurosurgery; Epilepsy/Seizure Disorders; **Hospital:** Primary Children's Med Ctr; **Address:** 100 N Medical Drive, Ste 2400, Salt Lake City, UT 84113; **Phone:** 801-662-5340; **Board Cert:** Neurological Surgery 2002; **Med School:** Canada 1984; **Resid:** Neurological Surgery, Univ Toronto 1990; **Fellow:** Pediatric Neurological Surgery, Hosp Sick Chldn/Univ Toronto 1992; **Fac Appt:** Prof NS, Univ Utah

Lillehei, Kevin O MD [NS] - **Spec Exp:** Neuro-Oncology; Pituitary Tumors; Peripheral Nerve Surgery; **Hospital:** Univ Colorado Hosp, Exempla Lutheran Med Ctr; **Address:** Univ Colorado Hosp, Dept Neurosurgery, 12631 E 17th Ave, Box C307, Aurora, CO 80045; **Phone:** 303-724-2280; **Board Cert:** Neurological Surgery 1989; **Med School:** Univ Minn 1979; **Resid:** Neurological Surgery, Univ Mich Med Ctr 1985; **Fac Appt:** Prof NS, Univ Colorado

Nazzaro, Jules M MD [NS] - **Spec Exp:** Parkinson's Disease; Movement Disorders; Stereotactic Radiosurgery; **Hospital:** Univ of Kansas Hosp; **Address:** Kansas University Medical Ctr, 3901 Rainbow Blvd, MS 3021, Kansas City, KS 66160; **Phone:** 913-588-5129; **Board Cert:** Neurological Surgery 1996; **Med School:** Albert Einstein Coll Med 1984; **Resid:** Neurological Surgery, NYU Med Ctr 1991; **Fellow:** Neurosurgical Oncology, Meml Sloan-Kettering Cancer Ctr 1992; **Fac Appt:** Assoc Prof NS, Univ Kans

Taylon, Charles MD [NS] - **Spec Exp:** Spinal Surgery-Cervical; Spinal Surgery-Low Back; Carpal Tunnel Syndrome; Trauma; **Hospital:** Creighton Univ Med Ctr; **Address:** Creighton Univ, Dept Surg, 601 N 30th St, Ste 3700, Omaha, NE 68131; **Phone:** 402-280-4497; **Board Cert:** Neurological Surgery 1984; **Med School:** Creighton Univ 1975; **Resid:** Neurological Surgery, Univ Wisc Hosps 1981; **Fac Appt:** Assoc Prof NS, Creighton Univ

Walker, Marion L MD [NS] - **Spec Exp:** Pediatric Neurosurgery; Spasticity & Movement Disorders; Hydrocephalus; Brain Tumors; **Hospital:** Primary Children's Med Ctr, Univ Utah Hosps and Clins; **Address:** Primary Children's Med Ctr, Div Ped Neurosurgery, 100 N Mario Capecchi Drive, Ste 1475, Salt Lake City, UT 84113-1103; **Phone:** 801-662-5340; **Board Cert:** Neurological Surgery 1979; Pediatric Neurological Surgery 1996; **Med School:** Univ Tenn Coll Med, Memphis 1969; **Resid:** Surgery, St Joseph's Hosp 1971; Neurological Surgery, St Joseph's Hosp-Barrow Neuro Inst 1976; **Fellow:** Pediatric Neurological Surgery, Hosp for Sick Chldn 1973; **Fac Appt:** Prof NS, Univ Utah

Winston, Ken R MD [NS] - **Spec Exp:** Pediatric Neurosurgery; Craniosynostosis; Epilepsy/Seizure Disorders; **Hospital:** Chldn's Hosp - Aurora, The, Univ Colorado Hosp; **Address:** 12631 E 17th Ave, Box C307, Aurora, CO 80045; **Phone:** 303-724-2305; **Board Cert:** Neurological Surgery 1973; **Med School:** Univ Tenn Coll Med, Memphis 1963; **Resid:** Surgery, Colorado Genl Hosp 1967; Neurological Surgery, Colorado Genl Hosp 1971; **Fac Appt:** Prof NS, Univ Colorado

Zimmerman, Christian G MD [NS] - **Spec Exp:** Spinal Surgery-Complex; Spinal Disorders-Degenerative; Trauma; **Hospital:** St Alphonsus Regl Med Ctr, St. Luke's Reg Med Ctr - Boise; **Address:** 1075 N Curtis Rd, Ste 200, Boise, ID 83706; **Phone:** 208-367-3500; **Board Cert:** Neurological Surgery 1996; Pain Medicine 1998; **Med School:** Univ MD Sch Med 1985; **Resid:** Surgery, Univ Md Hosp-Prince Georges Med Ctr 1987; Neurological Surgery, Oreg Hlth Sci Univ 1992; **Fellow:** Spinal Surgery, Barrow Neur Inst 1993

Southwest

Adelson, P David MD [NS] - **Spec Exp:** Pediatric Neurosurgery; Brain Injury; Epilepsy/Seizure Disorders; Spinal Cord Injury; **Hospital:** Phoenix Children's Hosp; **Address:** Phoenix Children's Hospital, Dept of Neurosurgery, 1919 E Thomas Rd, Phoenix, AZ 85106; **Phone:** 602-546-0923; **Board Cert:** Neurological Surgery 1997; Pediatric Neurological Surgery 1998; **Med School:** Columbia P&S 1986; **Resid:** Neurological Surgery, UCLA Med Ctr 1992; **Fellow:** Pediatric Neurological Surgery, Children's Hosp 1994; **Fac Appt:** Prof NS, Univ Ariz Coll Med

Al-Mefty, Ossama MD [NS] - **Spec Exp:** Skull Base Surgery; Brain Tumors; Cerebrovascular Surgery; **Hospital:** UAMS Med Ctr, Arkansas Chldns Hosp; **Address:** 4301 W Markham, Slot 507, Little Rock, AR 72205; **Phone:** 501-686-8757; **Board Cert:** Neurological Surgery 1980; **Med School:** Syria 1972; **Resid:** Surgery, Med Coll Ohio 1974; Neurological Surgery, West Va Med Ctr 1978; **Fac Appt:** Prof NS, Univ Ark

De Monte, Franco MD [NS] - **Spec Exp:** Skull Base Tumors & Surgery; Neuro-Oncology; **Hospital:** UT MD Anderson Cancer Ctr; **Address:** UT MD Anderson Cancer Ctr, Dept Neurosurgery, 1515 Holcombe Blvd, Ste 442, Houston, TX 77030; **Phone:** 713-792-2400; **Board Cert:** Neurological Surgery 1995; **Med School:** Canada 1985; **Resid:** Neurological Surgery, Univ Western Ontario 1991; **Fellow:** Skull Base Surgery, Loyola Univ-Stritch Sch Med 1992

Hankinson, Hal L MD [NS] - **Spec Exp:** Brain Tumors; **Hospital:** St Vincent Hosp - Santa Fe; **Address:** 465 St Michael's Drive, Ste 107, Sante Fe, NM 87505; **Phone:** 505-988-3233; **Board Cert:** Neurological Surgery 1977; **Med School:** Tulane Univ 1967; **Resid:** Neurological Surgery, UCSF Med Ctr 1975; **Fac Appt:** Clin Prof NS, Univ New Mexico

Harper, Richard L MD [NS] - **Spec Exp:** Spinal Surgery; Brain Tumors & Hemifacial Spasms; **Hospital:** Methodist Hosp - Houston; **Address:** 6560 Fannin St, Ste 1200, Houston, TX 77030; **Phone:** 713-790-1211; **Board Cert:** Neurological Surgery 1983; **Med School:** Baylor Coll Med 1971; **Resid:** Neurological Surgery, Baylor Hosps 1978; **Fac Appt:** Asst Clin Prof NS, Baylor Coll Med

Jimenez, David F MD [NS] - **Spec Exp:** Pediatric Neurosurgery; Craniosynostosis; Endoscopic Strip Craniectomy; Spinal Surgery; **Hospital:** Univ Hlth Syst-San Antonio, St Luke's Baptist Hosp; **Address:** Dept of Neurosurgery, 7703 Floyd Curl Drive, MC 7843, San Antonio, TX 78229-3900; **Phone:** 210-567-5625; **Board Cert:** Neurological Surgery 1995; **Med School:** Temple Univ 1985; **Resid:** Neurological Surgery, Temple Univ Hosp 1991; **Fellow:** Pediatric Neurological Surgery, Montefiore Med Ctr 1992; **Fac Appt:** Prof NS, Univ Tex, San Antonio

Kim, Daniel H MD [NS] - **Spec Exp:** Spinal Surgery; Peripheral Nerve Reconstruction; **Hospital:** St Luke's Episcopal Hosp-Houston; **Address:** Baylor Dept Neurosurgery, 1709 Dryden Rd, Ste 750, Houston, TX 77030; **Phone:** 713-798-4696; **Board Cert:** Neurological Surgery 1998; **Med School:** Tulane Univ 1989; **Resid:** Neurological Surgery, LSU Med Ctr 1995; **Fellow:** Spinal Surgery, Univ Fla 1998; **Fac Appt:** Prof NS, Baylor Coll Med

Neurological Surgery

Krisht, Ali F MD [NS] - **Spec Exp:** Skull Base Surgery; Meningioma; Vascular Neurosurgery; **Hospital:** UAMS Med Ctr; **Address:** 4301 W Markham St, slot# 788, Little Rock, AR 72205; **Phone:** 501-296-1463; **Board Cert:** Neurological Surgery 1999; **Med School:** Amer Univ Beirut 1985; **Resid:** Neurological Surgery, Emory Univ Affil Hosp 1994; **Fac Appt:** Prof NS, Univ Ark

Lang Jr, Frederick F MD [NS] - **Spec Exp:** Brain & Spinal Tumors; Neuro-Oncology; **Hospital:** UT MD Anderson Cancer Ctr; **Address:** Univ Texas MD Anderson Cancer Ctr, 1515 Holcombe Blvd, Unit 442, Houston, TX 77030; **Phone:** 713-792-6600; **Board Cert:** Neurological Surgery 2000; **Med School:** Yale Univ 1988; **Resid:** Neurological Surgery, NYU Med Ctr 1995; **Fellow:** Neurosurgical Oncology, MD Anderson Cancer Ctr 1996; **Fac Appt:** Prof NS, Univ Tex, Houston

Luerssen, Thomas G MD [NS] - **Spec Exp:** Pediatric Neurosurgery; Brain Injury-Traumatic; **Hospital:** Texas Chldns Hosp; **Address:** Texas Children's Hosp, Ped Neurosurgery, Clinical Care Center, Ste 1230, 6621 Fannin St, MC CC 1230.01, Houston, TX 77030-2399; **Phone:** 832-822-3950; **Board Cert:** Neurological Surgery 1985; Pediatric Neurological Surgery 2005; **Med School:** Indiana Univ 1976; **Resid:** Neurological Surgery, Indiana Univ Hosp 1981; **Fellow:** Pediatric Neurological Surgery, Chldns Hosp 1984; **Fac Appt:** Prof NS, Baylor Coll Med

Mapstone, Timothy B MD [NS] - **Spec Exp:** Brain Tumors-Adult & Pediatric; Pediatric Neurosurgery; Congenital Anomalies; **Hospital:** OU Med Ctr, Chldns Hosp OU Med Ctr; **Address:** Univ OK Hlth Sci Ctr, Dept Neurosurgery, 1000 N Lincoln Blvd, Ste 400, Oklahoma City, OK 73104; **Phone:** 405-271-4912; **Board Cert:** Neurological Surgery 1985; Pediatric Neurological Surgery 2005; **Med School:** Case West Res Univ 1977; **Resid:** Neurological Surgery, Univ Hosps 1983; **Fellow:** Research, Case West Reserve Univ; **Fac Appt:** Prof NS, Univ Okla Coll Med

Mickey, Bruce E MD [NS] - **Spec Exp:** Brain Tumors; Skull Base Surgery; **Hospital:** UT Southwestern Med Ctr at Dallas; **Address:** UTSW Med Ctr, Dept Neurosurgery, 5323 Harry Hines Blvd, Dallas, TX 75390-8855; **Phone:** 214-645-2300; **Board Cert:** Neurological Surgery 1987; **Med School:** Univ Tex SW, Dallas 1978; **Resid:** Neurological Surgery, Parkland Meml Hosp 1984; **Fellow:** Research, Righospitalet 1983; **Fac Appt:** Prof NS, Univ Tex SW, Dallas

Papadopoulos, Stephen M MD [NS] - **Spec Exp:** Spinal Surgery; Stereotactic Radiosurgery; **Hospital:** St Joseph's Hosp & Med Ctr - Phoenix; **Address:** Barrow Neurosurg Assocs, 2910 N 3rd Ave, Phoenix, AZ 85013; **Phone:** 602-406-3159; **Board Cert:** Neurological Surgery 1991; **Med School:** Univ Tex, Houston 1978; **Resid:** Neurological Surgery, Univ Mich Med Ctr 1988; **Fellow:** Spinal Surgery, Barrow Neuro Inst 1989

Samson, Duke S MD [NS] - **Spec Exp:** Vascular Neurosurgery; Cerebrovascular Disease; Arteriovenous Malformations; **Hospital:** UT Southwestern Med Ctr at Dallas, Parkland Hlth & Hosp Sys; **Address:** Univ Tex SW Med Ctr, Dept Neuro Surg, 5323 Harry Hines Blvd, Dallas, TX 75390-8855; **Phone:** 214-648-3529; **Board Cert:** Neurological Surgery 1978; **Med School:** Washington Univ, St Louis 1969; **Resid:** Neurological Surgery, Univ Texas SW Med Ctr 1975; **Fellow:** Neurological Surgery, Ctr Medico-Chirurgical Fech 1973; Neurological Surgery, Univ Zurich 1973; **Fac Appt:** Prof NS, Univ Tex SW, Dallas

Sawaya, Raymond MD [NS] - **Spec Exp:** Brain Tumors; **Hospital:** UT MD Anderson Cancer Ctr, Baylor Univ Medical Ctr; **Address:** MD Anderson Cancer Ctr, 1515 Holcombe Blvd, Unit 442, Houston, TX 77030; **Phone:** 713-563-8749; **Board Cert:** Neurological Surgery 1985; **Med School:** Lebanon 1974; **Resid:** Neurological Surgery, Univ Cincinnati Med Ctr 1980; Neurological Surgery, Johns Hopkins Med Ctr 1981; **Fellow:** Neuro-Oncology, Natl Inst Hlth 1982; **Fac Appt:** Prof NS, Univ Tex, Houston

Sklar, Frederick H MD [NS] - **Spec Exp:** Pediatric Neurosurgery; Craniofacial Surgery; Hydrocephalus; **Hospital:** Chldns Med Ctr of Dallas, Texas Scottish Rite Hosp for Chldn; **Address:** Center Pediatric Neurosurgery, 1935 Medical District Drive, Dallas, TX 75235; **Phone:** 214-456-6660; **Board Cert:** Neurological Surgery 1978; **Med School:** Johns Hopkins Univ 1970; **Resid:** Neurological Surgery, Johns Hopkins Hosp 1976; **Fac Appt:** Assoc Clin Prof NS, Univ Tex SW, Dallas

Sonntag, Volker MD [NS] - **Spec Exp:** Spinal Surgery; **Hospital:** St Joseph's Hosp & Med Ctr - Phoenix; **Address:** Barrow Neurosurgery Associates, 2910 N 3rd Ave, Phoenix, AZ 85013; **Phone:** 602-406-3458; **Board Cert:** Neurological Surgery 1980; **Med School:** Univ Ariz Coll Med 1971; **Resid:** Neurological Surgery, New England Med Ctr 1977; **Fac Appt:** Clin Prof NS, Univ Ariz Coll Med

Spetzler, Robert F MD [NS] - **Spec Exp:** Skull Base Tumors & Surgery; Cerebrovascular Surgery; **Hospital:** St Joseph's Hosp & Med Ctr - Phoenix; **Address:** Barrow Neurosurgical Assocs, 2910 N Third Ave, Phoenix, AZ 85013; **Phone:** 602-406-3489; **Board Cert:** Neurological Surgery 1979; **Med School:** Northwestern Univ 1971; **Resid:** Neurological Surgery, UCSF Med Ctr 1976; **Fac Appt:** Prof S, Univ Ariz Coll Med

Walsh, John W MD/PhD [NS] - **Spec Exp:** Pediatric Neurosurgery; Epilepsy; Craniofacial Surgery/Reconstruction; **Hospital:** Tulane Univ Hosp & Clin; **Address:** 1415 Tulane Ave, New Orleans, LA 70112; **Phone:** 504-988-8000; **Board Cert:** Neurological Surgery 1997; Pediatric Neurological Surgery 1996; **Med School:** UCLA 1969; **Resid:** Neurological Surgery, Childrens Hosp/Peter Bent Brigham Hosp 1974; **Fellow:** Neurological Surgery, Lahey Clin Fdn 1975; **Fac Appt:** Prof NS, Tulane Univ

Yonas, Howard MD [NS] - **Spec Exp:** Vascular Neurosurgery; Stroke; Skull Base Surgery; Trigeminal Neuralgia; **Hospital:** Univ Hosp of New Mexico; **Address:** 1 University of New Mexico, MSC10 5615, Albuquerque, NM 87131-0001; **Phone:** 505-272-9494; **Board Cert:** Neurological Surgery 1981; **Med School:** Ohio State Univ 1970; **Resid:** Neurological Surgery, Case West Res 1976; **Fellow:** Univ Pittsburgh 1978; **Fac Appt:** Prof NS, Univ New Mexico

West Coast and Pacific

Adler Jr, John R MD [NS] - **Spec Exp:** Stereotactic Radiosurgery; Brain Tumors; Acoustic Neuroma; **Hospital:** Stanford Univ Med Ctr; **Address:** Stanford Univ Med Ctr, Dept Neurosurg, 300 Pasteur Drive R Bldg - rm 205, Stanford, CA 94305-5327; **Phone:** 650-723-5573; **Board Cert:** Neurological Surgery 1990; **Med School:** Harvard Med Sch 1980; **Resid:** Neurological Surgery, Chldns Hosp 1987; Neurological Surgery, Mass Genl Hosp 1985; **Fellow:** Cerebrovascular Disease, Karolinska Inst 1986; **Fac Appt:** Prof NS, Stanford Univ

Amar, Arun P MD/PhD [NS] - **Spec Exp:** Interventional Neuroradiology; Stroke; Stroke Prevention; **Hospital:** USC Univ Hosp; **Address:** 1200 N State St, Ste 5046, Los Angeles, CA 90033; **Phone:** 323-442-5720; **Board Cert:** Neurological Surgery 2005; **Med School:** UCSF 1993; **Resid:** Neurological Surgery, USC Univ Hosp 2000; **Fellow:** Interventional Neuroradiology, USC Univ Hosp 2003; **Fac Appt:** Clin Prof NS, USC-Keck School of Medicine

Apuzzo, Michael L J MD [NS] - **Spec Exp:** Brain Tumors; Epilepsy/Seizure Disorders; Stereotactic Radiosurgery; **Hospital:** LAC & USC Med Ctr, USC Norris Cancer Hosp; **Address:** 1420 N San Pablo Street, PMBA106, Los Angeles, CA 90033-1029; **Phone:** 323-226-7421; **Board Cert:** Neurological Surgery 1975; **Med School:** Boston Univ 1965; **Resid:** Neurological Surgery, Hartford Hosp 1970; Neurological Surgery, Hartford Hosp 1973; **Fellow:** Neurological Physiology, Yale Univ Hosp 1972; **Fac Appt:** Prof NS, USC Sch Med

Neurological Surgery

Badie, Behnam MD [NS] - **Spec Exp:** Brain Tumors; **Hospital:** City of Hope Natl Med Ctr & Beckman Rsch; **Address:** 1500 E Duarte Rd, Duarte, CA 91010; **Phone:** 626-471-7100; **Board Cert:** Neurological Surgery 1998; **Med School:** UCLA 1989; **Resid:** Neurological Surgery, UCLA Med Ctr 1996; **Fac Appt:** Assoc Prof NS, UCLA

Berger, Mitchel S MD [NS] - **Spec Exp:** Brain & Spinal Cord Tumors; Pituitary Tumors; Neuro-Oncology; Pain Management; **Hospital:** UCSF Med Ctr; **Address:** UCSF Med Ctr, Dept Neuro-surgery, 505 Parnassus Avenue, M-786, San Francisco, CA 94143-0112; **Phone:** 415-353-3933; **Board Cert:** Neurological Surgery 1991; **Med School:** Univ Miami Sch Med 1979; **Resid:** Neuro-logical Surgery, UCSF Med Ctr 1984; **Fellow:** Neuro-Oncology, UCSF Med Ctr 1985; Pediatric Neu-rological Surgery, Hosp Sick Chldn 1986; **Fac Appt:** Prof NS, UCSF

Black, Keith L MD [NS] - **Spec Exp:** Brain Tumors; Pituitary Surgery; Trigeminal Neuralgia; **Hospital:** Cedars-Sinai Med Ctr; **Address:** Cedars Sinai Med Ctr, Dept Neurosugery, 8631 W 3rd St, Ste 800E, Los Angeles, CA 90048; **Phone:** 310-423-7900; **Board Cert:** Neurological Surgery 1990; **Med School:** Univ Mich Med Sch 1981; **Resid:** Neurological Surgery, Univ Michigan Med Ctr 1987; **Fac Appt:** Prof NS, UCLA-David Geffen Sch Med

Boggan, James E MD [NS] - **Spec Exp:** Skull Base Tumors & Surgery; Pediatric Neurosurgery; **Hospital:** UC Davis Med Ctr; **Address:** Dept Neurological Surgery, 4860 Y St, Ste 3740, Sacra-mento, CA 95817-2307; **Phone:** 916-734-2371; **Board Cert:** Neurological Surgery 1985; **Med School:** Univ Chicago-Pritzker Sch Med 1976; **Resid:** Neurological Surgery, UCSF Med Ctr 1982; **Fac Appt:** Prof NS, UC Davis

Burchiel, Kim J MD [NS] - **Spec Exp:** Pain Management; Stereotactic Radiosurgery; Epilepsy/Movement Disorders; **Hospital:** OR Hlth & Sci Univ; **Address:** OHSU, Dept Neurosurgery, 3303 SW Bond Ave, MC CH8N, Portland, OR 97239; **Phone:** 503-494-4314; **Board Cert:** Neuro-logical Surgery 1984; **Med School:** UCSD 1976; **Resid:** Neurological Surgery, Univ Wash Med Ctr 1982; **Fac Appt:** Prof NS, Oregon Hlth & Sci Univ

Chen, Thomas C MD [NS] - **Spec Exp:** Brain & Spinal Tumors; Brain Tumors-Metastatic; Gliomas; Microdiscectomy; **Hospital:** USC Norris Cancer Hosp, USC Univ Hosp; **Address:** USC Health Consultation Clinic 2, 1520 San Pablo St, rm 3800, Los Angeles, CA 90033; **Phone:** 323-442-5720; **Board Cert:** Neurological Surgery 2000; **Med School:** UCSF 1988; **Resid:** Neurologi-cal Surgery, USC Univ Hosp 1995; **Fellow:** Spinal Surgery, Med Coll Wisconsin 1997; **Fac Appt:** Assoc Prof NS, USC-Keck School of Medicine

Edwards, Michael S MD [NS] - **Spec Exp:** Brain Tumors-Pediatric; Pediatric Neurosurgery; Stereotactic Radiosurgery; **Hospital:** Lucile Packard Chldn's Hosp; **Address:** Pediatric Neurosurgery, 300 Pasteur Drive, Ste R211, MC 5327, Stanford, CA 94305-5327; **Phone:** 650-497-8775; **Board Cert:** Neurological Surgery 1980; Pediatric Neurological Surgery 2006; **Med School:** Tulane Univ 1970; **Resid:** Neurological Surgery, Oschner Fdn Hosp/Charity Hosp 1977; **Fellow:** Pediatric Neuro-Oncology, UCSF Med Ctr 1978; **Fac Appt:** Prof NS, Stanford Univ

Ellenbogen, Richard MD [NS] - **Spec Exp:** Pediatric Neurosurgery; Chiari's Deformity; Brain Tumors; **Hospital:** Chldns Hosp and Regl Med Ctr - Seattle, Univ Wash Med Ctr; **Address:** 4800 Sand Point Way NE, MS W-7729, Seattle, WA 98105; **Phone:** 206-987-2544; **Board Cert:** Neuro-logical Surgery 1992; Pediatric Neurological Surgery 1998; **Med School:** Brown Univ 1983; **Resid:** Neurological Surgery, Brigham Womens Hosp/Childrens Hosp 1989; **Fac Appt:** Prof NS, Univ Wash

Frazee, John G MD [NS] - **Spec Exp:** Vascular Neurosurgery; Spinal Surgery; Neuro-En-doscopy; **Hospital:** UCLA Ronald Reagan Med Ctr, VA Med Ctr - W Los Angeles; **Address:** UCLA Med Ctr, Div Neurosurgery, 750 Charles E Young Drive, Los Angeles, CA 90095-7039; **Phone:** 310-206-1231; **Board Cert:** Neurological Surgery 1984; **Med School:** Univ Rochester 1975; **Resid:** Neurological Surgery, UCLA Med Ctr 1982; **Fac Appt:** Clin Prof NS, UCLA

Giannotta, Steven L MD [NS] - **Spec Exp:** Aneurysm-Cerebral; Skull Base Tumors; Acoustic Neuroma; **Hospital:** USC Univ Hosp, LAC & USC Med Ctr; **Address:** 1520 San Pablo St, Ste 3800, Los Angeles, CA 90033; **Phone:** 323-442-5720; **Board Cert:** Neurological Surgery 1980; **Med School:** Univ Mich Med Sch 1972; **Resid:** Neurological Surgery, Univ Michigan Med Ctr 1978; **Fac Appt:** Prof NS, USC Sch Med

Gupta, Nalin MD/PhD [NS] - **Spec Exp:** Pediatric Neurosurgery; **Hospital:** UCSF Med Ctr; **Address:** 400 Parnassus Ave, rm A808, San Francisco, CA 94143; **Phone:** 415-353-7500; **Board Cert:** Neurological Surgery 2002; Pediatric Neurological Surgery 2003; **Med School:** Univ Toronto 1987; **Resid:** Neurological Surgery, Univ Ottawa 1989; Neurological Surgery, Univ Toronto 1997; **Fellow:** Pediatric Neurological Surgery, Hosp for Sick Chldn 1998; **Fac Appt:** Asst Prof NS, UCSF

Harsh IV, Griffith R MD [NS] - **Spec Exp:** Brain & Spinal Cord Tumors; Skull Base Tumors; Pituitary Tumors; Acoustic Neuroma; **Hospital:** Stanford Univ Med Ctr; **Address:** Stanford Center for Advanced Medicine, 875 Blake Wilbur Drive, MC 5826, Stanford, CA 94305; **Phone:** 650-736-9976; **Board Cert:** Neurological Surgery 1989; **Med School:** Harvard Med Sch 1980; **Resid:** Neurological Surgery, UCSF Med Ctr 1986; **Fellow:** Neuro-Oncology, UCSF Med Ctr 1987; **Fac Appt:** Prof NS, Stanford Univ

Levy, Michael L MD/PhD [NS] - **Spec Exp:** Pediatric Neurosurgery; **Hospital:** Rady Children's Hosp - San Diego, UCSD Med Ctr; **Address:** 8010 Frost St, Ste 502, San Diego, CA 92123; **Phone:** 858-966-8574; **Board Cert:** Neurological Surgery 1997; Pediatric Neurological Surgery 1998; **Med School:** UCSF 1986; **Resid:** Neurological Surgery, USC 1993; **Fellow:** Pediatric Neurological Surgery, Chldns Hosp 1995; Physiology; **Fac Appt:** Prof NS, USC Sch Med

Liau, Linda M MD/PhD [NS] - **Spec Exp:** Brain Tumors; Neuro-Oncology; **Hospital:** UCLA Ronald Reagan Med Ctr; **Address:** CHS 74-145, Box 956901, 10833 Le Conte Ave, Los Angeles, CA 90095-6901; **Phone:** 310-267-2621; **Board Cert:** Neurological Surgery 2002; **Med School:** Stanford Univ 1991; **Resid:** Neurological Surgery, UCLA Med Ctr 1998; **Fellow:** Neuro-Oncology, UCLA Med Ctr 1998; **Fac Appt:** Prof NS, UCLA

Liker, Mark A MD [NS] - **Spec Exp:** Spinal Surgery; Deep Brain Stimulation; **Hospital:** Henry Mayo Newhall Memorial Hosp, USC Univ Hosp; **Address:** 25751 McBean Pkwy, Ste 305, Valencia, CA 91355; **Phone:** 661-799-2542; **Board Cert:** Neurological Surgery 2005; **Med School:** SUNY Downstate 1995; **Resid:** Neurological Surgery, USC Med Ctr 2001; **Fellow:** Spinal Surgery, USC Med Ctr 1999; **Fac Appt:** Asst Prof NS, USC-Keck School of Medicine

Linskey, Mark E MD [NS] - **Spec Exp:** Brain Tumors; Stereotactic Radiosurgery; Skull Base Surgery; **Hospital:** UC Irvine Med Ctr, Chldns Hosp Orange Co; **Address:** UCI Med Ctr, Dept Neurosurgery-Route 81, 101 The City Drive S Bldg 56 - Ste 400, Orange, CA 92868-3298; **Phone:** 714-456-6392; **Board Cert:** Neurological Surgery 1996; **Med School:** Columbia P&S 1986; **Resid:** Neurological Surgery, Univ Pittsburgh Hlth Ctrs 1993; **Fellow:** Neuro-Oncology, Ludwig Inst Cancer Rsch/Univ Coll London 1994; Neuro-Oncology, Pittsburgh Cancer Inst/Univ Pittsburgh 1992; **Fac Appt:** Assoc Prof NS, UC Irvine

Liu, Charles Y MD [NS] - **Spec Exp:** Epilepsy; Skull Base Tumors & Surgery; Stereotactic Radiosurgery; Meningioma; **Hospital:** USC Univ Hosp; **Address:** 1520 San Pablo St, Ste 3800, Los Angeles, CA 90033; **Phone:** 323-442-5720; **Board Cert:** Neurological Surgery 2007; **Med School:** Yale Univ 1996; **Resid:** Neurological Surgery, LAC/USC Med Ctr 2001; **Fellow:** Spinal Surgery, LAC/USC Med Ctr 2003; **Fac Appt:** Asst Prof NS, USC-Keck School of Medicine

Mamelak, Adam N MD [NS] - **Spec Exp:** Brain Tumors; Epilepsy; Spinal Tumors; **Hospital:** Cedars-Sinai Med Ctr, Huntington Memorial Hosp; **Address:** Maxine Dunitz Neurosurgical Institute, 8631 W Third St, Ste 800-East, Los Angeles, CA 90048; **Phone:** 310-423-7900; **Board Cert:** Neurological Surgery 2000; **Med School:** Harvard Med Sch 1990; **Resid:** Neurological Surgery, UCSF Med Ctr 1994; **Fellow:** Epilepsy, UCSF Epilepsy Research Lab 1996

Marshall, Lawrence F MD [NS] - **Spec Exp:** Spinal Surgery; Spinal Cord Surgery; Brain Tumors; Head Injury; **Hospital:** UCSD Med Ctr; **Address:** UCSD Medical Ctr, Dept Neurosurgery, 200 W Arbor Drive, rm 8893, San Diego, CA 92103; **Phone:** 619-543-5540; **Board Cert:** Neurological Surgery 1977; **Med School:** Univ Mich Med Sch 1969; **Resid:** Neurological Surgery, Hosp U Penn 1975; **Fellow:** Neurological Pathology, Glasgow Univ Med Research 1976; **Fac Appt:** Prof NS, UCSD

Martin, Neil A MD [NS] - **Spec Exp:** Vascular Neurosurgery; **Hospital:** UCLA Ronald Reagan Med Ctr; **Address:** UCLA Med Ctr, Div Neuro Surgery, 10833 LeConte Ave, Box 95-7039, Los Angeles, CA 90095-7039; **Phone:** 310-825-5482; **Board Cert:** Neurological Surgery 1989; **Med School:** Med Coll VA 1978; **Resid:** Neurological Surgery, UCSF Med Ctr 1984; **Fellow:** Neurological Vascular Surgery, Barrow Neuro Inst 1985; **Fac Appt:** Prof NS, UCLA

Mayberg, Marc R MD [NS] - **Spec Exp:** Pituitary Surgery; Stroke/Cerebrovascular Disease; Skull Base Tumors; Acoustic Neuroma; **Hospital:** Swedish Med Ctr - Seattle; **Address:** Seattle Neuroscience Inst, 550 17th Ave, Ste 500, Seattle, WA 98122; **Phone:** 206-320-2800; **Board Cert:** Neurological Surgery 1988; **Med School:** Mayo Med Sch 1978; **Resid:** Neurological Surgery, Mass Genl Hosp 1984; **Fellow:** Neurological Surgery, Natl Hosp for Nervous Dis 1985

McDermott, Michael W MD [NS] - **Spec Exp:** Brain Tumors; Meningioma; Stereotactic Radiosurgery; Skull Base Tumors; **Hospital:** UCSF Med Ctr; **Address:** UCSF Dept Neurosurgery, 400 Parnassus Ave, rm A808, San Francisco, CA 94143; **Phone:** 415-353-7500; **Board Cert:** Neurological Surgery 2003; **Med School:** Univ Toronto 1982; **Resid:** Neurological Surgery, Univ British Columbia 1988; **Fellow:** Neuro-Oncology, UCSF Med Ctr 1990; **Fac Appt:** Prof NS, UCSF

Neuwelt, Edward A MD [NS] - **Spec Exp:** Neuro-Oncology; Brain Tumors; **Hospital:** OR Hlth & Sci Univ; **Address:** Oregon Hlth Sci Univ, Dept NS, 3181 SW Sam Jackson Pk Rd, MC-L603, Portland, OR 97239; **Phone:** 503-494-5626; **Board Cert:** Neurological Surgery 1980; **Med School:** Univ Colorado 1972; **Resid:** Neurological Surgery, Univ Tex SW Med Sch 1978; **Fellow:** Neuro-Oncology, Natl Canc Inst, NIH 1976; **Fac Appt:** Prof NS, Oregon Hlth & Sci Univ

Ott, Kenneth H MD [NS] - **Spec Exp:** Brain Tumors; Stereotactic Radiosurgery; **Hospital:** Scripps Meml Hosp - La Jolla; **Address:** Neurosurgical Medical Clinic, 2100 Fifth Ave, Ste 200, San Diego, CA 92101; **Phone:** 619-297-4481; **Board Cert:** Neurological Surgery 1980; **Med School:** UCSF 1970; **Resid:** Surgery, Mass Genl Hosp 1972; Neurological Surgery, Mass Genl Hosp 1976; **Fac Appt:** Assoc Clin Prof S, UCSD

Sekhar, Laligam N MD [NS] - **Spec Exp:** Aneurysm-Cerebral; Arteriovenous Malformations; Brain Tumors; Skull Base Tumors; **Hospital:** Harborview Med Ctr, Univ Wash Med Ctr; **Address:** Harborview Med Ctr, UW Dept Neurosurgery, 325 Ninth Ave, Box 359766, Seattle, WA 98104-2420; **Phone:** 206-744-9300; **Board Cert:** Neurological Surgery 1986; **Med School:** India 1975; **Resid:** Neurology, Univ Cincinnati Med Ctr 1977; Neurology, Univ Pittsburgh Med Ctr 1982; **Fellow:** Skull Base Surgery, Norstadt Krankenhaus 1983; Cerebrovascular Neurosurgery, Univ Zurich Hospital; **Fac Appt:** Prof NS, Univ Wash

Selden, Nathan R MD/PhD [NS] - **Spec Exp:** Pediatric Neurosurgery; Epilepsy; Spasticity & Movement Disorders; Chiari's Deformity; **Hospital:** OR Hlth & Sci Univ; **Address:** 3303 SW Bond Ave, MC CH8N, Portland, OR 97239; **Phone:** 503-494-4314; **Board Cert:** Neurological Surgery 2004; **Med School:** Harvard Med Sch 1993; **Resid:** Neurological Surgery, Univ Michigan Med Ctr 1999; **Fac Appt:** Assoc Prof NS, Oregon Hlth & Sci Univ

Shuer, Lawrence M MD [NS] - **Spec Exp:** Pediatric Neurosurgery; Craniosynostosis; Epilepsy; Chiari's Deformity; **Hospital:** Stanford Univ Med Ctr, Lucile Packard Chldn's Hosp; **Address:** Stanford Univ Med Ctr, Dept Neurosurgery, 300 Pasteur Drive, rm R229, Stanford, CA 94305; **Phone:** 650-723-5574; **Board Cert:** Neurological Surgery 1986; **Med School:** Univ Mich Med Sch 1978; **Resid:** Neurological Surgery, Stanford Univ 1984; **Fac Appt:** Prof NS, Stanford Univ

Silbergeld, Daniel MD [NS] - **Spec Exp:** Brain Tumors; Brain Tumors-Metastatic; Brain Mapping; **Hospital:** Univ Wash Med Ctr; **Address:** Univ Wash Med Ctr, Dept Neurosurg, 1959 NE Pacific, Box 356470, Seattle, WA 98195; **Phone:** 206-598-5637; **Board Cert:** Neurological Surgery 1995; **Med School:** Univ Cincinnati 1984; **Resid:** Neurological Surgery, Univ Wash Med Ctr 1990; Research, Univ Wash Med Ctr 1988; **Fellow:** Neuro-Oncology, Univ Wash Med Ctr 1991; Epilepsy, Univ Wash Med Ctr 1991; **Fac Appt:** Assoc Prof NS, Univ Wash

Steinberg, Gary K MD/PhD [NS] - **Spec Exp:** Aneurysm-Cerebral; Moya Moya; Arteriovenous Malformations; **Hospital:** Stanford Univ Med Ctr; **Address:** Stanford Univ Hosp, Dept Neurosurg, 300 Pasteur Drive, rm R281, Stanford, CA 94305-5327; **Phone:** 650-723-5575; **Board Cert:** Neurological Surgery 1989; **Med School:** Stanford Univ 1980; **Resid:** Neuropathology, Stanford Univ Med Ctr 1982; Neurological Surgery, Stanford Univ Med Ctr 1987; **Fellow:** Cerebrovascular Neurosurgery, Univ West Ontario 1985; **Fac Appt:** Prof NS, Stanford Univ

Sun, Peter P MD [NS] - **Spec Exp:** Pediatric Neurosurgery; Congenital Cranial Deformities; Brain Tumors; **Hospital:** Chldns Hosp - Oakland; **Address:** Children's Hospital, Dept Neurosurgery, 744 52nd St, Oakland, CA 94609; **Phone:** 510-428-3319; **Board Cert:** Neurological Surgery 2002; Pediatric Neurological Surgery 2006; **Med School:** Columbia P&S 1991; **Resid:** Neurological Surgery, UC Davis Med Ctr 1994; Neurological Surgery, Yale-New Haven Hosp 1996; **Fellow:** Neurological Surgery, NYU Med Ctr 1997; Pediatric Neurological Surgery, Childrens Hosp 1998; **Fac Appt:** Asst Clin Prof NS, UCSF

Yu, John S MD [NS] - **Spec Exp:** Brain Tumors; Spinal Tumors; Clinical Trials; Spinal Surgery; **Hospital:** Cedars-Sinai Med Ctr; **Address:** Maxine Dunitz Neurosurgical Institute, 8631 W 3rd St, Ste 800-East, Los Angeles, CA 90048; **Phone:** 310-423-7900; **Board Cert:** Neurological Surgery 2002; **Med School:** Harvard Med Sch 1990; **Resid:** Neurological Surgery, Mass General Hosp 1997

Cleveland Clinic

Neurological Institute

The Cleveland Clinic Neurological Institute is a fully integrated entity with a disease-specific focus, combining all physicians and other healthcare providers in neurology, neurosurgery, neuroradiology, the behavioral sciences and nursing who treat children and adults with neurological and neurobehavioral disorders. Our staff of more than 250 specialists sees one of the largest and most diverse patient populations in the country. Because of our clinical expertise, academic achievement and innovative research, the Cleveland Clinic Neurological Institute has earned an international reputation for excellence.

U.S.News & World Report's "America's Best Hospitals" survey has consistently ranked our Neurology and Neurosurgery programs among the Top 10 in the nation and best in Ohio. Our pediatric neurology/neurosurgery program has been ranked fourth in the nation.

Our unique clinical structure allows us to deliver coordinated, comprehensive, multidisciplinary care to our patients through more efficient treatment decision making and consultation for complex cases. Fully integrating specialties along disease lines creates an exciting synergy among Institute physicians who share similar clinical, research and educational interests, to the benefit of patients and physicians alike.

Major advances in the treatment of brain tumors, epilepsy, mood disorders, stroke, movement disorders, pain and spinal disorders are improving quality of life and survival for thousands of patients. For those diseases resistant to available treatments, we believe the innovative model of medicine created within the Neurological Institute will speed research and advances in treatment, resulting in better clinical care and more rapid breakthroughs in the full range of neurological and behavioral disorders.

Comprehensive Neurological Care

Cleveland Clinic offers expert diagnostic and treatment options for all neurologic conditions affecting children and adults, including:

- Alzheimer's disease
- ALS (Amyotrophic Lateral Sclerosis)
- Aneurysms
- Arteriovenous Malformations (AVMs)
- Back and Neck Disorders
- Brain and Spine Tumors
- Cerebral Palsy
- Chronic Pain Rehabilitation
- Congenital Disorders
- Craniofacial Disorders
- Epilepsy
- Headache
- Hydrocephalus
- Metastatic Tumors
- Mild Cognitive Impairment
- Multiple Sclerosis
- Movement Disorders
- Neonatal Disorders
- Neurofibromatosis
- Parkinson's Disease
- Pediatric Neurological Disorders
- Peripheral Neuropathies
- Pituitary Disorders
- Psychiatric Disorders
- Skull Base Disorders
- Sleep Disorders
- Stroke

For more information about the Cleveland Clinic Neurological Institute, to schedule a second opinion or to learn about assistance for out-of-town patients, call 800.890.2467 or visit www.clevelandclinic.org/neurotopdocs.

Cleveland Clinic Neurological Institute
9500 Euclid Avenue / AC311 | Cleveland OH 44195

PENN NEUROSURGERY

The Department of Neurosurgery at Penn provides comprehensive medical and surgical care for people with disorders of the brain, spinal cord and peripheral nervous system. One of the hallmarks of Penn's neurosurgery program is its integration of research and clinical practice, embracing new technologies and seeking the highest quality and best outcomes possible. More Penn neurosurgeons are listed in *The Best Doctors in America*® than are found at any other hospital or medical center in the Philadelphia region.

Penn Neurosurgery is a component of the Penn Comprehensive Neuroscience Center, which facilitates and strengthens the integration of Penn's world-class neuroscience programs within the areas of clinical care, research and education.

Penn's neurosurgical specialists, backed by the most extensive neurodiagnostic and imaging facilities in the region, perform more than 4,500 operations each year. The neurosurgical faculty all have a particular subspecialty focus, covering the entire spectrum of surgically-treated disorders of the nervous system.

Excellence and Expertise

The Penn Gamma Knife® **Center at Pennsylvania Hospital** offers power, precision and hope to patients suffering from brain tumors and other serious brain disorders. Gamma Knife radiosurgery is noninvasive, effective, and safe for treating conditions including benign or malignant brain tumors, blood vessel malformations and trigeminal neuralgia.

The Center for Functional and Restorative Neurosurgery at Pennsylvania Hospital performed more deep brain stimulation procedures for the treatment of Parkinson's disease and epilepsy in the past year than any other hospital or health system in the U.S.

The Center for Cranial Base Surgery offers expert evaluation and treatment of tumors of the head, neck, face and other complex skull base disorders. With the development of innovative and endoscopic surgical procedures and state-of-the-art imaging, many of these tumors, previously inaccessible, can now be successfully treated.

The Neuro-Oncology Program provides evaluation, diagnosis and treatment to patients with brain and spinal tumors and other cancer-related neurological central nervous system and peripheral nervous system problems. The program utilizes a patient-oriented team approach bringing together some of the nation's leading experts in the field.

The Neurosurgical Spine Center provides medical and surgical care for the most complex disorders of the spinal cord. Penn is a regional and national leader in providing quality spine care utilizing a multidisciplinary team approach, implementing the latest advances in techniques and technology.

The Neurovascular Center offers minimally invasive (endovascular) coiling and stent treatments of brain aneurysms, vascular malformations and atherosclerotic narrowing of the blood vessels of the brain, combining the skill sets of neurosurgeons and interventional neuroradiologists to obtain the best possible outcomes.

Programs

- Center for Brain Injury and Repair
- Center for Cranial Base Surgery
- Center for Functional and Restorative Neurosurgery
- Penn Gamma Knife® Center
- Neuro Intensive Care
- Neuro-Oncology Program
- Neurovascular Center
- Neurosurgical Spine Center

Gamma Knife and Leksell Gamma Knife are U.S. federally registered trademarks of Elekta Instrument S.A., Geneva, Switzerland.

Locations

Hospital of the University of Pennsylvania

Pennsylvania Hospital

Maimonides Medical Center
MAIMONIDES STROKE CENTER

Maimonides
Medical Center

4802 Tenth Avenue • Brooklyn, New York 11219
Phone: 718.283.7670 • Fax: 718.635.7223
www.maimonidesmed.org/stroke

The Maimonides Stroke Center is ranked among the top 5% in the nation, and the top two in New York State. There are several other stroke centers in Brooklyn, but the services at Maimonides are far more advanced than at any other institution.

After the onset of stroke symptoms, there is a three-hour window of opportunity for the administration of a clot-busting drug. With highly specialized training, experts at certified stroke centers can administer that drug to appropriate patients. But there is a nine-hour window of opportunity for an advanced treatment, and Maimonides is one of only a handful of hospitals in the New York metropolitan area with the capability to provide that treatment.

Dr. Jeffrey Farkas, Director of Interventional Neuroradiology, can insert a special instrument into a blood vessel, thread it up to the brain, and remove a stroke-causing blood clot. This procedure can greatly reduce stroke damage, and in some cases has completely reversed all symptoms. Dr. Farkas is among an elite few in the nation with significant experience utilizing this advanced technology for stroke patients.

Dr. Steven Rudolph, the neurologist Stroke Director at Maimonides, has been selected as investigator in two clinical trials for the newest medical stroke therapies. This distinction is bestowed only on the most respected clinicians in that specialty. These therapies, too, will be able to provide treatment up to nine hours after the onset of symptoms.

In addition, Maimonides has a multidisciplinary team of stroke experts that includes physicians and nurses from the Department of Emergency Medicine, providing the vital first line of defense in combating stroke. The ER at Maimonides is equipped with telemedicine, an interactive system that allows consultation with a stroke neurologist in real time, even when the doctor is at a remote location.

In our stroke unit and interventional neuroradiology suite, nurses are certified and experienced in these specialties, and they coordinate recovery plans that include numerous technicians and therapists.

Physicians at Maimonides are among the small percentage in the US who use computers to enter patient orders, thereby reducing the risk of errors, increasing efficiency, and speeding the healing process. Maimonides has appeared on the American Hospital Association's "Most Wired" and "Most Wireless" lists more often than any other health care institution in the metropolitan area. Advanced technology allows our doctors to focus more attention on caring for their patients.

Maimonides Medical Center
Passionate about medicine.
Compassionate about people.

www.maimonidesmed.org/stroke

MOUNT SINAI SCHOOL OF MEDICINE

THE MOUNT SINAI MEDICAL CENTER NEUROSURGERY
One Gustave L. Levy Place
Fifth Avenue and 100th Street
New York, NY 10029-6574
Physician Referral: 1-800-MD-SINAI (637-4624)
www.mountsinai.org

THE DEPARTMENT OF NEUROSURGERY at Mount Sinai, established in 1920, has earned a distinguished international reputation. Areas of clinical expertise include the treatment of skull base tumors, primary and metastatic brain tumors, pituitary adenomas and acoustic neuromas, and deep brain stimulation for movement disorders. The Department also provides advanced endovascular and microsurgical treatment of aneurysms, treatments for arteriovenous malformations and stroke, microvascular decompression for trigeminal neuralgia and hemifacial spasm, and advanced minimally invasive treatments of spine disease.

The Comprehensive Brain Tumor Program collaborates with The Tisch Cancer Institute and the Departments of Neurology, Radiation Oncology, Radiology, and Pathology to provide comprehensive therapies for primary and metastatic brain tumors. Each case is reviewed at our Tumor Board Conference by a team of specialists from each of these areas. We develop the most appropriate treatment plan that maximizes survival, and improves quality of life during and after treatment, and we maintain a close working relationship with local physicians, regularly communicating diagnostic findings and treatment recommendations. We have pioneered minimally invasive approaches using imaging technology, frameless stereotaxy, and skull base endoscopy, awake and asleep brain mapping, and advanced microneurosurgery. Stereotactic radiosurgery, a minimally invasive treatment that does not require open surgery, is frequently an option. Gene therapy and clinical trials are also available to selected patients.

The Neuroendocrine Program sees over 200 new pituitary tumor patients each year as well as over 300 follow-up patients. The ultimate in care is provided with medical therapy, micro- and endoscopic surgery, and stereotactic radiosurgery. Studies are under way to understand the cause of these adenomas, and to offer treatments that are least invasive and most effective.

The Minimally Invasive and Endoscopic Skull Base Surgery Program provides comprehensive, highly advanced treatment for lesions located near the complex structures at the base of the skull. This multidisciplinary program unites surgical specialists in neurosurgery, otolaryngology, head and neck cancer, craniofacial surgery, oral and maxillofacial surgery, and microvascular and reconstructive procedures. We have pioneered the development of minimally invasive techniques including, transnasal endoscopic tumor resection and stereotactic radiosurgery for complex skull base lesions. This program offers patients the benefit of a wide range of experts who are renowned for the treatment of pituitary adenomas, acoustic neuromas, meningiomas, chordomas, craniopharyngiomas, cholesterol granulomas, chondrosarcomas, and all the pathologies of the skull base.

The Cerebrovascular Program is a leader in rapidly evolving endovascular treatments for patients with intracranial aneurysms, arteriovenous malformations, stroke, intracranial stenosis, and other cerebrovascular diseases. Our team treats a high volume of patients using endovascular methods. Each patient is evaluated to determine whether minimally invasive techniques, such as stenting or coiling, can be used.

The Functional and Restorative Neurosurgery Program uses the latest technology to precisely target areas of abnormal activity in the brain and spinal cord. Our physicians are focused on developing minimally invasive neurosurgical techniques that either modulate neural function, replace lost neuronal populations, or halt the neurodegenerative process altogether. Currently, deep brain stimulation dominates this field, but many technologies with great potential are on the horizon. Our physicians have been honored by the Dystonia Medical Research Foundation for their pioneering work treating dystonia with deep brain stimulation. We also use cutting-edge techniques, such as gene therapy for the treatment of patients with Parkinson's disease, epilepsy, essential tremor, facial nerve disorders, and chronic pain syndromes.

The Neurosurgery Spinal Disorders Program offers comprehensive treatment for all disorders of the spinal column and spinal cord, including degenerative disorders (disc herniations, spinal stenosis, spinal instability), trauma, infections, congenital disorders (including scoliosis), and tumors. Our neurosurgeons have pioneered endoscopic, minimally invasive surgical approaches to treat disorders of the spine. These approaches have the potential to reduce postoperative pain and disability, speed recovery, shorten hospital stays, and facilitate an early return to normal activity.

NEUROSURGERY

About the Department of Neurosurgery:

The Department of Neurosurgery at NYU Langone Medical Center offers some of the most advanced surgical procedures available. In an environment of cutting-edge research and medical education, the Department's interdisciplinary team of physicians, nurses and allied health professionals are world renowned for their highly specialized training.

We specialize in the following areas:

CEREBROVASCULAR SURGERY

The Division of Cerebrovascular Surgery is a premier treatment center for brain aneurysms, giant intracranial aneurysms (aneurysms with a diameter greater than 25 mm), brain vascular malformations and cavernomas (blood-filled clusters of vessels).

BRAIN TUMOR

The Department of Neurosurgery at NYU Langone Medical Center specializes in both malignant and benign brain tumors, including tumors of the skull base. Our particular expertise includes glioblastoma, ependymoma, hemangioblastoma, other gliomas, meningiomas and especially vestibular schwannomas (acoustic neuromas).

EPILEPSY

The Comprehensive Epilepsy Center is the largest epilepsy center in the United States, offering the most advanced surgical and medical options in the treatment of epilepsy. Complementary management approaches such as diet alteration, yoga, biofeedback, meditation, lifestyle changes and other remedies are also offered to patients.

NEURO-CRITICAL CARE

The Division of Neuro-Critical Care provides intensive care and treatment of critical neurosurgical illnesses such as respiratory failure, hypotension, hypertension, coagulopathy (blood clotting disorder) as well as infections including pneumonia, sepsis, wound infections and meningitis. The Division also offers high-caliber care for patients with seizures and raised intracranial pressure, and hosts a dedicated group of physicians available 24 hours/day for immediate consultation in the intensive care unit.

NEUROSURGICAL TECHNOLOGY

Using the Leksell Gamma Knife, neurosurgeons at NYU Langone Medical Center remove deep-seated tumors, vascular malformations and other sites of dysfunction with outstanding results. Aided by three-dimensional MRI technology, the Knife is used by neurosurgeons to bombard its target with precise doses of radiation, while still preserving healthy tissue. The Medical Center is one of the only two hospitals on the East Coast to have the Knife.

The Department of Neurosurgery at NYU Langone Medical Center also provides state-of-the-art patient care and research through the following divisions:

- The Division of Facial Pain provides patients a careful, thorough examination and if required, nerve injections and minimally invasive surgery.

- The Division of Functional Neurosurgery offers diagnosis and treatment of Parkinson's disease and conditions that involve involuntary muscle contractions.

- The Division of Pediatric Neurosurgery provides treatment to children with brain and spinal cord tumors, congenital and development disorders.

- The Division of Peripheral Nerve Surgery focuses on the diagnosis and treatment of nerve compressions, nerve tremors, Brachial Plexus (never fiber) and nerve injuries.

- The Division of Spine Surgery provides treatment for spinal diseases such as degenerative diseases, spinal tumors, spinal trauma and spinal infections.

Neurology

A neurologist specializes in the diagnosis and treatment of all types of disease or impaired function of the brain, spinal cord, peripheral nerves, muscles and autonomic nervous system, as well as the blood vessels that relate to these structures. A child neurologist has special skills in the diagnosis and management of neurologic disorders of the neonatal period, infancy, early childhood and adolescence.

Training Required: Four years

NEUROLOGY

New England

Amato, Anthony A MD [N] - **Spec Exp:** Peripheral Neuropathy; Neuromuscular Disorders; Muscular Dystrophy; **Hospital:** Brigham & Women's Hosp; **Address:** Brigham & Women's Hosp, Dept Neurology, 75 Francis St, Boston, MA 02115; **Phone:** 617-732-8046; **Board Cert:** Neurology 1991; **Med School:** Univ Cincinnati 1986; **Resid:** Neurology, Wilford Hall USAF Med Ctr 1990; **Fellow:** Neuromuscular Medicine, Ohio State Med Ctr 1992; **Fac Appt:** Prof N, Harvard Med Sch

Armon, Carmel MD [N] - **Spec Exp:** Amyotrophic Lateral Sclerosis (ALS); Epilepsy/Seizure Disorders; Vascular Neurology; Sleep Medicine; **Hospital:** Baystate Med Ctr; **Address:** Baystate Neurology, 759 Chestnut St, Springfield, MA 01199; **Phone:** 413-794-7192; **Board Cert:** Neurology 1990; Clinical Neurophysiology 2002; Vascular Neurology 2005; Sleep Medicine 2007; **Med School:** Israel 1980; **Resid:** Neurology, Mayo Clinic 1988; **Fellow:** Neurology, Mayo Clinic 1989; Clinical Neurophysiology, Duke Univ Med Ctr 1991; **Fac Appt:** Prof N, Tufts Univ

Blumenfeld, Hal MD/PhD [N] - **Spec Exp:** Epilepsy/Seizure Disorders; **Hospital:** Yale-New Haven Hosp; **Address:** Yale Dept of Neurology, 40 Temple St, PO Box 208018, New Haven, CT 06520-8018; **Phone:** 203-785-3865; **Board Cert:** Neurology 2008; **Med School:** Columbia P&S 1992; **Resid:** Neurology, Mass Genl Hosp 1996; **Fellow:** Epilepsy, Yale-New Haven Hosp 1998; **Fac Appt:** Assoc Prof N, Yale Univ

Bromfield, Edward B MD [N] - **Spec Exp:** Epilepsy/Seizure Disorders; Sleep Disorders/Apnea; **Hospital:** Brigham & Women's Hosp, Mass Genl Hosp; **Address:** Brigham & Women's Hosp, Dept Neurology, Division of Epilepsy and EEG, 75 Francis St, Boston, MA 02115; **Phone:** 617-732-7547; **Board Cert:** Neurology 1989; **Med School:** Harvard Med Sch 1983; **Resid:** Neurology, New York Hosp 1987; **Fellow:** Epilepsy, Natl Inst Hlth/NINDS 1989; **Fac Appt:** Assoc Prof N, Harvard Med Sch

Caplan, Louis R MD [N] - **Spec Exp:** Stroke; **Hospital:** Beth Israel Deaconess Med Ctr - Boston; **Address:** Palmer 127 West Campus BIDMC, 330 Brookline Ave, Boston, MA 02215; **Phone:** 617-632-8911; **Board Cert:** Internal Medicine 1969; Neurology 1972; Vascular Neurology 2005; **Med School:** Univ MD Sch Med 1962; **Resid:** Neurology, Boston City Hosp 1969; **Fellow:** Neurology, Harvard Univ Affil Hosp 1970; **Fac Appt:** Prof N, Harvard Med Sch

Cole, Andrew J MD [N] - **Spec Exp:** Epilepsy/Seizure Disorders; Rasmussen's Syndrome; **Hospital:** Mass Genl Hosp; **Address:** Mass Genl Hosp-Epilepsy Svc, 55 Fruit St, rm Wang 735, Boston, MA 02214; **Phone:** 617-726-3311; **Board Cert:** Neurology 1987; **Med School:** Dartmouth Med Sch 1982; **Resid:** Neurology, Neuro Inst-McGill 1986; **Fellow:** Electroencephalography, Neuro Inst-McGill 1987; Neurological Surgery, Johns Hopkins Hosp 1988; **Fac Appt:** Asst Prof N, Harvard Med Sch

Feldmann, Edward MD [N] - **Spec Exp:** Cerebrovascular Disease; Stroke; **Hospital:** Rhode Island Hosp; **Address:** 110 Lockwood St, Ste 324, Providence, RI 02903; **Phone:** 401-444-8806; **Board Cert:** Neurology 1988; Vascular Neurology 2005; **Med School:** Harvard Med Sch 1983; **Resid:** Neurology, New York Hosp 1987; **Fellow:** Cerebrovascular Disease, Tufts New Eng Med Ctr 1988; **Fac Appt:** Prof N, Brown Univ

Flaherty, Alice W MD/PhD [N] - **Spec Exp:** Parkinson's Disease; Movement Disorders; Deep Brain Stimulation; Tourette's Syndrome; **Hospital:** Mass Genl Hosp, McLean Hosp; **Address:** Neurology Assocs, 15 Parkman St, WAC 715, Boston, MA 02114; **Phone:** 617-726-5532; **Board Cert:** Neurology 1999; **Med School:** Harvard Med Sch 1994; **Resid:** Neurology, Mass Genl Hosp 1998

Furie, Karen L MD [N] - **Spec Exp:** Stroke; Cerebrovascular Disease; **Hospital:** Mass Genl Hosp; **Address:** MGH Neurology Stroke Service, 15 Parkman St, WAC 835, Boston, MA 02114; **Phone:** 617-726-8459; **Board Cert:** Neurology 2006; Vascular Neurology 2008; **Med School:** Brown Univ 1990; **Resid:** Neurology, Rhode Island Hosp 1994; **Fellow:** Cerebrovascular Disease, Brown Univ 1995

Hafler, David A MD [N] - **Spec Exp:** Multiple Sclerosis; **Hospital:** Brigham & Women's Hosp; **Address:** Harvard Med Sch, 77 Ave Louis Pasteur, NRB 641-D, Boston, MA 02115; **Phone:** 617-525-5330; **Board Cert:** Neurology 1987; **Med School:** Univ Miami Sch Med 1978; **Resid:** Neurology, NY Hosp-Cornell Med Ctr 1982; **Fellow:** Neurological Immunology, Harvard Med Sch 1984; **Fac Appt:** Prof N, Harvard Med Sch

Jobst, Barbara C MD [N] - **Spec Exp:** Epilepsy/Seizure Disorders; Epilepsy in Women; **Hospital:** Dartmouth - Hitchcock Med Ctr; **Address:** One Medical Center Drive, Lebanon, NH 03756-1000; **Phone:** 603-653-6118; **Board Cert:** Neurology 2002; Clinical Neurophysiology 2005; **Med School:** Germany 1993; **Resid:** Neurology, Krankenhaus Barmherzigen Bruder 1996; Neurology, Dartmouth-Hitchcock Med Ctr 2000; **Fellow:** Epilepsy, Dartmouth-Hitchcock Med Ctr 2001; **Fac Appt:** Assoc Prof N, Dartmouth Med Sch

Jones Jr, H Royden MD [N] - **Spec Exp:** Neuromuscular Disorders; Amyotrophic Lateral Sclerosis (ALS); Myasthenia Gravis; Peripheral Neuropathy; **Hospital:** Lahey Clin; **Address:** Lahey Clinic, 41 Mall Rd, Burlington, MA 01805; **Phone:** 781-744-5126; **Board Cert:** Neurology 2004; Clinical Neurophysiology 2000; Neuromuscular Medicine 2006; **Med School:** Northwestern Univ 1962; **Resid:** Internal Medicine, Mayo Clinic 1965; Neurology, Mayo Clinic 1969; **Fellow:** Neurological Physiology, Mayo Clinic 1972; **Fac Appt:** Clin Prof N, Harvard Med Sch

Kase, Carlos S MD [N] - **Spec Exp:** Stroke; **Hospital:** Boston Med Ctr; **Address:** Boston Univ Sch of Med, 715 Albany St, Neurology C-329, Boston, MA 02118; **Phone:** 617-638-5102; **Board Cert:** Neurology 1980; Vascular Neurology 2005; **Med School:** Chile 1967; **Resid:** Neurology, Mass Genl Hosp 1973; Neurology, Mass Genl Hosp 1978; **Fac Appt:** Prof N, Boston Univ

Ropper, Allan MD [N] - **Spec Exp:** Trauma Neurology; Guillain-Barre Syndrome; **Hospital:** Brigham & Women's Hosp; **Address:** 75 Francis St, Box BB204, Boston, MA 02115; **Phone:** 617-732-8047; **Board Cert:** Internal Medicine 1977; Neurology 1980; **Med School:** Cornell Univ-Weill Med Coll 1974; **Resid:** Internal Medicine, UCSF Med Ctr 1976; Neurology, Mass Genl Hosp 1979; **Fac Appt:** Prof N, Tufts Univ

Samuels, Martin A MD [N] - **Spec Exp:** Neurologic Aspects of Systemic Disease; **Hospital:** Brigham & Women's Hosp; **Address:** Brigham & Women's Hosp, Dept Neurology, 75 Francis St, Neurology ASB-1, rm 158, Boston, MA 02115; **Phone:** 617-732-7432; **Board Cert:** Internal Medicine 1974; Neurology 1978; **Med School:** Univ Cincinnati 1971; **Resid:** Internal Medicine, Boston City Hosp 1975; Neurology, Mass Genl Hosp 1977; **Fellow:** Neurological Pathology, Mass Genl Hosp 1976; **Fac Appt:** Prof N, Harvard Med Sch

Saper, Clifford MD/PhD [N] - **Spec Exp:** Sleep Disorders/Apnea; **Hospital:** Beth Israel Deaconess Med Ctr - Boston; **Address:** 330 Brookline Ave, Neurology, Kirstein 406, Boston, MA 02215; **Phone:** 617-667-2622; **Board Cert:** Neurology 1982; **Med School:** Washington Univ, St Louis 1977; **Resid:** Neurology, NY Hosp 1981; **Fac Appt:** Prof N, Harvard Med Sch

Selkoe, Dennis MD [N] - **Spec Exp:** Alzheimer's Disease; **Hospital:** Brigham & Women's Hosp; **Address:** 77 Ave Louis Pasteur HIM 730 Bldg, Boston, MA 02115-5716; **Phone:** 617-525-5200; **Board Cert:** Neurology 1977; **Med School:** Univ VA Sch Med 1969; **Resid:** Neurology, Peter Bent Brigham 1975; **Fellow:** Neurological Biology, Chldns Hosp Med Ctr 1978; **Fac Appt:** Prof N, Harvard Med Sch

Neurology

Spencer, Susan S MD [N] - **Spec Exp:** Epilepsy/Seizure Disorders; **Hospital:** Yale-New Haven Hosp; **Address:** Yale Univ Sch Med, Dept Neurology, 333 Cedar St, Box 208018, New Haven, CT 06520-8018; **Phone:** 203-785-3865; **Board Cert:** Neurology 1980; Clinical Neurophysiology 1988; **Med School:** Univ Rochester 1974; **Resid:** Neurology, Yale-New Haven Hosp 1978; **Fellow:** Epilepsy, Yale New Haven Hosp 1980; **Fac Appt:** Prof N, Yale Univ

Weiner, Howard L MD [N] - **Spec Exp:** Multiple Sclerosis; Autoimmune Disease; **Hospital:** Brigham & Women's Hosp; **Address:** Harvard Inst Med-Ctr Neuro Disease, 77 Ave Louis Pasteur, Bldg HIM 730, Boston, MA 02115; **Phone:** 617-525-5300; **Board Cert:** Neurology 1978; **Med School:** Univ Colorado 1969; **Resid:** Internal Medicine, Beth Israel 1971; Neurology, Longwood Prog 1974; **Fellow:** Immunology, Univ Colo 1976; **Fac Appt:** Prof N, Harvard Med Sch

Young, Anne MD/PhD [N] - **Spec Exp:** Huntington's Disease; Parkinson's Disease; Movement Disorders; **Hospital:** Mass Genl Hosp; **Address:** Mass Genl Hosp, Dept Neurology, 55 Fruit Street, WAC 915, Boston, MA 02114; **Phone:** 617-726-2385; **Board Cert:** Neurology 1981; **Med School:** Johns Hopkins Univ 1973; **Resid:** Neurology, UCSF Med Ctr 1978; **Fac Appt:** Prof N, Harvard Med Sch

Mid Atlantic

Apatoff, Brian R MD/PhD [N] - **Spec Exp:** Multiple Sclerosis; Neuro-Immunology; **Hospital:** NY-Presby Hosp/Weill Cornell (page 66); **Address:** Multiple Sclerosis Inst, Ctr for Neurologic Disease, 401 E 55th St, New York, NY 10022; **Phone:** 212-593-6262; **Board Cert:** Neurology 1991; **Med School:** Univ Chicago-Pritzker Sch Med 1984; **Resid:** Neurology, Columbia Presby Med Ctr 1990; **Fellow:** Multiple Sclerosis, Neuro Inst-Columbia Univ 1992; **Fac Appt:** Assoc Prof N, Cornell Univ-Weill Med Coll

Baser, Susan M MD [N] - **Spec Exp:** Parkinson's Disease; Huntington's Disease; Dystonia; Movement Disorders; **Hospital:** Allegheny General Hosp; **Address:** Allegheny Neurology Assocs, 490 E North Ave Prof Bldg - Ste 500, Pittsburgh, PA 15212; **Phone:** 412-359-8860; **Board Cert:** Neurology 1990; **Med School:** Loyola Univ-Stritch Sch Med 1983; **Resid:** Neurology, Univ Pittsburgh 1987; **Fellow:** Neuropharmacology, Natl Inst Hlth 1990; **Fac Appt:** Assoc Prof N, Thomas Jefferson Univ

Bell, Rodney D MD [N] - **Spec Exp:** Stroke; **Hospital:** Thomas Jefferson Univ Hosp; **Address:** Thomas Jefferson Univ Dept Neurology, 900 Walnut St, Ste 200, Philadelphia, PA 19107; **Phone:** 215-955-6488; **Board Cert:** Internal Medicine 1975; Neurotology 1981; Vascular Neurology 2005; **Med School:** Oregon Hlth & Sci Univ 1971; **Resid:** Internal Medicine, Parkland Meml Hosp 1975; Neurology, Parkland Meml Hosp 1978; **Fac Appt:** Prof N, Thomas Jefferson Univ

Bergey, Gregory K MD [N] - **Spec Exp:** Epilepsy/Seizure Disorders; Epilepsy in Women; Epilepsy in Pregnancy; **Hospital:** Johns Hopkins Hosp (page 61); **Address:** Johns Hopkins Epilepsy Ctr, 601 N Caroline St, Meyer 2-147, Baltimore, MD 21287; **Phone:** 410-955-7337; **Board Cert:** Internal Medicine 1978; Neurology 1984; **Med School:** Univ Pennsylvania 1975; **Resid:** Internal Medicine, Yale-New Haven Hosp 1977; Neurology, Johns Hopkins Hosp 1981; **Fellow:** Neurological Physiology, Natl Inst Health 1983; **Fac Appt:** Prof N, Johns Hopkins Univ

Bressman, Susan MD [N] - **Spec Exp:** Parkinson's Disease; Movement Disorders; Dystonia; **Hospital:** Beth Israel Med Ctr - Petrie Division (page 57); **Address:** 10 Union Square East, Ste 5K, New York, NY 10003-3314; **Phone:** 212-844-8379; **Board Cert:** Neurology 1983; **Med School:** Columbia P&S 1977; **Resid:** Neurology, Columbia-Presby Med Ctr 1981; **Fellow:** Movement Disorders, Columbia-Presby Med Ctr 1983; **Fac Appt:** Prof N, Albert Einstein Coll Med

Brick, John MD [N] - **Spec Exp:** Epilepsy; **Hospital:** WV Univ Hosp - Ruby Memorial; **Address:** WV Univ-Dept Neurology, rm 7500 HSS, PO Box 9180, Morgantown, WV 26506-9180; **Phone:** 304-293-3527; **Board Cert:** Neurology 1982; **Med School:** W VA Univ 1977; **Resid:** Neurology, W Va Univ Hosp 1981; **Fellow:** Electroencephalography, Mayo Clinic 1983; **Fac Appt:** Prof N, W VA Univ

Brust, John C M MD [N] - **Spec Exp:** Stroke; Substance Abuse; Behavioral Neurology; **Hospital:** Harlem Hosp Ctr, NY-Presby Hosp/Columbia (page 66); **Address:** 506 Lenox Ave, rm 16-101, New York, NY 10037-1802; **Phone:** 212-939-4244; **Board Cert:** Neurology 2004; **Med School:** Columbia P&S 1962; **Resid:** Internal Medicine, Columbia Presby 1966; Neurology, Columbia Presby 1969; **Fac Appt:** Clin Prof N, Columbia P&S

Buchholz, David W MD [N] - **Spec Exp:** Migraine; Headache; **Hospital:** Johns Hopkins Hosp (page 61); **Address:** Johns Hopkins at Green Spring Station, 10753 Falls Rd, Ste 315, Lutherville, MD 21093; **Phone:** 410-583-2830; **Board Cert:** Neurology 1984; **Med School:** Univ Pennsylvania 1979; **Resid:** Neurology, Johns Hopkins Hosp 1983; **Fac Appt:** Assoc Prof N, Johns Hopkins Univ

Caronna, John J MD [N] - **Spec Exp:** Cerebrovascular Disease; Stroke; **Hospital:** NY-Presby Hosp/Weill Cornell (page 66); **Address:** Cornell Univ Dept Neurology, 520 E 70th St, Ste 607, New York, NY 10021; **Phone:** 212-746-2304; **Board Cert:** Neurology 1974; **Med School:** Cornell Univ-Weill Med Coll 1965; **Resid:** Internal Medicine, New York Hosp 1967; Neurology, New York Hosp 1971; **Fellow:** Neurology, New York Hosp/Cornell 1973; **Fac Appt:** Prof N, Cornell Univ-Weill Med Coll

Charney, Jonathan Z MD [N] - **Spec Exp:** Headache; Stroke; **Hospital:** Mount Sinai Med Ctr (page 64); **Address:** 1111 Park Ave, Ste 1H, New York, NY 10128-1234; **Phone:** 212-831-2886; **Board Cert:** Neurology 1977; **Med School:** NY Med Coll 1969; **Resid:** Neurology, Methodist Hosp-Baylor 1971; Neurology, Columbia-Presby Med Ctr 1973; **Fac Appt:** Asst Prof N, Mount Sinai Sch Med

Cook, Stuart D MD [N] - **Spec Exp:** Multiple Sclerosis; Infectious & Demyelinating Diseases; **Hospital:** UMDNJ-Univ Hosp-Newark; **Address:** 65 Bergen St, rm 1435, Newark, NJ 07101-1709; **Phone:** 973-972-9181; **Board Cert:** Neurology 1970; **Med School:** Univ VT Coll Med 1962; **Resid:** Neurology, Albert Einstein Coll Med 1968; **Fac Appt:** Prof N, UMDNJ-NJ Med Sch, Newark

Cornblath, David R MD [N] - **Spec Exp:** Peripheral Neuropathy; **Hospital:** Johns Hopkins Hosp (page 61); **Address:** 600 N Wolfe St Meyer 6-181A, Baltimore, MD 21287-6965; **Phone:** 410-955-2229; **Board Cert:** Neurology 1982; **Med School:** Case West Res Univ 1977; **Resid:** Neurology, Hosp Univ Penn 1981; **Fellow:** Neurology, Hosp Univ Penn 1982; **Fac Appt:** Prof N, Johns Hopkins Univ

Coyle, Patricia K MD [N] - **Spec Exp:** Multiple Sclerosis; Neuro-Immunology; Lyme Disease; Infections-Neurologic; **Hospital:** Stony Brook Univ Med Ctr; **Address:** Dept Neurology, HSC T-12, rm 020, Stonybrook Univ Med Ctr, East Setauket, NY 11794; **Phone:** 631-444-2599; **Board Cert:** Neurology 2004; **Med School:** Johns Hopkins Univ 1974; **Resid:** Neurology, Johns Hopkins Hosp 1978; **Fellow:** Neurological Immunology, Johns Hopkins Hosp 1980; **Fac Appt:** Prof N, SUNY Stony Brook

Dalakas, Marinos C MD [N] - **Spec Exp:** Neuromuscular Disorders; **Hospital:** Thomas Jefferson Univ Hosp; **Address:** Thomas Jefferson Univ Hosp, Neuromuscular Div, 900 Walnut St, Ste 200, Philadelphia, PA 19107; **Phone:** 215-955-7952; **Board Cert:** Neurology 1980; **Med School:** Greece 1972; **Resid:** Neurology, UMDNJ-Univ Hosp 1977; **Fellow:** Neuromuscular Medicine, Natl Inst Hlth 1980

Neurology

De Angelis, Lisa M MD [N] - **Spec Exp:** Neuro-Oncology; **Hospital:** Meml Sloan-Kettering Cancer Ctr; **Address:** 1275 York Avenue, New York, NY 10065; **Phone:** 212-639-7123; **Board Cert:** Neurology 1986; **Med School:** Columbia P&S 1980; **Resid:** Neurology, Neuro Inst-Presby Hosp 1984; **Fellow:** Neuro-Oncology, Neuro Inst-Presby Hosp 1985; Neuro-Oncology, Meml Sloan-Kettering Cancer Ctr 1986; **Fac Appt:** Prof N, Cornell Univ-Weill Med Coll

Devinsky, Orrin MD [N] - **Spec Exp:** Epilepsy; Tuberous Sclerosis; Behavioral Neurology; **Hospital:** NYU Langone Med Ctr (page 67), St Barnabas Med Ctr; **Address:** 223 E 34th St Fl Ground, New York, NY 10016-4972; **Phone:** 646-558-0803; **Board Cert:** Neurology 1987; Clinical Neurophysiology 1990; **Med School:** Harvard Med Sch 1982; **Resid:** Neurology, NY Hosp-Cornell Med Ctr 1986; **Fellow:** Epilepsy, Natl Inst Health 1988; **Fac Appt:** Prof N, NYU Sch Med

Dewberry, Robert G MD [N] - **Hospital:** Maryland Genl Hosp; **Address:** Maryland Genl Hosp, Div Neurology, 827 Linden Ave Fl Basement, Baltimore, MD 21201; **Phone:** 410-225-8290; **Board Cert:** Neurology 1992; **Med School:** Univ MD Sch Med 1987; **Resid:** Neurology, Barnes Hospital 1991; **Fellow:** Neuromuscular Disease, Univ Virginia Hosp 1993

Dichter, Marc A MD [N] - **Spec Exp:** Epilepsy/Seizure Disorders; **Hospital:** Hosp Univ Penn - UPHS (page 60); **Address:** Dept Neurology, 3W Gates Bldg, 3400 Spruce St, Philadelphia, PA 19104; **Phone:** 215-349-5166; **Board Cert:** Neurology 1978; **Med School:** NYU Sch Med 1969; **Resid:** Neurology, Beth Israel Hosp/Chldns Hosp/ Brigham Hosp 1975; **Fac Appt:** Prof N, Univ Pennsylvania

Drachman, Daniel B MD [N] - **Spec Exp:** Muscular Dystrophy; Neuromuscular Disorders; Myasthenia Gravis; Amyotrophic Lateral Sclerosis (ALS); **Hospital:** Johns Hopkins Hosp (page 61); **Address:** Johns Hopkins Med Ctr, 600 N Wolfe St, Meyer 5-119, Baltimore, MD 21287-7519; **Phone:** 410-955-5406; **Board Cert:** Neurology 1963; **Med School:** NYU Sch Med 1956; **Resid:** Neurology, Boston City Hosp 1959; Neuropathology, Mallory Inst Path/Boston City Hosp 1960; **Fellow:** Neurology, Harvard Med Sch 1960; **Fac Appt:** Prof N, Johns Hopkins Univ

Dromerick, Alexander MD [N] - **Spec Exp:** Stroke Rehabilitation; **Hospital:** Natl Rehab Hosp, Washington Hosp Ctr; **Address:** NRH-Neuroscience Rsch Ctr, 102 Irving St NW, Washington, DC 20010; **Phone:** 202-877-1000; **Board Cert:** Neurology 1992; **Med School:** Univ MD Sch Med 1986; **Resid:** Neurology, Hosp Univ Penn 1991; **Fellow:** Neurological Rehabilitation, Hosp Univ Penn 1992; Neurological Rehabilitation, Cornell-Burke Rehab Ctr 1993

Fahn, Stanley MD [N] - **Spec Exp:** Movement Disorders; Parkinson's Disease; **Hospital:** NY-Presby Hosp/Columbia (page 66); **Address:** Neurological Institute, 710 W 168th St Fl 3 - rm 350, New York, NY 10032; **Phone:** 212-305-5277; **Board Cert:** Neurology 1968; **Med School:** UCSF 1958; **Resid:** Neurology, Neuro Inst-Columbia 1962; **Fac Appt:** Prof N, Columbia P&S

Feinberg, Todd E MD [N] - **Spec Exp:** Alzheimer's Disease; Dementia; **Hospital:** Beth Israel Med Ctr - Petrie Division (page 57); **Address:** Beth Israel Med Ctr, Yarmon Neurobehavioral Ctr, First Ave at 16th St, New York, NY 10003; **Phone:** 212-420-4111; **Board Cert:** Psychiatry 1984; Neurology 1987; **Med School:** Mount Sinai Sch Med 1978; **Resid:** Psychiatry, Mt Sinai Med Ctr 1982; Neurology, Mt Sinai Med Ctr 1984; **Fellow:** Behavioral Neurology, Univ Florida 1986; **Fac Appt:** Clin Prof N, Albert Einstein Coll Med

Fink, Matthew E MD [N] - **Spec Exp:** Cerebrovascular Disease; Stroke; **Hospital:** NY-Presby Hosp/Weill Cornell (page 66); **Address:** NY Cornell Med Ctr Dept Neurology, 525 E 68th St, New York, NY 10065; **Phone:** 212-746-4564; **Board Cert:** Internal Medicine 1980; Neurology 1983; Vascular Neurology 2005; **Med School:** Univ Pittsburgh 1976; **Resid:** Internal Medicine, Boston Med Ctr 1980; Neurology, Columbia-Presby Hosp 1982; **Fac Appt:** Prof N, Cornell Univ

Foo, Sun-Hoo MD [N] - **Spec Exp:** Stroke; Headache; Parkinson's Disease; Dementia; **Hospital:** NYU Langone Med Ctr (page 67), NY Downtown Hosp; **Address:** 650 1st Ave, FL 4, New York, NY 10016-3240; **Phone:** 212-213-0270; **Board Cert:** Internal Medicine 1976; Neurology 1980; **Med School:** Taiwan 1972; **Resid:** Internal Medicine, St Vincent's Hosp 1976; Neurology, NYU Med Ctr 1979; **Fac Appt:** Prof N, NYU Sch Med

French, Jacqueline MD [N] - **Spec Exp:** Epilepsy/Seizure Disorders; **Hospital:** NYU Langone Med Ctr (page 67); **Address:** 223 E 34th St, New York, NY 10016; **Phone:** 646-558-0805; **Board Cert:** Neurology 1987; **Med School:** Brown Univ 1982; **Resid:** Neurology, Mount Sinai Hosp 1986; **Fellow:** Epilepsy, Mount Sinai Hosp 1988; Epilepsy, Yale-New Haven Hosp 1989; **Fac Appt:** Prof N, NYU Sch Med

Galetta, Steven MD [N] - **Spec Exp:** Neuro-Ophthalmology; Optic Nerve Disorders; Multiple Sclerosis; **Hospital:** Hosp Univ Penn - UPHS (page 60); **Address:** Hosp Univ Penn, Dept Neurology, 3W Gates Bldg, 3400 Spruce St, Philadelphia, PA 19104; **Phone:** 215-662-3381; **Board Cert:** Neurology 1988; **Med School:** Cornell Univ-Weill Med Coll 1983; **Resid:** Neurology, Hosp Univ Penn 1987; **Fellow:** Neuro-Ophthalmology, Bascom Palmer Eye Inst 1988; **Fac Appt:** Prof N, Univ Pennsylvania

Gendelman, Seymour MD [N] - **Spec Exp:** Parkinson's Disease; Dementia; Headache; **Hospital:** Mount Sinai Med Ctr (page 64); **Address:** 5 E 98th St Fl 7, Box 1139, New York, NY 10029-6501; **Phone:** 212-241-8172; **Board Cert:** Neurology 1971; **Med School:** Geo Wash Univ 1964; **Resid:** Neurology, Mt Sinai Hosp 1968; **Fac Appt:** Clin Prof N, Mount Sinai Sch Med

Gizzi, Martin S MD/PhD [N] - **Spec Exp:** Neuro-Ophthalmology; Balance Disorders; Progressive Supranuclear Palsy (PSP); Stroke; **Hospital:** JFK Med Ctr - Edison; **Address:** NJ Neuroscience Insitute, 65 James St, Edison, NJ 08820-3947; **Phone:** 732-321-7010; **Board Cert:** Neurology 1990; Vascular Neurology 2008; **Med School:** Univ Miami Sch Med 1985; **Resid:** Neurology, Mount Sinai Hosp 1989; **Fellow:** Neuro-Ophthalmology, Mount Sinai Hosp 1991; **Fac Appt:** Prof N, Seton Hall Univ Sch Hlth & Med Scis

Glass, Jon MD [N] - **Spec Exp:** Neuro-Oncology; Brain Tumors; Spinal Tumors; **Hospital:** Thomas Jefferson Univ Hosp; **Address:** 909 Walnut St Fl 2, Philadelphia, PA 19107; **Phone:** 215-503-7005; **Board Cert:** Neurology 1993; **Med School:** SUNY Downstate 1986; **Resid:** Neurology, Boston Univ 1990; **Fellow:** Neuro-Oncology, Mass Genl Hosp 1992; **Fac Appt:** Asst Prof N, NYU Sch Med

Golbe, Lawrence I MD [N] - **Spec Exp:** Parkinson's Disease; Progressive Supranuclear Palsy (PSP); Movement Disorders; **Hospital:** Robert Wood Johnson Univ Hosp - New Brunswick; **Address:** 97 Paterson St Fl 2 - rm 204, New Brunswick, NJ 08901-2160; **Phone:** 732-235-7733; **Board Cert:** Neurology 1984; **Med School:** NYU Sch Med 1978; **Resid:** Internal Medicine, Hahnemann Univ Hosp 1980; Neurology, Bellevue Hosp 1983; **Fac Appt:** Prof N, UMDNJ-RW Johnson Med Sch

Goodgold, Albert MD [N] - **Spec Exp:** Parkinson's Disease; Spinal Cord Disorders; Multiple Sclerosis; Movement Disorders; **Hospital:** NYU Langone Med Ctr (page 67); **Address:** 530 First Ave Fl 5 - Ste 5A, New York, NY 10016; **Phone:** 212-263-7205; **Med School:** Switzerland 1955; **Resid:** Neurology, Bellevue Hosp 1960; **Fac Appt:** Prof N, NYU Sch Med

Griffin, John W MD [N] - **Spec Exp:** Peripheral Neuropathy; Guillain-Barre Syndrome; Diabetic Polyneuropathy; **Hospital:** Johns Hopkins Hosp (page 61); **Address:** 600 N Wolfe St, Pathology, Rm 509, Baltimore, MD 21287; **Phone:** 410-955-2227; **Board Cert:** Internal Medicine 1974; Neurology 1976; **Med School:** Stanford Univ 1968; **Resid:** Internal Medicine, Johns Hopkins Hosp 1970; Neurology, Johns Hopkins Hosp 1973; **Fac Appt:** Prof N, Johns Hopkins Univ

Neurology

Hiesiger, Emile MD [N] - **Spec Exp:** Pain Management; Neuro-Oncology; **Hospital:** NYU Langone Med Ctr (page 67), VA Med Ctr - Manhattan; **Address:** 530 1st Ave, Ste 5A, New York, NY 10016-6402; **Phone:** 212-263-6123; **Board Cert:** Neurology 1983; **Med School:** NY Med Coll 1978; **Resid:** Neurology, NYU Med Ctr 1982; **Fellow:** Neurology, Meml Sloan-Kettering Cancer Ctr 1984; **Fac Appt:** Assoc Clin Prof N, NYU Sch Med

Hurtig, Howard MD [N] - **Spec Exp:** Parkinson's Disease; Movement Disorders; **Hospital:** Pennsylvania Hosp (page 60); **Address:** Pennsylvania Hosp Neurological Inst, 330 S 9th St Fl 3, Philadelphia, PA 19107; **Phone:** 215-829-6500; **Board Cert:** Neurology 1976; **Med School:** Tulane Univ 1966; **Resid:** Internal Medicine, New York Hosp 1968; Neurology, Hosp Univ Penn 1973; **Fac Appt:** Prof N, Univ Pennsylvania

Jordan, Barry D MD [N] - **Spec Exp:** Brain Injury; Sports Neurology; Concussion; Memory Disorders; **Hospital:** Burke Rehab Hosp; **Address:** Burke Rehabilitation Hosp, 785 Mamaroneck Ave, White Plains, NY 10605; **Phone:** 914-597-2332; **Board Cert:** Neurology 1989; **Med School:** Harvard Med Sch 1981; **Resid:** Neurology, New York Hosp 1986; **Fellow:** Hosp Spec Surgery 1987; UCLA Med Ctr 1998; **Fac Appt:** Assoc Prof N, Cornell Univ-Weill Med Coll

Kolodny, Edwin H MD [N] - **Spec Exp:** Pediatric Neurology; Inherited Disorders of Nervous System; Gaucher Disease; Fabry's Disease; **Hospital:** NYU Langone Med Ctr (page 67), Bellevue Hosp Ctr; **Address:** 403 E 34 St Fl 2, New York, NY 10016-6402; **Phone:** 212-263-8344; **Board Cert:** Neurology 1971; Clinical Genetics 1984; Clinical Biochemical Genetics 1987; **Med School:** NYU Sch Med 1962; **Resid:** Internal Medicine, Bellevue Hosp 1964; Neurology, Mass Genl Hosp 1967; **Fellow:** Neurological Pathology, Mass Genl Hosp 1966; Neurology, Nat Inst Neurol Dis & Stroke 1970; **Fac Appt:** Prof N, NYU Sch Med

Krauss, Gregory L MD [N] - **Spec Exp:** Epilepsy/Seizure Disorders; **Hospital:** Johns Hopkins Hosp (page 61); **Address:** Johns Hopkins Hosp, Dept Neurology, 600 N Wolfe St, Meyer 2-147, Baltimore, MD 21287; **Phone:** 410-955-2822; **Board Cert:** Neurology 1990; **Med School:** Oregon Hlth & Sci Univ 1985; **Resid:** Neurology, Johns Hopkins Hosp 1989; **Fellow:** Epilepsy, Johns Hopkins Hosp 1991; **Fac Appt:** Assoc Prof N, Johns Hopkins Univ

Krumholz, Allan MD [N] - **Spec Exp:** Epilepsy/Seizure Disorders; **Hospital:** Univ of MD Med Ctr; **Address:** Univ Maryland Med System, Dept Neurology, 16 S Eutaw St, Baltimore, MD 21201-1544; **Phone:** 410-328-6266; **Board Cert:** Neurology 1977; Clinical Neurophysiology 2006; **Med School:** Ros Franklin Univ/Chicago Med Sch 1970; **Resid:** Internal Medicine, Baltimore City Hosp 1972; Neurology, Johns Hopkins Hosp 1975; **Fellow:** Electroencephalography, Johns Hopkins Hosp 1980; **Fac Appt:** Prof N, Univ MD Sch Med

Kula, Roger W MD [N] - **Spec Exp:** Neuromuscular Disorders; Myasthenia Gravis; Syringomyelia & Spinal Cord Diseases; Chiari's Deformity; **Hospital:** N Shore Univ Hosp, Schneider Chldn's Hosp; **Address:** 865 Northern Blvd, Ste 302, Great Neck, NY 11021; **Phone:** 516-570-4400; **Board Cert:** Internal Medicine 1975; Neurology 1977; Neuromuscular Medicine 2008; **Med School:** Johns Hopkins Univ 1970; **Resid:** Internal Medicine, New York Hosp 1972; Neurology, UCSF Med Ctr 1974; **Fellow:** Neuromuscular Medicine, Natl Inst Hlth 1977; **Fac Appt:** Assoc Prof N, SUNY Hlth Sci Ctr

Kunschner, Lara MD [N] - **Spec Exp:** Neuro-Oncology; Brain Tumors; **Hospital:** Allegheny General Hosp; **Address:** 420 E North Ave, Ste 206, Pittsburgh, PA 15212; **Phone:** 412-359-8850; **Board Cert:** Neurology 1999; **Med School:** Univ Pittsburgh 1994; **Resid:** Neurology, Univ Michigan Hosps 1999; **Fellow:** Neuro-Oncology, MD Anderson Cancer Ctr 2000

Kuzniecky, Ruben MD [N] - **Spec Exp:** Epilepsy/Seizure Disorders; MRI; Developmental Disorders; **Hospital:** NYU Langone Med Ctr (page 67); **Address:** 223 E 34th St Fl Ground, New York, NY 10016; **Phone:** 646-558-0802; **Board Cert:** Neurology 1990; **Med School:** Argentina 1980; **Resid:** Neurology, McGill Univ 1986; **Fellow:** Epilepsy, McGill Univ 1988; **Fac Appt:** Prof N, NYU Sch Med

Labar, Douglas R MD/PhD [N] - **Spec Exp:** Epilepsy/Seizure Disorders; **Hospital:** NY-Presby Hosp/Weill Cornell (page 66); **Address:** NY Weill Cornell Med Ctr, 525 E 68th St, Ste K619, New York, NY 10021; **Phone:** 212-746-2359; **Board Cert:** Neurology 1987; **Med School:** Med Coll PA 1982; **Resid:** Neurology, Columbia Presby Med Ctr 1986; **Fellow:** Epilepsy, Columbia Presby Med Ctr 1988; **Fac Appt:** Prof N, Cornell Univ-Weill Med Coll

Lacomis, David MD [N] - **Spec Exp:** Amyotrophic Lateral Sclerosis (ALS); Muscle Disorders; Myasthenia Gravis; Neuromuscular Disorders; **Hospital:** UPMC Presby, Pittsburgh; **Address:** Dept Neurology -Kaufmann Med Bldg, 3471 Fifth Ave, Ste 810, Pittsburgh, PA 15213; **Phone:** 412-692-4917; **Board Cert:** Neurology 1992; Clinical Neurophysiology 2004; **Med School:** Penn State Univ-Hershey Med Ctr 1987; **Resid:** Neurology, Harvard Affil Hosp 1991; **Fellow:** Neuromuscular Disease, Univ Mass Med Ctr 1993; **Fac Appt:** Prof N, Univ Pittsburgh

Laterra, John J MD/PhD [N] - **Spec Exp:** Neuro-Oncology; Brain Tumors; **Hospital:** Johns Hopkins Hosp (page 61), Kennedy Krieger Inst; **Address:** Phipps 115, 600 N Wolfe St, Baltimore, MD 21287; **Phone:** 410-614-3853; **Board Cert:** Neurology 1990; **Med School:** Case West Res Univ 1984; **Resid:** Neurology, Univ Mich Hosps 1988; **Fellow:** Research, Johns Hopkins Hosp 1989; **Fac Appt:** Prof N, Johns Hopkins Univ

Latov, Norman MD/PhD [N] - **Spec Exp:** Peripheral Neuropathy; Neuro-Immunology; **Hospital:** NY-Presby Hosp/Weill Cornell (page 66); **Address:** 1305 York Ave Fl 2, New York, NY 10021; **Phone:** 646-962-3202; **Board Cert:** Neurology 1989; **Med School:** Univ Pennsylvania 1975; **Resid:** Internal Medicine, Boston City Hosp 1976; Neurology, Columbia-Presby Med Ctr 1979; **Fellow:** Immunology, Columbia-Presby Med Ctr 1981; **Fac Appt:** Prof N, Cornell Univ-Weill Med Coll

Levine, David N MD [N] - **Spec Exp:** Dementia; Stroke; Spinal Cord Disorders; **Hospital:** NYU Langone Med Ctr (page 67); **Address:** 400 E 34th St, Ste RIRM-311, New York, NY 10016-4901; **Phone:** 212-263-7744; **Board Cert:** Neurology 1976; **Med School:** Harvard Med Sch 1968; **Resid:** Neurology, Mass Genl Hosp 1974; **Fellow:** Neurology, Mass Genl Hosp 1976; **Fac Appt:** Prof N, NYU Sch Med

Levine, Steven R MD [N] - **Spec Exp:** Stroke; Cerebrovascular Disease; **Hospital:** Mount Sinai Med Ctr (page 64); **Address:** 5 E 98th St, Fl 7th, Box 1139, New York, NY 10029-6500; **Phone:** 212-241-1970; **Board Cert:** Neurology 1986; Vascular Neurology 2005; **Med School:** Med Coll Wisc 1981; **Resid:** Neurology, Univ Mich Hosps 1985; **Fellow:** Cerebrovascular Disease, Henry Ford Hosp 1987; **Fac Appt:** Prof N, Mount Sinai Sch Med

Liporace, Joyce D MD [N] - **Spec Exp:** Epilepsy in Women; Women's Health; Epilepsy in Pregnancy; **Hospital:** Riddle Meml Hosp; **Address:** Riddle Healthcare 2, 1088 Baltimore Pike, Ste 2205, Media, PA 19063; **Phone:** 610-744-2960; **Board Cert:** Neurological Surgery 1993; Clinical Neurophysiology 1999; **Med School:** Johns Hopkins Univ 1988; **Resid:** Neurology, Hosp U Penn 1992; **Fellow:** Clinical Neurophysiology, Hosp U Penn 1994; **Fac Appt:** Assoc Prof Med, Thomas Jefferson Univ

Neurology

Lipton, Richard MD [N] - **Spec Exp:** Headache; Clinical Trials; **Hospital:** Montefiore Med Ctr - Div. Weiler; **Address:** Montefiore Headache Center, 1575 Blondell Ave, Ste 225, Bronx, NY 10461-2662; **Phone:** 718-405-8360; **Board Cert:** Neurology 1985; **Med School:** Univ Chicago-Pritzker Sch Med 1980; **Resid:** Neurology, Montefiore Med Ctr 1984; **Fellow:** Neurological Physiology, Montefiore Med Ctr 1985; NeuroEpidemiology, Columbia Univ 1990; **Fac Appt:** Prof N, Albert Einstein Coll Med

Liu, Grant T MD [N] - **Spec Exp:** Pediatric Neuro-Ophthalmology; Neuro-Ophthalmology; **Hospital:** Hosp Univ Penn - UPHS (page 60), Chldns Hosp of Philadelphia, The; **Address:** Hosp Univ Penn, Dept Neurology, 3W Gates Bldg, 3400 Spruce St, Philadelphia, PA 19104; **Phone:** 215-349-8460; **Board Cert:** Neurology 1993; **Med School:** Columbia P&S 1988; **Resid:** Neurology, Harvard-Nolgwood Neurology Program 1992; **Fellow:** Neuro-Ophthalmology, Bascom Palmer Eye Inst 1993; **Fac Appt:** Assoc Prof N, Univ Pennsylvania

Logigian, Eric L MD [N] - **Spec Exp:** Neuromuscular Disorders; Electromyography; Lyme Disease; Peripheral Neuropathy; **Hospital:** Univ of Rochester Strong Meml Hosp, Highland Hosp of Rochester; **Address:** Univ Rochester, Dept of Neurology, 601 Elmwood Ave, Box 673, Rochester, NY 14642; **Phone:** 585-275-4568; **Board Cert:** Internal Medicine 1981; Neurology 1985; Clinical Neurophysiology 1999; **Med School:** Boston Univ 1978; **Resid:** Internal Medicine, Beth Israel Hosp 1981; Neurology, Mass Genl Hosp 1984; **Fellow:** Clinical Neurophysiology, Mass General Hosp 1985; **Fac Appt:** Prof N, Univ Rochester

Lublin, Fred D MD [N] - **Spec Exp:** Multiple Sclerosis; **Hospital:** Mount Sinai Med Ctr (page 64); **Address:** Dickinson Ctr for Multiple Sclerosis, 5 E 98th St, Box 1138, New York, NY 10029-6574; **Phone:** 212-241-6854; **Board Cert:** Neurology 1977; **Med School:** Jefferson Med Coll 1972; **Resid:** Neurology, New York Hosp/Cornell 1976; **Fac Appt:** Prof N, Mount Sinai Sch Med

McArthur, Justin C MD [N] - **Spec Exp:** AIDS/HIV; Multiple Sclerosis; **Hospital:** Johns Hopkins Hosp (page 61); **Address:** Johns Hopkins Hosp, Dept Neurology, 600 N Wolfe St, Meyer 6-113, Baltimore, MD 21287; **Phone:** 410-955-3730; **Board Cert:** Neurology 1986; Internal Medicine 1984; **Med School:** England, UK 1979; **Resid:** Internal Medicine, Johns Hopkins Hosp 1982; Neurology, Johns Hopkins Hosp 1985; **Fac Appt:** Prof N, Johns Hopkins Univ

McCluskey, Leo MD [N] - **Spec Exp:** Amyotrophic Lateral Sclerosis (ALS); **Hospital:** Hosp Univ Penn - UPHS (page 60); **Address:** 330 S 9th St, Philadelphia, PA 19107; **Phone:** 215-829-3053; **Board Cert:** Neurology 1986; **Med School:** Columbia P&S 1980; **Resid:** Internal Medicine, Univ Mich 1982; Neurology, Hosp Univ Penn 1985; **Fellow:** Neuromuscular Disease, Hosp Univ Penn 1986; **Fac Appt:** Assoc Prof N, Univ Pennsylvania

Miller, Aaron MD [N] - **Spec Exp:** Multiple Sclerosis; Alzheimer's Disease; Autoimmune Disease; **Hospital:** Mount Sinai Med Ctr (page 64), Maimonides Med Ctr (page 63); **Address:** Corinne Goldsmith Dickinson Ctr for MS, 5 E 98th St, Box 1138, New York, NY 10029; **Phone:** 212-241-6854; **Board Cert:** Internal Medicine 1972; Neurology 1977; **Med School:** NYU Sch Med 1968; **Resid:** Internal Medicine, Jacobi Med Ctr 1970; Neurology, Montefiore Med Ctr 1975; **Fellow:** Neurovirology, Johns Hopkins Hosp 1977; **Fac Appt:** Prof N, Mount Sinai Sch Med

Mitsumoto, Hiroshi MD [N] - **Spec Exp:** Amyotrophic Lateral Sclerosis (ALS); Neuromuscular Disorders; Clinical Trials; **Hospital:** NY-Presby Hosp/Columbia (page 66); **Address:** Neurological Inst, 710 W 168th St Fl 9 - rm 9001, New York, NY 10032; **Phone:** 212-305-1319; **Board Cert:** Neurology 1978; **Med School:** Japan 1968; **Resid:** Internal Medicine, Toho Univ Hosps 1972; Neurology, Univ Hosps 1976; **Fellow:** Neurological Pathology, Cleveland Clinic 1978; Neuromuscular Medicine, New England Med Ctr 1981; **Fac Appt:** Prof N, Columbia P&S

Mohr, JP MD [N] - **Spec Exp:** Aphasia; Stroke; Arteriovenous Malformations; Arteriovenous Malformations; **Hospital:** NY-Presby Hosp/Columbia (page 66); **Address:** Neurological Inst-Dept Neurology, 710 W 168 St, Ste 615, New York, NY 10032-2603; **Phone:** 212-305-8033; **Board Cert:** Neurology 1971; Vascular Neurology 2005; **Med School:** Univ VA Sch Med 1963; **Resid:** Neurology, Columbia Presby Med Ctr 1966; Neurology, Mass Genl Hosp 1968; **Fellow:** Neurology, Mass Genl Hosp 1969; **Fac Appt:** Clin Prof N, Columbia P&S

Nath, Avindra MD [N] - **Spec Exp:** Neurological Infections; AIDS/HIV; Multiple Sclerosis; **Hospital:** Johns Hopkins Hosp (page 61); **Address:** Johns Hopkins Dept Neuroscience, 600 Wolfe St, Room 509 Pathology, Baltimore, MD 21287; **Phone:** 443-287-4656; **Board Cert:** Neurology 1988; **Med School:** India 1982; **Resid:** Neurology, Univ Texas HSC 1986; **Fellow:** Neurological Immunology, Univ Texas 1988; Neurological Viral Immunology, Natl Inst Hlth 1990; **Fac Appt:** Prof N, Johns Hopkins Univ

Newman, Lawrence C MD [N] - **Spec Exp:** Headache; Pain-Facial; **Hospital:** St Luke's - Roosevelt Hosp Ctr - Roosevelt Div (page 57); **Address:** St Luke's-Roosevelt Hosp-Headache Inst, 1000 Tenth Ave Fl 1 - Ste 1C10, New York, NY 10019-1192; **Phone:** 212-523-5869; **Board Cert:** Neurology 2005; Headache Medicine 2006; **Med School:** Mexico 1983; **Resid:** Internal Medicine, Elmhurst Hosp 1986; Neurology, Montefiore Med Ctr 1989; **Fac Appt:** Assoc Prof N, Albert Einstein Coll Med

Olanow, C Warren MD [N] - **Spec Exp:** Parkinson's Disease; Movement Disorders; **Hospital:** Mount Sinai Med Ctr (page 64); **Address:** 5 E 98th St, New York, NY 10029; **Phone:** 212-241-8435; **Med School:** Univ Toronto 1965; **Resid:** Neurology, Toronto Genl Hosp 1968; Neurology, Columbia Presby Hosp 1970; **Fellow:** Neurological Anatomy, Columbia Presby Hosp 1971; **Fac Appt:** Prof N, Mount Sinai Sch Med

Pedley, Timothy A MD [N] - **Spec Exp:** Epilepsy/Seizure Disorders; **Hospital:** NY-Presby Hosp/Columbia (page 66); **Address:** The Neurological Inst, 710 W 168th St, rm 1406, New York, NY 10032; **Phone:** 212-305-6489; **Board Cert:** Neurology 1975; **Med School:** Yale Univ 1969; **Resid:** Neurology, Stanford Univ Hosp 1973; **Fellow:** Clinical Neurophysiology, Stanford Univ Hosp 1975; **Fac Appt:** Prof N, Columbia P&S

Petito, Frank A MD [N] - **Spec Exp:** Multiple Sclerosis; Headache; Lyme Disease; **Hospital:** NY-Presby Hosp/Weill Cornell (page 66); **Address:** 525 E 68th St, Ste 615, New York, NY 10065; **Phone:** 212-746-2309; **Board Cert:** Neurology 1974; **Med School:** Columbia P&S 1967; **Resid:** Neurology, New York Hosp 1971; **Fac Appt:** Prof N, Cornell Univ-Weill Med Coll

Posner, Jerome MD [N] - **Spec Exp:** Neuro-Oncology; Brain Tumors; **Hospital:** Meml Sloan-Kettering Cancer Ctr; **Address:** 1275 York Avenue, New York, NY 10065; **Phone:** 212-639-7047; **Board Cert:** Neurology 1962; **Med School:** Univ Wash 1955; **Resid:** Neurology, Univ WA Affil Hosp 1959; **Fellow:** Biochemistry, Univ WA Affil Hosp 1963; **Fac Appt:** Prof N, Cornell Univ-Weill Med Coll

Pula, Thaddeus MD [N] - **Spec Exp:** Neurophysiology; Electromyography; **Hospital:** Maryland Genl Hosp; **Address:** Maryland Genl Hosp, Div Neurology, 827 Linden Ave Fl Basement, Baltimore, MD 21201-4606; **Phone:** 410-225-8290; **Board Cert:** Neurology 1981; **Med School:** Univ MD Sch Med 1976; **Resid:** Internal Medicine, Mercy Hosp Med Ctr; **Fellow:** Neurology, Univ Maryland

Reich, Stephen G MD [N] - **Spec Exp:** Movement Disorders; Parkinson's Disease; Ataxia; Dystonia-Botox Therapy; **Hospital:** Univ of MD Med Ctr; **Address:** Univ Maryland Med System, Frenkil Bldg, 16 S Eutaw St Fl 3, Baltimore, MD 21201; **Phone:** 410-328-5858; **Board Cert:** Neurology 1989; **Med School:** Tulane Univ 1983; **Resid:** Neurology, Case West Res Univ Hosp 1987; **Fellow:** Movement Disorders, Johns Hopkins Hosp 1988; **Fac Appt:** Assoc Prof N, Univ MD Sch Med

Neurology

Relkin, Norman R MD/PhD [N] - **Spec Exp:** Alzheimer's Disease; Dementia; Memory Disorders; **Hospital:** NY-Presby Hosp/Weill Cornell (page 66); **Address:** Weill Cornell Memory Disorders Program, 428 E 72nd St, Ste 500, New York, NY 10021; **Phone:** 212-746-2441; **Board Cert:** Neurology 1992; **Med School:** Albert Einstein Coll Med 1987; **Resid:** Neurology, New York Hosp 1991; **Fellow:** Behavioral Neurology, New York Hosp-Cornell 1992; **Fac Appt:** Asst Prof N, Cornell Univ-Weill Med Coll

Rosenfeld, Myrna MD/PhD [N] - **Spec Exp:** Neuro-Oncology; Brain Tumors; **Hospital:** Hosp Univ Penn - UPHS (page 60); **Address:** Hosp Univ Penn, Dept Neurology, 3400 Spruce St, 3W Gates, Philadelphia, PA 19104; **Phone:** 215-746-4707; **Board Cert:** Neurology 1990; **Med School:** Northwestern Univ 1985; **Resid:** Neurology, Northwestern Univ Hosp 1987; Neurology, Univ Hosp Cleveland 1989; **Fellow:** Neuro-Oncology, Meml Sloan Kettering Cancer Ctr; **Fac Appt:** Assoc Prof N, Univ Pennsylvania

Rosenfeld, Steven S MD [N] - **Spec Exp:** Brain Tumors; Gliomas; Neuro-Oncology; **Hospital:** NY-Presby Hosp/Columbia (page 66); **Address:** Neurological Inst of NY-Brain Tumor Ctr, 710 W 168th St, rm 204, New York, NY 10032; **Phone:** 212-305-1718; **Board Cert:** Neurology 1994; **Med School:** Northwestern Univ 1985; **Resid:** Neurology, Duke Univ Med Ctr 1989; **Fellow:** Neuro-Oncology, Duke Univ Med Ctr 1990; **Fac Appt:** Prof N, Columbia P&S

Sage, Jacob MD [N] - **Spec Exp:** Parkinson's Disease; **Hospital:** Robert Wood Johnson Univ Hosp - New Brunswick; **Address:** UMDNJ, Dept Neurology, 97 Paterson St, New Brunswick, NJ 08901-2160; **Phone:** 732-235-7733; **Board Cert:** Neurology 1979; **Med School:** Univ Pittsburgh 1972; **Resid:** Neurology, Univ Pittsburgh Hosps 1978; **Fellow:** Neurological Chemistry, NY Hosp-Cornell 1980; **Fac Appt:** Prof N, UMDNJ-RW Johnson Med Sch

Schwartzman, Robert J MD [N] - **Spec Exp:** Reflex Sympathetic Dystrophy (RSD); Pain Management; **Hospital:** Hahnemann Univ Hosp; **Address:** Drexel Neurological Assocs, 219 N Broad St Fl 7, Philadelphia, PA 19107; **Phone:** 215-762-6915; **Board Cert:** Internal Medicine 1971; Neurology 1974; **Med School:** Univ Pennsylvania 1965; **Resid:** Internal Medicine, Duke Univ Hosp 1967; Neurology, Hosp Univ Penn 1969; **Fellow:** Neurology, NIH-Med Neur Br 1971; **Fac Appt:** Prof N, Drexel Univ Coll Med

Shefner, Jeremy M MD/PhD [N] - **Spec Exp:** Amyotrophic Lateral Sclerosis (ALS); Neuromuscular Disorders; **Hospital:** Univ Hosp - SUNY Upstate; **Address:** 750 E Adams Rd, Syracuse, NY 13210-1834; **Phone:** 315-464-4243; **Board Cert:** Neurology 1989; Clinical Neurophysiology 2004; **Med School:** Northwestern Univ 1983; **Resid:** Neurology, Harvard-Longwood Neur Trng 1988; **Fellow:** Neuromuscular Disease, Brigham & Womens Hosp 1990; **Fac Appt:** Prof N, SUNY Upstate Med Univ

Shoulson, Ira MD [N] - **Spec Exp:** Parkinson's Disease; Movement Disorders; Huntington's Disease; **Hospital:** Univ of Rochester Strong Meml Hosp; **Address:** 1351 Mount Hope Ave, Ste 218, Rochester, NY 14620; **Phone:** 585-275-2585; **Board Cert:** Internal Medicine 1974; Neurology 1980; **Med School:** Univ Rochester 1971; **Resid:** Internal Medicine, Strong Meml Hosp 1973; Neurology, Strong Meml Hosp 1977; **Fellow:** Neurology, Natl Inst Hlth 1975; **Fac Appt:** Prof N, Univ Rochester

Shulman, Lisa M MD [N] - **Spec Exp:** Movement Disorders; Movement Disorders-Botox Therapy; Parkinson's Disease; **Hospital:** Univ of MD Med Ctr; **Address:** 110 Paca St Fl 3, Baltimore, MD 21201; **Phone:** 410-328-2164; **Board Cert:** Neurology 1994; **Med School:** Univ Miami Sch Med 1988; **Resid:** Neurology, Jackson Meml Hosp 1992; **Fellow:** Movement Disorders, Jackson Meml Hosp 1994; **Fac Appt:** Assoc Prof N, Univ MD Sch Med

Silberstein, Stephen D MD [N] - **Spec Exp:** Headache; Migraine; Pain-Facial; **Hospital:** Thomas Jefferson Univ Hosp; **Address:** Jefferson Headache Center, 111 S 11th St, Gibbon Bldg, Philadelphia, PA 19107; **Phone:** 215-955-2243; **Board Cert:** Neurology 1975; Headache Medicine 2006; **Med School:** Univ Pennsylvania 1967; **Resid:** Internal Medicine, Hosp Univ Penn 1969; Neurology, Hosp Univ Penn 1975; **Fac Appt:** Clin Prof N, Temple Univ

Sirdofsky, Michael D MD [N] - **Spec Exp:** Neuromuscular Disorders; Electrodiagnosis; **Hospital:** Georgetown Univ Hosp; **Address:** Pasquerilla Health Care Bldg, Entrance 1 Fl 7, 3800 Resevoir Rd NW, Washington, DC 20007; **Phone:** 202-444-8525; **Board Cert:** Neurology 1981; **Med School:** Georgetown Univ 1976; **Resid:** Neurology, Georgetown Univ Hosp 1980; **Fac Appt:** Assoc Prof N, Georgetown Univ

Sperling, Michael R MD [N] - **Spec Exp:** Epilepsy; **Hospital:** Thomas Jefferson Univ Hosp; **Address:** Thomas Jefferson Univ Hosp, Dept Neurology, 900 Walnut St, Ste 200, Philadelphia, PA 19107; **Phone:** 215-955-1222; **Board Cert:** Neurology 1984; Clinical Neurophysiology 1999; **Med School:** Temple Univ 1978; **Resid:** Neurology, Mt Sinai Hosp 1982; **Fellow:** Epilepsy, UCLA Med Ctr 1984; **Fac Appt:** Prof N, Thomas Jefferson Univ

Stern, Matthew MD [N] - **Spec Exp:** Parkinson's Disease; Movement Disorders; Botox Therapy; **Hospital:** Pennsylvania Hosp (page 60), Hosp Univ Penn - UPHS (page 60); **Address:** Pennsylvania Hosp, Dept Neurology, 330 S 9th St Fl 3, Philadelphia, PA 19107; **Phone:** 215-829-6500; **Board Cert:** Neurology 1983; **Med School:** Duke Univ 1978; **Resid:** Neurology, Hosp Univ Penn 1982; **Fac Appt:** Prof N, Univ Pennsylvania

Swerdlow, Michael L MD [N] - **Spec Exp:** Myasthenia Gravis; Spinal Disorders; Multiple Sclerosis; **Hospital:** Montefiore Med Ctr - Div. Moses; **Address:** 3400 Bainbridge Ave, Bronx, NY 10467-2401; **Phone:** 718-920-4178; **Board Cert:** Neurology 1975; **Med School:** Univ Pennsylvania 1967; **Resid:** Internal Medicine, Mount Sinai Hosp 1969; Neurology, Albert Einstein Coll 1972; **Fellow:** Neurology, Natl Inst Hlth 1974; **Fac Appt:** Prof N, Albert Einstein Coll Med

Vas, George A MD [N] - **Spec Exp:** Stroke; Multiple Sclerosis; **Hospital:** SUNY Downstate Med Ctr, Kings County Hosp Ctr; **Address:** 450 Clarkson Ave, Ste A, Brooklyn, NY 11203-2056; **Phone:** 718-270-2502; **Board Cert:** Internal Medicine 1973; Neurology 1977; Clinical Neurophysiology 2002; **Med School:** Univ Pittsburgh 1970; **Resid:** Internal Medicine, New York Hosp 1972; Neurology, New York Hosp 1975; **Fac Appt:** Prof N, SUNY Downstate

Wechsler, Lawrence R MD [N] - **Spec Exp:** Cerebrovascular Disease; Stroke; **Hospital:** UPMC Presby, Pittsburgh, UPMC Shadyside; **Address:** UPMC Stroke Institute, 3471 Fifth Ave, Ste 810, Pittsburgh, PA 15213; **Phone:** 412-692-4920; **Board Cert:** Internal Medicine 1983; Neurology 1984; Clinical Neurophysiology 1994; Vascular Neurology 2005; **Med School:** Univ Pennsylvania 1978; **Resid:** Internal Medicine, Presby-Univ Hosp 1980; Neurology, Mass Genl Hosp 1983; **Fellow:** Clinical Neurophysiology, Mass Genl Hosp 1984; Cerebrovascular Disease, Mass Genl Hosp 1985; **Fac Appt:** Prof N, Univ Pittsburgh

Weinberg, Harold J MD [N] - **Spec Exp:** Headache; Spinal Disorders; Neuromuscular Disorders; Memory Disorders; **Hospital:** NYU Langone Med Ctr (page 67); **Address:** 650 1st Ave Fl 4, New York, NY 10016-3240; **Phone:** 212-213-9339; **Board Cert:** Neurology 1983; Electrodiagnostic Medicine 1989; **Med School:** Albert Einstein Coll Med 1978; **Resid:** Neurology, Columbia-Presby Med Ctr 1982; **Fellow:** Neuromuscular Medicine, Columbia-Presby Med Ctr 1982; **Fac Appt:** Clin Prof N, NYU Sch Med

Neurology

Weiner, William J MD [N] - **Spec Exp:** Movement Disorders; Parkinson's Disease; Huntington's Disease; Progressive Supranuclear Palsy (PSP); **Hospital:** Univ of MD Med Ctr; **Address:** Univ Maryland Med System, Dept Neurology, 22 S Greene St, rm N4W46, Baltimore, MD 21201; **Phone:** 410-328-2172; **Board Cert:** Neurology 1975; **Med School:** Univ IL Coll Med 1969; **Resid:** Neurology, Univ Minn 1971; Neurology, Rush-Presby Med Ctr 1973; **Fac Appt:** Prof N, Univ MD Sch Med

Wityk, Robert J MD [N] - **Spec Exp:** Stroke; Cerebrovascular Disease; **Hospital:** Johns Hopkins Hosp (page 61); **Address:** 601 N Caroline St, Ste 5073A, Baltimore, MD 21287; **Phone:** 410-955-2228; **Board Cert:** Internal Medicine 1988; Neurology 1992; **Med School:** Case West Res Univ 1985; **Resid:** Internal Medicine, UCSD Med Ctr 1988; Neurology, Mass Genl Hosp 1991; **Fellow:** Cardiovascular Disease, Tufts U-New Eng MC 1992; **Fac Appt:** Assoc Prof N, Johns Hopkins Univ

Zimmerman, Earl A MD [N] - **Spec Exp:** Memory Disorders; Alzheimer's Disease; Dementia; **Hospital:** Albany Med Ctr; **Address:** Albany Med Ctr-Neurology, 47 New Scotland Ave, MC 65, Albany, NY 12208; **Phone:** 518-262-0800; **Board Cert:** Neurology 1970; Internal Medicine 1970; **Med School:** Univ Pennsylvania 1963; **Resid:** Internal Medicine, Presbyterian Hosp 1965; Neurology, Neurological Inst 1968; **Fellow:** Endocrinology, Presbyterian Hosp 1972; **Fac Appt:** Prof N, Albany Med Coll

Southeast

Adams, David J MD [N] - **Spec Exp:** Diagnostic Problems; Hydrocephalus-normal pressure; Pseudotumor Cerebri; Autoimmune Disease; **Hospital:** Univ of Miami Hosp (page 71), Jackson Meml Hosp (page 70); **Address:** Univ Miami Dept Neurology, 1150 NW 14th St, Ste 609, Miami, FL 33136; **Phone:** 305-243-6732; **Board Cert:** Neurology 1977; **Med School:** Columbia P&S 1969; **Resid:** Neurology, Neurological Inst 1975; **Fac Appt:** Clin Prof N, Univ Miami Sch Med

Adams, Robert J MD [N] - **Spec Exp:** Stroke; **Hospital:** MUSC Med Ctr; **Address:** MUSC Stroke Center, 96 Jonathan Lucas St, Ste 307, Charleston, SC 29425; **Phone:** 843-792-7058; **Board Cert:** Neurology 1987; Vascular Neurology 2008; **Med School:** Univ Ark 1980; **Resid:** Neurology, Med Coll Georgia 1985; **Fac Appt:** Assoc Prof N, Med Coll GA

Ashizawa, Tetsuo MD [N] - **Spec Exp:** Movement Disorders; Myasthenia Gravis; Parkinson's Disease; Huntington's Disease; **Hospital:** Shands at Univ of FL; **Address:** Neurology @ Shands Med Plaza, 2000 SW Archer Rd Fl 3, Gainesville, FL 32608; **Phone:** 352-265-8408; **Board Cert:** Neurology 1980; **Med School:** Japan 1973; **Resid:** Neurology, Baylor Coll of Med Affil Hosp 1978; **Fellow:** Neuromuscular Disease, Baylor Coll of Med Affil Hosp 1978; **Fac Appt:** Prof N, Univ Fla Coll Med

Berger, Joseph MD [N] - **Spec Exp:** Multiple Sclerosis; AIDS/HIV; Infectious & Demyelinating Diseases; **Hospital:** Univ of Kentucky Chandler Hosp; **Address:** Univ Kentucky, Dept Neurology, Kentucky Clinic, Rm L-445, 740 S Limestone, Lexington, KY 40536; **Phone:** 859-323-5661; **Board Cert:** Neurology 1983; Internal Medicine 1977; **Med School:** Jefferson Med Coll 1974; **Resid:** Internal Medicine, Georgetown Univ Hosp 1977; Neurology, Jackson Meml Hosp 1981; **Fac Appt:** Prof N, Univ KY Coll Med

Bernad, Peter MD [N] - **Spec Exp:** Stroke; Headache; Migraine; Head Injury; **Hospital:** Inova Fairfax Hosp, G Washington Univ Hosp; **Address:** 2296 Opitz Blvd, Ste 360, Woodbridge, VA 22191; **Phone:** 703-878-0600; **Board Cert:** Internal Medicine 1979; Neurology 1981; **Med School:** McGill Univ 1974; **Resid:** Internal Medicine, USC Univ Hosp 1976; Neurology, Mass Genl Hosp-Harvard 1979; **Fellow:** Neuromuscular Disease, Natl Inst Hlth 1981; **Fac Appt:** Clin Prof N, Geo Wash Univ

Bertorini, Tulio E MD [N] - **Spec Exp:** Clinical Neurophysiology; Neuromuscular Diseases; Electromyography; **Hospital:** Methodist Univ Hosp - Memphis; **Address:** 1211 Union Ave, Ste 400, Memphis, TN 38104; **Phone:** 901-725-8920; **Board Cert:** Neurology 1977; **Med School:** Peru 1970; **Resid:** Neurology, Georgetown Univ Sch Med 1973; Neurology, VA Hosp/Armed Forces Inst Path 1974; **Fellow:** Electrodiagnosis, Mass Genl Hosp 1975; Clinical Neurophysiology, Natl Inst Neuro Comm Dis & Stroke/NIH 1977; **Fac Appt:** Prof N, Univ Tenn Coll Med, Memphis

Brooks, Benjamin R MD [N] - **Spec Exp:** Neuromuscular Disorders; Multiple Sclerosis; Neurotoxicology; **Hospital:** Carolinas Med Ctr, Levine Chldns Hosp; **Address:** 1010 Edgehill Rd N, Charlotte, NC 28207-1885; **Phone:** 704-446-4360; **Board Cert:** Internal Medicine 1974; Neurology 1978; **Med School:** Harvard Med Sch 1970; **Resid:** Neurology, Mass Genl Hosp 1974; Neurology, Natl Inst Neuro Disorders & Stroke-NIH 1976; **Fellow:** Neurovirology, Johns Hopkins Hosp 1978

Corbett, James MD [N] - **Spec Exp:** Neuro-Ophthalmology; Pseudotumor Cerebri; Neurosarcoidosis; Headache; **Hospital:** Univ Mississippi Med Ctr; **Address:** Univ Mississippi Med Ctr, Dept Neurology, 2500 N State St, Jackson, MS 39216-4505; **Phone:** 601-984-5501; **Board Cert:** Neurology 2004; **Med School:** Ros Franklin Univ/Chicago Med Sch 1966; **Resid:** Internal Medicine, Rhode Island Hosp 1968; Neurology, Univ Hosp-Case Western Reserve 1971; **Fac Appt:** Prof N, Univ Miss

De Long, Mahlon R MD [N] - **Spec Exp:** Parkinson's Disease; Movement Disorders; **Hospital:** Emory Univ Hosp; **Address:** Emory Univ Dept Neurology, 101 Woodruff Cir, Ste 6000, Atlanta, GA 30322; **Phone:** 404-712-8485; **Board Cert:** Neurology 1980; **Med School:** Harvard Med Sch 1966; **Resid:** Internal Medicine, Boston City Hosp 1968; Neurology, Johns Hopkins Hosp 1976; **Fellow:** Neurology, NIMH 1973; **Fac Appt:** Prof N, Emory Univ

DeKosky, Steven T MD [N] - **Spec Exp:** Alzheimer's Disease; Dementia; Behavioral Neurology; Geriatric Neurology; **Hospital:** Univ Virginia Med Ctr; **Address:** Univ Virgina School of Med, PO Box 800973, Charlottesville, VA 22908; **Phone:** 434-924-5118; **Board Cert:** Neurology 2004; **Med School:** Univ Fla Coll Med 1974; **Resid:** Internal Medicine, Johns Hopkins Hosp 1975; Neurology, Univ Florida 1978; **Fellow:** Neurological Chemistry, Univ Virginia Hosp 1979; **Fac Appt:** Prof N, Univ VA Sch Med

Dure IV, Leon S MD [N] - **Spec Exp:** Huntington's Disease; Tourette's Syndrome; Movement Disorders; **Hospital:** Univ of Ala Hosp at Birmingham; **Address:** 1600 7th Ave S CHB Bldg - Ste 314, Birmingham, AL 35233-0011; **Phone:** 205-996-7865; **Board Cert:** Child Neurology 1991; **Med School:** Baylor Coll Med 1984; **Resid:** Pediatrics, Columbia Presby Hosp 1986; Child Neurology, Texas Chldns Hosp 1989; **Fellow:** Child Neurology, Univ Michigan Affil Hosp 1990; **Fac Appt:** Assoc Prof N, Univ Alabama

Finkel, Alan G MD [N] - **Spec Exp:** Headache; Pain-Facial; Migraine; **Hospital:** Univ NC Hosps; **Address:** Univ North Carolina Dept Neurology, 3114 Bioinformatics Bldg, CB# 7025, Chapel Hill, NC 27599-7025; **Phone:** 919-966-2527; **Board Cert:** Neurology 1991; Pain Medicine 2003; Headache Medicine 2006; **Med School:** SUNY Buffalo 1985; **Resid:** Neurology, NC Meml HOsp 1989; **Fellow:** Pain & Headache Medicine, Univ NC; **Fac Appt:** Prof N, Univ NC Sch Med

Finkel, Michael F MD [N] - **Spec Exp:** Movement Disorders-Lower Limb; ADD/ADHD; Headache in Women; Trauma Neurology; **Hospital:** Physicians Regl Med Ctr; **Address:** Medical Surgical Specialists, 6101 Pine Ridge Rd, Naples, FL 34119; **Phone:** 239-348-4400; **Board Cert:** Neurology 1979; **Med School:** Washington Univ, St Louis 1973; **Resid:** Neurology, Strong Meml Hosp 1977

Neurology

Glass, Jonathan D MD [N] - **Spec Exp:** Neuro-Pathology; Amyotrophic Lateral Sclerosis (ALS); Peripheral Neuropathy; Neuromuscular Disorders; **Hospital:** Emory Univ Hosp, Grady Hlth Sys; **Address:** 1365 Clifton Rd NE, Ste A3100, Atlanta, GA 30322; **Phone:** 404-778-3444; **Board Cert:** Neurology 1990; Neuropathology 1997; **Med School:** Univ VT Coll Med 1985; **Resid:** Neurology, Johns Hopkins Univ 1989; **Fellow:** Neuropathology, Johns Hopkins Univ 1991; **Fac Appt:** Prof N, Emory Univ

Goldstein, Larry B MD [N] - **Spec Exp:** Stroke; Carotid Artery Disease; **Hospital:** Duke Univ Med Ctr, VA Med Ctr - Durham; **Address:** Duke Univ Med Ctr, Box 3651, Durham, NC 27710-0001; **Phone:** 919-684-3801; **Board Cert:** Neurology 1987; Vascular Neurology 2005; **Med School:** Mount Sinai Sch Med 1981; **Resid:** Neurology, Mt Sinai Hosp 1985; **Fellow:** Cerebrovascular Disease, Duke Univ Med Ctr 1986; **Fac Appt:** Prof N, Duke Univ

Gress, Daryl Ray MD [N] - **Spec Exp:** Critical Care; Stroke; **Hospital:** Univ Virginia Med Ctr; **Address:** Box 800394, Charlottesville, VA 22908; **Phone:** 434-924-8371; **Board Cert:** Neurology 1989; **Med School:** Washington Univ, St Louis 1982; **Resid:** Internal Medicine, Johns Hopkins Hosp 1984; Neurology, Mass Genl Hosp 1987; **Fellow:** Stroke, Mass Genl Hosp 1988

Haley Jr, Elliott C MD [N] - **Spec Exp:** Stroke; **Hospital:** Univ Virginia Med Ctr; **Address:** Univ VA Hlth Sys, Dept Neurology, PO Box 800394, Charlottesville, VA 22908; **Phone:** 434-982-6952; **Board Cert:** Internal Medicine 1978; Neurology 1985; Vascular Neurology 2008; **Med School:** Tulane Univ 1974; **Resid:** Internal Medicine, Univ Va Hosp 1978; Neurology, Univ Va Hosp 1982; **Fellow:** Cerebrovascular Disease, Mass Genl Hosp 1984; **Fac Appt:** Prof N, Univ VA Sch Med

Heilman, Kenneth M MD [N] - **Spec Exp:** Behavioral Neurology; Memory Disorders; Aphasia; Speech Disorders; **Hospital:** Shands at Univ of FL, Malcolm Randall VA Med Ctr; **Address:** Hlth Ctr Univ Fla Coll Med, Dept Neur, PO Box 100236, Gainesville, FL 32610-0236; **Phone:** 352-273-5550; **Board Cert:** Neurology 1973; **Med School:** Univ VA Sch Med 1963; **Resid:** Internal Medicine, Bellevue Hosp Ctr 1965; Neurology, Boston City Hosp 1970; **Fac Appt:** Prof N, Univ Fla Coll Med

Hess, David C MD [N] - **Spec Exp:** Stroke; Antiphospholipid Syndrome (APS); **Hospital:** Med Coll of GA Hosp and Clin (MCG Health Inc); **Address:** Med Coll Ga Dept Neurology, 1120 15th St, rm BI-3080, Augusta, GA 30912; **Phone:** 706-721-4581 x1; **Board Cert:** Internal Medicine 1986; Neurology 1990; Vascular Surgery 2008; **Med School:** Univ MD Sch Med 1983; **Resid:** Internal Medicine, Allegheny Genl Hosp 1985; Neurology, Med Coll Ga 1989; **Fellow:** Cerebrovascular Disease, Med Coll Ga 1990; **Fac Appt:** Prof N, Med Coll GA

Hurwitz, Barrie J MD [N] - **Spec Exp:** Multiple Sclerosis; Parkinson's Disease; Stroke/Cerebrovascular Disease; **Hospital:** Duke Univ Med Ctr; **Address:** Duke Univ Med Ctr, 122 Baker House, Box 3184, Durham, NC 27710; **Phone:** 919-684-4126; **Board Cert:** Neurology 1979; **Med School:** South Africa 1968; **Resid:** Internal Medicine, Johannesburg Genl Hosp 1973; Neurology, New York Hosp/Sloan Kettering Hosp 1977; **Fellow:** Neurology, New York Hosp-Cornell 1976; **Fac Appt:** Assoc Prof Med, Duke Univ

Janss, Anna J MD/PhD [N] - **Spec Exp:** Brain Tumors-Pediatric; Clinical Trials; Cancer Survivors-Late Effects of Therapy; **Hospital:** Chldns Hlthcare Atlanta @ Egleston; **Address:** Aflac Cancer & Blood Disorders Ctr, Outpatient Clin, Tower 1 Fl 4, 1405 Clifton Rd NE, Atlanta, GA 30322; **Phone:** 404-785-1200; **Board Cert:** Neurology 1993; **Med School:** Univ Iowa Coll Med 1988; **Resid:** Neurology, Hosp Univ Penn 1992; **Fellow:** Pediatric Neuro-Oncology, Chldns Hosp 1996; **Fac Appt:** Assoc Prof N, Emory Univ

Kirshner, Howard S MD [N] - **Spec Exp:** Stroke; Aphasia; Neuro-Rehabilitation; Dementia; **Hospital:** Vanderbilt Univ Med Ctr, Vanderbilt Stallworth Rehab Hosp Lp; **Address:** Vanderbilt Univ Med Ctr, Dept Neurology, A-0118 Med Ctr N, Nashville, TN 37232-2551; **Phone:** 615-936-1354; **Board Cert:** Neurology 1980; Vascular Neurology 2005; **Med School:** Harvard Med Sch 1972; **Resid:** Neurology, Mass Genl Hosp 1978; **Fellow:** Neurological Science, Natl Inst Hlth 1975; **Fac Appt:** Prof N, Vanderbilt Univ

Kurtzke, Robert N MD [N] - **Spec Exp:** Electromyography; Nerve/Muscle Disorders; **Hospital:** Inova Fairfax Hosp, Reston Hosp Ctr; **Address:** Neurology Ctr of Fairfax, 3020 Hamaker Ct, Ste 400, Fairfax, VA 22031-2220; **Phone:** 703-876-0800; **Board Cert:** Neurology 1990; Clinical Neurophysiology 2004; **Med School:** Georgetown Univ 1985; **Resid:** Neurology, Neurology Inst-Columbia Presby 1989; **Fellow:** Neuromuscular Disease, Duke Univ Med Ctr 1990

Lavin, Patrick J MD [N] - **Spec Exp:** Neuro-Ophthalmology; Eye Movement Disorders; Headache; Neuro-Otology; **Hospital:** Vanderbilt Univ Med Ctr; **Address:** Vanderbilt Dept Neurology, 1161 21st Ave S, A-0118 MCN, Nashville, TN 37232-2551; **Phone:** 615-936-0060; **Board Cert:** Neurology 1985; **Med School:** Ireland 1970; **Resid:** Internal Medicine, St Vincent Hosp Elm Pk 1973; Internal Medicine, Genl Hosp-Royal Infirm 1976; **Fellow:** Neurology, Case Western Reserve Univ 1981; Neuro-Ophthalmology, Case Western Reserve Univ 1983; **Fac Appt:** Prof N, Vanderbilt Univ

Montgomery Jr, Erwin B MD [N] - **Spec Exp:** Parkinson's Disease; **Hospital:** Univ of Ala Hosp at Birmingham; **Address:** 1720 7th Ave S, Ste 350SC, Birmingham, AL 53792; **Phone:** 205-996-2094; **Board Cert:** Neurology 1982; **Med School:** SUNY Buffalo 1976; **Resid:** Neurology, Wahington Univ Med Ctr 1980; **Fellow:** Neurological Physiology, Washington Univ Med Ctr 1981; **Fac Appt:** Prof N, Univ Wisc

Morgenlander, Joel Charles MD [N] - **Spec Exp:** Nerve/Muscle Disorders; **Hospital:** Duke Univ Med Ctr; **Address:** Duke Univ Med Ctr, Box 3394, Durham, NC 27710; **Phone:** 919-684-6887; **Board Cert:** Neurology 1992; **Med School:** Univ Pittsburgh 1986; **Resid:** Neurology, Duke Univ Med Ctr 1990; **Fellow:** Neuromuscular Disease, Duke Univ Med Ctr 1991; **Fac Appt:** Assoc Prof N, Duke Univ

Nabors III, Louis Burt MD [N] - **Spec Exp:** Neuro-Oncology; Brain Tumors; **Hospital:** Univ of Ala Hosp at Birmingham; **Address:** UAB, FOT 1020, 510 20th St S, Birmingham, AL 35294-0001; **Phone:** 205-934-1432; **Board Cert:** Neurology 1999; **Med School:** Univ Tenn Coll Med, Memphis 1991; **Resid:** Neurology, Univ Alabama; **Fellow:** Neuro-Oncology, Univ Alabama; **Fac Appt:** Assoc Prof N, Univ Alabama

Newman, Nancy Jean MD [N] - **Spec Exp:** Neuro-Ophthalmology; **Hospital:** Emory Univ Hosp; **Address:** Emory Eye Center, 1365B Clifton Rd NE, Ste 3600, Atlanta, GA 30322; **Phone:** 404-778-5360; **Board Cert:** Neurology 1989; **Med School:** Harvard Med Sch 1984; **Resid:** Neurology, Mass Genl Hosp 1988; **Fellow:** Neuro-Ophthalmology, Mass EE Infirmary 1989; **Fac Appt:** Prof N, Emory Univ

Nolan, Bruce A MD [N] - **Spec Exp:** Sleep Disorders/Apnea; **Hospital:** Jackson Meml Hosp (page 70); **Address:** Univ Miami Dept Neurology, 1501 NW 9th Ave, Miami, FL 33136; **Phone:** 305-243-5195; **Board Cert:** Neurology 1974; **Med School:** Wayne State Univ 1966; **Resid:** Neurology, Univ Miami Affil Hosp 1970; **Fac Appt:** Assoc Prof N, Univ Miami Sch Med

Oh, Shin Joong MD [N] - **Spec Exp:** Neuromuscular Disorders; Electromyography; **Hospital:** Univ of Ala Hosp at Birmingham; **Address:** Dept of Neurology, 1530 3rd Ave S SC Bldg - rm 200, Birmingham, AL 35294; **Phone:** 205-934-2121; **Board Cert:** Neurology 1973; Clinical Neurophysiology 2001; **Med School:** Korea 1960; **Resid:** Internal Medicine, Seoul National Univ Hosp 1964; Neurology, Georgetown Univ Hosp 1967; **Fellow:** NeuroEpidemiology, Univ Minnesota Hosps 1968; **Fac Appt:** Prof N, Univ Alabama

Patchell, Roy MD [N] - **Spec Exp:** Neuro-Oncology; Brain Tumors; Spinal Tumors; **Hospital:** Univ of Kentucky Chandler Hosp; **Address:** Univ Kentucky Neurosurgery, Chandler Med Ctr, 800 Rose St, MS 105, Lexington, KY 40536; **Phone:** 859-257-1532; **Board Cert:** Neurology 1984; **Med School:** Univ KY Coll Med 1979; **Resid:** Neurology, Johns Hopkins Hosp 1983; **Fellow:** Neuro-Oncology, Meml Sloan-Kettering Canc Ctr 1985; **Fac Appt:** Prof N, Univ KY Coll Med

Rothrock, John F MD [N] - **Spec Exp:** Headache; Stroke; **Hospital:** Univ of Ala Hosp at Birmingham; **Address:** UAB, Dept Neurology, SC 350, 7th Ave S, 35294-0017, Birmingham, AL 35249; **Phone:** 205-801-8986; **Board Cert:** Neurology 1984; **Med School:** Univ VA Sch Med 1977; **Resid:** Neurology, Univ Ariz Med Ctr 1981; **Fac Appt:** Prof N, Univ Alabama

Sacco, Ralph L MD [N] - **Spec Exp:** Stroke; Stroke Prevention; **Hospital:** Jackson Meml Hosp (page 70), Univ of Miami Hosp & Clins/Sylvester Comp Canc Ctr (page 70); **Address:** Univ of Miami-Dept of Neurology, 1120 NW 14th St Fl 13 - Ste 1352, Miami, FL 33136; **Phone:** 305-243-7519; **Board Cert:** Neurology 1989; **Med School:** Boston Univ 1983; **Resid:** Neurology, Columbia-Presby Med Ctr 1987; **Fellow:** Cerebrovascular Disease, Columbia-Presby Med Ctr 1989; **Fac Appt:** Prof N, Univ Miami Sch Med

Sadowsky, Carl H MD [N] - **Spec Exp:** Memory Disorders; Alzheimer's Disease; Dementia; **Hospital:** Columbia Hosp - W Palm Beach; **Address:** 4631 N Congress Ave, Ste 200, West Palm Beach, FL 33407-2234; **Phone:** 561-845-0500 x129; **Board Cert:** Neurology 1977; **Med School:** Cornell Univ 1971; **Resid:** Internal Medicine, Dartmouth-Hitchcock Med Ctr 1973; Neurology, Dartmouth-Hitchcock Med Ctr 1976; **Fac Appt:** Assoc Clin Prof N, Nova SE Univ, Coll Osteo Med

Schatz, Norman J MD [N] - **Spec Exp:** Neuro-Ophthalmology; Multiple Sclerosis & Visual Loss; Vision-Unexplained Loss; **Hospital:** Bascom Palmer Eye Inst (page 55), Univ of Miami Hosp (page 71); **Address:** 4701 N Meridian Ave, Adams Bldg - Ste 500A, Miami Beach, FL 33140; **Phone:** 305-532-2885; **Board Cert:** Neurology 1969; **Med School:** Hahnemann Univ 1961; **Resid:** Neurology, Jefferson Hosp 1965; **Fellow:** Neuro-Ophthalmology, Bascom Palmer Eye Inst 1966; **Fac Appt:** Clin Prof N, Univ Pennsylvania

Schiff, David MD [N] - **Spec Exp:** Brain Tumors; Spinal Cord Tumors; Neurologic Complications of Cancer; Neuro-Oncology; **Hospital:** Univ Virginia Med Ctr; **Address:** Univ VA, Div of Neuro-Oncology, PO Box 800432, Charlottesville, VA 22908; **Phone:** 434-982-4415; **Board Cert:** Neurology 1994; **Med School:** Harvard Med Sch 1988; **Resid:** Neurology, Harvard Longwood 1992; **Fellow:** Neuro-Oncology, Meml Sloan Kettering Cancer Ctr 1993; Mayo Clinic 1994; **Fac Appt:** Assoc Prof NS, Univ VA Sch Med

Sethi, Kapil D MD [N] - **Spec Exp:** Parkinson's Disease; Restless Legs Syndrome; Movement Disorders; Botox Therapy; **Hospital:** Med Coll of GA Hosp and Clin (MCG Health Inc); **Address:** Med Coll Georgia, Dept Neurology, 1429 Harper St, Augusta, GA 30912-0004; **Phone:** 706-721-2798; **Board Cert:** Neurology 1987; **Med School:** India 1976; **Resid:** Neurology, Pgimer 1981; Neurology, Med Coll Georgia 1985; **Fac Appt:** Prof N, Med Coll GA

Singer, Carlos MD [N] - **Spec Exp:** Parkinson's Disease; Movement Disorders; Botox Therapy; **Hospital:** Jackson Meml Hosp (page 70); **Address:** Univ Miami Dept Neurology, 1501 NW 9th Ave, Miami, FL 33136; **Phone:** 305-243-3876; **Board Cert:** Neurology 1981; Internal Medicine 1976; **Med School:** Venezuela 1972; **Resid:** Internal Medicine, Montefiore Hosp 1976; Neurology, Albert Einstein Affil Hosp 1979; **Fellow:** Electromyography, Jackson Meml Hosp 1981; Movement Disorders, Univ Miami 1989; **Fac Appt:** Prof N, Univ Miami Sch Med

Valenstein, Edward MD [N] - **Spec Exp:** Neuromuscular Disorders; Multiple Sclerosis; Amyotrophic Lateral Sclerosis (ALS); **Hospital:** Shands at Univ of FL; **Address:** 100 S Newell Drive, Box 100263, Gainesville, FL 32610; **Phone:** 352-265-8408; **Board Cert:** Neurology 1976; Clinical Neurophysiology 2006; **Med School:** Albert Einstein Coll Med 1967; **Resid:** Neurology, Boston City Hosp 1971; **Fac Appt:** Prof N, Univ Fla Coll Med

Watts, Ray L MD [N] - **Spec Exp:** Parkinson's Disease; Movement Disorders; **Hospital:** Univ of Ala Hosp at Birmingham; **Address:** Kirkland Clinic, 2000 6th Ave S Fl 5, Birmingham, AL 35233; **Phone:** 205-934-0683; **Board Cert:** Neurology 1985; **Med School:** Washington Univ, St Louis 1980; **Resid:** Neurology, Mass Genl Hosp 1984; **Fellow:** Electromyography, Mass Genl Hosp 1983; **Fac Appt:** Prof N, Univ Alabama

Wooten Jr, George F MD [N] - **Spec Exp:** Movement Disorders; Parkinson's Disease; Tremor & Dystonia; **Hospital:** Univ Virginia Med Ctr; **Address:** Univ VA Hlth Sys, Dept Neuro-McKim Hall, PO Box 800394, Charlottesville, VA 22908; **Phone:** 434-924-2706; **Board Cert:** Neurology 1977; **Med School:** Cornell Univ-Weill Med Coll 1970; **Resid:** Neurology, NY Hosp-Cornell 1977; **Fellow:** Pharmacology, Natl Inst Hlth-NIMH 1974; **Fac Appt:** Prof N, Univ VA Sch Med

Midwest

Adams Jr, Harold P MD [N] - **Spec Exp:** Stroke; Cerebrovascular Disease; **Hospital:** Univ Iowa Hosp & Clinics; **Address:** Univ Iowa Hosp, Dept Neurology, 200 Hawkins Drive, rm 2148-RCP, Iowa City, IA 52242; **Phone:** 319-356-4110; **Board Cert:** Neurology 2004; Vascular & Interventional Radiology 2005; **Med School:** Northwestern Univ 1970; **Resid:** Neurology, Univ Iowa Hosp 1974; **Fac Appt:** Prof N, Univ Iowa Coll Med

Ahlskog, J Eric MD/PhD [N] - **Spec Exp:** Parkinson's Disease; Movement Disorders; **Hospital:** Mayo Med Ctr & Clin - Rochester, St Mary's Hosp - Rochester; **Address:** Mayo Clinic, Dept Neurology, 200 First St SW, Rochester, MN 55905; **Phone:** 507-538-1038; **Board Cert:** Neurology 1984; **Med School:** Dartmouth Med Sch 1976; **Resid:** Internal Medicine, Univ Chicago Hosps Clins 1978; Neurology, Mayo Grad Sch Med 1981; **Fac Appt:** Prof N, Mayo Med Sch

Alberts, Mark J MD [N] - **Spec Exp:** Stroke/Cerebrovascular Disease; **Hospital:** Northwestern Meml Hosp; **Address:** 675 N St Clair, Galter Bldg Fl 20 - Ste 100, Chicago, IL 60611; **Phone:** 312-695-7950; **Board Cert:** Neurology 1987; Vascular Neurology 2005; **Med School:** Tufts Univ 1982; **Resid:** Neurology, Duke Univ Med Ctr 1986; **Fellow:** Cerebrovascular Disease, Duke Univ Med Ctr 1987; **Fac Appt:** Prof N, Northwestern Univ

Arnason, Barry G W MD [N] - **Spec Exp:** Multiple Sclerosis; Guillain-Barre Syndrome; Myasthenia Gravis; **Hospital:** Univ of Chicago Med Ctr; **Address:** 5841 S Maryland Ave, MC 2030, Chicago, IL 60637; **Phone:** 773-702-6222; **Board Cert:** Neurology 1971; **Med School:** Univ Manitoba 1957; **Resid:** Neurology, Mass Genl Hosp 1959; Neurology, Mass Genl Hosp 1962; **Fac Appt:** Prof N, Univ Chicago-Pritzker Sch Med

Barger, Geoffrey R MD [N] - **Spec Exp:** Neuro-Oncology; Brain Tumors; **Hospital:** Harper Univ Hosp; **Address:** Wayne State Univ Hlth Ctr, 4201 St Antoine, Ste 8D-UHC, Detroit, MI 48201; **Phone:** 313-745-4275; **Board Cert:** Neurology 1981; **Med School:** Jefferson Med Coll 1975; **Resid:** Neurology, Penn Hosp 1979; **Fellow:** Neuro-Oncology, Moffitt Hosp & Brain Tumor Ctr/UCSF 1982; **Fac Appt:** Assoc Prof N, Wayne State Univ

Bernstein, Richard A MD/PhD [N] - **Spec Exp:** Stroke/Cerebrovascular Disease; **Hospital:** Northwestern Meml Hosp; **Address:** Stroke Program, 710 N Lake Shore Drive, Abbott Hall Fl 11, Chicago, IL 60026; **Phone:** 312-503-4394; **Board Cert:** Neurology 2001; Vascular Neurology 2005; **Med School:** Cornell Univ-Weill Med Coll 1996; **Resid:** Neurology, Columbia-Presby Med Ctr 2000; **Fellow:** Neurovascular Medicine, UCSF Med Ctr 2001; Stroke, Stanford Med Ctr 2002; **Fac Appt:** Assoc Prof N, Northwestern Univ-Feinberg Sch Med

Broderick, Joseph P MD [N] - **Spec Exp:** Stroke; **Hospital:** Univ Hosp - Cincinnati; **Address:** Univ Cincinnati, Dept Neurology, 222 Piedmont Ave, Ste 3200, Cincinnati, OH 45219; **Phone:** 513-475-8730; **Board Cert:** Neurotology 1988; Vascular Neurology 2005; **Med School:** Univ Cincinnati 1982; **Resid:** Neurology, Mayo Clinic 1986; **Fac Appt:** Clin Prof N, Univ Cincinnati

Brown, Robert D MD [N] - **Spec Exp:** Stroke; Cerebrovascular Disease; **Hospital:** Mayo Med Ctr & Clin - Rochester; **Address:** Mayo Clinic, Dept Neurology, 200 First St SW, Rochester, MN 55905; **Phone:** 507-266-4143; **Board Cert:** Neurology 1994; Vascular Surgery 2008; **Med School:** Mayo Med Sch 1989; **Resid:** Neurology, Mayo Clinic 1991; **Fellow:** Cerebrovascular Disease, Mayo Clinic 1992; **Fac Appt:** Prof N, Mayo Med Sch

Burke, Allan M MD [N] - **Spec Exp:** Cerebrovascular Disease; Neurologic Imaging; **Hospital:** Northwestern Meml Hosp; **Address:** 233 E Erie St, Ste 500, Chicago, IL 60611-2912; **Phone:** 312-944-0063; **Board Cert:** Neurology 1982; Neuroimaging 2002; **Med School:** Columbia P&S 1976; **Resid:** Internal Medicine, NY Hosp 1978; Neurology, Columbia-Presby Med Ctr 1981; **Fellow:** Cerebrovascular Disease, Hosp Univ Penn 1983; **Fac Appt:** Assoc Clin Prof N, Northwestern Univ

Cascino, Terrence L MD [N] - **Spec Exp:** Neuro-Oncology; **Hospital:** Mayo Med Ctr & Clin - Rochester; **Address:** Mayo Clinic, Dept Neurology, 200 1st St SW, Rochester, MN 55905-0001; **Phone:** 507-284-2576; **Board Cert:** Neurology 1984; **Med School:** Loyola Univ-Stritch Sch Med 1972; **Resid:** Neurology, Mayo Clinic 1980; **Fellow:** Neuro-Oncology, Meml Sloan Kettering Cancer Ctr; **Fac Appt:** Assoc Prof N, Mayo Med Sch

Cohen, Jeffrey Alan MD [N] - **Spec Exp:** Multiple Sclerosis; Neuro-Immunology; **Hospital:** Cleveland Clin Fdn (page 56); **Address:** Cleveland Clin - Mellen Ctr, 9500 Euclid Ave, Ste U10, Cleveland, OH 44195; **Phone:** 216-445-8110; **Board Cert:** Neurology 1985; **Med School:** Univ Chicago-Pritzker Sch Med 1980; **Resid:** Neurology, Hosp Univ Penn 1984; **Fellow:** Neurological Immunology, Hosp Univ Penn 1987

Cutrer, F Michael MD [N] - **Spec Exp:** Headache; Pain-Facial; Migraine; **Hospital:** Mayo Med Ctr & Clin - Rochester, Rochester Methodist Hosp; **Address:** Mayo Clinic, Dept Neurology, 200 First St NW, Rochester, MN 55905-0001; **Phone:** 507-284-4409; **Board Cert:** Neurology 1993; **Med School:** Univ Miss 1988; **Resid:** Neurology, UCLA Med Ctr 1992; **Fellow:** Neurology, Mass Genl Hosp-Harvard 1994; **Fac Appt:** Assoc Prof N, Mayo Med Sch

Elias, Stanton B MD [N] - **Spec Exp:** Multiple Sclerosis; Myasthenia Gravis; **Hospital:** Henry Ford Hosp; **Address:** Henry Ford Hosp, Dept Neurology, 2799 W Grand Blvd, Fl K-11, Detroit, MI 48202-2689; **Phone:** 313-916-7207; **Board Cert:** Neurology 1979; **Med School:** Univ Pittsburgh 1972; **Resid:** Neurology, Duke Univ Med Ctr 1976; **Fellow:** Neurology, Duke Univ Med Ctr 1977

Farlow, Martin R MD [N] - **Spec Exp:** Alzheimer's Disease; Neurodegenerative Disorders; Multiple Sclerosis; **Hospital:** Indiana Univ Hosp, Wishard Hlth Srvs; **Address:** Dept Neurology, Clinical Bldg - rm 291, 541 Clinical Drive, Indianapolis, IN 46202; **Phone:** 317-274-2291; **Board Cert:** Neurology 1988; **Med School:** Indiana Univ 1979; **Resid:** Neurology, Indiana Univ Hosp 1983; **Fac Appt:** Prof N, Indiana Univ

Feldman, Eva L MD/PhD [N] - **Spec Exp:** Neuromuscular Disorders; Amyotrophic Lateral Sclerosis (ALS); Peripheral Neuropathy; **Hospital:** Univ Michigan Hlth Sys; **Address:** Univ Mich, Dept Neurology, 1500 E Med Ctr Drive, SPC 5322, rm 1324 Taubman, Ann Arbor, MI 48109-0322; **Phone:** 734-936-9020; **Board Cert:** Neurology 1988; **Med School:** Univ Mich Med Sch 1983; **Resid:** Neurology, Johns Hopkins Hosp 1987; **Fellow:** Neuromuscular Medicine, Univ Mich Hosps 1988; **Fac Appt:** Prof N, Univ Mich Med Sch

Furlan, Anthony J MD [N] - **Spec Exp:** Stroke; Thrombolytic Therapy; **Hospital:** Univ Hosps Case Med Ctr; **Address:** Dept Neurology, 11100 Euclid Ave, Fl 5, Hanna House, Cleveland, OH 44106; **Phone:** 216-844-3192; **Board Cert:** Neurology 1979; Vascular Neurology 2005; **Med School:** Loyola Univ-Stritch Sch Med 1973; **Resid:** Neurology, Cleveland Clinic 1977; **Fellow:** Cerebrovascular Disease, Mayo Clinic 1978; **Fac Appt:** Assoc Prof N, Ohio State Univ

Gilman, Sid MD [N] - **Spec Exp:** Parkinson's Disease/Movement Disorders; Alzheimer's Disease; Multiple Sclerosis; Epilepsy; **Hospital:** Univ Michigan Hlth Sys; **Address:** Univ Mich, Dept Neurology, 300 N Ingalls 3D15, Ann Arbor, MI 48109-0489; **Phone:** 734-936-1808; **Board Cert:** Neurology 1966; **Med School:** UCLA 1957; **Resid:** Neurology, Boston City Hosp-Harvard 1963; **Fellow:** Neurological Physiology, Boston City Hosp-Harvard 1965; **Fac Appt:** Prof N, Univ Mich Med Sch

Goetz, Christopher G MD [N] - **Spec Exp:** Movement Disorders; Parkinson's Disease; Dyskinesias; **Hospital:** Rush Univ Med Ctr; **Address:** 1725 W Harrison St, Ste 755, Chicago, IL 60612-3835; **Phone:** 312-563-2030; **Board Cert:** Neurology 1982; **Med School:** Rush Med Coll 1975; **Resid:** Neurology, Michael Reese Med Ctr 1977; Neurology, Rush-Presby-St Luke's Med Ctr 1979; **Fac Appt:** Prof N, Rush Med Coll

Hain, Timothy C MD [N] - **Spec Exp:** Neuro-Otology; Balance Disorders; Motion Sickness; **Hospital:** Northwestern Meml Hosp; **Address:** 645 N Michigan Ave, Ste 410, Chicago, IL 60611; **Phone:** 312-274-0197; **Board Cert:** Neurology 1983; **Med School:** Univ IL Coll Med 1978; **Resid:** Neurology, Univ Illinois Affil Hosp 1982; **Fellow:** Neurology, Johns Hopkins Hosp 1984; Ophthalmology, Johns Hopkins Hosp 1984; **Fac Appt:** Prof N, Northwestern Univ

Hecox, Kurt E MD [N] - **Spec Exp:** Pediatric Neurology; Epilepsy/Seizure Disorders; Hearing Loss; **Hospital:** Chldns Hosp - Wisconsin; **Address:** Dept Neurology, 9000 W Wisconsin Ave, rm CCC-540, PO Box 1997, Milwaukee, WI 53226; **Phone:** 414-266-3464; **Board Cert:** Clinical Neurophysiology 1977; **Med School:** UCSD 1971; **Resid:** Neurology, Univ Texas Southwestern Med Ctr 1975; **Fellow:** Pediatric Neurology, Children's Med Ctr/Parkland Hosp 1978; **Fac Appt:** Prof N, Med Coll Wisc

Josephson, David A MD [N] - **Spec Exp:** Electromyography; Epilepsy; Stroke; **Hospital:** St Vincent Indianapolis Hosp, Comm Hosp N - Indianapolis; **Address:** 8402 Harcourt Rd, Ste 615, Indianapolis, IN 46260; **Phone:** 317-355-1555; **Board Cert:** Neurology 2004; **Med School:** Indiana Univ 1971; **Resid:** Neurology, Univ Mich Med Ctr 1973; Neurology, Indiana Univ Med Ctr 1975; **Fac Appt:** Assoc Clin Prof N, Indiana Univ

Neurology

Kincaid, John C MD [N] - **Spec Exp:** Neuromuscular Disorders; Electromyography; Pain-Facial; **Hospital:** Indiana Univ Hosp; **Address:** Indiana Univ Hosp, 550 N University Blvd, Ste 1711, Indianapolis, IN 46202; **Phone:** 317-274-0311; **Board Cert:** Neurology 1982; Clinical Neurophysiology 2000; **Med School:** Indiana Univ 1975; **Resid:** Neurology, Indiana Univ 1979; **Fellow:** Electromyography, Mayo Clin 1980; **Fac Appt:** Prof N, Indiana Univ

Lisak, Robert P MD [N] - **Spec Exp:** Multiple Sclerosis; Myasthenia Gravis; Vasculitis; Demyelinating Neuropathy; **Hospital:** Harper Univ Hosp, Detroit Receiving Hospital; **Address:** Wayne State Univ Sch Med, 4201 St Antoine, Hlth Ctr 8D, Detroit, MI 48201; **Phone:** 313-745-4240; **Board Cert:** Neurology 1975; **Med School:** Columbia P&S 1965; **Resid:** Internal Medicine, Bronx Municipal Hosp-Einstein 1969; Neurology, Hosp Univ Penn 1972; **Fac Appt:** Prof N, Wayne State Univ

Logan, William R MD [N] - **Spec Exp:** Stroke; Cerebrovascular Disease; **Hospital:** St John's Mercy Med Ctr - St Louis; **Address:** St Johns Mercy Med Ctr, Tower B, 621 New Ballas Rd, Ste 5003, St Louis, MO 63141; **Phone:** 314-227-2020; **Board Cert:** Internal Medicine 1981; Neurology 1986; **Med School:** Univ Okla Coll Med 1978; **Resid:** Internal Medicine, Univ Missouri Hosps 1982; Neurology, Unix Texas Hlth Sci Ctr 1984

Luders, Hans MD/PhD [N] - **Spec Exp:** Epilepsy; **Hospital:** Univ Hosps Case Med Ctr; **Address:** University Hosps-Case Med Ctr, 11100 Euclid Ave, Dept Neurology, Lakeside Bldg - Ste 3200, Cleveland, OH 44106; **Phone:** 216-844-3650; **Board Cert:** Neurology 1985; **Med School:** Chile 1965; **Resid:** Neurology, Neur Inst-Kyushu Univ 1971; **Fellow:** Neurological Physiology, Mayo Grad Sch Med 1975; **Fac Appt:** Prof N, Ohio State Univ

Mahowald, Mark W MD [N] - **Spec Exp:** Sleep Disorders/Apnea; **Hospital:** Hennepin Cnty Med Ctr; **Address:** Minn Regional Sleep Disorders Ctr, 701 Park Ave S, Minneapolis, MN 55415; **Phone:** 612-873-6201; **Board Cert:** Neurology 1976; **Med School:** Univ Minn 1968; **Resid:** Neurology, Fairview Univ Med Ctr 1974; **Fac Appt:** Prof N, Univ Minn

Maraganore, Demetrius MD [N] - **Spec Exp:** Movement Disorders; Parkinson's Disease; **Hospital:** Evanston/Northshore Univ Hlth Syst, Glenbrook/NorthShore Univ Hlth Syst; **Address:** Neurology Dept, 2650 Ridge Ave Birch Bldg, Evanston, IL 60201; **Phone:** 847-570-2570; **Board Cert:** Neurology 1990; **Med School:** Northwestern Univ-Feinberg Sch Med 1985; **Resid:** Neurology, Mayo Clinic 1989; **Fellow:** Movement Disorders, Natl Hosp for Nervous Disorders 1990

Mesulam, Marel MD [N] - **Spec Exp:** Alzheimer's Disease; Tourette's Syndrome; Dementia; **Hospital:** Northwestern Meml Hosp; **Address:** 320 E Superior St, Chicago, IL 60611; **Phone:** 312-908-9339; **Board Cert:** Neurology 1977; **Med School:** Harvard Med Sch 1972; **Resid:** Neurology, Boston City Hosp 1976; **Fac Appt:** Prof N, Northwestern Univ

Mikkelsen, Tommy MD [N] - **Spec Exp:** Brain Tumors; Gliomas; **Hospital:** Henry Ford Hosp, William Beaumont Hosp; **Address:** Henry Ford Hospital, ER 3096, 2799 W Grand Blvd, Detroit, MI 48202; **Phone:** 313-916-8641; **Board Cert:** Neurology 2008; **Med School:** Univ Calgary 1983; **Resid:** Internal Medicine, Calgary General Hosp 1985; Neurology, Montreal Neurological Inst 1988; **Fellow:** Neuro-Oncology, Royal Victoria Hosp 1990; Neuro-Oncology, Ludwig Inst for Cancer Rsch 1992; **Fac Appt:** Assoc Prof N, Case West Res Univ

Mohammad, Yousef M MD [N] - **Spec Exp:** Headache; Migraine; Stroke; **Hospital:** Rush Univ Med Ctr; **Address:** Rush Professional Office Bldg, 1725 W Harrison St, Ste 1106, Chicago, IL 60612; **Phone:** 312-942-4500; **Board Cert:** Neurology 2004; **Med School:** Amer Univ Beirut 1989; **Resid:** Neurology, Wayne State Univ Affil Hosps 1996; **Fellow:** Stroke, Emory Univ 1999

Morris, John C MD [N] - **Spec Exp:** Alzheimer's Disease; **Hospital:** Barnes-Jewish Hosp; **Address:** Memory Diagnostic Ctr, 4488 Forest Park, Ste 160, St Louis, MO 63108-2215; **Phone:** 314-286-1967; **Board Cert:** Internal Medicine 1979; Neurology 1985; **Med School:** Univ Rochester 1974; **Resid:** Internal Medicine, Akron Genl Med Ctr 1979; Neurology, Cleveland Metro Genl Hosp 1982; **Fellow:** Neuropharmacology, Washington Univ 1985; **Fac Appt:** Prof N, Washington Univ, St Louis

Newton, Herbert B MD [N] - **Spec Exp:** Neuro-Oncology; Brain & Spinal Tumors; **Hospital:** Ohio St Univ Med Ctr, Arthur G James Cancer Hosp & Research Inst; **Address:** 320 W 10th Ave, Starling Loving Bldg, rm M410, Columbus, OH 43210; **Phone:** 614-293-8930; **Board Cert:** Neurology 1989; **Med School:** SUNY Buffalo 1984; **Resid:** Neurology, Univ Michigan Med Ctr 1988; **Fellow:** Neuro-Oncology, Meml Sloan-Kettering Cancer Ctr 1990; **Fac Appt:** Prof N, Ohio State Univ

Pascuzzi, Robert M MD [N] - **Spec Exp:** Neuromuscular Disorders; Amyotrophic Lateral Sclerosis (ALS); Myasthenia Gravis; **Hospital:** Indiana Univ Hosp, Wishard Hlth Srvs; **Address:** Clarian Hlth-Indiana Univ Sch Med, 545 Barnhill Drive, EH 125, Indianapolis, IN 46202; **Phone:** 317-274-4455; **Board Cert:** Neurology 2004; **Med School:** Indiana Univ 1979; **Resid:** Neurology, Univ Va Med Ctr 1983; **Fellow:** Neuromuscular Medicine, Univ Va Med Ctr 1985; **Fac Appt:** Prof N, Indiana Univ

Perlmutter, Joel S MD [N] - **Spec Exp:** Parkinson's Disease; Movement Disorders; Huntington's Disease; **Hospital:** Barnes-Jewish Hosp; **Address:** Wash Univ Sch Med, Dept Neurology, 660 S Euclid Ave, Box 8111, St Louis, MO 63110; **Phone:** 314-362-6908; **Board Cert:** Neurology 1985; **Med School:** Univ MO-Columbia Sch Med 1979; **Resid:** Neurology, Barnes Hosp-Wash Univ 1983; **Fellow:** Movement Disorders, Barnes Hosp-Wash Univ 1984; **Fac Appt:** Prof N, Washington Univ, St Louis

Pestronk, Alan MD [N] - **Spec Exp:** Neuromuscular Disorders; Peripheral Neuropathy; **Hospital:** Barnes-Jewish Hosp; **Address:** Washington Univ Sch Med, Dept Neurology, 660 S Euclid Ave, Box 8111, St Louis, MO 63110; **Phone:** 314-362-6981; **Board Cert:** Neurology 1978; **Med School:** Johns Hopkins Univ 1970; **Resid:** Neurology, Johns Hopkins Hosp 1974; **Fellow:** Neuromuscular Medicine, Johns Hopkins Hosp 1977; **Fac Appt:** Prof NPath, Washington Univ, St Louis

Petersen, Ronald C MD/PhD [N] - **Spec Exp:** Alzheimer's Disease; **Hospital:** Mayo Med Ctr & Clin - Rochester; **Address:** Mayo Clinic, Dept Neurology, 200 1st St SW, Rochester, MN 55905; **Phone:** 507-538-1038; **Board Cert:** Neurology 1986; **Med School:** Mayo Med Sch 1980; **Resid:** Neurology, Mayo Clinic 1984; **Fellow:** Behavioral Neurology, Beth Israel Med Ctr 1986; **Fac Appt:** Prof N, Mayo Med Sch

Reder, Anthony T MD [N] - **Spec Exp:** Multiple Sclerosis; Tetanus; Myasthenia Gravis; Reflex Sympathetic Dystrophy (RSD); **Hospital:** Univ of Chicago Med Ctr; **Address:** Ctr Advanced Medicine, 5758 S Maryland Ave, rm 4D, Chicago, IL 60637-1426; **Phone:** 773-702-6222; **Board Cert:** Neurology 1984; **Med School:** Univ Mich Med Sch 1978; **Resid:** Neurology, Univ Minn Hosps 1982; **Fellow:** Neurological Immunology, Univ Chicago 1984; **Fac Appt:** Assoc Prof N, Univ Chicago-Pritzker Sch Med

Reed, Robert L MD [N] - **Spec Exp:** Multiple Sclerosis; Stroke; **Hospital:** Good Samaritan Hosp - Cincinnati; **Address:** 111 Wellington Pl, Cincinnati, OH 45219; **Phone:** 513-241-2370; **Board Cert:** Neurology 1975; **Med School:** Univ Cincinnati 1966; **Resid:** Internal Medicine, Mayo Grad Sch Med 1970; Neurology, Mayo Grad Sch Med 1973

Rogers, Lisa R DO [N] - **Spec Exp:** Neuro-Oncology; Brain Tumors; Brain Radiation Toxicity; **Hospital:** Univ Michigan Hlth Sys; **Address:** Univ Michigan, Dept Neurology, 1914 Taubman Center, Ann Arbor, MI 48109-5316; **Phone:** 734-615-2994; **Board Cert:** Neurology 1982; **Med School:** Kirksville Coll Osteo Med 1976; **Resid:** Neurology, Cleveland Clin Fdn 1980; **Fellow:** Neuro-Oncology, Meml-Sloan Kettering Cancer Ctr 1982; **Fac Appt:** Prof N, Univ Mich Med Sch

Roos, Karen L MD [N] - **Spec Exp:** Infections-Neurologic; Encephalitis; **Hospital:** Indiana Univ Hosp, Wishard Hlth Srvs; **Address:** Indiana Univ Med Ctr, 550 N University Blvd, rm 1711, Indianapolis, IN 46202-5149; **Phone:** 317-278-6785; **Board Cert:** Neurology 1986; **Med School:** Hahnemann Univ 1981; **Resid:** Neurology, Univ Virginia Med Ctr 1985; **Fac Appt:** Prof N, Indiana Univ

Roos, Raymond MD [N] - **Spec Exp:** Amyotrophic Lateral Sclerosis (ALS); Multiple Sclerosis; Neuromuscular Disorders; **Hospital:** Univ of Chicago Med Ctr; **Address:** Univ Chicago, Dept Neurology, 5841 S Maryland Ave, MC-2030, Chicago, IL 60637; **Phone:** 773-702-7852; **Board Cert:** Neurology 1976; **Med School:** SUNY Downstate 1968; **Resid:** Neurology, Johns Hopkins Hosp 1974; **Fellow:** Neurology, Natl Inst Neur Dis & Stroke 1971; Neurological Viral Immunology, Johns Hopkins Hosp 1976; **Fac Appt:** Prof N, Univ Chicago-Pritzker Sch Med

Rubin, Susan M MD [N] - **Spec Exp:** Multiple Sclerosis in Women; Epilepsy in Pregnancy; Headache in Women; Migraine in Women; **Hospital:** Glenbrook/NorthShore Univ Hlth Syst, Evanston/Northshore Univ Hlth Syst; **Address:** Glenbrook Hosp, Dept Neurology, 2100 Pfingsten Rd, Glenview, IL 60026; **Phone:** 847-657-5875; **Board Cert:** Neurology 2006; **Med School:** Univ IL Coll Med 1988; **Resid:** Neurology, Northwestern Meml Hosp 1993; **Fellow:** Neurological Physiology, Northwestern Meml Hosp 1994; **Fac Appt:** Asst Clin Prof N, Northwestern Univ

Ruff, Robert L MD/PhD [N] - **Spec Exp:** Spinal Cord Injury; Neuro-Rehabilitation; Muscle Disorders; **Hospital:** VA Med Ctr - Cleveland; **Address:** Department of Neurology, 10701 East Blvd, Cleveland, OH 44106; **Phone:** 216-791-3800 x5230; **Board Cert:** Neurology 1982; Spinal Cord Injury Medicine 2002; **Med School:** Univ Wash 1976; **Resid:** Neurology, NY-Cornell Hosp 1980; **Fac Appt:** Prof N, Case West Res Univ

Saper, Joel R MD [N] - **Spec Exp:** Headache; Pain-Chronic after Head Injury; **Hospital:** Chelsea Comm Hosp; **Address:** Michigan Head Pain & Neurological Inst, 3120 Professional Drive, Ann Arbor, MI 48104; **Phone:** 734-677-6000; **Board Cert:** Neurology 1975; Pain Medicine 1996; Headache Medicine 2006; **Med School:** Univ IL Coll Med 1969; **Resid:** Neurology, Univ Mich Med Ctr 1973; **Fac Appt:** Clin Prof N, Mich State Univ

Siddique, Teepu MD [N] - **Spec Exp:** Amyotrophic Lateral Sclerosis (ALS); Muscular Dystrophy; Neurogenetics; **Hospital:** Northwestern Meml Hosp; **Address:** Northwestern Univ-Feinberg, Dept Neuro, 303 E Chicago Ave, Tarry Bldg, rm 13-715, Chicago, IL 60611-5935; **Phone:** 312-695-5886; **Board Cert:** Neurology 1980; **Med School:** Pakistan 1973; **Resid:** Neurology, UMDNJ Affil Hosp 1979; **Fellow:** Electromyography, Hosp Special Surg 1980; Neuromuscular Disease, Natl Inst Hlth 1981; **Fac Appt:** Prof N, Northwestern Univ

Swanson, Jerry W MD [N] - **Spec Exp:** Headache; Migraine; **Hospital:** Mayo Med Ctr & Clin - Rochester; **Address:** Mayo Clinic, Dept Neurology, 200 First St SW, Rochester, MN 55905-0001; **Phone:** 507-538-1036; **Board Cert:** Neurology 1984; Headache Medicine 2006; **Med School:** Northwestern Univ 1977; **Resid:** Neurology, Mayo Clinic 1982; **Fellow:** Electroencephalography, Mayo Clinic 1983; **Fac Appt:** Prof N, Mayo Med Sch

Taylor, Frederick R MD [N] - **Spec Exp:** Headache; Pain-Facial; **Hospital:** Methodist Hosp - Minnesota; **Address:** Park Nicollet Headache Clinic, 6490 Excelsior Blvd, Meadowbrook Bldg, Ste E-500, Minneapolis, MN 55426; **Phone:** 952-993-3432; **Board Cert:** Pediatrics 1982; Neurology 1985; Headache Medicine 2006; **Med School:** Univ New Mexico 1977; **Resid:** Pediatrics, Univ Wisc Hlth Sci Ctr 1980; Neurology, Univ Wisc Hlth Sci Ctr 1983; **Fellow:** Neurological Physiology, Univ Wisc Hlth Sci Ctr 1984

Vick, Nicholas A MD [N] - **Spec Exp:** Brain Tumors; Neuro-Oncology; **Hospital:** Evanston/Northshore Univ Hlth Syst; **Address:** Evanston Hosp, Dept Neurology, 2650 Ridge Ave, Evanston, IL 60201; **Phone:** 847-570-2570; **Board Cert:** Neurology 1971; **Med School:** Univ Chicago-Pritzker Sch Med 1965; **Resid:** Neurology, Univ Chicago Hosps 1968; **Fellow:** Neurology, Natl Inst Hlth 1970; **Fac Appt:** Prof N, Northwestern Univ

Vitek, Jerrold Lee MD/PhD [N] - **Spec Exp:** Parkinson's Disease/Movement Disorders; Tremor & Dystonia; **Hospital:** Cleveland Clin Fdn (page 56); **Address:** 9500 Euclid Ave, MC NC30, Cleveland, OH 44195; **Phone:** 216-445-0267; **Board Cert:** Neurology 1992; **Med School:** Univ Minn 1984; **Resid:** Neurology, Johns Hopkins Hosp 1988; **Fac Appt:** Prof N, Cleveland Cl Coll Med/Case West Res

Windebank, Anthony J MD [N] - **Spec Exp:** Peripheral Neuropathy; Amyotrophic Lateral Sclerosis (ALS); Multiple Sclerosis; **Hospital:** Mayo Med Ctr & Clin - Rochester; **Address:** Mayo Clin, Dept Neurology, 200 First St SW, Rochester, MN 55905; **Phone:** 507-284-2798; **Board Cert:** Neurology 1982; **Med School:** England, UK 1974; **Resid:** Internal Medicine, Radcliffe Infirm 1977; Neurology, Mayo Clin 1981; **Fellow:** Neurology, Mayo Clin 1982; **Fac Appt:** Prof N, Mayo Med Sch

Wright, Robert B MD [N] - **Spec Exp:** Myasthenia Gravis; Migraine; **Hospital:** Rush Univ Med Ctr; **Address:** 1725 W Harrison St, Ste 1118, Chicago, IL 60612-3841; **Phone:** 312-942-5936; **Board Cert:** Neurology 1988; **Med School:** Univ IL Coll Med 1982; **Resid:** Neurology, Rush Presby-St Luke's Med Ctr 1986; **Fellow:** Neuromuscular Medicine, Rush Presby-St Luke's Med Ctr 1987; **Fac Appt:** Asst Prof N, Rush Med Coll

Great Plains and Mountains

Barohn, Richard J MD [N] - **Spec Exp:** Peripheral Neuropathy; Myasthenia Gravis; Amyotrophic Lateral Sclerosis (ALS); **Hospital:** Univ of Kansas Hosp; **Address:** Univ Kansas Medical Ctr, Dept Neurology, 3901 Rainbow Blvd, MS 2012, Kansas City, KS 66160; **Phone:** 913-588-6970; **Board Cert:** Neurology 1987; Clinical Neurophysiology 2004; **Med School:** Univ MO-Kansas City 1980; **Resid:** Neurology, Lackland AFB 1985

Bromberg, Mark B MD/PhD [N] - **Spec Exp:** Peripheral Neuropathy; Neuromuscular Disorders; **Hospital:** Univ Utah Hosps and Clins; **Address:** 175 N Medical Drive, Clinical Neurosciences Center, Salt Lake City, UT 84132; **Phone:** 801-585-7575; **Board Cert:** Neurology 1988; Clinical Neurophysiology 2002; **Med School:** Univ Mich Med Sch 1982; **Resid:** Neurology, Univ Mich Med Ctr 1986; **Fellow:** Electromyography, Univ Mich Med Ctr 1987; Neuromuscular Disease, Univ Mich Med Ctr 1987; **Fac Appt:** Prof N, Univ Utah

Filley, Christopher M MD [N] - **Spec Exp:** Leukoencephalopathy; Alzheimer's Disease; Brain Injury-Traumatic; Multiple Sclerosis; **Hospital:** Univ Colorado Hosp, VA Med Ctr; **Address:** Univ CO, Neurology Dept, Behavioral Neurology Sect., 12631 E 17th Ave, MS B185, Aurora, CO 80045; **Phone:** 303-724-2187; **Board Cert:** Neurology 1984; Behavioral Neurology & Neuropsychiatry 2006; **Med School:** Johns Hopkins Univ 1979; **Resid:** Neurology, Univ Colorado Hosp 1983; **Fellow:** Behavioral Neurology, Boston VA Hosp 1984; **Fac Appt:** Prof N, Univ Colorado

Neurology

Kelly, James P MD [N] - **Spec Exp:** Brain Injury; Memory Disorders; Neurologic Rehabilitation; Brain Injury-Traumatic; **Hospital:** Univ Colorado Hosp; **Address:** PO Box 6510, Campus Box F727, Aurora, CO 80045; **Phone:** 720-848-2086; **Board Cert:** Neurology 1991; **Med School:** Northwestern Univ 1983; **Resid:** Neurology, Univ Colorado Med Ctr 1988; **Fellow:** Behavioral Neurology, Univ Colorado Med Ctr 1989; **Fac Appt:** Prof N, Univ Colorado

Kelts, K Alan MD/PhD [N] - **Spec Exp:** Pediatric Neurology; Sleep Disorders/Apnea; Neuromuscular Disorders; **Hospital:** Rapid City Reg Hosp; **Address:** Black Hills Neurology, 2929 5th St, Ste 240, Rapid City, SD 57701; **Phone:** 605-341-3770; **Board Cert:** Pediatrics 1977; Child Neurology 1978; **Med School:** Univ Rochester 1971; **Resid:** Pediatrics, Chldns & Univ Hosps 1973; Child Neurology, Colorado Med Ctr 1976; **Fellow:** Neuromuscular Disease, Muscular Dystrophy Assn 1975; **Fac Appt:** Clin Prof N, Univ SD Sch Med

Ringel, Steven MD [N] - **Spec Exp:** Neuromuscular Disorders; **Hospital:** Univ Colorado Hosp; **Address:** Univ CO Hosp, Neuromuscular Dept, 12631 E 17th Ave, Box B185, Denver, CO 80045; **Phone:** 303-714-2188; **Board Cert:** Neurology 1974; **Med School:** Univ Mich Med Sch 1968; **Resid:** Neurology, Rush-Presby-St Lukes Med Ctr 1972; **Fellow:** Neurology, Natl Inst Neuro Dis-NIH 1976; **Fac Appt:** Prof N, Univ Colorado

Vollmer, Timothy L MD [N] - **Spec Exp:** Multiple Sclerosis; Myasthenia Gravis; Vasculitis of the Nervous System; Stroke; **Hospital:** Univ Colorado Hosp; **Address:** Rocky Mountain MS Ctr-Anschutz, Mail Stop B185, 12631 E 17th Ave Fl 5, Aurora, CO 80045; **Phone:** 720-848-2080; **Board Cert:** Neurology 1991; **Med School:** Stanford Univ 1983; **Resid:** Neurology, Stanford Univ Hosp 1987; **Fellow:** Neurological Immunology, Stanford Univ 1986; **Fac Appt:** Prof N, Univ Colorado

Southwest

Ahern, Geoffrey L MD/PhD [N] - **Spec Exp:** Behavioral Neurology; Dementia; Alzheimer's Disease; **Hospital:** Univ Med Ctr - Tucson; **Address:** Univ Arizona, Dept Neurology, 1501 N Campbell Ave, Box 245093, Tucson, AZ 85724-5093; **Phone:** 520-694-8888; **Board Cert:** Neurology 1992; **Med School:** Yale Univ 1984; **Resid:** Neurology, Boston Univ Affil Hosps 1988; **Fellow:** Behavioral Neurology, Beth Israel Hosp 1990; **Fac Appt:** Prof N, Univ Ariz Coll Med

Burns, Richard S MD [N] - **Spec Exp:** Movement Disorders; Ataxia; Neurodegenerative Disorders; **Hospital:** St Joseph's Hosp & Med Ctr - Phoenix; **Address:** Barrow Neurological Institute, 500 W Thomas Rd, Ste 720, Phoenix, AZ 85013; **Phone:** 602-406-4931; **Board Cert:** Neurology 1985; **Med School:** Univ Minn 1969; **Resid:** Internal Medicine, Huntington Meml Hosp 1971; Neurology, UC Irvine Med Ctr 1978; **Fellow:** Clinical Pharmacology, Natl Inst Genl Med Sci 1980

Carter, John E MD [N] - **Spec Exp:** Neuro-Ophthalmology; **Hospital:** Univ Hlth Syst-San Antonio; **Address:** Univ Tex Hlth Sci Ctr, Div Neurology, 7703 Floyd Curl, rm 5.318T, MC 7883, San Antonio, TX 78229-3900; **Phone:** 210-567-5088; **Board Cert:** Neurology 1978; **Med School:** Univ Ark 1969; **Resid:** Neurology, Boston Univ Med Ctr 1978; Neuro-Ophthalmology, Tufts Univ 1979; **Fac Appt:** Assoc Prof N, Univ Tex, San Antonio

Couch Jr, James R MD/PhD [N] - **Spec Exp:** Headache; Stroke; **Hospital:** OU Med Ctr, VA Med Ctr - Oklahoma City; **Address:** 711 S L Young Blvd, Ste 210, Oklahoma City, OK 73104-5021; **Phone:** 405-271-3635; **Board Cert:** Neurology 1974; Clinical Neurophysiology 2002; Headache Medicine 2006; **Med School:** Baylor Coll Med 1965; **Resid:** Neurology, Washington Univ Med Ctr 1972; **Fellow:** Neuropharmacology, Natl Inst Hlth 1969; **Fac Appt:** Prof N, Univ Okla Coll Med

Coull, Bruce M MD [N] - **Spec Exp:** Stroke; Cerebrovascular Disease; **Hospital:** Univ Med Ctr
- Tucson; **Address:** 2800 E Ajo Way, Tucson, AZ 85713; **Phone:** 520-874-2700; **Board Cert:**
Neurology 1979; Vascular Neurology 2005; **Med School:** Univ Pittsburgh 1972; **Resid:** Neurology,
Stanford Univ Med Ctr 1976; **Fac Appt:** Prof N, Univ Ariz Coll Med

Dodick, David W MD [N] - **Spec Exp:** Headache; Migraine; **Hospital:** Mayo Clinic - Scottsdale, Mayo Clinic - Phoenix; **Address:** Mayo Clinic, Dept of Neurology, 5777 E Mayo Blvd, Ste 5E,
Phoenix, AZ 85054; **Phone:** 480-342-3078; **Board Cert:** Neurology 2006; Vascular Neurology
2005; Headache Medicine 2006; **Med School:** Dalhousie Univ 1990; **Resid:** Neurology, Mayo
Clinic 1994; **Fellow:** Headache, Sunnybrook Hlth Sci Ctr 1996; **Fac Appt:** Prof N, Mayo Med Sch

Doody, Rachelle Smith MD/PhD [N] - **Spec Exp:** Alzheimer's Disease; Memory Disorders;
Hospital: Methodist Hosp - Houston; **Address:** Alzheimer's & Memory Disorder Ctr, Dept of Neurology, Smith Tower Fl 18, 6550 Fanning, Ste 1801, Houston, TX 77030; **Phone:** 713-798-4734;
Board Cert: Neurology 1988; **Med School:** Baylor Coll Med 1983; **Resid:** Neurology, Baylor Coll
of Med Affil Hosp 1987; **Fac Appt:** Prof N, Baylor Coll Med

Ferrendelli, James A MD [N] - **Spec Exp:** Epilepsy/Seizure Disorders; Geriatric Neurology;
Hospital: Meml Hermann Hosp - Texas Med Ctr; **Address:** UT Houston Sch Med, Dept Neurology,
6431 Fannin St, Ste 7.102, Houston, TX 77030-1501; **Phone:** 713-500-7080; **Board Cert:** Neurology 1973; **Med School:** Univ Colorado 1962; **Resid:** Neurology, Cleveland Metro Genl Hosp
1968; **Fellow:** Neuropharmacology, Washington Univ Med Sch 1971; **Fac Appt:** Prof N, Univ Tex,
Houston

Fox, Peter Thornton MD [N] - **Spec Exp:** PET Imaging; **Hospital:** Univ Hlth Syst-San Antonio;
Address: Rsch Imaging Ctr, 7703 Floyd Curl Drive, MS 6240, San Antonio, TX 78229-3900;
Phone: 210-567-8150; **Board Cert:** Neurology 1985; **Med School:** Georgetown Univ 1979;
Resid: Neurology, Washington Univ 1983; **Fellow:** Radiotracer Imaging, Washington Univ 1984;
Fac Appt: Prof N, Univ Tex, San Antonio

Gilbert, Mark R MD [N] - **Spec Exp:** Brain Tumors; Neuro-Oncology; **Hospital:** UT MD Anderson Cancer Ctr; **Address:** Univ Tex MD Anderson Cancer Ctr, 1515 Holcombe Blvd, Unit 431, Houston, TX 77030; **Phone:** 713-792-4008; **Board Cert:** Internal Medicine 1985; Neurology 1990;
Med School: Johns Hopkins Univ 1982; **Resid:** Internal Medicine, Johns Hopkins Hosp 1985; Neurology, Johns Hopkins Hosp 1988; **Fellow:** Neuro-Oncology, Johns Hopkins Hosp 1988; **Fac Appt:**
Assoc Prof N, Univ Tex, Houston

Grotta, James C MD [N] - **Spec Exp:** Stroke; **Hospital:** Meml Hermann Hosp - Texas Med Ctr;
Address: UT Houston Med Sch, Dept Neur, 6410 Fannin St, Ste 1014, Houston, TX 77030; **Phone:**
832-325-7080; **Board Cert:** Neurology 1978; Vascular Neurology 2005; **Med School:** Univ VA
Sch Med 1971; **Resid:** Neurology, Univ Colorado Hlth Sci Ctr 1977; **Fellow:** Diagnostic Radiology,
Mass Genl Hosp 1979; **Fac Appt:** Prof N, Univ Tex, Houston

Harati, Yadollah MD [N] - **Spec Exp:** Neuromuscular Disorders; Amyotrophic Lateral Sclerosis
(ALS); Myasthenia Gravis; Nerve/Muscle Disorders; **Hospital:** St Luke's Episcopal Hosp-Houston; **Ad-
dress:** Baylor Neurology, Smith Tower, 6550 Fannin, Ste 1801, Houston, TX 77030; **Phone:** 713-
798-7411; **Board Cert:** Neurology 1978; **Med School:** Iran 1970; **Resid:** Neurology, Univ
Nebraska Affil Hosp 1974; Neurology, Baylor Coll of Med Affil Hosp 1975; **Fellow:** Neuromuscular
Disease, Baylor Coll of Med Affil Hosp 1976; **Fac Appt:** Prof N, Baylor Coll Med

Hart, Robert G MD [N] - **Spec Exp:** Stroke; **Hospital:** Univ Hlth Syst-San Antonio; **Address:**
Univ Tex Hlth & Sci Ctr, Dept Neurology, 7703 Floyd Curl, MC 7883, San Antonio, TX 78229-3901;
Phone: 210-592-0404; **Board Cert:** Neurology 1985; Vascular Neurology 2005; **Med School:**
Univ MO-Columbia Sch Med 1977; **Resid:** Neurology, Univ Hosp & Clinic 1981; **Fellow:** Stroke,
Oregon Hlth Sci Ctr 1982; **Fac Appt:** Prof N, Univ Tex, San Antonio

Infante, Ernesto MD [N] - **Spec Exp:** Neuromuscular Disorders; Movement Disorders; Headache; **Hospital:** Meml Hermann Hosp - Texas Med Ctr; **Address:** 6410 Fannin St, Ste 1014, UT Professional Building Fl 10, Houston, TX 77030; **Phone:** 832-325-7080; **Board Cert:** Neurology 1973; **Med School:** Spain 1964; **Resid:** Neurology, Univ Minn Hosps 1969; **Fellow:** Electromyography, Mayo Clinic 1970; **Fac Appt:** Assoc Clin Prof N, Univ Tex, Houston

Jankovic, Joseph MD [N] - **Spec Exp:** Movement Disorders; Parkinson's Disease; Tourette's Syndrome; **Hospital:** Methodist Hosp - Houston, St Luke's Episcopal Hosp-Houston; **Address:** Parkinson's Dis Ctr & Movement Disorders Clin, 6550 Fannin St, Smith Twr, Ste 1801, Houston, TX 77030; **Phone:** 713-798-5998; **Board Cert:** Neurology 1979; **Med School:** Univ Ariz Coll Med 1973; **Resid:** Neurology, Columbia-Presby Med Ctr 1977; **Fac Appt:** Prof N, Baylor Coll Med

Kent, Thomas Andrew MD [N] - **Spec Exp:** Stroke; Neuro-Psychiatry; **Hospital:** DeBakey VA Med Ctr-Houston; **Address:** 2002 Holcombe Blvd, MS 127, Houston, TX 77030; **Phone:** 713-794-7393; **Board Cert:** Psychiatry 1993; Neurology 2006; **Med School:** Univ Kans 1979; **Resid:** Psychiatry, Univ Kansas Affil Hosp 1983; Neurology, Univ Texas Affil Hosp 1985; **Fellow:** Psychopharmacology, Univ Kansas Affil Hosp 1983; **Fac Appt:** Prof N, Baylor Coll Med

Knoefel, Janice E MD [N] - **Spec Exp:** Geriatric Neurology; Neuro-Rehabilitation; **Hospital:** VA Med Ctr, Univ NM Hlth & Sci Ctr; **Address:** New Mexico VA Hlth Care System, 1501 San Pedro SE, MC 111K, Albuquerque, NM 87108-5153; **Phone:** 505-256-2795; **Board Cert:** Neurology 1983; **Med School:** Ohio State Univ 1977; **Resid:** Internal Medicine, Univ Cincinnati Med Ctr 1979; Neurology, Boston Univ Med Ctr 1982; **Fellow:** Geriatric Medicine, Boston Univ Med Ctr 1983; **Fac Appt:** Prof N, Univ New Mexico

Labiner, David M MD [N] - **Spec Exp:** Epilepsy; Seizure Disorders; **Hospital:** Univ Med Ctr - Tucson; **Address:** Univ Arizona HSC, Dept Neurology, 1501 N Campbell Ave, PO Box 245023, Tucson, AZ 85724-5023; **Phone:** 520-626-2006; **Board Cert:** Neurology 1992; **Med School:** Med Coll GA 1984; **Resid:** Neurology, Neuro Inst/Columbia 1988; **Fellow:** Epilepsy, Duke Univ Med Ctr 1989; **Fac Appt:** Prof N, Univ Ariz Coll Med

Levin, Victor A MD [N] - **Spec Exp:** Brain Tumors; Neuro-Oncology; Clinical Trials; **Hospital:** UT MD Anderson Cancer Ctr; **Address:** 1515 Holcombe Blvd, Unit #431, Houston, TX 77030-4009; **Phone:** 713-792-8297; **Board Cert:** Neurology 1976; **Med School:** Univ Wisc 1966; **Resid:** Neurology, Mass Genl Hosp 1972; **Fac Appt:** Prof Med, Univ Tex, Houston

Nicholl, Jeffrey S MD [N] - **Spec Exp:** Seizure Disorders; Epilepsy; **Hospital:** Tulane Univ Hosp & Clin; **Address:** Tulane Univ Sch Med Dept Neuro TB-52, 1440 Canal St, New Orleans, LA 70112; **Phone:** 504-988-2241; **Board Cert:** Neurology 1999; Psychiatry 1981; Clinical Neurophysiology 2001; Emergency Medicine 2004; **Med School:** Georgetown Univ 1974; **Resid:** Psychiatry, UCLA Neuro Psyc Inst 1979; Neurology, Tulane Univ 1997; **Fellow:** Clinical Neurophysiology, Tulane Univ 1998; Epilepsy, UCLA 2000; **Fac Appt:** Assoc Prof N, Tulane Univ

Oommen, Kalarickal J MD [N] - **Spec Exp:** Epilepsy; **Hospital:** Univ Med Ctr-Lubbock; **Address:** Texas Tech Univ Hlth Sciences Ctr, Dept Neurology, 3601 4th St, MS 8321, Lubbock, TX 79430; **Phone:** 806-725-4115; **Board Cert:** Neurology 1983; **Med School:** India 1973; **Resid:** Psychiatry, Arizona Hlth Sci Ctr 1979; Neurology, Arizona Hlth Sci Ctr 1982; **Fellow:** Electroencephalography, Med Coll Georgia 1983; **Fac Appt:** Prof N, Texas Tech Univ

Shapiro, William R MD [N] - **Spec Exp:** Neuro-Oncology; **Hospital:** St Joseph's Hosp & Med Ctr - Phoenix; **Address:** Barrow Neurology Clinics, 500 W Thomas Rd, Ste 300, Phoenix, AZ 85013; **Phone:** 602-406-6262; **Board Cert:** Neurology 1969; **Med School:** UCSF 1961; **Resid:** Internal Medicine, Univ Wash Hosp 1963; Neurology, NY Hosp-Cornell Med Ctr 1966; **Fellow:** Neuro-Oncology, Natl Inst Hlth 1969; **Fac Appt:** Prof N, Univ Ariz Coll Med

Suarez, Jose MD [N] - **Spec Exp:** Stroke; Critical Care; **Hospital:** St Luke's Episcopal Hosp-Houston; **Address:** Neurology Associates, Smith Tower, 6550 Fannin St Fl 18 - Ste 1801, Houston, TX 77030; **Phone:** 713-798-2273; **Board Cert:** Neurology 2008; Vascular Neurology 2005; **Med School:** Colombia 1988; **Resid:** Neurology, Case Western Reserve Univ Hosp 1996; **Fellow:** Neurocritical Care, Johns Hopkins Univ Hosp 1998; **Fac Appt:** Assoc Prof N, Baylor Coll Med

Wolinsky, Jerry S MD [N] - **Spec Exp:** Multiple Sclerosis; Clinical Trials; MRI; **Hospital:** Meml Hermann Hosp - Texas Med Ctr; **Address:** Univ Texas Med Sch, 6431 Fannin St, MSMB 7.044, Houston, TX 77030-1503; **Phone:** 713-500-7135; **Board Cert:** Neurology 1975; **Med School:** Univ IL Coll Med 1969; **Resid:** Neurology, UCSF Med Ctr 1973; **Fellow:** Neuropathology, VA Hosp 1975; **Fac Appt:** Prof N, Univ Tex, Houston

Yung, Wai-Kwan A MD [N] - **Spec Exp:** Neuro-Oncology; Brain Tumors; **Hospital:** UT MD Anderson Cancer Ctr; **Address:** 1515 Holcombe Blvd, Unit 431, Houston, TX 77030-4017; **Phone:** 713-794-1285; **Board Cert:** Neurology 1980; **Med School:** Univ Chicago-Pritzker Sch Med 1975; **Resid:** Neurology, UCSD Med Ctr 1978; **Fellow:** Neuro-Oncology, Meml Sloan Kettering Cancer Ctr 1981; **Fac Appt:** Prof N, Univ Tex, Houston

West Coast and Pacific

Adornato, Bruce T MD [N] - **Spec Exp:** Stroke; Peripheral Neuropathy; Sleep Disorders/Apnea; **Hospital:** Stanford Univ Med Ctr, VA Hlth Care Sys - Palo Alto; **Address:** 1101 Welch Rd, Ste C5, Palo Alto, CA 94304-1926; **Phone:** 650-324-4300; **Board Cert:** Internal Medicine 1975; Neurology 1978; **Med School:** UCSD 1972; **Resid:** Internal Medicine, UCSF-Moffitt Hosp 1974; Neurology, UCSF-Moffitt Hosp 1976; **Fellow:** Neurology, Natl Inst Hlth 1978; **Fac Appt:** Clin Prof N, Stanford Univ

Albers, Gregory W MD [N] - **Spec Exp:** Cerebrovascular Disease; Stroke; **Hospital:** Stanford Univ Med Ctr; **Address:** Stanford Univ Med Ctr, Dept Neurology, 701 Welch Rd, Ste 325, Palo Alto, CA 74304; **Phone:** 650-723-4448; **Board Cert:** Neurology 1990; Vascular Neurology 2008; **Med School:** UCSD 1984; **Resid:** Neurology, Standford Univ Med Ctr 1988; **Fellow:** Stroke, Standford Univ Med Ctr 1989; **Fac Appt:** Assoc Prof N, Stanford Univ

Aminoff, Michael J MD [N] - **Spec Exp:** Movement Disorders; Parkinson's Disease; **Hospital:** UCSF Med Ctr; **Address:** 505 Parnassus Ave, Fl 3 - rm M348, San Francisco, CA 94143-0216; **Phone:** 415-353-2904; **Board Cert:** Neurology 2004; Clinical Neurophysiology 2000; **Med School:** England, UK 1965; **Resid:** Internal Medicine, Univ London Hosps 1970; Neurology, Middlesex Hosp/Natl Hosp Queen Sq 1972; **Fac Appt:** Prof N, UCSF

Aurora, Sheena K MD [N] - **Spec Exp:** Headache; Migraine; Electromyography; Movement Disorders; **Hospital:** Swedish Med Ctr - Seattle; **Address:** Swedish Headache Ctr, 1101 Madison Med Tower, Ste 200, Seattle, WA 98104-1306; **Phone:** 206-215-2243; **Board Cert:** Neurology 2006; Electrodiagnostic Medicine 1998; Clinical Neurophysiology 1999; Headache Medicine 2006; **Med School:** India 1990; **Resid:** Neurology, Henry Ford Hosp 1997

Becker, Kyra J MD [N] - **Spec Exp:** Stroke/Cerebrovascular Disease; Neuro-Immunology; Stroke-Young Adults; **Hospital:** Harborview Med Ctr, Univ Wash Med Ctr; **Address:** Harborview Medical Ctr, Dept Neurology, 325 9th Ave, Box 359775, Seattle, WA 98104; **Phone:** 206-744-6285; **Board Cert:** Neurology 2006; Vascular Neurology 2005; **Med School:** Duke Univ 1989; **Resid:** Neurology, Johns Hopkins Hosp 1993; **Fellow:** Critical Care Neurology, Johns Hopkins Hosp 1995; Research, NIH-NINDS 1996; **Fac Appt:** Assoc Prof N, Univ Wash

Bourdette, Dennis MD [N] - **Spec Exp:** Multiple Sclerosis; Guillain-Barre Syndrome; Myasthenia Gravis; **Hospital:** OR Hlth & Sci Univ; **Address:** OHSU, Dept Neurology, 3181 SW Sam Jackson Park Rd, MS L226, Portland, OR 97239; **Phone:** 503-494-5759; **Board Cert:** Neurology 1985; **Med School:** UC Davis 1978; **Resid:** Neurology, Oregon Hlth Sci Univ Hosp 1982; **Fellow:** Neurological Immunology, VA Med Ctr 1985; **Fac Appt:** Prof N, Oregon Hlth & Sci Univ

Bowen, James MD [N] - **Spec Exp:** Multiple Sclerosis; **Hospital:** Swedish Med Ctr - Seattle; **Address:** Swedish Med Ctr, 550 17th Ave, Ste 540, Seattle, WA 98122; **Phone:** 206-320-2200; **Board Cert:** Neurology 1990; **Med School:** Johns Hopkins Univ 1982; **Resid:** Internal Medicine, Univ Washington Med Ctr 1984; Neurology, Univ Washington Med Ctr 1987; **Fac Appt:** Asst Clin Prof N, Univ Wash

Charles, Andrew C MD [N] - **Spec Exp:** Headache; Migraine; **Hospital:** UCLA Ronald Reagan Med Ctr; **Address:** UCLA Neurological Svcs, 300 Med Plaza, Ste B200, Los Angeles, CA 90095; **Phone:** 310-794-1195; **Board Cert:** Neurology 1992; **Med School:** UCLA 1986; **Resid:** Neurology, UCLA Med Ctr 1990; **Fellow:** Neurology, UCLA Med Ctr 1992; **Fac Appt:** Prof N, UCLA

Chui, Helena Chang MD [N] - **Spec Exp:** Stroke; Dementia; Alzheimer's Disease; **Hospital:** USC Univ Hosp, Rancho Los Amigos Natl Rehab Ctr; **Address:** Health Care Consultation Center II, 1510 San Pablo St, Ste 618, Los Angeles, CA 90033; **Phone:** 323-442-7591; **Board Cert:** Neurology 1984; **Med School:** Johns Hopkins Univ 1977; **Resid:** Neurology, Univ Iowa Med Ctr 1981; **Fellow:** Behavioral Neurology, Univ Iowa Med Ctr 1979; **Fac Appt:** Prof N, USC Sch Med

Cloughesy, Timothy F MD [N] - **Spec Exp:** Neuro-Oncology; Seizure Disorders; Brain Tumors; **Hospital:** UCLA Ronald Reagan Med Ctr; **Address:** UCLA Neurological Services, 710 Westwood Plaza, Ste 1-230, Los Angeles, CA 90095; **Phone:** 310-825-5321; **Board Cert:** Neurology 1993; **Med School:** Tulane Univ 1987; **Resid:** Neurology, UCLA Med Ctr 1991; **Fellow:** Neuro-Oncology, Meml Sloan-Kettering Canc Ctr; **Fac Appt:** Clin Prof N, UCLA

Corey-Bloom, Jody MD [N] - **Spec Exp:** Multiple Sclerosis; **Hospital:** UCSD Med Ctr; **Address:** Clin Chief Neurosis, Perlman Ambulatory Care Ctr, 9350 Campus Point Drive, La Jolla, CA 92037; **Phone:** 858-657-8540; **Board Cert:** Neurology 1993; **Med School:** UCSD 1986; **Resid:** Neurology, UCSD Med Ctr 1990; **Fellow:** Neurology, UCSD Med Ctr 1992; **Fac Appt:** Prof N, UCSD

Cummings, Jeffrey Lee MD [N] - **Spec Exp:** Neuro-Psychiatry; Alzheimer's Disease; Parkinson's Disease; **Hospital:** UCLA Ronald Reagan Med Ctr; **Address:** UCLA Med Ctr, Alzheimer's Disease Ctr, 10911 Weyburn Ave, Ste 200, Los Angeles, CA 90095-7226; **Phone:** 310-794-3665; **Board Cert:** Neurology 1979; **Med School:** Univ Wash 1974; **Resid:** Neurology, Boston Univ Sch Med 1978; **Fellow:** Behavioral Neurology and Psychiatry, Boston Univ Sch Med 1979; Neurological Pathology, The Natl Hosp 1980; **Fac Appt:** Assoc Prof N, UCLA

DeGiorgio, Christopher M MD [N] - **Spec Exp:** Epilepsy; Seizure Disorders; Neurocysticercosis; Parasitic Infections; **Hospital:** UCLA Ronald Reagan Med Ctr; **Address:** UCLA Med Ctr, Dept Neurology, 710 Westwood Plaza, rm 2145, Los Angeles, CA 90095; **Phone:** 310-794-1195; **Board Cert:** Neurology 1987; **Med School:** Loyola Univ-Stritch Sch Med 1981; **Resid:** Neurology, West Los Angeles VA Hosp 1985; **Fellow:** Epilepsy, UCLA Med Ctr 1987; **Fac Appt:** Assoc Prof N, UCLA

Engel, William King MD [N] - **Spec Exp:** Neuromuscular Disorders; **Hospital:** Good Samaritan Hosp - LA, USC Univ Hosp; **Address:** 637 S Lucas Ave Fl 3, Los Angeles, CA 90017; **Phone:** 213-975-9950; **Board Cert:** Neurology 1962; **Med School:** McGill Univ 1955; **Resid:** Neurology, Natl Inst Hlth 1959; Neurology, Natl Hosp 1960; **Fellow:** Neuromuscular Medicine, Natl Inst Hlth 1961; **Fac Appt:** Prof N, USC Sch Med

Engstrom, John W MD [N] - **Spec Exp:** Peripheral Neuropathy; Spinal Cord Disorders; **Hospital:** UCSF Med Ctr; **Address:** UCSF Med Ctr, Dept Neurology, 400 Parnassus Ave Fl 8, Box 0348, San Francisco, CA 94143; **Phone:** 415-353-2273; **Board Cert:** Internal Medicine 1984; Neurology 1991; Clinical Neurophysiology 2002; **Med School:** Stanford Univ 1981; **Resid:** Internal Medicine, Johns Hopkins Hosp 1984; Neurology, UCSF Med Ctr 1988; **Fellow:** Neurology, UCSF Med Ctr 1989; **Fac Appt:** Prof N, UCSF

Fisher, Mark Jay MD [N] - **Spec Exp:** Stroke; Cerebrovascular Disease; **Hospital:** UC Irvine Med Ctr; **Address:** UC Irvine Med Ctr, Dept Neurology, 101 The City Drive S, Shanbrom Hall, rm 121, Orange, CA 92868; **Phone:** 714-456-6856; **Board Cert:** Neurology 1981; Vascular Neurology 2005; **Med School:** Univ Cincinnati 1975; **Resid:** Neurology, UCLA-Wadsworth VA Hosp 1980; **Fac Appt:** Prof N, UC Irvine

Fisher, Robert S MD [N] - **Spec Exp:** Epilepsy/Seizure Disorders; **Hospital:** Stanford Univ Med Ctr; **Address:** 300 Pasteur Drive, rm A-343, Dept of Neurology, Stanford, CA 94305-5235; **Phone:** 650-498-3056; **Board Cert:** Neurology 1983; Clinical Neurophysiology 2002; **Med School:** Stanford Univ 1977; **Resid:** Internal Medicine, Stanford Univ 1979; Neurology, Johns Hopkins Hosp 1982

Goodin, Douglas MD [N] - **Spec Exp:** Multiple Sclerosis; **Hospital:** UCSF Med Ctr, VA Med Ctr - San Francisco; **Address:** UCSF MS Ctr, 400 Parnassus Ave Fl 8, San Francisco, CA 94117; **Phone:** 415-353-2069; **Board Cert:** Neurology 1985; **Med School:** UC Irvine 1978; **Resid:** Neurology, UCSF Med Ctr 1981; **Fac Appt:** Assoc Prof N, UCSF

Graves, Michael C MD [N] - **Spec Exp:** Amyotrophic Lateral Sclerosis (ALS); **Hospital:** UCLA Ronald Reagan Med Ctr; **Address:** UCLA Neurological Svcs, 300 Medical Plaza, Ste B200, Box 956975, Los Angeles, CA 90095-6975; **Phone:** 310-825-7266; **Board Cert:** Neurology 1977; **Med School:** Stanford Univ 1970; **Resid:** Internal Medicine, UCSD Med Ctr 1972; Neurology, Johns Hopkins Hosp 1975; **Fellow:** Rockefeller Univ Hosp; **Fac Appt:** Assoc Prof N, UCLA

Hauser, Stephen L MD [N] - **Spec Exp:** Multiple Sclerosis; Epilepsy; **Hospital:** UCSF Med Ctr; **Address:** UCSF MS Ctr, 400 Parnassus Ave Fl 8th, Box 0114, San Francisco, CA 94143-0164; **Phone:** 415-353-2069; **Board Cert:** Internal Medicine 1978; Neurology 1981; **Med School:** Harvard Med Sch 1975; **Resid:** Internal Medicine, NY Presby-Cornell 1977; Neurology, Mass Genl Hosp 1980; **Fellow:** Neurology, Harvard Univ 1980; **Fac Appt:** Prof N, UCSF

Heck, Christianne N MD [N] - **Spec Exp:** Epilepsy; **Hospital:** USC Univ Hosp; **Address:** Neurologic Care & Research Ctr, 1520 San Pablo St, Ste 3000, Los Angeles, CA 90033; **Phone:** 323-442-5710; **Board Cert:** Neurology 2001; **Med School:** USC-Keck School of Medicine 1991; **Resid:** Neurology, LAC/USC Med Ctr 1995; **Fellow:** Epilepsy, USC Med Ctr 1996; **Fac Appt:** Assoc Prof N, USC-Keck School of Medicine

Henderson, Victor W MD [N] - **Spec Exp:** Alzheimer's Disease; Dementia; Memory Disorders; **Hospital:** Stanford Univ Med Ctr; **Address:** Stanford Univ Hosp, Dept Neurology, 300 Pasteur Drive, rm A343, Stanford, CA 94305-5235; **Phone:** 650-723-5184; **Board Cert:** Neurology 1981; **Med School:** Johns Hopkins Univ 1976; **Resid:** Internal Medicine, Duke Univ Med Ctr 1977; Neurology, Barnes Hosp- Wash Univ 1980; **Fellow:** Behavioral Neurology, Aphasia Rsch Ctr-Boston Univ 1981; **Fac Appt:** Prof N, Stanford Univ

Langston, J William MD [N] - **Spec Exp:** Parkinson's Disease; Movement Disorders; Tremor; **Hospital:** Parkinson's Inst/Movement Disorders Trmt Ctr, The; **Address:** The Parkinsons Institute, 675 Almanor Ave, Sunnyvale, CA 94085; **Phone:** 408-542-5633; **Board Cert:** Neurology 1986; **Med School:** Univ MO-Columbia Sch Med 1967; **Resid:** Neurology, Stanford Univ 1974; **Fellow:** Electroencephalography, Stanford Univ

Neurology

Lutsep, Helmi L MD [N] - **Spec Exp:** Stroke/Cerebrovascular Disease; **Hospital:** OR Hlth & Sci Univ; **Address:** Oregon Stroke Ctr, Oregon HSU, 3181 SW Sam Jackson Park Rd, CR-131, Portland, OR 97239; **Phone:** 503-494-7225; **Board Cert:** Neurology 1994; Vascular Neurology 2005; **Med School:** Mayo Med Sch 1988; **Resid:** Neurology, Mayo Clinic 1992; **Fellow:** Behavioral Neurology, UC Davis Med Ctr 1995; Stroke, Stanford Univ Med Ctr 1996; **Fac Appt:** Prof N, Oregon Hlth & Sci Univ

Morrell, Martha J MD [N] - **Spec Exp:** Epilepsy; Epilepsy in Women; **Hospital:** Stanford Univ Med Ctr; **Address:** 300 Pasteur Drive, rm A-343, MC 5235, Stanford, CA 94305; **Phone:** 650-498-6648; **Board Cert:** Neurology 1989; Clinical Neurophysiology 2003; **Med School:** Stanford Univ 1984; **Resid:** Neurology, Hosp Univ Penn 1988; **Fellow:** Epilepsy, Graduate Hosp-Univ Penn 1990; **Fac Appt:** Prof N, Stanford Univ

Nutt Jr, John G MD [N] - **Spec Exp:** Movement Disorders; Parkinson's Disease; **Hospital:** OR Hlth & Sci Univ; **Address:** Oregon Health Science Univ, MC OP-32, 3181 SW Sam Jackson Park Rd, Portland, OR 97239; **Phone:** 503-494-7230; **Board Cert:** Neurology 1978; **Med School:** Baylor Coll Med 1970; **Resid:** Neurology, Univ Wash Med Ctr 1976; **Fellow:** Pharmacology, Natl Inst Neuro Disorders /Stroke 1978; **Fac Appt:** Prof N, Oregon Hlth & Sci Univ

Phuphanich, Surasak MD [N] - **Spec Exp:** Neuro-Oncology; Brain Tumors; Spinal Tumors; Lymphoma-Primary CNS; **Hospital:** Cedars-Sinai Med Ctr; **Address:** 8631 W 3rd St, Ste 410E, Los Angeles, CA 90048; **Phone:** 310-423-8100; **Board Cert:** Neurology 1983; **Med School:** Thailand 1975; **Resid:** Neurology, Univ Illinois Med Ctr 1981; **Fellow:** Neuro-Oncology, UCSF Med Ctr 1984

Raskin, Neil H MD [N] - **Spec Exp:** Headache; Migraine; **Hospital:** UCSF Med Ctr; **Address:** UCSF Neurology Faculty Pract., 400 Parnassus Ave Fl 8, Box 0348, San Francisco, CA 94143; **Phone:** 415-353-2273; **Board Cert:** Neurology 1969; **Med School:** Harvard Med Sch 1959; **Resid:** Internal Medicine, Bellevue Hosp Ctr 1961; Neurology, Neuro Inst/Columbia 1964; **Fellow:** Neurology, Neuro Inst/Columbia 1965; **Fac Appt:** Prof N, UCSF

Rosenbaum, Richard B MD [N] - **Spec Exp:** Neuromuscular Disorders; **Hospital:** OR Hlth & Sci Univ; **Address:** Oregon Clinic Neurology Department, 5050 NE Hoyt St, Ste 315, Portland, OR 97213-2975; **Phone:** 503-963-3100; **Board Cert:** Internal Medicine 1975; Neurology 1979; **Med School:** Harvard Med Sch 1971; **Resid:** Internal Medicine, Stanford Med Ctr 1973; Neurology, UCSF Med Ctr 1977; **Fac Appt:** Clin Prof N, Oregon Hlth & Sci Univ

Saver, Jeffrey Lawrence MD [N] - **Spec Exp:** Stroke; Stroke Prevention; Brain Tumors; **Hospital:** UCLA Ronald Reagan Med Ctr; **Address:** UCLA Stroke Ctr, 710 Westwood Plaza, rm 4126, Los Angeles, CA 90095; **Phone:** 310-794-6379; **Board Cert:** Neurology 2006; Vascular Neurology 2006; **Med School:** Harvard Med Sch 1986; **Resid:** Neurological Surgery, Harvard-Longwood Neuro Inst 1990; **Fellow:** Behavioral Neurology, Univ Iowa Hosps 1991; Cerebrovascular Disease, Rhode Island Hosp 1992; **Fac Appt:** Prof N, UCLA

Smith, Wade S MD/PhD [N] - **Spec Exp:** Stroke; Pain-Back & Shoulder; **Hospital:** UCSF Med Ctr; **Address:** UCSF, Dept Neurology, 505 Parnassus Ave, Ste M830, Box 0114, San Francisco, CA 94143; **Phone:** 415-353-1489; **Board Cert:** Neurology 2006; Vascular Neurology 2008; **Med School:** Univ Wash 1989; **Resid:** Neurology, UCSF-Moffitt Hosp 1993; **Fellow:** Critical Care Medicine, UCSF-Moffitt Hosp 1994; **Fac Appt:** Asst Clin Prof N, UCSF

Starr, Arnold MD [N] - **Spec Exp:** Hearing Disorders; Neurophysiology-Aging; Neurophysiology-Dementia; Hearing Disorders; **Hospital:** UC Irvine Med Ctr; **Address:** Dept Neurology, 1 Medical Plaza Drive, Irvine, CA 92697; **Phone:** 714-456-7239; **Board Cert:** Neurology 1970; **Med School:** NYU Sch Med 1957; **Resid:** Neurology, Boston City Hosp 1959; **Fellow:** Neurology, Natl Inst Hlth 1962; Clinical Neurophysiology, Inst Neurophysiology 1963; **Fac Appt:** Prof N, UC Irvine

Tanner, Caroline M MD/PhD [N] - **Spec Exp:** Parkinson's Disease; Movement Disorders; Dystonia; **Hospital:** Parkinson's Inst/Movement Disorders Trmt Ctr, The; **Address:** The Parkinson's Inst, 675 Almanor Ave, Sunnyvale, CA 94085; **Phone:** 408-734-2800; **Board Cert:** Neurology 1982; **Med School:** Loyola Univ-Stritch Sch Med 1976; **Resid:** Neurology, Rush-Presby-St Luke's Med Ctr 1980; **Fellow:** Neurological Pharmacology, Rush-Presby-St Luke's Med Ctr 1982

Taylor, Lynne P MD [N] - **Spec Exp:** Brain Tumors; Gliomas; **Hospital:** Virginia Mason Med Ctr; **Address:** Virginia Mason Medical Ctr, Neurology, 1100 9th Ave Fl 7, Seattle, WA 98111; **Phone:** 206-341-0420; **Board Cert:** Neurology 1987; **Med School:** Washington Univ, St Louis 1982; **Resid:** Neurology, Hosp U Penn 1986; **Fellow:** Neuro-Oncology, Meml Sloan Kettering Cancer Ctr 1988

Tetrud, James W MD [N] - **Spec Exp:** Movement Disorders; Parkinson's Disease; Tremor; **Hospital:** Parkinson's Inst/Movement Disorders Trmt Ctr, The; **Address:** The Parkinson's Institute, 675 Almanor Ave, Sunnyvale, CA 94085; **Phone:** 408-734-2800; **Board Cert:** Neurology 1981; **Med School:** NYU Sch Med 1973; **Resid:** Internal Medicine, VA Med Ctr-West Los Angeles 1974; Neurology, VA Med Ctr-West Los Angeles 1978

Weiner, Leslie P MD [N] - **Spec Exp:** Multiple Sclerosis; Amyotrophic Lateral Sclerosis (ALS); **Hospital:** USC Univ Hosp, LAC & USC Med Ctr; **Address:** Keck Sch Med, Dept Neurology, 2025 Zonal Ave, RMR - 506, Los Angeles, CA 90089; **Phone:** 323-442-3020; **Board Cert:** Neurology 1969; **Med School:** Univ Cincinnati 1961; **Resid:** Neurology, Baltimore City Hosp 1963; Neurology, Johns Hopkins Hosp 1965; **Fellow:** Neurology, Johns Hopkins Hosp 1969; **Fac Appt:** Prof N, USC Sch Med

Cleveland Clinic

Neurological Institute

The Cleveland Clinic Neurological Institute is a fully integrated entity with a disease-specific focus, combining all physicians and other healthcare providers in neurology, neurosurgery, neuroradiology, the behavioral sciences and nursing who treat children and adults with neurological and neurobehavioral disorders. Our staff of more than 250 specialists sees one of the largest and most diverse patient populations in the country. Because of our clinical expertise, academic achievement and innovative research, the Cleveland Clinic Neurological Institute has earned an international reputation for excellence.

U.S.News & World Report's "America's Best Hospitals" survey has consistently ranked our Neurology and Neurosurgery programs among the Top 10 in the nation and best in Ohio. Our pediatric neurology/neurosurgery program has been ranked fourth in the nation.

Our unique clinical structure allows us to deliver coordinated, comprehensive, multidisciplinary care to our patients through more efficient treatment decision making and consultation for complex cases. Fully integrating specialties along disease lines creates an exciting synergy among Institute physicians who share similar clinical, research and educational interests, to the benefit of patients and physicians alike.

Major advances in the treatment of brain tumors, epilepsy, mood disorders, stroke, movement disorders, pain and spinal disorders are improving quality of life and survival for thousands of patients. For those diseases resistant to available treatments, we believe the innovative model of medicine created within the Neurological Institute will speed research and advances in treatment, resulting in better clinical care and more rapid breakthroughs in the full range of neurological and behavioral disorders.

Comprehensive Neurological Care
Cleveland Clinic offers expert diagnostic and treatment options for all neurologic conditions affecting children and adults, including:

- Alzheimer's disease
- ALS (Amyotrophic Lateral Sclerosis)
- Aneurysms
- Arteriovenous Malformations (AVMs)
- Back and Neck Disorders
- Brain and Spine Tumors
- Cerebral Palsy
- Chronic Pain Rehabilitation
- Congenital Disorders
- Craniofacial Disorders
- Epilepsy
- Headache
- Hydrocephalus
- Metastatic Tumors
- Mild Cognitive Impairment
- Multiple Sclerosis
- Movement Disorders
- Neonatal Disorders
- Neurofibromatosis
- Parkinson's Disease
- Pediatric Neurological Disorders
- Peripheral Neuropathies
- Pituitary Disorders
- Psychiatric Disorders
- Skull Base Disorders
- Sleep Disorders
- Stroke

For more information about the Cleveland Clinic Neurological Institute, to schedule a second opinion or to learn about assistance for out-of-town patients, call 800.890.2467 or visit www.clevelandclinic.org/neurotopdocs.

Cleveland Clinic Neurological Institute
9500 Euclid Avenue / AC311 | Cleveland OH 44195

Continuum
NeuroSciences

Neurology and Neurosurgery Expertise

(800) 420-4004

The member hospitals of the Continuum Neurosciences consortium—St. Luke's and Roosevelt Hospitals, Beth Israel Medical Center and Long Island College Hospital of Brooklyn—are home to many international leaders in neurology, neurosurgery, neuro-radiology and endovascular neurosurgery. Each of the hospitals has clinicians who are nationally and internationally recognized for their accomplishments and attract patients from throughout the United States and other countries who are looking for innovative treatment programs delivered by physicians specializing in both clinical care and research. Our expertise includes treatments for:

- complex brain tumors, tumors of the skull base, spine and spinal cord; chordomas, meningiomas, acoustic neuromas, trigeminal neuralgias and hemifacial spasms
- headaches
- disorders of the brain, spinal cord, peripheral nerves and muscles
- stroke/cerebrovascular diseases
- epilepsy and seizures
- Parkinson's disease and other movement disorders
- neuro-ophthalmologic conditions
- neuro-oncology-related illnesses
- neuro-psychiatry/psychology-based conditions
- many adult and pediatric neurologic conditions

A few of our Centers of Excellence include:

St. Luke's and Roosevelt Hospitals

- The Hyman-Newman Institute for Neurology and Neurosurgery
- Center for Endovascular Surgery
- The Vascular Birthmarks Institute
- Vascular Malformations Center of NY
- Center for Cranial Base Surgery
- The Headache Institute
- The Stroke Center

Long Island College Hospital of Brooklyn

- Neurosurgery
- The Stroke Center
- The Center for Interventional Neurology
- The Neurodiagnostic Center

Beth Israel Medical Center

- Neurosurgery
- Peripheral Nerve Center
- The Alan and Barbara Mirken Department of Neurology
- The Betty and Morton Yarmon Stroke Center
- National Parkinson Foundation Center of Excellence
- ALS (Lou Gehrig's disease) Center sponsored by the ALS Association
- Internationally respected divisions of Adult and Pediatric Epilepsy
- Bachmann-Strauss Dystonia Center of Excellence

Beth Israel   **Roosevelt Hospital**   **St. Luke's Hospital**   **Long Island College Hospital**   **NY Eye & Ear Infirmary**

www.chpnyc.org

PENN NEUROLOGY

The University of Pennsylvania's history of excellence in the treatment of neurological diseases dates back to the establishment of the Department of Neurology in 1874. The Best Doctors in America® lists more neurologists and neurosurgeons from the Hospital of the University of Pennsylvania than from any other hospital or medical center in the Philadelphia region.

The Department of Neurology is a component of the Penn Comprehensive Neuroscience Center, which is dedicated to the advancement of the understanding of the brain, spine and peripheral nervous system, facilitating and strengthening the integration of Penn's world-class neuroscience programs within the areas of clinical care, research and education.

Excellence and Expertise

Recognized by the National Parkinson Foundation as one of its worldwide Centers of Excellence, the **Parkinson's Disease and Movement Disorders Center** is committed to providing exceptional patient care, education, social support services and ongoing research into the causes of Parkinson's disease. Research is an important and ongoing mission of the Center, which actively pursues the investigation of the disease as well as exploration of new medications.

The **Multiple Sclerosis Center Program** provides comprehensive evaluation, diagnosis and treatment for patients with MS and other demyelinating disorders of the central nervous system. The Center specializes in quality, state-of-the-art care with a personal approach. The comprehensive multidisciplinary team includes neurologists, nurse practitioners and specialists from other disciplines who are available

for consultation in the management of genitourinary complications, spasticity and pain. In addition to maintaining high standards for clinical service, the Penn MS program is a leader in MS training and in clinical and laboratory-based research.

The **Neuro-Oncology Program** has set the standard for the region and provides comprehensive evaluation, diagnosis and treatment to patients with brain and spinal tumors and other cancer-related neurological central nervous system and peripheral nervous system problems. The program utilizes a patient-oriented team approach and brings together some of the nation's leading experts in the field. Each patient's case is reviewed by a multidisciplinary team to ensure that the patient is offered the most up-to-date therapy that is appropriate for them. The goal is to provide the best chance for a cure while preserving quality of life for each patient.

The **Penn Epilepsy Center** provides the highest standard of care to patients with epilepsy and related problems. The Center offers a comprehensive, full continuum of care including state-of-the-art diagnostic techniques, cutting-edge research, medical treatments, surgery, and support services to patients with epilepsy. Both outpatient evaluation and inpatient care are available via this multidisciplinary, full-service facility.

The **Penn Stroke Center** provides emergent care to stroke patients 24 hours a day, seven days a week, 365 days per year. The Center employs state-of-the-art approaches to the diagnosis, treatment and prevention of stroke and critical neurologic conditions. Inpatients are cared for by physicians and nurses with

specialty training in neurological diseases in different settings, depending on their needs including the Neuroscience floor with telemetry and the Intermediate Neurological Care Unit. The new Neurological Intensive Care Unit is the most technologically advanced and sophisticated neuro-critical care unit in the nation, and is the only dedicated academic facility of its kind in the region.

Program

- Cognitive Neurology Program
- Center for Brain Injury and Repair
- Interventional Neuro Center
- Memory Disorders Clinic
- Multiple Sclerosis Center
- Neurological Intensive Care
- Neurogenetics Center
- Neuromuscular Disorders Program
- Neuro-Oncology Program
- Neuro-Ophthalmology Service
- Neuropsychology Service
- Parkinson's Disease and Movement Disorders Center
- Penn Epilepsy Center
- Penn Center for Sleep Disorders
- Penn Memory Center
- Stroke Center

**MOUNT SINAI
SCHOOL OF
MEDICINE**

THE MOUNT SINAI MEDICAL CENTER
NEUROLOGY
One Gustave L. Levy Place
Fifth Avenue and 100th Street
New York, NY 10029-6574
Physician Referral: 1-800-MD-SINAI (637-4624)
www.mountsinai.org

THE ESTELLE AND DANIEL MAGGIN DEPARTMENT OF NEUROLOGY provides compassionate and innovative care for a range of neurological disorders.

The Robert and John M. Bendheim Parkinson's and Movement Disorders Center is one of the world's leading multidisciplinary centers for the study of Parkinson's disease and related disorders, and serves as a forum for collaboration among internationally acclaimed neuroscientists. The Center offers state-of-the-art clinical care, translational research, and basic science programs aimed at discovering the cause of and cure for Parkinson's, dystonia, and other movement disorders. The Center incorporates a renowned deep-brain stimulation program and has played a major role in evaluating cell-based and gene therapies for the treatment of movement disorders.

The Corinne Goldsmith Dickinson Center for Multiple Sclerosis is an internationally recognized comprehensive center uniting the efforts of leading physicians and scientists from many disciplines to understand the causes and consequences of multiple sclerosis (MS). The Center provides services in all aspects of diagnosis, disease management, rehabilitation, and patient support, and the opportunity for patients to participate in potentially groundbreaking clinical trials.

The Clinical Program for Cerebrovascular Disorders comprises an outstanding team of medical experts who specialize in the most advanced approaches in the evaluation, treatment, and rehabilitation of patients with cerebrovascular diseases. Services include the early diagnosis of stroke, a specialized Neurointensive Care Unit, and an advanced inpatient stroke unit. Physicians are available at all times for emergency consultation with referring physicians.

The NeuroAIDS Program provides diagnosis and treatment for neurological disorders associated with HIV disease. This program is one of the few in the world to treat the various complications of the disease that affect the central and peripheral nervous systems in as many as 70 percent of patients.

The Epilepsy Center provides specific expertise in the diagnosis and treatment of epilepsy and related disorders. The Center encompasses outstanding epileptologists, a new modern inpatient epilepsy monitoring unit, and full outpatient EEG and diagnostic capabilities.

The ALS/Muscular Dystrophy Program provides diagnosis and treatment of muscular dystrophy and amyotrophic lateral sclerosis (ALS). Our clinical care team specializes in improving the quality of life for patients, and scientists engage in both clinical and laboratory research aimed at finding better treatment and cures.

THE ESTELLE AND DANIEL MAGGIN DEPARTMENT OF NEUROLOGY
The Mount Sinai Medical Center is renowned for its unique integration of outstanding patient care and cutting-edge research laboratories, which together work to find better treatment for Parkinson's disease, MS, stroke, and other neurological disorders. One of the nation's top programs for research and patient care, the department is led by some of the most prominent figures in American neurology and receives annual research grants of more than $20 million.

The Division of Neuromuscular Diseases provides unparalleled diagnosis, treatment, and compassionate care for patients with disorders in neuromuscular transmission, muscle diseases, and peripheral nerve problems.

Mount Sinai's Neurological Tumor Program is world-acclaimed for the treatment of pituitary adenomas, acoustic neuromas, meningiomas, and cancerous brain tumors. The program's multispecialty group of physicians works together to provide outstanding care through state-of-the-art surgical procedures, radiation therapy, chemotherapy, and supportive therapy. Our physicians have pioneered the treatment of tumors with stereotactic radiosurgery, as well as developed a number of experimental treatment protocols to improve patients' lives.

The Eye Movement and Vestibular Disorder Program at Mount Sinai is one of the finest in the world. Our physicians participate in NASA programs, employing equipment used to assess these disorders in space. Our scientists have helped to define the physiologic basis of these disorders, and are performing groundbreaking research for such problems as gait dysfunction and motion sickness.

NEUROLOGY

About the Department of Neurology:

The Department of Neurology at NYU Langone Medical Center evaluates and treats children and adults with a broad spectrum of neurological diseases. Specialty groups within the department deliver integrated care to patients with stroke, epilepsy, cerebrovacular diseases, behavioral disorders and dementia, brain tumors, genetic and degenerative diseases, nerve and muscle problems, headache and pain syndromes and movement disorders. NYU Langone Medical Center is home to the largest multiple sclerosis program in New York and the first primary Stroke Center in New York City.

We specialize in the following areas:

AUTONOMIC DISEASES

A specialized center in the Department of Neurology evaluates and treats children and adults with familial dysautonomia and other inherited or acquired autonomic nervous system diseases including orthostatic hypotension and rare forms of hereditary sensory neuropathy.

EPILEPSY

The Comprehensive Epilepsy Center at NYU Langone Medical Center offers the most advanced surgical and medical options in the treatment of epilepsy. Complementary management approaches such as diet alteration, lifestyle changes and other remedies are considered to be part of a comprehensive management plan. The Center's primary goal is to help patients with unmanageable epilepsy achieve complete control, or at least a reduction in the frequency of seizures and/or the medical side effects experienced to achieve the highest possible quality of life.

MULTIPLE SCLEROSIS

The Comprehensive Multiple Sclerosis (MS) Care Center provides state-of-the-art diagnostic evaluations and follow-up care to individuals with MS. The Center features an onsite team of highly trained professionals, as well as consulting services, to provide continuous and comprehensive care to patients.

NEUROGENETICS

The Division of Neurogenetics runs a full-service clinical facility, with a focus on inherited diseases of the nervous system. Services include diagnosis and management of inherited diseases, biochemical and molecular testing and genetic counseling.

NEURO-ONCOLOGY

The NYU Cancer Institute at NYU Langone Medical Center is home to one of the nation's leading brain and spinal cord tumor treatment programs, with medical experts experienced in neuro-oncology, neurosurgery, neuroradiology, and offers individualized patient-centered care for the treatment of tumors in the nervous system.

NEUROMUSCULAR DISEASES

The Neuromuscular Division offers multidisciplinary inpatient and outpatient programs in all aspects of neuromuscular diseases with a specific emphasis on the following: acquired peripheral neuropathy, Charcot Marie Tooth neuropathy, myasthenia gravis, Amyotrophic lateral sclerosis, spinal muscular atrophy and post-polio syndrome, muscular dystrophy and Lyme neuroborreliosis.

PARKINSON'S DISEASE

The Parkinson and Movement Disorders Center at NYU Langone Medical Center helps individuals and families living with Parkinson disease and other movement disorders to achieve the highest possible quality of life. The Center has an active research program that explores best treatments options for Parkinson's disease as well as an interdisciplinary care team for individuals and families.

STROKE CARE

The first primary stroke center in New York City, the multidisciplinary Comprehensive Stroke Care Center at NYU Langone Medical Center provides rapid diagnosis, immediate and effective intervention and early rehabilitation for victims of stroke. Specialists also provide public education for primary stroke prevention.

Nuclear Medicine

A nuclear medicine specialist employs the properties of radioactive atoms and molecules in the diagnosis and treatment of disease, and in research. Radiation detection and imaging instrument systems are used to detect disease as it changes the function and metabolism of normal cells, tissues and organs. A wide variety of diseases can be found in this way, usually before the structure of the organ involved by the disease can be seen to be abnormal by any other techniques. Early detection of coronary artery disease (including acute heart attack); early cancer detection and evaluation of the effect of tumor treatment; diagnosis of infection and inflammation anywhere in the body; and early detection of blood clot in the lungs, are all possible with these techniques. Unique forms of radioactive molecules can attack and kill cancer cells (e.g., lymphoma, thyroid cancer) or can relieve the severe pain of cancer that has spread to bone.

The nuclear medicine specialist has special knowledge in the biologic effects of radiation exposure, the fundamentals of the physical sciences and the principles and operation of radiation detection and imaging instrumentation systems.

Training required: Three years

Nuclear Medicine

Mid Atlantic

Alavi, Abass MD [NuM] - **Spec Exp:** Brain Tumors; Neurologic Imaging; PET Imaging-Brain; Brain Infections; **Hospital:** Hosp Univ Penn - UPHS (page 60), Chldns Hosp of Philadelphia, The; **Address:** Hosp Univ Penn, Div Nuclear Med, 3400 Spruce St, Donner Bldg rm 110, Philadelphia, PA 19104; **Phone:** 215-662-3014; **Board Cert:** Nuclear Medicine 1973; Internal Medicine 1972; **Med School:** Iran 1964; **Resid:** Internal Medicine, Albert Einstein Med Ctr/Phila VA Hosp 1969; Hematology, Hosp Univ Penn 1970; **Fellow:** Nuclear Medicine, Hosp Univ Penn 1973; **Fac Appt:** Prof Rad, Univ Pennsylvania

Carrasquillo, Jorge A MD [NuM] - **Spec Exp:** Radioimmunotherapy of Cancer; PET Imaging; **Hospital:** Meml Sloan-Kettering Cancer Ctr; **Address:** 1275 York Avenue, Nuclear Medicine Svc, Box 77, New York, NY 10065; **Phone:** 212-639-2459; **Board Cert:** Internal Medicine 1977; Nuclear Medicine 1982; **Med School:** Univ Puerto Rico 1974; **Resid:** Internal Medicine, Univ Dist Hosp 1977; Nuclear Medicine, Univ Wash Hosp 1982

Freeman, Leonard M MD [NuM] - **Spec Exp:** Nuclear Oncology; Gastrointestinal Disorders; PET Imaging; CT Scan; **Hospital:** Montefiore Med Ctr - Div. Moses; **Address:** 111 E 210th St, Bronx, NY 10467-2401; **Phone:** 718-920-6060; **Board Cert:** Diagnostic Radiology 1966; Nuclear Medicine 1972; Nuclear Radiology 1974; **Med School:** Ros Franklin Univ/Chicago Med Sch 1961; **Resid:** Diagnostic Radiology, Bronx Municipal Hosp 1965; **Fac Appt:** Prof NuM, Albert Einstein Coll Med

Goldsmith, Stanley J MD [NuM] - **Spec Exp:** Thyroid Cancer; Neuroendocrine Tumors; PET Imaging; Lymphoma; **Hospital:** NY-Presby Hosp/Weill Cornell (page 66); **Address:** 525 E 68th St Starr Bldg - rm 2-21, New York, NY 10021-9800; **Phone:** 212-746-4588; **Board Cert:** Internal Medicine 1969; Nuclear Medicine 1972; Endocrinology 1972; **Med School:** SUNY Downstate 1962; **Resid:** Internal Medicine, Kings Co Hosp 1967; **Fellow:** Endocrinology, Diabetes & Metabolism, Mt Sinai Hosp 1968; Nuclear Medicine, Bronx VA Hosp 1969; **Fac Appt:** Prof Rad, Cornell Univ-Weill Med Coll

Lamonica, Dominick M MD [NuM] - **Spec Exp:** Thyroid Cancer; **Hospital:** Roswell Park Cancer Inst; **Address:** Roswell Park Cancer Inst, Elm & Carlton St, Dept of Nuclear Medicine, Buffalo, NY 14263; **Phone:** 716-845-3282; **Board Cert:** Internal Medicine 2005; Nuclear Medicine 2006; **Med School:** Mount Sinai Sch Med 1987; **Resid:** Internal Medicine, Univ Hosp-SUNY Stony Brook 1991; Diagnostic Radiology, Nassau City Med Ctr 1992; **Fellow:** Nuclear Medicine, DVAMC North Port-SUNY Stony Brook 1994; Nuclear Medicine, SUNY Buffalo-RPCI 1995; **Fac Appt:** Asst Prof, SUNY Buffalo

Larson, Steven M MD [NuM] - **Spec Exp:** Thyroid Cancer; PET Imaging; **Hospital:** Meml Sloan-Kettering Cancer Ctr; **Address:** 1275 York Avenue, New York, NY 10065; **Phone:** 800-525-2225; **Board Cert:** Nuclear Medicine 1972; Internal Medicine 1973; **Med School:** Univ Wash 1965; **Resid:** Internal Medicine, Virginia Mason Hosp 1970; Nuclear Medicine, Natl Inst Hlth 1972; **Fac Appt:** Prof NuM, Cornell Univ-Weill Med Coll

Majd, Massoud MD [NuM] - **Spec Exp:** Pediatric Nuclear Medicine; **Hospital:** Chldns Natl Med Ctr; **Address:** 111 Michigan Ave NW, Washington, DC 20010-2978; **Phone:** 202-476-3698; **Board Cert:** Radiology 1972; Nuclear Medicine 1973; **Med School:** Iran 1960; **Resid:** Diagnostic Radiology, Georgetown Univ Hosp 1966; **Fac Appt:** Prof Rad, Geo Wash Univ

Mountz, James M MD/PhD [NuM] - **Spec Exp:** Neurologic Imaging; Brain Imaging; **Hospital:** UPMC Presby, Pittsburgh; **Address:** UPMC Hlth Sys, Presby Univ Hosp, 200 Lothrop St, PET Facility, rm B 932, Pittsburgh, PA 15213; **Phone:** 412-647-0104; **Board Cert:** Diagnostic Radiology 1985; Nuclear Medicine 1986; **Med School:** Case West Res Univ 1981; **Resid:** Diagnostic Radiology, Univ Michigan Hosps 1985; **Fellow:** Nuclear Medicine, Univ Michigan Hosps 1986; **Fac Appt:** Prof Rad, Univ Pittsburgh

Neumann, Ronald D MD [NuM] - **Hospital:** Natl Inst of Hlth - Clin Ctr; **Address:** NIH, Bldg 10, 1C-401, 9000 Rockville Drive, MSC 1180, Bethesda, MD 20892-1180; **Phone:** 301-496-6455; **Board Cert:** Nuclear Medicine 1979; **Med School:** Yale Univ 1974; **Resid:** Pathology, Yale-New Haven Hosp 1977; Nuclear Medicine, Yale-New Haven Hosp 1979

Sanger, Joseph J MD [NuM] - **Spec Exp:** Nuclear Cardiology; **Hospital:** NYU Langone Med Ctr (page 67); **Address:** NYU Med Ctr, 545 1st Ave, rm SC2-184, New York, NY 10016-6402; **Phone:** 212-263-3434; **Board Cert:** Nuclear Medicine 1981; **Med School:** NYU Sch Med 1977; **Resid:** Diagnostic Radiology, NYU Med Ctr 1979; **Fellow:** Nuclear Medicine, NYU Med Ctr 1981; **Fac Appt:** Assoc Clin Prof, NYU Sch Med

Strashun, Arnold M MD [NuM] - **Spec Exp:** Neurologic Imaging; Nuclear Cardiology; Thyroid Disorders; PET Imaging-Brain; **Hospital:** SUNY Downstate Med Ctr, Kings County Hosp Ctr; **Address:** SUNY Hlth Sci Ctr, Dept Radiology, 450 Clarkson Ave, Box 1198, Brooklyn, NY 11203; **Phone:** 718-270-1603; **Board Cert:** Internal Medicine 1977; Nuclear Medicine 1979; **Med School:** Baylor Coll Med 1974; **Resid:** Internal Medicine, Baylor Med Ctr 1975; Internal Medicine, Texas Med Ctr 1977; **Fellow:** Nuclear Medicine, VA Med Ctr 1978; Nuclear Medicine, Mount Sinai Hosp 1979; **Fac Appt:** Prof NuM, SUNY Downstate

Strauss, H William MD [NuM] - **Spec Exp:** Cardiac Imaging in Cancer Therapy; Thyroid Disorders; Cardiac Imaging; **Hospital:** Meml Sloan-Kettering Cancer Ctr; **Address:** 1275 York Avenue, New York, NY 10065; **Phone:** 212-639-7238; **Board Cert:** Nuclear Medicine 1988; **Med School:** SUNY Downstate 1965; **Resid:** Internal Medicine, Downstate Med Ctr 1967; Internal Medicine, Bellevue Hosp 1968; **Fellow:** Nuclear Medicine, Johns Hopkins Hosp 1970; **Fac Appt:** Prof NuM, Cornell Univ-Weill Med Coll

Van Heertum, Ronald L MD [NuM] - **Spec Exp:** PET Imaging; PET Imaging in Alzheimer's Disease; **Hospital:** NY-Presby Hosp/Columbia (page 66); **Address:** NY Presby Hosp, Dept Radiology, 622 W 168th St, Ste HP 3-320, New York, NY 10032; **Phone:** 212-305-7132; **Board Cert:** Diagnostic Radiology 1971; Nuclear Medicine 1973; **Med School:** UMDNJ-NJ Med Sch, Newark 1966; **Resid:** Diagnostic Radiology, St Vincents Hosp 1970; **Fellow:** Diagnostic Radiology, St Vincents Hosp Med Ctr 1971; Nuclear Medicine, SUNY-Upstate Med Ctr 1975; **Fac Appt:** Prof Rad, Columbia P&S

Wahl, Richard L MD [NuM] - **Spec Exp:** Radioimmunotherapy of Cancer; PET Imaging; PET Imaging-Breast; **Hospital:** Johns Hopkins Hosp (page 61); **Address:** Johns Hopkins Hosp, Radiology Dept, Nuclear Medicine Fl 3, 601 N Caroline St, JHOC-3223, Baltimore, MD 21287; **Phone:** 410-955-5465; **Board Cert:** Diagnostic Radiology 1982; Nuclear Radiology 1983; Nuclear Medicine 1985; **Med School:** Washington Univ, St Louis 1978; **Resid:** Diagnostic Radiology, Mallinckrodt Inst 1982; **Fellow:** Nuclear Radiology, Mallinckrodt Inst 1983; **Fac Appt:** Prof Rad, Johns Hopkins Univ

Nuclear Medicine

Southeast

Alazraki, Naomi P MD [NuM] - **Spec Exp:** Nuclear Oncology; **Hospital:** VA Med Ctr - Atlanta, Emory Univ Hosp; **Address:** VA Medical Ctr - Atlanta, 1670 Clairmont Rd, MC 115, Decatur, GA 30033; **Phone:** 404-728-7629; **Board Cert:** Nuclear Medicine 1972; Diagnostic Radiology 1972; **Med School:** Albert Einstein Coll Med 1966; **Resid:** Diagnostic Radiology, Univ Hospital 1971; **Fac Appt:** Prof, Emory Univ

Coleman, R Edward MD [NuM] - **Spec Exp:** PET Imaging; SPECT Imaging; Tumor Imaging; **Hospital:** Duke Univ Med Ctr; **Address:** Duke Univ Med Ctr, Erwin Rd, Box 3949, Durham, NC 27710-0001; **Phone:** 919-684-7244; **Board Cert:** Internal Medicine 1973; Nuclear Medicine 1973; **Resid:** Internal Medicine, Royal Victoria Hosp 1970; **Fellow:** Nuclear Medicine, Mallinckrodt Inst Radiology 1974; **Fac Appt:** Prof Rad

Sandler, Martin P MD [NuM] - **Spec Exp:** Nuclear Endocrinology; Cardiac Imaging; PET Imaging; **Hospital:** Vanderbilt Univ Med Ctr; **Address:** Vanderbilt Univ Med Ctr, 3300 MCN Bldg, 1161 21st Ave S, Nashville, TN 37232-2104; **Phone:** 615-322-0860; **Board Cert:** Nuclear Medicine 1983; **Med School:** South Africa 1972; **Resid:** Internal Medicine, Groote Schur Hosp; **Fellow:** Endocrinology, Diabetes & Metabolism, Vanderbilt Univ Med Ctr 1980; Nuclear Medicine, Vanderbilt Univ Med Ctr 1982; **Fac Appt:** Prof Rad, Vanderbilt Univ

Midwest

Dillehay, Gary L MD [NuM] - **Spec Exp:** Lymphoma; Bone Densitometry; PET Imaging; **Hospital:** Northwestern Meml Hosp; **Address:** Northwestern Meml Hosp, Dept Nuclear Medicine, 675 N St Clair St, Galter 8-110, Chicago, IL 60611; **Phone:** 312-926-0411; **Board Cert:** Nuclear Medicine 1985; Nuclear Radiology 1987; **Med School:** Mayo Med Sch 1979; **Resid:** Diagnostic Radiology, Northwestern Meml Hosp 1983; Nuclear Medicine, Northwestern Meml Hosp 1984

Neumann, Donald R MD [NuM] - **Spec Exp:** Nuclear Oncology; Nuclear Cardiology; Parathyroid Disease; Pheochromocytoma; **Hospital:** Cleveland Clin Fdn (page 56); **Address:** Cleveland Clinic, Dept Nuclear Medicine, 9500 Euclid Ave, MS Jb3, Cleveland, OH 44195; **Phone:** 216-444-2193; **Board Cert:** Diagnostic Radiology 1987; Nuclear Radiology 1990; **Med School:** Wright State Univ 1980; **Resid:** Diagnostic Radiology, Mount Sinai Med Ctr 1987; **Fellow:** Magnetic Resonance Imaging, Mount Sinai Med Ctr 1987

Siegel, Barry A MD [NuM] - **Spec Exp:** Cancer Detection & Staging; PET Imaging; Hyperthyroidism; **Hospital:** Barnes-Jewish Hosp, St Louis Chldns Hosp; **Address:** Mallinckrodt Inst of Radiology, 510 S Kingshighway Blvd, St Louis, MO 63110-1016; **Phone:** 314-362-2809; **Board Cert:** Nuclear Medicine 1973; Diagnostic Radiology 1977; Nuclear Radiology 1981; **Med School:** Washington Univ, St Louis 1969; **Resid:** Diagnostic Radiology, Mallinckrodt Inst Radiology 1973; **Fellow:** Nuclear Medicine, Mallinckrodt Inst Radiology 1973; **Fac Appt:** Prof Rad, Washington Univ, St Louis

Wiseman, Gregory MD [NuM] - **Spec Exp:** Lymphoma, Non-Hodgkin's; Multiple Myeloma; Radioimmunotherapy of Cancer; **Hospital:** Mayo Med Ctr & Clin - Rochester; **Address:** Mayo Clinic, Dept Nuc Med, 200 First St SW, Charlton Bldg, Rochester, MN 55905; **Phone:** 507-284-9599; **Board Cert:** Internal Medicine 1986; Hematology 1988; Nuclear Medicine 2002; **Med School:** Univ Utah 1983; **Resid:** Internal Medicine, Mayo Clinic 1986; Nuclear Medicine, Univ Washington Med Ctr 1992; **Fellow:** Hematology, Mayo Clinic 1989; Medical Oncology, Univ Washington 1991; **Fac Appt:** Asst Prof, Mayo Med Sch

Southwest

Podoloff, Donald MD [NuM] - **Spec Exp:** Prostate Cancer; Breast Cancer; Lymphoma; **Hospital:** UT MD Anderson Cancer Ctr; **Address:** UT MD Anderson Cancer Ctr, 1515 Holcombe Blvd, Box 57, Houston, TX 77030; **Phone:** 713-745-1160; **Board Cert:** Diagnostic Radiology 1973; Nuclear Medicine 1975; Nuclear Radiology 1975; **Med School:** SUNY Downstate 1964; **Resid:** Internal Medicine, Beth Israel Med Ctr 1968; Diagnostic Radiology, Wilford Hall USAF Med Ctr 1973; **Fac Appt:** Prof Rad, Univ Tex, Houston

West Coast and Pacific

Dae, Michael W MD [NuM] - **Spec Exp:** Nuclear Cardiology; Pediatric Nuclear Medicine; **Hospital:** UCSF Med Ctr; **Address:** UCSF, Dept Nuclear Med, 505 Parnassus Ave, Box 0252, San Francisco, CA 94143-0252; **Phone:** 415-353-1521; **Board Cert:** Pediatrics 1983; Nuclear Medicine 1984; **Med School:** Duke Univ 1976; **Resid:** Pediatrics, Chldns Hosp 1978; **Fellow:** Pediatric Cardiology, UCSF Med Ctr 1982; Nuclear Cardiology, UCSF Med Ctr 1983; **Fac Appt:** Prof, UCSF

Scheff, Alice M MD [NuM] - **Spec Exp:** PET Imaging; Thyroid Disorders; Neurologic Imaging; Cardiac Imaging; **Hospital:** Santa Clara Vly Med Ctr; **Address:** 751 S Bascom Ave, San Jose, CA 95128; **Phone:** 408-885-6970; **Board Cert:** Nuclear Medicine 1982; Nuclear Radiology 1983; **Med School:** Penn State Univ-Hershey Med Ctr 1978; **Resid:** Diagnostic Radiology, Penn State-Hershey Med Ctr 1982; Nuclear Medicine, Penn State-Hershey Med Ctr 1982; **Fellow:** Magnetic Resonance Imaging, Long Beach Meml Med Ctr 1993

Schelbert, Heinrich R MD/PhD [NuM] - **Spec Exp:** Nuclear Cardiology; Coronary Artery Disease; **Hospital:** UCLA Ronald Reagan Med Ctr, Santa Monica - UCLA Med Ctr & Ortho Hosp; **Address:** B2-085J CHS, Box 95648, Dept Molecular & Med Pharmacology, UCLA Med Ctr, Los Angeles, CA 90095-6948; **Phone:** 310-825-3076; **Board Cert:** Nuclear Medicine 1976; **Med School:** Germany 1964; **Resid:** Internal Medicine, Mercy Med Ctr 1968; Cardiovascular Disease, Univ Duesseldorf Sch Med 1972; **Fellow:** Nuclear Medicine, UCSD 1973; Cardiovascular Disease, UCSD 1969

Waxman, Alan D MD [NuM] - **Spec Exp:** PET Imaging-Brain; Thyroid Cancer; Cancer Detection & Staging; **Hospital:** Cedars-Sinai Med Ctr, USC Univ Hosp; **Address:** Cedars-Sinai Med Ctr, Taper Imaging, 8700 Beverly Blvd, rm 1251, Los Angeles, CA 90048-1804; **Phone:** 310-423-4216; **Board Cert:** Nuclear Medicine 1972; **Med School:** USC Sch Med 1963; **Resid:** Nuclear Medicine, Wadsworth VA Hosp 1965; **Fellow:** Internal Medicine, Natl Inst Hlth 1967; **Fac Appt:** Clin Prof, USC Sch Med

Obstetrics & Gynecology

An obstetrician/gynecologist possesses special knowledge, skills and professional capability in the medical and surgical care of the female reproductive system and associated disorders. This physician serves as a consultant to other physicians and as a primary physician for women.

Training Required: Four years *plus* two years in clinical practice before certification is complete.

Obstetrics & Gynecology

New England

Cramer, Daniel W MD [ObG] - **Spec Exp:** Ovarian Cancer; Ovarian Cancer-High Risk; **Hospital:** Brigham & Women's Hosp, Dana-Farber Cancer Inst; **Address:** Brigham & Women's Hosp, Ob/Gyn Epidemiology Ctr, 221 Longwood Ave, RFB 336, Boston, MA 02115; **Phone:** 617-732-4895; **Board Cert:** Obstetrics & Gynecology 1979; **Med School:** Univ Colorado 1970; **Resid:** Obstetrics & Gynecology, Boston Womens Hosp 1976; **Fellow:** Public Health, Harvard Med Sch 1982; **Fac Appt:** Prof ObG, Harvard Med Sch

Laufer, Marc MD [ObG] - **Spec Exp:** Adolescent Gynecology; Endometriosis; Congenital Anomalies-Gynecologic; Pediatric Gynecology; **Hospital:** Children's Hospital - Boston, Brigham & Women's Hosp; **Address:** Chldns Hosp, Dept of Ped Gynecology, 300 Longwood Ave, Boston, MA 02115; **Phone:** 617-355-5785; **Board Cert:** Obstetrics & Gynecology 2007; **Med School:** Univ Pennsylvania 1986; **Resid:** Obstetrics & Gynecology, Brigham & Womens Hosp/Mass Genl Hosp 1990; **Fellow:** Reproductive Endocrinology, Brigham & Womens Hosp/Chldns Hosp 1992; Gynecology, Chldns Hosp 1992; **Fac Appt:** Assoc Prof ObG, Harvard Med Sch

Noller, Kenneth L MD [ObG] - **Spec Exp:** DES-Exposed Females; Gynecology Only; Cervical Cancer; **Hospital:** Tufts Med Ctr; **Address:** Tufts New England Med Ctr, Box 324, 750 Washington St, Boston, MA 02111; **Phone:** 617-636-2382; **Board Cert:** Obstetrics & Gynecology 1991; **Med School:** Creighton Univ 1970; **Resid:** Obstetrics & Gynecology, Mayo Clinic 1974; **Fac Appt:** Prof ObG, Tufts Univ

Nour, Nawal M MD [ObG] - **Spec Exp:** Female Genital Cutting (FGC) Education; **Hospital:** Brigham & Women's Hosp; **Address:** Brigham & Women's Hosp, Dept Ob/Gyn, 75 Francis St, Connors Ctr, 3rd Fl, Boston, MA 02115; **Phone:** 617-732-4740; **Board Cert:** Obstetrics & Gynecology 2002; **Med School:** Harvard Med Sch 1994; **Resid:** Obstetrics & Gynecology, Brgham & Women's Hosp 1998

Reilly, Raymond J MD [ObG] - **Spec Exp:** Gynecologic Surgery; **Hospital:** Brigham & Women's Hosp; **Address:** 1 Brookline Pl, Ste 522, Brookline, MA 02445; **Phone:** 617-731-3400; **Board Cert:** Obstetrics & Gynecology 1969; **Med School:** Ireland 1958; **Resid:** Obstetrics & Gynecology, Johns Hopkins Hosp 1964; **Fac Appt:** Assoc Prof ObG, Harvard Med Sch

Mid Atlantic

Brodman, Michael MD [ObG] - **Spec Exp:** Incontinence-Female; Laparoscopic Surgery; Pelvic Organ Prolapse Repair; Uro-Gynecology; **Hospital:** Mount Sinai Med Ctr (page 64); **Address:** Div of Obstetrics & Gynecology, 5 E 98th St Fl 2, Box 1170, New York, NY 10029; **Phone:** 212-241-7952; **Board Cert:** Obstetrics & Gynecology 2006; **Med School:** Mount Sinai Sch Med 1982; **Resid:** Obstetrics & Gynecology, Mount Sinai Hosp 1986; **Fellow:** Pelvic Surgery, Mount Sinai Hosp 1987; **Fac Appt:** Assoc Prof ObG, Mount Sinai Sch Med

Carson, Donald G MD [ObG] - **Hospital:** Magee-Womens Hosp - UPMC; **Address:** Ob/Gyn Assocs of Pittsburgh, 3380 Boulevard of the Allies, Ste 1, Pittsburgh, PA 15213; **Phone:** 412-621-7575; **Board Cert:** Obstetrics & Gynecology 2006; **Med School:** Univ Pittsburgh 1977; **Resid:** Obstetrics & Gynecology, Magee-Women's Hosp 1981; **Fac Appt:** Clin Prof ObG, Univ Pittsburgh

De Cherney, Alan Hersh MD [ObG] - **Spec Exp:** Infertility-Female; Reproductive Endocrinology; **Hospital:** Natl Inst of Hlth - Clin Ctr; **Address:** NICHD, NIH, Bldg 10, CRC, 1 East, 10 Center Drive, rm 1-3140, MS 1109, Bethesda, MD 20892-5800; **Phone:** 301-770-9667; **Board Cert:** Obstetrics & Gynecology 1989; Reproductive Endocrinology 1979; **Med School:** Temple Univ 1967; **Resid:** Obstetrics & Gynecology, Hosp Univ Penn 1972; **Fac Appt:** Prof ObG, UCLA

Evans, Mark I MD [ObG] - **Spec Exp:** Prenatal Diagnosis; Multiple Gestation; Fetal Therapy; Reproductive Genetics; **Hospital:** Mount Sinai Med Ctr (page 64); **Address:** Comprehensive Genetics, 131 E 65th St, New York, NY 10021; **Phone:** 212-744-2590; **Board Cert:** Obstetrics & Gynecology 2006; Clinical Genetics 1984; **Med School:** SUNY Downstate 1978; **Resid:** Obstetrics & Gynecology, Lying-In Hosp 1982; **Fellow:** Clinical Genetics, Natl Inst Hlth 1984; **Fac Appt:** Prof ObG, Mount Sinai Sch Med

Goldstein, Martin S MD [ObG] - **Spec Exp:** Incontinence; Laparoscopic Surgery; Uterine Fibroids; Pelvic Organ Prolapse Repair; **Hospital:** Mount Sinai Med Ctr (page 64); **Address:** 40 E 84th St, New York, NY 10028-1314; **Phone:** 212-472-6500; **Board Cert:** Obstetrics & Gynecology 1980; **Med School:** SUNY Hlth Sci Ctr 1966; **Resid:** Obstetrics & Gynecology, Mount Sinai Hosp 1971; **Fac Appt:** Assoc Clin Prof ObG, Mount Sinai Sch Med

Lucente, Vincent R MD [ObG] - **Spec Exp:** Uro-Gynecology; Pelvic Floor Reconstruction; Incontinence-Female; **Hospital:** St Luke's Hosp - Bethlehem, Abington Mem Hosp; **Address:** Park Professional Bldg, 2200 W Hamilton St, Ste 111, Allentown, PA 18104; **Phone:** 610-435-9575; **Board Cert:** Obstetrics & Gynecology 2006; **Med School:** SUNY Stony Brook 1985; **Resid:** Obstetrics & Gynecology, N Shore Univ Hosp 1989; **Fellow:** Uro-Gynecology, Methodist Hosp 1990; **Fac Appt:** Clin Prof ObG, Temple Univ

Minkoff, Howard L MD [ObG] - **Spec Exp:** AIDS/HIV in Pregnancy-Consultation; Pregnancy-High Risk, Consultation; **Hospital:** Maimonides Med Ctr (page 63); **Address:** Maimonides Med Ctr, Dept Ob-Gyn, 4802 Tenth Ave, Brooklyn, NY 11219; **Phone:** 718-283-7973; **Board Cert:** Obstetrics & Gynecology 1995; Maternal & Fetal Medicine 1995; **Med School:** Penn State Univ-Hershey Med Ctr 1975; **Resid:** Obstetrics & Gynecology, Kings Co Hosp Ctr 1979; Obstetrics & Gynecology, SUNY Hlth Sci Ctr 1981; **Fellow:** Maternal & Fetal Medicine, Kings Co Hosp Ctr 1981; **Fac Appt:** Prof ObG, SUNY Hlth Sci Ctr

Plante, Lauren A MD [ObG] - **Spec Exp:** Pregnancy-High Risk; **Hospital:** Thomas Jefferson Univ Hosp; **Address:** 834 Chestnut St, Ste 400, Philadelphia, PA 19107-5113; **Phone:** 215-955-5000; **Board Cert:** Anesthesiology 2004; Obstetrics & Gynecology 2006; Maternal & Fetal Medicine 2006; Critical Care Medicine 1993; **Med School:** Albert Einstein Coll Med 1984; **Resid:** Anesthesiology, Montefiore Med Ctr 1989; Obstetrics & Gynecology, Hahnemann Univ Hosp 1994; **Fellow:** Critical Care Medicine, Montefiore Med Ctr 1990; Maternal & Fetal Medicine, Temple Univ Med Ctr 1998

Scher, Jonathan MD [ObG] - **Spec Exp:** Miscarriage-Recurrent; Pregnancy-High Risk; **Hospital:** Mount Sinai Med Ctr (page 64); **Address:** 1126 Park Ave, New York, NY 10128-1203; **Phone:** 212-427-7400; **Board Cert:** Obstetrics & Gynecology 1981; **Med School:** South Africa 1964; **Resid:** Obstetrics & Gynecology, Groote Schuur Hosp 1970; Obstetrics & Gynecology, Kings College Hosp 1972; **Fac Appt:** Asst Clin Prof ObG, Mount Sinai Sch Med

Wiesenfeld, Harold C MD [ObG] - **Spec Exp:** Infectious Diseases-Gynecologic; Sexually Transmitted Diseases; **Hospital:** Magee-Womens Hosp - UPMC; **Address:** Magee-Women's Hosp, Dept Ob/Gyn, 300 Halket St, Pittsburgh, PA 15213; **Phone:** 412-641-6412; **Board Cert:** Obstetrics & Gynecology 2006; **Med School:** McGill Univ 1987; **Resid:** Obstetrics & Gynecology, McGill Univ 1990; **Fac Appt:** Assoc Prof ObG, Univ Pittsburgh

Obstetrics & Gynecology

Witter, Frank R MD [ObG] - **Spec Exp:** Pregnancy-High Risk; Multiple Gestation; Lupus/SLE in Pregnancy; **Hospital:** Johns Hopkins Hosp - Baltimore (page 61); **Address:** 600 N Wolfe St, Nelson 2170, Baltimore, MD 21287; **Phone:** 410-955-1421; **Board Cert:** Obstetrics & Gynecology 1997; Maternal & Fetal Medicine 1997; **Med School:** Univ Chicago-Pritzker Sch Med 1976; **Resid:** Obstetrics & Gynecology, Johns Hopkins Hosp 1980; **Fellow:** Maternal & Fetal Medicine, Johns Hopkins Hosp 1982; Clinical Pharmacology, Johns Hopkins Hosp 1984; **Fac Appt:** Prof ObG, Johns Hopkins Univ

Young, Bruce MD [ObG] - **Spec Exp:** Infertility; Minimally Invasive Surgery; Twin to Twin Transfusion Syndrome (TTTS); Miscarriage-Recurrent; **Hospital:** NYU Med Ctr (page 68); **Address:** 530 1st Ave, HCC-5th Fl, Ste 5G, New York, NY 10016; **Phone:** 212-263-6359; **Board Cert:** Obstetrics & Gynecology 1970; Maternal & Fetal Medicine 1975; **Med School:** NYU Sch Med 1963; **Resid:** Obstetrics & Gynecology, New York Univ Med Ctr 1968; **Fellow:** Reproductive Endocrinology, New York Univ Med Ctr 1968; **Fac Appt:** Prof ObG, NYU Sch Med

Southeast

Duff, W Patrick MD [ObG] - **Spec Exp:** Pregnancy-High Risk; Infectious Disease; Maternal & Fetal Medicine; **Hospital:** Shands at Univ of FL; **Address:** Magnolia Park Women's Health, 3951 NW 48th Terr, Ste 101, Gainesville, FL 32606; **Phone:** 352-265-6200; **Board Cert:** Obstetrics & Gynecology 2003; Maternal & Fetal Medicine 2003; **Med School:** Georgetown Univ 1974; **Resid:** Obstetrics & Gynecology, Walter Reed Med Ctr 1978; **Fellow:** Maternal & Fetal Medicine, UT - San Antonio 1983; **Fac Appt:** Prof ObG, Univ S Fla Coll Med

Filip, Stanley J MD [ObG] - **Spec Exp:** Uterine Fibroids; Menopause Problems; Hysterectomy Alternatives; Endometriosis; **Hospital:** Duke Univ Med Ctr, Durham Regional Hosp; **Address:** 3116 N Duke St, Durham, NC 27704; **Phone:** 919-684-2471; **Board Cert:** Obstetrics & Gynecology 1985; **Med School:** Mount Sinai Sch Med 1979; **Resid:** Obstetrics & Gynecology, Univ Colo Hlth Scis Ctr 1983

Hager, W David MD [ObG] - **Spec Exp:** Infectious Diseases-Gynecologic; Sexually Transmitted Diseases; **Hospital:** Central Baptist Hosp; **Address:** 1720 Nicholasville Rd, Lexington, KY 40503; **Phone:** 859-278-0363; **Board Cert:** Obstetrics & Gynecology 1993; **Med School:** Univ KY Coll Med 1972; **Resid:** Obstetrics & Gynecology, Univ Kentucky Med Ctr 1976; **Fac Appt:** Prof ObG, Univ KY Coll Med

Kovac, S Robert MD [ObG] - **Spec Exp:** Pelvic Reconstruction; **Hospital:** Emory Univ Hosp, Grady Hlth Sys; **Address:** Emory Clinic A, Dept Ob/Gyn, 1365 Clifton Rd NE Fl 4, Atlanta, GA 30322; **Phone:** 404-778-3401; **Board Cert:** Obstetrics & Gynecology 1979; **Med School:** Univ MO-Columbia Sch Med 1964; **Resid:** Obstetrics & Gynecology, Barnes JewishHosp 1970; **Fellow:** Reconstructive Pelvic Surgery, Barnes Hosp 1969; **Fac Appt:** Prof ObG, Emory Univ

Morgan, Linda S MD [ObG] - **Spec Exp:** Gynecologic Cancer; Women's Health; **Hospital:** Shands at Univ of FL; **Address:** Univ of Florida, PO Box 100294, Dept Ob/Gyn, Gainesville, FL 32610; **Phone:** 352-392-4161; **Board Cert:** Obstetrics & Gynecology 2006; Gynecologic Oncology 2006; **Med School:** Med Coll PA Hahnemann 1975; **Resid:** Obstetrics & Gynecology, Shands Hosp 1979; **Fellow:** Gynecologic Oncology, Mass Genl Hosp 1981; **Fac Appt:** Prof ObG, Univ Fla Coll Med

Sanz, Luis E MD [ObG] - **Spec Exp:** Uro-Gynecology; Hysteroscopic Surgery; Vaginal Reconstructive Surgery; Pelvic Reconstruction; **Hospital:** Virginia Hosp Ctr - Arlington; **Address:** 1625 N George Mason Drive, Ste 475, Arlington, VA 22205; **Phone:** 703-717-4000; **Board Cert:** Obstetrics & Gynecology 1982; **Med School:** Georgetown Univ 1976; **Resid:** Obstetrics & Gynecology, Georgetown Univ Hosp 1980; **Fellow:** Advanced Pelvic Surgery, Georgetown Univ 1982; **Fac Appt:** Prof ObG, Georgetown Univ

Simpson, Joe Leigh MD [ObG] - **Spec Exp:** Prenatal Diagnosis; Ovarian Failure; Infertility/Genetics; **Hospital:** Mount Sinai Med Ctr - Miami; **Address:** Florida International University, University Park HLS 693, 11200 SW H St, Miami, FL 33199; **Phone:** 305-348-0613; **Board Cert:** Obstetrics & Gynecology 2004; Clinical Genetics 1982; **Med School:** Duke Univ 1968; **Resid:** Obstetrics & Gynecology, NY Hosp-Cornell Med Ctr 1973; **Fac Appt:** Prof ObG, Baylor Coll Med

Steege, John F MD [ObG] - **Spec Exp:** Laparoscopic Surgery; Endometriosis; Pain-Pelvic & Perineal; Gynecologic Surgery; **Hospital:** Univ NC Hosps; **Address:** Univ NC-Dept OB/GYN, CB 7570, Chapel Hill, NC 27599-7570; **Phone:** 919-966-7764; **Board Cert:** Obstetrics & Gynecology 1978; **Med School:** Yale Univ 1972; **Resid:** Obstetrics & Gynecology, Yale - New Haven Hosp 1976; **Fac Appt:** Prof ObG, Univ NC Sch Med

Underwood, Paul B MD [ObG] - **Spec Exp:** Pelvic Reconstruction; Women's Health over age 40; **Hospital:** MUSC Med Ctr; **Address:** 1280 Johnnie Dodds Blvd, Ste 200, Mt Pleasant, SC 29464; **Phone:** 843-881-1312; **Board Cert:** Obstetrics & Gynecology 1989; Gynecologic Oncology 1974; **Med School:** Med Univ SC 1959; **Resid:** Obstetrics & Gynecology, Med University SC 1964; **Fellow:** Gynecologic Oncology, MD Anderson Hosp 1967; **Fac Appt:** Prof ObG, Med Univ SC

Midwest

De Lia, Julian E MD [ObG] - **Spec Exp:** Fetal Surgery; Twin to Twin Transfusion Syndrome (TTTS); **Hospital:** Wheaton Franciscan Hlthcare-St Joseph-Milwaukee; **Address:** TTTS Inst, WFHC-St Joseph, 5000 W Chambers St, Milwaukee, WI 53210-1688; **Phone:** 414-447-3535; **Board Cert:** Obstetrics & Gynecology 1993; **Med School:** UMDNJ-NJ Med Sch, Newark 1972; **Resid:** Obstetrics & Gynecology, St Barnabas Med Ctar 1976; **Fac Appt:** Assoc Prof ObG, Med Coll Wisc

DeLancey, John O MD [ObG] - **Spec Exp:** Uro-Gynecology; Incontinence; Pelvic Organ Prolapse Repair; **Hospital:** Univ Michigan Hlth Sys; **Address:** Univ Mich Med Ctr, Dept ObGyn, 1500 E Med Ctr Drive, rm L4100-WH, Ann Arbor, MI 48109-0276; **Phone:** 734-763-6295; **Board Cert:** Obstetrics & Gynecology 1997; **Med School:** Univ Mich Med Sch 1977; **Resid:** Obstetrics & Gynecology, Univ Mich Med Ctr 1981; **Fac Appt:** Prof ObG, Univ Mich Med Sch

Gonik, Bernard MD [ObG] - **Spec Exp:** Maternal & Fetal Medicine; Infectious Disease; Prenatal Diagnosis; Vaccinations in Pregnancy; **Hospital:** Sinai-Grace Hosp - Detroit; **Address:** Womens Diagnostic Unit, 6071 W Outer Drive, Detroit, MI 48235-2624; **Phone:** 313-966-1880; **Board Cert:** Obstetrics & Gynecology 2006; Maternal & Fetal Medicine 2006; **Med School:** Mich State Univ 1978; **Resid:** Obstetrics & Gynecology, Univ Texas Med Sch 1982; **Fellow:** Maternal & Fetal Medicine, Univ Texas Med Sch 1985; **Fac Appt:** Prof ObG, Wayne State Univ

Hale, Douglass S MD [ObG] - **Spec Exp:** Uro-Gynecology; Pelvic Floor Reconstruction; Reconstructive Surgery; Robotic Surgery; **Hospital:** Methodist Hosp - Indianapolis; **Address:** Urogynecology Assocs, 1633 N Capital Ave, Ste 436, Indianapolis, IN 46202; **Phone:** 317-962-6600; **Board Cert:** Obstetrics & Gynecology 2006; **Med School:** Med Coll OH 1989; **Resid:** Obstetrics & Gynecology, T Jefferson Univ Hosp 1993; **Fellow:** Uro-Gynecology, Methodist Hosp 1995; Reconstructive Surgery, Methodist Hosp 1995; **Fac Appt:** Assoc Clin Prof ObG, Indiana Univ

Obstetrics & Gynecology

Karram, Mickey M MD [ObG] - **Spec Exp:** Uro-Gynecology; Pelvic Floor Reconstruction; Incontinence-Female; **Hospital:** Good Samaritan Hosp - Cincinnati; **Address:** Good Samaritan Hosp, 7759 University Drive, Ste D, Westchester, OH 45069; **Phone:** 513-463-2500; **Board Cert:** Obstetrics & Gynecology 1998; **Med School:** Egypt 1982; **Resid:** Obstetrics & Gynecology, Good Samaritan Hosp 1985; **Fellow:** Gynecologic Urology, Harbor Hosp-UCLA 1986; **Fac Appt:** Prof ObG, Univ Cincinnati

Levine, Elliot MD [ObG] - **Spec Exp:** Sexually Transmitted Diseases; Sexual Dysfunction; Vulvar & Vaginal Disorders; **Hospital:** Adv Illinois Masonic Med Ctr, Weiss Meml Hosp; **Address:** 4646 N Marine Drive, Ste 8A, Chicago, IL 60640; **Phone:** 773-564-5355; **Board Cert:** Obstetrics & Gynecology 1984; **Med School:** Ros Franklin Univ/Chicago Med Sch 1978; **Resid:** Obstetrics & Gynecology, Illinois Masonic Med Ctr 1982; **Fac Appt:** Asst Prof ObG, Rush Med Coll

Lipscomb, Gary H MD [ObG] - **Spec Exp:** Pregnancy-High Risk; Cervical Cancer; Uro-Gynecology; **Hospital:** Northwestern Meml Hosp; **Address:** 675 N St Clair Fl 14 - rm 200, Galter Pavilion, Chicago, IL 60611; **Phone:** 312-695-7382; **Board Cert:** Obstetrics & Gynecology 1997; **Med School:** Univ Tenn Coll Med, Memphis 1981; **Resid:** Obstetrics & Gynecology, Univ Tenn Affil Hosps 1985; **Fac Appt:** Prof ObG, Northwestern Univ

Merritt, Diane F MD [ObG] - **Spec Exp:** Adolescent Gynecology; Pediatric Gynecology; Endometriosis; **Hospital:** Barnes-Jewish Hosp, St Louis Chldns Hosp; **Address:** Washington Univ Sch Medicine, 660 S Euclid Ave, St Louis, MO 63110; **Phone:** 314-362-4211; **Board Cert:** Obstetrics & Gynecology 1984; **Med School:** NYU Sch Med 1975; **Resid:** Surgery, Barnes Hosp-Wash Univ 1977; Obstetrics & Gynecology, Barnes Hosp-Wash Univ 1980; **Fac Appt:** Prof ObG, Washington Univ, St Louis

Shulman, Lee MD [ObG] - **Spec Exp:** Prenatal Diagnosis; Breast Cancer Genetics; Ovarian Cancer Genetics; **Hospital:** Northwestern Meml Hosp, Rush Univ Med Ctr; **Address:** Northwestern Univ, Dept Ob/Gyn, 333 E Superior St, Ste 484, Chicago, IL 60611; **Phone:** 312-926-6622; **Board Cert:** Obstetrics & Gynecology 1999; Clinical Genetics 1990; **Med School:** Cornell Univ-Weill Med Coll 1983; **Resid:** Obstetrics & Gynecology, North Shore Univ Hosp 1987; **Fellow:** Reproductive Genetics, Univ Tenn Med Ctr 1989; **Fac Appt:** Prof ObG, Northwestern Univ

Great Plains and Mountains

Bury, Robert J MD [ObG] - **Spec Exp:** Infertility; Laser Surgery; Microsurgery; **Hospital:** St. Alexius Med Ctr - Bismarck; **Address:** Mid Dakota Clinic-Center for Women, PO Box 5538, Bismarck, ND 58506; **Phone:** 701-530-6000; **Board Cert:** Obstetrics & Gynecology 1981; **Med School:** Baylor Coll Med 1975; **Resid:** Obstetrics & Gynecology, Baylor Affil Hosp 1979; **Fac Appt:** Clin Prof ObG, Univ ND Sch Med

Byrne, Janice LB MD [ObG] - **Hospital:** Univ Utah Hosps and Clins; **Address:** 50 N Medical Drive, Salt Lake City, UT 84132; **Phone:** 801-581-2719; **Board Cert:** Obstetrics & Gynecology 2005; Clinical Genetics 2006; Maternal & Fetal Medicine 2005; **Med School:** Univ Tex SW, Dallas 1987; **Resid:** Obstetrics & Gynecology, Univ Utah Hosps & Clins 1991; **Fellow:** Clinical Genetics, Univ Utah Hosps & Clins 1993; Maternal & Fetal Medicine, Univ Utah Hosps & Clins 1994; **Fac Appt:** Assoc Clin Prof ObG, Univ Utah

America's Top Doctors® 9th Edition

Southwest

Carr, Bruce MD [ObG] - **Spec Exp:** Infertility-Female; **Hospital:** UT Southwestern Med Ctr - Dallas, Parkland Meml Hosp - Dallas; **Address:** 5323 Harry Hines Blvd, Outpatient Bldg Fl 6, Dallas, TX 75390-8865; **Phone:** 214-648-8846; **Board Cert:** Obstetrics & Gynecology 2000; Reproductive Endocrinology 2000; **Med School:** Univ Mich Med Sch 1971; **Resid:** Obstetrics & Gynecology, Parkland Meml Hosp 1975; **Fellow:** Reproductive Endocrinology, Univ Texas SW Med Ctr 1980; **Fac Appt:** Prof ObG, Univ Tex SW, Dallas

Cornella, Jeffrey L MD [ObG] - **Spec Exp:** Pelvic Reconstructive Surgery; Robotic Surgery; Laparoscopic Surgery; Vaginal Reconstruction; **Hospital:** Mayo Clinic - Scottsdale; **Address:** Mayo Clinic Scottsdale, 13400 E Shea Blvd, Scottsdale, AZ 85259; **Phone:** 480-342-2867; **Board Cert:** Obstetrics & Gynecology 1998; **Med School:** Washington Univ, St Louis 1981; **Resid:** Obstetrics & Gynecology, Mayo Clinic 1986; **Fellow:** Uro-Gynecology, UC Irvine 1987; **Fac Appt:** Prof ObG, Mayo Med Sch

Faro, Sebastian MD/PhD [ObG] - **Spec Exp:** Infections in Pregnancy; Infectious Diseases-Gynecologic; Sexually Transmitted Diseases; **Hospital:** Woman's Hosp TX, The, St Luke's Episcopal Hosp - Houston; **Address:** 7400 Fannin, Ste 840, Houston, TX 77054; **Phone:** 713-799-9091; **Board Cert:** Obstetrics & Gynecology 2006; **Med School:** Creighton Univ 1975; **Resid:** Obstetrics & Gynecology, Creighton Univ 1978; **Fac Appt:** Clin Prof ObG, Univ Tex, Houston

Young, Amy E MD [ObG] - **Hospital:** Baylor Univ Medical Ctr; **Address:** 6620 Main St, Ste 1450, Houston, TX 77030-2717; **Phone:** 713-798-7500; **Board Cert:** Obstetrics & Gynecology 2005; **Med School:** Univ Miss 1994; **Resid:** Obstetrics & Gynecology, Baylor Coll Med 1999

West Coast and Pacific

Eschenbach, David A MD [ObG] - **Spec Exp:** Gynecologic Surgery-Complex; Infectious Disease; Vulvar & Vaginal Disorders; **Hospital:** Univ Wash Med Ctr; **Address:** Univ Washington Women's Health Care, 4245 Roosevelt Way NE, Box 354765, Seattle, WA 98105-6920; **Phone:** 206-598-5500; **Board Cert:** Obstetrics & Gynecology 1975; **Med School:** Univ Wisc 1968; **Resid:** Obstetrics & Gynecology, Univ Wash Hosp 1973; **Fellow:** Infectious Disease, Univ Wash Hosp 1974; **Fac Appt:** Prof ObG, Univ Wash

Sweet, Richard L MD [ObG] - **Spec Exp:** Sexually Transmitted Diseases; Infectious Diseases-Gynecologic; Women's Health; Infections in Pregnancy; **Hospital:** UC Davis Med Ctr; **Address:** UC Davis Women's Center for Health, 4860 Y St, Ste 2500, Sacramento, CA 95817; **Phone:** 916-734-6670; **Board Cert:** Obstetrics & Gynecology 1975; **Med School:** Univ Mich Med Sch 1966; **Resid:** Obstetrics & Gynecology, Univ Mich Med Ctr 1973; **Fac Appt:** Prof ObG, UC Davis

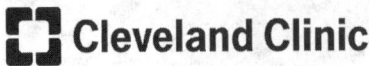
Cleveland Clinic

Obstetrics and Gynecology

Reproductive Endocrinology and Infertility: Our reproductive endocrinology and infertility program involves close collaboration between male and female infertility specialists, andrologists and embryologists. We offer all available treatment options including medications, artificial insemination, in vitro fertilization (IVF) and reproductive surgery. Our reproductive surgeons are nationally recognized experts in minimally invasive surgery and pioneered the world's first robotic surgery.

Urogynecology and Reconstructive Pelvic Surgery: This Center offers cutting-edge and traditional surgery for urinary incontinence and pelvic organ prolapse, along with medical and behavioral therapy.

Center for Female Pelvic Medicine and Reconstructive Surgery: Urogynecologist, urologists and colorectal surgeons in this center treat incontinence and prolapse via the abdominal, vaginal and laparoscopic routes. Pelvic floor subspecialists collaborate with each other, basic scientists, and physical therapists to advance research, education and healthcare for women suffering from pelvic floor disorders.

Maternal-Fetal Medicine/Obstetrics: Maternal-fetal medicine specialists provide comprehensive management for high-risk pregnancies throughout Northeast Ohio. Clinical services include genetic counseling, obstetrical ultrasound, fetal antepartum surveillance, prenatal diagnostic testing and consultation.

The Fetal Care Center: The Fetal Care team of perinatologists, neonatologists, and pediatric subspecialists and surgeons provides prenatal diagnosis for complex fetal abnormalities using state-of-the-art imaging techniques to develop a plan for pregnancy management, delivery and newborn care.

Menstrual Disorders, Fibroids and Hysteroscopic Services: This Center offers individualized evaluation for women with abnormal menstrual bleeding, post-menopausal bleeding and uterine fibroids. Clinicians utilize in-office minimally invasive and comfortable technology such as office flexible hysteroscopy and saline infusion sonography to evaluate uterine health. Therapies include medical management, Mirena intra-uterine system, endometrial ablation, myomectomy, hysterectomy, uterine fibroid embolization and sterilization. Our goal is to offer the most minimally invasive approach.

Gynecologic Oncology: Our gynecologic oncologists have garnered national and international recognition for expertise in complex reproductive cancers, clinical and basic research and preventive oncology. Cleveland Clinic gynecologists were among the first to treat early cervical and endometrial cancers laparoscopically. In performing less invasive surgical procedures, we always weigh curative potential against preservation of fertility. We offer oocyte, embryo and ovarian tissue cryopreservation for cancer patients.

Women's Health Center: The Cleveland Clinic Center for Specialized Women's Health offers a full range of specialized women's health services in one location. We manage menopause, hormone therapy, vulvar disorders, and premenstrual dysthymic disorder and hormonally exacerbated mood disorders. We offer evaluation and treatment for women with urinary incontinence, osteoporosis or breast concerns. Breast specialists in this center evaluate and treat breast cancer as well as benign breast disease.

For more information about the Cleveland Clinic Department of Obstetrics and Gynecology, to schedule a second opinion or to learn about assistance for out-of-town patients, call 800.890.2467 or visit www.clevelandclinic.org/obgyntopdocs.

Department of Obstetrics and Gynecology
9500 Euclid Avenue / AC311 | Cleveland OH 44195

PENN OB/GYN CARE

A Leader in Women's Health Care

Penn Ob/Gyn Care at Penn Medicine is committed to providing the highest quality and most advanced health care for women of all ages. From adolescence through the childbearing and menopausal years, patients receive comprehensive care from our high quality programs and services.

A leader in women's health care for more than two centuries, Penn Ob/Gyn Care offers a full range of specialized services and programs including:

- Advanced and robotic gynecologic surgery
- Bladder and pelvic floor health
- Fertility care
- Genetic counseling and prenatal diagnosis
- Gynecologic cancer care
- High-risk pregnancy care
- Obstetric and gynecology care
- Level III intensive care nurseries staffed by physicians from the Children's Hospital of Philadelphia

Penn combines the resources of a world-renowned health system with state-of-the-art research to provide excellence in patient care.

Obstetric Care at Penn

Expert maternity care

Penn obstetricians are consistently ranked among the best in the Philadelphia region and the nation. With over 9,000 births each year, Penn offers a wide array of specialized treatments and services.

Penn's maternal fetal medicine specialists provide expertise in prenatal diagnosis and treatment, obstetric care, fetal diagnosis and antepartum testing. Our specialists treat a variety of prenatal conditions including: heart disease, diabetes or other endocrine disorders, hypertension or pre-eclampisa, multiple gestation pregnancies, cervical insufficiency, placental problems and more.

Gynecologic Oncology

Innovators in cancer prevention and treatment

Penn's Division of Gynecologic Oncology is proud to be a pioneer in establishing and developing the subspecialty of gynecologic oncology. It continues to hold a national reputation for outstanding patient care and providing innovative treatment approaches. *U.S.News & World Report* consistently ranks Penn among the top in the nation for cancer and women's health services.

Penn Ovarian Cancer Research Center

The Center provides an infrastructure for ovarian cancer research and treatment and promotes interdisciplinary collaboration in the field of ovarian cancer research. Current research efforts include developing blood tests to detect ovarian cancer, advancing molecular imaging techniques, discovering ovarian cancer vaccines, and developing therapies for ovarian cancer with emphasis on immune and biological therapies.

Penn Fertility Care

Pioneers in fertility treatment and research

Penn Fertility Care is a pioneer in the development of infertility treatment and has been a national leader in research breakthroughs for over 40 years. Fertility procedures at Penn have advanced to where we now treat more than 1,000 couples each year and have helped bring thousands of healthy new lives into the world.

Our key fertility services include:
- Basic and advanced fertility evaluation and treatment
- Donor egg program for egg donors and recipients
- Reproductive surgery and assisted reproductive technologies including in vitro fertilization.
- PCOS Center and endometriosis treatment
- Preimplantation Genetic Diagnosis services

Urogynecology at Penn

Penn Urogynecology offers comprehensive, efficient, state-of-the-art urogynecology services for a variety of pelvic floor disorders. Our staff conducts national and international clinical trials, providing our physicians access to the most progressive therapies available.

We treat a variety of disorders including: urinary and stress incontinence, urge incontinence or overactive bladder, fecal incontinence, pelvic organ prolapse, fistulas, and benign conditions of the vagina and urethra.

Locations

Hospital of the University of Pennsylvania

Penn Presbyterian Medical Center

Pennsylvania Hospital

Penn Medicine at Radnor

Services also available at:

The Pavilions at Voorhees and satellite locations throughout New Jersey and Pennsylvania

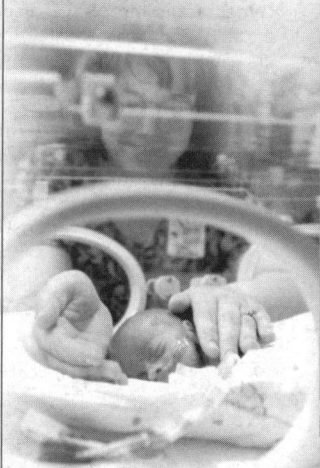

Hospital of the University of Pennsylvania | Penn Presbyterian Medical Center | Pennsylvania Hospital

MOUNT SINAI
SCHOOL OF
MEDICINE

THE MOUNT SINAI MEDICAL CENTER OBSTETRICS, GYNECOLOGY, AND REPRODUCTIVE SCIENCE

One Gustave L. Levy Place
Fifth Avenue and 100th Street
New York, NY 10029-6574
Physician Referral: 1-800-MD-SINAI (637-4624)
www.mountsinai.org

Building on more than a century of leadership in providing health care to women, the **DEPARTMENT OF OBSTETRICS, GYNECOLOGY, AND REPRODUCTIVE SCIENCE** at The Mount Sinai Medical Center offers special expertise in:

General obstetrics – Genetic counseling, prenatal care, labor and delivery management, and postpartum care. In addition to our talented physicians, other health care professionals are integrated into our practice, including genetic counselors, nutritionists, social workers, nurse midwives, childbirth educators, and lactation/breastfeeding specialists.

High-risk obstetrics – Advanced techniques in prenatal diagnosis and consultations in the management of complicated pregnancies. Our ultrasound unit is recognized for its expertise in fetal anatomy ultrasound assessments. The latest technology, including 4D imaging, is employed. Antepartum testing, including amniocentesis, chorionic villus sampling, and fetal blood sampling, are all routinely performed at Mount Sinai.

Reproductive endocrinology and infertility – Diagnosis and treatment of both female and male factor infertility. Treatment options for women include fertility medications, intrauterine insemination, in vitro fertilization, intracytoplasmic sperm injection, and ovum donation.

General gynecology – Cancer screening, management of abnormal Pap smears, family planning, and surgical management of fibroids, endometriosis, and other benign gynecologic conditions.

Gynecologic infectious diseases – Treatment and prevention of sexually transmitted infections and consultations on obstetrical and gynecological infections.

Gynecologic oncology – Care for women with cancers of the ovary, uterus, cervix, vulva, and vagina.

Minimally invasive surgery – For many conditions.

Urogynecology and reconstructive pelvic surgery – Lower urinary tract disorders.

INNOVATIVE APPROACHES TO PRENATAL CARE AND THE TREATMENT OF GYNECOLOGIC CANCERS

Known worldwide for excellence and innovative approaches to prenatal diagnosis and fetal therapy, Mount Sinai's Department of Obstetrics, Gynecology, and Reproductive Science has a long tradition of advancing clinical practice through patient-oriented research. Faculty members are pioneering work in diverse areas, including first- and second-trimester screening for fetal chromosomal abnormalities, vaccines for the prevention of sexually transmitted infections, minimally invasive surgical techniques, and new approaches to the diagnosis and treatment of gender-specific cancers.

Ophthalmology

An ophthalmologist has the knowledge and professional skills needed to provide comprehensive eye and vision care. Ophthalmologists are medically trained to diagnose, monitor and medically or surgically treat all ocular and visual disorders. This includes problems affecting the eye and its component structures, the eyelids, the orbit and the visual pathways. In so doing, an ophthalmologist prescribes vision services, including glasses and contact lenses.

Training Required: Four years

OPHTHALMOLOGY

New England

Aiello, Lloyd M MD [Oph] - **Spec Exp:** Diabetic Eye Disease/Retinopathy; **Hospital:** Beth Israel Deaconess Med Ctr - Boston; **Address:** Beetham Eye Inst-Joslin Diabetes Ctr, 1 Joslin Pl, Boston, MA 02215-5397; **Phone:** 617-732-2520; **Board Cert:** Ophthalmology 1966; **Med School:** Boston Univ 1960; **Resid:** Ophthalmology, Mass Eye & Ear Infirm 1964; **Fac Appt:** Assoc Clin Prof Oph, Harvard Med Sch

Dana, Reza MD [Oph] - **Spec Exp:** Corneal Disease & Transplant; Dry Eye Syndrome; Uveitis; **Hospital:** Mass Eye & Ear Infirmary; **Address:** Mass Eye & Ear Infirmary, 243 Charles St, Boston, MA 02114; **Phone:** 617-573-4331; **Board Cert:** Ophthalmology 2006; **Med School:** Johns Hopkins Univ 1989; **Resid:** Ophthalmology, Illinois Eye & Ear Infirm 1993; **Fellow:** Cornea & Ext Eye Disease, Wills Eye Hosp 1994; Uveitis, Mass Eye & Ear Infirm 1995; **Fac Appt:** Prof Oph, Harvard Med Sch

Duker, Jay S MD [Oph] - **Spec Exp:** Retinal Disorders; Retinal Disorders-Pediatric; Diabetic Eye Disease/Retinopathy; **Hospital:** Tufts Med Ctr; **Address:** New England Eye Ctr, 750 Washington St, Box 450, Boston, MA 02111; **Phone:** 617-636-4600; **Board Cert:** Ophthalmology 1989; **Med School:** Jefferson Med Coll 1984; **Resid:** Ophthalmology, Wills Eye Hosp 1988; **Fellow:** Vitreoretinal Surgery & Disease, Wills Eye Hosp 1990; **Fac Appt:** Assoc Prof Oph, Tufts Univ

Foster, C Stephen MD [Oph] - **Spec Exp:** Uveitis; Corneal Disease; Cataract Surgery; **Hospital:** Mass Eye & Ear Infirmary, Mount Auburn Hosp; **Address:** 5 Cambridge Ctr Fl 8, Cambridge, MA 02142; **Phone:** 866-353-6377; **Board Cert:** Ophthalmology 1976; **Med School:** Duke Univ 1969; **Resid:** Ophthalmology, Barnes Hosp 1975; **Fellow:** Cornea, Mass EE Infirm-Harvard 1976; Ocular Immunology, Mass EE Infirm-Harvard 1977; **Fac Appt:** Prof Oph, Harvard Med Sch

Hedges, Thomas R MD [Oph] - **Spec Exp:** Neuro-Ophthalmology; **Hospital:** Tufts Med Ctr; **Address:** New England Med Ctr, 750 Washington St, Box 450, Boston, MA 02111; **Phone:** 617-636-5488; **Board Cert:** Ophthalmology 1980; **Med School:** Tufts Univ 1975; **Resid:** Ophthalmology, Mass EE Infirm 1980; **Fellow:** Neuro-Ophthalmology, UCSF Med Ctr 1981; **Fac Appt:** Prof Oph, Tufts Univ

Hunter, David G MD/PhD [Oph] - **Spec Exp:** Pediatric Ophthalmology; Eye Muscle Disorders; Strabismus; Cataract-Pediatric; **Hospital:** Children's Hospital - Boston; **Address:** Chlds Hosp Boston, Dept Ophthalmology, 300 Longwood Ave Fegan 4 Bldg, Boston, MA 02115; **Phone:** 617-355-6401; **Board Cert:** Ophthalmology 2003; **Med School:** Baylor Coll Med 1987; **Resid:** Ophthalmology, Mass EE Infirm 1991; **Fellow:** Pediatric Ophthalmology, Wilmer Ophthalmic Inst 1992; **Fac Appt:** Assoc Prof Oph, Harvard Med Sch

Kornmehl, Ernest W MD [Oph] - **Spec Exp:** Laser Vision Surgery; Cornea & External Eye Disease; Dry Eye Syndrome; **Hospital:** Mass Eye & Ear Infirmary, Brigham & Women's Hosp; **Address:** Kornmehl Laser Eye Assoc, 54 Washington St, Wellesley, MA 02481; **Phone:** 877-870-2010; **Board Cert:** Ophthalmology 1989; **Med School:** SUNY Downstate 1984; **Resid:** Ophthalmology, Yale-New Haven Hosp 1988; **Fellow:** Cornea & Ext Eye Disease, Mass E&E Infirm 1990; **Fac Appt:** Assoc Clin Prof Oph, Tufts Univ

Miller, Joan W MD [Oph] - **Spec Exp:** Macular Degeneration; Retinal Disorders; **Hospital:** Mass Eye & Ear Infirmary; **Address:** Mass Eye & Ear Infirm, Ophthalmology, 243 Charles St, Boston, MA 02114; **Phone:** 617-573-3915; **Board Cert:** Ophthalmology 1991; **Med School:** Harvard Med Sch 1985; **Resid:** Ophthalmology, Mass Eye & Ear Infirm 1989; **Fellow:** Retina, Mass Eye & Ear Infirm 1991; **Fac Appt:** Assoc Prof Oph, Harvard Med Sch

Mitchell, Paul Ralph MD [Oph] - **Spec Exp:** Pediatric Ophthalmology; **Hospital:** CT Chldns Med Ctr, Hartford Hosp; **Address:** 366 Colt Hwy, Route 6, Farmington, CT 06032-2547; **Phone:** 860-409-0449; **Board Cert:** Ophthalmology 1977; **Med School:** Geo Wash Univ 1970; **Resid:** Ophthalmology, Wills Eye Hosp 1976; **Fellow:** Pediatric Ophthalmology, Chldns Hosp MC/Geo Wash 1977; **Fac Appt:** Asst Clin Prof Oph, Univ Conn

Rizzo III, Joseph F MD [Oph] - **Spec Exp:** Neuro-Ophthalmology; Retinal Disorders; **Hospital:** Mass Eye & Ear Infirmary; **Address:** Mass Eye and Ear Infirmary, 243 Charles St Fl 9, Boston, MA 02114; **Phone:** 617-573-3412; **Board Cert:** Neurology 1984; Ophthalmology 1987; **Med School:** Louisiana State U, New Orleans 1978; **Resid:** Neurology, Tufts-New Engl Med Ctr 1982; Ophthalmology, Boston Univ 1985; **Fellow:** Neuro-Ophthalmology, Harvard Univ 1986; **Fac Appt:** Assoc Prof Oph, Harvard Med Sch

Rubin, Peter A D MD [Oph] - **Spec Exp:** Oculoplastic Surgery; Orbital & Eyelid Tumors/Cancer; Eyelid Cancer & Reconstruction; Eyelid Cosmetic & Reconstructive Surgery; **Hospital:** Beth Israel Deaconess Med Ctr - Boston; **Address:** 44 Washington St, Brookline, MA 02445; **Phone:** 617-232-9600; **Board Cert:** Ophthalmology 1991; **Med School:** Yale Univ 1985; **Resid:** Ophthalmology, Manhattan EET Hosp 1989; **Fellow:** Oculoplastic Surgery, Mass EE Infirm 1990; **Fac Appt:** Assoc Prof Oph, Harvard Med Sch

Shingleton, Bradford J MD [Oph] - **Spec Exp:** Cataract Surgery; Glaucoma; **Hospital:** Mass Eye & Ear Infirmary; **Address:** Ophthalmic Consultants of Boston, 50 Stanford St, Ste 600, Boston, MA 02114; **Phone:** 617-314-2614; **Board Cert:** Ophthalmology 1982; **Med School:** Univ Mich Med Sch 1977; **Resid:** Ophthalmology, Mass E&E Infirm 1981; **Fellow:** Refractive Surgery, Mass E&E Infirm 1982; **Fac Appt:** Asst Clin Prof Oph, Harvard Med Sch

Tsai, James C MD [Oph] - **Spec Exp:** Glaucoma; **Hospital:** Yale-New Haven Hosp; **Address:** Yale Eye Center, 40 Temple St, New Haven, CT 06520-8061; **Phone:** 203-785-2020; **Board Cert:** Ophthalmology 2006; **Med School:** Stanford Univ 1989; **Resid:** Ophthalmology, Doheny Eye Inst/USC 1993; **Fellow:** Glaucoma, Bascom Palmer Eye Inst 1994; Glaucoma, Moorfields Eye Hosp 1995; **Fac Appt:** Prof Oph, Yale Univ

Walton, David S MD [Oph] - **Spec Exp:** Glaucoma-Pediatric; Cataract-Pediatric; Neuro-Ophthalmology; **Hospital:** Mass Eye & Ear Infirmary, Mass Genl Hosp; **Address:** 2 Longfellow Pl, Ste 201, Boston, MA 02114; **Phone:** 617-227-3011; **Board Cert:** Ophthalmology 1969; Pediatrics 1983; **Med School:** Duke Univ 1961; **Resid:** Ophthalmology, Mass EE Infirm 1967; **Fellow:** Glaucoma, Mass EE Infirm 1968; **Fac Appt:** Prof Oph, Harvard Med Sch

Mid Atlantic

Abramson, David H MD [Oph] - **Spec Exp:** Eye Tumors/Cancer; Orbital Tumors/Cancer; Retinoblastoma; Melanoma-Choroidal (eye); **Hospital:** Meml Sloan-Kettering Cancer Ctr; **Address:** 1275 York Avenue, New York, NY 10065; **Phone:** 800-525-2225; **Board Cert:** Ophthalmology 1975; **Med School:** Albert Einstein Coll Med 1969; **Resid:** Ophthalmology, Harkness Eye Inst 1974; **Fellow:** Ocular Oncology, Columbia-Presby Med Ctr 1975; **Fac Appt:** Clin Prof Oph, Cornell Univ-Weill Med Coll

Ophthalmology

Behrens, Myles MD [Oph] - **Spec Exp:** Neuro-Ophthalmology; **Hospital:** NY-Presby Hosp/Columbia (page 66); **Address:** 635 W 165th St, New York, NY 10032-3701; **Phone:** 212-305-5415; **Board Cert:** Ophthalmology 1971; **Med School:** Columbia P&S 1962; **Resid:** Internal Medicine, Columbia Presby Hosp 1964; Ophthalmology, Columbia Presby Hosp 1970; **Fellow:** Neuro-Ophthalmology, UCSF Med Ctr 1971; **Fac Appt:** Clin Prof Oph, Columbia P&S

Bressler, Neil M MD [Oph] - **Spec Exp:** Retinal Disorders; **Hospital:** Johns Hopkins Hosp (page 61); **Address:** Wilmer Eye Institute, 550 N Broadway, Ste 115, Baltimore, MD 21205; **Phone:** 410-955-8342; **Board Cert:** Ophthalmology 1987; **Med School:** Johns Hopkins Univ 1982; **Resid:** Internal Medicine, Johns Hopkins Hosp 1983; Ophthalmology, Mass Eye & Ear Infirm 1986; **Fellow:** Retina, Wilmer Inst/Johns Hopkins Hosp 1987; **Fac Appt:** Assoc Prof Oph, Johns Hopkins Univ

Brown, Gary C MD [Oph] - **Spec Exp:** Retinal Disorders; Retinal Vascular Diseases; **Hospital:** Wills Eye Hosp, Thomas Jefferson Univ Hosp; **Address:** 910 E Willow Grove Ave, Wyndmoor, PA 19038; **Phone:** 215-233-4300; **Board Cert:** Ophthalmology 2003; **Med School:** SUNY Upstate Med Univ 1975; **Resid:** Ophthalmology, Wills Eye Hosp 1979; **Fellow:** Vitreoretinal Disease, Wills Eye Hosp 1981; **Fac Appt:** Prof Oph, Jefferson Med Coll

Brucker, Alexander J MD [Oph] - **Spec Exp:** Retinal Disorders; Retina/Vitreous Surgery; Macular Degeneration; **Hospital:** Penn Presby Med Ctr - UPHS (page 60); **Address:** Univ Penn, Scheie Eye Inst, 51 N 39th St, rm 517, Philadelphia, PA 19104; **Phone:** 215-662-9702; **Board Cert:** Ophthalmology 1977; **Med School:** NY Med Coll 1972; **Resid:** Ophthalmology, Friedenwald Inst 1976; **Fellow:** Retina/Vitreous, Johns Hopkins Hosp 1977; **Fac Appt:** Prof Oph, Univ Pennsylvania

Campochiaro, Peter MD [Oph] - **Spec Exp:** Retina/Vitreous Surgery; **Hospital:** Johns Hopkins Hosp (page 61); **Address:** Wilmer Ophthalmological Inst, 600 N Wolfe St, 747 Maumenee, Baltimore, MD 21287-9277; **Phone:** 410-955-5106; **Board Cert:** Ophthalmology 1983; **Med School:** Johns Hopkins Univ 1978; **Resid:** Ophthalmology, Univ Virginia 1982; **Fellow:** Retina/Vitreous, John Hopkins Univ 1984; **Fac Appt:** Prof Oph, Johns Hopkins Univ

Caputo, Anthony R MD [Oph] - **Spec Exp:** Pediatric Ophthalmology; Strabismus; **Hospital:** Clara Maass Med Ctr; **Address:** 556 Eagle Rock Ave, Ste 203, Roseland, NJ 07068-1500; **Phone:** 973-228-3111; **Board Cert:** Ophthalmology 1976; **Med School:** Italy 1969; **Resid:** Ophthalmology, UMDNJ-Univ Hosp 1974; **Fellow:** Ophthalmology, Wills Eye Hosp 1975; **Fac Appt:** Prof Oph, UMDNJ-NJ Med Sch, Newark

Chang, Stanley MD [Oph] - **Spec Exp:** Diabetic Eye Disease/Retinopathy; Macular Disease/Degeneration; Retina/Vitreous Surgery; Retinal Disorders; **Hospital:** NY-Presby Hosp/Columbia (page 66); **Address:** 635 W 165th St, Box 20, New York, NY 10032; **Phone:** 212-305-9535; **Board Cert:** Ophthalmology 1979; **Med School:** Columbia P&S 1974; **Resid:** Ophthalmology, Mass Eye & Ear Infirm 1978; **Fellow:** Vitreoretinal Surgery, Bascom Palmer Eye Inst 1979; **Fac Appt:** Prof Oph, Columbia P&S

D'Amico, Donald MD [Oph] - **Spec Exp:** Diabetic Eye Disease/Retinopathy; Retinal Detachment; Retinal Disorders; **Hospital:** NY-Presby Hosp/Weill Cornell (page 66); **Address:** Weill Cornell Medical College, Dept of Ophthalmology, 1305 York Ave Fl 11th, New York, NY 10021; **Phone:** 646-962-2020; **Board Cert:** Ophthalmology 1982; **Med School:** Univ IL Coll Med 1977; **Resid:** Ophthalmology, Mass Eye & Ear Infirm 1981; **Fellow:** Vitreoretinal Surgery, Bascom Palmer Eye Inst 1982; **Fac Appt:** Prof Oph, Cornell Univ-Weill Med Coll

Del Priore, Lucian MD/PhD [Oph] - **Spec Exp:** Diabetic Eye Disease/Retinopathy; Macular Degeneration; Retinal Detachment; Retina-Artificial; **Hospital:** NY-Presby Hosp/Columbia (page 66), Lenox Hill Hosp (Manh Eye, Ear & Throat Hosp) (page 62); **Address:** Harkness Eye Inst, 635 W 165th St, New York, NY 10032; **Phone:** 212-305-9535; **Board Cert:** Ophthalmology 1989; **Med School:** Univ Rochester 1982; **Resid:** Ophthalmology, Wilmer Eye Inst/Johns HopkinsHosp 1987; **Fellow:** Glaucoma, Wilmer Eye Inst/Johns Hopkins Hosp 1988; Vitreoretinal Surgery, Wilmer Eye Inst/Johns Hopkins Hosp 1989; **Fac Appt:** Prof Oph, Columbia P&S

Della Rocca, Robert C MD [Oph] - **Spec Exp:** Orbital Tumors/Cancer; Eyelid Tumors/Cancer; Thyroid Eye Disease; Oculoplastic Surgery; **Hospital:** New York Eye & Ear Infirm (page 65), Sound Shore Med Ctr - Westchester; **Address:** 310 E 14th St, South Bldg, rm 319, New York, NY 10003; **Phone:** 212-979-4575; **Board Cert:** Ophthalmology 1975; **Med School:** Creighton Univ 1967; **Resid:** Ophthalmology, NY Eye & Ear Infirm 1973; **Fellow:** Oculoplastic Surgery, Albany Med Ctr

Dodick, Jack M MD [Oph] - **Spec Exp:** Cataract Surgery-Lens Implant; Laser Vision Surgery; **Hospital:** Lenox Hill Hosp (Manh Eye, Ear & Throat Hosp) (page 62), NYU Langone Med Ctr (page 67); **Address:** 535 Park Ave, New York, NY 10021-8167; **Phone:** 212-288-7638; **Board Cert:** Ophthalmology 1969; **Med School:** Univ Toronto 1963; **Resid:** Ophthalmology, Manhattan EE&T Hosp 1967; **Fellow:** Anterior Segment - External Disease, Westchester Co Med Ctr 1968; **Fac Appt:** Prof Oph, NYU Sch Med

Eagle, Ralph C MD [Oph] - **Spec Exp:** Ophthalmic Pathology; **Hospital:** Wills Eye Hosp; **Address:** Wills Eye Hosp, Dept Pathology, 840 Walnut St, Ste 1410, Philadelphia, PA 19107; **Phone:** 215-928-3280; **Board Cert:** Ophthalmology 1976; **Med School:** Univ Pennsylvania 1970; **Resid:** Ophthalmology, Scheie Eye Inst 1975; **Fellow:** Ophthalmic Pathology, Armed Forces Inst Path 1978; **Fac Appt:** Prof Oph, Jefferson Med Coll

Eggers, Howard M MD [Oph] - **Spec Exp:** Pediatric Ophthalmology; Strabismus-Adult & Pediatric; **Hospital:** NY-Presby Hosp/Columbia (page 66); **Address:** Harkness Eye Institute, 635 W 165th St, New York, NY 10032-3724; **Phone:** 212-305-5409; **Board Cert:** Ophthalmology 1978; **Med School:** Columbia P&S 1971; **Resid:** Ophthalmology, Harkness Inst - Presby Hosp 1975; **Fac Appt:** Prof Oph, Columbia P&S

Feldon, Steven E MD [Oph] - **Spec Exp:** Neuro-Ophthalmology; Orbital Surgery; Strabismus; **Hospital:** Univ of Rochester Strong Meml Hosp, Rochester Genl Hosp; **Address:** 601 Elmwood Ave, Box 659, Rochester, NY 14642; **Phone:** 585-275-1126; **Board Cert:** Ophthalmology 1979; **Med School:** Albert Einstein Coll Med 1973; **Resid:** Ophthalmology, Mass Eye & Ear Infirmary 1978; **Fellow:** Neuro-Ophthalmology, UCSF Med Ctr 1979; **Fac Appt:** Prof Oph, Univ Rochester

Finger, Paul T MD [Oph] - **Spec Exp:** Eye Tumors/Cancer; Melanoma-Choroidal (eye); Retinoblastoma; Orbital Tumors/Cancer; **Hospital:** New York Eye & Ear Infirm (page 65), NYU Langone Med Ctr (page 67); **Address:** The New York Eye Cancer Ctr, 115 E 61st St, New York, NY 10021-8183; **Phone:** 212-832-8170; **Board Cert:** Ophthalmology 1990; **Med School:** Tulane Univ 1982; **Resid:** Ophthalmology, Manhattan EET Hosp 1986; **Fellow:** Ocular Oncology, N Shore Univ Hosp 1987; **Fac Appt:** Clin Prof Oph, NYU Sch Med

Friberg, Thomas R MD [Oph] - **Spec Exp:** Retinal Disorders; Diabetic Eye Disease; Macular Degeneration; **Hospital:** UPMC Presby, Pittsburgh; **Address:** UPMC Eye Center, 203 Lothrop St, rm 824, Pittsburgh, PA 15213-2548; **Phone:** 412-647-2200; **Board Cert:** Ophthalmology 1979; **Med School:** Univ Minn 1973; **Resid:** Ophthalmology, Stanford Univ Med Ctr 1977; **Fellow:** Retina, Mass EE Infirmary 1978; Vitreoretinal Surgery, Duke Univ Med Ctr 1979; **Fac Appt:** Prof Oph, Univ Pittsburgh

Ophthalmology

Fuchs, Wayne MD [Oph] - **Spec Exp:** Diabetic Eye Disease/Retinopathy; Macular Disease/Degeneration; Retina/Vitreous Surgery; Retinal Disorders; **Hospital:** Mount Sinai Med Ctr (page 64), Lenox Hill Hosp (Manh Eye, Ear & Throat Hosp) (page 62); **Address:** 121 E 60th St, Ste 5B, New York, NY 10022-1186; **Phone:** 212-319-8205; **Board Cert:** Ophthalmology 1985; **Med School:** Mount Sinai Sch Med 1979; **Resid:** Ophthalmology, Mt Sinai Hosp 1983; **Fellow:** Vitreoretinal Surgery & Disease, NY Hosp-Cornell Med Ctr 1984; **Fac Appt:** Clin Prof Oph, Mount Sinai Sch Med

Gaasterland, Douglas E MD [Oph] - **Spec Exp:** Glaucoma; Laser Surgery; Anterior Segment Surgery; **Hospital:** Georgetown Univ Hosp; **Address:** 2 Wisconsin Cir, Ste 200, Chevy Chase, MD 20815; **Phone:** 301-215-7100; **Board Cert:** Ophthalmology 1971; **Med School:** Johns Hopkins Univ 1965; **Resid:** Ophthalmology, Yale-New Haven Hosp 1970; **Fellow:** Glaucoma, National Eye Inst-NIH 1971; **Fac Appt:** Clin Prof Oph, Georgetown Univ

Gallin, Pamela F MD [Oph] - **Spec Exp:** Pediatric Ophthalmology; Amblyopia; Strabismus; Tear Duct Problems; **Hospital:** NY-Presby Hosp/Columbia (page 66), Lenox Hill Hosp (Manh Eye, Ear & Throat Hosp) (page 62); **Address:** Columbia Presby Med Ctr, 635 W 165th St, Ste 224, New York, NY 10032-3701; **Phone:** 212-305-5407; **Board Cert:** Ophthalmology 1983; **Med School:** Washington Univ, St Louis 1978; **Resid:** Ophthalmology, Mount Sinai Med Ctr 1982; **Fellow:** Pediatric Ophthalmology, Chldns Natl Med Ctr 1983; Strabismus, Columbia-Presby Med Ctr 1983; **Fac Appt:** Clin Prof Oph, Columbia P&S

Gentile, Ronald MD [Oph] - **Spec Exp:** Retina/Vitreous Surgery; Diabetic Eye Disease; Macular Degeneration; Retinal Disorders; **Hospital:** New York Eye & Ear Infirm (page 65); **Address:** 2nd Ave at 14th St, South Bldg - Ste 319, New York, NY 10003-4201; **Phone:** 212-979-4120; **Board Cert:** Ophthalmology 2008; **Med School:** SUNY Downstate 1991; **Resid:** Ophthalmology, NY Eye & Ear Infirm 1995; **Fellow:** Vitreoretinal Surgery & Disease, Kresge Eye Inst 1998; **Fac Appt:** Assoc Prof Oph, NY Med Coll

Gibralter, Richard P MD [Oph] - **Spec Exp:** Cataract Surgery; Laser Vision Surgery; Cornea Transplant; Corneal Disease & Surgery; **Hospital:** Lenox Hill Hosp (Manh Eye, Ear & Throat Hosp) (page 62), New York Eye & Ear Infirm (page 65); **Address:** 154 E 71st St, New York, NY 10021-5123; **Phone:** 212-628-2202; **Board Cert:** Ophthalmology 1981; **Med School:** Mount Sinai Sch Med 1976; **Resid:** Ophthalmology, Manhattan EE&T Hosp 1980; **Fellow:** Cornea, Manhattan EE&T Hosp 1981; **Fac Appt:** Asst Prof Oph, NYU Sch Med

Goldberg, Morton MD [Oph] - **Spec Exp:** Macular Disease/Degeneration; Diabetic Eye Disease; Retinal Disorders; **Hospital:** Johns Hopkins Hosp (page 61); **Address:** Johns Hopkins Hosp, 600 N Wolfe St, Maumenee 713, Baltimore, MD 21287-9128; **Phone:** 410-955-6846; **Board Cert:** Ophthalmology 1968; **Med School:** Harvard Med Sch 1962; **Resid:** Ophthalmology, Wilmer Ophth Inst 1966; **Fellow:** Ophthalmology, Wilmer Ophth Inst 1967; Research, Johns Hopkins Hosp 1967; **Fac Appt:** Prof Oph, Johns Hopkins Univ

Guyton, David MD [Oph] - **Spec Exp:** Strabismus; Pediatric Ophthalmology; **Hospital:** Johns Hopkins Hosp (page 61); **Address:** Johns Hopkins Hosp, 600 N Wolfe, Wilmer 233, Baltimore, MD 21287; **Phone:** 410-955-8314; **Board Cert:** Ophthalmology 1977; **Med School:** Harvard Med Sch 1969; **Resid:** Ophthalmology, Johns Hopkins Hosp 1976; **Fellow:** Pediatric Ophthalmology, Baylor Coll Med 1977; **Fac Appt:** Prof Oph, Johns Hopkins Univ

Hall, Lisabeth S MD [Oph] - **Spec Exp:** Pediatric Ophthalmology; Strabismus; Eye Muscle Disorders; Cataract-Pediatric; **Hospital:** New York Eye & Ear Infirm (page 65), Lenox Hill Hosp (page 62); **Address:** 40 W 72nd St, New York, NY 10023; **Phone:** 212-979-4614; **Board Cert:** Ophthalmology 2009; **Med School:** SUNY Stony Brook 1992; **Resid:** Ophthalmology, Manhattan Eye & Ear Infirm 1996; **Fellow:** Pediatric Ophthalmology, Jules Stein Eye Inst 1997; **Fac Appt:** Asst Prof Oph, NY Med Coll

Haller, Julia Allison MD [Oph] - **Spec Exp:** Retina/Vitreous Surgery; Retinal Disorders; **Hospital:** Wills Eye Hosp; **Address:** 840 Walnut St, Ste 1510, Philadelphia, PA 19107; **Phone:** 215-928-3073; **Board Cert:** Ophthalmology 1987; **Med School:** Harvard Med Sch 1980; **Resid:** Ophthalmology, Wilmer Eye Inst/Johns Hopkins 1985; **Fellow:** Retina/Vitreous, Wilmer Eye Inst/Johns Hopkins 1986; **Fac Appt:** Prof Oph, Jefferson Med Coll

Handa, James T MD [Oph] - **Spec Exp:** Macular Degeneration; Melanoma-Choroidal (eye); Retinoblastoma; **Hospital:** Johns Hopkins Hosp (page 61); **Address:** Johns Hopkins-Wilmer Eye Inst, 1550 Orleans St, rm CRB-144, Baltimore, MD 21287; **Phone:** 410-955-3518; **Board Cert:** Ophthalmology 1991; **Med School:** Univ Pennsylvania 1986; **Resid:** Ophthalmology, Wills Eye Hosp 1990; **Fellow:** Retina/Vitreous, Duke Eye Ctr 1992; Ophthalmic Oncololgy, USC Sch Med 1993; **Fac Appt:** Assoc Prof Oph, Johns Hopkins Univ

Hersh, Peter MD [Oph] - **Spec Exp:** LASIK-Refractive Surgery; Cornea Transplant; Keratoconus; **Hospital:** Hackensack Univ Med Ctr; **Address:** 300 Frank W Burr Blvd, Ste 71, Teaneck, NJ 07666-6704; **Phone:** 201-883-0505; **Board Cert:** Ophthalmology 1987; **Med School:** Johns Hopkins Univ 1982; **Resid:** Internal Medicine, Lenox Hill Hosp 1983; Ophthalmology, Mass Eye & Ear Infirm 1986; **Fellow:** Cornea & Ext Eye Disease, Mass Eye & Ear Infirm 1987; **Fac Appt:** Prof Oph, UMDNJ-NJ Med Sch, Newark

Ho, Allen C MD [Oph] - **Spec Exp:** Retina/Vitreous Surgery; Macular Degeneration; Diabetic Eye Disease/Retinopathy; **Hospital:** Wills Eye Hosp, Abington Mem Hosp; **Address:** 910 E Willow Grove Ave, Mid Atlantic Retina, Wyndmoor, PA 19038; **Phone:** 215-233-4300; **Board Cert:** Ophthalmology 2004; **Med School:** Columbia P&S 1988; **Resid:** Ophthalmology, Wills Eye Hosp 1992; **Fellow:** Retina/Vitreous, Manhattan E&E Hosp 1994; **Fac Appt:** Prof Oph, Jefferson Med Coll

Iliff, Nicholas T MD [Oph] - **Spec Exp:** Oculoplastic Surgery; Orbital & Eyelid Tumors/Cancer; **Hospital:** Johns Hopkins Hosp (page 61); **Address:** Wilmer at Bayview Med Ctr, 4940 Eastern Ave, Baltimore, MD 21224; **Phone:** 410-550-2360; **Board Cert:** Ophthalmology 1978; **Med School:** Johns Hopkins Univ 1972; **Resid:** Ophthalmology, Johns Hopkins-Wilmer Inst 1977; **Fellow:** Retinal Surgery, Johns Hopkins-Wilmer Inst 1978; Oculoplastic & Reconstructive Surgery, Johns Hopkins-Wilmer Inst 1980; **Fac Appt:** Prof Oph, Johns Hopkins Univ

Jaafar, Mohamad S MD [Oph] - **Spec Exp:** Pediatric Ophthalmology; Strabismus-Adult & Pediatric; Glaucoma-Pediatric; **Hospital:** Chldns Natl Med Ctr, G Washington Univ Hosp; **Address:** Dept Ophthalmology, 111 Michigan Ave NW, Washington, DC 20010-2970; **Phone:** 202-476-3045; **Board Cert:** Ophthalmology 2008; **Med School:** Amer Univ Beirut 1978; **Resid:** Ophthalmology, Am Univ Beirut Med Ctr 1981; Ophthalmology, Washington Hosp Ctr 1994; **Fellow:** Pediatric Ophthalmology, Chldns Hosp 1982; Pediatric Ophthalmology, Baylor Coll Med 1983; **Fac Appt:** Prof Oph, Geo Wash Univ

Jabs, Douglas MD [Oph] - **Spec Exp:** Uveitis; **Hospital:** Mount Sinai Med Ctr (page 64); **Address:** 17 E 102 St Fl 8, New York, NY 10029; **Phone:** 212-241-6752; **Board Cert:** Ophthalmology 1982; Internal Medicine 1983; **Med School:** Johns Hopkins Univ 1977; **Resid:** Ophthalmology, Wilmer Eye Inst 1981; Internal Medicine, Johns Hopkins Hosp 1983; **Fellow:** Rheumatology, Johns Hoskins Hosp 1984; **Fac Appt:** Prof Oph, Mount Sinai Sch Med

Katowitz, James A MD [Oph] - **Spec Exp:** Oculoplastic & Orbital Surgery; Pediatric Ophthalmology; Corneal Disease & Surgery; **Hospital:** Chldns Hosp of Philadelphia, The, Hosp Univ Penn - UPHS (page 60); **Address:** Childrens Hosp, Div Ophthalmology, 34th St & Civic Center Blvd, Wood Bldg Fl 1, Philadelphia, PA 19104; **Phone:** 215-590-2791; **Board Cert:** Ophthalmology 1969; **Med School:** Univ Pennsylvania 1963; **Resid:** Ophthalmology, Hosp Univ Penn 1967; **Fellow:** Oculoplastic Surgery, Queen Victoria Hosp 1968; Oculoplastic Surgery, Moorfield Eye Hosp 1968; **Fac Appt:** Prof Oph, Univ Pennsylvania

Ophthalmology

Kidwell, Earl MD [Oph] - **Spec Exp:** Oculoplastic Surgery; **Hospital:** Howard Univ Hosp; **Address:** Ophthalmology Associates, 2041 Georgia Ave NW, Ste 2000, Washington, DC 20060; **Phone:** 202-865-1257; **Board Cert:** Ophthalmology 1978; **Med School:** Johns Hopkins Univ 1973; **Resid:** Ophthalmology, Johns Hopkins Hosp 1977; **Fellow:** Oculoplastic Surgery, Univ Miami Hosps 1978

Koller, Harold Paul MD [Oph] - **Spec Exp:** Pediatric Ophthalmology; Eye Muscle Surgery; Visual Perception & Learning Disorders; Strabismus; **Hospital:** Wills Eye Hosp, Abington Mem Hosp; **Address:** 1650 Huntington Pike, Ste 150, Meadowbrook, PA 19046-8001; **Phone:** 215-947-6660; **Board Cert:** Ophthalmology 1971; **Med School:** Tulane Univ 1964; **Resid:** Ophthalmology, Tulane Hosp Med Ctr 1968; **Fellow:** Pediatric Ophthalmology, Washington Chldn's Hosp 1970; **Fac Appt:** Clin Prof Oph, Thomas Jefferson Univ

Kupersmith, Mark MD [Oph] - **Spec Exp:** Neuro-Ophthalmology; **Hospital:** St Luke's - Roosevelt Hosp Ctr - Roosevelt Div (page 57); **Address:** 1000 10th Ave, New York, NY 10009; **Phone:** 212-870-9418; **Board Cert:** Ophthalmology 1981; Neurology 1981; **Med School:** Northwestern Univ 1974; **Resid:** Neurology, NYU Med Ctr 1978; Ophthalmology, NYU Med Ctr 1980; **Fac Appt:** Prof Oph, NYU Sch Med

Lewis, Hilel MD [Oph] - **Spec Exp:** Retinal Detachment; Diabetic Eye Disease/Retinopathy; Macular Disease/Degeneration; **Hospital:** NY-Presby Hosp/Columbia (page 66); **Address:** Edward Harkness Eye Inst, 635 W 165th St, rm 516, New York, NY 10032; **Phone:** 212-305-4606; **Board Cert:** Ophthalmology 1990; **Med School:** Mexico 1980; **Resid:** Ophthalmology, Jules Stein Eye Inst-UCLA 1986; **Fellow:** Ocular Pathology, Jules Stein Eye Inst-UCLA 1983; Vitreoretinal Surgery, Med Coll Wisconsin 1987; **Fac Appt:** Prof Oph, Columbia P&S

Liebmann, Jeffrey M MD [Oph] - **Spec Exp:** Glaucoma; Cataract Surgery; **Hospital:** New York Eye & Ear Infirm (page 65), Lenox Hill Hosp (Manh Eye, Ear & Throat Hosp) (page 62); **Address:** 121 E 60th St Fl 8, New York, NY 10022; **Phone:** 212-477-7540; **Board Cert:** Ophthalmology 1989; **Med School:** Boston Univ 1983; **Resid:** Ophthalmology, SUNY Downstate Med Ctr 1987; **Fellow:** Glaucoma, New York EE Infirmary 1988; **Fac Appt:** Clin Prof Oph, NYU Sch Med

Lisman, Richard D MD [Oph] - **Spec Exp:** Oculoplastic Surgery; Eyelid/Tear Duct Reconstruction; Eyelid Cosmetic & Reconstructive Surgery; Orbital Surgery; **Hospital:** NYU Langone Med Ctr (page 67), Lenox Hill Hosp (Manh Eye, Ear & Throat Hosp) (page 62); **Address:** 635 Park Ave, New York, NY 10021-6546; **Phone:** 212-585-1405; **Board Cert:** Ophthalmology 1981; **Med School:** NYU Sch Med 1976; **Resid:** Ophthalmology, Manhattan EE Hosp 1980; **Fellow:** Ophthalmic Plastic Surgery, NY Eye & Ear Infirmary 1981; Plastic Surgery, Manhattan EE&T Hosp 1982; **Fac Appt:** Clin Prof Oph, NYU Sch Med

Mackool, Richard J MD [Oph] - **Spec Exp:** Cataract Surgery; LASIK-Refractive Surgery; Lens Implants-Multifocal (Restor); Corneal Disease & Surgery; **Hospital:** New York Eye & Ear Infirm (page 65); **Address:** 31-27 41st St, Astoria, NY 11103; **Phone:** 718-728-3400; **Board Cert:** Ophthalmology 1975; **Med School:** Boston Univ 1968; **Resid:** Ophthalmology, New York EE Infirm 1973; **Fac Appt:** Clin Prof Oph, NYU Sch Med

Magramm, Irene MD [Oph] - **Spec Exp:** Pediatric Ophthalmology; Strabismus; Cataract Surgery; **Hospital:** Lenox Hill Hosp (Manh Eye, Ear & Throat Hosp) (page 62), New York Eye & Ear Infirm (page 65); **Address:** 225 E 64th St, New York, NY 10021; **Phone:** 212-644-5100; **Board Cert:** Ophthalmology 1987; **Med School:** Cornell Univ-Weill Med Coll 1981; **Resid:** Ophthalmology, North Shore Univ Hosp 1985; **Fellow:** Pediatric Ophthalmology, Manhattan EE&T Hosp 1986; **Fac Appt:** Asst Clin Prof Oph, Cornell Univ-Weill Med Coll

Maguire, Joseph MD [Oph] - **Spec Exp:** Retinal Disorders; **Hospital:** Wills Eye Hosp, Lankenau Hosp; **Address:** Walnut Towers Fl 10 - Ste 1020, 840 Walnut St, Philadelphia, PA 19107; **Phone:** 215-928-3300; **Board Cert:** Ophthalmology 1989; **Med School:** Jefferson Med Coll 1983; **Resid:** Ophthalmology, Wills Eye Hosp 1987; **Fellow:** Retina/Vitreous, Wills Eye Hosp 1989; Retina, Moorfields Hosp 1990; **Fac Appt:** Assoc Prof Oph, Thomas Jefferson Univ

Mandel, Eric R MD [Oph] - **Spec Exp:** LASIK-Refractive Surgery; Corneal Disease; PRK-Refractive Surgery; **Hospital:** New York Eye & Ear Infirm (page 65), Lenox Hill Hosp (page 62); **Address:** 211 E 70th St, New York, NY 10021-5106; **Phone:** 212-734-0111; **Board Cert:** Ophthalmology 1988; **Med School:** SUNY Stony Brook 1982; **Resid:** Ophthalmology, Lenox Hill Hosp 1986; **Fellow:** Cornea & Ext Eye Disease, Mass EE Infirm 1987

Medow, Norman MD [Oph] - **Spec Exp:** Cataract-Pediatric; Glaucoma-Pediatric; Corneal Disease-Pediatric; **Hospital:** Lenox Hill Hosp (Manh Eye, Ear & Throat Hosp) (page 62), NY-Presby Hosp/Weill Cornell (page 66); **Address:** 225 E 64th St, Ste 6, New York, NY 10021-6690; **Phone:** 212-644-5100; **Board Cert:** Ophthalmology 1975; **Med School:** SUNY Hlth Sci Ctr 1966; **Resid:** Ophthalmology, Manhattan EE&T Hosp 1972; **Fellow:** Cataract/Lens Implant Surgery, Charles Kelman, MD 1973; **Fac Appt:** Assoc Clin Prof Oph, Cornell Univ-Weill Med Coll

Miller, Neil MD [Oph] - **Spec Exp:** Neuro-Ophthalmology; Orbital Diseases; Thyroid Eye Disease; **Hospital:** Johns Hopkins Hosp (page 61); **Address:** Johns Hopkins - Wilmer Eye Inst, 600 N Wolfe St Maumenee Bldg - rm 127, Baltimore, MD 21287-0001; **Phone:** 410-955-8679; **Board Cert:** Ophthalmology 1976; **Med School:** Johns Hopkins Univ 1971; **Resid:** Ophthalmology, Johns Hopkins Hosp 1975; **Fellow:** Neuro-Ophthalmology, UCSF Med Ctr 1975; **Fac Appt:** Prof Oph, Johns Hopkins Univ

Mills, Monte D MD [Oph] - **Spec Exp:** Pediatric Ophthalmology; Eye Muscle Disorders; Strabismus; **Hospital:** Chldns Hosp of Philadelphia, The; **Address:** Chldns Hosp, Richard D Wood Bldg, 34th St and Civic Center Blvd, Wood Bldg Fl 1, Philadelphia, PA 19104; **Phone:** 215-590-2791; **Board Cert:** Ophthalmology 1993; **Med School:** Baylor Coll Med 1988; **Resid:** Ophthalmology, Mass E&E Infirm 1992; **Fellow:** Pediatric Ophthalmology, Chldns Hosp 1993; **Fac Appt:** Prof Oph, Univ Pennsylvania

Muldoon, Thomas O MD [Oph] - **Spec Exp:** Retina/Vitreous Surgery; Macular Disease/Degeneration; Diabetic Eye Disease/Retinopathy; **Hospital:** New York Eye & Ear Infirm (page 65); **Address:** 310 E 14th St, Ste 402, New York, NY 10003-4201; **Phone:** 212-979-4595; **Board Cert:** Ophthalmology 1971; **Med School:** Univ Rochester 1962; **Resid:** Surgery, St Lukes Hosp 1966; Ophthalmology, NY EE Infirm 1969; **Fellow:** Retinal Surgery, NY EE Infirm 1970; **Fac Appt:** Assoc Clin Prof Oph, NY Med Coll

Myers, Jonathan S MD [Oph] - **Spec Exp:** Glaucoma; **Hospital:** Wills Eye Hosp; **Address:** Wills Eye Inst, 840 Walnut St, Ste 1110, Philadelphia, PA 19107; **Phone:** 215-928-3197; **Board Cert:** Ophthalmology 2008; **Med School:** Univ Pennsylvania 1992; **Resid:** Ophthalmology, Wills Eye Hosp 1996; **Fellow:** Glaucoma, Duke Univ Med Ctr 1997; **Fac Appt:** Asst Prof Oph, Thomas Jefferson Univ

Nelson, Leonard B MD [Oph] - **Spec Exp:** Pediatric Ophthalmology; Strabismus; Eye Muscle Disorders; **Hospital:** Wills Eye Hosp; **Address:** Wills Eye Hospital, 840 Walnut St, Ste 1210, Philadelphia, PA 19107; **Phone:** 215-928-3244; **Board Cert:** Ophthalmology 1981; **Med School:** Harvard Med Sch 1976; **Resid:** Ophthalmology, Bellevue Hosp Ctr-NYU 1980; **Fellow:** Pediatric Ophthalmology, Chldns Hosp Med Ctr 1981; Ocular Disease, Johns Hopkins Hosp 1982; **Fac Appt:** Assoc Prof Oph, Jefferson Med Coll

Ophthalmology

Odel, Jeffrey G MD [Oph] - **Spec Exp:** Neuro-Ophthalmology; Retinal Disorders; Optic Nerve Disorders; **Hospital:** NY-Presby Hosp/Columbia (page 66); **Address:** Harkness Eye Institute, 635 W 165th St, rm 316, New York, NY 10032-3701; **Phone:** 212-305-5415; **Board Cert:** Ophthalmology 1981; **Med School:** Univ Rochester 1975; **Resid:** Ophthalmology, Mt Sinai Hosp 1981; **Fellow:** Ophthalmology, Bascom-Palmer Eye Inst 1977; Ophthalmology, Columbia Presby Med Ctr 1982; **Fac Appt:** Assoc Clin Prof Oph, Columbia P&S

Quigley, Harry A MD [Oph] - **Spec Exp:** Glaucoma; **Hospital:** Johns Hopkins Hosp (page 61); **Address:** 600 N Wolfe St, Maumenee B-110, Baltimore, MD 21287-9205; **Phone:** 410-955-6052; **Board Cert:** Ophthalmology 1976; **Med School:** Johns Hopkins Univ 1971; **Resid:** Ophthalmology, Wilmer Inst-Johns Hopkins Hosp 1975; **Fellow:** Ophthalmology, Bascom Palmer Eye Inst 1977; **Fac Appt:** Prof Oph, Johns Hopkins Univ

Quinn, Graham E MD [Oph] - **Spec Exp:** Pediatric Ophthalmology; Eye Growth/Development; **Hospital:** Chldns Hosp of Philadelphia, The; **Address:** Chldns Hosp of Philadelphia, Div Ophthalmology, 34th St & Civic Center Blvd, Wood Bldg Fl 1, Philadelphia, PA 19104-4399; **Phone:** 215-590-2791; **Board Cert:** Ophthalmology 1979; **Med School:** Duke Univ 1973; **Resid:** Pathology, Metro Genl Hosp 1975; Ophthalmology, Hosp Univ Penn 1978; **Fellow:** Pediatric Ophthalmology, Childrens Hosp 1979; **Fac Appt:** Prof Oph, Univ Pennsylvania

Regillo, Carl D MD [Oph] - **Spec Exp:** Retinal Disorders; **Hospital:** Wills Eye Hosp, Thomas Jefferson Univ Hosp; **Address:** 910 E Willow Grove Ave, Wyndmoor, PA 19038; **Phone:** 800-331-6634; **Board Cert:** Ophthalmology 2004; **Med School:** Harvard Med Sch 1988; **Resid:** Ophthalmology, Wills Eye Hosp 1992; **Fellow:** Retinal Surgery, Wills Eye Hosp 1994; **Fac Appt:** Prof Oph, Jefferson Med Coll

Reynolds, James D MD [Oph] - **Spec Exp:** Pediatric Ophthalmology; Strabismus; Retinopathy of Prematurity; **Hospital:** Women's & Chldn's Hosp of Buffalo, The; **Address:** Ross Eye Institute, 1176 Main St, Buffalo, NY 14209; **Phone:** 716-881-7900; **Board Cert:** Ophthalmology 1982; **Med School:** SUNY Buffalo 1978; **Resid:** Ophthalmology, Erie Co Med Ctr 1981; **Fellow:** Pediatric Ophthalmology, Pittsburgh EE Hospital 1982; **Fac Appt:** Prof Oph, SUNY Buffalo

Ritch, Robert MD [Oph] - **Spec Exp:** Glaucoma; **Hospital:** New York Eye & Ear Infirm (page 65); **Address:** 310 E 14th St, rm 304S, New York, NY 10003-4201; **Phone:** 212-477-7540; **Board Cert:** Ophthalmology 1977; **Med School:** Albert Einstein Coll Med 1972; **Resid:** Ophthalmology, Mt Sinai Hosp 1976; **Fellow:** Glaucoma, Mt Sinai Hosp 1978; **Fac Appt:** Clin Prof Oph, NY Med Coll

Schein, Oliver D MD [Oph] - **Spec Exp:** Cataract Surgery; Corneal Disease & Surgery; **Hospital:** Johns Hopkins Hosp (page 61); **Address:** Johns Hopkins Hosp, 600 N Wolfe St, Maumenee 317, Baltimore, MD 21287; **Phone:** 410-955-7677; **Board Cert:** Internal Medicine 1984; Ophthalmology 1990; **Med School:** Johns Hopkins Univ 1981; **Resid:** Internal Medicine, Johns Hopkins Hosp 1984; Ophthalmology, Mass Eye & Ear Infirm 1987; **Fellow:** Cornea & Ext Eye Disease, Mass Eye & Ear Infirm 1988; **Fac Appt:** Prof Oph, Johns Hopkins Univ

Schiff, William M MD [Oph] - **Spec Exp:** Macular Disease/Degeneration; Diabetic Eye Disease/Retinopathy; Retinal Detachment; **Hospital:** NY-Presby Hosp/Columbia (page 66), St Luke's - Roosevelt Hosp Ctr - Roosevelt Div (page 57); **Address:** Columbia Ophthalmic Consultants, 635 W 165th St, New York, NY 10032; **Phone:** 212-305-9535; **Board Cert:** Ophthalmology 2006; **Med School:** NYU Sch Med 1988; **Resid:** Ophthalmology, New York Eye & Ear Infirm 1994; **Fellow:** Retina/Vitreous, NY Hosp-Harkness Eye Inst 1996; **Fac Appt:** Assoc Prof Oph, Columbia P&S

Schuman, Joel S MD [Oph] - **Spec Exp:** Glaucoma; Cataract Surgery; **Hospital:** UPMC Presby, Pittsburgh, UPMC Shadyside; **Address:** Eye & Ear Institute, Ste 816, 203 Lothrop St, Pittsburgh, PA 15213; **Phone:** 412-647-2200; **Board Cert:** Ophthalmology 1990; **Med School:** Mount Sinai Sch Med 1984; **Resid:** Ophthalmology, Med Coll Virginia Hosps 1988; **Fellow:** Glaucoma, Mass EE Infirmary 1990; **Fac Appt:** Prof Oph, Univ Pittsburgh

Sergott, Robert C MD [Oph] - **Spec Exp:** Neuro-Ophthalmology; Optic Nerve Disorders; Glaucoma; Thyroid Eye Disease; **Hospital:** Thomas Jefferson Univ Hosp, Wills Eye Hosp; **Address:** Wills Eye Hosp, Dept Neuro-Opthalmology, 840 Walnut St Fl 9 - Ste 930, Philadelphia, PA 19107; **Phone:** 215-928-3130; **Board Cert:** Ophthalmology 1982; **Med School:** Johns Hopkins Univ 1975; **Resid:** Internal Medicine, Mary Imogene Bassett Hosp 1976; Ophthalmology, Jackson Meml Hosp 1980; **Fellow:** Ophthalmology, Jackson Meml Hosp 1980

Shabto, Uri MD [Oph] - **Spec Exp:** Retinopathy of Prematurity; Macular Disease/Degeneration; Diabetic Eye Disease/Retinopathy; **Hospital:** New York Eye & Ear Infirm (page 65), Beth Israel Med Ctr - Petrie Division (page 57); **Address:** 310 E 14th St South Bldg - Ste 419, New York, NY 10003-4201; **Phone:** 212-677-2000; **Board Cert:** Ophthalmology 1991; **Med School:** Harvard Med Sch 1986; **Resid:** Ophthalmology, NY Eye & Ear Infirm 1990; **Fellow:** Vitreoretinal Surgery, Montefiore Hosp 1991; **Fac Appt:** Asst Prof Oph, NYU Sch Med

Shields, Carol L MD [Oph] - **Spec Exp:** Orbital Tumors/Cancer; Melanoma-Choroidal (eye); Retinoblastoma; Pediatric Ophthalmology; **Hospital:** Wills Eye Hosp, Jefferson Hosp - Pittsburgh; **Address:** Wills Eye Hosp, Ocular Oncology Service, 840 Walnut St, Ste 1440, Phildelphia, PA 19107; **Phone:** 215-928-3105; **Board Cert:** Ophthalmology 1989; **Med School:** Univ Pittsburgh 1983; **Resid:** Ophthalmology, Willis Eye Hosp 1988; **Fellow:** Ophthalmic Pathology, Willis Eye Hosp 1988; Ophthalmic Oncololgy, Willis Eye Hosp 1989; **Fac Appt:** Prof Oph, Jefferson Med Coll

Shields, Jerry MD [Oph] - **Spec Exp:** Eye Tumors/Cancer; Pediatric Ophthalmology; Retinoblastoma; Melanoma-Choroidal (eye); **Hospital:** Wills Eye Hosp; **Address:** Wills Eye Hosp, Ocular Oncology Service, 840 Walnut St, Ste 1440, Philadelphia, PA 19107; **Phone:** 215-928-3105; **Board Cert:** Ophthalmology 1972; **Med School:** Univ Mich Med Sch 1964; **Resid:** Ophthalmology, Wills Eye Hosp 1970; **Fellow:** Ophthalmology, Wills Eye Hosp 1972; **Fac Appt:** Prof Oph, Thomas Jefferson Univ

Simon, John W MD [Oph] - **Spec Exp:** Pediatric Ophthalmology; Strabismus; **Hospital:** Albany Med Ctr, St Peter's Hosp - Albany; **Address:** 1220 New Scotland Rd, Ste 202, Slingerlands, NY 12159; **Phone:** 518-533-6502; **Board Cert:** Ophthalmology 1981; **Med School:** Mount Sinai Sch Med 1976; **Resid:** Ophthalmology, Mt Sinai Hosp 1980; **Fellow:** Pediatric Ophthalmology, Wills Eye Hosp 1981; **Fac Appt:** Prof Oph, Albany Med Coll

Stark, Walter J MD [Oph] - **Spec Exp:** Corneal Disease & Transplant; Cataract Surgery; Refractive Surgery; **Hospital:** Johns Hopkins Hosp (page 61); **Address:** Wilmer Eye Institute, 600 N Wolfe St Maumenee Bldg - rm 327, Baltimore, MD 21287-9238; **Phone:** 410-955-5490; **Board Cert:** Ophthalmology 1973; **Med School:** Univ Okla Coll Med 1967; **Resid:** Ophthalmology, Wilmer Inst-Johns Hopkins 1971; **Fac Appt:** Prof Oph, Johns Hopkins Univ

Stefanyszyn, Mary MD [Oph] - **Spec Exp:** Cosmetic Surgery-Eyes; Oculoplastic & Orbital Surgery; Eyelid Surgery; **Hospital:** Wills Eye Hosp; **Address:** Wills Eye Hosp, 840 Walnut St, Ste 912, Philadelphia, PA 19107; **Phone:** 215-928-3171; **Board Cert:** Ophthalmology 1983; **Med School:** Harvard Med Sch 1978; **Resid:** Ophthalmology, Wills Eye Hosp 1982; Ophthalmic Pathology, Armed Forces Inst of Pathology 1982; **Fellow:** Oculoplastic & Reconstructive Surgery, Wills Eye Hosp 1983; Orbital Surgery, Moorfields Eye Hosp 1985

Ophthalmology

Sterns, Gwen K MD [Oph] - **Spec Exp:** Geriatric Ophthalmology; Low Vision; **Hospital:** Rochester Genl Hosp, Univ of Rochester Strong Meml Hosp; **Address:** 1425 Portland Ave, Box 224, Ophthalmology Dept, Rochester, NY 14621; **Phone:** 585-922-4794; **Board Cert:** Ophthalmology 1976; **Med School:** Med Coll PA 1970; **Resid:** Ophthalmology, Nassau Co Med Ctr 1974; **Fellow:** Ophthalmology, Colum-Presby Eye Inst 1975

Vander, James F MD [Oph] - **Spec Exp:** Diabetic Eye Disease; Retinal Disorders; Macular Degeneration; **Hospital:** Wills Eye Hosp; **Address:** 910 E Willow Grove Ave, Mid Atlantic Retina, Wyndmoor, PA 19038-7910; **Phone:** 215-233-4300; **Board Cert:** Ophthalmology 1989; **Med School:** Univ Mich Med Sch 1984; **Resid:** Ophthalmology, Univ Michigan Med Ctr 1988; **Fellow:** Retina/Vitreous, Wills Eye Hosp 1990; **Fac Appt:** Prof Oph, Thomas Jefferson Univ

Walsh, Joseph B MD [Oph] - **Spec Exp:** Diabetic Eye Disease; Macular Degeneration; Retinal Disorders; **Hospital:** New York Eye & Ear Infirm (page 65), Beth Israel Med Ctr - Petrie Division (page 57); **Address:** 310 E 14th St Bldg S Fl 3, New York, NY 10003-4201; **Phone:** 212-979-4500; **Board Cert:** Ophthalmology 2005; **Med School:** Georgetown Univ 1966; **Resid:** Internal Medicine, Univ Hosp 1968; Ophthalmology, NY Eye & Ear Infirm 1973; **Fellow:** Retina, Montefiore Med Ctr 1974; **Fac Appt:** Prof Oph, NY Med Coll

Wang, Frederick MD [Oph] - **Spec Exp:** Pediatric Ophthalmology; Strabismus; Eye Muscle Disorders; **Hospital:** New York Eye & Ear Infirm (page 65), Montefiore Med Ctr - Div. Moses; **Address:** 30 E 40th St, Ste 405, New York, NY 10016-1201; **Phone:** 212-684-3980; **Board Cert:** Pediatrics 1978; Ophthalmology 1980; **Med School:** Albert Einstein Coll Med 1972; **Resid:** Pediatrics, Jacobi Med Ctr 1974; Ophthalmology, Albert Einstein 1979; **Fellow:** Pediatric Ophthalmology, Children's Hosp Natl Med Ctr 1980; **Fac Appt:** Clin Prof Oph, Albert Einstein Coll Med

Yannuzzi, Lawrence MD [Oph] - **Spec Exp:** Retina/Vitreous Surgery; Macular Disease/Degeneration; Diabetic Eye Disease; **Hospital:** Lenox Hill Hosp (Manh Eye, Ear & Throat Hosp) (page 62); **Address:** 460 Park Ave Fl 5, New York, NY 10021-4028; **Phone:** 212-861-9797; **Board Cert:** Ophthalmology 1970; **Med School:** Boston Univ 1964; **Resid:** Ophthalmology, Manhattan EE&T Hosp 1968; **Fellow:** Ophthalmology, Manhattan EE&T Hosp 1971; **Fac Appt:** Clin Prof Oph, Columbia P&S

Zaidman, Gerald MD [Oph] - **Spec Exp:** Laser Vision Surgery; Cornea Transplant; Cataract Surgery; **Hospital:** Westchester Med Ctr, Montefiore Med Ctr - Div. North; **Address:** Westchester Med Ctr, Macy Pavilion, Dept Opth, rm 1100, Valhalla, NY 10595; **Phone:** 914-493-1599; **Board Cert:** Ophthalmology 1981; **Med School:** Albert Einstein Coll Med 1975; **Resid:** Ophthalmology, Beth Abraham Hosp 1977; Ophthalmology, Lenox Hill Hosp 1980; **Fellow:** Cornea & Ext Eye Disease, Univ Pittsburgh 1982; **Fac Appt:** Assoc Prof Oph, NY Med Coll

Southeast

Alfonso, Eduardo MD [Oph] - **Spec Exp:** Corneal Disease & Surgery; Cornea Transplant & Artificial Cornea; Cataract Surgery; Eye Infections; **Hospital:** Bascom Palmer Eye Inst (page 55), Jackson Meml Hosp (page 70); **Address:** Bascom Palmer Eye Institute, 900 NW 17th St, Miami, FL 33136-1119; **Phone:** 305-326-6366; **Board Cert:** Ophthalmology 1985; **Med School:** Yale Univ 1980; **Resid:** Ophthalmology, Bascom Palmer Eye Inst 1984; **Fellow:** Cornea, Mass Eye & Ear Hosp 1986; Ophthalmological Pathology, Mass Eye & Ear Hosp 1986; **Fac Appt:** Prof Oph, Univ Miami Sch Med

Buckley, Edward G MD [Oph] - **Spec Exp:** Pediatric Ophthalmology; Strabismus; Cataract-Pediatric; **Hospital:** Duke Univ Med Ctr; **Address:** 2351 Erwin Rd, Durham, NC 27705; **Phone:** 919-684-6084; **Board Cert:** Ophthalmology 2007; **Med School:** Duke Univ 1977; **Resid:** Ophthalmology, Duke Univ Eye Ctr 1981; **Fellow:** Ophthalmology, Bascom Palmer Eye Inst 1983; **Fac Appt:** Prof Oph, Duke Univ

Budenz, Donald L MD [Oph] - **Spec Exp:** Glaucoma; **Hospital:** Bascom Palmer Eye Inst (page 55); **Address:** Bascom Palmer Eye Inst, 900 NW 17th St, Ste 341, Miami, FL 33136; **Phone:** 305-326-6384; **Board Cert:** Ophthalmology 2003; **Med School:** Harvard Med Sch 1987; **Resid:** Ophthalmology, Scheie Eye Inst 1991; **Fellow:** Glaucoma, Bascom Palmer Eye Inst 1992; **Fac Appt:** Assoc Prof Oph, Univ Miami Sch Med

Capo, Hilda MD [Oph] - **Spec Exp:** Pediatric Ophthalmology; Strabismus; Neuro-Ophthalmology; **Hospital:** Bascom Palmer Eye Inst (page 55); **Address:** Bascom Palmer Eye Institute, 900 NW 17th St, Miami, FL 33136; **Phone:** 305-326-6555; **Board Cert:** Ophthalmology 1989; **Med School:** Puerto Rico 1982; **Resid:** Ophthalmology, Univ Puerto Rico Affil Hosp 1987; **Fellow:** Neuro-Ophthalmology, NYU Med Ctr 1989; Pediatric Ophthalmology, Johns Hopkins Hosp 1988; **Fac Appt:** Clin Prof Oph, Univ Miami Sch Med

Culbertson, William MD [Oph] - **Spec Exp:** LASIK-Refractive Surgery; Corneal Disease & Surgery; Cataract Surgery; **Hospital:** Bascom Palmer Eye Inst (page 55); **Address:** Bascom Palmer Eye Institute, 900 NW 17th St, Miami, FL 33136-1119; **Phone:** 305-243-2020; **Board Cert:** Ophthalmology 1976; **Med School:** Emory Univ 1970; **Resid:** Ophthalmology, Vanderbilt Univ Hosp 1974; **Fellow:** Cornea & Ext Eye Disease, Bascom Palmer Eye Inst 1979; **Fac Appt:** Prof Oph, Univ Miami Sch Med

Dutton, Jonathan J MD/PhD [Oph] - **Spec Exp:** Oculoplastic Surgery; Eye Tumors/Cancer; Melanoma-Choroidal (eye); **Hospital:** Univ NC Hosps; **Address:** Univ North Carolina - Dept Ophthalmology, 130 Mason Farm Rd, 5156 Bioinformatics, CB 7040, Chapel Hill, NC 27599; **Phone:** 919-966-5296; **Board Cert:** Ophthalmology 1983; **Med School:** Washington Univ, St Louis 1977; **Resid:** Ophthalmology, Washington Univ Med Ctr 1982; **Fellow:** Oculoplastic Surgery, Univ Iowa Med Ctr 1983; **Fac Appt:** Prof Oph, Univ NC Sch Med

Flynn Jr, Harry W MD [Oph] - **Spec Exp:** Retina/Vitreous Surgery; Diabetic Eye Disease/Retinopathy; **Hospital:** Bascom Palmer Eye Inst (page 55), Univ of Miami Hosp & Clins/Sylvester Comp Canc Ctr (page 70); **Address:** Bascom Palmer Eye Institute, 900 NW 17th St, Miami, FL 33136-1119; **Phone:** 305-326-6118; **Board Cert:** Ophthalmology 1976; **Med School:** Univ VA Sch Med 1971; **Resid:** Ophthalmology, Univ Virginia Hosp 1975; **Fellow:** Retina, Pacific Med Ctr 1976; **Fac Appt:** Prof Oph, Univ Miami Sch Med

Forster, Richard K MD [Oph] - **Spec Exp:** Cornea Transplant; Cataract Surgery; **Hospital:** Bascom Palmer Eye Inst (page 55); **Address:** Bascom Palmer Eye Institute, 900 NW 17th St, Miami, FL 33136; **Phone:** 305-243-2020; **Board Cert:** Ophthalmology 1971; **Med School:** Boston Univ 1963; **Resid:** Ophthalmology, Bascom Palmer Eye Inst 1969; **Fellow:** Ophthalmology, Fl Proctor Fdn/UCSF 1970; **Fac Appt:** Prof Oph, Univ Miami Sch Med

Freedman, Sharon F MD [Oph] - **Spec Exp:** Pediatric Ophthalmology; Glaucoma-Pediatric; Strabismus; Retinopathy of Prematurity; **Hospital:** Duke Univ Med Ctr; **Address:** Duke Eye Center, DUMC 3082, Durham, NC 27710-0001; **Phone:** 919-684-4584; **Board Cert:** Ophthalmology 1991; **Med School:** Harvard Med Sch 1985; **Resid:** Ophthalmology, Mass Eye & Ear Infirm 1989; **Fellow:** Pediatric Ophthalmology, Childns Hosp 1990; Glaucoma, Duke Eye Ctr 1992; **Fac Appt:** Prof Oph, Duke Univ

Ophthalmology

Glaser, Joel MD [Oph] - **Spec Exp:** Neuro-Ophthalmology; Orbital Diseases; **Hospital:** Cleveland Clin - Weston, Univ of Miami Hosp (page 71); **Address:** 4701 N Meridian Ave, Adams Bldg - Ste 500 A, Miami Beach, FL 33140; **Phone:** 305-532-2885; **Board Cert:** Ophthalmology 1968; **Med School:** Duke Univ 1963; **Resid:** Ophthalmology, Univ Miami Med Coll 1965; **Fellow:** Neuro-Ophthalmology, UCSF Med Ctr 1970; **Fac Appt:** Prof Oph, Univ Miami Sch Med

Gorovoy, Mark S MD [Oph] - **Spec Exp:** Corneal Disease & Transplant; Cataract Surgery; Glaucoma; LASIK-Refractive Surgery; **Hospital:** Lee Memorial Hlth Systems; **Address:** 12381 S Cleveland Ave, Ste 300, Fort Myers, FL 33907; **Phone:** 239-939-1444; **Board Cert:** Ophthalmology 1982; **Med School:** Geo Wash Univ 1973; **Resid:** Ophthalmology, George Washington Univ Hosp 1980; **Fellow:** Cornea & Ext Eye Disease, Univ Florida 1982

Grossniklaus, Hans E MD [Oph] - **Spec Exp:** Ophthalmic Pathology; Melanoma-Choroidal (eye); Macular Disease/Degeneration; Retinal Disorders; **Hospital:** Emory Univ Hosp; **Address:** Emory Clinic - LF Montgomery Lab, 1365-B Clifton Rd NE, rm BT428, Atlanta, GA 30322; **Phone:** 404-778-4611; **Board Cert:** Ophthalmology 1985; Anatomic Pathology 1987; **Med School:** Ohio State Univ 1980; **Resid:** Ophthalmology, Case West Res Univ Hosp 1984; Pathology, Case West Res Univ Hosp 1987; **Fellow:** Ophthalmological Pathology, Johns Hopkins Hosp 1985; **Fac Appt:** Prof Oph, Emory Univ

Haik, Barrett MD [Oph] - **Spec Exp:** Eye Tumors/Cancer; Orbital Diseases; **Hospital:** St Jude Children's Research Hosp; **Address:** Univ Tenn Med Group, Ophthamology, 930 Madison Ave, Ste 200, Memphis, TN 38103-3452; **Phone:** 901-448-6650; **Board Cert:** Ophthalmology 1981; **Med School:** Louisiana State U, New Orleans 1976; **Resid:** Ophthalmology, Columbia-Presby/Harkness Eye Inst 1980; **Fac Appt:** Prof Oph, Univ Tenn Coll Med, Memphis

Hess, J Bruce MD [Oph] - **Spec Exp:** Pediatric Ophthalmology; Strabismus; **Hospital:** All Children's Hosp, Bayfront Med Ctr; **Address:** 880 6th St S, Ste 350, St Petersburg, FL 33701; **Phone:** 727-767-4393; **Board Cert:** Ophthalmology 1978; **Med School:** Baylor Coll Med 1971; **Resid:** Ophthalmology, Geisinger Med Ctr 1977; **Fellow:** Ophthalmology, Wills Eye Hosp 1978; **Fac Appt:** Assoc Prof Oph, Univ S Fla Coll Med

Holliday, James N MD/PhD [Oph] - **Spec Exp:** Glaucoma; Diabetic Eye Disease; Dry Eye Syndrome; Uveitis in Rheumatoid Disease; **Hospital:** St Francis Hosp - Memphis, Baptist Memorial Hospital - Memphis; **Address:** 4571 Summer Ave, Memphis, TN 38122; **Phone:** 901-680-0043; **Board Cert:** Ophthalmology 2005; **Med School:** Duke Univ 1987; **Resid:** Ophthalmology, UC Irvine Med Ctr 1992; **Fellow:** Anterior Segment - External Disease, Mayo Clinic 1993

Kerr, Natalie C MD [Oph] - **Spec Exp:** Pediatric Ophthalmology; Strabismus-Pediatric; Cataract-Pediatric; Genetic Disorders-Eye; **Hospital:** Le Bonheur Chldns Med Ctr, St Jude Children's Research Hosp; **Address:** Hamilton Eye Inst, 930 Madison Ave, Ste 200, Memphis, TN 38103; **Phone:** 901-448-6650; **Board Cert:** Ophthalmology 2003; **Med School:** Univ Fla Coll Med 1987; **Resid:** Ophthalmology, Univ Florida Affil Hosp 1991; **Fellow:** Pediatric Ophthalmology, Univ Tennessee Affil Hosp 1992; **Fac Appt:** Prof Oph, Univ Tenn Coll Med, Memphis

Lambert, Scott R MD [Oph] - **Spec Exp:** Pediatric Ophthalmology; Strabismus; Cataract-Pediatric; **Hospital:** Chldns Hlthcare Atlanta @ Egleston, Emory Univ Hosp; **Address:** Emory Eye Ctr, Dept Ped Opth, 1365 Clifton Rd B Bldg - Ste 4513, Atlanta, GA 30322; **Phone:** 404-778-3431; **Board Cert:** Ophthalmology 1989; **Med School:** Yale Univ 1983; **Resid:** Ophthalmology, UCSF Med Ctr 1987; **Fellow:** Pediatric Ophthalmology, Hosp for Sick Chldn 1988; Strabismus, Smith Kuttlewell 1988; **Fac Appt:** Prof Oph, Emory Univ

Lee, Paul P MD [Oph] - **Spec Exp:** Glaucoma; **Hospital:** Duke Univ Med Ctr; **Address:** Duke Univ Eye Ctr, DUMC Box 3082, 2351 Erwin Rd, Durham, NC 27710; **Phone:** 919-681-3937; **Board Cert:** Ophthalmology 1991; **Med School:** Univ Mich Med Sch 1986; **Resid:** Ophthalmology, Wilmer Eye Inst/Johns Hopkins 1990; **Fellow:** Glaucoma, Mass EE Infirm 1991; **Fac Appt:** Prof Oph, Duke Univ

McKeown, Craig A MD [Oph] - **Spec Exp:** Pediatric Ophthalmology; Strabismus-Adult & Pediatric; Eye Muscle Disorders; **Hospital:** Bascom Palmer Eye Inst (page 55); **Address:** Bascom Palmer Eye Institute, 900 NW 17th St, Miami, FL 33136; **Phone:** 305-243-2020; **Board Cert:** Ophthalmology 1982; **Med School:** Northwestern Univ 1971; **Resid:** Ophthalmology, Walter Reed Med Ctr 1980; **Fellow:** Pediatric Ophthalmology, Chldns Hosp Natl Med Ctr 1984; Pediatric Ophthalmology, Wilmer Inst-Johns Hospkins 1985; **Fac Appt:** Assoc Clin Prof Oph, Univ Miami Sch Med

Meredith, Travis A MD [Oph] - **Spec Exp:** Retina/Vitreous Surgery; Macular Degeneration; Diabetic Eye Disease/Retinopathy; **Hospital:** Univ NC Hosps; **Address:** 5151 Bio Informatics, CB#7040, Chapel Hill, NC 27599-7040; **Phone:** 919-966-5296; **Board Cert:** Ophthalmology 1976; **Med School:** Johns Hopkins Univ 1969; **Resid:** Ophthalmology, Wilmer Inst-Johns Hopkins 1971; Ophthalmology, Wilmer Inst-Johns Hopkins 1975; **Fellow:** Vitreoretinal Surgery, Med Coll Wisconsin 1976; **Fac Appt:** Prof Oph, Univ NC Sch Med

Murray, Timothy MD [Oph] - **Spec Exp:** Retinal Disorders; Eye Tumors/Cancer; **Hospital:** Bascom Palmer Eye Inst (page 55); **Address:** Bascom Palmer Eye Inst, 900 NW 17th St, rm 254, Miami, FL 33136-1119; **Phone:** 305-326-6166; **Board Cert:** Ophthalmology 1990; **Med School:** Johns Hopkins Univ 1985; **Resid:** Ophthalmology, UCSF Med Ctr 1989; **Fellow:** Ophthalmology, UCSF 1999; Ophthalmology, Med Coll Wisconsin 1991; **Fac Appt:** Prof Oph, Univ Miami Sch Med

Nussbaum, Julian MD [Oph] - **Spec Exp:** Diabetic Eye Disease/Retinopathy; Macular Degeneration; Retinopathy of Prematurity; **Hospital:** Med Coll of GA Hosp and Clin (MCG Health Inc); **Address:** Med Coll Georgia, 1120 15th St BA Bldg - rm 2701, Augusta, GA 30912; **Phone:** 706-721-1148; **Board Cert:** Ophthalmology 1981; **Med School:** Univ Miami Sch Med 1976; **Resid:** Internal Medicine, Jackson Memorial Hosp 1977; Ophthalmology, Med Coll Georgia 1980; **Fellow:** Vitreoretinal Surgery, Mass Eye & Ear Infirmary 1982; **Fac Appt:** Prof Oph, Med Coll GA

Palmberg, Paul F MD/PhD [Oph] - **Spec Exp:** Glaucoma; **Hospital:** Bascom Palmer Eye Inst (page 55); **Address:** Bascom Palmer Eye Inst, 900 NW 17th St, Miami, FL 33136; **Phone:** 305-243-2020; **Board Cert:** Ophthalmology 1976; **Med School:** Northwestern Univ 1970; **Resid:** Ophthalmology, Barnes Hosp 1974; Ophthalmology, Barnes Hosp 1977; **Fellow:** Glaucoma, Washington Univ 1976; **Fac Appt:** Prof Oph, Univ Miami Sch Med

Parrish, Richard K MD [Oph] - **Spec Exp:** Glaucoma; Cataract Surgery; Anterior Segment Surgery; **Hospital:** Bascom Palmer Eye Inst (page 55), Jackson Meml Hosp (page 70); **Address:** Bascom Palmer Eye Institute, 900 NW 17th St, Miami, FL 33136; **Phone:** 305-243-2020; **Board Cert:** Ophthalmology 1981; **Med School:** Indiana Univ 1976; **Resid:** Ophthalmology, Wills Eye Hosp 1980; **Fellow:** Glaucoma, Bascom Palmer Eye Inst 1982; **Fac Appt:** Prof Oph, Univ Miami Sch Med

Patrinely, James R MD [Oph] - **Spec Exp:** Ophthalmic Plastic Surgery; Eyelid Surgery; Orbital Surgery; **Hospital:** Methodist Hosp - Houston, St Luke's Episcopal Hosp-Houston; **Address:** 5147 N 9th Ave, Ste 203, Pensacola, FL 32504; **Phone:** 850-473-0990; **Board Cert:** Ophthalmology 2002; **Med School:** Vanderbilt Univ 1980; **Resid:** Ophthalmology, Bayloy College Med 1984; **Fellow:** Ophthalmological Pathology, Johns Hopkins Hosp 1985; Ophthalmic Plastic & Reconstructive Surgery, Univ Utah Med Ctr 1986; **Fac Appt:** Clin Prof Oph, Baylor Coll Med

Ophthalmology

Perez, Victor Lucas MD [Oph] - **Spec Exp:** Cornea & External Eye Disease; Cornea Transplant; Cataract Surgery-Lens Implant; Uveitis; **Hospital:** Bascom Palmer Eye Inst (page 55); **Address:** 900 NW 17 St, Miami, FL 33136; **Phone:** 305-243-2020; **Board Cert:** Ophthalmology 2001; **Med School:** Univ Puerto Rico 1991; **Resid:** Ophthalmology, Mass Eye & Ear Infirmary 2000; **Fellow:** Immunology, Brigham & Women's Hosp 1996; Cornea, Mass Eye & Ear Infirmary 2002; **Fac Appt:** Assoc Prof Oph, Univ Miami Sch Med

Pollard, Zane F MD [Oph] - **Spec Exp:** Pediatric Ophthalmology; Strabismus; Tear Duct Problems; **Hospital:** Chldns Hlthcare Atlanta - Scottish Rite, Piedmont Hosp; **Address:** 5445 Meridian Mark Rd, Ste 220, Atlanta, GA 30342-4722; **Phone:** 404-255-2419; **Board Cert:** Ophthalmology 1975; **Med School:** Tulane Univ 1966; **Resid:** Surgery, UCSF Med Ctr 1968; Ophthalmology, USC Med Ctr 1973; **Fellow:** Pediatric Ophthalmology, Wills Eye Hosp 1975

Rosenfeld, Philip J MD/PhD [Oph] - **Spec Exp:** Macular Disease/Degeneration; Diabetic Eye Disease/Retinopathy; Retinal Detachment; Retina/Vitreous Surgery; **Hospital:** Bascom Palmer Eye Inst (page 55); **Address:** Bascom Palmer Eye Institute, 900 NW 17th St, Miami, FL 33136; **Phone:** 305-243-2020; **Board Cert:** Ophthalmology 2008; **Med School:** Johns Hopkins Univ 1988; **Resid:** Ophthalmology, Mass Eye & Ear Infirm 1995; **Fellow:** Retina, Bascom Palmer Eye Inst 1996; **Fac Appt:** Prof Oph, Univ Fla Coll Med

Sherwood, Mark B MD [Oph] - **Spec Exp:** Glaucoma; **Hospital:** Shands at Univ of FL; **Address:** Shands at Univ Florida, Dept Ophthalmology, 1600 SW Archer Rd, Box 100284, Gainesville, FL 32610; **Phone:** 352-273-8708; **Med School:** England, UK 1976; **Resid:** Ophthalmology, Moorefield's Eye Hosp 1980; **Fellow:** Glaucoma, Wills Eye Hosp 1982; Glaucoma, Moorefield's Eye Hosp 1983; **Fac Appt:** Prof Oph, Univ Fla Coll Med

Sternberg Jr, Paul MD [Oph] - **Spec Exp:** Retina/Vitreous Surgery; Macular Degeneration; Eye Tumors/Cancer; **Hospital:** Vanderbilt Univ Med Ctr, Vanderbilt Children's Hosp; **Address:** Vanderbilt Eye Institute, 2311 Pierce Ave, Nashville, TN 37232-8808; **Phone:** 615-936-1453; **Board Cert:** Ophthalmology 1985; **Med School:** Univ Chicago-Pritzker Sch Med 1979; **Resid:** Ophthalmology, Johns Hopkins Hosp 1983; **Fellow:** Vitreoretinal Surgery, Duke Univ Med Ctr 1984; **Fac Appt:** Prof Oph, Vanderbilt Univ

Stulting, R Doyle MD [Oph] - **Spec Exp:** Laser Vision Surgery; Cataract Surgery; Corneal Disease & Transplant; **Hospital:** Emory Univ Hosp; **Address:** The Emory Clinic, Dept Ophthalmology, 1365 Clifton Rd NE, Ste 4500, Atlanta, GA 30322; **Phone:** 404-778-2020; **Board Cert:** Ophthalmology 1982; **Med School:** Duke Univ 1976; **Resid:** Internal Medicine, Barnes Hosp 1978; Ophthalmology, Bascom Palmer Eye Inst 1981; **Fellow:** Cornea, Emory Univ 1982; **Fac Appt:** Prof Oph, Emory Univ

Tse, David MD [Oph] - **Spec Exp:** Oculoplastic Surgery; Orbital Tumors/Cancer; Lacrimal Gland Disorders; Eyelid Tumors/Cancer; **Hospital:** Bascom Palmer Eye Inst (page 55), Jackson Meml Hosp (page 70); **Address:** Bascom Palmer Eye Inst, 900 NW 17th St, Miami, FL 33136-1119; **Phone:** 305-326-6086; **Board Cert:** Ophthalmology 2002; **Med School:** Univ Miami Sch Med 1976; **Resid:** Ophthalmology, LAC/USC Med Ctr 1981; **Fellow:** Oculoplastic Surgery, Univ Iowa Hosps 1982; **Fac Appt:** Prof Oph, Univ Miami Sch Med

Wang, Ming X MD/PhD [Oph] - **Spec Exp:** Laser Vision Surgery; Anterior Segment Surgery; Corneal Disease; **Hospital:** Saint Thomas Hosp - Nashville; **Address:** 1801 West End Ave, Palmer Plaza, Ste 1150, Nashville, TN 37203; **Phone:** 615-321-8881; **Board Cert:** Ophthalmology 1998; **Med School:** Harvard Med Sch 1991; **Resid:** Ophthalmology, Wills Eye Hosp 1996; **Fellow:** Refractive Surgery, Bascom Palmer Eye Inst 1997; **Fac Appt:** Asst Prof Oph, Vanderbilt Univ

Waring III, George O MD [Oph] - **Spec Exp:** LASIK-Refractive Surgery; Cataract Surgery; Lens Implants; **Hospital:** Northside Hosp; **Address:** 301 Perimeter Center N, Ste 600, Atlanta, GA 30346; **Phone:** 678-222-5102; **Board Cert:** Ophthalmology 1975; **Med School:** Baylor Coll Med 1967; **Resid:** Ophthalmology, Wills Eye Hosp 1973; **Fellow:** Cornea & Ext Eye Disease, Wills Eye Hosp 1974

Wilson Jr, Marion E MD [Oph] - **Spec Exp:** Cataract-Pediatric; Strabismus; Lens Implants-Pediatric; Pediatric Ophthalmology; **Hospital:** MUSC Chldns Hosp; **Address:** MUSC Storm Eye Inst, 167 Ashley Ave, PO Box 250676, Charleston, SC 29425; **Phone:** 843-792-7622; **Board Cert:** Ophthalmology 1987; **Med School:** Med Univ SC 1980; **Resid:** Ophthalmology, Natl Naval Med Ctr 1986; **Fellow:** Pediatric Ophthalmology, Chldns Hosp - Naval Med Ctr 1987; **Fac Appt:** Prof Oph, Med Univ SC

Wilson, Matthew W MD [Oph] - **Spec Exp:** Eye Tumors/Cancer; Retinoblastoma; Melanoma-Choroidal (eye); **Hospital:** St Jude Children's Research Hosp, Methodist Univ Hosp - Memphis; **Address:** Univ Tenn Med Grp, Ophthalmology, 930 Madison Ave, Ste 200, Memphis, TN 38103; **Phone:** 901-448-6650; **Board Cert:** Ophthalmology 2007; **Med School:** Emory Univ 1990; **Resid:** Ophthalmology, Emory Univ Med Ctr 1994; Ophthalmic Pathology, Emory Univ Med Ctr 1995; **Fellow:** Ocular Oncology, Moorfields Eye Hosp 1996; Ophthalmic Plastic & Reconstructive Surgery, Casey Eye Inst 1998; **Fac Appt:** Assoc Prof Oph, Univ Tenn Coll Med, Memphis

Yeatts, R Patrick MD [Oph] - **Spec Exp:** Oculoplastic Surgery; Orbital Tumors/Cancer; Eyelid Tumors/Cancer; Orbital Diseases; **Hospital:** Wake Forest Univ Baptist Med Ctr (page 72); **Address:** Wake Forest Univ Eye Ctr, Janeway Clinical Sciences Bldg Fl 6, Medical Ctr Blvd, Winston-Salem, NC 27157; **Phone:** 336-716-4091; **Board Cert:** Ophthalmology 1983; **Med School:** Wake Forest Univ 1978; **Resid:** Ophthalmology, Mayo Clinic 1982; **Fellow:** Oculoplastic & Reconstructive Surgery, Mass Eye & Ear Infirmary 1983; **Fac Appt:** Prof Oph, Wake Forest Univ

Midwest

Abrams, Gary W MD [Oph] - **Spec Exp:** Retina/Vitreous Surgery; **Hospital:** Hutzel Hosp - Detroit; **Address:** Kresge Eye Institute, 4717 St Antoine St, Detroit, MI 48201; **Phone:** 313-577-8900; **Board Cert:** Ophthalmology 1977; **Med School:** Univ Okla Coll Med 1968; **Resid:** Ophthalmology, Med Coll Wisc Affil Hosps 1976; **Fellow:** Vitreoretinal Surgery, Bascom Palmer Eye Inst 1978; **Fac Appt:** Prof Oph, Wayne State Univ

Albert, Daniel M MD [Oph] - **Spec Exp:** Eye Tumors/Cancer; Ophthalmic Pathology; **Hospital:** Univ WI Hosp & Clins; **Address:** 2880 University Ave, Madison, WI 53705; **Phone:** 608-263-7171; **Board Cert:** Ophthalmology 1969; **Med School:** Univ Pennsylvania 1962; **Resid:** Ophthalmology, Hosp Univ Penn 1966; Neuro-Ophthalmology, Natl Inst Hlth 1968; **Fellow:** Pathology, Armed Forces Inst Path 1969; **Fac Appt:** Prof Oph, Univ Wisc

Alward, Wallace MD [Oph] - **Spec Exp:** Glaucoma; **Hospital:** Univ Iowa Hosp & Clinics, VA Med Ctr - Iowa City; **Address:** 200 Hawkins Drive, Iowa City, IA 52242-1009; **Phone:** 319-356-3938; **Board Cert:** Ophthalmology 2006; **Med School:** Ohio State Univ 1976; **Resid:** Ophthalmology, Univ Louisville 1986; **Fellow:** Glaucoma, Univ Miami-Bascom Palmer Eye Inst 1987; **Fac Appt:** Prof Oph, Univ Iowa Coll Med

Archer, Steven M MD [Oph] - **Spec Exp:** Pediatric Ophthalmology; **Hospital:** Univ Michigan Hlth Sys; **Address:** Kellogg Eye Ctr, 1000 Wall St, Ann Arbor, MI 48105-1912; **Phone:** 734-764-7558; **Board Cert:** Ophthalmology 1986; **Med School:** Univ Chicago-Pritzker Sch Med 1978; **Resid:** Ophthalmology, Univ Chicago 1984; **Fellow:** Pediatric Ophthalmology, Indiana Univ 1986; **Fac Appt:** Asst Prof Oph, Univ Mich Med Sch

Ophthalmology

Augsburger, James MD [Oph] - **Spec Exp:** Eye Tumors/Cancer; Melanoma-Choroidal (eye); Retinoblastoma; **Hospital:** Univ Hosp - Cincinnati, Cincinnati Chldns Hosp Med Ctr; **Address:** Medical Arts Bldg, Ste 1500, 222 Piedmont Ave, rm ML 665-E, Cincinnati, OH 45267-0665; **Phone:** 513-475-7300; **Board Cert:** Ophthalmology 1979; **Med School:** Univ Cincinnati 1974; **Resid:** Ophthalmology, Univ Hosp-Cincinnati 1978; **Fellow:** Ocular Oncology, Wills Eye Hosp 1980; **Fac Appt:** Prof Oph, Univ Cincinnati

Azar, Dimitri T MD [Oph] - **Spec Exp:** Cornea Transplant; Cornea & External Eye Disease; Refractive Surgery; **Hospital:** Univ of IL at Chicago Eye & Ear Infirm, Univ of IL Med Ctr at Chicago; **Address:** Univ of Illinois, 30 N Michigan, Ste 410, Chicago, IL 60602; **Phone:** 312-996-2020; **Board Cert:** Ophthalmology 1991; **Med School:** Lebanon 1983; **Resid:** Ophthalmology, American Univ Med Ctr 1986; Ophthalmology, Mass E&E Infirm 1991; **Fellow:** Cornea & Ext Eye Disease, Mass E&E Infirm 1988; Cornea Research, Harvard Med Sch 1991

Baker, John D MD [Oph] - **Spec Exp:** Pediatric Ophthalmology; **Hospital:** Chldns Hosp of Michigan; **Address:** 2355 Monroe Blvd, Dearborn, MI 48124-3009; **Phone:** 313-561-1777; **Board Cert:** Ophthalmology 1974; **Med School:** Wayne State Univ 1967; **Resid:** Ophthalmology, Detroit Genl Hosp 1971; **Fellow:** Pediatric Ophthalmology, Chldns Natl Med Ctr 1972; **Fac Appt:** Clin Prof Oph, Wayne State Univ

Burke, Miles J MD [Oph] - **Spec Exp:** Pediatric Ophthalmology; Eye Muscle Surgery; Amblyopia & Vision Development; Tear Duct Problems; **Hospital:** Cincinnati Chldns Hosp Med Ctr, Jewish Hosp - Kenwood - Cincinnati; **Address:** 10475 Montgomery Rd, Ste 4F, Cincinnati, OH 45242-5200; **Phone:** 513-984-4949; **Board Cert:** Ophthalmology 1979; **Med School:** Univ Ariz Coll Med 1974; **Resid:** Ophthalmology, Univ Michigan Med Ctr 1978; **Fellow:** Pediatric Ophthalmology, Wills Eye Hosp 1979

Carter, Keith D MD [Oph] - **Spec Exp:** Oculoplastic & Orbital Surgery; Eyelid Surgery; Botox Therapy; **Hospital:** Univ Iowa Hosp & Clinics; **Address:** Univ Iowa, Dept Ophthalmology, 200 Hawkins Dr, PFP 11136-F, Iowa City, IA 52242; **Phone:** 319-356-2852; **Board Cert:** Ophthalmology 1988; **Med School:** Indiana Univ 1983; **Resid:** Ophthalmology, Univ Michigan Med Ctr 1987; **Fellow:** Oculoplastic Surgery, Univ Iowa 1988; **Fac Appt:** Prof Oph, Univ Iowa Coll Med

Del Monte, Monte A MD [Oph] - **Spec Exp:** Pediatric Ophthalmology; Strabismus-Adult & Pediatric; Glaucoma-Pediatric; Cataract-Pediatric; **Hospital:** Univ Michigan Hlth Sys; **Address:** Kellogg Eye Center, 1000 Wall St, Ann Arbor, MI 48105-1912; **Phone:** 734-764-3111; **Board Cert:** Ophthalmology 1982; **Med School:** Johns Hopkins Univ 1974; **Resid:** Pediatrics, Chldns Hosp Med Ctr 1977; Ophthalmology, Wilmer Eye Inst 1981; **Fellow:** Ophthalmology, Wilmer Eye Inst 1978; Pediatric Ophthalmology, Chldns Hosp 1981; **Fac Appt:** Prof Oph, Univ Mich Med Sch

Elner, Victor H MD/PhD [Oph] - **Spec Exp:** Eyelid Tumors/Cancer; Orbital Tumors/Cancer; **Hospital:** Univ Michigan Hlth Sys; **Address:** Kellogg Eye Ctr, 1000 Wall St, Ann Arbor, MI 48105; **Phone:** 734-763-9142; **Board Cert:** Ophthalmology 1983; Pathology 1988; **Med School:** Univ Chicago-Pritzker Sch Med 1979; **Resid:** Ophthalmology, Univ Chicago 1982; Pathology, Univ Chicago 1984; **Fellow:** Ophthalmological Pathology, Armed Forces Inst 1985; Ophthalmic Plastic & Reconstructive Surgery, Univ Wisconsin 1987; **Fac Appt:** Prof Oph, Univ Mich Med Sch

Feder, Robert S MD [Oph] - **Spec Exp:** Corneal Disease; LASIK-Refractive Surgery; Cataract Surgery; **Hospital:** Northwestern Meml Hosp; **Address:** 675 N St Clair St, Fl 15, Chicago, IL 60611-5975; **Phone:** 312-695-8150; **Board Cert:** Ophthalmology 1983; **Med School:** Northwestern Univ 1978; **Resid:** Ophthalmology, Barnes Hosp 1982; **Fellow:** Cornea & Ext Eye Disease, Univ Iowa Med Ctr 1983; **Fac Appt:** Assoc Prof Oph, Northwestern Univ

Greenwald, Mark MD [Oph] - **Spec Exp:** Pediatric Ophthalmology; **Hospital:** Univ of Chicago Med Ctr; **Address:** Dept Ophthalmology, 5841 S Maryland Ave, MC 2114, Chicago, IL 60637; **Phone:** 773-834-5685; **Board Cert:** Ophthalmology 1981; **Med School:** Harvard Med Sch 1976; **Resid:** Ophthalmology, Univ Illinois Hosp 1980; **Fellow:** Pediatric Ophthalmology, Chldns Hosp 1981; **Fac Appt:** Assoc Prof Oph, Univ Wash

Harbour, J William MD [Oph] - **Spec Exp:** Eye Tumors/Cancer; Melanoma-Choroidal (eye); Retinoblastoma; **Hospital:** Barnes-Jewish Hosp, St Louis Chldns Hosp; **Address:** 1600 S Brentwood, Ste 800, St Louis, MO 63144; **Phone:** 314-367-1278 x2156; **Board Cert:** Ophthalmology 2007; **Med School:** Johns Hopkins Univ 1990; **Resid:** Ophthalmology, Wills Eye Hosp 1994; **Fellow:** Retina/Vitreous, Bascom Palmer Eye Inst 1995; Ocular Oncology, UCSF Med Ctr 1996; **Fac Appt:** Prof Oph, Washington Univ, St Louis

Heckenlively, John R MD [Oph] - **Spec Exp:** Eye Diseases-Hereditary; Retinal Disorders; Opthalmic Genetics; **Hospital:** Univ Michigan Hlth Sys; **Address:** MI Kellogg Eye Ctr, 1000 Wall St, Ann Arbor, MI 48105; **Phone:** 734-763-2280; **Board Cert:** Ophthalmology 1977; **Med School:** Univ Colorado 1972; **Resid:** Ophthalmology, Univ KY 1976; **Fellow:** Vitreoretinal Disease, Jules Stein Eye Inst 1977; Johns Hopkins Hosp 1978; **Fac Appt:** Prof Oph, Univ Mich Med Sch

Heuer, Dale K MD [Oph] - **Spec Exp:** Glaucoma; **Hospital:** Froedtert Meml Lutheran Hosp; **Address:** The Eye Institute, 925 N 87th St, Milwaukee, WI 53226; **Phone:** 414-456-2020; **Board Cert:** Ophthalmology 1983; **Med School:** Northwestern Univ 1978; **Resid:** Ophthalmology, Med Coll Wisc Affil Hosp 1982; **Fellow:** Glaucoma, Bascom Palmer Eye Inst 1984; **Fac Appt:** Prof Oph, Med Coll Wisc

Holland, Edward J MD [Oph] - **Spec Exp:** Corneal Disease; Refractive Surgery; Cataract Surgery; **Hospital:** St Elizabeth Med Ctr (South Unit), Bethesda North Hosp; **Address:** 1945 CEI Drive, Cincinnati, OH 45242; **Phone:** 513-984-5133; **Board Cert:** Ophthalmology 1986; **Med School:** Loyola Univ-Stritch Sch Med 1981; **Resid:** Ophthalmology, Univ Minn Med Ctr 1985; **Fellow:** Cornea & Ext Eye Disease, Univ Iowa 1986; Ocular Immunology, Natl Eye Inst 1987; **Fac Appt:** Clin Prof Oph, Univ Cincinnati

John, Thomas MD [Oph] - **Spec Exp:** Cornea Transplant & Artificial Cornea; Amniotic Membrane Transplant; Cataract Surgery; Refractive Surgery; **Hospital:** Loyola Univ Med Ctr, Adv S Suburban Hosp; **Address:** 16532 S Oak Park Ave, Ste 201, Tinley Park, IL 60477; **Phone:** 708-429-2223; **Board Cert:** Ophthalmology 1987; **Med School:** India 1977; **Resid:** Ophthalmology, Hosp Univ Penn 1984; **Fellow:** Cornea & Ext Eye Disease, Univ Rochester Sch Med & Dentistry 1985; Cornea & Ext Eye Disease, Mass Eye & Ear Infirmary 1987; **Fac Appt:** Assoc Clin Prof Oph, Loyola Univ-Stritch Sch Med

Kaufman, Paul L MD [Oph] - **Spec Exp:** Glaucoma; **Hospital:** Univ WI Hosp & Clins; **Address:** Univ Wisconsin Hosp, Dept Ophthalmology, 3310 University Ave, Ste 206, Madison, WI 53705-2135; **Phone:** 608-263-7171; **Board Cert:** Ophthalmology 1976; **Med School:** NYU Sch Med 1967; **Resid:** Ophthalmology, Barnes Hosp 1973; **Fellow:** Ocular Pharmacology, Univ Uppsala 1975; **Fac Appt:** Prof Oph, Univ Wisc

Krachmer, Jay H MD [Oph] - **Spec Exp:** Corneal Disease; **Hospital:** Univ Minn Med Ctr, Fairview - Univ Campus; **Address:** Dept Ophthalmology, 420 Delaware St SE, MMC 88, Minneapolis, MN 55455; **Phone:** 612-625-4400; **Board Cert:** Ophthalmology 1972; **Med School:** Tulane Univ 1966; **Resid:** Ophthalmology, Univ Hosp 1970; **Fellow:** Cornea, Wills Eye Hosp 1974; **Fac Appt:** Prof Oph, Univ Minn

Ophthalmology

Krueger, Ronald MD [Oph] - **Spec Exp:** Corneal Disease; Refractive Surgery; **Hospital:** Cleveland Clin Fdn (page 56); **Address:** Cleveland Clinic Fdn - Cole Eye Inst, 9500 Euclid Ave, Desk i32, Cleveland, OH 44195; **Phone:** 216-444-8158; **Board Cert:** Ophthalmology 2003; **Med School:** UMDNJ-NJ Med Sch, Newark 1987; **Resid:** Ophthalmology, Columbia Presby Med Ctr 1991; **Fellow:** Refractive Surgery, Univ Okla Hlth Sci Ctr-McGee Eye Inst 1992; Cornea, USC-Doheny Eye Inst 1993

Kushner, Burton J MD [Oph] - **Spec Exp:** Pediatric Ophthalmology; Strabismus-Adult & Pediatric; **Hospital:** Univ WI Hosp & Clins; **Address:** Dept Ophth-UNW Hosp, 2870 University Ave, Ste 102, Madison, WI 53705; **Phone:** 608-263-7171; **Board Cert:** Ophthalmology 1975; **Med School:** Northwestern Univ 1969; **Resid:** Ophthalmology, Univ Wisc Hosp 1973; **Fellow:** Pediatric Ophthalmology, Bascom Palmer Eye Inst 1974; **Fac Appt:** Prof Oph, Univ Wisc

Lane, Stephen S MD [Oph] - **Spec Exp:** Laser Vision Surgery; Cataract Surgery; **Hospital:** United Hosp; **Address:** Associated Eye Care, 2950 Curve Crest Blvd, Stillwater, MN 55082; **Phone:** 651-275-3000; **Board Cert:** Ophthalmology 1986; **Med School:** Univ Minn 1980; **Resid:** Ophthalmology, MS Hershey Med Ctr 1984; **Fellow:** Cornea & Ext Eye Disease, Univ Minn 1984; **Fac Appt:** Clin Prof Oph, Univ Minn

Lichter, Paul R MD [Oph] - **Spec Exp:** Cataract Surgery; Glaucoma; **Hospital:** Univ Michigan Hlth Sys; **Address:** 1000 Wall St, WK Kellogg Eye Ctr, Ann Arbor, MI 48105; **Phone:** 734-763-5874; **Board Cert:** Ophthalmology 1970; **Med School:** Univ Mich Med Sch 1964; **Resid:** Ophthalmology, Univ Mich Med Ctr 1968; **Fellow:** Ophthalmology, UCSF Med Ctr 1969; **Fac Appt:** Prof Oph, Univ Mich Med Sch

Lindstrom, Richard L MD [Oph] - **Spec Exp:** Corneal Disease; Cataract Surgery; Refractive Surgery; **Hospital:** Abbott - Northwestern Hosp, Phillips Eye Inst; **Address:** 9801 DuPont Ave, Bloomington, MN 55443; **Phone:** 612-813-3600; **Board Cert:** Ophthalmology 1978; **Med School:** Univ Minn 1972; **Resid:** Ophthalmology, Univ Minn 1979; Ophthalmology, Univ Minn 1980; **Fellow:** Anterior Segment - External Disease, Mary Shields Eye Hosp; Glaucoma, Univ Hosps; **Fac Appt:** Prof Oph, Univ Minn

Lueder, Gregg T MD [Oph] - **Spec Exp:** Retinoblastoma; Eye Tumors-Pediatric; Pediatric Ophthalmology; **Hospital:** St Louis Chldns Hosp; **Address:** St Louis Children's Hospital, One Children's Pl, Ste 2S89, St Louis, MO 63110; **Phone:** 314-454-6026; **Board Cert:** Ophthalmology 2003; **Med School:** Univ Iowa Coll Med 1985; **Resid:** Pediatrics, St Louis Children's Hosp 1988; Ophthalmology, Univ Iowa Med Ctr 1991; **Fellow:** Pediatric Ophthalmology, Hosp for Sick Children 1993; **Fac Appt:** Assoc Prof Oph, Washington Univ, St Louis

Maguire, Leo J MD [Oph] - **Spec Exp:** Cornea Transplant; Refractive Surgery; **Hospital:** Mayo Med Ctr & Clin - Rochester; **Address:** Mayo Clin, Dept Ophthalmology, 200 First St SW, Rochester, MN 55905; **Phone:** 507-284-4152; **Board Cert:** Ophthalmology 1986; **Med School:** Jefferson Med Coll 1980; **Resid:** Ophthalmology, Univ Michigan Med Ctr 1984; **Fellow:** Cornea & Ext Eye Disease, LSU Eye Ctr 1986; **Fac Appt:** Assoc Prof Oph, Mayo Med Sch

Mets, Marilyn MD [Oph] - **Spec Exp:** Pediatric Ophthalmology; Ophthalmic Genetics; Strabismus; Retinal Disorders; **Hospital:** Children's Mem Hosp; **Address:** 2300 Children's Plaza, Box 70, Chicago, IL 60614; **Phone:** 773-880-4020; **Board Cert:** Ophthalmology 2005; **Med School:** Geo Wash Univ 1976; **Resid:** Ophthalmology, Cleveland Clinic Fdn 1980; **Fellow:** Pediatric Ophthalmology, Natl Chldns Hosp 1981; **Fac Appt:** Prof Oph, Northwestern Univ

Mieler, William F MD [Oph] - **Spec Exp:** Retina/Vitreous Surgery; Eye Tumors/Cancer; Macular Disease/Degeneration; **Hospital:** Univ of IL Med Ctr at Chicago, Weiss Meml Hosp; **Address:** Univ Chicago, Dept Opth & Vis Sci, 1855 E Taylor St, MS 648, Chicago, IL 60637; **Phone:** 773-702-3838; **Board Cert:** Ophthalmology 1984; **Med School:** Univ Wisc 1979; **Resid:** Ophthalmology, Bascom-Palmer Eye Inst 1983; **Fellow:** Vitreoretinal Surgery & Disease, Med Ctr Wisconsin Eye Inst 1984; Oculoplastic Surgery, Wills Eye Hosp 1986; **Fac Appt:** Prof Oph, Univ IL Coll Med

Mizen, Thomas R MD [Oph] - **Spec Exp:** Neuro-Ophthalmology; Optic Nerve Disorders; **Hospital:** Rush Univ Med Ctr; **Address:** 1725 W Harrison St, Ste 928, Chicago, IL 60612-3862; **Phone:** 312-942-3500; **Board Cert:** Ophthalmology 1986; **Med School:** Finch/Chicago Med Sch 1980; **Resid:** Ophthalmology, Rush-Presby-St Lukes Med Ctr 1984; **Fellow:** Neuro-Ophthalmology, Barnes Hosp/Wash Univ 1985; **Fac Appt:** Asst Prof Oph, Rush Med Coll

Nerad, Jeffrey MD [Oph] - **Spec Exp:** Orbital Tumors/Cancer; Eyelid Cancer & Reconstruction; Oculoplastic Surgery; **Address:** Cincinnati Eye Institute, 1945 CEI Drive, Cincinnati, OH 45242; **Phone:** 513-984-5133; **Board Cert:** Ophthalmology 1984; **Med School:** St Louis Univ 1979; **Resid:** Ophthalmology, St Louis Univ Med Ctr 1983; **Fellow:** Oculoplastic & Reconstructive Surgery, Univ Iowa 1984; **Fac Appt:** Prof Oph, Univ Iowa Coll Med

Nunery, William R MD [Oph] - **Spec Exp:** Orbital Surgery; Oculoplastic Surgery; Thyroid Eye Disease; **Hospital:** Univ of Louisville Hosp, Methodist Hosp - Indianapolis; **Address:** Oculofacial Plastic & Orbital Surgery, 8801 N Meridian St, Ste 207, Indianapolis, IN 46260; **Phone:** 502-889-1000; **Board Cert:** Ophthalmology 1980; **Med School:** Case West Res Univ 1975; **Resid:** Ophthalmology, Indiana Univ Hosp 1979; **Fellow:** Ophthalmic Plastic Surgery, Emory Univ 1980

Olitsky, Scott E MD [Oph] - **Spec Exp:** Pediatric Ophthalmology; Strabismus; **Hospital:** Chldns Mercy Hosps & Clinics; **Address:** Chldns Mercy Hosp, Dept Oph, 2401 Gillham Rd, Kansas City, MO 64108; **Phone:** 816-234-3046; **Board Cert:** Ophthalmology 2004; **Med School:** Jefferson Med Coll 1988; **Resid:** Ophthalmology, SUNY Buffalo Med Ctr 1992; **Fellow:** Pediatric Ophthalmology, Wills Eye Hosp 1993; **Fac Appt:** Prof Oph, Univ MO-Kansas City

Osher, Robert H MD [Oph] - **Spec Exp:** Cataract Surgery-Lens Implant; **Address:** 1945 CEI Drive, Cincinnati, OH 45242; **Phone:** 513-984-5133; **Board Cert:** Ophthalmology 1981; **Med School:** Univ Rochester 1976; **Resid:** Ophthalmology, Bascom Palmer Eye Inst 1980; **Fellow:** Ophthalmology, Wills Eye Hosp 1977; Ophthalmology, Bascom Palmer Eye Inst 1981; **Fac Appt:** Prof Oph, Univ Cincinnati

Pepose, Jay MD [Oph] - **Spec Exp:** LASIK-Refractive Surgery; Cataract Surgery; Corneal & External Eye Disease; **Hospital:** Barnes-Jewish Hosp, St John's Mercy Med Ctr - St Louis; **Address:** 1815 Clarkson Rd, Chesterfield, MO 63017; **Phone:** 636-728-0111; **Board Cert:** Ophthalmology 1989; **Med School:** UCLA 1982; **Resid:** Ophthalmology, Johns Hopkins Hosp 1987; **Fellow:** Cornea & Ext Eye Disease, Georgetown Univ Med Ctr 1988; **Fac Appt:** Prof Oph, Washington Univ, St Louis

Plager, David A MD [Oph] - **Spec Exp:** Pediatric Ophthalmology; Strabismus; Cataract-Pediatric; Glaucoma-Pediatric; **Hospital:** Riley Hosp for Children; **Address:** Riley Outpatient Ctr-Ophthalmology, 702 Barnhill Drive, Ste 3340, Indianapolis, IN 46202-5133; **Phone:** 317-274-8103; **Board Cert:** Ophthalmology 2006; **Med School:** Indiana Univ 1983; **Resid:** Ophthalmology, Indiana Univ Hosps 1987; **Fellow:** Pediatric Ophthalmology, Chldns Hosp Natl Med Ctr 1988; **Fac Appt:** Prof Oph, Indiana Univ

Ophthalmology

Pulido, Jose S MD [Oph] - **Spec Exp:** Retina/Vitreous Surgery; Eye Tumors/Cancer; **Hospital:** Mayo Med Ctr & Clin - Rochester; **Address:** 200 1st St SW, Rochester, MN 55905; **Phone:** 507-284-3721; **Board Cert:** Ophthalmology 1986; **Med School:** Tulane Univ 1981; **Resid:** Ophthalmology, Illinois Eye & Ear Infirm 1986; **Fellow:** Vitreoretinal Surgery & Disease, Bascom-Palmer Eye Inst 1987; Ocular Oncology, Wills Eye Hosp; **Fac Appt:** Prof Oph, Mayo Med Sch

Putterman, Allen M MD [Oph] - **Spec Exp:** Oculoplastic & Orbital Surgery; Cosmetic Surgery-Face & Eyes; Thyroid Eye Disease; **Hospital:** St Joseph Hosp, Univ of IL Med Ctr at Chicago; **Address:** 111 N Wabash Ave, Ste 1722, Chicago, IL 60602-2002; **Phone:** 312-372-2256; **Board Cert:** Ophthalmology 1971; **Med School:** Univ Wisc 1963; **Resid:** Ophthalmology, Michael Reese Hosp 1969; **Fellow:** Oculoplastic Surgery, Manhattan Eye/Ear Infirm 1970; **Fac Appt:** Prof Oph, Univ IL Coll Med

Rogers, Gary L MD [Oph] - **Spec Exp:** Strabismus-Adult & Pediatric; **Hospital:** Nationwide Chldn's Hosp; **Address:** 555 S 18th St, Ste 4C, Columbus, OH 43205; **Phone:** 614-224-6222; **Board Cert:** Ophthalmology 1974; **Med School:** Ohio State Univ 1968; **Resid:** Ophthalmology, Mt Sinai Hosp 1972; **Fellow:** Pediatric Ophthalmology, Chldns Hosp Natl Med Ctr 1974; **Fac Appt:** Clin Prof Oph, Ohio State Univ

Rosenberg, Michael A MD [Oph] - **Spec Exp:** Refractive Surgery; Cataract Surgery; Eye Muscle Surgery; **Hospital:** Northwestern Meml Hosp; **Address:** Northwestern Med Fac Fdn, 675 N St Clair St, Ste 15-150, Chicago, IL 60611-5967; **Phone:** 312-695-8150; **Board Cert:** Ophthalmology 1975; **Med School:** Northwestern Univ 1967; **Resid:** Ophthalmology, Bascom Palmer Eye Inst 1973; **Fellow:** Neuro-Ophthalmology, UCSF Med Ctr 1974; Refractive Surgery, Univ Monterrey 1998; **Fac Appt:** Assoc Clin Prof Oph, Northwestern Univ

Samuelson, Thomas W MD [Oph] - **Spec Exp:** Glaucoma; Cataract Surgery; Anterior Segment Surgery; Refractive Surgery; **Hospital:** Phillips Eye Inst, Regions Hosp - St Paul; **Address:** Minnesota Eye Consultants, 710 E 24th St, Ste 100, Minneapolis, MN 55404-3810; **Phone:** 612-813-3600; **Board Cert:** Ophthalmology 1991; **Med School:** Univ Minn 1985; **Resid:** Ophthalmology, Univ S Florida 1990; **Fellow:** Glaucoma, Wills Eye Hosp 1991; **Fac Appt:** Assoc Clin Prof Oph, Univ Minn

Schachat, Andrew P MD [Oph] - **Spec Exp:** Retina/Vitreous Surgery; Diabetic Eye Disease/Retinopathy; Melanoma-Choroidal (eye); **Hospital:** Cleveland Clin Fdn (page 56); **Address:** The Cleveland Clinic Fdn, Cole Eye Inst, 9500 Euclid Ave, Desk i30, Cleveland, OH 44195; **Phone:** 216-444-7963; **Board Cert:** Ophthalmology 1983; **Med School:** Johns Hopkins Univ 1979; **Resid:** Ophthalmology, Wilmer Inst-John Hopkins Hosp 1982; **Fellow:** Vitreoretinal Surgery & Disease, Wilmer Eye Inst-Johns Hopkins Hosp 1983; **Fac Appt:** Prof Oph

Stone, Edwin MD [Oph] - **Spec Exp:** Retinal Disorders; Eye Diseases-Hereditary; **Hospital:** Univ Iowa Hosp & Clinics; **Address:** Dept Ophthalmology, 200 Hawkins Dr, PFP 11136-F, Iowa City, IA 52242; **Phone:** 319-356-2852; **Board Cert:** Ophthalmology 1990; **Med School:** Baylor Coll Med 1985; **Resid:** Ophthalmology, Univ Iowa Hosps 1989; **Fellow:** Retina, Univ Iowa Hosps 1992; **Fac Appt:** Prof Oph, Univ Iowa Coll Med

Summers, C Gail MD [Oph] - **Spec Exp:** Eye Diseases-Hereditary; Albinism; **Hospital:** Univ Minn Med Ctr, Fairview - Univ Campus; **Address:** Dept Ophthalmology, 420 Delaware St SE, MMC 493, Minneapolis, MN 55455-0356; **Phone:** 612-625-4400; **Board Cert:** Ophthalmology 1984; **Med School:** Univ Minn 1979; **Resid:** Ophthalmology, Univ Minnesota Med Ctr 1983; **Fellow:** Pediatric Ophthalmology, Unin Minnesota Med Ctr 1984; **Fac Appt:** Prof Oph, Univ Minn

Traboulsi, Elias Iskan MD [Oph] - **Spec Exp:** Pediatric Ophthalmology; Glaucoma-Pediatric; **Hospital:** Cleveland Clin Fdn (page 56); **Address:** Cleveland Clinic Fdn, Cole Eye Inst, 9500 Euclid Ave, Desk i32, Cleveland, OH 44195; **Phone:** 216-444-4363; **Board Cert:** Clinical Genetics 1987; Ophthalmology 1991; **Med School:** Amer Univ Beirut 1982; **Resid:** Ophthalmology, American Univ Beirut Hosp 1985; Ophthalmology, Georgetown Hosp 1989; **Fellow:** Ophthalmology, Johns Hopkins Hosp 1986; Pediatric Ophthalmology, Chldns Hosp Natl Med Ctr 1990; **Fac Appt:** Prof Oph, Ohio State Univ

Trese, Michael T MD [Oph] - **Spec Exp:** Retina/Vitreous Surgery; Retinal Disorders-Pediatric; **Hospital:** William Beaumont Hosp, Chldns Hosp of Michigan; **Address:** 3535 W 13 Mile Rd, Ste 344, Royal Oak, MI 48073-6710; **Phone:** 248-288-2280; **Board Cert:** Ophthalmology 1981; **Med School:** Georgetown Univ 1976; **Resid:** Ophthalmology, Jules Stein Eye Inst-UCLA 1980; **Fellow:** Retina, Duke Univ Med Ctr 1981; **Fac Appt:** Assoc Clin Prof Oph, Wayne State Univ

Trobe, Jonathan Daniel MD [Oph] - **Spec Exp:** Neuro-Ophthalmology; Optic Nerve Disorders; **Hospital:** Univ Michigan Hlth Sys; **Address:** WK Kellogg Eye Ctr, 1000 Wall St, Ann Arbor, MI 48105-1912; **Phone:** 734-763-9142; **Board Cert:** Ophthalmology 1974; Neurology 1988; **Med School:** Harvard Med Sch 1968; **Resid:** Ophthalmology, Wills Eye Hosp 1972; Neurology, Jackson Meml Hosp/U Miami 1986; **Fellow:** Neuro-Ophthalmology, Bascom Palmer Eye Inst 1977; **Fac Appt:** Prof Oph, Univ Mich Med Sch

Tychsen, Lawrence MD [Oph] - **Spec Exp:** Pediatric Ophthalmology; Strabismus; Amblyopia; **Hospital:** St Louis Chldns Hosp, Barnes-Jewish Hosp; **Address:** Chldns Eye Care Ctr, 1 Children's Pl, Ste 2 South 89, St Louis, MO 63110; **Phone:** 314-454-6026; **Board Cert:** Ophthalmology 1984; **Med School:** Georgetown Univ 1979; **Resid:** Ophthalmology, Univ Iowa Hosp 1983; **Fellow:** Pediatric Ophthalmology, UCSF Med Ctr 1985; **Fac Appt:** Assoc Prof Oph, Washington Univ, St Louis

Weingeist, Thomas A MD/PhD [Oph] - **Spec Exp:** Retinal Disorders; Eye Tumors/Cancer; **Hospital:** Univ Iowa Hosp & Clinics; **Address:** Univ Iowa, Dept Ophthalmology, 200 Hawkins Drive, Iowa City, IA 52242; **Phone:** 319-356-2864; **Board Cert:** Ophthalmology 1976; **Med School:** Univ Iowa Coll Med 1972; **Resid:** Ophthalmology, Univ Iowa Hosp 1975; **Fellow:** Vitreoretinal Surgery, Univ Iowa 1976; **Fac Appt:** Prof Oph, Univ Iowa Coll Med

Williams, George A MD [Oph] - **Spec Exp:** Retinal Disorders; Macular Degeneration; **Hospital:** William Beaumont Hosp; **Address:** Associated Retinal Consultants, 3535 W 13 Mile Rd MOB Bldg - Ste 344, Royal Oak, MI 48073; **Phone:** 248-288-2280; **Board Cert:** Ophthalmology 2005; **Med School:** Northwestern Univ 1978; **Resid:** Ophthalmology, Med Coll Wisconsin 1982; **Fellow:** Retina/Vitreous, Med Coll Wisconsin 1984; **Fac Appt:** Clin Prof Oph, Univ Mich Med Sch

Wilson, Steven E MD [Oph] - **Spec Exp:** PRK-Refractive Surgery; Corneal Disease; **Hospital:** Cleveland Clin Fdn (page 56); **Address:** Cleveland Clinic Fdn - Cole Eye Inst, 9500 Euclid Ave, Ste I32, Cleveland, OH 44195; **Phone:** 216-444-5887; **Board Cert:** Ophthalmology 1990; **Med School:** UCSD 1984; **Resid:** Ophthalmology, Mayo Clinic 1988; **Fellow:** Refractive Surgery, Med Ctr Louisiana-LSU 1990; **Fac Appt:** Prof Oph, Case West Res Univ

Younge, Brian R MD [Oph] - **Spec Exp:** Neuro-Ophthalmology; Temporal Arteritis; Ocular Palsies; **Hospital:** Mayo Med Ctr & Clin - Rochester; **Address:** Mayo Clin, Dept Ophthalmology, 200 First St SW, Rochester, MN 55905-0001; **Phone:** 507-284-4567; **Board Cert:** Ophthalmology 1974; **Med School:** Univ Alberta 1965; **Resid:** Ophthalmology, Montreal Genl Hosp 1972; **Fellow:** Neuro-Ophthalmology, Mayo Clin 1974; **Fac Appt:** Prof Oph, Mayo Med Sch

Ophthalmology

Great Plains and Mountains

Anderson, Richard L MD [Oph] - **Spec Exp:** Orbital & Eyelid Tumors/Cancer; Eyelid Problems/Ptosis/Blepharospasm; Cosmetic Surgery-Face & Eyes; **Hospital:** Salt Lake Regional Med Ctr, Intermountain Shriners Hosp; **Address:** 1002 E South Temple, Ste 308, Salt Lake City, UT 84102-1525; **Phone:** 801-363-3355; **Board Cert:** Ophthalmology 1976; **Med School:** Univ Iowa Coll Med 1971; **Resid:** Ophthalmology, Univ Iowa Hosps-Clins 1975; **Fellow:** Oculoplastic & Reconstructive Surgery, Albany Med Ctr 1975; Oculoplastic & Reconstructive Surgery, UCSF Med Ctr 1976; **Fac Appt:** Prof PlS, Univ Utah

Crandall, Alan S MD [Oph] - **Spec Exp:** Glaucoma; Cataract Surgery; **Hospital:** Univ Utah Hosps and Clins; **Address:** Moran Eye Ctr- Univ Utah Hosp, 65 N Mario Cappecchi Drive, Salt Lake City, UT 84132; **Phone:** 801-581-2352; **Board Cert:** Ophthalmology 1977; **Med School:** Univ Utah 1973; **Resid:** Ophthalmology, Hosp Univ Penn 1976; **Fellow:** Glaucoma, Scheie Eye Inst; **Fac Appt:** Clin Prof Oph, Univ Utah

Durrie, Daniel MD [Oph] - **Spec Exp:** LASIK-Refractive Surgery; Corneal Disease; **Hospital:** Univ of Kansas Hosp; **Address:** 5520 College Blvd, Ste 201, Leawood, KS 66211; **Phone:** 913-491-3330; **Board Cert:** Ophthalmology 1979; **Med School:** Univ Nebr Coll Med 1975; **Resid:** Ophthalmology, Univ Nebr Med Coll Affil Hosp 1979; **Fellow:** Cornea, Filkins Eye Inst 1980; **Fac Appt:** Clin Prof Oph, Univ Kans

Gigantelli, James W MD [Oph] - **Spec Exp:** Orbital Tumors/Cancer; Eyelid Cancer & Reconstruction; Lymphoma-Ocular (eye); **Hospital:** Nebraska Med Ctr; **Address:** Univ Nebraska Med Ctr, Ophthalmology, 985540 Nebraska Medical Ctr, Omaha, NE 68198-5540; **Phone:** 402-559-4276; **Board Cert:** Ophthalmology 1991; **Med School:** Vanderbilt Univ 1985; **Resid:** Ophthalmology, Baylor Coll Med 1989; **Fellow:** Oculoplastic Surgery, Duke Unv Med Ctr 1990; **Fac Appt:** Assoc Prof Oph, Univ Nebr Coll Med

Southwest

Ellis Jr, George S MD [Oph] - **Spec Exp:** Pediatric Ophthalmology; Eye Muscle Disorders; **Hospital:** Children's Hospital - New Orleans, E Jefferson Genl Hosp; **Address:** Children's Hospital, 200 Henry Clay Ave, Ste 3106, New Orleans, LA 70118; **Phone:** 504-896-9426; **Board Cert:** Ophthalmology 1982; **Med School:** Tulane Univ 1977; **Resid:** Ophthalmology, Duke Univ-Eye Ctr 1982; Pediatric Ophthalmology, Hall Eye Clinic 1982; **Fellow:** Pediatric Ophthalmology, Chldns Hosp 1983; **Fac Appt:** Assoc Clin Prof Oph, Tulane Univ

Esmaeli-Azad, Bita MD [Oph] - **Spec Exp:** Orbital & Eyelid Tumors/Cancer; Eyelid Cancer & Reconstruction; Oculoplastic Surgery; **Hospital:** UT MD Anderson Cancer Ctr; **Address:** Dept of Head & Neck Surgery, Ophthalmology Section, 1515 Holcombe Blvd, Ste 1445, Houston, TX 77030; **Phone:** 713-792-6523; **Board Cert:** Ophthalmology 2006; **Med School:** Ros Franklin Univ/Chicago Med Sch 1990; **Resid:** Ophthalmology, Univ Michigan Affil Hosp 1994; **Fellow:** Ophthalmic Plastic & Reconstructive Surgery, Univ Toronto Affil Hosp 1996; **Fac Appt:** Assoc Prof Oph, Univ Tex, Houston

Eustis, Horatio S MD [Oph] - **Spec Exp:** Pediatric Ophthalmology; **Hospital:** Ochsner Fdn Hosp; **Address:** Ochsner Clinic, Dept Oph, 1514 Jefferson Hwy, Fl 10, New Orleans, LA 70121; **Phone:** 504-842-3995; **Board Cert:** Ophthalmology 1985; **Med School:** Louisiana State U, New Orleans 1980; **Resid:** Ophthalmology, LSU Eye Ctr 1984; **Fellow:** Pediatric Ophthalmology, Hosp Sick Chldn 1985; Pediatric Ophthalmology, Chldns Hosp; **Fac Appt:** Clin Prof Oph, Louisiana State U, New Orleans

Holladay, Jack T MD [Oph] - **Spec Exp:** LASIK-Refractive Surgery; PRK-Refractive Surgery; **Hospital:** Park Plaza Hosp; **Address:** Holladay LASIK Institute, 6802 Mapleridge, Ste 200, Houston, TX 77401; **Phone:** 713-668-7337; **Board Cert:** Ophthalmology 1979; **Med School:** Univ Tex, Houston 1974; **Resid:** Ophthalmology, Univ Texas Hlth Sci Ctr 1978; **Fac Appt:** Clin Prof Oph, Baylor Coll Med

Koch, Douglas D MD [Oph] - **Spec Exp:** Cataract Surgery; Refractive Surgery; **Hospital:** Methodist Hosp - Houston; **Address:** 7200 Cambridge St, Houston, TX 77030-2704; **Phone:** 713-798-6100; **Board Cert:** Ophthalmology 1982; **Med School:** Harvard Med Sch 1977; **Resid:** Ophthalmology, Baylor Coll Med 1981; **Fellow:** Cornea, Moorfields Eye Hosp 1982; Refractive Surgery, Baylor Coll Med 1982; **Fac Appt:** Prof Oph, Baylor Coll Med

Lambert, H Michael MD [Oph] - **Spec Exp:** Retina/Vitreous Surgery; Macular Disease/Degeneration; Diabetic Eye Disease/Retinopathy; **Hospital:** Methodist Hosp - Houston, St Luke's Episcopal Hosp-Houston; **Address:** 2727 Gramercy, Ste 200, Houston, TX 77025-1633; **Phone:** 713-799-9975; **Board Cert:** Ophthalmology 1983; **Med School:** Baylor Coll Med 1977; **Resid:** Ophthalmology, Wilford Hall USAF Med Ctr 1982; **Fellow:** Vitreoretinal Surgery, Duke Univ Eye Ctr 1983; **Fac Appt:** Assoc Clin Prof Oph, Baylor Coll Med

Lee, Andrew G MD [Oph] - **Spec Exp:** Neuro-Ophthalmology; Optic Nerve Disorders; Optic Nerve Tumors; **Hospital:** Methodist Hosp - Houston; **Address:** Methodist Hosp, Dept Ophthalmology, 6560 Fannin St, Ste 2100, Houston, TX 77030; **Phone:** 713-441-8821; **Board Cert:** Ophthalmology 2006; **Med School:** Univ VA Sch Med 1989; **Resid:** Ophthalmology, Cullen Eye Inst-Baylor 1993; **Fellow:** Neuro-Ophthalmology, Wilmer Eye Inst-Johns Hopkins 1994; **Fac Appt:** Prof Oph, Univ Iowa Coll Med

Lewis, Richard Alan MD [Oph] - **Spec Exp:** Eye Diseases-Hereditary; Ophthalmic Genetics; Retinal Disorders; **Hospital:** St Luke's Episcopal Hosp-Houston, Texas Chldns Hosp; **Address:** Cullen Eye Institute NC-206, Baylor College of Medicine, One Baylor Plaza, Houston, TX 77030; **Phone:** 713-798-6100; **Board Cert:** Ophthalmology 1976; **Med School:** Univ Mich Med Sch 1969; **Resid:** Ophthalmology, Univ Michigan Hosp 1973; **Fellow:** Retina, Univ Michigan Hosp 1974; Macular Disease, Bascom Palmer Eye Inst 1975; **Fac Appt:** Prof Oph, Baylor Coll Med

Mazow, Malcolm L MD [Oph] - **Spec Exp:** Strabismus-Adult & Pediatric; Pediatric Ophthalmology; **Hospital:** Meml Hermann Hosp - Texas Med Ctr; **Address:** 2855 Gramercy St, Fl 2nd, Houston, TX 77025; **Phone:** 713-668-6828; **Board Cert:** Ophthalmology 1967; **Med School:** Univ Tex Med Br, Galveston 1961; **Resid:** Ophthalmology, Univ Iowa Hosp 1965; **Fellow:** Strabismus, Univ Iowa Hosp 1966; **Fac Appt:** Clin Prof Oph, Univ Tex, Houston

McCulley, James P MD [Oph] - **Spec Exp:** Corneal & External Eye Disease; Laser Vision Surgery; Cataract Surgery; **Hospital:** UT Southwestern Med Ctr at Dallas, Univ Med Ctr-Lubbock; **Address:** Univ Tex SW Med Ctr, Dept Oph, 5323 Harry Hines Blvd, Dallas, TX 75390-9057; **Phone:** 214-645-2020; **Board Cert:** Ophthalmology 1974; **Med School:** Washington Univ, St Louis 1968; **Resid:** Ophthalmology, Mass EE Infirm 1973; **Fellow:** Cornea, Cornea Rsch-Retina Fdn 1974; Cornea, Mass EE Infirm 1974; **Fac Appt:** Prof Oph, Univ Tex SW, Dallas

Miller, Joseph M MD [Oph] - **Spec Exp:** Pediatric Ophthalmology; Strabismus; Amblyopia; **Hospital:** Univ Med Ctr - Tucson; **Address:** Univ Ariz, Dept Ophthalmology, 707 N Alvernon Way, Tucson, AZ 85711; **Phone:** 520-694-1460; **Board Cert:** Ophthalmology 1991; **Med School:** NE Ohio Univ 1985; **Resid:** Ophthalmology, Yale New Haven Hosp 1990; **Fellow:** Pediatric Ophthalmology, Johns Hopkins Hosp 1991; Refractive Surgery, Univ Arizona Hosp 2001; **Fac Appt:** Prof Oph, Univ Ariz Coll Med

Ophthalmology

Mims III, James Luther MD [Oph] - **Spec Exp:** Pediatric Ophthalmology; Strabismus-Adult & Pediatric; **Hospital:** Baptist Med Ctr - San Antonio, Methodist Chldns Hosp of South Texas; **Address:** 311 Camden St, Ste 511, San Antonio, TX 78215-2015; **Phone:** 210-225-0084; **Board Cert:** Ophthalmology 1977; **Med School:** Tulane Univ 1968; **Resid:** Ophthalmology, Wills Eye Hosp 1976; **Fellow:** Pediatric Ophthalmology, Wills Eye Hosp 1977; **Fac Appt:** Clin Prof Oph, Univ Tex, San Antonio

Pflugfelder, Stephen C MD [Oph] - **Spec Exp:** Corneal & External Eye Disease; Refractive Surgery; Cataract Surgery; Lens Implants; **Hospital:** Methodist Hosp - Houston; **Address:** Alkek Eye Ctr-Baylor College of Medicine, 7200B Cambridge, Houston, TX 77030; **Phone:** 713-798-6100; **Board Cert:** Ophthalmology 1987; **Med School:** SUNY Upstate Med Univ 1981; **Resid:** Ophthalmology, Baylor Coll of Med Affil Hosp 1985; **Fellow:** Cornea & Ext Eye Disease, Bascom Palmer Eye Inst 1986; **Fac Appt:** Prof Oph, Baylor Coll Med

Richard, James M MD [Oph] - **Spec Exp:** Pediatric Ophthalmology; Eye Muscle Surgery; **Hospital:** Chldns Hosp OU Med Ctr, Integris Baptist Med Ctr - OK; **Address:** 11013 Hefner Pointe Drive, Oklahoma City, OK 73120-5050; **Phone:** 405-751-2020; **Board Cert:** Ophthalmology 1979; **Med School:** Univ Okla Coll Med 1974; **Resid:** Ophthalmology, Baylor Coll Med 1978; **Fellow:** Pediatric Ophthalmology, Chldns Hosp 1979; Ophthalmology, Johns Hopkins Hosp 1980; **Fac Appt:** Clin Prof Oph, Univ Okla Coll Med

Schiffman, Jade S MD [Oph] - **Spec Exp:** Neuro-Ophthalmology; **Hospital:** UT MD Anderson Cancer Ctr; **Address:** MD Anderson Cancer, 1515 Holcombe Blvd Unit 1445, Houston, TX 77035; **Phone:** 713-792-3798; **Board Cert:** Neurology 1983; Ophthalmology 1991; **Med School:** SUNY Upstate Med Univ 1975; **Resid:** Neurology, Univ Miami Affil Hosp 1980; Ophthalmology, Univ California Affil Hosp 1989; **Fellow:** Neuro-Ophthalmology, Univ California Med Ctr 1981; **Fac Appt:** Prof Oph, Univ Tex, Houston

Siatkowski, R Michael MD [Oph] - **Spec Exp:** Pediatric Ophthalmology; Neuro-Ophthalmology; Retinopathy of Prematurity; Strabismus; **Hospital:** OU Med Ctr; **Address:** Dean Mcgee Eye Institute, 608 Stanton L Young Blvd, Oklahoma City, OK 73104; **Phone:** 405-271-1094; **Board Cert:** Ophthalmology 2003; **Med School:** Jefferson Med Coll 1987; **Resid:** Ophthalmology, St Francis Med Ctr 1991; **Fellow:** Neuro-Ophthalmology, Bascom Palmer Eye Inst 1992; Pediatric Ophthalmology, Bascom Palmer Eye Inst 1993; **Fac Appt:** Prof Oph, Univ Okla Coll Med

Soparkar, Charles MD [Oph] - **Spec Exp:** Eye Tumors/Cancer; Orbital & Eyelid Tumors/Cancer; Oculoplastic Surgery; **Hospital:** Methodist Hosp - Houston, Texas Chldns Hosp; **Address:** Plastic Eye Surg Assocs, 3730 Kirby Drive, Ste 900, Houston, TX 77098; **Phone:** 713-795-0705; **Board Cert:** Ophthalmology 2007; **Med School:** Univ Mass Sch Med 1990; **Resid:** Ophthalmology, Baylor Affil Hosps 1994; **Fellow:** Ophthalmic Oncololgy, Texas Med Ctr 1995; Ophthalmic Plastic Surgery, Texas Med Ctr 1995; **Fac Appt:** Asst Clin Prof Oph, Baylor Coll Med

Wallace III, Robert B MD [Oph] - **Spec Exp:** Refractive Surgery; Cataract Surgery; **Hospital:** St Francis Med Ctr; **Address:** 4110 Parliament Drive, Alexandria, LA 71303; **Phone:** 318-448-4488; **Board Cert:** Ophthalmology 1979; **Med School:** Tulane Univ 1974; **Resid:** Ophthalmology, Tulane Univ 1979; **Fac Appt:** Clin Prof Oph, Louisiana State U, New Orleans

Wilhelmus, Kirk R MD/PhD [Oph] - **Spec Exp:** Corneal & External Eye Disease; **Hospital:** Baylor Univ Medical Ctr; **Address:** Cullen Eye Inst, 7200 B Cambridge St, Houston, TX 77030; **Phone:** 713-798-6100; **Board Cert:** Ophthalmology 1981; **Med School:** Vanderbilt Univ 1975; **Resid:** Ophthalmology, Baylor Coll Med 1979; **Fellow:** Cornea & Ext Eye Disease, Moorfields Eye Hosp 1981; **Fac Appt:** Prof Oph, Baylor Coll Med

West Coast and Pacific

Abbott, Richard L MD [Oph] - **Spec Exp:** Cornea & External Eye Disease; **Hospital:** UCSF Med Ctr; **Address:** UCSF, Dept Ophthalmology, 8 Koret Way, K301, San Francisco, CA 94143-0730; **Phone:** 415-476-3705; **Board Cert:** Ophthalmology 1978; **Med School:** Geo Wash Univ 1971; **Resid:** Ophthalmology, Presby-Pacific Med Ctr 1977; **Fellow:** Cornea & Ext Eye Disease, Bascom Palmer Eye Inst 1978; **Fac Appt:** Clin Prof Oph, UCSF

Arnold, Anthony C MD [Oph] - **Spec Exp:** Neuro-Ophthalmology; **Hospital:** UCLA Ronald Reagan Med Ctr; **Address:** 100 Stein Plaza, Box 957000, Los Angeles, CA 90095-7005; **Phone:** 310-825-4344; **Board Cert:** Ophthalmology 2008; **Med School:** UCLA 1975; **Resid:** Ophthalmology, Jules Stein Eye Inst-UCLA 1979; **Fellow:** Neuro-Ophthalmology, Jules Stein Eye Inst-UCLA 1983; **Fac Appt:** Clin Prof Oph, UCLA

Baerveldt, George MD [Oph] - **Spec Exp:** Glaucoma; **Hospital:** UC Irvine Med Ctr; **Address:** UC Irvine Med Ctr, Dept Ophthalmology, 118 Med-Surg I, Irvine, CA 92697-4375; **Phone:** 949-824-2020; **Med School:** South Africa 1967; **Resid:** Ophthalmology, Univ of Witwatersrand 1975; **Fellow:** Neuro-Ophthalmology, SUNY Downstate Med Ctr 1975; **Fac Appt:** Prof Oph, UC Irvine

Baylis, Henry I MD [Oph] - **Spec Exp:** Oculoplastic Surgery; Eyelid Surgery; **Hospital:** UCLA Ronald Reagan Med Ctr, Hoag Meml Hosp Presby; **Address:** 1260 15 St, Ste 600, Santa Monica, CA 90404; **Phone:** 310-207-0300; **Board Cert:** Ophthalmology 1969; **Med School:** Univ Mich Med Sch 1960; **Resid:** Ophthalmology, UCLA Med Ctr 1966; **Fellow:** Oculoplastic Surgery, Manhattan EET Hosp 1967; **Fac Appt:** Clin Prof Oph, UCLA

Binder, Perry S MD [Oph] - **Spec Exp:** Refractive Surgery; **Hospital:** Sharp Meml Hosp; **Address:** 2500 6th Ave, Ste 307, San Diego, CA 92103; **Phone:** 619-702-7938; **Board Cert:** Ophthalmology 1975; **Med School:** Northwestern Univ 1969; **Resid:** Ophthalmology, USC Med Ctr 1973; **Fellow:** Cornea, Univ Fla Hosps 1974

Blumenkranz, Mark S MD [Oph] - **Spec Exp:** Retinal Disorders; Macular Degeneration; **Hospital:** Stanford Univ Med Ctr; **Address:** 1225 Crane St, Ste 202, Menlo Park, CA 94025; **Phone:** 650-323-0231; **Board Cert:** Ophthalmology 1980; **Med School:** Brown Univ 1975; **Resid:** Ophthalmology, Stanford Univ Hosp 1979; **Fellow:** Vitreoretinal Surgery, Bascom Palmer Eye Inst 1980; **Fac Appt:** Prof Oph, Stanford Univ

Borchert, Mark S MD [Oph] - **Spec Exp:** Pediatric Ophthalmology; Vision-Unexplained Loss; Optic Nerve Disorders; **Hospital:** Chldns Hosp - Los Angeles; **Address:** Chldns Hosp, Div Ophthalmology, MS 88, 4650 Sunset Blvd, Los Angeles, CA 90027-6062; **Phone:** 323-361-4510; **Board Cert:** Ophthalmology 1989; **Med School:** Baylor Coll Med 1983; **Resid:** Ophthalmology, LAC-USC Med Ctr 1987; **Fellow:** Neuro-Ophthalmology, Mass EE Infirm-Harvard 1988; **Fac Appt:** Assoc Prof Oph, USC Sch Med

Boxer Wachler, Brian S MD [Oph] - **Spec Exp:** LASIK-Refractive Surgery; Keratoconus; Corneal Disease & Surgery; **Address:** Boxer Wachler Vision Inst, 465 N Roxbury Drive, Ste 902, Los Angeles, CA 90210; **Phone:** 310-860-1900; **Board Cert:** Ophthalmology 1999; **Med School:** Dartmouth Med Sch 1993; **Resid:** Ophthalmology, St Louis Univ Eye Inst 1997; **Fellow:** Refractive Surgery, Univ Kansas Med Ctr 1998

Ophthalmology

Boxrud, Cynthia Ann MD [Oph] - **Spec Exp:** Oculoplastic Surgery; Eye Tumors/Cancer; Orbital Diseases; **Hospital:** UCLA Ronald Reagan Med Ctr, St John's Hlth Ctr, Santa Monica; **Address:** 2021 Santa Monica Blvd, Ste 700E, Santa Monica, CA 90404-2208; **Phone:** 310-829-9060; **Board Cert:** Ophthalmology 2008; **Med School:** Case West Res Univ 1986; **Resid:** Ophthalmology, NYU-Bellevue Hosp Ctr 1990; **Fellow:** Ophthalmic Oncololgy, New York Hosp-Cornell Med Ctr 1992; Ophthalmic Plastic Surgery, UCLA-Jules Stein Eye Inst 1993; **Fac Appt:** Asst Prof Oph, UCLA

Caprioli, Joseph MD [Oph] - **Spec Exp:** Glaucoma; Cataract Surgery; **Hospital:** UCLA Ronald Reagan Med Ctr; **Address:** UCLA-Jules Stein Eye Institute, 100 Stein Plaza Fl 2 - Ste 273, Los Angeles, CA 90095-7006; **Phone:** 310-794-9442; **Board Cert:** Ophthalmology 1985; **Med School:** SUNY Buffalo 1979; **Resid:** Ophthalmology, Yale-New Haven Hosp. 1983; **Fellow:** Glaucoma, Wills Eye Hosp 1984; **Fac Appt:** Prof Oph, UCLA

Caster, Andrew I MD [Oph] - **Spec Exp:** LASIK-Refractive Surgery; Laser Vision Surgery; Strabismus; Laser Surgery; **Hospital:** Cedars-Sinai Med Ctr; **Address:** 9100 Wilshire Blvd, Ste 265E, Beverly Hills, CA 90212; **Phone:** 310-274-1221; **Board Cert:** Ophthalmology 1986; **Med School:** Harvard Med Sch 1980; **Resid:** Ophthalmology, UCLA Jules Stein Eye Inst 1984

Char, Devron H MD [Oph] - **Spec Exp:** Eye Tumors/Cancer; Thyroid Eye Disease; Oculoplastic Surgery; **Hospital:** CA Pacific Med Ctr - Pacific Campus, UCSF Med Ctr; **Address:** 45 Castro St, Ste 309, San Francisco, CA 94114; **Phone:** 415-522-0700; **Board Cert:** Ophthalmology 1978; **Med School:** Univ Minn 1970; **Resid:** Internal Medicine, Mass Genl Hosp 1972; Ophthalmology, UCSF Med Ctr 1977; **Fellow:** Medical Oncology, Natl Cancer Inst 1974; Ophthalmology, UCSF Med Ctr 1978; **Fac Appt:** Prof Oph, Stanford Univ

Choy, Andrew MD [Oph] - **Spec Exp:** Eye Muscle Disorders; Oculoplastic & Orbital Surgery; **Hospital:** Long Beach Meml Med Ctr, Los Alamitos Med Ctr; **Address:** 4100 Long Beach Blvd, Ste 108, Long Beach, CA 90807-2619; **Phone:** 562-426-3925; **Board Cert:** Ophthalmology 1976; **Med School:** USC Sch Med 1969; **Resid:** Neurology, LAC-USC Med Ctr 1971; Ophthalmology, Bellevue Hosp Ctr-NYU 1974; **Fellow:** Strabismus, Columbia-Presby Med Ctr 1975; **Fac Appt:** Assoc Clin Prof Oph, UCLA

Cockerham, Kimberly P MD [Oph] - **Spec Exp:** Meningioma-Orbital (eye); Orbital Tumors/Cancer; Eyelid Cancer & Reconstruction; Neuro-Ophthalmology; **Hospital:** El Camino Hosp, Stanford Univ Med Ctr; **Address:** 762 Altos Oaks Drive, Ste 2, Los Altos, CA 94024; **Phone:** 650-559-9150; **Board Cert:** Ophthalmology 2004; **Med School:** Geo Wash Univ 1987; **Resid:** Ophthalmology, Walter Reed Army Med Ctr 1992; **Fellow:** Neuro-Ophthalmology, Walter Reed Army Med Ctr 1993; Neuro-Ophthalmology, Allegheny General Hosp 1995

Day, Susan H MD [Oph] - **Spec Exp:** Pediatric Ophthalmology; Strabismus; **Hospital:** CA Pacific Med Ctr - Pacific Campus; **Address:** 2340 Clay St, Ste 100, San Francisco, CA 94115; **Phone:** 415-202-1500; **Board Cert:** Ophthalmology 1980; **Med School:** Louisiana State U, New Orleans 1975; **Resid:** Ophthalmology, California Pacific Med Ctr 1979; **Fellow:** Pediatric Ophthalmology, Hosp Sick Chldn 1980

De Juan Jr, Eugene MD [Oph] - **Spec Exp:** Retina/Vitreous Surgery; **Hospital:** UCSF Med Ctr; **Address:** 400 Parnassus Ave, Box 0344, San Francisco, CA 94143; **Phone:** 415-353-2800; **Board Cert:** Ophthalmology 1985; **Med School:** Univ S Ala Coll Med 1979; **Resid:** Ophthalmology, Johns Hopkins Hosp 1983; **Fellow:** Vitreoretinal Surgery, Duke Univ Eye Ctr 1984; **Fac Appt:** Prof Oph, UCSF

Demer, Joseph L MD/PhD [Oph] - **Spec Exp:** Pediatric Ophthalmology; Strabismus; Nystagmus; **Hospital:** UCLA Ronald Reagan Med Ctr; **Address:** Jules Stein Eye Institute, 100 Stein Plaza, MC 700219, Los Angeles, CA 90095-7065; **Phone:** 310-825-5931; **Board Cert:** Ophthalmology 1988; **Med School:** Johns Hopkins Univ 1983; **Resid:** Ophthalmology, Baylor Coll Med 1987; **Fellow:** Pediatric Ophthalmology, Texas Chldns Hosp 1988; **Fac Appt:** Prof Oph, UCLA

Gorin, Michael B MD/PhD [Oph] - **Spec Exp:** Retinal Disorders; Macular Disease/Degeneration; Eye Diseases-Hereditary; **Hospital:** UCLA Ronald Reagan Med Ctr; **Address:** Dept Ophthalmology, Jules Stein Eye Inst, 100 Stein Plaza, Los Angeles, CA 90095-7000; **Phone:** 310-794-5400; **Board Cert:** Ophthalmology 1987; **Med School:** Univ Pennsylvania 1980; **Resid:** Ophthalmology, Jules Stein Eye Inst/UCLA 1986; **Fellow:** Medical Retina, Moorfields Eye Hosp 1987; **Fac Appt:** Prof Oph, UCLA-David Geffen Sch Med

Granet, David Bruce MD [Oph] - **Spec Exp:** Pediatric Ophthalmology; Eye Muscle Disorders; Strabismus; **Hospital:** UCSD Med Ctr, Rady Children's Hosp - San Diego; **Address:** UCSD-Shiley Eye Ctr, 9415 Campus Point Drive, La Jolla, CA 92093; **Phone:** 858-534-2020; **Board Cert:** Ophthalmology 2005; **Med School:** Yale Univ 1987; **Resid:** Ophthalmology, Bellevue Hosp-NYU 1991; **Fellow:** Pediatric Ophthalmology, Chldns Hosp 1993; **Fac Appt:** Assoc Prof Oph, UCSD

Humayun, Mark S MD/PhD [Oph] - **Spec Exp:** Retina/Vitreous Surgery; Retinal Disorders; Retinal Vascular Diseases; Diabetic Eye Disease/Retinopathy; **Hospital:** USC Univ Hosp; **Address:** Doheny Eye Inst, 1450 San Pablo St Fl 4, Los Angeles, CA 90033; **Phone:** 323-442-6522; **Board Cert:** Ophthalmology 2006; **Med School:** Duke Univ 1989; **Resid:** Ophthalmology, Duke Univ Hosp 1993; **Fellow:** Vitreoretinal Surgery, Johns Hopkins Univ Hosp 1995; **Fac Appt:** Prof Oph, USC-Keck School of Medicine

Irvine, John A MD [Oph] - **Spec Exp:** Corneal & External Eye Disease; **Hospital:** USC Univ Hosp; **Address:** USC-Doheny Eye Institute, 1450 San Pablo St, Ste 5703, Los Angeles, CA 90033; **Phone:** 323-442-6335; **Board Cert:** Ophthalmology 1989; **Med School:** USC Sch Med 1982; **Resid:** Ophthalmology, Mass EE Infirm/Harvard 1986; **Fellow:** Cornea & Ext Eye Disease, Mass EE Infirm 1987; **Fac Appt:** Prof Oph, USC Sch Med

Isenberg, Sherwin Jay MD [Oph] - **Spec Exp:** Strabismus; Pediatric Ophthalmology; **Hospital:** LAC - Harbor - UCLA Med Ctr, UCLA Ronald Reagan Med Ctr; **Address:** Jules Stein Eye Institute, 100 Stein Plaza, Los Angeles, CA 90095-7000; **Phone:** 310-825-8840; **Board Cert:** Ophthalmology 1978; **Med School:** UCLA 1973; **Resid:** Ophthalmology, Illinois Ear & Eye Infirm 1977; **Fellow:** Pediatric Ophthalmology, Chldns Hosp Natl Med Ctr 1978; **Fac Appt:** Prof Oph, UCLA

Iwach, Andrew G MD [Oph] - **Spec Exp:** Glaucoma; **Hospital:** UCSF Med Ctr, CA Pacific Med Ctr; **Address:** Glaucoma Ctr of San Francisco, 55 Stevenson St, San Francisco, CA 94105; **Phone:** 415-981-2020; **Board Cert:** Ophthalmology 1991; **Med School:** UCLA 1984; **Resid:** Ophthalmology, Stanford Univ Med Ctr 1988; **Fellow:** Glaucoma, UCSF Med Ctr 1989; **Fac Appt:** Assoc Prof Oph, UCSF

Kim, Jonathan W MD [Oph] - **Spec Exp:** Oculoplastic Surgery; Orbital Tumors/Cancer; **Hospital:** Stanford Univ Med Ctr; **Address:** 900 Blake Wilbur Drive, rm W3002, MC 5353, Palo Alto, CA 94304; **Phone:** 650-736-8098; **Board Cert:** Ophthalmology 2000; **Med School:** Univ Iowa Coll Med 1994; **Resid:** Ophthalmology, CA Pacific Med Ctr 1998; **Fellow:** Oculoplastic Surgery, Jules Stein Eye Inst/UCLA Med Ctr 2000; Orbital Surgery, Mass Eye & Ear Infirm 2004

Ophthalmology

Mahon, Kathleen M K MD [Oph] - **Spec Exp:** Pediatric Ophthalmology; Retinopathy of Prematurity; Eye Muscle Disorders; Glaucoma; **Hospital:** Sunrise Hosp & Med Ctr/Sunrise Chldn's Hosp, Univ Med Ctr - Las Vegas; **Address:** Nevada Eye & Ear, 9100 W Post Rd, Las Vegas, NV 89148; **Phone:** 702-896-6043; **Board Cert:** Ophthalmology 1980; **Med School:** Univ New Mexico 1975; **Resid:** Ophthalmology, Univ Florida Med Ctr 1979; **Fellow:** Pediatric Ophthalmology, Univ Tex Hlth Sci Ctr 1980; **Fac Appt:** Clin Prof Oph, Univ Nevada

Maloney, Robert K MD [Oph] - **Spec Exp:** Refractive Surgery; LASIK-Refractive Surgery; **Hospital:** UCLA Ronald Reagan Med Ctr; **Address:** Maloney Vision Inst, 10921 Wilshire Blvd, Ste 900, Los Angeles, CA 90024-4002; **Phone:** 310-208-3937; **Board Cert:** Ophthalmology 1991; **Med School:** UCSF 1985; **Resid:** Ophthalmology, Johns Hopkins Hosp 1989; **Fellow:** Refractive Surgery, Emory Univ Hosp 1991; **Fac Appt:** Clin Prof Oph, UCLA

Manche, Edward E MD [Oph] - **Spec Exp:** LASIK-Refractive Surgery; Corneal Disease & Transplant; PRK-Refractive Surgery; **Hospital:** Stanford Univ Med Ctr; **Address:** 900 Blake Wilbur Dr, rm W3002, Palo Alto, CA 94304-2201; **Phone:** 650-498-7020; **Board Cert:** Ophthalmology 2007; **Med School:** Albert Einstein Coll Med 1990; **Resid:** Ophthalmology, UMDNJ-NJ Med Sch 1994; **Fellow:** Cornea & Ext Eye Disease, Jules Stein Eye Inst-UCLA 1996; **Fac Appt:** Assoc Prof Oph, Stanford Univ

Mannis, Mark J MD [Oph] - **Spec Exp:** Cornea Transplant & Artificial Cornea; Refractive Surgery; **Hospital:** UC Davis Med Ctr; **Address:** UC Davis Med Ctr, Dept Ophthalmology, 4860 Y St, Ste 2400, Sacramento, CA 95817; **Phone:** 916-734-6602; **Board Cert:** Ophthalmology 1980; **Med School:** Univ Fla Coll Med 1975; **Resid:** Ophthalmology, Univ Washington 1979; **Fellow:** Cornea & Ext Eye Disease, Univ IA Hosps & Clins 1980; **Fac Appt:** Prof Oph, UC Davis

Marmor, Michael F MD [Oph] - **Spec Exp:** Retinal Disorders; Retinal Dystrophies; Electroretinograms (ERG); Macular Degeneration; **Hospital:** Stanford Univ Med Ctr; **Address:** California Vitreoretinal Ctr, 1225 Crane St, Ste 202, Menlo Park, CA 94025; **Phone:** 650-323-0231; **Board Cert:** Ophthalmology 1974; **Med School:** Harvard Med Sch 1966; **Resid:** Ophthalmology, Mass EE Infirm 1973; **Fellow:** Neurological Physiology, Natl Inst Mntl Hlth 1970; **Fac Appt:** Prof Oph, Stanford Univ

Masket, Samuel MD [Oph] - **Spec Exp:** Cataract Surgery; Cataract Surgery Revision; **Address:** 2080 Century Park E, Ste 911, Los Angeles, CA 90067; **Phone:** 310-229-1220; **Board Cert:** Ophthalmology 1974; **Med School:** NY Med Coll 1968; **Resid:** Ophthalmology, Metropolitan Hosp Ctr 1973; **Fellow:** Ophthalmology, Columbia Presby Med Ctr 1973; **Fac Appt:** Clin Prof Oph, UCLA

Mathers, William MD [Oph] - **Spec Exp:** Corneal & External Eye Disease; Refractive Surgery; **Hospital:** OR Hlth & Sci Univ; **Address:** Casey Eye Inst, 3375 SW Terwilliger Blvd, Portland, OR 97239-4197; **Phone:** 503-494-7674; **Board Cert:** Anesthesiology 1980; Ophthalmology 1987; **Med School:** Stanford Univ 1973; **Resid:** Anesthesiology, Stanford Univ Hosp 1977; Ophthalmology, Univ Wash Med Ctr 1985; **Fellow:** Cornea, Georgetown Univ Med Ctr 1986; **Fac Appt:** Prof Oph, Oregon Hlth & Sci Univ

Minckler, Donald S MD [Oph] - **Spec Exp:** Glaucoma; **Hospital:** UC Irvine Med Ctr; **Address:** UC Irvine Med Ctr, 118 Med Surge 1 Bldg 810, Irvine, CA 92697; **Phone:** 949-824-2020; **Board Cert:** Ophthalmology 2007; Pathology 1978; **Med School:** Oregon Hlth & Sci Univ 1964; **Resid:** Anatomic Pathology, Univ Wash Med Ctr 1970; Ophthalmology, Univ Wash Med Ctr 1973; **Fellow:** Pathology, Armed Forces Inst Path 1975; Glaucoma, Shaffer Assocs-UCSF 1982; **Fac Appt:** Prof Oph, USC Sch Med

Mondino, Bartly MD [Oph] - **Spec Exp:** Cornea & External Eye Disease; **Hospital:** UCLA Ronald Reagan Med Ctr; **Address:** 100 Stein Plaza, MC 700019, Los Angeles, CA 90095-7065; **Phone:** 310-825-5053; **Board Cert:** Ophthalmology 1976; **Med School:** Stanford Univ 1971; **Resid:** Ophthalmology, NY Hosp/Cornell Univ 1975; **Fellow:** Cornea & Ext Eye Disease, Univ Pittsburgh Eye & Ear Hosp 1976; **Fac Appt:** Prof Oph, UCLA

Murphree, A Linn MD [Oph] - **Spec Exp:** Pediatric Ophthalmology; Eye Diseases-Hereditary; Retinoblastoma; Orbital Tumors/Cancer; **Hospital:** Chldns Hosp - Los Angeles, USC Univ Hosp; **Address:** Chldns Hosp, Div Oph, 4650 Sunset Blvd, MS 88, Los Angeles, CA 90027-6016; **Phone:** 323-361-2347; **Board Cert:** Ophthalmology 1978; **Med School:** Baylor Coll Med 1972; **Resid:** Clinical Genetics, Baylor Heed 1973; Ophthalmology, Baylor Coll Med 1976; **Fellow:** Ophthalmology, Wilmer Inst/Johns Hopkins 1977; **Fac Appt:** Prof Oph, USC Sch Med

O'Brien, Joan M MD [Oph] - **Spec Exp:** Eye Tumors/Cancer; Retinoblastoma; **Hospital:** UCSF Med Ctr; **Address:** UCSF, Dept Ophthalmology, 533 Parnassus Ave Fl 5 - Ste 525, San Francisco, CA 94143; **Phone:** 415-476-3705; **Board Cert:** Ophthalmology 2007; **Med School:** Dartmouth Med Sch 1986; **Resid:** Ophthalmology, Mass Eye & Ear Infirm 1992; **Fellow:** Ophthalmic Pathology, Mass Eye & Ear Infirm 1989; UCSF Med Ctr 1993; **Fac Appt:** Prof Oph, UCSF

Palmer, Earl A MD [Oph] - **Spec Exp:** Strabismus; Retinopathy of Prematurity; **Hospital:** OR Hlth & Sci Univ; **Address:** Casey Eye Institute, 3375 SW Terwilliger Blvd, Portland, OR 97239-4197; **Phone:** 503-494-7675; **Board Cert:** Pediatrics 1975; Ophthalmology 1976; **Med School:** Duke Univ 1966; **Resid:** Pediatrics, Univ Colo Med Ctr 1968; Ophthalmology, Oregon Hlth & Sciences Univ 1974; **Fellow:** Pediatric Ophthalmology, Texas Chldns Hosp 1975; **Fac Appt:** Prof Oph, Oregon Hlth & Sci Univ

Paul, T Otis MD [Oph] - **Spec Exp:** Pediatric Ophthalmology; Strabismus; **Hospital:** CA Pacific Med Ctr - Pacific Campus, Chldns Hosp - Oakland; **Address:** 2100 Webster St, Ste 214, San Francisco, CA 94115; **Phone:** 415-923-3007; **Board Cert:** Ophthalmology 1974; **Med School:** UCLA 1967; **Resid:** Ophthalmology, Naval Hosp 1972; **Fellow:** Pediatric Ophthalmology, Ca Pacific Med Ctr 1974

Puliafito, Carmen A MD [Oph] - **Spec Exp:** Retinal Disorders; Macular Degeneration; **Hospital:** USC Univ Hosp; **Address:** Doheny Eye Inst, 1537 Norfolk St, Los Angeles, CA 90033; **Phone:** 323-442-1900; **Board Cert:** Ophthalmology 1983; **Med School:** Harvard Med Sch 1978; **Resid:** Ophthalmology, Mass Eye & Ear Infirm 1982; **Fellow:** Vitreoretinal Surgery, Mass Eye & Ear Infirm 1983; **Fac Appt:** Prof Oph, USC-Keck School of Medicine

Rao, Narsing A MD [Oph] - **Spec Exp:** Uveitis/AIDS; Eye Pathology; **Hospital:** USC Univ Hosp; **Address:** USC Doheny Eye Inst, 1450 San Pablo St, rm DVRZ 211, Los Angeles, CA 90033-4697; **Phone:** 323-442-6645; **Board Cert:** Pathology 1974; Ophthalmology 1977; **Med School:** India 1967; **Resid:** Pathology, Georgetown Hosp 1972; Ophthalmology, Georgetown Hosp 1975; **Fac Appt:** Prof Oph, USC Sch Med

Salz, James J MD [Oph] - **Spec Exp:** LASIK-Refractive Surgery; PRK-Refractive Surgery; Cataract Surgery; **Hospital:** Cedars-Sinai Med Ctr; **Address:** 240 S La Cienega Blvd, Ste 250, Beverly Hills, CA 90211; **Phone:** 323-653-3800; **Board Cert:** Ophthalmology 1971; **Med School:** Duke Univ 1965; **Resid:** Ophthalmology, LAC-USC Med Ctr 1969; **Fac Appt:** Clin Prof Oph, USC Sch Med

Savino, Peter J MD [Oph] - **Spec Exp:** Neuro-Ophthalmology; **Hospital:** UCSD Med Ctr; **Address:** Shiley Eye Ctr, 9415 Campus Point Drive, La Jolla, CA 92093-0946; **Phone:** 858-534-6290; **Board Cert:** Ophthalmology 1975; **Med School:** Italy 1968; **Resid:** Ophthalmology, Georgetown Med Ctr 1973; **Fellow:** Neuro-Ophthalmology, Bascom Palmer Eye Inst 1974; **Fac Appt:** Prof Oph, Thomas Jefferson Univ

Ophthalmology

Seibel, Barry S MD [Oph] - **Spec Exp:** Cataract Surgery; **Hospital:** Cedars-Sinai Med Ctr; **Address:** 11620 Wilshire Blvd, Ste 711, Los Angeles, CA 90025; **Phone:** 310-444-1134; **Board Cert:** Ophthalmology 1991; **Med School:** Univ Tex, Houston 1985; **Resid:** Ophthalmology, Hollywood Presby Med Ctr 1987; Ophthalmology, USC-Doheny Eye Clin 1989; **Fac Appt:** Asst Clin Prof Oph, UCLA

Seiff, Stuart R MD [Oph] - **Spec Exp:** Oculoplastic Surgery; Orbital Tumors/Cancer; **Hospital:** UCSF Med Ctr, CA Pacific Med Ctr; **Address:** 2100 Webster St, Ste 214, San Francisco, CA 94115; **Phone:** 415-923-3007; **Board Cert:** Ophthalmology 1986; **Med School:** UCSF 1980; **Resid:** Ophthalmology, UCSF Med Ctr 1984; **Fellow:** Ophthalmic Plastic & Reconstructive Surgery, UCLA Med Ctr 1985; Oculoplastic Surgery, Moorfield's Eye Hosp 1986; **Fac Appt:** Prof Oph, UCSF

Serafano, Donald N MD [Oph] - **Spec Exp:** LASIK-Refractive Surgery; Cataract Surgery; Lens Implants; **Hospital:** Los Alamitos Med Ctr, Long Beach Meml Med Ctr; **Address:** 10861 Cherry St, Ste 204, Box 250, Los Alamitos, CA 90720-5403; **Phone:** 562-598-3160; **Board Cert:** Ophthalmology 1978; **Med School:** Wayne State Univ 1971; **Resid:** Ophthalmology, Mayo Clinic 1978; **Fac Appt:** Assoc Clin Prof Oph, USC Sch Med

Smith, Ronald E MD [Oph] - **Spec Exp:** Corneal Disease; Uveitis; **Hospital:** USC Univ Hosp; **Address:** USC-Doheny Eye Institute, 1450 San Pablo Rd, Ste 5703, Los Angeles, CA 90033; **Phone:** 323-442-6335; **Board Cert:** Ophthalmology 1974; **Med School:** Johns Hopkins Univ 1967; **Resid:** Ophthalmology, Wilmer Oph Inst/Johns Hopkins 1973; **Fellow:** Research, Proctor Fdn/Univ California 1972; **Fac Appt:** Prof Oph, USC Sch Med

Steinert, Roger F MD [Oph] - **Spec Exp:** Refractive Surgery; Cataract Surgery; Cornea Transplant; **Hospital:** UC Irvine Med Ctr; **Address:** Gottschalk Med Plaza, 1 Medical Plaza Drive Fl 2, Irvine, CA 92697; **Phone:** 949-824-2020; **Board Cert:** Ophthalmology 1982; **Med School:** Harvard Med Sch 1977; **Resid:** Ophthalmology, Mass EE Infirm 1981; **Fac Appt:** Prof Oph, UC Irvine

Stout, John T MD/PhD [Oph] - **Spec Exp:** Retinal Disorders-Pediatric; Retinoblastoma; Retinopathy of Prematurity; **Hospital:** OR Hlth & Sci Univ, Providence St Vincent Med Ctr; **Address:** 3375 SW Terwilliger Blvd, Portland, OR 97239; **Phone:** 503-494-2435; **Board Cert:** Ophthalmology 1999; **Med School:** Baylor Coll Med 1989; **Resid:** Ophthalmology, Doheny Eye Inst 1993; **Fellow:** Ophthalmology, Moorfields Eye Hosp 1994; Retinal Surgery, Doheny Eye Inst 1995; **Fac Appt:** Assoc Prof Oph, Oregon Hlth & Sci Univ

Weiss, Avery H MD [Oph] - **Spec Exp:** Pediatric Ophthalmology; Strabismus; Amblyopia; **Hospital:** Chldns Hosp and Regl Med Ctr - Seattle; **Address:** 4800 Sand Point Way NE, MS W-4753, Seattle, WA 98105; **Phone:** 206-987-2177; **Board Cert:** Ophthalmology 1981; **Med School:** Univ Miami Sch Med 1974; **Resid:** Internal Medicine, Barnes Hosp 1976; Ophthalmology, Barnes Hosp 1980; **Fellow:** Research, Barnes Hosp 1977; Pediatric Ophthalmology, Chldns Hosp Natl Med Ctr 1981; **Fac Appt:** Assoc Prof Oph, Univ Wash

Wilson, David Jean MD [Oph] - **Spec Exp:** Eye Tumors/Cancer; Ophthalmic Pathology; **Hospital:** OR Hlth & Sci Univ, Legacy Health System; **Address:** 3375 SW Terwilliger Blvd, Portland, OR 97239; **Phone:** 503-494-7891; **Board Cert:** Ophthalmology 1987; **Med School:** Baylor Coll Med 1981; **Resid:** Ophthalmology, Univ Oregon 1985; **Fellow:** Ophthalmic Pathology, John Hopkins Hosp 1987; Retina/Vitreous, Mass Eye & Ear Infirm 1988; **Fac Appt:** Prof Oph, Oregon Hlth & Sci Univ

Wright, Kenneth W MD [Oph] - **Spec Exp:** Cataract Surgery-Lens Implant; Strabismus-Adult & Pediatric; Pediatric Eye Surgery-Ptosis; Pediatric Ophthalmology; **Hospital:** Cedars-Sinai Med Ctr; **Address:** 520 S San Vincente Blvd, Los Angeles, CA 90048; **Phone:** 310-652-6420; **Board Cert:** Ophthalmology 1983; **Med School:** Boston Univ 1977; **Resid:** Ophthalmology, LAC-USC Med Ctr 1981; **Fellow:** Pediatric Ophthalmology, Johns Hopkins Hosp 1981; Pediatric Ophthalmology, Chldns Hosp Natl Med Ctr 1982; **Fac Appt:** Clin Prof Oph, USC Sch Med

INTERNATIONALLY ACCLAIMED

Bascom Palmer Eye Institute is committed to the protection and preservation of the treasured gift of sight and is recognized as one of the world's finest and most progressive centers for ophthalmic care, vision research, and education. Each of our 65 clinical faculty members specializes in a specific area of ophthalmology and is board-certified by the American Board of Ophthalmology. In addition to providing care to more than 250,000 patients annually, all clinical faculty members have research and teaching responsibilities at the University of Miami Miller School of Medicine.

BASCOM PALMER EYE INSTITUTE RANKED #1 IN USA

Bascom Palmer continues to be ranked the nation's best ophthalmic hospital by board-certified ophthalmologists from across the United States. In 2009, it was ranked #1 in ophthalmology by *U.S. News & World Report* for the sixth consecutive year; and #1 in the nation for Clinical (Patient Care) and its Residency program by *Ophthalmology Times*.

BASCOM PALMER RESEARCHERS ADVANCE OPHTHALMIC CARE AND TREATMENT

Consistent with its mission to resolve diseases and disorders of the eye, the physicians and scientists of Bascom Palmer Eye Institute develop new theories, therapeutic techniques, and surgical instruments. Many of the institute's innovations have advanced the course of ophthalmic practices worldwide, including:

- Discovering a new treatment for wet macular degeneration and introducing the use of bevacizumab (Avastin) as a remarkable breakthrough therapy.
- Performing the nation's first modified osteo-odonto-keratoprosthesis using a blind patient's eyetooth to restore sight.
- Alerting ophthalmologists around the world of fungal infections affecting contact lens users, significantly reducing the number of new infections.
- Performing the first successful vitreous surgery – and inventing miniature surgical instrumentation required for this procedure.
- Unraveling the mystery of normal tension glaucoma.
- Establishing predictive tests and new treatments for complicated retinal detachments.

To schedule an appointment please call (800) 329-7000 or visit www.bascompalmer.org.

Miami:
900 NW 17th Street
Miami, FL 33136
(305) 326-6000

Palm Beach Gardens:
7101 Fairway Drive,
Palm Beach Gardens, FL 33418
(561) 515-1500

Naples:
311 9th Street North
Naples, FL 34102
(239) 659-3937

Plantation:
1000 South Pine Island Road
Plantation, FL 33324
(954) 465-2700

UHealth: Top-ranked doctors and hospitals providing the finest health care at more than 30 convenient South Florida locations, including our hospitals: University of Miami Hospital, Bascom Palmer Eye Institute, and Sylvester Comprehensive Cancer Center. UHealth is powered by the research and education of the University of Miami Miller School of Medicine.

Cleveland Clinic

Cole Eye Institute

Cleveland Clinic Cole Eye Institute is one of the few dedicated, comprehensive eye institutes in the world. We are here to serve the needs of patients and referring physicians for early, accurate diagnosis and excellent, effective patient care. Here, the lines between research and patient care blur. The belief that the two are interdependent and synergistic is the foundation for everything we do. We believe that this approach enhances diagnosis and advances treatment, to the benefit of our patients today and tomorrow.

Our Specialized, Experienced Staff

All of our ophthalmologists have advanced expertise in treating disorders and diseases of a specific part or parts of the eye. This specialized approach offers patients a higher level of care and the assurance that their physicians are experienced in treating even the most unusual eye problems.

- Retina and Vitreous Surgery: Age-related macular degeneration, diabetic retinopathy, inherited retinal diseases and infectious retinopathies.
- Cornea and External Diseases: Diseases of the eye's external surface and cornea, such as inflammatory, infectious and degenerative diseases of the cornea, conjunctiva and lens; corneal tumors; and contact lens-related problems.
- Glaucoma: All forms of this silent thief of sight.
- Neuro-Ophthalmology: Vision problems related to neurologic disorders such as stroke, multiple sclerosis and tumors.
- Oculoplastics and Orbital Surgery: Problems of the orbit and eyelids.
- Ocular Oncology: Primary and metastatic tumors of the eye and eyelids.
- Pediatric Ophthalmology: Strabismus, amblyopia and congenital cataracts.
- Refractive Surgery: Correction of nearsightedness, farsightedness and astigmatism.
- Uveitis: Internal ocular inflammation and infection-related immune system disturbances.

Emergency Services

A Cole Eye Institute ophthalmologist is on-call 24 hours a day for immediate consultation on or treatment of eye emergencies. When necessary, a complete surgical team can be assembled promptly to provide emergency treatment for the most serious cases.

For more information about the Cleveland Clinic Cole Eye Institute, to schedule a second opinion or to learn about assistance for out-of-town patients, call 800.890.2467 or visit www.clevelandclinic.org/eyetopdocs.

Cole Eye Institute | 9500 Euclid Avenue / AC311 | Cleveland OH 44195

Why choose Cole Eye Institute?

- Internationally recognized, subspecialty medical staff.
- Among the world's most advanced eye institutes, dedicated to comprehensive and highly specialized ophthalmologic care.
- One of the highest patient volumes in the United States.
- Aggressive research program that bridges the gap between laboratory and patient care and offers access to the latest clinical trials.
- State-of-the-art diagnostic technology and outpatient surgical center.
- We examine our clinical outcomes and objectively measure our success and make them publicly available at clevelandclinic.org/quality

MOUNT SINAI
SCHOOL OF
MEDICINE

THE MOUNT SINAI MEDICAL CENTER
OPHTHALMOLOGY
One Gustave L. Levy Place
Fifth Avenue and 100th Street
New York, NY 10029-6574
Physician Referral: 1-800-MD-SINAI (637-4624)
www.mountsinai.org

Specializing in the prevention, diagnosis, and treatment of eye disorders, the **DEPARTMENT OF OPHTHALMOLOGY** at Mount Sinai features faculty with wide experience in special eye problems. The Department provides comprehensive eye care for the full range of eye disorders and needs.

- Refractive errors
- Glaucoma
- Eye infections
- Corneal and external diseases of the eye
- Retinal disorders (diabetic retinopathy, macular degeneration, and inherited retinal diseases)
- Dry eyes (Sjögren's syndrome)
- Contact lenses
- Neuro-ophthalmic disorders (double vision and optic nerve problems)
- Trauma
- Orbital tumors and thyroid-related eye problems
- Pediatric eye care and strabismus
- Uveitis (inflammation inside the eye)

> **A PIONEERING METHOD OF CORRECTING FARSIGHTEDNESS**
> Mount Sinai ophthalmologists helped pioneer a new radiofrequency method of correcting farsightedness. Known as conductive keratoplasty (CK), the brief procedure is performed in the doctor's office with only topical anesthesia (eye drops). For most farsighted patients—especially those over age 40 whose eyes are naturally aging—the CK procedure eliminates the need for glasses.

The Department offers the full range of sophisticated diagnostic tests for evaluating patient conditions, including optical coherence tomography, fundus photography, fluorescein angiography, diagnostic ultrasound, electroretinography, visually evoked potentials, electro-oculography, computerized tomography, magnetic resonance imaging, corneal topography, and confocal microscopy, as well as state-of-the-art techniques for assessing glaucoma. These techniques include perimetry HRT II imaging and ultrasound biomicroscopy, a noninvasive method to achieve high-resolution imaging of the inside of the eye. In certain cases of glaucoma, it is the only noninvasive way to identify the exact cause of the condition and ascertain optimal treatment. These methods allow for faster, more accurate diagnosis and help determine the best treatment plan for each individual patient.

Our highly skilled eye surgeons perform cataract surgery, corneal transplants, refractive surgery, glaucoma surgery, strabismus surgery, ophthalmic plastic and reconstructive surgery, laser surgery, and vitreoretinal surgery for complicated retinal problems. We also offer minimally invasive procedures to treat eye disease, including non-laser refractive surgeries, small-incision cataract surgery, bladeless laser procedures, and Intacs for keratoconus.

NY Eye & Ear Infirmary

Continuum Health Partners, Inc.

THE NEW YORK EYE AND EAR INFIRMARY
310 East 14th Street
New York, New York 10003
Tel. 212.979.4000   Fax. 212.228.0664
http://www.nyee.edu

PROVIDING EXCEPTIONAL EYE CARE

The Department of Ophthalmology is the region's most comprehensive center for the delivery of primary through tertiary eye care. It is also by far the largest provider of eye care in the metropolitan area—with some 155,000 outpatient visits and 19,200 surgical cases performed each year. 375 board-certified ophthalmologists located throughout New York City and its tri-state area comprise the attending Medical Staff.

IN A HIGHLY SPECIALIZED SETTING

As a specialty hospital, the Infirmary is uniquely qualified to handle the most complicated cases. It serves as a nationwide referral center with a commitment to teaching, research, and high-technology based patient care. Computerized ocular imaging equipment includes the new combination of scanning laser ophthalmoscopy with optical coherence tomography, to provide highest resolution in-depth images which detect the smallest defects and assist in the earliest and most accurate diagnosis of diseases such as glaucoma and macular degeneration. Highly experienced staff using state-of-the-art instrumentation have made the Infirmary's 17 operating rooms a national benchmark in efficiency in eye surgery cases.

FOR PATIENTS OF ALL AGES

Staff at the Infirmary are sensitive to the specific needs of patients of all ages. Senior citizens are the vast majority of the Infirmary's 8,000 yearly cataract patients, as well as individuals receiving treatment for age-related macular degeneration. Young children are now 25 percent of the patient population, with conditions such as strabismus, acquired and congenital cataracts, corneal diseases and ocular trauma. For those rare cases of children who have a disease ordinarily associated with age, the Infirmary runs New York's only Pediatric Glaucoma Service. Active adults of all ages utilize the New York Metropolitan Eye Trauma Center and Oculoplastic and Orbital Surgery Services.

Ophthalmology Clinical Services

Ambulatory Care Services

Comprehensive Eye Care

Cornea & Refractive Surgery

Eye Trauma

Glaucoma

Low Vision

Neuro-Ophthalmology

Oculoplastic & Orbital Surgery

Ocular Tumor

Pediatric Ophthalmology & Strabismus

Retinal-Vitreal

Uveitis/Ocular Immunology

Facilities

Ambulatory Surgery Center

Metropolitan Eye Trauma Center

Retina Center

About The New York Eye and Ear Infirmary

Founded in 1820, it is the nation's first and foremost, continuously operating specialty hospital. More than 10 million people have sought treatment here since its inception.

Physician Referral
1.800.449.HOPE (4673)

Orthopaedic Surgery

An orthopaedic surgeon is trained in the preservation, investigation and restoration of the form and function of the extremities, spine and associated structures by medical, surgical and physical means.

An orthopaedic surgeon is involved with the care of patients whose musculoskeletal problems include congenital deformities, trauma, infections, tumors, metabolic disturbances of the musculoskeletal system, deformities, injuries and degenerative diseases of the spine, hands, feet, knee, hip, shoulder and elbow in children and adults. An orthopaedic surgeon is also concerned with primary and secondary muscular problems and the effects of central or peripheral nervous system lesions of the musculoskeletal system.

Note: *There are many Orthopaedic Surgeons who are trained in Sports Medicine and prefer to be listed under that heading; some trained in Sports Medicine prefer to be listed under Orthopaedics.*

Training Required: Five years (including general surgery training) *plus* two years in clinical practice before final certification is achieved.

ORTHOPAEDIC SURGERY

New England

Brick, Gregory MD [OrS] - **Spec Exp:** Hip Replacement; Knee Replacement; Spinal Surgery; **Hospital:** Brigham & Women's Hosp; **Address:** Brigham & Womens, Dept Orth Surg, 75 Francis St, Boston, MA 02115; **Phone:** 617-732-5386; **Med School:** New Zealand 1976; **Resid:** Surgery, Greenlane Hosp 1981; Orthopaedic Surgery, Middlemore Hosp 1984; **Fellow:** Joint Replacement Surgery, Brigham & Women's Hosp 1986; Spinal Surgery, Vanderbilt Univ Med Ctr 1987; **Fac Appt:** Assoc Clin Prof OrS, Harvard Med Sch

Browner, Bruce D MD [OrS] - **Spec Exp:** Fractures-Complex; Osteomyelitis; Bone Infections; Fractures-Non Union; **Hospital:** Univ of Conn Hlth Ctr, John Dempsey Hosp, Hartford Hosp; **Address:** Med Arts & Rsch Bldg, 263,Farmington Ave Fl 3 - Ste 2, Farmington, CT 06034-4037; **Phone:** 860-679-6650; **Board Cert:** Orthopaedic Surgery 1979; **Med School:** SUNY Downstate 1973; **Resid:** Orthopaedic Surgery, Albany Med Ctr 1978; **Fellow:** Trauma, Albany Med Ctr 1975; **Fac Appt:** Prof OrS, Univ Conn

Burke, Dennis MD [OrS] - **Spec Exp:** Knee Replacement; Hip Replacement; Reconstructive Surgery; **Hospital:** Mass Genl Hosp; **Address:** Mass General Hospital, Yawkey 3910, 55 Fruit St, Boston, MA 02114-2696; **Phone:** 617-726-3411; **Board Cert:** Orthopaedic Surgery 2009; **Med School:** Loyola Univ-Stritch Sch Med 1978; **Resid:** Surgery, Beth Israel Deaconess Med Ctr 1980; Orthopaedic Surgery, Mass Genl Hosp 1984

DiGiovanni, Christopher W MD [OrS] - **Spec Exp:** Foot & Ankle Surgery; **Hospital:** Rhode Island Hosp; **Address:** University Orthopedics Inc, 100 Butler Dr, Providence, RI 02906-4862; **Phone:** 401-330-1430; **Board Cert:** Orthopaedic Surgery 2001; **Med School:** Brown Univ 1991; **Resid:** Orthopaedic Surgery, Rhode Island Hosp 1997; **Fellow:** Joint Replacement Surgery, Hosp Spec Surgery 1998; Foot & Ankle Surgery, Harborview Med Ctr 1999; **Fac Appt:** Prof OrS, Brown Univ

Einhorn, Thomas A MD [OrS] - **Spec Exp:** Hip & Knee Replacement; Bone Disorders-Metabolic; Hip & Knee Reconstruction; **Hospital:** Boston Med Ctr; **Address:** Boston Medical Ctr, Doctors Office Bldg, 720 Harrison Ave, Ste 808, Boston, MA 02118-2393; **Phone:** 617-638-5633; **Board Cert:** Orthopaedic Surgery 1998; **Med School:** Cornell Univ-Weill Med Coll 1976; **Resid:** Orthopaedic Surgery, St Lukes-Roosevelt Hosp 1981; Pediatric Orthopaedic Surgery, Alfred DuPont Inst 1981; **Fellow:** Orthopaedic Surgery, Hosp Special Surgery 1982; **Fac Appt:** Prof OrS, Boston Univ

Endrizzi, Donald P MD [OrS] - **Spec Exp:** Shoulder Surgery; Rotator Cuff Surgery; Elbow Surgery; **Hospital:** Maine Med Ctr; **Address:** 33 Sewall St, Portland, M, ME 04102; **Phone:** 207-828-2100; **Board Cert:** Orthopaedic Surgery 2001; **Med School:** Columbia P&S 1982; **Resid:** Surgery, Columbia-Presby Med Ctr 1984; Orthopaedic Surgery, Columbia Presby Med Ctr 1987; **Fac Appt:** Assoc Clin Prof S, Univ VT Coll Med

Friedlaender, Gary E MD [OrS] - **Spec Exp:** Bone & Soft Tissue Tumors; Limb Surgery/Reconstruction; Fractures-Non Union; Tissue Banking; **Hospital:** Yale-New Haven Hosp; **Address:** Dept Orthopedic Surgery, Box 208071, New Haven, CT 06520-8071; **Phone:** 203-737-5656; **Board Cert:** Orthopaedic Surgery 1975; **Med School:** Univ Mich Med Sch 1969; **Resid:** Surgery, Michigan Med Ctr 1971; Orthopaedic Surgery, Yale-New Haven Hosp 1974; **Fellow:** Musculoskeletal Oncology, Mass Genl Hosp 1983; **Fac Appt:** Prof OrS, Yale Univ

Fulkerson, John P MD [OrS] - **Spec Exp:** Knee-Patella Problems; Arthroscopic Surgery-Knee; Shoulder Surgery; Sports Medicine; **Hospital:** Hartford Hosp; **Address:** 499 Farmington Ave Fl 3, Farmington, CT 06032; **Phone:** 860-549-8269; **Board Cert:** Orthopaedic Surgery 1980; **Med School:** Yale Univ 1972; **Resid:** Orthopaedic Surgery, Yale-New Haven Hosp 1978; **Fellow:** Sports Medicine, Hosp for Special Surg 1979; **Fac Appt:** Clin Prof OrS, Univ Conn

Gebhardt, Mark MD [OrS] - **Spec Exp:** Musculoskeletal Tumors; Bone Tumors; **Hospital:** Beth Israel Deaconess Med Ctr - Boston, Children's Hospital - Boston; **Address:** 330 Brookline Ave, Shapiro Bldg Fl 2nd, Boston, MA 02215; **Phone:** 617-667-3940; **Board Cert:** Orthopaedic Surgery 2007; **Med School:** Univ Cincinnati 1975; **Resid:** Surgery, Univ Pittsburg Med Ctr 1977; Orthopaedic Surgery, Harvard Affil Hosps 1982; **Fellow:** Pediatric Orthopaedic Surgery, Boston Chldns Hosp 1983; Orthopaedic Oncology, Mass Genl Hosp 1983; **Fac Appt:** Prof OrS, Harvard Med Sch

Green, Andrew MD [OrS] - **Spec Exp:** Shoulder Surgery; Elbow Surgery; Rotator Cuff Surgery; Arthroscopic Surgery; **Hospital:** Rhode Island Hosp, Miriam Hosp; **Address:** Univ Orthopedics Inc, 2 Dudley St, Ste 200, Providence, RI 02905-3248; **Phone:** 401-457-1533; **Board Cert:** Orthopaedic Surgery 2006; **Med School:** Columbia P&S 1987; **Resid:** Orthopaedic Surgery, Rhode Island Hosp 1992; **Fellow:** Pacific Med Ctr 1993; **Fac Appt:** Assoc Prof OrS, Brown Univ

Hornicek, Francis J MD/PhD [OrS] - **Spec Exp:** Bone Tumors; Sarcoma; Bone Tumors-Metastatic; Soft Tissue Tumors; **Hospital:** Mass Genl Hosp; **Address:** Orthopaedic Associates, 55 Fruit St, YAW 3700, Boston, MA 02114; **Phone:** 617-724-3700; **Board Cert:** Orthopaedic Surgery 2009; **Med School:** Univ Pittsburgh 1991; **Resid:** Orthopaedic Surgery, Jackson Meml Hosp 1996; **Fellow:** Orthopaedic Oncology, Mass Genl Hosp/Chldns Hosp 1997; **Fac Appt:** Assoc Prof OrS, Harvard Med Sch

Jokl, Peter MD [OrS] - **Spec Exp:** Knee Surgery; Sports Medicine; Shoulder Surgery; **Hospital:** Yale-New Haven Hosp; **Address:** Yale Sports Med, Dept Orthopaedics, 800 Howard Ave, New Haven, CT 06519-1369; **Phone:** 203-785-2579; **Board Cert:** Orthopaedic Surgery 1974; **Med School:** Yale Univ 1968; **Resid:** Orthopaedic Surgery, Yale-New Haven Hosp 1972; **Fac Appt:** Prof OrS, Yale Univ

Jupiter, Jesse B MD [OrS] - **Spec Exp:** Upper Extremity Trauma; Hand Surgery; **Hospital:** Mass Genl Hosp, Newton - Wellesley Hosp; **Address:** Yawkey Center, Ste 2100, 55 Fruit St, Boston, MA 02114-2621; **Phone:** 617-726-8530; **Board Cert:** Orthopaedic Surgery 1982; **Med School:** Yale Univ 1972; **Resid:** Surgery, Mass Genl Hosp 1976; Orthopaedic Surgery, Mass Genl Hosp 1979; **Fellow:** Hand Surgery, Univ Louisville 1981; Trauma, AO/ASIF 1980; **Fac Appt:** Prof OrS, Harvard Med Sch

Kasser, James MD [OrS] - **Spec Exp:** Pediatric Orthopaedic Surgery; **Hospital:** Children's Hospital - Boston; **Address:** Chldns Hosp, Dept Ortho Surgery, 300 Longwood Ave, Boston, MA 02115; **Phone:** 617-355-6617; **Board Cert:** Orthopaedic Surgery 2005; **Med School:** Tufts Univ 1976; **Resid:** Orthopaedic Surgery, Tufts Med Ctr 1981; **Fellow:** Pediatric Orthopaedic Surgery, Dupont Inst 1984; **Fac Appt:** Prof OrS, Harvard Med Sch

Kocher, Mininder S MD [OrS] - **Spec Exp:** Pediatric Orthopaedic Surgery; Bone Infections in Children; Limb Lengthening; Pediatric Sports Medicine; **Hospital:** Children's Hospital - Boston; **Address:** Children's Hosp, Dept Orthopaedic Surg, 319 Longwood Ave, Boston, MA 02115; **Phone:** 617-355-3501; **Board Cert:** Orthopaedic Surgery 2002; **Med School:** Duke Univ 1993; **Resid:** Orthopaedic Surgery, Beth Israel Hosp 1999; **Fellow:** Pediatric Orthopaedic Surgery, Chldns Hosp 1999; Sports Medicine, Steadman Hawkins Clin 2000; **Fac Appt:** Asst Prof OrS, Harvard Med Sch

Orthopaedic Surgery

Laurencin, Cato T MD/PhD [OrS] - **Spec Exp:** Shoulder & Knee Surgery; Sports Medicine; **Hospital:** Univ of Conn Hlth Ctr, John Dempsey Hosp; **Address:** Univ Conn Health Ctr, 263 Farmington Ave, Farmington, CT 06030-3800; **Phone:** 860-679-8384; **Board Cert:** Orthopaedic Surgery 2007; **Med School:** Harvard Med Sch 1987; **Resid:** Orthopaedic Surgery, Harvard Combined Program 1993; **Fellow:** Sports Medicine & Shoulder Surgery, Hosp for Special Surg 1994; **Fac Appt:** Prof OrS, Univ Conn

Marsh, James S MD [OrS] - **Spec Exp:** Pediatric Orthopaedic Surgery; **Hospital:** Yale-New Haven Hosp, Hosp of St Raphael; **Address:** 1200 Boston Post Rd, Ste 201B, Guilford, CT 06437; **Phone:** 203-453-1088; **Board Cert:** Orthopaedic Surgery 2000; **Med School:** Harvard Med Sch 1981; **Resid:** Orthopaedic Surgery, Stanford Univ 1986; **Fellow:** Pediatric Orthopaedic Surgery, Mass Genl Hosp 1987; **Fac Appt:** Assoc Prof OrS, Yale Univ

Ready, John E MD [OrS] - **Spec Exp:** Bone Cancer; Sarcoma-Soft Tissue; Hip & Knee Replacement in Bone Tumors; Hip & Knee Replacement; **Hospital:** Brigham & Women's Hosp, Dana-Farber Cancer Inst; **Address:** Brigham & Women's Hospital, Dept Orthopaedics, 75 Francis St, Boston, MA 02115; **Phone:** 617-732-5368; **Board Cert:** Orthopaedic Surgery 2002; **Med School:** Dalhousie Univ 1982; **Resid:** Orthopaedic Surgery, Dalhousie Univ Hosp 1987; **Fellow:** Orthopaedic Oncology, St Michael's Hosp 1988; Orthopaedic Oncology, Mass Genl Hosp/Childns Hosp 1989

Reilly, Donald T MD [OrS] - **Spec Exp:** Hip & Knee Replacement; **Hospital:** New England Bapt Hosp; **Address:** 125 Parker Hill Ave, Ste 550, Boston, MA 02120; **Phone:** 617-232-6025; **Board Cert:** Orthopaedic Surgery 1984; **Med School:** Case West Res Univ 1975; **Resid:** Orthopaedic Surgery, Harvard Combined Ortho 1981

Scott, Richard D MD [OrS] - **Spec Exp:** Hip Replacement; Knee Replacement; **Hospital:** Brigham & Women's Hosp, New England Bapt Hosp; **Address:** 125 Parker Hill Ave, Boston, MA 02120; **Phone:** 617-738-9151; **Board Cert:** Orthopaedic Surgery 1975; **Med School:** Temple Univ 1968; **Resid:** Orthopaedic Surgery, Mass Genl Hosp 1974; **Fellow:** Orthopaedic Surgery, Mass Genl Hosp 1974; **Fac Appt:** Prof OrS, Harvard Med Sch

Springfield, Dempsey MD [OrS] - **Spec Exp:** Bone Tumors; Soft Tissue Tumors; **Hospital:** Mass Genl Hosp; **Address:** 55 Fruit St, Ste YAW 3700, Boston, MA 02114-2621; **Phone:** 617-724-3700; **Board Cert:** Orthopaedic Surgery 2007; **Med School:** Univ Fla Coll Med 1971; **Resid:** Orthopaedic Surgery, Univ Florida/Shands 1978; **Fellow:** Orthopaedic Surgery, Univ Florida/Shands 1979

Thornhill, Thomas S MD [OrS] - **Spec Exp:** Hip & Knee Replacement; Arthritis; Shoulder & Elbow Surgery; **Hospital:** Brigham & Women's Hosp; **Address:** Brigham & Women's Hosp, Dept Orth Surg, 45 Francis St, Boston, MA 02115; **Phone:** 617-732-5322; **Board Cert:** Internal Medicine 1973; Orthopaedic Surgery 1979; **Med School:** Cornell Univ-Weill Med Coll 1970; **Resid:** Internal Medicine, Peter Brent Brigham Hosp 1972; Orthopaedic Surgery, Harvard Combined Prgm 1978; **Fellow:** Joint Replacement Surgery, Robert Breck Brigham Hosp; **Fac Appt:** Prof OrS, Harvard Med Sch

Tornetta III, Paul MD [OrS] - **Spec Exp:** Trauma; Fractures-Complex; Minimally Invasive Surgery; Fractures in the Elderly; **Hospital:** Boston Med Ctr; **Address:** Boston Medical Ctr, 850 Harrison Ave, Yawkey 3rd Fl, Boston, MA 02118; **Phone:** 617-414-4865; **Board Cert:** Orthopaedic Surgery 2006; **Med School:** SUNY Downstate 1987; **Resid:** Orthopaedic Surgery, Downstate Med Ctr 1992; **Fellow:** Trauma, Good Samaritan Hosp 1993; **Fac Appt:** Prof OrS, Boston Univ

Weinstein, James DO [OrS] - **Spec Exp:** Pain-Back; Spinal Tumors; **Hospital:** Dartmouth - Hitchcock Med Ctr; **Address:** DHMC, Dept Orthopaedic Surgery, One Medical Ctr Drive, Lebanon, NH 03756; **Phone:** 603-650-2225; **Board Cert:** Orthopaedic Surgery 2002; **Med School:** Chicago Coll Osteo Med 1973; **Resid:** Orthopaedic Surgery, Rush Presby-St Lukes Med Ctr 1983; **Fac Appt:** Prof OrS, Dartmouth Med Sch

Zarins, Bertram MD [OrS] - **Spec Exp:** Knee Injuries/ACL; Arthroscopic Surgery; Shoulder Injuries; Rotator Cuff Surgery; **Hospital:** Mass Genl Hosp; **Address:** MGH Sports Medicine, 175 Cambridge St Fl 4, Boston, MA 02114; **Phone:** 617-726-3421; **Board Cert:** Orthopaedic Surgery 1975; **Med School:** SUNY Upstate Med Univ 1967; **Resid:** Surgery, Johns Hopkins Hosp 1969; Orthopaedic Surgery, Harvard Ortho Prog 1973; **Fellow:** Sports Medicine, Mass Genl Hosp 1976; **Fac Appt:** Clin Prof OrS, Harvard Med Sch

Mid Atlantic

Albert, Todd J MD [OrS] - **Spec Exp:** Spinal Surgery; Spinal Surgery-Cervical; Spinal Deformity; **Hospital:** Thomas Jefferson Univ Hosp; **Address:** Rothman Institute, 925 Chesnut St Fl 5, Philadelphia, PA 19107; **Phone:** 800-321-9999; **Board Cert:** Orthopaedic Surgery 2006; **Med School:** Univ VA Sch Med 1987; **Resid:** Orthopaedic Surgery, Thomas Jefferson Univ Hosp 1992; **Fellow:** Spinal Surgery, Minnesota Spine Ctr 1993; **Fac Appt:** Prof OrS, Thomas Jefferson Univ

Balderston, Richard MD [OrS] - **Spec Exp:** Scoliosis; Spinal Surgery; Spinal Disc Replacement; **Hospital:** Pennsylvania Hosp (page 60); **Address:** 800 Spruce St, 3B Orthopaedics, Philadelphia, PA 19107; **Phone:** 215-829-2222; **Board Cert:** Orthopaedic Surgery 1985; **Med School:** Univ Pennsylvania 1977; **Resid:** Orthopaedic Surgery, Hosp Univ Penn 1982; **Fellow:** Spinal Surgery, Univ Minn Affil Hosp 1983; **Fac Appt:** Clin Prof OrS, Univ Pennsylvania

Bartolozzi, Arthur R MD [OrS] - **Spec Exp:** Sports Medicine; Arthroscopic Surgery-Knee; Knee Ligament Reconstruction; Shoulder Surgery; **Hospital:** Pennsylvania Hosp (page 60); **Address:** 800 Spruce St Fl 1, Philadelphia, PA 19107; **Phone:** 215-829-2222; **Board Cert:** Orthopaedic Surgery 2000; **Med School:** UCSD 1981; **Resid:** Orthopaedic Surgery, Hosp Univ Penn 1986; **Fellow:** Sports Medicine, UCLA Med Ctr 1987; **Fac Appt:** Assoc Clin Prof OrS, Univ Pennsylvania

Bauman, Phillip A MD [OrS] - **Spec Exp:** Foot & Ankle Surgery; Knee Surgery; Dance/Sports Medicine; Arthroscopic Surgery; **Hospital:** St Luke's - Roosevelt Hosp Ctr - Roosevelt Div (page 57), NY-Presby Hosp/Columbia (page 66); **Address:** Orthopaedic Assocs of NY, 343 W 58th St, rm 1, New York, NY 10019; **Phone:** 212-506-0228; **Board Cert:** Orthopaedic Surgery 2001; **Med School:** Columbia P&S 1981; **Resid:** Surgery, St Lukes-Roosevelt Hosp Ctr 1983; Orthopaedic Surgery, Columbia-Presby Med Ctr 1987; **Fac Appt:** Asst Prof OrS, Columbia P&S

Benevenia, Joseph MD [OrS] - **Spec Exp:** Limb Sparing Surgery; Bone Cancer; Sarcoma-Soft Tissue; **Hospital:** UMDNJ-Univ Hosp-Newark; **Address:** 90 Bergen St, Ste 1200, Newark, NJ 07103; **Phone:** 973-972-2153; **Board Cert:** Orthopaedic Surgery 2003; **Med School:** UMDNJ-NJ Med Sch, Newark 1984; **Resid:** Orthopaedic Surgery, UMDNJ-NJ Med Sch Hosp 1988; **Fellow:** Orthopaedic Oncology, Case Western Reserve Univ 1991; **Fac Appt:** Prof OrS, UMDNJ-NJ Med Sch, Newark

Betz, Randal R MD [OrS] - **Spec Exp:** Spinal Cord Injury-Pediatric; Praxis Functional Electrical Stim (FES); Scoliosis; Spinal Deformity-Pediatric; **Hospital:** Philadelphia Shriners Hosp; **Address:** Shriners Hospital for Children, 3351 N Broad St, Philadelphia, PA 19140; **Phone:** 215-430-4026; **Board Cert:** Orthopaedic Surgery 1998; Spinal Cord Injury Medicine 1998; **Med School:** Temple Univ 1977; **Resid:** Orthopaedic Surgery, Shriners Hospital 1980; Orthopaedic Surgery, Temple Univ Hospital 1982; **Fellow:** Pediatric Orthopaedic Surgery, DuPont Inst 1983; **Fac Appt:** Prof OrS, Temple Univ

Orthopaedic Surgery

Bigliani, Louis U MD [OrS] - **Spec Exp:** Shoulder Surgery; Sports Medicine; Arthroscopic Surgery; **Hospital:** NY-Presby Hosp/Columbia (page 66); **Address:** 622 W 168th St, rm 1130, New York, NY 10032-3720; **Phone:** 212-305-0998; **Board Cert:** Orthopaedic Surgery 1979; **Med School:** Loyola Univ-Stritch Sch Med 1973; **Resid:** Surgery, Roosevelt Hosp 1974; Orthopaedic Surgery, Columbia Presby Med Ctr 1977; **Fac Appt:** Prof OrS, Columbia P&S

Bitan, Fabien D MD [OrS] - **Spec Exp:** Spinal Surgery-Pediatric & Adult; Spinal Disc Replacement; Spinal Deformity; Spinal Disorders-Degenerative; **Hospital:** Lenox Hill Hosp (page 62); **Address:** Manhattan Orthopaedics, 130 E 77th St Fl 7, New York, NY 10075; **Phone:** 212-744-8114; **Med School:** France 1981; **Resid:** Orthopaedic Surgery, Hospital Beaujon 1987; Pediatric Orthopaedic Surgery, Hosp des Enfants Malades 1990; **Fellow:** Pediatric Orthopaedic Surgery, Hosp Special Surgery 1997; Spinal Surgery, Beth Israel Med Ctr 1998

Boachie-Adjei, Oheneba MD [OrS] - **Spec Exp:** Spinal Surgery; Scoliosis; **Hospital:** Hosp For Special Surgery (page 59); **Address:** Hospital for Special Surgery, 535 E 70th St, New York, NY 10021; **Phone:** 212-606-1948; **Board Cert:** Orthopaedic Surgery 2000; **Med School:** Columbia P&S 1980; **Resid:** Surgery, St Vincents Hosp 1982; Orthopaedic Surgery, Hosp Spec Surg 1986; **Fellow:** Orthopaedic Pathology, Hosp Spec Surg 1983; Spinal Surgery, Twin Cities Scoliosis Ctr/Minn Spine Ctr 1987; **Fac Appt:** Assoc Clin Prof S, Cornell Univ-Weill Med Coll

Booth Jr, Robert E MD [OrS] - **Spec Exp:** Knee Replacement & Revision; **Hospital:** Pennsylvania Hosp (page 60); **Address:** 800 Spruce St, Philadelphia, PA 19107; **Phone:** 215-829-2222; **Board Cert:** Orthopaedic Surgery 1978; **Med School:** Univ Pennsylvania 1971; **Resid:** Surgery, Penn Hosp 1973; Orthopaedic Surgery, Hosp Univ Penn 1977; **Fac Appt:** Clin Prof OrS, Univ Pennsylvania

Bronson, Michael J MD [OrS] - **Spec Exp:** Joint Replacement; Knee Replacement; Hip Replacement; Arthritis; **Hospital:** Mount Sinai Med Ctr (page 64), Lenox Hill Hosp (page 62); **Address:** Mt Sinai Med Ctr, Dept Orthopedic Surgery, 5 E 98th St, Box 1188, New York, NY 10029; **Phone:** 212-241-1640; **Board Cert:** Orthopaedic Surgery 1984; **Med School:** NY Med Coll 1976; **Resid:** Orthopaedic Surgery, Lenox Hill Hosp 1980; **Fellow:** Hip & Knee Surgery, Columbia-Presby Med Ctr 1981; **Fac Appt:** Assoc Clin Prof OrS, Mount Sinai Sch Med

Brushart, Thomas M MD [OrS] - **Spec Exp:** Hand Surgery; Peripheral Nerve Surgery; **Hospital:** Johns Hopkins Hosp (page 61); **Address:** 601 N Caroline St, rm 5221, Baltimore, MD 21287-0882; **Phone:** 410-955-9663; **Board Cert:** Orthopaedic Surgery 1985; Hand Surgery 2000; **Med School:** Harvard Med Sch 1978; **Resid:** Orthopaedic Surgery, Harvard Affil Hosps 1981; **Fellow:** Hand Surgery, Curtis Hand Ctr 1983; **Fac Appt:** Prof OrS, Johns Hopkins Univ

Buly, Robert L MD [OrS] - **Spec Exp:** Hip Replacement; Minimally Invasive Surgery; Arthritis; Knee Replacement; **Hospital:** Hosp For Special Surgery (page 59), NY-Presby Hosp/Weill Cornell (page 66); **Address:** Hospital for Special Surgery, 535 E 70th St, New York, NY 10021; **Phone:** 212-606-1971; **Board Cert:** Orthopaedic Surgery 2004; **Med School:** Cornell Univ-Weill Med Coll 1985; **Resid:** Orthopaedic Surgery, Hosp for Special Surg 1990; **Fellow:** Hip Surgery, Mueller Fdn 1991; Joint Reconstruction, Case Western Res/ Univ Hosp 1992; **Fac Appt:** Assoc Prof OrS, Cornell Univ-Weill Med Coll

Cammisa Jr, Frank P MD [OrS] - **Spec Exp:** Spinal Surgery; Spinal Disc Replacement; Minimally Invasive Spinal Surgery; Scoliosis; **Hospital:** Hosp For Special Surgery (page 59), NY-Presby Hosp/Weill Cornell (page 66); **Address:** 523 E 72nd St, Fl 3, New York, NY 10021; **Phone:** 212-606-1946; **Board Cert:** Orthopaedic Surgery 2001; **Med School:** Columbia P&S 1982; **Resid:** Surgery, Columbia-Presby Hosp 1983; Orthopaedic Surgery, Hosp for Special Surgery 1987; **Fellow:** Spinal Surgery, Jackson Meml Hosp 1988; **Fac Appt:** Assoc Prof OrS, Cornell Univ-Weill Med Coll

Cappuccino, Andrew MD [OrS] - **Spec Exp:** Spinal Surgery; Spinal Disc Replacement; **Hospital:** Kenmore Mercy Hosp; **Address:** Buffalo Spine Surgery, 46 Davison Ct, Lockport, NY 14094; **Phone:** 716-438-2976; **Board Cert:** Orthopaedic Surgery 2007; **Med School:** SUNY Buffalo 1988; **Resid:** Orthopaedic Surgery, Monmouth Med Ctr 1993; Pediatric Orthopaedic Surgery, Childrens Hosp 1992; **Fellow:** Orthopaedic Surgery, Johns Hopkins/Paul McAfee, MD 1994

Chu, Constance R MD [OrS] - **Spec Exp:** Sports Medicine; Knee Injuries/ACL; Cartilage Damage; **Hospital:** UPMC Montefiore, UPMC Shadyside; **Address:** Kaufmann Bldg, 3471 5th Ave, Ste 110, Pittsburgh, PA 15213; **Phone:** 412-687-3900; **Board Cert:** Orthopaedic Surgery 2002; **Med School:** Harvard Med Sch 1992; **Resid:** Orthopaedic Surgery, UCSD Med Ctr 1995; **Fellow:** Joint Replacement Surgery, Brigham & Women's Hosp 1999; **Fac Appt:** Assoc Prof OrS, Univ Pittsburgh

Craig, Edward V MD [OrS] - **Spec Exp:** Shoulder Arthroscopic Surgery; Shoulder Replacement; Sports Medicine; Elbow Surgery; **Hospital:** Hosp For Special Surgery (page 59), NY-Presby Hosp/Weill Cornell (page 66); **Address:** 535 E 70th St, New York, NY 10021-4892; **Phone:** 212-606-1966; **Board Cert:** Orthopaedic Surgery 1984; **Med School:** Columbia P&S 1973; **Resid:** Internal Medicine, Columbia-Presby Hosp 1976; Orthopaedic Surgery, Columbia-Presby Hosp 1980; **Fellow:** Shoulder Surgery, Columbia-Presby Hosp 1981; Hand Surgery, Columbia-Presby Hosp 1982; **Fac Appt:** Clin Prof OrS, Cornell Univ-Weill Med Coll

Crossett, Lawrence MD [OrS] - **Spec Exp:** Hip Surgery; Knee Surgery; **Hospital:** UPMC Presby, Pittsburgh, UPMC Shadyside; **Address:** Univ Pittsburgh Physicians, Orthopaedics, 5200 Centre Ave, Ste 415, Pittsburgh, PA 15232; **Phone:** 412-802-4100; **Board Cert:** Orthopaedic Surgery 2000; **Med School:** Temple Univ 1981; **Resid:** Orthopaedic Surgery, Temple Univ Hosp 1986; Orthopaedic Surgery, Shriners Children's Hosp 1984; **Fac Appt:** Assoc Prof OrS, Univ Pittsburgh

Davidson, Richard S MD [OrS] - **Spec Exp:** Limb Lengthening (Ilizarov Procedure); Limb Deformities; Foot Deformities; Clubfoot; **Hospital:** Chldns Hosp of Philadelphia, The; **Address:** Children's Hospital, Dept Orthopaedics, 34th St & Civic Ctr Blvd, Wood Center Fl 2, Philadelphia, PA 19104; **Phone:** 215-590-1527; **Board Cert:** Orthopaedic Surgery 1997; **Med School:** NYU Sch Med 1976; **Resid:** Orthopaedic Surgery, Hosp Special Surgery 1981; **Fellow:** Pediatric Orthopaedic Surgery, Hosp for Sick Children 1982; **Fac Appt:** Assoc Clin Prof OrS, Univ Pennsylvania

Delahay, John N MD [OrS] - **Spec Exp:** Pediatric Orthopaedic Surgery; Trauma; **Hospital:** Georgetown Univ Hosp; **Address:** 3800 Reservoir Rd NW, PHC Bldg, Ground FL, Washington, DC 20007; **Phone:** 202-444-1438; **Board Cert:** Orthopaedic Surgery 1975; **Med School:** Georgetown Univ 1969; **Resid:** Orthopaedic Surgery, Georgetown Univ Hosp 1974; **Fac Appt:** Prof OrS, Georgetown Univ

Deland, Jonathan T MD [OrS] - **Spec Exp:** Foot & Ankle Surgery; Sports Medicine; Arthritis; **Hospital:** Hosp For Special Surgery (page 59); **Address:** Hosp Spec Surg, Foot & Ankle Service, 535 E 70th St, New York, NY 10021-4099; **Phone:** 212-606-1665; **Board Cert:** Orthopaedic Surgery 2003; **Med School:** Columbia P&S 1980; **Resid:** Orthopaedic Surgery, St Luke's-Roosevelt Hosp Ctr 1982; Orthopaedic Surgery, Mass Genl Hosp 1987; **Fac Appt:** Asst Prof S, Cornell Univ-Weill Med Coll

Dines, David M MD [OrS] - **Spec Exp:** Shoulder Surgery; Sports Medicine; Shoulder Replacement; **Hospital:** Long Island Jewish Med Ctr, Hosp For Special Surgery (page 59); **Address:** 935 Northern Blvd, Ste 303, Great Neck, NY 11021-5309; **Phone:** 516-482-1037; **Board Cert:** Orthopaedic Surgery 1980; **Med School:** UMDNJ-NJ Med Sch, Newark 1974; **Resid:** Surgery, NY Hosp-Cornell Med Ctr 1976; Orthopaedic Surgery, Hosp Special Surg 1979; **Fac Appt:** Clin Prof OrS, Albert Einstein Coll Med

Donaldson III, William F MD [OrS] - **Spec Exp:** Spinal Surgery; **Hospital:** UPMC Presby, Pittsburgh; **Address:** Univ Pittsburgh Physicians, Orthopaedics, 3471 5th Ave, Ste 1010, Pittsburgh, PA 15213; **Phone:** 412-605-3218; **Board Cert:** Orthopaedic Surgery 2009; **Med School:** Rush Med Coll 1980; **Resid:** Surgery, Rush Presby-St Luke's Med Ctr 1981; Orthopaedic Surgery, Hosp Special Surg 1985; **Fellow:** Spinal Surgery, Hosp Special Surg 1986; **Fac Appt:** Assoc Prof OrS, Univ Pittsburgh

Dormans, John P MD [OrS] - **Spec Exp:** Bone Cancer; Spinal Surgery-Pediatric; Pediatric Orthopaedic Surgery; **Hospital:** Chldns Hosp of Philadelphia, The; **Address:** Dept Orthopaedic Surgery, 34th St & Civic Center Blvd, Wood Bldg Fl 2 - rm 2315, Philadelphia, PA 19104-4399; **Phone:** 215-590-1534; **Board Cert:** Orthopaedic Surgery 2002; **Med School:** Indiana Univ 1983; **Resid:** Orthopaedic Surgery, Michigan State Univ Hosps 1988; **Fellow:** Pediatric Orthopaedic Surgery, Hosp for Sick Children 1989; **Fac Appt:** Prof OrS, Univ Pennsylvania

Errico, Thomas J MD [OrS] - **Spec Exp:** Spinal Surgery; Spinal Disc Replacement; Scoliosis; **Hospital:** NYU Langone Med Ctr (page 67), Hosp For Joint Diseases (page 67); **Address:** 530 1st Ave, Ste 8U, New York, NY 10016-6402; **Phone:** 212-263-7182; **Board Cert:** Orthopaedic Surgery 1986; **Med School:** UMDNJ-NJ Med Sch, Newark 1978; **Resid:** Orthopaedic Surgery, NYU Med Ctr 1983; **Fellow:** Spinal Surgery, Toronto Genl Hosp 1984; **Fac Appt:** Assoc Prof OrS, NYU Sch Med

Feldman, David S MD [OrS] - **Spec Exp:** Limb Deformities; Spinal Surgery; Pediatric Orthopaedic Surgery; Scoliosis; **Hospital:** Hosp For Joint Diseases (page 67), NYU Langone Med Ctr (page 67); **Address:** 67 Irving Pl Fl 8, New York, NY 10003; **Phone:** 212-533-5310; **Board Cert:** Orthopaedic Surgery 2007; **Med School:** Albert Einstein Coll Med 1988; **Resid:** Orthopaedic Surgery, Hosp for Joint Diseases 1993; **Fellow:** Pediatric Surgery, Hosp For Sick Chldn 1994; **Fac Appt:** Asst Prof OrS, NYU Sch Med

Flatow, Evan MD [OrS] - **Spec Exp:** Rotator Cuff Surgery; Shoulder Injuries; Shoulder Replacement; Shoulder Arthroscopic Surgery; **Hospital:** Mount Sinai Med Ctr (page 64); **Address:** 5 E 98th St Fl 9, Box 1188, New York, NY 10029; **Phone:** 212-241-1663; **Board Cert:** Orthopaedic Surgery 2000; **Med School:** Columbia P&S 1981; **Resid:** Surgery, Roosevelt Hosp 1983; Orthopaedic Surgery, Columbia-Presby Med Ctr 1985; **Fellow:** Shoulder Surgery, Columbia-Presby Med Ctr 1987; **Fac Appt:** Prof OrS, Mount Sinai Sch Med

Frassica, Frank J MD [OrS] - **Spec Exp:** Bone Cancer; **Hospital:** Johns Hopkins Hosp (page 61), Univ of MD Med Ctr; **Address:** 601 N Caroline St, Ste 5215, Baltimore, MD 21287-0882; **Phone:** 410-955-9300; **Board Cert:** Orthopaedic Surgery 2001; **Med School:** Univ SC Sch Med 1982; **Resid:** Orthopaedic Surgery, Mayo Clinic 1987; **Fellow:** Orthopaedic Oncology, Mayo Clinic 1988; **Fac Appt:** Prof OrS, Johns Hopkins Univ

Fu, Freddie H MD [OrS] - **Spec Exp:** Sports Medicine; Knee Injuries/ACL; Shoulder Injuries; **Hospital:** UPMC Presby, Pittsburgh, UPMC South Side; **Address:** Presbyterian Univ Hosp, Kaufmann Bldg, 3471 5th Ave, Ste 1011, Pittsburgh, PA 15213; **Phone:** 412-432-3611; **Board Cert:** Orthopaedic Surgery 1984; **Med School:** Univ Pittsburgh 1977; **Resid:** Orthopaedic Surgery, Univ Pittsburgh Med Ctr 1982; **Fellow:** Orthopaedic Research, Univ Pittsburgh Med Ctr 1979; **Fac Appt:** Prof OrS, Univ Pittsburgh

Gladstone, James N MD [OrS] - **Spec Exp:** Shoulder & Knee Surgery; Cartilage Damage; Knee-Patella Problems; Arthritis; **Hospital:** Mount Sinai Med Ctr (page 64); **Address:** Mt Sinai Med Ctr, 5 E 98th St Fl 9, Box 1188, New York, NY 10029; **Phone:** 212-241-1645; **Board Cert:** Orthopaedic Surgery 2009; **Med School:** Tufts Univ 1990; **Resid:** Orthopaedic Surgery, Columbia-Presby Med Ctr 1995; **Fellow:** Sports Medicine, American Sports Med Inst 1996; **Fac Appt:** Assoc Prof OrS, Mount Sinai Sch Med

Glashow, Jonathan L MD [OrS] - **Spec Exp:** Sports Medicine; Shoulder Surgery; Knee Surgery; Arthroscopic Surgery; **Hospital:** Mount Sinai Med Ctr (page 64), Lenox Hill Hosp (page 62); **Address:** 737 Park Ave, Ste 1C, New York, NY 10021; **Phone:** 212-794-5096; **Board Cert:** Orthopaedic Surgery 2004; **Med School:** Cornell Univ-Weill Med Coll 1984; **Resid:** Orthopaedic Surgery, Lenox Hill Hosp 1989; **Fellow:** Arthroscopic Surgery, S Calif Ortho Inst 1990; Shoulder Surgery, Univ Texas Med Ctr 1990; **Fac Appt:** Assoc Clin Prof OrS, Mount Sinai Sch Med

Goldstein, Jeffrey A MD [OrS] - **Spec Exp:** Spinal Surgery; Minimally Invasive Spinal Surgery; Spinal Disc Replacement; **Hospital:** Hosp For Joint Diseases (page 67), NYU Langone Med Ctr (page 67); **Address:** 19 Beekman St Fl 5, New York, NY 10038; **Phone:** 212-513-7711; **Board Cert:** Orthopaedic Surgery 2004; **Med School:** SUNY Downstate 1990; **Resid:** Orthopaedic Surgery, Case West Univ Med Ctr 1995; **Fellow:** Spinal Surgery, Maryland Spine Ctr 1996; **Fac Appt:** Assoc Clin Prof OrS, NYU Sch Med

Grelsamer, Ronald P MD [OrS] - **Spec Exp:** Knee-Patella Problems; Sports Medicine; Knee Reconstruction; Arthritis-Hip & Knee; **Hospital:** Mount Sinai Med Ctr (page 64); **Address:** Mount Sinai Medical Ctr, Dept Orthopaedics, 5 E 98th St, Box 1188, New York, NY 10029-6574; **Phone:** 212-241-2914; **Board Cert:** Orthopaedic Surgery 2007; **Med School:** Columbia P&S 1979; **Resid:** Orthopaedic Surgery, Columbia Presby Med Ctr 1984; **Fellow:** Hip & Knee Surgery, Columbia Presby Med Ctr 1985; **Fac Appt:** Assoc Prof OrS, Mount Sinai Sch Med

Haas, Steven B MD [OrS] - **Spec Exp:** Knee Surgery; Knee Replacement; Minimally Invasive Surgery; **Hospital:** Hosp For Special Surgery (page 59); **Address:** Hospital for Special Surgery, 535 E 70th St Fl 3, New York, NY 10021; **Phone:** 212-606-1852; **Board Cert:** Orthopaedic Surgery 2004; **Med School:** Univ Rochester 1985; **Resid:** Orthopaedic Surgery, Hosp Special Surgery 1990; **Fellow:** Knee Surgery, Hosp Special Surgery 1991; **Fac Appt:** Assoc Prof OrS, Cornell Univ-Weill Med Coll

Hannafin, Jo A MD/PhD [OrS] - **Spec Exp:** Sports Medicine-Women; Shoulder Arthroscopic Surgery; Knee Injuries/Ligament Surgery; Ligament Reconstruction; **Hospital:** Hosp For Special Surgery (page 59), NY-Presby Hosp/Weill Cornell (page 66); **Address:** 535 E 70th St, New York, NY 10021-4872; **Phone:** 212-606-1469; **Board Cert:** Orthopaedic Surgery 2005; **Med School:** Albert Einstein Coll Med 1985; **Resid:** Orthopaedic Surgery, Montefiore Med Ctr 1990; **Fellow:** Sports Medicine, Hosp Special Surg-Cornell 1992; **Fac Appt:** Assoc Prof OrS, Cornell Univ-Weill Med Coll

Hausman, Michael R MD [OrS] - **Spec Exp:** Hand Reconstruction; Elbow Reconstruction; Reconstructive Microvascular Surgery; Arthroscopic Surgery; **Hospital:** Mount Sinai Med Ctr (page 64); **Address:** 5 E 98th St, Box 1188, New York, NY 10029-6501; **Phone:** 212-241-1658; **Board Cert:** Orthopaedic Surgery 2000; Hand Surgery 2000; **Med School:** Yale Univ 1979; **Resid:** Surgery, Yale-New Haven Hosp 1981; Orthopaedic Surgery, Yale-New Haven Hosp 1985; **Fellow:** Hand Surgery, Roosevelt Hosp 1987; **Fac Appt:** Assoc Clin Prof OrS, Mount Sinai Sch Med

Healey, John H MD [OrS] - **Spec Exp:** Bone Tumors; Hip & Knee Replacement in Bone Tumors; Sarcoma; Sarcoma-Soft Tissue; **Hospital:** Meml Sloan-Kettering Cancer Ctr, Hosp For Special Surgery (page 59); **Address:** 1275 York Avenue, New York, NY 10065; **Phone:** 800-525-2225; **Board Cert:** Orthopaedic Surgery 2007; **Med School:** Univ VT Coll Med 1978; **Resid:** Orthopaedic Surgery, Hosp Special Surg 1983; **Fellow:** Orthopaedic Oncology, Meml Sloan Kettering Cancer Ctr 1984; Orthopaedic Surgery, Hosp Special Surgery 1984; **Fac Appt:** Prof OrS, Cornell Univ-Weill Med Coll

Orthopaedic Surgery

Hecht, Andrew MD [OrS] - **Spec Exp:** Spinal Surgery; Spinal Disc Replacement; Minimally Invasive Spinal Surgery; **Hospital:** Mount Sinai Med Ctr (page 64); **Address:** Mount Sinai Med Ctr, Dept Orthopaedic Surg, 5 E 98th St Fl 9, Box 1188, New York, NY 10029; **Phone:** 212-241-0735; **Board Cert:** Orthopaedic Surgery 2003; **Med School:** Harvard Med Sch 1994; **Resid:** Orthopaedic Surgery, Mass Genl Hosp 1999; **Fellow:** Spinal Surgery, Emory Univ Spine Ctr 2001; **Fac Appt:** Asst Prof OrS, Mount Sinai Sch Med

Helfet, David L MD [OrS] - **Spec Exp:** Fractures-Complex; Fractures-Non Union; Fractures-Stress; Deformity Reconstruction; **Hospital:** Hosp For Special Surgery (page 59), NY-Presby Hosp/Weill Cornell (page 66); **Address:** 535 E 70th St, New York, NY 10021; **Phone:** 212-606-1888; **Board Cert:** Orthopaedic Surgery 1984; **Med School:** South Africa 1975; **Resid:** Surgery, Edendale Hosp 1977; Orthopaedic Surgery, Johns Hopkins Hosp 1981; **Fellow:** Orthopaedic Surgery, Inselspita Hosp 1981; Orthopaedic Surgery, UCLA Med Ctr 1982; **Fac Appt:** Prof OrS, Cornell Univ-Weill Med Coll

Herzenberg, John E MD [OrS] - **Spec Exp:** Limb Lengthening (Ilizarov Procedure); Limb Deformities; Pediatric Orthopaedic Surgery; Clubfoot; **Hospital:** Sinai Hosp - Baltimore; **Address:** Rubin Inst for Advanced Orthopaedics, 2401 W Belvedere Ave, Baltimore, MD 21215; **Phone:** 410-601-8700; **Board Cert:** Orthopaedic Surgery 2009; **Med School:** Boston Univ 1979; **Resid:** Orthopaedic Surgery, Duke Univ Med Ctr 1985; **Fellow:** Pediatric Orthopaedic Surgery, Hosp for Sick Children 1986

Hilibrand, Alan S MD [OrS] - **Spec Exp:** Spinal Surgery; Spinal Trauma; Spinal Surgery-Neck; Spinal Deformity; **Hospital:** Thomas Jefferson Univ Hosp, Atlantic City Medical Center- City Division; **Address:** Rothman Institute, 925 Chestnut St Fl 5, Philadelphia, PA 19107; **Phone:** 800-321-9999; **Board Cert:** Orthopaedic Surgery 2009; **Med School:** Yale Univ 1990; **Resid:** Orthopaedic Surgery, Univ Michigan Hlth System 1995; **Fellow:** Spinal Surgery, Cleveland Spine Inst 1996; **Fac Appt:** Prof OrS, Jefferson Med Coll

Hotchkiss, Robert MD [OrS] - **Spec Exp:** Hand Surgery; Wrist Surgery; Elbow Reconstruction; Dupuytren's Contracture; **Hospital:** Hosp For Special Surgery (page 59), NY-Presby Hosp/Weill Cornell (page 66); **Address:** 523 E 72nd St Fl 4, New York, NY 10021-4099; **Phone:** 212-606-1964; **Board Cert:** Orthopaedic Surgery 2000; Hand Surgery 2000; **Med School:** Johns Hopkins Univ 1980; **Resid:** Surgery, Johns Hopkins Hosp 1982; Orthopaedic Surgery, Johns Hopkins Hosp 1985; **Fellow:** Hand Surgery, Union Meml Hosp 1987; **Fac Appt:** Assoc Prof OrS, Cornell Univ-Weill Med Coll

Hozack, William J MD [OrS] - **Spec Exp:** Hip Surgery; Knee Surgery; Joint Replacement; **Hospital:** Thomas Jefferson Univ Hosp; **Address:** Rothman Institute, 925 Chestnut St Fl 5, Philadelphia, PA 19107; **Phone:** 800-321-9999; **Board Cert:** Orthopaedic Surgery 2000; **Med School:** McGill Univ 1981; **Resid:** Orthopaedic Surgery, Hosp Univ Penn 1986; **Fellow:** Joint Reconstruction, Penn Hosp/Thomas Jefferson Univ 1987; **Fac Appt:** Prof OrS, Jefferson Med Coll

Hume, Eric L MD [OrS] - **Spec Exp:** Hip Replacement; Knee Replacement; **Hospital:** Cooper Univ Hosp; **Address:** 3 Cooper Pl, Ste 408, Camden, NJ 08103; **Phone:** 856-963-3670; **Board Cert:** Orthopaedic Surgery 2007; **Med School:** SUNY Upstate Med Univ 1978; **Resid:** Orthopaedic Surgery, Jefferson Univ Hosp 1983; **Fac Appt:** Assoc Prof OrS, Thomas Jefferson Univ

Hungerford, Marc W MD [OrS] - **Spec Exp:** Knee Replacement & Revision; Hip Replacement & Revision; Cartilage Damage; **Hospital:** Mercy Med Ctr; **Address:** Mercy Medical Center, Joint Replacement & Trauma Ctr, 301 Saint Paul Pl, Baltimore, MD 21202; **Phone:** 410-539-2227; **Board Cert:** Orthopaedic Surgery 2001; **Med School:** Vanderbilt Univ 1992; **Resid:** Orthopaedic Surgery, Johns Hopkins Hosp 1997; **Fac Appt:** Asst Prof OrS, Johns Hopkins Univ

Johanson, Norman A MD [OrS] - **Spec Exp:** Hip & Knee Replacement; Joint Replacement; Juvenile Arthritis; Joint Replacement Revision; **Hospital:** Hahnemann Univ Hosp; **Address:** Drexel Orthopaedic Assocs, 216-220 N Broad St, Feinstein Bldg, Fl 2, Philadelphia, PA 19102; **Phone:** 215-762-2663; **Board Cert:** Orthopaedic Surgery 2007; **Med School:** Cornell Univ ; **Resid:** Orthopaedic Surgery, Hosp Special Surg; **Fellow:** Hosp Special Surg; **Fac Appt:** Prof OrS, Drexel Univ Coll Med

Johnson, Carl A MD [OrS] - **Spec Exp:** Knee Surgery; **Hospital:** Johns Hopkins Bayview Med Ctr (page 61), Johns Hopkins Hosp (page 61); **Address:** Johns Hopkins at Whitemarsh, 4924 Campbell Blvd, Ste 130, Nottingham, MD 21236; **Phone:** 443-442-2086; **Board Cert:** Orthopaedic Surgery 1983; **Med School:** Johns Hopkins Univ 1976; **Resid:** Surgery, Johns Hopkins Hosp 1978; Orthopaedic Surgery, Johns Hopkins Hosp 1981; **Fac Appt:** Assoc Prof OrS, Johns Hopkins Univ

Kaplan, Frederick S MD [OrS] - **Spec Exp:** Bone Disorders-Metabolic; Fibrodysplasia Ossificans Progressiv FOP; Progressive Osseous Heteroplasia POH; **Hospital:** Hosp Univ Penn - UPHS (page 60), Thomas Jefferson Univ Hosp; **Address:** Orthopaedic Inst, 3400 Spruce St, 2 Silverstein, MC 4283, Philadelphia, PA 19104; **Phone:** 215-349-8727; **Med School:** Johns Hopkins Univ 1976; **Resid:** Orthopaedic Surgery, Hosp U Penn 1981; **Fellow:** Orthopaedic Research, Hosp U Penn 1982; Musculoskeletal Disorders, Dr Michael Zasloff/U Penn 1991; **Fac Appt:** Prof OrS, Univ Pennsylvania

Keenan, Mary Ann MD [OrS] - **Spec Exp:** Neuro-Orthopaedic Surgery; Arthritis; Deformity Reconstruction; Heterotopic Ossification; **Hospital:** Hosp Univ Penn - UPHS (page 60), Pennsylvania Hosp (page 60); **Address:** Hosp Univ Penn, Dept Orthopaedic Surg, 3400 Spruce St, 2 Fl- Silverstein, Philadelphia, PA 19104; **Phone:** 215-662-3340; **Board Cert:** Orthopaedic Surgery 1997; **Med School:** Med Coll PA 1976; **Resid:** Orthopaedic Surgery, Albert Einstein Med Ctr 1981; **Fellow:** Arthritis Surgery, Rancho Los Amigos Med Ctr 1981; Neurological Orthopaedic Surgery, Rancho Los Amigos Med Ctr 1982; **Fac Appt:** Prof OrS, Univ Pennsylvania

Kenan, Samuel MD [OrS] - **Spec Exp:** Bone Tumors; Hip Replacement; Knee Replacement; **Hospital:** Hosp For Joint Diseases (page 67), NYU Langone Med Ctr (page 67); **Address:** 317 E 34th St Fl 9 - Ste 903, New York, NY 10016; **Phone:** 212-684-5511; **Med School:** Israel 1976; **Resid:** Orthopaedic Surgery, Hadassah Univ Hosp 1984; **Fellow:** Orthopaedic Pathology, Hosp for Joint Diseases 1987; **Fac Appt:** Prof OrS, NYU Sch Med

Krackow, Kenneth A MD [OrS] - **Spec Exp:** Knee Replacement; Knee Reconstruction; Hip Replacement & Revision; **Hospital:** Buffalo General Hosp; **Address:** Bufffalo General Hosp, Dept Orthopaedic Surgery, 100 High St, Ste B276, Buffalo, NY 14203; **Phone:** 716-859-1256; **Board Cert:** Orthopaedic Surgery 1993; **Med School:** Duke Univ 1971; **Resid:** Surgery, Johns Hopkins Hosp 1973; **Fellow:** Orthopaedic Surgery, Johns Hopkins Hosp 1976; **Fac Appt:** Prof OrS, SUNY Buffalo

Lackman, Richard D MD [OrS] - **Spec Exp:** Bone Cancer; Sarcoma; Limb Sparing Surgery; **Hospital:** Hosp Univ Penn - UPHS (page 60), Pennsylvania Hosp (page 60); **Address:** Hosp Univ Penn-Dept Orthopaedic Surg, 301 S 8th St, Garfield Duncan Bldg, Ste 2C, Philadelphia, PA 19104; **Phone:** 215-829-5022; **Board Cert:** Orthopaedic Surgery 1985; **Med School:** Univ Pennsylvania 1977; **Resid:** Orthopaedic Surgery, Hosp Univ Penn 1982; **Fellow:** Orthopaedic Oncology, Mayo Clinic 1983; **Fac Appt:** Assoc Prof OrS, Univ Pennsylvania

Lane, Joseph MD [OrS] - **Spec Exp:** Bone Disorders-Metabolic; Osteoporosis Spine-Kyphoplasty; Bone Cancer; **Hospital:** Hosp For Special Surgery (page 59), NY-Presby Hosp/Weill Cornell (page 66); **Address:** Hosp for Special Surgery, 535 E 70th St, New York, NY 10021; **Phone:** 212-606-1172; **Board Cert:** Orthopaedic Surgery 1974; **Med School:** Harvard Med Sch 1965; **Resid:** Surgery, Hosp Univ Penn 1967; Orthopaedic Surgery, Hosp Univ Penn 1973; **Fac Appt:** Prof OrS, Cornell Univ-Weill Med Coll

Orthopaedic Surgery

Lauerman, William MD [OrS] - **Spec Exp:** Spinal Deformity-Pediatric & Adult; Spinal Surgery; Pain-Back; Scoliosis; **Hospital:** Georgetown Univ Hosp; **Address:** 3800 Reservoir Rd NW, Spine Surgery Clinic-1 Gorman, Washington, DC 20007; **Phone:** 202-444-8766 x2; **Board Cert:** Orthopaedic Surgery 2001; **Med School:** Georgetown Univ 1982; **Resid:** Orthopaedic Surgery, Georgetown Univ Med Ctr 1987; **Fellow:** Orthopaedic Surgery, Univ Minn-Twin Cities Scoliosis Ctr 1988; **Fac Appt:** Prof OrS, Georgetown Univ

Leadbetter, Wayne MD [OrS] - **Spec Exp:** Knee-Patella Problems; Arthritis-Knee; **Hospital:** Sinai Hosp - Baltimore; **Address:** Ctr Joint Preservation & Reconstruction, Sinai Hosp, 2401 W Belvedere Ave, Baltimore, MD 21215; **Phone:** 410-601-8500; **Board Cert:** Orthopaedic Surgery 1977; **Med School:** Creighton Univ 1970; **Resid:** Surgery, Johns Hopkins Hosp 1972; Orthopaedic Surgery, Johns Hopkins Hosp 1976; **Fellow:** Orthopaedic Surgery, Jonhs Hopkins Hosp 1973; **Fac Appt:** Asst Clin Prof S, Uniformed Srvs Univ, Bethesda

Lee, Francis Y MD/PhD [OrS] - **Spec Exp:** Bone Tumors; Pediatric Orthopaedic Cancers; Pediatric Orthopaedic Surgery; **Hospital:** NYPresby-Morgan Stanley Children's Hosp (page 66), NYPresby Hosp/Columbia (page 66); **Address:** 3959 Broadway, Ste 800N, New York, NY 10032; **Phone:** 212-305-4565; **Board Cert:** Orthopaedic Surgery 2001; **Med School:** South Korea 1986; **Resid:** Orthopaedic Surgery, NJ Med Ctr 1997; **Fellow:** Orthopaedic Oncology, Harvard Med Sch 1998; Pediatric Orthopaedic Surgery, Hosp for Sick Chldn/Univ Toronto 1999; **Fac Appt:** Asst Prof OrS, Columbia P&S

Levine, Alan M MD [OrS] - **Spec Exp:** Bone Cancer; Spinal Surgery; **Hospital:** Sinai Hosp - Baltimore; **Address:** Sinai Hosp, Cancer Inst, 2401 W Belvedere Ave, Baltimore, MD 21215; **Phone:** 410-601-4606; **Board Cert:** Orthopaedic Surgery 1981; **Med School:** Yale Univ 1974; **Resid:** Orthopaedic Surgery, Yale-New Haven Hosp 1980; **Fellow:** Research, Natl Cancer Inst 1981; **Fac Appt:** Prof S, Univ MD Sch Med

Macaulay, William B MD [OrS] - **Spec Exp:** Hip Replacement; Knee Replacement; Minimally Invasive Surgery; Reconstructive Surgery; **Hospital:** NY-Presby Hosp/Columbia (page 66); **Address:** Columbia Orthopaedics, 161 Fort Washington Ave, Irving Pavilion Fl 2, New York, NY 10032; **Phone:** 212-305-6959; **Board Cert:** Orthopaedic Surgery 2001; **Med School:** Columbia P&S 1992; **Resid:** Orthopaedic Surgery, Univ Pittsburgh Med Ctr 1997; **Fellow:** Adult Reconstructive Surgery, Hosp for Special Surgery 1999; **Fac Appt:** Prof OrS, Columbia P&S

Malawer, Martin M MD [OrS] - **Spec Exp:** Bone Tumors; Limb Sparing Surgery; Pediatric Orthopaedic Surgery; Sarcoma; **Hospital:** Washington Hosp Ctr; **Address:** Washington Cancer Institute, 110 Irving St NW, Ste C2173, Washington, DC 20010; **Phone:** 202-877-3970; **Board Cert:** Orthopaedic Surgery 1993; **Med School:** NYU Sch Med 1969; **Resid:** Surgery, Bronx Muni Hosp 1972; Orthopaedic Surgery, Bellevue Hosp Ctr 1975; **Fellow:** Orthopaedic Oncology, Shands Hosp-Univ Florida 1978; **Fac Appt:** Prof OrS, Geo Wash Univ

McAfee, Paul C MD [OrS] - **Spec Exp:** Spinal Reconstructive Surgery; Spinal Disc Replacement; Scoliosis; **Hospital:** St Joseph Med Ctr; **Address:** Scoliosis & Spine Ctr, 7505 Osler Drive, Ste 104, Towson, MD 21204; **Phone:** 410-337-8888; **Board Cert:** Orthopaedic Surgery 2007; **Med School:** SUNY Upstate Med Univ 1979; **Resid:** Orthopaedic Surgery, SUNY Upstate Med Ctr 1984; **Fellow:** Spinal Surgery, Case West Res Univ Hosps 1986; **Fac Appt:** Assoc Prof OrS, Johns Hopkins Univ

McCann, Peter D MD [OrS] - **Spec Exp:** Shoulder Surgery; Elbow Surgery; **Hospital:** Beth Israel Med Ctr - Petrie Division (page 57); **Address:** 10 Union Square E, Ste 3M, New York, NY 10003; **Phone:** 212-844-6735; **Board Cert:** Orthopaedic Surgery 2009; **Med School:** Columbia P&S 1980; **Resid:** Surgery, St Vincent's Hosp 1982; Orthopaedic Surgery, Columbia-Presby Med Ctr 1985; **Fellow:** Shoulder Surgery, Columbia-Presby Med Ctr 1986; **Fac Appt:** Assoc Prof OrS, Albert Einstein Coll Med

McFarland, Edward G MD [OrS] - **Spec Exp:** Sports Medicine; Rotator Cuff Surgery; Shoulder Surgery; **Hospital:** Johns Hopkins Hosp (page 61); **Address:** 10753 Falls Rd, Ste 215, Lutherville, MD 21093; **Phone:** 410-583-2850; **Board Cert:** Orthopaedic Surgery 2001; **Med School:** Univ Louisville Sch Med 1982; **Resid:** Orthopaedic Surgery, Mayo Clinic 1987; **Fellow:** Sports Medicine, Kerlan-Jobe Orthopaedic Group 1989; **Fac Appt:** Assoc Prof OrS, Johns Hopkins Univ

Myerson, Mark MD [OrS] - **Spec Exp:** Foot & Ankle Surgery; **Hospital:** Mercy Med Ctr; **Address:** 301 St Paul Pl, Baltimore, MD 21202; **Phone:** 410-659-2800; **Board Cert:** Orthopaedic Surgery 1999; **Med School:** South Africa 1979; **Resid:** Surgery, Sinai Hospital 1981; Orthopaedic Surgery, Johns Hopkins Hosp 1985; **Fellow:** Foot & Ankle Surgery, Hospital Joint Disease

Neuwirth, Michael MD [OrS] - **Spec Exp:** Scoliosis; Spinal Surgery; **Hospital:** Beth Israel Med Ctr - Petrie Division (page 57); **Address:** Beth Israel Med Ctr - Spine Institute, 10 Union Square E, Ste 5P, New York, NY 10003-3314; **Phone:** 212-844-8692; **Board Cert:** Orthopaedic Surgery 1980; **Med School:** SUNY Hlth Sci Ctr 1974; **Resid:** Orthopaedic Surgery, Hosp for Joint Diseases 1978; **Fellow:** Spinal Surgery, Rush-Presby Med Ctr 1979; **Fac Appt:** Assoc Clin Prof OrS, NYU Sch Med

Nicholas, Stephen J MD [OrS] - **Spec Exp:** Sports Medicine; Shoulder & Knee Surgery; Arthroscopic Surgery; **Hospital:** Lenox Hill Hosp (page 62); **Address:** 130 E 77 St, New York, NY 10075; **Phone:** 212-737-3301; **Board Cert:** Orthopaedic Surgery 2005; **Med School:** NY Med Coll 1986; **Resid:** Orthopaedic Surgery, Hosp for Special Surgery 1991; **Fellow:** Sports Medicine, Lenox Hill Hosp 1992

O'Keefe, Regis J MD/PhD [OrS] - **Spec Exp:** Bone & Soft Tissue Tumors; Reconstructive Surgery; Bone Disorders-Metabolic; **Hospital:** Univ of Rochester Strong Meml Hosp, Highland Hosp of Rochester; **Address:** Univ Rochester, Dept Orthopaedic Surgery, 601 Elmwood Ave, Box 665, Rochester, NY 14642; **Phone:** 585-275-3100; **Board Cert:** Orthopaedic Surgery 2007; **Med School:** Harvard Med Sch 1985; **Resid:** Surgery, New Eng Deaconess Hosp/Harvard 1986; Orthopaedic Surgery, Univ Rochester 1992; **Fellow:** Orthopaedic Oncology, Mass Genl Hosp 1993; **Fac Appt:** Prof S, Univ Rochester

O'Leary, Patrick MD [OrS] - **Spec Exp:** Spinal Surgery; **Hospital:** Hosp For Special Surgery (page 59); **Address:** 1015 Madison Ave Fl 4, New York, NY 10021; **Phone:** 212-249-8100; **Board Cert:** Orthopaedic Surgery 1983; **Med School:** Ireland 1968; **Resid:** Surgery, Roosevelt Hosp 1972; Orthopaedic Surgery, Hosp Spec Surg-Cornell 1975; **Fellow:** Spinal Surgery, Univ Toronto Genl Ortho Hosp 1976; **Fac Appt:** Assoc Clin Prof OrS, Cornell Univ-Weill Med Coll

Padgett, Douglas E MD [OrS] - **Spec Exp:** Hip & Knee Replacement; Arthroscopic Surgery-Hip; Arthroscopic Surgery-Knee; Dance Medicine; **Hospital:** Hosp For Special Surgery (page 59); **Address:** Hosp for Special Surgery, 535 E 70 St, New York, NY 10021; **Phone:** 212-606-1642; **Board Cert:** Orthopaedic Surgery 2003; **Med School:** NY Med Coll 1982; **Resid:** Orthopaedic Surgery, Hosp Spec Surg 1989; **Fellow:** Orthopaedic Surgery, Rush Presby Med Ctr 1990; **Fac Appt:** Assoc Prof OrS, Cornell Univ-Weill Med Coll

Pellicci, Paul M MD [OrS] - **Spec Exp:** Hip Replacement-Young Adults; Hip Resurfacing; Knee Replacement; Joint Replacement; **Hospital:** Hosp For Special Surgery (page 59), NY-Presby Hosp/Weill Cornell (page 66); **Address:** 535 E 70th St, New York, NY 10021-4872; **Phone:** 212-606-1010; **Board Cert:** Orthopaedic Surgery 1982; **Med School:** Cornell Univ-Weill Med Coll 1975; **Resid:** Surgery, NY Hosp 1977; Orthopaedic Surgery, Hosp Spec Surg 1980; **Fellow:** Joint Replacement Surgery, Brigham & Womens Hosp 1981; **Fac Appt:** Prof OrS, Cornell Univ-Weill Med Coll

Orthopaedic Surgery

Ramsey, Matthew L MD [OrS] - **Spec Exp:** Shoulder Surgery; Elbow Surgery; Sports Medicine; **Hospital:** Thomas Jefferson Univ Hosp; **Address:** Rothman Institute, 925 Chestnut St Fl 5, Philadelphia, PA 19107; **Phone:** 800-321-9999; **Board Cert:** Orthopaedic Surgery 2009; **Med School:** SUNY Hlth Sci Ctr 1990; **Resid:** Orthopaedic Surgery, Thomas Jefferson Univ Hosp 1995; **Fellow:** Shoulder Surgery, Hosp Univ Penn 1996; **Fac Appt:** Assoc Prof OrS, Thomas Jefferson Univ

Ranawat, Chitranjan MD [OrS] - **Spec Exp:** Hip Replacement; Knee Replacement; **Hospital:** Hosp For Special Surgery (page 59); **Address:** Hospital for Special Surgery, 535 E 70th St Fl 6, New York, NY 10021; **Phone:** 646-797-8700; **Board Cert:** Orthopaedic Surgery 1969; **Med School:** India 1958; **Resid:** Surgery, MY Hosp 1963; Orthopaedic Surgery, Albany Med Ctr 1965; **Fellow:** Orthopaedic Surgery, Hosp Special Surg 1969; **Fac Appt:** Prof OrS, Cornell Univ-Weill Med Coll

Rechtine, Glenn MD [OrS] - **Spec Exp:** Spinal Surgery; **Hospital:** Univ of Rochester Strong Meml Hosp; **Address:** Strong Meml Hosp, Dept Orthopaedics, 601 Elmwood Ave, Box 665, Rochester, NY 14618; **Phone:** 585-275-2225; **Board Cert:** Orthopaedic Surgery 1982; **Med School:** Univ S Fla Coll Med 1975; **Resid:** Orthopaedic Surgery, Naval Regional Med Ctr 1980; **Fellow:** Spinal Surgery, Case West Res Univ 1981; **Fac Appt:** Prof OrS, Univ Rochester

Rodosky, Mark W MD [OrS] - **Spec Exp:** Sports Medicine; Shoulder Surgery; Rotator Cuff Surgery; **Hospital:** UPMC South Side; **Address:** UPMC Center for Sports Medicine, 3200 S Water St, Pittsburgh, PA 15203; **Phone:** 412-432-3621; **Board Cert:** Orthopaedic Surgery 2008; **Med School:** Mount Sinai Sch Med 1987; **Resid:** Surgery, Univ Pittsburgh Med Ctr 1993; **Fellow:** Orthopaedic Surgery, NY Presby-Columbia Presby Med Ctr 1994; **Fac Appt:** Asst Prof OrS, Univ Pittsburgh

Rosier, Randy MD/PhD [OrS] - **Spec Exp:** Bone Disorders-Metabolic; **Hospital:** Univ of Rochester Strong Meml Hosp; **Address:** Univ Rochester, Dept Orthopaedic Surgery, 601 Elmwood Ave, Box 665, Rochester, NY 14642; **Phone:** 585-275-3100; **Board Cert:** Orthopaedic Surgery 1998; **Med School:** Univ Rochester 1978; **Resid:** Orthopaedic Surgery, Univ Iowa Hosp 1984; **Fac Appt:** Prof OrS, Univ Rochester

Rothman, Richard H MD/PhD [OrS] - **Spec Exp:** Hip Replacement; Knee Replacement; Joint Replacement; **Hospital:** Thomas Jefferson Univ Hosp; **Address:** Rothman Institute, 925 Chestnut St Fl 5, Philadelphia, PA 19107; **Phone:** 800-321-9999; **Board Cert:** Orthopaedic Surgery 1970; **Med School:** Univ Pennsylvania 1962; **Resid:** Orthopaedic Surgery, Jefferson Hosp 1968; **Fac Appt:** Prof OrS, Jefferson Med Coll

Roye, David MD [OrS] - **Spec Exp:** Pediatric Orthopaedic Surgery; Scoliosis; Hip Disorders-Pediatric; **Hospital:** NY-Presby Hosp/Columbia (page 66), Greenwich Hosp; **Address:** Morgan Stanley Chlds Hosp NewYork-Presby, 3959 Broadway, 8 North, New York, NY 10032-1559; **Phone:** 212-305-5475; **Board Cert:** Orthopaedic Surgery 1981; **Med School:** Columbia P&S 1975; **Resid:** Orthopaedic Surgery, Columbia-Presby Med Ctr 1979; **Fellow:** Orthopaedic Surgery, Hosp for Sick Chldn 1980; **Fac Appt:** Prof OrS, Columbia P&S

Rozbruch, S Robert MD [OrS] - **Spec Exp:** Limb Lengthening; Limb Deformities; Limb Surgery/Reconstruction; Fractures-Complex & Non Union; **Hospital:** Hosp For Special Surgery (page 59), NY-Presby Hosp/Weill Cornell (page 66); **Address:** 535 E 70th St, New York, NY 10021; **Phone:** 212-606-1415; **Board Cert:** Orthopaedic Surgery 2009; **Med School:** Cornell Univ-Weill Med Coll 1990; **Resid:** Orthopaedic Surgery, Hosp Special Surgery 1995; **Fellow:** Trauma, Univ Bern Hosp 1997; Limb Lengthening, Intl Ctr Limb Length/Univ MD 1999; **Fac Appt:** Assoc Clin Prof OrS, Cornell Univ-Weill Med Coll

Salvati, Eduardo A MD [OrS] - **Spec Exp:** Hip Surgery; Hip & Knee Replacement; **Hospital:** Hosp For Special Surgery (page 59); **Address:** Hosp for Spec Surg, 535 E 70th Street, New York, NY 10021; **Phone:** 212-606-1472; **Board Cert:** Orthopaedic Surgery 1972; **Med School:** Argentina 1963; **Resid:** Orthopaedic Surgery, Univ Florence Ortho Clinic 1965; Orthopaedic Surgery, Hosp Buenos Aires 1969; **Fellow:** Hip Surgery, Hosp For Spec Surg 1972; **Fac Appt:** Clin Prof OrS, Cornell Univ-Weill Med Coll

Sandhu, Harvinder S MD [OrS] - **Spec Exp:** Minimally Invasive Surgery; Spinal Disc Replacement; Spinal Surgery; **Hospital:** Hosp For Special Surgery (page 59), NY-Presby Hosp/Weill Cornell (page 66); **Address:** 535 E 70th St, New York, NY 10021; **Phone:** 212-606-1798; **Board Cert:** Orthopaedic Surgery 2007; **Med School:** Northwestern Univ 1987; **Resid:** Orthopaedic Surgery, Univ Hosp-SUNY Hlth Sci Ctr 1992; **Fellow:** Spinal Surgery, UCLA Med Ctr 1993; **Fac Appt:** Assoc Prof OrS, Cornell Univ-Weill Med Coll

Schmidt, Richard G MD [OrS] - **Spec Exp:** Bone Tumors; Sarcoma-Soft Tissue; Limb Sparing Surgery; Bone Tumors-Metastatic; **Hospital:** Lankenau Hosp, Fox Chase Cancer Ctr (page 58); **Address:** Musculoskeletal Tumor Ctr, 15 N Presidential Blvd, Ste 300, Bala Cynwyd, PA 19004; **Phone:** 610-667-2663; **Board Cert:** Orthopaedic Surgery 1999; **Med School:** Penn State Univ-Hershey Med Ctr 1980; **Resid:** Orthopaedic Surgery, Hosp Univ Penn 1985; **Fellow:** Orthopaedic Oncology, Shands Hosp 1986

Scott, W Norman MD [OrS] - **Spec Exp:** Knee Injuries; Knee Replacement; Sports Medicine; **Hospital:** Lenox Hill Hosp (page 62), Franklin Hosp; **Address:** 210 E 64th St Fl 4, New York, NY 10065; **Phone:** 212-434-4301; **Board Cert:** Orthopaedic Surgery 1978; **Med School:** Cornell Univ-Weill Med Coll 1972; **Resid:** Surgery, St Lukes-Roosevelt Hosp Ctr 1974; Orthopaedic Surgery, Hosp Special Surg 1977; **Fac Appt:** Clin Prof OrS, Cornell Univ-Weill Med Coll

Sculco, Thomas P MD [OrS] - **Spec Exp:** Hip Replacement; Knee Replacement; Minimally Invasive Surgery; Joint Replacement; **Hospital:** Hosp For Special Surgery (page 59); **Address:** 535 E 70th St, Ste 238, New York, NY 10021-4872; **Phone:** 212-606-1475; **Board Cert:** Orthopaedic Surgery 1976; **Med School:** Columbia P&S 1969; **Resid:** Surgery, Roosevelt Hosp 1971; Orthopaedic Surgery, Hosp For Special Surgery 1974; **Fellow:** Orthopaedic Surgery, The London Hosp 1975; **Fac Appt:** Prof OrS, Cornell Univ-Weill Med Coll

Sherman, Orrin MD [OrS] - **Spec Exp:** Knee Injuries/ACL; Shoulder Surgery; Sports Medicine; Arthroscopic Surgery; **Hospital:** NYU Langone Med Ctr (page 67), Hosp For Joint Diseases (page 67); **Address:** 530 1st Ave, Ste 8U, New York, NY 10016-6402; **Phone:** 212-263-8961; **Board Cert:** Orthopaedic Surgery 2007; **Med School:** Geo Wash Univ 1978; **Resid:** Orthopaedic Surgery, NYU Med Ctr 1983; **Fellow:** Sports Medicine, So Cal Orthopedic Inst 1984; **Fac Appt:** Assoc Prof OrS, NYU Sch Med

Spivak, Jeffrey M MD [OrS] - **Spec Exp:** Spinal Surgery; Scoliosis; Sports Medicine Back Injuries; **Hospital:** Hosp For Joint Diseases (page 67), NYU Langone Med Ctr (page 67); **Address:** Hospital for Joint Diseases, Spine Ctr, 301 E 17th St, Ste 400, New York, NY 10003-3804; **Phone:** 212-598-6696; **Board Cert:** Orthopaedic Surgery 2006; **Med School:** Cornell Univ-Weill Med Coll 1986; **Resid:** Orthopaedic Surgery, Hosp for Joint Diseases 1992; **Fellow:** Spinal Surgery, Thomas Jefferson Univ Hosp 1993; **Fac Appt:** Asst Prof OrS, NYU Sch Med

Sponseller, Paul D MD [OrS] - **Spec Exp:** Cerebral Palsy; Scoliosis; Pediatric Orthopaedic Surgery; **Hospital:** Johns Hopkins Hosp (page 61); **Address:** 601 N Caroline St, Ste 5212, Baltimore, MD 21287-0882; **Phone:** 410-955-3136; **Board Cert:** Orthopaedic Surgery 2000; **Med School:** Univ Mich Med Sch 1980; **Resid:** Orthopaedic Surgery, Univ Wisc Hosp 1985; **Fellow:** Pediatric Orthopaedic Surgery, Children's Hosp 1986; **Fac Appt:** Prof OrS, Johns Hopkins Univ

Orthopaedic Surgery

Strongwater, Allan MD [OrS] - **Spec Exp:** Pediatric Orthopaedic Surgery; Cerebral Palsy; Deformity Reconstruction; **Hospital:** Hosp For Joint Diseases (page 67), NYU Langone Med Ctr (page 67); **Address:** 301 E 17th St, New York, NY 10003; **Phone:** 973-754-2414; **Board Cert:** Orthopaedic Surgery 2007; **Med School:** Rush Med Coll 1978; **Resid:** Orthopaedic Surgery, Yale-New Haven Hosp 1983; Pediatric Orthopaedic Surgery, Hosp Joint Diseases 1984; **Fac Appt:** Clin Prof OrS, NYU Sch Med

Stuchin, Steven MD [OrS] - **Spec Exp:** Hand Surgery; Arthritis; Hip & Knee Replacement; Hip Resurfacing; **Hospital:** Hosp For Joint Diseases (page 67), Lenox Hill Hosp (page 62); **Address:** 301 E 17th St, Ste 1402, New York, NY 10003-3804; **Phone:** 212-598-6708; **Board Cert:** Orthopaedic Surgery 1984; **Med School:** Columbia P&S 1976; **Resid:** Surgery, Roosevelt Hosp 1978; Orthopaedic Surgery, Hosp For Special Surg 1981; **Fellow:** Hand Surgery, Thomas Jefferson Univ Hosp 1982; **Fac Appt:** Assoc Prof OrS, NYU Sch Med

Vaccaro, Alexander R MD/PhD [OrS] - **Spec Exp:** Spinal Surgery; Spinal Trauma; Spinal Cord Injury; **Hospital:** Thomas Jefferson Univ Hosp; **Address:** Rothman Institute, 925 Chestnut St Fl 5, Philadelphia, PA 19107; **Phone:** 800-321-9999; **Board Cert:** Orthopaedic Surgery 2006; **Med School:** Georgetown Univ 1987; **Resid:** Orthopaedic Surgery, Thos Jefferson Univ Hosp 1992; **Fellow:** Spinal Surgery, UCSD Med Ctr 1993; **Fac Appt:** Prof OrS, Thomas Jefferson Univ

Wapner, Keith L MD [OrS] - **Spec Exp:** Foot & Ankle Surgery; Tendon Surgery; Arthritis; **Hospital:** Pennsylvania Hosp (page 60); **Address:** The Farm Journal Bldg Fl 5, 230 W Washington Square, Philadelphia, PA 19106-3500; **Phone:** 215-829-3668; **Board Cert:** Orthopaedic Surgery 1999; **Med School:** Temple Univ 1980; **Resid:** Surgery, Hosp Univ Penn 1981; Orthopaedic Surgery, Hosp Univ Penn 1985; **Fellow:** Joint Reconstruction, Ohio St Univ Med Ctr 1986; Foot & Ankle Surgery, UCSF Med Ctr 1987; **Fac Appt:** Clin Prof OrS, Univ Pennsylvania

Warren, Russell MD [OrS] - **Spec Exp:** Knee Injuries/Ligament Surgery; Shoulder Reconstruction; Shoulder Replacement; Rotator Cuff Surgery; **Hospital:** Hosp For Special Surgery (page 59), NY-Presby Hosp/Weill Cornell (page 66); **Address:** 535 E 70th St, New York, NY 10021-4892; **Phone:** 212-606-1178; **Board Cert:** Orthopaedic Surgery 1974; **Med School:** SUNY Upstate Med Univ 1966; **Resid:** Surgery, St Lukes Hosp 1968; Orthopaedic Surgery, Hosp For Special Surgery 1973; **Fellow:** Shoulder Surgery, Columbia-Presby Med Ctr 1977; **Fac Appt:** Prof OrS, Cornell Univ-Weill Med Coll

Weinfeld, Steven B MD [OrS] - **Spec Exp:** Foot & Ankle Surgery; Diabetic Leg/Foot; **Hospital:** Mount Sinai Med Ctr (page 64), Hackensack Univ Med Ctr; **Address:** 5 E 98th St Fl 9, Box 1188, New York, NY 10029; **Phone:** 212-241-1634; **Board Cert:** Orthopaedic Surgery 2009; **Med School:** Albany Med Coll 1990; **Resid:** Orthopaedic Surgery, Albany Med Ctr 1995; **Fellow:** Ankle and Foot Surgery, Union Meml Hosp 1996; **Fac Appt:** Assoc Prof OrS, Mount Sinai Sch Med

Westrich, Geoffrey H MD [OrS] - **Spec Exp:** Knee Replacement & Revision; Hip Replacement; Joint Replacement; **Hospital:** Hosp For Special Surgery (page 59); **Address:** Hospital for Special Surgery, 535 E 70th St, New York, NY 10021; **Phone:** 212-606-1510; **Board Cert:** Orthopaedic Surgery 1998; **Med School:** Tufts Univ 1990; **Resid:** Orthopaedic Surgery, Hosp for Special Surg 1995; **Fellow:** Trauma, Inselspital 1995; Adult Reconstructive Surgery, Hosp for Special Surg 1996; **Fac Appt:** Assoc Prof OrS, Cornell Univ-Weill Med Coll

Wetzel, F Todd MD [OrS] - **Spec Exp:** Spinal Surgery; Minimally Invasive Surgery; **Hospital:** Temple Univ Hosp, Jeanes Hosp; **Address:** Temple Univ Hosp Zone B Fl 5, 3509 N Broad St, Philadelphia, PA 19140; **Phone:** 215-707-2111; **Board Cert:** Orthopaedic Surgery 2001; **Med School:** Univ Pennsylvania 1981; **Resid:** Surgery, Yale-New Haven Hosp 1983; Orthopaedic Surgery, Yale Univ Affil Hosps 1986; **Fellow:** Spinal Surgery, Dr Henry LaRocca 1987; **Fac Appt:** Prof OrS, Temple Univ

Wickiewicz, Thomas L MD [OrS] - **Spec Exp:** Shoulder Surgery; Sports Medicine; Knee Injuries/ACL; Knee Ligament Reconstruction; **Hospital:** Hosp For Special Surgery (page 59), NY-Presby Hosp/Weill Cornell (page 66); **Address:** 535 E 70th St, New York, NY 10021; **Phone:** 212-606-1450; **Board Cert:** Orthopaedic Surgery 1984; **Med School:** UMDNJ-NJ Med Sch, Newark 1976; **Resid:** Orthopaedic Surgery, Hosp for Special Surg 1981; **Fellow:** Sports Medicine, UCLA Med Ctr 1982; **Fac Appt:** Clin Prof OrS, Cornell Univ-Weill Med Coll

Wiesel, Sam W MD [OrS] - **Spec Exp:** Spinal Surgery; **Hospital:** Georgetown Univ Hosp; **Address:** 3800 Reservoir Rd NW, PHC Bldg Fl Ground, Washington, DC 20007-2113; **Phone:** 202-444-8766 x2; **Board Cert:** Orthopaedic Surgery 1977; **Med School:** Univ Pennsylvania 1971; **Resid:** Orthopaedic Surgery, Hosp Univ Penn 1976; **Fellow:** Orthopaedic Surgery, Hosp Univ Penn 1973; **Fac Appt:** Prof OrS, Georgetown Univ

Williams, Gerald MD [OrS] - **Spec Exp:** Shoulder Reconstruction; Shoulder Cartilage Implant; Shoulder Replacement; Rotator Cuff Surgery; **Hospital:** Thomas Jefferson Univ Hosp, Methodist Hosp; **Address:** Rothman Institute, 925 Chestnut St Fl 5, Philadelphia, PA 19107; **Phone:** 800-321-9999; **Board Cert:** Orthopaedic Surgery 2003; **Med School:** Temple Univ 1984; **Resid:** Orthopaedic Surgery, Univ Texas San Antonio Affil Hosp 1989; **Fellow:** Shoulder Surgery, Univ Texas San Antonio Affil Hosp 1990; **Fac Appt:** Prof OrS, Thomas Jefferson Univ

Williams, Riley J MD [OrS] - **Spec Exp:** Cartilage Damage & Transplant; Shoulder Arthroscopic Surgery; Knee Injuries/ACL; Knee Surgery; **Hospital:** Hosp For Special Surgery (page 59), NY-Presby Hosp/Weill Cornell (page 66); **Address:** Hospital For Special Surgery, 535 E 70th St, New York, NY 10021; **Phone:** 212-606-1855; **Board Cert:** Orthopaedic Surgery 2000; **Med School:** Stanford Univ 1992; **Resid:** Orthopaedic Surgery, Hosp Special Surgery 1997; **Fellow:** Sports Medicine & Shoulder Surgery, Hosp Special Surgery 1998; **Fac Appt:** Assoc Prof OrS, Cornell Univ-Weill Med Coll

Wittig, James C MD [OrS] - **Spec Exp:** Bone Tumors; Sarcoma-Soft Tissue; Hip & Knee Replacement; Limb Sparing Surgery; **Hospital:** Mount Sinai Med Ctr (page 64), Hackensack Univ Med Ctr; **Address:** 5 E 98th St Fl 9, New York, NY 10029; **Phone:** 212-241-1807; **Board Cert:** Orthopaedic Surgery 2003; **Med School:** NYU Sch Med 1994; **Resid:** Orthopaedic Surgery, Columbia Presby Med Ctr 1999; **Fellow:** Orthopaedic Oncology, Washington Cancer Inst 2001; Orthopaedic Oncology, NIH 2001; **Fac Appt:** Assoc Prof OrS, Mount Sinai Sch Med

Zuckerman, Joseph D MD [OrS] - **Spec Exp:** Shoulder Surgery; Hip Replacement; Knee Replacement; Rotator Cuff Surgery; **Hospital:** Hosp For Joint Diseases (page 67), NYU Langone Med Ctr (page 67); **Address:** NYU Hosp for Joint Diseases, Dept Ortho Surg, 301 E 17th St Fl 14 - Ste 1402, New York, NY 10003; **Phone:** 212-598-6674; **Board Cert:** Orthopaedic Surgery 2007; **Med School:** Med Coll Wisc 1978; **Resid:** Orthopaedic Surgery, Univ WA Med Ctr 1983; **Fellow:** Arthritis Surgery, Brigham & Womans Hosp 1984; Shoulder Surgery, Mayo Clinic 1984; **Fac Appt:** Prof OrS, NYU Sch Med

Southeast

Beaty, James H MD [OrS] - **Spec Exp:** Pediatric Orthopaedic Surgery; Clubfoot; Fractures-Pediatric; **Hospital:** Le Bonheur Chldns Med Ctr, Baptist Memorial Hospital - Memphis; **Address:** Campbell Clin, 1400 S Germantown Rd, Germantown, TN 38138; **Phone:** 901-759-3125; **Board Cert:** Orthopaedic Surgery 2007; **Med School:** Univ Tenn Coll Med, Memphis 1976; **Resid:** Surgery, Baptist Meml Hosp 1979; Orthopaedic Surgery, Campbell Clin Fdn 1981; **Fellow:** Pediatric Orthopaedic Surgery, Alfred I Dupont Inst 1982; **Fac Appt:** Prof OrS, Univ Tenn Coll Med, Memphis

Orthopaedic Surgery

Berrey, B Hudson MD [OrS] - **Spec Exp:** Musculoskeletal Tumors; Bone Cancer; Soft Tissue Tumors; Sarcoma; **Hospital:** Shands Jacksonville, Wolfson Chldns Hosp; **Address:** Univ Florida Coll Med, Dept Orth Surg, 655 W Eighth St, Jacksonville, FL 32209; **Phone:** 904-244-5942; **Board Cert:** Orthopaedic Surgery 1982; **Med School:** Univ Tex Med Br, Galveston 1977; **Resid:** Orthopaedic Surgery, Tripler Army Med Ctr 1981; **Fellow:** Medical Oncology, Mass Genl Hosp/Harvard 1985; **Fac Appt:** Prof OrS, Univ Fla Coll Med

Boden, Scott D MD [OrS] - **Spec Exp:** Spinal Disorders; Spinal Surgery; Spinal Disc Replacement; Microdiscectomy; **Hospital:** Emory Univ Hosp; **Address:** 59 Executive Park S, Ste 3000, Atlanta, GA 30329; **Phone:** 404-778-7143; **Board Cert:** Orthopaedic Surgery 2005; **Med School:** Univ Pennsylvania 1986; **Resid:** Orthopaedic Surgery, George Washington Univ Hosp 1991; **Fellow:** Spinal Surgery, Case Western Res Univ Hosp 1992; **Fac Appt:** Prof OrS, Emory Univ

Cuckler, John MD [OrS] - **Spec Exp:** Hip Replacement & Revision; Knee Replacement & Revision; Knee Cartilage Transplant; Minimally Invasive Surgery; **Hospital:** Brookwood Med Ctr; **Address:** Alabama Spine & Joint Center, 513 Brookwood Blvd, Ste 375, Birmingham, AL 35209; **Phone:** 205-802-4577; **Board Cert:** Orthopaedic Surgery 1999; **Med School:** NYU Sch Med 1975; **Resid:** Orthopaedic Surgery, Hosp Univ Penn 1980; **Fellow:** Orthopaedic Surgery, Hosp Univ Penn; **Fac Appt:** Prof OrS, Univ Alabama

Curl, Walton W MD [OrS] - **Spec Exp:** Sports Medicine; **Hospital:** Wake Forest Univ Baptist Med Ctr (page 72); **Address:** Wake Forest Med Ctr, Comp Rehab, 131 Miller St, Winston-Salem, NC 27103; **Phone:** 336-716-8091; **Board Cert:** Orthopaedic Surgery 1980; **Med School:** Duke Univ 1973; **Resid:** Orthopaedic Surgery, Letterman Army Med Ctr 1978; **Fellow:** Sports Medicine, Keller Army Hosp 1979; **Fac Appt:** Prof OrS, Wake Forest Univ

DeOrio, James K MD [OrS] - **Spec Exp:** Ankle Replacement & Revision; Foot & Ankle Surgery; Foot Deformities; **Hospital:** Duke Univ Med Ctr; **Address:** Duke Univ Medical Ctr, Durham, NC 27710; **Phone:** 919-613-7797; **Board Cert:** Orthopaedic Surgery 1983; **Med School:** Geo Wash Univ 1977; **Resid:** Orthopaedic Surgery, Mayo Clinic 1982; **Fellow:** Orthopaedic Surgery, Chur Hosp 1983

Diduch, David R MD [OrS] - **Spec Exp:** Sports Medicine; Knee Reconstruction; Knee Injuries/ACL; Shoulder Reconstruction; **Hospital:** Univ Virginia Med Ctr; **Address:** Univ Virginia Dept Ortho Surg, Box 800159, Charlottesville, VA 22908; **Phone:** 434-243-0274; **Board Cert:** Orthopaedic Surgery 2008; Orthopaedic Sports Medicine 2009; **Med School:** Harvard Med Sch 1988; **Resid:** Orthopaedic Surgery, Univ Virginia Med Ctr 1994; **Fellow:** Sports Medicine, Insall-Scott-Kelly Inst 1995; **Fac Appt:** Prof OrS, Univ VA Sch Med

Eismont, Frank MD [OrS] - **Spec Exp:** Spinal Surgery; **Hospital:** Jackson Meml Hosp (page 70); **Address:** Univ Miami Sch Med, Dept Orth Surg, PO Box 016960, D-27, Miami, FL 33101; **Phone:** 305-243-3000; **Board Cert:** Orthopaedic Surgery 2007; **Med School:** Univ Rochester 1973; **Resid:** Orthopaedic Surgery, Case Western Res Univ Hosp 1978; **Fellow:** Spinal Surgery, Case Western Res Univ Hosp 1979; Spinal Surgery, PA Hosp 1980; **Fac Appt:** Prof OrS, Univ Miami Sch Med

Foster, Mark D MD [OrS] - **Spec Exp:** Spinal Surgery; Foot & Ankle Surgery; **Hospital:** New Hanover Reg Med Ctr; **Address:** Wilimington Orthopaedic Group, 2716 Ashton Drive, Wilmington, NC 28412; **Phone:** 910-763-7344; **Board Cert:** Orthopaedic Surgery 2003; **Med School:** Univ SC Sch Med 1983; **Resid:** Orthopaedic Surgery, Med Univ of SC 1988; **Fellow:** Foot & Ankle Surgery, Med Coll of WI 1989; Spinal Surgery, NC Spine Ctr 1994

Garrett, William MD [OrS] - **Spec Exp:** Sports Medicine; Shoulder & Knee Surgery; Shoulder & Knee Reconstruction; Rotator Cuff Surgery; **Hospital:** Duke Univ Med Ctr; **Address:** Duke Univ Med Ctr, Box 3338, Durham, NC 27710; **Phone:** 919-684-5678; **Board Cert:** Orthopaedic Surgery 2007; Orthopaedic Sports Medicine 2007; **Med School:** Duke Univ 1976; **Resid:** Orthopaedic Surgery, Duke Univ Med Ctr 1982; **Fac Appt:** Prof OrS, Duke Univ

Goldner, Richard MD [OrS] - **Spec Exp:** Upper Extremity Surgery; Hand Surgery; **Hospital:** Duke Univ Med Ctr; **Address:** DUMC, Box 3480, Durham, NC 27710; **Phone:** 919-613-7797; **Board Cert:** Orthopaedic Surgery 1982; Hand Surgery 2000; **Med School:** Duke Univ 1974; **Resid:** Orthopaedic Surgery, Univ Virginia 1980; Surgery, Duke Univ Med Ctr 1976; **Fellow:** Hand Surgery, Duke Univ Med Ctr 1981; **Fac Appt:** Assoc Prof OrS, Duke Univ

Jiranek, William A MD [OrS] - **Spec Exp:** Knee Replacement; Arthritis; Minimally Invasive Surgery; Hip Replacement; **Hospital:** Med Coll of VA Hosp; **Address:** MCV Dept Orthopaedic Surgery, PO Box 980153, Richmond, VA 23298-0153; **Phone:** 804-228-4155; **Board Cert:** Orthopaedic Surgery 2005; **Med School:** Univ VA Sch Med 1985; **Resid:** Orthopaedic Surgery, Tufts Combined Program 1991; **Fellow:** Orthopaedic Surgery, Mass Genl Hosp/Harvard 1992; **Fac Appt:** Assoc Prof OrS, Med Coll VA

Johnson, Darren L MD [OrS] - **Spec Exp:** Knee Injuries; Sports Medicine; Knee Ligament Reconstruction; Arthroscopic Surgery; **Hospital:** Univ of Kentucky Chandler Hosp; **Address:** Univ Kentucky, Dept Orthopaedic Surgery, 740 S Limestone, Ste K-401, Lexington, KY 40536-0284; **Phone:** 859-257-4969; **Board Cert:** Orthopaedic Surgery 2006; Orthopaedic Sports Medicine 2007; **Med School:** UCLA 1987; **Resid:** Orthopaedic Surgery, LAC-USC Med Ctr 1992; **Fellow:** Sports Medicine, Univ Pittsburgh 1993; **Fac Appt:** Prof OrS, Univ KY Coll Med

Karas, Spero G MD [OrS] - **Spec Exp:** Sports Medicine; Shoulder Reconstruction; Elbow Reconstruction; Knee Reconstruction; **Hospital:** Emory Univ Hosp; **Address:** Emory Healthcare Sports Medicine, 59 Executive Park S, Ste 1000, Atlanta, GA 30329; **Phone:** 404-778-7204; **Board Cert:** Orthopaedic Surgery 2002; **Med School:** Indiana Univ 1993; **Resid:** Orthopaedic Surgery, Duke Univ Med Ctr 1999; **Fellow:** Orthopaedic Surgery, Steadman Hawkins Clinic 2000; **Fac Appt:** Assoc Prof OrS, Emory Univ

Kneisl, Jeffrey S MD [OrS] - **Spec Exp:** Bone Cancer; Musculoskeletal Tumors; **Hospital:** Carolinas Med Ctr; **Address:** Carolinas Med Ctr, 1001 Blythe Blvd, Ste 602, Charlotte, NC 28203; **Phone:** 704-355-5982; **Board Cert:** Orthopaedic Surgery 2000; **Med School:** Northwestern Univ 1980; **Resid:** Orthopaedic Surgery, Northwestern Univ 1987; **Fellow:** Orthopaedic Oncology, Univ Chicago 1990

Kress, Kenneth J MD [OrS] - **Spec Exp:** Knee Replacement; Reconstructive Surgery; Sports Medicine; Robotic Surgery; **Hospital:** St Joseph's Hosp - Atlanta; **Address:** Resergens Orthopaedics, 5671 Peachtree Dunwoody Rd NE, Ste 700, Atlanta, GA 30342; **Phone:** 404-847-9999; **Board Cert:** Orthopaedic Surgery 2004; **Med School:** Cornell Univ 1985; **Resid:** Orthopaedic Surgery, Hosp for Special Surg 1990; **Fellow:** Knee Reconstruction, Dr John C Garrett 1991

Miller, Mark D MD [OrS] - **Spec Exp:** Sports Medicine; Knee Ligament Reconstruction; Knee Cartilage/Meniscus Transplants; Shoulder Arthroscopic Surgery; **Hospital:** Univ Virginia Med Ctr; **Address:** Univ Virginia Dept Ortho Surg, 400 Ray C Hunt Drive, Ste 330, Charlottesville, VA 22908; **Phone:** 434-982-4832; **Board Cert:** Orthopaedic Surgery 2006; Orthopaedic Sports Medicine 2007; **Med School:** Uniformed Srvs Univ, Bethesda 1987; **Resid:** Orthopaedic Surgery, Wilford Hall USAF Med Ctr 1992; **Fellow:** Shoulder Surgery, Univ Pittsburgh 1993; Sports Medicine, Univ Pittsburgh 1993; **Fac Appt:** Prof OrS, Univ VA Sch Med

Orthopaedic Surgery

Nunley, James MD [OrS] - **Spec Exp:** Arthritis; Ankle Replacement & Revision; Foot & Ankle Surgery; Hand & Wrist Surgery; **Hospital:** Duke Univ Med Ctr; **Address:** Duke University Med Ctr, Box 2923, Durham, NC 27710-0001; **Phone:** 919-613-7797; **Board Cert:** Orthopaedic Surgery 1981; **Med School:** Tulane Univ 1973; **Resid:** Orthopaedic Surgery, Duke Univ Med Ctr 1979; **Fellow:** Hand Surgery, Duke Univ Med Ctr 1980; **Fac Appt:** Prof OrS, Duke Univ

Paley, Dror MD [OrS] - **Spec Exp:** Limb Lengthening (Ilizarov Procedure); Limb Deformities; Pediatric Orthopaedic Surgery; **Hospital:** St Mary's Med Ctr - W Palm Bch; **Address:** 901 45 St Kimmel Bldg, West Palm Beach, FL 33407; **Phone:** 561-844-2555; **Board Cert:** Orthopaedic Surgery 2000; **Med School:** Univ Toronto 1979; **Resid:** Orthopaedic Surgery, Univ Toronto Hosp 1985; **Fellow:** Hand Surgery, SunnyBrook Hosp 1986; Pediatric Orthopaedic Surgery, Hosp for Sick Children 1987; **Fac Appt:** Assoc Prof S, Univ MD Sch Med

Pettrone, Frank A MD [OrS] - **Spec Exp:** Sports Medicine; Shoulder & Knee Surgery; **Hospital:** Virginia Hosp Ctr - Arlington; **Address:** Commonwealth Ortho & Rehabilitation, 1635 N George Mason Drive, Ste 310, Arlington, VA 22205-3616; **Phone:** 703-525-6100; **Board Cert:** Orthopaedic Surgery 1975; **Med School:** Georgetown Univ 1969; **Resid:** Orthopaedic Surgery, Georgetown Hosp 1974; **Fac Appt:** Clin Prof OrS, Georgetown Univ

Poehling, Gary G MD [OrS] - **Spec Exp:** Hand Surgery; Arthroscopic Surgery; Sports Medicine; **Hospital:** Wake Forest Univ Baptist Med Ctr (page 72); **Address:** Wake Forest Med Ctr, Comp Rehab, 131 Miller St, Winston-Salem, NC 27103; **Phone:** 336-716-8091; **Board Cert:** Orthopaedic Surgery 1977; **Med School:** Marquette Sch Med 1968; **Resid:** Surgery, Duke Univ Med Ctr 1970; Orthopaedic Surgery, Duke Univ Med Ctr 1976; **Fac Appt:** Prof OrS, Wake Forest Univ

Richardson, William J MD [OrS] - **Spec Exp:** Spinal Surgery; Spinal Deformity; Spinal Disc Replacement; Spinal Trauma; **Hospital:** Duke Univ Med Ctr; **Address:** DUMC, PO Box 3077, Durham, NC 27710; **Phone:** 919-613-7797; **Board Cert:** Orthopaedic Surgery 2010; **Med School:** Eastern VA Med Sch 1979; **Resid:** Orthopaedic Surgery, Duke Univ Med Ctr 1986; **Fellow:** Spinal Surgery, Totonto General Hosp 1987

Scarborough, Mark T MD [OrS] - **Spec Exp:** Bone Tumors; Sarcoma; **Hospital:** Shands at Univ of FL; **Address:** Shands Healthcare Univ FL, 3450 Hull Rd, Gainesville, FL 32607; **Phone:** 352-273-7000; **Board Cert:** Orthopaedic Surgery 2003; **Med School:** Univ Fla Coll Med 1985; **Resid:** Orthopaedic Surgery, Univ Texas Med Ctr 1990; **Fellow:** Orthopaedic Surgery, Mass Genl Hosp 1991; **Fac Appt:** Prof OrS, Univ Fla Coll Med

Schwartz, Herbert S MD [OrS] - **Spec Exp:** Bone Tumors-Metastatic; Bone Tumors; Pelvic Surgery-Complex; Musculoskeletal Tumors; **Hospital:** Vanderbilt Univ Med Ctr, Baptist Hosp - Nashville; **Address:** Vanderbilt Orthopaedic Institute, Medical Center East, South Tower, Ste 4200, Nashville, TN 37232-8774; **Phone:** 615-343-8612; **Board Cert:** Orthopaedic Surgery 2007; **Med School:** Univ Chicago-Pritzker Sch Med 1981; **Resid:** Orthopaedic Surgery, Univ Chicago Hosps 1986; **Fellow:** Orthopaedic Oncology, Mayo Clinic 1987; **Fac Appt:** Prof OrS, Vanderbilt Univ

Scully, Sean P MD [OrS] - **Spec Exp:** Bone Cancer; Sarcoma; Musculoskeletal Tumors; Knee Replacement & Revision; **Hospital:** Univ of Miami Hosp & Clins/Sylvester Comp Canc Ctr (page 70), Jackson Meml Hosp (page 70); **Address:** Univ Miami Hospital, 1400 NW 12th Ave, Ste 4035, Miami, FL 33136; **Phone:** 305-325-4683; **Board Cert:** Orthopaedic Surgery 2006; **Med School:** Univ Rochester 1980; **Resid:** Orthopaedic Surgery, Duke Univ Med Ctr 1985; **Fellow:** Orthopaedic Oncology, Mass General Hosp 1987; Research, Natl Inst Health 1988; **Fac Appt:** Prof OrS, Univ Miami Sch Med

Siegel, Herrick J MD [OrS] - **Spec Exp:** Bone Cancer; Sarcoma; Bone Tumors-Benign; Soft Tissue Tumors-Benign; **Hospital:** Univ of Ala Hosp at Birmingham, UAB Highlands Hosp; **Address:** 1313 13th St S, Birmingham, AL 35205; **Phone:** 205-975-0415; **Board Cert:** Orthopaedic Surgery 2005; **Med School:** NYU Sch Med 1995; **Resid:** Orthopaedic Surgery, USC 2000; **Fellow:** Orthopaedic Oncology, Mayo Clinic 2002; **Fac Appt:** Assoc Prof OrS, Univ Alabama

Spengler, Dan M MD [OrS] - **Spec Exp:** Spinal Surgery; **Hospital:** Vanderbilt Univ Med Ctr; **Address:** Vanderbilt Orthopedic Inst, Medical Ctr E, S Tower Rm#4200, Nashville, TN 37232-8774; **Phone:** 615-343-6364; **Board Cert:** Orthopaedic Surgery 1988; **Med School:** Univ Mich Med Sch 1966; **Resid:** Orthopaedic Surgery, Univ Mich Med Ctr 1968; Orthopaedic Surgery, Univ Mich Med Ctr 1973; **Fellow:** Orthopaedic Surgery, Case West Res Hosps 1974; **Fac Appt:** Prof OrS, Vanderbilt Univ

Spindler, Kurt P MD [OrS] - **Spec Exp:** Sports Medicine; Arthroscopic Surgery; **Hospital:** Vanderbilt Univ Med Ctr; **Address:** Vanderbilt Orthopaedic Inst, 1215 21st Ave S, Ste 3200, Med Ctr East, Nashville, TN 37232-8828; **Phone:** 615-322-7878; **Board Cert:** Orthopaedic Surgery 2004; Orthopaedic Sports Medicine 2007; **Med School:** Univ Pennsylvania 1985; **Resid:** Orthopaedic Surgery, Hosp Univ Penn 1990; **Fellow:** Sports Medicine, Cleveland Clinic Fdn 1991; **Fac Appt:** Prof OrS, Vanderbilt Univ

Taft, Timothy N MD [OrS] - **Spec Exp:** Sports Medicine; Knee Injuries/ACL; Shoulder Surgery; **Hospital:** Univ NC Hosps; **Address:** UNC Orthopaedics, CB # 7055, Bioinformatics Bldg, Chapel Hill, NC 27599-7055; **Phone:** 919-962-6637; **Board Cert:** Orthopaedic Surgery 1976; **Med School:** Univ MO-Columbia Sch Med 1969; **Resid:** Orthopaedic Surgery, UNC Hosps 1974; Orthopaedic Surgery, N Carolina Ortho Hosp 1972; **Fac Appt:** Prof OrS, Univ NC Sch Med

Uribe, John W MD [OrS] - **Spec Exp:** Shoulder & Elbow Surgery; Arthroscopic Surgery; Sports Medicine; **Hospital:** Doctors' Hosp, Jackson Meml Hosp (page 70); **Address:** 1150 Campo Sano Ave, Ste 200, Coral Gables, FL 33146-6960; **Phone:** 305-669-3320; **Board Cert:** Orthopaedic Surgery 1982; Orthopaedic Sports Medicine 2007; **Med School:** Univ NC Sch Med 1976; **Resid:** Orthopaedic Surgery, Jackson Meml Hosp 1981; **Fellow:** Sports Medicine, Hughston Sports Med Hosp 1985; **Fac Appt:** Assoc Prof OrS, Univ Miami Sch Med

Walling, Arthur K MD [OrS] - **Spec Exp:** Bone Tumors; Soft Tissue Tumors; Foot & Ankle Surgery; **Hospital:** Tampa Genl Hosp; **Address:** Florida Orthopaedic Inst, 13020 Telecom Pkwy N, Tampa, FL 33637; **Phone:** 813-978-9700; **Board Cert:** Orthopaedic Surgery 1982; **Med School:** Creighton Univ 1976; **Resid:** Orthopaedic Surgery, Univ South Florida Affil Hosps 1980; **Fellow:** Surgical Oncology, Univ Florida 1981; **Fac Appt:** Assoc Clin Prof OrS, Univ S Fla Coll Med

Ward, William G MD [OrS] - **Spec Exp:** Bone Tumors; Soft Tissue Tumors; Reconstructive Surgery; **Hospital:** Wake Forest Univ Baptist Med Ctr (page 72); **Address:** Wake Forest Med Ctr, Comprehensive Rehab, 131 Miller St, Winston-Salem, NC 27157; **Phone:** 336-716-8200; **Board Cert:** Orthopaedic Surgery 2004; **Med School:** Duke Univ 1975; **Resid:** Surgery, Duke Univ Med Ctr 1985; Orthopaedic Surgery, Duke Univ Med Ctr 1989; **Fellow:** Sports Medicine, Cleveland Clinic 1990; Orthopaedic Oncology, UCLA Med Ctr 1991; **Fac Appt:** Prof OrS, Wake Forest Univ

Webb, Lawrence MD [OrS] - **Spec Exp:** Trauma; Pelvic & Acetabular Fractures; Fractures-Complex & Non Union; **Hospital:** Wake Forest Univ Baptist Med Ctr (page 72); **Address:** Wake Forest Med Ctr, Dept of Orth Surgery, 1 Med Ctr Blvd, Winston-Salem, NC 27157-1070; **Phone:** 336-716-3606; **Board Cert:** Orthopaedic Surgery 2007; **Med School:** Temple Univ 1978; **Resid:** Orthopaedic Surgery, Bowman Gray Affil Hosp 1983; **Fellow:** Trauma, Harborview Med Ctr 1984; **Fac Appt:** Prof OrS, Wake Forest Univ

Orthopaedic Surgery

Weiner, Richard L MD [OrS] - **Spec Exp:** Knee Surgery; Shoulder Surgery; Hip Surgery; **Hospital:** St Mary's Med Ctr - W Palm Bch, Palm Beach Gardens Med Ctr; **Address:** 733 US Highway 1, North Palm Beach, FL 33408-4508; **Phone:** 561-840-1090; **Board Cert:** Orthopaedic Surgery 2004; **Med School:** Univ Pennsylvania 1986; **Resid:** Orthopaedic Surgery, UMDNJ-Univ Hosp 1991

Midwest

An, Howard MD [OrS] - **Spec Exp:** Spinal Surgery; Scoliosis; Spinal Microdiscectomy; **Hospital:** Rush Univ Med Ctr; **Address:** 1725 W Harrison, Ste 1063, Chicago, IL 60612; **Phone:** 312-243-4244; **Board Cert:** Orthopaedic Surgery 2002; **Med School:** Med Coll OH 1982; **Resid:** Orthopaedic Surgery, Med College Ohio Hosps 1988; **Fellow:** Spinal Surgery, Jefferson Med College 1989; **Fac Appt:** Prof OrS, Rush Med Coll

Bach Jr, Bernard R MD [OrS] - **Spec Exp:** Sports Medicine; Knee Surgery; Knee Injuries/ACL; **Hospital:** Rush Univ Med Ctr; **Address:** Midwest Orthopaedics, 1725 W Harrison St, Ste 1063, Chicago, IL 60612; **Phone:** 312-243-4244; **Board Cert:** Orthopaedic Surgery 2000; **Med School:** Univ Cincinnati 1979; **Resid:** Surgery, New Eng Deaconess Hosp 1981; Orthopaedic Surgery, Mass Genl Hosp 1984; **Fellow:** Sports Medicine, Hosp Special Surgery 1986; **Fac Appt:** Prof OrS, Rush Med Coll

Biermann, J Sybil MD [OrS] - **Spec Exp:** Sarcoma; Bone Cancer; Multiple Myeloma; Limb Sparing Surgery; **Hospital:** Univ Michigan Hlth Sys; **Address:** Univ Michigan Cancer Ctr, 1500 E Medical Ctr Drive, 7304 CCGC, Ann Arbor, MI 48109-5946; **Phone:** 734-647-8902; **Board Cert:** Orthopaedic Surgery 2006; **Med School:** Stanford Univ 1987; **Resid:** Orthopaedic Surgery, Univ Iowa Hosp 1992; **Fellow:** Orthopaedic Oncology, Univ Chicago Hosps 1993; **Fac Appt:** Assoc Prof OrS, Univ Mich Med Sch

Blaha, John D MD [OrS] - **Spec Exp:** Hip & Knee Replacement; **Hospital:** Univ Michigan Hlth Sys; **Address:** Univ Michigan, Dept Orthopaedic Surg, 1500 E Medical Ctr Dr, 2912 Taubman, Ann Arbor, MI 48109; **Phone:** 734-647-9961; **Board Cert:** Orthopaedic Surgery 1979; **Med School:** Univ Mich Med Sch 1973; **Resid:** Surgery, Univ Mich Hosp 1975; Orthopaedic Surgery, Univ Mich Hosp 1978; **Fellow:** Joint Replacement Surgery, Univ London 1980; **Fac Appt:** Prof OrS, Univ Mich Med Sch

Bohlman, Henry H MD [OrS] - **Spec Exp:** Spinal Surgery-Cervical; **Hospital:** Univ Hosps Case Med Ctr; **Address:** Univ Hosps of Cleveland, Dept Ortho Surg, 11100 Euclid Ave, Cleveland, OH 44106-1736; **Phone:** 216-844-1025; **Board Cert:** Orthopaedic Surgery 1972; **Med School:** Univ MD Sch Med 1964; **Resid:** Surgery, Univ Hosp 1966; Orthopaedic Surgery, Johns Hopkins Hosp 1970; **Fellow:** Spinal Surgery, Johns Hopkins Hosp 1968; **Fac Appt:** Prof OrS, Case West Res Univ

Bridwell, Keith MD [OrS] - **Spec Exp:** Spinal Deformity; Scoliosis; Spinal Surgery; **Hospital:** Barnes-Jewish Hosp, St Louis Chldns Hosp; **Address:** 1 Barnes Jewish Hosp Plaza, Ste 11300, West Pav, Dept Ortho Surg, Campus Box 8233, St Louis, MO 63110; **Phone:** 314-747-2560; **Board Cert:** Orthopaedic Surgery 1985; **Med School:** Washington Univ, St Louis 1977; **Resid:** Orthopaedic Surgery, Barnes Hosp-Wash Univ 1981; **Fellow:** Spinal Surgery, Rush Presby-St Lukes Med Ctr 1982; **Fac Appt:** Prof OrS, Washington Univ, St Louis

Buckwalter IV, Joseph A MD [OrS] - **Spec Exp:** Bone Cancer; Bone Tumors-Metastatic; Fractures-Complex; **Hospital:** Univ Iowa Hosp & Clinics; **Address:** Univ Iowa Hosps, Dept Orthopaedics, 200 Hawkins Drive, Iowa City, IA 52242; **Phone:** 319-356-2595; **Board Cert:** Orthopaedic Surgery 1980; **Med School:** Univ Iowa Coll Med 1974; **Resid:** Orthopaedic Surgery, Iowa Hosp 1979; **Fac Appt:** Prof OrS, Univ Iowa Coll Med

Callaghan, John J MD [OrS] - **Spec Exp:** Hip & Knee Replacement; Sports Medicine; **Hospital:** Univ Iowa Hosp & Clinics; **Address:** Dept Orthopaedics, 200 Hawkins Drive, Iowa City, IA 52242; **Phone:** 319-356-3110; **Board Cert:** Orthopaedic Surgery 2000; **Med School:** Loyola Univ-Stritch Sch Med 1978; **Resid:** Orthopaedic Surgery, Univ Iowa Hosp 1983; **Fellow:** Orthopaedic Surgery, Hosp Special Surg 1984; **Fac Appt:** Prof OrS, Univ Iowa Coll Med

Cheng, Edward Y MD [OrS] - **Spec Exp:** Bone & Soft Tissue Tumors; Reconstructive Surgery-Adult; **Hospital:** Univ Minn Med Ctr, Fairview - Univ Campus; **Address:** Dept Orthopedic Surgery, Univ Minnesota, 2450 Riverside Ave S, Ste R-200, Minneapolis, MN 55455; **Phone:** 612-273-1177; **Board Cert:** Orthopaedic Surgery 2003; **Med School:** Northwestern Univ 1983; **Resid:** Surgery, Northwestern Univ 1985; Orthopaedic Surgery, Beth Israel Hosp 1989; **Fellow:** Surgical Oncology, Mass Genl Hosp 1990; **Fac Appt:** Prof OrS, Univ Minn

Clohisy, Denis MD [OrS] - **Spec Exp:** Bone Cancer; **Hospital:** Univ Minn Med Ctr, Fairview - Univ Campus; **Address:** Dept Orthopaedic Surgery, 2450 Riverside Ave S, Ste R200, Minneapolis, MN 55454; **Phone:** 612-273-1177; **Board Cert:** Orthopaedic Surgery 2004; **Med School:** Northwestern Univ 1983; **Resid:** Orthopaedic Surgery, Univ Minn 1990; **Fellow:** Pathology, Wash Univ Med Ctr 1987; Musculoskeletal Oncology, Mass Genl Hosp/Harvard 1991; **Fac Appt:** Prof OrS, Univ Minn

Ebraheim, Nabil A MD [OrS] - **Spec Exp:** Trauma; Fractures-Complex; **Hospital:** Univ of Toledo Med Ctr; **Address:** Univ of Toledo Med Ctr, Orthopaedics, 3065 Arlington Ave, MS 1094, Toledo, OH 43614; **Phone:** 419-383-3761; **Board Cert:** Orthopaedic Surgery 2008; **Med School:** Egypt 1975; **Resid:** Surgery, St Clare's Hosp 1980; Orthopaedic Surgery, SUNY-Downstate Med Ctr 1983; **Fellow:** Trauma, Univ Maryland Hosps 1984; Orthopaedic Surgery, Hanover Trauma Ctr 1985; **Fac Appt:** Prof OrS, Univ Toledo, Med Univ OH

Gitelis, Steven MD [OrS] - **Spec Exp:** Bone Cancer; Soft Tissue Tumors; Limb Sparing Surgery; Hip Replacement; **Hospital:** Rush Univ Med Ctr; **Address:** 1725 W Harrison St, Ste 440, Chicago, IL 60612; **Phone:** 312-243-4244; **Board Cert:** Orthopaedic Surgery 1982; **Med School:** Rush Med Coll 1975; **Resid:** Orthopaedic Surgery, Rush Presby-St Lukes Med Ctr 1980; **Fellow:** Orthopaedic Oncology, Mayo Clinic; **Fac Appt:** Prof OrS, Rush Med Coll

Goitz, Henry MD [OrS] - **Spec Exp:** Sports Medicine; Arthroscopic Surgery; Knee Injuries/ACL; Rotator Cuff Surgery; **Hospital:** Henry Ford Hosp, Henry Ford Macomb Hosp-Mt Clemens; **Address:** Henry Ford Lakeside Med Ctr, 14500 Hall Rd, Sterling Heights, MI 48313; **Phone:** 586-247-3758; **Board Cert:** Orthopaedic Surgery 2006; **Med School:** UMDNJ-Rutgers Med Sch 1985; **Resid:** Orthopaedic Surgery, Univ Virginia Affil Hosp 1991; **Fellow:** Sports Medicine & Hand Surgery, Univ Virginia Affil Hosp 1991; Sports Medicine, American Sports Med Inst 1992

Goldberg, Victor M MD [OrS] - **Spec Exp:** Hip & Knee Replacement; Arthritis; **Hospital:** Univ Hosps Case Med Ctr; **Address:** Univ Hosps of Cleveland, Dept Ortho Surg, 11100 Euclid Ave, Cleveland, OH 44106; **Phone:** 216-844-3044; **Board Cert:** Orthopaedic Surgery 1983; **Med School:** SUNY Downstate 1964; **Resid:** Surgery, Univ Hosp 1966; Orthopaedic Surgery, Hosp Special Surg 1971; **Fac Appt:** Prof OrS, Case West Res Univ

Goldstein, Wayne MD [OrS] - **Spec Exp:** Hip Replacement; Knee Replacement; **Hospital:** Adv Luth Genl Hosp; **Address:** 9000 Waukegan Rd, Ste 200, Morton Grove, IL 60053; **Phone:** 847-375-3000; **Board Cert:** Orthopaedic Surgery 2007; **Med School:** Univ IL Coll Med 1978; **Resid:** Orthopaedic Surgery, Univ Ilinois Med Ctr 1983; **Fellow:** Arthritis Surgery, Brigham & Women's Hosp 1984; **Fac Appt:** Assoc Clin Prof OrS, Univ Chicago-Pritzker Sch Med

Orthopaedic Surgery

Graf, Ben K MD [OrS] - **Spec Exp:** Sports Medicine; **Hospital:** Univ WI Hosp & Clins; **Address:** 600 Highland Ave, rm K4-735, Madison, WI 53792-3228; **Phone:** 608-263-8850; **Board Cert:** Orthopaedic Surgery 2008; Orthopaedic Sports Medicine 2007; **Med School:** Univ Wisc 1979; **Resid:** Orthopaedic Surgery, Univ Wisc Hosps 1984; **Fellow:** Sports Medicine, Long Beach Meml Hosp 1985; **Fac Appt:** Assoc Prof S, Univ Wisc

Grant, Richard E MD [OrS] - **Spec Exp:** Hip & Knee Replacement; Spinal Surgery-Low Back; Sickle Cell Disease-Hip Surgery; **Hospital:** Univ Hosps Case Med Ctr; **Address:** Univ Hosps Cleveland, Dept Ortho Surgery, 11100 Euclid Ave, Cleveland, OH 44106; **Phone:** 216-844-1118; **Board Cert:** Orthopaedic Surgery 2007; **Med School:** Howard Univ 1976; **Resid:** Orthopaedic Surgery, Wilford Hall Med Ctr-Lackland 1984; **Fellow:** Joint Arthroplasty, Ohio State Univ Hosp 1985; Spinal Cord Injury Medicine, St Lukes/Baylor Univ 1986; **Fac Appt:** Prof OrS, Howard Univ

Hensinger, Robert N MD [OrS] - **Spec Exp:** Pediatric Orthopaedic Surgery; Spinal Surgery-Pediatric; **Hospital:** Univ Michigan Hlth Sys; **Address:** Univ Michigan Med Ctr, Dept Ortho Surg, 2912 Taubman Ctr, 1500 E Medical Ctr Dr, Ann Arbor, MI 48109-0328; **Phone:** 734-936-5780; **Board Cert:** Orthopaedic Surgery 2007; **Med School:** Univ Mich Med Sch 1964; **Resid:** Orthopaedic Surgery, Univ Michigan 1966; Orthopaedic Surgery, Univ Michigan 1971; **Fellow:** Pediatric Orthopaedic Surgery, AI DuPont Inst 1972; **Fac Appt:** Prof OrS, Univ Mich Med Sch

Iannotti, Joseph MD/PhD [OrS] - **Spec Exp:** Shoulder Surgery; Rotator Cuff Surgery; **Hospital:** Cleveland Clin Fdn (page 56); **Address:** Cleveland Clinic, Dept Orthopaedic Surg, 9500 Euclid Ave, Desk A41, Cleveland, OH 44195-5027; **Phone:** 216-445-5151; **Board Cert:** Orthopaedic Surgery 2007; **Med School:** Northwestern Univ 1979; **Resid:** Orthopaedic Surgery, Hosp Univ Penn 1984; **Fellow:** Orthopaedic Research, Hosp Univ Penn 1985; **Fac Appt:** Prof OrS, Cleveland Cl Coll Med/Case West Res

Irwin, Ronald B MD [OrS] - **Spec Exp:** Bone Cancer; Limb Sparing Surgery; Sarcoma-Soft Tissue; **Hospital:** Mount Clemens Regional Med Ctr; **Address:** Mount Clemens Regional Med Ctr, 1080 Harrington Blvd, Ste 201, Mount Clemens, MI 48043; **Phone:** 586-493-7575; **Board Cert:** Orthopaedic Surgery 1979; **Med School:** Univ Mich Med Sch 1971; **Resid:** Orthopaedic Surgery, William Beaumont Hosp 1978; **Fellow:** Orthopaedic Oncology, Mayo Clinic 1978

Joyce, Michael J MD [OrS] - **Spec Exp:** Bone & Soft Tissue Tumors; Fractures-Complex & Non Union; Musculoskeletal Tissue Banking; Pelvic & Acetabular Fractures; **Hospital:** Cleveland Clin Fdn (page 56); **Address:** Cleveland Clinic, Dept Orthopaedic Surgery, 9500 Euclid Ave, Desk A41, Cleveland, OH 44195-0001; **Phone:** 216-444-4282; **Board Cert:** Orthopaedic Surgery 1985; **Med School:** Univ Louisville Sch Med 1976; **Resid:** Surgery, Johns Hopkins Hosp 1978; Orthopaedic Surgery, Harvard Combined Program 1981; **Fellow:** Orthopaedic Oncology, Mass General Hosp 1982; Trauma, Univ Toronto-Sunnybrook Hosp 1983; **Fac Appt:** Assoc Clin Prof OrS, Case West Res Univ

Lenke, Lawrence G MD [OrS] - **Spec Exp:** Spinal Surgery; Spinal Deformity; Scoliosis; **Hospital:** Barnes-Jewish Hosp, St Louis Chldns Hosp; **Address:** Washington Univ Sch Med, 660 S Euclid Ave, Campus Box 8233, St Louis, MO 63110; **Phone:** 314-747-2500; **Board Cert:** Orthopaedic Surgery 2005; **Med School:** Northwestern Univ 1986; **Resid:** Orthopaedic Surgery, Barnes-Jewish Hosp 1990; **Fellow:** Spinal Surgery, Barnes-Jewish Hosp 1992; **Fac Appt:** Prof OrS, Washington Univ, St Louis

Lock, Terrence Ralph MD [OrS] - **Spec Exp:** Sports Medicine; Arthroscopic Surgery; Shoulder & Knee Reconstruction; **Hospital:** Henry Ford Hosp, Bon Secours Cottage Hosp; **Address:** Henry Ford Hosp, Ctr for Athletic Med, 625 2nd St, Detroit, MI 48202; **Phone:** 313-972-4085; **Board Cert:** Orthopaedic Surgery 2002; Orthopaedic Sports Medicine 2007; **Med School:** Wayne State Univ 1983; **Resid:** Orthopaedic Surgery, Wayne St Univ Sch Med 1988; **Fellow:** Sports Medicine, Mass Genl Hosp 1989

Manoli II, Arthur MD [OrS] - **Spec Exp:** Foot & Ankle Surgery; Reconstructive Surgery; **Hospital:** St Joseph Mercy Oakland Hosp; **Address:** 44555 Woodward Ave, Ste 503, Pontiac, MI 48341; **Phone:** 248-858-6773; **Board Cert:** Orthopaedic Surgery 2007; **Med School:** Univ Mich Med Sch 1970; **Resid:** Surgery, Oakwood Hosp 1972; Orthopaedic Surgery, Wayne St Univ Affil Hosps 1975; **Fellow:** Ankle and Foot Surgery, Univ Wash/Vanderbilt Univ 1990

McCarthy, James J MD [OrS] - **Spec Exp:** Lower Extremity Surgery in Children; Arthroscopic Surgery-Hip; Pediatric Orthopaedic Surgery; **Hospital:** Univ WI Hosp & Clins; **Address:** University Hospital, rm K4-735, 600 Highland Ave, Madison, WI 53792-3228; **Phone:** 608-263-5411; **Board Cert:** Orthopaedic Surgery 2009; **Med School:** Univ NC Sch Med 1991; **Resid:** Orthopaedic Surgery, Cleveland Clinic 1996; **Fellow:** Arthroscopic Surgery, Children's Hosp 1997; **Fac Appt:** Prof OrS, Univ Wisc

McDonald, Douglas J MD [OrS] - **Spec Exp:** Bone & Soft Tissue Tumors; Ewing's Sarcoma; Bone Cancer; Hip & Knee Reconstruction; **Hospital:** Barnes-Jewish Hosp; **Address:** Ctr Advanced Med, Orthopaedic Surg Ctr, 4921 Parkview Pl Fl 6 - Ste A, Box 8605, St Louis, MO 63110; **Phone:** 314-747-2500; **Board Cert:** Orthopaedic Surgery 2001; **Med School:** Univ Minn 1982; **Resid:** Orthopaedic Surgery, Mayo Clinic 1987; **Fellow:** Orthopaedic Oncology, Mayo Clinic 1988; **Fac Appt:** Prof OrS, Washington Univ, St Louis

Mott, Michael P MD [OrS] - **Spec Exp:** Bone Tumors; Musculoskeletal Tumors; Pediatric Orthopaedic Cancers; **Hospital:** Henry Ford Hosp; **Address:** Henry Ford Hosp, Dept Ortho Surg, 2799 W Grand Blvd Fl 12, Detroit, MI 48202; **Phone:** 313-916-1961; **Board Cert:** Orthopaedic Surgery 2007; **Med School:** Univ Mich Med Sch 1989; **Resid:** Orthopaedic Surgery, Wayne State Univ Affil Hosp 1994; **Fellow:** Musculoskeletal Oncology, Mass Genl Hosp 1995; Orthopaedic Oncology, Wayne State Univ 1996; **Fac Appt:** Assoc Prof OrS, Wayne State Univ

Muschler, George F MD [OrS] - **Spec Exp:** Hip Replacement; Knee Replacement; Fractures-Non Union; Fractures-Complex; **Hospital:** Cleveland Clin Fdn (page 56); **Address:** Cleveland Clinic, Dept Orthopaedic Surg, 9500 Euclid Ave, Desk A41, Cleveland, OH 44195-0001; **Phone:** 216-444-5338; **Board Cert:** Orthopaedic Surgery 2001; **Med School:** Northwestern Univ 1981; **Resid:** Orthopaedic Surgery, Univ Texas SW Med Ctr 1986; **Fellow:** Metabolic Bone Research, Hosp Special Surgery 1988; Musculoskeletal Oncology, Meml Sloan Kettering Cancer Ctr 1988; **Fac Appt:** Prof OrS, Cleveland Cl Coll Med/Case West Res

Nuber, Gordon MD [OrS] - **Spec Exp:** Shoulder Reconstruction; Rotator Cuff Surgery; Cartilage Damage; Arthroscopic Surgery-Knee; **Hospital:** Northwestern Meml Hosp; **Address:** Northwestern Orthopaedic Institute, 680 N Lakeshore Dr, Ste 1028, Chicago, IL 60611-4451; **Phone:** 312-664-6848; **Board Cert:** Orthopaedic Surgery 2007; **Med School:** Wayne State Univ 1978; **Resid:** Orthopaedic Surgery, Northwestern Meml Hosp 1983; **Fellow:** Sports Medicine, Natl Hlth Inst 1984; **Fac Appt:** Clin Prof OrS, Northwestern Univ

O'Driscoll, Shawn MD/PhD [OrS] - **Spec Exp:** Sports Medicine; Shoulder Surgery; Elbow Surgery; Cartilage Damage; **Hospital:** Mayo Med Ctr & Clin - Rochester; **Address:** Mayo Clinic, Gonda 14, 200 1st St SW, Rochester, MN 55905; **Phone:** 507-538-1284; **Board Cert:** Orthopaedic Surgery 2003; Orthopaedic Sports Medicine 2007; **Med School:** Univ Toronto 1980; **Resid:** Orthopaedic Surgery, Univ Toronto; **Fellow:** Arthroscopic Surgery, Toronto Western Hosp; Elbow & Shoulder Surgery, Mayo Clinic; **Fac Appt:** Prof OrS, Mayo Med Sch

Parsons III, Theodore W MD [OrS] - **Spec Exp:** Bone & Soft Tissue Tumors; Reconstructive Surgery-Adult; **Hospital:** Henry Ford Hosp; **Address:** Henry Ford Hosp, Dept Orthopaedics, 2799 West Grand, Detroit, MI 48202; **Phone:** 313-916-1964; **Board Cert:** Orthopaedic Surgery 2005; **Med School:** Uniformed Srvs Univ, Bethesda 1986; **Resid:** Orthopaedic Surgery, Wilford Hall USAF Med Ctr 1991; **Fellow:** Pediatric Oncology, Boston Chldns Hosp 1992; Orthopaedic Oncology, Mass Genl Hosp 1992; **Fac Appt:** Prof OrS, Wayne State Univ

Orthopaedic Surgery

Peabody, Terrance MD [OrS] - **Spec Exp:** Soft Tissue Tumors; Bone Tumors; Pediatric Orthopaedic Cancers; **Hospital:** Univ of Chicago Med Ctr; **Address:** Univ Chicago Hospital, 5841 S Maryland Ave, MC 3079, Chicago, IL 60637-1463; **Phone:** 773-702-3442; **Board Cert:** Orthopaedic Surgery 2004; **Med School:** UC Irvine 1985; **Resid:** Orthopaedic Surgery, UC Irvine Med Ctr 1990; **Fellow:** Orthopaedic Oncology, Univ Chicago Hosps 1991; **Fac Appt:** Prof S, Univ Chicago-Pritzker Sch Med

Pinzur, Michael S MD [OrS] - **Spec Exp:** Diabetes-Amputation; Foot & Ankle Surgery; Amputation Surgery; **Hospital:** Loyola Univ Med Ctr; **Address:** Loyola Univ Med Ctr, Dept Orth Surg, 2160 S 1st Ave, Maywood, IL 60153-3304; **Phone:** 708-216-4993; **Board Cert:** Orthopaedic Surgery 1980; **Med School:** Rush Med Coll 1974; **Resid:** Orthopaedic Surgery, Northwestern Meml Hosp 1979; **Fac Appt:** Prof OrS, Loyola Univ-Stritch Sch Med

Polly, David W MD [OrS] - **Spec Exp:** Spinal Surgery; Amputation Surgery; Scoliosis; **Hospital:** Univ Minn Med Ctr, Fairview - Univ Campus; **Address:** Univ Minnesota, Orthopaedic Dept, 2450 Riverside Ave S, rm 200, Minneapolis, MN 55454; **Phone:** 612-273-9400; **Board Cert:** Orthopaedic Surgery 2005; **Med School:** Uniformed Srvs Univ, Bethesda 1985; **Resid:** Orthopaedic Surgery, Walter Reed Army Med Ctr 1991; **Fellow:** Spinal Surgery, Univ Minn 1992

Riew, K Daniel MD [OrS] - **Spec Exp:** Spinal Surgery-Cervical; Minimally Invasive Spinal Surgery; Spinal Microdiscectomy; **Hospital:** Barnes-Jewish Hosp; **Address:** Ctr for Advanced Med-Spine Ctr, 4921 Parkview Pl, CAM Bldg Fl 12 - Ste A, St Louis, MO 63110; **Phone:** 314-747-2500; **Board Cert:** Internal Medicine 1987; Orthopaedic Surgery 2008; **Med School:** Case West Res Univ 1984; **Resid:** Internal Medicine, NY Hosp-Cornell Med Ctr 1987; Orthopaedic Surgery, George Wash Univ Med Ctr 1994; **Fellow:** Spinal Surgery, Case West Res Univ 1995; **Fac Appt:** Prof OrS, Washington Univ, St Louis

Rosenberg, Aaron G MD [OrS] - **Spec Exp:** Hip & Knee Replacement; Hip & Knee Reconstruction; **Hospital:** Rush Univ Med Ctr; **Address:** 1725 W Harrison St, Ste 1063, Chicago, IL 60612-3828; **Phone:** 312-432-2340; **Board Cert:** Orthopaedic Surgery 2007; **Med School:** Albany Med Coll 1978; **Resid:** Orthopaedic Surgery, Rush Presby-St Lukes Med Ctr 1983; **Fellow:** Arthritis Surgery, Mass Genl Hosp 1984; **Fac Appt:** Prof OrS, Rush Med Coll

Schafer, Michael F MD [OrS] - **Spec Exp:** Sports Medicine; Spinal Surgery; Scoliosis; **Hospital:** Northwestern Meml Hosp, Children's Mem Hosp; **Address:** 675 N St Clair Fl 17 - Ste 100, Galter Pavillion, Chicago, IL 60611-5968; **Phone:** 312-695-6800; **Board Cert:** Orthopaedic Surgery 1983; **Med School:** Univ Iowa Coll Med 1967; **Resid:** Orthopaedic Surgery, Northwestern Univ Hosp 1972; **Fellow:** Spinal Surgery, Natl Fdn Traveling Fellowship 1973; **Fac Appt:** Prof OrS, Northwestern Univ

Shelbourne, K Donald MD [OrS] - **Spec Exp:** Knee Surgery; Arthroscopic Surgery; Knee Rehabilitation (Non-Surgical); Knee Ligament Reconstruction; **Hospital:** Methodist Hosp - Indianapolis; **Address:** 1815 N Capitol Ave, Ste 600, Indianapolis, IN 46202-1288; **Phone:** 317-924-8636; **Board Cert:** Orthopaedic Surgery 1984; **Med School:** Indiana Univ 1976; **Resid:** Orthopaedic Surgery, Indiana Univ Hosp 1981; **Fellow:** Sports Medicine, Univ Wisconsin 1982; **Fac Appt:** Assoc Clin Prof OrS, Indiana Univ

Stulberg, S David MD [OrS] - **Spec Exp:** Hip & Knee Replacement; **Hospital:** Northwestern Meml Hosp; **Address:** 680 N Lake Shore Drive, Ste 924, Chicago, IL 60611; **Phone:** 312-664-6848; **Board Cert:** Orthopaedic Surgery 1977; **Med School:** Univ Mich Med Sch 1969; **Resid:** Orthopaedic Surgery, Mass Genl Hosp 1974; **Fellow:** Research, Toronto Hosp Sick Chldn 1976; **Fac Appt:** Prof OrS, Northwestern Univ

Swiontkowski, Marc F MD [OrS] - **Spec Exp:** Osteomyelitis; Fractures-Non Union; Trauma; Bone Infections; **Hospital:** Univ Minn Med Ctr, Fairview - Univ Campus; **Address:** Univ Minnesota, Orthopaedic Dept, 2450 Riverside Ave S, rm 102, Minneapolis, MN 55454; **Phone:** 612-273-9400; **Board Cert:** Orthopaedic Surgery 2008; **Med School:** USC Sch Med 1979; **Resid:** Orthopaedic Surgery, Univ Washington Med Ctr 1984; **Fac Appt:** Prof OrS, Univ Minn

Weinstein, Stuart L MD [OrS] - **Spec Exp:** Scoliosis; Hip Disorders & Dysplasia; Hip Disorders-Pediatric; Spinal Deformity; **Hospital:** Univ Iowa Hosp & Clinics; **Address:** Univ Iowa, Dept Orthopaedics, 200 Hawkins Drive, Iowa City, IA 52242-1009; **Phone:** 319-356-1872; **Board Cert:** Orthopaedic Surgery 2007; **Med School:** Univ Iowa Coll Med 1972; **Resid:** Orthopaedic Surgery, Univ Iowa Hosps 1976; **Fac Appt:** Prof OrS, Univ Iowa Coll Med

Wixson, Richard L MD [OrS] - **Spec Exp:** Hip & Knee Replacement; **Hospital:** Northwestern Meml Hosp; **Address:** 680 N Lake Shore Drive Fl 9 - rm 924, Chicago, IL 60611; **Phone:** 312-664-6848; **Board Cert:** Orthopaedic Surgery 1979; **Med School:** Univ Wisc 1972; **Resid:** Orthopaedic Surgery, Henry Ford Hosp 1977; Orthopaedic Surgery, New Eng Baptist Hosp 1979; **Fellow:** Orthopaedic Surgery, Mass Genl Hosp 1978; **Fac Appt:** Clin Prof OrS, Northwestern Univ

Yamaguchi, Ken MD [OrS] - **Spec Exp:** Shoulder Surgery; Elbow Surgery; Rotator Cuff Surgery; **Hospital:** Barnes-Jewish Hosp; **Address:** 660 Euclid Ave, CB 8233, St Louis, MO 63110-1036; **Phone:** 314-747-2534; **Board Cert:** Orthopaedic Surgery 2008; **Med School:** Geo Wash Univ 1989; **Resid:** Orthopaedic Surgery, George Wash Univ Med Ctr 1994; **Fellow:** Shoulder Surgery, Columbia Presby Med Ctr 1995; **Fac Appt:** Prof OrS, Washington Univ, St Louis

Yasko, Alan MD [OrS] - **Spec Exp:** Pediatric Orthopaedic Surgery; Pediatric Orthopaedic Cancers; Sarcoma; **Hospital:** Northwestern Meml Hosp, Children's Mem Hosp; **Address:** Dept Orthopaedics, 676 N St Clair St, Ste 1350, Chicago, IL 60611; **Phone:** 312-926-4444; **Board Cert:** Orthopaedic Surgery 2004; **Med School:** Northwestern Univ 1984; **Resid:** Orthopaedic Surgery, Case Western 1989; **Fellow:** Orthopaedic Oncology, Meml Sloan Kettering 1991; Metabolic Diseases, Hosp for Special Surgery 1991; **Fac Appt:** Prof S, Northwestern Univ-Feinberg Sch Med

Zdeblick, Thomas MD [OrS] - **Spec Exp:** Spinal Surgery; **Hospital:** Univ WI Hosp & Clins; **Address:** 600 Highland Ave, rm K4-739 CSC, Madison, WI 53792-7375; **Phone:** 608-265-3207; **Board Cert:** Orthopaedic Surgery 2002; **Med School:** Tufts Univ 1982; **Resid:** Orthopaedic Surgery, Case West Res Univ 1988; **Fellow:** Spinal Surgery, Johns Hopkins Univ 1989; **Fac Appt:** Prof OrS, Univ Wisc

Great Plains and Mountains

Coughlin, Michael J MD [OrS] - **Spec Exp:** Foot & Ankle Surgery; **Hospital:** St Alphonsus Regl Med Ctr; **Address:** 901 N Curtis Rd, Ste 503, Boise, ID 83706; **Phone:** 208-377-1000; **Board Cert:** Orthopaedic Surgery 1980; **Med School:** Oregon Hlth & Sci Univ 1974; **Resid:** Orthopaedic Surgery, UCSF Med Ctr 1978; **Fellow:** Foot & Ankle Surgery, Samuel Merrit Hosp 1979; **Fac Appt:** Clin Prof OrS, Oregon Hlth & Sci Univ

Garvin, Kevin L MD [OrS] - **Spec Exp:** Hip Surgery; Knee Surgery; Joint Replacement; **Hospital:** Nebraska Med Ctr; **Address:** Orthopaedic Clinic, 989265 Nebraska Medical Ctr Fl 2, Omaha, NE 68198-9265; **Phone:** 402-559-8000; **Board Cert:** Orthopaedic Surgery 2001; **Med School:** Med Coll Wisc 1982; **Resid:** Orthopaedic Surgery, Univ Arkansas Hosp 1987; **Fellow:** Hip Surgery, Hosp for Special Surgery 1988; **Fac Appt:** Prof OrS, Univ Nebr Coll Med

Orthopaedic Surgery

Millett, Peter J MD [OrS] - **Spec Exp:** Shoulder Surgery; Sports Medicine; Arthroscopic Surgery; **Hospital:** Vail Valley Med Ctr; **Address:** Steadman-Hawkins Clinic, 181 W Meadow Drive, Ste 400, Vail, CO 81657; **Phone:** 970-476-1100; **Board Cert:** Orthopaedic Surgery 2003; **Med School:** Dartmouth Med Sch 1995; **Resid:** Orthopaedic Surgery, Hosp Special Surgery 2000; **Fellow:** Sports Medicine, Steadman Hawkins Clinic 2001

Philippon, Marc J MD [OrS] - **Spec Exp:** Arthroscopic Surgery-Hip; Sports Medicine; **Hospital:** Vail Valley Med Ctr; **Address:** Steadman-Hawkins Clinic, 181 W Meadow Drive, Ste 400, Vail, CO 81657; **Phone:** 970-476-1100; **Board Cert:** Orthopaedic Surgery 1999; **Med School:** Canada 1990; **Resid:** Orthopaedic Surgery, Jackson Meml Hosp 1995; **Fac Appt:** , Univ Pittsburgh

Randall, R Lor MD [OrS] - **Spec Exp:** Bone Tumors; Sarcoma-Soft Tissue; Pediatric Orthopaedic Surgery; **Hospital:** Univ Utah Hosps and Clins, Primary Children's Med Ctr; **Address:** Ped Ortho Surg, Primary Chlds Med Ctr, 100 N Medical Drive, Ste 4550, SLC, UT 84113, Salt Lake City, UT 84113; **Phone:** 801-662-5600; **Board Cert:** Orthopaedic Surgery 2001; **Med School:** Yale Univ 1992; **Resid:** Orthopaedic Surgery, UCSF Med Ctr 1997; **Fellow:** Musculoskeletal Oncology, Univ WA Med Ctr 1998; **Fac Appt:** Assoc Prof OrS, Univ Utah

Rosenberg, Thomas D MD [OrS] - **Spec Exp:** Knee Surgery; Sports Medicine; **Hospital:** Ortho Spec Hosp, The (TOSH); **Address:** 1820 Sidewinder Drive, Park City, UT 84060; **Phone:** 435-655-6600; **Board Cert:** Orthopaedic Surgery 1979; **Med School:** Univ Utah 1973; **Resid:** Orthopaedic Surgery, Univ Utah Affil Hosps 1977; **Fellow:** Sports Medicine, Univ Wisconsin Hosp 1978

Saltzman, Charles L MD [OrS] - **Spec Exp:** Foot & Ankle Surgery; **Hospital:** Univ Utah Hosps and Clins; **Address:** Dept Orthopaedic Surgery, 590 Wakara Way, Salt Lake City, UT 84108; **Phone:** 801-587-5404; **Board Cert:** Orthopaedic Surgery 2004; **Med School:** Univ NC Sch Med 1985; **Resid:** Orthopaedic Surgery, Univ Michigan Med Ctr; **Fellow:** Orthopaedic Surgery, Mayo Clinic; **Fac Appt:** Prof OrS, Univ Utah

Steadman, J Richard MD [OrS] - **Spec Exp:** Knee-Microfracture Surgery; Sports Medicine; **Hospital:** Vail Valley Med Ctr; **Address:** Steadman-Hawkins Sports Medicine Clinic, 181 W Meadow Drive, Ste 400, Vail, CO 81657; **Phone:** 970-476-1100; **Board Cert:** Orthopaedic Surgery 1972; **Med School:** Univ Tex SW, Dallas 1963; **Resid:** Orthopaedic Surgery, Charity Hosp 1966; Orthopaedic Surgery, Louisiana St Univ Hosp 1967

Wiedel, Jerome D MD [OrS] - **Spec Exp:** Hip/Knee Replacement; Reconstructive Surgery; **Hospital:** Univ Colorado Hosp; **Address:** 1635 Aurora Ct, Ste 4100, PO Box 6510, MS F722, Aurora, CO 80045; **Phone:** 720-848-1900; **Board Cert:** Orthopaedic Surgery 1993; **Med School:** Univ Nebr Coll Med 1964; **Resid:** Orthopaedic Surgery, Univ Colorado Med Ctr 1971; **Fellow:** Reconstructive Surgery, Robert Jones-A Hunt Ortho Hosp 1972; **Fac Appt:** Prof OrS, Univ Colorado

Wilkins, Ross M MD [OrS] - **Spec Exp:** Bone Cancer; Bone Infections; Fractures-Non Union; **Hospital:** Presby - St Luke's Med Ctr; **Address:** 1601 E 19th Ave, Ste 3300, Denver, CO 80218; **Phone:** 303-837-0072; **Board Cert:** Orthopaedic Surgery 2007; **Med School:** Wayne State Univ 1978; **Resid:** Orthopaedic Surgery, Univ Colorado Med Ctr 1983; **Fellow:** Orthopaedic Oncology, Mayo Clinic 1984

Southwest

Agarwal, Animesh MD [OrS] - **Spec Exp:** Trauma; Fractures-Complex; **Hospital:** Univ Hlth Syst-San Antonio; **Address:** UTHSCSA Div of Orthopaedic Trauma, 7703 Floyd Curl Drive, MC 7774, San Antonio, TX 78229-3900; **Phone:** 210-592-0115; **Board Cert:** Orthopaedic Surgery 2000; **Med School:** Univ Tex, San Antonio 1992; **Resid:** Orthopaedic Surgery, Unix TX Med Ctr 1997; **Fellow:** Trauma, Grant Med Ctr 1998; **Fac Appt:** Assoc Prof OrS, Univ Tex, San Antonio

Aronson, James MD [OrS] - **Spec Exp:** Limb Lengthening (Ilizarov Procedure); Hip Disorders & Dysplasia; Clubfoot; Limb Deformities; **Hospital:** Arkansas Chldns Hosp; **Address:** Arkansas Chldns Hosp, Dept Orthopaedics, 800 Marshall St, Slot 839, Little Rock, AR 72202; **Phone:** 501-364-1468; **Board Cert:** Orthopaedic Surgery 2007; **Med School:** Univ Pittsburgh 1975; **Resid:** Surgery, Maine Med Ctr 1977; Orthopaedic Surgery, Duke Univ Med Ctr 1982; **Fellow:** Pediatric Orthopaedic Surgery, Alfred I DuPont Inst 1983; **Fac Appt:** Prof OrS, Univ Ark

Brodsky, James W MD [OrS] - **Spec Exp:** Foot & Ankle Surgery; **Hospital:** Baylor Univ Medical Ctr; **Address:** 411 N Washington Ave, Ste 7000, Dallas, TX 75246-1777; **Phone:** 214-823-7090; **Board Cert:** Orthopaedic Surgery 2008; **Med School:** Case West Res Univ 1979; **Resid:** Orthopaedic Surgery, Bellevue Hosp Ctr/NYU 1981; Orthopaedic Surgery, Baylor Coll Med 1984; **Fellow:** Foot & Ankle Surgery, Rancho Los Amigos/USC/LAC Hosp 1985; **Fac Appt:** Clin Prof OrS, Univ Tex SW, Dallas

Bucholz, Robert W MD [OrS] - **Spec Exp:** Hip & Knee Replacement; **Hospital:** UT Southwestern Med Ctr at Dallas, Parkland Hlth & Hosp Sys; **Address:** Dept Ortho Surg, 1801 Inwood Rd, Dallas, TX 75390-8882; **Phone:** 214-645-3300; **Board Cert:** Orthopaedic Surgery 2005; **Med School:** Yale Univ 1973; **Resid:** Orthopaedic Surgery, Yale-New Haven Hosp 1977; **Fac Appt:** Prof OrS, Univ Tex SW, Dallas

Cooper, Daniel E MD [OrS] - **Spec Exp:** Sports Medicine; Knee Injuries/ACL; Arthroscopic Surgery; Reconstructive Surgery; **Hospital:** Baylor Univ Medical Ctr, Mary Shiels Hosp; **Address:** The Carrell Clin, 9301 N Central Expwy, Ste 400, Dallas, TX 75231; **Phone:** 214-220-2468; **Board Cert:** Orthopaedic Surgery 2003; **Med School:** Univ Tex SW, Dallas 1984; **Resid:** Orthopaedic Surgery, Univ Texas Health Scis Ctr 1989; **Fellow:** Sports Medicine, Hospital for Special Surgery 1990

Gugenheim Jr, Joseph J MD [OrS] - **Spec Exp:** Limb Lengthening (Ilizarov Procedure); Limb Deformities; **Hospital:** Texas Ortho Hosp; **Address:** Foundren Orthopaedic Group, 7401 S Main St, Houston, TX 77030; **Phone:** 713-799-2300; **Board Cert:** Orthopaedic Surgery 1978; **Med School:** Northwestern Univ 1972; **Resid:** Orthopaedic Surgery, Baylor Univ Hosp 1976; **Fellow:** Pediatric Orthopaedic Surgery, Boston Chldns Hosp 1977; **Fac Appt:** Assoc Prof S, Baylor Coll Med

Hochschuler, Stephen H MD [OrS] - **Spec Exp:** Spinal Surgery; **Hospital:** Presby Hosp of Plano; **Address:** Texas Back Institute, 6020 W Parker Rd, Ste 200, Plano, TX 75093-7916; **Phone:** 972-608-5000; **Board Cert:** Orthopaedic Surgery 1978; **Med School:** Harvard Med Sch 1968; **Resid:** Surgery, Boston City Hosp 1971; Orthopaedic Surgery, Univ Texas SW Med Ctr 1976

Mabrey, Jay D MD [OrS] - **Spec Exp:** Knee Replacement & Revision; Hip Replacement & Revision; Arthroscopic Surgery-Hip; **Hospital:** Baylor Univ Medical Ctr; **Address:** Baylor Univ Med Ctr, Dept Orthopaedics, 3500 Gaston Ave Bldg Hob Fl 6, Dallas, TX 75246-9990; **Phone:** 214-820-3434; **Board Cert:** Orthopaedic Surgery 2009; **Med School:** Cornell Univ-Weill Med Coll 1981; **Resid:** Orthopaedic Surgery, Duke Univ MC 1987; Surgery, Duke Univ MC 1983; **Fellow:** Joint Replacement Surgery, Hosp Special Surg 1991; **Fac Appt:** Clin Prof OrS, Univ Tex SW, Dallas

Orthopaedic Surgery

Seltzer, Dana G MD [OrS] - **Spec Exp:** Sports Medicine; Trauma; Arthroscopic Surgery; **Hospital:** St Joseph's Hosp & Med Ctr - Phoenix; **Address:** 500 W Thomas Rd, Ste 850, Phoenix, AZ 85013; **Phone:** 602-406-2663; **Board Cert:** Orthopaedic Surgery 2007; **Med School:** USC Sch Med 1986; **Resid:** Orthopaedic Surgery, Univ Miami-Jackson Meml Hosp 1991; **Fellow:** Sports Medicine, Kerlan-Jobe Clinic 1992; Shoulder Surgery, UTSA 1993

Souryal, Tarek O MD [OrS] - **Spec Exp:** Sports Medicine; Knee Injuries/ACL; **Hospital:** Presby Hosp of Dallas; **Address:** 6901 Snider Plaza, Ste 200, Dallas, TX 75205; **Phone:** 214-369-7733; **Board Cert:** Orthopaedic Surgery 2001; **Med School:** Univ Tex, San Antonio 1982; **Resid:** Orthopaedic Surgery, UTSW Med Ctr 1987; **Fellow:** Sports Medicine, Sports Med Clin N Tex 1987; Sports Medicine, Hughston Ortho Clinic 1988; **Fac Appt:** Clin Prof OrS, Univ Tex SW, Dallas

Trick, Lorence W MD [OrS] - **Spec Exp:** Hip Replacement; Knee Replacement; **Hospital:** SW TX Meth Hosp, Univ Hlth Syst-San Antonio; **Address:** 4647 Medical Drive, San Antonio, TX 78229; **Phone:** 210-567-0924; **Board Cert:** Orthopaedic Surgery 1973; **Med School:** Geo Wash Univ 1967; **Resid:** Orthopaedic Surgery, Wilford Hall USAF Med Ctr 1972; **Fellow:** Orthopaedic Surgery, New Eng Baptist Med Ctr; **Fac Appt:** Clin Prof OrS, Univ Tex, San Antonio

Williams, Ronald P MD [OrS] - **Spec Exp:** Bone Tumors; **Hospital:** Univ Hlth Syst-San Antonio; **Address:** Dept of Orthopaedics, 7703 Floyd Curl Drive, MC 7774, San Antonio, TX 78229-3900; **Phone:** 210-567-5125; **Board Cert:** Orthopaedic Surgery 2003; **Med School:** Univ Tex, San Antonio 1984; **Resid:** Orthopaedic Surgery, Univ Kans Sch Med 1989; **Fellow:** Orthopaedic Oncology, Case West Res Univ 1990; **Fac Appt:** Prof OrS, Univ Tex, San Antonio

Wirth, Michael A MD [OrS] - **Spec Exp:** Shoulder Surgery; Shoulder Replacement; **Hospital:** Univ Hlth Syst-San Antonio; **Address:** Univ Tex Hlth Sci Ctr, Dept Orth, 7703 Floyd Curl Drive, MC 7774, San Antonio, TX 78229-3900; **Phone:** 210-567-5135; **Board Cert:** Orthopaedic Surgery 2004; **Med School:** Oregon Hlth & Sci Univ 1985; **Resid:** Orthopaedic Surgery, Univ Texas Hlth Sci Ctr 1990; **Fellow:** Shoulder Surgery, Charles Rockwood Jr MD 1991; **Fac Appt:** Prof OrS, Univ Tex, San Antonio

West Coast and Pacific

Anderson, Lesley J MD [OrS] - **Spec Exp:** Knee Injuries/ACL; Knee Cartilage/Meniscus Transplants; Cartilage Damage; Shoulder Injuries; **Hospital:** CA Pacific Med Ctr; **Address:** 2100 Webster St, Ste 309, San Francisco, CA 94115; **Phone:** 415-923-3029; **Board Cert:** Orthopaedic Surgery 2007; **Med School:** Penn State Univ-Hershey Med Ctr 1976; **Resid:** Orthopaedic Surgery, UCLA Med Ctr 1983; **Fellow:** Sports Medicine/Knee Surgery, Blazina Ortho Clinic 1984; **Fac Appt:** Asst Clin Prof OrS, UCSF

Bos, Gary D MD [OrS] - **Spec Exp:** Musculoskeletal Tumors; Sarcoma; Reconstructive Surgery; **Hospital:** Yakima Valley Mem Hosp; **Address:** 16th Avenue Station, 1470 16th Ave, Yakima, WA 98902; **Phone:** 509-574-3300; **Board Cert:** Orthopaedic Surgery 2008; **Med School:** Univ Chicago-Pritzker Sch Med 1978; **Resid:** Orthopaedic Surgery, Case West Reserve 1984; **Fellow:** Orthopaedic Surgery, Case West Reserve 1980; Orthopaedic Oncology, Mayo Clinic 1985

Brien, Earl Warren MD [OrS] - **Spec Exp:** Bone & Soft Tissue Tumors; **Hospital:** Cedars-Sinai Med Ctr; **Address:** 444 S San Vicente Blvd, Ste 603, Los Angeles, CA 90048; **Phone:** 310-423-9887; **Board Cert:** Orthopaedic Surgery 2006; **Med School:** Howard Univ 1986; **Resid:** Orthopaedic Surgery, LAC-King Drew Med Ctr 1992; **Fellow:** Musculoskeletal Disorders, Memorial Sloan Kettering 1993; Metabolic Bone Research, Hosp for Special Surgery 1994

Cannon Jr, Wayne Dilworth MD [OrS] - **Spec Exp:** Sports Medicine; Knee Surgery; **Hospital:** UCSF Med Ctr; **Address:** 1701 Divisadero St, Ste 240, San Francisco, CA 94115-1351; **Phone:** 415-353-7566; **Board Cert:** Orthopaedic Surgery 1972; **Med School:** Columbia P&S 1963; **Resid:** Surgery, St Vincents Hosp 1965; Orthopaedic Surgery, NY Ortho Hosp 1970; **Fellow:** Orthopaedic Surgery, Royal Natl Ortho Hosp 1971; **Fac Appt:** Clin Prof OrS, UCSF

Carragee, Eugene J MD [OrS] - **Spec Exp:** Spinal Surgery; Spinal Disc Replacement; **Hospital:** Stanford Univ Med Ctr; **Address:** Stanford Univ, Orthopaedics/Spine Clin, 450 Broadway St A Bldg, Redwood City, CA 94304; **Phone:** 650-725-5905; **Board Cert:** Orthopaedic Surgery 2005; **Med School:** Stanford Univ 1982; **Resid:** Internal Medicine, Stanford Univ Hosp 1984; Orthopaedic Surgery, Stanford Univ Hosp 1988; **Fac Appt:** Prof OrS, Stanford Univ

Chambers, Richard Byron MD [OrS] - **Spec Exp:** Diabetes-Amputation; **Hospital:** Rancho Los Amigos Natl Rehab Ctr; **Address:** 7601 E Imperial Hwy, Surgery Dept, Downey, CA 90242; **Phone:** 562-401-7166; **Board Cert:** Orthopaedic Surgery 1977; **Med School:** Columbia P&S 1971; **Resid:** Surgery, NY Hosp; Orthopaedic Surgery, Hosp Special Surg

Conrad, Ernest U MD [OrS] - **Spec Exp:** Pediatric Orthopaedic Surgery; Bone Tumors; Sarcoma; **Hospital:** Chldns Hosp and Regl Med Ctr - Seattle, Univ Wash Med Ctr; **Address:** 1959 NE Pacific St, Box 356500, Seattle, WA 98195; **Phone:** 206-543-3690; **Board Cert:** Orthopaedic Surgery 2009; **Med School:** Univ VA Sch Med 1979; **Resid:** Orthopaedic Surgery, Hosp for Special Surgery 1984; **Fellow:** Orthopaedic Oncology, Univ Fla Coll Med 1985; Pediatric Orthopaedic Surgery, Hosp for Sick Chldn 1986; **Fac Appt:** Prof OrS, Univ Wash

Copp, Steven N MD [OrS] - **Spec Exp:** Foot & Ankle Surgery; Hip & Knee Replacement; **Hospital:** Scripps Green Hosp; **Address:** Scripps Clinic, Dept Orthopedic Surgery, 10666 N Torrey Pines Rd, La Jolla, CA 92037; **Phone:** 858-554-9773; **Board Cert:** Orthopaedic Surgery 2002; **Med School:** UCSD 1983; **Resid:** Orthopaedic Surgery, UCSD Med Ctr 1988

Delamarter, Rick B MD [OrS] - **Spec Exp:** Spinal Surgery; Minimally Invasive Spinal Surgery; Spinal Disc Replacement; Spinal Reconstructive Surgery; **Hospital:** St John's Hlth Ctr, Santa Monica; **Address:** Spine Institute of Santa Monica, 1301 20th St, Ste 400, Santa Monica, CA 90404; **Phone:** 310-828-7757; **Board Cert:** Orthopaedic Surgery 2000; **Med School:** Oregon Hlth & Sci Univ 1981; **Resid:** Orthopaedic Surgery, UCLA Med Ctr 1986; **Fac Appt:** Assoc Prof S, UCLA

Di Cesare, Paul E MD [OrS] - **Spec Exp:** Reconstructive Surgery; Knee Replacement & Revision; Hip Replacement; Hip Resurfacing; **Hospital:** UC Davis Med Ctr; **Address:** UC Davis Medical Group-Orthopaedic Surg, 550 W Ranch View Drive, Rocklin, CA 95765; **Phone:** 916-734-2700; **Board Cert:** Orthopaedic Surgery 2005; **Med School:** USC Sch Med 1986; **Resid:** Orthopaedic Surgery, LAC-USC Med Ctr 1991; **Fellow:** Hip Surgery, Muller Fdn 1992; **Fac Appt:** Prof OrS, UC Davis

Dillingham, Michael F MD [OrS] - **Spec Exp:** Sports Medicine; **Hospital:** Stanford Univ Med Ctr, CA Pacific Med Ctr; **Address:** 500 Arguello St, Ste 100, Redwood City, CA 94063; **Phone:** 650-851-4900; **Board Cert:** Orthopaedic Surgery 1977; Physical Medicine & Rehabilitation 1979; **Med School:** Stanford Univ 1971; **Resid:** Orthopaedic Surgery, Standford Univ Med Ctr 1975; Physical Medicine & Rehabilitation, Santa Clara Valley Med Ctr 1977; **Fellow:** Spinal Surgery, Santa Clara Valley Med Ctr 1976; **Fac Appt:** Clin Prof OrS, Stanford Univ

Dorr, Lawrence Douglas MD [OrS] - **Spec Exp:** Hip & Knee Replacement; **Hospital:** Good Samaritan Hosp - LA; **Address:** Dorr Arthritis Institute, 637 S Lucas Ave, Ste 500, Los Angeles, CA 90017; **Phone:** 213-977-2280; **Board Cert:** Orthopaedic Surgery 1978; **Med School:** Univ Iowa Coll Med 1967; **Resid:** Orthopaedic Surgery, LAC-USC Med Ctr 1976; **Fellow:** Joint Replacement Surgery, Hosp Special Surgery 1977

Eckardt, Jeffrey J MD [OrS] - **Spec Exp:** Bone Tumors; Soft Tissue Tumors; Limb Sparing Surgery; **Hospital:** Santa Monica - UCLA Med Ctr & Ortho Hosp, UCLA Ronald Reagan Med Ctr; **Address:** UCLA Med Ctr, Dept Ortho Surg/Oncology, 1250 16th St Tower # 745, Santa Monica, CA 90404; **Phone:** 310-319-3816; **Board Cert:** Orthopaedic Surgery 1981; **Med School:** Cornell Univ-Weill Med Coll 1971; **Resid:** Orthopaedic Surgery, UCLA Med Ctr 1979; **Fellow:** Orthopaedic Oncology, Mayo Clinic 1980; **Fac Appt:** Prof OrS, UCLA

Finerman, Gerald MD [OrS] - **Spec Exp:** Sports Medicine; Hip & Knee Replacement; **Hospital:** UCLA Ronald Reagan Med Ctr, Santa Monica - UCLA Med Ctr & Ortho Hosp; **Address:** 1245 16 St, Ste 202, Santa Monica, CA 90404; **Phone:** 310-825-6019; **Board Cert:** Orthopaedic Surgery 1971; **Med School:** Johns Hopkins Univ 1962; **Resid:** Surgery, Johns Hopkins Hosp 1964; Orthopaedic Surgery, Johns Hopkins Hosp 1969; **Fac Appt:** Prof OrS, UCLA

Garfin, Steven R MD [OrS] - **Spec Exp:** Spinal Surgery; **Hospital:** UCSD Med Ctr; **Address:** UCSD, Dept Orthopedic Surgery, 9350 Campus Pointe Drive, Ste 1B, La Jolla, CA 92037; **Phone:** 858-657-8200; **Board Cert:** Orthopaedic Surgery 1982; **Med School:** Univ Minn 1972; **Resid:** Orthopaedic Surgery, UCSD Med Ctr 1979; **Fellow:** Spinal Surgery, Pennsylvania Hosp 1981; **Fac Appt:** Prof OrS, UCSD

Goodman, Stuart B MD/PhD [OrS] - **Spec Exp:** Arthritis; Joint Replacement; Reconstructive Surgery; **Hospital:** Stanford Univ Med Ctr, Lucile Packard Chldn's Hosp; **Address:** Stanford Univ, Div Ortho Surgery, 450 Broadway St, MC 6110, Redwood City, CA 94063; **Phone:** 650-721-7662; **Board Cert:** Orthopaedic Surgery 2008; **Med School:** Univ Toronto 1978; **Resid:** Orthopaedic Surgery, Univ Toronto 1984; **Fellow:** Orthopaedic Surgery, Univ Toronto 1985; **Fac Appt:** Prof OrS, Stanford Univ

Hansen, Sigvard MD [OrS] - **Spec Exp:** Ankle Replacement & Revision; Deformity Reconstruction; Neuromuscular Disorders; Foot & Ankle Surgery; **Hospital:** Harborview Med Ctr, Univ Wash Med Ctr; **Address:** Foot & Ankle Institute, 325 9th Ave, Box 359799, Seattle, WA 98104; **Phone:** 206-744-4830; **Board Cert:** Orthopaedic Surgery 1972; **Med School:** Univ Wash 1961; **Resid:** Orthopaedic Surgery, Univ Washington Affil Hosps 1969; **Fellow:** Orthopaedic Surgery, Sheffield Chldns Hosp 1970; **Fac Appt:** Prof OrS, Univ Wash

Johnson, Eric E MD [OrS] - **Spec Exp:** Pelvic & Acetabular Fractures; Limb Lengthening; **Hospital:** UCLA Ronald Reagan Med Ctr; **Address:** UCLA Med Ctr-Dept Orthopedic Surgery, 10833 Le Conte Ave, rm 62-266 CHF, Los Angeles, CA 90095-6902; **Phone:** 310-206-1169; **Board Cert:** Orthopaedic Surgery 1985; **Med School:** Univ Utah 1976; **Resid:** Surgery, Univ Utah 1978; Orthopaedic Surgery, UCLA Med Ctr 1981; **Fac Appt:** Prof OrS, UCLA

Lowenberg, David W MD [OrS] - **Spec Exp:** Osteomyelitis; Limb Lengthening (Ilizarov Procedure); Fractures-Complex & Non Union; Limb Deformities; **Hospital:** CA Pacific Med Ctr; **Address:** Dept of Orthopaedic Surgery, 2100 Webster St, Ste 117, San Francisco, CA 94115; **Phone:** 415-600-3835; **Board Cert:** Orthopaedic Surgery 2003; **Med School:** UCLA 1985; **Resid:** Orthopaedic Surgery, UCSF Med Ctr 1990; **Fac Appt:** Assoc Prof OrS, UCSF

Luck Jr, James V MD [OrS] - **Spec Exp:** Hemophilia Related Disease; Hip & Knee Replacement; Musculoskeletal Tumors; **Hospital:** Santa Monica - UCLA Med Ctr & Ortho Hosp; **Address:** 2400 S Flower St, Fl 3, Los Angeles, CA 90007-2660; **Phone:** 213-749-8255; **Board Cert:** Orthopaedic Surgery 2000; **Med School:** USC Sch Med 1967; **Resid:** Orthopaedic Surgery, Orthopaedic Hosp 1973; **Fellow:** Orthopaedic Oncology, Orthopaedic Hosp 1974; Reconstructive Surgery, Rancho Los Amigos 1974; **Fac Appt:** Prof OrS, UCLA

Mandelbaum, Bert R MD [OrS] - **Spec Exp:** Sports Medicine; Knee Injuries/ACL; Cartilage Damage; **Hospital:** St John's Hlth Ctr, Santa Monica; **Address:** Santa Monica Orthopaedic Group, 220 Santa Monica Blvd Fl 4, Santa Monica, CA 90404; **Phone:** 310-829-2663; **Board Cert:** Orthopaedic Surgery 1999; **Med School:** Washington Univ, St Louis 1980; **Resid:** Orthopaedic Surgery, Johns Hopkins Hosp 1985

Matsen, Frederick MD [OrS] - **Spec Exp:** Shoulder Replacement; Elbow Replacement; Rotator Cuff Surgery; **Hospital:** Univ Wash Med Ctr; **Address:** Bone & Joint Ctr, UWMC-Roosevelt, 4245 Roosevelt Way NE, Box 354740, Seattle, WA 98105; **Phone:** 206-598-4288; **Board Cert:** Orthopaedic Surgery 1978; **Med School:** Baylor Coll Med 1968; **Resid:** Orthopaedic Surgery, Univ Washington Med Ctr 1974; **Fac Appt:** Prof OrS, Univ Wash

O'Donnell, Richard John MD [OrS] - **Spec Exp:** Bone Cancer; Sarcoma-Soft Tissue; Pediatric Orthopaedic Cancers; **Hospital:** UCSF Med Ctr; **Address:** 1600 Divisadero St Fl 4, San Francisco, CA 94115; **Phone:** 415-885-3800; **Board Cert:** Orthopaedic Surgery 1999; **Med School:** Harvard Med Sch 1989; **Resid:** Orthopaedic Surgery, Mass Genl Hosp 1995; **Fellow:** Musculoskeletal Oncology, Univ WA Med Ctr 1996; **Fac Appt:** Assoc Prof OrS, UCSF

Oppenheim, William L MD [OrS] - **Spec Exp:** Limb Lengthening; Scoliosis; Clubfoot/Foot Deformities in Children; Pediatric Orthopaedic Surgery; **Hospital:** UCLA Ronald Reagan Med Ctr; **Address:** 10833 Le Conte Ave, UCLA Med Ctr-Div Orth—Rm 76-134CHS, Los Angeles, CA 90024-1300; **Phone:** 310-206-6345; **Board Cert:** Orthopaedic Surgery 1980; **Med School:** Georgetown Univ 1970; **Resid:** Orthopaedic Surgery, Univ Washington Hosp 1978; **Fellow:** Pediatric Orthopaedic Surgery, Orthopaedic Hosp UCLA 1979; **Fac Appt:** Prof OrS, UCLA

Patzakis, Michael J MD [OrS] - **Spec Exp:** Osteomyelitis; Fractures-Non Union; Joint Infections; **Hospital:** USC Univ Hosp; **Address:** 1200 N State St GNH3900, Los Angeles, CA 90033-1029; **Phone:** 323-226-7201; **Board Cert:** Orthopaedic Surgery 1983; **Med School:** Ohio State Univ 1963; **Resid:** Orthopaedic Surgery, LAC-USC Med Ctr 1968; **Fellow:** Rheumatology, Univ CO Med Ctr 1969; **Fac Appt:** Prof OrS, USC Sch Med

Peterson, Davis C MD [OrS] - **Spec Exp:** Spinal Surgery; Scoliosis; Trauma; **Hospital:** Providence Alaska Med Ctr, Alaska Regl Hosp; **Address:** 3260 Providence Drive, Ste 200, Anchorage, AK 99508-4603; **Phone:** 907-563-3145; **Board Cert:** Orthopaedic Surgery 2009; **Med School:** Baylor Coll Med 1980; **Resid:** Orthopaedic Surgery, Madigan Army Med Ctr 1986; **Fellow:** Spinal Surgery, St Luke's Med Ctr 1990

Sangeorzan, Bruce J MD [OrS] - **Spec Exp:** Foot & Ankle Surgery; Trauma; Ankle Replacement & Revision; **Hospital:** Harborview Med Ctr, Univ Wash Med Ctr; **Address:** 908 Jefferson St, Box 359799, Seattle, WA 98104-2499; **Phone:** 206-744-4830; **Board Cert:** Orthopaedic Surgery 2000; **Med School:** Wayne State Univ 1981; **Resid:** Orthopaedic Surgery, Wayne State Univ 1986; **Fellow:** Trauma, Univ Wash 1986; Foot & Ankle Reconstruction, Univ Wash 1987; **Fac Appt:** Prof OrS, Univ Wash

Schmalzried, Thomas P MD [OrS] - **Spec Exp:** Hip Replacement; **Hospital:** St Vincent's Med Ctr - Los Angeles; **Address:** The Joint Replacement Institute, 2200 W 3rd St, Ste 400, Los Angeles, CA 90057; **Phone:** 213-484-7600; **Board Cert:** Orthopaedic Surgery 2004; **Med School:** UCLA 1984; **Resid:** Orthopaedic Surgery, UCLA Med Ctr 1990; **Fellow:** Orthopaedic Surgery, UCLA Med Ctr 1987; Hip Surgery, Mass Genl Hosp/Harvard 1991; **Fac Appt:** Asst Prof OrS, UCLA

Orthopaedic Surgery

Schurman, David J MD [OrS] - **Spec Exp:** Hip & Knee Replacement; Sports Medicine; Bone Infections; **Hospital:** Stanford Univ Med Ctr; **Address:** 450 Broadway St, MC 6342, Stamford Med Outpatient Ctr, Dept of Orthopaedic Surgery, Redwood City, CA 94063; **Phone:** 650-721-7661; **Board Cert:** Orthopaedic Surgery 1994; **Med School:** Columbia P&S 1965; **Resid:** Surgery, Mount Sinai Hosp 1967; Orthopaedic Surgery, UCLA Med Ctr 1972; **Fellow:** Arthritis Surgery, UCLA Med Ctr 1973; **Fac Appt:** Prof OrS, Stanford Univ

Singer, Daniel I MD [OrS] - **Spec Exp:** Hand Surgery; Bone Cancer; Hand & Upper Extremity Tumors; **Hospital:** Queen's Med Ctr - Honolulu; **Address:** Queen's Physicians' Office Blg 1, 1380 Lusitana St, Ste 615, Honolulu, HI 96813-2442; **Phone:** 808-521-8109; **Board Cert:** Orthopaedic Surgery 2008; Hand Surgery 2008; **Med School:** Boston Univ 1979; **Resid:** Surgery, Univ Conn Hlth Ctr 1981; Orthopaedic Surgery, Univ Hawaii 1984; **Fellow:** Hand Surgery, Thomas Jefferson Univ Med Ctr 1985; Microvascular Surgery, St Vincent's Hosp 1986; **Fac Appt:** Asst Prof OrS, Univ Hawaii JA Burns Sch Med

Teitz, Carol C MD [OrS] - **Spec Exp:** Sports Injuries; Arthroscopic Surgery-Knee; Musculoskeletal Injuries in Dancers; Pain-Back; **Hospital:** Univ Wash Med Ctr; **Address:** UW Sports Medicine Clinic, Bank of America Edmundson Pavilion, 3950 Montlake Blvd NE, rm 148, Seattle, WA 98195; **Phone:** 206-543-1552; **Board Cert:** Orthopaedic Surgery 1981; Orthopaedic Sports Medicine 2007; **Med School:** Yale Univ 1974; **Resid:** Orthopaedic Surgery, Univ Wash Affil Hosps 1980; **Fellow:** Arthroscopic Surgery, J McGinty MD, Newton-Wellesley Hosp 1993; **Fac Appt:** Prof OrS, Univ Wash

Thordarson, David B MD [OrS] - **Spec Exp:** Foot & Ankle Surgery-Complex; Reconstructive Surgery; Trauma; **Hospital:** USC Univ Hosp; **Address:** USC Orthopaedic Surgery Assocs, 1520 San Pablo St, Ste 2000, Los Angeles, CA 90033; **Phone:** 323-442-5860; **Board Cert:** Orthopaedic Surgery 2003; **Med School:** UCLA 1984; **Resid:** Orthopaedic Surgery, UCLA Med Ctr 1989; **Fellow:** Foot & Ankle Surgery, UCLA-Kaiser 1990; **Fac Appt:** Prof OrS, USC-Keck School of Medicine

Tolo, Vernon T MD [OrS] - **Spec Exp:** Pediatric Orthopaedic Surgery; Spinal Deformity-Pediatric; Skeletal Dysplasia; **Hospital:** Chldns Hosp - Los Angeles, USC Univ Hosp; **Address:** Chldns Hosp LA, Orthopaedic Surgery, 4650 W Sunset Blvd, MS 69, Los Angeles, CA 90027-6062; **Phone:** 323-361-4658; **Board Cert:** Orthopaedic Surgery 1977; **Med School:** Johns Hopkins Univ 1968; **Resid:** Orthopaedic Surgery, Johns Hopkins Hosp 1975; **Fellow:** Pediatric Orthopaedic Surgery, Hosp Sick Chldn 1976; **Fac Appt:** Prof OrS, USC Sch Med

Vail, Thomas P MD [OrS] - **Spec Exp:** Hip & Knee Replacement; Hip Resurfacing; Arthritis; Osteonecrosis; **Hospital:** UCSF Med Ctr; **Address:** 400 Parnassus Ave, Lower Plaza Level, San Francisco, CA 94143; **Phone:** 415-353-2808; **Board Cert:** Orthopaedic Surgery 2005; **Med School:** Loyola Univ-Stritch Sch Med 1985; **Resid:** Thoracic Surgery, Duke Univ Med Ctr 1987; Orthopaedic Surgery, Duke Univ Med Ctr 1991; **Fellow:** Reconstructive Surgery, North Amer/Euro Trav Prgm 1992; **Fac Appt:** Prof OrS, UCSF

Wang, Jeffrey C MD [OrS] - **Spec Exp:** Spinal Surgery; **Hospital:** UCLA Ronald Reagan Med Ctr, Santa Monica - UCLA Med Ctr & Ortho Hosp; **Address:** UCLA Spine Center, 1250 16th St, Ste 745, Santa Monica, CA 90404; **Phone:** 310-319-3334; **Board Cert:** Orthopaedic Surgery 2009; **Med School:** Univ Pittsburgh 1991; **Resid:** Orthopaedic Surgery, Orthopaedic Hosp UCLA 1996; **Fellow:** Spinal Cord Injury Medicine, Case Western Reserve Univ 1997; **Fac Appt:** Prof OrS, UCLA

Watkins III, Robert G MD [OrS] - **Spec Exp:** Spinal Surgery; Spinal Disc Replacement; **Address:** 13160 Mindanao Way, Ste 325, Marina Del Rey, CA 90292; **Phone:** 310-448-7890; **Board Cert:** Orthopaedic Surgery 2007; **Med School:** Univ Tenn Coll Med, Memphis 1969; **Resid:** Orthopaedic Surgery, LAC-USC Med Ctr 1978; **Fellow:** Spinal Surgery, Jones-Hunt Orth Hosp 1979; **Fac Appt:** Assoc Prof OrS, USC Sch Med

Yoo, Jung MD [OrS] - **Spec Exp:** Spinal Surgery; **Hospital:** OR Hlth & Sci Univ; **Address:** 3181 SW Sam Jackson Park Rd, MC OP-31, Portland, OR 97239; **Phone:** 503-494-6406; **Board Cert:** Orthopaedic Surgery 2004; **Med School:** Univ Chicago-Pritzker Sch Med 1984; **Resid:** Orthopaedic Surgery, Case Western Reserve Univ 1990; **Fellow:** Orthopaedic Surgery, SUNY Hlth Sci Ctr 1991; **Fac Appt:** Prof OrS, Oregon Hlth & Sci Univ

◼️ Cleveland Clinic

Orthopaedic Surgery

The Cleveland Clinic Department of Orthopaedic Surgery has a long history of excellence and innovation in treating musculoskeletal injuries and diseases. For the past several years, *U.S.News & World Report* has consistently ranked the Department of Orthopaedic Surgery among the nation's top five orthopaedic programs.

Foot and Ankle: All specialists and surgeons in the Cleveland Clinic Foot and Ankle Center have extensive training in the diagnosis and care of foot and ankle disorders. Our orthopaedic surgeons, podiatrists, nurse clinicians, certified pedorthists and technicians deliver state-of-the-art care exclusively for the foot and ankle.

Joint Replacement: Cleveland Clinic's Center for Adult Reconstruction treats osteoarthritis and rheumatoid arthritis of the hip and knee, and fractures of these joints, and performs joint replacement, resurfacing and revision surgery. At the frontier of surgical innovation our experienced surgeons offer the most advanced implants and minimally invasive techniques to restore patient mobility.

Pediatrics: Cleveland Clinic's Center for Pediatric Orthopaedics handles more than 14,000 outpatient visits each year. Our physicians offer expertise in the management of all musculoskeletal conditions, in children, including spinal deformity, scoliosis, hip dysplasia, clubfoot, fractures and growth plate injuries, neuromuscular disorders and sports injuries. They also perform leg lengthening and limb deformity correction.

Research and Education

The Cleveland Clinic Orthopaedic and Rheumatologic Research Center (ORRC) is a unique collaboration that taps into the synergy between Orthopaedic Surgery, Rheumatology and Biomedical Engineering. The Center's mission is to advance the health and treatment of people with disorders of the musculoskeletal system through basic and applied scientific investigation, and to train future leaders in musculoskeletal care, research and education. Recent developments, such as harvesting bone marrow cells to generate new bone tissue and research collaboration with other leading institutions, help to advance patient care.

Center for Spine Health: Cleveland Clinic's Center for Spine Health diagnoses and treats more than 13,000 patients annually. The center brings together the expertise of specialists in neurosurgery, orthopaedic surgery and non-surgical spine care. The Center for Spine Health integrates functions of research and clinical practice with education.

Trauma: Cleveland Clinic has been a leader in the treatment of fracture non-union and in the development of methods to improve outcomes through advanced bone-grafting techniques.

Center for Musculoskeletal Tumors: As one of the largest multi-disciplinary centers of its kind, we offer expertise in treating bone and soft tissue sarcomas, and performing limb salvage.

For more information about the Cleveland Clinic Department of Orthopaedic Surgery, to schedule a second opinion, or to learn about assistance for out-of-town patients, call 800.890.2467 or visit www.clevelandclinic.org/orthotopdocs.

Department of Orthopaedic Surgery
9500 Euclid Avenue / AC311 | Cleveland OH 44195

Penn Medicine

Philadelphia, PA 19104
800.789.PENN
PennMedicine.org

PENN ORTHOPAEDICS

Penn Orthopaedics, a leader in treating patients with musculo-skeletal injuries and disorders from the most common to the most complex, provides comprehensive, quality care that ranks among the very best in the nation. Our multidisciplinary team of surgeons and staff use the latest technology and techniques to get people – grandparents and professional athletes alike – back in motion.

Programs

Penn Orthopaedics offers special-ized services and programs to treat a wide range of orthopaedic problems, including:

- Hand
- Hip and knee replacements
- Neuro-orthopaedics
- Orthopaedic oncology
- Shoulder and elbow
- Spine
- Sports medicine
- Trauma

Leadership

As recognized clinical leaders, our doctors offer state-of-the-art treatment options, including:

- Advanced minimally invasive joint replacement procedures, such as one- and two-incision hip replacements.
- Upper extremity services dedicated to the treatment of shoulder, elbow, wrist and hand disorders.
- Treatment for malignant and benign tumors of the bone and soft tissue.

- Neuro-orthopaedic procedures to restore range of motion for patients with permanent disabilities following stroke, head injury or cerebral palsy.

Our physicians serve on the boards of the nation's premiere orthopaedic organizations and publish articles in many of the leading orthopaedic journals in the world.

Also a noted research group, Penn Orthopaedics is helping to create the next generation of orthopaedic care, in areas including tissue engineering, tendon healing and biomechanics of the shoulder and spine. Additionally, we are one of the most prominent recipients of orthopaedic grants from the National Institutes of Health.

Expertise

Penn Orthopaedics is consistently recognized as a national leader in outstanding care. Many of our surgeons are listed among the *Best Doctors in America®*, and a number of our physicians are listed annually in *Philadelphia* magazine's "Top Docs" issue.

Locations

Hospital of the University of Pennsylvania

Penn Presbyterian Medical Center

Pennsylvania Hospital

Penn Sports Medicine Center at Weightman Hall

Penn Medicine at Bucks County

Penn Medicine at Cherry Hill

Penn Medicine at Radnor

For an appointment, call 800-789-PENN.

MOUNT SINAI
SCHOOL OF
MEDICINE

THE MOUNT SINAI MEDICAL CENTER
ORTHOPAEDICS
One Gustave L. Levy Place
Fifth Avenue and 100th Street
New York, NY 10029-6574
Physician Referral: 1-800-MD-SINAI (637-4624)
www.mountsinai.org

Beyond its reputation for depth and breadth of expertise, **THE LENI AND PETER W. MAY DEPARTMENT OF ORTHOPAEDICS** is known for personalized care. The faculty and staff invest the time to get to know their patients as individuals, ensuring that they receive direct care from subspecialty-trained orthopedists. The faculty share expertise in surgery of the foot and ankle, knee, hip, hand, elbow, shoulder, and spine; total joint replacement; microvascular surgery; cancer surgery; and minimally invasive surgery. Taking a whole-patient approach to care, they work in close collaboration with specialists in geriatrics, neurology, oncology, pathology, and rehabilitation medicine.

Investigation and Innovation – Recent years have seen successive refinements in the techniques of orthopedic surgery at Mount Sinai, including the design and composition of the prostheses used in joint replacements that have led to improved postoperative function. Faculty members have also been instrumental in the design and perfection of hip and shoulder prostheses. Additionally, Mount Sinai has broadened the applications of arthroscopic surgery—the fiberoptic technology that first heralded the arrival of minimally invasive surgery.

Mount Sinai orthopedic scientists are known for their studies of "wear and tear" diseases of the skeletal system. Researchers are currently investigating bone wear at the microscopic level, rotator cuff degeneration, the effects of microgravity on aging of bones and tissue, how joints of the foot degenerate, methods of determining bone strength, and how genetic alterations change the skeleton's function.

Use of Cutting-Edge Techniques – Mount Sinai uses innovative, minimally invasive approaches for joint replacement and fracture repair. The Department's oncology service is renowned for saving limbs with both bone and joint malignancies.

The Sports Service is one of few departments in the country that provides patients the option of arthroscopic surgery of the hip. Patients have the ability to return to activities faster and with less pain with this minimally invasive procedure. Our arthroscopists also specialize in cartilage preservation techniques, including cartilage transplantation, allowing patients to preserve their own joints and delaying the need for joint replacement surgery.

GROUNDBREAKING PROCEDURES ENHANCE QUALITY OF LIFE

Today at Mount Sinai, arthroscopy is used to repair not only the knee but virtually every joint. Converting what used to be major open surgery to outpatient procedures has dramatically shortened rehabilitation and return-to-work times. More significantly, it has allowed many more patients to get help for painful, function-limiting conditions. That is the case for many elderly or frail patients who are physically unable to undergo major surgery. The fact that such procedures are now more widely accessible is enhancing the quality of life for many patients and allowing them to lead more active lives.

NYU Hospital for Joint Diseases
NYU LANGONE MEDICAL CENTER

301 East 17th Street
(at Second Avenue)
New York, NY 10003
212-598-6000 FAX: 212-260-1203
www.nyuhjd.org

ORTHOPAEDIC SERVICES

About Orthopaedic Services, Department of Orthopaedic Surgery:

The Department of Orthopaedic Surgery caters to the unique treatment needs of today's patients. Expert physicians combine their experience and research with the latest technology to provide care of bone and joint problems that affect patients' ability to function. Areas of specialty include: sports medicine, adult reconstructive services, joint replacement, spine, hand, shoulder and elbow, foot and ankle, pediatric orthopeadics, trauma and fractures and oncology.

We specialize in the following areas:

BONE HEALING

The Bone Healing Center is dedicated to the evaluation and treatment of complex problem fractures. The Center is pioneering new technologies and procedures to help patients facing a long and difficult recovery due to complex fracture reconstruction or problems with fracture healing.

DANCE INJURIES

From young students and dancers to seasoned professionals and members of internationally acclaimed companies, the Harkness Center for Dance Injuries offers many subsidized and free services for the dance community, including clinics staffed by orthopaedists and dance physical therapists. The Center also offers state-of-the-art research, rehabilitation technology and free injury prevention screenings and lectures.

FOOT AND ANKLE

The Diabetes Foot and Ankle Center focuses on the prevention of foot and ankle problems and their recurrence. Dedicated medical professionals provide the most advanced treatment for those complications.

HIP CARE

Our Hip Center is dedicated to treating a wide range of conditions that affect the hip, whether they are developmental, traumatic or degenerative, and allows doctors to see the issues from a broad perspective.

IMMEDIATE CARE

The Samuels Orthopaedic Immediate Care Center is New York City's only walk-in orthopaedic clinic. Staffed by members of the Department of Orthopaedic Surgery, the Center, or "I-Care", uses state-of-the-art diagnostic equipment to evaluate and treat all urgent orthopaedic problems, including hand and foot injuries, hip, arm or leg fractures, dislocation or joint injury, sprains, and bone or joint infection.

JOINT REPLACEMENT

At The Joint Replacement Center, patients have access to physicians and surgeons highly specialized in treating degenerative joint conditions. The Center is one of the most active in the world, performing more than 2,500 joint replacements annually and its surgeons are know for their expertise in knee, hip and shoulder replacements, complex joint revisions, as well as minimally invasive surgeries.

OCCUPATIONAL AND INDUSTRIAL ORTHOPAEDICS

The Occupational and Industrial Orthopaedic Center provides clinical, educational, research and consulting services in the prevention and treatment of musculoskeletal injuries and disorders that arise from work or from the work environment.

PEDIATRIC ORTHOPAEDIC SERVICES

The Department's skilled specialists provide orthopaedic care for children with neuromuscular diseases such as cerebral palsy, spina bifida and muscular dystrophies and congenital conditions such as clubfoot, hip dysplasia and limb deformities.

SPINE

The Spine Center provides comprehensive treatment of adult and pediatric spine disorders including lower back pain, neck pain, scoliosis, osteoporosis and the most complex spine problems. The Center performs minimally invasive spinal fusions and is designated as one of the first in the country to successfully perform artificial disc implantation.

Wake Forest University Baptist
MEDICAL CENTER ®

Orthopaedic Services

Medical Center Boulevard • Winston-Salem, NC 27157 • 336-716-2011
Health On-Call® (Patient Access) 1-800-446-2255
Physician-To-Physician Calls (PAL®) 1-800-277-7654
wfubmc.edu/ortho

Wake Forest University Baptist Medical Center offers comprehensive programs in all facets of adult and pediatric bone and joint care including joint preservation, resurfacing and replacement, sports medicine, pediatrics, spine, hand and upper extremity, foot and ankle, and innovative therapies that are setting the standards for orthopaedics.

PROGRAM HIGHLIGHTS

The **Comprehensive Joint Replacement Program** employs the most advanced technologies and surgical techniques for hips and knees as well as specialized after-surgery care. Our surgeons perform a number of procedures that offer joint patients a quicker recovery, less pain and more precise placement, such as hip arthroscopy, hip resurfacing, anterior approach hip replacement, and robotic arm assisted partial knee replacement.

The **Hand and Upper Extremity Program** has nationally and internationally recognized experts with experience in a broad range of diseases and conditions. Our specialists treat complex nerve disorders, peripheral neurotization, brachial plexus injuries, congenital conditions and traumatic injuries, as well as perform micro-vascular reconstruction and joint replacements. We have the area's only certified hand surgeons.

The **Sports Medicine Program** is comprised of the region's most well-trained physicians and therapists working collaboratively to provide a comprehensive, evidence-based approach. The orthopaedic surgery and family medicine team utilizes an individualized approach to treating athletes and people of all ages whose physical abilities have been limited by injury, degenerative disease or aging. Our sports medicine specialists serve as the team doctors for Wake Forest University, Winston-Salem State University and local professional and high school athletes.

A TEAM APPROACH

Our physical therapy programs support the orthopaedic team in all areas including inpatient services, musculoskeletal, joints, sports medicine, spine, hand and upper extremity, foot and ankle, and pediatrics.

The Wake Forest Institute for Regenerative Medicine is leading the way in the use of patients' own cells to develop tissues and organs in the laboratory. Our orthopaedic surgeons and researchers are working with the Institute on multiple projects that will benefit patients with orthopaedic injuries. Those projects include the development of ligament and meniscus replacements, technologies to improve nerve regeneration, and methods of bone regeneration.

The **Pediatric Orthopaedics Program** has experts with specialty training in acquired and congenital disorders of children and draw patients nationwide and worldwide. The program offers multidisciplinary treatment for cerebral palsy. Surgeons here are pioneers in the use of Botox® injections for treating spasticity disorders and are leaders in treating spinal deformities and hip disorders in children.

The **Orthopaedic Oncology Program** has a comprehensive team of specialists who provide the most advanced diagnostic technologies and treatment modalities available for patients with benign or malignant bone and soft tissue tumors.

To make an appointment or find a specialist, call Health On-Call® at 1-800-446-2255.

Otolaryngology

An otolaryngologist-head and neck surgeon provides comprehensive medical and surgical care for patients with diseases and disorders that affect the ears, nose, throat, the respiratory and upper alimentary systems and related structures of the head and neck.

An otolaryngologist diagnoses and provides medical and/or surgical therapy or prevention of diseases, allergies, neoplasms, deformities, disorders and/or injuries of the ears, nose, sinuses, throat, respiratory and upper alimentary systems, face, jaws and the other head and neck systems. Head and neck oncology, facial plastic and reconstructive surgery and the treatment of disorders of hearing and voice are fundamental areas of expertise.

Training Required: Five years

Certification in the following subspecialty requires additional training and examination.

Plastic Surgery within the Head and Neck: An otolaryngologist with additional training in plastic and reconstructive procedures within the head, face, neck and associated structures, including cutaneous head and neck oncology and reconstruction, management of maxillofacial trauma, soft tissue repair and neural surgery.

Facial Plastic and Reconstructive Surgery is not a recognized ABMS subspecialty. However this designation has been included because the certification process is meaningful and rigorous. It is awarded to those doctors who hold a current ABMS certification in Otolaryngology, but those board certified in Plastic Surgery, Ophthalmology, or Dermatology are also eligible. Certification requires a post-graduate fellowship in Facial Plastic and Reconstructive Surgery followed by a written examination.

This field is diverse and involves a wide age range of patients, from the newborn to the aged. While both cosmetic and reconstructive surgeries are practiced, there are many additional procedures which interface with them.

OTOLARYNGOLOGY

New England

Bhattacharyya, Neil MD [Oto] - **Spec Exp:** Head & Neck Surgery; **Hospital:** Brigham & Women's Hosp, Dana-Farber Cancer Inst; **Address:** Brigham and Women's Hospital, 45 Francis St, Boston, MA 02115-6105; **Phone:** 617-525-6540; **Board Cert:** Otolaryngology 1998; **Med School:** Univ IL Coll Med 1992; **Resid:** Otolaryngology, Mass Eye & Ear Infirm 1997

Deschler, Daniel G MD [Oto] - **Spec Exp:** Head & Neck Cancer; Head & Neck Reconstruction; Salivary Gland Tumors & Surgery; Voice after Laryngeal Cancer Surgery; **Hospital:** Mass Eye & Ear Infirmary, Mass Genl Hosp; **Address:** Mass Eye & Ear Infirmary, Head & Neck Surgery, 243 Charles St, Boston, MA 02114; **Phone:** 617-573-4100; **Board Cert:** Otolaryngology 1996; **Med School:** Harvard Med Sch 1990; **Resid:** Otolaryngology, UCSF Med Ctr 1995; **Fellow:** Head & Neck Surgical Oncology, Hahneman U Med Ctr 1996; **Fac Appt:** Assoc Prof Oto, Harvard Med Sch

Gliklich, Richard E MD [Oto] - **Spec Exp:** Cosmetic Surgery-Face & Neck; Rhinoplasty; Skin Laser Surgery-Resurfacing; **Hospital:** Mass Eye & Ear Infirmary; **Address:** Mass Eye & Ear Infirmary, 243 Charles St Fl 9, Boston, MA 02114; **Phone:** 617-573-4105; **Board Cert:** Otolaryngology 1994; Facial Plastic & Reconstr Surgery 1996; **Med School:** Harvard Med Sch 1988; **Resid:** Otolaryngology, Mass E&E Infirmary 1993; **Fellow:** Facial Plastic Surgery, Mass E&E Infirmary 1994; **Fac Appt:** Assoc Prof Oto, Harvard Med Sch

Grillone, Gregory A MD [Oto] - **Spec Exp:** Laryngeal Disorders; Voice Disorders; Laryngeal Cancer; Head & Neck Cancer & Surgery; **Hospital:** Boston Med Ctr; **Address:** Boston Univ Med Ctr, Dept Otolaryngology, 830 Harrison Ave, Boston, MA 02118; **Phone:** 617-638-8124; **Board Cert:** Otolaryngology 1988; **Med School:** Mount Sinai Sch Med 1983; **Resid:** Oncology, Boston Univ Med Ctr 1988; **Fac Appt:** Asst Prof Oto, Boston Univ

Grundfast, Kenneth MD [Oto] - **Spec Exp:** Hearing Loss; Pediatric Otolaryngology; Chronic Ear Disease; **Hospital:** Boston Med Ctr, Boston VA Med Ctr; **Address:** Boston Medical Center, 830 Harrison Ave, Ste 1400, Boston, MA 02119; **Phone:** 617-638-8124; **Board Cert:** Otolaryngology 1977; **Med School:** SUNY Upstate Med Univ 1969; **Resid:** Surgery, Sibley Meml Hosp 1974; Otolaryngology, Boston-Affil Hosps 1977; **Fellow:** Pediatric Otolaryngology, Chldns Hosp 1978; **Fac Appt:** Prof Oto, Boston Univ

Hadlock, Theresa MD [Oto] - **Spec Exp:** Facial Paralysis; **Hospital:** Mass Eye & Ear Infirmary; **Address:** Mass Eye & Ear Infirmary, Facial Plastic Ste, 243 Charles St, Boston, MA 02114; **Phone:** 617-573-3641; **Board Cert:** Otolaryngology 2002; **Med School:** Harvard Med Sch 1994; **Resid:** Otolaryngology, Mass Eye & Ear Infirm 1998; **Fellow:** Facial Plastic Surgery, Mass Eye & Ear Infirm 1999; **Fac Appt:** Asst Prof Oto, Harvard Med Sch

Kveton, John MD [Oto] - **Spec Exp:** Ear Disorders; Cochlear Implants; Acoustic Neuroma; **Hospital:** Yale-New Haven Hosp, Hosp of St Raphael; **Address:** 46 Prince St, Ste 601, New Haven, CT 06519-1634; **Phone:** 203-752-1726; **Board Cert:** Otolaryngology 1982; Neurotology 2004; **Med School:** St Louis Univ 1978; **Resid:** Otolaryngology, Yale-New Haven Hosp 1982; **Fellow:** Neurotology, The Otology Group 1983; **Fac Appt:** Clin Prof Oto, Yale Univ

McKenna, Michael J MD [Oto] - **Spec Exp:** Skull Base Surgery; Otology; Neuro-Otology; **Hospital:** Mass Eye & Ear Infirmary; **Address:** Massachusetts Eye & Ear Infirmary, 243 Charles St, Boston, MA 02114-3002; **Phone:** 617-573-3672; **Board Cert:** Otolaryngology 1988; Neurotology 2004; **Med School:** USC Sch Med 1982; **Resid:** Otolaryngology, Mass Eye & Ear Infirm 1988; **Fellow:** Neurotology, Otologic Med Group 1989; **Fac Appt:** Prof Oto, Harvard Med Sch

Otolaryngology

Metson, Ralph MD [Oto] - **Spec Exp:** Sinus Disorders/Surgery; **Hospital:** Mass Eye & Ear Infirmary; **Address:** Zero Emerson Pl, Ste 2D, Boston, MA 02114; **Phone:** 617-227-4366; **Board Cert:** Otolaryngology 1985; **Med School:** UCSD 1979; **Resid:** Otolaryngology, UCLA Med Ctr 1985; **Fac Appt:** Assoc Clin Prof Oto, Harvard Med Sch

Nadol, Joseph B MD [Oto] - **Spec Exp:** Ear Disorders/Surgery; Hearing Disorders; Cochlear Implants; **Hospital:** Mass Eye & Ear Infirmary, Mass Genl Hosp; **Address:** Mass Eye & Ear Infirmary, 243 Charles St, Boston, MA 02114-3096; **Phone:** 617-573-3632; **Board Cert:** Otolaryngology 1975; Neurotology 2005; **Med School:** Johns Hopkins Univ 1970; **Resid:** Surgery, Beth Israel Hosp 1972; Otolaryngology, Mass Eye & Ear Infirmary 1975; **Fac Appt:** Prof Oto, Harvard Med Sch

Randolph, Gregory W MD [Oto] - **Spec Exp:** Thyroid Disorders; Thyroid Cancer; Parathyroid Disease; **Hospital:** Mass Eye & Ear Infirmary; **Address:** Mass Eye & Ear Infirmary, 243 Charles St Fl 2, Boston, MA 02114; **Phone:** 617-573-4115; **Board Cert:** Otolaryngology 1993; **Med School:** Cornell Univ-Weill Med Coll 1987; **Resid:** Otolaryngology, Mass E&E Infirmary 1992; **Fellow:** Thyroid Oncology, Mass E&E Infirmary 1993; **Fac Appt:** Asst Prof Oto, Harvard Med Sch

Rauch, Steven D MD [Oto] - **Spec Exp:** Hearing & Balance Disorders; Meniere's Disease; Neuro-Otology; **Hospital:** Mass Eye & Ear Infirmary; **Address:** Mass Eye & Ear Infirmary, Dept Otolary, 243 Charles St, Boston, MA 02114; **Phone:** 617-573-3644; **Board Cert:** Otolaryngology 1984; **Med School:** Univ Cincinnati 1979; **Resid:** Surgery, U Mass Med Ctr 1981; Otolaryngology, Mass E&E Infirm 1984; **Fac Appt:** Assoc Prof Oto, Harvard Med Sch

Rebeiz, Elie E MD [Oto] - **Spec Exp:** Head & Neck Surgery; **Hospital:** Tufts Med Ctr; **Address:** Tufts Medical Ctr, Dept Otolaryngology, 750 Washington St, Boston, MA 02111; **Phone:** 617-636-1664; **Board Cert:** Otolaryngology 2000; **Med School:** Lebanon 1984; **Resid:** Otolaryngology, Amer Univ Med Ctr 1988; **Fellow:** Otolaryngology, Mass E&E Infirm 1990; **Fac Appt:** Prof Oto, Tufts Univ

Sasaki, Clarence T MD [Oto] - **Spec Exp:** Head & Neck Cancer; Skull Base Surgery; Voice Disorders; Swallowing Disorders; **Hospital:** Yale-New Haven Hosp, Hosp of St Raphael; **Address:** Yale Sch Med, Dept Otolaryngology, 333 Cedar St, Box 208041, New Haven, CT 06520-8041; **Phone:** 203-785-2592; **Board Cert:** Otolaryngology 1973; **Med School:** Yale Univ 1966; **Resid:** Surgery, Mary Hitchcock Hosp 1968; Otolaryngology, Yale-New Haven Hosp 1973; **Fellow:** Head and Neck Surgery, Univ of Milan 1978; Skull Base Surgery, Univ Zurich 1982; **Fac Appt:** Prof Oto, Yale Univ

Vining, Eugenia M MD [Oto] - **Spec Exp:** Sinus Disorders/Surgery; Skull Base Tumors; Sinus Tumors; **Hospital:** Yale-New Haven Hosp, Hosp of St Raphael; **Address:** 46 Prince St, Ste 601, New Haven, CT 06519; **Phone:** 203-752-1726; **Board Cert:** Otolaryngology 1993; **Med School:** Yale Univ 1987; **Resid:** Otolaryngology, Yale-New Haven Hosp 1991; Otolaryngology, Yale-New Haven Hosp 1992; **Fellow:** Sinus Surgery, Univ Penn 1993

Zeitels, Steven MD [Oto] - **Spec Exp:** Laryngeal Disorders; Voice Disorders; Laryngeal Cancer; Head & Neck Cancer & Surgery; **Hospital:** Mass Genl Hosp; **Address:** Mass Genl Hosp, 1 Bowdoin Square Fl 11, Boston, MA 02114; **Phone:** 617-726-0218; **Board Cert:** Otolaryngology 1988; **Med School:** Boston Univ 1982; **Resid:** Surgery, Univ Hosp-Boston City Hosp 1983; Otolaryngology, Boston Univ-Tufts Univ 1987; **Fellow:** Head and Neck Surgery, Boston VA Med Ctr 1988; **Fac Appt:** Prof S, Harvard Med Sch

Mid Atlantic

Arriaga, Moises A MD [Oto] - **Spec Exp:** Hearing Loss; Acoustic Neuroma; Balance Disorders; Otology & Neuro-Otology; **Hospital:** Allegheny General Hosp, UPMC Mercy, Pittsburgh; **Address:** 420 E North Ave, Ste 402, Pittsburgh, PA 15212; **Phone:** 412-359-6690; **Board Cert:** Otolaryngology 1990; Neurotology 2004; **Med School:** Brown Univ 1985; **Resid:** Otolaryngology, Univ Pittsburgh Med Ctr 1990; **Fellow:** Neurotology, House Ear Clinic 1991; **Fac Appt:** Assoc Clin Prof Oto, Univ Pittsburgh

Aviv, Jonathan MD [Oto] - **Spec Exp:** Voice Disorders; Swallowing Disorders; Vocal Cord Disorders; Endoscopy; **Hospital:** Mount Sinai Med Ctr (page 64); **Address:** 210 E 86th St Fl 9, New York, NY 10028; **Phone:** 212-722-5570; **Board Cert:** Otolaryngology 1990; **Med School:** Columbia P&S 1985; **Resid:** Surgery, Mt Sinai Med Ctr 1987; Otolaryngology, Mt Sinai Med Ctr 1990; **Fellow:** Otolaryngology, Mt Sinai Med Ctr 1991; **Fac Appt:** Prof Oto, Columbia P&S

Blitzer, Andrew MD/DDS [Oto] - **Spec Exp:** Voice Disorders; Swallowing Disorders; Nasal & Sinus Surgery; Botox Therapy; **Hospital:** St Luke's - Roosevelt Hosp Ctr - Roosevelt Div (page 57); **Address:** 425 W 59th St Fl 10, New York, NY 10019-1104; **Phone:** 212-262-9500; **Board Cert:** Otolaryngology 1977; **Med School:** Mount Sinai Sch Med 1973; **Resid:** Surgery, Beth Israel Med Ctr 1974; Otolaryngology, Mt Sinai Hosp 1977; **Fac Appt:** Clin Prof Oto, Columbia P&S

Carrau, Ricardo L MD [Oto] - **Spec Exp:** Skull Base Tumors & Surgery; Nasal & Sinus Cancer & Surgery; Swallowing Disorders; **Hospital:** UPMC Presby, Pittsburgh; **Address:** Eye & Ear Institute, 200 Lothrop St, Ste 500, Pittsburgh, PA 15213; **Phone:** 412-647-2100; **Board Cert:** Otolaryngology 1987; **Med School:** Univ Puerto Rico 1981; **Resid:** Surgery, University Hosp 1984; Head and Neck Surgery, University Hosp 1987; **Fellow:** Head & Neck Oncology, Univ Pittsburgh Med Ctr 1990; **Fac Appt:** Assoc Prof Oto, Univ Pittsburgh

Chalian, Ara A MD [Oto] - **Spec Exp:** Head & Neck Cancer; Head & Neck Reconstruction; Thyroid Cancer; Reconstructive Surgery; **Hospital:** Hosp Univ Penn - UPHS (page 60); **Address:** Hosp Univ Penn, Dept Otolaryngology, 3400 Spruce St, Silverstein Bldg, Philadelphia, PA 19104; **Phone:** 215-349-5559; **Board Cert:** Otolaryngology 1994; **Med School:** Indiana Univ 1988; **Resid:** Surgery, Indiana Univ Hosp 1990; Otolaryngology, Indiana Univ Hosp 1993; **Fellow:** Molecular Biology, Hosp U Penn 1994; Head and Neck Surgery, Hosp U Penn 1995; **Fac Appt:** Assoc Prof Oto, Univ Pennsylvania

Close, Lanny G MD [Oto] - **Spec Exp:** Skull Base Surgery; Head & Neck Cancer; Sinus Disorders/Surgery; Endoscopic Sinus Surgery; **Hospital:** NY-Presby Hosp/Columbia (page 66); **Address:** 16 E 60th St, Ste 470, New York, NY 10022; **Phone:** 212-326-8475; **Board Cert:** Otolaryngology 1977; **Med School:** Baylor Coll Med 1972; **Resid:** Surgery, Johns Hopkins Hosp 1974; Otolaryngology, Baylor Affil Hosps 1977; **Fellow:** Head and Neck Surgery, MD Anderson Cancer Ctr 1979; **Fac Appt:** Prof Oto, Columbia P&S

Costantino, Peter D MD [Oto] - **Spec Exp:** Skull Base Tumors; Head & Neck Cancer; Craniofacial Surgery/Reconstruction; **Hospital:** St Luke's - Roosevelt Hosp Ctr - Roosevelt Div (page 57), NY-Presby Hosp/Columbia (page 66); **Address:** 1000 W 10th Ave, Ste 5G-80, New York, NY 10019-1104; **Phone:** 212-523-6756; **Board Cert:** Otolaryngology 1990; Facial Plastic & Reconstr Surgery 2000; **Med School:** Northwestern Univ 1984; **Resid:** Surgery, Northwestern Meml Hosp 1986; Otolaryngology, Northwestern Meml Hosp 1989; **Fellow:** Head and Neck Surgery, Northwestern Meml Hosp 1990; Skull Base Surgery, Univ Pittsburgh 1991; **Fac Appt:** Prof Oto, Columbia P&S

Otolaryngology

Davidson, Bruce J MD [Oto] - **Spec Exp:** Head & Neck Cancer; Thyroid Disorders; **Hospital:** Georgetown Univ Hosp; **Address:** Georgetown Univ Med Ctr, Dept Otolaryngology-Head & Neck Surgery, 3800 Reservoir Rd NW Gorman Bldg Fl 1, Washington, DC 20007; **Phone:** 202-444-8186; **Board Cert:** Otolaryngology 1993; **Med School:** W VA Univ 1987; **Resid:** Otolaryngology, Georgetown Univ Med Ctr 1992; **Fellow:** Otolaryngology, Memorial Sloan-Kettering Cancer Ctr 1994; **Fac Appt:** Asst Prof Oto, Georgetown Univ

Edelstein, David R MD [Oto] - **Spec Exp:** Endoscopic Sinus Surgery; Nasal Reconstruction; Rhinoplasty; Sleep Disorders/Apnea; **Hospital:** Lenox Hill Hosp (Manh Eye, Ear & Throat Hosp) (page 62), Lenox Hill Hosp (page 62); **Address:** 1421 3rd Ave Fl 4, New York, NY 10028; **Phone:** 212-452-1500; **Board Cert:** Otolaryngology 1985; **Med School:** Boston Univ 1980; **Resid:** Otolaryngology, Mount Sinai Hosp 1984; **Fac Appt:** Clin Prof Oto, Cornell Univ-Weill Med Coll

Feghali, Joseph G MD [Oto] - **Spec Exp:** Ear Disorders/Surgery; Acoustic Neuroma; Hearing Disorders; Neuro-Otology; **Hospital:** Montefiore Med Ctr - Div. Moses; **Address:** 182 E 210th St, Bronx, NY 10467; **Phone:** 718-881-3277; **Board Cert:** Otolaryngology 1990; **Med School:** Lebanon 1978; **Resid:** Otolaryngology, American Univ Beirut 1982; Otolaryngology, Montefiore Med Ctr 1990; **Fellow:** Otology & Neurotology, House Ear Inst 1983; Neurological Surgery, Meml Sloan Kettering Cancer Ctr 1984; **Fac Appt:** Clin Prof Oto, Albert Einstein Coll Med

Fried, Marvin P MD [Oto] - **Spec Exp:** Endoscopic Sinus Surgery; Head & Neck Tumors; Laryngeal & Voice Disorders; Sinus Disorders/Surgery; **Hospital:** Montefiore Med Ctr - Div. Moses, Montefiore Med Ctr - Div. Weiler; **Address:** 3400 Bainbridge Ave Fl 3, Bronx, NY 10467; **Phone:** 718-920-4646; **Board Cert:** Otolaryngology 1975; **Med School:** Tufts Univ 1969; **Resid:** Surgery, Jewish Hosp 1971; Otolaryngology, Barnes Hosp 1975; **Fellow:** Stroke, Washington Univ 1976; **Fac Appt:** Prof Oto, Albert Einstein Coll Med

Genden, Eric M MD [Oto] - **Spec Exp:** Head & Neck Cancer & Surgery; Head & Neck Cancer Reconstruction; Airway Reconstruction; Thyroid & Parathyroid Cancer & Surgery; **Hospital:** Mount Sinai Med Ctr (page 64); **Address:** Mt Sinai Dept Otolaryngology, 1 Gustave L Levy Pl, Box 1191, New York, NY 10029; **Phone:** 212-241-9410; **Board Cert:** Otolaryngology 1999; Facial Plastic & Reconstr Surgery 2000; **Med School:** Mount Sinai Sch Med 1992; **Resid:** Otolaryngology, Barnes Jewish Hosp 1998; **Fellow:** Head and Neck Surgery, Mt Sinai Med Ctr 1999; **Fac Appt:** Assoc Prof Oto, Mount Sinai Sch Med

Gold, Scott D MD [Oto] - **Spec Exp:** Endoscopic Sinus Surgery; Sinus Disorders/Surgery; **Hospital:** Beth Israel Med Ctr - Petrie Division (page 57), Mount Sinai Med Ctr (page 64); **Address:** 36A E 36th St, Ste 200, New York, NY 10016-3401; **Phone:** 212-889-8575; **Board Cert:** Otolaryngology 1983; **Med School:** Mount Sinai Sch Med 1979; **Resid:** Otolaryngology, Mt Sinai Med Ctr 1983; **Fac Appt:** Asst Clin Prof Oto, Mount Sinai Sch Med

Goldenberg, David MD [Oto] - **Spec Exp:** Head & Neck Cancer & Surgery; Thyroid & Parathyroid Cancer & Surgery; Salivary Gland Tumors & Surgery; **Hospital:** Penn State Milton S Hershey Med Ctr; **Address:** MSHMC-Otolaryngololgy/ENT, 500 University Ave, MC HU25, Hershey, PA 17033-0850; **Phone:** 717-531-5215; **Med School:** Israel 1995; **Resid:** Otolaryngology, Rambam Med Ctr; **Fellow:** Head & Neck Surgical Oncology, Johns Hopkins Med Ctr; **Fac Appt:** Assoc Prof S, Penn State Univ-Hershey Med Ctr

Grandis, Jennifer R MD [Oto] - **Spec Exp:** Head & Neck Cancer; **Hospital:** UPMC Presby, Pittsburgh, Magee-Womens Hosp - UPMC; **Address:** Univ Pittsburgh Med Ctr EELB, 200 Lothrop St, Ste 500, Pittsburgh, PA 15213; **Phone:** 412-647-5280; **Board Cert:** Otolaryngology 1994; **Med School:** Univ Pittsburgh 1987; **Resid:** Otolaryngology, Univ Pittsburgh Med Ctr 1993; **Fac Appt:** Prof Oto, Univ Pittsburgh

Hammerschlag, Paul E MD [Oto] - **Spec Exp:** Cochlear Implants; Hearing Loss; Meniere's Disease; Balance Disorders; **Hospital:** NYU Langone Med Ctr (page 67), New York Eye & Ear Infirm (page 65); **Address:** 650 First Ave, New York, NY 10016-3240; **Phone:** 212-889-2600; **Board Cert:** Otolaryngology 1978; **Med School:** Albert Einstein Coll Med 1972; **Resid:** Surgery, Virginia Mason Hosp 1974; Otolaryngology, Mass Eye & Ear Infirm 1978; **Fellow:** Otolaryngology, Mass Eye & Ear Infirm 1978; **Fac Appt:** Assoc Clin Prof Oto, NYU Sch Med

Har-El, Gady MD [Oto] - **Spec Exp:** Head & Neck Cancer; Thyroid & Parathyroid Surgery; Skull Base Surgery; **Hospital:** Lenox Hill Hosp (page 62), Lenox Hill Hosp (Manh Eye, Ear & Throat Hosp) (page 62); **Address:** 186 E 76th St Fl 2, New York, NY 10021; **Phone:** 212-434-2323; **Board Cert:** Otolaryngology 1992; **Med School:** Israel 1982; **Resid:** Otolaryngology, SUNY Downstate Med Ctr 1991; **Fac Appt:** Prof Oto, SUNY Hlth Sci Ctr

Hicks Jr, Wesley L MD/DDS [Oto] - **Spec Exp:** Head & Neck Cancer & Surgery; Reconstructive Surgery; **Hospital:** Roswell Park Cancer Inst; **Address:** Roswell Park Cancer Inst, Dept Head & Neck Surgery, Elm & Carlton Sts, Buffalo, NY 14263; **Phone:** 716-845-3158; **Board Cert:** Otolaryngology 1993; **Med School:** SUNY Buffalo 1984; **Resid:** Otolaryngology, Manhattan Eye Ear & Throat Hosp 1988; Otolaryngology, New York Hosp/Meml Sloan Kettering Cancer Ctr 1989; **Fellow:** Head and Neck Surgery, Stanford Univ Med Ctr 1990; **Fac Appt:** Prof Oto, SUNY Buffalo

Hirsch, Barry MD [Oto] - **Spec Exp:** Hearing Loss; Ear Infections; Ear Tumors; Skull Base Tumors; **Hospital:** UPMC Presby, Pittsburgh; **Address:** 200 Lothrop St, Ste 500, Ear Nose Throat Inst, Dept Otolaryngology, Pittsburgh, PA 15213; **Phone:** 412-647-2100; **Board Cert:** Otolaryngology 1982; Neurotology 2005; **Med School:** Univ Pennsylvania 1977; **Resid:** Otolaryngology, Univ Pittsburgh Med Ctr 1982; **Fellow:** Neurotology, Univ Pittsburgh 1985; Neurotology, Univ Zurich 1986; **Fac Appt:** Prof Oto, Univ Pittsburgh

Hoffman, Ronald MD [Oto] - **Spec Exp:** Cochlear Implants; Balance Disorders; Ear Disorders/Surgery; **Hospital:** New York Eye & Ear Infirm (page 65); **Address:** 310 14th St Fl 6th, New York, NY 10003; **Phone:** 212-614-8388; **Board Cert:** Otolaryngology 1976; **Med School:** Jefferson Med Coll 1971; **Resid:** Otolaryngology, NYU Med Ctr 1976; **Fellow:** Otology & Neurotology, Lenox Hill Hosp 1977; **Fac Appt:** Prof Oto, Albert Einstein Coll Med

Holliday, Michael J MD [Oto] - **Spec Exp:** Neuro-Otology; Skull Base Surgery; Otology; **Hospital:** Johns Hopkins Hosp (page 61), Johns Hopkins Bayview Med Ctr (page 61); **Address:** Johns Hopkins Hosp-Otology Division, 601 N Caroline St Fl 6, Baltimore, MD 21287; **Phone:** 410-955-3492; **Board Cert:** Otolaryngology 1976; **Med School:** Marquette Sch Med 1969; **Resid:** Otolaryngology, Johns Hopkins Hosp 1976; **Fellow:** Neurotology, Univ Zurich 1979; **Fac Appt:** Assoc Prof Oto, Johns Hopkins Univ

Hopping, Steven B MD [Oto] - **Spec Exp:** Cosmetic Surgery-Face; Hair Restoration/Transplant; **Hospital:** G Washington Univ Hosp; **Address:** The Center for Cosmetic Surgery, 2440 M St NW, Ste 205, Washington, DC 20037-1449; **Phone:** 202-785-3175; **Board Cert:** Otolaryngology 1980; Facial Plastic & Reconstr Surgery 1986; Hair Restoration Surgery 1990; **Med School:** Univ Cincinnati 1975; **Resid:** Surgery, George Washington Hosp 1977; Otolaryngology, Maa E&E Infirmary 1980; **Fellow:** Plastic Surgery, Mass E&E Infirmary 1981; **Fac Appt:** Clin Prof S, Geo Wash Univ

Hurst, Michael K MD/DDS [Oto] - **Spec Exp:** Nasal Allergy; Sleep Disorders/Apnea; Thyroid Surgery; **Hospital:** WV Univ Hosp - Ruby Memorial, Monongalia Genl Hosp; **Address:** 1188 Pineview Drive, Morgantown, WV 26505; **Phone:** 304-599-3959; **Board Cert:** Otolaryngology 1994; **Med School:** Marshall Univ 1988; **Resid:** Otolaryngology, Univ West Virginia Hosps 1993; Head and Neck Surgery, Univ West Virginia Hosps 1993; **Fac Appt:** Assoc Prof Oto, W VA Univ

Otolaryngology

Jacobs, Joseph B MD [Oto] - **Spec Exp:** Endoscopic Sinus Surgery; Sinus Disorders/Surgery; Sinus Surgery-Revision; **Hospital:** NYU Langone Med Ctr (page 67); **Address:** NYU Med Ctr, 530 1st Ave, Ste 3C, New York, NY 10016-6402; **Phone:** 212-263-7398; **Board Cert:** Otolaryngology 1978; **Med School:** Albert Einstein Coll Med 1974; **Resid:** Otolaryngology, NYU Med Ctr 1978; **Fellow:** Plastic Reconstructive Surgery, UCLA Med Ctr 1979; **Fac Appt:** Prof Oto, NYU Sch Med

Johnson, Jonas T MD [Oto] - **Spec Exp:** Head & Neck Surgery; Head & Neck Cancer; Sleep Disorders/Apnea/Snoring; Parotid Gland Tumors; **Hospital:** UPMC Montefiore, Magee-Womens Hosp - UPMC; **Address:** Univ Physicians UPMC, Eye & Ear Inst, 200 Lothrop St, Ste 300, Pittsburgh, PA 15213; **Phone:** 412-647-2100; **Board Cert:** Otolaryngology 1977; **Med School:** SUNY Upstate Med Univ 1972; **Resid:** Surgery, Med Coll Virginia Hosps 1974; Otolaryngology, SUNY-Univ Hosp 1977; **Fac Appt:** Prof Oto, Univ Pittsburgh

Josephson, Jordan S MD [Oto] - **Spec Exp:** Rhinoplasty Revision; Endoscopic Sinus Surgery; Nasal & Sinus Disorders; Sleep Apnea; **Hospital:** Lenox Hill Hosp (Manh Eye, Ear & Throat Hosp) (page 62), Lenox Hill Hosp (page 62); **Address:** 111 E 77th St, New York, NY 10021-1802; **Phone:** 212-717-1773; **Board Cert:** Otolaryngology 1988; **Med School:** SUNY Downstate 1983; **Resid:** Otolaryngology, LI Jewish Med Ctr 1988; **Fellow:** Sinus Surgery, Johns Hopkins Hosp 1989

Keane, William M MD [Oto] - **Spec Exp:** Head & Neck Cancer & Surgery; Thyroid Cancer; **Hospital:** Thomas Jefferson Univ Hosp; **Address:** Thomas Jefferson Hosp, 925 Chestnut St Fl 6, Philadelphia, PA 19107; **Phone:** 215-955-6760; **Board Cert:** Otolaryngology 1978; **Med School:** Harvard Med Sch 1970; **Resid:** Surgery, Strong Meml Hosp 1972; Otolaryngology, Univ Penn Hosp 1977; **Fac Appt:** Prof Oto, Thomas Jefferson Univ

Kennedy, David W MD [Oto] - **Spec Exp:** Sinus Disorders/Surgery; Skull Base Tumors & Surgery; Endoscopic Sinus Surgery; Minimally Invasive Transnasal Surgery; **Hospital:** Hosp Univ Penn - UPHS (page 60), Pennsylvania Hosp (page 60); **Address:** Hosp Univ Penn, Dept Oto/Head & Neck Surg, 3400 Spruce St Ravdin Bldg Fl 5, Philadelphia, PA 19104-4229; **Phone:** 215-662-6971; **Board Cert:** Otolaryngology 1978; **Med School:** Ireland 1972; **Resid:** Surgery, Johns Hopkins Hosp 1974; Otolaryngology, Johns Hopkins Hosp 1978; **Fac Appt:** Prof Oto, Univ Pennsylvania

Koch, Wayne Martin MD [Oto] - **Spec Exp:** Head & Neck Cancer; Sinus Tumors; **Hospital:** Johns Hopkins Hosp (page 61); **Address:** Johns Hopkins Hosp, Dept Otolaryngology, 601 N Caroline St, rm 6221, Baltimore, MD 21287; **Phone:** 410-955-4906; **Board Cert:** Otolaryngology 1987; **Med School:** Univ Pittsburgh 1982; **Resid:** Otolaryngology, Tufts-Boston Univ Hosps 1987; **Fellow:** Surgical Oncology, Johns Hopkins Hosp 1989; **Fac Appt:** Assoc Prof Oto, Johns Hopkins Univ

Koufman, Jamie A MD [Oto] - **Spec Exp:** Voice Disorders; Laryngeal Disorders; **Hospital:** New York Eye & Ear Infirm (page 65); **Address:** 200 W 57th St, Ste 1203, New York, NY 10019; **Phone:** 212-463-8014; **Board Cert:** Otolaryngology 1978; **Med School:** Boston Univ 1973; **Resid:** Surgery, Hartford Hosp 1975; Otolaryngology, Boston Univ Med Ctr 1978

Kraus, Dennis H MD [Oto] - **Spec Exp:** Head & Neck Cancer; Skull Base Tumors; Thyroid & Parathyroid Surgery; **Hospital:** Meml Sloan-Kettering Cancer Ctr; **Address:** 1275 York Avenue, New York, NY 10065; **Phone:** 800-525-2225; **Board Cert:** Otolaryngology 1990; **Med School:** Univ Rochester 1985; **Resid:** Surgery, Cleveland Clinic 1987; Otolaryngology, Cleveland Clinic 1990; **Fellow:** Head and Neck Surgery, Meml Sloan Kettering Cancer Ctr 1991; **Fac Appt:** Prof Oto, Cornell Univ-Weill Med Coll

Krespi, Yosef P MD [Oto] - **Spec Exp:** Nasal & Sinus Cancer & Surgery; Sleep Disorders/Apnea; Head & Neck Cancer & Surgery; Snoring/Sleep Apnea; **Hospital:** St Luke's - Roosevelt Hosp Ctr - Roosevelt Div (page 57); **Address:** 425 W 59th St Fl 10, New York, NY 10019-1128; **Phone:** 212-262-4444; **Board Cert:** Otolaryngology 1981; **Med School:** Israel 1973; **Resid:** Surgery, Mt Sinai Hosp 1976; Otolaryngology, Mt Sinai Hosp 1980; **Fellow:** Surgery, Northwestern Meml Hosp 1981; **Fac Appt:** Clin Prof Oto, Columbia P&S

Kuhel, William I MD [Oto] - **Spec Exp:** Head & Neck Surgery; Thyroid Surgery; Parathyroid Surgery; **Hospital:** NY-Presby Hosp/Weill Cornell (page 66), Hosp For Special Surgery (page 59); **Address:** 1305 York Ave Fl 5, New York, NY 10021; **Phone:** 646-962-6325; **Board Cert:** Otolaryngology 1988; **Med School:** Univ Mich Med Sch 1983; **Resid:** Surgery, St Vincent's Hosp 1985; Otolaryngology, Indiana Univ 1988; **Fellow:** Head and Neck Surgery, MD Anderson Hosp 1989; **Fac Appt:** Assoc Clin Prof Oto, Cornell Univ-Weill Med Coll

Lalwani, Anil K MD [Oto] - **Spec Exp:** Ear Disorders/Surgery; Facial Nerve Disorders; Pediatric Otolaryngology; Skull Base Surgery; **Hospital:** NYU Langone Med Ctr (page 67); **Address:** 540 1st Ave, Ste 8S, New York, NY 10016; **Phone:** 212-263-7167; **Board Cert:** Otolaryngology 1992; **Med School:** Univ Mich Med Sch 1985; **Resid:** Surgery, Duke Univ Med Ctr 1987; Otolaryngology, UCSF Med Ctr 1991; **Fellow:** Skull Base Surgery, UCSF Med Ctr 1992; **Fac Appt:** Prof Oto, NYU Sch Med

Lawson, William MD [Oto] - **Spec Exp:** Sinus Disorders/Surgery; Cosmetic Surgery-Face; Head & Neck Cancer; Skull Base Surgery; **Hospital:** Mount Sinai Med Ctr (page 64); **Address:** 5 E 98th St Fl 8, Box 1191, New York, NY 10029-6501; **Phone:** 212-241-9410; **Board Cert:** Otolaryngology 1974; **Med School:** NYU Sch Med 1965; **Resid:** Surgery, Bronx VA Hosp 1967; Otolaryngology, Mt Sinai Hosp 1973; **Fellow:** Otolaryngology, Mt Sinai Hosp 1970; **Fac Appt:** Prof Oto, Mount Sinai Sch Med

Linstrom, Christopher MD [Oto] - **Spec Exp:** Cochlear Implants; Acoustic Neuroma; Encephalocele; Cholesteatoma; **Hospital:** New York Eye & Ear Infirm (page 65), St Vincent Cath Med Ctrs - Manhattan; **Address:** NY Eye & Ear Infirmary, Dept Otolaryngology, 310 E 14th St Fl 6, New York, NY 10003-4201; **Phone:** 212-979-4200; **Board Cert:** Otolaryngology 1987; **Med School:** McGill Univ 1982; **Resid:** Surgery, Geo Wash Med Ctr 1984; Otolaryngology, NY Hosp 1987; **Fellow:** Otology & Neurotology, Michigan Ear Inst 1989; **Fac Appt:** Assoc Prof Oto, NY Med Coll

Minor, Lloyd B MD [Oto] - **Spec Exp:** Balance Disorders; Neuro-Otology; Meniere's Disease; **Hospital:** Johns Hopkins Hosp (page 61); **Address:** 601 N Caroline St, rm 6210, Baltimore, MD 21287; **Phone:** 410-955-3403; **Board Cert:** Otolaryngology 1993; Neurotology 2004; **Med School:** Brown Univ 1982; **Resid:** Otolaryngology, Univ Chicago Hosps 1992; **Fellow:** Otolaryngology, Ear Foundation/Baptist Hosp 1993; **Fac Appt:** Prof Oto, Johns Hopkins Univ

Moscatello, Augustine L MD [Oto] - **Spec Exp:** Nasal & Sinus Disorders; Head & Neck Surgery; **Hospital:** Westchester Med Ctr; **Address:** 1055 Sawmill River Rd, Ste 101, Ardsley, NY 10502; **Phone:** 914-693-7636; **Board Cert:** Otolaryngology 1987; **Med School:** Mount Sinai Sch Med 1982; **Resid:** Surgery, Mt Sinai Hosp 1987; Otolaryngology, Mt Sinai Hosp 1987; **Fac Appt:** Assoc Prof Oto, NY Med Coll

Niparko, John MD [Oto] - **Spec Exp:** Ear Disorders/Surgery; Neuro-Otology; **Hospital:** Johns Hopkins Hosp (page 61); **Address:** Johns Hopkins Hosp, Dept Otolaryngology, 601 N Caroline St, rm 6223, Baltimore, MD 21287-0910; **Phone:** 410-955-2689; **Board Cert:** Otolaryngology 1986; Neurotology 2004; **Med School:** Univ Mich Med Sch 1980; **Resid:** Surgery, William Beaumont Hosp 1982; Otolaryngology, Univ Michigan Hosp 1986; **Fellow:** Otolaryngology, Univ Michigan Hosp; **Fac Appt:** Prof Oto, Johns Hopkins Univ

Otolaryngology

O'Malley Jr, Bert W MD [Oto] - **Spec Exp:** Head & Neck Cancer; Sinus Tumors; Skull Base Tumors; **Hospital:** Hosp Univ Penn - UPHS (page 60); **Address:** Hosp Univ Penn, Dept Otolaryngology, 3400 Spruce St, 5 Ravdin, Philadelphia, PA 19104; **Phone:** 215-615-4325; **Board Cert:** Otolaryngology 1995; **Med School:** Univ Tex SW, Dallas 1988; **Resid:** Surgery, UTSW Med Ctr/Parkland Meml Hosp 1989; Otolaryngology, Baylor Coll Med 1993; **Fellow:** Head & Neck Oncology, Univ Pittsburgh 1994; Skull Base Surgery, Univ Pittsburgh 1995; **Fac Appt:** Prof Oto, Univ Pennsylvania

Papel, Ira D MD [Oto] - **Spec Exp:** Rhinoplasty; Cosmetic Surgery-Face; Reconstructive Surgery-Face; Skin Cancer/Facial Reconstruction; **Hospital:** Greater Baltimore Med Ctr, Johns Hopkins Hosp (page 61); **Address:** 1838 Greene Tree Rd, Ste 370, Baltimore, MD 21208; **Phone:** 410-486-3400; **Board Cert:** Otolaryngology 1986; Facial Plastic & Reconstr Surgery 1991; **Med School:** Boston Univ 1981; **Resid:** Otolaryngology, Johns Hopkins Hosp 1986; **Fellow:** Facial Plastic Surgery, UCSF Med Ctr 1987; **Fac Appt:** Assoc Prof Oto, Johns Hopkins Univ

Parisier, Simon C MD [Oto] - **Spec Exp:** Cochlear Implants; Hearing Loss; Ear Disorders/Surgery; Cholesteatoma; **Hospital:** New York Eye & Ear Infirm (page 65); **Address:** NY Eye & Ear Infirmary - Otolaryngology, 310 E 14th St, 6th Fl - Window 5, New York, NY 10003-4297; **Phone:** 212-979-4542; **Board Cert:** Otolaryngology 1967; **Med School:** Boston Univ 1961; **Resid:** Otolaryngology, Mount Sinai Hosp 1966; **Fac Appt:** Prof Oto, NY Med Coll

Persky, Mark S MD [Oto] - **Spec Exp:** Head & Neck Cancer; Skull Base Tumors; Thyroid Cancer; **Hospital:** Beth Israel Med Ctr - Petrie Division (page 57); **Address:** 10 Union Square East, Ste 4J, New York, NY 10003; **Phone:** 212-844-8648; **Board Cert:** Otolaryngology 1976; **Med School:** SUNY Upstate Med Univ 1972; **Resid:** Otolaryngology, Bellevue Hosp 1976; **Fellow:** Head and Neck Surgery, Beth Israel Med Ctr 1977; **Fac Appt:** Clin Prof Oto, Albert Einstein Coll Med

Picken, Catherine A MD [Oto] - **Spec Exp:** Head & Neck Reconstruction; Thyroid Disorders; Sinus Disorders/Surgery; **Hospital:** Georgetown Univ Hosp; **Address:** 2440 M St NW, Ste 620, Washington, DC 20006; **Phone:** 202-785-5000; **Board Cert:** Otolaryngology 1989; **Med School:** Northwestern Univ 1979; **Resid:** Surgery, Natl Heart Lung Blood Inst 1983; Otolaryngology, Georgetown Univ Hosp 1989; **Fac Appt:** Assoc Prof Oto, Georgetown Univ

Quatela, Vito C MD [Oto] - **Spec Exp:** Facial Plastic Surgery; Rhinoplasty; **Hospital:** Univ of Rochester Strong Meml Hosp, Rochester Genl Hosp; **Address:** 973 East Ave, Ste 101, Rochester, NY 14607; **Phone:** 585-244-1000; **Board Cert:** Otolaryngology 1985; Facial Plastic & Reconstr Surgery 1991; **Med School:** Northwestern Univ 1979; **Resid:** Surgery, Med Ctr Hosp Vermont 1984; Otolaryngology, Northwestern Univ Hosp 1985; **Fellow:** Facial Plastic Surgery, Tulane Univ 1986; Facial Plastic Surgery, Oregon Hlth Science Univ 1987; **Fac Appt:** Assoc Clin Prof Oto, Univ Rochester

Rassekh, Christopher MD [Oto] - **Spec Exp:** Laryngeal Cancer-Organ Preservation; Skull Base Tumors; Salivary Gland Tumors & Surgery; **Hospital:** WV Univ Hosp - Ruby Memorial, Monongalia Genl Hosp; **Address:** West Virginia Univ, Dept Otolaryngology, Robin C Byrd Hlth Scis Ctr, Head & Neck Surgery, PO Box 9200, Morgantown, WV 26506-9200; **Phone:** 304-293-3233; **Board Cert:** Otolaryngology 1993; **Med School:** Univ Iowa Coll Med 1986; **Resid:** Otolaryngology, Univ Iowa Med Ctr 1992; **Fellow:** Head and Neck Surgery, Univ Pittsburgh Med Ctr 1993; **Fac Appt:** Assoc Prof Oto, W VA Univ

Roland Jr, J Thomas MD [Oto] - **Spec Exp:** Acoustic Neuroma; Cochlear Implants; Neuro-Otology; Facial Nerve Disorders; **Hospital:** NYU Langone Med Ctr (page 67), Bellevue Hosp Ctr; **Address:** 550 First Avenue, Ste 8S, New York, NY 10016; **Phone:** 212-263-5565; **Board Cert:** Otolaryngology 1993; Neurotology 2004; **Med School:** Temple Univ 1983; **Resid:** Otolaryngology, NYU Med Ctr 1992; **Fellow:** Neurotology, NYU Med Ctr 1993; **Fac Appt:** Assoc Prof Oto, NYU Sch Med

Rosen, Clark A MD [Oto] - **Spec Exp:** Voice Disorders; **Hospital:** UPMC Mercy, Pittsburgh; **Address:** UPMC The Voice Ctr, 1400 Locust St, D Bldg Fl 2 - Ste 2100, Pittsburgh, PA 15219; **Phone:** 412-647-2100; **Board Cert:** Otolaryngology 1995; **Med School:** Rush Med Coll 1989; **Resid:** Otolaryngology, Oregon Hlth Sci Univ 1994; **Fellow:** Otolaryngology, Univ Tenn Med Ctr 1995; **Fac Appt:** Assoc Prof Oto, Univ Pittsburgh

Sataloff, Robert T MD [Oto] - **Spec Exp:** Neuro-Otology; Voice Disorders; Laryngeal Disorders; Throat Disorders; **Hospital:** Hahnemann Univ Hosp, St Christopher's Hosp for Chldn; **Address:** 1721 Pine Street, Philadelphia, PA 19103-6701; **Phone:** 215-545-3322; **Board Cert:** Otolaryngology 1980; **Med School:** Jefferson Med Coll 1975; **Resid:** Otolaryngology, Univ Mich Hosp 1980; **Fellow:** Neurotology, Univ Mich Hosp 1981; **Fac Appt:** Prof Oto, Drexel Univ Coll Med

Schaefer, Steven D MD [Oto] - **Spec Exp:** Sinus Disorders/Surgery; Head & Neck Surgery; Endoscopic Sinus Surgery; **Hospital:** New York Eye & Ear Infirm (page 65), Beth Israel Med Ctr - Petrie Division (page 57); **Address:** NY Eye & Ear Infirm, Dept Otolaryngology, 310 E 14th St, New York, NY 10003-4201; **Phone:** 212-979-4200; **Board Cert:** Otolaryngology 1978; **Med School:** UC Irvine 1972; **Resid:** Surgery, UCLA Med Ctr 1974; Otolaryngology, Stanford Med Ctr 1977; **Fac Appt:** Prof Oto, NY Med Coll

Schantz, Stimson P MD [Oto] - **Spec Exp:** Head & Neck Surgery; Head & Neck Cancer; Thyroid Cancer; **Hospital:** New York Eye & Ear Infirm (page 65), Beth Israel Med Ctr - Petrie Division (page 57); **Address:** 310 E 14th St Fl 6N, New YorkNew York, NY 10003; **Phone:** 212-979-4535; **Board Cert:** Surgery 2005; **Med School:** Univ Cincinnati 1975; **Resid:** Surgery, Georgetown Univ Med CtrGeorgetown Univ Med Ctr 1982; Otolaryngology, Univ Illinois Eye & Ear Infirm 1980; **Fellow:** Surgical Oncology, MD Anderson Cancer Ctr 1984; **Fac Appt:** Prof Oto, NY Med Coll

Schley, W Shain MD [Oto] - **Spec Exp:** Nasal & Sinus Disorders; Throat Disorders; Voice Disorders; Sleep Disorders; **Hospital:** NY-Presby Hosp/Weill Cornell (page 66); **Address:** 449 E 68th St Fl 2 - Ste DS 10, New York, NY 10065; **Phone:** 212-746-2223; **Board Cert:** Otolaryngology 1973; **Med School:** Emory Univ 1966; **Resid:** Surgery, Roosevelt Hosp 1968; Otolaryngology, New York Hosp 1973; **Fac Appt:** Assoc Clin Prof Oto, Cornell Univ-Weill Med Coll

Setzen, Michael MD [Oto] - **Spec Exp:** Nasal & Sinus Surgery; Rhinoplasty; Sleep Disorders/Apnea; Snoring/Sleep Apnea; **Hospital:** N Shore Univ Hosp, St Francis Hosp - The Heart Ctr (page 69); **Address:** 600 Northern Blvd, Ste 312, Great Neck, NY 11021-5200; **Phone:** 516-829-0045; **Board Cert:** Otolaryngology 1982; **Med School:** South Africa 1974; **Resid:** Surgery, Cleveland Clinic Fdn 1978; Otolaryngology, Barnes Jewish Hosp 1982; **Fac Appt:** Assoc Clin Prof Oto, NYU Sch Med

Shapshay, Stanley M MD [Oto] - **Spec Exp:** Laryngeal Cancer; Vocal Cord Disorders; Sleep Apnea; **Hospital:** Albany Med Ctr; **Address:** University Ear, Nose & Throat Ctr, 35 Hackett Blvd, Albany, NY 12208-3420; **Phone:** 518-262-5575; **Board Cert:** Otolaryngology 1975; **Med School:** Med Coll VA 1968; **Resid:** Surgery, New England Med Ctr 1971; Otolaryngology, Boston Med Ctr 1975; **Fellow:** Surgery, Serafimer Hosp/Karolinska Med Sch 1972; **Fac Appt:** Prof Oto, Albany Med Coll

Snyderman, Carl H MD [Oto] - **Spec Exp:** Skull Base Tumors & Surgery; Sinus Tumors; Head & Neck Cancer; Endoscopic Surgery; **Hospital:** UPMC Presby, Pittsburgh; **Address:** Eye Ear Inst, Dept of Otolaryngology, 200 Lothrop St, Ste 500, Pittsburgh, PA 15213; **Phone:** 412-647-2100; **Board Cert:** Otolaryngology 1987; **Med School:** Univ Chicago-Pritzker Sch Med 1982; **Resid:** Otolaryngology, Eye-Ear Hosp/Univ Pittsburgh 1987; **Fellow:** Skull Base Surgery, Eye-Ear Hosp/Univ Pittsburgh 1988; **Fac Appt:** Prof Oto, Univ Pittsburgh

Otolaryngology

Stewart, Michael G MD [Oto] - **Spec Exp:** Nasal & Sinus Disorders; Sleep Disorders/Apnea; Head & Neck Surgery; **Hospital:** NY-Presby Hosp/Weill Cornell (page 66); **Address:** Weill Cornell Physicians, 1305 York Ave Fl 5th, New York, NY 10011; **Phone:** 646-962-6673; **Board Cert:** Otolaryngology 1995; **Med School:** Johns Hopkins Univ 1988; **Resid:** Otolaryngology, Baylor Coll Med 1994; **Fac Appt:** Prof Oto, Cornell Univ-Weill Med Coll

Strome, Marshall MD [Oto] - **Spec Exp:** Sleep Disorders/Apnea; Voice Disorders; Head & Neck Cancer; Swallowing Disorders; **Hospital:** St Luke's - Roosevelt Hosp Ctr - St Luke's Hosp (page 57); **Address:** 110 E 59th St, Ste 10A, New York, NY 10022; **Phone:** 212-223-1333; **Board Cert:** Otolaryngology 1970; **Med School:** Univ Mich Med Sch 1964; **Resid:** Surgery, Harper Hosp 1966; Otolaryngology, Univ Michigan Hosp 1970; **Fac Appt:** Prof Oto

Strome, Scott MD [Oto] - **Spec Exp:** Microsurgery; Head & Neck Cancer; Head & Neck Reconstruction; **Hospital:** Univ of MD Med Ctr; **Address:** 16 S Eutaw St, Ste 500, Baltimore, MD 21201; **Phone:** 410-328-6467; **Board Cert:** Otolaryngology 1998; **Med School:** Harvard Med Sch 1991; **Resid:** Otolaryngology, Univ Michigan 1997; **Fellow:** Head and Neck Surgery, Allegheny Genl Hosp 1998; Microvascular Surgery, Allegheny Genl Hosp 1998; **Fac Appt:** Prof Oto, Univ MD Sch Med

Sulica, Radu Lucian MD [Oto] - **Spec Exp:** Laryngeal & Vocal Cord Surgery; Voice Disorders; Vocal Cord Disorders; Botox Therapy; **Hospital:** NY-Presby Hosp/Weill Cornell (page 66); **Address:** Weill Cornell Otorhinolaryngology, 1305 York Ave Fl 5, New York, NY 10021; **Phone:** 646-962-4734; **Board Cert:** Otolaryngology 2000; **Med School:** Georgetown Univ 1993; **Resid:** Surgery, Georgetown Univ Hosp 1995; Otolaryngology, Georgetown Univ Hosp 1999; **Fellow:** Laryngology, St Lukes Roosevelt 2000; **Fac Appt:** Assoc Prof Oto, Cornell Univ-Weill Med Coll

Urken, Mark MD [Oto] - **Spec Exp:** Head & Neck Cancer & Surgery; Head & Neck Cancer Reconstruction; Thyroid & Parathyroid Cancer & Surgery; Salivary Gland Tumors; **Hospital:** Beth Israel Med Ctr - Petrie Division (page 57); **Address:** Inst for Head, Neck & Thyroid Cancer, 10 Union Square E, Ste 5B, New York, NY 10003-3314; **Phone:** 212-844-8775; **Board Cert:** Otolaryngology 1986; **Med School:** Univ VA Sch Med 1981; **Resid:** Otolaryngology, Mt Sinai Hosp 1986; **Fellow:** Microvascular Surgery, Mercy Hosp 1987; **Fac Appt:** Prof Oto, Albert Einstein Coll Med

Waner, Milton MD [Oto] - **Spec Exp:** Pediatric Facial Plastic Surgery; Hemangiomas/Birthmarks; Vascular Malformations; **Hospital:** St Luke's - Roosevelt Hosp Ctr - St Luke's Hosp (page 57), Beth Israel Med Ctr - Petrie Division (page 57); **Address:** Vascular Birthmark Institute, 126 W 60th St, New York, NY 10023; **Phone:** 212-636-3970; **Med School:** South Africa 1977; **Resid:** Surgery, Univ of Witwatersrand 1980; Otolaryngology, Univ of Witwatersrand 1984; **Fellow:** Otolaryngology, Univ Cincinnatti Med Ctr 1985

Weinstein, Gregory MD [Oto] - **Spec Exp:** Head & Neck Cancer; Laryngeal Cancer; **Hospital:** Hosp Univ Penn - UPHS (page 60); **Address:** Hosp Univ Penn, Dept Otolaryngology, 3400 Spruce St, 5 Ravdin, Philadelphia, PA 19104; **Phone:** 215-349-5390; **Board Cert:** Otolaryngology 1990; **Med School:** NY Med Coll 1985; **Resid:** Otolaryngology, Univ Iowa Hosp 1990; **Fellow:** Head & Neck Oncology, UC Davis Med Ctr 1991; **Fac Appt:** Assoc Prof Oto, Univ Pennsylvania

Woo, Peak MD [Oto] - **Spec Exp:** Voice Disorders; Laryngeal Disorders; Laryngeal Cancer; **Hospital:** Mount Sinai Med Ctr (page 64); **Address:** 300 Central Park West, Ste 1-H, New York, NY 10024; **Phone:** 212-580-1004; **Board Cert:** Otolaryngology 1983; **Med School:** Boston Univ 1978; **Resid:** Otolaryngology, Boston Univ Med Ctr 1983; **Fac Appt:** Clin Prof Oto, Mount Sinai Sch Med

Zalzal, George MD [Oto] - **Spec Exp:** Airway Disorders; Laryngeal & Tracheal Disorders; Ear Disorders/Surgery; **Hospital:** Chldns Natl Med Ctr; **Address:** Childrens Natl Med Ctr, Dept Oto-laryngology, 111 Michigan Ave NW Fl 1 - rm 1000, Washington, DC 20010; **Phone:** 202-476-2159; **Board Cert:** Otolaryngology 1996; **Med School:** Lebanon 1979; **Resid:** Otolaryngology, American Univ Hosp 1983; **Fellow:** Pediatric Otolaryngology, Univ Cincinnati 1985; **Fac Appt:** Prof Ped, Geo Wash Univ

Southeast

Balkany, Thomas J MD [Oto] - **Spec Exp:** Ear Disorders/Surgery; Neuro-Otology; Cochlear Implants; Hearing Loss; **Hospital:** Jackson Meml Hosp (page 70); **Address:** Univ Miami Dept Oto-laryngology, PO Box 016960, Miami, FL 33101; **Phone:** 305-243-2000; **Board Cert:** Otolaryngology 1977; Neurotology 2004; **Med School:** Univ Miami Sch Med 1972; **Resid:** Surgery, St Joseph Hosp 1974; Otolaryngology, Colorado Med Ctr 1977; **Fellow:** Otology & Neurotology, House Ear Inst 1978; **Fac Appt:** Clin Prof Oto, Univ Miami Sch Med

Becker, Ferdinand F MD [Oto] - **Spec Exp:** Cosmetic Surgery-Face; **Hospital:** Indian River Med Ctr; **Address:** 5070 N A1A, Ste A, Vero Beach, FL 32963-1229; **Phone:** 772-234-3700; **Board Cert:** Otolaryngology 1972; **Med School:** Tulane Univ 1965; **Resid:** Surgery, Charity Hosp 1969; Otolaryngology, Charity Hosp 1972; **Fac Appt:** Asst Clin Prof Oto, Univ Fla Coll Med

Bolger, William E MD [Oto] - **Spec Exp:** Nasal & Sinus Surgery; Encephalocele; **Hospital:** Mayo - Jacksonville; **Address:** Mayo Clinic, Otolaryngology Dept, 4500 San Pablo Rd, Davis E-3B, Jacksonville, FL 32224; **Phone:** 904-953-2217; **Board Cert:** Otolaryngology 1992; **Med School:** Uniformed Srvs Univ, Bethesda 1986; **Resid:** Otolaryngology, Willford Hall USAF Med Ctr 1991; **Fellow:** Rhinoplasty & Sinus Surgery, Hosp Univ Penn 1992

Browne, J Dale MD [Oto] - **Spec Exp:** Head & Neck Cancer; Thyroid Cancer; Skull Base Sur-gery; Head & Neck Reconstruction; **Hospital:** Wake Forest Univ Baptist Med Ctr (page 72); **Ad-dress:** Wake Forest Baptist Med Ctr, Dept Otolaryngology, Medical Center Blvd, Winston Salem, NC 27103; **Phone:** 336-716-4161; **Board Cert:** Otolaryngology 1987; **Med School:** Med Coll GA 1982; **Resid:** Otolaryngology, NC Baptist Hosp 1987; **Fellow:** Otolaryngology, Univ Hosp 1991; **Fac Appt:** Prof Oto, Wake Forest Univ

Bumpous, Jeffrey MD [Oto] - **Spec Exp:** Head & Neck Cancer; Head & Neck Reconstruction; Thyroid & Parathyroid Cancer & Surgery; **Hospital:** Univ of Louisville Hosp, Norton Hosp; **Address:** 401 E Chestnut St, Ste 710, Louisville, KY 40202-1845; **Phone:** 502-583-8303; **Board Cert:** Oto-laryngology 1994; **Med School:** Univ Louisville Sch Med 1988; **Resid:** Otolaryngology, Univ Louisville Hosp 1993; **Fellow:** Head and Neck Surgery, Univ Pittsburgh 1994; **Fac Appt:** Prof Oto, Univ Louisville Sch Med

Cassisi, Nicholas J MD [Oto] - **Spec Exp:** Head & Neck Cancer; Voice Disorders; **Hospital:** Shands at Univ of FL; **Address:** Shands Healthcare at Univ FL, 1600 SW Archer Rd, Box 100383, Gainesville, FL 32610; **Phone:** 352-265-8989; **Board Cert:** Otolaryngology 1971; **Med School:** Univ Miami Sch Med 1965; **Resid:** Surgery, Jackson Meml Hosp 1967; Otolaryngology, Barnes Hosp-Washington Univ 1971; **Fac Appt:** Prof Oto, Univ Fla Coll Med

Civantos, Francisco J MD [Oto] - **Spec Exp:** Head & Neck Cancer; **Hospital:** Univ of Miami Hosp & Clins/Sylvester Comp Canc Ctr (page 70); **Address:** Sylvester CAncer Ctr, Otolaryn-gology, 1475 NW 12th Ave, Ste 4027, Miami, FL 33136; **Phone:** 205-243-5276; **Board Cert:** Otolaryngology 1992; **Med School:** Columbia P&S 1986; **Resid:** Otolaryngology, Univ Illinois Coll Med 1991; **Fellow:** Head & Neck Oncology, Vanderbilt Univ 1992; **Fac Appt:** Assoc Prof Oto, Univ Miami Sch Med

Otolaryngology

Couch, Marion E MD [Oto] - **Spec Exp:** Head & Neck Cancer; Thyroid Cancer; **Hospital:** Univ NC Hosps; **Address:** Univ N Carolina Sch Med, Dept Otolaryngology, CB 7070, Chapel Hill, NC 27599-7070; **Phone:** 919-966-3342; **Board Cert:** Otolaryngology 1997; **Med School:** Rush Med Coll 1990; **Resid:** Surgery, Johns Hopkins Hosp 1991; Otolaryngology, Johns Hopkins Hosp 1995; **Fac Appt:** Assoc Prof Oto, Univ NC Sch Med

Day, Terrence A MD [Oto] - **Spec Exp:** Head & Neck Cancer; Reconstructive Microvascular Surgery; Skull Base Surgery; Facial Plastic & Reconstructive Surgery; **Hospital:** MUSC Med Ctr; **Address:** MUSC, Dept Otolaryngology, 135 Rutledge Ave, Ste 1130, Box MSC550, Charleston, SC 29425; **Phone:** 843-792-0719; **Board Cert:** Otolaryngology 1996; **Med School:** Univ Okla Coll Med 1989; **Resid:** Otolaryngology, LSU Med Ctr 1995; **Fellow:** Head & Neck Surgical Oncology, UC Davis Med Ctr 1996; Maxillofacial Surgery, Univ Hosp 1994; **Fac Appt:** Assoc Prof Oto, Med Univ SC

Farrior, Edward MD [Oto] - **Spec Exp:** Rhinoplasty; Ear Reshaping (Otoplasty); Facial Plastic Surgery; **Hospital:** Tampa Genl Hosp; **Address:** 2908 W Azeele St, Tampa, FL 33609-3109; **Phone:** 813-875-3223; **Board Cert:** Otolaryngology 1987; Facial Plastic & Reconstr Surgery 1992; **Med School:** Univ VA Sch Med 1982; **Resid:** Otolaryngology, Univ Mich Hosps 1987; **Fellow:** Facial Plastic & Reconstr Surgery, Tampa Genl Hosp 1988; **Fac Appt:** Assoc Clin Prof S, Univ S Fla Coll Med

Farrior, Joseph Brown MD [Oto] - **Spec Exp:** Otosclerosis/Stapedectomy; Hearing Loss; Meniere's Disease; Otology; **Hospital:** St Joseph's Hosp - Tampa, Tampa Genl Hosp; **Address:** Farrior Ear Clinic, 2727 Martin Luther King Jr Blvd, Ste 520, Tampa, FL 33607; **Phone:** 800-342-3277; **Board Cert:** Otolaryngology 1981; **Med School:** Emory Univ 1975; **Resid:** Surgery, Johns Hopkins Hosp 1977; Otolaryngology, Johns Hopkins Hosp 1981; **Fellow:** Otolaryngology, Farrior Clin/St Josephs Hosp 1980; **Fac Appt:** Assoc Clin Prof Oto, Univ S Fla Coll Med

Goodwin, W Jarrard MD [Oto] - **Spec Exp:** Head & Neck Cancer; **Hospital:** Univ of Miami Hosp & Clins/Sylvester Comp Canc Ctr (page 70), Jackson Meml Hosp (page 70); **Address:** Dept Otolaryngology, 1475 NW 12th Ave, Ste 4037, Miami, FL 33136-1015; **Phone:** 305-243-4387; **Board Cert:** Otolaryngology 1978; **Med School:** Albany Med Coll 1972; **Resid:** Surgery, Univ Miami/Jackson Hosp Meml Hosp 1974; Otolaryngology, Univ Miami/Jackson Hosp 1977; **Fellow:** Head & Neck Surgical Oncology, MD Anderson Hosp 1980; **Fac Appt:** Prof Oto, Univ Miami Sch Med

Kesser, Bradley W MD [Oto] - **Spec Exp:** Aural Atresia Repair; Neurotology; **Hospital:** Univ Virginia Med Ctr; **Address:** Univ VA Dept Otolaryngology, PO Box 800713, Charlottesville, VA 22908; **Phone:** 434-924-2040; **Board Cert:** Otolaryngology 1999; **Med School:** Univ VA Sch Med 1993; **Resid:** Otolaryngology, Univ Va Med Ctr 1998; **Fellow:** Otology & Neurotology, House Ear Clinic 2000; **Fac Appt:** Asst Prof Oto, Univ VA Sch Med

Kuhn, Frederick MD [Oto] - **Spec Exp:** Endoscopic Sinus Surgery; Allergic Fungal Sinusitis; Rhinoplasty Revision; **Hospital:** Meml Hlth Univ Med Ctr - Savannah, St Joseph's-Candler Hosp; **Address:** Georgia Nasal & Sinus Inst, 4750 Waters Ave, Ste 112, Savannah, GA 31404; **Phone:** 912-355-1070; **Board Cert:** Otolaryngology 1972; **Med School:** Univ Okla Coll Med 1966; **Resid:** Surgery, Univ Oklahoma Hosp 1967; Surgery, St Lukes Hosp 1968; **Fellow:** Otolaryngology, Barnes Hosp/Wash Univ 1972

Lambert, Paul R MD [Oto] - **Spec Exp:** Neuro-Otology; Acoustic Neuroma; Meniere's Disease; Cholesteatoma; **Hospital:** MUSC Med Ctr; **Address:** MUSC, Dept Otolaryngology, 135 Rutledge Ave, Box 250550, Charleston, SC 29425; **Phone:** 843-792-3531; **Board Cert:** Otolaryngology 1981; Neurotology 2004; **Med School:** Duke Univ 1976; **Resid:** Surgery, UCLA Med Ctr 1978; Otolaryngology, UCLA Med Ctr 1981; **Fellow:** Neurotology, Otologic Med Group 1982; **Fac Appt:** Prof Oto, Med Univ SC

America's Top Doctors® 9th Edition

Lanza, Donald C MD [Oto] - **Spec Exp:** Skull Base Tumors; Sinus Disorders/Surgery; Rhinitis; Graves' Disease-Eye; **Hospital:** St Anthony's Hosp - St Petersburg, All Children's Hosp; **Address:** 900 Carillon Pkwy, Ste 200, St. Petersburg, FL 33716-1108; **Phone:** 727-573-0074; **Board Cert:** Otolaryngology 1990; **Med School:** SUNY Hlth Sci Ctr 1985; **Resid:** Surgery, Albany Med Ctr 1987; Otolaryngology, Albany Med Ctr 1990; **Fellow:** Rhinology, Johns Hopkins Univ 1990; Rhinology, Univ Penn 1991

Levine, Paul A MD [Oto] - **Spec Exp:** Head & Neck Cancer; Head & Neck Reconstruction; Skull Base Tumors; **Hospital:** Univ Virginia Med Ctr; **Address:** Dept Otolaryngology, PO Box 800713, Charlottesville, VA 22908; **Phone:** 434-924-5593; **Board Cert:** Otolaryngology 1978; **Med School:** Albany Med Coll 1973; **Resid:** Otolaryngology, Yale-New Haven Hosp 1977; **Fellow:** Head and Neck Surgery, Stanford Med Ctr 1978; **Fac Appt:** Prof Oto, Univ VA Sch Med

Mangat, Devinder S MD [Oto] - **Spec Exp:** Cosmetic & Reconstructive Surgery-Face; **Hospital:** St Elizabeth Med Ctr (South Unit); **Address:** 133 Barnwood Drive, Edgewood, KY 41017; **Phone:** 513-984-3223; **Board Cert:** Otolaryngology 1978; Facial Plastic & Reconstr Surgery 1991; **Med School:** Univ KY Coll Med 1973; **Resid:** Surgery, Univ KY Med Ctr 1975; Otolaryngology, Univ Okla Hlth Scis Ctr 1978; **Fellow:** Facial Plastic Surgery, McCullough Clinic 1979; **Fac Appt:** Assoc Prof Oto, Univ Cincinnati

Mattox, Douglas E MD [Oto] - **Spec Exp:** Neuro-Otology; Meniere's Disease; Hearing Loss; **Hospital:** Emory Univ Hosp, Chldns Hlthcare Atlanta - Scottish Rite; **Address:** Emory Univ Hospital, Dept Otolaryngology, 1365 Clifton Rd NE A Bldg - Ste 2100, Atlanta, GA 30322; **Phone:** 404-778-3381; **Board Cert:** Otolaryngology 1977; Neurotology 2004; **Med School:** Yale Univ 1973; **Resid:** Otolaryngology, Stanford Univ Hosp 1977; **Fellow:** Neurotology, Ugo Fisch, MD 1985; **Fac Appt:** Prof Oto, Emory Univ

McCaffrey, Thomas V MD [Oto] - **Spec Exp:** Head & Neck Cancer; Thyroid Cancer; Tracheal Surgery; **Hospital:** H Lee Moffitt Cancer Ctr & Research Inst, Tampa Genl Hosp; **Address:** H Lee Moffitt Cancer Ctr, Dept Otolaryngology-HNS, 12902 Magnolia Drive, Tampa, FL 33612; **Phone:** 813-745-8463; **Board Cert:** Otolaryngology 1980; **Med School:** Loyola Univ-Stritch Sch Med 1974; **Resid:** Surgery, Mayo Affil Hosps 1976; Otolaryngology, Mayo Affil Hosps 1980; **Fac Appt:** Prof Oto, Univ S Fla Coll Med

Netterville, James L MD [Oto] - **Spec Exp:** Head & Neck Surgery; Head & Neck Cancer; Vocal Cord Disorders; Skull Base Tumors; **Hospital:** Vanderbilt Univ Med Ctr, Vanderbilt Children's Hosp; **Address:** Vanderbilt Univ Med Ctr, Dept Oto, 7209 Med Ctr East, South Twr, 1215 21st Ave S, Nashville, TN 37232-8605; **Phone:** 615-343-8840; **Board Cert:** Otolaryngology 1985; **Med School:** Univ Tenn Coll Med, Memphis 1980; **Resid:** Surgery, Methodist Hosp 1982; Otolaryngology, Univ Tenn Med Ctr 1985; **Fellow:** Surgical Oncology, Univ Iowa 1986; **Fac Appt:** Prof Oto, Vanderbilt Univ

Osguthorpe, John D MD [Oto] - **Spec Exp:** Head & Neck Cancer; Thyroid & Parathyroid Cancer & Surgery; Nasal & Sinus Disorders; Salivary Gland Tumors & Surgery; **Hospital:** MUSC Med Ctr, E Cooper Reg Med Ctr; **Address:** MUSC Med Ctr-Dept Otolaryngology, 135 Rutledge Ave, MS S50, Charleston, SC 29425; **Phone:** 843-792-3533; **Board Cert:** Otolaryngology 1978; **Med School:** Univ Utah 1973; **Resid:** Surgery, UCLA Med Ctr 1975; Otolaryngology, UCLA Med Ctr 1978; **Fellow:** Skull Base Surgery, Univ Zurich 1989; **Fac Appt:** Prof Oto, Med Univ SC

Peters, Glenn E MD [Oto] - **Spec Exp:** Thyroid & Parathyroid Cancer & Surgery; **Hospital:** Univ of Ala Hosp at Birmingham; **Address:** UAB Med Ctr, Div of Head & Neck Surgery, 1530 3rd Ave S, Ste BDB 563, Birmingham, AL 35294-0012; **Phone:** 205-934-9767; **Board Cert:** Otolaryngology 1985; **Med School:** Louisiana State U, New Orleans 1980; **Resid:** Surgery, Baptist Med Ctr 1982; Otolaryngology, Univ Alabama Hosp 1984; **Fellow:** Head & Neck Surgical Oncology, Johns Hopkins Hosp 1987; **Fac Appt:** Prof S, Univ Alabama

Otolaryngology

Pillsbury, Harold C MD [Oto] - **Spec Exp:** Cochlear Implants; Neuro-Otology; Ear Disorders/Surgery; **Hospital:** Univ NC Hosps; **Address:** 170 Manning Drive, Physicians Bldg, Box CB 7070, Chapel Hill, NC 27599-7070; **Phone:** 919-966-8926; **Board Cert:** Otolaryngology 1978; Neurotology 2004; **Med School:** Geo Wash Univ 1972; **Resid:** Surgery, Univ NC Hosp 1973; Otolaryngology, NC Meml Hosp 1976; **Fac Appt:** Prof Oto, Univ NC Sch Med

Pitman, Karen MD [Oto] - **Spec Exp:** Head & Neck Cancer & Surgery; Thyroid & Parathyroid Cancer & Surgery; Sentinel Node Surgery; **Hospital:** Univ Mississippi Med Ctr; **Address:** Univ Mississippi Med Ctr, 2500 N State St, Jackson, MS 39216; **Phone:** 601-984-5160; **Board Cert:** Otolaryngology 1995; **Med School:** Uniformed Srvs Univ, Bethesda 1987; **Resid:** Otolaryngology, Naval Med Ctr 1994; **Fellow:** Head & Neck Oncology, Univ Pittsburgh 1996; **Fac Appt:** Prof Oto, Univ Miss

Poole, Michael D MD/PhD [Oto] - **Spec Exp:** Pediatric Otolaryngology; Ear Infections; Sleep Disorders/Apnea; Sinus Disorders; **Hospital:** Meml Hlth Univ Med Ctr - Savannah, St Joseph's-Candler Hosp; **Address:** Georgia Ear Institute, 3700 Waters Ave, Savannah, GA 31404; **Phone:** 912-356-1515; **Board Cert:** Otolaryngology 1986; **Med School:** Univ NC Sch Med 1981; **Resid:** Otolaryngology, NC Meml Hosp 1986; **Fac Appt:** Prof Oto, Mercer Univ Sch Med

Postma, Gregory N MD [Oto] - **Spec Exp:** Voice Disorders; **Hospital:** Med Coll of GA Hosp and Clin (MCG Health Inc); **Address:** Med Coll Georgia, Voice & Swallowing Center, 1120 15th St, BP-4109, Augusta, GA 30912; **Phone:** 706-721-6100; **Board Cert:** Otolaryngology 1994; **Med School:** Hahnemann Univ 1984; **Resid:** Otolaryngology, Oakland Naval Hosp 1992; Otolaryngology, Univ N Carolina Hosps 1993; **Fellow:** Otolaryngology, Vanderbilt Univ 1996; **Fac Appt:** Prof Oto, Med Coll GA

Senior, Brent A MD [Oto] - **Spec Exp:** Sinus Disorders/Surgery; Nasal Allergy; Sleep Disorders; **Hospital:** Univ NC Hosps; **Address:** UNC-Chapel Hill, Dept Oto-H&N Surg, 17D Manning CB 7070 Drive, Box G120, Chapel Hill, NC 27599-7070; **Phone:** 919-966-6483; **Board Cert:** Otolaryngology 1996; **Med School:** Univ Mich Med Sch 1990; **Resid:** Otolaryngology, Boston Univ/Tufts Univ 1995; **Fellow:** Sinus Surgery, Univ Penn 1996; **Fac Appt:** Prof Oto, Univ NC Sch Med

Shockley, William W MD [Oto] - **Spec Exp:** Facial Plastic & Reconstructive Surgery; Rhinoplasty; Salivary Gland Surgery; Thyroid Surgery; **Hospital:** Univ NC Hosps; **Address:** UNC Otolaryngology-Head & Neck Surgery, Campus Box 7070, 107 Manning Drive, Chapel Hill, NC 27599-7070; **Phone:** 919-966-6483; **Board Cert:** Otolaryngology 1981; Facial Plastic & Reconstr Surgery ; **Med School:** Indiana Univ 1976; **Resid:** Otolaryngology, Univ Cincinnati Hosps 1981; **Fellow:** Head and Neck Surgery, H&N Surg Assoc 1982; **Fac Appt:** Prof Oto, Univ NC Sch Med

Sillers, Michael J MD [Oto] - **Spec Exp:** Nasal & Sinus Disorders; Sinus Disorders/Surgery; **Hospital:** St Vincent's Hosp - Birmingham, Brookwood Med Ctr; **Address:** Alabama Nasal & Sinus Ctr, 7191 Cahaba Valley Rd, Ste 301, Birmingham, AL 35242; **Phone:** 205-980-2091; **Board Cert:** Otolaryngology 1994; **Med School:** Univ Alabama 1988; **Resid:** Otolaryngology, Univ Alabama Hosp 1993; **Fellow:** Sinus Surgery, Med Coll Georgia 1994; **Fac Appt:** Asst Prof S, Univ Alabama

Silverstein, Herbert MD [Oto] - **Spec Exp:** Ear Disorders/Surgery; Meniere's Disease; **Hospital:** Sarasota Meml Hosp; **Address:** Silverstein Institute, 1901 Floyd St, Sarasota, FL 34239; **Phone:** 941-366-9222; **Board Cert:** Otolaryngology 1967; **Med School:** Temple Univ 1961; **Resid:** Surgery, Hosp Univ Penn 1963; Otolaryngology, Mass EE Infirm 1966; **Fac Appt:** Clin Prof S, Univ S Fla Coll Med

Stringer, Scott P MD [Oto] - **Spec Exp:** Nasal & Sinus Disorders; Head & Neck Cancer; Thyroid & Parathyroid Cancer & Surgery; **Hospital:** Univ Mississippi Med Ctr; **Address:** Dept Otolaryngology, 2500 N State St, Jackson, MS 39216-4505; **Phone:** 601-984-5160; **Board Cert:** Otolaryngology 1987; **Med School:** Univ Tex SW, Dallas 1982; **Resid:** Surgery, Univ Tex SW Med Ctr 1984; Otolaryngology, Univ Tex SW Med Ctr 1987; **Fac Appt:** Prof Oto, Univ Miss

Terris, David J MD [Oto] - **Spec Exp:** Thyroid Surgery; Thyroid Cancer; Parathyroid Disease; Minimally Invasive Thyroid Surgery; **Hospital:** Med Coll of GA Hosp and Clin (MCG Health Inc), Doctors Hosp; **Address:** MCG Health System-Dept of Otolaryngology, 1120 15th St, rm BP4109, Augusta, GA 30912; **Phone:** 706-721-4400; **Board Cert:** Otolaryngology 1994; **Med School:** Duke Univ 1988; **Resid:** Surgery, Stanford Univ Med Ctr 1989; Otolaryngology, Stanford Univ Med Ctr 1993; **Fellow:** Head and Neck Surgery, Stanford Univ Med Ctr 1994; **Fac Appt:** Prof Oto, Med Coll GA

Tucci, Debara Lyn MD [Oto] - **Spec Exp:** Skull Base Surgery; Middle Ear Disorders; Otology; Hearing Disorders; **Hospital:** Duke Univ Med Ctr; **Address:** 3556 Stead-Blue Zone, South Hospital, Durham, NC 27710; **Phone:** 919-684-6968; **Board Cert:** Otolaryngology 1990; Neurotology 2004; **Med School:** Univ VA Sch Med 1985; **Resid:** Otolaryngology, Univ Va Hlth Sci Ctr 1990; **Fellow:** Otology & Neurotology, Univ Mich Med Ctr 1992; **Fac Appt:** Assoc Prof S, Duke Univ

Valentino, Joseph MD [Oto] - **Spec Exp:** Head & Neck Cancer; Reconstructive Microvascular Surgery; Thyroid Cancer; **Hospital:** Univ of Kentucky Chandler Hosp; **Address:** 740 S Limestone St, rm B-317, Lexington, KY 40536-0284; **Phone:** 859-257-5405; **Board Cert:** Otolaryngology 1993; **Med School:** UMDNJ-RW Johnson Med Sch 1987; **Resid:** Otolaryngology, Univ Minn 1992; **Fellow:** Otolaryngology, Univ Iowa Coll Med 1993; **Fac Appt:** Assoc Prof Oto, Univ KY Coll Med

Wazen, Jack J MD [Oto] - **Spec Exp:** Skull Base Surgery; Meniere's Disease; Acoustic Neuroma; Hearing & Balance Disorders; **Hospital:** Sarasota Meml Hosp; **Address:** Silverstein Institute, 1901 Floyd St, Sarasota, FL 34239; **Phone:** 941-366-9222; **Board Cert:** Otolaryngology 1983; **Med School:** Lebanon 1978; **Resid:** Surgery, St Lukes Hosp 1980; Otolaryngology, Columbia Presby Hosp 1983; **Fellow:** Neurotology, Ear Rsch Fdn 1984; **Fac Appt:** Assoc Clin Prof Oto, Columbia P&S

Weissler, Mark C MD [Oto] - **Spec Exp:** Head & Neck Cancer; Laryngeal & Tracheal Disorders; Voice Disorders; **Hospital:** Univ NC Hosps; **Address:** G106 Physicians Office Bldg, 170 Manning Drive, #CB 7070, Chapel Hill, NC 27599-7070; **Phone:** 919-966-6483; **Board Cert:** Otolaryngology 1985; **Med School:** Boston Univ 1980; **Resid:** Surgery, Mass Genl Hosp 1982; Otolaryngology, Mass Eye & Ear Infirm 1985; **Fellow:** Head & Neck Oncology, Univ Cincinnati 1986; **Fac Appt:** Prof Oto, Univ NC Sch Med

Yarbrough, Wendell G MD [Oto] - **Spec Exp:** Head & Neck Cancer; **Hospital:** Vanderbilt Univ Med Ctr; **Address:** Vanderbilt Otolaryngology, 1215 21st Ave S, Ste 7209, Nashville, TN 37232-8605; **Phone:** 615-343-8840; **Board Cert:** Otolaryngology 1995; **Med School:** Univ NC Sch Med 1989; **Resid:** Otolaryngology, Univ NC Hosps 1994; **Fellow:** Surgical Oncology, Univ NC Hosps 1996; **Fac Appt:** Assoc Prof Oto, Vanderbilt Univ

Otolaryngology

Midwest

Arts, H Alexander MD [Oto] - **Spec Exp:** Skull Base Tumors & Surgery; Neuro-Otology; Hearing Loss; Cochlear Implants; **Hospital:** Univ Michigan Hlth Sys; **Address:** Univ Michigan Health Systems, Dept Otolaryngology, 1500 E Medical Ctr Dr, 1904 Taubman Ctr, Ann Arbor, MI 48109; **Phone:** 734-936-8006; **Board Cert:** Otolaryngology 1992; Neurotology 2004; **Med School:** Baylor Coll Med 1983; **Resid:** Surgery, Univ Washington Med Ctr 1985; Otolaryngology, Univ Washington Med Ctr 1990; **Fellow:** Neurotology, Univ Virginia 1991; **Fac Appt:** Prof Oto, Univ Mich Med Sch

Baim, Howard M MD [Oto] - **Spec Exp:** Head & Neck Surgery; Sleep Disorders/Apnea; Sinus Disorders; **Hospital:** Adv Illinois Masonic Med Ctr, Highland Park/North Shore Univ Hlth Syst; **Address:** 2532 N Lincoln Ave, Chicago, IL 60614-2468; **Phone:** 773-883-1177; **Board Cert:** Otolaryngology 1978; **Med School:** Univ IL Coll Med 1973; **Resid:** Surgery, Illinois Met Grp Hosps 1975; Otolaryngology, Illinois EE Infirmary 1978; **Fac Appt:** Asst Clin Prof Oto, Univ IL Coll Med

Baker, Shan Ray MD [Oto] - **Spec Exp:** Cosmetic Surgery-Face & Neck; Reconstructive Surgery; **Hospital:** Univ Michigan Hlth Sys; **Address:** Ctr Facial & Cosmetic Surgery, 19900 Haggerty Rd, Ste 103, Livonia, MI 48152-1054; **Phone:** 734-432-7634; **Board Cert:** Otolaryngology 1977; Facial Plastic & Reconstr Surgery 1990; **Med School:** Univ Iowa Coll Med 1971; **Resid:** Surgery, UCSD Med Ctr 1973; Otolaryngology, Univ Iowa Hosps 1977; **Fac Appt:** Prof Oto, Univ Mich Med Sch

Bastian, Robert W MD [Oto] - **Spec Exp:** Voice Disorders; Swallowing Disorders; Laryngeal Disorders; **Hospital:** Adv Good Samaritan Hosp; **Address:** Bastian Voice Inst, 3010 Highland Parkway, Ste 550, Downers Grove, IL 60515-5500; **Phone:** 630-724-1100; **Board Cert:** Otolaryngology 1983; **Med School:** Washington Univ, St Louis 1978; **Resid:** Surgery, Barnes Hosp 1979; Otolaryngology, Barnes Hosp 1983; **Fellow:** Otolaryngology, Hosp Foch 1983

Beatty, Charles W MD [Oto] - **Spec Exp:** Otology & Neuro-Otology; Acoustic Neuroma; Meniere's Disease; Cochlear Implants; **Hospital:** Mayo Med Ctr & Clin - Rochester; **Address:** Mayo Clinic, Dept Otolaryngology, 200 First St SW Fl W5, Rochester, MN 55905; **Phone:** 507-284-8532; **Board Cert:** Otolaryngology 1982; **Med School:** Univ Iowa Coll Med 1977; **Resid:** Otolaryngology, Mayo Clinic 1982; **Fac Appt:** Prof Oto, Mayo Med Sch

Benninger, Michael S MD [Oto] - **Spec Exp:** Voice Disorders; Nasal & Sinus Disorders; Sinus Disorders/Surgery; **Hospital:** Cleveland Clin Fdn (page 56); **Address:** Cleveland Clinic Main Campus, MC A71, 9500 Euclid Ave, Cleveland, OH 44195; **Phone:** 216-444-6686; **Board Cert:** Otolaryngology 1988; **Med School:** Case West Res Univ 1983; **Resid:** Surgery, Cleveland Clin Fdn 1985; Otolaryngology, Cleveland Clin Fdn 1988; **Fac Appt:** Prof S, Cleveland Cl Coll Med/Case West Res

Bojrab, Dennis I MD [Oto] - **Spec Exp:** Otology & Neuro-Otology; Facial Nerve Disorders; Skull Base Tumors; **Hospital:** Providence Hosp - Southfield, William Beaumont Hosp; **Address:** Michigan Ear Inst, 30055 Northwestern Hwy, Ste 101, Farmington Hills, MI 48334; **Phone:** 248-865-4444; **Board Cert:** Otolaryngology 1985; Neurotology 2005; **Med School:** Indiana Univ 1979; **Resid:** Surgery, Butterworth Hosp 1981; Otolaryngology, Univ Indiana Sch Med 1984; **Fellow:** Skull Base Surgery, Vanderbilt Univ Med Ctr 1985; **Fac Appt:** Prof Oto, Wayne State Univ

Bradford, Carol MD [Oto] - **Spec Exp:** Head & Neck Cancer; Melanoma-Head & Neck; Skin Cancer-Head & Neck; **Hospital:** Univ Michigan Hlth Sys; **Address:** University of Michigan Health System, 1500 E Medical Center Drive, rm 1904-TC, Ann Arbor, MI 48109-0312; **Phone:** 734-936-8029; **Board Cert:** Otolaryngology 1993; **Med School:** Univ Mich Med Sch 1986; **Resid:** Otolaryngology, Univ Michigan Med Ctr 1992; **Fellow:** Head and Neck Surgery, Univ Michigan Med Ctr 1988; **Fac Appt:** Prof Oto, Univ Mich Med Sch

Branham, Gregory H MD [Oto] - **Spec Exp:** Cosmetic & Reconstructive Surgery-Face; Nasal Surgery; Botox Therapy; Skin Laser Surgery-Resurfacing; **Hospital:** Washington Univ Med Ctr, Barnes-Jewish Hosp; **Address:** 605 Old Ballas Rd, Ste 100, St Louis, MO 63141; **Phone:** 314-432-7760; **Board Cert:** Otolaryngology 1989; Facial Plastic & Reconstr Surgery 1993; **Med School:** Washington Univ, St Louis 1983; **Resid:** Otolaryngology, St Louis Univ Hosp 1989; **Fellow:** Facial Plastic & Reconstr Surgery, Washington Univ Affil Hosp 1990; **Fac Appt:** Assoc Prof Oto, St Louis Univ

Burkey, Brian MD [Oto] - **Spec Exp:** Parotid Gland Tumors; Head & Neck Cancer; Reconstructive Microvascular Surgery; **Hospital:** Cleveland Clin Fdn (page 56); **Address:** Head & Neck Institute, Desk A71, The Cleveland Clinic, 9500 Euclid Ave, Cleveland, OH 44195; **Phone:** 216-445-8838; **Board Cert:** Otolaryngology 1992; **Med School:** Univ VA Sch Med 1986; **Resid:** Otolaryngology, Univ Mich Med Ctr 1991; **Fellow:** Microsurgery, Ohio State Univ 1991; **Fac Appt:** Assoc Prof Oto, Vanderbilt Univ

Caldarelli, David D MD [Oto] - **Spec Exp:** Laryngeal & Vocal Cord Surgery; Sinus Disorders/Surgery; Ear Disorders/Surgery; Meniere's Disease; **Hospital:** Rush Univ Med Ctr; **Address:** 1725 W Harrison St, Ste 308, Chicago, IL 60612; **Phone:** 312-733-4341; **Board Cert:** Otolaryngology 1970; **Med School:** Univ IL Coll Med 1965; **Resid:** Surgery, Presby-St Lukes Hosp 1967; Otolaryngology, Univ Illinois Eye/Ear Infirm 1970; **Fac Appt:** Prof Oto, Rush Med Coll

Campbell, Bruce H MD [Oto] - **Spec Exp:** Head & Neck Cancer; Thyroid Surgery; **Hospital:** Froedtert Meml Lutheran Hosp, Chldns Hosp - Wisconsin; **Address:** Med Coll Wisc-Dept Oto, 9200 W Wisconsin Ave, Milwaukee, WI 53226; **Phone:** 414-805-5583; **Board Cert:** Otolaryngology 1986; **Med School:** Rush Med Coll 1980; **Resid:** Otolaryngology, Med Coll Wisconsin 1985; **Fellow:** Head and Neck Surgery, MD Anderson Cancer Ctr 1987; **Fac Appt:** Prof Oto, Med Coll Wisc

Corey, Jacquelynne P MD [Oto] - **Spec Exp:** Nasal & Sinus Disorders; Allergy; Voice Disorders; **Hospital:** Univ of Chicago Med Ctr; **Address:** 5841 S Maryland Ave, MC 1035, Chicago, IL 60637; **Phone:** 773-702-1865; **Board Cert:** Otolaryngology 1985; **Med School:** Univ IL Coll Med 1979; **Resid:** Otolaryngology, Rush Presby-St Lukes Med Ctr 1984; **Fac Appt:** Assoc Prof Oto, Univ Chicago-Pritzker Sch Med

Driscoll, Colin L W MD [Oto] - **Spec Exp:** Acoustic Neuroma; Cochlear Implants; Skull Base Tumors; **Hospital:** Mayo Med Ctr & Clin - Rochester; **Address:** Mayo Clinic, Dept Otolaryngology, 200 First St SW, W5, Rochester, MN 55905-0001; **Phone:** 507-284-4065; **Board Cert:** Otolaryngology 1998; **Med School:** Univ New Mexico 1992; **Resid:** Otolaryngology, Mayo Clinic 1997; **Fellow:** Neurotology, UCSF Med Ctr 1998; Skull Base Surgery, UCSF Med Ctr 1999; **Fac Appt:** Assoc Prof Oto, Mayo Med Sch

Ford, Charles N MD [Oto] - **Spec Exp:** Voice Disorders; Laryngeal Disorders; **Hospital:** Univ WI Hosp & Clins; **Address:** Univ of WI Hosp & Clinics, 600 Highland Avenue-K4-714, Madison, WI 53792-3284; **Phone:** 608-263-0192; **Board Cert:** Otolaryngology 1971; **Med School:** Univ Louisville Sch Med 1965; **Resid:** Otolaryngology, Henry Ford Hosp 1970; **Fac Appt:** Prof Oto, Univ Wisc

Friedman, Michael MD [Oto] - **Spec Exp:** Sleep Disorders/Apnea/Snoring; Thyroid & Parathyroid Surgery; Sinus Disorders/Surgery; **Hospital:** Adv Illinois Masonic Med Ctr, Rush Univ Med Ctr; **Address:** 30 N Michigan St, Ste 1107, Chicago, IL 60602-3747; **Phone:** 312-236-3642; **Board Cert:** Otolaryngology 1977; **Med School:** Univ IL Coll Med 1972; **Resid:** Surgery, Illinois Masonic Hosp 1974; Otolaryngology, Univ Illinois Med Ctr 1977; **Fac Appt:** Prof Oto, Rush Med Coll

Otolaryngology

Funk, Gerry F MD [Oto] - **Spec Exp:** Head & Neck Cancer; Head & Neck Reconstruction; Head & Neck Trauma; **Hospital:** Univ Iowa Hosp & Clinics; **Address:** UIHC, Dept Otolaryngology, 200 Hawkins Drive, Iowa City, IA 52242-1009; **Phone:** 319-356-2165; **Board Cert:** Otolaryngology 1992; **Med School:** Univ Chicago-Pritzker Sch Med 1986; **Resid:** Surgery, LAC-USC Med Ctr 1987; Otolaryngology, LAC-USC Med Ctr 1991; **Fellow:** Head and Neck Surgery, Univ Iowa Hosp 1992; **Fac Appt:** Prof Oto, Univ Iowa Coll Med

Gantz, Bruce MD [Oto] - **Spec Exp:** Cochlear Implants; Neuro-Otology; Skull Base Surgery; **Hospital:** Univ Iowa Hosp & Clinics; **Address:** Univ Hosp & Clins, Dept Otolaryngology, 200 Hawkins Drive, rm 21201PFP, Iowa City, IA 52242-1078; **Phone:** 319-356-2173; **Board Cert:** Otolaryngology 1980; Neurotology 2004; **Med School:** Univ Iowa Coll Med 1974; **Resid:** Otolaryngology, Univ Iowa Hosps 1980; **Fellow:** Neurotology, Univ Zurich 1982; **Fac Appt:** Prof Oto, Univ Iowa Coll Med

Goebel, Joel Alan MD [Oto] - **Spec Exp:** Dizziness; Hearing Disorders; Otology & Neuro-Otology; **Hospital:** Barnes-Jewish Hosp, St Louis Chldns Hosp; **Address:** Barnes Jewish Hosp South, 660 S Euclid, Box 8115, St Louis, MO 63110; **Phone:** 314-362-7509; **Board Cert:** Otolaryngology 1985; **Med School:** Washington Univ, St Louis 1980; **Resid:** Otolaryngology, Barnes Hosp/Wash Univ 1985; **Fac Appt:** Prof Oto, Washington Univ, St Louis

Hartig, Gregory K MD [Oto] - **Spec Exp:** Head & Neck Cancer; Skull Base Tumors; **Hospital:** Univ WI Hosp & Clins; **Address:** 600 Highland Ave, rm K4/720, Madison, WI 53792-7375; **Phone:** 608-263-6190; **Board Cert:** Otolaryngology 1994; **Med School:** Univ Mich Med Sch 1988; **Resid:** Otolaryngology, Univ Mich Med Ctr 1993; **Fellow:** Univ Penn Med Ctr 1994; **Fac Appt:** Prof Oto, Univ Mich Med Sch

Haughey, Bruce H MD [Oto] - **Spec Exp:** Reconstructive Surgery-Face; Head & Neck Cancer; Head & Neck Reconstruction; **Hospital:** Barnes-Jewish Hosp, St Louis Chldns Hosp; **Address:** Barnes Jewish Hosp South, 660 S Euclid Ave, Box 8115, St Louis, MO 63110; **Phone:** 314-362-7509; **Board Cert:** Otolaryngology 1984; **Med School:** New Zealand 1976; **Resid:** Surgery, Univ Auckland 1981; Otolaryngology, Univ Iowa Med Ctr 1984; **Fellow:** Otolaryngology, Univ Iowa Med Ctr 1985; **Fac Appt:** Prof Oto, Washington Univ, St Louis

Hilger, Peter A MD [Oto] - **Spec Exp:** Head & Neck Surgery; Facial Plastic Surgery; **Hospital:** Regions Hosp - St Paul, Fairview Southdale Hosp; **Address:** Centennial Lakes Med Bldg, 7373 France Ave S, Ste 410, Edina, MN 55435; **Phone:** 952-844-0404; **Board Cert:** Otolaryngology 1979; **Med School:** Univ Minn 1974; **Resid:** Surgery, Univ Minn Hosp 1975; Otolaryngology, Univ Minn Hosp 1979; **Fellow:** Plastic Surgery, Mass Eye & Ear Infirm 1980; **Fac Appt:** Asst Prof Oto, Univ Minn

Hoffman, Henry T MD [Oto] - **Spec Exp:** Voice Disorders; Head & Neck Cancer; Salivary Gland Tumors & Surgery; **Hospital:** Univ Iowa Hosp & Clinics; **Address:** Univ Iowa Hosp & Clins-Dept Oto, 200 Hawkins Drive, Iowa City, IA 52242; **Phone:** 319-356-2166; **Board Cert:** Otolaryngology 1985; **Med School:** UCSD 1980; **Resid:** Otolaryngology, Univ Iowa Hosp & Clinics 1985; **Fellow:** Head & Neck Oncology, Univ Michigan Hosp 1989; **Fac Appt:** Clin Prof Oto, Univ Iowa Coll Med

Hogikyan, Norman D MD [Oto] - **Spec Exp:** Voice Disorders; Vocal Cord Disorders; Swallowing Disorders; Airway Disorders; **Hospital:** Univ Michigan Hlth Sys; **Address:** University og Michigan Health System, Taubman Ctr, rm 1904, 1500 E Medical Ctr Drive, Ann Arbor, MI 48109; **Phone:** 734-436-7633; **Board Cert:** Otolaryngology 1995; **Med School:** Univ Mich Med Sch 1988; **Resid:** Otolaryngology, Barnes Jewish Med Ctr 1994; **Fellow:** Otolaryngology, Loyola Univ Med Ctr 1995; **Fac Appt:** Assoc Prof Oto, Univ Mich Med Sch

Hotaling, Andrew J MD [Oto] - **Spec Exp:** Pediatric Otolaryngology; Sleep Disorders/Apnea; Neck Masses; Ear Infections; **Hospital:** Loyola Univ Med Ctr, Children's Mem Hosp; **Address:** Loyola Univ Med Ctr, 2160 S 1st Ave Bldg 105 - rm 1870, Maywood, IL 60153-5590; **Phone:** 708-216-9183; **Board Cert:** Otolaryngology 1985; **Med School:** Case West Res Univ 1979; **Resid:** Surgery, Case Western 1981; Otolaryngology, Northwestern Meml Hosp 1984; **Fellow:** Pediatric Otolaryngology, Univ Pittsburgh Med Ctr 1985; **Fac Appt:** Prof Oto, Loyola Univ-Stritch Sch Med

Jones, Paul J MD [Oto] - **Spec Exp:** Pediatric Otolaryngology; **Hospital:** Rush Univ Med Ctr; **Address:** 1725 W Harrison St, Ste 918, Chicago, IL 60612; **Phone:** 312-942-2175; **Board Cert:** Otolaryngology 1989; **Med School:** Rush Med Coll 1983; **Resid:** Otolaryngology, Rush Presby-St Lukes Med Ctr 1988; **Fac Appt:** Asst Prof Oto, Rush Med Coll

Kartush, Jack MD [Oto] - **Spec Exp:** Ear Disorders/Surgery; Balance Disorders; **Hospital:** Providence Hosp - Southfield; **Address:** Michigan Ear Inst, 30055 Northwestern Hwy, Ste 101, Farmington Hills, MI 48334; **Phone:** 248-865-4444; **Board Cert:** Otolaryngology 1984; **Med School:** Univ Mich Med Sch 1978; **Resid:** Otolaryngology, Univ Mich Med Ctr 1984; **Fellow:** Neurotology, Univ Mich Med Ctr 1985; **Fac Appt:** Assoc Clin Prof Oto, Wayne State Univ

Kern, Robert C MD [Oto] - **Spec Exp:** Head & Neck Cancer; Sinus Disorders/Surgery; Rhinoplasty; Head & Neck Surgery; **Hospital:** Northwestern Meml Hosp, Stroger Hosp of Cook Co; **Address:** Northwestern Medical Faculty Fdn, 675 N St Clair St, Ste 15-200, Chicago, IL 60611; **Phone:** 312-695-8182; **Board Cert:** Otolaryngology 1990; **Med School:** Jefferson Med Coll 1985; **Resid:** Otolaryngology, Wayne State Affil Hosp 1990; **Fellow:** Research, Natl Inst Hlth 1991; **Fac Appt:** Prof Oto, Northwestern Univ

Lavertu, Pierre MD [Oto] - **Spec Exp:** Thyroid Cancer; Head & Neck Cancer; Skull Base Tumors; **Hospital:** Univ Hosps Case Med Ctr; **Address:** Univ Hosps, Dept Oto-Head & Neck Surg, 11100 Euclid Ave, Cleveland, OH 44106-5045; **Phone:** 216-844-4773; **Board Cert:** Otolaryngology 1981; **Med School:** Univ Montreal 1976; **Resid:** Otolaryngology, Univ Montreal Med Ctr 1981; **Fellow:** Head and Neck Surgery, Univ Montreal Med Ctr 1982; Head and Neck Surgery, Cleveland Clinic 1983; **Fac Appt:** Prof Oto, Case West Res Univ

Leonetti, John P MD [Oto] - **Spec Exp:** Skull Base Tumors & Surgery; Acoustic Neuroma; Neuro-Otology; **Hospital:** Loyola Univ Med Ctr; **Address:** Loyola University Medical Ctr, Dept Otolaryngology, 2160 S First Ave Bldg 105 - rm 1870, Maywood, IL 60153; **Phone:** 708-216-4804; **Board Cert:** Otolaryngology 1987; **Med School:** Loyola Univ-Stritch Sch Med 1982; **Resid:** Otolaryngology, Loyola Univ Med Ctr 1987; Research, House Ear Inst 1987; **Fellow:** Neurotology, Barnes Jewish Hosp 1988; **Fac Appt:** Prof Oto, Loyola Univ-Stritch Sch Med

Marentette, Lawrence J MD [Oto] - **Spec Exp:** Skull Base Tumors & Surgery; Facial Plastic & Reconstructive Surgery; **Hospital:** Univ Michigan Hlth Sys; **Address:** Univ Michigan Hlth Sys, Dept Oto, 1500 E Med Ctr Drive, 1904 Taubman Ctr, Ann Arbor, MI 48109; **Phone:** 734-936-8051; **Board Cert:** Otolaryngology 1981; Facial Plastic & Reconstr Surgery 1995; **Med School:** Wayne State Univ 1976; **Resid:** Otolaryngology, Wayne State Univ 1980; **Fellow:** Maxillofacial Surgery, Univ of Zurich 1985; **Fac Appt:** Prof Oto, Univ Mich Med Sch

Miyamoto, Richard T MD [Oto] - **Spec Exp:** Neuro-Otology; Acoustic Neuroma; Middle Ear Disorders; Cochlear Implants; **Hospital:** Indiana Univ Hosp, Riley Hosp for Children; **Address:** 702 Barnhill Drive, Ste 0860, Indianapolis, IN 46202; **Phone:** 317-274-3556; **Board Cert:** Otolaryngology 1975; Neurotology 2004; **Med School:** Univ Mich Med Sch 1970; **Resid:** Surgery, Butterworth Hosp 1972; Otolaryngology, Indiana Univ Hosps 1975; **Fellow:** Otology & Neurotology, Otologic Med Grp 1978; **Fac Appt:** Prof Oto, Indiana Univ

Otolaryngology

Naclerio, Robert M MD [Oto] - **Spec Exp:** Head & Neck Surgery; Pediatric Otolaryngology; Sinus Disorders/Surgery; **Hospital:** Univ of Chicago Med Ctr; **Address:** Univ Chicago Hosps, 5841 S Maryland Ave, MC 1035, AMB E102E, Chicago, IL 60637; **Phone:** 773-702-0080; **Board Cert:** Otolaryngology 1983; **Med School:** Baylor Coll Med 1976; **Resid:** Surgery, Johns Hopkins Hosp 1978; Otolaryngology, Baylor Coll Med 1980; **Fellow:** Clinical Immunology, Johns Hopkins Hosp 1982; **Fac Appt:** Prof Oto, Univ Chicago-Pritzker Sch Med

Olsen, Kerry D MD [Oto] - **Spec Exp:** Head & Neck Cancer & Surgery; Esthesioneuroblastoma; Salivary Gland Tumors & Surgery; Skull Base Tumors; **Hospital:** Mayo Med Ctr & Clin - Rochester; **Address:** Mayo Clinic, Dept Otolaryngology, 200 1st St SW, Rochester, MN 55905-0001; **Phone:** 507-284-3542; **Board Cert:** Otolaryngology 1981; **Med School:** Mayo Med Sch 1976; **Resid:** Otolaryngology, Mayo Clinic 1981; **Fac Appt:** Prof Oto, Mayo Med Sch

Ozer, Enver MD [Oto] - **Spec Exp:** Head & Neck Cancer; Head & Neck Surgery; **Hospital:** Ohio St Univ Med Ctr; **Address:** 456 W 10th Ave, Ste 4A, Columbus, OH 43210; **Phone:** 614-293-8074; **Med School:** Turkey 1994; **Resid:** Otolaryngology, Marmara Univ Med Sch 1996; Head and Neck Surgery, Marmara Univ Med Sch 2000; **Fellow:** Head & Neck Oncology, Ohio St Univ Med Ctr 2005; **Fac Appt:** Asst Prof Oto, Ohio State Univ

Paparella, Michael M MD [Oto] - **Spec Exp:** Hearing Disorders; Neuro-Otology; Meniere's Disease; **Hospital:** Univ Minn Med Ctr, Fairview - Riverside Campus; **Address:** 701 25th Ave S, Ste 200, Minneapolis, MN 55454-1443; **Phone:** 612-339-2836; **Board Cert:** Otolaryngology 1963; **Med School:** Univ Mich Med Sch 1957; **Resid:** Otolaryngology, Henry Ford Hosp 1961; **Fac Appt:** Clin Prof Oto, Univ Minn

Pelzer, Harold J MD/DDS [Oto] - **Spec Exp:** Head & Neck Cancer; Swallowing Disorders; **Hospital:** Northwestern Meml Hosp; **Address:** Northwestern Medical Faculty Fdn, 675 N St Clair St, Ste 15-200, Chicago, IL 60611; **Phone:** 312-695-8182; **Board Cert:** Otolaryngology 1985; **Med School:** Northwestern Univ 1979; **Resid:** Surgery, Northwestern Meml Hosp 1983; **Fellow:** Head and Neck Surgery, Northwestern Meml Hosp 1985; **Fac Appt:** Assoc Prof Oto, Northwestern Univ

Pensak, Myles L MD [Oto] - **Spec Exp:** Skull Base Tumors; Facial Paralysis; Hearing & Balance Disorders; **Hospital:** Univ Hosp - Cincinnati, Good Samaritan Hosp - Cincinnati; **Address:** Univ Medical Arts Building, 222 Piedmont Ave, Ste 5200, Cincinnati, OH 45219; **Phone:** 513-475-8400; **Board Cert:** Otolaryngology 1983; Neurotology 2004; **Med School:** NY Med Coll 1978; **Resid:** Surgery, Upstate Med Ctr 1980; Otolaryngology, Yale Univ 1983; **Fellow:** Otology & Neurotology, The Otology Group 1984; **Fac Appt:** Prof Oto, Univ Cincinnati

Petruzzelli, Guy MD/PhD [Oto] - **Spec Exp:** Head & Neck Cancer & Surgery; Skull Base Tumors; Thyroid Cancer; **Hospital:** Rush Univ Med Ctr; **Address:** Rush Univ Med Ctr, 1725 W Harrison St, Ste 218, Chicago, IL 60612; **Phone:** 312-942-6100; **Board Cert:** Otolaryngology 1993; **Med School:** Rush Med Coll 1987; **Resid:** Otolaryngology, Univ Pittsburgh Med Ctr 1992; **Fellow:** Head & Neck Oncology, Univ Pittsburgh Med Ctr 1993; Skull Base Surgery, Univ Pittsburgh Ctr Cranial Base Surg; **Fac Appt:** Prof Oto, Rush Med Coll

Piccirillo, Jay MD [Oto] - **Spec Exp:** Sleep Disorders/Apnea; Sinus Disorders/Surgery; **Hospital:** Barnes-Jewish Hosp; **Address:** Barnes Jewish Hosp South, 660 S Euclid, Box 8115, St Louis, MO 63110; **Phone:** 314-362-7509; **Board Cert:** Otolaryngology 1990; **Med School:** Univ VT Coll Med 1985; **Resid:** Otolaryngology, Albany Med Ctr 1990; **Fellow:** Yale Univ 1992; **Fac Appt:** Asst Prof Oto, Washington Univ, St Louis

Siegel, Gordon J MD [Oto] - **Spec Exp:** Head & Neck Cancer; Nasal & Sinus Disorders; **Hospital:** Northwestern Meml Hosp; **Address:** 3 E Huron St Fl 1, Chicago, IL 60611-2705; **Phone:** 312-988-7777; **Board Cert:** Otolaryngology 1984; **Med School:** Ros Franklin Univ/Chicago Med Sch 1978; **Resid:** Otolaryngology, Northwestern Univ Affil Hosp 1982; **Fac Appt:** Asst Clin Prof Oto, Northwestern Univ

Stankiewicz, James MD [Oto] - **Spec Exp:** Endoscopic Sinus Surgery; Rhinosinusitis; Nasal & Sinus Disorders; **Hospital:** Loyola Univ Med Ctr; **Address:** Loyola Univ Med Ctr, Dept Oto, 2160 S First Ave, Maywood, IL 60153-5590; **Phone:** 708-216-8563; **Board Cert:** Otolaryngology 1978; **Med School:** Univ Chicago-Pritzker Sch Med 1974; **Resid:** Otolaryngology, Univ Chicago Hosp 1978; **Fac Appt:** Prof Oto, Loyola Univ-Stritch Sch Med

Stenson, Kerstin M MD [Oto] - **Spec Exp:** Head & Neck Cancer; Head & Neck Cancer Reconstruction; Trauma; Vocal Cord Disorders; **Hospital:** Univ of Chicago Med Ctr; **Address:** 5841 S Maryland Ave, MC 1035, Chicago, IL 60637-1463; **Phone:** 773-702-1865; **Board Cert:** Otolaryngology 1994; **Med School:** Ros Franklin Univ/Chicago Med Sch 1988; **Resid:** Otolaryngology, Univ Illinois Affil Hosp 1993; **Fellow:** Head & Neck Oncology, Univ Michigan 1994; Microvascular Surgery, Univ Michigan 1994; **Fac Appt:** Prof S, Univ Chicago-Pritzker Sch Med

Szachowicz II, Edward H MD [Oto] - **Spec Exp:** Cosmetic Surgery-Face; Rhinoplasty; Liposuction & Body Contouring; **Hospital:** Abbott - Northwestern Hosp; **Address:** Centennial Lakes Med Bldg, 7373 France Ave S, Ste 508, Edina, MN 55435-4538; **Phone:** 952-835-5665; **Board Cert:** Otolaryngology 1984; **Med School:** Univ IL Coll Med 1979; **Resid:** Surgery, Fairview Univ Med Ctr 1980; Otolaryngology, Fairview Univ Med Ctr 1984; **Fellow:** Facial Plastic Surgery, Fairview Univ Med Ctr 1986; **Fac Appt:** Asst Clin Prof Oto, Univ Minn

Teknos, Theodoros N MD [Oto] - **Spec Exp:** Head & Neck Cancer; Thyroid Cancer; Facial Plastic & Reconstructive Surgery; Reconstructive Microvascular Surgery; **Hospital:** Ohio St Univ Med Ctr; **Address:** 456 W 10th Ave, Ste 4A, Columbus, OH 43210; **Phone:** 614-293-8074; **Board Cert:** Otolaryngology 1997; **Med School:** Harvard Med Sch 1991; **Resid:** Otolaryngology, Mass Eye & Ear Hosp 1996; **Fellow:** Head and Neck Surgery, Vanderbilt Univ Med Ctr 1997; **Fac Appt:** Assoc Prof Oto, Univ Mich Med Sch

Telian, Steven A MD [Oto] - **Spec Exp:** Cochlear Implants; Ear Disorders/Surgery; Acoustic Neuroma; **Hospital:** Univ Michigan Hlth Sys; **Address:** Univ Mich Med Ctr, Dept Otolaryngology-Head & Neck Surgery, 1500 E Med Ctr Drive, 1904 Taubman Ctr, Ann Arbor, MI 48109-0312; **Phone:** 734-936-8006; **Board Cert:** Otolaryngology 1985; Neurotology 2004; **Med School:** Univ Pennsylvania 1980; **Resid:** Otolaryngology, Hosp Univ Penn 1985; **Fellow:** Neurotology, Univ Mich Med Ctr 1986; **Fac Appt:** Prof Oto, Univ Mich Med Sch

Toriumi, Dean MD [Oto] - **Spec Exp:** Rhinoplasty; Cosmetic Surgery-Face; Reconstructive Plastic Surgery; **Hospital:** Univ of IL Med Ctr at Chicago; **Address:** 60 E Delaware Pl, Ste 1460, Chicago, IL 60611; **Phone:** 312-255-8812; **Board Cert:** Otolaryngology 1988; **Med School:** Rush Med Coll 1981; **Resid:** Surgery, Univ Illinois Med Ctr 1985; Otolaryngology, Northwestern Univ Med Sch 1987; **Fellow:** Facial Plastic Surgery, Tulane Med Sch 1988; Facial Plastic Surgery, Virginia Mason Med Ctr 1989; **Fac Appt:** Assoc Prof Oto, Univ IL Coll Med

Wackym, P Ashley MD [Oto] - **Spec Exp:** Cochlear Implants; Acoustic Neuroma; Head & Neck Surgery; **Hospital:** Froedtert Meml Lutheran Hosp, Chldns Hosp - Wisconsin; **Address:** Dept Otolaryngology, 9200 W Wisconsin Ave, Milwaukee, WI 53226; **Phone:** 414-805-5625; **Board Cert:** Otolaryngology 1992; Neurotology 2004; **Med School:** Vanderbilt Univ 1985; **Resid:** Neurological Surgery, UCLA Med Ctr 1987; Head and Neck Surgery, UCLA Med Ctr 1991; **Fellow:** Otology & Neurotology, Univ Iowa 1992; Neurological Science, UCLA Med Ctr 1995; **Fac Appt:** Prof Oto, Med Coll Wisc

Otolaryngology

Wiet, Richard J MD [Oto] - **Spec Exp:** Acoustic Neuroma; Hearing Loss; Otosclerosis/Stapedectomy; Cochlear Implants; **Hospital:** Hinsdale Hosp, Northwestern Meml Hosp; **Address:** Ear Institute of Chicago, 11 Salt Creek Rd, Ste 101, Hinsdale, IL 60521; **Phone:** 630-789-3110; **Board Cert:** Otolaryngology 1976; Neurotology 2004; **Med School:** Loyola Univ-Stritch Sch Med 1971; **Resid:** Otolaryngology, Cincinnati Med Ctr 1976; **Fellow:** Neurotology, Univ Zurich/Ear Fdn 1979; **Fac Appt:** Clin Prof Oto, Northwestern Univ

Wilson, Keith M MD [Oto] - **Spec Exp:** Head & Neck Cancer & Surgery; Voice Disorders; **Hospital:** Univ Hosp - Cincinnati; **Address:** Univ Cincinnati Medical Ctr, 222 Piedmont Ave, Ste 5200, Cincinnati, OH 45219-4222; **Phone:** 513-475-8400; **Board Cert:** Otolaryngology 1992; **Med School:** Cornell Univ-Weill Med Coll 1986; **Resid:** Otolaryngology, St Louis Univ Med Ctr 1991; **Fellow:** Head & Neck Surgical Oncology, Ohio State Med Ctr 1992; **Fac Appt:** Assoc Prof Oto, Univ Cincinnati

Wolf, Gregory T MD [Oto] - **Spec Exp:** Head & Neck Cancer; Laryngeal Cancer; **Hospital:** Univ Michigan Hlth Sys; **Address:** Univ Mich Med Ctr, Dept Oto-HNS, 1500 E Med Ctr, Taubman Ctr, rm 1904, Ann Arbor, MI 48109-0312; **Phone:** 734-936-8029; **Board Cert:** Otolaryngology 1978; **Med School:** Univ Mich Med Sch 1973; **Resid:** Surgery, Georgetown Univ Hosp 1975; Otolaryngology, SUNY Upstate Med Ctr 1978; **Fac Appt:** Prof Oto, Univ Mich Med Sch

Woodson, B Tucker MD [Oto] - **Spec Exp:** Sleep Disorders/Apnea; **Hospital:** Froedtert Meml Lutheran Hosp, Chldns Hosp - Wisconsin; **Address:** Froedtert West ENT Clinic, 9200 W Wisconsin Ave, Milwaukee, WI 53226-3522; **Phone:** 414-805-7667; **Board Cert:** Otolaryngology 1988; **Med School:** Univ MO-Columbia Sch Med 1983; **Resid:** Surgery, Henry Ford Hosp 1984; Otolaryngology, Henry Ford Hosp 1988; **Fac Appt:** Assoc Prof Oto, Med Coll Wisc

Woodson, Gayle Ellen MD [Oto] - **Spec Exp:** Voice Disorders; Swallowing Disorders; **Hospital:** St John's Hosp - Springfield, Memorial Med Ctr-Springfield; **Address:** Div Otolaryngology, PO Box 19662, Springfield, IL 62794-9662; **Phone:** 217-545-6099; **Board Cert:** Otolaryngology 1981; **Med School:** Baylor Coll Med 1975; **Resid:** Surgery, Johns Hopkins Hosp 1978; Otolaryngology, Baylor Coll Med 1981; **Fellow:** Laryngology, Inst Laryngology and Otology 1982; **Fac Appt:** Prof Oto, Southern IL Univ

Young, Nancy MD [Oto] - **Spec Exp:** Cochlear Implants; Cholesteatoma; Hearing Loss; Baha Implant; **Hospital:** Children's Mem Hosp, Glenbrook/NorthShore Univ Hlth Syst; **Address:** Children's Memorial, Div Otolaryngology, 2300 Children's Plaza, Box 265, Chicago, IL 60614; **Phone:** 773-880-3020; **Board Cert:** Otolaryngology 1987; **Med School:** NYU Sch Med 1982; **Resid:** Surgery, Montefiore Med Ctr 1984; Otolaryngology, Northwestern Univ Hosp 1987; **Fellow:** Neurotology, Hinsdale Hosp 1988; **Fac Appt:** Assoc Prof Oto, Northwestern Univ

Yueh, Bevan MD [Oto] - **Spec Exp:** Head & Neck Cancer; Hearing Loss; **Hospital:** Univ Minn Med Ctr, Fairview - Univ Campus; **Address:** Dept Otolaryngology/Head & Neck Surgery, MMC 396, 420 Delaware St, Minneapolis, MN 55455-0932; **Phone:** 612-625-2410; **Board Cert:** Otolaryngology 1995; **Med School:** Stanford Univ 1989; **Resid:** Otolaryngology, Johns Hopkins Hosp 1994; **Fellow:** Otolaryngology, Johns Hopkins Hosp 1995; **Fac Appt:** Assoc Prof Oto, Univ Minn

Great Plains and Mountains

Abaza, Mona M MD [Oto] - **Spec Exp:** Voice Disorders; Swallowing Disorders; **Hospital:** Univ Colorado Hosp; **Address:** 1635 Aurora Ct, Aurora, CO 80045; **Phone:** 720-848-2820; **Board Cert:** Otolaryngology 1999; **Med School:** Med Coll PA Hahnemann 1991; **Resid:** Otolaryngology, Univ TX Hlth Sci Ctr 1998; **Fellow:** Research, Natl Insts of Deafness & Communicative Disorders 1994; Laryngology, Jefferson Univ Hosp 1999; **Fac Appt:** Assoc Prof Oto, Univ Colorado

Chowdhury, Khalid MD [Oto] - **Spec Exp:** Skull Base Tumors & Surgery; Craniofacial Surgery; Cosmetic Surgery-Face; **Hospital:** Presby - St Luke's Med Ctr, Chldn's Hosp - Aurora, The; **Address:** Center for Craniofacial Surgery, 1601 E 19th Ave, Ste 3000, Denver, CO 80218; **Phone:** 303-839-5155; **Board Cert:** Otolaryngology 1990; Facial Plastic & Reconstr Surgery 1995; **Med School:** Univ Saskatchewan 1982; **Resid:** Surgery, Univ Saskatchewan Hosp 1985; Otolaryngology, McGill Univ Hosps 1989; **Fellow:** Craniofacial Surgery, Univ Bern Hosp 1990; Facial Plastic & Reconstr Surgery, Univ Bern Hosp 1990; **Fac Appt:** Assoc Prof Oto, Univ Colorado

Denenberg, Steven M MD [Oto] - **Spec Exp:** Cosmetic Surgery-Face; Rhinoplasty; **Hospital:** Nebraska Meth Hosp, Alegent Hlth - Bergan Mercy Med Ctr; **Address:** 7640 Pacific St, Omaha, NE 68114-5421; **Phone:** 402-391-7640; **Board Cert:** Otolaryngology 1984; Facial Plastic & Reconstr Surgery 1992; **Med School:** Univ Nebr Coll Med 1980; **Resid:** Otolaryngology, Stanford Univ Med Ctr 1984; **Fellow:** Facial Plastic Surgery, McCollough Ctr 1985; **Fac Appt:** Asst Clin Prof Oto, Univ Nebr Coll Med

Jenkins, Herman A MD [Oto] - **Spec Exp:** Ear Disorders/Surgery; Neuro-Otology; Acoustic Neuroma; Cochlear Implants; **Hospital:** Univ Colorado Hosp, Chldn's Hosp - Aurora, The; **Address:** Univ Colorado Hosp, Dept Otolaryngology, PO Box 6510, MS F737, Aurora, CO 80045; **Phone:** 720-848-2820; **Board Cert:** Otolaryngology 1977; Neurotology 2004; **Med School:** Vanderbilt Univ 1970; **Resid:** Surgery, UCLA Med Ctr 1972; Otolaryngology, UCLA Med Ctr 1977; **Fellow:** Neurotology, Univ Hosp 1980; **Fac Appt:** Prof Oto, Univ Colorado

Kingdom, Todd T MD [Oto] - **Spec Exp:** Nasal & Sinus Disorders; Endoscopic Sinus Surgery; Skull Base Surgery; **Hospital:** Univ Colorado Hosp, Natl Jewish Med & Rsch Ctr; **Address:** Univ Colorado Hospital, PO Box 6510, MS F737, Aurora, CO 80045; **Phone:** 720-848-2820; **Board Cert:** Otolaryngology 1997; **Med School:** Emory Univ 1991; **Resid:** Otolaryngology, UCSF Med Ctr 1996; **Fac Appt:** Assoc Prof Oto, Univ Colorado

Leopold, Donald Arthur MD [Oto] - **Spec Exp:** Olfactory Disorders; Sinus Disorders/Surgery; **Hospital:** Nebraska Med Ctr; **Address:** Univ Nebr, Dept Oto-Head & Neck Surg, 981225 Nebraska Med Ctr, Omaha, NE 68198-1225; **Phone:** 402-559-5208; **Board Cert:** Otolaryngology 1978; Facial Plastic & Reconstr Surgery 1991; **Med School:** Ohio State Univ 1973; **Resid:** Surgery, St Luke's Med Ctr 1974; Otolaryngology, Univ Iowa Affil Hosp 1978; **Fac Appt:** Prof Oto, Univ Nebr Coll Med

Lydiatt, Daniel D MD/DDS [Oto] - **Spec Exp:** Head & Neck Cancer; **Hospital:** Methodist Hosp - Omaha, Nebraska Med Ctr; **Address:** 981225 Nebraska Medical Ctr, Omaha, NE 68198-1225; **Phone:** 402-559-6500; **Board Cert:** Otolaryngology 1992; **Med School:** Univ Nebr Coll Med 1983; **Resid:** Otolaryngology, Univ Nebraska Med Ctr 1990; **Fellow:** Head and Neck Surgery, MD Anderson Med Ctr 1991; **Fac Appt:** Assoc Prof Oto, Univ Nebr Coll Med

Lydiatt, William M MD [Oto] - **Spec Exp:** Head & Neck Cancer; Thyroid Cancer; Salivary Gland Tumors & Surgery; **Hospital:** Nebraska Med Ctr, Nebraska Meth Hosp; **Address:** 981225 Nebraska Medical Ctr, Omaha, NE 68198-1225; **Phone:** 402-559-6500; **Board Cert:** Otolaryngology 1994; **Med School:** Univ Nebr Coll Med 1988; **Resid:** Otolaryngology, Univ Nebraska Med Ctr 1993; **Fellow:** Head and Neck Surgery, Meml Sloan Kettering Cancer Ctr 1995; **Fac Appt:** Prof Oto, Univ Nebr Coll Med

Shelton, Clough MD [Oto] - **Spec Exp:** Facial Nerve Disorders; Acoustic Neuroma; Hearing & Balance Disorders; Cochlear Implants; **Hospital:** Univ Utah Hosps and Clins; **Address:** Univi Utah Sch Med, 50 N Medical Drive, 1900 East, Ste 3C120, Salt Lake City, UT 84132; **Phone:** 801-585-5450; **Board Cert:** Otolaryngology 1986; Neurotology 2004; **Med School:** Univ Tex SW, Dallas 1981; **Resid:** Otolaryngology, Stanford Univ Med Ctr 1986; **Fellow:** Neurotology, Otologic Med Group 1987; **Fac Appt:** Prof Oto, Univ Utah

Otolaryngology

Song, John I MD [Oto] - **Spec Exp:** Head & Neck Cancer; Skull Base Tumors; Swallowing Disorders; **Hospital:** Univ Colorado Hosp; **Address:** Univ Colorado Hosp, Otolaryngology, 12605 E 16th Ave, MS F737, PO Box 6510, Denver, CO 80219; **Phone:** 720-848-2820; **Board Cert:** Otolaryngology 1998; **Med School:** NYU Sch Med 1991; **Resid:** Otolaryngology, UCLA Med Ctr 1997; **Fellow:** Head and Neck Surgery, Univ Pittsburgh Med Ctr 1998; **Fac Appt:** Asst Prof Oto, Univ Colorado

Southwest

Clark, Keith F MD [Oto] - **Spec Exp:** Pediatric Otolaryngology; Airway Reconstruction; Voice Disorders; Vocal Cord Disorders-Botox Therapy; **Hospital:** St Anthony Hosp -Oklahoma City; **Address:** 535 NW 9th St, Ste 300, Oklahoma City, OK 73102; **Phone:** 405-272-6027; **Board Cert:** Otolaryngology 1983; **Med School:** Univ Mich Med Sch 1978; **Resid:** Otolaryngology, Univ Iowa Med Ctr 1983

Clayman, Gary Lee MD/DMD [Oto] - **Spec Exp:** Thyroid Cancer & Surgery; Salivary Gland Tumors & Surgery; Head & Neck Cancer; Thyroid & Parathyroid Surgery; **Hospital:** UT MD Anderson Cancer Ctr; **Address:** Univ TX/MD Anderson Cancer Center, 1515 Holcombe Blvd, Box 1445, Houston, TX 77030-4009; **Phone:** 713-792-8837; **Board Cert:** Otolaryngology 1992; **Med School:** NE Ohio Univ 1986; **Resid:** Surgery, Hennepin Co Med Ctr 1987; Otolaryngology, Univ Minn Med Ctr 1991; **Fellow:** Head and Neck Surgery, MD Anderson Cancer Ctr 1993; **Fac Appt:** Prof Oto, Univ Tex, Houston

Daspit, C Phillip MD [Oto] - **Spec Exp:** Hearing & Balance Disorders; Cochlear Implants; Chronic Ear Disease; **Hospital:** St Joseph's Hosp & Med Ctr - Phoenix; **Address:** 222 W Thomas Rd, Ste 114, Phoenix, AZ 85013; **Phone:** 602-279-5444; **Board Cert:** Otolaryngology 1977; **Med School:** Louisiana State U, New Orleans 1968; **Resid:** Surgery, UCSF Med Ctr 1973; Otolaryngology, Ft Miley VA Hosp 1977; **Fellow:** Otology & Neurotology, House Ear Inst 1978; Skull Base Surgery, House Ear Inst 1978; **Fac Appt:** Clin Prof S, Univ Ariz Coll Med

Donovan, Donald T MD [Oto] - **Spec Exp:** Head & Neck Cancer; Voice Disorders; Vocal Cord Disorders; Thyroid Disorders; **Hospital:** Methodist Hosp - Houston, St Luke's Episcopal Hosp-Houston; **Address:** 6550 Fannin St, Ste 1701, Houston, TX 77030; **Phone:** 713-798-3380; **Board Cert:** Otolaryngology 1981; **Med School:** Baylor Coll Med 1976; **Resid:** Surgery, Baylor Affil Hosps 1978; Otolaryngology, Baylor Affil Hosps 1981; **Fellow:** Head and Neck Surgery, Columbia-Presby Med Ctr 1982; **Fac Appt:** Prof Oto, Baylor Coll Med

Dornhoffer, John L MD [Oto] - **Spec Exp:** Hearing & Balance Disorders; Neurotology; Hearing Loss; **Hospital:** UAMS Med Ctr; **Address:** UAMS, Dept Otolaryngology, Head & Neck Surgery, 4301 W Markham St, #543, Little Rock, AR 72205; **Phone:** 501-686-5878; **Board Cert:** Otolaryngology 1994; **Med School:** Univ Kans 1988; **Resid:** Otolaryngology, UAMS Med Ctr 1992; **Fellow:** Otology, Univ of Zurich Affil Hosp 1994; Otology, Univ of Wuzburg Affil Hosp 1994; **Fac Appt:** Prof Oto, Univ Ark

Gianoli, Gerard MD [Oto] - **Spec Exp:** Dizziness; Hearing Loss; Ear Disorders; **Hospital:** North Oaks Med Ctr; **Address:** 17050 Medical Center Drive, Ste 315, The Ear & Balance Institute, Baton Rouge, LA 70816-3249; **Phone:** 225-293-6973; **Board Cert:** Otolaryngology 1993; Neurotology 2004; **Med School:** Tulane Univ 1986; **Resid:** Pediatrics, Tulane Univ 1988; Otolaryngology, Tulane Univ 1992; **Fellow:** Otology & Neurotology, Michigan Ear Inst; **Fac Appt:** Assoc Clin Prof Oto, Tulane Univ

Hanna, Ehab YN MD [Oto] - **Spec Exp:** Skull Base Tumors & Surgery; Head & Neck Cancer & Surgery; **Hospital:** UT MD Anderson Cancer Ctr; **Address:** Univ Tex MD Anderson Cancer Ctr, 1515 Holcolmbe Blvd, Unit 1445, Houston, TX 77030; **Phone:** 713-745-1815; **Board Cert:** Otolaryngology 1994; **Med School:** Egypt 1982; **Resid:** Otolaryngology, Cleveland Clinic 1989; Otolaryngology, Cleveland Clinic 1993; **Fellow:** Otolaryngology, Univ Pittsburgh Med Ctr 1994; **Fac Appt:** Prof Oto, Univ Tex, Houston

Hayden, Richard E MD [Oto] - **Spec Exp:** Head & Neck Surgery; Facial Plastic & Reconstructive Surgery; Microvascular Surgery; **Hospital:** Mayo Clinic - Phoenix; **Address:** Mayo Clinic, Dept Otolaryngology, 5777 E Mayo Blvd, Phoenix, AZ 85054; **Phone:** 480-342-2912; **Board Cert:** Otolaryngology 1978; **Med School:** McGill Univ 1974; **Resid:** Otolaryngology, Univ Toronto Affil Hosp 1978; **Fellow:** Head & Neck Oncology, MD Anderson Hosp 1979; Radiation Oncology, Princess Margaret Hosp 1980; **Fac Appt:** Prof Oto, Mayo Med Sch

Johnson Jr, Calvin M MD [Oto] - **Spec Exp:** Ear Disorders/Surgery; Nasal Surgery; Cosmetic Surgery-Face; **Address:** Hedgewood Surgical Ctr, 2427 St Charles Ave, New Orleans, LA 70130; **Phone:** 504-895-7642; **Board Cert:** Otolaryngology 1974; **Med School:** Tulane Univ 1967; **Resid:** Surgery, Tulane Univ Sch Med 1971; Otolaryngology, Tulane Univ Sch Med 1974; **Fellow:** Facial Plastic Surgery, Amer Academy Facial Plastic & Recon Surg 1975

Macias, John D MD [Oto] - **Spec Exp:** Otology; Neuro-Otology; Cochlear Implants; Hearing Loss; **Hospital:** Banner Good Samaritan Regl Med Ctr - Phoenix, Phoenix Children's Hosp; **Address:** 1515 N 9th St, Ste B, Phoenix, AZ 85006-2523; **Phone:** 602-257-4228; **Board Cert:** Otolaryngology 1994; Neurotology 2005; **Med School:** Stanford Univ 1988; **Resid:** Otolaryngology, Univ Iowa Hosps & Clins 1993; **Fellow:** Otology & Neurotology, Ear Fdn/Otology Grp 1994

Medina, Jesus E MD [Oto] - **Spec Exp:** Head & Neck Cancer & Surgery; **Hospital:** OU Med Ctr; **Address:** OU Physicians, Dept Otolaryngology, 825 NE 10th St, Ste 4200, Oklahoma City, OK 73104; **Phone:** 405-271-7559; **Board Cert:** Otolaryngology 1980; **Med School:** Peru 1974; **Resid:** Surgery, Wayne St Univ Affil Hosp 1977; Otolaryngology, Wayne St Univ Affil Hosp 1980; **Fellow:** Head and Neck Surgery, Univ Tex Cancer Ctrs 1981; **Fac Appt:** Prof Oto, Univ Okla Coll Med

Myers, Jeffrey N MD/PhD [Oto] - **Spec Exp:** Head & Neck Cancer; Melanoma-Head & Neck; Tongue Cancer; **Hospital:** UT MD Anderson Cancer Ctr; **Address:** Univ Texas MD Anderson Cancer Ctr, 1515 Holcombe Blvd, Box 441, Houston, TX 77030; **Phone:** 713-745-2667; **Board Cert:** Otolaryngology 1997; **Med School:** Univ Pennsylvania 1991; **Resid:** Otolaryngology, Univ Pittsburgh Med Ctr 1996; **Fellow:** Head & Neck Surgical Oncology, MD Anderson Cancer Ctr 1997; **Fac Appt:** Assoc Prof Oto, Univ Tex, Houston

Nuss, Daniel W MD [Oto] - **Spec Exp:** Head & Neck Cancer; Skull Base Tumors & Surgery; **Hospital:** Our Lady of the Lake Regl Med Ctr; **Address:** Our Lady of the Lake Regl Med Ctr, 7777 Hennessy Blvd, Ste 409, Baton Rouge, LA 70808; **Phone:** 225-765-1765; **Board Cert:** Otolaryngology 1987; **Med School:** Louisiana State U, New Orleans 1981; **Resid:** Surgery, Charity Hosp 1983; Otolaryngology, LSU Med Ctr 1987; **Fellow:** Surgical Oncology, MD Anderson Hosp & Tumor Inst 1984; Head and Neck Surgery, Ctr Cranial Base Surg-Univ Pittsburgh 1991; **Fac Appt:** Prof Oto, Louisiana State U, New Orleans

Otto, Randal A MD [Oto] - **Spec Exp:** Head & Neck Cancer; Thyroid & Parathyroid Cancer & Surgery; Sinus Disorders/Surgery; **Hospital:** Univ Hlth Syst-San Antonio, Audie L Murphy Meml Vets Hosp; **Address:** 7703 Floyd Curl Drive, MS 7777, San Antonio, TX 78229-3900; **Phone:** 210-567-5655; **Board Cert:** Otolaryngology 1987; **Med School:** Univ MO-Columbia Sch Med 1981; **Resid:** Pathology, Queens Med Ctr 1982; Otolaryngology, Univ of Missouri 1987; **Fac Appt:** Prof Oto, Univ Tex, San Antonio

Otolaryngology

Stasney, C Richard MD [Oto] - **Spec Exp:** Voice Disorders; Vocal Cord Disorders; Laryngeal Disorders; **Hospital:** Methodist Hosp - Houston; **Address:** Texas ENT Consultants, 6550 Fannin St, Ste 2025, Houston, TX 77030; **Phone:** 713-796-2001; **Board Cert:** Otolaryngology 1974; **Med School:** Baylor Coll Med 1969; **Resid:** Surgery, Baylor Affil Hosps 1971; Otolaryngology, Baylor Affil Hosps 1974; **Fac Appt:** Clin Prof Oto, Cornell Univ-Weill Med Coll

Suen, James Y MD [Oto] - **Spec Exp:** Head & Neck Cancer; Vascular Lesions-Head & Neck; Laryngeal Disorders; Thyroid Cancer; **Hospital:** UAMS Med Ctr, Arkansas Chldns Hosp; **Address:** Univ Hosp Arkansas Med Scis, 4301 W Markham St, Slot 543, Little Rock, AR 72205; **Phone:** 501-686-8224; **Board Cert:** Otolaryngology 1973; **Med School:** Univ Ark 1966; **Resid:** Surgery, Univ Arkansas Med Ctr 1970; Otolaryngology, Univ Arkansas Med Ctr 1973; **Fellow:** Head and Neck Surgery, MD Anderson Cancer Ctr-Tumor Inst 1974; **Fac Appt:** Prof Oto, Univ Ark

Weber, Randal S MD [Oto] - **Spec Exp:** Skin Cancer; Thyroid & Parathyroid Cancer & Surgery; Salivary Gland Tumors & Surgery; Head & Neck Cancer; **Hospital:** UT MD Anderson Cancer Ctr; **Address:** 1515 Holcombe Blvd, Unit 441, Houston, TX 77030-4009; **Phone:** 713-745-0497; **Board Cert:** Otolaryngology 1985; **Med School:** Univ Tenn Coll Med, Memphis 1976; **Resid:** Surgery, Baylor Coll Med 1982; Otolaryngology, Baylor Coll Med 1985; **Fellow:** Head and Neck Surgery, MD Anderson Cancer Ctr 1986; **Fac Appt:** Prof Oto, Univ Tex, Houston

Weber, Samuel C MD [Oto] - **Spec Exp:** Thyroid Cancer; Parathyroid Cancer; Nasal & Sinus Cancer & Surgery; Head & Neck Surgery; **Hospital:** St Luke's Episcopal Hosp-Houston, Methodist Chldns Hosp of South Texas; **Address:** 6624 Fannin St, Ste 1480, Houston, TX 77030-2385; **Phone:** 713-795-5343; **Board Cert:** Otolaryngology 1972; **Med School:** Univ Tenn Coll Med, Memphis 1965; **Resid:** Surgery, Baylor Coll Med 1971; Otolaryngology, Baylor Coll Med 1972; **Fac Appt:** Clin Prof Oto, Univ Tex, San Antonio

West Coast and Pacific

Berke, Gerald S MD [Oto] - **Spec Exp:** Head & Neck Surgery; Head & Neck Cancer; Voice Disorders; Laryngeal Disorders; **Hospital:** UCLA Ronald Reagan Med Ctr; **Address:** 200 UCLA Med Plaza, Ste 550, Los Angeles, CA 90095; **Phone:** 310-825-5179; **Board Cert:** Otolaryngology 1984; **Med School:** USC Sch Med 1978; **Resid:** Otolaryngology, LAC-USC Med Ctr 1979; **Fellow:** Head and Neck Surgery, UCLA Med Ctr 1984; **Fac Appt:** Prof Oto, UCLA

Brackmann, Derald E MD [Oto] - **Spec Exp:** Ear Disorders/Surgery; Facial Nerve Disorders; Acoustic Neuroma; Otosclerosis Surgery/Stapedectomy; **Hospital:** St Vincent's Med Ctr - Los Angeles, USC Univ Hosp; **Address:** House Clinic, 2100 W 3rd St, Fl 1st, Los Angeles, CA 90057-1902; **Phone:** 213-483-9930; **Board Cert:** Otolaryngology 1971; Neurotology 2005; **Med School:** Univ IL Coll Med 1962; **Resid:** Otolaryngology, LAC/USC Med Ctr 1970; **Fellow:** Otology & Neurotology, House Ear Clinic 1971; **Fac Appt:** Clin Prof Oto, USC-Keck School of Medicine

Cohen, James I MD [Oto] - **Hospital:** VA Medical Center - Portland; **Address:** Portland VAMC P3-OC, 3710 US Veteran's Hospital Rd, Portland, OR 97239; **Phone:** 503-220-8262; **Board Cert:** Otolaryngology 1984; **Med School:** Univ Manitoba 1978; **Resid:** Surgery, Univ Minn Med Ctr 1980; Otolaryngology, Univ Minn Med Ctr 1984; **Fellow:** Head & Neck Surgical Oncology, MD Anderson Cancer Ctr 1985; **Fac Appt:** Prof Oto, Oregon Hlth & Sci Univ

Courey, Mark S MD [Oto] - **Spec Exp:** Laryngeal Disorders; Swallowing Disorders; Laryngeal Cancer; **Hospital:** UCSF - Mt Zion Med Ctr, UCSF Med Ctr; **Address:** UCSF Voice & Swallowing Ctr, 2330 Post St, Ste 526, San Francisco, CA 94115; **Phone:** 415-885-7700; **Board Cert:** Otolaryngology 1993; **Med School:** SUNY Buffalo 1987; **Resid:** Otolaryngology, SUNY-Buffalo Med Ctr 1992; **Fellow:** Laryngology, Vanderbilt Univ 1993; **Fac Appt:** Prof Oto, UCSF

De la Cruz, Antonio MD [Oto] - **Spec Exp:** Otosclerosis/Stapedectomy; Acoustic Neuroma; Otology; **Hospital:** St Vincent's Med Ctr - Los Angeles, Torrance Memorial Med Ctr; **Address:** 2100 W 3rd St Fl 1, Los Angeles, CA 90057; **Phone:** 213-483-9930; **Board Cert:** Otolaryngology 1973; **Med School:** Costa Rica 1967; **Resid:** Surgery, Univ Miami Med Ctr 1970; Otolaryngology, Univ Miami Med Ctr 1973; **Fellow:** Otology & Neurotology, House Ear Clinic 1974; **Fac Appt:** Clin Prof Oto, USC Sch Med

Donald, Paul MD [Oto] - **Spec Exp:** Skull Base Tumors & Surgery; Head & Neck Cancer; **Hospital:** UC Davis Med Ctr; **Address:** 2521 Stockton Blvd, rm 7200, Sacramento, CA 95817; **Phone:** 916-734-2832; **Board Cert:** Otolaryngology 1973; **Med School:** Univ British Columbia Fac Med 1964; **Resid:** Surgery, St Pauls Hosp 1969; Otolaryngology, Univ Iowa Hosp 1973; **Fac Appt:** Prof Oto, UC Davis

Eisele, David W MD [Oto] - **Spec Exp:** Salivary Gland Tumors & Surgery; Head & Neck Cancer; Thyroid Cancer; **Hospital:** UCSF Med Ctr; **Address:** UCSF, Dept Head & Neck Surgery, 2380 Sutter St Fl 2nd, Box 1703, San Francisco, CA 94115-1703; **Phone:** 415-885-7528; **Board Cert:** Otolaryngology 1988; **Med School:** Cornell Univ-Weill Med Coll 1982; **Resid:** Surgery, Univ Wash Med Ctr 1984; Otolaryngology, Univ Wash Med Ctr 1988; **Fac Appt:** Prof Oto, UCSF

Fee Jr, Willard E MD [Oto] - **Spec Exp:** Head & Neck Cancer; Parotid Gland Tumors; Thyroid Cancer; **Hospital:** Stanford Univ Med Ctr; **Address:** Stanford Cancer Ctr, 875 Lake Wilbur Dr, CC-2227, Stanford, CA 94305-5826; **Phone:** 650-498-6000; **Board Cert:** Otolaryngology 1974; **Med School:** Univ Colorado 1969; **Resid:** Surgery, Wadsworth VA Hosp 1971; Otolaryngology, UCLA Med Ctr 1974; **Fac Appt:** Prof Oto, Stanford Univ

Flint, Paul W MD [Oto] - **Spec Exp:** Voice Disorders; Laryngeal Disorders; **Hospital:** OR Hlth & Sci Univ; **Address:** Oregon Health & Science Univ, 3181 SW Sam Jackson Park Rd, PV01, Portland, OR 97239; **Phone:** 503-494-0619; **Board Cert:** Otolaryngology 1989; **Med School:** Baylor Coll Med 1983; **Resid:** Surgery, Univ Washington 1985; Otolaryngology, Univ Washington 1989; **Fellow:** Otolaryngology, Guys Hosp 1989; **Fac Appt:** Prof Oto, Oregon Hlth & Sci Univ

Futran, Neal D MD/DMD [Oto] - **Spec Exp:** Head & Neck Cancer & Surgery; Head & Neck Cancer Reconstruction; Skull Base Tumors & Surgery; **Hospital:** Univ Wash Med Ctr, Harborview Med Ctr; **Address:** U Wash Med Ctr, Oto Office, 1959 NE Pacific St, Box 356515, Seattle, WA 98195-6515; **Phone:** 206-543-3060; **Board Cert:** Otolaryngology 1993; **Med School:** SUNY Downstate 1987; **Resid:** Surgery, Kings Co-SUNY Downstate 1985; Otolaryngology, Univ Rochester Med Ctr 1992; **Fellow:** Microvascular Surgery, Mt Sinai Hosp 1993; **Fac Appt:** Prof Oto, Univ Wash

Harris, Jeffrey P MD/PhD [Oto] - **Spec Exp:** Neuro-Otology; Hearing & Balance Disorders; Skull Base Surgery; **Hospital:** UCSD Med Ctr, VA San Diego Hlthcre Sys; **Address:** UCSD Med Ctr, 200 W Arbor Drive, MC 8895, San Diego, CA 92103-8895; **Phone:** 858-657-8590; **Board Cert:** Otolaryngology 1979; Neurotology 2004; **Med School:** Univ Pennsylvania 1974; **Resid:** Otolaryngology, Mass EE Infirmary 1979; **Fellow:** Neurological Surgery, Univ Zurich Med Ctr 1983; **Fac Appt:** Prof S, UCSD

Jackler, Robert K MD [Oto] - **Spec Exp:** Neuro-Otology; Skull Base Surgery; Ear Tumors; **Hospital:** Stanford Univ Med Ctr; **Address:** Stanford Univ Med Ctr, Dept Head & Neck Surg, 801 Welch Rd, Stanford, CA 94305-5739; **Phone:** 650-725-6500; **Board Cert:** Otolaryngology 1984; Neurotology 2004; **Med School:** Boston Univ 1979; **Resid:** Otolaryngology, UCSF Med Ctr 1984; **Fellow:** Otolaryngology, Oto Med Grp 1985; **Fac Appt:** Prof Oto, Stanford Univ

Otolaryngology

Kaplan, Michael J MD [Oto] - **Spec Exp:** Head & Neck Surgery; Skull Base Surgery; Head & Neck Cancer; **Hospital:** Stanford Univ Med Ctr; **Address:** Stanford Cancer Ctr, Dept Otolaryngology, 801 Welch Rd Fl 2, Stanford, CA 94305-5739; **Phone:** 650-498-6000; **Board Cert:** Otolaryngology 1982; **Med School:** Harvard Med Sch 1977; **Resid:** Surgery, Beth Israel-Chldns Hosps 1979; Otolaryngology, Mass EE Infirm 1982; **Fellow:** Head and Neck Surgery, Univ Virginia 1984; **Fac Appt:** Prof Oto, Stanford Univ

Keller, Gregory S MD [Oto] - **Spec Exp:** Cosmetic Surgery-Face; **Hospital:** Santa Barbara Cottage Hosp, UCLA Ronald Reagan Med Ctr; **Address:** 221 W Pueblo St, Ste A, Santa Barbara, CA 93105; **Phone:** 805-687-6408; **Board Cert:** Otolaryngology 1976; **Med School:** Univ IL Coll Med 1971; **Resid:** Surgery, Cottage Hosp 1973; Otolaryngology, Univ Illinois 1976; **Fac Appt:** Assoc Clin Prof S, UCLA

Larrabee Jr, Wayne F MD [Oto] - **Spec Exp:** Cosmetic Surgery-Face; Eyelid Surgery; Rhinoplasty; Nasal Surgery; **Hospital:** Swedish Med Ctr - Seattle; **Address:** Facial Plastic Surgery Ctr, 600 Broadway Ste 280, Seattle, WA 98122-5371; **Phone:** 206-386-3550; **Board Cert:** Otolaryngology 1979; Facial Plastic & Reconstr Surgery 1999; **Med School:** Tulane Univ 1971; **Resid:** Surgery, Charity Hosp 1976; Otolaryngology, Tulane Univ Med Ctr 1979; **Fac Appt:** Clin Prof Oto, Univ Wash

McMenomey, Sean O MD [Oto] - **Spec Exp:** Otology & Neuro-Otology; Skull Base Tumors & Surgery; Head & Neck Surgery; Stereotactic Radiosurgery; **Hospital:** OR Hlth & Sci Univ, Providence St Vincent Med Ctr; **Address:** Oregon Hlth & Sci Univ, Dept Otolaryngology, 3181 SW Sam Jackson Park Rd, MC PV-01, Portland, OR 97239; **Phone:** 503-494-8135; **Board Cert:** Otolaryngology 1993; Neurotology 2004; **Med School:** St Louis Univ 1987; **Resid:** Otolaryngology, Oregon Hlth Sci Ctr 1992; **Fellow:** Otology & Neurotology, Baptist Hosp 1993; **Fac Appt:** Assoc Prof Oto, Oregon Hlth & Sci Univ

Powell, Nelson B MD/DDS [Oto] - **Spec Exp:** Sleep Disorders/Apnea; Maxillofacial Surgery; **Hospital:** Stanford Univ Med Ctr; **Address:** 750 Welch Rd, Ste 317, Palo Alto, CA 94304; **Phone:** 650-328-0511; **Board Cert:** Otolaryngology 1984; **Med School:** Univ Wash 1979; **Resid:** Surgery, Stanford Univ Hosp & Clinics 1980; Otolaryngology, Stanford Univ Hosp 1983; **Fac Appt:** Clin Prof S, Stanford Univ

Rice, Dale MD [Oto] - **Spec Exp:** Head & Neck Cancer; Sinus Disorders/Surgery; **Hospital:** USC Univ Hosp, USC Norris Cancer Hosp; **Address:** USC Keck Sch Med, 1200 N State St, rm 4316, Los Angeles, CA 90033-1029; **Phone:** 323-442-5790; **Board Cert:** Otolaryngology 1976; **Med School:** Univ Mich Med Sch 1968; **Resid:** Surgery, Univ Mich Med Ctr 1970; Otolaryngology, Univ Mich Med Ctr 1976; **Fac Appt:** Prof Oto, USC Sch Med

Senders, Craig W MD [Oto] - **Spec Exp:** Pediatric Otolaryngology; Cleft Palate/Lip; Endoscopic Sinus Surgery; Sleep Disorders/Apnea; **Hospital:** UC Davis Med Ctr; **Address:** UC Davis, Dept Oto-Head & Neck Surg, 2521 Stockton Blvd, Ste 7200, Sacramento, CA 95817; **Phone:** 916-734-5400; **Board Cert:** Otolaryngology 1984; **Med School:** Oregon Hlth & Sci Univ 1979; **Resid:** Otolaryngology, Univ Iowa Hosps & Clins 1983; **Fellow:** Maxillofacial Surgery, Univ Iowa Hosps & Clins 1984; **Fac Appt:** Prof Oto, UC Davis

Shindo, Maisie L MD [Oto] - **Spec Exp:** Head & Neck Cancer & Surgery; Thyroid Cancer; Laryngeal Cancer; Parathyroid Cancer; **Hospital:** OR Hlth & Sci Univ; **Address:** Thyroid & Parathyroid Clinic, 3181 SW Sam Jackson Park Rd, Ste 250, Physicians Pavilion, PV-01, Portland, OR 97239-3098; **Phone:** 503-494-2544; **Board Cert:** Otolaryngology 1989; **Med School:** Univ Saskatchewan 1984; **Resid:** Otolaryngology, LAC-USC Med Ctr 1989; **Fellow:** Head and Neck Surgery, Northwestern Univ 1991; **Fac Appt:** Prof Oto, Oregon Hlth & Sci Univ

Singer, Mark I MD [Oto] - **Spec Exp:** Head & Neck Surgery; Head & Neck Cancer; Melanoma; **Hospital:** CA Pacific Med Ctr; **Address:** 2340 Clay St Fl 2, San Francisco, CA 94115; **Phone:** 415-600-2450; **Board Cert:** Otolaryngology 1976; **Med School:** Columbia P&S 1970; **Resid:** Surgery, Northwestern Meml Hosp 1973; Otolaryngology, Northwestern Meml Hosp 1976; **Fellow:** Oncology, Northwestern Meml Hosp 1976

Sinha, Uttam K MD [Oto] - **Spec Exp:** Head & Neck Cancer; Voice Disorders; **Hospital:** USC Univ Hosp, House Ear Inst; **Address:** 1200 N State St, rm 4136, Los Angeles, CA 90033; **Phone:** 323-226-7315; **Board Cert:** Otolaryngology 1998; **Med School:** India 1985; **Resid:** Otolaryngology, LAC-USC Med Ctr 1995; **Fellow:** Microvascular Surgery, Mount Sinai Med Ctr 1996; Laryngology 1997; **Fac Appt:** Assoc Prof Oto, USC Sch Med

Wax, Mark K MD [Oto] - **Spec Exp:** Facial Nerve Disorders; Skull Base Tumors & Surgery; Facial Plastic & Reconstructive Surgery; Microvascular Surgery; **Hospital:** OR Hlth & Sci Univ; **Address:** Oregon Hlth Scis Univ, Dept Ototlaryngology, 3181 SW Sam Jackson Park Rd, Ste PV-01, Portland, OR 97201; **Phone:** 503-494-5355; **Board Cert:** Otolaryngology 1985; Facial Plastic & Reconstr Surgery 1987; **Med School:** Univ Toronto 1980; **Resid:** Otolaryngology, Univ Toronto 1985; Surgery, Cedars-Sinai Med Ctr 1983; **Fellow:** Head and Neck Surgery, St Michaels Hosp 1991; **Fac Appt:** Prof Oto, Oregon Hlth & Sci Univ

Weisman, Robert A MD [Oto] - **Spec Exp:** Head & Neck Cancer; Clinical Trials; Thyroid & Parathyroid Cancer & Surgery; Head & Neck Cancer Reconstruction; **Hospital:** UCSD Med Ctr; **Address:** Moores-UCSD Cancer Center, 3855 Health Sciences Drive, MC 0987, La Jolla, CA 92093-0987; **Phone:** 858-822-6197; **Board Cert:** Otolaryngology 1978; **Med School:** Washington Univ, St Louis 1973; **Resid:** Head and Neck Surgery, UCLA Med Ctr 1978; **Fac Appt:** Prof S, UCSD

Weymuller, Ernest MD [Oto] - **Spec Exp:** Head & Neck Cancer; Sinus Disorders/Surgery; **Hospital:** Univ Wash Med Ctr; **Address:** 1959 NE Pacific St, Box 356161, Seattle, WA 98195-6161; **Phone:** 206-598-4022; **Board Cert:** Otolaryngology 1973; **Med School:** Harvard Med Sch 1966; **Resid:** Surgery, Vanderbilt Univ Hosp 1968; Otolaryngology, Mass Eye and Ear Infirm 1973; **Fac Appt:** Prof Oto, Univ Wash

Cleveland Clinic

Head and Neck Institute

The specialists at the Cleveland Clinic Head and Neck Institute have been recognized nationally and internationally as leaders in this multidisciplinary field. The Institute is composed of specialists with extensive training in all areas, including:

Audiology: Audiologists provide the non-medical management of hearing disorders including comprehensive audiologic evaluation and treatment through the use of assistive listening devices, hearing aids, Baha Hearing Systems, and cochlear implants.

Facial Plastic and Reconstructive Surgery: Surgeons perform a broad range of procedures, from office-based treatments including Botox and Restylane injections to operative procedures ranging from rhinoplasty and facelifts to major facial reconstructive surgery, including the world's first near-total face transplant.

The Cleveland Clinic Head and Neck Institute has been routinely recognized among the best programs in the United States by *U.S.News & World Report* magazine.

With more than 30 full-time faculty members caring for adult and pediatric patients with routine or complex ear, nose and throat disorders, the Institute is one of the largest otolaryngology programs in the United States.

Head and Neck Surgery: Evaluation and treatment of both benign and malignant head and neck tumors. Patients are seen in a team fashion by surgeons, radiation therapists and oncologists to facilitate optimal treatment.

Laryngotracheal Reconstruction: Laryngeal airway obstruction, esophageal reflux, tracheal aspiration, and voice preservation and rehabilitation and removal of upper and lower respiratory foreign bodies.

The Voice Center: The Voice Center represents a dedicated center of excellence to uniquely serve the voice disordered population, with special focus on the professional voice user.

Nasal and Sinus Disorders: Treatment of a wide variety of sinonasal conditions, including rhinosinusitus, nasal polyps, fungal sinusitis, septal deviation, nasal obstruction and inhalant allergies. Minimally invasive, computer-aided, endoscopic techniques for revision sinus surgery, CSF leaks and neoplasms of the nose, sinuses and skull base.

Otology-Neurotology: Care of all forms of otologic disorders, including middle and posterior cranial fossa surgery for cerebellopontine and skull base tumors. Immune-mediated inner ear disease (deafness), Meniere's disease and cochlear implantation are also handled here.

Pediatric Otolaryngology: Treatment of all forms of pediatric otolaryngologic disorders, with support from Cleveland Clinic Children's Hospital, a pediatric intensive care unit and numerous other pediatric specialists on staff.

Speech-Language Pathology: Comprehensive evaluation and treatment for all speech, language, voice, cognitive and swallowing disorders. Services are provided to pediatric through geriatric patient populations via an interdisciplinary medical care model.

Vestibular and Balance Disorders: Diagnosis and vestibular rehabilitation from dizziness, disequilibrium.

For more information about the Cleveland Clinic Head and Neck Institute, to schedule a second opinion or to learn about assistance for out-of-town patients, call 800.890.2467 or visit www.clevelandclinic.org/headandnecktopdocs.

Head and Neck Institute | 9500 Euclid Avenue / AC311 | Cleveland OH 44195

MOUNT SINAI SCHOOL OF MEDICINE

THE MOUNT SINAI MEDICAL CENTER
OTOLARYNGOLOGY – EAR, NOSE, AND THROAT
One Gustave L. Levy Place
Fifth Avenue and 100th Street
New York, NY 10029-6574
Physician Referral: 1-800-MD-SINAI (637-4624)
www.mountsinai.org

Mount Sinai's **DEPARTMENT OF OTOLARYNGOLOGY** is consistently ranked among the top ear, nose, and throat centers nationwide. The Department is one of the oldest and most respected otolaryngology departments in the US. All of its physicians are board-certified specialists dedicated to healing disorders of the ear, nose, throat, head, and neck. The Department provides the following services:

Robotic Surgery – The Department is spearheading the use of robotic surgery to treat head and neck cancers. The DaVinci Surgical System®, a cutting-edge technology, magnifies the surgical field and gives surgeons greater visualization, dexterity, and precision during an operation, resulting in less-invasive surgical techniques and reduced scarring while also improving outcomes.

Endoscopic Surgery – This technique enables surgeons to remove tumors of the voice box, skull base, and neck without external incisions. Many patients are treated on an outpatient basis.

Cranial Base Surgery – Surgeons at Mount Sinai have developed techniques to remove skull base tumors endoscopically through the nose, leaving no visible sign of surgery. Interdisciplinary teams provide expertise in the diagnosis and treatment of tumors, vascular lesions, and trauma at the base of the brain.

Thyroid and Parathyroid Surgery – Minimally invasive thyroidectomy and parathyroidectomy can be performed through a one-inch incision. We believe that a team approach involving an experienced surgeon, a dedicated endocrinologist, and a team of physicians trained in nuclear medicine is of critical importance for the treatment of thyroid cancers.

Audiology – All aspects of audiology are covered at Mount Sinai, including the performance and interpretation of audiograms, brain stem-evoked potentials, otoacoustic emission testing, neonatal hearing screening, and evaluations for assisted listening devices.

Facial Plastic and Cosmetic Surgery – Our reconstructive facial surgeons and specialists in facial cosmetic surgery use state-of-the-art endoscopic techniques.

Head and Neck Reconstructive Surgery – The Department has some of the most experienced reconstructive surgeons in the world, specializing in microvascular free tissue transfer.

Hearing, Facial Nerve, and Balance Disorders – Multidisciplinary teams provide treatment for a broad range of adult and pediatric neuro-otologic and otologic disorders.

Maxillofacial Prosthodontics – Mount Sinai offers complete services to restore speech and chewing abilities and minimize cosmetic defects.

Nasal and Sinus Surgery – Renowned rhinologists treat all inflammatory and infectious diseases of the nose and sinuses.

Oral and Maxillofacial Surgery – Our team provides all treatment options for patients with congenital, acquired, or traumatic problems of the oral cavity, jaws, and associated structures.

Additionally, The Grabscheid Voice Center offers the highest level of medical care for the professional voice, along with a profound understanding of the special medical, psychological, and professional needs of singers, actors, and lecturers.

A NATIONALLY RENOWNED HEAD AND NECK CANCER TEAM
Mount Sinai's multi-disciplinary head and neck cancer team has gained national recognition for its expertise and innovation in the management of head, neck, and skull-base cancer. Mount Sinai has a nationally recognized team of experts in minimally invasive and endoscopic head and neck surgery. The team comprises a group of surgeons and oncologists focused on curative treatment for head and neck malignancies. The expert team works to treat tumors of the oral cavity, jaw, and larynx and preserve each patient's quality of life. Speech and swallowing rehabilitation therapists work with patients to help them recover. Mount Sinai is on the cutting edge of head and neck cancer therapy, reconstruction, and rehabilitation.

NY Eye & Ear Infirmary

Continuum Health Partners, Inc.

THE NEW YORK EYE AND EAR INFIRMARY

310 East 14th Street
New York, New York 10003
Tel. 212.979.4000   Fax. 212.228.0664
http://www.nyee.edu

PROVIDING EXCEPTIONAL CARE OF THE EAR, NOSE, THROAT, AND HEAD & NECK

Established in 1820 the Department of Otolaryngology/Head & Neck Surgery is the first training program in this specialty in the Western Hemisphere. Over nearly two centuries the department has evolved to be an international referral center for the medical and surgical treatment of diseases of the ear, nose, and throat.

OUTSTANDING SERVICES:

Ear Institute (Otology – Neuro-otology): Specializing in the care of chronic ear disease including hearing loss, cochlear implantation, dizziness, tinnitus, intra cranial tumors and facial nerve disorders. Our advanced otologic and vestibular diagnostic labs assist physicians in treatment.

Facial Plastic Surgery: In-office or ambulatory procedures utilizing computer imaging, new techniques and materials produce outstanding results with minimal incisions, rapid recovery and a natural, youthful appearance.

Facial Paralysis: Comprehensive center treating all causes and offering reconstruction of the paralyzed face.

Head & Neck Oncology: A multi-disciplinary team including board-certified surgeons, medical & radiation oncologists, nutritionists and rehabilitation specialists insure rapid recovery from complex, life-saving surgical procedures and return to daily activities.

Pediatric Otolaryngology: Treating children has long been a priority at the Infirmary. Pediatric care ranges from middle ear infection, tonsil and adenoid disease, and neck masses to complex sinus and airway diseases.

Rhinology and Sinus Surgery: Internationally known specialists utilize minimally invasive techniques to treat disorders from sinusitis to intra cranial tumors.

Thyroid Center: A comprehensive program to streamline the diagnosis and treatment of thyroid diseases and cancers. A highly skilled team of surgeons, endocrinologists and radiologists manage the patient's care.

Voice & Swallowing Institute: Combining the expertise of physicians, speech pathologists and a voice physiologist to diagnose and treat voice problems – not only for performing artists but also for teachers, stockbrokers, receptionists, salespeople – anyone for whom voice is an important part of life.

Otolaryngology Clinical Services

General Otolaryngology *plus*
Facial Plastic & Reconstructive Surgery
Cochlear Implantation
Voice & Vocal Dynamics
Head & Neck Oncology
Laryngology
Otology & Neuro-otology
Pediatric Otolaryngology
Rhinology & Sinus Surgery
Swallowing Disorders
Thyroid Center

Facilities

Ambulatory Care Services
Faculty Practice
Teaching Practice
Hearing Aid Dispensary
Vestibular Rehabilitation

About The New York Eye and Ear Infirmary

The Infirmary is the nation's oldest, continuously operating specialty hospital and one of the most experienced in terms of the number of patients it treats and complexity of its cases. Each year the otolaryngology department performs more than 6,000 surgeries and sees more than 70,000 visits from outpatients

Physician Referral
1.800.449.HOPE (4673)

OTOLARYNGOLOGY

About the Department of Otolaryngology:

The Department of Otolaryngology at NYU Langone Medical Center provides the highest quality treatment for the full spectrum of ear, nose, throat, head and neck disorders. The Department also has one of the leading Head and Neck Surgery programs in the country, delivering the most advanced patient care and innovative research.

We specialize in the following areas:

COCHLEAR IMPLANTS

At the Cochlear Implant Center at NYU Langone Medical Center, patients undergo extensive assessments, device programming and speech rehabilitation. Patients are offered both pre- and post-operative speech and language evaluation and therapy. The Center was the first in the U.S. to use a multichannel cochlear implant in a profoundly deaf adult and the first in the northeast to perform an auditory brainstem implant.

FACIAL PLASTIC AND RECONSTRUCTIVE SURGERY

The Division of Facial Plastic and Reconstructive Surgery provides care for patients requiring facial reconstructive surgery for a wide variety of facial deformities or those patients seeking facial cosmetic surgery. Specialties of the Division include functional and aesthetic rhinoplasty, facial rejuvenation surgery, injectable fillers, Botulinum Toxin (Botox) for facial spasm or wrinkles and chemical peels and microdermabrasion.

GENERAL OTOLARYNGOLOGY AND SLEEP SURGERY

The Division of General Otolaryngology provides care for adult patients suffering from voice, sleep, allergy and nasal breathing disorders, as well as patients falling within the broad scope of general otolaryngology. Otolaryngology services specific to children are provided through the Division of Pediatric Otolaryngology.

HEAD AND NECK SURGERY AND ONCOLOGY

The Division of Head and Neck Surgery and Oncology at NYU Langone Medical Center provides state-of-the-art multidisciplinary care for patients with cancer of the head and neck including cancer of the: larynx, oral cavity, throat, nasal cavity and sinuses, salivary glands and lymph nodes in the neck. In addition, the Division also provides microvascular reconstruction, treatment for thyroid neoplasms and anterior cranial base surgery.

VOICE AND SWALLOWING DISORDERS

The only center of its kind in New York City, the Voice Center at NYU Langone Medical Center provides comprehensive diagnosis, treatment and therapy for voice and swallowing disorders. Disorders treated at the Center include: sore throat, chronic cough, hoarseness, voice loss, swallowing dysfunction, benign growths and cancerous tumors, vocal cord paralysis, the aging voice, recurrent or chronic laryngitis, gastroesophageal reflux and injuries related to overuse and misuse of the voice.

The Department of Otolaryngology also provides state-of-the-art patient care and research through the following divisions:

- The Division of Audiology at NYU Langone Medical Center offers treatment for patients suffering with hearing or balance disorders.

- The Division of Head and Neck Speech Pathology at NYU Langone Medical Center provides treatment for voice, speech or swallowing problems.

- The Division of Rhinology at NYU Langone Medical Center provides treatment for all diseases of the paranasal sinuses, nose and related structures.

- Skull Base Surgery at NYU Langone Medical Center offers a minimally invasive and advanced surgical approach to the tumors of the anterior and posterior skull base.

Pain Medicine

subspecialty of Anesthesiology, Neurology, and in Physical Medicine and Rehabilitation or Psychiatry

Some physicians who have their primary board certification in anesthesiology, neurology, physical medicine and rehabilitation, or psychiatry have completed additional training and passed an examination in the subspecialty called pain management. These doctors provide a high level of care, either as a primary physician or consultant, for patients experiencing problems with acute, chronic and/or cancer pain in both hospital and ambulatory settings.

For more information about the main specialties of these physicians, see **Anesthesiology, Neurology, Physical Medicine** and **Rehabilitation** or **Psychiatry** section(s).

Training Required: Number of years required for primary specialty *plus* additional training and examination

PAIN MEDICINE

New England

Abrahm, Janet L MD [PM] - **Spec Exp:** Palliative Care; Pain-Cancer; **Hospital:** Dana-Farber Cancer Inst, Brigham & Women's Hosp; **Address:** Dana-Farber Cancer Institute, 44 Binney St, Shields-Warren 420, Boston, MA 02115; **Phone:** 617-632-6464; **Board Cert:** Internal Medicine 1976; Medical Oncology 1981; Hematology 1978; Hospice & Palliative Medicine 2008; **Med School:** UCSF 1973; **Resid:** Internal Medicine, Mass Genl Hosp 1975; Internal Medicine, Moffitt Hosp-UCSF 1977; **Fellow:** Hematology, Mass Genl Hosp 1976; Hematology & Oncology, Hosp Univ Penn 1980; **Fac Appt:** Assoc Prof Med, Harvard Med Sch

Berde, Charles Benjamin MD/PhD [PM] - **Spec Exp:** Pain Management-Pediatric; Critical Care; Reflex Sympathetic Dystrophy (RSD); **Hospital:** Children's Hospital - Boston, Spaulding Rehab Hosp; **Address:** Chldns Hosp, Dept Anes, 300 Longwood Ave, Bader 3, Boston, MA 02115; **Phone:** 617-355-7040; **Board Cert:** Pediatrics 1988; Anesthesiology 1988; Pain Medicine 2004; **Med School:** Stanford Univ 1980; **Resid:** Pediatrics, Chldns Hosp 1983; Anesthesiology, Mass Genl Hosp 1985; **Fellow:** Pediatric Anesthesiology, Chldns Hosp 1985; **Fac Appt:** Prof Ped, Harvard Med Sch

Billings, J Andrew MD [PM] - **Spec Exp:** Palliative Care; Pain Management; Pain-Cancer; **Hospital:** Mass Genl Hosp; **Address:** 55 Fruit St, FND 600, Boston, MA 02114; **Phone:** 617-724-9197; **Board Cert:** Internal Medicine 1975; Hospice & Palliative Medicine 2001; **Med School:** Harvard Med Sch 1972; **Resid:** Internal Medicine, Univ California Hosps 1975; **Fellow:** Internal Medicine, Mass Genl Hosp 1977; **Fac Appt:** Assoc Prof Med, Harvard Med Sch

Loder, Elizabeth W MD [PM] - **Spec Exp:** Headache; Migraine; **Hospital:** Brigham & Women's Hosp, Faulkner Hosp; **Address:** 1153 Centre St, Ste 4970, Boston, MA 02130; **Phone:** 617-983-7580; **Board Cert:** Internal Medicine 2000; **Med School:** Univ ND Sch Med 1985; **Resid:** Internal Medicine, Faulkner Hosp 1989; **Fellow:** Pain Medicine, Graham Headache Ctr 1990; **Fac Appt:** Asst Prof Med, Harvard Med Sch

Ross, Edgar L MD [PM] - **Hospital:** Brigham & Women's Hosp; **Address:** Brigham & Women's Dept of Pain Medicine, 850 Boylston St, Ste 320, Chestnut Hill, MA 02467; **Phone:** 617-732-9060; **Board Cert:** Anesthesiology 1984; Pain Medicine 2004; **Med School:** Wayne State Univ 1980; **Resid:** Anesthesiology, Case West Univ Hosps 1983; **Fellow:** Pain Medicine, Case West Univ Hosps 1984; **Fac Appt:** Asst Prof Anes, Harvard Med Sch

Mid Atlantic

Cope, Doris K MD [PM] - **Hospital:** UPMC St Margaret; **Address:** UPMC St Margaret Pain Med Ctr, 200 Delafield Ave, Ste 2070, Pittsburgh, PA 15215; **Phone:** 412-784-5343; **Board Cert:** Anesthesiology 1989; Pain Medicine 2007; **Med School:** Med Coll GA 1982; **Resid:** Anesthesiology, Univ S Alabama 1986; **Fac Appt:** Prof Anes, Univ Pittsburgh

De Leon-Casasola, Oscar A MD [PM] - **Spec Exp:** Pain-Acute; Pain-Chronic; Pain-Cancer; **Hospital:** Roswell Park Cancer Inst; **Address:** Roswell Park Cancer Inst, Dept Anesthesia/Pain Medicine, Elm & Carlton Sts, Buffalo, NY 14263; **Phone:** 716-845-4595; **Board Cert:** Anesthesiology 1991; Critical Care Medicine 1993; Pain Medicine 2005; **Med School:** Guatemala 1982; **Resid:** Surgery, SUNY-Downstate Med Ctr 1986; Anesthesiology, Univ Buffalo 1989; **Fac Appt:** Prof Anes, SUNY Buffalo

Diwan, Sudhir MD [PM] - **Spec Exp:** Pain-after Spinal Intervention; Pain-Musculoskeletal; Pain-Neuropathic; Pain-Cancer; **Hospital:** NY-Presby Hosp/Weill Cornell (page 66); **Address:** 1305 York Ave Fl 10, Box 120, New York, NY 10021; **Phone:** 646-962-7246; **Board Cert:** Anesthesiology 2001; Pain Medicine 2002; **Med School:** India 1983; **Resid:** Surgery, St Luke's-Roosevelt Hosp Ctr 1994; Anesthesiology, St Luke's-Roosevelt Hosp Ctr 1997; **Fellow:** Pain Medicine, NY Presby Hosp 1998; **Fac Appt:** Assoc Prof Anes, Cornell Univ-Weill Med Coll

Dubois, Michel MD [PM] - **Spec Exp:** Pain-Back & Neck; Pain-Neuropathic; **Hospital:** NYU Langone Med Ctr (page 67), Bellevue Hosp Ctr; **Address:** 317 E 34th St, Ste 902, New York, NY 10016-4974; **Phone:** 212-201-1004; **Board Cert:** Anesthesiology 1985; Pain Medicine 2004; **Med School:** France 1974; **Resid:** Anesthesiology, Georgetown Univ Hosp 1980; **Fellow:** Pain Medicine, Georgetown Univ Hosp 1983; **Fac Appt:** Prof Anes, NYU Sch Med

Gharibo, Christopher G MD [PM] - **Spec Exp:** Pain-Back & Neck; Pain-Neuropathic; Pain-Chronic; Complex Regional Pain Syndrome-CRPS; **Hospital:** NYU Langone Med Ctr (page 67), Hosp For Joint Diseases (page 67); **Address:** 301 E 17th St, Ste 1001, New York, NY 10003; **Phone:** 212-598-6174; **Board Cert:** Anesthesiology 1997; Pain Medicine 1998; **Med School:** UMDNJ-NJ Med Sch, Newark 1992; **Resid:** Anesthesiology, NYU Med Ctr 1995; **Fellow:** Pain Medicine, Jefferson Univ Hosp 1997; **Fac Appt:** Asst Prof Anes, NYU Sch Med

Jain, Subhash MD [PM] - **Spec Exp:** Pain-Cancer; Pain-Pelvic; Reflex Sympathetic Dystrophy (RSD); Pain-Neuropathic; **Hospital:** Beth Israel Med Ctr - Petrie Division (page 57); **Address:** 360 S 72nd St, Ste C, New York, NY 10021; **Phone:** 212-439-6100; **Board Cert:** Anesthesiology 1994; Pain Medicine 1998; **Med School:** India 1968; **Resid:** Surgery, St Vincent Med Ctr 1977; Anesthesiology, New York Hosp 1979; **Fellow:** Pain Medicine, New York Hosp/Meml Sloan Kettering Cancer Ctr 1980; **Fac Appt:** Assoc Prof Anes, Cornell Univ-Weill Med Coll

Kreitzer, Joel MD [PM] - **Spec Exp:** Pain-Back; Pain-Cancer; Pain-Neuropathic; **Hospital:** Mount Sinai Med Ctr (page 64), Mount Sinai Hosp of Queens (page 64); **Address:** Upper East Side Pain Medicine, 1540 York Ave, New York, NY 10028; **Phone:** 212-288-2180; **Board Cert:** Anesthesiology 1990; Pain Medicine 2004; **Med School:** Albert Einstein Coll Med 1985; **Resid:** Anesthesiology, Mt Sinai Hosp 1989; **Fellow:** Pain Medicine, Mt Sinai Hosp 1989; **Fac Appt:** Assoc Clin Prof Anes, Mount Sinai Sch Med

Ngeow, Jeffrey MD [PM] - **Spec Exp:** Pain-Musculoskeletal-Spine & Neck; Acupuncture; Reflex Sympathetic Dystrophy (RSD); Pain-Neuropathic; **Hospital:** Hosp For Special Surgery (page 59); **Address:** 535 E 70th St, New York, NY 10021-4872; **Phone:** 212-606-1059; **Board Cert:** Anesthesiology 1980; Pain Medicine 2005; **Med School:** England, UK 1971; **Resid:** Anesthesiology, Peter Bent Brigham Hosp 1977; **Fellow:** Pain Medicine, Tufts New England Med Ctr 1978; **Fac Appt:** Assoc Clin Prof Anes, Cornell Univ-Weill Med Coll

Portenoy, Russell MD [PM] - **Spec Exp:** Pain-Cancer; Palliative Care; **Hospital:** Beth Israel Med Ctr - Petrie Division (page 57); **Address:** Beth Israel Med Ctr, Dept Pain Medicine/Palliative Care, First Ave at 16th St, New York, NY 10003; **Phone:** 212-844-1403; **Board Cert:** Neurology 1985; Hospice & Palliative Medicine 2008; **Med School:** Univ MD Sch Med 1980; **Resid:** Neurology, Montefiore Med Ctr 1984; **Fellow:** Pain Medicine, Meml Sloan-Kettering Cancer Ctr 1985; **Fac Appt:** Prof N, Albert Einstein Coll Med

Raja, Srinivasa MD [PM] - **Spec Exp:** Pain-Neuropathic; Herpetic Neuralgia (Shingles); Reflex Sympathetic Dystrophy (RSD); **Hospital:** Johns Hopkins Hosp (page 61); **Address:** 600 N Wolfe St Bldg Osler Fl 2 - rm 292, Baltimore, MD 21287; **Phone:** 410-955-7246; **Board Cert:** Anesthesiology 1982; Pain Medicine 2004; **Med School:** India 1974; **Resid:** Anesthesiology, Univ Washington Med Ctr 1979; **Fellow:** Pain Medicine, Univ Virginia Hosp 1981; **Fac Appt:** Prof Anes, Johns Hopkins Univ

Pain Medicine

Staats, Peter MD [PM] - **Spec Exp:** Pain-Cancer; Pain-Back; **Hospital:** Riverview Med Ctr, CentraState Med Ctr; **Address:** Metzger Staats Pain Mgmt, 160 Avenue at the Commons, Ste 1, Shrewsbury, NJ 07702; **Phone:** 732-380-0200; **Board Cert:** Anesthesiology 1994; Pain Medicine 2005; **Med School:** Univ Mich Med Sch 1989; **Resid:** Anesthesiology, Johns Hopkins Hosp 1993; **Fellow:** Pain Medicine, Johns Hopkins Hosp 1994

Weinberger, Michael L MD [PM] - **Spec Exp:** Pain-Cancer; Pain-Back; **Hospital:** NY-Presby Hosp/Columbia (page 66); **Address:** 630 W 168th St, PH5, rm 500, New York, NY 10032-3720; **Phone:** 212-305-7114; **Board Cert:** Internal Medicine 1986; Anesthesiology 1990; Pain Medicine 2004; Hospice & Palliative Medicine 2006; **Med School:** Columbia P&S 1983; **Resid:** Internal Medicine, St Vincent's Hosp 1986; Anesthesiology, Columbia-Presby Med Ctr 1989; **Fellow:** Pain Medicine, Meml Sloan Kettering Cancer Ctr 1990; **Fac Appt:** Assoc Prof Anes, Columbia P&S

Southeast

Anghelescu, Doralina L MD [PM] - **Spec Exp:** Pain Management-Pediatric; Pain-Cancer; **Hospital:** St Jude Children's Research Hosp; **Address:** St Jude Chldn's Rsch Hosp, Anesthesiology, 262 Danny Thomas Pl, MS 130, Memphis, TN 38105; **Phone:** 901-495-4034; **Board Cert:** Anesthesiology 1998; Pain Medicine 2001; **Med School:** Romania 1985; **Resid:** Anesthesiology, Univ N Mex Hosp 1997; **Fellow:** Pain Medicine, Chldns Natl Med Ctr 1998; Pain Medicine, Univ NMex Hosp 1999

Baumann, Patricia L MD [PM] - **Hospital:** Emory Univ Hosp Midtown, Emory Univ Hosp; **Address:** 550 Peachtree St NE Fl 7 - Ste 7085, Atlanta, GA 30308; **Phone:** 404-686-2410; **Board Cert:** Anesthesiology 1993; Pain Medicine 2005; **Med School:** Emory Univ 1988; **Resid:** Anesthesiology, Emory Univ Med Ctr 1992; **Fac Appt:** Asst Prof Anes, Emory Univ

Rauck, Richard L MD [PM] - **Spec Exp:** Pain-Cancer; Spinal Cord Stimulation; Complex Regional Pain Syndrome-CRPS; **Hospital:** Forsyth Med Ctr, Wake Forest Univ Baptist Med Ctr (page 72); **Address:** Carolinas Pain Institute, 145 Kimel Park Drive, Ste 330, Winston-Salem, NC 27103; **Phone:** 336-765-6181; **Board Cert:** Anesthesiology 1987; Pain Medicine 2005; **Med School:** Bowman Gray 1982; **Resid:** Anesthesiology, Univ Cincinnati Hosp 1985; **Fellow:** Pain Medicine, Univ Cincinnati Hosp 1986; **Fac Appt:** Assoc Prof Anes, Wake Forest Univ

Midwest

Abram, Stephen E MD [PM] - **Hospital:** Froedtert Meml Lutheran Hosp; **Address:** Pain Management Ctr/Tosa Ctr, 1155 N Mayfair Rd, Wauwatosa, WI 53226; **Phone:** 414-456-7600; **Board Cert:** Anesthesiology 2001; Pain Medicine 2004; **Med School:** Jefferson Med Coll 1970; **Resid:** Anesthesiology, Mary Hitchcock Meml Hosp 1973; **Fac Appt:** Prof Anes, Med Coll Wisc

Amin, Sandeep D MD [PM] - **Spec Exp:** Headache-Supraorbital Stimulation; Complex Regional Pain Syndrome-CRPS; Pain-Cancer; Pain-after Spinal Intervention; **Hospital:** Rush Univ Med Ctr, Rush Oak Park Hosp; **Address:** Rush Pain Ctr, 1725 W Harrison St, Ste 550, Chicago, IL 60612; **Phone:** 312-942-6631; **Board Cert:** Anesthesiology 1998; Pain Medicine 2000; **Med School:** India 1991; **Resid:** Anesthesiology, Univ Illinois Hosps 1997; **Fellow:** Pain Medicine, Univ Illinois Hosps 1998; Pain Medicine, Johns Hopkins Hosp 1999; **Fac Appt:** Prof Anes, Rush Med Coll

America's Top Doctors® 9th Edition

Benedetti, Costantino MD [PM] - **Spec Exp:** Pain-Cancer; Palliative Care; Pain-Acute; Pain-Chronic; **Hospital:** Ohio St Univ Med Ctr, Arthur G James Cancer Hosp & Research Inst; **Address:** Ohio State Univ Med Ctr, 300 W 10th Ave, Ste 519, Columbus, OH 43210; **Phone:** 614-293-6599; **Board Cert:** Hospice & Palliative Medicine 1997; **Med School:** Italy 1972; **Resid:** Anesthesiology, Univ Colorado Hosp 1975; Anesthesiology, Univ Wash Med Ctr 1976; **Fellow:** Pain Medicine, Univ Wash Med Ctr 1978; **Fac Appt:** Clin Prof Anes, Ohio State Univ

Benzon, Honorio T MD [PM] - **Spec Exp:** Pain-Back; Complex Regional Pain Syndrome-CRPS; Pain-Neuropathic; Pain-Cancer; **Hospital:** Northwestern Meml Hosp; **Address:** 675 N Saint Clair St Fl 20, Ste 20-100, Chicago, IL 60611-3015; **Phone:** 312-695-2500; **Board Cert:** Anesthesiology 1995; Pain Medicine 2004; **Med School:** Philippines 1971; **Resid:** Anesthesiology, Univ Cincinnati Med Ctr 1975; Anesthesiology, Northwestern Meml Hosp 1976; **Fellow:** Research, Brigham & Womens Hosp 1986; **Fac Appt:** Prof Anes, Northwestern Univ

Covington, Edward C MD [PM] - **Spec Exp:** Pain-Chronic; **Hospital:** Cleveland Clin Fdn (page 56); **Address:** 9500 Euclid Ave, Desk C21, Cleveland, OH 44195; **Phone:** 216-444-5964; **Board Cert:** Psychiatry 1978; Addiction Psychiatry 1998; Pain Medicine 2001; **Med School:** Univ Tenn Coll Med, Memphis 1970; **Resid:** Psychiatry, Mayo Clinic 1975

Green, Carmen R MD [PM] - **Spec Exp:** Pain Care-Racial/Ethnic Disparities; **Hospital:** Univ Michigan Hlth Sys; **Address:** Univ Mich Hlth Sys, Dept Anesthesiology, rm 1H247 Univ Hosp, 1500 E Med Ctr Drive, SPC5048, Ann Arbor, MI 48109-5048; **Phone:** 734-936-4240; **Board Cert:** Anesthesiology 1996; Pain Medicine 1998; **Med School:** Mich State Univ 1987; **Resid:** Anesthesiology, Univ Mich Med Ctr 1989; **Fellow:** Pain Medicine, Univ Mich Med Ctr 1992; **Fac Appt:** Asst Prof Anes, Univ Mich Med Sch

Harden, R Norman MD [PM] - **Spec Exp:** Pain-Back; Reflex Sympathetic Dystrophy (RSD); Fibromyalgia; Headache; **Hospital:** Rehab Inst of Chicago; **Address:** 980 N Michigan Ave, Ste 800, Chicago, IL 60611; **Phone:** 312-238-7800; **Med School:** Med Coll GA 1984; **Resid:** Neurology, Univ South Carolina Med Ctr 1985; **Fellow:** Pain Medicine, Rehab Inst-Georgia 1989; **Fac Appt:** Asst Prof PMR, Northwestern Univ

Huntoon, Marc MD [PM] - **Spec Exp:** Pain-Cancer; Pain-after Spinal Intervention; Palliative Care; **Hospital:** Mayo Med Ctr & Clin - Rochester; **Address:** Mayo Clinic - Pain Medicine, 200 First St SW, Rochester, MN 55905; **Phone:** 507-266-9240; **Board Cert:** Anesthesiology 2003; Pain Medicine 2004; Hospice & Palliative Medicine 2004; **Med School:** Wayne State Univ 1985; **Resid:** Anesthesiology, Naval Hosp Med Ctr 1991; **Fellow:** Pain Medicine, Naval Hosp Med Ctr 1992

Robbins, Lawrence D MD [PM] - **Spec Exp:** Headache; Migraine; Psychopharmacology; Pain Management; **Address:** 1535 Lake Cook Rd, Ste 506, Northbrook, IL 60062-1451; **Phone:** 847-480-9399; **Board Cert:** Pain Medicine 1995; **Med School:** Univ IL Coll Med 1981; **Resid:** Neurology, Univ Illinois Med Ctr 1985; **Fellow:** Pain Medicine, Diamond Headache Clinic 1986; **Fac Appt:** Asst Prof N, Rush Med Coll

Rosenquist, Richard W MD [PM] - **Spec Exp:** Complex Regional Pain Syndrome-CRPS; Pain-Back; Pain-Facial; Headache; **Hospital:** Univ Iowa Hosp & Clinics, VA Med Ctr - Iowa City; **Address:** Center Pain Medicine-Dept Anesthesia, 200 Hawkins Drive, Iowa City, IA 52242; **Phone:** 319-356-2320; **Board Cert:** Anesthesiology 1988; Pain Medicine 2004; **Med School:** Northwestern Univ 1984; **Resid:** Anesthesiology, Northwestern Univ Med Ctr 1987; **Fellow:** Anesthesiology & Pain Management, Emory Univ 1988; **Fac Appt:** Prof Anes, Univ Iowa Coll Med

Pain Medicine

Suresh, Santhanam MD [PM] - **Hospital:** Children's Mem Hosp; **Address:** Chldns Meml Hosp, Dept Anesthesia, 2300 Children's Plaza, Box 19, Chicago, IL 60614; **Phone:** 773-880-4006; **Board Cert:** Pediatrics 2004; Anesthesiology 2001; Pain Medicine 2009; **Med School:** India 1983; **Resid:** Pediatrics, Cook Co Hosp 1988; Anesthesiology, Loyola Univ Med Ctr 1990; **Fellow:** Pediatric Anesthesiology, Northwestern Meml Hosp 1991; **Fac Appt:** Prof Anes, Northwestern Univ-Feinberg Sch Med

Swarm, Robert A MD [PM] - **Spec Exp:** Pain-Acute; Pain-Chronic; Pain-Cancer; **Hospital:** Barnes-Jewish Hosp; **Address:** Ctr for Advanced Med-Pain Mngmt Ctr, 4921 Parkview Pl, Ste 10A, MS 90-35-706, St Louis, MO 63110; **Phone:** 314-362-8820; **Board Cert:** Anesthesiology 1990; Pain Medicine 2004; **Med School:** Washington Univ, St Louis 1983; **Resid:** Surgery, Barnes Hosp 1986; Anesthesiology, Barnes Hosp 1989; **Fellow:** Pain Medicine, Univ Sydney; **Fac Appt:** Assoc Prof Anes, Washington Univ, St Louis

Weisman, Steven J MD [PM] - **Spec Exp:** Pain Management-Pediatric; Palliative Care-Pediatric; Complex Regional Pain Syndrome-CRPS; Pain-Cancer; **Hospital:** Chldns Hosp - Wisconsin; **Address:** Chldns Hosp Wisconsin, 9000 W Wisconsin Ave, MS 792, Milwaukee, WI 53226-3518; **Phone:** 414-266-2775; **Board Cert:** Pediatrics 1982; Pediatric Hematology-Oncology 1984; Anesthesiology 1996; **Med School:** Albert Einstein Coll Med 1978; **Resid:** Pediatrics, Chldns Hosp 1981; Anesthesiology, Univ Conn Hlth Ctr 1994; **Fellow:** Pediatric Hematology-Oncology, Indiana Univ Sch Med 1984; **Fac Appt:** Prof Anes, Med Coll Wisc

Great Plains and Mountains

Fine, Perry G MD [PM] - **Spec Exp:** Pain-Cancer; Palliative Care; Pain-Chronic; **Hospital:** Univ Utah Hosps and Clins; **Address:** 546 S Chipeta Way, Ste 200, Salt Lake City, UT 84108; **Phone:** 801-581-7246; **Board Cert:** Anesthesiology 1985; Pain Medicine 2004; **Med School:** Med Coll VA 1981; **Resid:** Anesthesiology, Univ Utah Hlth Sci Ctr 1984; **Fellow:** Pain Medicine, Univ Toronto 1985; **Fac Appt:** Prof Anes, Univ Utah

Weinstein, Sharon M MD [PM] - **Spec Exp:** Pain-Cancer; Palliative Care; **Hospital:** Univ Utah Hosps and Clins; **Address:** Huntsman Cancer Institute, 2000 Circle of Hope, Salt Lake City, UT 84112; **Phone:** 801-585-0112; **Board Cert:** Neurology 1993; Pain Medicine 2000; **Med School:** Albert Einstein Coll Med 1986; **Resid:** Neurology, Montefiore Med Ctr 1990; **Fellow:** Pain Medicine, Meml Sloan Kettering Cancer Ctr 1991; **Fac Appt:** Assoc Prof Anes, Univ Utah

Southwest

Burton, Allen W MD [PM] - **Spec Exp:** Pain-Cancer; Palliative Care; **Hospital:** UT MD Anderson Cancer Ctr; **Address:** MD Anderson Cancer Ctr, Dept Anesth, 1400 Holcombe Blvd, Unit 409, Houston, TX 77030; **Phone:** 713-745-7246; **Board Cert:** Anesthesiology 1996; Pain Medicine 1998; **Med School:** Baylor Coll Med 1991; **Resid:** Anesthesiology, Brigham & Women's Hosp 1995; **Fellow:** Pain Medicine, U Texas Med Branch Hosp 1998; **Fac Appt:** Assoc Prof Anes, Univ Tex Med Br, Galveston

Driver, Larry C MD [PM] - **Spec Exp:** Pain-Cancer; Palliative Care; **Hospital:** UT MD Anderson Cancer Ctr; **Address:** UT MD Anderson Cancer Ctr, Dept Pain Medicine, 1400 Holcombe Blvd, Unit 409, Houston, TX 77030; **Phone:** 713-745-7246; **Board Cert:** Anesthesiology 1992; Pain Medicine 2002; **Med School:** Univ Tex, San Antonio 1980; **Resid:** Anesthesiology, Univ Colorado Hlth Sci Ctr 1984; **Fellow:** Pain Medicine, MD Anderson Cancer Ctr 1999; **Fac Appt:** Assoc Prof Anes, Univ Tex, Houston

Racz, Gabor MD [PM] - **Spec Exp:** Pain-after Spinal Intervention; Reflex Sympathetic Dystrophy (RSD); Pain-Back, Head & Neck; Headache/Facial Pain; **Hospital:** Univ Med Ctr-Lubbock; **Address:** 3601 4th St, rm 1C282, Lubbock, TX 79430-0002; **Phone:** 806-743-3112; **Board Cert:** Anesthesiology 1993; Pain Medicine 2004; **Med School:** England, UK 1962; **Resid:** Anesthesiology, SUNY Upstate Med Ctr 1969; **Fac Appt:** Prof Anes, Texas Tech Univ

Ramamurthy, Somayaji MD [PM] - **Spec Exp:** Pain-Back; Pain-Chronic; **Hospital:** Univ Hlth Syst-San Antonio; **Address:** Univ Tex Hlth Sci Ctr, Dept Anes, 7703 Floyd Curl Drive, MC 7838, San Antonio, TX 78229-3900; **Phone:** 210-567-4543; **Board Cert:** Anesthesiology 1972; Pain Medicine 2004; **Med School:** India 1965; **Resid:** Anesthesiology, Cook Co Hosp 1970; **Fac Appt:** Prof Anes, Univ Tex, San Antonio

Walsh, Nicolas E MD [PM] - **Spec Exp:** Pain-Back; Trauma Rehabilitation; Post Polio Syndrome (PPS); **Hospital:** Univ Hlth Syst-San Antonio, Audie L Murphy Meml Vets Hosp; **Address:** Univ Tex Hlth Sci Ctr, Rehab Med (7798), 7703 Floyd Curl Drive, San Antonio, TX 78229-3901; **Phone:** 210-567-5350; **Board Cert:** Physical Medicine & Rehabilitation 1983; Pain Medicine 2000; **Med School:** Univ Colorado 1979; **Resid:** Physical Medicine & Rehabilitation, Univ Tex Hlth Sci Ctr 1982; **Fac Appt:** Prof PMR, Univ Tex, San Antonio

West Coast and Pacific

Anderson, Corrie TM MD [PM] - **Spec Exp:** Pain Management-Pediatric; Pain-Pediatric Cancer; **Hospital:** Chldns Hosp and Regl Med Ctr - Seattle, Univ Wash Med Ctr; **Address:** Chldns Hosp & Regl Med Ctr, Dept Anesth, 4800 Sands Point Way NE, rm W9825, Seattle, WA 98105; **Phone:** 206-987-2704; **Board Cert:** Anesthesiology 1994; Pain Medicine 2007; **Med School:** Stanford Univ 1982; **Resid:** Pediatrics, Chldns Hosp 1985; Anesthesiology, Brigham & Womens Hosp 1987; **Fellow:** Pediatric Anesthesiology, Chldns Hosp 1988; **Fac Appt:** Prof Anes, Univ Wash

Audell, Laura G MD [PM] - **Spec Exp:** Complex Regional Pain Syndrome-CRPS; Reflex Sympathetic Dystrophy (RSD); Herpetic Neuralgia (Shingles); Spinal Cord Disorders; **Hospital:** Cedars-Sinai Med Ctr; **Address:** 444 S San Vincente, Ste 1101, Los Angeles, CA 90048; **Phone:** 310-423-9600; **Board Cert:** Internal Medicine 1988; Anesthesiology 1988; Pain Medicine 2007; **Med School:** Univ Wash 1982; **Resid:** Internal Medicine, UCLA-Hosps 1985; Anesthesiology, UCLA-Hosps 1987; **Fellow:** Pain Medicine, UCLA-Hosps 1988

Ferrante, F Michael MD [PM] - **Spec Exp:** Pain-Back & Neck; Reflex Sympathetic Dystrophy (RSD); Botox for Pain; Pain-Neuropathic; **Hospital:** Santa Monica - UCLA Med Ctr & Ortho Hosp, UCLA Ronald Reagan Med Ctr; **Address:** UCLA Pain Program, 1245 16th St, Ste 225, Santa Monica, CA 90404; **Phone:** 310-319-2241; **Board Cert:** Internal Medicine 1985; Anesthesiology 1987; Pain Medicine 2004; **Med School:** NY Med Coll 1980; **Resid:** Internal Medicine, Emroy Univ Affil Hosp 1983; Anesthesiology, Emroy Univ Affil Hosp 1986; **Fellow:** Infectious Disease, Barnes Hosp-Wash Univ 1984; Pain Medicine, Brigham & Womens Hosp 1987; **Fac Appt:** Prof Anes, UCLA

Fishman, Scott M MD [PM] - **Spec Exp:** Pain-Cancer; Pain-Chronic; **Hospital:** UC Davis Med Ctr; **Address:** UC Davis Med Ctr, Pain Management Clinic, 4860 Y St, Ste 2700, Sacramento, CA 95817; **Phone:** 916-734-6824; **Board Cert:** Psychiatry 1998; Pain Medicine 1995; **Med School:** Univ Mass Sch Med 1990; **Resid:** Internal Medicine, Greenwich Hosp 1993; Psychiatry, Mass Genl Hosp 1996; **Fellow:** Pain Medicine, Mass Genl Hosp 1995; **Fac Appt:** Prof Anes, UC Davis

Pain Medicine

Fitzgibbon, Dermot R MD [PM] - **Spec Exp:** Pain-Cancer; **Hospital:** Univ Wash Med Ctr; **Address:** Univ Wash Med Ctr, Dept Anesthesiology, 1959 NE Pacific St, Box 356540, Seattle, WA 98195; **Phone:** 206-598-4260; **Board Cert:** Anesthesiology 1996; Pain Medicine 1998; **Med School:** Ireland 1983; **Resid:** Anesthesiology, St Vincent's Hosp 1992; Anesthesiology, Univ Washington Med Ctr 1995; **Fellow:** Pain Medicine, Univ Wash-Pain Mngmt Clinic 1994; **Fac Appt:** Assoc Prof Anes, Univ Wash

Mackey, Sean MD/PhD [PM] - **Hospital:** Stanford Univ Med Ctr; **Address:** Stanford Univ Pain Management Clinic, 300 Pasteur DR, A408, MC 5340, Stanford, CA 94305; **Phone:** 650-723-6238; **Board Cert:** Anesthesiology 1999; Pain Medicine 2000; **Med School:** Univ Ariz Coll Med 1994; **Resid:** Anesthesiology, Stanford Univ Med Ctr 1998; **Fellow:** Pain Medicine, Stanford Univ Med Ctr 1999; **Fac Appt:** Assoc Prof Anes, Stanford Univ

Prager, Joshua P MD [PM] - **Spec Exp:** Complex Regional Pain Syndrome-CRPS; **Hospital:** UCLA Ronald Reagan Med Ctr; **Address:** 100 UCLA Med Plaza, Ste 760, Los Angeles, CA 90095; **Phone:** 310-264-7246 x100; **Board Cert:** Internal Medicine 1984; Anesthesiology 1987; Pain Medicine 2004; **Med School:** Stanford Univ 1981; **Resid:** Internal Medicine, UCLA Med Ctr 1984; Anesthesiology, Mass Genl Hosp 1986; **Fac Appt:** Asst Clin Prof Anes, UCLA

Ready, L Brian MD [PM] - **Spec Exp:** Pain-Cancer; **Hospital:** Allenmore Hosp; **Address:** 1901 S Union Ave, Ste A244, Tacoma, WA 98405; **Phone:** 253-459-6509; **Med School:** Canada 1967; **Resid:** Anesthesiology, Univ Washington Med Ctr 1975

Rosner, Howard L MD [PM] - **Spec Exp:** Pain-after Spinal Intervention; Pain-Cancer; Pain-Back; **Hospital:** Cedars-Sinai Med Ctr; **Address:** 444 S San Vincente Blvd, Ste 1101, Cedars-Sinai Med Ctr,Mark Goodson Bldg, Los Angeles, CA 90048; **Phone:** 310-423-9612; **Board Cert:** Anesthesiology 1989; Pain Medicine 2004; **Med School:** Univ Miami Sch Med 1980; **Resid:** Anesthesiology, Mass Genl Hosp 1983; **Fellow:** Pain Medicine, Columbia-Presby Med Ctr 1984

Rowbotham, Michael C MD [PM] - **Spec Exp:** Reflex Sympathetic Dystrophy (RSD); Pain-Nerve Injury; Herpetic Neuralgia (Shingles); **Hospital:** UCSF - Mt Zion Med Ctr; **Address:** 2255 Post St, San Francisco, CA 94115; **Phone:** 415-885-7246; **Board Cert:** Neurology 1989; **Med School:** UCSF 1979; **Resid:** Neurology, Boston Univ 1986; Neurology, UCSF Med Ctr 1987; **Fellow:** Neurological Pharmacology, UCSF Med Ctr 1980; Pain Medicine, UCSF Med Ctr 1989; **Fac Appt:** Assoc Prof N, UCSF

Slatkin, Neal E MD [PM] - **Spec Exp:** Pain-Cancer; Palliative Care; **Address:** Hospice of the Valley, 4850 Union Ave, San Jose, CA 95124-5156; **Phone:** 408-559-5600; **Board Cert:** Neurology 1982; Pain Medicine 2000; **Med School:** SUNY Stony Brook 1976; **Resid:** Neurology, Bellevue Hosp Ctr-NYU 1978; Neurology, Med Coll Va Hosps 1981; **Fellow:** Neurology, Med Coll Va 1982; Neuro-Oncology, Meml Sloan-Kettering Cancer Ctr 1984; **Fac Appt:** Asst Clin Prof Med, USC-Keck School of Medicine

Wallace, Mark Steven MD [PM] - **Spec Exp:** Pain-Chronic; Pain-Cancer; Palliative Care; **Hospital:** UCSD Med Ctr; **Address:** 9350 Campus Point Drive, MC 7651, La Jolla, CA 92037; **Phone:** 858-657-6035; **Board Cert:** Anesthesiology 1992; Pain Medicine 2005; **Med School:** Creighton Univ 1987; **Resid:** Anesthesiology, Univ Maryland Hosp 1991; **Fellow:** Pain Medicine, UCSD Med Ctr 1994

Pathology

A pathologist deals with the causes and nature of disease and contributes to diagnosis, prognosis and treatment through knowledge gained by the laboratory application of the biologic, chemical and physical sciences.

A pathologist uses information gathered from the microscopic examination of tissue specimens, cells and body fluids, and from clinical laboratory tests on body fluids and secretions for the diagnosis, exclusion and monitoring of disease.

Training Required: Five to seven years

Certification in the following subspecialty requires additional training and examination.

Dermatopathology: A dermatopathologist has the expertise to diagnose and monitor diseases of the skin including infectious, immunologic, degenerative and neoplastic diseases. This entails the examination and interpretation of specially prepared tissue sections, cellular scrapings and smears of skin lesions by means of routine and special (electron and flourescent) microscopes.

PATHOLOGY

New England

Bhan, Atul Kumar MD [Path] - **Spec Exp:** Immunopathology; Liver Pathology; Liver Cancer; **Hospital:** Mass Genl Hosp; **Address:** Mass Genl Hosp, Dept Path, 55 Fruit St, Warren 501, Boston, MA 02114-2620; **Phone:** 617-726-2588; **Board Cert:** Anatomic Pathology 1976; Immunopathology 1985; **Med School:** India 1965; **Resid:** Pathology, Boston Univ Hosp 1971; Pathology, Chldns Univ Hosp 1974; **Fac Appt:** Prof Path, Harvard Med Sch

Connolly, James Leo MD [Path] - **Spec Exp:** Breast Pathology; Breast Cancer; **Hospital:** Beth Israel Deaconess Med Ctr - Boston, Brigham & Women's Hosp; **Address:** Beth Israel Deaconess Med Ctr, Dept Path, 330 Brookline Ave, rm ES 112, Boston, MA 02215-5400; **Phone:** 617-667-4344; **Board Cert:** Anatomic Pathology 1980; **Med School:** Vanderbilt Univ 1974; **Resid:** Anatomic Pathology, Beth Israel Hosp 1978; **Fac Appt:** Prof Path, Harvard Med Sch

DeLellis, Ronald A MD [Path] - **Spec Exp:** Thyroid Cancer; Endocrine Pathology; **Hospital:** Rhode Island Hosp, Miriam Hosp; **Address:** Rhode Island Hospital, Dept Pathology, 593 Eddy St, Providence, RI 02903-4923; **Phone:** 401-444-5154; **Board Cert:** Anatomic Pathology 1972; **Med School:** Tufts Univ 1966; **Resid:** Anatomic Pathology, Natl Inst Hlth 1971; **Fellow:** Pathology, Univ Hosp 1973; **Fac Appt:** Prof Path, Brown Univ

Fletcher, Christopher MD [Path] - **Spec Exp:** Soft Tissue Tumors; Sarcoma; Surgical Pathology; **Hospital:** Brigham & Women's Hosp, Dana-Farber Cancer Inst; **Address:** Brigham & Women's Hospital, Dept Pathology, 75 Francis St, Boston, MA 02115-6110; **Phone:** 617-732-8558; **Med School:** England, UK 1981; **Resid:** Pathology, St Thomas Hosp 1985; **Fellow:** Pathology, St Thomas Hosp 1986; **Fac Appt:** Prof Path, Harvard Med Sch

Harris, Nancy L MD [Path] - **Spec Exp:** Lymphoma; Hematopathology; **Hospital:** Mass Genl Hosp; **Address:** Mass Genl Hosp, Dept Path, 55 Fruit St, Warren 211, Boston, MA 02114; **Phone:** 617-726-5155; **Board Cert:** Anatomic Pathology 1978; Clinical Pathology 1978; **Med School:** Stanford Univ 1970; **Resid:** Pathology, Beth Israel Hosp 1978; **Fellow:** Immunopathology, Mass Genl Hosp 1980; **Fac Appt:** Prof Path, Harvard Med Sch

Kaufman, Richard Max MD [Path] - **Spec Exp:** Transfusion Medicine; **Hospital:** Brigham & Women's Hosp, Dana-Farber Cancer Inst; **Address:** Brigham and Women's Hospital, 75 Francis St, Boston, MA 02115-6110; **Phone:** 617-732-4749; **Board Cert:** Clinical Pathology 2000; Blood Banking Transfusion Medicine 2002; **Med School:** Washington Univ, St Louis 1992; **Resid:** Pathology, Washington Univ 2000; **Fellow:** Blood Banking Transfusion Medicine, Washington Univ 2001; **Fac Appt:** Asst Prof Path, Harvard Med Sch

Mark, Eugene J MD [Path] - **Spec Exp:** Pulmonary Pathology; Cardiac Pathology; Forensic Pathology; **Hospital:** Mass Genl Hosp; **Address:** Mass Genl Hosp, Dept Path, 55 Fruit St, Warren 246, Boston, MA 02114; **Phone:** 617-726-8891; **Board Cert:** Anatomic & Clinical Pathology 1973; Dermatopathology 1975; **Med School:** Harvard Med Sch 1967; **Resid:** Pathology, Mass Genl Hosp 1972; **Fellow:** Pathology, Kantonspital 1966; **Fac Appt:** Prof Path, Harvard Med Sch

Odze, Robert D MD [Path] - **Spec Exp:** Gastrointestinal Pathology; Liver Pathology; Esophageal Cancer; **Hospital:** Brigham & Women's Hosp; **Address:** Brigham & Women's Hosp, Dept Pathology, 75 Francis St, Boston, MA 02115; **Phone:** 617-732-7549; **Board Cert:** Anatomic Pathology 1990; **Med School:** McGill Univ 1984; **Resid:** Surgery, McGill Univ 1987; Pathology, McGill Univ 1990; **Fellow:** Gastrointestinal Pathology, New England Deaconess Med Ctr 1991; **Fac Appt:** Assoc Prof Path, Harvard Med Sch

Rennke, Helmut G MD [Path] - **Spec Exp:** Kidney Pathology; **Hospital:** Brigham & Women's Hosp; **Address:** Brigham & Womens Hosp, Dept Pathology, 75 Francis St Emory Bldg, Boston, MA 02115; **Phone:** 617-732-6518; **Board Cert:** Anatomic Pathology 1980; **Med School:** Chile 1971; **Resid:** Pathology, Boston City Hosp 1974; Pathology, Peter Bent Brigham Hosp 1977; **Fac Appt:** Prof Path, Harvard Med Sch

Schnitt, Stuart J MD [Path] - **Spec Exp:** Breast Pathology; Breast Cancer; **Hospital:** Beth Israel Deaconess Med Ctr - Boston; **Address:** Beth Israel Deaconess Med Ctr, Dept Pathology, 330 Brookline Ave, rm ES 112, Boston, MA 02215-5400; **Phone:** 617-667-4344; **Board Cert:** Anatomic & Clinical Pathology 1983; **Med School:** Albany Med Coll 1979; **Resid:** Anatomic Pathology, Beth Israel Deaconess Med Ctr 1983; **Fellow:** Surgical Pathology, Beth Israel Deaconess Med Ctr 1984; **Fac Appt:** Assoc Prof Path, Harvard Med Sch

Smith, Thomas W MD [Path] - **Spec Exp:** Neuropathology; **Hospital:** UMass Meml - Univ Campus; **Address:** Univ Mass Dept Pathology, Div Neuropathology, 55 Lake Ave N, Worcester, MA 01655; **Phone:** 508-856-2331; **Board Cert:** Neuropathology 1999; **Med School:** Cornell Univ 1972; **Resid:** Neuropathology, Peter Bent Brigham Hosp 1976; Radiology, Mass General Hosp 1977; **Fellow:** Anatomic Pathology, Peter Bent Brigham Hosp 1978; **Fac Appt:** Prof Path, Univ Mass Sch Med

Young, Robert H MD [Path] - **Spec Exp:** Ovarian Cancer; Gynecologic Cancer; **Hospital:** Mass Genl Hosp; **Address:** Mass Genl Hosp, Dept Pathology, 55 Fruit St, Warren 215, Boston, MA 02114; **Phone:** 617-726-8892; **Board Cert:** Anatomic Pathology 1980; **Med School:** Ireland 1974; **Resid:** Pathology, Mass Genl Hosp 1979; Pathology, Dublin Univ 1977; **Fac Appt:** Prof Path, Harvard Med Sch

Mid Atlantic

Bagg, Adam MD [Path] - **Spec Exp:** Hematopathology; Leukemia & Lymphoma; Myelodysplastic Syndromes; **Hospital:** Hosp Univ Penn - UPHS (page 60); **Address:** Hosp Univ Penn, Dept Pathology & Lab Med, 3400 Spruce St, Phildelphia, PA 19104; **Phone:** 215-662-4280; **Board Cert:** Clinical Pathology 1992; Hematology 1999; **Med School:** South Africa 1981; **Resid:** Internal Medicine, Univ Witwatersrand 1992; Clinical Pathology, Georgetown Univ 1992; **Fellow:** Hematopathology, Georgetown Univ 1993; **Fac Appt:** Prof Path, Univ Pennsylvania

Brooks, John S MD [Path] - **Spec Exp:** Tumor Pathology; Sarcoma; Bone & Soft Tissue Pathology; **Hospital:** Pennsylvania Hosp (page 60), Hosp Univ Penn - UPHS (page 60); **Address:** Pennsylvania Hospital, Preston 6 FL, 800 Spruce St, Philadelphia, PA 19107; **Phone:** 215-829-3541; **Board Cert:** Anatomic Pathology 1978; Immunopathology 1983; **Med School:** Thomas Jefferson Univ 1974; **Resid:** Pathology, Hosp Univ Penn 1978; **Fellow:** Immunopathology, Hosp Univ Penn 1978; **Fac Appt:** Prof Path, Univ Pennsylvania

Burger, Peter MD [Path] - **Spec Exp:** Brain Tumors; Neuro-Pathology; **Hospital:** Johns Hopkins Hosp (page 61); **Address:** Johns Hopkins Hosp-Dept Pathology, 600 N Wolfe St, rm 710, Baltimore, MD 21287; **Phone:** 410-955-8378; **Board Cert:** Anatomic Pathology 1976; Neuropathology 1976; **Med School:** Northwestern Univ 1966; **Resid:** Anatomic Pathology, Duke Univ Med Ctr 1973; **Fellow:** Neuropathology, Duke Univ Med Ctr 1973

Crawford, James M MD/PhD [Path] - **Spec Exp:** Liver Pathology; Gastrointestinal Pathology; Gastrointestinal Cancer; **Hospital:** N Shore Univ Hosp; **Address:** NS-LIJ Laboratories, 10 Nevada Drive, Lake Success, NY 11042-1114; **Phone:** 516-719-1060; **Board Cert:** Anatomic Pathology 1987; **Med School:** Duke Univ 1982; **Resid:** Pathology, Brigham & Women's Hosp 1984; **Fellow:** Gastrointestinal Pathology, Brigham & Women's Hosp 1987; **Fac Appt:** Prof Path, Univ Fla Coll Med

Pathology

Demetris, Anthony J MD [Path] - **Spec Exp:** Transplant Pathology; Liver Pathology; **Hospital:** UPMC Montefiore; **Address:** UPMC - Montefiore, 3459 5th Ave, rm E741, Pittsburgh, PA 15213; **Phone:** 412-647-2067; **Board Cert:** Anatomic & Clinical Pathology 1987; **Med School:** Univ Pittsburgh 1982; **Resid:** Anatomic & Clinical Pathology, Univ Pittsburgh Med Ctr 1986; **Fac Appt:** Prof Path, Univ Pittsburgh

Ehya, Hormoz MD [Path] - **Spec Exp:** Cytopathology; Breast Pathology; Lung Pathology; **Hospital:** Fox Chase Cancer Ctr (page 58); **Address:** Fox Chase Cancer Center, 333 Cottman Ave, rm C427, Philadelphia, PA 19111-2497; **Phone:** 215-728-5389; **Board Cert:** Anatomic Pathology 1979; Cytopathology 1989; **Med School:** Iran 1974; **Resid:** Pathology, Univ Miss Med Ctr 1979; **Fellow:** Cytopathology, Meml Sloan-Kettering Cancer Ctr 1980

Epstein, Jonathan MD [Path] - **Spec Exp:** Bladder Cancer; Prostate Cancer; Urologic Pathology; **Hospital:** Johns Hopkins Hosp (page 61); **Address:** 401 N Broadway, Weinberg 2242, Baltimore, MD 21231; **Phone:** 410-955-5043; **Board Cert:** Anatomic Pathology 1986; **Med School:** Boston Univ 1981; **Resid:** Pathology, Johns Hopkins Hosp 1985; **Fellow:** Pathology, Meml Sloan Kettering Cancer Ctr 1984; **Fac Appt:** Prof Path, Johns Hopkins Univ

Fogt, Franz MD/PhD [Path] - **Spec Exp:** Gastrointestinal Pathology; **Hospital:** Penn Presby Med Ctr - UPHS (page 60); **Address:** Presbyterian Medical Ctr, Dept Pathology, 551 Wright Saunders Bldg, Philadelphia, PA 19104; **Phone:** 215-662-8077; **Board Cert:** Anatomic & Clinical Pathology 1995; **Med School:** Germany 1988; **Resid:** Anatomic & Clinical Pathology, New England Deaconess Hosp 1995; **Fellow:** Gastrointestinal Pathology, New England Deaconess Hosp 1996; **Fac Appt:** Assoc Prof Path, Univ Pennsylvania

Gottlieb, Geoffrey J MD [Path] - **Spec Exp:** Dermatopathology; Melanoma; **Address:** Ackerman Academy Dermatopathology, 145 E 32nd St Fl 10, New York, NY 10016; **Phone:** 212-889-6225; **Board Cert:** Anatomic Pathology 1979; Dermatopathology 1982; **Med School:** Cornell Univ-Weill Med Coll 1976; **Resid:** Pathology, NY Hosp-Cornell Med Ctr 1979; **Fellow:** Dermatopathology, NYU Med Ctr 1982

Gupta, Prabodh K MD [Path] - **Spec Exp:** Lung Pathology; Cervical Cancer; Fine Needle Aspiration Biopsy; **Hospital:** Hosp Univ Penn - UPHS (page 60); **Address:** Hosp Univ Penn - Cytopathology, 3400 Spruce St, 6 Founders, Philadelphia, PA 19104; **Phone:** 215-662-3238; **Board Cert:** Anatomic Pathology 1975; Cytopathology 1989; **Med School:** India 1965; **Resid:** Pathology, All India Inst Med Scis 1967; **Fellow:** Pathology, Mass Genl Hosp 1968; Cytopathology, Johns Hopkins Hosp 1969; **Fac Appt:** Prof Path, Univ Pennsylvania

Heller, Debra S MD [Path] - **Spec Exp:** Gynecologic Pathology; Pediatric Pathology; Perinatal Pathology; **Hospital:** UMDNJ-Univ Hosp-Newark; **Address:** UMDNJ-NJ Med Sch Dept Pathology, 185 S Orange Ave, Newark, NJ 07101; **Phone:** 973-972-0751; **Board Cert:** Anatomic Pathology 1988; Obstetrics & Gynecology 2008; Pediatric Pathology 1999; **Med School:** NY Med Coll 1977; **Resid:** Obstetrics & Gynecology, Beth Israel Med Ctr 1981; Anatomic Pathology, Mt Sinai Med Ctr 1988; **Fellow:** Pediatric Pathology, Mt Sinai Med Ctr 1987; Gynecologic Pathology, Mt Sinai Med Ctr 1989; **Fac Appt:** Prof Path, UMDNJ-NJ Med Sch, Newark

Hoda, Syed A MD [Path] - **Spec Exp:** Breast Cancer; Surgical Pathology; **Hospital:** NY-Presby Hosp/Weill Cornell (page 66); **Address:** 525 E 68th St, 1028 Starr, New York, NY 10021-4870; **Phone:** 212-746-2700; **Board Cert:** Anatomic & Clinical Pathology 1990; Cytopathology 1991; Pathology 2001; **Med School:** Pakistan 1984; **Resid:** Anatomic & Clinical Pathology, Tulane Univ Affil Hosps 1990; **Fellow:** Cytopathology, Meml Sloan Kettering Cancer Ctr 1991; Pathology, Meml Sloan Kettering Cancer Ctr 1992; **Fac Appt:** Clin Prof Path, Cornell Univ-Weill Med Coll

Hruban, Ralph H MD [Path] - **Spec Exp:** Gastrointestinal Pathology; Pancreatic Cancer; **Hospital:** Johns Hopkins Hosp (page 61); **Address:** Johns Hopkins Hosp, Dept Pathology, 401 N Broadway Bldg Weinberg - rm 2242, Baltimore, MD 21231; **Phone:** 410-955-9132; **Board Cert:** Anatomic Pathology 1990; **Med School:** Johns Hopkins Univ 1985; **Resid:** Pathology, Johns Hopkins Hosp 1990; **Fellow:** Meml Sloan Kettering Cancer Ctr 1989; **Fac Appt:** Prof Path, Johns Hopkins Univ

Jaffe, Elaine S MD [Path] - **Spec Exp:** Lymphoma; Hematopathology; **Hospital:** Natl Inst of Hlth - Clin Ctr; **Address:** NIH/NCI - Lab Pathology, 10 Center Drive Bldg 10 - rm 2B42, Bethesda, MD 20892-1500; **Phone:** 301-496-0183; **Board Cert:** Anatomic Pathology 1974; **Med School:** Univ Pennsylvania 1969; **Resid:** Pathology, Clinical Ctr/NIH 1972; **Fellow:** Hematopathology, Natl Cancer Inst 1974; **Fac Appt:** Clin Prof Path, Geo Wash Univ

Jones, Robert V MD [Path] - **Spec Exp:** Neuro-Pathology; Brain Tumors; **Hospital:** Georgetown Univ Hosp; **Address:** GWUMC, Dept Path, 2300 Eye St NW, Ross Hall, Ste 502, Washington, DC 20037; **Phone:** 202-994-3391; **Board Cert:** Anatomic & Clinical Pathology 1981; Neuropathology 1994; **Med School:** Univ VA Sch Med 1977; **Resid:** Anatomic & Clinical Pathology, Walter Reed AMC 1981; **Fellow:** Neurological Pathology, ARmed Forces Inst Path 1990; **Fac Appt:** Assoc Prof Path, Geo Wash Univ

Kahn, Leonard B MD [Path] - **Spec Exp:** Bone Pathology; Head & Neck Pathology; Soft Tissue Tumors; **Hospital:** Long Island Jewish Med Ctr, N Shore Univ Hosp; **Address:** 270-05 76th Ave, rm B67, New Hyde Park, NY 11040-1433; **Phone:** 718-470-7491; **Board Cert:** Anatomic Pathology 1980; **Med School:** South Africa 1960; **Resid:** Pathology, Univ Cape Town 1966; **Fellow:** Pathology, Washington Univ 1969; **Fac Appt:** Prof Path, Albert Einstein Coll Med

Katzenstein, Anna-Luise A MD [Path] - **Spec Exp:** Lung Cancer; Pulmonary Pathology; Interstitial Lung Disease; **Hospital:** Univ Hosp - SUNY Upstate, Crouse Hosp; **Address:** SUNY Upstate Medical Univ, 766 Irving Ave, Weiskotten, rm 2106, Syracuse, NY 13210; **Phone:** 315-464-7125; **Board Cert:** Anatomic Pathology 1976; **Med School:** Johns Hopkins Univ 1971; **Resid:** Pathology, Univ Hosp 1975; **Fellow:** Surgical Pathology, Barnes Hosp-Wash Univ 1976; **Fac Appt:** Prof Path, SUNY Upstate Med Univ

Knowles, Daniel M MD [Path] - **Spec Exp:** Lymph Node Pathology; Bone Marrow Pathology; Lymphoma; **Hospital:** NY-Presby Hosp/Weill Cornell (page 66); **Address:** Cornell-Weill Med Coll-Dept Pathology, 1300 York Ave, rm C302, New York, NY 10021; **Phone:** 212-746-6464; **Board Cert:** Anatomic Pathology 1978; Immunopathology 1984; **Med School:** Univ Chicago-Pritzker Sch Med 1973; **Resid:** Anatomic Pathology, Columbia-Presby Med Ctr 1975; **Fellow:** Immunopathology, Rockefeller Univ 1977; **Fac Appt:** Prof Path, Cornell Univ-Weill Med Coll

Kurman, Robert J MD [Path] - **Spec Exp:** Gynecologic Pathology; Ovarian Cancer; Uterine Cancer; **Hospital:** Johns Hopkins Hosp (page 61); **Address:** Johns Hopkins Hosp, Dept Pathology, 401 N Broadway, Weinberg-2242, Baltimore, MD 21231; **Phone:** 410-955-0471; **Board Cert:** Anatomic Pathology 1972; Obstetrics & Gynecology 1980; **Med School:** SUNY Upstate Med Univ 1968; **Resid:** Pathology, Peter Bent Brigham Hosp/Mass Genl Hosp 1977; Obstetrics & Gynecology, LAC Hosp/USC 1978; **Fellow:** Obstetrics & Gynecology, Harvard Univ 1973; **Fac Appt:** Prof Path, Johns Hopkins Univ

Li Volsi, Virginia A MD [Path] - **Spec Exp:** Endocrine Cancers; Thyroid Cancer; Gynecologic Cancer; **Hospital:** Hosp Univ Penn - UPHS (page 60); **Address:** Hosp Univ Penn - Pathology, 3400 Spruce St 6 Founders Bldg - Ste 6030, Philadelphia, PA 19104; **Phone:** 215-662-6545; **Board Cert:** Anatomic Pathology 1974; **Med School:** Columbia P&S 1969; **Resid:** Anatomic Pathology, Presbyterian Hosp 1974; **Fac Appt:** Prof Path, Univ Pennsylvania

McNutt, N Scott MD [Path] - **Spec Exp:** Dermatopathology; **Hospital:** Rockefeller Univ; **Address:** Rockefeller Univ, Krueger Laboratory, 1230 York Ave, Box 175, New York, NY 10065; **Phone:** 212-327-8000; **Board Cert:** Anatomic Pathology 1973; Dermatopathology 1979; **Med School:** Harvard Med Sch 1966; **Resid:** Pathology, Mass Genl Hosp 1970; **Fellow:** Pathology, Mass Genl Hosp 1972

Melamed, Jonathan MD [Path] - **Spec Exp:** Prostate Cancer; Tumor Banking-Prostate; **Hospital:** NYU Langone Med Ctr (page 67); **Address:** NYU Medical Ctr, Dept Pathology, TH-461, 560 First Ave, New York, NY 10016; **Phone:** 212-263-8927; **Board Cert:** Anatomic & Clinical Pathology 1992; **Med School:** South Africa 1985; **Resid:** Pathology, Lenox Hill Hosp 1991; **Fellow:** Pathology, Meml Sloan Kettering Cancer Ctr 1992; Urologic Pathology, Meml Sloan Kettering Cancer Ctr 1993; **Fac Appt:** Assoc Prof Path, NYU Sch Med

Mies, Carolyn MD [Path] - **Spec Exp:** Breast Cancer; **Hospital:** Hosp Univ Penn - UPHS (page 60); **Address:** Hosp Univ Penn-Surgical Pathology, 3400 Spruce St, Founders 6, Philadelphia, PA 19104; **Phone:** 215-662-6503; **Board Cert:** Anatomic Pathology 1984; **Med School:** Rush Med Coll 1980; **Resid:** Pathology, Tufts-New England Med Ctr 1982; Pathology, New England Deaconess Hosp 1984; **Fellow:** Surgical Pathology, Meml Sloan Kettering Cancer Ctr 1986; **Fac Appt:** Assoc Prof Path, Univ Pennsylvania

Montgomery, Elizabeth A MD [Path] - **Spec Exp:** Barrett's Esophagus; Esophageal Cancer; Gastrointestinal Pathology; **Hospital:** Johns Hopkins Hosp (page 61); **Address:** Johns Hopkins Univ, Dept Pathology, 401 N Broadway Weinberg Bldg - rm 2242, Baltimore, MD 21231; **Phone:** 410-614-2308; **Board Cert:** Anatomic Pathology 1988; Cytopathology 1994; **Med School:** Geo Wash Univ 1984; **Resid:** Pathology, Walter Reed AMC 1988; **Fac Appt:** Assoc Prof Path, Johns Hopkins Univ

Orazi, Attilio MD [Path] - **Spec Exp:** Hematopathology; Bone Marrow Pathology; Lymph Node Pathology; **Hospital:** NY-Presby Hosp/Weill Cornell (page 66); **Address:** NY Presby-Cornell Medical Ctr, 525 E 68th St, Starr Pavilion, rm 715, New York, NY 10021; **Phone:** 212-746-2050; **Board Cert:** Anatomic Pathology 1997; Hematology 1998; **Med School:** Italy 1979; **Resid:** Internal Medicine, Leicester Royal Infirmary 1982; Histopathology, Northampton Genl Hosp 1983; **Fellow:** Anatomic Pathology, Natl Cancer Inst 1985; **Fac Appt:** Prof Path, Cornell Univ-Weill Med Coll

Patchefsky, Arthur S MD [Path] - **Spec Exp:** Breast Cancer; Pulmonary Pathology; Sarcoma; **Hospital:** Fox Chase Cancer Ctr (page 58); **Address:** Fox Chase Cancer Center, 333 Cottman Ave, rm C4333, Philadelphia, PA 19111; **Phone:** 215-728-5390; **Board Cert:** Anatomic Pathology 1969; **Med School:** Hahnemann Univ 1963; **Resid:** Pathology, John Hopkins Hosp 1966; Pathology, Hosp Univ Penn 1967; **Fellow:** Pathology, Meml Sloan Kettering Cancer Ctr 1968; **Fac Appt:** Prof Path, Thomas Jefferson Univ

Reuter, Victor E MD [Path] - **Spec Exp:** Prostate Cancer; Genitourinary Pathology; Bladder Cancer; Urologic Pathology; **Hospital:** Meml Sloan-Kettering Cancer Ctr; **Address:** Memorial Sloan Kettering Cancer Ctr, Dept Pathology, 1275 York Ave, New York, NY 10021; **Phone:** 212-639-8225; **Board Cert:** Anatomic & Clinical Pathology 1983; **Med School:** Dominican Republic 1978; **Resid:** Anatomic Pathology, Thos Jefferson Univ Hosp 1981; Clinical Pathology, Thos Jefferson Univ Hosp 1983; **Fellow:** Surgical Pathology, Meml Sloan Kettering Cancer Ctr 1985; **Fac Appt:** Prof Path, Cornell Univ-Weill Med Coll

Rosen, Paul P MD [Path] - **Spec Exp:** Breast Pathology; Breast Cancer; **Hospital:** NY-Presby Hosp/Weill Cornell (page 66); **Address:** New York Presbyterian, Dept Pathology, 525 E 68th St, Starr 1031, New York, NY 10065; **Phone:** 212-746-6482; **Board Cert:** Anatomic & Clinical Pathology 1969; Pathology 1998; **Med School:** Columbia P&S 1964; **Resid:** Pathology, Presby Hosp 1966; Pathology, VA Hosp 1968; **Fellow:** Pathology, Meml Hosp Cancer Ctr 1970; **Fac Appt:** Prof Path, Cornell Univ-Weill Med Coll

Rosenblum, Marc K MD [Path] - **Spec Exp:** Neuropathology; Brain Tumors; **Hospital:** Meml Sloan-Kettering Cancer Ctr; **Address:** 1275 York Avenue, New York, NY 10065; **Phone:** 212-639-5905; **Board Cert:** Anatomic Pathology 1984; Pathology 1998; Neuropathology 1988; **Med School:** Univ Miami Sch Med 1979; **Resid:** Anatomic Pathology, Mt Sinai Med Ctr 1984; **Fellow:** Pathology, Meml Sloan-Kettering Cancer Ctr 1985; Neurological Pathology, Bellevue-NYU Med Ctr 1987; **Fac Appt:** Prof Path, Cornell Univ-Weill Med Coll

Ross, Jeffrey S MD [Path] - **Spec Exp:** Urologic Cancer; Prostate Cancer; Breast Cancer; **Hospital:** Albany Med Ctr; **Address:** Albany Med Coll, Dept Path, 47 New Scotland Ave, MC 81, Albany, NY 12208; **Phone:** 518-262-5471; **Board Cert:** Anatomic & Clinical Pathology 1974; **Med School:** SUNY Buffalo 1970; **Resid:** Pathology, Mass Genl Hosp 1974; **Fellow:** Pathology, Harvard Med Sch 1974; **Fac Appt:** Prof Path, Albany Med Coll

Sanchez, Miguel A MD [Path] - **Spec Exp:** Breast Cancer; Thyroid Cancer; **Hospital:** Englewood Hosp & Med Ctr; **Address:** Englewood Hosp & Med Ctr, Dept Pathology, 350 Engle St, Englewood, NJ 07631-1898; **Phone:** 201-894-3423; **Board Cert:** Anatomic Pathology 1975; Clinical Pathology 1979; Cytopathology 1991; **Med School:** Spain 1969; **Resid:** Pathology, Englewood Hosp 1972; Pathology, Temple Univ 1973; **Fellow:** Pathology, Meml Sloan Kettering Cancer Ctr 1974; Clinical Pathology, St Vincents Hosp 1975; **Fac Appt:** Assoc Prof Path, Mount Sinai Sch Med

Schiller, Alan L MD [Path] - **Spec Exp:** Bone & Joint Pathology; Soft Tissue Pathology; Bone Tumors; **Hospital:** Mount Sinai Med Ctr (page 64); **Address:** Mt Sinai Sch Med, Dept Pathology, 1 Gustave Levy Pl, Box 1194, New York, NY 10029-6500; **Phone:** 212-241-8014; **Board Cert:** Anatomic Pathology 1973; **Med School:** Ros Franklin Univ/Chicago Med Sch 1967; **Resid:** Pathology, Mass Genl Hosp 1972; **Fac Appt:** Prof Path, Mount Sinai Sch Med

Silverberg, Steven G MD [Path] - **Spec Exp:** Gynecologic Pathology; Breast Pathology; Urologic Pathology; Endocrine Pathology; **Hospital:** Univ of MD Med Ctr; **Address:** Univ Maryland Med Ctr, Dept Pathology, 22 S Greene St, Baltimore, MD 21201; **Phone:** 410-328-5072; **Board Cert:** Anatomic Pathology 1969; **Med School:** Johns Hopkins Univ 1962; **Resid:** Pathology, Yale-New Haven Hosp 1965; **Fellow:** Surgical Pathology, Meml Sloan Kettering Cancer Ctr 1966; **Fac Appt:** Prof Path, Univ MD Sch Med

Silverman, Jan F MD [Path] - **Spec Exp:** Breast Cancer; Lung Cancer; Gastrointestinal Pathology; Fine Needle Aspiration Biopsy; **Hospital:** Allegheny General Hosp, West Penn Hosp - Forbes Campus; **Address:** Allegheny Gen Hosp-Dept Lab Medicine, 320 E North Ave, Pittsburgh, PA 15212; **Phone:** 412-359-6886; **Board Cert:** Anatomic & Clinical Pathology 1975; Cytopathology 1989; **Med School:** Med Coll VA 1970; **Resid:** Pathology, Med Coll Virginia 1975; **Fellow:** Surgical Pathology, Med Coll Virginia 1975; **Fac Appt:** Prof Path, Drexel Univ Coll Med

Swerdlow, Steven H MD [Path] - **Spec Exp:** Lymphoma; Hematopathology; Transplant Pathology; **Hospital:** UPMC Presby, Pittsburgh; **Address:** Div Hematopathology, 200 Lothrop St, Ste G-300, Pittsburgh, PA 15213-2536; **Phone:** 412-647-5191; **Board Cert:** Anatomic Pathology 2005; Clinical Pathology 2005; **Med School:** Harvard Med Sch 1975; **Resid:** Pathology, Beth Israel Hosp 1979; **Fellow:** Hematopathology, Vanderbilt Univ 1981; Hematopathology, St Bartholmew's Hosp 1983; **Fac Appt:** Prof Path, Univ Pittsburgh

Tomaszewski, John E MD [Path] - **Spec Exp:** Kidney Pathology; Lung Pathology; Uterine Cancer; Genitourinary Pathology; **Hospital:** Hosp Univ Penn - UPHS (page 60); **Address:** Hosp Univ Penn, Dept Pathology & Lab Med, 3400 Spruce St, 6 Founders Bldg, Ste 6042, Philadelphia, PA 19104; **Phone:** 215-662-6852; **Board Cert:** Anatomic Pathology 1982; Immunopathology 1983; **Med School:** Univ Pennsylvania 1977; **Resid:** Pathology, Hosp Univ Penn 1982; **Fellow:** Surgical Pathology, Hosp Univ Penn 1983; **Fac Appt:** Prof Path, Univ Pennsylvania

Pathology

Tornos, Carmen MD [Path] - **Spec Exp:** Gynecologic Cancer; Breast Cancer; Ovarian Cancer; **Hospital:** Stony Brook Univ Med Ctr; **Address:** Stony Brook Univ Hosp, Dept Pathology, Level 2, rm 766, Stony Brook, NY 11794; **Phone:** 631-444-2222; **Board Cert:** Anatomic & Clinical Pathology 1989; **Med School:** Spain 1977; **Resid:** Hematology, Ciudad Sanitaria Valle de Hebron 1982; Anatomic & Clinical Pathology, Univ Texas HSC 1989; **Fellow:** Surgical Pathology, MD Anderson Cancer Ctr 1990; **Fac Appt:** Prof Path, SUNY Stony Brook

Travis, William MD [Path] - **Spec Exp:** Pulmonary Pathology; Lung Cancer; Interstitial Lung Disease; **Hospital:** Meml Sloan-Kettering Cancer Ctr; **Address:** 1275 York Avenue, Pathology Dept, New York, NY 10065; **Phone:** 800-525-2225; **Board Cert:** Anatomic & Clinical Pathology 1985; **Med School:** Univ Fla Coll Med 1981; **Resid:** Anatomic Pathology, New England Deaconess Hosp 1983; Clinical Pathology, Mayo Clinic 1985; **Fellow:** Surgical Pathology, Mayo Clinic 1986

Yousem, Samuel A MD [Path] - **Spec Exp:** Pulmonary Pathology; Transplant-Lung (Pathology); Lung Cancer; **Hospital:** UPMC Presby, Pittsburgh; **Address:** Dept Pathology, A-610, UPMC-Presbyterian Campus, 200 Lothrop St, Pittsburgh, PA 15213; **Phone:** 412-647-6193; **Board Cert:** Anatomic Pathology 1985; Cytopathology 1997; **Med School:** Univ MD Sch Med 1981; **Resid:** Pathology, Stanford Univ Med Ctr 1983; **Fellow:** Surgical Pathology, Stanford Univ Med Ctr 1984; **Fac Appt:** Prof Path, Univ Pittsburgh

Zagzag, David MD/PhD [Path] - **Spec Exp:** Neuropathology; Brain Tumors; Tumor Banking-Brain; **Hospital:** NYU Langone Med Ctr (page 67), Bellevue Hosp Ctr; **Address:** NYU Med Ctr, Dept Pathology, 550 First Ave, Div Neuropathology, NB-4N30, New York, NY 10016; **Phone:** 212-263-6449; **Board Cert:** Anatomic Pathology 1993; Neuropathology 1993; **Med School:** France 1984; **Resid:** Surgical Pathology, NYU Med Ctr 1990; **Fellow:** Neurological Pathology, NYU Med Ctr 1992; **Fac Appt:** Assoc Prof Path, NYU Sch Med

Southeast

Banks, Peter MD [Path] - **Spec Exp:** Hematopathology; Lymphoma; **Hospital:** Carolinas Med Ctr; **Address:** Dept Pathology, 1000 Blythe Blvd, 4th Fl Pathology Lab, Charlotte, NC 28203; **Phone:** 704-355-2251; **Board Cert:** Anatomic Pathology 2008; **Med School:** Harvard Med Sch 1971; **Resid:** Pathology, National Cancer Inst 1974; Pathology, Duke Univ Med Ctr 1975; **Fellow:** Surgical Pathology, Univ Minn Med Ctr 1976; **Fac Appt:** Prof Path, Univ NC Sch Med

Bostwick, David MD [Path] - **Spec Exp:** Urologic Pathology; Prostate Cancer; Bladder Cancer; Gastrointestinal Pathology; **Address:** 4355 Innslake Drive, Glen Allen, VA 23060; **Phone:** 804-967-9225; **Board Cert:** Anatomic Pathology 2003; **Med School:** Univ MD Sch Med 1979; **Resid:** Pathology, Stanford Univ Med Ctr 1981; **Fellow:** Surgical Pathology, Stanford Univ Med Ctr 1984

Braylan, Raul MD [Path] - **Spec Exp:** Hematopathology; Leukemia; Lymphoma; **Hospital:** Shands at Univ of FL; **Address:** Univ Florida, Dept Hematopathology, PO Box 100275, Gainesville, FL 32610; **Phone:** 352-265-9900; **Board Cert:** Anatomic Pathology 1972; **Med School:** Argentina 1960; **Resid:** Anatomic Pathology, Mt Sinai Hosp 1965; Anatomic Pathology, Einstein Affil Hosps 1967; **Fellow:** Anatomic Pathology, Meml Sloan Kettering Cancer Hosp 1968; Hematopathology, Univ Chicago Hosps 1973; **Fac Appt:** Prof Path, Univ Fla Coll Med

Chesney, Carolyn M MD [Path] - **Spec Exp:** Hematopathology; Bleeding/Coagulation Disorders; **Hospital:** Baptist Memorial Hospital - Memphis; **Address:** Dept of Pathology-Coag Lab, 6019 Walnut Grove, Memphis, TN 38120; **Phone:** 901-226-5650; **Board Cert:** Internal Medicine 1972; Hematology 1999; **Med School:** Vanderbilt Univ 1968; **Resid:** Internal Medicine, Vanderbilt Univ Hosp 1970; **Fellow:** Hematology, Mass Genl Hosp 1972; **Fac Appt:** Prof Med, Univ Tenn Coll Med, Memphis

Cote, Richard J MD [Path] - **Spec Exp:** Lymph Node Pathology; Bladder Cancer; Breast Cancer; **Hospital:** Univ of Miami Hosp (page 71); **Address:** 1611 NW 12th Ave, Holtz Bldg - rm 2046, Miami, FL 33136; **Phone:** 305-585-6103; **Board Cert:** Anatomic Pathology 1987; **Med School:** Univ Chicago-Pritzker Sch Med 1980; **Resid:** Pathology, New York Hosp-Cornell 1987; **Fellow:** Pathology, Meml Sloan-Kettering Cancer Ctr 1990; **Fac Appt:** Prof Path, USC-Keck School of Medicine

Faye-Petersen, Ona MD [Path] - **Spec Exp:** Perinatal Pathology; Fetal Pathology; Neonatal Pathology; Pediatric Pathology; **Hospital:** Univ of Ala Hosp at Birmingham, UAB Highlands Hosp; **Address:** UAB Hospital, 1802 6th Ave S, Birmingham, AL 35249; **Phone:** 205-975-8880; **Board Cert:** Anatomic & Clinical Pathology 1987; Pediatric Pathology 1991; **Med School:** Univ Colorado 1980; **Resid:** Pathology, Presby-Denver Hosp 1985; **Fellow:** Surgical Pathology, Meml Sloan Ketter Cancer Ctr 1986; Pediatric Pathology, Mt Sinai Hosp 1987; **Fac Appt:** Assoc Prof Path, Univ Alabama

Lage, Janice MD [Path] - **Spec Exp:** Obstetric Pathology; Gynecologic Pathology; Breast Pathology; **Hospital:** MUSC Med Ctr; **Address:** MUSC Med Ctr, Dept Path, 165 Ashley Ave, Ste 309, Box 250908, Charleston, SC 29425; **Phone:** 843-792-3121; **Board Cert:** Anatomic Pathology 2001; **Med School:** Washington Univ, St Louis 1980; **Resid:** Pathology, Barnes Hosp/Wash Univ 1982; Obstetrics & Gynecology, Barnes Hosp/Wash Univ 1983; **Fellow:** Surgical Pathology, Barnes Hosp/Wash Univ 1984; **Fac Appt:** Prof Path, Med Univ SC

Masood, Shahla MD [Path] - **Spec Exp:** Breast Cancer; Breast Pathology; **Hospital:** Shands Jacksonville; **Address:** Univ of Florida, Dept Pathology, 655 W 8th St, Jacksonville, FL 32209-6511; **Phone:** 904-244-4387; **Board Cert:** Anatomic & Clinical Pathology 1998; Cytopathology 1990; **Med School:** Iran 1973; **Resid:** Anatomic Pathology, Univ Hosp 1977; **Fac Appt:** Prof Path, Univ Fla Coll Med

McCurley, Thomas L MD [Path] - **Spec Exp:** Hematopathology; Immunopathology; **Hospital:** Vanderbilt Univ Med Ctr, VA Med Ctr - Nashville; **Address:** Vanderbilt Univ Hosp, Dept Pathology, 21st & Garland Ave, Nashville, TN 37232-0001; **Phone:** 615-343-9167; **Board Cert:** Anatomic & Clinical Pathology 1981; Immunopathology 1986; Hematology 1999; **Med School:** Vanderbilt Univ 1974; **Resid:** Internal Medicine, UCSF Med Ctr 1976; Pathology, Vanderbilt Univ Med Ctr 1981; **Fellow:** Hematopathology, Vanderbilt Univ 1984; **Fac Appt:** Assoc Prof Path, Vanderbilt Univ

Mills, Stacey E MD [Path] - **Spec Exp:** Breast Pathology; Ear, Nose & Throat Cancer; Surgical Pathology; **Hospital:** Univ Virginia Med Ctr; **Address:** Univ VA Hlth System, Dept Pathology, PO Box 800214, Charlottesville, VA 22908-0214; **Phone:** 434-982-4406; **Board Cert:** Anatomic Pathology 1999; **Med School:** Univ VA Sch Med 1977; **Resid:** Pathology, Univ Virginia Med Ctr 1980; **Fellow:** Pathology, Univ Virginia 1981; **Fac Appt:** Prof Path, Univ VA Sch Med

Nicosia, Santo MD [Path] - **Spec Exp:** Ovarian Cancer; **Hospital:** H Lee Moffitt Cancer Ctr & Research Inst; **Address:** 12901 Bruce B Downs Blvd, MDC Box 11, Tampa, FL 33612-4742; **Phone:** 813-974-3133; **Board Cert:** Anatomic Pathology 1978; Cytopathology 1990; **Med School:** Italy 1967; **Resid:** Anatomic Pathology, Michael Reese Hosp 1972; **Fellow:** Hosp Univ Penn 1973; **Fac Appt:** Prof Path, Univ S Fla Coll Med

Norenberg, Michael D MD [Path] - **Spec Exp:** Liver Pathology; Parkinson's Disease; **Hospital:** Jackson Meml Hosp (page 70); **Address:** Jackson Meml Hosp, Dept Pathology, 1611 NW 12th Ave Holtz Ctr, rm 2142, Miami, FL 33136; **Phone:** 305-585-7017; **Board Cert:** Anatomic Pathology 1972; Neuropathology 1974; **Med School:** Univ Rochester 1965; **Resid:** Pathology, Strong Meml Hosp 1970; **Fellow:** Neuropathology, Strong Meml Hosp 1972; **Fac Appt:** Prof Path, Univ Miami Sch Med

Pathology

Page, David L MD [Path] - **Spec Exp:** Breast Cancer; **Hospital:** Vanderbilt Univ Med Ctr; **Address:** Vanderbilt Univ, 1161 21st Ave S, rm C 3309, Nashville, TN 37232-2561; **Phone:** 615-322-3759; **Board Cert:** Anatomic Pathology 1972; Dermatopathology 1974; **Med School:** Johns Hopkins Univ 1966; **Resid:** Pathology, Mass Genl Hosp 1969; Pathology, Johns Hopkins Hosp 1972; **Fac Appt:** Prof Path, Vanderbilt Univ

Petito, Carol K MD [Path] - **Spec Exp:** Neuro-Pathology; **Hospital:** Jackson Meml Hosp (page 70); **Address:** Univ Miami Dept Pathology (R-5), 1550 NW 10th Ave, PAP Bldg, rm 417, Miami, FL 33136; **Phone:** 305-243-3584; **Board Cert:** Anatomic Pathology 1973; Neuropathology 1973; **Med School:** Columbia P&S 1967; **Resid:** Pathology, NY Hosp-Cornell Med Ctr 1970; Neuropathology, Armed Forces Inst; **Fac Appt:** Prof Path, Univ Miami Sch Med

Sewell, C Whitaker MD [Path] - **Spec Exp:** Breast Pathology; Surgical Pathology; **Hospital:** Emory Univ Hosp; **Address:** Emory Univ Hosp, Dept Pathology, 1364 Clifton Rd NE, rm H185C, Atlanta, GA 30322; **Phone:** 404-712-5947; **Board Cert:** Anatomic Pathology 1974; Clinical Pathology 1974; **Med School:** Emory Univ 1969; **Resid:** Pathology, Emory Univ Hosp 1974; **Fac Appt:** Prof Path, Emory Univ

Weiss, Sharon A W MD [Path] - **Spec Exp:** Soft Tissue Pathology; Surgical Pathology; Sarcoma; **Hospital:** Emory Univ Hosp; **Address:** Emory Univ Hosp, Dept Pathology, 1364 Clifton Rd NE, rm H176, Atlanta, GA 30322; **Phone:** 404-712-0708; **Board Cert:** Anatomic Pathology 1974; **Med School:** Johns Hopkins Univ 1971; **Resid:** Pathology, Johns Hopkins Hosp 1975; **Fac Appt:** Prof Path, Emory Univ

Midwest

Allred, D Craig MD [Path] - **Spec Exp:** Breast Cancer; Breast Pathology; Breast Cancer Risk Assessment; **Hospital:** Barnes-Jewish Hosp; **Address:** Washington Univ Sch Med, Path & Immunology, 660 S Euclid Ave, Box 8118, St Louis, MO 63110; **Phone:** 314-362-6313; **Board Cert:** Anatomic Pathology 1984; **Med School:** Univ Utah 1979; **Resid:** Anatomic Pathology, Univ Conn Hlth Ctr 1983; **Fellow:** Immunopathology, Univ Conn Hlth Ctr 1982; **Fac Appt:** Prof Path, Baylor Coll Med

Appelman, Henry MD [Path] - **Spec Exp:** Gastrointestinal Pathology; Liver Pathology; **Hospital:** Univ Michigan Hlth Sys; **Address:** Univ Michigan, Dept Pathology, 1500 E Med Ctr Drive, Ann Arbor, MI 48109-0054; **Phone:** 734-936-6770; **Board Cert:** Anatomic & Clinical Pathology 1966; **Med School:** Univ Mich Med Sch 1961; **Resid:** Pathology, Univ Mich Med Ctr 1966; **Fac Appt:** Prof Path, Univ Mich Med Sch

Balla, Andre K MD/PhD [Path] - **Spec Exp:** Prostate Cancer; Gynecologic Pathology; Tumor Banking; **Hospital:** Univ of IL Med Ctr at Chicago; **Address:** Univ Illinois Chicago, Dept Path, 840 S Wood St, rm 130, MC 847, Chicago, IL 60612; **Phone:** 312-996-3879; **Board Cert:** Anatomic & Clinical Pathology 1988; **Med School:** Brazil 1972; **Resid:** Pathology, Hahnemann Univ Hosp 1988; **Fellow:** Clinical Immunology, Scripps Clin Rsch Fdn 1981; **Fac Appt:** Prof Path, Univ IL Coll Med

Behm, Frederick G MD [Path] - **Spec Exp:** Hematopathology; **Hospital:** Univ of IL Med Ctr at Chicago; **Address:** Univ Illinois Chicago, Dept Pathology, 130 CSN, MC 847, 840 S Wood St, Chicago, IL 60612-7335; **Phone:** 312-996-3150; **Board Cert:** Anatomic & Clinical Pathology 1980; Hematology 1983; **Med School:** Med Coll Wisc 1974; **Resid:** Pathology, Med Coll Va Hosps 1979; **Fac Appt:** Prof Path, Univ IL Coll Med

Bell, Debra A MD [Path] - **Spec Exp:** Gynecologic Pathology; Ovarian Cancer; **Hospital:** Mayo Med Ctr & Clin - Rochester; **Address:** Mayo Clinic-Pathology Dept, 200 First St SW, Rochester, MN 55905; **Phone:** 507-284-1800; **Board Cert:** Anatomic Pathology 1980; Cytopathology 1989; **Med School:** Albany Med Coll 1976; **Resid:** Pathology, NYU Med Ctr 1981; **Fellow:** Cytopathology, Meml Sloan Kettering Cancer Ctr 1982; **Fac Appt:** Assoc Prof Path, Mayo Med Sch

Cho, Kathleen R MD [Path] - **Spec Exp:** Gynecologic Pathology; Ovarian Cancer; Cervical Cancer; **Hospital:** Univ Michigan Hlth Sys; **Address:** Univ Michigan Med Sch, 109 Zina Pitcher Pl, rm 1506, Ann Arbor, MI 48109-2200; **Phone:** 734-764-1549; **Board Cert:** Anatomic Pathology 1990; **Med School:** Vanderbilt Univ 1984; **Resid:** Pathology, Johns Hopkins Hosp 1988; **Fellow:** Gynecologic Pathology, Johns Hopkins Hosp 1990; **Fac Appt:** Prof Path, Univ Mich Med Sch

Cohen, Michael B MD [Path] - **Spec Exp:** Urologic Cancer; Cytopathology; **Hospital:** Univ Iowa Hosp & Clinics, VA Med Ctr - Iowa City; **Address:** Univ Iowa - Dept Pathology, 200 Hawkins Drive, C670GH, Iowa City, IA 52242; **Phone:** 319-384-9609; **Board Cert:** Anatomic Pathology 2008; Cytopathology 1996; **Med School:** Albany Med Coll 1982; **Resid:** Pathology, UCSF Hosps & Clinics 1986; **Fellow:** Cytopathology, UCSF Hosps & Clinics 1987; **Fac Appt:** Prof Path, Univ Iowa Coll Med

Gambetti, Pierluigi MD [Path] - **Spec Exp:** Neuro-Pathology; Neurodegenerative Disorders; Creutzfeldt-Jakob Disease (CJD); **Hospital:** Univ Hosps Case Med Ctr; **Address:** Case Western Reserve Univ, Inst Path, 2085 Adelbert Rd, rm 419, Cleveland, OH 44106; **Phone:** 216-368-0587; **Board Cert:** Neuropathology 1981; **Med School:** Italy 1960; **Resid:** Neurology, Univ Bologna Med Ctr 1963; **Fellow:** Neurological Pathology, Institut Bunge 1965; Neurological Pathology, Hosp Univ Penn 1968; **Fac Appt:** Prof Path, Case West Res Univ

Goldblum, John R MD [Path] - **Spec Exp:** Soft Tissue Pathology; Esophageal Cancer; Gastrointestinal Pathology; Sarcoma; **Hospital:** Cleveland Clin Fdn (page 56); **Address:** Cleveland Clinic, Anatomic Pathology L25, 9500 Euclid Ave, Cleveland, OH 44195; **Phone:** 216-444-8238; **Board Cert:** Anatomic Pathology 1993; **Med School:** Univ Mich Med Sch 1989; **Resid:** Anatomic Pathology, Univ Michigan Hosps 1993; **Fac Appt:** Prof Path, Cleveland Cl Coll Med/Case West Res

Greenson, Joel K MD [Path] - **Spec Exp:** Liver Cancer; Gastrointestinal Pathology; Liver Pathology; **Hospital:** Univ Michigan Hlth Sys; **Address:** Univ Michigan Hospitals, Dept Pathology, 1500 E Medical Center Drive, rm 2G332, Ann Arbor, MI 48109-0054; **Phone:** 734-936-6799; **Board Cert:** Anatomic & Clinical Pathology 1988; **Med School:** Univ Mich Med Sch 1984; **Resid:** Pathology, Cedars-Sinai Med Ctr 1988; **Fellow:** Gastrointestinal Pathology, Johns Hopkins Hosp 1990; **Fac Appt:** Prof Path, Univ Mich Med Sch

Kurtin, Paul J MD [Path] - **Spec Exp:** Lymph Node Pathology; Bone Marrow Pathology; Lymphoma; **Hospital:** Mayo Med Ctr & Clin - Rochester; **Address:** Mayo Clinic - Div Hematopathology, 200 First St SW, Hilton 1156A, Rochester, MN 55905; **Phone:** 507-284-4939; **Board Cert:** Anatomic & Clinical Pathology 1983; Hematology 1988; **Med School:** Med Coll Wisc 1979; **Resid:** Anatomic & Clinical Pathology, Vanderbilt Univ Med Ctr 1983; **Fellow:** Hematopathology, Brigham & Women's Hosp 1984; Surgical Pathology, Brigham & Women's Hosp 1986; **Fac Appt:** Prof Path, Mayo Med Sch

Mitros, Frank A MD [Path] - **Spec Exp:** Liver Pathology; Gastrointestinal Pathology; Surgical Pathology; **Hospital:** Univ Iowa Hosp & Clinics; **Address:** Univ Iowa Hosp & Clins, Dept Pathology, 200 Hawkins Dr, 5244B RCP, Iowa City, IA 52242; **Phone:** 319-356-1760; **Board Cert:** Anatomic Pathology 1979; **Med School:** UMDNJ-NJ Med Sch, Newark 1969; **Resid:** Pathology, Univ Chicago Hosps 1976; **Fac Appt:** Prof Path, Univ Iowa Coll Med

Pathology

Myers, Jeffrey L MD [Path] - **Spec Exp:** Lung Cancer; Lung Pathology; **Hospital:** Univ Michigan Hlth Sys; **Address:** Univ Michigan, 2G332 UH, CCC 1500 E Med Ctr Dr, Fl B1-Rm363, Ann Arbor, MI 48109-5912; **Phone:** 734-647-8902; **Board Cert:** Anatomic Pathology 1986; **Med School:** Washington Univ, St Louis 1981; **Resid:** Anatomic Pathology, Barnes Jewish Hosp 1984; **Fellow:** Surgical Pathology, U Alabama Med Ctr 1985; **Fac Appt:** Prof Path, Univ Mich Med Sch

Nascimento, Antonio G MD [Path] - **Spec Exp:** Bone & Soft Tissue Pathology; Head & Neck Pathology; **Hospital:** Mayo Med Ctr & Clin - Rochester; **Address:** Mayo Clinic - Dept Pathology, 200 First St SW, Rochester, MN 55905; **Phone:** 507-284-1187; **Board Cert:** Anatomic Pathology 1979; **Med School:** Brazil ; **Resid:** Pathology, Univ Mississippi Med Ctr; **Fellow:** Anatomic Pathology, Meml Sloan-Kettering Cancer Ctr; Surgical Pathology, Mayo Clinic

Perry, Arie MD [Path] - **Spec Exp:** Neuro-Pathology; Brain Tumors; **Hospital:** Washington Univ Med Ctr; **Address:** Washington Univ Sch Med, Dept Path-Div Neuropath, Box 8118, 660 S Euclid Ave, St Louis, MO 63110; **Phone:** 314-362-7426; **Board Cert:** Anatomic & Clinical Pathology 1995; Neuropathology 1997; **Med School:** Univ Tex SW, Dallas 1990; **Resid:** Pathology, Univ Tex SW 1994; **Fellow:** Surgical Pathology, Mayo Clinic 1995; Neurological Pathology, Mayo Clinic 1998; **Fac Appt:** Assoc Prof Path, Washington Univ, St Louis

Petras, Robert E MD [Path] - **Spec Exp:** Gastrointestinal Pathology; **Hospital:** Western Reserve Care Sys; **Address:** Ameripath GI Institute, 7730 First Pl, Ste A, Oakwood Village, OH 44146; **Phone:** 440-703-2100; **Board Cert:** Anatomic & Clinical Pathology 2004; **Med School:** Ohio State Univ 1978; **Resid:** Anatomic & Clinical Pathology, Cleveland Clinic 1982; **Fellow:** Gastrointestinal Pathology, St Marks Hosp; **Fac Appt:** Assoc Prof Path, NE Ohio Univ

Rubin, Brian P MD [Path] - **Spec Exp:** Bone & Soft Tissue Pathology; Sarcoma; **Hospital:** Cleveland Clin Fdn (page 56); **Address:** Cleveland Clinic, Dept Anatomic Pathology, L25, 9500 Euclid Ave, Cleveland, OH 44195; **Phone:** 216-445-5551; **Board Cert:** Anatomic Pathology 1999; **Med School:** Cornell Univ-Weill Med Coll 1995; **Resid:** Pathology, Brigham & Womens Hosp 2000; **Fac Appt:** Asst Prof Path, Univ Wash

Scheithauer, Bernd W MD [Path] - **Spec Exp:** Brain Tumors; Pituitary Tumors; Neuro-Pathology; Pituitary Disorders; **Hospital:** Mayo Med Ctr & Clin - Rochester; **Address:** Dept Pathology, 200 First St SW, Rochester, MN 55905; **Phone:** 507-284-8350; **Board Cert:** Anatomic Pathology 1979; Neuropathology 1979; **Med School:** Loma Linda Univ 1973; **Resid:** Anatomic Pathology, Stanford Univ Med Ctr 1976; Neuropathology, Stanford Univ Med Ctr 1978; **Fellow:** Surgical Pathology, Stanford Univ Med Ctr 1979; **Fac Appt:** Prof Path, Mayo Med Sch

Suster, Saul M MD [Path] - **Spec Exp:** Lung Cancer; Mediastinal Tumors; Surgical Pathology; **Hospital:** Froedtert Meml Lutheran Hosp; **Address:** Med College of Wisconsin, Dept Pathology, Dynacare Lab Bldg, rm 226, 9200 W Wisconsin Ave, Milwaukee, WI 53226; **Phone:** 414-805-6968; **Board Cert:** Anatomic & Clinical Pathology 1988; **Med School:** Ecuador 1976; **Resid:** Anatomic Pathology, Tel Aviv Univ Med Ctr 1984; Anatomic & Clinical Pathology, Mt Sinai Med Ctr 1988; **Fellow:** Surgical Pathology, Yale-New Haven Hosp 1990; **Fac Appt:** Prof Path, Med Coll Wisc

Ulbright, Thomas M MD [Path] - **Spec Exp:** Testicular Cancer; Gynecologic Pathology; **Hospital:** Indiana Univ Hosp; **Address:** Clarion Pathology Laboratory, 350 W 11th St, rm 4014, Indianapolis, IN 46202; **Phone:** 317-491-6498; **Board Cert:** Anatomic Pathology 1980; **Med School:** Washington Univ, St Louis 1975; **Resid:** Pathology, Barnes Jewish Hosp 1978; Surgical Pathology, Barnes Jewish Hosp 1979; **Fellow:** Gynecologic Pathology, St Johns Mercy Med Ctr 1980; **Fac Appt:** Prof Path, Indiana Univ

Great Plains and Mountains

De Masters, Bette K MD [Path] - **Spec Exp:** Neuro-Pathology; Brain Tumors; **Hospital:** Univ Colorado Hosp, Chldn's Hosp - Aurora, The; **Address:** Univ CO Hlth Sci Ctr, Dept Pathology, Box 6511, MS 8104, Aurora, CO 80045-0508; **Phone:** 303-724-3704; **Board Cert:** Anatomic & Clinical Pathology 1982; Neuropathology 1985; **Med School:** Univ Wisc 1977; **Resid:** Internal Medicine, Presby Hosp 1979; Pathology, Univ Colo Med Sch 1982; **Fellow:** Neurological Pathology, Univ Colo/Univ Kansas 1984; **Fac Appt:** Prof Path, Univ Colorado

Rodgers III, George M MD/PhD [Path] - **Spec Exp:** Hematopathology; Anemia-Cancer Related; Bleeding/Coagulation Disorders; **Hospital:** Univ Utah Hosps and Clins; **Address:** Univ Utah Med Ctr - Div Hematology, 30 N 1900 E, rm 5C402, Salt Lake City, UT 84132; **Phone:** 801-585-3229; **Board Cert:** Internal Medicine 1979; Hematology 1982; Pathology 1984; **Med School:** Tulane Univ 1976; **Resid:** Internal Medicine, Baylor Affil Hosps 1979; **Fellow:** Hematology, UCSF Med Ctr 1982; **Fac Appt:** Prof Med, Univ Utah

Thor, Ann D MD [Path] - **Spec Exp:** Breast Cancer; Gynecologic Cancer; **Hospital:** Univ Colorado Hosp; **Address:** Univ CO Hlth Sci Ctr, Dept Pathology, Box 6511, MS B216, Aurora, CO 80045-0508; **Phone:** 303-724-3704; **Board Cert:** Anatomic Pathology 1987; Cytopathology 1989; **Med School:** Vanderbilt Univ 1981; **Resid:** Pathology, Vanderbilt Univ 1983; **Fellow:** Immunopathology, Natl Cancer Inst 1986; Gynecologic Pathology, Mass Genl Hosp 1990; **Fac Appt:** Prof Path, Univ Colorado

Weisenburger, Dennis MD [Path] - **Spec Exp:** Hematopathology; Lymphoma; **Hospital:** Nebraska Med Ctr; **Address:** Univ Nebraska Med Ctr, Dept Pathology, 983135 Nebraska Medical Center, Omaha, NE 68198-3135; **Phone:** 402-559-7688; **Board Cert:** Anatomic & Clinical Pathology 1979; **Med School:** Univ Minn 1974; **Resid:** Anatomic Pathology, Univ Iowa Hosps 1978; **Fellow:** Hematopathology, City of Hope Natl Med Ctr 1980; **Fac Appt:** Prof Path, Univ Nebr Coll Med

Southwest

Bruner, Janet M MD [Path] - **Spec Exp:** Brain Tumors; Neuro-Pathology; **Hospital:** UT MD Anderson Cancer Ctr; **Address:** MD Anderson Cancer Ctr, 1515 Holcombe Blvd, Ste 85, Houston, TX 77030; **Phone:** 713-792-6127; **Board Cert:** Anatomic Pathology 1982; Neuropathology 1984; **Med School:** Med Coll OH 1979; **Resid:** Anatomic & Clinical Pathology, Med Coll Ohio Hosp 1982; **Fellow:** Neurological Pathology, Baylor Coll Med 1984

Cagle, Philip MD [Path] - **Spec Exp:** Pulmonary Pathology; Lung Cancer; Mesothelioma; **Hospital:** Methodist Hosp - Houston; **Address:** Methodist Hospital, Dept Pathology, 6565 Fannin St, Ste 227, Houston, TX 77030; **Phone:** 713-441-6478; **Board Cert:** Anatomic & Clinical Pathology 1985; **Med School:** Univ Tenn Coll Med, Memphis 1981; **Fac Appt:** Prof Path, Baylor Coll Med

Foucar, M Kathryn MD [Path] - **Spec Exp:** Leukemia; Lymph Node Pathology; Bone Marrow Pathology; **Hospital:** Univ NM Hlth & Sci Ctr; **Address:** TriCore Reference Lab, Hematopathology, 1001 Woodward Pl NE, Albuquerque, NM 87102; **Phone:** 505-938-8456; **Board Cert:** Anatomic & Clinical Pathology 1978; **Med School:** Ohio State Univ 1974; **Resid:** Anatomic Pathology, Univ NM Health & Sci Ctr 1976; Anatomic Pathology, Univ Minn Med Ctr 1978; **Fellow:** Surgical Pathology, Univ Minn Med Ctr 1979; **Fac Appt:** Prof Path, Univ New Mexico

Grogan, Thomas M MD [Path] - **Spec Exp:** Immunopathology; Lymphoma; **Hospital:** Univ Med Ctr - Tucson; **Address:** AHSC, Dept Pathology, 1501 N Campbell Ave, rm 5211, Tucson, AZ 85724; **Phone:** 520-626-7477; **Board Cert:** Anatomic Pathology 1976; **Med School:** Geo Wash Univ 1971; **Resid:** Pathology, Letterman Army Med Ctr 1976; **Fellow:** Immunopathology, Stanford Univ Sch Med 1979; **Fac Appt:** Prof Path, Univ Ariz Coll Med

Pathology

Hamilton, Stanley R MD [Path] - **Spec Exp:** Surgical Pathology; Gastrointestinal Pathology; Liver Pathology; **Hospital:** UT MD Anderson Cancer Ctr; **Address:** Univ Texas MD Anderson Cancer Ctr, 1515 Holcombe Blvd, Unit 085, Houston, TX 77030-4009; **Phone:** 713-792-2040; **Board Cert:** Anatomic & Clinical Pathology 1978; **Med School:** Indiana Univ 1973; **Resid:** Pathology, Johns Hopkins Hosp 1978; **Fellow:** St Marks Hosp 1979; **Fac Appt:** Prof Path, Univ Tex, Houston

Kinney, Marsha C MD [Path] - **Spec Exp:** Hematopathology; Lymphoma; Leukemia; **Hospital:** Univ Hlth Syst-San Antonio; **Address:** Univ Tex Hlth & Sci Ctr, Dept Path, 7703 Floyd Curl Drive, MC 775, San Antonio, TX 78229-3900; **Phone:** 210-567-4072; **Board Cert:** Anatomic & Clinical Pathology 1985; Hematology 1998; **Med School:** Univ Tex SW, Dallas 1981; **Resid:** Pathology, Vanderbilt Univ Med Ctr 1985; **Fellow:** Hematopathology, Vanderbilt Univ Med Ctr 1988; **Fac Appt:** Prof Path, Univ Tex, San Antonio

Leslie, Kevin O MD [Path] - **Spec Exp:** Pulmonary Pathology; Lung Cancer; Surgical Pathology; **Hospital:** Mayo Clinic - Scottsdale; **Address:** Mayo Clinic, Scottsdale, 13400 E Shea Blvd, Scottsdale, AZ 85259; **Phone:** 480-301-8021; **Board Cert:** Anatomic & Clinical Pathology 1982; **Med School:** Albert Einstein Coll Med 1976; **Resid:** Anatomic & Clinical Pathology, Univ Colorado Health Sci Ctr 1982; **Fellow:** Surgical Pathology, Stanford Univ Med Ctr 1983; **Fac Appt:** Prof Path, Mayo Med Sch

Moran, Cesar A MD [Path] - **Spec Exp:** Lung Cancer; Mediastinal Tumors; Mesothelioma; **Hospital:** UT MD Anderson Cancer Ctr; **Address:** MD Anderson Cancer Ctr, Dept Pathology, 1515 Holcombe Blvd, rm G1-3738, Houston, TX 77030; **Phone:** 713-792-8134; **Board Cert:** Anatomic Pathology 1992; **Med School:** Guatemala 1981; **Resid:** Anatomic Pathology, Mt Sinai Med Ctr 1988; **Fellow:** Surgical Pathology, Yale-New Haven Med Ctr 1989; **Fac Appt:** Prof Path, Univ Tex, Houston

Prieto, Victor G MD/PhD [Path] - **Spec Exp:** Dermatopathology; Melanoma; Skin Cancer; **Hospital:** UT MD Anderson Cancer Ctr; **Address:** MD Anderson Cancer Ctr, Dept Pathology, 1515 Holcombe Blvd, Box 85, Houston, TX 77030-4000; **Phone:** 713-792-0918; **Board Cert:** Anatomic Pathology 1995; Dermatopathology 1997; **Med School:** Spain 1986; **Resid:** Pathology, New York Hosp-Cornell Med Ctr 1993; **Fellow:** Pathology, Meml Sloan Kettering Cancer Ctr 1995; Dermatopathology, New York Hosp-Cornell Med Ctr 1996; **Fac Appt:** Prof Path, Univ Tex, Houston

Rashid, Asif MD/PhD [Path] - **Spec Exp:** Gastrointestinal Pathology; Liver Pathology; **Hospital:** UT MD Anderson Cancer Ctr; **Address:** MD Anderson Cancer Ctr, Dept Pathology, 1515 Holcombe Blvd, Box 85, Houston, TX 77030; **Phone:** 713-745-1101; **Board Cert:** Anatomic Pathology 1994; **Med School:** Pakistan 1984; **Resid:** Anatomic Pathology, Mass Genl Hosp 1993; **Fellow:** Anatomic Pathology, Mass Genl Hosp 1994; Anatomic Pathology, Johns Hopkins Med Inst 1996

Roberts, William C MD [Path] - **Spec Exp:** Cardiac Pathology; **Hospital:** Baylor Univ Medical Ctr; **Address:** Baylor Univ Med Ctr, Heart & Vascular Inst, 3500 Gaston Ave, Ste H-030, Dallas, TX 75246-2017; **Phone:** 214-820-7911; **Board Cert:** Anatomic Pathology 1965; **Med School:** Emory Univ 1958; **Resid:** Anatomic Pathology, Natl Heart Inst-NIH 1962; Internal Medicine, Johns Hopkins Hosp 1963; **Fellow:** Cardiovascular Disease, Natl Heart Inst-NIH 1964

Sahin, Aysegul MD [Path] - **Spec Exp:** Breast Cancer; **Hospital:** UT MD Anderson Cancer Ctr; **Address:** 1515 Holcombe Blvd, Box 0085, Houston, TX 77030; **Phone:** 713-794-1500; **Board Cert:** Pathology 1987; **Med School:** Turkey 1980; **Resid:** Pathology, Oregon Hlth Sci Univ 1986; **Fellow:** Surgical Pathology, Univ Iowa Hosps & Clins 1987; **Fac Appt:** Prof Path, Univ Tex, Houston

Silva, Elvio G MD [Path] - **Spec Exp:** Gynecologic Pathology; Gynecologic Cancer; **Hospital:** UT MD Anderson Cancer Ctr, Cedars-Sinai Med Ctr; **Address:** MD Anderson Cancer Ctr, Dept Pathology, 1515 Holcombe Blvd, Unit 85, Houston, TX 77030; **Phone:** 713-792-3154; **Board Cert:** Anatomic Pathology 2007; **Med School:** Argentina 1969; **Resid:** Pathology, National Univ Med Ctr 1975; Anatomic Pathology, Univ Toronto 1978; **Fellow:** Surgical Pathology, MD Anderson Cancer Ctr 1979; **Fac Appt:** Prof Path

Walker, David H MD [Path] - **Spec Exp:** Infections-Emerging; Tropical Diseases; Biodefense; **Hospital:** UTMB - John Sealy Hospital; **Address:** UT Med Br Galveston, Dept Path, 301 University Blvd, Galveston, TX 77555-0609; **Phone:** 409-772-3989; **Board Cert:** Anatomic & Clinical Pathology 1974; **Med School:** Vanderbilt Univ 1969; **Resid:** Anatomic & Clinical Pathology, Peter Bent Brigham Hosp 1973; **Fellow:** Pathology, Harvard Univ 1973; **Fac Appt:** Prof Path, Univ Tex Med Br, Galveston

Wheeler, Thomas M MD [Path] - **Spec Exp:** Thyroid Disorders; Thyroid Cancer; **Hospital:** Ben Taub Genl Hosp; **Address:** Baylor Coll Med, Dept Pathology, One Baylor Plaza, rm T203, Houston, TX 77030; **Phone:** 713-798-4664; **Board Cert:** Anatomic & Clinical Pathology 1999; Cytopathology 1990; **Med School:** Baylor Coll Med 1977; **Resid:** Pathology, Baylor Coll Med 1981; **Fac Appt:** Prof Path, Baylor Coll Med

West Coast and Pacific

Amin, Mahul MD [Path] - **Spec Exp:** Genitourinary Pathology; Bladder Cancer; **Hospital:** Cedars-Sinai Med Ctr; **Address:** Cedars Sinai Hosp, 8700 Beverly Blvd, Ste 8728, Los Angeles, CA 90048; **Phone:** 310-423-6631; **Board Cert:** Anatomic & Clinical Pathology 1996; **Med School:** India 1983; **Resid:** Pathology, Henry Ford Hosp 1992; **Fellow:** Surgical Pathology, MD Anderson Cancer Ctr 1993; **Fac Appt:** Prof Path, Emory Univ

Arber, Daniel A MD [Path] - **Spec Exp:** Bone Marrow Pathology; Lymph Node Pathology; Spleen Pathology; **Hospital:** Stanford Univ Med Ctr, Lucile Packard Chldn's Hosp; **Address:** Clinic Laboratories, Stanford Univ Med Ctr, 300 Pasteur Drive, rm H1507, MC 5627, Stanford, CA 94305; **Phone:** 650-725-5604; **Board Cert:** Anatomic & Clinical Pathology 1991; Hematology 1993; **Med School:** Univ Tex, San Antonio 1986; **Resid:** Anatomic & Clinical Pathology, Scott & White Meml Hosp 1991; **Fellow:** Hematopathology, City of Hope Natl Med Ctr 1993; **Fac Appt:** Prof Path, Stanford Univ

Bastian, Boris C MD [Path] - **Spec Exp:** Melanoma; Skin Cancer; **Hospital:** UCSF Med Ctr; **Address:** UCSF Comprehensive Cancer Center, Box 0808, San Francisco, CA 94143; **Phone:** 415-476-5132; **Med School:** Germany 1988; **Resid:** Dermatology, University of Wurzburg 1994; **Fellow:** Hematology, Ludwig-Maximilian-University 1989; **Fac Appt:** Asst Prof D, UCSF

Bollen, Andrew W MD [Path] - **Spec Exp:** Neuro-Pathology; Brain Tumors; Brain Infections; **Hospital:** UCSF Med Ctr, San Francisco Genl Hosp; **Address:** Dept Pathology/Neuropathology, 505 Parnassus Ave, M551, Box 0102, San Francisco, CA 94143-0511; **Phone:** 415-476-5236; **Board Cert:** Neuropathology 1992; Anatomic Pathology 1992; Clinical Pathology 1993; **Med School:** UCSD 1985; **Resid:** Anatomic Pathology, UCSF Med Ctr 1991; **Fellow:** Neuropathology, UCSF Med Ctr 1989; **Fac Appt:** Prof Path, UCSF

Chandrasoma, Parakrama T MD [Path] - **Spec Exp:** Gastrointestinal Pathology; Gastrointestinal Cancer; Neuro-Pathology; **Hospital:** LAC & USC Med Ctr; **Address:** LAC-USC Med Ctr, Dept Path, Clinic Tower Fl 7 - rm A7A127, 1100 N State St, Los Angeles, CA 90033; **Phone:** 323-226-4600; **Board Cert:** Anatomic Pathology 1982; **Med School:** Sri Lanka 1971; **Resid:** Anatomic Pathology, Univ Sri Lanka 1978; Anatomic Pathology, LAC-USC Med Ctr 1982; **Fac Appt:** Prof Path, USC Sch Med

Pathology

Chang, Karen L MD [Path] - **Spec Exp:** Leukemia; **Hospital:** City of Hope Natl Med Ctr & Beckman Rsch; **Address:** 1500 E Duarte Rd, Duarte, CA 91010-3012; **Phone:** 626-256-4673 x62456; **Board Cert:** Anatomic & Clinical Pathology 1992; **Med School:** Mount Sinai Sch Med 1985; **Resid:** Anatomic Pathology, Stanford Univ Med Ctr 1988; Clinical Pathology, Stanford Univ Med Ctr 1991; **Fellow:** Surgical Pathology, Stanford Univ Med Ctr 1989

Cochran, Alistair J MD [Path] - **Spec Exp:** Melanoma; Dermatopathology; **Hospital:** UCLA Ronald Reagan Med Ctr; **Address:** UCLA Med Ctr, Dept Path & Med, 10833 Le Conte Ave, rm 13145CHS, MC 173216, Los Angeles, CA 90095-1713; **Phone:** 310-825-2743; **Med School:** Scotland, UK 1959; **Resid:** Dermatopathology, Western Infirmary 1968; Pathology, Western Infirmary 1968; **Fellow:** Immunology, Karolinska Inst 1970; **Fac Appt:** Prof Path, UCLA

Dubeau, Louis MD/PhD [Path] - **Spec Exp:** Ovarian Cancer; Breast Cancer; **Hospital:** USC Norris Cancer Hosp; **Address:** USC Norris Cancer Ctr, Dept Pathology, 1441 Eastlake Ave, rm 6338, Los Angeles, CA 90033-1048; **Phone:** 323-865-0720; **Board Cert:** Anatomic Pathology 1984; **Med School:** McGill Univ 1979; **Resid:** Anatomic Pathology, McGill Univ Med Ctr 1984; **Fac Appt:** Prof Path, USC Sch Med

Ferrell, Linda MD [Path] - **Spec Exp:** Liver Pathology; **Hospital:** UCSF Med Ctr; **Address:** UCSF Med Ctr, Dept Pathology, 505 Parnassus Ave, rm M590, Box 0102, San Francisco, CA 94143-0102; **Phone:** 415-353-1090; **Board Cert:** Anatomic Pathology 1982; **Med School:** Univ Kans 1977; **Resid:** Anatomic Pathology, Univ Kansas Med Ctr 1979; Anatomic Pathology, UCSF Med Ctr 1981; **Fac Appt:** Prof Path, UCSF

Fishbein, Michael C MD [Path] - **Spec Exp:** Cardiovascular Pathology; Pulmonary Pathology; **Hospital:** UCLA Ronald Reagan Med Ctr; **Address:** 10833 Le Conte Ave, Los Angeles, CA 90095-1732; **Phone:** 310-825-9731; **Board Cert:** Anatomic & Clinical Pathology 1975; **Med School:** Univ IL Coll Med 1971; **Resid:** Anatomic & Clinical Pathology, UCLA-Harbor General Hosp 1975; **Fellow:** Pathology, Heart Lung Inst-NIH 1975; **Fac Appt:** Prof Path, UCLA

Govindarajan, Sugantha MD [Path] - **Spec Exp:** Liver Pathology; **Hospital:** Rancho Los Amigos Natl Rehab Ctr; **Address:** Rancho Los Amigos Natl Rehab Ctr, 7601 E Imperial Hwy, Bldg JPI - rm B170, Dept Pathology, Downey, CA 90242; **Phone:** 562-401-8996; **Board Cert:** Anatomic Pathology 1976; **Med School:** India 1969; **Resid:** Pathology, St Lukes Hosp 1976; **Fellow:** Pathology, Cleveland Clinic 1977; **Fac Appt:** Prof Path, USC Sch Med

Hammar, Samuel P MD [Path] - **Spec Exp:** Lung Cancer; Pulmonary Pathology; **Hospital:** Harrison Meml Hosp; **Address:** Diagnostic Specialties Laboratory, 700 Lebo Blvd, Bremerton, WA 98310; **Phone:** 360-479-7707; **Board Cert:** Anatomic & Clinical Pathology 1975; **Med School:** Univ Wash 1970

Hendrickson, Michael MD [Path] - **Spec Exp:** Gynecologic Cancer; Gynecologic Pathology; **Hospital:** Stanford Univ Med Ctr; **Address:** Stanford Univ Med Ctr, Surg Path Lab, 300 Pasteur Drive, rm H2110, MC 5324, Stanford, CA 94305; **Phone:** 650-723-7211; **Board Cert:** Anatomic Pathology 1975; **Med School:** Stanford Univ 1971; **Resid:** Anatomic Pathology, Stanford Univ Med Sch 1974; **Fac Appt:** Prof Path, Stanford Univ

Kanel, Gary MD [Path] - **Spec Exp:** Liver Disease; **Hospital:** USC Univ Hosp; **Address:** USC Univ Hosp, Dept Pathology, 1500 San Pablo St Fl 2, Los Angeles, CA 90033; **Phone:** 323-226-7127; **Board Cert:** Anatomic & Clinical Pathology 1979; **Med School:** Tufts Univ 1974; **Resid:** Pathology, Tufts-New England Med Ctr 1976; Pathology, Univ Chicago Hosp 1977; **Fellow:** Pathology, Tufts-New England Med Ctr 1979; **Fac Appt:** Prof Path, USC Sch Med

Kempson, Richard L MD [Path] - **Spec Exp:** Breast Pathology; Gynecologic Pathology; **Hospital:** Stanford Univ Med Ctr; **Address:** 300 Pasteur Drive, Ste H2110, Stanford, CA 94305-5243; **Phone:** 650-723-7211; **Board Cert:** Anatomic Pathology 1963; **Med School:** Tulane Univ 1955; **Resid:** Surgical Pathology, Barnes Hosp 1963; **Fellow:** Anatomic Pathology, Tulane Univ Med Ctr 1962; **Fac Appt:** Prof Path, Stanford Univ

Koss, Michael N MD [Path] - **Spec Exp:** Pulmonary Pathology; Lung Cancer; Kidney Pathology; **Hospital:** USC Norris Cancer Hosp, USC Univ Hosp; **Address:** 2222 Ocean View Ave, Ste 212, 2011 Zonal Ave, Los Angeles, CA 90057; **Phone:** 213-381-2260; **Board Cert:** Anatomic Pathology 1979; **Med School:** Stanford Univ 1970; **Resid:** Pathology, Columbia Presby Med Ctr 1974; **Fellow:** Renal Pathology, Columbia Presby Med Ctr 1975; Pulmonary Pathology, Armed Forces Inst Path 1978; **Fac Appt:** Prof Path, USC Sch Med

Le Boit, Philip E MD [Path] - **Spec Exp:** Cutaneous Lymphoma; Skin Cancer; Dermatopathology; **Hospital:** UCSF Med Ctr; **Address:** UCSF - Dermatopathology Section, 1701 Divisadero St, rm 350, San Francisco, CA 94115; **Phone:** 415-353-7546; **Board Cert:** Anatomic Pathology 1983; Dermatopathology 1983; Clinical Pathology 1986; **Med School:** Albany Med Coll 1979; **Resid:** Anatomic Pathology, UCSF Med Ctr 1981; Clinical Pathology, Mt Sinai Hosp 1982; **Fellow:** Dermatopathology, New York Hosp-Cornell Med Ctr 1983; **Fac Appt:** Prof Path, UCSF

Ljung, Britt-Marie E MD [Path] - **Spec Exp:** Breast Cancer; Cytopathology; Fine Needle Aspiration Biopsy; **Hospital:** UCSF - Mt Zion Med Ctr; **Address:** UCSF - Dept Pathology, 1600 Divisadero St, Box 1785, rm r-200, San Francisco, CA 94143-1785; **Phone:** 415-353-7320; **Board Cert:** Anatomic Pathology 1985; Cytopathology 1989; **Med School:** Sweden 1975; **Resid:** Pathology, Karolinska Hosp 1979; Anatomic Pathology, UCLA Med Ctr 1983; **Fac Appt:** Prof Path, UCSF

Mischel, Paul S MD [Path] - **Spec Exp:** Neuro-Pathology; Brain Tumors; **Hospital:** UCLA Ronald Reagan Med Ctr; **Address:** UCLA Med Ctr, Div Neuropathology, 10833 Le Conte Ave, rm 13-317 CHS, Los Angeles, CA 90095-1732; **Phone:** 310-825-0377; **Board Cert:** Anatomic Pathology 1997; Neuropathology 1997; **Med School:** Cornell Univ-Weill Med Coll 1991; **Resid:** Anatomic & Clinical Pathology, UCLA Med Center 1996; **Fellow:** Neurological Pathology, UCLA 1995; Research, Howard Hughes Med Inst/UCSF 1998; **Fac Appt:** Prof Path, UCLA

Nathwani, Bharat N MD [Path] - **Spec Exp:** Hematopathology; Leukemia; Lymphoma; **Hospital:** LAC & USC Med Ctr; **Address:** LAC & USC Med Ctr, Dept Pathology, 1200 N State St, rm 2422, Los Angeles, CA 90033-4526; **Phone:** 323-226-7064; **Board Cert:** Anatomic Pathology 1977; **Med School:** India 1969; **Resid:** Pathology, JJ Group-Grant Med Ctr 1972; Pathology, Rush-Presby-St Lukes Med Ctr 1974; **Fellow:** Hematopathology, City Hope Natl Med Ctr 1975; **Fac Appt:** Prof Path, USC Sch Med

Rutgers, Joanne MD [Path] - **Spec Exp:** Gynecologic Cancer; Cytopathology; Gastrointestinal Pathology; **Hospital:** Long Beach Meml Med Ctr; **Address:** 2801 Atlantic Ave, Dept of Pathology, Long Beach, CA 90806; **Phone:** 562-933-0717; **Board Cert:** Clinical Pathology 1992; Anatomic Pathology 1985; Cytopathology 1997; **Med School:** UCSD 1981; **Resid:** Pathology, Montefiore Med Ctr 1983; Pathology, NYU Med Ctr 1985; **Fellow:** Gynecologic Pathology, Mass Genl Hosp 1989; **Fac Appt:** Assoc Clin Prof Path, UCLA

Sibley, Richard K MD [Path] - **Spec Exp:** Kidney Pathology; Breast Pathology; Liver Pathology; **Hospital:** Stanford Univ Med Ctr; **Address:** Stanford Univ Med Ctr, Surg Path Lab, 300 Pasteur Drive, rm H2110, MC 5243, Stanford, CA 94305; **Phone:** 650-723-7211; **Board Cert:** Anatomic Pathology 1975; **Med School:** Univ Tex SW, Dallas 1971; **Resid:** Anatomic Pathology, Univ Chicago Hosps 1974; **Fellow:** Stanford Univ Med Ctr 1975; **Fac Appt:** Prof Path, Stanford Univ

Pathology

Triche, Timothy J MD/PhD [Path] - **Spec Exp:** Pediatric Pathology; Pediatric Cancers; Sarcoma; **Hospital:** Chldns Hosp - Los Angeles; **Address:** Chldns Hosp of Los Angeles, Dept Path, 4650 Sunset Blvd, MS 43, Los Angeles, CA 90027; **Phone:** 323-361-4516; **Board Cert:** Anatomic Pathology 1975; **Med School:** Tulane Univ 1971; **Resid:** Anatomic Pathology, Barnes Hosp-Wash Univ 1973; Surgical Pathology, Barnes Hosp 1974; **Fellow:** Pathology, Natl Cancer Inst 1975; **Fac Appt:** Prof Path, USC Sch Med

True, Lawrence D MD [Path] - **Spec Exp:** Urologic Pathology; Prostate Cancer; Bladder Cancer; **Hospital:** Univ Wash Med Ctr; **Address:** Univ Wash Med Ctr, Dept Anatomic Path, 1959 NE Pacific St, rm NE110, Box 356100, Seattle, WA 98195-6100; **Phone:** 206-598-6400; **Board Cert:** Anatomic Pathology 1981; **Med School:** Tulane Univ 1971; **Resid:** Pathology, Univ Colo Hlth Sci Ctr 1980; **Fac Appt:** Prof Path, Univ Wash

Warnke, Roger A MD [Path] - **Spec Exp:** Lymphoma; Hematopathology; **Hospital:** Stanford Univ Med Ctr; **Address:** Stanford Hosp, 300 Pasteur Drive, Pathology, rm L235, Stanford, CA 94305-5324; **Phone:** 650-725-5167; **Board Cert:** Anatomic Pathology 1975; **Med School:** Washington Univ, St Louis 1971; **Resid:** Pathology, Stanford Univ Med Ctr 1974; **Fellow:** Surgical Pathology, Stanford Univ Med Ctr 1975; Immunology, Stanford Univ Med Ctr 1976; **Fac Appt:** Prof Path, Stanford Univ

Weiss, Lawrence M MD [Path] - **Spec Exp:** Lymphoma; Hematopathology; Adrenal Pathology; **Hospital:** City of Hope Natl Med Ctr & Beckman Rsch; **Address:** City of Hope Natl Med Ctr, Div Pathology, 1500 E Duarte Rd, Duarte, CA 91010-0269; **Phone:** 626-359-8111 x62456; **Board Cert:** Anatomic Pathology 1985; **Med School:** Univ MD Sch Med 1981; **Resid:** Pathology, Brigham & Women's Hosp 1983; **Fellow:** Surgical Pathology, Stanford Univ Hosp 1984

Wilczynski, Sharon P MD/PhD [Path] - **Spec Exp:** Gynecologic Cancer; Breast Cancer; Ovarian Cancer; Clinical Trials; **Hospital:** City of Hope Natl Med Ctr & Beckman Rsch; **Address:** City Hope Natl Med Ctr-Dept of Pathology, 1500 E Duarte Blvd, Duarte, CA 91010; **Phone:** 626-256-4673 x62456; **Board Cert:** Anatomic & Clinical Pathology 1985; Cytopathology 1991; **Med School:** Med Coll PA Hahnemann 1981; **Resid:** Pathology, Hosp Univ Penn 1983; Anatomic & Clinical Pathology, Long Beach Meml Hosp 1985; **Fac Appt:** Prof Path, USC-Keck School of Medicine

Pediatrics

A pediatrician is concerned with the physical, emotional and social health of children from birth to young adulthood. Care encompasses a broad spectrum of health services ranging from preventive health-care to the diagnosis and treatment of acute and chronic diseases.

A pediatrician deals with biological, social and environmental influences on the developing child, and with the impact of disease and dysfunction on development.

Training Required: Three years

Pediatric Allergy and Immunology: An allergist-immunologist is trained in evaluation, physical and laboratory diagnosis and management of disorders involving the immune system. Selected examples of such conditions include asthma, anaphylaxis, rhinitis, eczema and adverse reactions to drugs, foods and insect stings as well as immune deficiency diseases (both acquired and congenital), defects in host defense and problems related to autoimmune disease, organ transplantation or malignancies of the immune system. As our understanding of the immune system develops, the scope of this specialty is widening.

Training Required: Prior certification in pediatrics *plus* two years in allergy/immunology. (Training programs are available at some medical centers to provide individuals with expertise in both allergy/immunology and pediatric pulmonology. Such individuals are candidates for dual certification.)

(continued on next page)

Certification in one of the following subspecialties requires additional training and examination.

Pediatric Cardiology: A pediatric cardiologist provides comprehensive care to patients with cardiovascular problems. This specialist is skilled in selecting, performing and evaluating the structural and functional assessment of the heart and blood vessels and the clinical evaluation of cardiovascular disease.

Pediatric Critical Care Medicine: A pediatrician who cares for children who are victims of life threatening disorders such as severe accidents, shock and diabetic acidosis.

Pediatric Endocrinology: A pediatrician who provides expert care to infants, children and adolescents who have diseases that result from an abnormality in the endocrine glands (glands which secrete hormones). These diseases include diabetes mellitus, growth failure, unusual size for age, early or late pubertal development, birth defects, the genital anomalies and disorders of the thyroid, the adrenal and pituitary glands.

Pediatric Gastroenterology: A pediatrician who specializes in the diagnosis and treatment of diseases of the digestive systems of infants, children and adolescents. This specialist treats conditions such as abdominal pain, ulcers, diarrhea, cancer and jaundice and performs complex diagnostic and therapeutic procedures using lighted scopes to see internal organs.

Pediatric Hematology-Oncology: A pediatrician trained in the combination of pediatrics, hematology and oncology to recognize and manage pediatric blood disorders and cancerous diseases.

Pediatric Infectious Diseases: A pediatrician trained to care for children in the diagnosis, treatment and prevention of infectious diseases. This specialist can apply specific knowledge to effect a better outcome for pediatric infections with complicated courses, underlying diseases that predispose to unusual or severe infections, unclear diagnoses, uncommon diseases and complex or investigational treatments.

Pediatric Nephrology: A pediatrician who deals with the normal and abnormal development and maturation of the kidney and urinary tract, the mechanisms by which the kidney can be damaged, the evaluation and treatment of renal diseases, fluid and electrolyte abnormalities, hypertension and renal replacement therapy.

Pediatric Otolaryngology: A pediatric otolaryngologist has special expertise in the management of infants and children with disorders that include congenital and acquired conditions involving the aerodigestive tract, nose and paranasal sinuses, the ear and other areas of the head and neck. The pediatric otolaryngologist has special skills in the diagnosis, treatment and management of childhood disorders of voice, speech, language and hearing.

Pediatric Pulmonology: A pediatrician dedicated to the prevention and treatment of all respiratory diseases affecting infants, children and young adults. This specialist is knowledgeable about the growth and development of the lung, assessment of respiratory function in infants and children and experienced in a variety of invasive and noninvasive diagnostic techniques.

Pediatric Rheumatology: A pediatrician who treats diseases of joints, muscle, bones and tendons. A pediatric rheumatologist diagnoses and treats arthritis, back pain, muscle strains, common athletic injuries and "collagen" diseases.

Pediatric Surgery: A surgeon with expertise in the management of surgical conditions in premature and newborn infants, children and adolescents.

PEDIATRICS

New England

Ferber, Richard A MD [Ped] - **Spec Exp:** Sleep Disorders; **Hospital:** Children's Hospital - Boston; **Address:** Children's Hosp, 9 Hope Ave, Waltham, MA 02453; **Phone:** 617-355-6663; **Board Cert:** Pediatrics 1980; Sleep Medicine 1980; **Med School:** Harvard Med Sch 1970; **Resid:** Pediatrics, Chldns Hosp 1974; **Fellow:** Psychiatry, Chldns Hosp 1978; Psychosomatic Medicine, Chldns Hosp 1979; **Fac Appt:** Assoc Prof N, Harvard Med Sch

Palfrey, Judith S MD [Ped] - **Spec Exp:** Special Health Care Needs (CSHCN); Developmental Disorders; **Hospital:** Children's Hospital - Boston; **Address:** Children's Hosp, 300 Longwood Ave, Boston, MA 02115; **Phone:** 617-355-4662; **Board Cert:** Pediatrics 1976; Developmental-Behavioral Pediatrics 2002; **Med School:** Columbia P&S 1971; **Resid:** Pediatrics, Montefiore Med Ctr 1974; **Fac Appt:** Prof Ped, Harvard Med Sch

Rappaport, Leonard MD [Ped] - **Spec Exp:** Developmental & Behavioral Disorders; **Hospital:** Children's Hospital - Boston; **Address:** Childrens Hosp Fegan 10, 300 Longwood Ave, Boston, MA 02115; **Phone:** 617-355-4683; **Board Cert:** Pediatrics 1983; Developmental-Behavioral Pediatrics 2002; **Med School:** Yale Univ 1977; **Resid:** Pediatrics, Chldns Hosp 1980; **Fellow:** Developmental-Behavioral Pediatrics, Chldns Hosp 1982; **Fac Appt:** Prof Ped, Harvard Med Sch

Shaywitz, Sally E MD [Ped] - **Spec Exp:** Learning Disorders-Studies Only; Dyslexia-Studies Only; **Hospital:** Yale-New Haven Hosp; **Address:** Yale Univ Dept Pediatrics, 333 Cedar St, PO Box 208064, New Haven, CT 06520-8064; **Phone:** 203-785-4641; **Board Cert:** Pediatrics 1971; **Med School:** Albert Einstein Coll Med 1966; **Resid:** Pediatrics, Albert Einstein Coll Med 1970; **Fellow:** Pediatrics, Bronx Muni Hosp Ctr 1968; Behavioral Pediatrics, Albert Einstein Coll Med 1970; **Fac Appt:** Prof Ped, Yale Univ

Mid Atlantic

Berlin Jr, Cheston M MD [Ped] - **Spec Exp:** Phenylketonuria (PKU); Tourette's Syndrome; **Hospital:** Penn State Milton S Hershey Med Ctr; **Address:** Penn State Univ Coll Med, Pediatrics, PO Box 850, Hershey, PA 17033; **Phone:** 717-531-8006; **Board Cert:** Pediatrics 1982; **Med School:** Harvard Med Sch 1962; **Resid:** Pediatrics, Childrens Hosp 1967; **Fac Appt:** Prof Ped, Penn State Univ-Hershey Med Ctr

Burgess, David B MD [Ped] - **Spec Exp:** Developmental & Behavioral Disorders; ADD/ADHD; Autism; **Hospital:** Chldns Hosp of Philadelphia, The; **Address:** Children's Hosp Philadelphia, Specialty Care Ctr, 4009 Black Horse Pike, Mays Landing, NJ 08330; **Phone:** 609-677-7895; **Board Cert:** Pediatrics 1978; Developmental-Behavioral Pediatrics 2004; **Med School:** Univ Wisc 1973; **Resid:** Pediatrics, Charity Hosp 1977; **Fellow:** Child Development, JFK Child Dev Ctr, Univ Colorado 1980; **Fac Appt:** Assoc Clin Prof Ped, Univ Pennsylvania

Gartner Jr, J Carlton MD [Ped] - **Spec Exp:** Diagnostic Problems; Multisystem Disorders; **Hospital:** Alfred I duPont Hosp for Children; **Address:** Alfred I duPont Hosp for Children, 1600 Rockland Rd, rm 3D 228, Wilmington, DE 19803; **Phone:** 302-651-5946; **Board Cert:** Pediatrics 2007; **Med School:** Johns Hopkins Univ 1971; **Resid:** Pediatrics, Childrens Hosp 1974; **Fac Appt:** Prof Ped, Thomas Jefferson Univ

Hofkosh, Dena MD [Ped] - **Spec Exp:** Developmental & Behavioral Disorders; Developmental Disorders; **Hospital:** Chldns Hosp of Pittsburgh - UPMC; **Address:** Childrens Hosp Pittsburgh, Dept Pediatrics, 45th St & Penn Ave, Pittsburgh, PA 15201; **Phone:** 412-692-6541; **Board Cert:** Pediatrics 1984; Neurodevelopmental Disabilities 2001; **Med School:** NYU Sch Med 1979; **Resid:** Pediatrics, Univ Pittsburgh Med Ctr 1982; **Fellow:** Ambulatory Pediatrics, Univ Pittsburgh Med Ctr 1984; **Fac Appt:** Prof Ped, Univ Pittsburgh

Morton, D Holmes MD [Ped] - **Spec Exp:** Genetic Disorders; Rare Disorders; **Hospital:** Lancaster Genl Hosp; **Address:** Clinic For Special Children, 535 Bunker Hill Rd, PO Box 128, Strasburg, PA 17579; **Phone:** 717-687-9407; **Board Cert:** Pediatrics 1987; **Med School:** Harvard Med Sch 1983; **Resid:** Pediatrics, Childrens Hosp 1986; **Fellow:** Research, Childrens Hosp 1988

Oeffinger, Kevin MD [Ped] - **Spec Exp:** Cancer Survivors-Late Effects of Therapy; **Hospital:** Meml Sloan-Kettering Cancer Ctr; **Address:** 1275 York Ave, Box 396, New York, NY 10065; **Phone:** 800-525-2225; **Board Cert:** Family Medicine 2000; **Med School:** Univ Tex, San Antonio 1984; **Resid:** Family Medicine, Baylor Coll Med 1985; **Fellow:** Family Medicine, Fam Practice Faculty Dev Ctr 1999; Natl Cancer Inst 2000

Vining, Eileen P MD [Ped] - **Spec Exp:** Pediatric Neurology; Epilepsy; Rasmussen's Syndrome; **Hospital:** Johns Hopkins Hosp (page 61); **Address:** Johns Hopkins Hospital, 600 N Caroline St, Baltimore, MD 21287; **Phone:** 410-955-9100; **Board Cert:** Pediatrics 1977; **Med School:** Johns Hopkins Univ 1972; **Resid:** Pediatrics, Chldns Hosp 1974; **Fellow:** Developmental-Behavioral Pediatrics, JFK Inst/Johns Hopkins Hosp 1976; **Fac Appt:** Assoc Prof Ped, Johns Hopkins Univ

Zitelli, Basil MD [Ped] - **Spec Exp:** Complex Diagnosis; **Hospital:** Chldns Hosp of Pittsburgh - UPMC; **Address:** Childrens Hospital Drive, 45th St & Penn Ave, Faculty Pavilion Fl 3, Pittsburgh, PA 15201; **Phone:** 412-692-5135; **Board Cert:** Pediatrics 1976; **Med School:** Univ Pittsburgh 1971; **Resid:** Pediatrics, Johns Hopkins Hosp 1976; **Fellow:** Pediatrics, Johns Hopkins Hosp 1978; **Fac Appt:** Prof Ped, Univ Pittsburgh

Southeast

Hershorin, Eugene R MD [Ped] - **Spec Exp:** ADD/ADHD; Developmental & Mood Disorders; **Hospital:** Jackson Meml Hosp (page 70); **Address:** 8932 SW 97th Ave, Ste 10, Miami, FL 33176; **Phone:** 305-270-5050; **Board Cert:** Pediatrics 1980; Developmental-Behavioral Pediatrics 2004; **Med School:** Penn State Univ-Hershey Med Ctr 1976; **Resid:** Pediatrics, Chldn's Hosp 1979; **Fac Appt:** Assoc Prof Ped, Univ Miami Sch Med

Midwest

Berman, Brian W MD [Ped] - **Spec Exp:** Sickle Cell Disease; Thrombotic Disorders; Hemophilia; **Hospital:** Rainbow Babies & Chldns Hosp; **Address:** Rainbow Babies & Chldn's Hosp, 11100 Euclid Ave, MS RBC6019, Cleveland, OH 44106-6019; **Phone:** 216-844-3752; **Board Cert:** Pediatrics 1989; Pediatric Hematology-Oncology 1989; **Med School:** Temple Univ 1975; **Resid:** Pediatrics, St Chris Hosp for Chldn 1978; **Fellow:** Pediatric Hematology-Oncology, Yale-New Haven Hosp 1980; **Fac Appt:** Prof Ped, Case West Res Univ

Bull, Marilyn J MD [Ped] - **Spec Exp:** Developmental Disorders; Down Syndrome; Birth Defects; **Hospital:** Riley Hosp for Children; **Address:** 702 Barnhill Drive, rm 1601, Indianapolis, IN 46202; **Phone:** 317-274-4846; **Board Cert:** Pediatrics 1973; Clinical Genetics 1982; Neurodevelopmental Disabilities 2001; **Med School:** Univ Mich Med Sch 1968; **Resid:** Pediatrics, Childrens Meml Hosp 1972; **Fellow:** Genetics, Boston Floating Hosp 1973; **Fac Appt:** Prof Ped, Indiana Univ

Pediatrics

Fost, Norman C MD [Ped] - **Spec Exp:** Ethics; **Hospital:** Univ WI Hosp & Clins; **Address:** Dept Pediatrics 4108, 600 Highland Ave, Madison, WI 53792-4108; **Phone:** 608-265-6050; **Board Cert:** Pediatrics 1970; **Med School:** Yale Univ 1964; **Resid:** Pediatrics, Johns Hopkins Hosp 1971; **Fellow:** Pediatrics, Harvard Sch Public Hlth 1973; **Fac Appt:** Prof Ped, Univ Wisc

Jacob, Molly MD [Ped] - **Spec Exp:** Asthma; ADD/ADHD; Nutrition; **Hospital:** Children's Mem Hosp, Adv Illinois Masonic Med Ctr; **Address:** 3000 N Halstead Ave, Ste 825, Chicago, IL 60657; **Phone:** 773-463-0136; **Board Cert:** Pediatrics 1980; **Med School:** India 1968; **Resid:** Pediatrics, Ill Masonic Med Ctr 1979; **Fellow:** Ambulatory Pediatrics, Ill Masonic Med Ctr 1979; **Fac Appt:** Asst Clin Prof Ped, Univ IL Coll Med

Kaplan, Lawrence Charles MD [Ped] - **Spec Exp:** Developmental Delay; Angelman Syndrome; Prader-Willi Syndrome; Asperger's Syndrome; **Hospital:** Univ WI Hosp & Clins; **Address:** Univ Wisconsin, Waisman Ctr, 1500 Highland Ave, rm 151, Madison, WI 53705; **Phone:** 608-263-3301; **Board Cert:** Pediatrics 1986; Neurodevelopmental Disabilities 2009; **Med School:** Univ VT Coll Med 1981; **Resid:** Pediatrics, Children's Hosp 1984; **Fellow:** Developmental-Behavioral Pediatrics, Children's Hosp 1986; Cerebral Palsy, Children's Hosp 1987; **Fac Appt:** Prof Ped, Univ Wisc

Lantos, John D MD [Ped] - **Spec Exp:** Ethics Issues in Pediatrics; Palliative Care; Ethics Issues in Neonatalogy; **Hospital:** Chldns Mercy Hosps & Clinics; **Address:** Childrens Mercy Bioethics Center, 2401 Gilham Rd, Kansas City, MO 64108; **Phone:** 816-234-3317; **Board Cert:** Pediatrics 1986; **Med School:** Univ Pittsburgh 1981; **Resid:** Pediatrics, Chldns Natl Med Ctr 1984; **Fellow:** Clinical Ethics, Univ Chicago Hosps 1987; **Fac Appt:** Prof Ped, Univ MO-Kansas City

Southwest

Infante, Anthony J MD/PhD [Ped] - **Spec Exp:** Immune Deficiencies-Primary; Autoimmune Disease; Myasthenia Gravis; **Hospital:** Univ Hlth Syst-San Antonio, Christus Santa Rosa Hosp-City Ctr; **Address:** 7703 Floyd Curl Drive, MS 7811, San Antonio, TX 78229-3900; **Phone:** 210-704-2187; **Board Cert:** Pediatrics 2004; **Med School:** Indiana Univ 1978; **Resid:** Pediatrics, Mayo Clinic 1980; **Fellow:** Pediatric Immunology, Mayo Clinic 1981; Immunology, Stanford Univ Hosp 1983; **Fac Appt:** Prof Ped, Univ Tex, San Antonio

Kleinerman, Eugenie S MD [Ped] - **Spec Exp:** Ewing's Sarcoma; Cancer Survivors-Late Effects of Therapy; **Hospital:** UT MD Anderson Cancer Ctr; **Address:** MD Anderson Cancer Ctr, Dept Pediatrics, 1515 Holcombe Blvd, Unit 87, Houston, TX 77030; **Phone:** 713-792-8110; **Board Cert:** Pediatrics 1980; **Med School:** Duke Univ 1975; **Resid:** Pediatrics, Chldns Hosp-Natl Med Ctr 1978; **Fellow:** Immunology, Natl Cancer Inst 1981; **Fac Appt:** Prof Ped, Univ Tex, Houston

West Coast and Pacific

Berkowitz, Carol D MD [Ped] - **Spec Exp:** Child Abuse; **Hospital:** LAC - Harbor - UCLA Med Ctr; **Address:** LAC-Harbor-UCLA Med Ctr, 1000 W Carson St, Box 437, Torrance, CA 90509-2910; **Phone:** 310-222-3091; **Board Cert:** Pediatrics 2000; Pediatric Emergency Medicine 2006; **Med School:** Columbia P&S 1969; **Resid:** Pediatrics, Roosevelt Hosp 1972; **Fac Appt:** Clin Prof Ped, UCLA

Feldman, Kenneth W MD [Ped] - **Spec Exp:** Child Abuse; **Hospital:** Chldns Hosp and Regl Med Ctr - Seattle; **Address:** Odessa Brown Chldns Clin, 2101 E Yesler Way, Ste 100, Seattle, WA 98122; **Phone:** 206-987-7225; **Board Cert:** Pediatrics 1975; **Med School:** Univ Wisc 1970; **Resid:** Pediatrics, Chldns Regl Med Ctr 1974; **Fac Appt:** Clin Prof Ped, Univ Wash

Jones Jr, Kenneth Lyons MD [Ped] - **Spec Exp:** Genetic Disorders; Dysmorphology; **Hospital:** UCSD Med Ctr; **Address:** 9500 Gilman Drive, San Diego, CA 92093-0828; **Phone:** 858-246-0047; **Board Cert:** Pediatrics 1971; **Med School:** Hahnemann Univ 1966; **Resid:** Pediatrics, Chldns Ortho Hosp 1969; **Fac Appt:** Prof Ped, UCSD

Zeltzer, Lonnie K MD [Ped] - **Spec Exp:** Pain Management; Complementary Medicine; **Hospital:** Mattel Chldns Hosp at UCLA; **Address:** UCLA Pediatric Pain Program, 10833 Le Conte Ave, #22-464 MDCC, Los Angeles, CA 90095-1752; **Phone:** 310-825-0731; **Board Cert:** Pediatrics 1976; **Med School:** Univ Cincinnati 1970; **Resid:** Pediatrics, Univ Ariz Hosp 1973; **Fellow:** Adolescent Medicine, Chldns Hosp 1976; **Fac Appt:** Prof Ped, UCLA

PEDIATRIC ALLERGY & IMMUNOLOGY

New England

Klein, Robert B MD [PA&I] - **Spec Exp:** Asthma; **Hospital:** Rhode Island Hosp; **Address:** Rhode Island Hosp, Dept of Pediatrics, 593 Eddy St, Providence, RI 02903; **Phone:** 401-793-8560; **Board Cert:** Pediatrics 1976; Allergy & Immunology 1977; **Med School:** Switzerland 1971; **Resid:** Pediatrics, Dartmouth/Hitchcock Med Ctr 1974; **Fellow:** Allergy & Immunology, UCLA 1976; **Fac Appt:** Prof Ped, Brown Univ

Mid Atlantic

Ehrlich, Paul M MD [PA&I] - **Spec Exp:** Asthma; Food Allergy; **Hospital:** New York Eye & Ear Infirm (page 65), NYU Langone Med Ctr (page 67); **Address:** 35 E 35th St, Ste 202, New York, NY 10016-3823; **Phone:** 212-685-4225; **Board Cert:** Pediatrics 1975; Allergy & Immunology 1977; **Med School:** NYU Sch Med 1970; **Resid:** Pediatrics, Bellevue Hosp Ctr 1973; **Fellow:** Allergy & Immunology, Walter Reed Army Med Ctr 1976; **Fac Appt:** Assoc Clin Prof Ped, NYU Sch Med

Josephs, Shelby H MD [PA&I] - **Spec Exp:** Food Allergy; **Hospital:** Georgetown Univ Hosp; **Address:** 6410 Rockledge Drive, Ste 304, Bethesda, MD 20871; **Phone:** 301-530-7907; **Board Cert:** Pediatrics 1979; Allergy & Immunology 1985; **Med School:** Duke Univ 1975; **Resid:** Pediatrics, Chldns Hosp 1977; Allergy & Immunology, Duke Univ Med Ctr 1979; **Fac Appt:** Assoc Clin Prof Ped, Georgetown Univ

Kamani, Naynesh R MD [PA&I] - **Spec Exp:** Stem Cell Transplant; Immunotherapy; Bone Marrow Transplant; **Hospital:** Chldns Natl Med Ctr; **Address:** Chldns Natl Med Ctr, Div Hematology, 111 Michigan Ave NW, Washington, DC 20010; **Phone:** 202-476-2800; **Board Cert:** Pediatrics 1983; Pediatric Allergy & Immunology 1983; Diagnostic Lab Immunology 1986; **Med School:** Ethiopia 1975; **Resid:** Pediatrics, Downstate Med Ctr-Kings Co Hosp 1981; **Fellow:** Pediatric Allergy & Immunology, Chldns Hosp 1983; **Fac Appt:** Prof Ped, Geo Wash Univ

Sampson, Hugh MD [PA&I] - **Spec Exp:** Food Allergy; Eczema; Atopic Dermatitis; **Hospital:** Mount Sinai Med Ctr (page 64); **Address:** Mt Sinai Sch Med, Dept Peds, 1 Gustave Levy Pl, Box 1198, New York, NY 10029-6500; **Phone:** 212-241-5548; **Board Cert:** Pediatrics 1980; Allergy & Immunology 1981; **Med School:** SUNY Buffalo 1975; **Resid:** Pediatrics, Chldns Meml Hosp 1979; **Fellow:** Allergy & Immunology, Duke Univ Med Ctr 1980; **Fac Appt:** Prof Ped, Mount Sinai Sch Med

Pediatric Allergy & Immunology

Schuberth, Kenneth Charles MD [PA&I] - **Spec Exp:** Allergy; Asthma; **Hospital:** Johns Hopkins Hosp (page 61), Greater Baltimore Med Ctr; **Address:** 10807 Falls Rd, Ste 200, Lutherville, MD 21093; **Phone:** 410-321-9393; **Board Cert:** Pediatrics 1979; Allergy & Immunology 1983; **Med School:** Johns Hopkins Univ 1973; **Resid:** Pediatrics, Johns Hopkins Hosp 1978; **Fellow:** Allergy & Immunology, Johns Hopkins Hosp 1980; **Fac Appt:** Assoc Prof Ped, Johns Hopkins Univ

Sicherer, Scott H MD [PA&I] - **Spec Exp:** Food Allergy; Drug Sensitivity; Eczema; **Hospital:** Mount Sinai Med Ctr (page 64); **Address:** 1 Gustave Levy Pl, Box 1198, New York, NY 10029-6500; **Phone:** 212-241-5548; **Board Cert:** Pediatrics 2008; Allergy & Immunology 2007; **Med School:** Johns Hopkins Univ 1990; **Resid:** Pediatrics, Mt Sinai Hosp 1994; **Fellow:** Allergy & Immunology, Johns Hopkins Hosp 1997; **Fac Appt:** Assoc Prof Ped, Mount Sinai Sch Med

Skoner, David Peter MD [PA&I] - **Spec Exp:** Asthma & Allergy; Rhinitis; **Hospital:** Allegheny General Hosp; **Address:** Allegheny Genl Hosp, Div Asthma Allergy & Immunology, 320 E North Ave, Fl 7 - South Tower, Pittsburgh, PA 15212; **Phone:** 412-359-6640; **Board Cert:** Pediatrics 1985; Allergy & Immunology 1985; **Med School:** Temple Univ 1980; **Resid:** Pediatrics, Chldns Hosp Med Ctr 1983; **Fellow:** Allergy & Immunology, Chldns Hosp 1985; **Fac Appt:** Prof Ped, Drexel Univ Coll Med

Sly, R Michael MD [PA&I] - **Spec Exp:** Asthma; Allergy; Atopic Dermatitis; **Hospital:** Chldns Natl Med Ctr; **Address:** Children's Natl Med Ctr, Dept Allergy, Pulmonary, Sleep Med, 111 Michigan Ave NW, Ste 1030, Washington, DC 20010-2970; **Phone:** 202-476-2128; **Board Cert:** Pediatric Allergy & Immunology 1967; Pediatrics 1980; Allergy & Immunology 1987; **Med School:** Washington Univ, St Louis 1960; **Resid:** Pediatrics, St Louis Chldns Hosp 1962; Pediatrics, Univ Kentucky Med Ctr 1963; **Fellow:** Pediatric Allergy & Immunology, UCLA Med Ctr 1967; **Fac Appt:** Prof Ped, Geo Wash Univ

Spergel, Jonathan MD/PhD [PA&I] - **Spec Exp:** Atopic Dermatitis; Food Allergy; Asthma; **Hospital:** Chldns Hosp of Philadelphia, The; **Address:** 3550 Market St Fl 3, Philadelphia, PA 19104; **Phone:** 215-590-2549; **Board Cert:** Pediatrics 2003; Allergy & Immunology 2006; **Med School:** Mount Sinai Sch Med 1992; **Resid:** Pediatrics, Yale New Haven Hosp 1994; **Fellow:** Allergy & Immunology, Chldn's Hosp 1995; **Fac Appt:** Assoc Prof Ped, Univ Pennsylvania

Wood, Robert A MD [PA&I] - **Spec Exp:** Food Allergy; Asthma; **Hospital:** Johns Hopkins Hosp (page 61); **Address:** 600 N Wolfe St, CMSC-1102, Baltimore, MD 21287; **Phone:** 410-955-5883; **Board Cert:** Pediatrics 1987; Allergy & Immunology 1997; **Med School:** Univ Rochester 1982; **Resid:** Pediatrics, Johns Hopkins Hosp 1985; **Fellow:** Allergy & Immunology, Johns Hopkins Hosp 1988; **Fac Appt:** Prof Ped, Johns Hopkins Univ

Southeast

Burks Jr, Arvil Wesley MD [PA&I] - **Spec Exp:** Asthma; Allergic Rhinitis; Food Allergy; Anaphylaxis; **Hospital:** Duke Univ Med Ctr; **Address:** Duke Univ Med Ctr, Box 2644, Durham, NC 27710; **Phone:** 919-668-4000; **Board Cert:** Pediatrics 1985; Allergy & Immunology 1985; **Med School:** Univ Ark 1980; **Resid:** Pediatrics, Ark Chldns Hosp 1983; **Fellow:** Allergy & Immunology, Duke Univ Med Ctr 1985; **Fac Appt:** Prof Ped, Duke Univ

Kelly, Cynthia S MD [PA&I] - **Spec Exp:** Asthma; Rhinitis; Sinusitis; **Hospital:** Chldns Hosp of King's Daughters; **Address:** Chlds Hosp of The Kings Daughters, 601 Childrens Lane, Norfolk, VA 23507; **Phone:** 757-668-8255; **Board Cert:** Pediatrics 2004; Allergy & Immunology 2007; **Med School:** Wayne State Univ 1985; **Resid:** Pediatrics, Univ Mich 1987; **Fellow:** Allergy & Immunology, UCLA Med Ctr 1988; Pediatric Infectious Disease, Vanderbilt Univ 1989; **Fac Appt:** Assoc Prof Ped, Eastern VA Med Sch

Ownby, Dennis R MD [PA&I] - **Spec Exp:** Food Allergy; Anaphylaxis; **Hospital:** Med Coll of GA Hosp and Clin (MCG Health Inc); **Address:** Allergy & Immunology, 1120 15th St Bldg BG - rm 1019, Augusta, GA 30912-0004; **Phone:** 706-721-2390; **Board Cert:** Pediatrics 1977; Pediatric Allergy & Immunology 2006; Clinical & Laboratory Immunology 1986; **Med School:** Med Coll OH 1972; **Resid:** Pediatrics, Duke Univ Med Ctr 1974; **Fellow:** Pediatric Allergy & Immunology, Duke Univ Med Ctr 1977; **Fac Appt:** Prof Ped, Med Coll GA

Sleasman, John W MD [PA&I] - **Spec Exp:** Infectious Disease; Immunodeficiency Disorders; **Hospital:** All Children's Hosp; **Address:** All Childrens Hosp, Div Ped Immun/Rheumatology, 801 6th St S, Box 9350, St Petersburg, FL 33701; **Phone:** 727-767-4150; **Board Cert:** Pediatrics 1988; Diagnostic Lab Immunology 1990; **Med School:** Univ Tenn Coll Med, Memphis 1981; **Resid:** Pediatrics, Shands Hosp 1984; **Fellow:** Pediatric Infectious Disease, Shands Hosp 1987; Immunology, Dana Farber Cancer Inst 1988

Midwest

Lemanske Jr, Robert F MD [PA&I] - **Spec Exp:** Asthma; Allergy; Immune Deficiency; **Hospital:** Univ WI Hosp & Clins; **Address:** 600 Highland Ave, rm K4/916 CSC, Madison, WI 53792; **Phone:** 608-265-2206; **Board Cert:** Pediatrics 1980; Allergy & Immunology 1981; **Med School:** Univ Wisc 1975; **Resid:** Pediatrics, Univ Wisc Hosp 1978; **Fellow:** Allergy & Immunology, Univ Wisc Hosp 1980; Allergy & Immunology, Natl Inst Hlth 1983; **Fac Appt:** Prof Ped, Univ Wisc

Pongracic, Jacqueline MD [PA&I] - **Spec Exp:** Latex Allergy; Asthma; Food Allergy; **Hospital:** Children's Mem Hosp, Northwestern Meml Hosp; **Address:** 2300 Children's Plaza, Box 60, Chicago, IL 60614; **Phone:** 773-327-3710; **Board Cert:** Internal Medicine 1988; Allergy & Immunology 2001; **Med School:** Northwestern Univ 1985; **Resid:** Internal Medicine, North Shore Univ Hosp 1988; **Fellow:** Allergy & Immunology, Johns Hopkins Hosp 1991; **Fac Appt:** Asst Prof Ped, Northwestern Univ

Strunk, Robert C MD [PA&I] - **Spec Exp:** Asthma; **Hospital:** St Louis Chldns Hosp; **Address:** 660 S Euclid Ave, Box 8116, St Louis, MO 63110; **Phone:** 314-454-2694; **Board Cert:** Pediatrics 1974; Allergy & Immunology 1987; **Med School:** Northwestern Univ 1968; **Resid:** Pediatrics, Cincinnati Chldns Hosp 1970; **Fellow:** Pediatric Allergy & Immunology, Boston Chldns Hosp 1974; **Fac Appt:** Prof Ped, Washington Univ, St Louis

Wolf, Raoul MD [PA&I] - **Spec Exp:** Asthma; Allergy; Immune Deficiency; **Hospital:** Univ of Chicago Med Ctr, La Rabida Chlds Hosp; **Address:** Dept Allergy & Immunology, E 65th St at Lake Michigan, Chicago, IL 60649; **Phone:** 773-753-8637; **Board Cert:** Pediatrics 1980; Allergy & Immunology 1983; **Med School:** South Africa 1969; **Resid:** Pediatrics, Baragwanath Hosp 1973; Pediatrics, Transvaal Meml Hosp Chldn 1976; **Fellow:** Allergy & Immunology, Chldns Hosp Med Ctr 1979; **Fac Appt:** Prof Ped, Univ Chicago-Pritzker Sch Med

Great Plains and Mountains

Bock, Samuel A MD [PA&I] - **Spec Exp:** Asthma up to age 50; Allergy up to age 50; Food Allergy; **Hospital:** Boulder Community Hospital, Natl Jewish Med & Rsch Ctr; **Address:** Boulder Asthma & Allergy Clinics, 3950 Broadway, Boulder, CO 80304; **Phone:** 303-444-5991; **Board Cert:** Pediatrics 1977; Allergy & Immunology 1977; **Med School:** Univ MD Sch Med 1972; **Resid:** Pediatrics, Colo Med Ctr/Natl Jewish Med Ctr 1974; **Fellow:** Allergy & Immunology, Colo Med Ctr/Natl Jewish Med Ctr 1976; **Fac Appt:** Clin Prof Ped, Univ Colorado

Pediatric Allergy & Immunology

Gelfand, Erwin W MD [PA&I] - **Spec Exp:** Immune Deficiency; Asthma; Allergy; **Hospital:** Natl Jewish Med & Rsch Ctr, Chldn's Hosp - Aurora, The; **Address:** National Jewish Health, 1400 Jackson St, Denver, CO 80206; **Phone:** 303-398-1196; **Board Cert:** Pediatrics 1972; **Med School:** McGill Univ 1966; **Resid:** Pediatrics, Montreal Childrens Hosp 1968; Pediatrics, Childrens Hosp Med Ctr 1969; **Fellow:** Immunology, Childrens Hosp Med Ctr 1971; **Fac Appt:** Prof Ped, Univ Colorado

Leung, Donald YM MD/PhD [PA&I] - **Spec Exp:** Atopic Dermatitis; Asthma; **Hospital:** Natl Jewish Med & Rsch Ctr, Chldn's Hosp - Aurora, The; **Address:** 1400 Jackson St, Bldg K - Ste 926I, Denver, CO 80206; **Phone:** 303-398-1379; **Board Cert:** Pediatrics 1982; Allergy & Immunology 1983; Clinical & Laboratory Immunology 1990; **Med School:** Univ Chicago-Pritzker Sch Med 1977; **Resid:** Pediatrics, Chldn's Hosp 1979; **Fellow:** Allergy & Immunology, Chldn's Hosp 1981; **Fac Appt:** Prof Ped, Univ Colorado

Southwest

Bahna, Sami L MD [PA&I] - **Spec Exp:** Food Allergy; Asthma; Eczema; **Hospital:** Louisiana State Univ Hosp; **Address:** LSU Hlth Scis Ctr, Dept Pediatrics, 1501 Kings Hwy, Shreveport, LA 71103; **Phone:** 318-675-7625; **Board Cert:** Pediatrics 1980; Allergy & Immunology 1981; **Med School:** Egypt 1964; **Resid:** Pediatrics, Univ Maryland Hosp 1975; **Fellow:** Allergy & Immunology, Harbor-UCLA Med Ctr 1978; **Fac Appt:** Prof Ped, Louisiana State U, New Orleans

Shearer, William T MD/PhD [PA&I] - **Spec Exp:** AIDS/HIV; Immune Deficiency; **Hospital:** Texas Chldns Hosp; **Address:** Dept Allergy & Immunology, 6621 Fannin St Fl 3, MC FC 330.01, Houston, TX 77030-2399; **Phone:** 832-824-1319; **Board Cert:** Pediatrics 1986; Allergy & Immunology 1989; Clinical & Laboratory Immunology 1986; **Med School:** Washington Univ, St Louis 1970; **Resid:** Pediatrics, Chldns Hosp-Wash Univ 1972; **Fellow:** Allergy & Immunology, Barnes Hosp-Wash Univ 1974; **Fac Appt:** Prof Ped, Baylor Coll Med

West Coast and Pacific

Church, Joseph A MD [PA&I] - **Spec Exp:** AIDS/HIV; Immune Deficiency; **Hospital:** Chldns Hosp - Los Angeles; **Address:** Childrens Hosp LA, MS75, Clinical Immunology & Allergy, 4650 W Sunset Blvd, Los Angeles, CA 90027; **Phone:** 323-361-2501; **Board Cert:** Pediatrics 1977; Allergy & Immunology 1977; **Med School:** UMDNJ-NJ Med Sch, Newark 1972; **Resid:** Pediatrics, Chldns Hosp/Natl Med Ctr 1974; **Fellow:** Allergy & Immunology, Georgetown Med Ctr 1976; **Fac Appt:** Prof Ped, USC Sch Med

Cowan, Morton J MD [PA&I] - **Spec Exp:** Immunodeficiency Disorders; Stem Cell Transplant-Fetal; Bone Marrow Transplant; **Hospital:** UCSF Med Ctr; **Address:** UCSF Med Ctr, Peds BMT Program, 505 Parnassus Ave, rm M659, San Francisco, CA 94143-1278; **Phone:** 415-476-2188; **Board Cert:** Pediatrics 1981; Allergy & Immunology 1983; **Med School:** Univ Pennsylvania 1970; **Resid:** Surgery, Duke Univ Med Ctr 1972; Pediatrics, UCSF Med Ctr 1977; **Fellow:** Research, Natl Inst Hlth 1975; Immunology, UCSF Med Ctr 1979; **Fac Appt:** Prof Ped, UCSF

Epstein, Stuart MD [PA&I] - **Spec Exp:** Asthma & Allergy; Food Allergy; **Hospital:** Cedars-Sinai Med Ctr; **Address:** 9735 Wilshire Blvd, Ste 121, Beverly Hills, CA 90212-2101; **Phone:** 310-274-6853; **Board Cert:** Allergy & Immunology 1999; **Med School:** Univ IL Coll Med 1978; **Resid:** Pediatrics, Cedars Sinai Med Ctr 1980; **Fellow:** Pediatrics, UC Irvine 1981; Pediatrics, USC Med Ctr 1982; **Fac Appt:** Assoc Clin Prof Ped, UCLA

Fanous, Yvonne F MD [PA&I] - **Spec Exp:** Asthma & Allergy; Cystic Fibrosis; Immune Deficiency; **Hospital:** Loma Linda Univ Med Ctr; **Address:** 11370 Anderson St, Ste B-100, Loma Linda, CA 92354; **Phone:** 909-558-2388; **Board Cert:** Pediatrics 1983; Allergy & Immunology 1985; **Med School:** Egypt 1973; **Resid:** Pediatrics, Texas Tech Univ Hosp 1980; Pediatrics, Loma Linda Univ 1981; **Fellow:** Allergy & Immunology, UC Irvine 1983; **Fac Appt:** Assoc Prof A&I, Loma Linda Univ

Stiehm, E Richard MD [PA&I] - **Spec Exp:** Immune Deficiency; Allergy; Pediatric Rheumatology; **Hospital:** UCLA Ronald Reagan Med Ctr; **Address:** UCLA Chldn's Hosp, 10833 Le Conte Ave, rm 12-430, Los Angeles, CA 90095-3075; **Phone:** 310-825-6481; **Board Cert:** Pediatrics 1964; Allergy & Immunology 1974; Diagnostic Lab Immunology 1986; **Med School:** Univ Wisc 1957; **Resid:** Pediatrics, Babies Hosp 1963; **Fellow:** Allergy & Immunology, Univ Wisc 1959; Allergy & Immunology, UCSF 1965; **Fac Appt:** Prof Ped, UCLA

Wara, Diane W MD [PA&I] - **Spec Exp:** AIDS/HIV; Immune Deficiency; **Hospital:** UCSF Med Ctr; **Address:** 505 Parnassus Ave, Box 0107, UCSF Dept Pediatrics, RM M-679, San Francisco, CA 94143; **Phone:** 415-476-2865; **Board Cert:** Pediatrics 1974; Allergy & Immunology 1975; **Med School:** UC Irvine 1969; **Resid:** Pediatrics, UCSF Med Ctr 1972; **Fellow:** Immunology, UCSF Med Ctr 1975; **Fac Appt:** Prof Ped, UCSF

PEDIATRIC CARDIOLOGY

New England

Lang, Peter MD [PCd] - **Spec Exp:** Interventional Cardiology; Cardiac Catheterization; **Hospital:** Children's Hospital - Boston; **Address:** Children's Hosp, Dept Cardiology, 300 Longwood Ave, Boston, MA 02114; **Phone:** 617-355-8539; **Board Cert:** Pediatrics 1977; Pediatric Cardiology 1979; **Med School:** Mount Sinai Sch Med 1972; **Resid:** Pediatrics, Babies Hosp-Presby Med Ctr 1975; **Fellow:** Pediatric Cardiology, Chldns Hospital Med Ctr 1978; **Fac Appt:** Assoc Prof Ped, Harvard Med Sch

Lock, James E MD [PCd] - **Spec Exp:** Interventional Cardiology; Angioplasty-Pulmonary Artery; Cardiac Catheterization; Fetal Surgery; **Hospital:** Children's Hospital - Boston; **Address:** Chldns Hosp, Dept Cardiology, 300 Longwood Ave, Farley 2, Boston, MA 02115-5724; **Phone:** 617-355-7313; **Board Cert:** Pediatrics 1978; Pediatric Cardiology 1981; **Med School:** Stanford Univ 1973; **Resid:** Pediatrics, Univ Minn Hosp 1975; Pediatric Cardiology, Univ Minn Hosp 1977; **Fellow:** Cardiovascular Disease, Hosp Sick Chldn 1979; **Fac Appt:** Prof Ped, Harvard Med Sch

Newburger, Jane MD [PCd] - **Spec Exp:** Kawasaki Disease; Cholesterol/Lipid Disorders; Congenital Heart Disease; **Hospital:** Children's Hospital - Boston, Brigham & Women's Hosp; **Address:** Chldns Hosp, Dept Ped Cardiology, 300 Longwood Ave, Farley Bldg Fl 2, Boston, MA 02115-5724; **Phone:** 617-355-5427; **Board Cert:** Pediatrics 1979; Pediatric Cardiology 1983; **Med School:** Harvard Med Sch 1974; **Resid:** Pediatrics, Chldns Hosp Med Ctr 1976; **Fellow:** Pediatric Cardiology, Chldns Hosp Med Ctr 1979; **Fac Appt:** Prof Ped, Harvard Med Sch

Walsh, Edward P MD [PCd] - **Spec Exp:** Arrhythmias; **Hospital:** Children's Hospital - Boston; **Address:** Chldns Hosp, Dept Cardiology, 300 Longwood Ave Bader Bldg Fl 2, Boston, MA 02115; **Phone:** 617-355-6328; **Board Cert:** Pediatrics 1985; Pediatric Cardiology 1985; **Med School:** Univ Pennsylvania 1979; **Resid:** Pediatrics, Chldns Hosp 1982; **Fellow:** Pediatric Cardiology, Chldns Hosp 1985; **Fac Appt:** Assoc Prof Ped, Harvard Med Sch

Pediatric Cardiology

Mid Atlantic

Beerman, Lee B MD [PCd] - **Spec Exp:** Congenital Heart Disease-Adult & Child; Arrhythmias; **Hospital:** Chldns Hosp of Pittsburgh - UPMC; **Address:** Chldns Hosp-Heart Ctr, 45th St & Penn Ave, Pittsburgh, PA 15201; **Phone:** 412-692-5540; **Board Cert:** Pediatrics 1979; Pediatric Cardiology 1979; **Med School:** Univ Pittsburgh 1974; **Resid:** Pediatrics, Chldns Hosp 1977; **Fellow:** Pediatric Cardiology, Chldns Hosp 1979; **Fac Appt:** Prof Ped, Univ Pittsburgh

Biancaniello, Thomas MD [PCd] - **Spec Exp:** Congenital Heart Disease; Fetal Echocardiography; Interventional Cardiology; Cardiac Catheterization; **Hospital:** Stony Brook Univ Med Ctr, Schneider Chldn's Hosp; **Address:** Stony Brook Univ Hosp, Dept Pediatrics, HSC T11, 040, Stony Brook, NY 11794-8111; **Phone:** 631-444-5437; **Board Cert:** Pediatrics 1979; Pediatric Cardiology 1981; **Med School:** NY Med Coll 1975; **Resid:** Pediatrics, North Shore Univ Hosp 1977; **Fellow:** Pediatric Cardiology, Cincinnati Chldns Hosp 1980; **Fac Appt:** Prof Ped, SUNY Stony Brook

Bierman, Fredrick MD [PCd] - **Spec Exp:** Fetal Echocardiography; Kawasaki Disease; Congenital Heart Disease; Echocardiography; **Hospital:** Schneider Chldn's Hosp; **Address:** Chldns Heart Ctr, Schneider Chldns Hosp, 269-01 76th Ave, rm 139, New Hyde Park, NY 11040; **Phone:** 718-470-7350; **Board Cert:** Pediatrics 1978; Pediatric Cardiology 1981; **Med School:** SUNY Downstate 1973; **Resid:** Pediatrics, Mount Sinai Med Ctr 1976; **Fellow:** Pediatric Cardiology, Harvard Chldns Hosp 1979; **Fac Appt:** Prof Ped, Albert Einstein Coll Med

Brenner, Joel I MD [PCd] - **Spec Exp:** Congenital Heart Disease; **Hospital:** Johns Hopkins Hosp (page 61); **Address:** Johns Hopkins Hosp, Pediatric Cardiology, 600 N Wolfe St, Brady 522, Baltimore, MD 21287; **Phone:** 410-955-5987; **Board Cert:** Pediatrics 1975; Pediatric Cardiology 1977; **Med School:** NY Med Coll 1970; **Resid:** Pediatrics, NY Hosp 1972; **Fellow:** Pediatric Cardiology, Yale-New Haven Hosp 1974; **Fac Appt:** Assoc Prof Ped, Johns Hopkins Univ

Cooper, Rubin MD [PCd] - **Spec Exp:** Congenital Heart Disease; Rheumatic Heart Disease; Kawasaki Disease; **Hospital:** NYPresby-Morgan Stanley Children's Hosp (page 66), NY Hosp Queens; **Address:** 525 E 68th St, Ste F695B, New York, NY 10021; **Phone:** 212-746-3561; **Board Cert:** Pediatrics 1976; Pediatric Cardiology 1979; **Med School:** NY Med Coll 1971; **Resid:** Pediatrics, Strong Meml Hosp 1973; **Fellow:** Pediatric Cardiology, Strong Meml Hosp 1975; **Fac Appt:** Prof Ped, Cornell Univ-Weill Med Coll

Gelb, Bruce D MD [PCd] - **Spec Exp:** Transplant Medicine-Heart; Marfan's Syndrome; Noonan Syndrome; **Hospital:** Mount Sinai Med Ctr (page 64); **Address:** 1 Gustave Levy Pl, Box 1201, New York, NY 10029; **Phone:** 212-241-8592; **Board Cert:** Pediatric Cardiology 2006; **Med School:** Univ Rochester 1984; **Resid:** Pediatrics, NY Presby Hosp 1987; **Fellow:** Pediatric Cardiology, Baylor College Med 1991; **Fac Appt:** Prof Ped, Mount Sinai Sch Med

Gewitz, Michael MD [PCd] - **Spec Exp:** Neonatal Cardiology; Kawasaki Disease; Echocardiography; Heart Failure; **Hospital:** Westchester Med Ctr, Vassar Bros Med Ctr; **Address:** Maria Fareri Children's Hospital, Rte 100, Munger Pavillion, Ste 618, Valhalla, NY 10595; **Phone:** 914-594-4370; **Board Cert:** Pediatrics 1979; Pediatric Cardiology 1981; **Med School:** Hahnemann Univ 1974; **Resid:** Pediatrics, Chldns Hosp 1976; Pediatrics, Hosp Sick Chldn 1977; **Fellow:** Pediatric Cardiology, Yale-New Haven Hosp 1979; **Fac Appt:** Prof Ped, NY Med Coll

Hellenbrand, William E MD [PCd] - **Spec Exp:** Interventional Cardiology; **Hospital:** NYPresby-Morgan Stanley Children's Hosp (page 66), Robert Wood Johnson Univ Hosp - New Brunswick; **Address:** Morgan Stanley Chlds Hosp, 3959 Broadway Fl 2N - rm 255, New York, NY 10032; **Phone:** 212-342-0610; **Board Cert:** Pediatrics 1975; Pediatric Cardiology 1977; **Med School:** SUNY Downstate 1970; **Resid:** Pediatrics, Yale-New Haven Hosp 1972; **Fellow:** Pediatric Cardiology, Yale-New Haven Hosp 1976; **Fac Appt:** Prof Ped, Columbia P&S

Hsu, Daphne MD [PCd] - **Spec Exp:** Interventional Cardiology; Heart Failure; Transplant Medicine-Heart; **Hospital:** Montefiore Med Ctr - Div. Moses, Jacobi Med Ctr; **Address:** Chldn's Hosp at Montefiore, 3415 Bainbridge Ave, Bronx, NY 10467; **Phone:** 718-741-2315; **Board Cert:** Pediatrics 1988; Pediatric Cardiology 2003; **Med School:** Yale Univ 1982; **Resid:** Pediatrics, Columbia Babies & Chldn's Hosp 1985; **Fellow:** Pediatric Cardiology, Columbia Babies & Chldn's Hosp 1988; **Fac Appt:** Prof Ped, Albert Einstein Coll Med

Parness, Ira A MD [PCd] - **Spec Exp:** Echocardiography; Congenital Heart Disease; Fetal Echocardiography; **Hospital:** Mount Sinai Med Ctr (page 64); **Address:** 1 Gustave Levy Pl, Box 1201, New York, NY 10029-6500; **Phone:** 212-241-8662; **Board Cert:** Pediatrics 1984; Pediatric Cardiology 1985; **Med School:** SUNY Downstate 1979; **Resid:** Pediatrics, Brookdale Hosp 1982; **Fellow:** Pediatric Cardiology, Chldns Hosp 1985; **Fac Appt:** Assoc Prof Ped, Mount Sinai Sch Med

Radtke, Wolfgang MD [PCd] - **Spec Exp:** Interventional Cardiology; Cardiac Catheterization; Congenital Heart Disease-Adult & Child; **Hospital:** Alfred I duPont Hosp for Children; **Address:** Nemours Cardiac Ctr, 1600 Rockland Rd, Wilmington, DE 19803; **Phone:** 302-651-6600; **Board Cert:** Pediatrics 2002; Pediatric Cardiology 2004; **Med School:** Germany 1980; **Resid:** Pediatrics, Kiel Univ Chldns Hosp 1985; **Fellow:** Pediatric Cardiology, Chldns Hosp 1988; **Fac Appt:** Prof Ped, Jefferson Med Coll

Steinherz, Laurel MD [PCd] - **Spec Exp:** Cardiac Effects of Cancer/Cancer Therapy; **Hospital:** Meml Sloan-Kettering Cancer Ctr, NY-Presby Hosp/Weill Cornell (page 66); **Address:** 1275 York Avenue, New York, NY 10065; **Phone:** 212-639-8103; **Board Cert:** Pediatrics 1976; Pediatric Cardiology 1978; **Med School:** Albert Einstein Coll Med 1970; **Resid:** Pediatrics, Chldns Hosp 1972; **Fellow:** Pediatric Cardiology, NY Hosp-Cornell Med Ctr 1975; **Fac Appt:** Prof Ped, Cornell Univ-Weill Med Coll

Velvis, Harm MD [PCd] - **Spec Exp:** Cardiac Catheterization; Congenital Heart Disease; Heart Disease in Down Syndrome; **Hospital:** Albany Med Ctr, St Peter's Hosp - Albany; **Address:** Capital Dist Ped Cardio Assoc, 319 S Manning Blvd, Ste 203, Albany, NY 12208-1743; **Phone:** 518-489-3292; **Board Cert:** Pediatric Cardiology 2002; **Med School:** Netherlands 1980; **Resid:** Pediatrics, Albany Med Ctr 1987; **Fellow:** Pediatric Cardiology, UCSF Med Ctr 1990; **Fac Appt:** Assoc Clin Prof Ped, Albany Med Coll

Walsh, Christine A MD [PCd] - **Spec Exp:** Arrhythmias; Congenital Heart Disease; Syncope; **Hospital:** Montefiore Med Ctr - Div. Moses, Montefiore Med Ctr - Div. Weiler; **Address:** 3415 Bainbridge Ave, Bronx, NY 10467-2401; **Phone:** 718-741-2343; **Board Cert:** Pediatrics 1978; Pediatric Cardiology 1983; Pediatric Critical Care Medicine 2003; **Med School:** Yale Univ 1973; **Resid:** Pediatrics, Columbia-Presby Med Ctr 1976; **Fellow:** Pediatric Cardiology, Columbia-Presby Med Ctr 1978; Pharmacology, Columbia P&S 1980; **Fac Appt:** Prof Ped, Albert Einstein Coll Med

Weinberg, Paul M MD [PCd] - **Spec Exp:** Cardiac Pathology; Cardiac MRI; **Hospital:** Chldns Hosp of Philadelphia, The; **Address:** Chldns Hosp, Div Cardiology, 34th St & Civic Ctr Blvd, Philadelphia, PA 19104; **Phone:** 215-590-3274; **Board Cert:** Pediatrics 1974; Pediatric Cardiology 1975; **Med School:** Jefferson Med Coll 1969; **Resid:** Pediatrics, Chldns Hosp 1971; Cardiology & Pathology, Chldns Hosp Med Ctr 1977; **Fellow:** Pediatric Cardiology, Chldns Hosp 1973; **Fac Appt:** Prof Ped, Univ Pennsylvania

Pediatric Cardiology

Southeast

Bricker, John T MD [PCd] - **Spec Exp:** Transplant Medicine-Heart; Congenital Heart Disease-Adult & Child; **Hospital:** Univ of Kentucky Chandler Hosp; **Address:** 800 Rose St, MN 150, Lexington, KY 40536-0298; **Phone:** 859-323-5481 x297; **Board Cert:** Pediatrics 1981; Pediatric Cardiology 1997; **Med School:** Ohio State Univ 1976; **Resid:** Pediatrics, Tex Chldns Hosp 1980; **Fellow:** Pediatric Cardiology, Tex Chldns Hosp 1983; **Fac Appt:** Prof Ped, Univ KY Coll Med

Colvin, Edward V MD [PCd] - **Spec Exp:** Congenital Heart Disease-Adult & Child; Fetal Echocardiography; Transplant Medicine-Heart; **Hospital:** Univ of Ala Hosp at Birmingham, Children's Hospital - Birmingham; **Address:** 320 Hillman Bldg, 620 20th St S, Birmingham, AL 35233; **Phone:** 205-934-3460; **Board Cert:** Pediatrics 1982; Pediatric Cardiology 1985; **Med School:** Univ Alabama 1977; **Resid:** Pediatrics, Chldns Hosp 1980; **Fellow:** Pediatric Cardiology, Baylor Coll Med 1983; **Fac Appt:** Prof Ped, Univ Alabama

Epstein, Michael L MD [PCd] - **Spec Exp:** Congenital Heart Disease; **Hospital:** All Children's Hosp; **Address:** All Children's Hosp, 801 Sixth St S, Box 9500, St Petersburg, FL 33701; **Phone:** 727-767-6941; **Board Cert:** Pediatrics 1976; Pediatric Cardiology 1981; **Med School:** Univ Tex Med Br, Galveston 1971; **Resid:** Pediatrics, Univ Ariz Hlth Sci Ctr 1974; **Fellow:** Pediatric Cardiology, Univ Minn Hosp 1979; **Fac Appt:** Prof Ped, Univ S Fla Coll Med

Fish, Frank A MD [PCd] - **Spec Exp:** Arrhythmias-Pediatric & Adult; Congenital Heart Disease-Adult; Pacemakers; Cardiac Electrophysiology; **Hospital:** Vanderbilt Children's Hosp, Vanderbilt Univ Med Ctr; **Address:** Vanderbilt Chldns Hosp, Div Pediatric Cardiology, 2200 Children's Way, 5230 DOT, Nashville, TN 37232-9119; **Phone:** 615-322-7447; **Board Cert:** Pediatrics 1987; Pediatric Cardiology 2006; **Med School:** Indiana Univ 1983; **Resid:** Pediatrics, Indiana Univ Hosp 1986; **Fellow:** Pediatric Cardiology, Vanderbilt Univ Med Ctr 1989; Cardiac Electrophysiology, Chldns Meml Hosp 1990; **Fac Appt:** Assoc Prof Ped, Vanderbilt Univ

Fricker, Frederick Jay MD [PCd] - **Spec Exp:** Transplant Medicine-Heart; **Hospital:** Shands at Univ of FL; **Address:** Shands Hlthcre, Div Pediatric Cardiology, 1600 SW Archer Rd, Box 100296, Gainesville, FL 32610-0296; **Phone:** 352-273-7770; **Board Cert:** Pediatrics 1975; Pediatric Cardiology 1981; **Med School:** Loyola Univ-Stritch Sch Med 1970; **Resid:** Pediatrics, Chldns Hosp 1973; **Fellow:** Pediatric Cardiology, Chldns Hosp 1977; **Fac Appt:** Prof Ped, Univ Fla Coll Med

Gullquist, Scott D MD [PCd] - **Hospital:** VCU Med Ctr; **Address:** 1200 E Broad St Fl 5, West Hosp, North Wing, Richmond, VA 23298; **Phone:** 804-828-5745; **Board Cert:** Pediatrics 1999; Pediatric Cardiology 2002; **Med School:** Georgetown Univ 1987; **Resid:** Pediatrics, Chldns Hosp 1990; Pediatric Cardiology, Chldns Hosp 1993; **Fac Appt:** Assoc Prof Ped, Med Coll VA

Moskowitz, William B MD [PCd] - **Spec Exp:** Patent Foramen Ovale; **Hospital:** Med Coll of VA Hosp; **Address:** Childrens Heart Ctr, Med Coll Virginia, 1200 E Broad St, PO Box 980543, Richmond, VA 23298; **Phone:** 804-828-9143; **Board Cert:** Pediatrics 1983; Pediatric Cardiology 1985; **Med School:** Univ S Fla Coll Med 1978; **Resid:** Pediatrics, Chldns Hosp 1981; **Fellow:** Pediatric Cardiology, Chldns Hosp 1984; **Fac Appt:** Prof Ped, Med Coll VA

Young, Ming-Lon MD [PCd] - **Spec Exp:** Arrhythmias; **Hospital:** Jackson Meml Hosp (page 70), Univ of Miami Hosp & Clins/Sylvester Comp Canc Ctr (page 70); **Address:** Univ Miami, Dept Peds, PO Box 016960 (R-76), Miami, FL 33101-6960; **Phone:** 305-585-6683; **Board Cert:** Pediatrics 1985; Pediatric Cardiology 1985; **Med School:** Taiwan 1976; **Resid:** Preventive Medicine, Johns Hopkins Hosp 1979; Pediatrics, St Agnes Hosp 1981; **Fellow:** Pediatric Cardiology, Univ Miami Hosps 1985; **Fac Appt:** Prof Ped, Univ Miami Sch Med

Zahn, Evan M MD [PCd] - **Spec Exp:** Interventional Cardiology; Ventricular Septal Defect (Amplatzer R); Congenital Heart Disease; **Hospital:** Miami Children's Hosp, Baptist Hosp of Miami; **Address:** Miami Childrens Hosp, 3100 SW 62nd Ave, Ambulatory Care Bldg, 2nd Fl, Miami, FL 33155-5009; **Phone:** 305-662-8301 x5; **Board Cert:** Pediatric Cardiology 2007; **Med School:** NY Med Coll 1986; **Resid:** Pediatrics, Univ Colorado Hosp 1989; **Fellow:** Interventional Cardiology, Hosp for Sick Children 1992

Midwest

Ackerman, Michael J MD [PCd] - **Spec Exp:** Long QT Interval Syndrome; Sudden Infant Death Syndrome (SIDS); Hypertrophic Cardiomyopathy (HCM); **Hospital:** Mayo Med Ctr & Clin - Rochester; **Address:** Mayo Clin, Dept Ped Cardiology, 200 First St SW, Rochester, MN 55905; **Phone:** 507-284-0101; **Board Cert:** Pediatric Cardiology 2002; **Med School:** Mayo Med Sch 1995; **Resid:** Pediatric & Adolescent Medicine, Mayo Clin 1998; **Fellow:** Pediatric Cardiology, Mayo Clin 2000; **Fac Appt:** Assoc Prof Ped, Mayo Med Sch

Agarwala, Brojendra MD [PCd] - **Spec Exp:** Congenital Heart Disease; **Hospital:** Univ of Chicago Med Ctr; **Address:** 5841 S Maryland Ave, rm C-104, MC 405, Chicago, IL 60637; **Phone:** 773-702-6172; **Board Cert:** Pediatrics 1970; Pediatric Cardiology 1978; **Med School:** India 1965; **Resid:** Pediatrics, St Vincent Hosp Med Ctr 1969; **Fellow:** Pediatric Cardiology, NYU Med Ctr 1972; **Fac Appt:** Prof Ped, Univ Chicago-Pritzker Sch Med

Beekman III, Robert H MD [PCd] - **Spec Exp:** Interventional Cardiology; Cardiac Catheterization; **Hospital:** Cincinnati Chldns Hosp Med Ctr; **Address:** Cincinnati Chldns Hosp Med Ctr, Div Cardiology, 3333 Burnet Ave, MC 2003, Cincinnati, OH 45229-3026; **Phone:** 513-636-7072; **Board Cert:** Pediatrics 1981; Pediatric Cardiology 1983; **Med School:** Duke Univ 1976; **Resid:** Pediatrics, UCLA Med Ctr 1979; **Fellow:** Pediatric Cardiology, Univ Mich Hosp 1981; **Fac Appt:** Prof Ped, Univ Cincinnati

Caldwell, Randall L MD [PCd] - **Spec Exp:** Transplant Medicine-Heart; Echocardiography; Congenital Heart Disease; **Hospital:** Riley Hosp for Children, Clarian Hlth Ptrs; **Address:** 702 Barnhill Drive, RR-127, Indianapolis, IN 46202-5128; **Phone:** 317-274-8906; **Board Cert:** Pediatrics 1976; Pediatric Cardiology 1978; **Med School:** Indiana Univ 1971; **Resid:** Pediatrics, Indiana Med Ctr 1974; **Fellow:** Pediatric Cardiology, Indiana Med Ctr 1978; **Fac Appt:** Prof Ped, Indiana Univ

Cetta Jr, Frank MD [PCd] - **Spec Exp:** Congenital Heart Disease-Adult; Congenital Heart Disease; **Hospital:** Mayo Med Ctr & Clin - Rochester; **Address:** Mayo Clin, Gonda 6-138 NW, 200 First St SW, Rochester, MN 55905; **Phone:** 507-266-0676; **Board Cert:** Pediatric Cardiology 2004; **Med School:** Loyola Univ-Stritch Sch Med 1987; **Resid:** Internal Medicine & Pediatrics, Loyola Med Ctr 1991; **Fac Appt:** Assoc Prof Ped, Mayo Med Sch

Dick, Macdonald MD [PCd] - **Spec Exp:** Congenital Heart Disease; **Hospital:** Mott Chldns Hosp; **Address:** C.S. Motts Chldns Hosp, Dept Ped Cardio, 1500 E Med Ctr Drive, rm L1242, Box 0204, Ann Arbor, MI 48109; **Phone:** 734-936-7418; **Board Cert:** Pediatrics 1989; Pediatric Cardiology 2007; **Med School:** Univ VA Sch Med 1967; **Resid:** Pediatrics, Univ Va Hosp 1971; **Fellow:** Pediatric Cardiology, Chldns Hosp Med Ctr 1974; **Fac Appt:** Prof Ped, Univ Mich Med Sch

Driscoll, David J MD [PCd] - **Spec Exp:** Exercise Physiology; Klippel-Trenaunay Syndrome; Cardiomyopathy; **Hospital:** Mayo Med Ctr & Clin - Rochester; **Address:** Mayo Clinic - Pediatric Cardiology, 200 First St SW, Rochester, MN 55905-0001; **Phone:** 507-284-3297; **Board Cert:** Pediatrics 1976; Pediatric Cardiology 2006; **Med School:** Marquette Sch Med 1970; **Resid:** Pediatrics, Milwaukee Chldns Hosp 1972; Pediatrics, Milwaukee Chldns Hosp 1975; **Fellow:** Pediatric Cardiology, Baylor Coll Med 1978; **Fac Appt:** Prof Ped, Mayo Med Sch

Pediatric Cardiology

Hardin, Joel T MD [PCd] - **Spec Exp:** Fetal Cardiology; Echocardiography; Cardiac Intensive Care; **Hospital:** Loyola Univ Med Ctr; **Address:** Loyola Univ Med Ctr, 2160 S 1st Ave, Maguire, Chicago, IL 60153-3328; **Phone:** 708-327-9103; **Board Cert:** Pediatrics 2005; Pediatric Cardiology 2009; **Med School:** Univ Tenn Coll Med, Memphis 1987; **Resid:** Pediatrics, Chldns Hosp/Wash Univ 1990; **Fellow:** Pediatric Cardiology, Chldns Hosp/Wash Univ 1993; **Fac Appt:** Assoc Prof Ped, Loyola Univ-Stritch Sch Med

Hijazi, Ziyad M MD [PCd] - **Spec Exp:** Interventional Cardiology; Congenital Heart Disease; Coarctation of the Aorta; **Hospital:** Univ of Chicago Med Ctr; **Address:** 1653 W Congress Pkwy, Ste 770 Jones, Chicago, IL 60612; **Phone:** 312-942-8941; **Board Cert:** Pediatric Cardiology 2007; **Med School:** Jordan 1982; **Resid:** Pediatrics, Yale-New Haven Hosp 1988; **Fellow:** Pediatric Cardiology, Yale-New Haven Hosp 1991; **Fac Appt:** Prof Ped, Univ Chicago-Pritzker Sch Med

Latson, Larry A MD [PCd] - **Spec Exp:** Congenital Heart Disease; Interventional Cardiology; **Hospital:** Cleveland Clin Fdn (page 56); **Address:** Ped Cardiology, 9500 Euclid Ave, Desk M41, Cleveland, OH 44195; **Phone:** 216-445-6532; **Board Cert:** Pediatrics 1981; Pediatric Cardiology 1983; Pediatric Critical Care Medicine 2003; **Med School:** Baylor Coll Med 1976; **Resid:** Pediatrics, Baylor Coll Med 1978; **Fellow:** Pediatric Cardiology, Baylor Coll Med 1981; **Fac Appt:** Prof Ped, Case West Res Univ

O'Laughlin, Martin P MD [PCd] - **Spec Exp:** Cardiac Catheterization; Congenital Heart Disease-Adult & Child; Interventional Cardiology; **Hospital:** Chldns Mercy Hosps & Clinics, St Luke's Hosp of Kansas City; **Address:** 4400 Broadway, Ste 400, Kansas City, MO 64111; **Phone:** 816-931-5440; **Board Cert:** Pediatrics 1985; Pediatric Cardiology 2003; **Med School:** Columbia P&S 1980; **Resid:** Pediatrics, Baylor Coll Med 1984; **Fellow:** Pediatric Cardiology, Texas Chldns Hosp/Baylor 1987

Pahl, Elfriede MD [PCd] - **Spec Exp:** Transplant Medicine-Heart; Heart Failure; Congenital Heart Disease; Kawasaki Disease; **Hospital:** Children's Mem Hosp; **Address:** Children's Memorial Hosp, Ped Cardiology, 2300 Children's Plaza, Box 21, Chicago, IL 60614-3394; **Phone:** 773-880-6388; **Board Cert:** Pediatrics 1987; Pediatric Cardiology 2003; **Med School:** Northwestern Univ 1983; **Resid:** Pediatrics, Chldns Meml Hosp 1986; **Fellow:** Pediatric Cardiology, Chldns Hosp of Pittsburgh 1988; **Fac Appt:** Prof Ped, Northwestern Univ

Porter, Co-burn MD [PCd] - **Spec Exp:** Arrhythmias; Arrhythmias-Fetal; Transplant Medicine-Heart; **Hospital:** St Mary's Hosp - Rochester; **Address:** Mayo Clinic, Dept Ped Cardiology, 200 First St SW, Rochester, MN 55905-0001; **Phone:** 507-284-3297; **Board Cert:** Pediatrics 1977; Pediatric Cardiology 1983; **Med School:** Creighton Univ 1972; **Resid:** Pediatrics, Univ Colo Hlth Sci Ctr 1975; **Fellow:** Pediatric Cardiology, Baylor Coll Med 1977; Pediatric Cardiology, Baylor Coll Med 1981; **Fac Appt:** Prof Ped, Mayo Med Sch

Rocchini, Albert P MD [PCd] - **Spec Exp:** Congenital Heart Disease; Interventional Cardiology; Hypertension in Obesity; **Hospital:** Univ Michigan Hlth Sys; **Address:** Mott Chldns Hosp, Dept Ped Cardiology, 1500 E Med Ctr Drive, rm L1242, Box 0204, Ann Arbor, MI 48109-0204; **Phone:** 734-936-8993; **Board Cert:** Pediatrics 1989; Pediatric Cardiology 1989; **Med School:** Univ Pittsburgh 1972; **Resid:** Pediatrics, Univ Minn 1974; **Fellow:** Pediatric Cardiology, Chldns Hosp 1977; **Fac Appt:** Prof Ped, Univ Mich Med Sch

Great Plains and Mountains

Minich, Lois LuAnn MD [PCd] - **Spec Exp:** Echocardiography; **Hospital:** Primary Children's Med Ctr; **Address:** Dept Ped Cardiology, 100 N Medical Drive, Ste 1500, Salt Lake City, UT 84113; **Phone:** 801-662-5400; **Board Cert:** Pediatric Cardiology 2007; **Med School:** W VA Univ 1986; **Resid:** Pediatrics, Fletcher Allen Health Care 1989; **Fellow:** Pediatric Cardiology, Univ Michigan Hosps 1992

Southwest

Dreyer, William J MD [PCd] - **Spec Exp:** Congenital Heart Disease; Transplant Medicine-Heart; **Hospital:** Texas Chldns Hosp; **Address:** Texas Chldns Hosp, 6621 Fannin St, MC 19345-C, Houston, TX 77030; **Phone:** 832-826-5659; **Board Cert:** Pediatrics 1987; Pediatric Cardiology 2006; **Med School:** Univ Fla Coll Med 1981; **Resid:** Pediatrics, UCSF Med Ctr 1984; **Fellow:** Pediatric Cardiology, Baylor Coll Med 1988; **Fac Appt:** Assoc Prof Ped, Baylor Coll Med

Friedman, Richard A MD [PCd] - **Spec Exp:** Cardiac Electrophysiology; **Hospital:** Texas Chldns Hosp; **Address:** Texas Children's Hospital, 6621 Fannin St, MC 19345-C, Houston, TX 77030-2303; **Phone:** 832-826-5600; **Board Cert:** Pediatrics 1986; Pediatric Cardiology 2003; **Med School:** Univ Pittsburgh 1980; **Resid:** Pediatrics, Baylor Affil Hosps 1983; **Fellow:** Pediatric Cardiology, Baylor Affil Hosps 1985; **Fac Appt:** Assoc Prof Ped, Baylor Coll Med

Gillette, Paul C MD [PCd] - **Spec Exp:** Arrhythmias; **Hospital:** Cook Chldns Med Ctr, Harris Methodist Hosp - Fort Worth; **Address:** Pediatric Cardiology, 209 Bonnie Brae St, Ste 100, Denton, TX 76201; **Phone:** 940-243-0104; **Board Cert:** Pediatrics 1974; Pediatric Cardiology 1975; **Med School:** Med Univ SC 1969; **Resid:** Pediatrics, Baylor Coll Med 1972; **Fellow:** Pediatric Cardiology, Baylor Coll Med 1974

Mahony, Lynn MD [PCd] - **Spec Exp:** Congenital Heart Disease; Marfan's Syndrome; Congestive Heart Failure; **Hospital:** Chldns Med Ctr of Dallas; **Address:** 1935 Motor District Drive, Dallas, TX 75235; **Phone:** 214-456-2333; **Board Cert:** Pediatrics 1979; Pediatric Cardiology 1997; **Med School:** Stanford Univ 1975; **Resid:** Pediatrics, Stanford Univ 1978; **Fellow:** Pediatric Cardiology, UCSF Med Ctr 1981; **Fac Appt:** Prof Ped, Univ Tex SW, Dallas

Moodie, Douglas S MD [PCd] - **Spec Exp:** Marfan's Syndrome; Congenital Heart Disease-Adult & Child; **Hospital:** Ochsner Fdn Hosp; **Address:** Ochsner Chldns Health Ctr, 1315 Jefferson Hwy, New Orleans, LA 70121; **Phone:** 504-842-4827; **Board Cert:** Pediatrics 1977; Pediatric Cardiology 1977; **Med School:** Med Coll Wisc 1972; **Resid:** Pediatrics, Mayo Clinic 1974; **Fellow:** Pediatric Cardiology, Mayo Clinic 1977

Rogers Jr, James H MD [PCd] - **Spec Exp:** Congenital Heart Disease; **Hospital:** Christus Santa Rosa Children's Hosp, Univ Hlth Syst-San Antonio; **Address:** Chldns Heart Network, 1901 Babcock Rd, Ste 301, San Antonio, TX 78229; **Phone:** 210-341-7722; **Board Cert:** Pediatrics 1976; Pediatric Cardiology 1977; **Med School:** Med Coll GA 1971; **Resid:** Pediatrics, Wilford Hall USAF Med Ctr 1974; **Fellow:** Pediatric Cardiology, Med Coll Georgia 1976; **Fac Appt:** Clin Prof Ped, Univ Tex, San Antonio

Pediatric Cardiology

West Coast and Pacific

Bernstein, Daniel MD [PCd] - **Spec Exp:** Transplant Medicine-Heart; **Hospital:** Lucile Packard Chldn's Hosp, Stanford Univ Med Ctr; **Address:** Lucile Packard Chldns Hosp, Div Ped Card, 750 Welch Rd, Ste 305, Palo Alto, CA 94304-1510; **Phone:** 650-723-7913; **Board Cert:** Pediatrics 1984; Pediatric Cardiology 1985; **Med School:** NYU Sch Med 1978; **Resid:** Pediatrics, Montefiore Hosp-Einstein 1982; **Fellow:** Pediatric Cardiology, UCSF 1986; **Fac Appt:** Prof Ped, Stanford Univ

Boucek Jr, Robert J MD [PCd] - **Spec Exp:** Congenital Heart Disease; Transplant Medicine-Heart; **Hospital:** Chldns Hosp and Regl Med Ctr - Seattle; **Address:** 4800 Sand Point Way NE, MS G0035, Seattle, WA 98105; **Phone:** 206-987-2015; **Board Cert:** Pediatrics 1974; Pediatric Cardiology 1977; **Med School:** Tulane Univ 1969; **Resid:** Pediatrics, Duke Univ Med Ctr 1971; **Fellow:** Ambulatory Pediatrics, US Naval Hosp 1973; Pediatric Cardiology, Vanderbilt Med Ctr 1976; **Fac Appt:** Prof Ped, Univ Wash

Perry, Stanton Bruce MD [PCd] - **Spec Exp:** Interventional Cardiology; **Hospital:** Lucile Packard Chldn's Hosp; **Address:** L Packard Chldn's Hosp, Ped Cardiology, 750 Welch Rd, Ste 305, Palo Alto, CA 94304; **Phone:** 650-723-7913; **Board Cert:** Pediatrics 1986; **Med School:** Iceland 1978; **Resid:** Pediatrics, St Louis Chldn's Hosp 1983; **Fellow:** Pediatric Cardiology, Chldn's Hosp 1984; **Fac Appt:** Assoc Prof Ped, Stanford Univ

Teitel, David F MD [PCd] - **Hospital:** UCSF Med Ctr; **Address:** UCSF, Dept Ped Cardiology, 400 Parnassus Ave Fl 2nd, San Francisco, CA 94143-0544; **Phone:** 415-353-2008; **Board Cert:** Pediatrics 1980; Pediatric Cardiology 2004; **Med School:** Univ Toronto 1975; **Resid:** Pediatrics, Chldns Hosp 1980; **Fellow:** Pediatric Cardiology, UCSF Med Ctr 1982; **Fac Appt:** Prof Ped, UCSF

PEDIATRIC CRITICAL CARE MEDICINE

New England

Fleisher, Gary R MD [PCCM] - **Spec Exp:** Infectious Disease; Trauma; **Hospital:** Children's Hospital - Boston; **Address:** Chldns Hosp, Dept Med, 300 Longwood Ave Hunnewell Bldg - rm 258, Boston, MA 02115-5724; **Phone:** 617-355-5022; **Board Cert:** Emergency Medicine 2001; Pediatrics 1992; Pediatric Emergency Medicine 2007; **Med School:** Jefferson Med Coll 1973; **Resid:** Pediatrics, Chldns Hosp 1976; Pediatrics, Chldns Hosp 1977; **Fellow:** Infectious Disease, Chldns Hosp 1979; **Fac Appt:** Prof Ped, Harvard Med Sch

Mid Atlantic

Fuhrman, Bradley P MD [PCCM] - **Hospital:** Women's & Chldn's Hosp of Buffalo, The; **Address:** Chldns Hosp Buffalo, Dept Ped Critical Care, 219 Bryant St, Buffalo, NY 14222-2006; **Phone:** 716-878-7442; **Board Cert:** Pediatrics 1992; Pediatric Critical Care Medicine 2003; Neonatal-Perinatal Medicine 1979; Pediatric Cardiology 1979; **Med School:** NYU Sch Med 1971; **Resid:** Pediatrics, Univ Minnesota Med Ctr 1973; **Fellow:** Pediatric Cardiology, Univ Minnesota 1974; Neonatal-Perinatal Medicine, Univ Minnesota 1979; **Fac Appt:** Prof Ped, SUNY Buffalo

Thompson, Ann Ellen MD [PCCM] - **Spec Exp:** Mechanical Ventilation; Critical Care; Respiratory Failure; **Hospital:** Chldns Hosp of Pittsburgh - UPMC; **Address:** Chldns Hosp, Dept Ped Crit Care, Childrens Drive, 45th & Penn, Pittsburgh, PA 15201; **Phone:** 412-692-5164; **Board Cert:** Anesthesiology 1980; Pediatrics 1992; Pediatric Critical Care Medicine 2003; **Med School:** Tufts Univ 1974; **Resid:** Pediatrics, Chldns Hosp 1977; Anesthesiology, Hosp Univ Penn 1980; **Fellow:** Pediatric Critical Care Medicine, Chldns Hosp 1979; **Fac Appt:** Prof Ped, Univ Pittsburgh

Southeast

Anand, Kanwaljeet Singh MD/PhD [PCCM] - **Spec Exp:** Pain Management; Critical Care; **Hospital:** Le Bonheur Chldns Med Ctr, St Jude Children's Research Hosp; **Address:** 50 N Dunlap St, Memphis, TN 38103-2893; **Phone:** 901-287-5925; **Board Cert:** Pediatric Critical Care Medicine 2004; **Med School:** India 1981; **Resid:** Pediatrics, Chldns Hosp 1991; Neonatal-Perinatal Medicine, John Radcliffe Hosp 1985; **Fellow:** Pediatric Critical Care Medicine, Mass Genl Hosp 1993; **Fac Appt:** Prof Ped, Univ Tenn Coll Med, Memphis

Midwest

Sarnaik, Ashok P MD [PCCM] - **Spec Exp:** Critical Care; Perinatal Medicine; **Hospital:** Chldns Hosp of Michigan; **Address:** Chldns Hosp, Div Crit Care Med, 3901 Beaubien St, Carl's Bldg - Ste 4134, Detroit, MI 48201-2119; **Phone:** 313-745-5629; **Board Cert:** Pediatrics 1975; Neonatal-Perinatal Medicine 1979; Pediatric Critical Care Medicine 2003; **Med School:** India 1969; **Resid:** Pediatrics, JJ Hosp-Bombay Univ 1971; Pediatrics, Chldns Hosp Mich 1974; **Fellow:** Neonatal-Perinatal Medicine, Chldns Hosp Mich 1975; **Fac Appt:** Prof Ped, Wayne State Univ

Great Plains and Mountains

Dean, Jonathan M MD [PCCM] - **Hospital:** Primary Children's Med Ctr; **Address:** Pediatric ICU, 100 N Medical Drive, Salt Lake City, UT 84113; **Phone:** 801-587-7572; **Board Cert:** Pediatrics 1981; Pediatric Critical Care Medicine 2003; **Med School:** Northwestern Univ 1977; **Resid:** Pediatrics, Children's Hosp 1981; **Fellow:** Pediatric Critical Care Medicine, Johns Hopkins Hosp 1983; **Fac Appt:** Prof Ped, Univ Utah

Southwest

Perez Fontan, J Julio MD [PCCM] - **Spec Exp:** Respiratory Failure; **Hospital:** UT Southwestern Med Ctr at Dallas, Chldns Med Ctr of Dallas; **Address:** UT SW Med Ctr, Dept Peds, 5323 Harry Hines Blvd, Dallas, TX 75390-9063; **Phone:** 214-648-9618; **Board Cert:** Pediatrics 1987; Pediatric Critical Care Medicine 2003; **Med School:** Spain 1977; **Resid:** Pediatrics, Chldns Hosp/Univ Barcelona 1981; **Fellow:** Critical Care Medicine, UCSF Med Ctr 1984; **Fac Appt:** Prof Ped, Univ Tex SW, Dallas

Taylor, Richard P MD [PCCM] - **Hospital:** Univ Hlth Syst-San Antonio; **Address:** Dept Ped Critical Care, 7703 Floyd Curl Drive, MC 7829, San Antonio, TX 78229; **Phone:** 210-562-5816; **Board Cert:** Internal Medicine 1988; Pediatric Critical Care Medicine 2004; **Med School:** Univ Tex Med Br, Galveston 1984; **Resid:** Internal Medicine, St Joseph Mercy Hosp 1988; Pediatrics, UNiv Michigan Med Ctr 1988; **Fellow:** Pediatric Critical Care Medicine, Univ Michigan Med Ctr 1995; **Fac Appt:** Assoc Prof Ped

Thomas, James A MD [PCCM] - **Hospital:** Chldns Med Ctr of Dallas; **Address:** Children's Medical Ctr of Dallas, PICU, 1935 Medical District Drive, Dallas, TX 75235; **Phone:** 214-456-5095; **Board Cert:** Pediatric Critical Care Medicine 2004; Pediatrics 2007; **Med School:** Stanford Univ 1989; **Resid:** Pediatrics, Children's Hosp 1992; **Fellow:** Pediatric Critical Care Medicine, U Texas SW Med Ctr 1996

Pediatric Critical Care Medicine

West Coast and Pacific

Schwarz, Adam J MD [PCCM] - **Hospital:** Chldns Hosp Orange Co; **Address:** Chldns Hosp of Orange, 455 S Main St, Orange, CA 92868; **Phone:** 714-532-8620; **Board Cert:** Pediatric Critical Care Medicine 2004; **Med School:** Stanford Univ 1990; **Resid:** Pediatrics, Stanford Med Ctr 1993; **Fellow:** Pediatric Critical Care Medicine, Harbor-UCLA Med Ctr 1996; **Fac Appt:** Assoc Clin Prof Ped

Zimmerman, Jerry John MD [PCCM] - **Spec Exp:** Inflammation in Critical Illness; Sepsis; Septic Shock; **Hospital:** Chldns Hosp and Regl Med Ctr - Seattle, Harborview Med Ctr; **Address:** Seattle Chldn's Hosp, 4800 Sand Point Way NE, MS W8866, Seattle, WA 98105-0371; **Phone:** 206-987-3862; **Board Cert:** Pediatrics 1992; Pediatric Critical Care Medicine 2003; **Med School:** Univ Wisc 1979; **Resid:** Pediatrics, Univ Wisconsin Hosp 1982; **Fellow:** Pediatric Critical Care Medicine, Childrens Natl Med Ctr 1984; **Fac Appt:** Prof Ped, Univ Wash

PEDIATRIC ENDOCRINOLOGY

New England

Casella, Samuel Joseph MD [PEn] - **Spec Exp:** Thyroid Disorders; Growth/Development Disorders; **Hospital:** Dartmouth - Hitchcock Med Ctr; **Address:** Dartmouth-Hitchcock Med Ctr, Dept Ped Endo, One Medical Center Drive, Lebanon, NH 03756; **Phone:** 603-653-9877; **Board Cert:** Pediatrics 1985; Pediatric Endocrinology 1986; **Med School:** SUNY Upstate Med Univ 1981; **Resid:** Pediatrics, Upstate Med Ctr 1984; **Fellow:** Pediatric Endocrinology, NC Meml Hosp-Univ NC 1986; **Fac Appt:** Assoc Prof Ped, Johns Hopkins Univ

Gordon, Catherine M MD [PEn] - **Spec Exp:** Bone Disorders-Metabolic; **Hospital:** Children's Hospital - Boston; **Address:** Children's Hospital, Ped Endocrinology, 300 Longwood Ave, Boston, MA 02115; **Phone:** 617-355-7476; **Board Cert:** Pediatric Endocrinology 2007; Adolescent Medicine 2001; **Med School:** Univ NC Sch Med 1991; **Resid:** Pediatrics, Children's Hosp 1994; **Fellow:** Pediatric Endocrinology, Children's Hosp 1996; **Fac Appt:** Assoc Prof Ped, Harvard Med Sch

Levitsky, Lynne Lipton MD [PEn] - **Spec Exp:** Diabetes; Growth/Development Disorders; Cushing's Syndrome; **Hospital:** Mass Genl Hosp; **Address:** Mass Genl Hosp, Ped Endo, 32 Fruit St, YAW-6800, Boston, MA 02114-2696; **Phone:** 617-726-2909; **Board Cert:** Pediatrics 1971; Pediatric Endocrinology 1978; **Med School:** Yale Univ 1966; **Resid:** Pediatrics, Chldns Hosp 1968; **Fellow:** Pediatric Endocrinology, Univ Maryland Hosp 1970; **Fac Appt:** Assoc Prof Ped, Harvard Med Sch

Ludwig, David S MD/PhD [PEn] - **Spec Exp:** Obesity; Nutrition; **Hospital:** Children's Hospital - Boston; **Address:** Chldns Hosp, Div Endocrinology, 333 Longwood Ave Fl 6 - rm 624, Boston, MA 02115; **Phone:** 617-355-7476; **Board Cert:** Pediatric Endocrinology 2003; **Med School:** Stanford Univ 1990; **Resid:** Pediatrics, Chldns Hosp 1993; **Fellow:** Pediatric Endocrinology, Chldns Hosp 1995; **Fac Appt:** Asst Prof Ped, Harvard Med Sch

Rivkees, Scott A MD [PEn] - **Spec Exp:** Thyroid Disorders; Adrenal Disorders; **Hospital:** Yale-New Haven Hosp; **Address:** Yale Dept Pediatrics, 464 Congress Ave, PO Box 208081, New Haven, CT 06520-8081; **Phone:** 203-764-9199; **Board Cert:** Pediatrics 1987; Pediatric Endocrinology 2005; **Med School:** UMDNJ-NJ Med Sch, Newark 1982; **Resid:** Pediatrics, Mass Genl Hosp 1985; **Fellow:** Pediatric Endocrinology, Mass Genl Hosp 1986; **Fac Appt:** Prof Ped, Yale Univ

Spack, Norman P MD [PEn] - **Spec Exp:** Diabetes; Growth Disorders; Transgender Issues; **Hospital:** Children's Hospital - Boston; **Address:** Childrens Hosp, Div Endocrinology, 300 Longwood Ave, Boston, MA 02115; **Phone:** 617-355-7476; **Board Cert:** Pediatrics 1975; Pediatric Endocrinology 2003; **Med School:** Univ Rochester 1969; **Resid:** Pediatrics, Boston City Hosp/Chldns Hosp 1972; **Fellow:** Adolescent Medicine, Chldns Hosp 1975; Pediatric Endocrinology, Chldns Hosp 1978; **Fac Appt:** Assoc Prof Ped, Harvard Med Sch

Tamborlane, William V MD [PEn] - **Spec Exp:** Diabetes; **Hospital:** Yale-New Haven Hosp; **Address:** Yale Pediatric Endocrinology, 333 Cedar St, rm 3091-LMP, New Haven, CT 06510-3289; **Phone:** 203-764-6747; **Board Cert:** Pediatrics 1978; Pediatric Endocrinology 1986; **Med School:** Georgetown Univ 1972; **Resid:** Pediatrics, Georgetown Univ Hosp 1975; **Fellow:** Pediatric Endocrinology, Yale-New Haven Hosp 1977; **Fac Appt:** Prof Ped, Yale Univ

Mid Atlantic

Alter, Craig A MD [PEn] - **Spec Exp:** Diabetes; Growth Disorders; Thyroid Disorders; Pubertal Disorders; **Hospital:** Chldns Hosp of Philadelphia, The; **Address:** Children's Hosp of Philadelphia, Dept Pediatric Endocrinology, 34th & Civic Ctr Blvd, Philadelphia, PA 19104; **Phone:** 215-590-3174; **Board Cert:** Pediatrics 2005; Pediatric Endocrinology 2003; **Med School:** Harvard Med Sch 1987; **Resid:** Pediatrics, Boston Children's Hosp 1990; **Fellow:** Pediatric Endocrinology, Children's Hosp 1993; **Fac Appt:** Assoc Prof Ped, Univ Pennsylvania

Arslanian, Silva MD [PEn] - **Spec Exp:** Diabetes; Obesity; **Hospital:** Chldns Hosp of Pittsburgh - UPMC; **Address:** Dept Weight Management, 45th St & Penn Ave, Pittsburgh, PA 15201; **Phone:** 412-692-6935; **Board Cert:** Pediatrics 1983; Pediatric Endocrinology 1983; **Med School:** Lebanon 1978; **Resid:** Pediatrics, American Univ Hosp 1980; **Fellow:** Pediatric Endocrinology, Chldns Hosp 1983; **Fac Appt:** Prof Ped, Univ Pittsburgh

Becker, Dorothy J MD [PEn] - **Spec Exp:** Diabetes; **Hospital:** Chldns Hosp of Pittsburgh - UPMC; **Address:** Children's Hospital Drive, Div Endocrinology, 45th St & Penn, Pittsburgh, PA 15201; **Phone:** 412-692-5172; **Board Cert:** Pediatrics 1978; Pediatric Endocrinology 1978; **Med School:** South Africa 1964; **Resid:** Pediatrics, Univ Capetown 1972; Endocrinology, Diabetes & Metabolism, Univ Capetown 1974; **Fellow:** Pediatric Endocrinology, Univ Pittsburgh 1976; **Fac Appt:** Prof Ped, Univ Pittsburgh

De Luca, Francesco MD [PEn] - **Spec Exp:** Growth Disorders; Metabolic Syndrome; Osteoporosis; Diabetes; **Hospital:** St Christopher's Hosp for Chldn; **Address:** St Christophers Hosp for Children, Endocrinology Section, Ste 3303, Erie Ave & Front St, Philadelphia, PA 19134; **Phone:** 215-427-8100; **Board Cert:** Pediatrics 2002; Pediatric Endocrinology 2003; **Med School:** Italy 1983; **Resid:** Pediatrics, Cath Univ Sacred Heart Affil Hosp; Pediatrics, Albert Einstein Med Ctr; **Fellow:** Pediatric Endocrinology, St Christophers Hosp; Pediatric Endocrinology, Natl Inst Hlth; **Fac Appt:** Assoc Prof Ped, Drexel Univ Coll Med

Levine, Michael A MD [PEn] - **Spec Exp:** Bone Disorders-Metabolic; Osteoporosis; **Hospital:** Chldns Hosp of Philadelphia, The; **Address:** Childrens Hosp Philadelphia, Div Endocrinology, 34th St & Civic Center Blvd, Philadelphia, PA 19104; **Phone:** 215-590-3174; **Board Cert:** Internal Medicine 1979; Endocrinology, Diabetes & Metabolism 1981; **Med School:** Hahnemann Univ 1976; **Resid:** Internal Medicine, Johns Hopkins Hosp 1979; **Fellow:** Endocrinology, Natl Inst Hlth 1981; Genetics, Natl Inst Hlth 1981; **Fac Appt:** Prof Med, Univ Pennsylvania

Pediatric Endocrinology

New, Maria I MD [PEn] - **Spec Exp:** Adrenal Disorders; Growth/Development Disorders; **Hospital:** Mount Sinai Med Ctr (page 64); **Address:** Mount Sinai Medical Ctr, 1 Gustave L Levy Pl, Box 1198, New York, NY 10029; **Phone:** 212-241-8210; **Board Cert:** Pediatrics 1960; **Med School:** Univ Pennsylvania 1954; **Resid:** Pediatrics, New York Hosp 1957; **Fellow:** Pediatric Endocrinology, New York Hosp 1958; Endocrinology, Diabetes & Metabolism, New York Hosp 1964; **Fac Appt:** Prof Ped, Cornell Univ-Weill Med Coll

Oberfield, Sharon E MD [PEn] - **Spec Exp:** Adrenal Disorders; Neuroendocrine Growth Disorders; Growth Disorders; **Hospital:** NYPresby-Morgan Stanley Children's Hosp (page 66); **Address:** 630 W 168th St PH East Bldg - Ste 522, New York, NY 10032; **Phone:** 212-305-6559; **Board Cert:** Pediatrics 1979; Pediatric Endocrinology 2000; **Med School:** Cornell Univ-Weill Med Coll 1974; **Resid:** Pediatrics, NY Hosp-Cornell 1976; **Fellow:** Pediatric Endocrinology, NY Hosp-Cornell 1979; **Fac Appt:** Prof Ped, Columbia P&S

Plotnick, Leslie Parker MD [PEn] - **Spec Exp:** Diabetes; Growth Disorders; Thyroid Disorders; Pubertal Disorders; **Hospital:** Johns Hopkins Hosp (page 61); **Address:** Johns Hopkins Hospital, Dept Pediatric Endocrinology, Baltimore, MD 21287; **Phone:** 410-955-6463; **Board Cert:** Pediatrics 1975; Pediatric Endocrinology 1978; **Med School:** Univ MD Sch Med 1970; **Resid:** Pediatrics, Johns Hopkins Hosp 1972; **Fellow:** Pediatric Endocrinology, Johns Hopkins Hosp 1974; **Fac Appt:** Prof Ped, Johns Hopkins Univ

Sklar, Charles A MD [PEn] - **Spec Exp:** Cancer Survivors-Late Effects of Therapy; Growth Disorders in Childhood Cancer; Pituitary Disorders; **Hospital:** Meml Sloan-Kettering Cancer Ctr; **Address:** 1275 York Avenue, New York, NY 10065; **Phone:** 800-525-2225; **Board Cert:** Pediatrics 1979; Pediatric Endocrinology 1980; **Med School:** USC Sch Med 1974; **Resid:** Pediatrics, Childrens Hosp 1976; **Fellow:** Pediatric Endocrinology, UCSF Med Ctr 1979; **Fac Appt:** Assoc Prof Ped, Cornell Univ-Weill Med Coll

Sperling, Mark A MD [PEn] - **Spec Exp:** Diabetes; Growth/Development Disorders; Hypoglycemia; Thyroid Disorders; **Hospital:** Chldns Hosp of Pittsburgh - UPMC, UPMC Presby, Pittsburgh; **Address:** Chldns Hosp Pittsburgh, Endocrinology, 3705 5th Ave DeSoto Bldg Fl 4A - Ste 400, Pittsburgh, PA 15213-2524; **Phone:** 412-692-5172; **Board Cert:** Pediatrics 1986; Pediatric Endocrinology 1986; **Med School:** Australia 1962; **Resid:** Internal Medicine, Prince Henry Hosp 1964; Pediatrics, Royal Chldns Hosp 1968; **Fellow:** Pediatric Endocrinology, Chldns Hosp 1970; **Fac Appt:** Prof Ped, Univ Pittsburgh

Stanley, Charles MD [PEn] - **Spec Exp:** Hyperinsulinism-Congenital; Hypoglycemia; **Hospital:** Chldns Hosp of Philadelphia, The; **Address:** Chldns Hosp, Div Endocrinology, 34th St & Civic Ctr Blvd, Philadelphia, PA 19104; **Phone:** 215-590-3174; **Board Cert:** Pediatrics 1976; Pediatric Endocrinology 1978; **Med School:** Univ VA Sch Med 1970; **Resid:** Pediatrics, Children's Hosp 1972; **Fellow:** Pediatric Endocrinology, Children's Hosp 1976; **Fac Appt:** Prof Ped, Univ Pennsylvania

Southeast

Diamond, Frank B MD [PEn] - **Spec Exp:** Growth Disorders; Obesity; Calcium Disorders in Newborn; **Hospital:** All Children's Hosp, Tampa Genl Hosp; **Address:** All Children's Hosp, 801 6th St S, ACH Box 6900, St Petersburg, FL 33701; **Phone:** 727-767-4237; **Board Cert:** Pediatrics 1979; Pediatric Endocrinology 1980; **Med School:** Penn State Univ-Hershey Med Ctr 1974; **Resid:** Pediatrics, Chldns Hosp-Univ Alabama 1976; **Fellow:** Pediatric Endocrinology, Chldns Hosp-Univ Penn 1978; **Fac Appt:** Prof Ped, Univ S Fla Coll Med

Freemark, Michael S MD [PEn] - **Spec Exp:** Thyroid Disorders; Growth Disorders; Pubertal Disorders; Diabetes; **Hospital:** Duke Univ Med Ctr, Durham Regional Hosp; **Address:** DUMC, Box 3080, 3000 Erwin Rd, Lenox Baker Bldg, Ste 200, Durham, NC 27705; **Phone:** 919-684-8350; **Board Cert:** Pediatrics 1980; Pediatric Endocrinology 1983; **Med School:** Duke Univ 1976; **Resid:** Pediatrics, Duke Univ Med Ctr 1979; **Fellow:** Pediatric Endocrinology, Duke Univ Med Ctr 1983; Pediatric Endocrinology, Hospital Necker Enfants Malades 1993; **Fac Appt:** Prof Ped, Duke Univ

Friedman, Nancy E MD [PEn] - **Spec Exp:** Calcium Disorders; Bone Disorders-Metabolic; Growth/Development Disorders; Cancer Survivors-Late Effects of Therapy; **Hospital:** Duke Univ Med Ctr; **Address:** Duke Consultative Services, 3480 Wake Forest Rd, Ste 310, Raleigh, NC 27609; **Phone:** 919-684-4000; **Board Cert:** Pediatrics 1979; Pediatric Endocrinology 2003; **Med School:** Med Coll VA 1975; **Resid:** Pediatrics, Childrens Hosp Med Ctr 1977; Pediatrics, Childrens Meml Hosp 1978; **Fellow:** Endocrinology, Diabetes & Metabolism, Michael Reese Hosp 1980; **Fac Appt:** Asst Clin Prof Ped, Duke Univ

Key Jr, L Lyndon MD [PEn] - **Spec Exp:** Osteopetrosis; Osteoporosis-Juvenile; **Hospital:** MUSC Med Ctr; **Address:** MUSC Med Ctr, Dept Pediatrics, 135 Rutledge Ave, MSC 561, Charleston, SC 29425; **Phone:** 843-876-1417; **Board Cert:** Pediatrics 1983; Pediatric Endocrinology 1983; **Med School:** Univ NC Sch Med 1977; **Resid:** Pediatrics, Duke Univ Med Ctr 1980; **Fellow:** Endocrinology, Chldns Hosp 1983; **Fac Appt:** Prof Ped, Med Univ SC

Meacham, Lillian R MD [PEn] - **Spec Exp:** Growth Disorders in Childhood Cancer; Cancer Survivors-Late Effects of Therapy; **Hospital:** Chldns Hlthcare Atlanta @ Egleston, Emory Univ Hosp; **Address:** Emory Childrens Ctr, 2015 Uppergate Drive, Atlanta, GA 30322; **Phone:** 404-778-2400; **Board Cert:** Pediatrics 2006; Pediatric Endocrinology 2006; **Med School:** Emory Univ 1984; **Resid:** Pediatrics, Emory Univ Hosp 1987; **Fellow:** Pediatric Endocrinology, Emory Univ Hosp 1990; **Fac Appt:** Assoc Prof Ped, Emory Univ

Schwartz, Robert P MD [PEn] - **Hospital:** Wake Forest Univ Baptist Med Ctr (page 72); **Address:** Wake Forest Univ Sch Med-Dept Pediatrics, Med Ctr Blvd, Winston-Salem, NC 27157-0001; **Phone:** 336-716-3199; **Board Cert:** Pediatrics 1994; Pediatric Endocrinology 2002; **Med School:** Univ Fla Coll Med 1968; **Resid:** Pediatrics, Charlotte Meml Hosp 1970; Pediatrics, Duke Univ Med Ctr 1971; **Fellow:** Pediatric Endocrinology, Duke Univ Med Ctr 1971; Pediatric Endocrinology, Duke Univ Med Ctr 1974; **Fac Appt:** Prof Ped, Wake Forest Univ

Silverstein, Janet H MD [PEn] - **Spec Exp:** Diabetes; Growth/Development Disorders; Obesity; **Hospital:** Shands at Univ of FL; **Address:** Univ Florida - Shands Hlthcare, 1600 SW Archer Rd, Box 100296, Gainesville, FL 32610-3003; **Phone:** 352-334-1390; **Board Cert:** Pediatrics 1975; Pediatric Endocrinology 2004; **Med School:** Univ Pennsylvania 1970; **Resid:** Pediatrics, Chldns Hosp 1972; Pediatrics, Chldns Hosp 1975; **Fellow:** Pediatric Endocrinology, Duke Univ Med Ctr 1977; **Fac Appt:** Prof Ped, Univ Fla Coll Med

Midwest

Allen, David Bruce MD [PEn] - **Spec Exp:** Growth Disorders; Pubertal Disorders; Diabetes; **Hospital:** Univ WI Hosp & Clins; **Address:** Univ Wisc American Fam Chldn's Hosp, H4/448 CSC-Pediatrics, 600 Highland Ave, Madison, WI 53792-4108; **Phone:** 608-263-5835; **Board Cert:** Pediatrics 1986; Pediatric Endocrinology 2004; **Med School:** Duke Univ 1980; **Resid:** Pediatrics, Univ Wisc Hosp 1985; **Fellow:** Pediatric Endocrinology, Univ Wisc Hosp 1988; **Fac Appt:** Prof Ped, Univ Wisc

Pediatric Endocrinology

Eugster, Erica A MD [PEn] - **Spec Exp:** Pubertal Disorders; Turner Syndrome; Growth/Development Disorders; Sex Development Disorders; **Hospital:** Riley Hosp for Children; **Address:** Riley Chldns Hosp, 702 Barnhill Drive, Pediatric Endocrinology, rm 5960, Indianapolis, IN 46202; **Phone:** 317-274-3889; **Board Cert:** Pediatrics 2002; Pediatric Endocrinology 2005; **Med School:** Med Coll PA 1990; **Resid:** Pediatrics, Marshfield Clin-St Josephs Hosp 1994; **Fellow:** Pediatric Endocrinology, Univ Minn Hosp 1997; **Fac Appt:** Prof Ped, Indiana Univ

Gutai, James MD [PEn] - **Hospital:** Chldns Hosp of Michigan, Marquette Genl Hosp; **Address:** Morris J Hood Comp Diabetes Ctr, 4201 St Antoine St, Univ Hlth Ctr, Box 247, Detroit, MI 48201; **Phone:** 313-577-0133; **Board Cert:** Pediatrics 1977; Pediatric Endocrinology 1980; **Med School:** Temple Univ 1970; **Resid:** Pediatrics, Johns Hopkins Hosp 1976; **Fellow:** Pediatric Endocrinology, Johns Hopkins Hosp 1976; **Fac Appt:** Prof Ped, Wayne State Univ

Levy, Richard Alshuler MD [PEn] - **Spec Exp:** Growth Disorders; Pituitary Disorders; Thyroid Disorders; **Hospital:** Rush Copley Med Ctr, Ingalls Meml Hosp; **Address:** 1725 W Harrison St, Ste 328, Chicago, IL 60612-3863; **Phone:** 312-942-8989; **Board Cert:** Internal Medicine 1976; Pediatrics 1983; Endocrinology 1985; Pediatric Endocrinology 1986; **Med School:** Louisiana State U, New Orleans 1971; **Resid:** Internal Medicine, Univ Mass Med Ctr 1977; Pediatrics, Beth Israel Hosp 1978; **Fellow:** Endocrinology, Diabetes & Metabolism, Barnes Jewish Hosp 1982; **Fac Appt:** Asst Prof Ped, Rush Med Coll

Menon, Ram K MD [PEn] - **Spec Exp:** Growth/Development Disorders; Diabetes; **Hospital:** Univ Michigan Hlth Sys; **Address:** Univ Mich Med Ctr, 1500 E Med Ctr Drive, MPB Bldg-SPC5178, Ann Arbor, MI 48109; **Phone:** 734-764-5175; **Board Cert:** Pediatrics 2002; Pediatric Endocrinology 2003; **Med School:** India 1979; **Resid:** Pediatrics, All India Inst of Med Sci 1984; **Fellow:** Pediatric Endocrinology, Chldn's Hosp 1989; **Fac Appt:** Assoc Prof Ped, Univ Mich Med Sch

Mirmira, Raghu G MD [PEn] - **Spec Exp:** Diabetes; **Hospital:** Riley Hosp for Children; **Address:** Riley Hosp Chldn-Endocrinology, 702 Barnhill Drive, rm 5900, Indianapolis, IN 46202; **Phone:** 317-274-3889; **Board Cert:** Endocrinology, Diabetes & Metabolism 2008; **Med School:** Univ Chicago-Pritzker Sch Med 1993; **Resid:** Internal Medicine, UCSF Med Ctr 1995; **Fellow:** Endocrinology, Diabetes & Metabolism, UCSF 1998; **Fac Appt:** Assoc Prof Ped, Indiana Univ

Rogers, Douglas G MD [PEn] - **Spec Exp:** Diabetes; Growth/Development Disorders; Thyroid Disorders; **Hospital:** Cleveland Clin Fdn (page 56); **Address:** Div Pediatric Endocrinology, 9500 Euclid Ave, Box A120, Cleveland, OH 44195-0001; **Phone:** 216-445-8048; **Board Cert:** Pediatrics 1984; Pediatric Endocrinology 1986; **Med School:** Ros Franklin Univ/Chicago Med Sch 1978; **Resid:** Pediatrics, Cardinal Glennon Chldns Hosp 1981; **Fellow:** Endocrinology, Diabetes & Metabolism, St Louis Chldns Hosp 1985

Rosenfield, Robert L MD [PEn] - **Spec Exp:** Polycystic Ovarian Syndrome; Pubertal Disorders; Menstrual Disorders; **Hospital:** Univ of Chicago Med Ctr; **Address:** 5758 S Maryland Ave, MC 505, Chicago, IL 60637-1463; **Phone:** 773-702-6169; **Board Cert:** Pediatrics 1986; Pediatric Endocrinology 1986; **Med School:** Northwestern Univ 1960; **Resid:** Pediatrics, Chldns Hosp 1963; **Fellow:** Pediatric Endocrinology, Chldns Hosp 1968; **Fac Appt:** Prof Ped, Univ Chicago-Pritzker Sch Med

White, Neil H MD [PEn] - **Spec Exp:** Diabetes; Hypoglycemia; **Hospital:** St Louis Chldns Hosp; **Address:** St Louis Chldn's Hosp, One Children's Pl, CB 8116, St Louis, MO 63110-1010; **Phone:** 314-454-6051; **Board Cert:** Pediatrics 1981; Pediatric Endocrinology 1983; **Med School:** Albert Einstein Coll Med 1975; **Resid:** Pediatrics, St Louis Chldns Hosp 1977; **Fellow:** Endocrinology, Diabetes & Metabolism, Washington Univ 1979; **Fac Appt:** Prof Ped, Washington Univ, St Louis

Zimmerman, Donald MD [PEn] - **Spec Exp:** Growth Disorders in Childhood Cancer; Thyroid Cancer; Thyroid Disorders; Growth/Development Disorders; **Hospital:** Children's Mem Hosp; **Address:** Children's Memorial Hosp, 2300 Children's Plaza, Div Endocrinology, Box 54, Chicago, IL 60614; **Phone:** 773-327-7740; **Board Cert:** Internal Medicine 1977; Endocrinology 1979; Pediatrics 1983; Pediatric Endocrinology 2001; **Med School:** Univ IL Coll Med 1974; **Resid:** Internal Medicine, Johns Hopkins Hosp 1977; Pediatrics, Mayo Clinic 1981; **Fellow:** Endocrinology, Diabetes & Metabolism, Mayo Clinic 1980; **Fac Appt:** Prof Ped, Northwestern Univ

Great Plains and Mountains

Foster, Carol M MD [PEn] - **Spec Exp:** Diabetes; Growth/Development Disorders; Pubertal Disorders; **Hospital:** Primary Children's Med Ctr, Univ Utah Hosps and Clins; **Address:** Utah Diabetes Ctr, 615 Arapeen Drive, Ste 100, Salt Lake City, UT 84108; **Phone:** 801-581-7761; **Board Cert:** Pediatrics 1983; Pediatric Endocrinology 1983; **Med School:** Washington Univ, St Louis 1978; **Resid:** Pediatrics, Univ Utah Hlth Scis Ctr 1981; **Fellow:** Pediatric Endocrinology, Natl Inst Hlth 1984; **Fac Appt:** Prof Med, Univ Utah

Kappy, Michael S MD/PhD [PEn] - **Spec Exp:** Growth/Development Disorders; Thyroid Disorders; Pubertal Disorders; **Hospital:** Chldn's Hosp - Aurora, The; **Address:** Chldns Hosp-Dept Ped Endocrinology, 13123 E 16th Ave, Box B265, Aurora, CO 80045; **Phone:** 720-777-6128; **Board Cert:** Pediatrics 1972; Pediatric Endocrinology 1980; **Med School:** Univ Wisc 1967; **Resid:** Pediatrics, Univ Colorado Med Ctr 1972; **Fellow:** Pediatric Endocrinology, Johns Hopkins Hosp 1980; **Fac Appt:** Prof Ped, Univ Colorado

Klingensmith, Georgeanna MD [PEn] - **Spec Exp:** Diabetes; **Hospital:** Chldn's Hosp - Aurora, The; **Address:** Barbara Davis Ctr for Childhood Diabetes, MS B140, PO Box 6511, Aurora, CO 80045-0511; **Phone:** 303-724-2323; **Board Cert:** Pediatrics 1976; Pediatric Endocrinology 2000; **Med School:** Duke Univ 1971; **Resid:** Pediatrics, Childrens Hosp 1973; **Fellow:** Pediatric Endocrinology, Johns Hopkins Hosp 1976; Pediatric Endocrinology, Childrens Hosp 1974; **Fac Appt:** Prof Ped, Univ Colorado

West Coast and Pacific

Geffner, Mitchell E MD [PEn] - **Spec Exp:** Growth Disorders; Pubertal Disorders; Thyroid Disorders; Pituitary Disorders; **Hospital:** Chldns Hosp - Los Angeles; **Address:** Chlds Hosp LA, Div Endocrinology, 4650 Sunset Blvd, MS 61, Los Angeles, CA 90027; **Phone:** 323-361-2185; **Board Cert:** Pediatrics 1980; Pediatric Endocrinology 2006; **Med School:** Albert Einstein Coll Med 1975; **Resid:** Pediatrics, LAC-USC Med Ctr 1979; **Fellow:** Pediatric Endocrinology, UCLA Med Ctr 1982; **Fac Appt:** Prof Ped, USC Sch Med

Wilson, Darrell M MD [PEn] - **Spec Exp:** Diabetes; Growth Disorders; **Hospital:** Stanford Univ Med Ctr, Lucile Packard Chldn's Hosp; **Address:** Stanford Univ Med Ctr - Pediatrics, 300 Pasteur Rd, Ste G-313, MC 5208, Stanford, CA 94305-5208; **Phone:** 650-723-5791; **Board Cert:** Pediatrics 1982; Pediatric Endocrinology 2003; **Med School:** UCSD 1977; **Resid:** Pediatrics, Stanford Univ Med Ctr 1980; **Fellow:** Endocrinology, Diabetes & Metabolism, Stanford Univ Med Ctr 1984; **Fac Appt:** Prof Ped, Stanford Univ

Pediatric Gastroenterology

New England

Jonas, Maureen M MD [PGe] - **Spec Exp:** Liver Disease; Transplant Medicine-Liver; Hepatitis; **Hospital:** Children's Hospital - Boston, Brigham & Women's Hosp; **Address:** Children's Hospital, Dept Ped Gastroenterology, 300 Longwood Ave, Boston, MA 02115; **Phone:** 617-355-5837; **Board Cert:** Pediatrics 1982; Pediatric Gastroenterology 2005; Pediatric Transplant Hepatology 2006; **Med School:** Univ Miami Sch Med 1977; **Resid:** Pediatrics, Chldns Hosp 1980; **Fellow:** Pediatric Gastroenterology, Chldns Hosp 1982; **Fac Appt:** Assoc Prof Ped, Harvard Med Sch

Kleinman, Ronald E MD [PGe] - **Spec Exp:** Transplant Medicine-Liver; Nutrition; **Hospital:** Mass Genl Hosp, N Shore Children's Hosp; **Address:** Mass Genl Hosp, Div Ped GI/Nutrition, 55 Fruit St, VBK 107, Boston, MA 02114; **Phone:** 617-726-8705; **Board Cert:** Pediatrics 1992; Pediatric Gastroenterology 2005; **Med School:** NY Med Coll 1972; **Resid:** Pediatrics, Montefiore Med Ctr 1977; **Fellow:** Pediatric Gastroenterology, Mass Genl Hosp 1980; **Fac Appt:** Prof Ped, Harvard Med Sch

Mid Atlantic

Baker Jr, Robert D MD/PhD [PGe] - **Spec Exp:** Gastroesophageal Reflux Disease (GERD); Cystic Fibrosis; Nutrition; **Hospital:** Women's & Chldn's Hosp of Buffalo, The; **Address:** Childrens Hospital, Div Gastroenterology, 219 Bryant St, Buffalo, NY 14222-2006; **Phone:** 716-878-7793; **Board Cert:** Pediatrics 1978; Pediatric Gastroenterology 2005; **Med School:** Temple Univ 1972; **Resid:** Pediatrics, Buffalo Chldns Hosp 1975; **Fellow:** Gastroenterology, Mass Genl Hosp/Chldns Hosp Med Ctr 1983; Nutritional Biochemistry, MIT 1984; **Fac Appt:** Prof Ped, SUNY Buffalo

Baker, Susan S MD/PhD [PGe] - **Spec Exp:** Nutrition; Obesity; Liver Disease; **Hospital:** Women's & Chldn's Hosp of Buffalo, The; **Address:** Childrens Hospital, Div Gastroenterology, 219 Bryant St, Buffalo, NY 14201-2099; **Phone:** 716-878-7793; **Board Cert:** Pediatrics 1978; Pediatric Gastroenterology 2005; **Med School:** Temple Univ 1972; **Resid:** Pediatrics, Buffalo Chldns Hosp 1975; **Fellow:** Nutrition, MIT 1981; Gastroenterology, Mass Genl Hosp/Harvard 1984; **Fac Appt:** Prof Ped, SUNY Buffalo

Baldassano, Robert N MD [PGe] - **Spec Exp:** Inflammatory Bowel Disease; Ulcerative Colitis; Crohn's Disease; **Hospital:** Chldns Hosp of Philadelphia, The; **Address:** Chldns Hosp of Philadelphia, GI/Nutrition, 324 S 34th St, Philadelphia, PA 19104-4399; **Phone:** 215-590-3630; **Board Cert:** Pediatrics 1989; Pediatric Gastroenterology 2000; **Med School:** SUNY Downstate 1984; **Resid:** Pediatrics, Childrens Hosp 1988; **Fellow:** Pediatric Gastroenterology, Childrens Hosp 1991; **Fac Appt:** Assoc Prof Ped, Univ Pennsylvania

Baldridge, Alan D MD [PGe] - **Spec Exp:** Inflammatory Bowel Disease; Celiac Disease; **Hospital:** St Christopher's Hosp for Chldn; **Address:** St Christophers Hosp for Children, Gastroenterology Section, Erie Ave at Front St, Philadelphia, PA 19134; **Phone:** 215-427-6778; **Board Cert:** Pediatrics 2008; Pediatric Gastroenterology 2005; **Med School:** Med Coll VA 1988; **Resid:** Pediatrics, Boston City Hosp 1991; **Fellow:** Pediatric Gastroenterology, Mass Genl Hosp 1994; **Fac Appt:** Asst Prof Med, Drexel Univ Coll Med

Benkov, Keith J MD [PGe] - **Spec Exp:** Inflammatory Bowel Disease/Crohn's; Liver Disease; Celiac Disease; **Hospital:** Mount Sinai Med Ctr (page 64), Englewood Hosp & Med Ctr; **Address:** Mt Sinai Div Ped Gastroenterology, 5 E 98th St Fl 10, New York, NY 10029; **Phone:** 212-241-5415; **Board Cert:** Pediatrics 1984; Pediatric Gastroenterology 2005; **Med School:** Mount Sinai Sch Med 1979; **Resid:** Pediatrics, Mt Sinai Hosp 1982; **Fellow:** Pediatric Gastroenterology, Mt Sinai Hosp 1984; **Fac Appt:** Assoc Prof Ped, Mount Sinai Sch Med

Fasano, Alessio MD [PGe] - **Spec Exp:** Celiac Disease; Diarrheal Diseases; Nutrition; **Hospital:** Univ of MD Med Ctr; **Address:** 20 Penn St, rm 351, Baltimore, MD 21201; **Phone:** 410-328-6749; **Med School:** Italy ; **Resid:** Pediatrics, Univ Naples; **Fellow:** Univ Naples; **Fac Appt:** Prof Ped, Univ MD Sch Med

Hillemeier, A Craig MD [PGe] - **Spec Exp:** Gastroesophageal Reflux Disease (GERD); Inflammatory Bowel Disease/Crohn's; **Hospital:** Penn State Milton S Hershey Med Ctr, Penn State Chldns Hosp; **Address:** Hershey Medical Ctr, 500 University Drive, MC H085, Hershey, PA 17033-0850; **Phone:** 717-531-6700; **Board Cert:** Pediatrics 1981; Pediatric Gastroenterology 2005; **Med School:** Loyola Univ-Stritch Sch Med 1976; **Resid:** Pediatrics, Loyola Univ Stritch 1978; **Fellow:** Pediatric Gastroenterology, Yale New Haven Med Ctr 1982; **Fac Appt:** Prof Ped, Penn State Univ-Hershey Med Ctr

Levy, Joseph MD [PGe] - **Spec Exp:** Celiac Disease; Irritable Bowel Syndrome; Gastroesophageal Reflux Disease (GERD); Nutrition in Autism; **Hospital:** NYU Langone Med Ctr (page 67); **Address:** 160 E 32nd St Fl 2, New York, NY 10016; **Phone:** 212-263-5407; **Board Cert:** Pediatrics 1981; Pediatric Gastroenterology 2005; **Med School:** Israel 1973; **Resid:** Pediatrics, Beth Israel Med Ctr 1977; **Fellow:** Research, Columbia-Presby Med Ctr 1975; Pediatric Gastroenterology, Columbia-Presby Med Ctr 1979; **Fac Appt:** Prof Ped, NYU Sch Med

Newman, Leonard MD [PGe] - **Spec Exp:** Inflammatory Bowel Disease; Celiac Disease; **Hospital:** Westchester Med Ctr, Montefiore Med Ctr - Div. North; **Address:** NY Med College, Dept Ped, Munger Pavillion - rm 123, Valhalla, NY 10595; **Phone:** 914-367-0000; **Board Cert:** Pediatrics 1975; Pediatric Gastroenterology 1990; **Med School:** NY Med Coll 1970; **Resid:** Pediatrics, UCSD Med Ctr 1972; Pediatrics, NY Med Coll 1973; **Fellow:** Gastroenterology, Bronx Lebanon Hosp/Einstein 1974; **Fac Appt:** Prof Ped, NY Med Coll

Oliva-Hemker, Maria M MD [PGe] - **Spec Exp:** Inflammatory Bowel Disease/Crohn's; Ulcerative Colitis; Malabsorption Syndrome; **Hospital:** Johns Hopkins Hosp (page 61); **Address:** Johns Hopkins Hosp, Ped GI & Nutrition, 600 N Wolfe St, Brady 320, Baltimore, MD 21287-2631; **Phone:** 410-955-8765; **Board Cert:** Pediatrics 2007; Pediatric Gastroenterology 2007; **Med School:** Johns Hopkins Univ 1986; **Resid:** Pediatrics, Johns Hopkins Hosp 1989; **Fellow:** Gastroenterology, Johns Hopkins Hosp 1992; **Fac Appt:** Assoc Prof Ped, Johns Hopkins Univ

Piccoli, David A MD [PGe] - **Spec Exp:** Liver Disease; **Hospital:** Chldns Hosp of Philadelphia, The; **Address:** Chlds Hosp of Philadelphia, Div Gastroenterology/Nutrition, 34th St and Civic Ctr Blvd, Ste 9S20C, Philadelphia, PA 19104; **Phone:** 215-590-1678; **Board Cert:** Pediatrics 1984; Pediatric Gastroenterology 2005; **Med School:** Harvard Med Sch 1979; **Resid:** Pediatrics, Chldns Hosp Med Ctr 1983; **Fellow:** Gastroenterology, Chldns Hosp 1986; **Fac Appt:** Prof Ped, Univ Pennsylvania

Schwarz, Kathleen B MD [PGe] - **Spec Exp:** Hepatitis B & C; Transplant Medicine-Liver; Liver Disease; **Hospital:** Johns Hopkins Hosp (page 61); **Address:** Johns Hopkins Pediatric GI, 600 N Wolfe St, Brady 320, Baltimore, MD 21287-0005; **Phone:** 410-955-8769; **Board Cert:** Pediatrics 1977; Pediatric Gastroenterology 2005; Pediatric Transplant Hepatology 2006; **Med School:** Washington Univ, St Louis 1972; **Resid:** Pediatrics, St Louis Chldns Hosp 1974; **Fellow:** Pediatric Gastroenterology, St Louis Chldns Hosp 1976; **Fac Appt:** Prof Ped, Johns Hopkins Univ

Pediatric Gastroenterology

Schwarz, Steven M MD [PGe] - **Spec Exp:** Gastroesophageal Reflux Disease (GERD); Nutrition; Endoscopy; **Hospital:** SUNY Downstate Med Ctr, Beth Israel Med Ctr- Kings Hwy Div (page 57); **Address:** Children's Hosp at SUNY Downstate, 445 Lenox Rd, Box 49, Brooklyn, NY 11203; **Phone:** 718-270-4714; **Board Cert:** Pediatrics 1979; Pediatric Gastroenterology 2005; **Med School:** Columbia P&S 1974; **Resid:** Pediatrics, Columbia-Presby Med Ctr 1977; **Fellow:** Pediatric Gastroenterology, Stanford Univ Med Ctr 1978; Pediatric Gastroenterology, Columbia-Presby Med Ctr 1980; **Fac Appt:** Prof Ped, SUNY Downstate

Spivak, William MD [PGe] - **Spec Exp:** Inflammatory Bowel Disease/Crohn's; Ulcerative Colitis; Gastroesophageal Reflux Disease (GERD); Feeding Disorders; **Hospital:** NY-Presby Hosp/Weill Cornell (page 66), Lenox Hill Hosp (page 62); **Address:** 177 E 87th St, Ste 305, New York, NY 10128; **Phone:** 212-369-7700; **Board Cert:** Pediatrics 1981; Pediatric Gastroenterology 2005; **Med School:** Albert Einstein Coll Med 1976; **Resid:** Pediatrics, Jacobi Med Ctr 1979; **Fellow:** Gastroenterology, Childrens Hosp 1982; Research, Brigham & Womens Hosp 1982; **Fac Appt:** Clin Prof Ped, Cornell Univ-Weill Med Coll

Squires, Robert H MD [PGe] - **Spec Exp:** Liver Disease; **Hospital:** Chldns Hosp of Pittsburgh - UPMC; **Address:** Children's Hosp Pittsburgh, Pediatric Gastroenterology, 45th St & Penn Ave Fl 5 - Ste 5000, Pittsburgh, PA 15201; **Phone:** 412-692-5180; **Board Cert:** Pediatrics 1981; Pediatric Gastroenterology 2005; Pediatric Transplant Hepatology 2006; **Med School:** Univ Tex Med Br, Galveston 1977; **Resid:** Pediatrics, Children's Hosp 1979; **Fellow:** Pediatric Gastroenterology, Children's Hosp 1982; **Fac Appt:** Prof Ped, Univ Pittsburgh

Suchy, Frederick J MD [PGe] - **Spec Exp:** Hepatitis; Liver Disease; Neonatal Cholestasis; **Hospital:** Mount Sinai Med Ctr (page 64); **Address:** Mount Sinai Medical Ctr, 1 Gustave Levy Pl, Box 1198, New York, NY 10029; **Phone:** 212-241-6933; **Board Cert:** Pediatrics 1982; Pediatric Gastroenterology 2005; Pediatric Transplant Hepatology 2006; **Med School:** Univ Cincinnati 1974; **Resid:** Pediatrics, Chldns Hosp Med Ctr 1978; **Fellow:** Pediatric Gastroenterology, Chldns Hosp Med Ctr 1981; **Fac Appt:** Prof Ped, Mount Sinai Sch Med

Treem, William R MD [PGe] - **Spec Exp:** Liver Disease; Inflammatory Bowel Disease; Celiac Disease; **Hospital:** SUNY Downstate Med Ctr, Beth Israel Med Ctr- Kings Hwy Div (page 57); **Address:** SUNY Downstate Med Ctr, Dept Peds, 445 Lennox Rd, Box 49, Brooklyn, NY 11203; **Phone:** 718-270-4714; **Board Cert:** Pediatrics 1982; Pediatric Gastroenterology 2005; **Med School:** Stanford Univ 1977; **Resid:** Pediatrics, Chldns Hosp 1980; **Fellow:** Pediatric Gastroenterology, Univ Penn Hosp 1985; **Fac Appt:** Prof Ped, SUNY Downstate

Southeast

Hill, Ivor D MD [PGe] - **Spec Exp:** Celiac Disease; Inflammatory Bowel Disease; Malabsorption Syndrome; Diarrheal Diseases; **Hospital:** Wake Forest Univ Baptist Med Ctr (page 72); **Address:** Wake Forest Univ Sch Med, Div Ped Gastro, Medical Center Blvd, Winston-Salem, NC 27157; **Phone:** 336-716-3009; **Board Cert:** Pediatrics 2007; Pediatric Gastroenterology 2003; **Med School:** South Africa 1972; **Resid:** Pediatrics, Addington Hosp 1976; Pediatrics, Red Cross Chldns Hosp 1977; **Fellow:** Pediatric Gastroenterology, Red Cross Chlds Hosp 1980; **Fac Appt:** Prof Ped, Wake Forest Univ

Novak, Donald A MD [PGe] - **Spec Exp:** Liver Disease; **Hospital:** Shands at Univ of FL; **Address:** Univ Florida Pediatrics, Div Gastroenterology/Hepatology, 720 SW 2nd Ave, Ste 405, Gainesville, FL 32601; **Phone:** 352-733-0094; **Board Cert:** Pediatrics 2004; Pediatric Gastroenterology 2007; **Med School:** Univ S Fla Coll Med 1981; **Resid:** Pediatrics, Univ South Fla 1984; **Fellow:** Pediatric Gastroenterology, Childrens Hosp 1987; **Fac Appt:** Prof Ped, Univ Fla Coll Med

Thompson, John F MD [PGe] - **Spec Exp:** Inflammatory Bowel Disease/Crohn's; Short Bowel Syndrome; Transplant Medicine-Bowel; **Hospital:** Jackson Meml Hosp (page 70); **Address:** Jackson Meml Hospital, Dept Pediatrics, Div GI & Nutrition, 1601 NW 12th Ave, rm 3005A, MC D820, Miami, FL 33136; **Phone:** 305-243-6426; **Board Cert:** Pediatrics 1983; Pediatric Gastroenterology 2005; **Med School:** Loyola Univ-Stritch Sch Med 1977; **Resid:** Pediatrics, Wylers Chldns Hosp-Univ Chicago 1980; **Fellow:** Pediatric Gastroenterology, Babies Hosp-Columbia Univ 1985; **Fac Appt:** Prof Ped, Univ Miami Sch Med

Ulshen, Martin H MD [PGe] - **Spec Exp:** Liver Disease; Inflammatory Bowel Disease; Irritable Bowel Syndrome; **Hospital:** Duke Univ Med Ctr; **Address:** Duke Univ Med Ctr, Box 102375, Durham, NC 27710; **Phone:** 919-684-5068; **Board Cert:** Pediatrics 1993; Pediatric Gastroenterology 2005; **Med School:** Univ Rochester 1969; **Resid:** Pediatrics, Univ Colorado Med Ctr 1974; **Fellow:** Pediatric Gastroenterology, Univ Colorado Med Ctr 1975; Pediatric Gastroenterology, Chldns Hosp 1977; **Fac Appt:** Prof Ped, Duke Univ

Midwest

Berman, James MD [PGe] - **Spec Exp:** Inflammatory Bowel Disease/Crohn's; Nutrition; Ulcerative Colitis; **Hospital:** Loyola Univ Med Ctr, Adv Luth Genl Hosp; **Address:** Loyola Univ Med Ctr, Dept Ped Gastro, 2160 S 1st Ave Bldg 105 - rm 3346, Maywood, IL 60153-3304; **Phone:** 708-327-9073; **Board Cert:** Pediatrics 1986; Pediatric Gastroenterology 2005; **Med School:** Univ Pittsburgh 1981; **Resid:** Pediatrics, Chldns Hosp 1984; **Fellow:** Pediatric Gastroenterology, Mass Genl Hosp/Chldns Hosp 1987; **Fac Appt:** Asst Prof Ped, Loyola Univ-Stritch Sch Med

Cohen, Mitchell B MD [PGe] - **Spec Exp:** Inflammatory Bowel Disease; Diarrheal Diseases; Celiac Disease; **Hospital:** Cincinnati Chldns Hosp Med Ctr; **Address:** Chldns Hosp Med Ctr, 3333 Burnet Ave, MLC 2010, Cincinnati, OH 45229; **Phone:** 513-636-4415; **Board Cert:** Pediatrics 1981; Pediatric Gastroenterology 2005; **Med School:** Mount Sinai Sch Med 1977; **Resid:** Pediatrics, Johns Hopkins Hosp 1980; **Fellow:** Pediatric Gastroenterology, Chldns Hosp Med Ctr 1986; **Fac Appt:** Prof Ped, Univ Cincinnati

El-Youssef, Mounif MD [PGe] - **Spec Exp:** Liver Disease; **Hospital:** Mayo Med Ctr & Clin - Rochester; **Address:** Mayo Clin, Div Ped Gastroenterology, 200 First St SW, Rochester, MN 55905; **Phone:** 507-284-2141; **Board Cert:** Pediatric Gastroenterology 2005; **Med School:** Belgium 1982; **Resid:** Pediatrics, Cleveland Clin 1987; **Fellow:** Pediatric Gastroenterology, Harvard Med Sch 1990

Gunasekaran, T S MD [PGe] - **Spec Exp:** Gastroesophageal Reflux Disease (GERD); Esophageal Disorders; Inflammatory Bowel Disease; Pain-Abdominal Recurrent; **Hospital:** Adv Luth Genl Hosp, Loyola Univ Med Ctr; **Address:** Lutheran Genl Chldns Hosp, Dept Ped GI, 1675 Dempster St, Park Ridge, IL 60068; **Phone:** 847-723-7700; **Board Cert:** Pediatric Gastroenterology 2007; **Med School:** India 1977; **Resid:** Pediatrics 1982; Pediatrics 1987; **Fellow:** Pediatric Gastroenterology, BC Childrens Hosp 1992; **Fac Appt:** Assoc Clin Prof Ped, Loyola Univ-Stritch Sch Med

Kirschner, Barbara S MD [PGe] - **Spec Exp:** Ulcerative Colitis; Pain-Abdominal Recurrent; Inflammatory Bowel Disease/Crohn's; **Hospital:** Univ of Chicago Med Ctr; **Address:** Comer Childrens Hosp, 5839 S Maryland Ave, Ste C-474, MC 4065, Chicago, IL 60637; **Phone:** 773-702-6418; **Board Cert:** Pediatrics 1972; Pediatric Gastroenterology 2005; **Med School:** Med Coll PA 1967; **Resid:** Pediatrics, Univ Chicago Hosps 1970; **Fellow:** Pediatric Gastroenterology, Univ Chicago Hosps 1977; **Fac Appt:** Prof Ped, Univ Chicago-Pritzker Sch Med

Pediatric Gastroenterology

Molleston, Jean P MD [PGe] - **Spec Exp:** Liver Disease; Inflammatory Bowel Disease/Crohn's; Transplant Medicine-Liver; **Hospital:** Riley Hosp for Children, Clarian North Med Ctr; **Address:** Indiana Univ-Riley Chldns Hosp, Div Ped Gastroenterology, 702 Barnhill Drive, rm ROC 4210, Indianapolis, IN 46202-5225; **Phone:** 317-274-3774; **Board Cert:** Pediatric Gastroenterology 2003; Pediatric Transplant Hepatology 2006; **Med School:** Washington Univ, St Louis 1986; **Resid:** Pediatrics, Chldns Hosp 1988; **Fellow:** Pediatric Gastroenterology, Washington Univ 1991; **Fac Appt:** Clin Prof Ped, Indiana Univ

Rothbaum, Robert J MD [PGe] - **Spec Exp:** Inflammatory Bowel Disease; **Hospital:** St Louis Chldns Hosp, Barnes-Jewish Hosp; **Address:** 1 Children's Pl, NWT Bldg Fl 9, Box 8116, St Louis, MO 63110; **Phone:** 314-454-6173; **Board Cert:** Pediatrics 1981; Pediatric Gastroenterology 2005; **Med School:** Univ Chicago-Pritzker Sch Med 1976; **Resid:** Pediatrics, St Louis Chldns Hosp 1978; **Fellow:** Ambulatory Pediatrics, St Louis Chldns Hosp 1979; Pediatric Gastroenterology, Chldns Hosp Med Ctr 1982; **Fac Appt:** Prof Ped, Washington Univ, St Louis

Rudolph, Colin D MD [PGe] - **Spec Exp:** Feeding Disorders; Nutrition; Gastrointestinal Motility Disorders; Gastrointestinal Functional Disorders; **Hospital:** Chldns Hosp - Wisconsin; **Address:** 8701 Watertown Plank Rd, Milwaukee, WI 53226; **Phone:** 414-266-3690; **Board Cert:** Pediatrics 1987; Pediatric Gastroenterology 2005; **Med School:** Case West Res Univ 1982; **Resid:** Pediatrics, Chldn's Hosp 1984; **Fellow:** Pediatric Gastroenterology, UCSF Med Ctr 1986; **Fac Appt:** Assoc Prof Ped, Univ Wisc

Whitington, Peter F MD [PGe] - **Spec Exp:** Transplant Medicine-Liver; Liver Disease; **Hospital:** Children's Mem Hosp; **Address:** Chldns Meml Hosp, Div Ped Gastro, 2300 Children's Plaza, Box 57, Chicago, IL 60614; **Phone:** 773-880-4643; **Board Cert:** Pediatrics 1977; Pediatric Gastroenterology 2005; Pediatric Transplant Hepatology 2006; **Med School:** Univ Tenn Coll Med, Memphis 1971; **Resid:** Pediatrics, Univ Tenn Hosp 1975; **Fellow:** Gastroenterology, Johns Hopkins Hosp 1977; Gastroenterology, Univ Wisconsin Affil Hosp 1978; **Fac Appt:** Prof Ped, Northwestern Univ

Wyllie, Robert MD [PGe] - **Spec Exp:** Inflammatory Bowel Disease/Crohn's; Ulcerative Colitis; **Hospital:** Cleveland Clin Fdn (page 56); **Address:** Cleveland Clinic, 9500 Euclid Ave, Desk A111, Cleveland, OH 44195; **Phone:** 216-444-2237; **Board Cert:** Pediatrics 1982; Pediatric Gastroenterology 2005; **Med School:** Indiana Univ 1976; **Resid:** Pediatrics, Indiana Univ Med Ctr 1979; **Fellow:** Pediatric Gastroenterology, Indiana Univ Med Ctr 1980

Great Plains and Mountains

Hoffenberg, Edward J MD [PGe] - **Spec Exp:** Inflammatory Bowel Disease/Crohn's; Celiac Disease; **Hospital:** Chldn's Hosp - Aurora, The, Univ Colorado Hosp; **Address:** Chldns Hosp-Div Gastroenterology, 13123 E 16th Ave, Box B290, Denver, CO 80045; **Phone:** 303-861-6669; **Board Cert:** Pediatric Endocrinology 2000; **Med School:** Case West Res Univ 1986; **Resid:** Pediatrics, Rainbow Babie's & Chldns Hosp 1989; **Fellow:** Pediatric Gastroenterology, Chldn's Hosp 1992; **Fac Appt:** Assoc Prof Ped, Univ Colorado

Krebs, Nancy F MD [PGe] - **Spec Exp:** Obesity; Nutrition; **Hospital:** Chldn's Hosp - Aurora, The; **Address:** Chldn's Hosp, Hlth Ctr, 13123 E 16th Ave, Box B270, Aurora, CO 80045; **Phone:** 303-724-3260; **Board Cert:** Pediatrics 1999; Pediatric Gastroenterology 2003; **Med School:** Univ Colorado 1987; **Resid:** Pediatrics, Univ Colorado Hlth Sci Ctr 1990; **Fellow:** Pediatric Gastroenterology, Univ Colorado Hlth Sci Ctr 1992; Nutrition, Univ Colorado Hlth Sci Ctr 1993; **Fac Appt:** Prof Ped, Univ Colorado

Narkewicz, Michael R MD [PGe] - **Spec Exp:** Transplant Medicine-Liver; Liver Disease; **Hospital:** Chldn's Hosp - Aurora, The; **Address:** Children's Hospital, Dept Liver Disease and Nutrition, 13123 E 16th Ave, Aurora, CO 80045; **Phone:** 720-777-6669; **Board Cert:** Pediatrics 1988; Pediatric Gastroenterology 2005; Pediatric Transplant Hepatology 2006; **Med School:** Univ VT Coll Med 1983; **Resid:** Pediatrics, Univ Colorado Med Ctr 1986; **Fellow:** Pediatric Gastroenterology, Univ Colorado Med Ctr 1989; **Fac Appt:** Prof Ped, Univ Colorado

Vanderhoof, Jon A MD [PGe] - **Spec Exp:** Nutrition; Short Bowel Syndrome; Probiotics; **Hospital:** Boys Town Natl Rsch Hosp, Children's Hosp - Omaha; **Address:** Boystown Hospital & Clinic, 14040 Hospital Rd, Boystown, NE 68010; **Phone:** 402-778-6820; **Board Cert:** Pediatrics 1993; Pediatric Gastroenterology 2005; **Med School:** Univ Nebr Coll Med 1972; **Resid:** Pediatrics, Univ Nebr Coll Med 1974; **Fellow:** Pediatric Gastroenterology, UCLA Med Ctr 1976; **Fac Appt:** Prof Ped, Univ Nebr Coll Med

Southwest

Rhoads, J Marc MD [PGe] - **Spec Exp:** Diarrheal Diseases; Inflammatory Bowel Disease; Intestinal Disorders; **Hospital:** Meml Hermann Hosp - Texas Med Ctr; **Address:** Univ Texas Hlth Sci Ctr, Dept Pediatrics-Gastroenterology, 6431 Fannin St, MS 3.137, Houston, TX 77030; **Phone:** 832-325-6516; **Board Cert:** Pediatrics 1986; Pediatric Gastroenterology 2005; **Med School:** Johns Hopkins Univ 1980; **Resid:** Pediatrics, UCLA Med Ctr 1983; **Fellow:** Pediatric Gastroenterology, Hosp for Sick Chldn 1986; **Fac Appt:** Prof Ped, Univ Tex, Houston

West Coast and Pacific

Christie, Dennis L MD [PGe] - **Hospital:** Chldns Hosp and Regl Med Ctr - Seattle; **Address:** Chldns Hosp Med Ctr, Div Gastroenterology, 4800 Sand Point Way NE, MS 7830, Seattle, WA 98105-3901; **Phone:** 206-987-2521; **Board Cert:** Pediatrics 1992; Pediatric Gastroenterology 2005; **Med School:** Northwestern Univ 1968; **Resid:** Pediatrics, Univ Wash Med Ctr 1971; **Fellow:** Pediatric Gastroenterology, UCLA Ctr Hlth Sci 1976; **Fac Appt:** Prof Ped, Univ Wash

Dubinsky, Marla C MD [PGe] - **Spec Exp:** Inflammatory Bowel Disease; Crohn's Disease; Ulcerative Colitis; Clinical Trials; **Hospital:** Cedars-Sinai Med Ctr; **Address:** 8635 W 3rd St, Ste 1165W, Los Angeles, CA 90048; **Phone:** 310-423-7100; **Board Cert:** Pediatrics 2004; Pediatric Gastroenterology 2001; **Med School:** Canada 1993; **Fac Appt:** Asst Prof Ped, UCLA

Heyman, Melvin Bernard MD [PGe] - **Spec Exp:** Inflammatory Bowel Disease/Crohn's; Short Bowel Syndrome; Gastroesophageal Reflux Disease (GERD); **Hospital:** UCSF Med Ctr; **Address:** UCSF, Dept Ped Gastroenterology, 500 Parnassus Ave, Ste MU 406E, Box 0136, San Francisco, CA 94143-0136; **Phone:** 415-476-5892; **Board Cert:** Pediatrics 1981; Pediatric Gastroenterology 2005; **Med School:** UCLA 1976; **Resid:** Pediatrics, LAC-USC Med Ctr 1979; **Fellow:** Gastroenterology, UCLA Med Ctr 1981; Nutrition, Human Nutrition Res Ctr 1990; **Fac Appt:** Prof Ped, UCSF

McDiarmid, Suzanne V MD [PGe] - **Spec Exp:** Transplant Medicine-Liver; Transplant Medicine-Intestine; Transplant Immunology; **Hospital:** UCLA Ronald Reagan Med Ctr; **Address:** UCLA Med Ctr, 18033 Leconte Ave, Room MDCC 12-328, Los Angeles, CA 90095; **Phone:** 310-206-6134; **Board Cert:** Pediatrics 1984; Pediatric Gastroenterology 2000; **Med School:** New Zealand 1976; **Resid:** Pediatrics, UCLA Med Center 1980; **Fac Appt:** Prof Ped, UCLA

Pediatric Gastroenterology

Sinatra, Frank R MD [PGe] - **Spec Exp:** Liver Disease; **Hospital:** Women's & Children's Hosp-LA, Chldns Hosp - Los Angeles; **Address:** Women's & Children's Hospital, 1240 N Mission Rd, rm L902, Los Angeles, CA 90033; **Phone:** 323-226-3691; **Board Cert:** Pediatrics 1992; Pediatric Gastroenterology 2005; **Med School:** USC Sch Med 1971; **Resid:** Pediatrics, Chldns Hosp 1974; **Fellow:** Gastroenterology, Stanford Univ Med Ctr 1976; **Fac Appt:** Prof Ped, USC Sch Med

PEDIATRIC HEMATOLOGY-ONCOLOGY

New England

Albritton, Karen H MD [PHO] - **Spec Exp:** Sarcoma; **Hospital:** Dana-Farber Cancer Inst; **Address:** Dana Farber Cancer Inst, 44 Binney St, Smith 338, Boston, MA 02115; **Phone:** 617-582-7976; **Board Cert:** Pediatric Hematology-Oncology 2002; Medical Oncology 2001; **Med School:** Univ Tex, San Antonio 1992; **Resid:** Internal Medicine & Pediatrics, Univ NC Hosps 1996; **Fellow:** Hematology & Oncology, Univ NC Hosps 2000

Altman, Arnold MD [PHO] - **Spec Exp:** Leukemia; **Hospital:** CT Chldns Med Ctr; **Address:** CT Childrens Med Ctr, Hematology/Oncology, 282 Washington St, Ste 2J, Hartford, CT 06106; **Phone:** 860-545-9630; **Board Cert:** Pediatrics 1971; Pediatric Hematology-Oncology 1974; **Med School:** Johns Hopkins Univ 1965; **Resid:** Pediatrics, Chldns Hosp Med Ctr 1970; **Fellow:** Pediatric Hematology-Oncology, Chldns Hosp Med Ctr 1972; **Fac Appt:** Prof Ped, Univ Conn

Diller, Lisa R MD [PHO] - **Spec Exp:** Neuroblastoma; Cancer Survivors-Late Effects of Therapy; **Hospital:** Dana-Farber Cancer Inst; **Address:** Dana-Farber Cancer Inst, 44 Binney St, Shields Warren 312, Boston, MA 02115; **Phone:** 617-632-5642; **Board Cert:** Pediatric Hematology-Oncology 2007; **Med School:** UCSD 1985; **Resid:** Pediatrics, Chldns Hosp 1988; **Fellow:** Pediatric Hematology-Oncology, Chldns Hosp-Dana Farber Cancer Inst 1991; **Fac Appt:** Assoc Prof Ped, Harvard Med Sch

Grier, Holcombe E MD [PHO] - **Spec Exp:** Bone Cancer; Ewing's Sarcoma; **Hospital:** Dana-Farber Cancer Inst, Children's Hospital - Boston; **Address:** Dana Farber Cancer Inst, 44 Binney St, SW350, Boston, MA 02115; **Phone:** 617-632-3971; **Board Cert:** Pediatrics 1983; Internal Medicine 1980; Pediatric Hematology-Oncology 2005; **Med School:** Univ Pennsylvania 1976; **Resid:** Pediatrics, NC Meml Hosp 1980; Internal Medicine, NC Meml Hosp 1980; **Fellow:** Pediatric Oncology, Dana Farber Chldn's Hosp 1984; **Fac Appt:** Assoc Prof Ped, Harvard Med Sch

Homans, Alan C MD [PHO] - **Spec Exp:** Leukemia; **Hospital:** Fletcher Allen Health Care-Med Ctr Campus; **Address:** Vermont Childrens Hosp, 111 Colchester Ave, Smith 5-rm 559, Burlington, VT 05401; **Phone:** 802-847-2850; **Board Cert:** Pediatrics 1985; Pediatric Hematology-Oncology 1987; **Med School:** Ohio State Univ 1979; **Resid:** Pediatrics, Med Ctr Hosp 1981; Pediatrics, Univ Mass Med Ctr 1982; **Fellow:** Pediatric Hematology-Oncology, Rhode Island Hosp 1985; **Fac Appt:** Prof Ped, Univ VT Coll Med

Kieran, Mark W MD/PhD [PHO] - **Spec Exp:** Brain Tumors; Neuro-Oncology; **Hospital:** Dana-Farber Cancer Inst, Children's Hospital - Boston; **Address:** Dana Farber Cancer Inst, 44 Binney St, Shields Warren Ste 331, Boston, MA 02115; **Phone:** 617-632-4386; **Board Cert:** Pediatric Hematology-Oncology 2004; **Med School:** Univ Calgary 1986; **Resid:** Pediatrics, Montreal Chldns Hosp 1992; **Fellow:** Pediatric Hematology-Oncology, Chldns Hosp 1995; **Fac Appt:** Asst Prof Ped, Harvard Med Sch

America's Top Doctors® 9th Edition

Kretschmar, Cynthia S MD [PHO] - **Spec Exp:** Brain Tumors; Neuroblastoma; Drug Discovery & Development; **Hospital:** Tufts Med Ctr; **Address:** Floating Hosp, Div Pediatric Hem/Onc, 750 Washington St, NEMC 14, Boston, MA 02111; **Phone:** 617-636-5535; **Board Cert:** Pediatrics 1984; Pediatric Hematology-Oncology 1987; **Med School:** Yale Univ 1978; **Resid:** Pediatrics, Yale-New Haven Hosp 1981; **Fellow:** Pediatric Hematology-Oncology, Dana Farber Cancer Inst 1984; **Fac Appt:** Prof Ped, Tufts Univ

Sallan, Stephen MD [PHO] - **Spec Exp:** Pediatric Cancers; Leukemia; **Hospital:** Children's Hospital - Boston; **Address:** Dana Farber Cancer Inst, Dept Ped Oncology, 44 Binney St, Ste 1642, Boston, MA 02115; **Phone:** 617-632-3316; **Board Cert:** Pediatrics 1972; **Med School:** Wayne State Univ 1967; **Resid:** Pediatrics, Chldns Hosp 1969; Pediatrics, Hosp Sick Chldn 1970; **Fellow:** Pediatric Oncology, Chldns Hosp Med Ctr 1975; **Fac Appt:** Prof Ped, Harvard Med Sch

Schwartz, Cindy Lee MD [PHO] - **Spec Exp:** Hodgkin's Disease; Bone Cancer; Cancer Survivors-Late Effects of Therapy; **Hospital:** Rhode Island Hosp; **Address:** RI Hospital, Dept Ped-Div Ped Hem/Onc, 593 Eddy St, MPS, rm 117, Providence, RI 02903-4923; **Phone:** 401-444-5171; **Board Cert:** Pediatrics 1985; Pediatric Hematology-Oncology 2009; **Med School:** Brown Univ 1979; **Resid:** Pediatrics, Johns Hopkins Hosp 1982; **Fellow:** Pediatric Hematology-Oncology, Johns Hopkins Hosp 1985; **Fac Appt:** Prof Med, Brown Univ

van Hoff, Jack MD [PHO] - **Spec Exp:** Brain Tumors; Clinical Trials; **Hospital:** Dartmouth - Hitchcock Med Ctr; **Address:** DHMC, Dept Pediatric Hem/Onc, One Medical Center Drive, Lebanon, NH 03756; **Phone:** 603-650-5541; **Board Cert:** Pediatrics 1985; Pediatric Hematology-Oncology 1987; **Med School:** UMDNJ-NJ Med Sch, Newark 1981; **Resid:** Pediatrics, Yale New Haven Hosp 1984; **Fellow:** Pediatric Hematology-Oncology, Yale New Haven Hosp 1986

Weinstein, Howard J MD [PHO] - **Spec Exp:** Bone Marrow Transplant; Leukemia; Lymphoma; **Hospital:** Mass Genl Hosp, Dana-Farber Cancer Inst; **Address:** 55 Fruit St, Yawkey 8B-8893, Boston, MA 02114-2622; **Phone:** 617-724-3315; **Board Cert:** Pediatrics 1977; **Med School:** Univ MD Sch Med 1972; **Resid:** Pediatrics, Mass Genl Hosp 1974; **Fellow:** Pediatric Hematology-Oncology, Dana Farber Cancer Inst/Chldns Hosp 1977; **Fac Appt:** Prof Ped, Harvard Med Sch

Mid Atlantic

Adamson, Peter C MD [PHO] - **Spec Exp:** Drug Development; Clinical Trials; Rhabdomyosarcoma; Pediatric Cancers; **Hospital:** Chldns Hosp of Philadelphia, The; **Address:** Chldns Hosp of Philadelphia, 34th St & Civic Ctr Blvd Abramson Bldg, Philadelphia, PA 19104; **Phone:** 215-590-2299; **Board Cert:** Pediatric Hematology-Oncology 2005; **Med School:** Cornell Univ-Weill Med Coll 1984; **Resid:** Pediatrics, Chldns Hosp 1987; **Fellow:** Pediatric Hematology-Oncology, Natl Cancer Inst 1990; **Fac Appt:** Assoc Prof Pharm, Univ Pennsylvania

Aledo, Alexander MD [PHO] - **Spec Exp:** Leukemia; Lymphoma; Bone Tumors; **Hospital:** NY-Presby Hosp/Weill Cornell (page 66), NY Hosp Queens; **Address:** 525 E 68th St, rm P695, New York, NY 10021-4870; **Phone:** 212-746-3447; **Board Cert:** Pediatrics 2002; Pediatric Hematology-Oncology 2004; **Med School:** NYU Sch Med 1984; **Resid:** Pediatrics, NY Hosp 1987; **Fellow:** Pediatric Hematology-Oncology, Meml Sloan Kettering Cancer Ctr 1990; **Fac Appt:** Assoc Clin Prof Ped, Cornell Univ-Weill Med Coll

Pediatric Hematology-Oncology

Arceci, Robert J MD/PhD [PHO] - **Spec Exp:** Leukemia; Histiocytoma; Bone Marrow Transplant; **Hospital:** Johns Hopkins Hosp (page 61); **Address:** Kimmel Cancer Ctr, Bunting-Blaustein Bldg, 1650 Orleans St, I-207, Baltimore, MD 21231-1000; **Phone:** 410-502-7519; **Board Cert:** Pediatrics 1987; Pediatric Hematology-Oncology 2005; **Med School:** Univ Rochester 1981; **Resid:** Pediatrics, Chldns Hosp 1983; **Fellow:** Pediatric Hematology-Oncology, Chldns Hosp/Dana Farber Cancer Ctr 1986; **Fac Appt:** Prof Ped, Johns Hopkins Univ

Brecher, Martin L MD [PHO] - **Spec Exp:** Brain Tumors; Lymphoma; Hodgkin's Disease; Leukemia; **Hospital:** Roswell Park Cancer Inst, Women's & Chldn's Hosp of Buffalo, The; **Address:** Roswell Park Cancer Inst, Dept Pediatrics, Elm & Carlton Sts, Buffalo, NY 14263; **Phone:** 716-845-2333; **Board Cert:** Pediatrics 1977; Pediatric Hematology-Oncology 1978; **Med School:** SUNY Buffalo 1972; **Resid:** Pediatrics, Buffalo Chldns Hosp 1975; **Fellow:** Hematology & Oncology, Buffalo Chldns Hosp/Roswell Park Cancer Inst 1977; **Fac Appt:** Prof Ped, SUNY Buffalo

Bussel, James MD [PHO] - **Spec Exp:** Autoimmune Disease; Bleeding/Coagulation Disorders; **Hospital:** NY-Presby Hosp/Weill Cornell (page 66), Lenox Hill Hosp (page 62); **Address:** 525 E 68th St, rm P-695, New York, NY 10021; **Phone:** 212-746-3474; **Board Cert:** Pediatrics 1979; Pediatric Hematology-Oncology 1981; **Med School:** Columbia P&S 1975; **Resid:** Pediatrics, Chldns Hosp 1978; **Fellow:** Pediatric Hematology-Oncology, NY Presby Hosp/Cornell 1981; **Fac Appt:** Prof Ped, Cornell Univ-Weill Med Coll

Cairo, Mitchell S MD [PHO] - **Spec Exp:** Bone Marrow Transplant; Leukemia; Lymphoma; **Hospital:** NYPresby-Morgan Stanley Children's Hosp (page 66); **Address:** Babies/Chldns Hosp-Presby Med Ctr, 3959 Broadway, CHN 10-03, New York, NY 10032; **Phone:** 212-305-8316; **Board Cert:** Pediatrics 1980; Pediatric Hematology-Oncology 1982; **Med School:** UCSF 1976; **Resid:** Pediatrics, UCLA Med Ctr 1979; **Fellow:** Pediatric Hematology-Oncology, Indiana Univ Med Ctr 1981; **Fac Appt:** Prof Ped, Columbia P&S

Carroll, William L MD [PHO] - **Spec Exp:** Leukemia; **Hospital:** NYU Langone Med Ctr (page 67); **Address:** NYU Med Ctr, Div Ped Hem/Onc, 160 E 32nd St Fl 2, New York, NY 10016; **Phone:** 212-263-9947; **Board Cert:** Pediatrics 1984; Pediatric Hematology-Oncology 1987; **Med School:** UC Irvine 1978; **Resid:** Pediatrics, Chldns Hosp Med Ctr 1981; **Fellow:** Pediatric Hematology-Oncology, Stanford Univ 1987; **Fac Appt:** Prof Ped, NYU Sch Med

Chen, Allen R MD/PhD [PHO] - **Spec Exp:** Bone Marrow Transplant; Hodgkin's Disease; Immunotherapy; Graft vs Host Disease; **Hospital:** Johns Hopkins Hosp (page 61); **Address:** Johns Hopkins Hosp, Div Peds Oncology, 1650 Orleans St, CRB 2M53, Baltimore, MD 21231; **Phone:** 410-955-7385; **Board Cert:** Pediatrics 2002; Pediatric Hematology-Oncology 2006; **Med School:** Duke Univ 1986; **Resid:** Pediatrics, Chldns Hosp Med Ctr 1989; **Fellow:** Pediatric Hematology-Oncology, Fred Hutchinson Canc Ctr 1993; Bone Marrow Transplant, Fred Hutchinson Canc Ctr 1994; **Fac Appt:** Assoc Prof Ped, Johns Hopkins Univ

Civin, Curt I MD [PHO] - **Spec Exp:** Pediatric Cancers; Leukemia; Bone Marrow Transplant; **Hospital:** Univ of MD Med Ctr; **Address:** Univ Maryland Office of Assoc Dean, 655 W Baltimore St, rm 14-023, Baltimore, MD 21201; **Phone:** 410-706-1181; **Board Cert:** Pediatrics 1979; Pediatric Hematology-Oncology 1980; **Med School:** Harvard Med Sch 1974; **Resid:** Pediatrics, Chldns Hosp 1976; **Fellow:** Pediatric Hematology-Oncology, Natl Cancer Inst 1979; **Fac Appt:** Prof Ped, Univ MD Sch Med

Drachtman, Richard A MD [PHO] - **Spec Exp:** Pediatric Cancers; Sickle Cell Disease; **Hospital:** Robert Wood Johnson Univ Hosp - New Brunswick, Jersey Shore Univ Med Ctr; **Address:** Cancer Inst of New Jersey, 195 Little Albany St, New Brunswick, NJ 08903-2681; **Phone:** 732-235-5437; **Board Cert:** Pediatric Hematology-Oncology 2007; **Med School:** Ros Franklin Univ/Chicago Med Sch 1984; **Resid:** Pediatrics, N Shore Univ Hosp 1988; **Fellow:** Pediatric Hematology-Oncology, Mount Sinai Hosp 1991; **Fac Appt:** Prof Ped, UMDNJ-RW Johnson Med Sch

Dunkel, Ira J MD [PHO] - **Spec Exp:** Retinoblastoma; Brain & Spinal Cord Tumors; Brain Tumors; Pediatric Cancers; **Hospital:** Meml Sloan-Kettering Cancer Ctr; **Address:** 1275 York Avenue, New York, NY 10065; **Phone:** 800-525-2225; **Board Cert:** Pediatric Hematology-Oncology 2007; **Med School:** Duke Univ 1985; **Resid:** Pediatrics, Duke Univ Med Ctr 1988; **Fellow:** Pediatric Hematology-Oncology, Memorial-Sloan Kettering 1992; **Fac Appt:** Asst Prof Ped, Cornell Univ-Weill Med Coll

Felix, Carolyn A MD [PHO] - **Spec Exp:** Leukemia; Leukemia in Infants; **Hospital:** Chldns Hosp of Philadelphia, The; **Address:** Chldns Hosp of Philadelphia, 34th St & Civic Ctr Blvd Abramson Bldg, Philadelphia, PA 19104; **Phone:** 215-590-2831; **Board Cert:** Pediatrics 1987; Pediatric Hematology-Oncology 1987; **Med School:** Boston Univ 1981; **Resid:** Pediatrics, Chldns Hosp 1984; **Fellow:** Pediatric Hematology-Oncology, Natl Cancer Inst-Pediatric Br 1987; **Fac Appt:** Assoc Prof Ped, Univ Pennsylvania

Frantz, Christopher N MD [PHO] - **Spec Exp:** Solid Tumors; Neuroblastoma; Leukemia; **Hospital:** Alfred I duPont Hosp for Children, Christiana Care Hlth Svs; **Address:** Alfred I duPont Hosp for Chldn, 1600 Rockland Rd, Box 269, Wilmington, DE 19899; **Phone:** 302-651-5500; **Board Cert:** Pediatrics 1977; Pediatric Hematology-Oncology 2005; **Med School:** Albert Einstein Coll Med 1971; **Resid:** Pediatrics, Chldns Hosp 1976; **Fellow:** Pediatric Hematology-Oncology, Chldns Hosp/Dana Farber Cancer Inst 1979

Garvin, James H MD/PhD [PHO] - **Spec Exp:** Brain Tumors; Pediatric Cancers; Bone Marrow Transplant; **Hospital:** NYPresby-Morgan Stanley Children's Hosp (page 66); **Address:** 161 Fort Washington Ave Fl 7 - rm 708, New York, NY 10032-3729; **Phone:** 212-305-8685; **Board Cert:** Pediatrics 1982; Pediatric Hematology-Oncology 1984; **Med School:** Jefferson Med Coll 1976; **Resid:** Pediatrics, Chldns Hosp 1978; Pediatrics, Middlesex Hosp 1979; **Fellow:** Pediatric Hematology-Oncology, Dana Farber Cancer Inst/Childrens Hosp 1982; **Fac Appt:** Clin Prof Ped, Columbia P&S

Giardina, Patricia J V MD [PHO] - **Spec Exp:** Thalassemia; **Hospital:** NY-Presby Hosp/Weill Cornell (page 66); **Address:** 525 E 68th St, Payson Pavilion 695, New York, NY 10065; **Phone:** 212-746-3404; **Board Cert:** Pediatrics 1973; Pediatric Hematology-Oncology 1974; **Med School:** NY Med Coll 1968; **Resid:** Pediatrics, New York Hosp 1971; **Fellow:** Pediatric Hematology-Oncology, New York Hosp-Cornell 1974; **Fac Appt:** Clin Prof Ped, Cornell Univ-Weill Med Coll

Grupp, Stephan A MD [PHO] - **Spec Exp:** Stem Cell Transplant; Neuroblastoma; Bone Marrow Transplant; **Hospital:** Chldns Hosp of Philadelphia, The; **Address:** Childrens Hosp - Oncology, 34th St & Civic Ctr Blvd Abramson Bldg, Philadelphia, PA 19104; **Phone:** 215-590-2821; **Board Cert:** Pediatric Hematology-Oncology 2002; **Med School:** Univ Cincinnati 1987; **Resid:** Pediatrics, Chldns Hosp 1990; **Fellow:** Pediatric Hematology-Oncology, Dana Farber Cancer Inst/Chldns Hosp 1992; **Fac Appt:** Asst Prof Ped, Univ Pennsylvania

Guarini, Ludovico MD [PHO] - **Spec Exp:** Leukemia; Solid Tumors; Sickle Cell Disease; **Hospital:** Maimonides Med Ctr (page 63); **Address:** 6300 8th Ave, Brooklyn, NY 11220; **Phone:** 718-765-2671; **Board Cert:** Pediatrics 1984; Pediatric Hematology-Oncology 2007; **Med School:** Italy 1974; **Resid:** Pediatrics, Beth Israel Hosp 1981; **Fellow:** Pediatric Hematology-Oncology, Columbia-Presby Med Ctr 1984; **Fac Appt:** Assoc Prof Ped, Mount Sinai Sch Med

Halpern, Steven MD [PHO] - **Spec Exp:** Leukemia & Lymphoma; Brain Tumors; Hodgkin's Disease; Hemophilia; **Hospital:** Hackensack Univ Med Ctr; **Address:** 30 Prospect Ave, Ste TCI, Hackensack, NJ 07601; **Phone:** 201-996-5437; **Board Cert:** Pediatrics 1981; Pediatric Hematology-Oncology 1982; **Med School:** Ros Franklin Univ/Chicago Med Sch 1976; **Resid:** Pediatrics, St Christophers Hosp for Children 1979; **Fellow:** Pediatric Hematology-Oncology, Childrens Hosp 1982; **Fac Appt:** Asst Prof Ped, UMDNJ-NJ Med Sch, Newark

Pediatric Hematology-Oncology

Harris, Michael B MD [PHO] - **Spec Exp:** Leukemia & Lymphoma; Bone Tumors; Cancer Survivors-Late Effects of Therapy; **Hospital:** Hackensack Univ Med Ctr; **Address:** Tomorrows Chldns Inst, JM Sanzari Chldns Hosp, 30 Prospect Ave, Imus 1-TCI, rm PC116, Hackensack, NJ 07601; **Phone:** 201-996-5437; **Board Cert:** Pediatrics 1974; Pediatric Hematology-Oncology 1974; **Med School:** Albert Einstein Coll Med 1969; **Resid:** Pediatrics, Chldns Hosp 1971; **Fellow:** Pediatric Hematology-Oncology, Chldns Hosp 1974; **Fac Appt:** Prof Ped, UMDNJ-NJ Med Sch, Newark

Helman, Lee Jay MD [PHO] - **Spec Exp:** Solid Tumors; **Hospital:** Natl Inst of Hlth - Clin Ctr; **Address:** National Cancer Inst, NIH, 31 Center Drive, rm 3A11, Bethesda, MD 20892-2440; **Phone:** 301-496-4257; **Board Cert:** Internal Medicine 1983; Medical Oncology 1985; **Med School:** Univ MD Sch Med 1980; **Resid:** Internal Medicine, Barnes Hosp 1983; **Fellow:** Oncology, Natl Inst Hlth 1986

Hinkle, Andrea S MD [PHO] - **Spec Exp:** Cancer Survivors-Late Effects of Therapy; **Hospital:** Univ of Rochester Strong Meml Hosp; **Address:** Golisano Childrens Hosp at Strong, 601 Elmwood Ave, Box 667, Rochester, NY 14642; **Phone:** 585-275-8138; **Board Cert:** Pediatrics 2006; Pediatric Hematology-Oncology 2008; **Med School:** Brown Univ 1987; **Resid:** Pediatrics, Boston City Hosp 1991; **Fellow:** Pediatric Hematology-Oncology, Chldns Natl Med Ctr 1994; **Fac Appt:** Asst Prof Ped, Univ Rochester

Hoots, William K MD [PHO] - **Spec Exp:** Hemophilia; **Hospital:** Natl Inst of Hlth - Clin Ctr; **Address:** Nat Inst Hlth-Clin Ctr, 6701 Rockledge Drive, rm 93116, Bethesda, MD 20892; **Phone:** 301-435-0080; **Board Cert:** Pediatrics 1980; Pediatric Hematology-Oncology 1980; **Med School:** Univ NC Sch Med 1975; **Resid:** Pediatrics, Chldns Med Ctr 1978; **Fellow:** Pediatric Hematology-Oncology, Univ NC Med Ctr 1980; **Fac Appt:** Prof Ped, Univ Tex, Houston

Jakacki, Regina I MD [PHO] - **Spec Exp:** Neuro-Oncology; Clinical Trials; Palliative Care; **Hospital:** Chldns Hosp of Pittsburgh - UPMC; **Address:** Children's Hospital Pittsburgh, 45th & Penn Drive, Pittsburgh, PA 15201; **Phone:** 412-692-7056; **Board Cert:** Pediatric Hematology-Oncology 2007; **Med School:** Univ Pennsylvania 1985; **Resid:** Pediatrics, Childrens Hosp 1988; **Fellow:** Pediatric Hematology-Oncology, Childrens Hosp 1991; **Fac Appt:** Assoc Prof Ped, Univ Pittsburgh

Kamen, Barton A MD/PhD [PHO] - **Spec Exp:** Drug Development; Leukemia; **Hospital:** Robert Wood Johnson Univ Hosp - New Brunswick; **Address:** Cancer Inst of New Jersey, 195 Little Albany St, rm 3507, New Brunswick, NJ 08903; **Phone:** 732-235-8864; **Board Cert:** Pediatrics 1981; Pediatric Hematology-Oncology 1987; **Med School:** Case West Res Univ 1976; **Resid:** Pediatrics, Yale-New Haven Hosp 1978; **Fellow:** Pediatric Hematology-Oncology, Yale-New Haven Hosp 1980; **Fac Appt:** Prof Ped, UMDNJ-RW Johnson Med Sch

Korones, David N MD [PHO] - **Spec Exp:** Brain Tumors; Palliative Care; Pediatric Cancers; **Hospital:** Univ of Rochester Strong Meml Hosp; **Address:** Golisano Childrens Hosp at Strong, 601 Elmwood Ave, Box 777, Rochester, NY 14642-8777; **Phone:** 585-275-2981; **Board Cert:** Pediatrics 1987; Pediatric Hematology-Oncology 2006; Hospice & Palliative Medicine 2002; **Med School:** Vanderbilt Univ 1983; **Resid:** Pediatrics, Strong Meml Hosp 1986; **Fellow:** Pediatrics, Yale Univ 1988; Pediatric Hematology-Oncology, Strong Meml Hosp 1991; **Fac Appt:** Assoc Prof Ped, Univ Rochester

Kushner, Brian H MD [PHO] - **Spec Exp:** Neuroblastoma; Bone Marrow Transplant; Immunotherapy; **Hospital:** Meml Sloan-Kettering Cancer Ctr; **Address:** 1275 York Avenue, New York, NY 10065; **Phone:** 800-525-2225; **Board Cert:** Pediatrics 1983; Pediatric Hematology-Oncology 1987; **Med School:** Johns Hopkins Univ 1976; **Resid:** Pediatrics, Columbia-Presby Med Ctr 1978; Pediatrics, NY Hosp 1979; **Fellow:** Pediatric Hematology-Oncology, Boston Chldns Hosp 1980; Pediatric Hematology-Oncology, Meml Sloan Kettering Cancer Ctr 1986; **Fac Appt:** Prof Ped, Cornell Univ-Weill Med Coll

Lange, Beverly J MD [PHO] - **Spec Exp:** Leukemia; Brain & Spinal Cord Tumors; Cognitive Rehabilitation; **Hospital:** Chldns Hosp of Philadelphia, The; **Address:** Chldns Hosp Phila, Medical Oncology, 34th St & Civic Ctr Blvd, Wood Center, 4th Fl, Philadelphia, PA 19104; **Phone:** 215-590-2249; **Board Cert:** Pediatrics 1976; Pediatric Hematology-Oncology 1997; **Med School:** Temple Univ 1971; **Resid:** Pediatrics, Philadelphia Genl Hosp 1973; **Fellow:** Pediatric Oncology, Chldns Hosp; **Fac Appt:** Prof Ped, Univ Pennsylvania

Lipton, Jeffrey M MD/PhD [PHO] - **Spec Exp:** Bone Marrow Failure Disorders; Stem Cell Transplant; Bone Marrow Transplant; **Hospital:** Schneider Chldn's Hosp; **Address:** Div Hem-Onc & Stem Cell Transplant, 269-01 76th Ave, rm 255, MC-07670, New Hyde Park, NY 11040-1433; **Phone:** 718-470-3460; **Board Cert:** Pediatrics 1981; **Med School:** St Louis Univ 1975; **Resid:** Pediatrics, Boston Chldns Hosp 1977; **Fellow:** Pediatric Hematology-Oncology, Boston Chldns Hosp/Dana Farber Cancer Inst 1979; **Fac Appt:** Prof Ped, Albert Einstein Coll Med

Luchtman-Jones, Lori MD [PHO] - **Spec Exp:** Leukemia; Bleeding/Coagulation Disorders; **Hospital:** Chldns Natl Med Ctr; **Address:** Chldn's Natl Med Ctr, 111 Michigan Ave NW Fl 4 - Ste 4043, Washington, DC 20010; **Phone:** 202-476-2140; **Board Cert:** Pediatric Hematology-Oncology 2004; **Med School:** UCSD 1987; **Resid:** Pediatrics, UCSD School Med 1990; **Fellow:** Pediatric Hematology-Oncology, Washington Univ 1995; **Fac Appt:** Asst Prof Ped, Washington Univ, St Louis

Maris, John M MD [PHO] - **Spec Exp:** Neuroblastoma; Clinical Trials; **Hospital:** Chldns Hosp of Philadelphia, The; **Address:** Chldns Hosp Philadelphia - Oncology, 34th St & Civic Ctr Blvd Abramson Bldg, Philadelphia, PA 19104-4318; **Phone:** 215-590-5244; **Board Cert:** Pediatric Hematology-Oncology 2004; **Med School:** Univ Pennsylvania 1989; **Resid:** Pediatrics, Chldns Hosp 1992; **Fellow:** Pediatric Hematology-Oncology, Chldns Hosp 1996

Meek, Rita S MD [PHO] - **Hospital:** Alfred I duPont Hosp for Children, Christiana Care Hlth Svs; **Address:** Dupont Hosp for Chldn, Div Hem/Oncology, 1600 Rockland Rd, Wilmington, DE 19899; **Phone:** 302-651-5500; **Board Cert:** Pediatrics 1979; Pediatric Hematology-Oncology 1980; **Med School:** Geo Wash Univ 1974; **Resid:** Pediatrics, Childns Hosp Natl Med Ctr 1977; **Fellow:** Pediatric Hematology-Oncology, Chldns Hosp Natl Med Ctr 1979; **Fac Appt:** Assoc Clin Prof Ped, Jefferson Med Coll

Meyers, Paul A MD [PHO] - **Spec Exp:** Pediatric Cancers; Bone Tumors; Sarcoma; **Hospital:** Meml Sloan-Kettering Cancer Ctr, NY-Presby Hosp/Weill Cornell (page 66); **Address:** 1275 York Avenue, New York, NY 10065; **Phone:** 800-525-2225; **Board Cert:** Pediatrics 1978; Pediatric Hematology-Oncology 1978; **Med School:** Mount Sinai Sch Med 1973; **Resid:** Pediatrics, Mt Sinai Hosp 1976; **Fellow:** Pediatric Hematology-Oncology, NY Hosp-Cornell Med Ctr 1979; **Fac Appt:** Prof Ped, Cornell Univ-Weill Med Coll

O'Reilly, Richard MD [PHO] - **Spec Exp:** Bone Marrow Transplant; **Hospital:** Meml Sloan-Kettering Cancer Ctr, NY-Presby Hosp/Weill Cornell (page 66); **Address:** 1275 York Avenue, New York, NY 10065; **Phone:** 800-525-2225; **Board Cert:** Pediatrics 1974; **Med School:** Univ Rochester 1968; **Resid:** Pediatrics, Chldrns Hosp 1972; **Fellow:** Infectious Disease, Chldrns Hosp 1973; **Fac Appt:** Prof Ped, Cornell Univ-Weill Med Coll

Parker, Robert MD [PHO] - **Spec Exp:** Pediatric Cancers; Bleeding/Coagulation Disorders; Platelet Disorders; Lymphoma; **Hospital:** Stony Brook Univ Med Ctr; **Address:** Stony Brook Univ Hosp, Dept Peds, HSC T-11, Rm 029, Stony Brook, NY 11794-8111; **Phone:** 631-444-7720; **Board Cert:** Pediatrics 1983; Pediatric Hematology-Oncology 1984; **Med School:** Brown Univ 1976; **Resid:** Internal Medicine, Roger Williams Med Ctr 1977; Pediatrics, Rhode Island Hosp 1979; **Fellow:** Pediatric Hematology-Oncology, Natl Cancer Inst 1981; Hematology, Natl Cancer Inst 1984; **Fac Appt:** Prof Ped, SUNY Stony Brook

Pediatric Hematology-Oncology

Rausen, Aaron R MD [PHO] - **Spec Exp:** Leukemia & Lymphoma; Bone Tumors; Retinoblastoma; **Hospital:** NYU Langone Med Ctr (page 67), Lenox Hill Hosp (page 62); **Address:** NYU Medical Ctr, 160 E 32nd St Fl 2, New York, NY 10016; **Phone:** 212-263-7144; **Board Cert:** Pediatrics 1960; Pediatric Hematology-Oncology 1974; **Med School:** SUNY Downstate 1954; **Resid:** Pediatrics, Bellevue Hosp 1956; Pediatrics, Mount Sinai 1959; **Fellow:** Hematology, Chldns Hosp 1961; **Fac Appt:** Prof Ped, NYU Sch Med

Reaman, Gregory MD [PHO] - **Spec Exp:** Leukemia; Lymphoma; Cancer Survivors-Late Effects of Therapy; **Hospital:** Chldns Natl Med Ctr; **Address:** 111 Michigan Ave NW, Washington, DC 20010-2916; **Phone:** 202-476-2800; **Board Cert:** Pediatrics 1978; Pediatric Hematology-Oncology 1978; **Med School:** Loyola Univ-Stritch Sch Med 1973; **Resid:** Hematology, Montreal Chldns Hosp 1975; Pediatrics, Montreal Chldns Hosp 1976; **Fellow:** Pediatric Oncology, Natl Cancer Inst 1979; **Fac Appt:** Prof Ped, Geo Wash Univ

Rheingold, Susan R MD [PHO] - **Spec Exp:** Leukemia; Clinical Trials; **Hospital:** Chldns Hosp of Philadelphia, The; **Address:** Chldns Hosp Phila - Div Oncology, 34th & Civic Ctr Blvd, Philadelphia, PA 19104; **Phone:** 215-590-3025; **Board Cert:** Pediatrics 2003; Pediatric Hematology-Oncology 2008; **Med School:** Univ Pennsylvania 1992; **Resid:** Pediatrics, Johns Hopkins Hosp 1995; **Fellow:** Pediatric Hematology-Oncology, Chldns Hosp 1999; **Fac Appt:** Asst Prof Ped, Univ Pennsylvania

Ritchey, A Kim MD [PHO] - **Spec Exp:** Leukemia; Bleeding/Coagulation Disorders; **Hospital:** Chldns Hosp of Pittsburgh - UPMC; **Address:** Chldns Hosp, Div Hematology/Oncology, 3705 Fifth Ave, Desoto Wing 4B, Ste 385, Pittsburgh, PA 15213; **Phone:** 412-692-5055; **Board Cert:** Pediatrics 1977; Pediatric Hematology-Oncology 2007; **Med School:** Univ Cincinnati 1972; **Resid:** Pediatrics, Johns Hopkins Hosp 1975; **Fellow:** Pediatric Hematology-Oncology, Yale-New Haven Hosp 1980; **Fac Appt:** Prof Ped, Univ Pittsburgh

Shafer, Frank E MD [PHO] - **Spec Exp:** Bleeding/Coagulation Disorders; Anemia; Thrombotic Disorders; Hemophilia; **Hospital:** St Christopher's Hosp for Chldn, St Luke's Hosp - Bethlehem; **Address:** St Christophers Hosp, Hematology, Erie Ave at Front St Fl 2, Philadelphia, PA 19134-1095; **Phone:** 215-427-5096; **Board Cert:** Pediatrics 2007; Pediatric Hematology-Oncology 2007; **Med School:** Creighton Univ 1983; **Resid:** Pediatrics, Univ Colo HSC 1986; **Fellow:** Pediatric Hematology-Oncology, Chldns Natl Med Ctr 1990; **Fac Appt:** Assoc Prof Ped, Drexel Univ Coll Med

Steinherz, Peter G MD [PHO] - **Spec Exp:** Leukemia & Lymphoma; Pediatric Cancers; Wilms' Tumor; **Hospital:** Meml Sloan-Kettering Cancer Ctr, NY-Presby Hosp/Weill Cornell (page 66); **Address:** 1275 York Avenue, New York, NY 10065; **Phone:** 800-525-2225; **Board Cert:** Pediatrics 1973; Pediatric Hematology-Oncology 1978; **Med School:** Albert Einstein Coll Med 1968; **Resid:** Pediatrics, NY Hosp-Cornell 1971; **Fellow:** Pediatric Hematology-Oncology, NY Hosp-Cornell 1975; **Fac Appt:** Prof Ped, Cornell Univ-Weill Med Coll

Weinblatt, Mark E MD [PHO] - **Spec Exp:** Leukemia & Lymphoma; Sickle Cell Disease; Bleeding/Coagulation Disorders; Thalassemia; **Hospital:** Winthrop - Univ Hosp; **Address:** Winthrop Univ Hosp, 120 Mineola Blvd, Ste 460, Mineola, NY 11501; **Phone:** 516-663-9400; **Board Cert:** Pediatrics 1980; Pediatric Hematology-Oncology 1982; **Med School:** Albert Einstein Coll Med 1976; **Resid:** Pediatrics, Jacobi Med Ctr 1979; **Fellow:** Pediatric Hematology-Oncology, Children's Hosp 1981; **Fac Appt:** Prof Ped, SUNY Stony Brook

Weiner, Michael MD [PHO] - **Spec Exp:** Hodgkin's Disease; Lymphoma; Leukemia; **Hospital:** NY-Presby Hosp/Columbia (page 66); **Address:** 161 Fort Washington Ave, Irving Pavilion-FL 7, New York, NY 10032-3710; **Phone:** 212-305-9770; **Board Cert:** Pediatrics 1980; Pediatric Hematology-Oncology 1980; **Med School:** SUNY Hlth Sci Ctr 1972; **Resid:** Pediatrics, Montefiore Med Ctr 1974; **Fellow:** Pediatric Hematology-Oncology, NYU Med Ctr 1976; Pediatric Hematology-Oncology, Johns Hopkins Hosp 1977; **Fac Appt:** Prof Ped, Columbia P&S

Wexler, Leonard MD [PHO] - **Spec Exp:** Rhabdomyosarcoma; Bone Cancer; Gastrointestinal Stromal Tumors; Sarcoma-Soft Tissue; **Hospital:** Meml Sloan-Kettering Cancer Ctr; **Address:** 1275 York Avenue, New York, NY 10065; **Phone:** 800-525-2225; **Board Cert:** Pediatrics 2000; Pediatric Hematology-Oncology 2000; **Med School:** Boston Univ 1985; **Resid:** Pediatrics, Montefiore Med Ctr 1988; **Fellow:** Pediatric Hematology-Oncology, National Cancer Inst 1991; **Fac Appt:** Assoc Prof Ped, Columbia P&S

Wolfe, Lawrence C MD [PHO] - **Spec Exp:** Leukemia; Neuro-Oncology; Cancer Survivors-Late Effects of Therapy; Transfusion Medicine; **Hospital:** Long Island Jewish Med Ctr; **Address:** LIJ Medical Ctr, Div Pediatric Hematology/Oncology, 269-01 76th Ave, New Hyde Park, NY 11040; **Phone:** 718-470-3460; **Board Cert:** Pediatrics 1981; Pediatric Hematology-Oncology 1987; **Med School:** Harvard Med Sch 1976; **Resid:** Pediatrics, Chldns Hosp 1978; **Fellow:** Pediatric Hematology-Oncology, Chldns Hosp 1991

Southeast

Barredo, Julio C MD [PHO] - **Spec Exp:** Cancer Survivors-Late Effects of Therapy; Clinical Trials; **Hospital:** Univ of Miami Hosp & Clins/Sylvester Comp Canc Ctr (page 70); **Address:** Dept Pediatrics, R131 PO Box 016960, Miami, FL 33136; **Phone:** 305-585-5635; **Board Cert:** Pediatric Hematology-Oncology 2007; **Med School:** Peru 1982; **Resid:** Pediatrics, Kings Co Hosp 1987; **Fellow:** Pediatric Hematology-Oncology, Chldns Hosp/USC 1988; **Fac Appt:** Prof Ped, Univ Miami Sch Med

Bertolone, Salvatore MD [PHO] - **Spec Exp:** Bone Marrow Transplant; Kasabach-Merritt Syndrome (KMS); Sickle Cell Disease; **Hospital:** Kosair Chldn's Hosp, Norton Hosp; **Address:** Kosair Childrens Hosp, Dept Ped Hem/Onc, 601 Floyd St, rm 403, Louisville, KY 40202-3820; **Phone:** 502-629-7750; **Board Cert:** Pediatrics 1975; Pediatric Hematology-Oncology 1976; **Med School:** Univ Louisville Sch Med 1970; **Resid:** Pediatrics, Univ Louisville 1972; **Fellow:** Pediatric Hematology-Oncology, Univ Colorado 1974; **Fac Appt:** Prof Ped, Univ Louisville Sch Med

Blatt, Julie MD [PHO] - **Spec Exp:** Neuroblastoma; Cancer Survivors-Late Effects of Therapy; **Hospital:** Univ NC Hosps; **Address:** UNC, Dept Ped Hematology Oncology, CB 7236, Chapel Hill, NC 27599-7236; **Phone:** 919-966-1178; **Board Cert:** Pediatrics 1981; Pediatric Hematology-Oncology 1982; **Med School:** Johns Hopkins Univ 1976; **Resid:** Pediatrics, Columbia-Presby Hosp 1978; **Fellow:** Pediatric Oncology, Natl Cancer Inst 1982; **Fac Appt:** Prof Ped, Univ NC Sch Med

Castellino, Sharon M MD [PHO] - **Spec Exp:** Cancer Survivors-Late Effects of Therapy; Leukemia; Lymphoma; **Hospital:** Brenner Chldn's Hosp; **Address:** Wake Forest Univ Baptist Med Ctr, Div Pediatric Hematology/Oncology, Medical Center Blvd, Winston-Salem, NC 27157; **Phone:** 336-716-4324; **Board Cert:** Pediatrics 2003; Pediatric Hematology-Oncology 2006; **Med School:** Duke Univ 1992; **Resid:** Pediatrics, Childrens Hosp 1994; Pediatrics, Duke Univ Med Ctr 1995; **Fellow:** Pediatric Hematology-Oncology, Duke Univ 1997; **Fac Appt:** Asst Prof Ped, Wake Forest Univ

Frangoul, Haydar A MD [PHO] - **Spec Exp:** Stem Cell Transplant; **Hospital:** Vanderbilt Univ Med Ctr; **Address:** Ped Hem/Onc Clinic, 2200 Children's Way, Nashville, TN 37232-6310; **Phone:** 615-936-1762; **Board Cert:** Pediatric Hematology-Oncology 2008; **Med School:** Amer Univ Beirut 1990; **Resid:** Pediatrics, Duke Univ Med Ctr 1993; **Fellow:** Pediatric Hematology-Oncology, Duke Univ Med Ctr 1994; **Fac Appt:** Assoc Prof Ped, Vanderbilt Univ

Pediatric Hematology-Oncology

Friedman, Debra L MD [PHO] - **Spec Exp:** Cancer Survivors-Late Effects of Therapy; Hodgkin's Disease; Retinoblastoma; **Hospital:** Vanderbilt Children's Hosp, Vanderbilt Univ Med Ctr; **Address:** Vanderbilt Univ Med Ctr, 2525 West End Ave Fl 6 - Ste 600, Nashville, TN 37232; **Phone:** 615-322-4708; **Board Cert:** Pediatric Hematology-Oncology 2006; **Med School:** UMDNJ-RW Johnson Med Sch 1991; **Resid:** Pediatrics, Chldns Hosp 1994; **Fellow:** Pediatric Hematology-Oncology, Chldns Hosp 1997; **Fac Appt:** Asst Prof Ped, Vanderbilt Univ

Friedman, Henry S MD [PHO] - **Spec Exp:** Neuro-Oncology; Brain & Spinal Cord Tumors; **Hospital:** Duke Univ Med Ctr; **Address:** Preston Robert Tisch, Brain Tumor Ctr at Duke, DUMC, Box 3624, Durham, NC 27710; **Phone:** 919-684-5301; **Board Cert:** Pediatrics 1982; Pediatric Hematology-Oncology 1982; **Med School:** SUNY Upstate Med Univ 1977; **Resid:** Pediatrics, SUNY Upstate Med Ctr 1980; **Fellow:** Pediatric Hematology-Oncology, Duke Univ Med Ctr 1983; **Fac Appt:** Prof Ped, Duke Univ

Furman, Wayne L MD [PHO] - **Spec Exp:** Neuroblastoma; Liver Cancer; Drug Development; **Hospital:** St Jude Children's Research Hosp; **Address:** St Jude Children's Research Hospital, 332 N Lauderdale St, MS 260, Memphis, TN 38105; **Phone:** 901-595-2800; **Board Cert:** Pediatrics 1985; Pediatric Hematology-Oncology 1987; **Med School:** Ohio State Univ 1979; **Resid:** Pediatrics, Children's Hosp 1983; **Fellow:** Pediatric Hematology-Oncology, St Jude Chldn's Rsch Hosp 1985; **Fac Appt:** Prof Ped, Univ Tenn Coll Med, Memphis

Gajjar, Amar J MD [PHO] - **Spec Exp:** Brain Tumors; Medulloblastoma; Neuro-Oncology; Drug Development; **Hospital:** St Jude Children's Research Hosp; **Address:** St Judes Children's Hosp, Dept Oncology, 262 Danny Thomas Pl, rm C6024, MS 260, Memphis, TN 38105-2794; **Phone:** 901-495-4599; **Board Cert:** Pediatric Hematology-Oncology 2007; **Med School:** India 1984; **Resid:** Pediatrics, All Chldns Hosp 1989; **Fellow:** Hematology & Oncology, St Jude Chldns Hosp 1990; **Fac Appt:** Prof Ped, Univ Tenn Coll Med, Memphis

Godder, Kamar MD/PhD [PHO] - **Spec Exp:** Stem Cell Transplant; Leukemia; Palliative Care; **Hospital:** Med Coll of VA Hosp; **Address:** PO Box 980121, Richmond, VA 23219; **Phone:** 804-828-9605; **Board Cert:** Pediatric Hematology-Oncology 2005; **Med School:** Israel 1980; **Resid:** Pediatrics, Hadassah-Mt Scopus 1984; **Fellow:** Pediatric Hematology-Oncology, Meml Sloan Kettering Cancer Ctr 1988; **Fac Appt:** Prof Ped, Va Commonwealth Univ Sch Med

Gold, Stuart H MD [PHO] - **Spec Exp:** Leukemia; Brain Tumors; Cancer Survivors-Late Effects of Therapy; **Hospital:** Univ NC Hosps; **Address:** Univ of NC at Chapel Hill, Dept Ped Hem-Onc, CB# 7236 POB 1185A Bldg, Chapel Hill, NC 27599-7236; **Phone:** 919-966-1178; **Board Cert:** Pediatrics 1986; Pediatric Hematology-Oncology 1987; **Med School:** Vanderbilt Univ 1981; **Resid:** Pediatrics, Univ Colorado Hlth Sci Ctr 1984; **Fellow:** Pediatric Hematology-Oncology, Univ Colorado Hlth Sci Ctr 1989; **Fac Appt:** Prof Ped, Univ NC Sch Med

Green, Daniel M MD [PHO] - **Spec Exp:** Wilms' Tumor; Fertility in Cancer Survivors; Cancer Survivors-Late Effects of Therapy; **Hospital:** St Jude Children's Research Hosp; **Address:** Dept Epidemiology & Cancer Control, St Jude Chldn's Rsch Hosp, 332 N Lauderdale St, MS 735, Memphis, TN 38105-2794; **Phone:** 901-595-5915; **Board Cert:** Pediatrics 1986; Pediatric Hematology-Oncology 1997; **Med School:** St Louis Univ 1973; **Resid:** Pediatrics, Boston City Hosp 1975; **Fellow:** Pediatric Hematology-Oncology, Chldns Hosp Med Ctr 1978

Hudson, Melissa M MD [PHO] - **Spec Exp:** Cancer Survivors-Late Effects of Therapy; Hodgkin's Disease; **Hospital:** St Jude Children's Research Hosp; **Address:** St Jude Children's Research Hosp, 262 Danny Thomas Pl, MS 735, Memphis, TN 38105; **Phone:** 901-495-3384; **Board Cert:** Pediatrics 1988; Pediatric Hematology-Oncology 2006; **Med School:** Univ Tex SW, Dallas 1983; **Resid:** Pediatrics, Univ Texas Affil Hosps 1986; **Fellow:** Pediatric Hematology-Oncology, MD Anderson Cancer Ctr 1989

Johnston, J Martin MD [PHO] - **Spec Exp:** Leukemia; Lymphoma; Hemophilia; **Hospital:** Meml Hlth Univ Med Ctr - Savannah; **Address:** Backus Children's Hosp Outpatient Ctr, 4700 Waters Ave, PO Box 23089, Savannah, GA 31403-3089; **Phone:** 912-350-8194; **Board Cert:** Pediatric Hematology-Oncology 2002; **Med School:** Duke Univ 1984; **Resid:** Pediatrics, Univ Utah Med Ctr 1988; **Fellow:** Pediatric Hematology-Oncology, Barnes Jewish Hosp 1991

Kane, Javier R MD [PHO] - **Spec Exp:** Palliative Care; **Hospital:** St Jude Children's Research Hosp; **Address:** St Jude Chldns Rsch Hosp, Dept Oncology, 262 Danny Thomas Pl, MS 260, Memphis, TN 38105-2794; **Phone:** 901-495-4152; **Board Cert:** Pediatrics 2007; Pediatric Hematology-Oncology 2004; **Med School:** Mexico 1986; **Resid:** Pediatrics, Austin Med Ed Prog 1992; **Fellow:** Pediatric Hematology-Oncology, Univ Tennessee

Keller Jr, Frank G MD [PHO] - **Spec Exp:** Leukemia; Hodgkin's Disease; **Hospital:** Chldns Hlthcare Atlanta @ Egleston; **Address:** Emory Childrens Ctr-Aflac Cancer Ctr, 2015 Uppergate Drive NE Fl 4, Atlanta, GA 30322; **Phone:** 404-785-1200; **Board Cert:** Pediatric Hematology-Oncology 2002; **Med School:** Univ NC Sch Med 1986; **Resid:** Pediatrics, Vanderbilt Univ Med Ctr 1990; **Fellow:** Pediatric Hematology-Oncology, Duke Univ Med Ctr 1993; **Fac Appt:** Assoc Prof Ped, Emory Univ

Kreissman, Susan G MD [PHO] - **Spec Exp:** Neuroblastoma; Clinical Trials; **Hospital:** Duke Univ Med Ctr; **Address:** Duke Univ Med Ctr, Box 2916, Durham, NC 27710; **Phone:** 919-684-3401; **Board Cert:** Pediatric Hematology-Oncology 2004; **Med School:** Mount Sinai Sch Med 1985; **Resid:** Pediatrics, Chldns Hosp 1988; **Fellow:** Pediatric Hematology-Oncology, Chldns Hosp/Dana Farber Cancer Inst 1991; **Fac Appt:** Assoc Prof Ped, Duke Univ

Kurtzberg, Joanne MD [PHO] - **Spec Exp:** Stem Cell Transplant; Bone Marrow Transplant; **Hospital:** Duke Univ Med Ctr; **Address:** Duke Univ Med Ctr, Box 3350, Durham, NC 27710; **Phone:** 919-668-1100; **Board Cert:** Pediatrics 1982; Pediatric Hematology-Oncology 1982; **Med School:** NY Med Coll 1976; **Resid:** Pediatrics, Dartmouth Med Ctr 1977; Pediatrics, Upstate Med Ctr 1979; **Fellow:** Pediatric Hematology-Oncology, Upstate Med Ctr 1980; Pediatric Hematology-Oncology, Duke Med Ctr 1983; **Fac Appt:** Prof Ped, Duke Univ

Kuttesch, John F MD [PHO] - **Spec Exp:** Brain Tumors; Brain Tumors-Recurrent; **Hospital:** Vanderbilt Children's Hosp; **Address:** Vanderbilt Pediatric Hem/Oncology, 2220 Pierce Ave, Rm 397 PRB, Nashville, TN 37232-6310; **Phone:** 615-936-1762; **Board Cert:** Pediatric Hematology-Oncology 2007; **Med School:** Univ Tex, Houston 1985; **Resid:** Pediatrics, Vanderbilt Univ Med Ctr 1988; **Fellow:** Pediatric Hematology-Oncology, St Judes Chldns Hosp 1992; **Fac Appt:** Assoc Prof Ped, Vanderbilt Univ

Laver, Joseph MD [PHO] - **Spec Exp:** Stem Cell Transplant; Lymphoma, Non-Hodgkin's; **Hospital:** St Jude Children's Research Hosp; **Address:** St. Jude's Chldns Rsch Hosp, rm C-7045E, MS 282, 262 Danny Thomas Pl, Memphis, TN 38105-3678; **Phone:** 901-595-3532; **Board Cert:** Pediatrics 1985; Pediatric Hematology-Oncology 1987; **Med School:** Israel 1979; **Resid:** Pediatrics, Assaf Harofeh Med Ctr 1979; **Fellow:** Pediatric Hematology-Oncology, Meml Sloan Kettering 1985

Moscow, Jeffrey A MD [PHO] - **Spec Exp:** Pediatric Cancers; **Hospital:** Univ of Kentucky Chandler Hosp; **Address:** Univ Kentucky - Kentucky Clinic, 740 S Limestone, rm J457, Lexington, KY 40536-0001; **Phone:** 859-257-4554; **Board Cert:** Pediatrics 1988; Pediatric Hematology-Oncology 2007; **Med School:** Dartmouth Med Sch 1982; **Resid:** Pediatrics, Univ Texas SW Med Ctr 1985; **Fellow:** Pediatric Hematology-Oncology, Natl Cancer Inst 1986; **Fac Appt:** Prof Ped, Univ KY Coll Med

Pediatric Hematology-Oncology

Neuberg, Ronnie W MD [PHO] - **Spec Exp:** Pediatric Cancers; Gene Therapy; Clinical Trials; Brain Tumors; **Hospital:** Palmetto Richland Mem Hosp, MUSC Chldns Hosp; **Address:** Palmetto Health Richland, 7 Richland Medical Park Drive, Ste 7215, Columbia, SC 29203; **Phone:** 803-434-3533; **Board Cert:** Pediatrics 1982; Pediatric Hematology-Oncology 1982; **Med School:** SUNY Buffalo 1977; **Resid:** Pediatrics, Chldns Hosp 1980; **Fellow:** Pediatric Hematology-Oncology, SUNY Upstate Med Ctr 1982; **Fac Appt:** Assoc Prof Ped, Univ SC Sch Med

Nieder, Michael L MD [PHO] - **Spec Exp:** Bone Marrow Transplant; **Hospital:** All Children's Hosp; **Address:** 801 6th St S, Dept 7865, St Petersburg, FL 33701-4816; **Phone:** 727-767-6856; **Board Cert:** Pediatrics 1986; Pediatric Hematology-Oncology 1987; **Med School:** Univ IL Coll Med 1982; **Resid:** Pediatrics, Children's Meml Hosp 1985; **Fellow:** Pediatric Hematology-Oncology, Children's Meml Hosp 1988; **Fac Appt:** Prof Ped, Univ S Fla Coll Med

Olson, Thomas A MD [PHO] - **Spec Exp:** Platelet Disorders; Sarcoma; Brain Tumors; **Hospital:** Chldns Hlthcare Atlanta @ Egleston; **Address:** Emory Childrens Ctr-Aflac Cancer Ctr, 2015 Uppergate Drive NE Fl 4, Atlanta, GA 30322; **Phone:** 404-785-1200; **Board Cert:** Pediatrics 1982; Pediatric Hematology-Oncology 1984; **Med School:** Loyola Univ-Stritch Sch Med 1978; **Resid:** Pediatrics, Walter Reed AMC 1981; **Fellow:** Pediatric Hematology-Oncology, Walter Reed AMC 1983; **Fac Appt:** Assoc Prof Ped, Emory Univ

Pui, Ching-Hon MD [PHO] - **Spec Exp:** Leukemia; Lymphoma; **Hospital:** St Jude Children's Research Hosp; **Address:** St Jude Chldns Rsch Hosp, 332 N Lauderdale St, Memphis, TN 38105; **Phone:** 901-495-3335; **Board Cert:** Pediatrics 1980; Pediatric Hematology-Oncology 1982; **Med School:** Taiwan 1976; **Resid:** Pediatrics, St Jude Chldns Rsch Hosp 1979; **Fellow:** Hematology & Oncology, St Jude Chldns Rsch Hosp 1981; **Fac Appt:** Prof Ped, Univ Tenn Coll Med, Memphis

Rosoff, Philip M MD [PHO] - **Spec Exp:** Cancer Survivors-Late Effects of Therapy; Down Syndrome; Leukemia; **Hospital:** Duke Univ Med Ctr; **Address:** Duke Univ Med Ctr, Box 2916, Durham, NC 27710-0001; **Phone:** 919-684-3401; **Board Cert:** Pediatrics 1984; Pediatric Hematology-Oncology 2002; **Med School:** Case West Res Univ 1978; **Resid:** Pediatrics, Chldns Hosp 1980; **Fellow:** Pediatric Hematology-Oncology, Chldns Hosp/Dana Farber Cancer Inst 1984; **Fac Appt:** Assoc Prof Ped, Duke Univ

Sandler, Eric MD [PHO] - **Spec Exp:** Bone Marrow Transplant; Leukemia; Clinical Trials; **Hospital:** Wolfson Chldns Hosp; **Address:** 807 Childrens Way, Jacksonville, FL 32207; **Phone:** 904-390-3793; **Board Cert:** Pediatric Hematology-Oncology 2007; Pediatrics 2008; **Med School:** Univ VT Coll Med 1985; **Resid:** Pediatrics, UCSF Med Ctr 1988; **Fellow:** Pediatric Hematology-Oncology, Univ Fla Med Sch 1991; **Fac Appt:** Assoc Prof Ped, Mayo Med Sch

Sandlund Jr, John T MD [PHO] - **Spec Exp:** Lymphoma, Non-Hodgkin's; Leukemia & Lymphoma; Ataxia Telangiectasia; **Hospital:** St Jude Children's Research Hosp, Le Bonheur Chldns Med Ctr; **Address:** St Jude Children's Research Hosp, 262 Danny Thomas Pl, MS 260, Memphis, TN 38105; **Phone:** 901-595-2153; **Board Cert:** Pediatrics 1986; Pediatric Hematology-Oncology 1987; **Med School:** Ohio State Univ 1980; **Resid:** Pediatrics, Columbus Chldns Hosp 1983; **Fellow:** Hematology, Natl Cancer Inst 1986; Research, Natl Cancer Inst 1987

Santana, Victor M MD [PHO] - **Spec Exp:** Solid Tumors; **Hospital:** St Jude Children's Research Hosp; **Address:** St Jude Chldn's Rsch Hosp, Dept Oncology, 226 Danny Thomas Pl, rm C6041, MS 260, Memphis, TN 38105-2794; **Phone:** 901-495-2424; **Board Cert:** Pediatrics 1982; Pediatric Hematology-Oncology 1984; **Med School:** Puerto Rico 1978; **Resid:** Pediatrics, Johns Hopkins Hosp 1981; **Fellow:** Pediatric Hematology-Oncology, Johns Hopkins Hosp 1984

Shearer, Patricia C MD [PHO] - **Spec Exp:** Wilms' Tumor; Cancer Survivors-Late Effects of Therapy; **Hospital:** Shands at Univ of FL; **Address:** Univ Florida HSC, Div Ped Hem/Oncology, PO Box 100296, Gainesville, FL 32610; **Phone:** 352-392-5633; **Board Cert:** Pediatric Hematology-Oncology 2007; **Med School:** Louisiana State U, New Orleans 1986; **Resid:** Pediatrics, Johns Hopkins Hosp 1989; **Fellow:** Hematology & Oncology, St Jude Chldns Rsch Hosp 1992

Tebbi, Cameron MD [PHO] - **Spec Exp:** Hemophilia; Hodgkin's Disease; Leukemia; Sickle Cell Disease; **Hospital:** St Josephs Chldns Hosp, Tampa Genl Hosp; **Address:** 3001 W Martin Luther King Jr Blvd, Tampa, FL 33607; **Phone:** 813-870-4286; **Board Cert:** Pediatrics 1974; Pediatric Hematology-Oncology 1980; **Med School:** Iran 1968; **Resid:** Pediatrics, Cincinnati Chldns Hosp 1972; Pediatric Hematology-Oncology, MD Anderson Cancer Inst 1972; **Fellow:** Pediatric Hematology-Oncology, St Louis Chldns Hosp 1973; Medical Oncology, Ontario Cancer Inst 1974

Wang, Winfred C MD [PHO] - **Spec Exp:** Sickle Cell Disease; Bone Marrow Failure Disorders; Anemia-Aplastic; **Hospital:** St Jude Children's Research Hosp, Le Bonheur Chldns Med Ctr; **Address:** St Jude Chldn Rsch Hosp, 262 Danny Thomas Pl, rm R5036, Memphis, TN 38105-2729; **Phone:** 901-595-3497; **Board Cert:** Pediatrics 1972; Pediatric Hematology-Oncology 1974; **Med School:** Univ Chicago-Pritzker Sch Med 1967; **Resid:** Pediatrics, Montefiore Med Ctr 1969; Pediatrics, Kauikeolani Chldns Hosp 1970; **Fellow:** Pediatric Hematology-Oncology, UCSF 1975; **Fac Appt:** Prof Ped, Univ Tenn Coll Med, Memphis

Whitlock, James A MD [PHO] - **Spec Exp:** Leukemia; Drug Development; **Hospital:** Vanderbilt Children's Hosp, Vanderbilt Univ Med Ctr; **Address:** Vanderbilt Univ Med Ctr, Dept Peds, 2220 Pierce Ave, rm 397 PRB, Nashville, TN 37232-6310; **Phone:** 615-936-1762; **Board Cert:** Pediatric Hematology-Oncology 2007; **Med School:** Vanderbilt Univ 1984; **Resid:** Pediatrics, Vanderbilt Univ Med Ctr 1987; **Fellow:** Pediatric Hematology-Oncology, Vanderbilt Univ Med Ctr 1990; **Fac Appt:** Assoc Prof Ped, Vanderbilt Univ

Woods, William G MD [PHO] - **Spec Exp:** Leukemia; Neuroblastoma; **Hospital:** Chldns Hlthcare Atlanta @ Egleston, Chldns Hlthcare Atlanta - Scottish Rite; **Address:** AFLAC Cancer Ctr & Blood Disorders Svc, 2015 Uppergate Drive, rm 404, Atlanta, GA 30322; **Phone:** 404-785-6170; **Board Cert:** Pediatrics 1976; Pediatric Hematology-Oncology 1978; **Med School:** Univ Pennsylvania 1972; **Resid:** Pediatrics, Univ Minnesota Hosps 1975; **Fellow:** Hematology, Univ Minnesota Hosps 1977; **Fac Appt:** Prof Ped, Emory Univ

Midwest

Arndt, Carola A MD [PHO] - **Spec Exp:** Sarcoma; Brain Tumors; Stem Cell Transplant; **Hospital:** Mayo Med Ctr & Clin - Rochester; **Address:** Mayo Clinic, Dept Pediatrics, 200 1st St SW, Rochester, MN 55905; **Phone:** 507-284-2652; **Board Cert:** Pediatrics 1982; Pediatric Hematology-Oncology 1987; **Med School:** Boston Univ 1978; **Resid:** Pediatrics, Naval Reg Med Ctr 1981; **Fellow:** Pediatric Hematology-Oncology, Natl Inst Hlth 1984

Beyer, Eric C MD/PhD [PHO] - **Spec Exp:** Stem Cell Transplant; Bleeding/Coagulation Disorders; Pediatric Cancers; Anemia; **Hospital:** Univ of Chicago Med Ctr; **Address:** University of Chicago Hospitals, 5841 S Maryland Ave, MC-4060, Chicago, IL 60637; **Phone:** 773-702-8547; **Board Cert:** Pediatrics 1987; **Med School:** UCSD 1982; **Resid:** Pediatrics, Children's Hosp 1984; **Fellow:** Hematology & Oncology, Dana Farber Cancer Inst 1987; **Fac Appt:** Prof Ped, Univ Chicago-Pritzker Sch Med

Pediatric Hematology-Oncology

Boxer, Laurence MD [PHO] - **Spec Exp:** Congenital Neutropenia-Severe; Anemias & Red Cell Disorders; Thrombotic Disorders; Anemia-Aplastic; **Hospital:** Univ Michigan Hlth Sys; **Address:** Univ Michigan, L-2110 Womens Hosp, 1500 E Medical Ctr Dr, Box 0238, Ann Arbor, MI 48109-0238; **Phone:** 734-764-7127; **Board Cert:** Pediatrics 1971; Pediatric Hematology-Oncology 1974; **Med School:** Stanford Univ 1966; **Resid:** Pediatrics, Yale-New Haven Hosp 1968; Pediatrics, Stanford Univ Hosp 1969; **Fellow:** Hematology, Chldns Hosp-Harvard 1974; **Fac Appt:** Prof Ped, Univ Mich Med Sch

Camitta, Bruce M MD [PHO] - **Spec Exp:** Leukemia; Anemia-Aplastic; Bone Marrow Transplant; **Hospital:** Chldns Hosp - Wisconsin; **Address:** Midwest Childrens Cancer Ctr, 8701 Watertown Plank Rd, Ste 3018, Milwaukee, WI 53226; **Phone:** 414-456-4170; **Board Cert:** Pediatrics 1971; Pediatric Hematology-Oncology 1976; **Med School:** Johns Hopkins Univ 1966; **Resid:** Pediatrics, Chldns Hosp 1968; Pediatrics, Johns Hopkins Hosp 1969; **Fellow:** Pediatric Hematology-Oncology, Chldns Hosp 1973; **Fac Appt:** Prof Ped, Med Coll Wisc

Castle, Valerie P MD [PHO] - **Spec Exp:** Neuroblastoma; Bleeding/Coagulation Disorders; Cancer Survivors-Late Effects of Therapy; **Hospital:** Univ Michigan Hlth Sys; **Address:** Univ Mich Comp Cancer Ctr, 1500 E Med Ctr Drive, Desk B1-358, Ann Arbor, MI 48109-0911; **Phone:** 734-936-9814; **Board Cert:** Pediatric Hematology-Oncology 2006; **Med School:** McMaster Univ 1983; **Resid:** Pediatrics, McMaster Univ Med Ctr 1986; **Fellow:** Pediatric Hematology-Oncology, Univ Mich Hosps 1989; **Fac Appt:** Prof Ped, Univ Mich Med Sch

Cohn, Susan L MD [PHO] - **Spec Exp:** Neuroblastoma; **Hospital:** Univ of Chicago Med Ctr; **Address:** Univ Chicago, 5841 S Maryland Ave, MC 4060, Chicago, IL 60637-1470; **Phone:** 773-702-2571; **Board Cert:** Pediatrics 1985; Pediatric Hematology-Oncology 1987; **Med School:** Univ IL Coll Med 1980; **Resid:** Pediatrics, Michael Reese Hosp 1984; **Fellow:** Hematology & Oncology, Chldns Meml Hosp 1985; **Fac Appt:** Prof Ped, Univ Chicago-Pritzker Sch Med

Corey, Seth J MD [PHO] - **Spec Exp:** Bone Marrow Failure Disorders; Leukemia; Myelodysplastic Syndromes; Ataxia Telangiectasia; **Hospital:** Children's Mem Hosp; **Address:** Robert Lurie Comp Cancer Ctr, Lurie 5-107, 303 E Superior St, Chicago, IL 60611; **Phone:** 312-503-6694; **Board Cert:** Pediatrics 1986; Pediatric Hematology-Oncology 2004; **Med School:** Tulane Univ 1982; **Resid:** Pediatrics, St Louis Chldns Hosp 1985; **Fellow:** Hematology & Oncology, Tufts Med Sch 1992; Research, Boston Chldns-Dana Farber Ctr 1989; **Fac Appt:** Prof Ped, Northwestern Univ-Feinberg Sch Med

Croop, James M MD/PhD [PHO] - **Spec Exp:** Rhabdomyosarcoma; Clinical Trials; **Hospital:** Riley Hosp for Children; **Address:** Riley Hosp for Children, Hem/Onc, 702 Barnhill Drive, ROC 4340, Indianapolis, IN 46202; **Phone:** 317-274-8784; **Board Cert:** Pediatrics 1985; Pediatric Hematology-Oncology 2005; **Med School:** Univ Pennsylvania 1980; **Resid:** Pediatrics, Childrens Hosp 1983; **Fellow:** Pediatric Hematology-Oncology, Childrens Hosp 1985; **Fac Appt:** Prof Ped, Indiana Univ

Davies, Stella M MD/PhD [PHO] - **Spec Exp:** Leukemia; Bone Marrow Transplant; Stem Cell Transplant; **Hospital:** Cincinnati Chldns Hosp Med Ctr; **Address:** Cincinnati Chldns Hosp Med Ctr, 3333 Burnet Ave, MLC 7015, Cincinnati, OH 45229-3039; **Phone:** 513-636-2469; **Med School:** England, UK 1981; **Resid:** Pediatrics, Univ Newcastle Med Ctr 1985; **Fellow:** Pediatric Hematology-Oncology, Univ Minn Med Ctr 1993; **Fac Appt:** Prof Ped, Univ Cincinnati

DeBaun, Michael R MD [PHO] - **Spec Exp:** Sickle Cell Disease; **Hospital:** St Louis Chldns Hosp; **Address:** St Louis Children's Hospital, One Children's Pl, Box 8116, St Louis, MO 63110; **Phone:** 314-454-6018; **Board Cert:** Pediatrics 2008; Pediatric Hematology-Oncology 2002; **Med School:** Stanford Univ 1987; **Resid:** Pediatrics, St Louis Children's Hosp 1990; **Fellow:** Pediatric Hematology-Oncology, St Louis Children's Hosp 1993; **Fac Appt:** Assoc Prof Ped, Washington Univ, St Louis

Fallon, Robert J MD/PhD [PHO] - **Spec Exp:** Lymphoma; Hodgkin's Disease; Stem Cell Transplant; **Hospital:** Riley Hosp for Children; **Address:** Riley Childrens Hospital, 702 Barnhill Drive, rm Riley 4340, Indianapolis, IN 46202; **Phone:** 317-274-8784; **Board Cert:** Internal Medicine 1983; Medical Oncology 1985; **Med School:** NYU Sch Med 1980; **Resid:** Internal Medicine, Brigham & Womens Hosp 1983; **Fellow:** Hematology & Oncology, Brigham & Womens Hosp/Dana Farber Cancer Inst 1985; **Fac Appt:** Prof Ped, Indiana Univ

Ferrara, James MD [PHO] - **Spec Exp:** Bone Marrow Transplant; Graft vs Host Disease; Inflammatory Cytokines; **Hospital:** Univ Michigan Hlth Sys; **Address:** Univ Michigan Comprehensive Cancer Ctr, 1500 E Medical Center Drive, Ste 6308, Ann Arbor, MI 48109-0942; **Phone:** 734-615-1340; **Board Cert:** Pediatrics 2005; Pediatric Hematology-Oncology 2006; **Med School:** Georgetown Univ 1980; **Resid:** Pediatrics, Children's Hosp 1982; **Fellow:** Pediatric Hematology-Oncology, Children's Hosp 1985; **Fac Appt:** Prof Ped, Univ Mich Med Sch

Friebert, Sarah E MD [PHO] - **Spec Exp:** Palliative Care; Cancer Survivors-Late Effects of Therapy; **Hospital:** Children's Hosp & Med Ctr- Akron; **Address:** Children's Hosp Med Ctr of Akron, One Perkins Sq Fl 5, Akron, OH 44308; **Phone:** 330-543-3343; **Board Cert:** Pediatrics 2004; Pediatric Hematology-Oncology 2008; **Med School:** Case West Res Univ 1993; **Resid:** Pediatrics, Chldns Hosp 1996; **Fellow:** Pediatric Hematology-Oncology, Rainbow Babies-Chldns Hosp 1999; **Fac Appt:** Asst Prof Ped, NE Ohio Univ

Goldman, Stewart MD [PHO] - **Spec Exp:** Neuro-Oncology; Brain Tumors; Clinical Trials; **Hospital:** Children's Mem Hosp; **Address:** Childrens Meml Hosp, Div Hem/Onc, 2300 Childrens Plaza, Box 30, Chicago, IL 60614; **Phone:** 773-880-3004; **Board Cert:** Pediatric Hematology-Oncology 2004; **Med School:** Loyola Univ-Stritch Sch Med 1985; **Resid:** Pediatrics, Univ Chicago Hosps 1988; **Fellow:** Pediatric Hematology-Oncology, Univ Chicago Hosps 1991

Haut, Paul R MD [PHO] - **Spec Exp:** Stem Cell Transplant; Bone Marrow Transplant; Leukemia; **Hospital:** Riley Hosp for Children; **Address:** Riley Hospital for Children, 702 Barnhill Drive, rm 4340, Indianapolis, IN 46202; **Phone:** 317-274-2143; **Board Cert:** Pediatric Hematology-Oncology 2008; **Med School:** Univ Ark 1990; **Resid:** Pediatrics, Arkansas Children's Hosp 1994; **Fellow:** Pediatric Hematology-Oncology, Children's Meml Hosp 1997; **Fac Appt:** Assoc Prof Ped, Indiana Univ

Hayani, Ammar MD [PHO] - **Spec Exp:** Leukemia; Solid Tumors; **Hospital:** Adv Christ Med Ctr, Central DuPage Hosp; **Address:** Hope Children's Hospital, 4440 W 95th St, Oak Lawn, IL 60453-2600; **Phone:** 708-684-4094; **Board Cert:** Pediatric Hematology-Oncology 2005; **Med School:** Syria 1982; **Resid:** Pediatrics, Louisiana State Univ Hosp 1987; **Fellow:** Pediatric Hematology-Oncology, Baylor Coll Med Affil Hosp 1991

Hayashi, Robert J MD [PHO] - **Spec Exp:** Bone Marrow Transplant; Cancer Survivors-Late Effects of Therapy; Leukemia; **Hospital:** St Louis Chldns Hosp; **Address:** St Louis Chldns Hosp, Div Ped Hem Onc, One Children's Pl, Ste 9 South, Campus Box 8116, St Louis, MO 63110; **Phone:** 314-454-6018; **Board Cert:** Pediatrics 2007; Pediatric Hematology-Oncology 2007; **Med School:** Washington Univ, St Louis 1986; **Resid:** Pediatrics, St Louis Childrens Hosp 1989; **Fellow:** Pediatric Hematology-Oncology, Johns Hopkins Hosp 1992; **Fac Appt:** Assoc Prof Ped, Washington Univ, St Louis

Hetherington, Maxine MD [PHO] - **Spec Exp:** Brain Tumors; **Hospital:** Chldns Mercy Hosps & Clinics; **Address:** Childrens Mercy Hosptial, 2401 Gillham Rd, Kansas City, MO 64108; **Phone:** 816-234-3265; **Board Cert:** Pediatrics 1983; Pediatric Hematology-Oncology 1987; **Med School:** Univ Tenn Coll Med, Memphis 1978; **Resid:** Pediatrics, Childrens Med Ctr 1981; **Fellow:** Pediatric Hematology-Oncology, Univ Texas Hlth Sci Ctr 1987; **Fac Appt:** Assoc Prof Ped, Univ MO-Kansas City

Pediatric Hematology-Oncology

Hilden, Joanne M MD [PHO] - **Spec Exp:** Brain Tumors; Leukemia & Lymphoma; Bone Tumors; Soft Tissue Tumors; **Hospital:** St Vincent Indianapolis Hosp; **Address:** Peyton Manning Children's Hospital, at St Vincent, 8402 Harcourt Rd, Ste 603, Indianapolis, IN 46260; **Phone:** 317-338-4673; **Board Cert:** Pediatrics 2006; Pediatric Hematology-Oncology 2002; Hospice & Palliative Medicine 2008; **Med School:** Univ Minn 1988; **Resid:** Pediatrics, Univ Minn Med Ctr 1991; **Fellow:** Pediatric Hematology-Oncology, Univ Minn Med Ctr 1994; **Fac Appt:** Assoc Prof Ped, Indiana Univ

Hord, Jeffrey D MD [PHO] - **Spec Exp:** Hematologic Malignancies; Bone Marrow Failure Disorders; Sickle Cell Disease; Pediatric Cancers; **Hospital:** Children's Hosp & Med Ctr- Akron; **Address:** Akron Childrens Hosp, Hematology/Oncology, One Perkins Square, Akron, OH 44308; **Phone:** 330-543-8580; **Board Cert:** Pediatric Hematology-Oncology 2004; **Med School:** Univ KY Coll Med 1989; **Resid:** Pediatrics, Childrens Hosp 1992; **Fellow:** Pediatric Hematology-Oncology, Vanderbilt Univ Med Ctr 1995; **Fac Appt:** Prof Ped, NE Ohio Univ

Hutchinson, Raymond MD [PHO] - **Spec Exp:** Leukemia; Hodgkin's Disease; **Hospital:** Univ Michigan Hlth Sys; **Address:** Univ Michigan Hosp, 1500 E Med Ctr Drive, rm L2110, Flr 1-Recep B1, Ann Arbor, MI 48109-5238; **Phone:** 734-763-6336; **Board Cert:** Pediatrics 1979; Pediatric Hematology-Oncology 1980; **Med School:** Harvard Med Sch 1973; **Resid:** Pediatrics, New England Med Ctr 1975; **Fellow:** Pediatric Hematology-Oncology, Childrens Hosp 1978; **Fac Appt:** Prof Ped, Univ Mich Med Sch

Lusher, Jeanne M MD [PHO] - **Hospital:** Chldns Hosp of Michigan; **Address:** Children's Hospital Michigan, Div Hem/Onc, 3901 Beaubien Blvd, Detroit, MI 48201; **Phone:** 313-745-5515; **Board Cert:** Pediatrics 1986; Pediatric Hematology-Oncology 1986; **Med School:** Univ Cincinnati 1960; **Resid:** Pediatrics, Charity Hosp/Tulane Univ 1963; **Fellow:** Hematology & Oncology, Charity Hosp/Tulane Univ 1965; Hematology & Oncology, Saint Louis Children's Hosp 1966; **Fac Appt:** Prof Ped, Wayne State Univ

Manera, Ricarchito B MD [PHO] - **Spec Exp:** Leukemia; Brain Tumors; Lymphoma; **Hospital:** Loyola Univ Med Ctr; **Address:** Loyola University Med Ctr, 2160 S First Ave, Maywood, IL 60611; **Phone:** 708-327-9136; **Board Cert:** Pediatrics 2003; Pediatric Hematology-Oncology 2004; **Med School:** Philippines 1984; **Resid:** Pediatrics, Bronx-Lebanon Hosp Ctr 1995; **Fellow:** Pediatric Hematology-Oncology, MD Anderson Cancer Ctr 1994; Pediatric Hematology-Oncology, Columbia-Presby Med Ctr 1996; **Fac Appt:** Assoc Prof Ped, Loyola Univ-Stritch Sch Med

Morgan, Elaine MD [PHO] - **Spec Exp:** Leukemia; Palliative Care; Ethics; **Hospital:** Children's Mem Hosp; **Address:** Children's Meml Hosp, Div Hem/Onc, 2300 Children's Plaza, Box 30, Chicago, IL 60614; **Phone:** 773-880-4562; **Board Cert:** Pediatrics 1976; Pediatric Hematology-Oncology 1978; Hospice & Palliative Medicine 2005; **Med School:** Univ Pennsylvania 1971; **Resid:** Pediatrics, Chldns Hosp 1974; **Fellow:** Pediatric Hematology-Oncology, Chldns Hosp Med Ctr 1975; Pediatric Hematology-Oncology, Chldns Meml Med Ctr 1976; **Fac Appt:** Prof Ped, Northwestern Univ-Feinberg Sch Med

Nachman, James MD [PHO] - **Spec Exp:** Leukemia & Lymphoma; Bone Tumors; Hodgkin's Disease; **Hospital:** Univ of Chicago Med Ctr; **Address:** Univ Chicago Hosps, 5841 S Maryland Ave, rm C-429, MC 4060, Chicago, IL 60637; **Phone:** 773-702-6808; **Board Cert:** Pediatrics 1979; Pediatric Hematology-Oncology 1980; **Med School:** Johns Hopkins Univ 1974; **Resid:** Pediatrics, Chldns Meml Hosp 1977; Pediatrics, Fell-Wylers Chldns Hosp 1980; **Fellow:** Pediatric Hematology-Oncology, Chldns Meml Hosp 1979; **Fac Appt:** Prof Ped, Univ Chicago-Pritzker Sch Med

Neglia, Joseph MD [PHO] - **Spec Exp:** Cancer Survivors-Late Effects of Therapy; **Hospital:** Univ Minn Med Ctr, Fairview - Univ Campus; **Address:** Univ Minnesota-Div Ped Hem/Oncology, 420 Delaware St SE, MMC 484, Minneapolis, MN 55455; **Phone:** 612-626-2778; **Board Cert:** Pediatrics 1986; Pediatric Hematology-Oncology 1987; **Med School:** Loma Linda Univ 1981; **Resid:** Pediatrics, Baylor Coll Med 1984; **Fellow:** Pediatric Hematology-Oncology, Univ Minn Hosp 1987; **Fac Appt:** Prof Ped, Univ Minn

O'Dorisio, M Sue MD/PhD [PHO] - **Spec Exp:** Neuroblastoma; Medulloblastoma; Neuroendocrine Tumors; **Hospital:** Univ Iowa Hosp & Clinics; **Address:** UIHC Pediatrics Hema/Oncology, 200 Hawkins Drive, rm 2520 JCP, Iowa City, IA 52242; **Phone:** 319-356-7873; **Board Cert:** Pediatrics 2007; Pediatric Hematology-Oncology 2007; **Med School:** Ohio State Univ 1985; **Resid:** Pediatrics, Chldns Hosp 1988; **Fellow:** Pediatric Hematology-Oncology, Chldns Hosp 1992; **Fac Appt:** Prof Ped, Univ Iowa Coll Med

Plautz, Gregory E MD [PHO] - **Spec Exp:** Brain Tumors; Leukemia & Lymphoma; Wilms' Tumor; Cancer Survivors-Late Effects of Therapy; **Hospital:** Cleveland Clin Fdn (page 56); **Address:** Cleveland Clinic Fdn - Div Ped Hem Onc, 9500 Euclid Ave, MC S20, Cleveland, OH 44195; **Phone:** 216-445-3800; **Board Cert:** Pediatric Hematology-Oncology 2005; **Med School:** Indiana Univ 1984; **Resid:** Pediatrics, Johns Hopkins Hosp 1987; **Fellow:** Pediatric Hematology-Oncology, Univ Michigan Affil Hosp 1990; **Fac Appt:** Assoc Prof S, Case West Res Univ

Puccetti, Diane M MD [PHO] - **Spec Exp:** Brain Tumors; Neuro-Oncology; Cancer Survivors-Late Effects of Therapy; **Hospital:** Univ WI Hosp & Clins; **Address:** Univ Wisconsin Childrens Hosp, 600 Highland Ave, MC 4672, Madison, WI 53792; **Phone:** 608-263-6420; **Board Cert:** Pediatric Hematology-Oncology 2007; **Med School:** Med Coll OH 1985; **Resid:** Pediatrics, UC-Irvine Med Ctr 1986; Pediatrics, Med Coll Ohio 1988; **Fellow:** Pediatric Hematology-Oncology, Riley Hosp Chldn 1991; **Fac Appt:** Assoc Clin Prof Ped, Univ Wisc

Razzouk, Bassem I MD [PHO] - **Spec Exp:** Leukemia; Clinical Trials; **Hospital:** St Vincent Indianapolis Hosp; **Address:** St Vincent Hosp & Hlth Services, Center for Cancer & Blood Diseases, 2001 W 86th St, Indianapolis, IN 46260; **Phone:** 317-338-4673; **Board Cert:** Pediatric Hematology-Oncology 2004; **Med School:** Lebanon 1987; **Resid:** Pediatrics, American Univ Med Ctr 1990; Pediatrics, SUNY Hlth Sci Ctr 1992; **Fellow:** Hematology & Oncology, St Jude Chldns Rsch Hosp 1995

Salvi, Sharad MD [PHO] - **Spec Exp:** Leukemia; Bleeding/Coagulation Disorders; Anemia; **Hospital:** Adv Christ Med Ctr, Central DuPage Hosp; **Address:** Hope Chldns Hosp, 4440 W 95th St, Oak Lawn, IL 60453; **Phone:** 708-684-4094; **Board Cert:** Pediatrics 1982; Pediatric Hematology-Oncology 1982; **Med School:** India 1974; **Resid:** Pediatrics, Lincoln Meml Hosp 1979; **Fellow:** Pediatric Hematology-Oncology, Chldns Hosp/Roswell Park Meml Cancer Inst 1981

Sencer, Susan F MD [PHO] - **Spec Exp:** Pediatric Cancers; Complementary Medicine; **Hospital:** Chldns Hosp and Clinics - Minneapolis; **Address:** Chldns Specialty Clinic, Hem/Onc Clin, 2525 Chicago Ave S, Fl 4 - Ste 4150, Minneapolis, MN 55404; **Phone:** 612-813-5940; **Board Cert:** Pediatric Hematology-Oncology 2007; **Med School:** Univ Minn 1984; **Resid:** Pediatrics, Univ Minnesota Affil Hosp 1988; **Fellow:** Pediatric Hematology-Oncology, Univ Minnesota Affil Hosp 1991

Shapiro, Amy D MD [PHO] - **Spec Exp:** Hemophilia; **Hospital:** St Vincent Indianapolis Hosp; **Address:** Indiana Hemophilia & Thrombosis Ctr, 8402 Harcourt Rd, Ste 500, Indianapolis, IN 46260; **Phone:** 317-871-0000; **Board Cert:** Pediatrics 1986; Pediatric Hematology-Oncology 1987; **Med School:** NYU Sch Med 1980; **Resid:** Pediatrics, Univ Colo Hlth Sci Ctr 1982; **Fellow:** Pediatric Hematology-Oncology, Univ Colo Hlth Sci Ctr 1983

Pediatric Hematology-Oncology

Sondel, Paul M MD [PHO] - **Spec Exp:** Immunotherapy; Stem Cell Transplant; Pediatric Cancers; **Hospital:** Univ WI Hosp & Clins; **Address:** 600 Highland Ave, K4-448 Clin Sci Ctr, Madison, WI 53792-4672; **Phone:** 608-263-6200; **Board Cert:** Pediatrics 1981; **Med School:** Harvard Med Sch 1977; **Resid:** Pediatrics, Univ Wisconsin Hosp 1980; **Fellow:** Research, Sidney Farber Cancer Inst/Harvard 1977; **Fac Appt:** Prof Ped, Univ Wisc

Tannous, Raymond MD [PHO] - **Spec Exp:** Wilms' Tumor; Leukemia & Lymphoma; Pain-Cancer; **Hospital:** Univ Iowa Hosp & Clinics; **Address:** Univ Iowa Hosps & Clinics, Dept Peds, 200 Hawkins Drive, rm 2528 JCP, Iowa City, IA 52242; **Phone:** 319-356-1905; **Board Cert:** Pediatrics 1976; Pediatric Hematology-Oncology 1978; **Med School:** France 1972; **Resid:** Pediatrics, St Jude Chldns Rsch Hosp 1976; **Fellow:** Pediatric Hematology-Oncology, St Jude Chldns Rsch Hosp 1977; **Fac Appt:** Assoc Prof Ped, Univ Iowa Coll Med

Valentino, Leonard Anthony MD [PHO] - **Spec Exp:** Bleeding/Coagulation Disorders; Thrombotic Disorders; Hemophilia; **Hospital:** Rush Univ Med Ctr, Rush Copley Med Ctr; **Address:** 1653 W Congress Pkwy, Chicago, IL 60612-3828; **Phone:** 312-942-5983; **Board Cert:** Pediatrics 2007; Pediatric Hematology-Oncology 2005; **Med School:** Creighton Univ 1984; **Resid:** Pediatrics, Univ Illinios Med Ctr 1987; **Fellow:** Pediatric Hematology-Oncology, UCLA Med Ctr 1990; **Fac Appt:** Assoc Prof Ped, Rush Med Coll

Vik, Terry A MD [PHO] - **Spec Exp:** Neuroblastoma; Clinical Trials; Cancer Survivors-Late Effects of Therapy; Leukemia; **Hospital:** Riley Hosp for Children; **Address:** Riley Hosp Children, 702 Barnhill Drive, Riley 4340, Indianapolis, IN 46202; **Phone:** 317-274-2143; **Board Cert:** Pediatrics 1987; Pediatric Hematology-Oncology 2004; **Med School:** Johns Hopkins Univ 1983; **Resid:** Pediatrics, UCLA Med Ctr 1986; **Fellow:** Pediatric Hematology-Oncology, Chldns Hosp 1989; **Fac Appt:** Assoc Clin Prof Ped, Indiana Univ

Yaddanapudi, Ravindranath MD [PHO] - **Spec Exp:** Leukemia; **Hospital:** Chldns Hosp of Michigan; **Address:** Children's Hospital Michigan, Div Hem/Onc, 3901 Beaubien Blvd, Detroit, MI 48201; **Phone:** 313-745-5515; **Board Cert:** Pediatrics 1970; Pediatric Hematology-Oncology 1974; **Med School:** India 1964; **Resid:** Pathology, Western Penn Hosp 1967; Pediatrics, Children's Hosp 1969; **Fellow:** Pediatric Hematology-Oncology, Children's Hosp Michigan 1971; **Fac Appt:** Prof Ped, Wayne State Univ

Great Plains and Mountains

Abromowitch, Minnie MD [PHO] - **Hospital:** Children's Hosp - Omaha; **Address:** Children's Hosp-Dept Ped Hem Oncology, 8200 Dodge St, Omaha, NE 68114; **Phone:** 402-955-3950; **Board Cert:** Pediatrics 1980; Pediatric Hematology-Oncology 1982; **Med School:** Canada 1972; **Resid:** Pediatrics, Hospital for Sick Children 1976; **Fellow:** Pediatric Hematology-Oncology, Univ Manitoba 1978; Pediatric Hematology-Oncology, St Jude Chldns Research Hosp 1980; **Fac Appt:** Assoc Prof Ped, Univ Nebr Coll Med

Bruggers, Carol S MD [PHO] - **Spec Exp:** Brain Tumors; Clinical Trials; **Hospital:** Primary Children's Med Ctr; **Address:** Primary Children's Medical Ctr, 100 N Medical Drive, Salt Lake City, UT 84113; **Phone:** 801-662-4700; **Board Cert:** Pediatrics 2008; Pediatric Hematology-Oncology 2008; **Med School:** Mich State Univ 1984; **Resid:** Pediatrics, Univ Colorado Health Sci Ctr 1987; **Fellow:** Pediatric Hematology-Oncology, Duke Univ Med Ctr 1991; **Fac Appt:** Prof Ped, Univ Utah

Coccia, Peter F MD [PHO] - **Spec Exp:** Bone Marrow Transplant; Leukemia & Lymphoma; Solid Tumors; **Hospital:** Nebraska Med Ctr, Children's Hosp - Omaha; **Address:** Univ Nebr Med Ctr, Dept Pediatrics, 982168 Nebraska Med Ctr, Omaha, NE 68198-2168; **Phone:** 402-559-7257; **Board Cert:** Clinical Pathology 1972; Hematology 1975; Pediatrics 1976; Pediatric Hematology-Oncology 1976; **Med School:** SUNY Upstate Med Univ 1968; **Resid:** Pathology, Upstate Med Ctr 1970; Pediatrics, Univ Minn 1973; **Fellow:** Pediatric Hematology-Oncology, Univ Minn 1974; **Fac Appt:** Prof Ped, Univ Nebr Coll Med

Manco-Johnson, Marilyn MD [PHO] - **Spec Exp:** Hemophilia; Thrombotic Disorders; **Hospital:** Chldn's Hosp - Aurora, The, Univ Colorado Hosp; **Address:** Univ Colorado, Hemophilia Ctr, Box 6507, MS F416, Aurora, CO 80045-0507; **Phone:** 303-724-0365; **Board Cert:** Pediatrics 1979; Pediatric Hematology-Oncology 1980; **Med School:** Jefferson Med Coll 1974; **Resid:** Pediatrics, Univ Colorado Affil Hosps 1977; **Fellow:** Pediatric Hematology-Oncology, Chldn's Hosp/Colorado Med Ctr 1981; **Fac Appt:** Prof Ped, Univ Colorado

Odom, Lorrie F MD [PHO] - **Spec Exp:** Leukemia; Solid Tumors; Cancer Survivors-Late Effects of Therapy; **Hospital:** Presby - St Luke's Med Ctr, Sky Ridge Med Ctr; **Address:** Rocky Mountain Ped Hem Onc, 1601 E 19th Ave, Ste 6600, Denver, CO 80218; **Phone:** 303-832-2344; **Board Cert:** Pediatrics 1974; Pediatric Hematology-Oncology 1976; **Med School:** Univ Colorado 1969; **Resid:** Pediatrics, Chldns Hosp 1972; **Fellow:** Pediatric Hematology-Oncology, Dana-Farber Cancer Inst 1974; Pediatric Hematology-Oncology, Univ Colorado Med Ctr 1975; **Fac Appt:** Clin Prof Ped, Univ Colorado

Southwest

Abella, Esteban MD [PHO] - **Spec Exp:** Leukemia; Anemia-Aplastic; Neuroblastoma; Bone Marrow Transplant; **Hospital:** Banner Desert Med Ctr, St Joseph's Hosp & Med Ctr - Phoenix; **Address:** 1432 S Dobson, Ste 107, Mesa, AZ 85202; **Phone:** 480-833-1123; **Board Cert:** Pediatric Hematology-Oncology 2009; **Med School:** Dominican Republic 1985; **Resid:** Pediatrics, Chldns Hosp Michigan 1988; **Fellow:** Pediatric Hematology-Oncology, Chldns Hosp Michigan/Wayne St Univ 1991

Berg, Stacey MD [PHO] - **Spec Exp:** Drug Discovery & Development; Brain Tumors; Solid Tumors; **Hospital:** Texas Chldns Hosp; **Address:** Texas Chldns Cancer Ctr, Ped Hem-Onc, 6621 Fannin St, MC 3-3320, Houston, TX 77030; **Phone:** 832-824-4240; **Board Cert:** Pediatrics 2007; Pediatric Hematology-Oncology 2007; **Med School:** Univ Pittsburgh 1985; **Resid:** Pediatrics, Chldns Hosp 1988; **Fellow:** Pediatric Hematology-Oncology, Natl Inst Hlth 1991; **Fac Appt:** Prof Ped, Baylor Coll Med

Blaney, Susan MD [PHO] - **Spec Exp:** Brain Tumors; Neuro-Oncology; Drug Development; Clinical Trials; **Hospital:** Texas Chldns Hosp; **Address:** 6621 Fannin St #CC 1410.00, Houston, TX 77030; **Phone:** 832-822-1482; **Board Cert:** Pediatric Hematology-Oncology 2005; **Med School:** Med Coll OH 1984; **Resid:** Pediatrics, Letterman AMC 1987; **Fellow:** Pediatric Oncology, Walter Reed AMC 1990; **Fac Appt:** Prof Ped, Baylor Coll Med

Buchanan, George R MD [PHO] - **Spec Exp:** Sickle Cell Disease; Thrombotic Disorders; Hemophilia; Leukemia; **Hospital:** Chldns Med Ctr of Dallas; **Address:** Univ Texas SW Med Ctr, Peds Hem Onc, 5323 Harry Hines Blvd, MC 9063, Dallas, TX 75390-9063; **Phone:** 214-456-2978; **Board Cert:** Pediatrics 1975; Pediatric Hematology-Oncology 2000; **Med School:** Univ Chicago-Pritzker Sch Med 1970; **Resid:** Pediatrics, Chldn's Meml Hosp 1973; **Fellow:** Hematology & Oncology, Chldn's Meml Hosp 1975; **Fac Appt:** Prof Ped, Univ Tex SW, Dallas

Pediatric Hematology-Oncology

Dreyer, ZoAnn E MD [PHO] - **Spec Exp:** Cancer Survivors-Late Effects of Therapy; Leukemia in Infants; **Hospital:** Texas Chldns Hosp; **Address:** Texas Childrens Hosp, Clinical Care Ctr, 6701 Fannin Fl 14, MC CC1400, Houston, TX 77030; **Phone:** 832-822-4242; **Board Cert:** Pediatrics 1988; Pediatric Hematology-Oncology 2005; **Med School:** UC Davis 1982; **Resid:** Pediatrics, Baylor Affil Hosps 1985; **Fellow:** Pediatric Hematology-Oncology, Baylor Coll Med 1988; **Fac Appt:** Assoc Prof Ped, Baylor Coll Med

Goldman, Stanton C MD [PHO] - **Spec Exp:** Leukemia; Lymphoma; Stem Cell Transplant; **Hospital:** Med City Dallas Hosp; **Address:** 7777 Forest Ln, Ste D400, Dallas, TX 75230; **Phone:** 972-566-6647; **Board Cert:** Pediatric Hematology-Oncology 2004; **Med School:** Boston Univ 1990; **Resid:** Pediatrics, Chldns Natl Med Ctr 1996; **Fellow:** Pediatric Hematology-Oncology, Johns Hopkins Hosp

Graham, Michael L MD [PHO] - **Spec Exp:** Bone Marrow Transplant; Leukemia; Stem Cell Transplant; **Hospital:** Univ Med Ctr - Tucson; **Address:** Univ Arizona Hlth Science Ctr, 1501 N Campbell Ave, rm 4341, Box 245073, Tucson, AZ 85724-5073; **Phone:** 520-626-6527; **Board Cert:** Pediatrics 1980; Pediatric Hematology-Oncology 1984; **Med School:** Brown Univ 1975; **Resid:** Pediatrics, Johns Hopkins Hosp 1978; Pediatric Hematology-Oncology, Johns Hopkins Hosp 1980; **Fellow:** Medical Oncology, Yale-New Haven Hosp 1982; **Fac Appt:** Assoc Prof Ped, Univ Ariz Coll Med

Meyer, William H MD [PHO] - **Spec Exp:** Sarcoma; Pediatric Cancers; **Hospital:** Chldns Hosp OU Med Ctr; **Address:** OU Childrens Physicians, 940 NE 13th St, J Everett Tower, Fl 3 (Rm MRI 3000), Oklahoma City, OK 73104; **Phone:** 405-271-4412; **Board Cert:** Pediatrics 1980; Pediatric Hematology-Oncology 1980; **Med School:** Jefferson Med Coll 1974; **Resid:** Pediatrics, Wilmington Med Ctr 1977; **Fellow:** Pediatric Hematology-Oncology, Johns Hopkins Hosp 1980; **Fac Appt:** Prof Ped, Univ Okla Coll Med

Scher, Charles D MD [PHO] - **Spec Exp:** Sickle Cell Disease; Pediatric Cancers; Leukemia; **Hospital:** Tulane Univ Hosp & Clin; **Address:** Tulane Univ Hosp, Dept Pediatrics, 1430 Tulane Ave, Box SL-37, New Orleans, LA 70112; **Phone:** 504-988-5412; **Board Cert:** Pediatrics 1972; **Med School:** Univ Pennsylvania 1965; **Resid:** Pediatrics, Bronx Muni Hosp Ctr 1967; Pediatrics, Chldns Hosp Med Ctr 1972; **Fellow:** Pediatric Hematology-Oncology, Chldns Hosp Med Ctr 1974; **Fac Appt:** Prof Ped, Tulane Univ

Tomlinson, Gail E MD [PHO] - **Spec Exp:** Cancer Survivors-Late Effects of Therapy; Cancer Genetics; Liver Cancer; Kidney Cancer; **Hospital:** Christus Santa Rosa Children's Hosp, Univ Hlth Syst-San Antonio; **Address:** UT HSC at San Antonio, 7703 Floyd Curl Drive, San Antonio, TX 78229; **Phone:** 210-704-3405; **Board Cert:** Pediatrics 2008; Pediatric Hematology-Oncology 2002; **Med School:** Geo Wash Univ 1984; **Resid:** Pediatrics, Chldns Hosp Natl Med Ctr 1987; **Fellow:** Pediatric Hematology-Oncology, MD Anderson Cancer Ctr 1989; Pediatric Hematology-Oncology, Univ Texas SW Med Ctr 1992; **Fac Appt:** Prof Ped, Univ Tex, San Antonio

Winick, Naomi J MD [PHO] - **Spec Exp:** Leukemia; **Hospital:** Chldns Med Ctr of Dallas; **Address:** Ctr for Cancer & Blood Disorders, 1935 Motor St Brides Bldg Fl 3, Dallas, TX 75235-7794; **Phone:** 214-456-2382; **Board Cert:** Pediatrics 1984; Pediatric Hematology-Oncology 1987; **Med School:** Northwestern Univ 1978; **Resid:** Pediatrics, Babies Hosp-Columbia Presbyterian Med Ctr 1981; **Fellow:** Pediatric Hematology-Oncology, Sloan-Kettering Cancer Ctr 1983; **Fac Appt:** Prof Ped, Univ Tex SW, Dallas

West Coast and Pacific

Andrews, Robert G MD [PHO] - **Spec Exp:** Bone Marrow Transplant; Leukemia; Lymphoma; **Hospital:** Chldns Hosp and Regl Med Ctr - Seattle; **Address:** Fred Hutchinson Cancer Rsch Ctr, FHCRC, Box 358080, PO Box 19024, Seattle, WA 98109-1024; **Phone:** 206-667-5000; **Board Cert:** Pediatrics 1984; Pediatric Hematology-Oncology 1984; **Med School:** Univ Minn 1976; **Resid:** Pediatrics, New England Med Ctr 1979; **Fellow:** Pediatric Hematology-Oncology, Children's Hosp Med Ctr 1983; **Fac Appt:** Assoc Prof Ped, Univ Wash

Ducore, Jonathan M MD [PHO] - **Spec Exp:** Brain Tumors; Bone & Soft Tissue Tumors; Bleeding/Coagulation Disorders; **Hospital:** UC Davis Med Ctr; **Address:** UC Davis Med Ctr, Dept Pediatrics, Div Pediatric Hematology/Oncology, 2516 Stockton Blvd, Sacramento, CA 95817; **Phone:** 916-734-2781; **Board Cert:** Pediatrics 1978; Pediatric Hematology-Oncology 1978; **Med School:** Duke Univ 1973; **Resid:** Pediatrics, Chldns Med Ctr 1975; **Fellow:** Pediatric Hematology-Oncology, Univ Colorado Med Ctr 1977; Cancer Research, Natl Cancer Inst 1980; **Fac Appt:** Assoc Prof Ped, UC Davis

Finklestein, Jerry Z MD [PHO] - **Spec Exp:** Cancer Survivors-Late Effects of Therapy; Anemias & Red Cell Disorders; **Hospital:** Long Beach Meml Med Ctr, LAC - Harbor - UCLA Med Ctr; **Address:** 2653 Elm Ave, Ste 200, Long Beach, CA 90806-1652; **Phone:** 562-492-1062; **Board Cert:** Pediatrics 1980; Pediatric Hematology-Oncology 1974; **Med School:** McGill Univ 1963; **Resid:** Pediatrics, Montreal Chldns Hosp 1966; **Fellow:** Pediatric Hematology-Oncology, LA Chldns Hosp 1968; **Fac Appt:** Clin Prof Ped, UCLA

Finlay, Jonathan MD [PHO] - **Spec Exp:** Brain Tumors; **Hospital:** Chldns Hosp - Los Angeles, Chldns Hosp - Oakland; **Address:** Chldns Hosp-LA, Ped Hematology/Oncology, 4650 Sunset Blvd, MS 54, Los Angeles, CA 90027-6016; **Phone:** 323-361-8147; **Board Cert:** Pediatrics 1984; Pediatric Hematology-Oncology 1987; **Med School:** England, UK 1973; **Resid:** Pediatrics, Univ Birmingham 1975; Pediatrics, Christie Hosp 1976; **Fellow:** Pediatric Allergy & Immunology, Univ Wisconsin Hosp 1978; Pediatric Hematology-Oncology, Univ Wisconsin Hosp 1980; **Fac Appt:** Prof Ped, USC-Keck School of Medicine

Geyer, J Russell MD [PHO] - **Spec Exp:** Brain Tumors; **Hospital:** Chldns Hosp and Regl Med Ctr - Seattle, Univ Wash Med Ctr; **Address:** Chldns Hosp & Reg Med Ctr - Div Hem/Onc, 4800 Sands Point Way NE, MS B-6553, Seattle, WA 98105; **Phone:** 206-987-2106; **Board Cert:** Pediatrics 1983; Pediatric Hematology-Oncology 1987; **Med School:** Wayne State Univ 1977; **Resid:** Pediatrics, Chldns Hosp Michigan 1980; **Fellow:** Pediatric Hematology-Oncology, Univ Michigan Med Ctr 1981; **Fac Appt:** Prof Ped, Univ Wash

Glader, Bertil MD/PhD [PHO] - **Spec Exp:** Genetic Disorders-Blood; Hemophilia; **Hospital:** Lucile Packard Chldn's Hosp; **Address:** 770 Welch Rd Fl 2 - rm 261, Palo Alto, CA 94304; **Phone:** 650-497-8953; **Board Cert:** Pediatrics 1982; Pediatric Hematology-Oncology 2005; Hematology 1983; **Med School:** Northwestern Univ 1968; **Resid:** Pediatrics, Chldns Hosp Med Ctr 1973; **Fellow:** Hematology, Chldns Hosp Med Ctr 1975; **Fac Appt:** Prof Ped, Stanford Univ

Hawkins, Douglas MD [PHO] - **Spec Exp:** Bone Tumors; Ewing's Sarcoma; Leukemia; Rhabdomyosarcoma; **Hospital:** Chldns Hosp and Regl Med Ctr - Seattle; **Address:** Children's Hosp & Regl Med Ctr, 4800 Sand Point Way NE, Box 5371, MS B6553, Seattle, WA 98105; **Phone:** 206-987-2106; **Board Cert:** Pediatric Hematology-Oncology 2004; **Med School:** Harvard Med Sch 1990; **Resid:** Pediatrics, Univ Washington Med Ctr 1993; **Fellow:** Pediatric Hematology-Oncology, Fred Hutchinson Cancer Research Ctr 1996

Pediatric Hematology-Oncology

Horn, Biljana N MD [PHO] - **Spec Exp:** Bone Marrow Transplant; Brain Tumors; Stem Cell Transplant; Immunotherapy; **Hospital:** UCSF Med Ctr; **Address:** UCSF Med Ctr, Pediatric BMT Program, 505 Parnassus Ave, rm M-659, San Francisco, CA 94143; **Phone:** 415-476-2188; **Board Cert:** Pediatrics 2006; Pediatric Hematology-Oncology 2004; **Med School:** Croatia 1983; **Resid:** Pediatrics, Rainbow Babies & Chldns Hosp 1991; **Fellow:** Pediatric Hematology-Oncology, Natl Cancer Inst 1994; Pediatric Neuro-Oncology, UCSF 1998; **Fac Appt:** Assoc Prof Ped, UCSF

Kadota, Richard P MD [PHO] - **Spec Exp:** Bone Marrow Transplant; Brain Tumors; Clinical Trials; **Hospital:** Rady Children's Hosp - San Diego; **Address:** Children's Hospital San Diego, 3020 Children's Way, MC 5035, San Diego, CA 92123; **Phone:** 858-966-5811; **Board Cert:** Pediatrics 1984; Pediatric Hematology-Oncology 1984; **Med School:** Northwestern Univ 1979; **Resid:** Pediatrics, Mayo Clinic 1983; **Fellow:** Pediatric Hematology-Oncology, Mayo Clinic 1985; **Fac Appt:** Clin Prof Ped, UCSD

Kapoor, Neena MD [PHO] - **Spec Exp:** Bone Marrow Transplant; **Hospital:** Chldns Hosp - Los Angeles; **Address:** Chlds Hosp LA-Rsch Immunology/BMT, 4650 Sunset Blvd, MS 62, Los Angeles, CA 90027; **Phone:** 323-361-2546; **Board Cert:** Pediatrics 1978; **Med School:** India 1972; **Resid:** Pediatrics, Rhode Island Hosp 1976; **Fellow:** Pediatric Hematology-Oncology, Meml Sloan-Kettering Cancer Ctr 1978; **Fac Appt:** Prof Ped, USC Sch Med

Link, Michael P MD [PHO] - **Spec Exp:** Stem Cell Transplant; **Hospital:** Lucile Packard Chldn's Hosp, Stanford Univ Med Ctr; **Address:** 1000 Welch Rd, Ste 300, Palo Alto, CA 94304; **Phone:** 650-723-5535; **Board Cert:** Pediatrics 1979; Pediatric Hematology-Oncology 1980; **Med School:** Stanford Univ 1974; **Resid:** Pediatrics, Chldns Hosp Med Ctr 1976; **Fellow:** Hematology & Oncology, Dana Farber Cancer Inst 1979; **Fac Appt:** Prof Ped, Stanford Univ

Marina, Neyssa MD [PHO] - **Spec Exp:** Sarcoma; Cancer Survivors-Late Effects of Therapy; Germ Cell Tumors; **Hospital:** Lucile Packard Chldn's Hosp; **Address:** Pediatric Hematology & Oncology, 725 Walsh Rd-Clinic E, Palo Alto, CA 94304; **Phone:** 650-497-8953; **Board Cert:** Pediatrics 1987; Pediatric Hematology-Oncology 2005; **Med School:** Puerto Rico 1983; **Resid:** Pediatrics, Univ Pediatric Hosp 1986; **Fellow:** Pediatric Hematology-Oncology, St Jude Children's Hosp 1989; **Fac Appt:** Prof Ped, Stanford Univ

Matthay, Katherine K MD [PHO] - **Spec Exp:** Neuroblastoma; Bone Marrow & Stem Cell Transplant; **Hospital:** UCSF Med Ctr; **Address:** UCSF, Dept Ped Onc, 505 Parnassus Ave, Box 0106, San Francisco, CA 94143; **Phone:** 415-476-0603; **Board Cert:** Pediatrics 1979; Pediatric Hematology-Oncology 1980; **Med School:** Univ Pennsylvania 1973; **Resid:** Pediatrics, Univ Colorado 1976; **Fellow:** Pediatric Hematology-Oncology, UCSF 1979; **Fac Appt:** Prof Ped, UCSF

Nicholson, Henry Stacy MD [PHO] - **Spec Exp:** Brain Tumors; Cancer Survivors-Late Effects of Therapy; **Hospital:** Doernbecher Chldns Hosp/OHSU, OR Hlth & Sci Univ; **Address:** OR Hlth Scis Univ, 707 SW Gaines Rd, CDRCP, Portland, OR 97239; **Phone:** 503-494-4265; **Board Cert:** Pediatric Hematology-Oncology 2007; **Med School:** Med Coll GA 1985; **Resid:** Pediatrics, Chldns National Med Ctr 1988; **Fellow:** Pediatric Hematology-Oncology, Chldns National Med Ctr 1991; **Fac Appt:** Prof Ped, Oregon Hlth & Sci Univ

Pendergrass, Thomas W MD [PHO] - **Spec Exp:** Sarcoma; Leukemia & Lymphoma; Retinoblastoma; **Hospital:** Chldns Hosp and Regl Med Ctr - Seattle, Univ Wash Med Ctr; **Address:** Children's Hosp Regional Med Ctr, 4800 Sandpoint Way NE, Box 5371, MS B6553, Seattle, WA 98105; **Phone:** 206-987-2106; **Board Cert:** Pediatrics 1978; **Med School:** Univ Tenn Coll Med, Memphis 1971; **Resid:** Pediatrics, Children's Memorial Hosp 1973; **Fellow:** Pediatric Hematology-Oncology, Children's Hosp Med Ctr 1977; **Fac Appt:** Prof Ped, Univ Wash

America's Top Doctors® 9th Edition

Rosenthal, Joseph MD [PHO] - **Spec Exp:** Bone Marrow Transplant; Clinical Trials; **Hospital:** City of Hope Natl Med Ctr & Beckman Rsch; **Address:** City of Hope Med Ctr, 1500 E Duarte Rd, Duarte, CA 91010; **Phone:** 626-256-4673 x68442; **Board Cert:** Pediatrics 2003; Pediatric Hematology-Oncology 2004; **Med School:** Israel 1984; **Resid:** Pediatrics, Soroka Med Ctr 1988; Pediatrics, Chldn Hosp 1995; **Fellow:** Pediatric Hematology-Oncology, Univ Colorado Affil Hosp 1991; Pediatric Hematology-Oncology, Chldn Hosp 1994; **Fac Appt:** Assoc Prof Ped, USC-Keck School of Medicine

Russo, Carolyn MD [PHO] - **Spec Exp:** Brain Tumors; Cancer Survivors-Late Effects of Therapy; Palliative Care; **Hospital:** Kaiser Permanente Santa Clara Med Ctr; **Address:** 710 Lawrence Expwy, Dept 160, Santa Clara, CA 95051; **Phone:** 408-554-9810; **Board Cert:** Pediatric Hematology-Oncology 2005; **Med School:** UCLA 1984; **Resid:** Pediatrics, Harbor-UCLA Med Ctr 1987; **Fellow:** Pediatric Hematology-Oncology, Stanford Med Ctr 1990

Sakamoto, Kathleen M MD [PHO] - **Spec Exp:** Leukemia; Pediatric Cancers; Bone Marrow Transplant; **Hospital:** Mattel Chldns Hosp at UCLA; **Address:** Mattel Chldns Hosp UCLA, Div Hem-Onc, 10833 Le Conte Ave, rm A2140, Los Angeles, CA 90095-1752; **Phone:** 310-825-6708; **Board Cert:** Pediatrics 2007; Pediatric Hematology-Oncology 2007; **Med School:** Univ Cincinnati 1985; **Resid:** Pediatrics, Chldn's Hosp 1988; **Fellow:** Pediatric Hematology-Oncology, Chldn's Hosp 1991; **Fac Appt:** Prof Ped, UCLA

Siegel, Stuart E MD [PHO] - **Spec Exp:** Leukemia & Lymphoma; Infections in Cancer Patients; Psychosocial Support in Childhood Cancer; Solid Tumors; **Hospital:** Chldns Hosp - Los Angeles, Ventura Cnty Med Ctr; **Address:** Childrens Hospital, 4650 Sunset Blvd, MS 54, Los Angeles, CA 90027-6062; **Phone:** 323-361-2205; **Board Cert:** Pediatrics 1973; Pediatric Hematology-Oncology 1976; **Med School:** Boston Univ 1967; **Resid:** Pediatrics, Univ Minnesota Hosps 1969; **Fellow:** Pediatric Hematology-Oncology, Natl Cancer Inst 1972; **Fac Appt:** Prof Ped, USC-Keck School of Medicine

Wilkinson, Robert W MD [PHO] - **Hospital:** Kapiolani Med Ctr for Women & Chldn; **Address:** Kapiolani Med Ctr for Women & Children, 1319 Punahou St, Ste 1050, Honolulu, HI 96826; **Phone:** 808-942-8144; **Board Cert:** Pediatrics 1986; Pediatric Hematology-Oncology 1986; **Med School:** Tulane Univ 1967; **Resid:** Pediatrics, LAC-USC Med Ctr 1971; **Fellow:** Pediatric Hematology-Oncology, LAC-USC Med Ctr 1972; **Fac Appt:** Assoc Prof Ped, Univ Hawaii JA Burns Sch Med

PEDIATRIC INFECTIOUS DISEASE

New England

Andiman, Warren A MD [PInf] - **Spec Exp:** AIDS/HIV; Viral Infections; Lyme Disease; Infectious Mononucleosis; **Hospital:** Yale-New Haven Hosp; **Address:** 333 Cedar St, rm 418 LSOG, Box 208064, New Haven, CT 06520-8064; **Phone:** 203-785-4730; **Board Cert:** Pediatrics 1975; **Med School:** Albert Einstein Coll Med 1969; **Resid:** Pediatrics, Babies Hosp-Columbia Presby 1971; **Fellow:** Pediatric Infectious Disease, Yale Univ Sch Med 1973; **Fac Appt:** Prof Ped, Yale Univ

Baltimore, Robert MD [PInf] - **Spec Exp:** Neonatal Infections; Hospital Acquired Infections; Tuberculosis; **Hospital:** Yale-New Haven Hosp; **Address:** Yale Univ Sch Med, Dept Pediatrics, 333 Cedar St, Box 208064, New Haven, CT 06520-8064; **Phone:** 203-785-4655; **Board Cert:** Pediatrics 1975; Pediatric Infectious Disease 2008; **Med School:** SUNY Buffalo 1968; **Resid:** Pediatrics, Univ Chicago Hosps 1971; **Fellow:** Infectious Disease, Boston City Hosp-Harvard 1976; **Fac Appt:** Prof Ped, Yale Univ

Pediatric Infectious Disease

Durbin Jr, William Applebee MD [PInf] - **Hospital:** UMass Meml - Univ Campus; **Address:** 55 Lake Ave N, Worcester, MA 01655; **Phone:** 508-856-2650; **Board Cert:** Pediatrics 1978; Pediatric Infectious Disease 2002; **Med School:** Columbia P&S 1972; **Resid:** Pediatrics, Boston Chldns Hosp 1977; **Fellow:** Infectious Disease, Boston Chldns Hosp/Beth Israel 1979; **Fac Appt:** Prof Ped, Univ Mass Sch Med

Jenson, Hal B MD [PInf] - **Spec Exp:** Viral Infections; Tumor Virology; Vaccines; **Hospital:** Baystate Med Ctr; **Address:** 759 Chestnut St, Springfield, MA 01199; **Phone:** 419-794-5588; **Board Cert:** Pediatrics 1985; Pediatric Infectious Disease 2002; **Med School:** Geo Wash Univ 1979; **Resid:** Pediatrics, Rainbow Babies-Chldns Hosp. 1983; **Fellow:** Pediatric Infectious Disease, Yale Univ Sch Med 1985; **Fac Appt:** Prof Ped, Tufts Univ

Raszka Jr, William V MD [PInf] - **Hospital:** Fletcher Allen Health Care- Med Ctr Campus; **Address:** U Vermont Coll of Medicine, Pediatrics, D 201A Given Bldg, 89 Beaumont Ave, Burlington, VT 05405; **Phone:** 802-847-8200; **Board Cert:** Pediatric Infectious Disease 2002; **Med School:** Boston Univ 1985; **Resid:** Pediatrics, Tripler Army Med Ctr 1988; **Fellow:** Pediatric Infectious Disease, Uniformed Servs Hlth Ctr 1993; **Fac Appt:** Prof Ped, Univ VT Coll Med

Shapiro, Eugene D MD [PInf] - **Spec Exp:** Lyme Disease; Vaccines; **Hospital:** Yale-New Haven Hosp; **Address:** Yale Univ, Dept Pediatrics, 333 Cedar St, Box 208064, New Haven, CT 06520-8064; **Phone:** 203-688-4518; **Board Cert:** Pediatrics 1980; Pediatric Infectious Disease 2002; **Med School:** UCSF 1976; **Resid:** Pediatrics, Chldns Hosp 1979; **Fellow:** Pediatric Infectious Disease, Chldns Hosp 1981; Research, Yale Univ 1983; **Fac Appt:** Prof Ped, Yale Univ

Mid Atlantic

Borkowsky, William MD [PInf] - **Spec Exp:** AIDS/HIV; **Hospital:** NYU Langone Med Ctr (page 67), Bellevue Hosp Ctr; **Address:** 550 1st Ave, Dept Pediatrics, New York, NY 10016; **Phone:** 212-263-6513; **Board Cert:** Pediatrics 1979; Pediatric Infectious Disease 2002; **Med School:** NYU Sch Med 1972; **Resid:** Pediatrics, Bellevue Hosp Ctr 1975; **Fellow:** Infectious Disease, Bellevue Hosp Ctr-NYU 1978; **Fac Appt:** Prof Ped, NYU Sch Med

Green, Michael D MD [PInf] - **Spec Exp:** Infections-Transplant; **Hospital:** Chldns Hosp of Pittsburgh - UPMC; **Address:** University of Pittsburgh Physicians, 3520 Fifth Ave Keystone Bldg, Pittsburgh, PA 15213; **Phone:** 412-692-7885; **Board Cert:** Pediatrics 1987; Pediatric Infectious Disease 2002; **Med School:** Univ IL Coll Med 1983; **Resid:** Pediatrics, Children's Hosp 1986; **Fellow:** Pediatric Infectious Disease, Children's Hosp 1989; **Fac Appt:** Assoc Prof Ped, Univ Pittsburgh

Kotloff, Karen MD [PInf] - **Spec Exp:** Diarrheal Diseases; Infectious Disease; Sexually Transmitted Diseases; **Hospital:** Univ of MD Med Ctr; **Address:** Ctr for Vaccine Development, 685 W Baltimore St HSF Bldg - Ste 480, Baltimore, MD 21201; **Phone:** 410-706-5328; **Board Cert:** Pediatrics 1985; Pediatric Infectious Disease 2002; **Med School:** Temple Univ 1979; **Resid:** Pediatrics, Chldn's Hosp 1983; **Fellow:** Pediatric Infectious Disease, Univ Maryland Med Ctr 1986; **Fac Appt:** Prof Ped, Univ MD Sch Med

Krilov, Leonard MD [PInf] - **Spec Exp:** Infections-Respiratory; Infections in Int'l Adopted Children; Chronic Fatigue Syndrome; Lyme Disease; **Hospital:** Winthrop - Univ Hosp; **Address:** 120 Mineola Blvd, Ste 210, Mineola, NY 11501; **Phone:** 516-663-9570; **Board Cert:** Pediatrics 1983; Pediatric Infectious Disease 2001; **Med School:** Columbia P&S 1978; **Resid:** Pediatrics, Johns Hopkins Hosp 1981; **Fellow:** Pediatric Infectious Disease, Chldns Hosp 1984; **Fac Appt:** Prof Ped, SUNY Stony Brook

Long, Sarah S MD [PInf] - **Spec Exp:** Whooping Cough; Vaccines; Antibiotic Resistance; **Hospital:** St Christopher's Hosp for Chldn; **Address:** St Christopher's Hosp for Children, Erie Ave at Front St, Ste 1112, Philadelphia, PA 19134; **Phone:** 215-427-5201; **Board Cert:** Pediatrics 2002; Pediatric Infectious Disease 2002; **Med School:** Jefferson Med Coll 1970; **Resid:** Pediatrics, St Christophers Hosp Chldn 1973; **Fellow:** Pediatric Infectious Disease, Temple Univ Sch Med 1975; **Fac Appt:** Prof Ped, Drexel Univ Coll Med

Michaels, Marian G MD [PInf] - **Spec Exp:** AIDS/HIV; Infections in Immunocompromised Patients; **Hospital:** Chldns Hosp of Pittsburgh - UPMC, Magee-Womens Hosp - UPMC; **Address:** Children's Hosp Pittsburgh, Div Infectious Disease, 3705 Fifth Ave, Pittsburgh, PA 15213; **Phone:** 412-692-7438; **Board Cert:** Pediatrics 2005; Pediatric Infectious Disease 2002; **Med School:** Univ Pennsylvania 1985; **Resid:** Pediatrics, Children's Hosp 1988; Pediatrics, Hosp for Sick Children 1989; **Fellow:** Pediatric Infectious Disease, Univ Pittsburgh 1992; **Fac Appt:** Assoc Prof Ped, Univ Pittsburgh

Munoz, Jose Luis MD [PInf] - **Spec Exp:** Lyme Disease; Immune Deficiency; Tick-borne Diseases; **Hospital:** Westchester Med Ctr; **Address:** Pediatric Infectious Disease, 19 Bradhurst Ave, Ste 1400, Hawthorne, NY 10532; **Phone:** 914-493-8333; **Board Cert:** Pediatric Infectious Disease 2002; **Med School:** Yale Univ 1978; **Resid:** Pediatrics, Yale New Haven Hosp 1981; **Fellow:** Pediatric Infectious Disease, Univ Rochester 1984; **Fac Appt:** Assoc Prof Ped, NY Med Coll

Offit, Paul A MD [PInf] - **Spec Exp:** Vaccines; **Hospital:** Chldns Hosp of Philadelphia, The; **Address:** Children's Hospital of Philadelphia, Abramson Bldg, 34th St & Civic Center Blvd, Ste 1202D, Philadelphia, PA 19104; **Phone:** 215-590-2017; **Board Cert:** Pediatrics 1982; **Med School:** Univ MD Sch Med 1977; **Resid:** Pediatrics, Children's Hosp 1980; **Fac Appt:** Assoc Clin Prof Ped, Univ Pennsylvania

Saiman, Lisa MD [PInf] - **Spec Exp:** Cystic Fibrosis Infection; Fungal Infections; Tick-borne Diseases; Tuberculosis; **Hospital:** NYPresby-Morgan Stanley Children's Hosp (page 66); **Address:** Columbia University, 650 W 168th St Fl 4 PH4 W - rm 470, New York, NY 10032; **Phone:** 212-305-0635; **Board Cert:** Pediatrics 1987; Pediatric Infectious Disease 2002; **Med School:** Albert Einstein Coll Med 1983; **Resid:** Pediatrics, Babies Hosp/NY Presby 1986; **Fellow:** Infectious Disease, Babies Hosp/NY Presby 1989; **Fac Appt:** Assoc Clin Prof Ped, Columbia P&S

Singh, Nalini MD [PInf] - **Hospital:** Chldns Natl Med Ctr; **Address:** Div Infectious Disease, 111 Michigan Ave NW, Ste 35 West Wing, rm 100, Washington, DC 20010; **Phone:** 202-476-5051; **Board Cert:** Pediatrics 1982; Pediatric Infectious Disease 2005; **Med School:** India 1973; **Resid:** Pediatrics, Univ Mass Med Ctr 1979; **Fellow:** Infectious Disease, Natl Inst Hlth 1981; **Fac Appt:** Assoc Prof Ped, Geo Wash Univ

Southeast

Clements III, Dennis A MD/PhD [PInf] - **Spec Exp:** Vaccines; Latino Health Issues; International Health; **Hospital:** Duke Univ Med Ctr; **Address:** Duke Univ Med Center, rm 90519, Durham, NC 27708; **Phone:** 919-681-7714; **Board Cert:** Pediatrics 1978; **Med School:** Univ Rochester 1973; **Resid:** Pediatrics, Duke Univ Med Ctr 1976; **Fellow:** Pediatric Infectious Disease, Duke Univ Med Ctr 1988; **Fac Appt:** Prof Ped, Duke Univ

Edwards, Kathryn M MD [PInf] - **Spec Exp:** Vaccines; Clinical Trials; **Hospital:** Vanderbilt Univ Med Ctr; **Address:** Vanderbilt Univ, Peds Infectious Disease, 1161 21st Ave S, CCC-5311, Med Ctr N, Nashville, TN 37232-2581; **Phone:** 615-322-8299; **Board Cert:** Pediatrics 1978; Pediatric Infectious Disease 2005; **Med School:** Univ Iowa Coll Med 1973; **Resid:** Pediatrics, Childrens Meml Hosp 1976; **Fellow:** Pediatric Infectious Disease, Childrens Meml Hosp 1980; **Fac Appt:** Prof Ped, Vanderbilt Univ

Pediatric Infectious Disease

Emmanuel, Patricia MD [PInf] - **Spec Exp:** Infections in Immunocompromised Patients; AIDS/HIV; Congenital Infections; **Hospital:** Tampa Genl Hosp, All Children's Hosp; **Address:** 17 Davis Blvd, Ste 200, Tampa, FL 33606; **Phone:** 813-259-8800; **Board Cert:** Pediatrics 2005; Pediatric Infectious Disease 2002; **Med School:** Univ Fla Coll Med 1986; **Resid:** Pediatrics, Univ S Florida Affil Hosp 1989; **Fellow:** Infectious Disease, Univ S Florida Affil Hosp 1993; **Fac Appt:** Assoc Prof Ped, Univ S Fla Coll Med

Givner, Laurence B MD [PInf] - **Spec Exp:** Streptococcal Infections; Rocky Mountain Spotted Fever; **Hospital:** Wake Forest Univ Baptist Med Ctr (page 72), Brenner Chldrn's Hosp; **Address:** Wake Forest Univ Sch Med, Dept Ped, Medical Center Blvd, Winston-Salem, NC 27157-0001; **Phone:** 336-716-6568; **Board Cert:** Pediatrics 1984; Pediatric Infectious Disease 2002; **Med School:** Univ MD Sch Med 1978; **Resid:** Pediatrics, Univ Maryland 1982; **Fellow:** Infectious Disease, Baylor Coll Med 1984; **Fac Appt:** Prof Ped, Wake Forest Univ

Ingram, David MD [PInf] - **Hospital:** WakeMed New Bern; **Address:** WakeMed-Andrews Ctr, 3024 New Bern Ave, Ste 307, Raleigh, NC 27610; **Phone:** 919-350-2800; **Board Cert:** Pediatrics 1980; Pediatric Infectious Disease 2002; **Med School:** Yale Univ 1967; **Resid:** Pediatrics, Yale-New Haven Hosp 1971; **Fellow:** Pediatric Infectious Disease, Chldns Hosp Med Ctr 1973; **Fac Appt:** Prof Ped, Univ NC Sch Med

McKinney Jr, Ross E MD [PInf] - **Spec Exp:** Infections in Immunocompromised Patients; Fevers of Unknown Origin; AIDS/HIV; **Hospital:** Duke Univ Med Ctr; **Address:** Duke Univ Med Ctr, Box 3461, Durham, NC 27710; **Phone:** 919-668-9000; **Board Cert:** Pediatrics 1983; Pediatric Infectious Disease 2002; **Med School:** Univ Rochester 1979; **Resid:** Pediatrics, Duke Univ Med Ctr 1982; **Fellow:** Pediatric Infectious Disease, Duke Univ Med Ctr 1985; **Fac Appt:** Assoc Prof Ped, Duke Univ

Mitchell, Charles D MD [PInf] - **Spec Exp:** AIDS/HIV; Viral Infections; **Hospital:** Jackson Meml Hosp (page 70); **Address:** Univ Miami Div Ped Inf Disease, PO Box 016960 (D4-4), Miami, FL 33101; **Phone:** 305-243-2700; **Board Cert:** Pediatrics 1986; Pediatric Infectious Disease 2002; **Med School:** Univ Tex Med Br, Galveston 1977; **Resid:** Pediatrics, Univ Minn Hosp 1981; **Fellow:** Pediatric Infectious Disease, Univ Minn Hosp 1984; **Fac Appt:** Clin Prof Ped, Univ Miami Sch Med

Scott, Gwendolyn B MD [PInf] - **Spec Exp:** AIDS/HIV; **Hospital:** Jackson Meml Hosp (page 70), Univ of Miami Hosp & Clins/Sylvester Comp Canc Ctr (page 70); **Address:** Univ Miami Div Ped Inf Disease, 1580 NW 10th Ave, rm 286 (D4-4), Miami, FL 33136; **Phone:** 305-243-6522; **Board Cert:** Pediatrics 1978; Pediatric Infectious Disease 2002; **Med School:** UCSF 1972; **Resid:** Pediatrics, San Francisco Genl Hosp 1973; Pediatrics, Univ Maryland Hosp 1975; **Fellow:** Pediatric Infectious Disease, Univ Miami Hosp 1978; **Fac Appt:** Prof Ped, Univ Miami Sch Med

Midwest

Alexander, Kenneth MD/PhD [PInf] - **Spec Exp:** HPV-Human Papilloma Virus; Infections in Immunocompromised Patients; Fevers of Unknown Origin; Antibiotic Resistance; **Hospital:** Univ of Chicago Med Ctr; **Address:** 5841 S Maryland Ave, MC 6054, Chicago, IL 60637; **Phone:** 773-702-6176; **Board Cert:** Pediatric Infectious Disease 2005; **Med School:** Med Coll GA 1989; **Resid:** Pediatrics, Chldn's Hosp 1992; **Fellow:** Pediatric Infectious Disease, Duke Univ Hosp 1995; **Fac Appt:** Assoc Prof Ped, Univ Chicago-Pritzker Sch Med

Bernstein, David I MD [PInf] - **Spec Exp:** Vaccines; Viral Infections; **Hospital:** Cincinnati Chldns Hosp Med Ctr; **Address:** Cincinnatti Children's Hosp, Dept Infectious Diseases, 3333 Burnet Ave, Cincinnati, OH 45229-3039; **Phone:** 513-636-7625; **Board Cert:** Pediatrics 1982; **Med School:** SUNY Buffalo 1977; **Resid:** Pediatrics, Tufts-New Englan Med Ctr 1981; **Fellow:** Infectious Disease, UCLA Med Ctr 1981; **Fac Appt:** Prof Ped, Univ Cincinnati

Kleiman, Martin B MD [PInf] - **Spec Exp:** Histoplasmosis; Blastomycosis; Meningitis; AIDS/HIV; **Hospital:** Riley Hosp for Children; **Address:** 702 Barnhill Drive, Ste ROC4380, Indianapolis, IN 46202; **Phone:** 317-274-7260; **Board Cert:** Pediatrics 1973; Pediatric Infectious Disease 2002; **Med School:** SUNY Upstate Med Univ 1968; **Resid:** Pediatrics, Upstate Med Ctr 1971; **Fellow:** Infectious Disease, Johns Hopkins Hosp 1976; **Fac Appt:** Prof Ped, Indiana Univ

McAuley, James B MD [PInf] - **Spec Exp:** Tuberculosis; Parasitic Infections; Travel Medicine; Congenital Infections; **Hospital:** Rush Univ Med Ctr; **Address:** 1725 W Harrison St, Ste 718, Chicago, IL 60612; **Phone:** 312-563-2683; **Board Cert:** Pediatrics 2004; Internal Medicine 1989; Infectious Disease 2002; Pediatric Infectious Disease 2005; **Med School:** Northwestern Univ 1985; **Resid:** Internal Medicine & Pediatrics, Univ Chicago Hosp 1989; **Fellow:** Infectious Disease, Univ Chicago Hosp 1990; Public Health, Ctrs for Disease Control 1992; **Fac Appt:** Assoc Prof Ped, Rush Med Coll

Shulman, Stanford MD [PInf] - **Spec Exp:** Kawasaki Disease; Streptococcal Infections; **Hospital:** Children's Mem Hosp, Northwestern Meml Hosp; **Address:** 2300 Children's Plaza, Box 20, Chicago, IL 60614-3318; **Phone:** 773-880-4187; **Board Cert:** Pediatrics 1972; Pediatric Infectious Disease 2002; **Med School:** Univ Chicago-Pritzker Sch Med 1967; **Resid:** Pediatrics, Univ Chicago Hosps 1970; **Fellow:** Infectious Disease, Shands Hosp 1973; **Fac Appt:** Prof Ped, Northwestern Univ

Wald, Ellen MD [PInf] - **Spec Exp:** Urinary Tract Infections; Infections-Respiratory; Meningitis; **Hospital:** Chldns Hosp - Wisconsin; **Address:** Dept Pediatrics, Box 4108, 600 Highland Ave, Madison, WI 57392; **Phone:** 608-263-8558; **Board Cert:** Pediatrics 1973; Pediatric Infectious Disease 2002; **Med School:** SUNY Downstate 1968; **Resid:** Pediatrics, Kings Co Hosp 1971; **Fellow:** Infectious Disease, Univ Maryland Hosp 1973; **Fac Appt:** Prof Ped, Univ Wisc

Southwest

Baker, Carol J MD [PInf] - **Spec Exp:** Streptococcal Infections; Neonatal Infections; Vaccines; **Hospital:** Texas Chldns Hosp, Ben Taub Genl Hosp; **Address:** Baylor Coll Med, Dept Peds, One Baylor Plaza, rm 302 A, MC BCM320, Houston, TX 77030; **Phone:** 713-798-4790; **Board Cert:** Pediatrics 1973; Pediatric Infectious Disease 2009; **Med School:** Baylor Coll Med 1968; **Resid:** Pediatrics, Baylor Coll Med 1971; **Fellow:** Pediatric Infectious Disease, Baylor Coll Med 1973; Infectious Disease, Boston City Hosp/Harvard Med Sch 1974; **Fac Appt:** Prof Ped, Baylor Coll Med

Jacobs, Richard F MD [PInf] - **Spec Exp:** Viral Infections; Drug Discovery & Development; Neonatal Infections; **Hospital:** Arkansas Chldns Hosp, UAMS Med Ctr; **Address:** 800 Marshall St, Slot 512-11, Little Rock, AR 72202-3591; **Phone:** 501-364-1416; **Board Cert:** Pediatrics 1982; Pediatric Infectious Disease 2002; **Med School:** Univ Ark 1977; **Resid:** Pediatrics, Ark Chldns Hosp 1980; **Fellow:** Infectious Disease, Univ Washington 1982; **Fac Appt:** Prof Ped, Univ Ark

Kaplan, Sheldon MD [PInf] - **Spec Exp:** Pneumococcal Infections; Meningitis; **Hospital:** Texas Chldns Hosp; **Address:** Div Infectious Disease, 6621 Fannin St, MC 3-2371, Houston, TX 77030; **Phone:** 832-824-4330; **Board Cert:** Pediatrics 1978; Pediatric Infectious Disease 2002; **Med School:** Univ MO-Columbia Sch Med 1973; **Resid:** Pediatrics, St Louis Chldns Hosp 1975; **Fellow:** Pediatric Infectious Disease, St Louis Chldns Hosp 1977; **Fac Appt:** Prof Ped, Baylor Coll Med

Kline, Mark MD [PInf] - **Spec Exp:** AIDS/HIV; **Hospital:** Texas Chldns Hosp; **Address:** Texas Children's Hosp, 6621 Fannin St, MC CCC1210, Houston, TX 77030; **Phone:** 832-822-1038; **Board Cert:** Pediatrics 1987; Pediatric Infectious Disease 2002; **Med School:** Baylor Coll Med 1981; **Resid:** Pediatrics, Baylor Coll Med 1985; **Fellow:** Pediatric Infectious Disease, Baylor Coll Med 1987; **Fac Appt:** Prof Ped, Baylor Coll Med

Pediatric Infectious Disease

McCracken Jr, George H MD [PInf] - **Spec Exp:** Meningitis; Antibiotic Resistance; **Hospital:** UT Southwestern Med Ctr at Dallas; **Address:** Dept Pediatric Infectious Disease, 1935 Medical District Drive, Dallas, TX 75235; **Phone:** 214-456-6500; **Board Cert:** Pediatrics 1966; Pediatric Infectious Disease 2002; **Med School:** Cornell Univ-Weill Med Coll 1962; **Resid:** Pediatrics, NY-Cornell Med Ctr 1965; Pediatrics, Univ Texas SW Med Ctr 1966

West Coast and Pacific

Bradley, John S MD [PInf] - **Spec Exp:** Meningitis; Brain Infections; **Hospital:** Rady Children's Hosp - San Diego, UCSD Med Ctr; **Address:** 3020 Children's Way, MC 5041, San Diego, CA 92123; **Phone:** 858-966-7785; **Board Cert:** Pediatrics 1981; Pediatric Infectious Disease 2002; **Med School:** UC Davis 1976; **Resid:** Pediatrics, UC Davis Med Ctr 1980; **Fellow:** Pediatric Infectious Disease, Stanford Univ Hosp 1981; **Fac Appt:** Assoc Clin Prof Ped, UCSD

Bryson, Yvonne J MD [PInf] - **Spec Exp:** AIDS/HIV; Herpes Simplex; **Hospital:** UCLA Ronald Reagan Med Ctr; **Address:** 10833 Le Conte Ave, MDCC, rm 22-442, Los Angeles, CA 90095-1752; **Phone:** 310-825-5235; **Board Cert:** Pediatrics 1976; **Med School:** Univ Tex SW, Dallas 1970; **Resid:** Pediatrics, UCSD Med Ctr 1974; **Fellow:** Infectious Disease, UCSD Med Ctr 1976; **Fac Appt:** Prof Ped, UCLA

Mason, Wilbert H MD [PInf] - **Spec Exp:** Kawasaki Disease; **Hospital:** Chldns Hosp - Los Angeles, USC Univ Hosp; **Address:** Chldns Hosp, Div Inf Dis, 4650 West Sunset Blvd, MS 5, Los Angeles, CA 90027-6062; **Phone:** 323-361-2509; **Board Cert:** Pediatrics 1975; Pediatric Infectious Disease 2002; **Med School:** UC Irvine 1970; **Resid:** Pediatrics, Chldns Hosp 1973; **Fellow:** Infectious Disease, Chldns Hosp 1974; **Fac Appt:** Assoc Clin Prof Ped, USC Sch Med

Petru, Ann MD [PInf] - **Spec Exp:** AIDS/HIV; **Hospital:** Chldns Hosp - Oakland; **Address:** Childrens Hosp, Div Infectious Disease, 747 52nd St, Oakland, CA 94609; **Phone:** 510-428-3336; **Board Cert:** Pediatrics 1983; Pediatric Infectious Disease 2002; **Med School:** UCSF 1978; **Resid:** Pediatrics, Chldns Hosp Med Ctr 1982; **Fellow:** Pediatric Infectious Disease, Chldns Hosp Med Ctr 1983; **Fac Appt:** Asst Clin Prof Med, UCSF

PEDIATRIC NEPHROLOGY

Mid Atlantic

Dabbagh, Shermine MD [PNep] - **Spec Exp:** Kidney Disease; Kidney Failure-Chronic; Transplant Medicine-Kidney; **Hospital:** Alfred I duPont Hosp for Children; **Address:** Dupont Hosp for Children, Div Nephrology, 1600 Rockland Rd, PO Box 269, Wilmington, DE 19899; **Phone:** 302-651-4426; **Board Cert:** Pediatrics 1985; Pediatric Nephrology 1985; **Med School:** Lebanon 1979; **Resid:** Pediatrics, Univ Virginia Hosp 1981; **Fellow:** Pediatric Nephrology, Univ Wisconsin 1984

Ellis, Demetrius MD [PNep] - **Spec Exp:** Transplant Medicine-Kidney; Hypertension; **Hospital:** Chldns Hosp of Pittsburgh - UPMC; **Address:** Children's Hospital, Dept Nephrology, 45th St & Penn Ave, rm 412, Pittsburgh, PA 15201; **Phone:** 412-692-5182; **Board Cert:** Pediatrics 1978; Pediatric Nephrology 1979; **Med School:** SUNY Buffalo 1973; **Resid:** Pediatrics, Chldns Hosp 1975; **Fellow:** Pediatric Nephrology, Chldns Hosp-Natl Med Ctr 1977; **Fac Appt:** Prof Ped, Univ Pittsburgh

Fivush, Barbara A MD [PNep] - **Spec Exp:** Transplant Medicine-Kidney; **Hospital:** Johns Hopkins Hosp (page 61); **Address:** Johns Hopkins Hosp-Div Nephrology, 200 N Wolfe St, rm 3055, Baltimore, MD 21287; **Phone:** 410-955-2467; **Board Cert:** Pediatrics 1984; Pediatric Nephrology 2003; **Med School:** Boston Univ 1978; **Resid:** Pediatrics, Johns Hopkins Hosp 1981; **Fellow:** Pediatric Nephrology, Johns Hopkins Hosp 1983; Pediatric Nephrology, Chldns Hosp Natl Med Ctr 1984; **Fac Appt:** Assoc Prof Ped, Johns Hopkins Univ

Kaplan, Bernard S MD [PNep] - **Spec Exp:** Hemolytic Uremic Syndrome; Polycystic Kidney Disease; **Hospital:** Chldns Hosp of Philadelphia, The; **Address:** Chldns Hosp of Philadelphia, Div Nephrology, 34 St & Civic Ctr Blvd, rm 2143, Philadelphia, PA 19104; **Phone:** 215-590-2449; **Board Cert:** Pediatrics 1972; Pediatric Nephrology 1974; **Med School:** South Africa 1964; **Resid:** Pediatrics, Baragwanath Hosp, Transvaal Meml Hosp 1970; Nephrology, Royal Victoria Hosp 1973; **Fellow:** Nephrology, Montreal Chldns Hosp 1972; **Fac Appt:** Prof Ped, Univ Pennsylvania

Mendley, Susan MD [PNep] - **Spec Exp:** Transplant Medicine-Kidney; Hypertension; Dialysis Care; Glomerulonephritis; **Hospital:** Univ of MD Med Ctr; **Address:** Univ Maryland Med System, 22 S Greene St, Pediatric Nephrol N5W67, Baltimore, MD 21201; **Phone:** 410-328-5303; **Board Cert:** Internal Medicine 1988; Nephrology 2000; **Med School:** Boston Univ 1984; **Resid:** Internal Medicine, Univ Chicago Hosps 1987; **Fellow:** Nephrology, Univ Chicago 1990; Pediatric Nephrology, Chldns Meml Hosp/Northwestern Univ 1991; **Fac Appt:** Assoc Prof Ped, Univ MD Sch Med

Nash, Martin MD [PNep] - **Spec Exp:** Nephrotic Syndrome; Kidney Failure; Urinary Abnormalities; **Hospital:** NYPresby-Morgan Stanley Children's Hosp (page 66); **Address:** Morgan Stanley Chlds Hosp of NY-Presby, 3959 Broadway, rm 701, New York, NY 10032-1559; **Phone:** 212-305-5825; **Board Cert:** Pediatrics 1969; Nephrology 1974; **Med School:** Duke Univ 1964; **Resid:** Internal Medicine, Georgetown Univ Hosp 1965; Pediatrics, Columbia-Presby Med Ctr 1967; **Fellow:** Pediatric Nephrology, Montefiore Med Ctr 1971; **Fac Appt:** Clin Prof Ped, Columbia P&S

Roskes, Saul David MD [PNep] - **Hospital:** Johns Hopkins Hosp (page 61); **Address:** 10807 Falls Rd, Ste 200, Lutherville, MD 21093; **Phone:** 410-321-9393; **Board Cert:** Pediatrics 1970; Pediatric Nephrology 1976; **Med School:** Johns Hopkins Univ 1963; **Resid:** Pediatrics, Bronx Muni Hosp Ctr 1965; Pediatrics, Johns Hopkins Hosp 1968; **Fac Appt:** Assoc Prof Ped, Johns Hopkins Univ

Southeast

Chandar, Jayanthi J MD [PNep] - **Spec Exp:** Kidney Disease; Transplant Medicine-Kidney; Renal Replacement Therapy; **Hospital:** Jackson Meml Hosp (page 70); **Address:** Univ Miami Div Ped Nephrology, PO Box 016960 (M-714), Miami, FL 33101; **Phone:** 305-585-6726; **Board Cert:** Pediatrics 2005; Pediatric Nephrology 2003; **Med School:** India 1983; **Resid:** Pediatrics, Jackson Memorial Hosp 1987; **Fellow:** Pediatric Nephrology, Jackson Memorial Hosp 1993; **Fac Appt:** Assoc Prof Ped, Univ Miami Sch Med

Garin, Eduardo H MD [PNep] - **Hospital:** Shands at Univ of FL; **Address:** Shands Healthcare, Dept Ped Nephrology, 1600 SW Archer Rd, rm HD214, Box 100296, Gainesville, FL 32610; **Phone:** 352-392-4434; **Board Cert:** Pediatrics 1976; Pediatric Nephrology 1976; **Med School:** Chile 1970; **Resid:** Pediatrics, Univ Hosp and Clins 1973; **Fellow:** Pediatric Nephrology, Shands Hosp Univ FL 1975; **Fac Appt:** Prof Ped, Univ S Fla Coll Med

Pediatric Nephrology

Neiberger, Richard E MD/PhD [PNep] - **Spec Exp:** Kidney Disease-Genetic; **Hospital:** Shands at Univ of FL; **Address:** Univ Florida College of Medicine, Div Pediatric Nephrology, 1600 SW Archer Rd, Gainesville, FL 32610; **Phone:** 352-392-4434; **Board Cert:** Pediatrics 2006; Nephrology 2006; **Med School:** Univ Louisville Sch Med 1982; **Resid:** Pediatrics, Montefiore Med Ctr 1985; **Fellow:** Pediatric Nephrology, Montefiore Med Ctr 1988; **Fac Appt:** Assoc Prof Ped, Univ Fla Coll Med

Wyatt, Robert J MD [PNep] - **Spec Exp:** Kidney Disease-Autoimmune; Berger's Disease (IgA Nephropathy); **Hospital:** Le Bonheur Chldns Med Ctr; **Address:** Univ Tennessee, Dept Peds, 777 Washington Ave, Ste P110, Memphis, TN 38105; **Phone:** 901-448-2070; **Board Cert:** Pediatrics 1978; Pediatric Nephrology 1979; **Med School:** Med Coll GA 1973; **Resid:** Pediatrics, Kentucky Med Ctr 1976; **Fellow:** Pediatric Nephrology, Cincinnati Chldns Hosp 1979; **Fac Appt:** Prof Ped, Univ Tenn Coll Med, Memphis

Zilleruelo, Gaston E MD [PNep] - **Spec Exp:** Transplant Medicine-Kidney; Nephrotic Syndrome; Congenital Anomalies-Genitourinary; **Hospital:** Jackson Meml Hosp (page 70), Broward General Med Ctr; **Address:** Univ Miami, Dept Peds-Div Nephrology, PO Box 016960 (M-714), Miami, FL 33136; **Phone:** 305-585-6726; **Board Cert:** Pediatrics 1979; Pediatric Nephrology 1991; **Med School:** Chile 1969; **Resid:** Pediatrics, L Calvo-Mackenna Chldns Hosp 1972; Pediatrics, Jackson Meml Hosp 1977; **Fellow:** Pediatric Nephrology, Jackson Meml Hosp 1979; **Fac Appt:** Prof Ped, Univ Miami Sch Med

Midwest

Andreoli, Sharon MD [PNep] - **Spec Exp:** Kidney Failure; Kidney Failure-Chronic; Osteodystrophy; Glomerulonephritis; **Hospital:** Riley Hosp for Children, Indiana Univ Hosp; **Address:** 699 West Drive, rm RR230, Indianapolis, IN 46202; **Phone:** 317-278-0854; **Board Cert:** Pediatrics 1983; Pediatric Nephrology 1985; **Med School:** Indiana Univ 1978; **Resid:** Pediatrics, James W Riley Hosp 1981; **Fellow:** Pediatric Nephrology, Univ Minnesota 1981; Pediatric Nephrology, Indiana Univ 1984; **Fac Appt:** Prof Ped, Indiana Univ

Avner, Ellis D MD [PNep] - **Spec Exp:** Polycystic Kidney Disease; Kidney Disease-Genetic; **Hospital:** Chldns Hosp - Wisconsin; **Address:** 999 N 92nd Ave, Milwaukee, WI 53226; **Phone:** 414-337-7702; **Board Cert:** Pediatrics 1980; Pediatric Nephrology 1982; **Med School:** Univ Pennsylvania 1975; **Resid:** Pediatrics, Chldns Hosp Med Ctr 1978; **Fellow:** Pediatric Nephrology, Chldns Hosp Med Ctr 1980; **Fac Appt:** Prof Ped, Med Coll Wisc

Bunchman, Timothy E MD [PNep] - **Spec Exp:** Lupus/SLE; **Hospital:** DeVos Children's Hosp; **Address:** DeVos Ped Nephrology/Transplant, 221 Michigan St NE, Ste 406, MC 083, Grand Rapids, MI 49503; **Phone:** 616-391-3788; **Board Cert:** Pediatrics 1986; Pediatric Nephrology 2003; **Med School:** Loyola Univ-Stritch Sch Med 1981; **Resid:** Internal Medicine & Pediatrics, St Louis Univ 1982; Pediatrics, St Louis Univ 1984; **Fellow:** Pediatric Nephrology, Mayo Clinic 1986; Pediatric Nephrology, Univ Minn 1987; **Fac Appt:** Prof Ped, Univ Mich Med Sch

Cohn, Richard MD [PNep] - **Spec Exp:** Transplant Medicine-Kidney; Nephrotic Syndrome; Kidney Disease-Chronic; **Hospital:** Children's Mem Hosp; **Address:** Childrens Meml Hosp, 2300 Children's Plaza, Box 37, Chicago, IL 60614-3394; **Phone:** 773-327-3930; **Board Cert:** Pediatrics 1978; Pediatric Nephrology 1979; **Med School:** Albert Einstein Coll Med 1972; **Resid:** Pediatrics, Johns Hopkins Hosp 1975; **Fellow:** Pediatric Nephrology, Univ Minnesota Hosp 1978; **Fac Appt:** Prof Ped, Northwestern Univ

Friedman, Aaron L MD [PNep] - **Spec Exp:** Hypertension; Transplant Medicine-Kidney; Growth Disorders; **Hospital:** Univ Minn Med Ctr, Fairview - Univ Campus; **Address:** Univ Minnesota Chldns Hosp Fairview, MMC 391, 420 Delaware St SE, Minneapolis, MN 55455; **Phone:** 612-626-2802; **Board Cert:** Pediatrics 1979; Pediatric Nephrology 2003; **Med School:** SUNY Upstate Med Univ 1974; **Resid:** Pediatrics, Univ Wisconsin Med Ctr 1976; **Fellow:** Pediatric Nephrology, Univ Wisconsin 1980; **Fac Appt:** Prof Ped, Univ Minn

Kashtan, Clifford E MD [PNep] - **Spec Exp:** Transplant Medicine-Kidney; Kidney Disease-Genetic; **Hospital:** Univ Minn Med Ctr, Fairview - Univ Campus; **Address:** Univ Minn Amplatz Chldns Hosp, 420 Delaware St SEd, MMC 491, Minneapolis, MN 55455; **Phone:** 612-626-2922; **Board Cert:** Pediatrics 1983; Pediatric Nephrology 2003; **Med School:** Wayne State Univ 1978; **Resid:** Pediatrics, Boston City Hosp 1981; **Fellow:** Pediatric Nephrology, Mass Genl Hosp 1984; Pediatric Nephrology, Univ Minnesota Hosp 1987; **Fac Appt:** Prof Ped, Univ Minn

Langman, Craig MD [PNep] - **Spec Exp:** Kidney Stones; Osteoporosis-Juvenile; Oxalosis; **Hospital:** Children's Mem Hosp, Evanston/Northshore Univ Hlth Syst; **Address:** Children's Meml Hosp, 2300 N Children's Plaza, Box 37, Chicago, IL 60614-3394; **Phone:** 773-327-3930; **Board Cert:** Pediatrics 1982; Pediatric Nephrology 1992; **Med School:** Hahnemann Univ 1977; **Resid:** Pediatrics, Chldns Hosp 1979; **Fellow:** Pediatric Nephrology, Chldns Hosp 1981; **Fac Appt:** Prof Ped, Northwestern Univ

Nevins, Thomas E MD [PNep] - **Spec Exp:** Kidney Failure-Chronic; Transplant Medicine-Kidney; Hypertension; Dialysis Care; **Hospital:** Univ Minn Med Ctr, Fairview - Univ Campus; **Address:** Fairview Univ Med Ctr, Dept Peds, 420 Delaware St SE, MMC-491, Minneapolis, MN 55455-0374; **Phone:** 612-626-2922; **Board Cert:** Pediatrics 1975; Pediatric Nephrology 1992; **Med School:** Washington Univ, St Louis 1969; **Resid:** Pediatrics, Univ Minnesota Hosps 1972; **Fellow:** Nephrology, Univ Minnesota Hosps 1978; **Fac Appt:** Prof Ped, Univ Minn

Warady, Bradley MD [PNep] - **Spec Exp:** Dialysis Care; Transplant Medicine-Kidney; Kidney Disease-Chronic; **Hospital:** Chldns Mercy Hosps & Clinics; **Address:** Chldns Mercy Hosps & Clins, Dept Ped Nephrology, 2401 Gillham Rd, Kansas City, MO 64108; **Phone:** 816-234-3010; **Board Cert:** Pediatrics 1984; Pediatric Nephrology 1985; **Med School:** Univ IL Coll Med 1979; **Resid:** Pediatrics, Chldns Mercy Hosp 1982; **Fellow:** Pediatric Nephrology, Colorado Univ Med Ctr 1984; **Fac Appt:** Prof Ped, Univ MO-Kansas City

West Coast and Pacific

Alexander, Steven R MD [PNep] - **Spec Exp:** Kidney Failure; Transplant Medicine-Kidney; Nephrotic Syndrome; **Hospital:** Lucile Packard Chldn's Hosp; **Address:** Stanford Univ Med Ctr, Dept Peds, 300 Pasteur Drive, rm G306, Stanford, CA 94305-5208; **Phone:** 650-723-7903; **Board Cert:** Pediatrics 1986; Pediatric Nephrology 1986; **Med School:** Baylor Coll Med 1971; **Resid:** Pediatrics, Baylor Affil Hosps 1976; **Fellow:** Pediatric Nephrology, Baylor Affil Hosps 1978; **Fac Appt:** Prof Ped, Stanford Univ

Ettenger, Robert B MD [PNep] - **Spec Exp:** Transplant Medicine-Kidney; Hypertension in Children; Urinary Tract Infections; Kidney Disease; **Hospital:** UCLA Ronald Reagan Med Ctr, Mattel Chldns Hosp at UCLA; **Address:** Mattel Chldns Hosp, Dept Ped Nephrology, Le Conte Ave, Box 951752, Los Angeles, CA 90095; **Phone:** 310-206-6987; **Board Cert:** Pediatrics 1986; Pediatric Nephrology 1986; **Med School:** Univ Pennsylvania 1968; **Resid:** Pediatrics, St Christophers Hosp Chldn 1971; **Fellow:** Pediatric Nephrology, Chldns Hosp 1975; **Fac Appt:** Prof Ped, UCLA

Pediatric Nephrology

Flynn, Joseph T MD [PNep] - **Spec Exp:** Hypertension; Dialysis Care; **Hospital:** Chldns Hosp and Regl Med Ctr - Seattle; **Address:** Children's Hospital, Ped Nephrology, PO Box 5371, MS A-7931, Seattle, WA 98105; **Phone:** 206-987-2524; **Board Cert:** Pediatric Nephrology 2008; **Med School:** SUNY Upstate Med Univ 1987; **Resid:** Pediatrics, St Christophers Hosp 1990; **Fellow:** Pediatric Nephrology, St Christophers Hosp 1993; **Fac Appt:** Prof Ped, Univ Wash

Jordan, Stanley C MD [PNep] - **Spec Exp:** Transplant Medicine-Kidney; **Hospital:** Cedars-Sinai Med Ctr; **Address:** Cedars Sinai Med Ctr, Div Ped Nephrology, 8635 W 3rd St, Ste 590W, Los Angeles, CA 90048; **Phone:** 310-423-2624; **Board Cert:** Pediatrics 1978; Pediatric Nephrology 1979; Clinical & Laboratory Immunology 1988; **Med School:** Univ NC Sch Med 1973; **Resid:** Pediatrics, UCLA Med Ctr 1976; Pediatric Nephrology, UCLA Med Ctr 1977; **Fellow:** Renal Immunology, Scripps Clinic 1978; Dialysis & Tranplantation, Chldns Hosp 1980; **Fac Appt:** Prof Ped, UCLA

McDonald, Ruth A MD [PNep] - **Spec Exp:** Transplant Medicine-Kidney; Kidney Disease; **Hospital:** Chldns Hosp and Regl Med Ctr - Seattle; **Address:** 4800 Sand Point Way NE, MS A-7931, Seattle, WA 98105; **Phone:** 206-987-2524; **Board Cert:** Pediatric Nephrology 2005; **Med School:** Univ Minn 1987; **Resid:** Pediatrics, Chldns Hosp & Med Ctr 1990; **Fellow:** Pediatric Nephrology, Chldns Hosp & Med Ctr 1993; **Fac Appt:** Assoc Prof Ped, Univ Wash

PEDIATRIC OTOLARYNGOLOGY

New England

Cunningham, Michael J MD [PO] - **Spec Exp:** Head & Neck Tumors; Sinus Disorders; Hemangiomas; Vascular Malformations; **Hospital:** Mass Eye & Ear Infirmary, Mass Genl Hosp; **Address:** Mass Eye & Ear Infirmary, 243 Charles St, Boston, MA 02114; **Phone:** 617-573-4250; **Board Cert:** Otolaryngology 1988; **Med School:** Univ Rochester 1981; **Resid:** Pediatrics, Mass General Hosp 1983; Otolaryngology, U Pittsburgh Eye & Ear Hosp 1988; **Fellow:** Pediatric Otolaryngology, Mass Eye & Ear Infirm 1989; **Fac Appt:** Assoc Prof Oto, Harvard Med Sch

Healy, Gerald MD [PO] - **Hospital:** Children's Hospital - Boston; **Address:** Chldns Hosp, Dept Otolaryngology, 300 Longwood Ave, LO-367, Boston, MA 02115; **Phone:** 617-355-5064; **Board Cert:** Otolaryngology 1972; **Med School:** Boston Univ 1967; **Resid:** Surgery, Boston Univ Hosps 1969; Otolaryngology, Boston Univ Hosps 1972; **Fac Appt:** Prof Oto, Harvard Med Sch

McGill, Trevor J MD [PO] - **Spec Exp:** Head & Neck Tumors; Cholesteatoma; Lymphatic Malformations-Head & Neck; Hemangiomas; **Hospital:** Children's Hospital - Boston; **Address:** Childrens Hosp, Dept Otolaryngology, 300 Longwood Ave, MS LO-367, Boston, MA 02115; **Phone:** 617-355-8589; **Board Cert:** Otolaryngology 1988; **Med School:** Ireland 1967; **Resid:** Otolaryngology, Royal Natl Throat Nose & Ear Hosp 1974; **Fellow:** Otolaryngology, Mass Eye & Ear Infirm 1976; **Fac Appt:** Prof Oto, Harvard Med Sch

Mid Atlantic

April, Max M MD [PO] - **Spec Exp:** Sinus Disorders; Neck Masses; Laryngeal Disorders; Tonsil/Adenoid Disorders; **Hospital:** NY-Presby Hosp/Weill Cornell (page 66), Long Island Jewish Med Ctr; **Address:** Weill-Cornell Medical Ctr, Dept Otolaryngology, 1305 York Ave Fl 5, New York, NY 10021; **Phone:** 646-962-2225; **Board Cert:** Otolaryngology 1990; **Med School:** Boston Univ 1985; **Resid:** Otolaryngology, Boston Univ Med Ctr 1990; **Fellow:** Pediatric Otolaryngology, Johns Hopkins Hosp 1991; **Fac Appt:** Clin Prof Oto, Cornell Univ-Weill Med Coll

Casselbrant, Margaretha L MD/PhD [PO] - **Spec Exp:** Ear Infections; **Hospital:** Chldns Hosp of Pittsburgh - UPMC; **Address:** Children's Hospital, Dept Otolaryngology, 3705 Fifth Ave Fl 3, Pittsburgh, PA 15213; **Phone:** 412-692-5460; **Board Cert:** Otolaryngology 1992; **Med School:** Sweden 1973; **Resid:** Otolaryngology, Malmo Genl Hosp-Univ of Lund 1978; **Fellow:** Otolaryngology, Univ Pittsburgh 1982; **Fac Appt:** Prof Oto, Univ Pittsburgh

Dolitsky, Jay MD [PO] - **Spec Exp:** Ear Infections; Neck Masses; Tonsil/Adenoid Disorders; Sleep Disorders; **Hospital:** New York Eye & Ear Infirm (page 65); **Address:** 404 Park Ave S Fl 12, New York, NY 10016; **Phone:** 212-679-3499; **Board Cert:** Otolaryngology 1990; **Med School:** SUNY Downstate 1981; **Resid:** Otolaryngology, Manhattan EET Hosp 1990; **Fellow:** Pediatric Otolaryngology, Children's Hosp 1992; **Fac Appt:** Assoc Prof Oto, NY Med Coll

Goldsmith, Ari J MD [PO] - **Spec Exp:** Voice Disorders; Airway Disorders; Hearing Loss; Sleep Apnea; **Hospital:** Long Island Coll Hosp (page 57); **Address:** LICH-Dept Otolaryngology, 134 Atlantic Ave, Brooklyn, NY 11201-5502; **Phone:** 718-780-1498; **Board Cert:** Otolaryngology 1994; **Med School:** Albert Einstein Coll Med 1988; **Resid:** Otolaryngology, LI Jewish Hosp 1993; **Fellow:** Pediatric Otolaryngology, Chldns Hosp 1994; **Fac Appt:** Assoc Prof Oto, SUNY Hlth Sci Ctr

Haddad Jr, Joseph MD [PO] - **Spec Exp:** Ear Infections; Sinus Disorders; Cleft Palate/Lip; **Hospital:** NYPresby-Morgan Stanley Children's Hosp (page 66); **Address:** Morgan Stanley Chldns Hosp of NY-Presby, 3959 Broadway, Ste 501N, New York, NY 10032-1559; **Phone:** 212-305-8933; **Board Cert:** Otolaryngology 1988; **Med School:** NYU Sch Med 1983; **Resid:** Surgery, Columbia-Presby Hosp 1985; Otolaryngology, Columbia-Presby Hosp 1988; **Fellow:** Pediatric Otolaryngology, Chldns Hosp 1990; **Fac Appt:** Clin Prof Oto, Columbia P&S

Harley, Earl H MD [PO] - **Spec Exp:** Infectious Disease; **Hospital:** Georgetown Univ Hosp; **Address:** Georgetown Univ Hosp, 3800 Reservoir Rd NW, Gorman Bldg Fl 1, Washington, DC 20007; **Phone:** 202-444-8186; **Board Cert:** Otolaryngology 1984; **Med School:** Howard Univ 1971; **Resid:** Pediatrics, San Diego Naval Hosp 1973; Otolaryngology, Oakland Naval Hosp 1984; **Fellow:** Pediatric Otolaryngology, Chldn's Hosp Natl Med Ctr 1988; Pediatric Otolaryngology, Mass EE Infirm/Harvard Med Sch 1989; **Fac Appt:** Asst Prof Oto, Georgetown Univ

Jones, Jacqueline MD [PO] - **Spec Exp:** Sinus Disorders/Surgery; Ear Infections; **Hospital:** NY-Presby Hosp/Weill Cornell (page 66), Lenox Hill Hosp (page 62); **Address:** 1175 Park Ave, Ste 1A, New York, NY 10128; **Phone:** 212-996-2559; **Board Cert:** Otolaryngology 1989; **Med School:** Cornell Univ-Weill Med Coll 1984; **Resid:** Otolaryngology, Hosp Univ Penn 1989; **Fellow:** Pediatric Otolaryngology, Chldns Hosp 1990; **Fac Appt:** Assoc Prof Oto, Cornell Univ-Weill Med Coll

Kazahaya, Ken MD [PO] - **Spec Exp:** Cochlear Implants; Skull Base Surgery; Otology; Sinus Disorders; **Hospital:** Chldns Hosp of Philadelphia, The, Hosp Univ Penn - UPHS (page 60); **Address:** Children's Hosp of Philadelphia, Div Pediatric Otolaryngology, 34th St & Civic Ctr Blvd Wood Bldg Fl 1, Philadelphia, PA 19104; **Phone:** 215-590-3440; **Board Cert:** Otolaryngology 1999; **Med School:** Univ Pennsylvania 1993; **Resid:** Otolaryngology, Hosp U Penn 1998; **Fellow:** Pediatric Otolaryngology, Children's Hosp 2000; **Fac Appt:** Asst Prof Oto, Univ Pennsylvania

Rosenfeld, Richard M MD [PO] - **Spec Exp:** Sinus Disorders/Surgery; Head & Neck Surgery; Ear Disorders/Surgery; **Hospital:** Long Island Coll Hosp (page 57), SUNY Downstate Med Ctr; **Address:** Univ Otolaryngologists, 134 Atlantic Ave, Brooklyn, NY 11201; **Phone:** 718-780-1498; **Board Cert:** Otolaryngology 1989; **Med School:** SUNY Buffalo 1984; **Resid:** Otolaryngology, Mount Sinai Med Ctr 1989; **Fellow:** Pediatric Otolaryngology, Chldn's Hosp 1991; **Fac Appt:** Prof Oto, SUNY Downstate

Pediatric Otolaryngology

Tunkel, David E MD [PO] - **Spec Exp:** Laryngeal Disorders; Otology; Head & Neck Surgery; **Hospital:** Johns Hopkins Hosp (page 61), Greater Baltimore Med Ctr; **Address:** 601 N Caroline St, rm 6161, Baltimore, MD 21287; **Phone:** 410-955-1559; **Board Cert:** Otolaryngology 1990; **Med School:** Johns Hopkins Univ 1984; **Resid:** Surgery, Johns Hopkins Hosp 1986; Otolaryngology, Johns Hopkins Hosp 1990; **Fellow:** Pediatric Otolaryngology, Chldns Natl Med Ctr 1991; **Fac Appt:** Assoc Prof Oto, Johns Hopkins Univ

Ward, Robert MD [PO] - **Spec Exp:** Airway Disorders; Sinus Disorders/Surgery; Choanal Atresia; **Hospital:** NY-Presby Hosp/Weill Cornell (page 66), Lenox Hill Hosp (Manh Eye, Ear & Throat Hosp) (page 62); **Address:** Weill Cornell Med Ctr, Otolaryngology, 1305 York Ave Fl 5, New York, NY 10021; **Phone:** 646-962-2224; **Board Cert:** Otolaryngology 1986; **Med School:** Cornell Univ-Weill Med Coll 1981; **Resid:** Surgery, NY Hosp 1983; Otolaryngology, NY Hosp 1986; **Fellow:** Pediatric Otolaryngology, Chldns Hosp 1986; **Fac Appt:** Assoc Clin Prof Oto, Cornell Univ-Weill Med Coll

Southeast

Darrow, David H MD/DDS [PO] - **Spec Exp:** Airway Disorders; Sinus Disorders; Otology; Neck Masses; **Hospital:** Chldns Hosp of King's Daughters; **Address:** Chldns Hosp of Kings Daughters, Div Otolaryngology, 601 Childrens Lane, Norfolk, VA 23507; **Phone:** 757-668-9327; **Board Cert:** Otolaryngology 1994; **Med School:** Duke Univ 1987; **Resid:** Otolaryngology, UCSD Med Ctr 1993; **Fellow:** Pediatric Otolaryngology, Chldns Meml Hosp 1994; **Fac Appt:** Assoc Prof Oto, Eastern VA Med Sch

Drake, Amelia F MD [PO] - **Spec Exp:** Head & Neck Surgery; **Hospital:** Univ NC Hosps; **Address:** 170 Manning Drive, Physicians Bldg, Box CB 7070, Chapel Hill, NC 27599; **Phone:** 919-966-6483; **Board Cert:** Otolaryngology 1987; **Med School:** Univ NC Sch Med 1981; **Resid:** Otolaryngology, Univ Michigan Hosps 1986; **Fac Appt:** Prof Oto, Univ NC Sch Med

Eavey, Roland D MD [PO] - **Spec Exp:** Ear Reconstruction/Microtia; Ear Disorders/Surgery; **Hospital:** Vanderbilt Children's Hosp; **Address:** 1215 21st Ave S, Med Ctr East 6310, Nashville, TN 37232-8605; **Phone:** 615-936-0708; **Board Cert:** Pediatrics 1982; Otolaryngology 1981; **Med School:** Univ Pennsylvania 1975; **Resid:** Pediatrics, Chldns Hosp 1977; Surgery, Kaiser Hosp 1978; **Fellow:** Otolaryngology, Mass EE Infirm 1981; **Fac Appt:** Prof Oto, Vanderbilt Univ

Orobello Jr, Peter W MD [PO] - **Spec Exp:** Sinus Disorders; Ear Disorders; Cochlear Implants; Airway Reconstruction; **Hospital:** All Children's Hosp, St Josephs Chldns Hosp; **Address:** 801 6th St S, Box 7535, St Petersburg, FL 33701; **Phone:** 727-329-5400; **Board Cert:** Otolaryngology 1988; **Med School:** Univ Cincinnati 1983; **Resid:** Surgery, Univ Cincinnati Med Ctr 1984; Otolaryngology, Univ Cincinnati Med Ctr 1988; **Fellow:** Pediatric Otolaryngology, Johns Hopkins Hosp 1989; **Fac Appt:** Asst Clin Prof Ped, Univ S Fla Coll Med

Midwest

Arjmand, Ellis MD/PhD [PO] - **Spec Exp:** Hearing Loss; Cochlear Implants; **Hospital:** Cincinnati Chldns Hosp Med Ctr; **Address:** Children's Hospital, Dept Otolaryngology, 3333 Burnet Ave, ML 2018, Cincinnati, OH 45229; **Phone:** 513-636-4355; **Board Cert:** Otolaryngology 1994; **Med School:** Northwestern Univ 1986; **Resid:** Otolaryngology, Barnes Jewish Hosp 1993; **Fellow:** Pediatric Otolaryngology, Barnes Jewish Hosp 1994; **Fac Appt:** Assoc Prof Oto, Univ Cincinnati

Arnold, James E MD [PO] - **Spec Exp:** Airway Disorders; Otology; Ear Tumors; **Hospital:** Rainbow Babies & Chldns Hosp, Univ Hosps Case Med Ctr; **Address:** 11100 Euclid Ave, Lakeside Bldg Fl 4, Cleveland, OH 44106-2602; **Phone:** 216-844-5031; **Board Cert:** Otolaryngology 1982; **Med School:** Univ Tex, San Antonio 1977; **Resid:** Otolaryngology, Fitzsimons Army Med Ctr 1982; **Fellow:** Pediatric Otolaryngology, Childrens Hosp 1987; **Fac Appt:** Prof Oto, Case West Res Univ

Belenky, Walter MD [PO] - **Spec Exp:** Cochlear Implants; Airway Disorders; **Hospital:** Chldns Hosp of Michigan; **Address:** Chldns Hosp, Dept Ped Oto, 3901 Beaubien Fl 3, Detroit, MI 48201; **Phone:** 313-745-9048; **Board Cert:** Otolaryngology 1970; **Med School:** Univ Mich Med Sch 1963; **Resid:** Surgery, William Beaumont Hosps 1965; Otolaryngology, Wayne Affil Hosp 1968

Cotton, Robin MD [PO] - **Spec Exp:** Tracheal Surgery; Head & Neck Surgery; Airway Reconstruction; **Hospital:** Cincinnati Chldns Hosp Med Ctr; **Address:** Cincinnati Chldns Hosp, 3333 Burnet Ave, ML 2018, Cincinnati, OH 45229-3039; **Phone:** 513-636-4355; **Board Cert:** Otolaryngology 1972; **Med School:** England, UK 1965; **Resid:** Otolaryngology, Univ Birmingham 1968; Otolaryngology, Univ Toronto Med Ctr 1972; **Fellow:** Head and Neck Surgery, Univ Cincinnati Med Ctr 1973; **Fac Appt:** Prof Oto, Univ Cincinnati

Holinger, Lauren D MD [PO] - **Spec Exp:** Airway Disorders; Swallowing Disorders; Cough-Chronic; Voice Disorders; **Hospital:** Children's Mem Hosp; **Address:** Chldns Meml Hosp, Dept Otolaryngology, 2300 N Childrens Plaza, Box 25, Chicago, IL 60614-3394; **Phone:** 773-880-4457; **Board Cert:** Otolaryngology 1975; **Med School:** Ros Franklin Univ/Chicago Med Sch 1971; **Resid:** Surgery, Univ Colorado Affil Hosp 1972; Otolaryngology, Univ Colorado Affil Hosp 1975; **Fellow:** Pediatric Otolaryngology, Chldns Meml Hosp 1976; **Fac Appt:** Prof Oto, Northwestern Univ

Katz, Robert L MD [PO] - **Spec Exp:** Ear Infections; Sinus Disorders/Surgery; Hearing Loss; **Hospital:** Cleveland Clin Fdn (page 56); **Address:** 29800 Bainbridge Rd, Solon, OH 44139-2202; **Phone:** 440-519-6950; **Board Cert:** Otolaryngology 1968; **Med School:** Case West Res Univ 1963; **Resid:** Surgery, Mount Sinai Hosp 1965; Otolaryngology, Mass EE Infirm/Chldns Hosp 1968; **Fac Appt:** Clin Prof Oto, Case West Res Univ

Miller, Robert P MD [PO] - **Spec Exp:** Ear Disorders/Surgery; Airway Disorders; Sinus Disorders; Tonsil/Adenoid Disorders; **Hospital:** Adv Luth Genl Hosp, Children's Mem Hosp; **Address:** 8780 W Golf Rd, Ste 200, Niles, IL 60714; **Phone:** 847-674-5585; **Board Cert:** Otolaryngology 1978; **Med School:** Loyola Univ-Stritch Sch Med 1974; **Resid:** Otolaryngology, Univ Illinois Hosps 1978; **Fellow:** Pediatric Otolaryngology, Chldns Hosp Med Ctr 1987; **Fac Appt:** Asst Clin Prof Oto, Univ IL Coll Med

Myer III, Charles M MD [PO] - **Spec Exp:** Airway Disorders; Head & Neck Tumors; Neck Masses; **Hospital:** Cincinnati Chldns Hosp Med Ctr, Univ Hosp - Cincinnati; **Address:** Cincinnati Chldns Hosp, Dept Oto, 3333 Burnet Ave Bldg C Fl 3 - Ste 375, Cincinnati, OH 45229; **Phone:** 513-636-4355; **Board Cert:** Otolaryngology 1984; **Med School:** Univ Alabama 1978; **Resid:** Otolaryngology, Univ Cincinnati Med Ctr 1984; **Fellow:** Pediatric Otolaryngology, Chldns Hosp 1985; **Fac Appt:** Prof Oto, Univ Cincinnati

Great Plains and Mountains

Chan, Kenny H MD [PO] - **Spec Exp:** Ear Infections; Sinusitis; **Hospital:** Chldn's Hosp - Aurora, The, Parker Adventist Hosp; **Address:** Chldns Hosp, Dept Otolaryngology, 13123 E 16th Ave, Box B455, Aurora, CO 80045; **Phone:** 720-777-8501; **Board Cert:** Otolaryngology 1984; **Med School:** Loma Linda Univ 1977; **Resid:** Surgery, Oregon Hlth Sci Univ 1978; Otolaryngology, Loma Linda Univ Hosp 1983; **Fellow:** Pediatric Otolaryngology, Chldns Hosp 1987; **Fac Appt:** Prof Oto, Univ Colorado

Pediatric Otolaryngology

Lusk, Rodney P MD [PO] - **Spec Exp:** Cochlear Implants; Sinus Disorders/Surgery; Sleep Disorders/Apnea; **Hospital:** Boys Town Natl Rsch Hosp, Children's Hosp - Omaha; **Address:** Boystown National Research Hosp, 555 N 30th St, Omaha, NE 68131; **Phone:** 402-498-6502; **Board Cert:** Otolaryngology 1982; **Med School:** Univ MO-Columbia Sch Med 1977; **Resid:** Head and Neck Surgery, Univ Iowa Hosp & Clinics 1982; **Fellow:** Pediatric Otolaryngology, Chldns Hosp 1983

Southwest

Bower, Charles MD [PO] - **Spec Exp:** Airway Disorders; Sleep Disorders/Apnea; Sinus Disorders/Surgery; **Hospital:** Arkansas Chldns Hosp; **Address:** Arkansas Chldns Hosp, Dept Ped Oto, 800 Marshall St, Slot 836, Little Rock, AR 72202-3510; **Phone:** 501-364-1047; **Board Cert:** Otolaryngology 1990; **Med School:** Univ Ark 1985; **Resid:** Otolaryngology, Univ Ark Med Ctr 1991; **Fellow:** Pediatric Otolaryngology, Chldns Hosp 1992; **Fac Appt:** Assoc Prof Oto, Univ Ark

Duncan III, Newton O MD [PO] - **Spec Exp:** Sinus Disorders; Airway Disorders; Head & Neck Surgery; **Hospital:** Texas Chldns Hosp, Methodist Hosp - Houston; **Address:** Childrens Ear Nose & Throat, 6550 Fannin St, Ste 2001, Houston, TX 77030-2709; **Phone:** 713-796-2001; **Board Cert:** Otolaryngology 1986; **Med School:** Baylor Coll Med 1978; **Resid:** Surgery, Baylor Coll Med 1983; Otolaryngology, Baylor Coll Med 1986; **Fellow:** Pediatric Otolaryngology, Univ Wash 1991; Pediatric Otolaryngology, Royal Alexandra Hosp Chld 1992; **Fac Appt:** Asst Clin Prof Oto, Baylor Coll Med

Friedman, Ellen M MD [PO] - **Spec Exp:** Airway Disorders; Lymphatic Malformations-Head & Neck; **Hospital:** Texas Chldns Hosp; **Address:** 67010 Fannin, Ste 540, MC CC6102, Houston, TX 77030; **Phone:** 832-822-3250; **Board Cert:** Otolaryngology 1981; **Med School:** Albert Einstein Coll Med 1975; **Resid:** Surgery, Montefiore Hosp 1976; Otolaryngology, Washington Hosp Ctr 1979; **Fellow:** Pediatric Otolaryngology, Boston Chldns Hosp; **Fac Appt:** Prof Oto, Baylor Coll Med

West Coast and Pacific

Crockett, Dennis M MD [PO] - **Spec Exp:** Head & Neck Cancer; Airway Disorders; **Hospital:** USC Univ Hosp; **Address:** 26726 Crown Valley Pkwy, Ste 200, Mission Viejo, CA 92691; **Phone:** 949-364-4361; **Board Cert:** Otolaryngology 1985; **Med School:** USC Sch Med 1979; **Resid:** Otolaryngology, LAC-USC Med Ctr 1984; **Fellow:** Pediatrics, Boston Chldns Hosp 1985; **Fac Appt:** Assoc Prof Oto, USC Sch Med

Geller, Kenneth Allen MD [PO] - **Spec Exp:** Airway Disorders; Sinus Disorders/Surgery; Head & Neck Cancer; Pediatric Airway Disorders; **Hospital:** Chldns Hosp - Los Angeles, Huntington Memorial Hosp; **Address:** Chldns Hosp, Div Otolaryngology, 4650 Sunset Blvd, MS 58, Los Angeles, CA 90027; **Phone:** 323-361-2145; **Board Cert:** Otolaryngology 1978; **Med School:** USC Sch Med 1972; **Resid:** Surgery, Wadsworth VA Hosp 1975; Otolaryngology, UCLA Hlth Scis Ctr 1978; **Fellow:** Pediatric Otolaryngology, Chldns Hosp 1979; **Fac Appt:** Assoc Clin Prof Oto, USC Sch Med

Inglis, Andrew MD [PO] - **Spec Exp:** Airway Disorders; Voice Disorders; **Hospital:** Chldns Hosp and Regl Med Ctr - Seattle; **Address:** Children's Hospital & Medical Ctr, 4800 Sand Point Way NE, MS W6640, Seattle, WA 98105-0371; **Phone:** 206-987-2105; **Board Cert:** Otolaryngology 1987; **Med School:** Med Coll PA Hahnemann 1981; **Resid:** Surgery, Virginia Mason Hosp 1983; Otolaryngology, Univ Washington Hosps 1987; **Fellow:** Pediatric Otolaryngology, Royal Alexandria Hosp Chldn 1987; **Fac Appt:** Assoc Prof Oto, Univ Wash

Richardson, Mark A MD [PO] - **Spec Exp:** Sinus Disorders; Airway Disorders; Lymphatic Malformations-Head & Neck; **Hospital:** Doernbecher Chldns Hosp/OHSU, Providence St Vincent Med Ctr; **Address:** 3181 SW Sam Jackson Park Rd, MC PV01, Portland, OR 97239; **Phone:** 503-494-5350; **Board Cert:** Otolaryngology 1979; **Med School:** Med Univ SC 1975; **Resid:** Otolaryngology, Med Univ Hosp 1979; **Fellow:** Pediatric Otolaryngology, Chldns Hosp Med Ctr 1980; **Fac Appt:** Prof Oto, Oregon Hlth & Sci Univ

Rosbe, Kristina W MD [PO] - **Spec Exp:** Airway Disorders; Sinus Disorders/Surgery; Cochlear Implants; Neck Masses; **Hospital:** UCSF Med Ctr; **Address:** UCSF Med Ctr, Dept Otolaryngology, 400 Parnassus Ave Fl 7th, Box 0342, San Francisco, CA 94143-0342; **Phone:** 415-353-2757; **Board Cert:** Orthopaedic Surgery 1999; **Med School:** Dartmouth Med Sch 1993; **Resid:** Surgery, Univ N Carolina Hosps 1994; Otolaryngology, Univ N Carolina Hosps 1998; **Fellow:** Pediatric Otolaryngology, Chldns Hosp 2000; **Fac Appt:** Assoc Prof Ped, UCSF

PEDIATRIC PULMONOLOGY

New England

Lapey, Allen MD [PPul] - **Spec Exp:** Cystic Fibrosis; Asthma; Food Allergy; **Hospital:** Mass Genl Hosp; **Address:** 275 Cambridge St, Ste 530, Boston, MA 02114; **Phone:** 617-726-8707; **Board Cert:** Pediatrics 1972; Allergy & Immunology 1979; Pediatric Pulmonology 2003; **Med School:** Univ Rochester 1966; **Resid:** Pediatrics, Chldns Hosp 1968; **Fellow:** Pediatric Pulmonology, Mass Genl Hosp 1972; Allergy & Immunology, Mass Genl Hosp 1972; **Fac Appt:** Asst Clin Prof Ped, Harvard Med Sch

Mid Atlantic

Borowitz, Drucy S MD [PPul] - **Spec Exp:** Cystic Fibrosis; **Hospital:** Women's & Chldn's Hosp of Buffalo, The; **Address:** Women & Childrens Hospital, The Lung Center, 219 Bryant St, Buffalo, NY 14222; **Phone:** 716-878-7561; **Board Cert:** Pediatrics 1984; Pediatric Gastroenterology 2007; **Med School:** Cornell Univ-Weill Med Coll 1979; **Resid:** Pediatrics, UCSF Med Ctr 1982; **Fellow:** Nutrition, UCSF Med Ctr 1983; **Fac Appt:** Clin Prof Ped, SUNY Buffalo

Dozor, Allen J MD [PPul] - **Spec Exp:** Asthma; Cystic Fibrosis; **Hospital:** Westchester Med Ctr; **Address:** NY Med College, Munger Pavilion, Pediatric Pulmonology, Ste 106, Valhalla, NY 10595-1600; **Phone:** 914-493-7585; **Board Cert:** Pediatrics 1981; Pediatric Pulmonology 2003; **Med School:** Penn State Univ-Hershey Med Ctr 1977; **Resid:** Pediatrics, St Vincent's Hosp & Med Ctr 1980; **Fellow:** Pediatric Pulmonology, Chldns Hosp 1982; **Fac Appt:** Prof Ped, NY Med Coll

Kattan, Meyer MD [PPul] - **Spec Exp:** Asthma; Cystic Fibrosis; Chronic Lung Disease; **Hospital:** NY-Presby Hosp/Columbia (page 66), Englewood Hosp & Med Ctr; **Address:** 3959 Broadway, CHC 7-701, New York, NY 10032; **Phone:** 212-305-5122; **Board Cert:** Pediatrics 1980; Pediatric Pulmonology 2003; **Med School:** McGill Univ 1973; **Resid:** Pediatrics, Chldns Hosp 1975; Pediatrics, Hosp for Sick Chldn 1976; **Fellow:** Pulmonary Disease, Hosp for Sick Chldn 1978; **Fac Appt:** Prof Ped, Columbia P&S

Kurland, Geoffrey MD [PPul] - **Spec Exp:** Transplant Medicine-Lung; **Hospital:** Chldns Hosp of Pittsburgh - UPMC; **Address:** Children's Hospital Drive, Dept Pediatric Pulmonology, 45th St & Penn, Pittsburgh, PA 15201; **Phone:** 412-692-5630; **Board Cert:** Pediatrics 1978; Allergy & Immunology 1979; Pediatric Pulmonology 2003; **Med School:** Stanford Univ 1973; **Resid:** Pediatrics, Stanford Affil Hosps 1976; **Fellow:** Allergy & Immunology, Stanford Affil Hosps 1978; **Fac Appt:** Prof Ped, Univ Pittsburgh

Pediatric Pulmonology

Loughlin, Gerald M MD [PPul] - **Spec Exp:** Sleep Disorders/Apnea; Swallowing Disorders; Asthma & Chronic Lung Disease; Breathing Disorders; **Hospital:** NY-Presby Hosp/Weill Cornell (page 66); **Address:** Cornell Med Coll, Dept Peds, 525 E 68th St, rm M-622, New York, NY 10021-4870; **Phone:** 212-746-4111; **Board Cert:** Pediatrics 1993; Pediatric Pulmonology 2003; **Med School:** Univ Rochester 1973; **Resid:** Pediatrics, Univ Ariz Med Ctr 1973; **Fellow:** Pediatric Pulmonology, Univ Ariz Med Ctr 1977; **Fac Appt:** Prof Ped, Cornell Univ-Weill Med Coll

Marcus, Carole L MD [PPul] - **Spec Exp:** Sleep Disorders/Apnea; **Hospital:** Chldns Hosp of Philadelphia, The; **Address:** Chldns Hosp of Philadelphia, Wood Bldg 5FL, 34th St & Civic Ctr Blvd, Philadelphia, PA 19104; **Phone:** 215-590-3749; **Board Cert:** Pediatrics 2000; Pediatric Pulmonology 2000; **Med School:** South Africa 1982; **Resid:** Pediatrics, LIJ/SUNY Brooklyn Med Ctr 1986; **Fellow:** Pediatric Pulmonology, Chldns Hosp 1991; **Fac Appt:** Assoc Prof Ped, Univ Pennsylvania

Mcgrath-Morrow, Sharon A MD [PPul] - **Spec Exp:** Lung Injury-Neonatal; Bronchopulmonary Dysplasia; Ataxia Telangiectasia; Swallowing Disorders; **Hospital:** Johns Hopkins Hosp (page 61); **Address:** Johns Hopkins Ped Pulmonology, Rubenstein Childrens Hlth Bldg, 200 N Wolfe St, Ste 3029, Baltimore, MD 21287; **Phone:** 410-955-2035; **Board Cert:** Pediatrics 2007; Pediatric Pulmonology 2007; **Med School:** Univ VA Sch Med 1985; **Resid:** Pediatrics, Johns Hopkins Hosp 1988; **Fellow:** Pulmonary Critical Care Medicine, Johns Hopkins 1992; **Fac Appt:** Assoc Prof Ped, Johns Hopkins Univ

Orenstein, David M MD [PPul] - **Spec Exp:** Cystic Fibrosis; **Hospital:** Chldns Hosp of Pittsburgh - UPMC; **Address:** Children's Hospital Drive, Dept Pediatric Pulmonology, 45th St & Penn, Pittsburgh, PA 15213; **Phone:** 412-692-5630; **Board Cert:** Pediatrics 1979; Pediatric Pulmonology 2004; **Med School:** Case West Res Univ 1973; **Resid:** Pediatrics, Rainbow Babies & Chldn's Hosp 1976; **Fellow:** Pediatric Pulmonology, Rainbow Babies & Chldn's Hosp 1978; **Fac Appt:** Prof Ped, Univ Pittsburgh

Panitch, Howard B MD [PPul] - **Spec Exp:** Chronic Obstructive Lung Disease (COPD); Cystic Fibrosis; **Hospital:** Chldns Hosp of Philadelphia, The; **Address:** Div Pulmonology, 34th St & Civic Center Blvd, Wood Bldg Fl 5, Philadelphia, PA 19104; **Phone:** 215-590-3749; **Board Cert:** Pediatrics 1987; Pediatric Pulmonology 2004; **Med School:** Univ Pittsburgh 1982; **Resid:** Pediatrics, Children's Hosp 1985; **Fellow:** Pediatric Pulmonology, St Christopher's Hosp 1988; **Fac Appt:** Assoc Prof Ped, Univ Pennsylvania

Quittell, Lynne MD [PPul] - **Spec Exp:** Cystic Fibrosis; Asthma; **Hospital:** NYPresby-Morgan Stanley Children's Hosp (page 66); **Address:** Morgan Stanley Chlds Hosp of NY-Presby, 3959 Broadway Fl 7, New York, NY 10032-1551; **Phone:** 212-305-5122; **Board Cert:** Pediatrics 1986; Pediatric Pulmonology 2004; **Med School:** Israel 1981; **Resid:** Pediatrics, Schneider Chldns Hosp 1984; **Fellow:** Pediatric Pulmonology, St Christopher's Hosp 1988; **Fac Appt:** Assoc Prof Ped, Columbia P&S

Zeitlin, Pamela L MD [PPul] - **Spec Exp:** Cystic Fibrosis; **Hospital:** Johns Hopkins Hosp (page 61), Mt Washington Ped Hosp; **Address:** 200 N Wolfe St, Baltimore, MD 21287; **Phone:** 410-955-2035; **Board Cert:** Pediatrics 1988; Pediatric Pulmonology 2000; **Med School:** Yale Univ 1983; **Resid:** Pediatrics, Johns Hopkins Hosp 1986; **Fellow:** Pediatric Pulmonology, Johns Hopkins Hosp 1989; **Fac Appt:** Prof Ped, Johns Hopkins Univ

Southeast

Murphy, Thomas M MD [PPul] - **Spec Exp:** Cystic Fibrosis; Asthma; Pneumonia; **Hospital:** Duke Univ Med Ctr; **Address:** Duke Univ Med Ctr, Box 2994, Durham, NC 27710; **Phone:** 919-684-3364; **Board Cert:** Internal Medicine 1976; Pediatrics 2003; Pediatric Pulmonology 2004; **Med School:** Univ Rochester 1973; **Resid:** Internal Medicine, Georgetown Univ Hosp 1976; **Fellow:** Pediatric Pulmonology, Georgetown Univ Hosp 1978; **Fac Appt:** Assoc Prof Ped, Duke Univ

Rubin, Bruce MD [PPul] - **Spec Exp:** Asthma; Cystic Fibrosis; Mucus Clearance Disorders; Cough-Chronic; **Hospital:** Wake Forest Univ Baptist Med Ctr (page 72), Brenner Chldrn's Hosp; **Address:** Wake Forest, Dept Pediatrics, Medical Center Blvd, Winston-Salem, NC 27157; **Phone:** 336-713-4500; **Board Cert:** Pediatrics 1984; Pediatric Pulmonology 2005; **Med School:** Tulane Univ 1979; **Resid:** Pediatrics, Tulane Univ 1981; **Fellow:** Pediatric Pulmonary & Critical Care, Hosp for Sick Children 1983; **Fac Appt:** Prof Ped, Wake Forest Univ

Sallent, Jorge A MD [PPul] - **Spec Exp:** Chronic Lung Disease of Infancy; Asthma & Chronic Lung Disease; Lung Injuries-RSV related; **Hospital:** St Mary's Med Ctr - W Palm Bch, Palms - West Hosp; **Address:** Pediatric Respiratory Ctr, 500 US Highway 1, Lake Park, FL 33403-3598; **Phone:** 561-863-0105; **Board Cert:** Pediatrics 1984; Pediatric Pulmonology 2003; **Med School:** Dominican Republic 1978; **Resid:** Pediatrics, Orlando Regional Med Ctr 1983; **Fellow:** Pediatric Pulmonology, Univ Florida 1986; **Fac Appt:** Asst Prof Ped, Univ Fla Coll Med

Sherman, James MD [PPul] - **Spec Exp:** Asthma; Airway Disorders; Cough-Chronic; **Hospital:** Carilion Roanoke Meml Hosp; **Address:** 102 Highland Ave, Ste 203, Roanoke, VA 24013; **Phone:** 540-985-9835; **Board Cert:** Pediatrics 1981; Pediatric Pulmonology 2003; **Med School:** Univ S Fla Coll Med 1975; **Resid:** Pediatrics, SUNY Upstate Med Ctr 1977; Pediatrics, Tampa Genl Hosp- Univ So Florida 1978; **Fellow:** Pediatric Pulmonology, Rainbow Babies & Children's Hosp 1981; **Fac Appt:** Prof Ped, Univ Fla Coll Med

Midwest

Givan, Deborah C MD [PPul] - **Spec Exp:** Sleep Disorders/Apnea; Apnea in Infants; Asthma; **Hospital:** Riley Hosp for Children; **Address:** Childrens Sleep Disorder Ctr, Riley Hospital for Children, 702 Barnhill Drive, ROC 4270, Indianapolis, IN 46202; **Phone:** 317-274-7208; **Board Cert:** Pediatrics 1982; Pediatric Pulmonology 2003; Sleep Medicine 1997; **Med School:** Indiana Univ 1977; **Resid:** Pediatrics, Meethodist Hosp 1980; **Fellow:** Pediatric Pulmonology, Riley Chldns Hosp 1981; Pediatric Pulmonology, Texas Chldns Hosp 1982; **Fac Appt:** Clin Prof Ped, Indiana Univ

Green, Thomas P MD [PPul] - **Spec Exp:** Respiratory Failure; Breathing Disorders; **Hospital:** Children's Mem Hosp, Evanston/Northshore Univ Hlth Syst; **Address:** Dept Pulm-Crit Care Med, 2300 Chldns Pl, Box 86, Chicago, IL 60614; **Phone:** 773-880-8150; **Board Cert:** Pediatrics 1992; Pediatric Pulmonology 2002; Pediatric Critical Care Medicine 2003; **Med School:** Stanford Univ 1974; **Resid:** Pediatrics, Univ Minn Med Ctr 1977; **Fellow:** Pharmacology, Univ Minn Med Ctr 1979; Pediatric Pulmonology, Univ Minn Med Ctr 1994; **Fac Appt:** Prof Ped, Northwestern Univ

Kemp, James S MD [PPul] - **Spec Exp:** Sudden Infant Death Syndrome (SIDS); Breathing Disorders; Sleep Disorders; **Hospital:** St Louis Chldns Hosp; **Address:** One Children's Place, Ste 2C, St Louis, MO 63141; **Phone:** 314-454-2694; **Board Cert:** Pediatrics 1981; Sleep Medicine 2007; **Med School:** Creighton Univ 1976; **Resid:** Pediatrics, Cardinal Glennon Chldns Hosp 1978; Pediatrics, Baylor Univ 1979; **Fellow:** Pediatric Pulmonology, Texas Chldns Hosp 1988; **Fac Appt:** Assoc Prof Ped, Washington Univ, St Louis

Pediatric Pulmonology

Kim, Young-Jee MD [PPul] - **Spec Exp:** Asthma; Rare Lung Disease-Pediatric; Pulmonary Complications-Cancer Therapy; Pulmonary Complications-Sickle Cell Dis; **Hospital:** Riley Hosp for Children; **Address:** Riley Chldns Hosp - Dept Ped Pulm, 702 Barnhill Rd, ROC-rm 4270, Indianapolis, IN 46202-5128; **Phone:** 317-274-7208; **Board Cert:** Pediatric Pulmonology 2006; **Med School:** South Korea 1986; **Resid:** Pediatrics, Duke Univ Med Ctr 1995; **Fellow:** Pediatric Pulmonology, Yale Univ Med Sch 1991; Pediatric Pulmonology, Riley Hosp Chldn 1998; **Fac Appt:** Assoc Clin Prof Ped, Indiana Univ

Konstan, Michael W MD [PPul] - **Spec Exp:** Cystic Fibrosis; Asthma; **Hospital:** Rainbow Babies & Chldns Hosp; **Address:** Div Ped Pulmonology, 11100 Euclid Ave, Ste 3001, MS 6006, Cleveland, OH 44106-2624; **Phone:** 216-844-1997; **Board Cert:** Pediatrics 1986; Pediatric Pulmonology 2004; **Med School:** Case West Res Univ 1982; **Resid:** Pediatrics, Chldn's Hosp 1985; **Fellow:** Pediatric Pulmonology, Rainbow Babies & Chldns Hosp 1988; **Fac Appt:** Prof Ped, Case West Res Univ

Kurachek, Stephen MD [PPul] - **Spec Exp:** Critical Care; Asthma; **Hospital:** Chldns Hosp and Clinics - Minneapolis; **Address:** 2545 Chicago Ave S, Ste 617, Minneapolis, MN 55404; **Phone:** 612-863-3226; **Board Cert:** Pediatrics 1985; Pediatric Pulmonology 2004; Pediatric Critical Care Medicine 2003; **Med School:** Univ Miami Sch Med 1978; **Resid:** Pediatrics, Univ Hosp 1981; **Fellow:** Pulmonary Disease, Boston Chldns Hosp 1984; **Fac Appt:** Asst Clin Prof Ped, Univ Minn

Stern, Robert C MD [PPul] - **Spec Exp:** Cystic Fibrosis; Lung Disease; **Hospital:** Rainbow Babies & Chldns Hosp; **Address:** Div Pediatric Pulmonology, 11100 Euclid Ave, rm 3001, Cleveland, OH 44106-1736; **Phone:** 216-844-3267; **Board Cert:** Pediatrics 1968; Pediatric Pulmonology 2002; **Med School:** Albert Einstein Coll Med 1963; **Resid:** Pediatrics, Univ Hosp 1965; Pediatrics, Bronx Muni Hosp Ctr 1966; **Fellow:** Pediatric Pulmonology, Univ Hosp 1968; **Fac Appt:** Prof Ped, Case West Res Univ

Great Plains and Mountains

Accurso, Frank J MD [PPul] - **Spec Exp:** Cystic Fibrosis; **Hospital:** Chldn's Hosp - Aurora, The; **Address:** Chldn's Hosp, 13123 E 16th Ave, Box B395, Aurora, CO 80045; **Phone:** 720-777-2522; **Board Cert:** Pediatrics 1980; Pediatric Pulmonology 2003; **Med School:** Albert Einstein Coll Med 1974; **Resid:** Pediatrics, Univ Colo Hlth Sci Ctr 1977; **Fellow:** Pulmonary Disease, Univ Colo Hlth Sci Ctr 1980; **Fac Appt:** Prof Ped, Univ Colorado

Larsen, Gary L MD [PPul] - **Hospital:** Natl Jewish Med & Rsch Ctr, Chldn's Hosp - Aurora, The; **Address:** Mational Jewish Health, 1400 Jackson St, rm J303, Denver, CO 80206-2761; **Phone:** 303-398-1617; **Board Cert:** Pediatrics 1976; Pediatric Pulmonology 2003; **Med School:** Columbia P&S 1971; **Resid:** Pediatrics, Univ Colorado Med Ctr 1974; **Fellow:** Pediatric Pulmonology, Univ Colorado Med Ctr 1978; **Fac Appt:** Prof Ped, Univ Colorado

Southwest

Fan, Leland Lane MD [PPul] - **Spec Exp:** Interstitial Lung Disease; **Hospital:** Texas Chldns Hosp; **Address:** 6701 Fannin St, MC CCC 1040.01, Houston, TX 77030; **Phone:** 832-822-3300; **Board Cert:** Pediatrics 1978; Pediatric Pulmonology 2003; Pediatric Critical Care Medicine 2003; **Med School:** Baylor Coll Med 1973; **Resid:** Pediatrics, UCSF Med Ctr 1975; Pediatrics, Univ Colo Hlth Sci Ctr 1976; **Fellow:** Pediatric Pulmonary & Critical Care, Univ Colo Hlth Sci Ctr 1978; **Fac Appt:** Prof Ped, Baylor Coll Med

Morgan, Wayne J MD [PPul] - **Spec Exp:** Cystic Fibrosis; Asthma; **Hospital:** Univ Med Ctr - Tucson, Tucson Med Ctr; **Address:** Univ Arizona Hlth Sci Ctr, Div Pediatric Pulmonology, 1501 N Campbell Ave, Box 245073, Tucson, AZ 85724; **Phone:** 520-626-7780; **Board Cert:** Pediatrics 1982; Pediatric Pulmonology 2003; **Med School:** McGill Univ 1976; **Resid:** Pediatrics, Montreal Chldns Hosp 1980; **Fellow:** Pediatric Pulmonology, Univ Ariz Hlth Sci 1982; **Fac Appt:** Prof Ped, Univ Ariz Coll Med

Warren, Robert H MD [PPul] - **Spec Exp:** Muscular Dystrophy; Pulmonary Rehabilitation; **Hospital:** Arkansas Chldns Hosp; **Address:** Arkansas Chldns Hosp, Pulmonary Med, 1 Children's Way, Little Rock, AR 72202; **Phone:** 501-364-1006; **Board Cert:** Pediatrics 1973; Pediatric Pulmonology 2003; **Med School:** Univ Ark 1967; **Resid:** Pediatrics, LSU Med Ctr 1971; **Fellow:** Pediatric Pulmonology, Tulane Univ Sch Med; **Fac Appt:** Assoc Prof Ped, Univ Ark

West Coast and Pacific

Cooper, Dan M MD [PPul] - **Hospital:** Chldns Hosp Orange Co; **Address:** 455 S Main St, Orange, CA 92868; **Phone:** 714-532-7983; **Board Cert:** Pediatrics 1980; Pediatric Pulmonology 2002; **Med School:** UCSF 1974; **Resid:** Internal Medicine, Hadassah Hosp; Pediatrics, Children's Hosp Med Ctr; **Fellow:** Pediatric Pulmonology, Babies' Hosp-Columbia Univ; **Fac Appt:** Prof Ped, UC Irvine

Keens, Thomas G MD [PPul] - **Spec Exp:** Sudden Infant Death Syndrome (SIDS); Breathing Disorders; **Hospital:** Chldns Hosp - Los Angeles; **Address:** Chldns Hosp, Div Pulmonology, 4650 W Sunset Blvd, Box 127, Los Angeles, CA 90027-6062; **Phone:** 323-361-2101; **Board Cert:** Pediatrics 1978; Neonatal-Perinatal Medicine 1983; Pediatric Pulmonology 2003; **Med School:** UCSD 1972; **Resid:** Pediatrics, Chldns Hosp 1975; **Fellow:** Pediatric Pulmonology, Hosp Sick Chldn 1977; **Fac Appt:** Prof Ped, USC Sch Med

Platzker, Arnold CG MD [PPul] - **Spec Exp:** Asthma; Chronic Lung Disease; Cystic Fibrosis; HIV and Lung Disease; **Hospital:** Chldns Hosp - Los Angeles, Mattel Chldns Hosp at UCLA; **Address:** Chldns Hosp, Div Ped Pulmonology, 4650 Sunset Blvd, Box 83, Los Angeles, CA 90027-6062; **Phone:** 323-361-2101; **Board Cert:** Pediatrics 1967; Neonatal-Perinatal Medicine 1975; Pediatric Pulmonology 2002; **Med School:** Tufts Univ 1962; **Resid:** Pediatrics, City Hosp 1964; Pediatrics, Stanford Univ Med Ctr 1966; **Fellow:** Pediatric Pulmonology, UCSF Med Ctr 1971; Neonatal-Perinatal Medicine, UCSF Med Ctr 1971; **Fac Appt:** Prof Ped, USC Sch Med

Ramsey, Bonnie W MD [PPul] - **Spec Exp:** Cystic Fibrosis; **Hospital:** Chldns Hosp and Regl Med Ctr - Seattle; **Address:** 4800 Sand Point Way NE, MS A-5937, Seattle, WA 98105; **Phone:** 206-987-2024; **Board Cert:** Pediatrics 1981; Pediatric Pulmonology 2007; **Med School:** Harvard Med Sch 1976; **Resid:** Pediatrics, Chldns Hosp 1978; Pediatrics, Chldns Hosp 1979; **Fellow:** Pediatric Critical Care Medicine, Chldns Hosp 1981; **Fac Appt:** Prof Ped, Univ Wash

Redding, Gregory MD [PPul] - **Spec Exp:** Asthma; Chest Wall Deformities; Interstitial Lung Disease; **Hospital:** Chldns Hosp and Regl Med Ctr - Seattle; **Address:** Pulmonary Div, 4800 Sand Point Way NE, MS A-5937, Seattle, WA 98105; **Phone:** 206-987-2174; **Board Cert:** Pediatrics 1992; Pediatric Pulmonology 2003; **Med School:** Stanford Univ 1974; **Resid:** Pediatrics, Harbor-UCLA Affil Hosps 1977; **Fellow:** Pediatric Pulmonology, Univ Colo Affil Hosps 1979; **Fac Appt:** Prof Ped, Univ Wash

Wall, Michael A MD [PPul] - **Spec Exp:** Cystic Fibrosis; **Hospital:** OR Hlth & Sci Univ; **Address:** 3181 SW Sam Jackson Park Rd, Portland, OR 97239; **Phone:** 503-494-8023; **Board Cert:** Pediatrics 1992; Pediatric Pulmonology 2003; **Med School:** Univ NC Sch Med 1973; **Resid:** Pediatrics, Mass Genl Hosp 1976; **Fellow:** Pulmonary Disease, Chldns Hosp 1978; **Fac Appt:** Prof Ped, Oregon Hlth & Sci Univ

PEDIATRIC RHEUMATOLOGY

New England

McCarthy, Paul L MD [PRhu] - **Spec Exp:** Lupus/SLE; Juvenile Arthritis; Dermatomyositis; Vasculitis; **Hospital:** Yale-New Haven Hosp; **Address:** Yale Schl Med, 333 Cedar St, Box 208064, New Haven, CT 06520-3206; **Phone:** 203-688-2475; **Board Cert:** Pediatrics 1974; Pediatric Rheumatology 2007; **Med School:** Georgetown Univ 1969; **Resid:** Pediatrics, Chldns Hosp 1972; **Fellow:** Pediatrics, Chldns Hosp 1974; **Fac Appt:** Prof Ped, Yale Univ

Mid Atlantic

Finkel, Terri H MD [PRhu] - **Spec Exp:** Juvenile Arthritis; Lupus/SLE; Vasculitis; **Hospital:** Chldns Hosp of Philadelphia, The; **Address:** Chldns Hosp of Philadelphia, Div Rheum, 34th St & Civic Ctr Blvd, Chldns Seashore House, rm 236, Philadelphia, PA 19104; **Phone:** 215-590-2547; **Board Cert:** Pediatrics 1988; Pediatric Rheumatology 2002; **Med School:** Stanford Univ 1982; **Resid:** Pediatrics, Univ Colorado Med Ctr 1985; **Fellow:** Pediatric Rheumatology, Natl Jewish Med Ctr 1990; **Fac Appt:** Assoc Prof Ped, Univ Pennsylvania

Goldsmith, Donald P MD [PRhu] - **Spec Exp:** Arthritis; Juvenile Arthritis; Vasculitis; **Hospital:** St Christopher's Hosp for Chldn; **Address:** St Christophers Hosp for Children, Rheumatology Section, Erie Ave at Front St Fl 3rd, Philadelphia, PA 19134; **Phone:** 215-427-5051; **Board Cert:** Pediatrics 1974; Allergy & Immunology 1975; Pediatric Rheumatology 2007; **Med School:** Univ VT Coll Med 1967; **Resid:** Pediatrics, St Christophers Hosp for Chldn 1973; **Fellow:** Allergy Immunology & Rheumatology, St Christophers Hosp for Chldn 1975; **Fac Appt:** Prof Ped, Drexel Univ Coll Med

Haines, Kathleen A MD [PRhu] - **Spec Exp:** Juvenile Arthritis; Lupus/SLE; Immune Deficiency; **Hospital:** Hackensack Univ Med Ctr, NYU Langone Med Ctr (page 67); **Address:** Hackensack Univ Med Ctr, Don Imus Pediatric Ctr, 30 Prospect Ave Fl 3, Hackensack, NJ 07601; **Phone:** 201-996-5306; **Board Cert:** Pediatrics 1980; Allergy & Immunology 1981; Pediatric Rheumatology 2007; **Med School:** Albert Einstein Coll Med 1975; **Resid:** Pediatrics, New York Hosp 1977; **Fellow:** Allergy & Immunology, New York Hosp 1980; Rheumatology, NYU Med Sch 1982; **Fac Appt:** Assoc Prof Ped, UMDNJ-NJ Med Sch, Newark

Ilowite, Norman T MD [PRhu] - **Spec Exp:** Juvenile Arthritis; Lyme Disease; Lupus/SLE; Vasculitis; **Hospital:** Montefiore Med Ctr - Div. Moses; **Address:** Montefiore Children's Hosp, Rheumatology, 3415 Bainbridge Ave, Bronx, NY 10467; **Phone:** 718-741-2456; **Board Cert:** Pediatrics 1985; Clinical & Laboratory Immunology 1990; Pediatric Rheumatology 2007; **Med School:** SUNY Downstate 1979; **Resid:** Pediatrics, Chldns Hosp Natl Med Ctr 1982; **Fellow:** Pediatric Rheumatology, Univ WA Med Ctr 1984; **Fac Appt:** Prof Ped, Albert Einstein Coll Med

Lehman, Thomas MD [PRhu] - **Spec Exp:** Arthritis; Scleroderma; Lupus/SLE; Rheumatoid Arthritis; **Hospital:** Hosp For Special Surgery (page 59), NY-Presby Hosp/Weill Cornell (page 66); **Address:** 535 E 70th St, New York, NY 10021-4872; **Phone:** 212-606-1151; **Board Cert:** Pediatrics 1979; Pediatric Rheumatology 2007; **Med School:** Jefferson Med Coll 1974; **Resid:** Pediatrics, Chldns Hosp 1976; Pediatrics, UCSF Med Ctr 1977; **Fellow:** Pediatric Rheumatology, Chldns Hosp 1979; Rheumatology, Natl Inst Hlth 1983; **Fac Appt:** Prof Ped, Cornell Univ-Weill Med Coll

Sherry, David D MD [PRhu] - **Spec Exp:** Pain-Musculoskeletal; Reflex Sympathetic Dystrophy (RSD); Juvenile Arthritis; Lupus/SLE; **Hospital:** Chldns Hosp of Philadelphia, The; **Address:** Chldns Hosp of Phildelphia, Div Rheum, 34th St & Civic Ctr Blvd, rm 236, Chldns Seashore House, Philadelphia, PA 19104; **Phone:** 215-590-2547; **Board Cert:** Pediatrics 1981; Pediatric Rheumatology 2007; **Med School:** Texas Tech Univ 1977; **Resid:** Pediatrics, Duke Univ Med Ctr 1980; **Fellow:** Pediatric Rheumatology, Univ British Columbia 1982; **Fac Appt:** Prof Ped, Univ Pennsylvania

Sills, Edward M MD [PRhu] - **Spec Exp:** Juvenile Arthritis; Lupus/SLE; Dermatomyositis; **Hospital:** Johns Hopkins Hosp (page 61); **Address:** Johns Hopkins Hosp, 200 N Wolfe St, Ste 2-127, Baltimore, MD 21205; **Phone:** 410-955-6145; **Board Cert:** Pediatrics 1968; **Med School:** NYU Sch Med 1963; **Resid:** Pediatrics, Bronx Muni Hosp 1967; **Fac Appt:** Assoc Prof Ped, Johns Hopkins Univ

Southeast

Passo, Murray H MD [PRhu] - **Hospital:** MUSC Med Ctr; **Address:** MUSC, Dept Pediatrics, Div Pediatric Rheumatology, 135 Rutledge Ave, MSC 561, Charleston, SC 29425-5610; **Phone:** 843-792-5696; **Board Cert:** Pediatrics 1979; Pediatric Rheumatology 2007; **Med School:** Indiana Univ 1974; **Resid:** Pediatrics, Riley Chldns Hosp 1977; **Fellow:** Rheumatology, Indiana Univ Hosps 1979

Schanberg, Laura E MD [PRhu] - **Spec Exp:** Rheumatic Diseases of Childhood; Fibromyalgia; **Hospital:** Duke Univ Med Ctr; **Address:** Duke Univ Med Ctr, Box 3212, Durham, NC 27710; **Phone:** 919-684-6627; **Board Cert:** Pediatric Rheumatology 2007; **Med School:** Duke Univ 1984; **Resid:** Pediatrics, Duke Univ Med Ctr 1987; **Fellow:** Pediatric Rheumatology, Duke Univ Med Ctr 1991; **Fac Appt:** Asst Prof Ped, Duke Univ

Midwest

Klein-Gitelman, Marisa MD [PRhu] - **Spec Exp:** Lupus/SLE; Juvenile Arthritis; **Hospital:** Children's Mem Hosp; **Address:** Chldns Meml Hosp, 2300 Children's Plaza, Box 50, Chicago, IL 60614; **Phone:** 773-880-4360; **Board Cert:** Pediatrics 2006; Pediatric Rheumatology 2002; **Med School:** Washington Univ, St Louis 1985; **Resid:** Pediatrics, Columbia-Presby Med Ctr 1989; **Fellow:** Pediatric Rheumatology, New England Med Ctr 1993; **Fac Appt:** Assoc Prof Ped, Northwestern Univ

Wagner-Weiner, Linda MD [PRhu] - **Spec Exp:** Lupus/SLE; Juvenile Arthritis; Vasculitis; **Hospital:** Univ of Chicago Med Ctr; **Address:** 5841 S Maryland, rm C101, MC NC504, Chicago, IL 60637; **Phone:** 773-702-2246; **Board Cert:** Pediatrics 1984; Pediatric Rheumatology 2007; **Med School:** Rush Med Coll 1979; **Resid:** Pediatrics, Univ Chicago Hosps 1982; **Fellow:** Pediatric Rheumatology, Univ Chicago/La Rabida Chldns Hosp 1984; **Fac Appt:** Assoc Prof Ped, Univ Chicago-Pritzker Sch Med

Pediatric Rheumatology

Southwest

Myones, Barry Lee MD [PRhu] - **Spec Exp:** Vasculitis; Kawasaki Disease; Dermatomyositis; Scleroderma; **Hospital:** Texas Chldns Hosp; **Address:** Ped Rheumatology Ctr, 6701 Fannin St Fl 11, Houston, TX 77030; **Phone:** 832-824-3830; **Board Cert:** Pediatrics 1983; Pediatric Rheumatology 2007; **Med School:** Albany Med Coll 1977; **Resid:** Pediatrics, Duke Univ Med Ctr 1980; **Fellow:** Pediatric Rheumatology, Chldns Hosp-Stanford 1983; Rheumatology, Univ N Carolina 1988; **Fac Appt:** Assoc Clin Prof Ped, Baylor Coll Med

Warren, Robert W MD [PRhu] - **Spec Exp:** Juvenile Arthritis; Lupus/SLE; **Hospital:** Texas Chldns Hosp; **Address:** Texas Childrens Hosp, Pediatric Rheumatology Ctr, 6701 Fannin St Fl 11, Houston, TX 77030-2303; **Phone:** 832-824-3830; **Board Cert:** Pediatrics 1983; Allergy & Immunology 1983; Pediatric Rheumatology 2007; **Med School:** Washington Univ, St Louis 1978; **Resid:** Pediatrics, Duke Univ Med Ctr 1980; **Fellow:** Rheumatology, Duke Univ Med Ctr 1983; **Fac Appt:** Assoc Prof Ped, Baylor Coll Med

Wilking, Andrew MD [PRhu] - **Spec Exp:** Arthritis; Lupus/SLE; Dermatomyositis; **Hospital:** Texas Chldns Hosp, Driscoll Chldn's Hosp; **Address:** Tex Chldns Hosp, 6621 Fannin, MC 3-2290, Houston, TX 77030; **Phone:** 832-824-3826; **Board Cert:** Pediatrics 1985; **Med School:** Columbia P&S 1978; **Resid:** Pediatrics, Babies Hosp 1981; **Fellow:** Pediatric Rheumatology, Tex Chldns Hosp 1983; **Fac Appt:** Prof Ped, Baylor Coll Med

West Coast and Pacific

Emery, Helen M MD [PRhu] - **Spec Exp:** Rheumatic Diseases of Childhood; **Hospital:** Chldns Hosp and Regl Med Ctr - Seattle, Univ Wash Med Ctr; **Address:** Chldns Hosp & Regl Med Ctr, Ped Rheum, 4800 Sand Point Way NE, MS R-5420, PO Box 5371, Seattle, WA 98105; **Phone:** 206-987-2057; **Board Cert:** Pediatrics 1992; Pediatric Rheumatology 2007; **Med School:** Australia 1971; **Resid:** Pediatrics, Chldns Orth Hosp-Univ Wash 1975; **Fellow:** Pediatric Rheumatology, Chldns Orth Hosp-Univ Wash 1977; **Fac Appt:** Prof Ped, Univ Wash

PEDIATRIC SURGERY

New England

Jennings, Russell W MD [PS] - **Spec Exp:** Fetal Surgery; Pediatric Cardiac Surgery; Robotic Surgery; **Hospital:** Children's Hospital - Boston, Brigham & Women's Hosp; **Address:** Chldns Hosp, Fegan 3, 300 Longwood Ave, Boston, MA 02115; **Phone:** 617-355-3038; **Board Cert:** Surgery 2005; Pediatric Surgery 2007; **Med School:** UCSF 1986; **Resid:** Surgery, UCSF Med Ctr 1991; **Fellow:** Fetal Surgery, Fetal Trmt Ctr/UCSF Med Ctr 1994; Pediatric Surgery, Chldns Hosp 1996; **Fac Appt:** Asst Prof S, Harvard Med Sch

Latchaw, Laurie MD [PS] - **Spec Exp:** Thoracic Surgery; Cancer Surgery; Lung Disease in Newborns; Neonatal Surgery; **Hospital:** Dartmouth - Hitchcock Med Ctr; **Address:** DHMC, Clinic 6M, One Medical Center Drive, Lebanon, NH 03756; **Phone:** 603-653-9883; **Board Cert:** Surgery 2001; Pediatric Surgery 2003; **Med School:** Rush Med Coll 1976; **Resid:** Surgery, Univ Texas 1981; **Fellow:** Pediatric Surgery, Montreal Chldns Hosp 1983; **Fac Appt:** Assoc Prof S, Dartmouth Med Sch

Lillehei, Craig W MD [PS] - **Spec Exp:** Transplant-Kidney; Transplant-Liver; Transplant-Lung; **Hospital:** Children's Hospital - Boston; **Address:** Chldns Hosp, Dept Surgery-Fagen Bldg, 300 Longwood Ave Fl 3, Boston, MA 02115; **Phone:** 617-355-3039; **Board Cert:** Surgery 2006; Pediatric Surgery 2007; Surgical Critical Care 2001; **Med School:** Harvard Med Sch 1976

Mayer Jr, John E MD [PS] - **Spec Exp:** Pediatric Cardiothoracic Surgery; **Hospital:** Children's Hospital - Boston; **Address:** Chldns Hosp, Dept Cardiac Surg, 300 Longwood Ave, Bader 273, Boston, MA 02115; **Phone:** 617-355-8258; **Board Cert:** Thoracic Surgery 2001; **Med School:** Yale Univ 1972; **Resid:** Surgery, Univ Minn Med Ctr 1979; **Fellow:** Cardiothoracic Surgery, Univ Minn Med Ctr 1981; **Fac Appt:** Prof S, Harvard Med Sch

Moss, R Lawrence MD [PS] - **Spec Exp:** Congenital Anomalies; Cancer Surgery; Minimally Invasive Surgery; **Hospital:** Yale-New Haven Hosp; **Address:** Dept Surgery-Ped Surgery, PO Box 208062, rm FMB132, New Haven, CT 06520-8062; **Phone:** 203-785-2701; **Board Cert:** Surgery 1999; Pediatric Surgery 2003; Surgical Critical Care 2000; **Med School:** UCSD 1986; **Resid:** Surgery, Virginia Mason Med Ctr 1991; Surgical Critical Care, Chldns Mem Hosp 1992; **Fellow:** Pediatric Surgery, Chldns Mem Hosp 1994; **Fac Appt:** Prof S, Yale Univ

Shamberger, Robert C MD [PS] - **Spec Exp:** Inflammatory Bowel Disease; Critical Care; Cancer Surgery; **Hospital:** Children's Hospital - Boston; **Address:** Children's Hosp-Dept Surgery, 300 Longwood Ave, Fegan - 3, Boston, MA 02115; **Phone:** 617-355-8326; **Board Cert:** Surgery 2002; Surgical Critical Care 1999; Pediatric Surgery 2003; **Med School:** Harvard Med Sch 1975; **Resid:** Surgery, Massachusetts Genl Hosp 1978; Pediatric Surgery, Children's Hosp 1985; **Fellow:** Surgical Oncology, NCI-Surgical Branch 1980; **Fac Appt:** Prof S, Harvard Med Sch

Tracy Jr, Thomas F MD [PS] - **Spec Exp:** Thoracic Surgery; Endoscopic Surgery; Fetal Surgery; Hirschsprung's Disease; **Hospital:** Rhode Island Hosp; **Address:** 2 Dudley St, Ste 180, Providence, RI 02905; **Phone:** 401-421-1939; **Board Cert:** Surgery 2006; Pediatric Surgery 2006; **Med School:** Israel 1981; **Resid:** Surgery, Med Coll Virginia 1986; **Fellow:** Pediatric Surgery, Columbia Presby Med Ctr 1988; **Fac Appt:** Prof S, Brown Univ

Mid Atlantic

Adzick, N Scott MD [PS] - **Spec Exp:** Fetal Surgery; Congenital Hyperinsulinism; Neonatal Surgery; Twin to Twin Transfusion Syndrome (TTTS); **Hospital:** Chldns Hosp of Philadelphia, The; **Address:** 34th St & Civic Center Blvd, Wood Bldg - Ste 5113, Philadelphia, PA 19104-4399; **Phone:** 215-590-2727; **Board Cert:** Surgery 2006; Pediatric Surgery 2007; **Med School:** Harvard Med Sch 1979; **Resid:** Surgery, Mass Genl Hosp 1986; Pediatric Surgery, Chldns Hosp 1988; **Fellow:** Research, UCSF Med Ctr 1985; **Fac Appt:** Prof S, Univ Pennsylvania

Alexander, Frederick MD [PS] - **Spec Exp:** Inflammatory Bowel Disease; Solid Tumors; Congenital Anomalies-Gastrointestinal; **Hospital:** Hackensack Univ Med Ctr; **Address:** Joseph M Sanzari Chldns Hosp-HUMC, 30 Prospect Ave, Ste PC311, Hackensack, NJ 07601; **Phone:** 201-996-2921; **Board Cert:** Pediatric Surgery 1999; **Med School:** Columbia P&S 1977; **Resid:** Surgery, Brigham-Womens Hosp 1984; **Fellow:** Pediatric Surgery, Chldns Hosp 1986; **Fac Appt:** Clin Prof S

Colombani, Paul M MD [PS] - **Spec Exp:** Thoracic Surgery; Transplant-Kidney; Transplant-Liver; Cancer Surgery; **Hospital:** Johns Hopkins Hosp (page 61); **Address:** 600 N Wolfe St, Harvey 319, Baltimore, MD 21287; **Phone:** 410-955-2717; **Board Cert:** Surgery 2003; Pediatric Surgery 2003; **Med School:** Univ KY Coll Med 1976; **Resid:** Surgery, Geo Wash Univ Hosp 1981; **Fellow:** Pediatric Surgery, Johns Hopkins Hosp 1983; **Fac Appt:** Prof S, Johns Hopkins Univ

Pediatric Surgery

Dolgin, Stephen MD [PS] - **Spec Exp:** Neonatal Surgery; Ulcerative Colitis; Laparoscopy & Thoracostomy; Inflammatory Bowel Disease/Crohn's; **Hospital:** Schneider Chldn's Hosp, N Shore Univ Hosp; **Address:** Schneider Children's Hosp, Pediatric Surgery, 269-01 76th Ave, New Hyde Park, NY 11040; **Phone:** 718-470-3636; **Board Cert:** Surgery 2000; Pediatric Surgery 2003; Surgical Critical Care 2000; **Med School:** NYU Sch Med 1977; **Resid:** Surgery, Peter Bent Brigham Hosp 1982; **Fellow:** Pediatric Surgery, Chldns Meml Hosp 1984; **Fac Appt:** Prof S, Albert Einstein Coll Med

Eichelberger, Martin R MD [PS] - **Spec Exp:** Trauma; **Hospital:** Chldns Natl Med Ctr; **Address:** Childrens National Med Ctr, 111 Michigan Ave NW, Washington, DC 20010; **Phone:** 202-476-2778; **Board Cert:** Pediatric Surgery 2003; **Med School:** Hahnemann Univ 1971; **Resid:** Surgery, Case-Western Res Hosp 1978; **Fellow:** Pediatric Surgery, Chldns Hosp 1980; **Fac Appt:** Prof S, Geo Wash Univ

Flake, Alan W MD [PS] - **Spec Exp:** Fetal Surgery; Stem Cell Transplant-Fetal; Neonatal Surgery; **Hospital:** Chldns Hosp of Philadelphia, The; **Address:** Dept Pediatric Surgery, 34th St & Civic Center Blvd, Wood Bldg - Ste 5113, Philadelphia, PA 19104; **Phone:** 215-590-2727; **Board Cert:** Surgery 2000; Pediatric Surgery 1999; **Med School:** Univ Ark 1981; **Resid:** Surgery, UCSF Med Ctr 1988; **Fellow:** Pediatric Surgery, Chldns Hosp Med Ctr 1990; **Fac Appt:** Prof S, Univ Pennsylvania

Ginsburg, Howard B MD [PS] - **Spec Exp:** Neonatal Surgery; Tumor Surgery; Pediatric Urology; Gastrointestinal Surgery; **Hospital:** NYU Langone Med Ctr (page 67), Bellevue Hosp Ctr; **Address:** NYU Medical Ctr, Div Pediatric Surgery, 530 1st Ave, Ste 10W, New York, NY 10016-6402; **Phone:** 212-263-7391; **Board Cert:** Pediatric Surgery 2001; **Med School:** Univ Cincinnati 1972; **Resid:** Surgery, NYU-Bellvue Hosp 1977; Pediatric Surgery, Columbia-Presby Med Ctr 1979; **Fellow:** Pediatric Surgery, Mass Genl Hosp 1980; **Fac Appt:** Assoc Prof S, NYU Sch Med

Gittes, George K MD [PS] - **Spec Exp:** Gastrointestinal Surgery; **Hospital:** Chldns Hosp of Pittsburgh - UPMC; **Address:** Childrens Hosp Pittsburgh, Dept Surgery, Childrn's Hosp Drive, 45th St & Penn Ave, rm 7147, Pittsburgh, PA 15201; **Phone:** 412-692-7291; **Board Cert:** Surgery 2003; Pediatric Surgery 2007; **Med School:** Harvard Med Sch 1987; **Resid:** Surgery, UCSF Med Ctr 1994; **Fellow:** Pediatric Surgery, Childrens Mercy Hosp 1995; **Fac Appt:** Prof S, Univ Pittsburgh

Glick, Philip L MD [PS] - **Spec Exp:** Robotic Surgery; Neonatal Surgery; Pediatric Cancers; Chest Wall Deformities; **Hospital:** Women's & Chldn's Hosp of Buffalo, The, Roswell Park Cancer Inst; **Address:** Childrens Hospital, Dept Pediatric Surg, 219 Bryant St, Buffalo, NY 14222-2006; **Phone:** 716-878-7449; **Board Cert:** Surgery 2006; Pediatric Surgery 1997; Surgical Critical Care 1999; **Med School:** UCSF 1979; **Resid:** Surgery, UCSF Med Ctr 1985; **Fellow:** Fetal Surgery, UCSF Med Ctr 1984; Pediatric Surgery, Chldns Hosp Med Ctr 1988; **Fac Appt:** Prof S, SUNY Buffalo

Kane, Timothy D MD [PS] - **Spec Exp:** Minimally Invasive Surgery; Chest Wall Deformities; Neonatal Surgery; **Hospital:** Chldns Hosp of Pittsburgh - UPMC; **Address:** Chldns Hosp Pittsburgh - Dept Surg, 3705 Fifth Ave 4A485, Pittsburgh, PA 15213; **Phone:** 412-692-7282; **Board Cert:** Surgery 2001; Pediatric Surgery 2004; **Med School:** SUNY Upstate Med Univ 1992; **Resid:** Surgery, Univ Cincinnati Hosp 1999; **Fellow:** Pediatric Surgery, UAB Chldns Hosp 2001; **Fac Appt:** Asst Prof S, Univ Pittsburgh

La Quaglia, Michael MD [PS] - **Spec Exp:** Cancer Surgery; Neuroblastoma; Liver Tumors; Colon & Rectal Cancer; **Hospital:** Meml Sloan-Kettering Cancer Ctr, NY-Presby Hosp/Weill Cornell (page 66); **Address:** 1275 York Ave, Ste H1315, New York, NY 10065; **Phone:** 212-639-7002; **Board Cert:** Surgery 2003; Pediatric Surgery 2007; **Med School:** UMDNJ-NJ Med Sch, Newark 1976; **Resid:** Surgery, Mass Genl Hosp 1983; **Fellow:** Cardiothoracic Surgery, Broadgreen Ctr 1984; Pediatric Surgery, Chldns Hosp 1985; **Fac Appt:** Prof S, Cornell Univ-Weill Med Coll

Nance, Michael L MD [PS] - **Spec Exp:** Trauma; Critical Care; Brain Injury; Congenital Anomalies; **Hospital:** Chldns Hosp of Philadelphia, The; **Address:** Chldns Hosp of Philadelphia, Dept Surgery, 34th & Civic Ctr Blvd, Philadelphia, PA 19104; **Phone:** 215-590-5932; **Board Cert:** Surgery 2005; Pediatric Surgery 2007; **Med School:** Louisiana State U, New Orleans 1988; **Resid:** Surgery, Hosp U Penn 1995; **Fellow:** Surgical Critical Care, Hosp U Penn 1996; Pediatric Surgery, Chldns Hosp Philadelphia 1997; **Fac Appt:** Assoc Prof PS, Univ Pennsylvania

Quaegebeur, Jan M MD [PS] - **Spec Exp:** Arterial Switch; Heart Valve Surgery; Congenital Heart Surgery; Pediatric Cardiac Surgery; **Hospital:** NYPresby-Morgan Stanley Children's Hosp (page 66); **Address:** Morgan Stanley Chlds Hosp of NY-Presby, 3959 Broadway, Ste 276, New York, NY 10032; **Phone:** 212-305-5975; **Med School:** Belgium 1969; **Resid:** Surgery, St Michel Clinic 1973; **Fellow:** Thoracic Surgery, Baylor Coll Med 1974; Thoracic Surgery, Univ Hosp 1978; **Fac Appt:** Prof S, Columbia P&S

Schwartz, Marshall Z MD [PS] - **Spec Exp:** Gastrointestinal Surgery; Neonatal Surgery; Transplant-Kidney; Inflammatory Bowel Disease; **Hospital:** St Christopher's Hosp for Chldn, St Luke's Hosp - Bethlehem; **Address:** St Christopher's Hosp for Chldn, Dept of Surgery, Erie at Front St, Ste 2204, Philadelphia, PA 19134; **Phone:** 215-427-5446; **Board Cert:** Surgery 1998; Pediatric Surgery 1999; **Med School:** Univ Minn 1970; **Resid:** Surgery, Univ Minnesota Hosp 1972; Pediatric Surgery, Chldns Hosp Med Ctr - Harvard Med Sch 1974; **Fellow:** Surgery, Univ Minnesota Hosp 1975; **Fac Appt:** Prof S, Jefferson Med Coll

Shlasko, Edward MD [PS] - **Spec Exp:** Laparoscopic Surgery; Robotic Surgery; Thoracic Surgery; **Hospital:** Maimonides Med Ctr (page 63); **Address:** Maimonides, Dept Ped Surgery, 921 49th St, Brooklyn, NY 11219-2923; **Phone:** 718-283-7384; **Board Cert:** Surgery 1999; Pediatric Surgery 2001; **Med School:** Columbia P&S 1985; **Resid:** Surgery, Mt Sinai Hosp 1991; **Fellow:** Surgical Oncology, NIH-NCI Surg Branch 1989; Pediatric Surgery, SUNY Hlth Sci Ctr 1993; **Fac Appt:** Assoc Prof S, Mount Sinai Sch Med

Spray, Thomas L MD [PS] - **Spec Exp:** Cardiac Surgery-Adult & Pediatric; Transplant-Heart & Lung; Neonatal & Infant Cardiac Surgery; Congenital Heart Disease-Adult; **Hospital:** Chldns Hosp of Philadelphia, The, Hosp Univ Penn - UPHS (page 60); **Address:** Dept Surgery, 34th St & Civic Center Blvd, Ste 12NW10, Philadelphia, PA 19104; **Phone:** 215-590-2708; **Board Cert:** Thoracic Surgery 2004; **Med School:** Duke Univ 1973; **Resid:** Surgery, Duke Univ Med Ctr 1975; Cardiothoracic Surgery, Duke Univ Med Ctr 1983; **Fac Appt:** Prof S, Univ Pennsylvania

Stolar, Charles J H MD [PS] - **Spec Exp:** Pediatric Cancers; Neonatal Surgery; Diaphragmatic Hernia; **Hospital:** NYPresby-Morgan Stanley Children's Hosp (page 66); **Address:** Morgan Stanley Chldns Hosp NY-Presby, 3959 Broadway, Fl 2 - rm 215 North, New York, NY 10032; **Phone:** 212-342-8586; **Board Cert:** Surgery 2001; Pediatric Surgery 2007; **Med School:** Georgetown Univ 1974; **Resid:** Surgery, Univ Illinois Hosp 1980; **Fellow:** Pediatric Surgery, Chldns Hosp Natl Med Ctr 1982; **Fac Appt:** Prof S, Columbia P&S

Velcek, Francisca T MD [PS] - **Spec Exp:** Anorectal Malformations; Pediatric Gynecology; Neonatal Surgery; Hernia; **Hospital:** Lenox Hill Hosp (page 62), Long Island Coll Hosp (page 57); **Address:** 965 5th Ave, New York, NY 10021; **Phone:** 212-744-9396; **Board Cert:** Surgery 1974; Pediatric Surgery 2007; **Med School:** Philippines 1966; **Resid:** Surgery, St Clares Hosp 1971; Pediatric Surgery, SUNY Downstate Med Ctr 1975; **Fellow:** Pediatric Surgery, SUNY Downstate Med Ctr 1973; **Fac Appt:** Prof S, SUNY Hlth Sci Ctr

Pediatric Surgery

Southeast

Bond, Sheldon J MD [PS] - **Spec Exp:** Pediatric Cancers; Fetal Surgery; Trauma; **Hospital:** Kosair Chldn's Hosp; **Address:** University Pediatric Surgery Assocs, 234 E Gray St, Ste 766, Louisville, KY 40202; **Phone:** 502-583-7337; **Board Cert:** Surgery 1998; Pediatric Surgery 1999; Surgical Critical Care 2001; **Med School:** Med Coll Wisc 1983; **Resid:** Surgery, Univ Louisville Med Ctr 1989; **Fellow:** Fetal Surgery, UCSF Med Ctr; Pediatric Surgery, Chldns Natl Med Ctr 1991; **Fac Appt:** Prof S, Univ Louisville Sch Med

Davidoff, Andrew M MD [PS] - **Spec Exp:** Neuroblastoma; Cancer Surgery; **Hospital:** St Jude Children's Research Hosp, Le Bonheur Chldns Med Ctr; **Address:** St Jude Chldns Rsch Hosp, Dept Surg, 262 Danny Thomas Pl, MS 133, Memphis, TN 38105; **Phone:** 901-495-4060; **Board Cert:** Surgery 2005; Pediatric Surgery 2007; **Med School:** Univ Pennsylvania 1987; **Resid:** Surgery, Duke Med Ctr 1994; **Fellow:** Pediatric Surgery, Chldns Hosp 1996; **Fac Appt:** Assoc Prof S, Univ Tenn Coll Med, Memphis

Fallat, Mary E MD [PS] - **Spec Exp:** Trauma; Burn Care; **Hospital:** Kosair Chldn's Hosp, Univ of Louisville Hosp; **Address:** University Pediatric Surgery Assocs, 234 E Gray St, Ste 766, Louisville, KY 40202; **Phone:** 502-583-7337; **Board Cert:** Surgery 2005; Pediatric Surgery 1997; **Med School:** SUNY Upstate Med Univ 1979; **Resid:** Surgery, Univ Louisville Med Ctr 1985; **Fellow:** Research, Mass Genl Hosp 1983; Pediatric Surgery, Chldns Natl Med Ctr 1987; **Fac Appt:** Prof S, Univ Louisville Sch Med

Georgeson, Keith E MD [PS] - **Spec Exp:** Hirschsprung's Disease; Minimally Invasive Surgery; Gastroesophageal Reflux Disease (GERD); **Hospital:** Children's Hospital - Birmingham; **Address:** Chlds Hosp of Alabama, Dept Ped Surgery, 1600 7th Ave S, Ste ACC300, Birmingham, AL 35233-1711; **Phone:** 205-939-9688; **Board Cert:** Surgery 2000; Pediatric Surgery 2007; **Med School:** Loma Linda Univ 1969; **Resid:** Surgery, Loma Linda Univ Med Ctr 1973; Pediatric Surgery, Chldn's Hosp Mich 1975; **Fac Appt:** Prof S, Univ Alabama

Morgan III, Walter M MD [PS] - **Spec Exp:** Germ Cell Tumors; Neuroblastoma; Bone Cancer; Congenital Anomalies; **Hospital:** Vanderbilt Children's Hosp, Vanderbilt Univ Med Ctr; **Address:** Vanderbilt Children's Hosp-Dept Ped Surgery, 2200 Children's Way, Ste 4150, Nashville, TN 37232-9780; **Phone:** 615-936-1050; **Board Cert:** Pediatric Surgery 2001; **Med School:** Vanderbilt Univ 1982; **Resid:** Surgery, Johns Hopkins Hosp 1988; **Fellow:** Pediatric Surgery, Johns Hopkins Hosp 1990; **Fac Appt:** Asst Prof S, Vanderbilt Univ

Nakayama, Don K MD [PS] - **Spec Exp:** Neonatal Surgery; Minimally Invasive Surgery; **Hospital:** Med Ctr of Central GA; **Address:** 777 Hemlock St, MSC 140, Macon, GA 31201; **Phone:** 478-633-1367; **Board Cert:** Surgery 2003; Pediatric Surgery 2005; **Med School:** UCSF 1978; **Resid:** Surgery, UCSF Hosps 1984; **Fellow:** Pediatric Surgery, Childrens Hosp 1986; **Fac Appt:** Prof S, Mercer Univ Sch Med

Nuss, Donald MD [PS] - **Spec Exp:** Chest Wall Deformities; Minimally Invasive Surgery; **Hospital:** Chldns Hosp of King's Daughters; **Address:** Chldns Surg Specialty Grp, 601 Childrens Ln, Ste Pectus, Norfolk, VA 23507; **Phone:** 757-668-7703; **Board Cert:** Surgery 1973; Pediatric Surgery 2007; **Med School:** South Africa 1963; **Resid:** Surgery, Mayo Clinic 1971; Pediatric Surgery, Red Cross Chldns Hosp 1973; **Fac Appt:** Prof S, Eastern VA Med Sch

Paidas, Charles N MD [PS] - **Spec Exp:** Pediatric Cancers; Chest Wall Deformities; Transplant Surgery-Pediatric; Hernia; **Hospital:** Tampa Genl Hosp, Univ of S FL - Tampa; **Address:** Tampa Genl Hosp, Div Ped Surgery, 1 Tampa General Cir, rm G-441, Tampa, FL 33606; **Phone:** 813-259-0929; **Board Cert:** Surgery 1999; Pediatric Surgery 2001; Surgical Critical Care 2002; **Med School:** NY Med Coll 1981; **Resid:** Surgery, NY Med Coll Affil Hosps 1987; **Fellow:** Pediatric Surgery, Johns Hopkins Hosp 1991; **Fac Appt:** Prof S, Univ S Fla Coll Med

Rice, Henry MD [PS] - **Spec Exp:** Neonatal Surgery; Cancer Surgery; **Hospital:** Duke Univ Med Ctr; **Address:** Duke Univ Med Ctr, Dept Ped Surg, DUMC, Box 3815, Durham, NC 27710; **Phone:** 919-681-5077; **Board Cert:** Surgery 2006; Pediatric Surgery 2000; **Med School:** Yale Univ 1988; **Resid:** Surgery, Univ Wash Affil Hosps 1996; **Fellow:** Pediatric Surgery, Chldns Hosp of Buffalo 1998; **Fac Appt:** Assoc Prof S, Duke Univ

Ricketts, Richard R MD [PS] - **Spec Exp:** Neonatal Surgery; Cancer Surgery; Gastrointestinal Surgery; **Hospital:** Chldns Hlthcare Atlanta @ Egleston; **Address:** 1975 Century Blvd, Ste 6, Atlanta, GA 30345; **Phone:** 404-982-9938; **Board Cert:** Surgery 2004; Pediatric Surgery 2001; **Med School:** Northwestern Univ 1973; **Resid:** Surgery, LAC-USC Med Ctr 1978; **Fellow:** Pediatric Surgery, Chldns Meml Hosp 1980; **Fac Appt:** Prof S, Emory Univ

Rodgers, Bradley M MD [PS] - **Spec Exp:** Thoracic Surgery; Neonatal Surgery; Minimally Invasive Surgery; **Hospital:** Univ Virginia Med Ctr; **Address:** U VA Chldns Hosp, Dept Surgery, PO Box 800709, Charlottesville, VA 22908; **Phone:** 434-924-2673; **Board Cert:** Surgery 1997; Pediatric Surgery 2005; Thoracic Surgery 1975; **Med School:** Johns Hopkins Univ 1966; **Resid:** Surgery, Duke Univ Med Ctr 1968; Cardiothoracic Surgery, Duke Univ Med Ctr 1973; **Fellow:** Pediatric Surgery, Chldns Hosp 1974; **Fac Appt:** Prof S, Univ VA Sch Med

Shochat, Stephen J MD [PS] - **Spec Exp:** Cancer Surgery; Chest Wall Deformities; **Hospital:** St Jude Children's Research Hosp; **Address:** St Jude Childrens Research Hosp, Dept Surgery, 262 Danny Thomas Pl, Memphis, TN 38105; **Phone:** 901-495-4060; **Board Cert:** Surgery 1969; Thoracic Surgery 1975; Pediatric Surgery 2005; **Med School:** Med Coll VA 1963; **Resid:** Surgery, Barnes Hosp 1968; Pediatric Surgery, Boston Chldns Hosp 1970; **Fellow:** Thoracic Surgery, George Washington Univ Med Ctr 1974; **Fac Appt:** Prof S, Univ Tenn Coll Med, Memphis

Stylianos, Steven MD [PS] - **Spec Exp:** Trauma; Neonatal Surgery; Chest Wall Deformities; **Hospital:** Miami Children's Hosp; **Address:** Miami Childrens Hosp, 3200 SW 60th Court, Ste 201, Miami, FL 33155; **Phone:** 305-662-8320; **Board Cert:** Surgery 2002; Pediatric Surgery 2003; **Med School:** NYU Sch Med 1983; **Resid:** Surgery, Columbia-Presby Med Ctr 1988; Pediatric Surgery, Chldns Hosp 1992; **Fellow:** Pediatric Trauma, New England Med Ctr 1990; **Fac Appt:** Assoc Prof S, Univ Miami Sch Med

Midwest

Aiken, John J MD [PS] - **Spec Exp:** Tumor Surgery; Chest Wall Deformities; Hernia; Solid Tumors; **Hospital:** Chldns Hosp - Wisconsin; **Address:** 999 N 92nd St, Ste C-320, Milwaukee, WI 53226; **Phone:** 414-266-6550; **Board Cert:** Surgery 2004; Pediatric Surgery 2000; **Med School:** Univ Cincinnati 1984; **Resid:** Surgery, Mass Genl Hosp 1991; **Fellow:** Pediatric Surgery, Chldns Hosp 1993; **Fac Appt:** Assoc Prof S, Med Coll Wisc

Arensman, Robert MD [PS] - **Spec Exp:** Congenital Anomalies; **Hospital:** Alexian Brothers Med Ctr; **Address:** 1555 Barrington Rd DOB 1 Bldg - Ste 415, Hoffman Estates, IL 60196; **Phone:** 847-490-4222; **Board Cert:** Pediatric Surgery 1999; **Med School:** Univ IL Coll Med 1969; **Resid:** Surgery, Univ Illinois Med Ctr 1972; Surgery, Univ Illinois Med Ctr 1976; **Fellow:** Pediatric Surgery, Chldns Natl Med Ctr 1978

Barksdale Jr, Edward M MD [PS] - **Spec Exp:** Gastrointestinal Surgery; Nutrition in Bowel Disorders; Neuroblastoma; Minimally Invasive Surgery; **Hospital:** Rainbow Babies & Chldns Hosp; **Address:** Rainbow Babies & Children's Hosp, 11100 Euclid Ave, rm 122, Cleveland, OH 44106; **Phone:** 216-844-8623; **Board Cert:** Surgery 2002; Pediatric Surgery 2003; **Med School:** Harvard Med Sch 1984; **Resid:** Surgery, Mass Genl Hosp 1992; Pediatric Surgery, Chldns Hosp 1994; **Fellow:** Surgical Research, Mass Genl Hosp 1989; **Fac Appt:** Prof S, Ohio State Univ

Pediatric Surgery

Bove, Edward L MD [PS] - **Spec Exp:** Pediatric Cardiothoracic Surgery; Hypoplastic Left Heart Syndrome; Congenital Heart Surgery; **Hospital:** Univ Michigan Hlth Sys; **Address:** CS Mott Chldns Hosp, Dept Surg, 1500 E Med Ctr Drive, S144 CVC/SPC 5864, Ann Arbor, MI 48109-5864; **Phone:** 734-936-4980; **Board Cert:** Thoracic Surgery 1998; **Med School:** Albany Med Coll 1972; **Resid:** Surgery, Univ Mich Med Ctr 1976; Thoracic Surgery, Univ Mich Med Ctr 1979; **Fellow:** Pediatric Cardiac Surgery, Hosp Sick Chldn 1980; **Fac Appt:** Prof S, Univ Mich Med Sch

Caniano, Donna MD [PS] - **Hospital:** Nationwide Chldn's Hosp; **Address:** 555 S 18th St, OCC, 6G, Columbus, OH 43205; **Phone:** 614-722-3900; **Board Cert:** Surgery 2001; Pediatric Surgery 2007; **Med School:** Albany Med Coll 1976; **Resid:** Surgery, Albany Med Ctr 1981; **Fellow:** Pediatric Surgery, Columbus Chldn's Hosp 1983; **Fac Appt:** Prof S, Ohio State Univ

Coran, Arnold G MD [PS] - **Spec Exp:** Esophageal Surgery & Replacement; Hirschsprung's Disease; Neonatal Surgery; Colon & Rectal Surgery; **Hospital:** Mott Chldns Hosp; **Address:** Mott Children's Hospital, 1500 E Medical Ctr Drive, Ste F3970, Box 0245, Ann Arbor, MI 48109-0245; **Phone:** 734-764-4151; **Board Cert:** Surgery 1969; Thoracic Surgery 1970; Pediatric Surgery 1993; **Med School:** Harvard Med Sch 1963; **Resid:** Surgery, Peter Bent Brigham Hosp 1968; Surgery, Chldns Hosp 1968; **Fellow:** Neonatal Metabolism, Univ Oslo; **Fac Appt:** Prof S, Univ Mich Med Sch

Crombleholme, Timothy M MD [PS] - **Spec Exp:** Fetal Surgery; Twin to Twin Transfusion Syndrome (TTTS); **Hospital:** Cincinnati Chldns Hosp Med Ctr, Univ Hosp - Cincinnati; **Address:** Fetal Care Center of Cincinnati, 3333 Burnet Ave, Cincinnati, OH 45229; **Phone:** 513-636-9608; **Board Cert:** Surgery 2003; Pediatric Surgery 2007; **Med School:** Tufts Univ 1984; **Resid:** Surgery, UCSF Med Ctr 1991; **Fellow:** Pediatric Surgery, Tufts-New England Med Ctr 1993; **Fac Appt:** Prof S, Univ Cincinnati

Duncan, Brian W MD [PS] - **Spec Exp:** Pediatric Cardiac Surgery; Neonatal & Infant Cardiac Surgery; Transplant-Heart-Pediatric; **Hospital:** Cleveland Clin Fdn (page 56); **Address:** 9500 Euclid Ave, MC M41, Cleveland, OH 44195; **Phone:** 216-297-8276; **Board Cert:** Surgery 2004; Thoracic Surgery 2006; **Med School:** Indiana Univ 1985; **Resid:** Surgery, Mass General Hosp 1992; Thoracic Surgery, Mass General Hosp 1995; **Fellow:** Surgical Research, UCSF Med Ctr; **Fac Appt:** Prof S, Cleveland Cl Coll Med/Case West Res

Ehrlich, Peter F MD [PS] - **Spec Exp:** Pediatric Cancers; Wilms' Tumor; Thyroid Cancer; **Hospital:** Mott Chldns Hosp, Mich State Univ-Hurley Med Ctr; **Address:** Mott Children's Hospital, 1500 E Medical Center Drive, rm F3970, Ann Arbor, MI 48109-0245; **Phone:** 734-764-4151; **Board Cert:** Surgery 1997; Pediatric Surgery 2000; **Med School:** Canada 1989; **Resid:** Surgery, Univ Toronto Med Ctr 1996; **Fellow:** Pediatric Surgery, Children's Natl Med Ctr 1998; **Fac Appt:** Assoc Clin Prof S, Univ Mich Med Sch

Holterman, Mark J MD [PS] - **Spec Exp:** Minimally Invasive Surgery; Neonatal Surgery; Transplant-Liver; Transplant-Bowel; **Hospital:** Univ of IL Med Ctr at Chicago; **Address:** Dept Pediatric Surgery, 840 S Wood St, Ste 416, MC 958, Chicago, IL 60612; **Phone:** 312-413-7707; **Board Cert:** Surgery 2001; Pediatric Surgery 2007; **Med School:** Univ VA Sch Med 1988; **Resid:** Surgery, Univ Virginia Hosp 1993; **Fellow:** Pediatric Surgery, Chldns Hosp & Med Ctr 1993; **Fac Appt:** Assoc Prof S, Univ IL Coll Med

Ilbawi, Michel N MD [PS] - **Spec Exp:** Cardiac Surgery; Congenital Anomalies; Cardiovascular Surgery; **Hospital:** Adv Christ Med Ctr, Adv Luth Genl Hosp; **Address:** Hope Chldns Hosp at Adv Christ Med Ctr, 4440 W 95th St, Oak Lawn, IL 60453; **Phone:** 708-684-3029; **Board Cert:** Thoracic Surgery 2007; **Med School:** Lebanon 1971; **Resid:** Surgery, American Univ Hosp 1975; Thoracic Surgery, Univ Hosps 1977; **Fellow:** Thoracic Surgery, Chldns Meml Hosp 1978; **Fac Appt:** Clin Prof S, Univ IL Coll Med

Liu, Donald C MD [PS] - **Spec Exp:** Minimally Invasive Surgery; Cancer Surgery; Gastrointestinal Surgery; Inflammatory Bowel Disease/Chron's; **Hospital:** Univ of Chicago Med Ctr; **Address:** 5841 S Maryland Ave, MC 4062, Chicago, IL 60637; **Phone:** 773-702-6175; **Board Cert:** Surgery 2005; Pediatric Surgery 2007; **Med School:** Thomas Jefferson Univ 1990; **Resid:** Surgery, Hosp Univ Penn 1995; **Fellow:** Pediatric Surgery, Univ Michigan Affil Hosp 1997; **Fac Appt:** Prof S, Univ Chicago-Pritzker Sch Med

Lobe, Thom E MD [PS] - **Spec Exp:** Minimally Invasive Surgery; Robotic Surgery; Pediatric Urology; **Hospital:** Iowa Methodist Med Ctr; **Address:** Blank Children's Hospital, 1212 Pleasant St, Ste 300, Des Moines, IA 50309; **Phone:** 515-241-6000; **Board Cert:** Surgery 2000; Pediatric Surgery 2001; **Med School:** Univ MD Sch Med 1975; **Resid:** Surgery, Ohio State Univ Med Ctr 1979; Pediatric Surgery, Childrens Hosp 1981

Mavroudis, Constantine MD [PS] - **Spec Exp:** Congenital Heart Disease; Transplant-Heart & Lung; Coronary Artery Surgery; **Hospital:** Cleveland Clin Fdn (page 56); **Address:** 9500 Euclid Ave, Ped Cardiology, M41, Cleveland, OH 44195; **Phone:** 216-445-5015; **Board Cert:** Surgery 2000; Thoracic Surgery 2000; **Med School:** Univ VA Sch Med 1973; **Resid:** Surgery, UCSF Med Ctr 1979; **Fellow:** Thoracic Surgery, UCSF Med Ctr 1977; **Fac Appt:** Prof S, Northwestern Univ

Oldham, Keith T MD [PS] - **Spec Exp:** Neonatal Surgery; Thoracic Surgery; Gastrointestinal Surgery; **Hospital:** Chldns Hosp - Wisconsin; **Address:** 999 N 92nd St, Ste 320, Milwaukee, WI 53226; **Phone:** 414-266-6550; **Board Cert:** Surgery 2000; Pediatric Surgery 1991; Surgical Critical Care 1995; **Med School:** Med Coll VA 1976; **Resid:** Surgery, Univ Wash Med Ctr 1981; **Fellow:** Pediatric Surgery, Univ Cincinnati Chldns Hosp 1983; **Fac Appt:** Prof S, Med Coll Wisc

Pena, Alberto MD [PS] - **Spec Exp:** Imperforate Anus; Anorectal Malformations; Colon & Rectal Surgery; **Hospital:** Cincinnati Chldns Hosp Med Ctr; **Address:** Cincinnati Chlds Hosp Med Ctr, 3333 Burnet Ave, MLC 2023, Cincinnati, OH 45229; **Phone:** 513-636-3240; **Med School:** Mexico 1962; **Resid:** Surgery, Military Hosp 1966; **Fellow:** Pediatric Surgery, Childrens Hosp 1971; Cardiovascular Surgery, Childrens Hosp 1969

Rescorla, Frederick J MD [PS] - **Spec Exp:** Neonatal Surgery; Cancer Surgery; Head & Neck Cancer; Trauma; **Hospital:** Riley Hosp for Children; **Address:** 702 Barnhill Drive, Ste 2500, Indianapolis, IN 46202; **Phone:** 317-274-4681; **Board Cert:** Surgery 2004; Surgical Critical Care 1998; Pediatric Surgery 2007; **Med School:** Univ Wisc 1981; **Resid:** Surgery, Indiana Univ Med Ctr 1986; Pediatric Surgery, Indiana Univ Med Ctr 1988; **Fac Appt:** Prof S, Indiana Univ

Reynolds, Marleta MD [PS] - **Spec Exp:** Critical Care; Trauma; Congenital Anomalies; Pediatric Cancers; **Hospital:** Children's Mem Hosp; **Address:** Chldns Meml Hosp, Dept Ped Surg, 2300 Children's Plaza, Box 63, Chicago, IL 60614; **Phone:** 773-880-4292; **Board Cert:** Surgery 2001; Thoracic Surgery 2006; Pediatric Surgery 2003; **Med School:** Tulane Univ 1976; **Resid:** Surgery, Tulane Univ Affil Hosp 1981; Pediatric Surgery, Chldns Meml Hosp 1983; **Fellow:** Cardiothoracic Surgery, Northwestern Univ 1985; **Fac Appt:** Prof S, Northwestern Univ

Pediatric Surgery

Sato, Thomas T MD [PS] - **Spec Exp:** Neonatal Surgery; Congenital Anomalies; Laparoscopy & Thoracostomy; **Hospital:** Chldns Hosp - Wisconsin; **Address:** 999 N 92nd St, Ste C320, Milwaukee, WI 53226; **Phone:** 414-266-6550; **Board Cert:** Surgery 2006; Pediatric Surgery 2007; **Med School:** USC Sch Med 1988; **Resid:** Surgery, Univ Wash Med Ctr 1995; **Fellow:** Surgery, Harborview Med Ctr 1993; Pediatric Surgery, Chldns Natl Med Ctr 1997; **Fac Appt:** Prof S, Med Coll Wisc

Warner, Brad MD [PS] - **Spec Exp:** Gastrointestinal Surgery; Neonatal Surgery; Cancer Surgery; **Hospital:** St Louis Chldns Hosp; **Address:** 1 Children's Pl, Ste 5S40, St. Louis, MO 63110; **Phone:** 314-454-6066; **Board Cert:** Surgery 1998; Pediatric Surgery 2001; **Med School:** Univ MO-Kansas City 1982; **Resid:** Surgery, Univ Cincinnati Med Ctr 1989; **Fellow:** Pediatric Surgery, Chldns Hosp Med Ctr 1991; **Fac Appt:** Prof S, Univ Cincinnati

Great Plains and Mountains

Bensard, Denis D MD [PS] - **Spec Exp:** Endoscopic Surgery; Trauma; Minimally Invasive Surgery; Critical Care; **Hospital:** Denver Health Med Ctr; **Address:** Denver Health Medical Ctr, Director Pediatric Surgery & Trauma, 777 Bannock St, Denver, CO 80204; **Phone:** 317-338-8857; **Board Cert:** Surgery 2002; Pediatric Surgery 2005; Surgical Critical Care 2003; **Med School:** Univ Colorado 1986; **Resid:** Surgery, Univ Colorado Med Ctr 1992; **Fellow:** Pediatric Surgery, Ohio State Univ 1995; **Fac Appt:** Asst Clin Prof S, Univ Colorado

Karrer, Frederick M MD [PS] - **Spec Exp:** Liver Surgery; Transplant-Liver; Critical Care; Neonatal Surgery; **Hospital:** Chldn's Hosp - Aurora, The, Denver Health Med Ctr; **Address:** Children's Hospital, Dept Surgery, 13123 E 16th Ave, Box B323, Aurora, CO 80045; **Phone:** 720-777-6571; **Board Cert:** Surgery 2007; Pediatric Surgery 1997; Surgical Critical Care 1998; **Med School:** Univ Nebr Coll Med 1979; **Resid:** Surgery, Univ Ariz Med Ctr 1984; Pediatric Surgery, Chldns Meml Hosp 1988; **Fellow:** Transplant Surgery, Univ Pittsburgh Affil Hosp 1986; **Fac Appt:** Prof S, Univ Colorado

Meyers, Rebecka L MD [PS] - **Spec Exp:** Transplant-Liver; Tumor Surgery; Biliary Surgery; Pancreatic Surgery; **Hospital:** Primary Children's Med Ctr, Univ Utah Hosps and Clins; **Address:** Primary Chlds Med Ctr, Dept Ped Surg, 100 N Mario Capecchi Drive, Ste 2600, Salt Lake City, UT 84113-1103; **Phone:** 801-662-2950; **Board Cert:** Surgery 2003; Pediatric Surgery 2005; **Med School:** Oregon Hlth & Sci Univ 1985; **Resid:** Surgery, UCSF Med Ctr 1990; **Fellow:** Research, Cardio Rsch Inst-UCSF 1992; Pediatric Surgery, St Christophers Hosp for Chldn 1994; **Fac Appt:** Assoc Prof S, Univ Utah

Ziegler, Moritz M MD [PS] - **Spec Exp:** Hirschsprung's Disease; Gastrointestinal Surgery; Neuroblastoma; Tumor Surgery; **Hospital:** Chldn's Hosp - Aurora, The, Univ Colorado Hosp; **Address:** Chldns Hosp, Dept Surgery, 13123 E 16th Ave, Box 323, Aurora, CO 80045; **Phone:** 720-777-6524; **Board Cert:** Surgery 1975; Pediatric Surgery 2007; **Med School:** Univ Mich Med Sch 1968; **Resid:** Surgery, Univ Penn Hosp 1975; Pediatric Surgery, Chldns Hosp 1977; **Fellow:** Surgical Oncology, Amer Oncologic Hosp 1975; **Fac Appt:** Prof S, Univ Colorado

Southwest

Black, C Thomas MD [PS] - **Spec Exp:** Neonatal Surgery; Minimally Invasive Surgery; Chest Wall Deformities; **Hospital:** Cook Chldns Med Ctr; **Address:** Ped. Surg. Assocs Ft. Worth, 901 7th Ave Ste 210, Fort Worth, TX 76104; **Phone:** 817-336-7881; **Board Cert:** Pediatric Surgery 2007; Surgery 2005; **Med School:** Baylor Coll Med 1979; **Resid:** Surgery, Baylor College Affil Hosp 1984; **Fellow:** Pediatric Surgery, Riley Childrens Hospital 1985; Pediatric Surgery-ECMO, Chldn's Meml Hosp 1987

Foglia, Robert P MD [PS] - **Spec Exp:** Congenital Anomalies; Burn Care; **Hospital:** Chldns Med Ctr of Dallas; **Address:** 1935 Medical District Drive, Ste B3250, Dallas, TX 75235; **Phone:** 214-456-6040; **Board Cert:** Surgery 2002; Pediatric Surgery 1995; Surgical Critical Care 1993; **Med School:** Georgetown Univ 1974; **Resid:** Surgery, UCLA Med Ctr 1981; **Fellow:** Pediatric Surgery, Chldns Hosp Natl Med Ctr 1983; **Fac Appt:** Prof S, Univ Tex SW, Dallas

Jackson, Richard J MD [PS] - **Spec Exp:** Pediatric Cancers; Neonatal Surgery; Robotic Surgery; **Hospital:** Cook Chldns Med Ctr; **Address:** 1433 W Humbolt, Fort Worth, TX 76104; **Phone:** 682-885-7080; **Board Cert:** Surgery 1997; Pediatric Surgery 2001; Surgical Critical Care 1998; **Med School:** W VA Univ 1983; **Resid:** Surgery, W Va Univ Hosps 1988; Pediatric Surgery, Chldns Hosp 1989; **Fellow:** Surgical Critical Care, Chldns Hosp-Univ Pittsburgh 1990; Pediatric Surgery, Chldns Hosp-Univ Pittsburgh 1992

Nuchtern, Jed MD [PS] - **Spec Exp:** Thoracic Surgery; Cancer Surgery; Laparoscopic Surgery; **Hospital:** Texas Chldns Hosp, Ben Taub Genl Hosp; **Address:** Texas Children's Hosp, 6621 Fannin St, MC CC650, Houston, TX 77030; **Phone:** 832-822-3135; **Board Cert:** Surgery 2003; Surgical Critical Care 2002; Pediatric Surgery 2007; **Med School:** Harvard Med Sch 1985; **Resid:** Surgery, Univ Washington 1992; Pediatric Surgery, Baylor Coll Med 1995; **Fellow:** Cellular Molecular Biology, Natl Inst Hlth 1990; **Fac Appt:** Prof S, Baylor Coll Med

Skinner, Michael A MD [PS] - **Spec Exp:** Endocrine Cancers; Thyroid Cancer; **Hospital:** UT Southwestern Med Ctr at Dallas; **Address:** UT Southwestern Med Ctr at Dallas, 1935 Medical District Drive, Ste B3250, Dallas, TX 75235; **Phone:** 214-456-6040; **Board Cert:** Surgery 2000; Pediatric Surgery 2003; **Med School:** Rush Med Coll 1984; **Resid:** Surgery, Duke Univ Med Ctr 1991; **Fellow:** Pediatric Surgery, Indiana Univ 1993; **Fac Appt:** Assoc Prof S, Univ Tex SW, Dallas

West Coast and Pacific

Albanese, Craig T MD [PS] - **Spec Exp:** Fetal Surgery; Laparoscopic Surgery; Twin to Twin Transfusion Syndrome (TTTS); **Hospital:** Lucile Packard Chldn's Hosp; **Address:** 780 Welch Rd, Ste 206, MC 5733, Palo Alto, CA 94304; **Phone:** 650-723-6439; **Board Cert:** Surgery 2000; Pediatric Surgery 2003; **Med School:** SUNY Hlth Sci Ctr 1986; **Resid:** Surgery, Mt Sinai Med Ctr 1991; **Fellow:** Pediatric Surgery, Chldns Hosp 1994; **Fac Appt:** Prof S, Stanford Univ

Farmer, Diana MD [PS] - **Spec Exp:** Pediatric Cancers; **Hospital:** CA Pacific Med Ctr - Pacific Campus, UCSF Med Ctr; **Address:** 400 Parnassus Ave, rm A123, San Francisco, CA 94143; **Phone:** 415-476-2538; **Board Cert:** Surgery 2001; Pediatric Surgery 2005; **Med School:** Univ Wash 1983; **Resid:** Surgery, UCSF 1993; **Fellow:** Pediatric Surgery, Chldn's Hosp 1995; **Fac Appt:** Assoc Prof S, UCSF

Ford, Henri R MD [PS] - **Spec Exp:** Minimally Invasive Surgery; Trauma; **Hospital:** Chldns Hosp - Los Angeles; **Address:** 4650 Sunset Blvd, MS 100, Los Angeles, CA 90027; **Phone:** 323-361-2104; **Board Cert:** Surgery 2002; Pediatric Surgery 2005; **Med School:** Harvard Med Sch 1984; **Resid:** Surgery, NY Hosp 1991; **Fellow:** Pediatric Surgery, Chldns Hosp Pittsburgh 1995

Hilfiker, Mary L MD/PhD [PS] - **Hospital:** Rady Children's Hosp - San Diego; **Address:** 8010 Frost St, Ste 414, San Diego, CA 92123; **Phone:** 858-966-7711; **Board Cert:** Surgery 2004; Pediatric Surgery 2007; **Med School:** Wright State Univ 1988; **Resid:** Surgery, U New Mexico Med Ctr 1993; **Fellow:** Pediatric Surgery, SUNY-Children's Hosp 1995; **Fac Appt:** Assoc Clin Prof S, UCSD

Pediatric Surgery

Krummel, Thomas M MD [PS] - **Spec Exp:** Minimally Invasive Surgery; Robotic Surgery; Fetal Surgery; **Hospital:** Lucile Packard Chldn's Hosp, Stanford Univ Med Ctr; **Address:** Dept Surgery, 701B Welch Rd, Ste 225, MC 5784, Stanford, CA 94305-5784; **Phone:** 650-498-4292; **Board Cert:** Surgery 2004; Pediatric Surgery 2007; **Med School:** Univ Wisc 1977; **Resid:** Surgery, Med Coll Va Hosp 1983; Pediatric Surgery, Chldns Hosp 1985; **Fellow:** Fetal Surgery, UCSF Med Ctr 1985; **Fac Appt:** Prof S, Stanford Univ

Sawin, Robert S MD [PS] - **Spec Exp:** Pediatric Cancers; Thoracic Surgery; Neonatal Surgery-Gastrointestinal; **Hospital:** Chldns Hosp and Regl Med Ctr - Seattle; **Address:** Chldns Hosp & Regl Med Ctr, 4800 Sand Point Way NE, Box 5371, Seattle, WA 98105-0371; **Phone:** 206-987-2039; **Board Cert:** Surgery 1999; Surgical Critical Care 2001; Pediatric Surgery 1999; **Med School:** Univ Pittsburgh 1982; **Resid:** Surgery, Brigham Women's Hosp 1987; **Fellow:** Pediatric Surgery, Chldns Hosp 1989; **Fac Appt:** Prof S, Univ Wash

Stein, James E MD [PS] - **Hospital:** Chldns Hosp - Los Angeles; **Address:** Children's Hospital of LA, 4650 Sunset Blvd, MS 100, Los Angeles, CA 90027; **Phone:** 323-361-2322; **Board Cert:** Surgery 2004; Pediatric Surgery 2005; **Med School:** Tufts Univ 1986; **Resid:** Surgery, Tufts New England Med Ctr 1993; **Fellow:** Pediatric Surgery, Royal Chldns Hosp 1994; Pediatric Surgery, Babies Hosp/Columbia Presby 1996; **Fac Appt:** Assoc Prof S, USC Sch Med

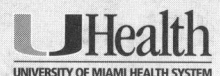

INTERNATIONALLY ACCLAIMED

Bascom Palmer Eye Institute is committed to the protection and preservation of the treasured gift of sight and is recognized as one of the world's finest and most progressive centers for ophthalmic care, vision research, and education. Each of our 65 clinical faculty members specializes in a specific area of ophthalmology and is board-certified by the American Board of Ophthalmology. In addition to providing care to more than 250,000 patients annually, all clinical faculty members have research and teaching responsibilities at the University of Miami Miller School of Medicine.

BASCOM PALMER EYE INSTITUTE RANKED #1 IN USA

Bascom Palmer continues to be ranked the nation's best ophthalmic hospital by board-certified ophthalmologists from across the United States. In 2009, it was ranked #1 in ophthalmology by *U.S. News & World Report* for the sixth consecutive year; and #1 in the nation for Clinical (Patient Care) and its Residency program by *Ophthalmology Times*.

PEDIATRIC OPHTHALMOLOGISTS DIAGNOSE AND TREAT CHILDHOOD EYE DISEASE AND DISORDERS

Bascom Palmer Eye Institute is one of only a few centers giving special attention to the diverse ophthalmic needs of children from infancy through adolescence – a critical time when clear vision plays an important role in mental, physical, and social development. As a major referral center serving the southeastern United States, Caribbean, and South America, we treat approximately 7,000 children annually in our children's clinic designed specifically for pediatric care. Our outpatient clinic is specifically designed to meet the unique ophthalmic and social needs of children with visual deficiencies as well as adults with strabismus. The clinic's diagnostic and treatment services encompass common eye disorders of childhood, such as amblyopia and strabismus, as well as rare disorders affecting infants and children. With the support of the extensive resources of the entire Bascom Palmer Eye Institute, we specialize in the blinding and visually-impairing diseases of childhood including congenital cataracts, congenital glaucoma, retinopathy of prematurity, detached retinas, ocular infections, hereditary disorders and tumors.

To schedule an appointment please call (800) 329-7000 or visit www.bascompalmer.org.

Miami:
900 NW 17th Street
Miami, FL 33136
(305) 326-6000

Palm Beach Gardens:
7101 Fairway Drive,
Palm Beach Gardens, FL 33418
(561) 515-1500

Naples:
311 9th Street North
Naples, FL 34102
(239) 659-3937

Plantation:
1000 South Pine Island Road
Plantation, FL 33324
(954) 465-2700

Cleveland Clinic

Children's Hospital

Cleveland Clinic Children's Hospital is ranked among the top pediatric hospitals in the United States, with more that 80 pediatricians recognized as "Best Doctors in America." Our specialists are nationally recognized for sophisticated diagnosis and innovative care of complex or chronic medical conditions affecting infants, children and adolescents as well as nationally funded research initiatives that are leading to advanced treatments for young patients.

- Our Center for Pediatric and Congenital Heart Disease, the largest and most experienced in Northern Ohio, is known for groundbreaking catheter and surgical treatments.
- Our pediatric digestive disease specialists, also the largest and most experienced in Northern Ohio, utilize breakthrough technology to diagnose and treat gastrointestinal problems.
- As part of Cleveland Clinic's Neurological Institute, our pediatric epilepsy specialists offer highly specialized diagnosis and surgery for different seizure disorders.
- Children's Hospital oncologists are national leaders in the treatment of childhood leukemia and other cancers.
- A comprehensive Fetal Care Center with maternal-fetal medicine specialists who diagnose fetal problems and treat them in the womb or immediately after birth.

In addition, Cleveland Clinic Children's Hospital has the only comprehensive pediatric transplant center in Northern Ohio, offering heart, lung, liver and kidney transplantation and follow-up.

Cleveland Clinic Children's Hospital

More than 250 Cleveland Clinic pediatricians and pediatric specialists offer advanced specialty and subspecialty care and rehabilitation for acute illnesses and injuries, as well as chronic and disabling conditions. Children with serious or complex medical problems such as congenital heart disease, cancer, epilepsy and digestive disorders are treated at our Main Campus. Our Shaker Campus is home to the Cleveland Clinic Children's Hospital for Rehabilitation, The Center for Autism and developmental, behavioral, therapeutic and rehabilitation programs that promote functional independence in children.

Our Pediatric ICU offers outstanding outcomes, saving many more young lives than similar centers, largely due to the 24-hour presence of seasoned critical care specialists. Our Pediatric Critical Care Transport Service transferred over 1,300 patients to our Children's Hospital from Ohio and surrounding states in 2008.

Our expertise in specialty pediatrics extends into the realm of long-term care for developmental, behavioral and rehabilitation needs. The Cleveland Clinic Children's Hospital for Rehabilitation, Shaker Campus, serves pediatric patients with chronic or complex medical conditions as one of just a handful of freestanding accredited pediatric rehabilitation hospitals in the country, and the only one in Ohio.

For more information about the Cleveland Clinic Children's Hospital, to schedule a second opinion or to learn about assistance for out-of-town patients, call 800.890.2467 or visit www.clevelandclinic.org/childrenstopdocs.

Children's Hospital | 9500 Euclid Avenue / AC311 | Cleveland OH 44195

The Maimonides Infants & Children's Hospital is a NACHRI-certi-fied children's hospital-within-a-hospital. Offering over 30 sub-spe-cialty divisions as well as primary care, the Pediatrics program is unrivaled in the region and serves one of the largest pediatric populations in the nation.

Steven Shelov, MD, head of the Children's Hospital and author of several bestselling books on childrearing, has built a family-cen-tered pediatrics program in a state-of-the-art medical environ-ment, where babies, children and adolescents receive the best and most appropriate care. For most children, this involves pre-venting illness and promoting healthy growth. For those whose problems are more complicated, Maimonides specialists can treat every manner of childhood disorder no matter how rare or com-plex. The level and quality of critical care provided is evidenced by the demand for the Maimonides Pediatric Transport Program, through which critically ill children from other hospitals are trans-ferred to Maimonides.

In recognition of its excellence in obstetrics and pediatrics, Maimonides was designated a Regional Perinatal Center by the New York State Department of Health.

Pediatric Specialties include:

Allergy	Infectious Disease
Behavioral & Developmental	Neonatology
Pediatrics	Nephrology
Cardiology	Neurology
Critical Care Medicine	Ophthalmology
Dentistry & Dental Surgery	Orthopedic Surgery
Emergency Medicine	Otolaryngology
Endocrinology	Psychiatry/Psychology
Gastroenterology	Pulmonology
Genetics	Rheumatology
Hematology/Oncology	Surgery
Immunology	Urology

Physicians at Maimonides are among the small percentage in the US who use comput-ers to enter patient orders, thereby reducing the risk of errors, increasing efficiency, and speeding the heal-ing process. Maimonides has appeared on the American Hospital Association's "Most Wired" and "Most Wireless" lists more often than any other health care institution in the metropolitan area. Advanced technology allows our doctors to focus more attention on caring for their patients.

**Maimonides Medical Center
Passionate about medicine.
Compassionate about people.**

www.maimonidesmed.org/pediatrics

NYU **Langone Medical Center**

550 First Avenue (at 31St Street)
New York, NY 10016
Physician Referral:
(888)7-NYU-MED (888-769-8633)
www.med.nyu.edu

PEDIATRIC CARDIOLOGY

About the Division of Pediatric Cardiology, Department of Pediatrics:

The Division of Pediatric Cardiology at the Cardiac and Vascular Institute at NYU Langone Medical Center is at the forefront of innovation in both research and clinical care. A growing emphasis on minimally invasive surgical techniques for infants, children, adolescents and young adults with a wide range of heart problems allows for quicker recoveries and shorter hospital stays. The Division's staff is vigilant in helping children stay in contact with their parents during their stay at the Medical Center, as well welcoming parents to stay overnight in their child's room on the pediatric floor whenever possible. Social workers and child life experts are always on hand to give families the information and support they need to cope with their child's disease during and after their stay at the Medical Center.

We specialize in the following areas:

CARDIOTHORACIC SURGERY
The Division offers corrective procedures for all types of congenital and acquired heart disease.

PEDIATRIC CARDIAC CRITICAL CARE
NYU Langone Medical Center provides intensive care for children with heart disease. Our staff of pediatric cardiologist, neonatologists, cardiac anesthesiologists, respiratory therapists and pediatric intensive care nurse are experienced, highly skilled and compassionate.

PEDIATRIC CARDIAC ELECTROPHYSIOLOGY
Specialists within the Division provide a wide array of diagnostic and therapeutic services including arrhythmia detection and pacemaker placement.

PEDIATRIC CARDIOPULMONARY EXERCISE LABORATORY
The lab assesses the cardio-respiratory response of exercise in children as young as three and four years old. It features some of the most sophisticated equipment in the region for measuring oxygen consumption, cardiac output and lung capacity.

PEDIATRIC INTERVENTIONAL CARDIAC CATHETERIZATION
The Division offers the treatment of serious heart conditions in a nonsurgical setting, sometimes used in combination with open-heart surgery.

PEDIATRIC NON-INVASIVE CARDIAC IMAGING
The Division of Pediatric Cardiology at the Cardiac and Vascular Institute at NYU Langone Medical Center offer echocardiography and magnetic resonance imaging (MRI) to diagnose and monitor a wide range of cardiac abnormalities.

NYU Langone Medical Center

550 First Avenue (at 31St Street)
New York, NY 10016
Physician Referral:
(888)7-NYU-MED (888-769-8633)
www.med.nyu.edu

PEDIATRIC EMERGENCY MEDICINE

About the Division of Pediatric Emergency Medicine, Department of Pediatrics:

The Division of Pediatric Emergency Medicine at NYU Langone Medical Center offers patients compassionate and state-of-the-art medical care. The dedicated pediatric emergency medicine trained doctors are experts in managing emergencies specific to infants, children, adolescents and young adults.

We specialize in the following areas:

PEDIATRIC EMERGENCY MEDICINE
The Tisch Hospital Pediatric Emergency Medicine Program at NYU Langone Medical Center provides the highest level of state-of-the-art care to all pediatric patients. Ill and injured children seeking care receive treatment in an area that is child friendly and family focused. The pediatric sub-specialty physicians and pediatric surgical physicians are available for consultation in the Emergency Department 24 hours a day, 365 days a year.

PEDIATRIC EMERGENCY SERVICES
Pediatric Emergency Services (PES) at Bellevue Hospital Center, an affiliate of NYU Langone Medical Center, is dedicated to the care of acutely ill and injured children. Each year approximately 25,000 children and young adults are evaluated in the PES which is staffed around the clock by board-certified pediatric emergency medicine physicians and nurses who specialize in the emergency care of children. The PES manages patients with a wide range of medical, surgical and psychiatric problems, including asthma, appendicitis, child abuse, orthopaedic injuries, major trauma, poisoning and suicide.

PEDIATRIC TRANSPORT
The Pediatric Transport Program at NYU Langone Medical Center transfers critically ill pediatric patients from outlying facilities to the Medical Center. In-house teams are available 24 hours a day, 7 days a week to allow a rapid response for medical transports. Patients are transported from more than 50 hospitals. The transport team assembled includes personnel with expertise in respiratory therapy and pediatric critical care nursing, in addition to the highest level of physician staff as appropriate. Patients are provided with the most advanced care from the beginning of the transport at the referring facility to their final destination, where they are cared for by physicians in a comprehensive network of sub-specialties.

NYU Langone Medical Center

550 First Avenue (at 31St Street)
New York, NY 10016
Physician Referral:
(888)7-NYU-MED (888-769-8633)
www.med.nyu.edu

PEDIATRIC GASTROENTEROLOGY

About the Division of Pediatric Gastroenterology, Department of Pediatrics:

The Division of Gastroenterology within the Department of Pediatrics at NYU Langone Medical Center is dedicated to providing the highest quality medical care and state-of-the-art techniques in the evaluation and management of gastrointestinal, liver and nutritional disorders from infancy to young adulthood. With access to the latest in endoscopic procedures performed at one of the country's leading academic medical centers, patients receive comprehensive and multidisciplinary treatments for a wide range of conditions. Physicians in the Division are particularly adept at providing family-centered, integrated care with a focus on the physical and psychological well-being of the child.

We specialize in the following areas:

CLINICAL CARE

Most children will occasionally experience one or more gastrointestinal symptoms during their childhood years. Some children, however, develop recurrent symptoms, which interrupt their normal lives and are the presenting features of important, treatable diseases. Experts within the Division of Pediatric Gastroenterology use the latest techniques to pinpoint problems and to determine the most effective therapy. At NYU Langone Medical Center, a vast range of therapeutic services are available, as well as access to clinical nutrition services, pediatric rehabilitation and some of the country's best surgeons.

SPECIALTY CARE

Pediatric gastroenterologists at NYU Langone Medical Center evaluate and treat a variety of disorders including: abdominal pain, celiac spruce, congenital bowel dysfunction, congenital liver disorders and chronic liver disease, chronic constipation, feeding problems in infants, failure to thrive, food allergies, lactose intolerance, gastrointestinal bleeding, gastroesophageal reflux, hepatitis, malabsorption syndromes, pancreatitis, peptic ulcer disease, ulcerative colitis and Crohn disease.

NYU **Langone Medical Center**

550 First Avenue (at 31St Street)
New York, NY 10016
Physician Referral:
(888)7-NYU-MED (888-769-8633)
www.med.nyu.edu

PEDIATRIC HEMATOLOGY/ONCOLOGY PROGRAM

About the Division of Pediatric Hematology/Oncology, Department of Pediatrics:

The Division of Pediatric Hematology and Oncology at NYU Langone Medical Center is an academically oriented program that is committed to providing modern, family-centered and highly personalized care to children with cancer and blood disorders. To provide the most modern, effective therapy for children, teams of specialists at the Medical Center deliver personalized care in a healing environment that promotes the physical, emotional and spiritual well-being of children and their families, using the tools of modern biology to identify the causes of childhood cancer and blood disorders and rapidly translate scientific discovery into better treatments for all children.

We specialize in the following areas:

HEMATOLOGIC MALIGNANCIES
The Pediatric Hematologic Malignancies Program at NYU Langone Medical Center offers new treatments for childhood acute lymphoblastic leukemia (ALL). Investigators at the Medical Center currently lead nationwide clinical trials for children and young adults with newly diagnosed leukemia as well as recurrent diseases, and actively participate in a number of clinical trials offering new treatment agents.

PEDIATRIC NEURO-ONCOLOGY
The Pediatric Neuro-Oncology program at NYU Langone Medical Center provides comprehensive care for infants, children, adolescents and young adults with primary central nervous system slow-growing and malignant tumors. Doctors offer a multidisciplinary approach to provide the safest and most effective curative treatment for patients with newly diagnosed and recurrent tumors.

THE PEDIATRIC SPECIAL HEMATOLOGY LABORATORY
The Pediatric Special Hematology Laboratory at NYU Langone Medical Center provides comprehensive homeostasis and red cell testing. Test procedures incorporate the latest developments in the field and have been adapted so that small quantities of blood can be drawn from pediatric patients. The Laboratory provides fast, precise test information that leads to effective treatments while maintaining rigorous quality control standards.

PSYCHOSOCIAL SERVICES
To help children and families cope with their disease and to prevent later psychological trauma, behavioral health professionals at NYU Langone Medical Center are committed to a holistic approach to patient care. Among the services provided are art therapy, relaxation training, play therapy, psychiatric evaluation, neuropsychological assessment, individual and group counseling and patient education.

VASCULAR ANOMALIES
The Vascular Anomalies Program at the Stephen D. Hassenfeld Children's Center for Cancer and Blood Disorders at NYU Langone Medical Center attracts nearly 500 new patients every year with vascular lesions that range from simple birthmarks to large disfiguring masses. The Program provides expert care to patients by a multidisciplinary team that includes hematologists, radiologists, plastic surgeons, and other healthcare professionals.

NYU Langone Medical Center

550 First Avenue (at 31St Street)
New York, NY 10016
Physician Referral:
(888)7-NYU-MED (888-769-8633)
www.med.nyu.edu

PEDIATRIC INFECTIOUS DISEASES

About the Division of Pediatric Infectious Diseases, Department of Pediatrics:

The Division of Pediatric Infectious Diseases (PID) at Bellevue Hospital Center, an affiliate of NYU Langone Medical Center, offers one of the largest programs in New York City for mothers and children with HIV infection. Initiated in 1982, this program furthers the understanding of the transmission of HIV from mothers to children and contributes to their improved care and longevity. The Division was one of the first NIH-funded Pediatric AIDS Clinical Trials Group sites and has cared for almost 500 HIV-infected children. Additionally, PID treats patients with other infectious diseases such as herpes viruses, respiratory viruses, hepatitis, bacterial, fungal and parasitic infections (tropical and local). We are also experienced in travel medicine and congenital infectious diseases.

We specialize in the following areas:

ADOLESCENT HIV CLINIC

The Bellevue Adolescent Clinic provides free, confidential HIV testing, pre- and post-test counseling, complete medical evaluations, comprehensive medical care and, if requested, referrals to clinical trials for HIV-positive teenagers. NYU Langone Medical Center was designated a Reaching for Excellence in Adolescent Care and Health (REACH) site, an NIH/HRSA-funded project. The clinic's primary objective is to increase the understanding of the natural history of HIV in teens and disease management.

INFECTIOUS DISEASES CLINIC

The Pediatric Infectious Diseases Clinic is one of the major providers of care for women and children at risk for HIV infection and other infectious diseases. Medical services are provided for children by the PID Clinic attending physicians, postdoctoral fellows and a pediatrician, with a dermatologist and pedodontist available. The clinic screens mothers for risk factors and provides counseling, testing and follow-up care for those receiving prenatal care.

PEDIATRICS INFECTIOUS DISEASE

Children requiring intravenous infusions during the course of their illness are cared for at the Pediatric Infectious Disease Day Hospital. The hospital also provides the medical, nursing, psychological and social support services these children require. Pediatrics patients can also use the hospital for non-acute care outside of regular clinic hours.

TB CLINIC

The TB Clinic evaluates approximately 200 new cases of latent and active tuberculosis a year and is a referral center for TB in the city. The Clinic is staffed by residents, a pediatric nurse practitioner, two PID attending physicians with particular expertise and experience with tuberculosis.

VIRAL HEPATITIS CLINIC

The Viral Hepatitis Clinic meets twice a week in Bellevue Hospital and follows approximately 250 children with chronic hepatitis C infection. The Clinic is a referral center for viral hepatitis infections in children and is the principal referral center for the NYC Pediatric Viral Hepatitis Network, a consortium of health facilities that is funded by the NY City Council.

NYU Langone Medical Center

550 First Avenue (at 31St Street)
New York, NY 10016
Physician Referral:
(888)7-NYU-MED (888-769-8633)
www.med.nyu.edu

PEDIATRIC PULMONOLOGY

About Pediatric Pulmonology, Department of Pediatrics:

On the forefront of technology, pediatric lung care specialists at NYU Langone Medical Center, including pediatric surgeons and pulmonologists, utilize minimally invasive techniques and state-of-the-art equipment to provide complete pediatric general surgical and thoracic services, as well as medical pulmonary care, for infants, children and adolescents. This includes surgical and specialized medical care for congenital and acquired lung problems, surgery in premature infants, tumor surgery and surgery on the lungs, esophageal surgery and the repair of chest wall deformities, as well as bronchoscopy for evaluation of airway lesions and infection. With more than a decade of experience in using minimally invasive techniques and state-of-the-art instruments to treat patients, the team of pediatricians performs procedures with minimal discomfort, little scarring and limited hospitalization. We also offer expertise in caring for the child with chronic respiratory failure, using both invasive and noninvasive ventilatory support and a variety of airway clearance devices.

We specialize in the following:

COMPREHENSIVE CARE
Because NYU Langone Medical Center is committed to comprehensive care through an interdisciplinary approach, its pediatric lung specialists are able to join forces with other centers, departments and divisions within the Medical Center. Pulmonary care at the NYU Infant Apnea/SIDS Program of Neonatology within the Department of Pediatrics, for example, is specifically designed and dedicated to the identification and treatment of infants with apnea and infants who are at an increased risk for sudden infant death syndrome (SIDS). The Program consists of physicians and nurses specially trained in this area, while providing testing and treatment for apnea and identification of high risk infants. Physicians and nurses also supply extensive education to the surrounding community and around-the-clock support to families of high-risk infants.

NYU **Langone Medical Center**

550 First Avenue (at 31St Street)
New York, NY 10016
Physician Referral:
(888)7-NYU-MED (888-769-8633)
www.med.nyu.edu

PEDIATRIC RHEUMATOLOGY

About the Division of Pediatric Rheumatology, Department of Pediatrics:

The Division of Pediatric Rheumatology at NYU Langone Medical Center is devoted to the complete care of children with rheumatic disease. In conjunction with a multidisciplinary therapeutic team of specialists, the Medical Center treats children with a variety of rheumatologic conditions including juvenile idiopathic arthritis (JIA), systemic lupus erythematosus, juvenile dermatomyositis and others. Through early diagnosis and appropriately intensive treatment, the staff at the Medical Center works to control the disease process as quickly and safely as possible in order to return children to their normal activities.

We specialize in the following areas:

JUEVENILLE IDIOPATHIC ARTHRITIS

An umbrella term for several different patterns of arthritis in children, juvenile idiopathic arthritis (JIA) refers to arthritic disorders caused by an autoimmune reaction. Pediatric Rheumatologists at NYU Langone Medical Center are experts in diagnosing and treating the different types of JIA. Each treatment is tailored to the individual patient with healthy and open communication between the doctors and family. Although JIA is not curable at present, rheumatologists have learned that aggressive, early treatment with methotrexate and injections of corticosteroids into the joints can actually prevent significant damage. The increased use of methotrexate in combination with new discovered biologic agents, such as Etanercept and Infliximab, gives even greater reason for optimism. Juvenile arthritis, once a cripple of children, is fast becoming a highly manageable disease.

PEDIATRICS OFARTHRITIS

Arthritis is the term used to describe inflammation and swelling of the tissues in a joint. Perhaps surprisingly, viruses are the most common cause of arthritis in children. This type of arthritis is usually temporary and passes quickly without permanent damage. However, a bacterial joint infection is a more urgent matter. Called septic arthritis, this painful condition requires urgent care to prevent the spread of infection and the possibility of permanent damage to the joint. At its first sign, the Medical Center's expert staff is quick to take steps to fight the infection at its source.

NYU **Langone Medical Center**

550 First Avenue (at 31St Street)
New York, NY 10016
Physician Referral:
(888)7-NYU-MED (888-769-8633)
www.med.nyu.edu

PEDIATRIC SURGERY

About the Division of Pediatric Surgery, Department of Surgery:

The Division of Pediatric Surgery at NYU Langone Medical Center provides comprehensive pediatric surgical care that starts even before the child is admitted and may continue long after the child is discharged. In addition to the highly skilled surgeons and surgical nurses, the Medical Center offers a wide array of Child Life Services to help children and their families become familiar with the hospital environment and lessen fears that often accompany a hospital stay.

We specialize in the following areas:

SURGICAL EXPERTISE
NYU Langone Medical Center is renowned for its achievements in the full spectrum of pediatric surgical specialties, including transplants, neurosurgery, thoracic surgery, cancer surgery, urological, abdominal surgery and reconstructive surgery, among others. NYU Langone Medical Center surgeons are experts at using minimally invasive techniques to treat a broad range of medical problems, resulting in shorter hospitals stays and faster recoveries.

CHILD LIFE SERVICES
The pediatric unit at Tisch Hospital is home to a Child Life Program that focuses on creating a supportive environment for children undergoing surgery. The program offers a total care approach for the child and support services for the families. The following child life services are available to the children and their families.

PEDIATRIC LIBRARY AND COMPUTER CENTER
A great variety of children's books, videos and audiotapes are available in the pediatric library, which also houses two computers with Internet access.

PRE-ADMISSION ORIENTATION AND INFORMATION
Informational packets are made available to families during pre-admission testing. Parents and their children are also encouraged to attend an orientation session with a member of the Child Life Program staff.

TEEN ESTEEM WORKSHOP SERIES
This workshop series addresses the special needs of teenagers who are living with chronic or life-threatening illnesses.

THERAPEUTIC PLAY
Therapists use arts and crafts, music, horticulture, games and cooking to keep children entertained and engaged throughout their hospital stay. Foster grandparents are also on hand to comfort, console and entertain children whose parents can not be present during the day. A group of specially trained dogs and their owners also regularly visit with eligible children.

Brenner Children's Hospital
Wake Forest University Baptist Medical Center

Medical Center Boulevard • Winston-Salem, NC 27157
336-716-2011
Health On-Call® (Patient Access) 1-800-446-2255
Physician-To-Physician Calls (PAL®) 1-877-716-1999
brennerchildrens.org

AN OPTIMAL PLACE FOR HEALING

Building on its tradition of excellence, Brenner Children's Hospital is housed in a state-of-the-art, 160-bed pediatric facility—an innovative environment designed to meet the complex needs of young patients and their families. Brenner Children's holistic care approach, outstanding facility, medical excellence and depth of pediatric subspecialty expertise—including western North Carolina's only Level IV neonatal intensive care nursery—have made it the resource for children's health in this region.

FAMILY-CENTERED

The pediatric tower exemplifies the gold standard for quality care and comfort, with spacious private rooms that encourage parents to room-in, a rooftop garden and play area, soothing quiet areas and interactive play centers. A Ronald McDonald Family Room—one of the first in the world—offers parents a comfortable place for respite and refreshment.

HOLISTIC CARE

Brenner Children's Hospital reflects a "whole child" philosophy. Every effort is made to meet emotional, spiritual and social needs as children receive expert medical care. Child Life specialists help patients and families cope with issues of hospitalization and illness.

COMMITTED TO CHILDREN'S HEALTH

Staffed by Wake Forest University School of Medicine faculty, Brenner Children's Hospital is committed to children's health research. Examples include the National Institutes of Health (NIH) Pediatric Heart Network. Brenner Children's Hospital joins other children's hospitals in the nation conducting clinical trials on patients with heart defects.

To make an appointment or find a specialist at Brenner Children's Hospital, call Health On-Call®️ at 1-800-446-2255.

PEDIATRIC EXPERTISE

- Brenner Children's Hospital is the region's only full service pediatric facility. More than 120 pediatric specialists and subspecialists provide expert care for critically ill children from NC, WV, TN, VA and SC.

- Brenner Children's Hospital offers children highly specialized, minimally invasive procedures often not available elsewhere in the Southeast, such as outpatient heart surgery for patent ductus arteriosus. Pediatric specialists manage every aspect of care.

- The neonatal intensive care nursery (the region's only Level IV nursery) at Brenner Children's Hospital participates in research to find new therapies and treatments.

- Brenner Children's houses the area's only pediatric Emergency Department, where children receive emergency care designed specifically for them.

- The Wake Forest Baptist ECMO (heart/lung) unit is one of only a few centers in the U.S. that supports newborns and children.

- Brenner Children's is one of eight centers in the United States participating in the National Institutes of Health (NIH) Pediatric Heart Network, which searches for the best ways to care for patients with heart defects.

- Our pediatric oncologists and nurses participate in a national Children's Oncology Group, a group of national researchers who evaluate current therapies used in treating children with cancer. This ensures that our children have access to the best cancer treatments available.

KNOWLEDGE MAKES ALL THE DIFFERENCE.

Physical Medicine & Rehabilitation

Physical medicine and rehabilitation, also referred to as rehabilitation medicine, is the medical specialty concerned with diagnosing, evaluating and treating patients with physical disabilities. These disabilities may arise from conditions affecting the musculoskeletal system such as neck and back pain, sports injuries, or other painful conditions affecting the limbs, for example carpal tunnel syndrome. Alternatively, the disabilities may result from neurological trauma or disease such as spinal cord injury, head injury or stroke.

A physician certified in physical medicine and rehabilitation is often called a physiatrist. The primary goal of the physiatrist is to achieve maximal restoration of physical, psychological, social and vocational function through comprehensive rehabilitation. Pain management is often an important part of the role of the physiatrist. For diagnosis and evaluation, a physiatrist may include the techniques of electromyography to supplement the standard history, physical, X-ray and laboratory examinations. The physiatrist has expertise in the appropriate use of therapeutic exercise, prosthetics (artificial limbs), orthotics and mechanical and electrical devices.

Training Required: Four years *plus* one year clinical practice.

Certification in the following subspecialty requires additional training and examination.

Spinal Cord Injury Medicine: A physician who addresses the prevention, diagnosis, treatment and management of traumatic spinal cord injury and non-traumatic etiologies of spinal cord dysfunction by working in an interdisciplinary manner. Care is provided to patients of all ages on a lifelong basis and covers related medical, physical, psychological and vocational disabilities and complications.

PHYSICAL MEDICINE & REHABILITATION

New England

Glenn, Mel B MD [PMR] - **Spec Exp:** Brain Injury Rehabilitation; Spasticity Management; **Hospital:** Spaulding Rehab Hosp, Mass Genl Hosp; **Address:** Spaulding Rehab Hospital, 125 Nashua St, Boston, MA 02114; **Phone:** 617-573-2625; **Board Cert:** Physical Medicine & Rehabilitation 1982; **Med School:** NYU Sch Med 1978; **Resid:** Physical Medicine & Rehabilitation, NYU Med Ctr 1981; **Fellow:** Spinal Cord Injury Medicine, NYU Med Ctr 1982; **Fac Appt:** Assoc Prof PMR, Harvard Med Sch

Richter, Edwin MD [PMR] - **Spec Exp:** Neuro-Rehabilitation; Musculoskeletal Injuries; Amputee Rehabilitation; Lymphedema; **Hospital:** Stamford Hosp; **Address:** 32 Strawberry Hill Ct Fl 4 - Ste 9, Stamford, CT 06902; **Phone:** 203-316-0610; **Board Cert:** Physical Medicine & Rehabilitation 1992; **Med School:** NYU Sch Med 1987; **Resid:** Physical Medicine & Rehabilitation, NYU Med Ctr 1991; **Fac Appt:** Asst Clin Prof PMR, NYU Sch Med

Silver, Julie K MD [PMR] - **Spec Exp:** Post Polio Syndrome/Rehabilitation; **Hospital:** UMass Memorial Med Ctr; **Address:** Harvard Health Publication, Countway Library, 2nd Fl, 10 Shattuck St, Boston, MA 02115; **Phone:** 508-871-2389; **Board Cert:** Physical Medicine & Rehabilitation 2006; **Med School:** Georgetown Univ 1991; **Resid:** Physical Medicine & Rehabilitation, Natl Rehab Hosp 1995; **Fac Appt:** Asst Prof PMR, Harvard Med Sch

Webster, Harry C MD [PMR] - **Spec Exp:** Pediatric Rehabilitation; Cerebral Palsy; Muscular Dystrophy; Spasticity Management; **Hospital:** Tufts Med Ctr; **Address:** Tufts Medical Ctr, 800 Washington St, Box 387, Boston, MA 02111; **Phone:** 617-636-5626; **Board Cert:** Pediatrics 1983; Physical Medicine & Rehabilitation 1987; **Med School:** UCSF 1977; **Resid:** Pediatrics, Children's Hosp 1980; Physical Medicine & Rehabilitation, Tufts Med Ctr 1987; **Fac Appt:** Asst Prof PMR, Tufts Univ

Zafonte, Ross DO [PMR] - **Spec Exp:** Brain Injury Rehabilitation; Spinal Cord Injury; **Hospital:** Spaulding Rehab Hosp; **Address:** Spaulding Rehab Hospital, 125 Nashua St, rm A55, Boston, MA 02114; **Phone:** 617-573-2754; **Board Cert:** Physical Medicine & Rehabilitation 1990; **Med School:** Nova SE Univ, Coll Osteo Med 1985; **Resid:** Physical Medicine & Rehabilitation, Mt Sinai Med Ctr 1989; **Fac Appt:** Clin Prof PMR, Boston Univ

Mid Atlantic

Ahn, Jung Hwan MD [PMR] - **Spec Exp:** Spinal Cord Injury; Stroke Rehabilitation; Neurologic Rehabilitation; **Hospital:** NYU Langone Med Ctr (page 67); **Address:** 400 E 34th St, rm 421, New York, NY 10016-4901; **Phone:** 212-263-6122; **Board Cert:** Physical Medicine & Rehabilitation 1980; Spinal Cord Injury Medicine 1998; **Med School:** South Korea 1970; **Resid:** Obstetrics & Gynecology, Elmhurst City Hosp - Mt Sinai 1976; Physical Medicine & Rehabilitation, NYU Med Ctr 1979; **Fellow:** Spinal Cord Injury Medicine, NYU Med Ctr 1980; **Fac Appt:** Clin Prof PMR, NYU Sch Med

Aseff, John N MD [PMR] - **Spec Exp:** Electrodiagnosis; Pain-Soft Tissue; **Hospital:** Natl Rehab Hosp, Washington Hosp Ctr; **Address:** National Rehabilitation Hosp, 102 Irving St NW, Washington, DC 20010; **Phone:** 202-877-1916; **Board Cert:** Physical Medicine & Rehabilitation 1978; **Med School:** Ohio State Univ 1973; **Resid:** Surgery, Univ Hosps Cleveland 1975; Physical Medicine & Rehabilitation, Ohio State Univ Hosps 1977; **Fac Appt:** Assoc Clin Prof PMR, Georgetown Univ

Bach, John MD [PMR] - **Spec Exp:** Neuromuscular Disorders; Amyotrophic Lateral Sclerosis (ALS); Post Polio Syndrome/Rehabilitation; **Hospital:** UMDNJ-Univ Hosp-Newark; **Address:** 150 Bergen St, Ste B403, Newark, NJ 07103; **Phone:** 973-972-7195; **Board Cert:** Physical Medicine & Rehabilitation 1986; **Med School:** UMDNJ-NJ Med Sch, Newark 1976; **Resid:** Physical Medicine & Rehabilitation, NYU Med Ctr 1980; **Fellow:** Neuromuscular Disease, Univ Hosp 1983; **Fac Appt:** Prof PMR, UMDNJ-NJ Med Sch, Newark

Ballard, Pamela H MD [PMR] - **Spec Exp:** Spinal Cord Injury; Spasticity Management; Neuromuscular Disorders; **Hospital:** Natl Rehab Hosp; **Address:** 102 Irving St NW, Washington, DC 20010; **Phone:** 202-877-1621; **Board Cert:** Physical Medicine & Rehabilitation 1991; Spinal Cord Injury Medicine 1999; **Med School:** Howard Univ 1986; **Resid:** Physical Medicine & Rehabilitation, Sinai Hosp 1990

Braddom, Randall L MD [PMR] - **Spec Exp:** Electromyography; Pain-Neck; Pain-Low Back; Musculoskeletal Disorders; **Hospital:** Riverview Med Ctr; **Address:** Orthopaedic, Sports Medicine & Rehab Ctr, 80 Oak Hill Rd, rm 368, Red Bank, NJ 07701; **Phone:** 732-741-2313; **Board Cert:** Physical Medicine & Rehabilitation 1974; **Med School:** Ohio State Univ 1968; **Resid:** Physical Medicine & Rehabilitation, Ohio State Univ Hosp 1973; **Fac Appt:** Clin Prof PMR, UMDNJ-NJ Med Sch, Newark

De Lateur, Barbara J MD [PMR] - **Spec Exp:** Frailty Syndrome; **Hospital:** Johns Hopkins Bayview Med Ctr (page 61); **Address:** Johns Hopkins Bayview Med Ctr, Rehab, AA Bldg Fl 01 - rm 1661, Baltimore, MD 21224; **Phone:** 410-550-5299; **Board Cert:** Physical Medicine & Rehabilitation 1970; **Med School:** Univ Wash 1963; **Resid:** Physical Medicine & Rehabilitation, Univ Wash Hosp 1968; **Fac Appt:** Prof PMR, Johns Hopkins Univ

Dillard, James N MD [PMR] - **Spec Exp:** Pain Management; Acupuncture; Complementary Medicine; Nutrition; **Hospital:** Stamford Hosp; **Address:** 110 E 59th St, Ste 10A, New York, NY 10022; **Phone:** 212-265-4038; **Board Cert:** Physical Medicine & Rehabilitation 2005; **Med School:** Rush Med Coll 1990; **Resid:** Physical Medicine & Rehabilitation, Columbia-Presby Med Ctr 1994; **Fac Appt:** Asst Clin Prof PMR, Columbia P&S

Esquenazi, Alberto M MD [PMR] - **Spec Exp:** Amputee Rehabilitation; Mobility Evaluation & Treatment; Post Polio Syndrome/Rehabilitation; **Hospital:** MossRehab Hosp; **Address:** Moss Rehab Hosp, 60 Township Line Rd, Philadelphia, PA 19027; **Phone:** 215-663-6676; **Board Cert:** Physical Medicine & Rehabilitation 1986; **Med School:** Mexico 1981; **Resid:** Physical Medicine & Rehabilitation, Temple Univ 1985; **Fellow:** Gait and Prosthetics, Moss Rehab Hosp 1986; **Fac Appt:** Prof PMR, Jefferson Med Coll

Evans, Sarah H MD [PMR] - **Spec Exp:** Pediatric Rehabilitation; **Hospital:** Chldns Natl Med Ctr; **Address:** Children's National Medical Ctr, Pediatric Rehabilitation, 111 Michigan Ave NW, Washington, DC 20010; **Phone:** 202-476-3080; **Board Cert:** Physical Medicine & Rehabilitation 1992; Pediatrics 2002; Pediatric Rehabilitation Medicine 2003; **Med School:** Univ MD Sch Med 1984; **Resid:** Pediatrics, Univ Colorado Hlth Sci Ctr 1987; **Fellow:** Physical Medicine & Rehabilitation, Univ Colorado Hlth Sci Ctr 1988; Pediatric Rehabilitation Medicine, Chldns Hosp 1989; **Fac Appt:** Assoc Prof PMR, Univ Colorado

Feinberg, Joseph Hunt MD [PMR] - **Spec Exp:** Peripheral Neuropathy; Spinal Rehabilitation; Electrodiagnosis; Sports Medicine; **Hospital:** Hosp For Special Surgery (page 59), Kessler Inst for Rehab - W Orange; **Address:** 523 E 72nd St Fl 2, New York, NY 10021-4872; **Phone:** 212-606-1568; **Board Cert:** Physical Medicine & Rehabilitation 1991; **Med School:** Albany Med Coll 1983; **Resid:** Surgery, Mt Sinai Hosp 1985; Physical Medicine & Rehabilitation, Rusk Inst Rehab 1990; **Fellow:** Orthopaedic Pathology, Hosp Spec Surg 1986; Orthopaedic Biomechanics, Univ Iowa Hosp & Clins 1987; **Fac Appt:** Assoc Prof PMR, Cornell Univ-Weill Med Coll

Physical Medicine & Rehabilitation

Flanagan, Steven R MD [PMR] - **Spec Exp:** Brain Injury Rehabilitation; Stroke Rehabilitation; **Hospital:** NYU Langone Med Ctr (page 67), Hosp For Joint Diseases (page 67); **Address:** 400 E 34th St, New York, NY 10016; **Phone:** 212-263-6105; **Board Cert:** Physical Medicine & Rehabilitation 2003; **Med School:** UMDNJ-NJ Med Sch, Newark 1988; **Resid:** Physical Medicine & Rehabilitation, Mt Sinai Hosp 1992; **Fac Appt:** Prof PMR, NYU Sch Med

Fried, Guy W MD [PMR] - **Spec Exp:** Brain Injury Rehabilitation; Spinal Cord Injury; Neurogenic Bladder; **Hospital:** Magee Rehab Hosp; **Address:** 1513 Race St, Philadelphia, PA 19102-1177; **Phone:** 215-587-3394; **Board Cert:** Physical Medicine & Rehabilitation 1990; Spinal Cord Injury Medicine 1999; Pain Medicine 2000; **Med School:** Yale Univ 1985; **Resid:** Physical Medicine & Rehabilitation, Thomas Jefferson Univ Hosp 1988; Preventive Medicine, Thomas Jefferson Univ Hosp 1989; **Fac Appt:** Asst Prof PMR, Thomas Jefferson Univ

Kirshblum, Steven C MD [PMR] - **Spec Exp:** Spinal Cord Injury; **Hospital:** Kessler Inst for Rehab - W Orange, St Barnabas Med Ctr; **Address:** Kessley Institute, 1199 Pleasant Valley Way, West Orange, NJ 07052-1424; **Phone:** 973-731-3600 x2258; **Board Cert:** Physical Medicine & Rehabilitation 1991; Spinal Cord Injury Medicine 1998; **Med School:** Univ Hlth Scis, Chicago Med Sch 1986; **Resid:** Physical Medicine & Rehabilitation, Mount Sinai Med Ctr 1990; **Fac Appt:** Prof PMR, UMDNJ-NJ Med Sch, Newark

Lutz, Gregory MD [PMR] - **Spec Exp:** Spinal Rehabilitation; Sports Medicine; Pain-Low Back; **Hospital:** Hosp For Special Surgery (page 59), Univ Med Ctr - Princeton; **Address:** 523 E 72nd St Fl 2, New York, NY 10021-4898; **Phone:** 212-606-1648; **Board Cert:** Physical Medicine & Rehabilitation 2003; **Med School:** Georgetown Univ 1988; **Resid:** Physical Medicine & Rehabilitation, Mayo Clinic 1992; **Fellow:** Sports Medicine, Hosp For Spec Surg 1993; **Fac Appt:** Assoc Prof PMR, Cornell Univ-Weill Med Coll

Ma, Dong M MD [PMR] - **Spec Exp:** Electromyography; Musculoskeletal Disorders; **Hospital:** NYU Rusk Inst (page 68), NYU Langone Med Ctr (page 67); **Address:** 400 E 34th St, rm 211, New York, NY 10016; **Phone:** 212-263-6338; **Board Cert:** Physical Medicine & Rehabilitation 1979; **Med School:** South Korea 1968; **Resid:** Physical Medicine & Rehabilitation, NYU Med Ctr 1975; **Fellow:** Physical Medicine & Rehabilitation, NYU Med Ctr 1977; **Fac Appt:** Clin Prof PMR, NYU Sch Med

Marino, Ralph J MD [PMR] - **Spec Exp:** Spinal Cord Injury; **Hospital:** Thomas Jefferson Univ Hosp; **Address:** 132 S 10th St, 375 Main Bldg, Philadelphia, PA 19107; **Phone:** 215-955-1200; **Board Cert:** Physical Medicine & Rehabilitation 1988; Spinal Cord Injury Medicine 2000; **Med School:** Jefferson Med Coll 1982; **Resid:** Physical Medicine & Rehabilitation, Thos Jefferson Univ Hosp 1987; **Fac Appt:** Assoc Prof PMR, Jefferson Med Coll

Mayer, Nathaniel H MD [PMR] - **Spec Exp:** Motor Control Analysis; Spasticity Management; Brain Injury Rehabilitation; **Hospital:** MossRehab Hosp; **Address:** Drucker Brain Injury Ctr, 60 E Township Line Rd, Elkins Park, PA 19027; **Phone:** 215-663-6681; **Board Cert:** Physical Medicine & Rehabilitation 1976; **Med School:** Albert Einstein Coll Med 1968; **Resid:** Physical Medicine & Rehabilitation, Temple Univ Hosp 1973; **Fac Appt:** Prof PMR, Temple Univ

Munin, Michael C MD [PMR] - **Spec Exp:** Spasticity Management; Amputee Rehabilitation; Hip Surgery Rehabilitation; Electrodiagnosis; **Hospital:** UPMC Shadyside, UPMC Inst Rehab & Rsch; **Address:** UPMC Shadyside, 3471 Fifth Ave, Kaufman Bldg Ste 1103, Pittsburgh, PA 15213; **Phone:** 412-692-4400; **Board Cert:** Physical Medicine & Rehabilitation 2003; **Med School:** Jefferson Med Coll 1988; **Resid:** Physical Medicine & Rehabilitation, Thomas Jefferson Univ Hosp 1992; **Fac Appt:** Assoc Prof PMR, Univ Pittsburgh

Ragnarsson, Kristjan T MD [PMR] - **Spec Exp:** Spinal Cord Injury; Brain Injury Rehabilitation; Pain-Back & Neck; **Hospital:** Mount Sinai Med Ctr (page 64); **Address:** 5 E 98th St Fl 6, New York, NY 10029-6501; **Phone:** 212-659-9370; **Board Cert:** Physical Medicine & Rehabilitation 1976; **Med School:** Iceland 1969; **Resid:** Physical Medicine & Rehabilitation, NYU Med Ctr 1974; **Fellow:** Spinal Cord & Brain Injury Rehab, NYU Med Ctr 1975; **Fac Appt:** Prof PMR, Mount Sinai Sch Med

Ried, Stephanie R MD [PMR] - **Spec Exp:** Pediatric Rehabilitation; **Hospital:** Shriners Hosp for Chldn-Phila; **Address:** Shriners Hosp for Children, Dept Physical Med & Rehab, 3551 N Broad St, Philadelphia, PA 19140; **Phone:** 215-430-4000; **Board Cert:** Pediatrics 2003; Physical Medicine & Rehabilitation 2006; Pediatric Rehabilitation Medicine 2006; Spinal Cord Injury Medicine 2007; **Med School:** Univ Mich Med Sch 1986; **Resid:** Pediatrics, Baylor Affil Hosps 1989; Physical Medicine & Rehabilitation, Univ Michigan Med Ctr 1992; **Fac Appt:** Asst Prof PMR, Temple Univ

Schwartz, L Matthew MD [PMR] - **Spec Exp:** Lymphedema; Pain-Cancer; Cancer Rehabilitation; Musculoskeletal Disorders; **Hospital:** Montgomery Rehab Hosp; **Address:** Montgomery Rehab Hosp, Medical Office, 8601 Stenton Ave, Wyndmoor, PA 19038; **Phone:** 215-233-6226; **Board Cert:** Physical Medicine & Rehabilitation 1992; Pain Medicine 2003; **Med School:** UMDNJ-NJ Med Sch, Newark 1987; **Resid:** Physical Medicine & Rehabilitation, Hosp U Penn 1989; Physical Medicine & Rehabilitation, Thos Jefferson Univ Hosp 1991; **Fac Appt:** Clin Prof PMR, Univ Pennsylvania

Stubblefield, Michael MD [PMR] - **Spec Exp:** Cancer Rehabilitation; Pain-Cancer; Pain-Musculoskeletal; Pain-Neuropathic; **Hospital:** Meml Sloan-Kettering Cancer Ctr; **Address:** 1275 York Avenue, New York, NY 10065; **Phone:** 212-639-7834; **Board Cert:** Internal Medicine 2001; Physical Medicine & Rehabilitation 2002; Electrodiagnostic Medicine 2003; **Med School:** Columbia P&S 1996; **Resid:** Internal Medicine, Columbia Presby Med Ctr 2001; Physical Medicine & Rehabilitation, Columbia Presby Med Ctr 2001; **Fac Appt:** Asst Prof PMR, Cornell Univ-Weill Med Coll

Southeast

Cardenas, Diana D MD [PMR] - **Spec Exp:** Spinal Cord Injury; Spina Bifida; Neurogenic Bladder; Urinary Tract Infections; **Hospital:** Univ of Miami Hosp & Clins/Sylvester Comp Canc Ctr (page 70), Jackson Meml Hosp (page 70); **Address:** Univ Miami, Dept Rehab Medicine, 1120 NW 14 St, Ste 958, Miami, FL 33136; **Phone:** 305-243-9516; **Board Cert:** Physical Medicine & Rehabilitation 1977; Electrodiagnostic Medicine 1989; **Med School:** Univ Tex SW, Dallas 1973; **Resid:** Physical Medicine & Rehabilitation, Univ Wash Affil Hosps 1976; **Fac Appt:** Prof PMR, Univ Miami Sch Med

Creamer, Michael DO [PMR] - **Spec Exp:** Spinal Cord Injury; Pain Management; Electrodiagnosis; **Hospital:** Orlando Regl Med Ctr, Florida Hosp - Orlando; **Address:** 100 W Gore St, Ste 203, Orlando, FL 32806-1041; **Phone:** 407-649-8707; **Board Cert:** Physical Medicine & Rehabilitation 1992; Spinal Cord Injury Medicine 1998; Pain Medicine 2000; **Med School:** Chicago Coll Osteo Med 1987; **Resid:** Physical Medicine & Rehabilitation, Rehab Inst Chicago 1991; **Fac Appt:** Asst Prof Med, Univ Fla Coll Med

Diamond, Paul T MD [PMR] - **Spec Exp:** Neuro-Rehabilitation; Geriatric Rehabilitation; **Hospital:** Univ Virginia Med Ctr; **Address:** Univ of Virginia Hlth Sci Ctr, Dept Rehabilitation, 545 Ray C Hunt Drive, Ste 240, Charlottesville, VA 22903; **Phone:** 434-243-5622; **Board Cert:** Internal Medicine 1989; Physical Medicine & Rehabilitation 2003; **Med School:** Univ VA Sch Med 1986; **Resid:** Internal Medicine, Johns Hospkins Bayview Hosp 1989; Physical Medicine & Rehabilitation, Sinai/Johns Hopkins Hosp 1992; **Fac Appt:** Assoc Prof PMR, Univ VA Sch Med

Physical Medicine & Rehabilitation

Gater Jr, David R MD/PhD [PMR] - **Spec Exp:** Spinal Cord Injury; Exercise Physiology; Electrodiagnosis; **Hospital:** Hunter Holmes McGuire VA Med Ctr, VCU Med Ctr; **Address:** 1201 Broadrock Blvd, Richmond, VA 23249; **Phone:** 804-675-5000 x5455; **Board Cert:** Physical Medicine & Rehabilitation 2007; Spinal Cord Injury Medicine 1999; Electrodiagnostic Medicine 1998; **Med School:** Univ Ariz Coll Med 1992; **Resid:** Physical Medicine & Rehabilitation, UC Davis Med Ctr 1994; **Fac Appt:** Prof PMR, Va Commonwealth Univ Sch Med

Jackson, Amie B MD [PMR] - **Spec Exp:** Spinal Cord Injury; **Hospital:** Univ of Ala Hosp at Birmingham, Children's Hospital - Birmingham; **Address:** Univ of Alabama at Birmingham, Spain Rehab Center, 1717 6th Ave S, rm 190, Birmingham, AL 35233; **Phone:** 205-934-3330; **Board Cert:** Physical Medicine & Rehabilitation 1990; **Med School:** Univ Alabama 1984; **Resid:** Physical Medicine & Rehabilitation, Univ Alabama Med Ctr 1987; **Fac Appt:** Prof PMR, Univ Alabama

King Jr, Richard W MD [PMR] - **Spec Exp:** Cancer Rehabilitation; Lymphedema; Soft Tissue Radiation Necrosis; Soft Tissue Radiation Necrosis-Breast; **Hospital:** WellStar Windy Hill Hosp, WellStar Cobb Hosp; **Address:** HyOx Medical Treatment Ctr, 2550 Windy Hill Rd, Ste 110, Marietta, GA 30067; **Phone:** 678-303-3200; **Board Cert:** Physical Medicine & Rehabilitation 1988; Undersea & Hyperbaric Medicine 2002; **Med School:** Emory Univ 1979; **Resid:** Physical Medicine & Rehabilitation, Emory Univ Hosp 1987; **Fac Appt:** Asst Clin Prof PMR, Emory Univ

Leslie, Donald P MD [PMR] - **Spec Exp:** Brain/Spinal Cord Injury; **Hospital:** Shepherd Ctr - Atlanta; **Address:** Shepherd Center, 2020 Peachtree Rd NW, Atlanta, GA 30309; **Phone:** 404-352-2020; **Board Cert:** Physical Medicine & Rehabilitation 1989; **Med School:** Univ Tenn Coll Med, Memphis 1972; **Resid:** Internal Medicine, Mayo Clinic 1975; Physical Medicine & Rehabilitation, Emory Univ Hosp 1986

McKinley, William MD [PMR] - **Spec Exp:** Spinal Cord Injury; **Hospital:** Hunter Holmes McGuire VA Med Ctr; **Address:** 417 N 11th St, Dept Phys, Med & Rehab Nelson Bldg Fl 6, Richmond, VA 23249; **Phone:** 804-828-4097; **Board Cert:** Physical Medicine & Rehabilitation 1990; Spinal Cord Injury Medicine 1998; **Med School:** Albany Med Coll 1985; **Resid:** Physical Medicine & Rehabilitation, Med Coll Va 1989; **Fac Appt:** Prof PMR, Va Commonwealth Univ Sch Med

Nelson, Maureen R MD [PMR] - **Spec Exp:** Pediatric Rehabilitation; Brachial Plexus Palsy; Electrodiagnosis; **Hospital:** Carolinas Med Ctr, Levine Chldns Hosp; **Address:** Carolinas Rehab, Dept PM&R, 1001 Blythe Blvd, Charlotte, NC 28203; **Phone:** 704-381-8895; **Board Cert:** Physical Medicine & Rehabilitation 1990; Pediatric Rehabilitation Medicine 2003; **Med School:** Univ IL Coll Med 1985; **Resid:** Physical Medicine & Rehabilitation, Univ Tex Hlth Scis Ctr 1989; **Fellow:** Pediatric Rehabilitation Medicine, Alfred I Dupont Inst 1990; **Fac Appt:** Assoc Clin Prof PMR, Univ NC Sch Med

Stewart, Paula JB MD [PMR] - **Spec Exp:** Lymphedema; Brain Tumors; Spinal Cord Tumors; Cancer Rehabilitation; **Hospital:** Healthsouth Lakeshore Rehab Hosp; **Address:** Healthsouth Lakeshore Rehab Hosp, 3800 Ridgeway Drive, Birmingham, AL 35209; **Phone:** 205-868-2347; **Board Cert:** Physical Medicine & Rehabilitation 1996; Spinal Cord Injury Medicine 2000; **Med School:** Univ Minn 1987; **Resid:** Physical Medicine & Rehabilitation, Mayo Clinic 1991

Midwest

Chen, David MD [PMR] - **Spec Exp:** Spinal Cord Injury; **Hospital:** Rehab Inst of Chicago; **Address:** 345 E Superior St, Ste 1146, Chicago, IL 60611; **Phone:** 312-238-0764; **Board Cert:** Physical Medicine & Rehabilitation 1992; Spinal Cord Injury Medicine 1998; **Med School:** Univ IL Coll Med 1987; **Resid:** Physical Medicine & Rehabilitation, Northwestern Med Sch 1991; **Fac Appt:** Asst Prof PMR, Northwestern Univ

Cheville, Andrea L MD [PMR] - **Spec Exp:** Lymphedema; Cancer Rehabilitation; Pain-Cancer; **Hospital:** Mayo Med Ctr & Clin - Rochester; **Address:** Mayo Clinic, Dept Physical Med & Rehab, 200 1st St SW, Rochester, MN 55905; **Phone:** 507-284-2747; **Board Cert:** Physical Medicine & Rehabilitation 2008; Pain Medicine 2004; **Med School:** Harvard Med Sch 1993; **Resid:** Physical Medicine & Rehabilitation, UMDNJ Med Ctr 1997; **Fellow:** Pain & Palliative Care, Meml Sloan Kettering Cancer Ctr 1999; **Fac Appt:** Asst Prof PMR, Mayo Med Sch

Clairmont, Albert C MD [PMR] - **Spec Exp:** Spasticity Management; Electrodiagnosis; **Hospital:** Ohio St Univ Med Ctr; **Address:** 480 Medical Center Drive, 1011 Dodd Hall, Columbus, OH 43210; **Phone:** 614-293-4837; **Board Cert:** Physical Medicine & Rehabilitation 1985; Pediatrics 1985; **Med School:** Jamaica 1974; **Resid:** Pediatrics, Columbus Chldns Hosp 1981; Physical Medicine & Rehabilitation, Ohio St Univ Hosps 1983; **Fac Appt:** Assoc Clin Prof PMR, Ohio State Univ

Colachis III, Samuel C MD [PMR] - **Spec Exp:** Spinal Cord Injury; Electrodiagnosis; **Hospital:** Ohio St Univ Med Ctr; **Address:** 480 Medical Center Drive, 1011 Dodd Hall, Columbus, OH 43210; **Phone:** 614-293-4837; **Board Cert:** Physical Medicine & Rehabilitation 1988; Spinal Cord Injury Medicine 2003; **Med School:** USC Sch Med 1984; **Resid:** Physical Medicine & Rehabilitation, Ohio State Univ Hosps 1987; **Fellow:** Electrodiagnosis, Ohio State Univ Hosps 1988; **Fac Appt:** Assoc Prof PMR, Ohio State Univ

DePompolo, Robert W MD [PMR] - **Spec Exp:** Cancer Rehabilitation; Lymphedema; **Hospital:** St Mary's Hosp - Rochester, Mayo Med Ctr & Clin - Rochester; **Address:** Mayo Clinic, Dept Phys Med & Rehab, 200 1st St SW, Rochester, MN 55905; **Phone:** 507-255-8972; **Board Cert:** Physical Medicine & Rehabilitation 1981; **Med School:** Wayne State Univ 1977; **Resid:** Physical Medicine & Rehabilitation, Univ Minnesota Affil Hosp 1980

Dillingham, Timothy R MD [PMR] - **Spec Exp:** Electrodiagnosis; Electromyography; Amputee Rehabilitation; **Hospital:** Froedtert Meml Lutheran Hosp; **Address:** Dept Physical Med & Rehab, 9200 W Wisconsin Ave, rm 2103, Milwaukee, WI 53226; **Phone:** 414-805-7343; **Board Cert:** Physical Medicine & Rehabilitation 1991; **Med School:** Univ Wash 1986; **Resid:** Physical Medicine & Rehabilitation, Univ Wash Affil Hosps 1990; **Fac Appt:** Prof PMR, Med Coll Wisc

Feldman, Joseph L MD [PMR] - **Spec Exp:** Lymphedema; **Hospital:** Evanston/Northshore Univ Hlth Syst; **Address:** 2650 Ridge Ave, rm 2204, Evanston, IL 60201-1718; **Phone:** 847-570-2066; **Board Cert:** Physical Medicine & Rehabilitation 1971; **Med School:** Univ IL Coll Med 1965; **Resid:** Physical Medicine & Rehabilitation, Univ of Ilinois Med Ctr 1969; **Fac Appt:** Asst Prof PMR, Northwestern Univ

Frost, Frederick S MD [PMR] - **Spec Exp:** Spinal Cord Injury; Stroke Rehabilitation; Geriatric Rehabilitation; **Hospital:** Cleveland Clin Fdn (page 56); **Address:** Cleveland Clinic Fdn, 9500 Euclid Ave, MC C21, Cleveland, OH 44195; **Phone:** 216-445-2006; **Board Cert:** Physical Medicine & Rehabilitation 1988; Spinal Cord Injury Medicine 1998; **Med School:** Northwestern Univ 1983; **Resid:** Physical Medicine & Rehabilitation, Northwestern Meml Hosp 1987; **Fellow:** Spinal Cord Injury Medicine, Rehab Inst Chicago; **Fac Appt:** Asst Prof PMR, Cleveland Cl Coll Med/Case West Res

Gamble, Gail L MD [PMR] - **Spec Exp:** Lymphedema; Head & Neck Cancer; Bone Tumors-Metastatic; **Hospital:** Rehab Inst of Chicago; **Address:** Rehab Inst of Chicago, 345 E Superior St, Chicago, IL 60611; **Phone:** 312-238-7670; **Board Cert:** Physical Medicine & Rehabilitation 1985; **Med School:** Mayo Med Sch 1979; **Resid:** Physical Medicine & Rehabilitation, Mayo Clinic 1983

Gittler, Michelle S MD [PMR] - **Spec Exp:** Spinal Cord Injury; Amputee Rehabilitation; **Hospital:** Schwab Rehab Hosp, Univ of Chicago Med Ctr; **Address:** 1401 S California Blvd, Chicago, IL 60608; **Phone:** 773-522-5853; **Board Cert:** Physical Medicine & Rehabilitation 2003; Spinal Cord Injury Medicine 2008; **Med School:** Univ IL Coll Med 1988; **Resid:** Physical Medicine & Rehabilitation, Rehab Inst Chicago 1992; **Fac Appt:** Assoc Clin Prof S, Univ Chicago-Pritzker Sch Med

Physical Medicine & Rehabilitation

Haig, Andrew MD [PMR] - **Spec Exp:** International Health; Pain-Back & Neck; Electrodiagnosis; **Hospital:** Univ Michigan Hlth Sys, VA Med Ctr - Ann Arbor; **Address:** Univ Michigan Spine Program, 325 E Eisenhower, Burlington Bldg - Ste 100, Ann Arbor, MI 48108-3346; **Phone:** 734-763-4200; **Board Cert:** Physical Medicine & Rehabilitation 1987; Pain Medicine 2002; **Med School:** Med Coll Wisc 1983; **Resid:** Physical Medicine & Rehabilitation, Northwestern Univ 1986; **Fac Appt:** Prof PMR, Univ Mich Med Sch

Keen, Mary MD [PMR] - **Spec Exp:** Pediatric Rehabilitation; Spasticity Management; Neurodevelopmental Disability; Autism; **Hospital:** Marianjoy Rehab Hosp, Central DuPage Hosp; **Address:** Marianjoy Rehab Medical Clinic, 26 W 171 Roosevelt Rd, Wheaton, IL 60187; **Phone:** 630-909-7005; **Board Cert:** Physical Medicine & Rehabilitation 1984; Pediatrics 2005; Neurodevelopmental Disabilities 2001; Pediatric Rehabilitation Medicine 2003; **Med School:** Northwestern Univ 1979; **Resid:** Physical Medicine & Rehabilitation, Univ Wash Med Ctr 1983; Pediatrics, Loyola Univ Med Ctr 1990; **Fac Appt:** Assoc Clin Prof Ped, Loyola Univ-Stritch Sch Med

Kirschner, Kristi MD [PMR] - **Spec Exp:** Spina Bifida-Adult; Neuromuscular Disorders; Women's Health/Disabilities; **Hospital:** Rehab Inst of Chicago, Northwestern Meml Hosp; **Address:** Rehab Inst of Chicago, 345 E Superior St Fl 11, Chicago, IL 60611-2654; **Phone:** 312-238-4744; **Board Cert:** Physical Medicine & Rehabilitation 1991; **Med School:** Northwestern Univ-Feinberg Sch Med 1986; **Resid:** Physical Medicine & Rehabilitation, Rehab Inst of Chicago/Northwestern Univ 1990; **Fellow:** Clinical Ethics, Maclean Ctr/Univ Chicago 1995; **Fac Appt:** Prof PMR, Northwestern Univ-Feinberg Sch Med

Kuiken, Todd A MD/PhD [PMR] - **Spec Exp:** Amputee Rehabilitation; Prosthesis Control; Gait Disorders; **Hospital:** Rehab Inst of Chicago; **Address:** Rehab Inst of Chicago, 345 E Superior St, rm 1309, Chicago, IL 60611; **Phone:** 312-238-8072; **Board Cert:** Physical Medicine & Rehabilitation 2006; **Med School:** Northwestern Univ 1990; **Resid:** Physical Medicine & Rehabilitation, Rehab Inst Chicago 1995; **Fac Appt:** Assoc Prof PMR, Northwestern Univ

La Ban, Myron M MD [PMR] - **Spec Exp:** Pain-Back; Electromyography; Neuromuscular Disorders; **Hospital:** William Beaumont Hosp; **Address:** 3535 W Thirteen Mile Rd, Ste 437, Royal Oak, MI 48073; **Phone:** 248-288-2237; **Board Cert:** Physical Medicine & Rehabilitation 1967; **Med School:** Univ Mich Med Sch 1961; **Resid:** Physical Medicine & Rehabilitation, Univ Ohio Hosps 1965; **Fac Appt:** Clin Prof PMR, Ohio State Univ

Leonard Jr, James A MD [PMR] - **Spec Exp:** Amputee Rehabilitation; Electrodiagnosis; **Hospital:** Univ Michigan Hlth Sys; **Address:** Univ Michigan, Dept Physical Med & Rehab, 325 E Eisenhower Pkwy, Ste 100, Ann Arbor, MI 48108; **Phone:** 734-936-7175; **Board Cert:** Physical Medicine & Rehabilitation 1977; **Med School:** Univ Mich Med Sch 1972; **Resid:** Physical Medicine & Rehabilitation, Univ Mich Med Ctr 1975; **Fac Appt:** Clin Prof PMR, Univ Mich Med Sch

Mysiw, W Jerry MD [PMR] - **Spec Exp:** Brain Injury Rehabilitation; **Hospital:** Ohio St Univ Med Ctr; **Address:** 480 Medical Center Drive, 1011 Dodd Hall, Columbus, OH 43210-1245; **Phone:** 614-293-4837; **Board Cert:** Physical Medicine & Rehabilitation 1985; **Med School:** Ohio State Univ 1981; **Resid:** Physical Medicine & Rehabilitation, Ohio State Univ Med Ctr 1984; **Fac Appt:** Assoc Prof PMR, Ohio State Univ

Nobunaga, Austin MD [PMR] - **Spec Exp:** Spinal Cord Injury; Electrodiagnosis; **Hospital:** Univ Hosp - Cincinnati; **Address:** Drake Center, 151 W Galbraith Rd, South Pavillion, Cincinnati, OH 45216; **Phone:** 513-418-2707; **Board Cert:** Physical Medicine & Rehabilitation 1990; Spinal Cord Injury Medicine 1999; **Med School:** Univ Mich Med Sch 1985; **Resid:** Physical Medicine & Rehabilitation, Rehab Inst Chicago 1989

Press, Joel MD [PMR] - **Spec Exp:** Sports Medicine; Pain-Back; Musculoskeletal Injuries; **Hospital:** Rehab Inst of Chicago; **Address:** Ctr for Spine, Sports & Occup Rehab, 1030 N Clark St, Ste 500, Chicago, IL 60610; **Phone:** 312-238-7767; **Board Cert:** Physical Medicine & Rehabilitation 1989; **Med School:** Univ IL Coll Med 1984; **Resid:** Physical Medicine & Rehabilitation, Northwestern Meml Hosp 1988; **Fac Appt:** Assoc Clin Prof PMR, Northwestern Univ

Roth, Elliot MD [PMR] - **Spec Exp:** Stroke Rehabilitation; Neurologic Rehabilitation; Geriatric Rehabilitation; **Hospital:** Rehab Inst of Chicago, Northwestern Meml Hosp; **Address:** Rehab Inst Chicago, 345 E Superior St, Chicago, IL 60611-2654; **Phone:** 312-238-4637; **Board Cert:** Physical Medicine & Rehabilitation 1987; **Med School:** Northwestern Univ 1982; **Resid:** Physical Medicine & Rehabilitation, Northwestern Univ 1985; **Fellow:** Physical Medicine & Rehabilitation, Rehab Inst Chicago 1986; **Fac Appt:** Prof PMR, Northwestern Univ

Sisung, Charles MD [PMR] - **Spec Exp:** Rheumatic Diseases of Childhood; Trauma Rehabilitation; Burn Care; **Hospital:** Rehab Inst of Chicago; **Address:** 345 E Superior St, rm 1158, Chicago, IL 60611; **Phone:** 312-238-1246; **Board Cert:** Pediatrics 2004; Physical Medicine & Rehabilitation 1991; Pediatric Rehabilitation Medicine 2003; **Med School:** Univ Mich Med Sch 1981; **Resid:** Pediatrics, Mott Chldns Hosp/Univ Mich 1984; Physical Medicine & Rehabilitation, Schwab Rehab Hosp 1989; **Fellow:** Pediatric Rheumatology, Univ Chicago Hosps 1991; **Fac Appt:** Asst Prof PMR, Northwestern Univ

Sliwa, James A DO [PMR] - **Spec Exp:** Post Polio Syndrome/Rehabilitation; Multiple Sclerosis; Pain-Back; **Hospital:** Rehab Inst of Chicago; **Address:** Rehab Inst Chicago, 345 E Superior St, rm 1108, Chicago, IL 60611-3015; **Phone:** 312-238-4093; **Board Cert:** Physical Medicine & Rehabilitation 2005; **Med School:** Chicago Coll Osteo Med 1980; **Resid:** Physical Medicine & Rehabilitation, Rehab Inst 1984; **Fac Appt:** Prof PMR, Northwestern Univ

Smith, Joanne MD [PMR] - **Spec Exp:** Pain-Pelvic; Pain-Back; **Hospital:** Rehab Inst of Chicago, Northwestern Meml Hosp; **Address:** Rehab Inst of Chicago, 345 E Superior St, Ste 1507, Chicago, IL 60611; **Phone:** 312-238-0815; **Board Cert:** Physical Medicine & Rehabilitation 2003; **Med School:** Mich State Univ 1988; **Resid:** Physical Medicine & Rehabilitation, Northwestern Univ 1992; **Fac Appt:** Asst Prof PMR, Northwestern Univ

Volshteyn, Oksana MD [PMR] - **Spec Exp:** Spinal Cord Injury; Amputee Rehabilitation; **Hospital:** Rehab Inst St. Louis, Barnes-Jewish Hosp; **Address:** 4444 Forest Park, Box 8518, St Louis, MO 63108; **Phone:** 314-362-4503; **Board Cert:** Physical Medicine & Rehabilitation 1986; Spinal Cord Injury Medicine 1999; **Med School:** Russia 1976; **Resid:** Physical Medicine & Rehabilitation, Barnes Jewish Hosp 1985; **Fac Appt:** Assoc Prof N, Washington Univ, St Louis

Great Plains and Mountains

Mason, Kristin D MD [PMR] - **Spec Exp:** Neurologic Rehabilitation; Electrodiagnosis; Musculoskeletal Injuries; **Hospital:** Swedish Med Ctr - Englewood; **Address:** Rehab Assocs Colorado, 8515 Pearl St, Ste 100, Thornton, CO 80229; **Phone:** 303-286-2888; **Board Cert:** Physical Medicine & Rehabilitation 2003; **Med School:** Baylor Coll Med 1988; **Resid:** Physical Medicine & Rehabilitation, Rehab Inst Chicago 1992

Matthews, Dennis J MD [PMR] - **Spec Exp:** Brain Injury Rehabilitation; Neuromuscular Disorders; Cerebral Palsy; **Hospital:** Chldn's Hosp - Aurora, The; **Address:** Chldns Hosp, Dept Rehabilitation, 13123 E 16th Ave, Box 285, Aurora, CO 80045; **Phone:** 720-777-3907; **Board Cert:** Physical Medicine & Rehabilitation 1979; Pediatric Rehabilitation Medicine 2003; Neuromuscular Medicine 2008; **Med School:** Univ Colorado 1975; **Resid:** Physical Medicine & Rehabilitation, Univ Minnesota Hosps 1978; **Fellow:** Research, Univ Minnesota Hosps 1978; **Fac Appt:** Assoc Prof PMR, Univ Colorado

Physical Medicine & Rehabilitation

Southwest

Barber, Douglas B MD [PMR] - **Spec Exp:** Spinal Cord Injury; **Hospital:** VA Healthcare Syst N TX-Dallas; **Address:** Dept Rehab Medicine (7798), 7703 Floyd Curl Drive, San Antonio, TX 78229-3900; **Phone:** 210-567-5353; **Board Cert:** Physical Medicine & Rehabilitation 1992; Spinal Cord Injury Medicine 1999; **Med School:** Univ Tex, Houston 1987; **Resid:** Physical Medicine & Rehabilitation, Univ TX Hlth Scis Ctr 1991; **Fac Appt:** Assoc Prof PMR, Univ Tex, San Antonio

Currie, Donald M MD [PMR] - **Spec Exp:** Pediatric Rehabilitation; Neuro-Rehabilitation; **Hospital:** Christus Santa Rosa Children's Hosp, Univ Hlth Syst-San Antonio; **Address:** Univ Hosp, 4502 Medical Drive, MS 64-1, San Antonio, TX 78229; **Phone:** 210-358-0500; **Board Cert:** Physical Medicine & Rehabilitation 1978; **Med School:** Univ Tex SW, Dallas 1972; **Resid:** Physical Medicine & Rehabilitation, Baylor Univ Med Ctr 1975; Physical Medicine & Rehabilitation, Univ Washington Affil Hosp 1977; **Fac Appt:** Prof PMR, Univ Tex, San Antonio

Dumitru, Daniel MD/PhD [PMR] - **Spec Exp:** Electrodiagnosis; **Hospital:** Univ Hlth Syst-San Antonio; **Address:** Univ Tex Hlth Sci Ctr, Dept Rehab Med, 7703 Floyd Curl Drive, San Antonio, TX 78229-3900; **Phone:** 210-358-0770; **Board Cert:** Physical Medicine & Rehabilitation 1984; **Med School:** Univ Cincinnati 1980; **Resid:** Physical Medicine & Rehabilitation, VA Hosp 1983; **Fac Appt:** Prof PMR, Univ Tex, San Antonio

Francisco, Gerard E MD [PMR] - **Spec Exp:** Spasticity Management; Brain Injury Rehabilitation; Stroke Rehabilitation; **Hospital:** TIRR, Memorial Hermann SE Hosp; **Address:** The Inst of Rehab & Research, 1333 Moursund St, Houston, TX 77030-3405; **Phone:** 713-797-5246; **Board Cert:** Physical Medicine & Rehabilitation 2005; **Med School:** Philippines 1989; **Resid:** Physical Medicine & Rehabilitation, UMDNJ-Univ Hosp 1994; **Fellow:** Physical Medicine & Rehabilitation, Baylor Coll Med 1995; **Fac Appt:** Clin Prof PMR, Univ Tex, Houston

Harris, David K MD [PMR] - **Spec Exp:** Spinal Rehabilitation; Spinal Cord Injury; Pain-Back; Pain-Spine; **Hospital:** St David's Med Ctr, Seton Med Ctr; **Address:** Spine and Sports Solutions, 4613 Bee Caves Rd, Ste 105, Austin, TX 78746; **Phone:** 512-892-0490; **Board Cert:** Physical Medicine & Rehabilitation 2004; Spinal Cord Injury Medicine 1998; Pain Medicine 2004; **Med School:** Univ Tex SW, Dallas 1988; **Resid:** Physical Medicine & Rehabilitation, Univ Colorado Hlth Sci Ctr 1992

Ivanhoe, Cindy MD [PMR] - **Spec Exp:** Brain Injury Rehabilitation; Spasticity Management; Movement Disorders; **Hospital:** TIRR, Meml Med Ctr-Livingston; **Address:** 2211 Norfolk, Ste 220, Houston, TX 77048; **Phone:** 713-942-7300; **Board Cert:** Physical Medicine & Rehabilitation 2003; **Med School:** Mexico 1984; **Resid:** Physical Medicine & Rehabilitation, Univ Ill Coll Med 1992; **Fellow:** Brain Injury, Baylor Coll Med 1993; **Fac Appt:** Asst Prof PMR, Baylor Coll Med

Kevorkian, Charles G MD [PMR] - **Spec Exp:** Stroke Rehabilitation; Neuromuscular Disorders; Electrodiagnosis; **Hospital:** St Luke's Episcopal Hosp-Houston; **Address:** Dept Physical Med & Rehab, 6624 Fannin St, Ste 2330, Houston, TX 77030-2335; **Phone:** 713-798-4061; **Board Cert:** Physical Medicine & Rehabilitation 1980; **Med School:** Australia 1972; **Resid:** Physical Medicine & Rehabilitation, Prince Henry Hosp 1976; Physical Medicine & Rehabilitation, Mayo Clinic 1979; **Fac Appt:** Assoc Prof PMR, Baylor Coll Med

King, John C MD [PMR] - **Spec Exp:** Stroke Rehabilitation; Pain-Chronic; Spinal Cord Injury; Electrodiagnosis; **Hospital:** Univ Hlth Syst-San Antonio; **Address:** Dept Rehab Med, 7703 Floyd Curl Drive, MC 7798, San Antonio, TX 78229-3900; **Phone:** 210-567-5345; **Board Cert:** Physical Medicine & Rehabilitation 1987; Spinal Cord Injury Medicine 2000; Pain Medicine 2002; **Med School:** Oral Roberts Sch Med 1983; **Resid:** Physical Medicine & Rehabilitation, Baylor Coll Med 1986; **Fac Appt:** Prof PMR, Univ Tex, San Antonio

West Coast and Pacific

Carter, Gregory T MD [PMR] - **Spec Exp:** Neuromuscular Disorders; Muscular Dystrophy; Amyotrophic Lateral Sclerosis (ALS); Charcot Marie Tooth Disease; **Hospital:** Providence Centralia Hosp, Univ Wash Med Ctr; **Address:** 1800 Cooks Hill Rd, Ste E, Centralia, WA 98531; **Phone:** 360-330-8626; **Board Cert:** Physical Medicine & Rehabilitation 1991; Neuromuscular Medicine 2006; **Med School:** Loyola Univ-Stritch Sch Med 1986; **Resid:** Physical Medicine & Rehabilitation, UC Davis Med Ctr 1990; **Fellow:** Neuromuscular Medicine, UC Davis Med Ctr 1991; **Fac Appt:** Clin Prof PMR, Univ Wash

Herring, Stanley A MD [PMR] - **Spec Exp:** Sports Medicine; Pain-Back; Spinal Rehabilitation; **Hospital:** Harborview Med Ctr; **Address:** 325 9th Ave, Box 359721, Seattle, WA 98104; **Phone:** 206-744-0401; **Board Cert:** Physical Medicine & Rehabilitation 1983; **Med School:** Univ Tex SW, Dallas 1979; **Resid:** Physical Medicine & Rehabilitation, Univ Washington Med Ctr 1982; **Fac Appt:** Clin Prof PMR, Univ Wash

Jaffe, Kenneth M MD [PMR] - **Spec Exp:** Brain Injury Rehabilitation; Spinal Cord Injury; Limb Deficiency-Arthrogryposis; Trauma Rehabilitation; **Hospital:** Harborview Med Ctr, Chldns Hosp and Regl Med Ctr - Seattle; **Address:** 325 Ninth Ave NE, Box 359740, Harborview Med Ctr., Seattle, WA 98104; **Phone:** 206-774-4954; **Board Cert:** Pediatrics 1980; Physical Medicine & Rehabilitation 1982; **Med School:** Harvard Med Sch 1975; **Resid:** Pediatrics, Univ Wash-Chldns Hosp 1980; Physical Medicine & Rehabilitation, Univ Wash Affil Hosp 1982; **Fac Appt:** Prof PMR, Univ Wash

Kraft, George H MD [PMR] - **Spec Exp:** Multiple Sclerosis; Spinal Cord Injury; Electrodiagnosis; **Hospital:** Univ Wash Med Ctr, Harborview Med Ctr; **Address:** 1959 NE Pacific St, Box 356490, Seattle, WA 98195; **Phone:** 206-598-3344; **Board Cert:** Physical Medicine & Rehabilitation 1969; Spinal Cord Injury Medicine 1998; **Med School:** Ohio State Univ 1963; **Resid:** Physical Medicine & Rehabilitation, UCSF-Moffitt Hosp 1965; Physical Medicine & Rehabilitation, Ohio State Univ Med Ctr 1967; **Fac Appt:** Prof PMR, Univ Wash

Massagli, Teresa L MD [PMR] - **Spec Exp:** Spinal Cord Injury-Pediatric; Brain Injury Rehabilitation-Pediatric; **Hospital:** Chldns Hosp and Regl Med Ctr - Seattle; **Address:** Seattle Children's Hosp, 4800 Sand Point Way NE, PO Box 5371, MS W6847, Seattle, WA 98105-3916; **Phone:** 206-987-2180; **Board Cert:** Pediatrics 1987; Physical Medicine & Rehabilitation 1989; Spinal Cord Injury Medicine 1998; **Med School:** Yale Univ 1982; **Resid:** Pediatrics, Yale-New Haven Hosp 1985; **Fellow:** Physical Medicine & Rehabilitation, Univ Washington 1988; **Fac Appt:** Prof PMR, Univ Wash

Robinson, Lawrence R MD [PMR] - **Spec Exp:** Electrodiagnosis; Electromyography; Botox Therapy; **Hospital:** Harborview Med Ctr, Univ Wash Med Ctr; **Address:** Box 356380, University of Washington, Seattle, WA 98195; **Phone:** 206-744-2523; **Board Cert:** Physical Medicine & Rehabilitation 1987; **Med School:** Baylor Coll Med 1982; **Resid:** Physical Medicine & Rehabilitation, Northwestern Meml Hosp 1985; **Fac Appt:** Prof PMR, Univ Wash

Saal, Jeffrey A MD [PMR] - **Spec Exp:** Pain-Lower Back (IDET procedure); Spinal Rehabilitation; Sports Medicine; **Address:** 500 Arguello St, Ste 100, Redwood City, CA 94063; **Phone:** 650-851-4900; **Board Cert:** Internal Medicine 1978; Physical Medicine & Rehabilitation 1982; **Med School:** Tulane Univ 1975; **Resid:** Internal Medicine, VA Med Ctr 1978; Physical Medicine & Rehabilitation, Stanford Univ Affil Hosps 1981; **Fac Appt:** Assoc Clin Prof PMR, UC Irvine

Cleveland Clinic

Physical Medicine and Rehabilitation

A strong, comprehensive rehabilitation program can help patients regain lost skills, improve function, relearn tasks and maximize independence. Cleveland Clinic Department of Physical Medicine and Rehabilitation, part of the Neurological Institute, offers patients several competitive edges – high quality physical, occupational and speech therapy programs, innovative treatments and interdisciplinary teamwork. Cleveland Clinic rehabilitation professionals work with patients who have suffered a variety of injuries or who have neuromuscular diseases or other conditions that greatly influence quality of life.

Cleveland Clinic rehabilitation therapists are trained in Neuro-Developmental Treatment (NDT), an advanced therapeutic approach designed for people with neurological challenges, such as stroke. Cleveland Clinic has more NDT-trained therapists than any other center in the region.

Rehabilitation physicians are highly regarded and provide medical directorship service to more than 55 acute inpatient rehabilitation beds throughout Greater Cleveland. Consulting services are provided to inpatient, outpatient and sub-acute settings. If the need arises, patients have quick access to any number of Cleveland Clinic medical specialists, an important benefit to patients with multiple or complex medical problems.

For more information about the Cleveland Clinic Department of Physical Medicine and Rehabilitation, to schedule a second opinion or to learn about assistance for out-of-town patients, call 800.890.2467 or visit www.clevelandclinic.org/rehabtopdocs.

Physical Medicine and Rehabilitation
9500 Euclid Avenue / AC311 | Cleveland OH 44195

Primary Conditions We Treat:
- Brain injury, brain tumors, stroke, and aneurysms
- Spinal cord injury
- Cancer
- Parkinson's Disease
- Post-Heart Transplant
- MS and Transverse Myelitis

We also offer:
- Return-to-Work Services
- Drivers Evaluation & Rehabilitation
- Orthotic and Prosthetic Services
- Golf Performance Assessment
- Low Vision Assistance
- Hand and Upper Extremity Rehabilitation
- Chronic Pain Rehabilitation
- Aquatic Rehabilitation
- Vestibular Rehabilitation
- Custom Orthotic and Prosthetic Fabrication

MOUNT SINAI
SCHOOL OF
MEDICINE

THE MOUNT SINAI MEDICAL CENTER
REHABILITATION MEDICINE

One Gustave L. Levy Place
Fifth Avenue and 100th Street
New York, NY 10029-6574
Physician Referral: 1-800-MD-SINAI (637-4624)
www.mountsinai.org

THE DEPARTMENT OF REHABILITATION MEDICINE at Mount Sinai is a Center of Excellence in the delivery of complete care for people with disabilities. A wide range of comprehensive patient care services is available for individuals with spinal cord injuries, brain injuries, and a variety of neuromuscular, musculoskeletal, and chronic conditions. We are accredited by the Commission on Accreditation of Rehabilitation Facilities (CARF) for our inpatient spinal cord and brain injury programs—the only such accredited programs at non-VA hospitals in New York City—as well as for our comprehensive rehabilitation medicine program.

Pivotal to successful rehabilitation, the multidisciplinary team approach at Mount Sinai takes advantage all areas of expertise to provide the highest quality of coordinated care. Our experienced professionals evaluate each patient and meet regularly to develop and implement individualized treatment plans in partnership with patients and their families. Our goal is to make each individual with a disability maximally self-sufficient and mobile, and able to return to community life.

The Mount Sinai Rehabilitation Center team is led by Kristjan T. Ragnarsson, MD, whose leadership and innovative approach to patient care has had a major impact in the field of rehabilitation medicine. The Center includes physicians, primary rehabilitation nurses, nurse practitioners, and professional staff in physical therapy, occupational therapy, speech therapy, nutrition, social work, psychology, therapeutic recreation, and vocational counseling. Special rehabilitation medicine programs include the following:

• **The Spinal Cord Injury Rehabilitation Program** provides comprehensive care to individuals with spinal cord injuries. This includes a full range of innovative medical and rehabilitation services. For example, our "Do It" program is a unique outpatient program that facilitates community integration.

• **The Brain Injury Rehabilitation Program** provides comprehensive care to individuals with brain injuries. It is well recognized that the treatment of individuals with cognitive and behavioral challenges is critical to community integration. Our program contains specialists uniquely qualified to meet these challenges.

• **The Sports Therapy Center** is a comprehensive outpatient physical and occupational therapy facility offering individualized treatments for people with a variety of musculoskeletal conditions. It is conveniently located in midtown Manhattan.

MODEL SYSTEMS OF CARE

The Department of Rehabilitation Medicine provides comprehensive services that serve as national models of care.

• Consistently ranked among the top rehabilitation centers by *U.S. News & World Report*.

• One of 14 programs designated by the National Institute of Disability and Rehabilitation Research (NIDRR) as a Model System of Care for Spinal Cord Injury, the only such designated program in New York State.

• One of 16 programs designated by NIDRR as a Model System of Care for Traumatic Brain Injury, the only such designated program in New York State.

• The only NIDRR-designated Research and Training Center for Traumatic Brain Injury Intervention.

• The first CDC Injury Control Research Center focusing on traumatic brain injury research.

Rusk Institute of Rehabilitation Medicine

NYU LANGONE MEDICAL CENTER

400 East 34th Street
(between 1st Avenue and FDR Drive)
New York, NY 10016
At NYU Hospital for Joint Diseases
301 East 17th Street (at 2nd Avenue):
New York, NY 10003
(212) 598-6252: www.ruskinstitute.org

About the Institute:

The Rusk Institute of Rehabilitation Medicine at NYU Langone Medical Center is the world's first university-affiliated facility devoted entirely to rehabilitation medicine. The Institute is the largest center of its kind for the treatment of adults and children with disabilities. Founded in 1948 by Dr. Howard Rusk, it has been voted as the best rehabilitation hospital in New York and among the top ten in the country since 1989, when *U.S. News & World Report.*

We specialize in the following areas:

The Rusk Institute of Rehabilitation provides patients with access to a continuum rehabilitation care depending on their individual medical needs, including acute hospital-based inpatient programs, outpatient programs and specialty clinics.

INPATIENT FACILITIES:

The Brain Injury Program provides a structured therapeutic program tailored to meet the medical and rehabilitative needs of patients who have sustained a brain injury or neurological illness. Specialized limb deficiency programs are available to patients who have undergone amputations.

The Medically Complex Conditions Unit offers individualized treatment programs for patients with a variety of medically complex conditions such as spinal cord injuries, multiple sclerosis, Parkinson's disease, amputations and pain syndrome.

Specialized pediatric therapy programs are available to newborns, children and young adults, including communication programs, educational services, occupational therapy, physical therapy, psychology and speech-language pathology services.

The Joan and Joel Smilow Cardiac Rehabilitation & Prevention Center provides personalized cardiac rehabilitation.

The NYUHJD Orthopaedic Rehabilitation Unit provides rehabilitation of musculoskeletal disorders and injuries.

The William Randolph Hearst Foundation Stroke Rehabilitation Unit treats all aspects of stroke rehabilitation.

OUTPATIENT FACILITIES:

The Adult Physical Therapy Outpatient Unit offers evaluation and treatment for musculoskeletal and neurological disorders through individual and group programs.

The Chest Physical Therapy Program provides programs to individuals with lung congestion, secretion retention or areas of lung collapse.

Occupational therapists work with individuals to devise a comprehensive treatment program to help them regain their independence in daily tasks.

The Outpatient Rehabilitation Psychology Service is the largest of its kind on the East coast, providing care to patients with neurological and medical conditions on an outpatient basis.

The Physical Therapy Department provides an array of outpatient programs designed to address concerns associated with pregnancy, osteoporosis, pelvic floor dysfunction and some cancers.

The Speech-Language Pathology Department offers rehabilitation services to patients with communication disorders due to neurological problems.

The Swallowing Disorders Center is dedicated to the diagnosis and therapeutic management of swallowing and feeding disorders.

The Vestibular Rehabilitation Program is the first program of its kind in the tri-state area, providing diagnosis and treatment for patients suffering from dizziness and imbalance.

The Vocational Services Department provides individuals with disabilities with the competencies needed to return to school, work and to lead a productive lifestyle.

SPECIALTY CLINICS:

The Adult Spasticity Clinic provides examination and treatment to patients with spasticity, resulting from cerebral palsy, traumatic brain injury, spinal cord injury, multiple sclerosis and stroke.

Patients with **neuromuscular disease** receive physical and occupational therapies, vocational counseling, equipment and seating and mobility services.

Plastic Surgery

A plastic surgeon deals with the repair, reconstruction or replacement of physical defects of form or function involving the skin, musculoskeletal system, craniomaxillofacial structures, hand, extremities, breast and trunk and external genitalia. He/she uses aesthetic surgical principles not only to improve undesirable qualities of normal structures (commonly called "cosmetic surgery") but in all reconstructive procedures as well.

A plastic surgeon possesses special knowledge and skill in the design and surgery of grafts, flaps, free tissue transfer and replantation. Competence in the management of complex wounds, the use of implantable materials, and in tumor surgery is required.

Training Required: Five to seven years

Certification in one of the following subspecialties requires additional training and examination.

Plastic Surgery within the Head and Neck: A plastic surgeon with additional training in plastic and reconstructive procedures within the head, face, neck and associated structures, including cutaneous head and neck oncology and reconstruction, management of maxillofacial trauma, soft tissue repair and neural surgery.

The field is diverse and involves a wide age range of patients, from the newborn to the aged. While both cosmetic and reconstructive surgery are practiced, there are many additional procedures which interface with them.

Surgery of the Hand (see Hand Surgery)

PLASTIC SURGERY

New England

Collins, Dale MD [PlS] - **Spec Exp:** Breast Cancer; Breast Reconstruction; **Hospital:** Dartmouth - Hitchcock Med Ctr; **Address:** Div Plastic Surgery, 1 Medical Center Drive, Lebanon, NH 03756; **Phone:** 603-653-3500; **Board Cert:** Plastic Surgery 2007; **Med School:** Emory Univ 1989; **Resid:** Plastic Surgery, Washington Univ Med Ctr 1994; **Fellow:** Microsurgery, Washington Univ Med Ctr 1995; **Fac Appt:** Prof S, Dartmouth Med Sch

Constantian, Mark B MD [PlS] - **Spec Exp:** Rhinoplasty; Rhinoplasty Revision; Cosmetic Surgery-Face; Breast Surgery; **Hospital:** St Joseph Hosp, Southern NH Med Ctr; **Address:** 19 Tyler St, Ste 302, Nashua, NH 03060-2951; **Phone:** 603-880-7700; **Board Cert:** Plastic Surgery 1979; **Med School:** Univ VA Sch Med 1972; **Resid:** Surgery, Boston Univ Med Ctr 1976; **Fellow:** Plastic Reconstructive Surgery, Medical Coll VA 1978

Eriksson, Elof K MD [PlS] - **Spec Exp:** Abdominoplasty; Cosmetic Surgery-Breast; Facial Plastic & Reconstructive Surgery; **Hospital:** Brigham & Women's Hosp, Children's Hospital - Boston; **Address:** Brigham & Women's Hosp, Div Plas Surg, 75 Francis St, Boston, MA 02115; **Phone:** 617-732-5093; **Board Cert:** Plastic Surgery 1980; **Med School:** Sweden 1969; **Resid:** Surgery, Chicago Affil Hosps 1977; **Fellow:** Plastic Surgery, Med Coll Va 1979; **Fac Appt:** Prof PlS, Harvard Med Sch

Feldman, Joel MD [PlS] - **Spec Exp:** Cosmetic Surgery-Face; Burns-Reconstructive Plastic Surgery; **Hospital:** Mount Auburn Hosp, Mass Genl Hosp; **Address:** 300 Mt Auburn St, Ste 304, Cambridge, MA 02138; **Phone:** 617-661-5998; **Board Cert:** Surgery 1975; Plastic Surgery 1977; **Med School:** Harvard Med Sch 1969; **Resid:** Surgery, Mass Genl Hosp 1974; Plastic Surgery, Johns Hopkins Hosp 1976; **Fac Appt:** Assoc Clin Prof PlS, Harvard Med Sch

Gallico III, G Gregory MD [PlS] - **Spec Exp:** Liposuction & Body Contouring; Rhinoplasty; Abdominoplasty; Breast Surgery; **Hospital:** Mass Genl Hosp, Mass Eye & Ear Infirmary; **Address:** 170 Commonwealth Ave, Boston, MA 02116; **Phone:** 617-267-5553; **Board Cert:** Plastic Surgery 1982; **Med School:** Harvard Med Sch 1973; **Resid:** Surgery, Mass Genl Hosp 1980; Plastic Surgery, Mass Genl Hosp 1981; **Fellow:** Immunology, Oxford Univ Med Sch 1977; **Fac Appt:** Assoc Clin Prof S, Harvard Med Sch

May Jr, James W MD [PlS] - **Spec Exp:** Cosmetic Surgery; Breast Reconstruction; Hand Surgery; **Hospital:** Mass Genl Hosp; **Address:** Mass Genl Hosp, 15 Parkman St, WACC 435, Boston, MA 02114; **Phone:** 617-726-8220; **Board Cert:** Surgery 1975; Plastic Surgery 1977; **Med School:** Northwestern Univ 1969; **Resid:** Plastic Surgery, Mass Genl Hosp 1975; **Fellow:** Hand Surgery, Univ Louisville 1975; **Fac Appt:** Prof S, Harvard Med Sch

Meara, John MD/DMD [PlS] - **Spec Exp:** Cleft Palate/Lip; Craniofacial Surgery-Pediatric; **Hospital:** Children's Hospital - Boston; **Address:** Department of Plastic Surgery, 300 Longwood Ave, Hunnewell 158, Boston, MA 02115; **Phone:** 617-355-4401; **Board Cert:** Plastic Surgery 2001; Otolaryngology 1998; **Med School:** Univ Mich Med Sch 1990; **Resid:** Plastic Surgery, Brigham & Womens & The Chldns Hosps 1999; Otolaryngology, Mass Eye & Ear Infirmary 1997; **Fellow:** Craniofacial Surgery, Royal Chldns Hosp 2000; **Fac Appt:** Assoc Prof PlS, Harvard Med Sch

Mulliken, John B MD [PlS] - **Spec Exp:** Pediatric Plastic Surgery; Cleft Palate/Lip; Vascular Malformations; **Hospital:** Children's Hospital - Boston; **Address:** Chldns Hosp, Div Plas Surg, 300 Longwood Ave, Hunnewell-1, Boston, MA 02115-5724; **Phone:** 617-355-7686; **Board Cert:** Surgery 1972; Plastic Surgery 1975; **Med School:** Columbia P&S 1964; **Resid:** Surgery, Mass Genl Hosp 1970; Plastic Surgery, Johns Hopkins Hosp 1974; **Fac Appt:** Prof S, Harvard Med Sch

Orgill, Dennis MD [PlS] - **Spec Exp:** Wound Healing/Care; Burns-Reconstructive Plastic Surgery; **Hospital:** Brigham & Women's Hosp; **Address:** Brigham & Women's Hosp, Dept Plas Surg, 75 Francis St, Boston, MA 02115; **Phone:** 617-732-5456; **Board Cert:** Surgery 2000; Plastic Surgery 1994; **Med School:** Harvard Med Sch 1985; **Resid:** Surgery, Brigham & Women's Hosp 1990; **Fellow:** Plastic Surgery, Brigham & Women's Hosp 1992; **Fac Appt:** Prof S, Harvard Med Sch

Persing, John A MD [PlS] - **Spec Exp:** Craniofacial Surgery; Vascular Malformations; Cosmetic Surgery; Cosmetic Surgery; **Hospital:** Yale-New Haven Hosp; **Address:** Yale Plastic Surgery, 330 Cedar St Boardroom Bldg Fl 3, New Haven, CT 06519-3218; **Phone:** 203-785-2570; **Board Cert:** Plastic Surgery 1985; Neurological Surgery 1986; **Med School:** Univ VT Coll Med 1974; **Resid:** Surgery, Univ Arizona Med Ctr 1976; Neurological Surgery, Univ Virginia Med Ctr 1982; **Fellow:** Plastic Surgery, Univ Virginia Med Ctr 1984; **Fac Appt:** Prof PlS, Yale Univ

Slavin, Sumner MD [PlS] - **Spec Exp:** Breast Reconstruction; Cosmetic Surgery-Face; Liposuction & Body Contouring; **Hospital:** Beth Israel Deaconess Med Ctr - Boston; **Address:** 1101 Beacon St, Ste 7E, Brookline, MA 02446; **Phone:** 617-277-7010; **Board Cert:** Plastic Surgery 1983; **Med School:** Univ VT Coll Med 1973; **Resid:** Surgery, Beth Israel Hosp 1978; Plastic Surgery, NYU Med Ctr 1980; **Fellow:** Hand & Microvascular Surgery, Bellevue Hosp-NYU Med Ctr 1981; **Fac Appt:** Assoc Clin Prof S, Harvard Med Sch

Stadelmann, Wayne K MD [PlS] - **Spec Exp:** Melanoma-Head & Neck; Breast Reconstruction; Breast Augmentation; **Hospital:** Concord Hospital, Elliot Hosp; **Address:** 248 Pleasant St, Ste 201, Concord, NH 03301; **Phone:** 603-224-5200; **Board Cert:** Plastic Surgery 1999; **Med School:** Univ Chicago-Pritzker Sch Med 1990; **Resid:** Surgery, Univ Chicago Hosps 1994; Plastic Surgery, Univ S Florida/H Lee Moffit Cancer Ctr 1997

Stahl, Richard S MD [PlS] - **Spec Exp:** Breast Reconstruction; Chest Wall Reconstruction; Abdominal Wall Reconstruction; Cosmetic Surgery-Breast; **Hospital:** Yale-New Haven Hosp, Hosp of St Raphael; **Address:** 5 Durham Rd, Guilford, CT 06437; **Phone:** 203-458-4440; **Board Cert:** Surgery 2001; Plastic Surgery 1984; **Med School:** Vanderbilt Univ 1976; **Resid:** Surgery, Yale New Haven Hosp 1981; **Fellow:** Plastic Surgery, Emory Univ Med Ctr 1983; **Fac Appt:** Clin Prof S, Yale Univ

Stotland, Mitchell A MD [PlS] - **Spec Exp:** Cleft Palate/Lip; Craniofacial Surgery-Pediatric; Pediatric Plastic Surgery; **Hospital:** Dartmouth - Hitchcock Med Ctr; **Address:** DHMC, Dept Plastic Surgery, 1 Medical Center Drive, Lebanon, NH 03756-1000; **Phone:** 603-650-8068; **Board Cert:** Plastic Surgery 2000; **Med School:** McGill Univ 1989; **Resid:** Surgery, McGill Univ Med Ctr 1994; Plastic Surgery, UCLA Med Ctr 1997; **Fac Appt:** Assoc Prof S, Dartmouth Med Sch

Sullivan, Patrick K MD [PlS] - **Spec Exp:** Cosmetic Surgery-Face; Cosmetic Surgery-Breast; Rhinoplasty; **Hospital:** Rhode Island Hosp; **Address:** 235 Plain St, Ste 502, Providence, RI 02905; **Phone:** 401-831-8300; **Board Cert:** Otolaryngology 1985; Plastic Surgery 1989; **Med School:** Mayo Med Sch 1979; **Resid:** Otolaryngology, Univ Colo Hlth Scis Ctr 1984; Plastic Surgery, Rhode Island Hosp 1986; **Fellow:** Craniofacial Surgery, Dr Paul Tessier & Dr Hugo Obwegeser 1987; **Fac Appt:** Assoc Prof PlS, Brown Univ

Plastic Surgery

Mid Atlantic

Ascherman, Jeffrey MD [PlS] - **Spec Exp:** Cosmetic Surgery; Craniofacial Surgery; Breast Cosmetic & Reconstructive Surgery; **Hospital:** NY-Presby Hosp/Columbia (page 66), New York Eye & Ear Infirm (page 65); **Address:** 161 Ft Washington Ave, Ste 607, New York, NY 10032-3713; **Phone:** 212-305-9612; **Board Cert:** Plastic Surgery 2007; **Med School:** Columbia P&S 1988; **Resid:** Surgery, Columbia-Presby Med Ctr 1991; Plastic Surgery, Columbia-Presby Med Ctr 1994; **Fellow:** Craniofacial Surgery, Hosp Necke-Enfants Malades 1995; **Fac Appt:** Assoc Prof S, Columbia P&S

Aston, Sherrell MD [PlS] - **Spec Exp:** Cosmetic Surgery-Face; Rhinoplasty; Cosmetic Surgery-Breast; Liposuction & Body Contouring; **Hospital:** Lenox Hill Hosp (page 62), NYU Langone Med Ctr (page 67); **Address:** 728 Park Ave, New York, NY 10021; **Phone:** 212-249-6000; **Board Cert:** Surgery 1974; Plastic Surgery 1978; **Med School:** Univ VA Sch Med 1968; **Resid:** Surgery, UCLA Med Ctr 1973; Plastic Surgery, NY Univ 1975; **Fellow:** Surgery, Johns Hopkins Hosp 1970; **Fac Appt:** Prof PlS, NYU Sch Med

Attinger, Christopher E MD [PlS] - **Spec Exp:** Limb Surgery/Reconstruction; Diabetic Leg/Foot; Wound Healing/Care; Lower Limb Reconstruction; **Hospital:** Georgetown Univ Hosp; **Address:** Georgetown Univ Hosp-Wound Healing Ctr, 3800 Resorvoir Rd NW 1 Bles Bldg, Washington, DC 20007; **Phone:** 202-444-6161; **Board Cert:** Plastic Surgery 1992; **Med School:** Yale Univ 1981; **Resid:** Surgery, Brigham & Women's Hosp 1986; Plastic Surgery, NYU Med Ctr 1989; **Fellow:** Vascular Surgery, Brigham & Women's Hosp 1987; Hand Surgery, NYU Med Ctr 1990; **Fac Appt:** Prof PlS, Georgetown Univ

Baker, Daniel MD [PlS] - **Spec Exp:** Cosmetic Surgery-Face; Reconstructive Surgery-Face; Rhinoplasty; **Hospital:** Lenox Hill Hosp (Manh Eye, Ear & Throat Hosp) (page 62); **Address:** 65 E 66th St, New York, NY 10021; **Phone:** 212-734-9695; **Board Cert:** Plastic Surgery 1978; **Med School:** Columbia P&S 1968; **Resid:** Surgery, UCSF Med Ctr 1975; Plastic Surgery, NYU Med Ctr 1977; **Fellow:** Head and Neck Surgery, NYU Med Ctr/St Vincents Hosp 1978; **Fac Appt:** Assoc Prof PlS, NYU Sch Med

Baker, Stephen B MD/DDS [PlS] - **Spec Exp:** Craniofacial Surgery/Reconstruction; Facial Trauma/Fractures; Eyelid Surgery; Cleft Palate/Lip; **Hospital:** Virginia Hosp Ctr - Arlington, Inova Fairfax Hosp; **Address:** Georgetown Univ-Dept Plastic Surgery, 3800 Reservoir Rd NW, PHC-1, Washington, DC 20007; **Phone:** 202-444-9302; **Board Cert:** Plastic Surgery 2002; **Med School:** Univ Pennsylvania 1993; **Resid:** Oral & Maxillofacial Surgery, Hosp U Penn 1996; Plastic Surgery, Hosp U Penn 2000; **Fellow:** Craniofacial Surgery, Children's Hosp 2001; **Fac Appt:** Assoc Prof PlS, Georgetown Univ

Bartlett, Scott P MD [PlS] - **Spec Exp:** Craniofacial Surgery/Reconstruction; Pediatric Plastic Surgery; Facial Plastic & Reconstructive Surgery; **Hospital:** Hosp Univ Penn - UPHS (page 60), Chldns Hosp of Philadelphia, The; **Address:** 10 Penn Tower, 3400 Spruce St, Philadelphia, PA 19104-4227; **Phone:** 215-662-2096; **Board Cert:** Plastic Surgery 1987; **Med School:** Washington Univ, St Louis 1975; **Resid:** Surgery, Mass Genl Hosp 1983; Plastic Surgery, Mass Genl Hosp 1985; **Fellow:** Craniofacial Surgery, Hosp Univ Penn 1986; **Fac Appt:** Prof PlS, Univ Pennsylvania

Boyajian, Michael J MD [PlS] - **Spec Exp:** Pediatric Plastic Surgery; **Hospital:** Chldns Natl Med Ctr; **Address:** 111 Michigan Ave NW, Ste 4W-100, Washington, DC 20010-2978; **Phone:** 202-476-2150; **Board Cert:** Plastic Surgery 1984; **Med School:** NYU Sch Med 1976; **Resid:** Surgery, Univ Colo Med Ctr 1979; Surgery, Univ Cincinnati Hosp 1981; **Fellow:** Plastic Surgery, Brigham & Women's Hosp 1983; Craniofacial Surgery, Chldns Hosp 1983; **Fac Appt:** Asst Prof PlS, Geo Wash Univ

Bucky, Louis P MD [PlS] - **Spec Exp:** Cosmetic Surgery-Face; Cosmetic Surgery-Breast; Liposuction & Body Contouring; Breast Reconstruction; **Hospital:** Pennsylvania Hosp (page 60), Hosp Univ Penn - UPHS (page 60); **Address:** 230 W Washington Square, Ste 101, Philadelphia, PA 19106; **Phone:** 215-829-6320; **Board Cert:** Plastic Surgery 1997; **Med School:** Harvard Med Sch 1986; **Resid:** Surgery, Mass Genl Hosp 1992; Plastic Surgery, Mass Genl Hosp 1994; **Fellow:** Microsurgery, Meml Sloan Kettering Cancer Ctr 1995; Craniofacial Surgery, Miami Chldns Hosp 1996; **Fac Appt:** Assoc Prof S, Univ Pennsylvania

Chiu, David T W MD [PlS] - **Spec Exp:** Hand & Microvascular Surgery; Cosmetic Surgery-Face; Peripheral Nerve Surgery; **Hospital:** NYU Langone Med Ctr (page 67), Lenox Hill Hosp (page 62); **Address:** 900 Park Ave, New York, NY 10021-0231; **Phone:** 212-879-8880; **Board Cert:** Plastic Surgery 1982; Hand Surgery 2000; **Med School:** Columbia P&S 1973; **Resid:** Surgery, Barnes Jewish Hosp 1977; Plastic Surgery, Columbia-Presby Med Ctr 1979; **Fellow:** Hand Surgery, NYU Med Ctr 1980; **Fac Appt:** Prof S, NYU Sch Med

Cordeiro, Peter G MD [PlS] - **Spec Exp:** Reconstructive Surgery; Breast Reconstruction; Facial Plastic & Reconstructive Surgery; **Hospital:** Meml Sloan-Kettering Cancer Ctr, Lenox Hill Hosp (Manh Eye, Ear & Throat Hosp) (page 62); **Address:** 1275 York Avenue, New York, NY 10065; **Phone:** 800-525-2225; **Board Cert:** Surgery 1998; Plastic Surgery 1994; **Med School:** Harvard Med Sch 1983; **Resid:** Surgery, New Eng Deaconess Hosp-Harvard 1989; Plastic Surgery, NYU Med Ctr 1991; **Fellow:** Microsurgery, Meml Sloan-Kettering Cancer Ctr. 1992; Craniofacial Surgery, Univ Miami 1992; **Fac Appt:** Prof S, Cornell Univ-Weill Med Coll

Cutting, Court MD [PlS] - **Spec Exp:** Cleft Palate/Lip; Reconstructive Plastic Surgery; Rhinoplasty; Craniofacial Surgery/Reconstruction; **Hospital:** NYU Langone Med Ctr (page 67); **Address:** 333 E 34th St, Ste 1K, New York, NY 10016-6481; **Phone:** 212-447-6229; **Board Cert:** Otolaryngology 1980; Plastic Surgery 1986; **Med School:** Univ Chicago-Pritzker Sch Med 1975; **Resid:** Otolaryngology, Univ Iowa Hosps 1980; Plastic Surgery, NYU Med Ctr 1983; **Fellow:** Craniofacial Surgery, NYU Med Ctr 1984; **Fac Appt:** Prof PlS, NYU Sch Med

Dagum, Alexander B MD [PlS] - **Spec Exp:** Reconstructive Plastic Surgery; Cleft Palate/Lip; Hand Surgery; Microsurgery; **Hospital:** Stony Brook Univ Med Ctr; **Address:** SUNY Health Science Ctr, T19-060, Box 8191, Stony Brook, NY 11794-8191; **Phone:** 631-444-8210; **Board Cert:** Plastic Surgery 2003; Hand Surgery 2004; **Med School:** Canada 1987; **Resid:** Surgery, Univ Ottawa Civic Hosp 1988; Plastic Surgery, Univ Toronto Med Ctr 1993; **Fellow:** Microsurgery, Univ Toronto Med Ctr 1984; Hand Surgery, Stony Brook Univ Hosp 1995; **Fac Appt:** Prof S, SUNY Stony Brook

Deleyiannis, Frederic W B MD [PlS] - **Spec Exp:** Head & Neck Reconstruction; Maxillofacial Surgery; Craniofacial Surgery; Pediatric Plastic Surgery; **Hospital:** UPMC Presby, Pittsburgh, Chldns Hosp of Pittsburgh - UPMC; **Address:** Falk Medical Bldg, 3601 Fifth Ave, Ste 6B, Pittsburgh, PA 15213; **Phone:** 412-648-9670; **Board Cert:** Otolaryngology 2000; Plastic Surgery 2003; **Med School:** Yale Univ 1992; **Resid:** Otolaryngology, Univ Washington Med Ctr 1999; Plastic Surgery, Univ Pittsburgh Med Ctr 2002; **Fellow:** Head and Neck Surgery, Univ Oviedo Med Ctr 2000; **Fac Appt:** Assoc Prof PlS, Univ Pittsburgh

Dufresne, Craig R MD [PlS] - **Spec Exp:** Craniofacial Surgery; Cosmetic Surgery; **Hospital:** Inova Fairfax Hosp, Sibley Mem Hosp; **Address:** 5530 Wisconsin Ave, Ste 1235, Chevy Chase, MD 20815; **Phone:** 301-654-9151; **Board Cert:** Plastic Surgery 1986; **Med School:** Columbia P&S 1977; **Resid:** Surgery, Johns Hopkins Hosp 1982; Plastic Surgery, NYU Med Ctr 1984; **Fellow:** Craniofacial Surgery, NYU Med Ctr 1985; **Fac Appt:** Clin Prof PlS, Georgetown Univ

Fox, James W MD [PlS] - **Spec Exp:** Breast Cancer & Surgery; Breast Reconstruction; **Hospital:** Thomas Jefferson Univ Hosp; **Address:** 840 Walnut St Fl 15, Philadelphia, PA 19107; **Phone:** 215-625-6630; **Board Cert:** Plastic Surgery 1978; **Med School:** Jefferson Med Coll 1970; **Resid:** Surgery, Jefferson Hosp 1974; **Fellow:** Plastic Surgery, Univ Virginia Med Ctr 1976; **Fac Appt:** Prof S, Jefferson Med Coll

Glat, Paul M MD [PlS] - **Spec Exp:** Pediatric & Adult Plastic Surgery; Burns-Reconstructive Plastic Surgery; Craniofacial Surgery; Cleft Palate/Lip; **Hospital:** St Christopher's Hosp for Chldn, Bryn Mawr Hosp; **Address:** St Christopher's Hosp for Children, Eire Ave at Font St, Ste 2204, Philadelphia, PA 19134; **Phone:** 866-472-6009; **Board Cert:** Plastic Surgery 1999; **Med School:** NYU Sch Med 1988; **Resid:** Surgery, NYU Med Ctr 1994; Plastic Surgery, NYU Med Ctr 1996; **Fellow:** Craniofacial Surgery, Univ Penn 1997; **Fac Appt:** Assoc Prof PlS, Drexel Univ Coll Med

Hidalgo, David MD [PlS] - **Spec Exp:** Cosmetic Surgery-Face; Cosmetic Surgery-Breast; Rhinoplasty; Reconstructive Surgery; **Hospital:** NY-Presby Hosp/Weill Cornell (page 66), Lenox Hill Hosp (page 62); **Address:** 655 Park Ave Fl 1, New York, NY 10021-5937; **Phone:** 212-517-9777; **Board Cert:** Plastic Surgery 1987; **Med School:** Georgetown Univ 1978; **Resid:** Surgery, NYU Med Ctr 1983; Plastic Surgery, NYU Med Ctr 1985; **Fellow:** Microsurgery, NYU Med Ctr 1986; **Fac Appt:** Clin Prof S, Cornell Univ-Weill Med Coll

Hoffman, Lloyd A MD [PlS] - **Spec Exp:** Cosmetic Surgery-Face; Liposuction; Breast Reconstruction; **Hospital:** NY-Presby Hosp/Columbia (page 66), Lenox Hill Hosp (page 62); **Address:** 12A E 68th St, New York, NY 10021; **Phone:** 212-861-1640; **Board Cert:** Plastic Surgery 1989; **Med School:** Northwestern Univ 1978; **Resid:** Surgery, New York Hosp 1983; Plastic Surgery, NYU Med Ctr 1986; **Fellow:** Hand Surgery, NYU Med Ctr 1987; **Fac Appt:** Assoc Prof PlS, Cornell Univ-Weill Med Coll

Hurwitz, Dennis J MD [PlS] - **Spec Exp:** Body Contouring; Cosmetic Surgery-Face; Rhinoplasty; Breast Reconstruction; **Hospital:** Magee-Womens Hosp - UPMC, Chldns Hosp of Pittsburgh - UPMC; **Address:** 3109 Forbes Ave, Ste 500, Pittsburgh, PA 15213; **Phone:** 412-802-6100; **Board Cert:** Plastic Surgery 2005; **Med School:** Univ MD Sch Med 1970; **Resid:** Surgery, Dartmouth Med Ctr 1975; Plastic Surgery, Univ Pittsburgh Med Ctr 1977; **Fac Appt:** Prof S, Univ Pittsburgh

Imber, Gerald MD [PlS] - **Spec Exp:** Cosmetic Surgery-Face; Eyelid Surgery; **Hospital:** NY-Presby Hosp/Weill Cornell (page 66); **Address:** 1009 5th Ave, New York, NY 10028; **Phone:** 212-472-1800; **Board Cert:** Plastic Surgery 1976; **Med School:** SUNY Downstate 1966; **Resid:** Surgery, LI Jewish Med Ctr 1972; Plastic Surgery, NY Hosp 1974; **Fac Appt:** Asst Clin Prof S, Cornell Univ-Weill Med Coll

Leipziger, Lyle S MD [PlS] - **Spec Exp:** Cosmetic Surgery-Face & Eyes; Cosmetic Surgery-Breast; Breast Reconstruction; Liposuction & Body Contouring; **Hospital:** N Shore Univ Hosp, Long Island Jewish Med Ctr; **Address:** 825 Northern Blvd Fl 3, Great Neck, NY 11021; **Phone:** 516-465-8787; **Board Cert:** Plastic Surgery 1994; **Med School:** Cornell Univ-Weill Med Coll 1985; **Resid:** Plastic Surgery, New York Hosp 1990; **Fellow:** Craniofacial Surgery, Johns Hopkins Hosp 1991; **Fac Appt:** Asst Prof S, Albert Einstein Coll Med

Levin, L Scott MD [PlS] - **Spec Exp:** Toe-to-Hand Transfer; Reconstructive Microvascular Surgery; Microsurgery; **Hospital:** Penn Presby Med Ctr - UPHS (page 60); **Address:** Univ Penn Hlth System-Orth Surgery Dept, 2 Silverstein, 3400 Spruce St, Philadelphia, PA 19104; **Phone:** 215-349-5803; **Board Cert:** Plastic Surgery 1993; Hand Surgery 2004; Orthopaedic Surgery 2004; **Med School:** Temple Univ 1982; **Resid:** Orthopaedic Surgery, Duke Univ Med Ctr 1988; Plastic Surgery, Duke Univ Med Ctr 1989; **Fac Appt:** Prof S, Duke Univ

Little, John W MD [PlS] - **Spec Exp:** Cosmetic Surgery-Face; **Hospital:** Georgetown Univ Hosp, G Washington Univ Hosp; **Address:** 1145 19th St NW, Ste 802, Washington, DC 20036; **Phone:** 202-467-6700; **Board Cert:** Surgery 1975; Plastic Surgery 1977; **Med School:** Harvard Med Sch 1969; **Resid:** Surgery, Case Western Reserve Affil Hosps 1974; Plastic Surgery, Case Western Reserve Affil Hosps 1975; **Fellow:** Plastic Surgery, Jackson Meml Hosp 1977; **Fac Appt:** Clin Prof PlS, Georgetown Univ

Loree, Thom R MD [PlS] - **Spec Exp:** Head & Neck Cancer; Thyroid Cancer; Reconstructive Surgery; **Hospital:** Roswell Park Cancer Inst, Millard Fillmore Gates Cir Hosp; **Address:** Roswell Park Cancer Inst, Dept Head & Neck Surgery, Elm & Carlton Sts, Buffalo, NY 14263; **Phone:** 716-845-3158; **Board Cert:** Surgery 1997; Plastic Surgery 2004; **Med School:** Geo Wash Univ 1982; **Resid:** Surgery, St Lukes-Roosevelt Hosp 1987; Plastic Surgery, St Lukes-Roosevelt Hosp 1989; **Fellow:** Head & Neck Surgical Oncology, Meml Sloan-Kettering Cancer Ctr 1990; **Fac Appt:** Assoc Prof S, SUNY Buffalo

Losee, Joseph E MD [PlS] - **Spec Exp:** Pediatric Plastic Surgery; Cleft Lip/Palate; Craniofacial Surgery/Reconstruction; **Hospital:** Chldns Hosp of Pittsburgh - UPMC; **Address:** Childrens Hosp Pittsburgh, Div Pediatric Plastic Surgery, 4401 Penn Ave Fl 3, Pittsburgh, PA 15224; **Phone:** 412-692-8650; **Board Cert:** Plastic Surgery 2001; **Med School:** Univ Rochester 1994; **Resid:** Plastic Surgery, Strong Meml Hosp 1999; **Fellow:** Pediatric Plastic Surgery, Childrens Hosp 2000; Craniofacial Surgery, Univ Pennsylvania 2000; **Fac Appt:** Assoc Prof S, Univ Pittsburgh

Low, David W MD [PlS] - **Spec Exp:** Microsurgery; Cosmetic & Reconstructive Surgery; Vascular Malformations; Cleft Palate/Lip; **Hospital:** Hosp Univ Penn - UPHS (page 60), Chldns Hosp of Philadelphia, The; **Address:** Hosp Univ Penn - Div Plastic Surg, 3400 Spruce St, 10 Penn Tower, Philadelphia, PA 19104; **Phone:** 215-662-2040; **Board Cert:** Plastic Surgery 1991; **Med School:** Harvard Med Sch 1980; **Resid:** Surgery, Hosp U Penn 1986; **Fellow:** Plastic Reconstructive Surgery, Hosp U Penn 1989; **Fac Appt:** Assoc Prof S, Univ Pennsylvania

Mackay, Donald R MD/DDS [PlS] - **Spec Exp:** Craniofacial Surgery; Cleft Palate/Lip; Cosmetic Surgery-Face; Reconstructive Surgery; **Hospital:** Penn State Milton S Hershey Med Ctr; **Address:** MS Hershey Med Ctr Plastic Surgery, 500 University Drive, MC H071, PO Box 850, Hershey, PA 17033; **Phone:** 717-531-8952; **Board Cert:** Plastic Surgery 2006; **Med School:** South Africa 1980; **Resid:** Plastic Surgery, Univ Teaching Hosps 1984; Plastic Surgery, MS Hershey Med Ctr 1995; **Fac Appt:** Prof PlS, Penn State Univ-Hershey Med Ctr

Manders, Ernest K MD [PlS] - **Spec Exp:** Facial Nerve Disorders; **Hospital:** UPMC Presby, Pittsburgh, Magee-Womens Hosp - UPMC; **Address:** 3550 Terrace St, Ste 668, Scaife Hall, Div Plastic Surgery, Pittsburgh, PA 15261; **Phone:** 412-648-9670; **Board Cert:** Surgery 1998; Plastic Surgery 1982; **Med School:** Harvard Med Sch 1972; **Resid:** Surgery, Univ Michigan Med Ctr 1979; Plastic Surgery, Univ Michigan Med Ctr 1981; **Fellow:** Viral Oncology, Natl Insts of Allergy-Infectious Disease 1975; **Fac Appt:** Prof S, Univ Pittsburgh

Manson, Paul MD [PlS] - **Spec Exp:** Cosmetic Surgery; Facial Trauma/Fractures; Skin Cancer; **Hospital:** Johns Hopkins Hosp (page 61), Univ of MD Med Ctr; **Address:** 601 N Caroline St, McElderry-8152F, Baltimore, MD 21287; **Phone:** 410-955-9470; **Board Cert:** Plastic Surgery 1979; **Med School:** Northwestern Univ 1968; **Resid:** Surgery, New Eng Deaconess Hosp 1971; Plastic Surgery, Johns Hopkins Hosp 1978; **Fellow:** Surgery, Lahey Clinic 1974; **Fac Appt:** Prof PlS, Johns Hopkins Univ

Plastic Surgery

Matarasso, Alan MD [PlS] - **Spec Exp:** Cosmetic Surgery-Face & Eyes; Rhinoplasty; Liposuction; Abdominoplasty; **Hospital:** Lenox Hill Hosp (Manh Eye, Ear & Throat Hosp) (page 62), New York Eye & Ear Infirm (page 65); **Address:** 1009 Park Ave, New York, NY 10028-0936; **Phone:** 212-249-7500; **Board Cert:** Plastic Surgery 1986; **Med School:** Univ Miami Sch Med 1979; **Resid:** Surgery, Montefiore Med Ctr 1983; Plastic Surgery, Montefiore Med Ctr 1985; **Fellow:** Plastic Surgery, Manhattan EET Hosp/NYU 1985; **Fac Appt:** Clin Prof PlS, Albert Einstein Coll Med

McCarthy, Joseph G MD [PlS] - **Spec Exp:** Craniofacial Surgery-Pediatric; Reconstructive Surgery-Face; Cosmetic Surgery-Face; **Hospital:** NYU Langone Med Ctr (page 67), Lenox Hill Hosp (Manh Eye, Ear & Throat Hosp) (page 62); **Address:** 722 Park Ave, New York, NY 10021-4954; **Phone:** 212-628-4420; **Board Cert:** Surgery 1972; Plastic Surgery 1974; **Med School:** Columbia P&S 1964; **Resid:** Surgery, Columbia-Presby Med Ctr 1971; Plastic Surgery, NYU Med Ctr 1973; **Fac Appt:** Prof S, NYU Sch Med

Mehrara, Babak J MD [PlS] - **Spec Exp:** Breast Reconstruction; Cancer Reconstruction; Microsurgery; Reconstructive Surgery-Face; **Hospital:** Meml Sloan-Kettering Cancer Ctr; **Address:** 1275 York Ave, New York, NY 10021; **Phone:** 212-639-8639; **Board Cert:** Plastic Surgery 2003; **Med School:** Columbia P&S 1993; **Resid:** Surgery, NYU Med Ctr 1996; Plastic Surgery, NYU Med Ctr 2001; **Fellow:** Microsurgery, UCLA Med Ctr 2002; **Fac Appt:** Assoc Prof S, Cornell Univ-Weill Med Coll

Napoli, Joseph A MD/DDS [PlS] - **Spec Exp:** Cleft Palate/Lip; Maxillofacial Surgery; Craniofacial Surgery-Pediatric; Facial Tumors; **Hospital:** Alfred I duPont Hosp for Children; **Address:** Al duPont Hosp for Children, Div Plastic Surgery, 1600 Rockland Rd, Wilmington, DE 19803; **Phone:** 302-651-6301; **Board Cert:** Plastic Surgery 2004; **Med School:** Columbia P&S 1987; **Resid:** Oral & Maxillofacial Surgery, Columbia-Presby Med Ctr 1985; Plastic Reconstructive Surgery, Dartmouth-Hitchcock Med Ctr 2001; **Fellow:** Craniofacial Surgery, Royal Chldns Hosp 2002; Pediatric Plastic Surgery, Royal Chldns Hosp 2002; **Fac Appt:** Asst Prof S, Jefferson Med Coll

Noone, R Barrett MD [PlS] - **Spec Exp:** Breast Reconstruction; Cosmetic Surgery; **Hospital:** Bryn Mawr Hosp, Lankenau Hosp; **Address:** 888 Glenbrook Ave, Bryn Mawr, PA 19010-2506; **Phone:** 610-527-4833; **Board Cert:** Surgery 1972; Plastic Surgery 1974; **Med School:** Univ Pennsylvania 1965; **Resid:** Surgery, Hosp Univ Penn 1971; Plastic Surgery, Hosp Univ Penn 1973; **Fac Appt:** Clin Prof S, Univ Pennsylvania

Pitman, Gerald H MD [PlS] - **Spec Exp:** Cosmetic Surgery-Face; Liposuction; Abdominoplasty; **Hospital:** Lenox Hill Hosp (Manh Eye, Ear & Throat Hosp) (page 62), NYU Langone Med Ctr (page 67); **Address:** 170 E 73rd St, New York, NY 10021-4352; **Phone:** 212-517-2600; **Board Cert:** Plastic Surgery 1978; **Med School:** Univ Pennsylvania 1968; **Resid:** Surgery, Columbia-Presby Hosp 1975; Plastic Surgery, NYU Med Ctr 1977; **Fellow:** Microsurgery, NYU Med Ctr 1981; **Fac Appt:** Clin Prof PlS, NYU Sch Med

Posnick, Jeffrey C MD/DMD [PlS] - **Spec Exp:** Cosmetic Surgery-Face; Craniofacial Surgery/Reconstruction; Maxillofacial Surgery; **Hospital:** Georgetown Univ Hosp; **Address:** 5530 Wisconsin Ave, Ste 1250, Chevy Chase, MD 20815; **Phone:** 301-986-9475; **Board Cert:** Plastic Surgery 1988; **Med School:** Vanderbilt Univ 1979; **Resid:** Surgery, Mass Genl Hosp 1983; Plastic Surgery, Eastern Virginia Med Sch 1986; **Fellow:** Craniofacial Surgery, Hosp Univ Penn/Chldns Hosp 1983; **Fac Appt:** Clin Prof PlS, Georgetown Univ

Serletti, Joseph M MD [PlS] - **Spec Exp:** Breast Reconstruction; Reconstructive Surgery; Cosmetic Surgery; **Hospital:** Hosp Univ Penn - UPHS (page 60); **Address:** Hosp Univ Penn, 3400 Spruce St, 10 Penn Tower, Philadelphia, PA 19104; **Phone:** 215-662-3743; **Board Cert:** Plastic Surgery 2003; **Med School:** Univ Rochester 1982; **Resid:** Surgery, U Rochester Med Ctr 1986; Plastic Surgery, U Rochester Med Ctr 1988; **Fellow:** Reconstructive Surgery, Johns Hopkins Hosp 1990; **Fac Appt:** Prof PlS, Univ Pennsylvania

Seyfer, Alan MD [PlS] - **Spec Exp:** Chest Wall Reconstruction; Cleft Palate/Lip; Hand Surgery; **Hospital:** W Reed Army Med Ctr; **Address:** USUHS-School of Medicine, 4301 Jones Bridge Rd, Bethesda, MD 20814; **Phone:** 301-295-0441; **Board Cert:** Hand Surgery 1999; Plastic Surgery 1982; **Med School:** Louisiana State U, New Orleans 1973; **Resid:** Surgery, Fitzsimons AMC 1978; Plastic Surgery, Walter Reed AMC 1981; **Fellow:** Hand Surgery, Duke Univ Med Ctr 1980; **Fac Appt:** Prof S, Uniformed Srvs Univ, Bethesda

Siebert, John W MD [PlS] - **Spec Exp:** Facial Plastic & Reconstructive Surgery; Microsurgery; Cosmetic Surgery-Face; **Hospital:** NYU Langone Med Ctr (page 67), Lenox Hill Hosp (Manh Eye, Ear & Throat Hosp) (page 62); **Address:** 630 Park Ave, New York, NY 10065; **Phone:** 212-737-8300; **Board Cert:** Plastic Surgery 1991; **Med School:** Univ Wisc 1981; **Resid:** Surgery, Mass Genl Hosp 1986; Plastic Surgery, NYU Med Ctr 1988; **Fellow:** Microsurgery, NYU Med Ctr 1989; **Fac Appt:** Assoc Prof S, NYU Sch Med

Silver, Lester MD [PlS] - **Spec Exp:** Cleft Palate/Lip; Pediatric Plastic Surgery; **Hospital:** Mount Sinai Med Ctr (page 64); **Address:** 5 E 98th St, Box 1259, New York, NY 10029-6574; **Phone:** 212-241-1968; **Board Cert:** Plastic Surgery 1978; **Med School:** Ros Franklin Univ/Chicago Med Sch 1960; **Resid:** Surgery, Montefiore Med Ctr 1966; Plastic Surgery, Mt Sinai Med Ctr 1969; **Fac Appt:** Prof PlS, Mount Sinai Sch Med

Slezak, Sheri MD [PlS] - **Spec Exp:** Breast Reconstruction; **Hospital:** Univ of MD Med Ctr; **Address:** Univ Maryland, Dept Plastic Surgery, 22 S Greene St, rm S8D12, Baltimore, MD 21201; **Phone:** 410-328-2360; **Board Cert:** Plastic Surgery 1991; **Med School:** Harvard Med Sch 1980; **Resid:** Surgery, Columbia-Presby Med Ctr 1985; Plastic Surgery, Johns Hopkins Hosp 1989; **Fac Appt:** Assoc Prof PlS, Univ MD Sch Med

Spence, Robert J MD [PlS] - **Spec Exp:** Burns-Reconstructive Plastic Surgery; Burn Care; Tissue Banking; Scleroderma; **Hospital:** Good Samaritan Hosp; **Address:** 5601 Loch Raven Blvd, Baltimore, MD 21239; **Phone:** 443-444-2876; **Board Cert:** Plastic Surgery 1981; **Med School:** Johns Hopkins Univ 1972; **Resid:** Surgery, Johns Hopkins Hops 1974; Surgery, Hershey Med Ctr 1978; **Fellow:** Plastic Surgery, Johns Hopkins Hosp 1980; **Fac Appt:** Assoc Prof S, Johns Hopkins Univ

Spinelli, Henry M MD [PlS] - **Spec Exp:** Cosmetic Surgery-Face; Craniofacial Surgery/Reconstruction; Oculoplastic & Orbital Surgery; **Hospital:** NY-Presby Hosp/Weill Cornell (page 66), Lenox Hill Hosp (Manh Eye, Ear & Throat Hosp) (page 62); **Address:** 875 Fifth Ave, New York, NY 10021-4952; **Phone:** 212-570-6235; **Board Cert:** Ophthalmology 1987; Plastic Surgery 1993; **Med School:** NYU Sch Med 1981; **Resid:** Ophthalmology, Manhattan EET Hosp 1985; Plastic Reconstructive Surgery, NYU-Bellevue Hosp 1990; **Fellow:** Craniofacial Surgery, NYU Med Ctr 1991; **Fac Appt:** Clin Prof S, Cornell Univ-Weill Med Coll

Staffenberg, David A MD [PlS] - **Spec Exp:** Craniofacial Surgery/Reconstruction; Pediatric Plastic Surgery; Ear Reconstruction/Microtia; Cosmetic Surgery-Face; **Hospital:** Montefiore Med Ctr - Div. Moses; **Address:** 1625 Poplar St, Bronx, NY 10467; **Phone:** 718-405-8337; **Board Cert:** Plastic Surgery 1999; **Med School:** NY Med Coll 1989; **Resid:** Surgery, Maimonides Med Ctr 1995; Plastic Surgery, Emory Univ Med Ctr 1997; **Fellow:** Craniofacial Surgery, UCLA Med Ctr 1998; **Fac Appt:** Assoc Prof PlS, Albert Einstein Coll Med

Sultan, Mark MD [PlS] - **Spec Exp:** Breast Reconstruction; Cosmetic Surgery-Breast; Cosmetic Surgery-Face; **Hospital:** St Luke's - Roosevelt Hosp Ctr - Roosevelt Div (page 57); **Address:** 1100 Park Ave, New York, NY 10128; **Phone:** 212-360-0700; **Board Cert:** Plastic Surgery 1992; **Med School:** Columbia P&S 1982; **Resid:** Surgery, Columbia-Presby Hosp 1987; Plastic Surgery, Columbia-Presby Hosp 1990; **Fellow:** Head and Neck Surgery, Emory Univ Hosp 1989; **Fac Appt:** Assoc Prof S, Columbia P&S

Plastic Surgery

Tabbal, Nicolas MD [PlS] - **Spec Exp:** Rhinoplasty; Cosmetic Surgery-Face; Eyelid Surgery; **Hospital:** Lenox Hill Hosp (Manh Eye, Ear & Throat Hosp) (page 62), NYU Langone Med Ctr (page 67); **Address:** 521 Park Ave, New York, NY 10021-8140; **Phone:** 212-644-5800; **Board Cert:** Plastic Surgery 1980; **Med School:** Lebanon 1972; **Resid:** Surgery, Am Univ Med Ctr 1976; Plastic Surgery, Akron City Hosp 1979; **Fellow:** Surgery, Upstate Med Ctr 1977; Reconstructive Micro-surgery, NYU Med Ctr 1980

Taub, Peter J MD [PlS] - **Spec Exp:** Pediatric Plastic Surgery; Craniofacial Surgery; Cosmetic Surgery; Maxillofacial Surgery; **Hospital:** Mount Sinai Med Ctr (page 64), Westchester Med Ctr; **Address:** Mount Sinai Medical Ctr, 5 E 98th St Fl 15, Box 1259, New York, NY 10029-6574; **Phone:** 212-241-4410; **Board Cert:** Surgery 2000; Plastic Surgery 2003; **Med School:** Albert Einstein Coll Med 1993; **Resid:** Surgery, Mt Sinai Med Ctr 1999; Plastic Surgery, UCLA Med Ctr 2001; **Fellow:** Craniofacial Surgery, UCLA Med Ctr 2002; **Fac Appt:** Assoc Prof PlS, Mount Sinai Sch Med

Thorne, Charles MD [PlS] - **Spec Exp:** Cosmetic Surgery-Face & Breast; Ear Reconstruction/Mi-crotia; Craniofacial Surgery; Pediatric Plastic Surgery; **Hospital:** NYU Langone Med Ctr (page 67), Lenox Hill Hosp (Manh Eye, Ear & Throat Hosp) (page 62); **Address:** 812 Park Ave, New York, NY 10021-2759; **Phone:** 212-794-0044; **Board Cert:** Plastic Surgery 1991; **Med School:** UCLA 1981; **Resid:** Surgery, Mass Genl Hosp 1986; Plastic Surgery, NYU Med Ctr 1988; **Fellow:** Cranio-facial Surgery, NYU Med Ctr 1989; **Fac Appt:** Assoc Prof PlS, NYU Sch Med

Ting, Jess MD [PlS] - **Spec Exp:** Reconstructive Microvascular Surgery; Hand Surgery; Nerve Surgery & Transplantation; Breast Reconstruction; **Hospital:** Mount Sinai Med Ctr (page 64); **Address:** Dept of Surgery Mount Sinai Sch Med, 5 E 98th St, Box 1259, New York, NY 10029; **Phone:** 212-241-4410; **Board Cert:** Plastic Surgery 2002; Hand Surgery 2003; **Med School:** Co-lumbia P&S 1995; **Resid:** Surgery, Columbia Presby Med Ctr 1998; Plastic Surgery, Univ Pittsburgh Med Ctr 2000; **Fellow:** Hand Surgery, Hosp Special Surgery 2001; **Fac Appt:** Asst Prof S, Mount Sinai Sch Med

Vander Kolk, Craig Alan MD [PlS] - **Spec Exp:** Cosmetic Surgery; Cleft Palate/Lip; Cranio-facial Surgery/Reconstruction; **Hospital:** Mercy Med Ctr; **Address:** 227 St Paul Pl Fl 6, Baltimore, MD 21202; **Phone:** 410-332-9700; **Board Cert:** Plastic Surgery 1989; **Med School:** Univ Mich Med Sch 1980; **Resid:** Surgery, Univ Mich Med Ctr 1983; Plastic Surgery, Univ Mich Med Ctr 1986; **Fellow:** Hand Surgery, St Vincents Hosp 1985; Craniofacial Surgery, Chldns Hosp 1987; **Fac Appt:** Assoc Prof PlS, Johns Hopkins Univ

Whitaker, Linton A MD [PlS] - **Spec Exp:** Cosmetic Surgery-Face; Craniofacial Surgery/Re-construction; Facial Tumors; Eyelid Surgery; **Hospital:** Hosp Univ Penn - UPHS (page 60), Chldns Hosp of Philadelphia, The; **Address:** Hosp Univ Penn-10 Penn Tower, 3400 Spruce St, Philadelphia, PA 19104; **Phone:** 215-662-2048; **Board Cert:** Surgery 1970; Plastic Surgery 1978; **Med School:** Tulane Univ 1962; **Resid:** Surgery, Dartmouth Affl Hosp 1969; Plastic Surgery, Hosp Univ Penn 1971; **Fac Appt:** Prof PlS, Univ Pennsylvania

Zide, Barry M MD/DMD [PlS] - **Spec Exp:** Facial Surgery-Chin & Lip; Hemangiomas/Birth-marks; Facial Plastic & Reconstructive Surgery; Craniofacial Surgery-Pediatric; **Hospital:** NYU Lan-gone Med Ctr (page 67); **Address:** 420 E 55th St, Ste 1D, New York, NY 10022-5140; **Phone:** 212-421-2424; **Board Cert:** Plastic Surgery 1981; **Med School:** Tufts Univ 1973; **Resid:** Surgery, Stanford Med Ctr 1976; Plastic Surgery, U NC Hosp 1978; **Fellow:** Head & Neck Oncology, Roswell Park Cancer Inst 1979; Craniofacial Surgery, NYU Med Ctr 1980; **Fac Appt:** Prof PlS, NYU Sch Med

Southeast

Allen, Robert J MD [PlS] - **Spec Exp:** Breast Reconstruction; **Hospital:** Roper Hosp, New York Eye & Ear Infirm (page 65); **Address:** 125 Doughty St, Ste 590, Charleston, SC 29403; **Phone:** 888-890-3437; **Board Cert:** Plastic Surgery 1985; **Med School:** Med Univ SC 1976; **Resid:** Surgery, LSU Med Ctr 1982; Plastic Surgery, LSU Med Ctr 1981; **Fellow:** Microsurgery, NYU Med Ctr 1983; **Fac Appt:** Assoc Clin Prof PlS, Louisiana State U, New Orleans

Argenta, Louis C MD [PlS] - **Spec Exp:** Pediatric Plastic Surgery; Craniofacial Surgery; Wound Healing/Care; **Hospital:** Wake Forest Univ Baptist Med Ctr (page 72); **Address:** WFU Bapt Med Ctr, Dept Plastic Surg, Medical Center Blvd, Winston-Salem, NC 27157-1075; **Phone:** 336-716-4171; **Board Cert:** Plastic Surgery 1982; **Med School:** Univ Mich Med Sch 1969; **Resid:** Surgery, Univ Mich Hosp 1977; Plastic Surgery, Univ Mich Hosp 1979; **Fellow:** Craniofacial Surgery, Hosp Foch 1982; **Fac Appt:** Prof PlS, Wake Forest Univ

Beasley, Michael MD [PlS] - **Spec Exp:** Breast Reconstruction & Augmentation; Liposuction; Body Contouring; **Hospital:** Presby Hosp - Charlotte; **Address:** 2215 Randolph Rd, Charlotte, NC 28207-1523; **Phone:** 704-372-6846; **Board Cert:** Plastic Surgery 1989; **Med School:** Univ NC Sch Med 1980; **Resid:** Surgery, NC Meml Hosp 1985; Plastic Surgery, Emory Univ Hosp 1987; **Fellow:** Plastic Surgery, St Joseph's Hosp 1987; **Fac Appt:** Clin Prof PlS, Univ NC Sch Med

Bermant, Michael A MD [PlS] - **Spec Exp:** Gynecomastia & Cosmetic Breast Surgery; Ear Reshaping (Otoplasty); Liposuction & Body Contouring; Abdominoplasty; **Hospital:** CJW Med Ctr; **Address:** 11601 Ironbridge Rd, Ste 201, Chester, VA 23831; **Phone:** 804-748-7737; **Board Cert:** Plastic Surgery 1991; **Med School:** Northwestern Univ 1978; **Resid:** Surgery, St Vincents Hosp 1982; Plastic Surgery, St Louis Univ Med Ctr 1984; **Fellow:** Microsurgery, NYU Med Ctr 1985

Burstein, Fernando D MD [PlS] - **Spec Exp:** Craniofacial Surgery-Pediatric; Cosmetic Surgery-Face; Maxillofacial Surgery; Rhinoplasty; **Hospital:** Chldns Hlthcare Atlanta - Scottish Rite, Northside Hosp; **Address:** 975 Johnson Ferry Rd NE, Ste 100, Atlanta, GA 30342; **Phone:** 404-256-1311; **Board Cert:** Otolaryngology 1986; Plastic Surgery 1991; **Med School:** Univ Kans 1980; **Resid:** Otolaryngology, UCLA Med Ctr 1986; Plastic Surgery, Yale Univ 1988; **Fellow:** Craniofacial Surgery, UCLA Med Ctr 1989; **Fac Appt:** Assoc Clin Prof PlS, Emory Univ

Carraway, James Howard MD [PlS] - **Spec Exp:** Oculoplastic Surgery; Cosmetic Surgery-Face; Eyelid Surgery; Breast Surgery; **Hospital:** Sentara Leigh Hosp; **Address:** 5589 Greenwich Rd, Ste 100, Virginia Beach, VA 23462; **Phone:** 757-557-0300; **Board Cert:** Surgery 1972; Plastic Surgery 1974; **Med School:** Univ VA Sch Med 1962; **Resid:** Surgery, Norfolk Med Ctr 1970; Plastic Surgery, Eastern VA Med Ctr 1973; **Fellow:** Plastic Surgery, Glasgow Royal Infirmary 1970; **Fac Appt:** Prof PlS, Eastern VA Med Sch

Cruse, C Wayne MD [PlS] - **Spec Exp:** Burns-Reconstructive Plastic Surgery; Cancer Reconstruction; **Hospital:** Tampa Genl Hosp, H Lee Moffitt Cancer Ctr & Research Inst; **Address:** 12902 Magnolia Dr, Ste 4035, Tampa, FL 33612; **Phone:** 813-745-1968; **Board Cert:** Plastic Surgery 1981; **Med School:** Univ Louisville Sch Med 1972; **Resid:** Surgery, Univ S Fla Hosp 1977; Plastic Surgery, Univ KY Hosp-Chandler Med Ctr 1979; **Fac Appt:** Prof S, Univ S Fla Coll Med

Fix, R Jobe MD [PlS] - **Spec Exp:** Breast Reconstruction; Hand Surgery; Microsurgery; **Hospital:** Univ of Ala Hosp at Birmingham, Children's Hospital - Birmingham; **Address:** Univ of Alabama Hosp, Div Plastic Surg, 510 S 20th St, FOT-Ste 1102, Birmingham, AL 35294; **Phone:** 205-934-3358; **Board Cert:** Surgery 1997; Plastic Surgery 1991; Hand Surgery 2001; **Med School:** Univ Nebr Coll Med 1982; **Resid:** Surgery, Valley Med Ctr 1987; Plastic Surgery, Univ Ala Hosp 1989; **Fac Appt:** Prof PlS, Univ Alabama

Plastic Surgery

Georgiade, Gregory MD [PlS] - **Spec Exp:** Breast Reconstruction; Cleft Palate/Lip; **Hospital:** Duke Univ Med Ctr; **Address:** Duke Univ Med Ctr, Box 3960, Durham, NC 27710; **Phone:** 919-684-3039; **Board Cert:** Plastic Surgery 1981; Surgery 2001; **Med School:** Duke Univ 1973; **Resid:** Surgery, Duke Univ Med Ctr 1978; Plastic Surgery, Duke Univ Med Ctr 1980; **Fac Appt:** Prof S, Duke Univ

Gregory, Richard O MD [PlS] - **Spec Exp:** Skin Laser Surgery; Cosmetic Surgery-Face; Facial Rejuvenation; **Hospital:** Florida Hosp Celebration Hlth, Florida Hosp - Orlando; **Address:** 400 Celebration Pl, Ste A320, Celebration, FL 34747; **Phone:** 407-303-4250; **Board Cert:** Plastic Surgery 1981; **Med School:** Indiana Univ 1971; **Resid:** Surgery, Duke Univ Med Ctr 1977; Plastic Surgery, Duke Univ Med Ctr 1979; **Fellow:** Hand Surgery, Univ Louisville Hlth Sci Ctr 1979; **Fac Appt:** Assoc Clin Prof PlS, Univ S Fla Coll Med

Grotting, James S MD [PlS] - **Spec Exp:** Cosmetic Surgery-Face & Body; Cosmetic Surgery-Breast; Breast Reconstruction; **Hospital:** UAB Highlands Hosp, St Vincent's Hosp - Birmingham; **Address:** One Inverness Center Pkwy, Ste 100, Birmingham, AL 35242-4865; **Phone:** 205-930-1600; **Board Cert:** Plastic Surgery 1986; **Med School:** Univ Minn 1978; **Resid:** Surgery, Univ Wash Affil Hosp 1983; Plastic Surgery, UCSF Med Ctr 1985; **Fac Appt:** Clin Prof PlS, Univ Alabama

Hagan, Kevin Francis MD [PlS] - **Spec Exp:** Reconstructive Surgery; Breast Surgery; Cosmetic Surgery; **Hospital:** Vanderbilt Univ Med Ctr; **Address:** Vanderbilt Univ Med Ctr, Dept Plastic Surg, D-4207 Med Ctr N, Nashville, TN 37232; **Phone:** 615-936-3574; **Board Cert:** Plastic Surgery 1983; **Med School:** Johns Hopkins Univ 1974; **Resid:** Surgery, Med Coll VA Hosps 1979; Plastic Surgery, UCSF Med Ctr 1982; **Fellow:** Microsurgery, Dr Harry Buncke Med Clinic 1980; **Fac Appt:** Assoc Prof PlS, Vanderbilt Univ

Hester Jr, T Roderick MD [PlS] - **Spec Exp:** Cosmetic Surgery-Face; Breast Reconstruction; **Hospital:** Emory Univ Hosp; **Address:** Paces Plastic Surgery, 3200 Dunwood Circle, Ste 6340, Atlanta, GA 30327-1610; **Phone:** 404-351-0051; **Board Cert:** Plastic Surgery 1980; Surgery 1973; **Med School:** Emory Univ 1967; **Resid:** Surgery, Emory Affil Hosps 1972; Plastic Reconstructive Surgery, Emory Affil Hosps 1978; **Fac Appt:** Assoc Prof PlS, Emory Univ

Hultman, C Scott MD [PlS] - **Spec Exp:** Breast Reconstruction; Burns-Reconstructive Plastic Surgery; Reconstructive Plastic Surgery; Cosmetic Surgery; **Hospital:** Univ NC Hosps; **Address:** UNC Div Plastic & Reconstructive Surgery, CB 7195, Chapel Hill, NC 27599-7195; **Phone:** 919-966-2300; **Board Cert:** Surgery 1999; Plastic Surgery 2001; Surgical Critical Care 2002; **Med School:** Univ Pittsburgh 1990; **Resid:** Surgery, Univ NC Hosps 1996; Plastic Surgery, Emory Univ Med Ctr 2000; **Fellow:** Surgical Critical Care, Univ N Carolina 1998; **Fac Appt:** Assoc Prof S, Univ NC Sch Med

Hunstad, Joseph P MD [PlS] - **Spec Exp:** Facial Plastic & Reconstructive Surgery; Body Contouring after Weight Loss; **Hospital:** Carolinas Med Ctr-Univ; **Address:** 8605 Cliff Cameron Drive, Ste 100, Charlotte, NC 28269; **Phone:** 704-549-0500; **Board Cert:** Plastic Surgery 1989; **Med School:** Mich State Univ 1981; **Resid:** Surgery, Butterworth Hosp 1984; Plastic Surgery, Grand Rapids Area Med Ed Ct 1986; **Fellow:** Reconstructive Microsurgery, MECOM MicSurg Inst 1987

Kelly, Kevin J MD/DDS [PlS] - **Spec Exp:** Craniofacial Surgery; Cosmetic Surgery; Maxillofacial Surgery; **Hospital:** Vanderbilt Univ Med Ctr; **Address:** Vanderbilt Univ Med Ctr, Dept Plastic Surgery, 1161 21st Ave S, rm D4207, Nashville, TN 37232-2345; **Phone:** 615-322-2350; **Board Cert:** Plastic Surgery 1991; **Med School:** SUNY Downstate 1982; **Resid:** Surgery, Albany Med Ctr 1986; Plastic Surgery, Albany Med Ctr 1988; **Fellow:** Craniofacial Surgery, Johns Hopkins Med Ctr 1989; **Fac Appt:** Assoc Prof PlS, Vanderbilt Univ

Mast, Bruce A MD [PlS] - **Spec Exp:** Breast Reconstruction & Augmentation; Body Contouring; Cosmetic Surgery-Face; Wound Healing/Care; **Hospital:** North Florida Regl Med Ctr, Shands at Alachua Gen Hosp; **Address:** 4340 Newberry Rd, Ste 301, Gainesville, FL 32607; **Phone:** 352-271-5367; **Board Cert:** Surgery 1995; Plastic Surgery 2008; **Med School:** UMDNJ-RW Johnson Med Sch 1987; **Resid:** Surgery, Med Coll Virginia 1993; Plastic Surgery, Univ Pittsburgh 1995; **Fac Appt:** Asst Clin Prof PlS, Univ Fla Coll Med

Matthews, David C MD [PlS] - **Spec Exp:** Craniofacial Surgery/Reconstruction; **Hospital:** Carolinas Med Ctr, Presby Hosp - Charlotte; **Address:** 1719 South Blvd, Ste B, Charlotte, NC 28203-2747; **Phone:** 704-375-2955; **Board Cert:** Plastic Surgery 1983; **Med School:** Univ Cincinnati 1974; **Resid:** Surgery, Hosp Univ Penn 1980; Plastic Surgery, Hosp Univ Penn 1982; **Fellow:** Craniofacial Surgery, Royal Melbourne Hosp; **Fac Appt:** Clin Prof PlS, Univ NC Sch Med

Maxwell, G Patrick MD [PlS] - **Spec Exp:** Cosmetic Surgery-Breast; Cosmetic Surgery-Face; Breast Reconstruction; **Hospital:** Baptist Hosp - Nashville, Centennial Med Ctr; **Address:** 2020 21st Ave S, Nashville, TN 37212; **Phone:** 615-932-7700; **Board Cert:** Plastic Surgery 1981; **Med School:** Vanderbilt Univ 1972; **Resid:** Surgery, Johns Hopkins Hosp 1976; Plastic Surgery, Johns Hopkins Hosp 1979; **Fellow:** Microsurgery, Davies Med Ctr 1975; **Fac Appt:** Asst Clin Prof PlS, Vanderbilt Univ

McCraw, John MD [PlS] - **Spec Exp:** Breast Reconstruction; **Hospital:** Univ Mississippi Med Ctr; **Address:** Univ Mississippi Med Ctr, Div Plastic Surg, 2500 N State St, Jackson, MS 39216; **Phone:** 601-815-1343; **Board Cert:** Surgery 1972; Plastic Surgery 1974; **Med School:** Univ MO-Columbia Sch Med 1966; **Resid:** Orthopaedic Surgery, Duke U Med Ctr 1969; Surgery, Univ Florida Med Ctr 1971; **Fellow:** Plastic Surgery, Univ Florida Med Ctr 1973; **Fac Appt:** Prof PlS, Univ Miss

Molnar, Joseph MD/PhD [PlS] - **Spec Exp:** Burns-Reconstructive Plastic Surgery; Reconstructive Microvascular Surgery; Hand Surgery; **Hospital:** Wake Forest Univ Baptist Med Ctr (page 72); **Address:** Wake Forest Univ Sch Med, Dept Plastic Surg, Medical Ctr Blvd, Winston-Salem, NC 27157-1075; **Phone:** 336-716-0432; **Board Cert:** Plastic Surgery 2005; Hand Surgery 2000; **Med School:** Ohio State Univ 1977; **Resid:** Surgery, Univ Wash Med Ctr 1989; Plastic Surgery, Med Coll VA 1992; **Fellow:** Microsurgery, Med Coll Wisc 1199; Hand Surgery, Med Coll Wisc 1994; **Fac Appt:** Asst Prof PlS, Wake Forest Univ

Morgan, Raymond F MD [PlS] - **Spec Exp:** Cosmetic Surgery; Laser Surgery; Hand Surgery; **Hospital:** Univ Virginia Med Ctr; **Address:** Univ VA Hlth Sys, Dept Plas Surg, PO Box 800376, Charlottesville, VA 22908; **Phone:** 434-924-2413; **Board Cert:** Plastic Surgery 1983; Hand Surgery 2005; **Med School:** W VA Univ 1976; **Resid:** Surgery, Johns Hopkins Hosp 1980; Plastic Surgery, Johns Hopkins Hosp 1982; **Fellow:** Hand Surgery, Union Meml Hosp; **Fac Appt:** Prof PlS, Univ VA Sch Med

Ramirez, Oscar M MD [PlS] - **Spec Exp:** Cosmetic Surgery-Face; Facial Implants (Endoscopic); Breast Reduction; **Address:** 4800 N Federal Hwy, Ste C101, Boca Raton, FL 33431; **Phone:** 561-367-9101; **Board Cert:** Plastic Surgery 1985; **Med School:** Peru 1976; **Resid:** Surgery, Franklin Sq Hosp 1982; Plastic Surgery, Univ Pittsburgh Affil Hosps 1984; **Fellow:** Craniofacial Surgery, Manuel Gea Gonzalez Hosp 1984; **Fac Appt:** Asst Clin Prof S, Johns Hopkins Univ

Smith Jr, David J MD [PlS] - **Spec Exp:** Breast Reconstruction; Burns-Reconstructive Plastic Surgery; **Hospital:** Univ of S FL - Tampa; **Address:** Div Plastic Surg, 2 Tampa General Circle Fl 7, Tampa, FL 33606; **Phone:** 813-259-0929; **Board Cert:** Plastic Surgery 1981; **Med School:** Indiana Univ 1973; **Resid:** Surgery, Emory Univ-Grady Hosp 1988; Plastic Surgery, Inidana Univ 1980; **Fellow:** Hand Surgery, Univ Louisville 1979; **Fac Appt:** Prof S, Univ S Fla Coll Med

Plastic Surgery

Smith, Paul D MD [PlS] - **Spec Exp:** Facial Plastic Surgery; Reconstructive Surgery-Face; Breast Reconstruction & Augmentation; **Hospital:** H Lee Moffitt Cancer Ctr & Research Inst; **Address:** 2 Tampa Genl Cir Fl 7, Tampa, FL 33606-3589; **Phone:** 813-259-0964; **Board Cert:** Plastic Surgery 2002; **Med School:** Univ IL Coll Med 1994; **Resid:** Surgery, Univ IL Med Ctr 1999; **Fellow:** Plastic Surgery, Univ Texas SW Med Ctr 2001; **Fac Appt:** Prof PlS, Univ S Fla Coll Med

Stuzin, James M MD [PlS] - **Spec Exp:** Cosmetic Surgery-Face; Eyelid Surgery; Skin Laser Surgery-Resurfacing; **Hospital:** Mercy Hosp; **Address:** 3225 Aviation Ave, Ste 100, Coconut Grove, FL 33133; **Phone:** 305-854-8828; **Board Cert:** Plastic Surgery 1989; **Med School:** Univ Fla Coll Med 1978; **Resid:** Surgery, Univ Wash Affil Hosp 1983; Plastic Surgery, NYU Med Ctr 1986; **Fellow:** Craniofacial Surgery, UCLA Med Ctr 1987

Thaller, Seth MD/DMD [PlS] - **Spec Exp:** Facial Plastic & Reconstructive Surgery; **Hospital:** Jackson Meml Hosp (page 70); **Address:** 1611 NW 12th Ave, Ste 3019, Miami, FL 33136-1005; **Phone:** 305-585-5285; **Board Cert:** Otolaryngology 1985; Plastic Surgery 1987; **Med School:** Univ Louisville Sch Med 1975; **Resid:** Otolaryngology, Mass Eye & Ear Infirmary 1983; Plastic Surgery, Montefiore Med Ctr 1985; **Fellow:** Surgery, UCLA Med Ctr 1986; **Fac Appt:** Prof PlS, Univ Miami Sch Med

Tobin, Gordon R MD [PlS] - **Spec Exp:** Reconstructive Plastic Surgery; Transplant-Hand; Cosmetic Surgery; Pelvic Reconstruction After Cancer; **Hospital:** Univ of Louisville Hosp, Jewish Hosp HlthCre Svcs Inc; **Address:** 401 E Chestnut St, Ste 790, Louisville, KY 40202; **Phone:** 502-583-8303; **Board Cert:** Plastic Surgery 1978; **Med School:** UCSF 1969; **Resid:** Surgery, Univ Ariz Affil Hosps 1975; Plastic Surgery, Univ Ariz Affil Hosps 1976; **Fellow:** Pediatric Plastic Surgery, Univ Miami 1973; Cosmetic Plastic Surgery, Univ Miami 1973; **Fac Appt:** Prof PlS, Univ Louisville Sch Med

Vasconez, Henry C MD [PlS] - **Spec Exp:** Craniofacial Surgery/Reconstruction; Pediatric Plastic Surgery; Breast Reconstruction; Cosmetic Surgery; **Hospital:** Univ of Kentucky Chandler Hosp; **Address:** 740 S Limestone St, Ste K454, Lexington, KY 40536; **Phone:** 859-257-7171; **Board Cert:** Plastic Surgery 1989; **Med School:** Ecuador 1978; **Resid:** Surgery, Cook Co Hosp 1984; Plastic Surgery, Emory Univ Med Ctr 1986; **Fellow:** Craniofacial Surgery, Baylor Med Ctr/International Craniofacial Inst 1987; **Fac Appt:** Prof S, Univ KY Coll Med

Vasconez, Luis O MD [PlS] - **Spec Exp:** Cosmetic Surgery-Face; Breast Reconstruction; **Hospital:** Univ of Ala Hosp at Birmingham; **Address:** 510 20th St S, FOT 1102, Birmingham, AL 35294-3411; **Phone:** 205-934-3245; **Board Cert:** Surgery 1970; Plastic Surgery 1971; **Med School:** Washington Univ, St Louis 1962; **Resid:** Surgery, Strong Meml Hosp 1970; Plastic Surgery, Shands Hosp-Univ FL 1969; **Fac Appt:** Prof S, Univ Alabama

Wilhelmi, Bradon J MD [PlS] - **Spec Exp:** Cosmetic Surgery; Hand Surgery; Plastic & Reconstructive Surgery; **Hospital:** Norton Hosp, Univ of Louisville Hosp; **Address:** University Surgical Assocs, 401 E Chestnut St, Ste 710, Louisville, KY 40202; **Phone:** 502-583-8303; **Board Cert:** Plastic Surgery 2001; Hand Surgery 2002; **Med School:** Rush Med Coll 1992; **Resid:** Surgery, Northwestern Univ 1996; Plastic Surgery, Univ Texas Med Ctr 1998; **Fellow:** Hand & Microvascular Surgery, Mass General Hosp 1999; **Fac Appt:** Prof PlS, Univ Louisville Sch Med

Wolfe, S Anthony MD [PlS] - **Spec Exp:** Craniofacial Surgery/Reconstruction; Maxillofacial Surgery; Cosmetic Surgery; **Hospital:** South Miami Hosp, Miami Children's Hosp; **Address:** 6280 Sunset Drive, Ste 400, Miami, FL 33143; **Phone:** 305-662-4111; **Board Cert:** Surgery 1973; Plastic Surgery 1978; **Med School:** Harvard Med Sch 1965; **Resid:** Surgery, Peter Bent Brigham Hosp 1972; Plastic Surgery, Jackson Meml Hosp 1974; **Fac Appt:** Assoc Clin Prof PlS, Univ Miami Sch Med

Yu, Jack C MD/DMD [PlS] - **Spec Exp:** Facial Plastic & Reconstructive Surgery; Facial Tumors; Craniofacial Surgery; Cleft Palate/Lip; **Hospital:** Med Coll of GA Hosp and Clin (MCG Health Inc); **Address:** Med College Of Georgia Health Inc, Dept Plastic Surgery, HB 5040, Augusta, GA 30912; **Phone:** 706-721-2198; **Board Cert:** Plastic Surgery 2004; Surgery 2003; **Med School:** Univ Pennsylvania 1985; **Resid:** Surgery, Hosp U Penn 1991; Plastic Surgery, Hosp U Penn 1993; **Fellow:** Craniofacial Surgery, Children's Hosp Philadelphia 1994; **Fac Appt:** Prof PlS, Med Coll GA

Midwest

Bauer, Bruce S MD [PlS] - **Spec Exp:** Cleft Palate/Lip; Vascular Birthmarks; Ear Reconstruction/Microtia; Pigmented Lesions; **Hospital:** Highland Park/North Shore Univ Hlth Syst, Children's Mem Hosp; **Address:** Highland Park Hosp, 777 Park Avenue West, rm 3454, Highland Park, IL 60035; **Phone:** 847-926-5856; **Board Cert:** Plastic Surgery 1980; **Med School:** Northwestern Univ 1974; **Resid:** Surgery, Northwestern Meml Hosp 1977; Plastic Surgery, Northwestern Meml Hosp 1979; **Fac Appt:** Clin Prof S, Northwestern Univ

Bentz, Michael L MD [PlS] - **Spec Exp:** Pediatric Plastic Surgery; Facial Deformities/Reconstruction; Hand Surgery; Hand Reconstruction; **Hospital:** Univ WI Hosp & Clins, Meriter Hosp; **Address:** Univ Wisconsin Hosp, 600 Highland Ave, CSC, rm G5-361, Madison, WI 53792-3236; **Phone:** 608-263-1367; **Board Cert:** Surgery 1998; Plastic Surgery 1994; **Med School:** Temple Univ 1984; **Resid:** Surgery, Temple Univ Hosp 1989; Plastic Surgery, Univ Pittsburgh Med Ctr 1992; **Fellow:** Research, Univ Pittsburgh 1990; **Fac Appt:** Prof S, Univ Wisc

Billmire, David A MD [PlS] - **Spec Exp:** Cleft Palate/Lip; Reconstructive Plastic Surgery; **Hospital:** Cincinnati Chldns Hosp Med Ctr, Univ Hosp - Cincinnati; **Address:** 3333 Burnet Ave, MC 2020, Cincinnati, OH 45229; **Phone:** 513-636-7181; **Board Cert:** Plastic Surgery 1985; **Med School:** Ohio State Univ 1975; **Resid:** Surgery, Univ Hosp 1982; Plastic Surgery, Univ Hosp 1984; **Fellow:** Craniofacial Surgery, Texas Craniofacial Fdn 1985; **Fac Appt:** Assoc Clin Prof S, Univ Cincinnati

Brandt, Keith Eric MD [PlS] - **Spec Exp:** Breast Reconstruction; Reconstructive Surgery; Microsurgery; Hand & Wrist Surgery; **Hospital:** Barnes-Jewish Hosp, Barnes-Jewish West County Hosp; **Address:** 4921 Parkview Pl, Ste 6G, St Louis, MO 63110-1010; **Phone:** 314-362-7388; **Board Cert:** Surgery 1999; Plastic Surgery 2003; Hand Surgery 2005; **Med School:** Univ Tex, Houston 1983; **Resid:** Surgery, Univ Nebraska Med Ctr 1989; Plastic Surgery, Univ Tennessee 1991; **Fellow:** Hand Surgery, Wash Univ 1992; Microsurgery, Wash Univ 1993; **Fac Appt:** Prof S, Washington Univ, St Louis

Buchman, Steven R MD [PlS] - **Spec Exp:** Pediatric Plastic Surgery; Craniofacial Surgery-Pediatric; Craniofacial Surgery; **Hospital:** Mott Chldns Hosp, Univ Michigan Hlth Sys; **Address:** Mott Children's Hospital, 1500 E Med Ctr Drive, rm 7894, Ann Arbor, MI 48109-5219; **Phone:** 734-763-8063; **Board Cert:** Plastic Surgery 2005; **Med School:** Univ VA Sch Med 1985; **Resid:** Surgery, Hosp Univ Penn 1990; Plastic Surgery, Hosp Univ Penn 1992; **Fellow:** Craniofacial Surgery, UCLA Med Ctr 1993; **Fac Appt:** Prof PlS, Univ Mich Med Sch

Canady, John MD [PlS] - **Spec Exp:** Cleft Palate/Lip; Craniofacial Surgery; Pediatric Plastic Surgery; **Hospital:** Univ Iowa Hosp & Clinics; **Address:** Dept Plastic Surg & Otolaryngology, 200 Hawkins Drive, rm 21262 PFP, Iowa City, IA 52242; **Phone:** 319-356-2168; **Board Cert:** Otolaryngology 1988; Plastic Surgery 1992; **Med School:** Univ Iowa Coll Med 1983; **Resid:** Otolaryngology, Univ Iowa Hosp 1988; Plastic Surgery, Univ Kansas Med Ctr 1990; **Fac Appt:** Prof PlS, Univ Iowa Coll Med

Plastic Surgery

Carstens, Michael H MD [PlS] - **Spec Exp:** Pediatric Plastic Surgery; Cleft Palate/Lip; Vascular Birthmarks; Ear Reconstruction/Microtia; **Hospital:** Cardinal Glennon Mem Children's Hosp, St Louis Univ Hosp; **Address:** St Louis Univ Div Plastic Surgery, 3635 Vista Ave Fl 3, St Louis, MO 63110; **Phone:** 314-268-4010; **Board Cert:** Plastic Surgery 2006; **Med School:** Stanford Univ 1981; **Resid:** Surgery, Boston Univ Med Ctr 1987; **Fellow:** Plastic Reconstructive Surgery, Univ Pittsburgh 1989; Craniofacial Surgery, Univ Pittsburgh 1990; **Fac Appt:** Prof PlS, St Louis Univ

Cederna, Paul S MD [PlS] - **Spec Exp:** Burns-Reconstructive Plastic Surgery; Cosmetic Surgery; Microsurgery; **Hospital:** Univ Michigan Hlth Sys; **Address:** 2130 Taubman Ctr, 1500 E Med Ctr Drive, Ann Arbor, MI 48109-0340; **Phone:** 734-998-6022; **Board Cert:** Plastic Surgery 2009; **Med School:** Univ Mich Med Sch 1989; **Resid:** Surgery, Univ Iowa Hosp & Clin 1994; **Fellow:** Microsurgery, Univ Iowa Hosp & Clin 1995; Plastic Surgery, Univ Michigan Hosps 1997; **Fac Appt:** Assoc Prof PlS, Univ Mich Med Sch

Coleman, John J MD [PlS] - **Spec Exp:** Cancer Reconstruction; Breast Reconstruction; Head & Neck Surgery; Pediatric Plastic Surgery; **Hospital:** Indiana Univ Hosp, Riley Hosp for Children; **Address:** 545 Barnhill Dr, Emerson Hall, Ste 232, Indianapolis, IN 46202-5120; **Phone:** 317-274-8106; **Board Cert:** Surgery 1998; Plastic Surgery 1981; **Med School:** Harvard Med Sch 1973; **Resid:** Surgery, Emory Univ Affil Hosp 1978; Plastic Surgery, Emory Univ Affil Hosp 1979; **Fellow:** Surgical Oncology, Univ Maryland Med Ctr 1981; **Fac Appt:** Prof S, Indiana Univ

Hammond, Dennis C MD [PlS] - **Spec Exp:** Breast Surgery; Breast Reduction; **Hospital:** Spectrum Hlth Blodgett Campus; **Address:** 4070 Lake Drive SE, Ste 202, Grand Rapids, MI 49546; **Phone:** 616-464-4420; **Board Cert:** Plastic Surgery 1994; **Med School:** Univ Mich Med Sch 1985; **Resid:** Surgery, Blodgett Meml Med Ctr 1988; Plastic Reconstructive Surgery, Grand Rapids Area Med Educ Ctr 1990; **Fellow:** Plastic Surgery, Baptist Hosp 1991; Hand & Microvascular Surgery, Med Coll Wisconsin 1992; **Fac Appt:** Prof PlS, Univ Mich Med Sch

Kane, Alex A MD [PlS] - **Spec Exp:** Pediatric Plastic Surgery; Craniofacial Surgery; Cleft Palate/Lip; **Hospital:** St Louis Chldns Hosp, Barnes-Jewish Hosp; **Address:** St Louis Children's Hospital, 6600 S Euclid, Box 8283, St Louis, MO 63110; **Phone:** 314-454-4894; **Board Cert:** Plastic Surgery 2001; **Med School:** Dartmouth Med Sch 1991; **Resid:** Surgery, Barnes Jewish Hosp 1994; Plastic Surgery, Barnes Jewish Hosp 1998; **Fellow:** Craniofacial Surgery, Chang-Gung Meml Hosp 1999; Craniofacial Imaging, Natl Lab for Diagnostic Research 1999; **Fac Appt:** Asst Prof S, Washington Univ, St Louis

Kuzon Jr, William M MD/PhD [PlS] - **Spec Exp:** Facial Paralysis Reconstruction; Abdominal Wall Reconstruction; Gender Reassignment Surgery; **Hospital:** Univ Michigan Hlth Sys, VA Med Ctr; **Address:** Univ Michigan, Dept Surgery, 1500 E Med Ctr Drive, 2130 Taubman Ctr, Ann Arbor, MI 48109-0340; **Phone:** 734-936-5890; **Board Cert:** Plastic Surgery 2006; **Med School:** Univ Rochester 1981; **Resid:** Plastic Surgery, Univ Toronto Med Ctr 1990; **Fellow:** Microvascular Surgery, Univ Toronto Med Ctr 1991; Hand & Microvascular Surgery, Univ Pittsburgh Med Ctr 1992; **Fac Appt:** Prof PlS, Univ Mich Med Sch

Lee, Raphael MD [PlS] - **Spec Exp:** Reconstructive Surgery; Burns-Reconstructive Plastic Surgery; Cosmetic Surgery Face & Body; Eyelid Surgery; **Hospital:** Univ of Chicago Med Ctr; **Address:** 5841 S Maryland Ave, MC 6035, Chicago, IL 60637-1463; **Phone:** 773-702-6302; **Board Cert:** Plastic Surgery 1989; **Med School:** Temple Univ 1975; **Resid:** Surgery, Univ Chicago Hosp 1981; Plastic Surgery, Mass Genl Hosp 1983; **Fellow:** Research, Harvard Med School 1979; **Fac Appt:** Prof PlS, Univ Chicago-Pritzker Sch Med

MacKinnon, Susan E MD [PlS] - **Spec Exp:** Nerve Surgery & Transplantation; Hand Surgery; Reconstructive Surgery; Peripheral Nerve Surgery; **Hospital:** Barnes-Jewish Hosp; **Address:** Washington Univ Sch Med, 660 S Euclid Ave, Box 8238, St Louis, MO 63110; **Phone:** 314-362-4586; **Med School:** Canada 1975; **Resid:** Surgery, Queens Univ-Kingston 1978; Plastic Surgery, Univ Toronto Med Ctr 1980; **Fellow:** Neurological Surgery, Univ Toronto Med Ctr 1981; Hand Surgery, Union Meml Hosp 1982; **Fac Appt:** Prof S, Washington Univ, St Louis

Marsh, Jeffrey L MD [PlS] - **Spec Exp:** Cleft Palate/Lip; Craniofacial Surgery/Reconstruction; Pediatric Plastic Surgery; **Hospital:** St John's Mercy Med Ctr - St Louis; **Address:** 621 S New Ballas Rd, Ste 260A, St Louis, MO 63141; **Phone:** 314-251-4772; **Board Cert:** Plastic Surgery 1979; **Med School:** Johns Hopkins Univ 1970; **Resid:** Surgery, UCLA Med Ctr 1975; Plastic Surgery, Univ Va Hosp 1977; **Fellow:** Craniofacial Surgery, Cannisburn Hosp; Craniofacial Surgery, Clinic Belvedere Hosp; **Fac Appt:** Clin Prof PlS, St Louis Univ

Mustoe, Thomas A MD [PlS] - **Spec Exp:** Cosmetic Surgery-Face; Cosmetic Surgery-Breast; Rhinoplasty; **Hospital:** Northwestern Meml Hosp; **Address:** NW Med Faculty Fdn-Plastic Surgery, 675 N St Clair St Fl 19 - Ste 250, Chicago, IL 60611-5975; **Phone:** 312-695-6022; **Board Cert:** Otolaryngology 1983; Plastic Surgery 1987; **Med School:** Harvard Med Sch 1978; **Resid:** Surgery, Brigham & Womens Hosp 1980; Otolaryngology, Mass Eye & Ear Infirm 1983; **Fellow:** Plastic Surgery, Brigham & Womens Hosp 1985; **Fac Appt:** Prof S, Northwestern Univ

Ness, John A MD [PlS] - **Hospital:** Northern Meml Hlth Care; **Address:** Wayzata Plastic Surgery, 319 Barry Ave, Ste 300, Wayzata, MN 55391; **Phone:** 952-473-1111; **Board Cert:** Otolaryngology 1992; Plastic Surgery 2009; **Med School:** Univ Minn 1986; **Resid:** Otolaryngology, Loyola U- Stritch Sch Med 1991; **Fellow:** Facial Plastic & Reconstr Surgery, UC Davis 1993; Craniofacial Surgery, Australian Craniofacial Inst 1996; **Fac Appt:** Asst Prof PlS, Univ Minn

Neumeister, Michael W MD [PlS] - **Spec Exp:** Hand Surgery; Microsurgery; Breast Reconstruction & Augmentation; Cleft Lip/Palate; **Hospital:** Memorial Med Ctr-Springfield; **Address:** SIU Div Plastic Surgery, PO Box 19653, Springfield, IL 62794; **Phone:** 217-545-6314; **Board Cert:** Plastic Surgery 2005; Hand Surgery 2006; **Med School:** Univ Toronto 1988; **Resid:** Surgery, Dalhousie Univ Affil Hosp 1991; Plastic Surgery, Univ Manitoba Affil Hosp 1994; **Fellow:** Microsurgery, Brigham & Womens Hosp; Hand & Microvascular Surgery, Southern Illinois Univ; **Fac Appt:** Prof S, Southern IL Univ

Patel, Pravin K MD [PlS] - **Spec Exp:** Pediatric Plastic Surgery; Craniofacial Surgery; Cleft Lip/Palate; Reconstructive Surgery-Complex; **Hospital:** Children's Mem Hosp, Shriners Hosp for Children-Chicago; **Address:** Childrens Memorial Hosp, Div Plastic Surgery, 2300 Childrens Plaza, Box 93, Chicago, IL 60707-3361; **Phone:** 773-327-2440; **Board Cert:** Plastic Surgery 2009; **Med School:** Hahnemann Univ 1985; **Resid:** Surgery, Mayo Clinic 1989; Plastic Surgery, Northwestern Univ 1993; **Fellow:** Craniofacial Surgery, UCLA Med Ctr 1994; **Fac Appt:** Assoc Prof S, Northwestern Univ-Feinberg Sch Med

Polley, John W MD [PlS] - **Spec Exp:** Craniofacial Surgery; Pediatric Plastic Surgery; Maxillofacial Surgery; **Hospital:** Rush Univ Med Ctr; **Address:** Rush Univ Med Ctr, Plastic Surgery, 1725 W Harrison St, Ste 425, Professional Bldg, Chicago, IL 60612-3841; **Phone:** 312-563-3000; **Board Cert:** Plastic Surgery 1992; **Med School:** Northwestern Univ 1983; **Resid:** Surgery, Mich State Univ Med Ctr 1986; Plastic Surgery, Mich State Univ Med Ctr 1988; **Fellow:** Craniofacial Surgery, Chang Gung Meml Hosp 1989; Hosp for Sick Chldn 1990; **Fac Appt:** Prof PlS, Rush Med Coll

Puckett, Charles L MD [PlS] - **Spec Exp:** Cosmetic & Reconstructive Surgery; Breast Surgery; **Hospital:** Univ of Missouri Hosp & Clins, Columbia Regional Hosp; **Address:** 1 Hospital Drive, Ste M349, Columbia, MO 65212-5276; **Phone:** 573-882-2275; **Board Cert:** Surgery 1972; Plastic Surgery 1977; **Med School:** Wake Forest Univ 1966; **Resid:** Surgery, Duke Univ Med Ctr 1971; Plastic Surgery, Duke Univ Med Ctr 1976; **Fac Appt:** Prof S, Univ MO-Columbia Sch Med

Plastic Surgery

Rees, Riley S MD [PIS] - **Spec Exp:** Wound Healing/Care; Melanoma; **Hospital:** Univ Michigan Hlth Sys, VA Med Ctr - Ann Arbor; **Address:** University of Michigan, 2130 Taubman Ctr, 1500 E Med Ctr Drive, Box 0340, Ann Arbor, MI 48109-0340; **Phone:** 734-615-3435; **Board Cert:** Plastic Surgery 1981; **Med School:** Univ Utah 1972; **Resid:** Surgery, LSU Med Ctr 1978; Plastic Surgery, Vanderbilt Univ Med Ctr 1980; **Fac Appt:** Prof S, Univ Mich Med Sch

Sanger, James R MD [PIS] - **Spec Exp:** Reconstructive Surgery; Hand Surgery; Microsurgery; **Hospital:** Froedtert Meml Lutheran Hosp, Chldns Hosp - Wisconsin; **Address:** Med Coll Wisc, Dept Plastic Surg, 8700 Watertown Plank Rd, Milwaukee, WI 53226; **Phone:** 414-805-5451; **Board Cert:** Plastic Surgery 1982; Hand Surgery 1999; **Med School:** Univ Wisc 1974; **Resid:** Surgery, LAC-Harbor UCLA Med Ctr 1979; Plastic Surgery, Med Coll Wisc Affil Hosps 1981; **Fellow:** Hand Surgery, Med Coll Wisc Affil Hosps 1982; **Fac Appt:** Prof PIS, Med Coll Wisc

Siemionow, Maria MD/PhD [PIS] - **Spec Exp:** Microsurgery; Peripheral Nerve Surgery; Reconstructive Plastic Surgery; Transplant-Face; **Hospital:** Cleveland Clin Fdn (page 56); **Address:** Cleveland Clin Fdn, 9500 Euclid Ave, Desk A60, Cleveland, OH 44195; **Phone:** 216-445-2405; **Med School:** Poland 1974; **Resid:** Surgery, Inst Orth & Rehab Med; **Fellow:** Plastic Surgery, Univ Hosp; Microsurgery, Univ Louisville Hosp

Sood, Rajiv MD [PIS] - **Spec Exp:** Burns-Reconstructive Plastic Surgery; Pediatric Hand Surgery; Breast Cosmetic & Reconstructive Surgery; Cosmetic Surgery; **Hospital:** Indiana Univ Hosp, Riley Hosp for Children; **Address:** Indiana Univ Med Ctr, 1001 W 10th St, Dunlap Bldg Fl 4, Richard Fairbanks Burn Ctr, Indianapolis, IN 46202; **Phone:** 317-278-1022; **Board Cert:** Plastic Surgery 1994; Hand Surgery 2006; **Med School:** Albany Med Coll 1984; **Resid:** Surgery, Temple Univ Hosp 1989; **Fellow:** Plastic Surgery, Cleveland Clinic Fdn 1991; Hand Surgery, Union Meml Hosp 1992; **Fac Appt:** Prof S, Indiana Univ

Vogt, Peter MD [PIS] - **Spec Exp:** Cosmetic Surgery; **Hospital:** Mercy Hosp - Coon Rapids, Unity Hosp - Fridley; **Address:** 319 Barry Ave S, Ste 300, Wayzata, MN 55391; **Phone:** 952-473-1111; **Board Cert:** Plastic Surgery 1974; **Med School:** Univ Manitoba 1965; **Resid:** Surgery, Montreal Genl Hosp 1970; Plastic Surgery, Winnipeg Hlth Scis Ctr 1973

Walton Jr, Robert L MD [PIS] - **Spec Exp:** Cosmetic Surgery-Face; Nasal Reconstruction; Breast Reconstruction; **Hospital:** Univ of Chicago Med Ctr, Resurrection Hlth Care St Joseph Hosp; **Address:** 60 E Delaware, Ste 1430, Chicago, IL 60611-1495; **Phone:** 312-337-7795; **Board Cert:** Plastic Surgery 1980; **Med School:** Univ Kans 1972; **Resid:** Surgery, Johns Hopkins Hosp 1974; Plastic Surgery, Yale-New Haven Hosp 1978; **Fellow:** Hand Surgery, Hartford Hosp 1978

Wilkins, Edwin G MD [PIS] - **Spec Exp:** Breast Reconstruction; Lower Limb Reconstruction; Microsurgery; **Hospital:** Univ Michigan Hlth Sys; **Address:** Univ Mich, Div Plastic Surg, 1500 E Med Ctr Drive, rm 2130 Taubman Ctr, Ann Arbor, MI 48109-5340; **Phone:** 734-998-6022; **Board Cert:** Plastic Surgery 1991; **Med School:** Wake Forest Univ 1981; **Resid:** Surgery, Charlotte Meml Hosp 1986; Plastic Surgery, Vanderbilt Univ Med Ctr 1988; **Fellow:** Reconstructive Microsurgery, Univ Louisville Sch Med 1989; **Fac Appt:** Assoc Prof PIS, Univ Mich Med Sch

Yetman, Randall MD [PIS] - **Spec Exp:** Breast Reconstruction; Melanoma; **Hospital:** Cleveland Clin Fdn (page 56); **Address:** 9500 Euclid Ave, Desk A60, Cleveland, OH 44195; **Phone:** 216-444-6908; **Board Cert:** Plastic Surgery 1984; **Med School:** Univ Miami Sch Med 1975; **Resid:** Surgery, Montefiore Med Ctr 1979; Plastic Surgery, NY Cornell Med Ctr 1981; **Fellow:** Plastic Surgery, Cleveland Clin Fdn 1982

Young, Vernon L MD [PlS] - **Spec Exp:** Breast Augmentation; Skin Laser Surgery-Resurfacing; Body Contouring after Weight Loss; **Address:** 969 N Mason Rd, Ste 170, St Louis, MO 63141; **Phone:** 314-628-8200; **Board Cert:** Plastic Surgery 1981; **Med School:** Univ KY Coll Med 1970; **Resid:** Surgery, Univ KY Med Ctr 1977; Plastic Surgery, Barnes Hosp-Wash Univ 1979; **Fac Appt:** Prof S, Washington Univ, St Louis

Zins, James MD [PlS] - **Spec Exp:** Cosmetic Surgery-Face; Maxillofacial Surgery; Craniofacial Surgery; **Hospital:** Cleveland Clin Fdn (page 56); **Address:** Department of Plastic Surgery, 9500 Euclid Ave, Desk A-60, Cleveland, OH 44195; **Phone:** 216-444-6901; **Board Cert:** Plastic Surgery 1985; **Med School:** Univ Pennsylvania 1974; **Resid:** Surgery, Hosp Univ Penn 1980; Plastic Surgery, Hosp Univ Penn 1982; **Fellow:** Craniofacial Surgery, Hosp Univ Penn 1978; Maxillofacial Surgery, Hosp Sick Chldn 1983

Great Plains and Mountains

Grossman, John A MD [PlS] - **Spec Exp:** Cosmetic Surgery; **Hospital:** Rose Med Ctr, Cedars-Sinai Med Ctr; **Address:** 4600 Hale Pkwy, Ste 100, Denver, CO 80220; **Phone:** 303-320-5566; **Board Cert:** Surgery 1974; Plastic Surgery 1976; **Med School:** Cornell Univ-Weill Med Coll 1967; **Resid:** Surgery, Boston City Hosp 1973; Plastic Surgery, Univ Colo Hlth Scis Ctr 1975; **Fellow:** Surgery, Harvard Med Sch 1973

Southwest

Barone, Constance M MD [PlS] - **Spec Exp:** Cosmetic Surgery; Breast Augmentation; Rhinoplasty; Craniofacial Surgery; **Hospital:** Christus Santa Rosa Med Ctr Hosp, Univ Hlth Syst-San Antonio; **Address:** 2829 Babcock Rd, Ste 615, San Antonio, TX 78229; **Phone:** 210-614-0400; **Board Cert:** Plastic Surgery 1991; **Med School:** Mount Sinai Sch Med 1982; **Resid:** Surgery, Temple Univ Hosp 1987; Plastic Surgery, NYU Med Ctr 1989; **Fellow:** Craniofacial Surgery, Montefiore-Weiler Einstein Div 1992; **Fac Appt:** Prof NS, Univ Tex, San Antonio

Barton Jr, Fritz MD [PlS] - **Spec Exp:** Cosmetic Surgery-Face; Liposuction & Body Contouring; **Hospital:** Baylor Univ Medical Ctr; **Address:** Dallas Plastic Surgery Institute, 9101 N Central Expresswy, Ste 600, Fl 6th, Dallas, TX 75231; **Phone:** 214-821-9355; **Board Cert:** Surgery 1975; Plastic Surgery 1977; **Med School:** Univ Tex SW, Dallas 1967; **Resid:** Surgery, Parkland Meml Hosp 1974; Plastic Reconstructive Surgery, NYU Med Ctr 1976; **Fac Appt:** Prof PlS, Univ Tex SW, Dallas

Beals, Stephen P MD [PlS] - **Spec Exp:** Craniofacial Surgery; Pediatric Plastic Surgery; Cosmetic Surgery-Face; **Hospital:** St Joseph's Hosp & Med Ctr - Phoenix, Phoenix Children's Hosp; **Address:** 500 W Thomas Rd, Ste 960, Phoenix, AZ 85013-4223; **Phone:** 602-266-9066; **Board Cert:** Plastic Surgery 1986; **Med School:** Wayne State Univ 1978; **Resid:** Surgery, William Beaumont Hosp 1983; Plastic Surgery, Phoenix Plastic Surgery Inst 1985; **Fellow:** Craniofacial Surgery, Hospital for Sick Chldn 1985; **Fac Appt:** Asst Prof PlS, Mayo Med Sch

Burns, A Jay MD [PlS] - **Spec Exp:** Cosmetic Surgery; Skin Laser Surgery; Vascular Birthmarks; **Hospital:** Baylor Univ Medical Ctr, Chldns Med Ctr of Dallas; **Address:** 9101 N Central Expressway St, Ste 600, Dallas, TX 75231; **Phone:** 214-823-1978; **Board Cert:** Plastic Surgery 1990; **Med School:** Univ Tex SW, Dallas 1981; **Resid:** Surgery, Univ Utah Hosp 1986; Plastic Surgery, Univ Tex SW Med Ctr 1988; **Fellow:** Vascular Anomalies, Chldns Hosp 1988; **Fac Appt:** Asst Prof PlS, Univ Tex SW, Dallas

Plastic Surgery

Butler, Charles E MD [PlS] - **Spec Exp:** Breast Cosmetic & Reconstructive Surgery; **Hospital:** UT MD Anderson Cancer Ctr; **Address:** Univ Texas- M.D. Anderson Cancer Ctr, 1515 Holcombe Blvd, Ste 443, P.O. Box 301402, Houston, TX 77030; **Phone:** 713-794-1247; **Board Cert:** Plastic Surgery 2010; Surgery 2008; **Med School:** Univ Pennsylvania 1990; **Resid:** Surgery, Mass Genl Hosp 1993; Plastic Surgery, Brigham & Women's Hosp 1995; **Fellow:** Research, Brigham & Women's Hosp 1998; **Fac Appt:** Prof PlS, Case West Res Univ

Byrd, H Stephenson MD [PlS] - **Spec Exp:** Cosmetic Surgery-Face; Craniofacial Surgery; Pediatric Plastic Surgery; **Hospital:** Baylor Univ Medical Ctr; **Address:** 9101 N Central Expresswy, Ste 600, Fl 6th, Dallas, TX 75231; **Phone:** 214-821-9662; **Board Cert:** Plastic Surgery 1980; **Med School:** Univ Tex Med Br, Galveston 1972; **Resid:** Surgery, Univ Utah Med Ctr 1977; Plastic Surgery, Dallas Co Hosp-Parkland Meml 1979; **Fac Appt:** Clin Prof PlS, Univ Tex SW, Dallas

Friedland, Jack A MD [PlS] - **Spec Exp:** Cleft Palate/Lip; Cosmetic Surgery-Face & Body; Cosmetic Surgery-Breast; Rhinoplasty; **Hospital:** Scottsdale Hlthcare - Shea, St Joseph's Hosp & Med Ctr - Phoenix; **Address:** 7425 E Shea Blvd, Ste 103, Scottsdale, AZ 85260-6411; **Phone:** 480-905-1700; **Board Cert:** Surgery 1971; Plastic Surgery 1975; **Med School:** Northwestern Univ 1965; **Resid:** Surgery, NYU Med Ctr 1970; Plastic Reconstructive Surgery, NYU Med Ctr 1974; **Fac Appt:** Assoc Prof PlS, Mayo Med Sch

Gunter, Jack MD [PlS] - **Spec Exp:** Rhinoplasty; Rhinoplasty Revision; **Hospital:** Presby Hosp of Dallas; **Address:** 8144 Walnut Hill Lane, Ste 170, Dallas, TX 75231-4218; **Phone:** 214-369-8123; **Board Cert:** Otolaryngology 1969; Plastic Surgery 1981; **Med School:** Univ Okla Coll Med 1963; **Resid:** Surgery, Univ Ark Med Ctr 1965; Otolaryngology, Tulane Univ Hosp 1968; **Fellow:** Mercy Hosp 1969; Plastic Surgery, Univ Mich Hosp 1980; **Fac Appt:** Clin Prof PlS, Univ Tex SW, Dallas

Hamra, Sameer T MD [PlS] - **Spec Exp:** Cosmetic Surgery-Face; Rhinoplasty; **Hospital:** Mary Shiels Hosp; **Address:** 9301 N Central Expresswy, Ste 551, Tower 2, Dallas, TX 75231; **Phone:** 214-754-9001; **Board Cert:** Surgery 1970; Plastic Surgery 1977; **Med School:** Univ Okla Coll Med 1963; **Resid:** Surgery, Univ Okla 1968; Plastic Surgery, NYU Med Ctr 1973; **Fellow:** Surgery, Univ Lausanne 1966; **Fac Appt:** Clin Prof S, Univ Tex SW, Dallas

Kelly, John M MD [PlS] - **Spec Exp:** Cosmetic Surgery-Face; Breast Surgery; Liposuction; **Hospital:** Integris Baptist Med Ctr - OK; **Address:** 3301 NW 63rd St, Oklahoma City, OK 73116-3705; **Phone:** 405-842-9732; **Board Cert:** Surgery 1970; Plastic Surgery 1978; **Med School:** Univ Ark 1963; **Resid:** Surgery, Univ Virginia Hosp 1969; Plastic Surgery, Johns Hopkins Hosp 1971; **Fac Appt:** Clin Prof S, Univ Okla Coll Med

Kenkel, Jeffrey M MD [PlS] - **Spec Exp:** Body Contouring; Body Contouring after Weight Loss; **Hospital:** UT Southwestern Med Ctr at Dallas; **Address:** 1801 Inwood Rd Fl 5, Dallas, TX 75390; **Phone:** 214-645-2353; **Board Cert:** Plastic Surgery 2008; **Med School:** Georgetown Univ 1990; **Resid:** Surgery, Georgetown Univ Med Ctr 1994; Plastic Surgery, UT Southwestern Med Ctr 1996; **Fac Appt:** Prof PlS, Univ Tex SW, Dallas

Meltzer, Toby R MD [PlS] - **Spec Exp:** Gender Reassignment Surgery; Penile Inversion Technique; Breast Augmentation; **Hospital:** Scottsdale Hlthcare - Osborn; **Address:** 7025 N Scottsdale Rd, Ste 302, Scottsdale, AZ 85253; **Phone:** 866-876-6329; **Board Cert:** Plastic Surgery 1992; **Med School:** Louisiana State U, New Orleans 1983; **Resid:** Surgery, Charity Hosp Louisiana 1988; Plastic Surgery, Univ Michigan Med Ctr 1990; **Fellow:** Burn Surgery, Wayne State Univ 1987; **Fac Appt:** Asst Clin Prof S, Univ Ariz Coll Med

Menick, Frederick J MD [PlS] - **Spec Exp:** Reconstructive Surgery-Face; Nasal Reconstruction; Cancer Reconstruction; Cosmetic Surgery; **Hospital:** St Joseph's Hosp - Tucson; **Address:** 1102 N Eldorado Pl, Tucson, AZ 85712; **Phone:** 520-881-4525; **Board Cert:** Plastic Surgery 1983; **Med School:** Yale Univ 1970; **Resid:** Surgery, Stanford Med Ctr; Surgery, Univ Ariz Med Ctr 1979; **Fellow:** Plastic Surgery, Queen Victoria Hosp/Univ Miami 1982; **Fac Appt:** Assoc Clin Prof S, Univ Ariz Coll Med

Rappaport, Norman H MD [PlS] - **Spec Exp:** Cosmetic Surgery; Botox Therapy; **Hospital:** St Luke's Episcopal Hosp-Houston, Methodist Hosp - Houston; **Address:** 6560 Fannin St, Ste 1812, Houston, TX 77030-2775; **Phone:** 713-790-4500; **Board Cert:** Plastic Surgery 1981; **Med School:** Hahnemann Univ 1975; **Resid:** Surgery, Abingdon Meml Hosp 1978; Plastic Surgery, Baylor Coll Med 1978; **Fellow:** Plastic Surgery, Hosp U Penn 1980; **Fac Appt:** Assoc Clin Prof S, Baylor Coll Med

Robb, Geoffrey L MD [PlS] - **Spec Exp:** Breast Reconstruction; Head & Neck Cancer Reconstruction; Facial Plastic & Reconstructive Surgery; **Hospital:** UT MD Anderson Cancer Ctr, St Luke's Episcopal Hosp-Houston; **Address:** 1515 Holcombe Blvd, Unit 443, Houston, TX 77030; **Phone:** 713-794-1247; **Board Cert:** Otolaryngology 1979; Plastic Surgery 1986; **Med School:** Univ Miami Sch Med 1974; **Resid:** Otolaryngology, Naval Reg Med Ctr 1979; Plastic Surgery, Univ Pittsburgh 1985; **Fellow:** Microvascular Surgery, Univ Pittsburgh 1986; **Fac Appt:** Prof PlS, Univ Tex, Houston

Rohrich, Rod J MD [PlS] - **Spec Exp:** Nasal Surgery; Rhinoplasty; Breast Reconstruction; Wound Healing/Care; **Hospital:** UT Southwestern Med Ctr at Dallas, Baylor Univ Medical Ctr; **Address:** Univ Tex SW Med Ctr, Plastic Surgery, 1801 Inwood Rd, Dallas, TX 75390-9132; **Phone:** 214-645-3119; **Board Cert:** Plastic Surgery 1987; Hand Surgery 1990; **Med School:** Baylor Coll Med 1979; **Resid:** Plastic Surgery, Univ Mich Hosp 1985; Plastic Surgery, Radcliffe Infirm/Oxford 1983; **Fellow:** Hand Surgery, Mass Genl Hosp-Harvard 1987; **Fac Appt:** Prof PlS, Univ Tex SW, Dallas

Schusterman, Mark A MD [PlS] - **Spec Exp:** Breast Reconstruction; Cancer Reconstruction; Cosmetic Surgery-Face & Breast; **Hospital:** St Luke's Episcopal Hosp-Houston, Park Plaza Hosp; **Address:** 1200 Binz St, Ste 1200, Houston, TX 77030; **Phone:** 713-794-0368; **Board Cert:** Plastic Surgery 1989; **Med School:** Univ Louisville Sch Med 1980; **Resid:** Surgery, Univ Hosp 1985; Pediatric Surgery, Univ Pittsburgh Med Ctr 1987; **Fellow:** Microsurgery, Univ Pittsburgh Med Ctr 1988; **Fac Appt:** Clin Prof PlS, Baylor Coll Med

Stal, Samuel MD [PlS] - **Spec Exp:** Pediatric Plastic Surgery; Craniofacial Surgery; Cleft Palate/Lip; Maxillofacial Surgery; **Hospital:** Texas Chldns Hosp; **Address:** Texas Children's Hosp, 6621 Fannin St, MC CCC 620.10, Houston, TX 77030; **Phone:** 832-822-3180; **Board Cert:** Otolaryngology 1981; Plastic Surgery 1982; **Med School:** Loyola Univ-Stritch Sch Med 1974; **Resid:** Otolaryngology, Univ Chicago Hosps 1979; Plastic Surgery, Baylor College Med 1981; **Fellow:** Craniofacial Surgery, Enfant Malade Hosp 1982; **Fac Appt:** Prof Oto, Baylor Coll Med

Tebbetts, John B MD [PlS] - **Spec Exp:** Breast Augmentation; Rhinoplasty; Liposuction; **Hospital:** Mary Shiels Hosp, Baylor Univ Medical Ctr; **Address:** 2801 Lemmon Ave W, Ste 300, Dallas, TX 75204-2398; **Phone:** 214-220-2712; **Board Cert:** Surgery 1978; Plastic Surgery 1980; **Med School:** Univ Tex Med Br, Galveston 1972; **Resid:** Surgery, Univ Utah Med Ctr 1977; Plastic Surgery, Dallas Co Hospital-Parkland Meml Hosp 1979; **Fac Appt:** Asst Clin Prof PlS, Univ Tex SW, Dallas

Plastic Surgery

Yuen, James C MD [PlS] - **Spec Exp:** Hand Reconstruction; Breast Reconstruction; Head & Neck Cancer Reconstruction; Chest Wall Reconstruction; **Hospital:** UAMS Med Ctr; **Address:** 4301 W Markham, Ste 720, Little Rock, AR 72205; **Phone:** 501-686-8711; **Board Cert:** Surgery 2001; Plastic Surgery 2004; **Med School:** Med Coll VA 1985; **Resid:** Surgery, West Va Med Ctr 1990; Plastic Reconstructive Surgery, Duke Univ Med Ctr 1993; **Fellow:** Hand & Microvascular Surgery, Kleinert Inst of Hand & Microsurgery 1991; **Fac Appt:** Assoc Prof S, Univ Ark

West Coast and Pacific

Alter, Gary J MD [PlS] - **Spec Exp:** Genitourinary Reconstruction; Gender Reassignment Surgery; Genital Enhancement; **Hospital:** Cedars-Sinai Med Ctr, UCLA Ronald Reagan Med Ctr; **Address:** 416 N Bedford Drive, Ste 400, Beverly Hills, CA 90210-4318; **Phone:** 310-275-5566; **Board Cert:** Urology 1981; Plastic Surgery 2007; **Med School:** UCLA 1973; **Resid:** Urology, Baylor Med Ctr 1979; Plastic Surgery, Mayo Clinic 1992; **Fellow:** Genitourinary Surgery, Eastern Va Med Sch 1992; **Fac Appt:** Clin Prof PlS, UCLA

Andersen, James S MD [PlS] - **Spec Exp:** Breast Reconstruction; Head & Neck Reconstruction; Microsurgery; **Hospital:** City of Hope Natl Med Ctr & Beckman Rsch, Huntington Memorial Hosp; **Address:** City of Hope National Cancer Ctr, Div Plastic Surgery, 1500 E Duarte Rd, Duarte, CA 91010; **Phone:** 626-471-7100; **Board Cert:** Plastic Surgery 1994; **Med School:** Jefferson Med Coll 1983; **Resid:** Surgery, Hosp U Penn 1989; Plastic Surgery, Hosp U Penn 1991; **Fellow:** Microsurgery, USC Med Ctr 1992; **Fac Appt:** Assoc Clin Prof S, USC Sch Med

Brent, Burton D MD [PlS] - **Spec Exp:** Ear Reconstruction/Microtia; **Hospital:** El Camino Hosp; **Address:** 2995 Woodside Rd, Ste 300, Woodside, CA 94062-2401; **Phone:** 650-851-5300; **Board Cert:** Plastic Surgery 1974; **Med School:** Ros Franklin Univ/Chicago Med Sch 1963; **Resid:** Surgery, University Hosp 1970; Plastic Surgery, Loyola Univ Med Ctr 1973; **Fellow:** Plastic Surgery, Canniesburn Hosp; **Fac Appt:** Assoc Clin Prof PlS, Stanford Univ

Brink, Robert Ross MD [PlS] - **Spec Exp:** Cosmetic Surgery; **Hospital:** Peninsula Med Ctr; **Address:** 66 Bovet Rd, Ste 101, San Mateo, CA 94402-3126; **Phone:** 650-570-6066; **Board Cert:** Plastic Surgery 1980; **Med School:** Univ Mich Med Sch 1970; **Resid:** Surgery, UC Davis Med Ctr 1977; Plastic Surgery, UCSF Med Ctr 1979

Chang, James MD [PlS] - **Spec Exp:** Reconstructive Surgery; Facial Nerve Disorders; Peripheral Nerve Surgery; Hand Reconstruction-Pediatric; **Hospital:** Stanford Univ Med Ctr; **Address:** Stanford Univ Med Ctr, 770 Welch Rd, Ste 400, Palo Alto, CA 94304; **Phone:** 650-723-5824; **Board Cert:** Plastic Surgery 2009; Hand Surgery 2002; **Med School:** Yale Univ 1993; **Resid:** Plastic Surgery, Stanford Univ Med Ctr 1998; **Fellow:** Hand Surgery, UCLA Med Ctr 2000; **Fac Appt:** Prof PlS, Stanford Univ

Cohen, Steven R MD [PlS] - **Spec Exp:** Craniofacial Surgery-Pediatric; Craniofacial Surgery/Reconstruction; **Hospital:** Rady Children's Hosp - San Diego, UCSD Med Ctr; **Address:** 8899 Univ Center Ln, Ste 350, San Diego, CA 92122; **Phone:** 858-453-7224; **Board Cert:** Plastic Surgery 1992; **Med School:** Geo Wash Univ 1980; **Resid:** Surgery, Columbia-Presby Med Ctr 1982; Surgery, Dartmouth-Hitchcock Med Ctr 1987; **Fellow:** Plastic Surgery, Hosp Univ Penn 1989; Craniofacial Surgery, UCLA Med Ctr 1990

Daniel, Rollin K MD [PlS] - **Spec Exp:** Cosmetic Surgery-Face; Rhinoplasty; **Hospital:** Hoag Meml Hosp Presby; **Address:** 1441 Avocado Ave, Ste 308, Newport Beach, CA 92660; **Phone:** 949-721-0494; **Board Cert:** Plastic Surgery 1977; **Med School:** Columbia P&S 1972; **Resid:** Plastic Surgery, McGill Univ Affil Hosps 1975; Hand Surgery, Univ Louisville Hosp 1976; **Fellow:** Craniofacial Surgery, Toronto Genl Hosp

Evans, Gregory R MD [PlS] - **Spec Exp:** Cosmetic Surgery-Face & Eyes; Cosmetic Surgery-Breast; Facial Plastic & Reconstructive Surgery; **Hospital:** UC Irvine Med Ctr; **Address:** Univ Calif Irvine, 200 S Manchester Ave, Ste 650, Orange, CA 92868; **Phone:** 714-456-5253; **Board Cert:** Surgery 2001; Plastic Surgery 2008; **Med School:** Univ SC Sch Med 1985; **Resid:** Surgery, USC Med Ctr 1990; Plastic Surgery, Johns Hopkins Hosp 1993; **Fac Appt:** Prof PlS, UC Irvine

Fisher, Garth MD [PlS] - **Spec Exp:** Cosmetic Surgery-Face; Cosmetic Surgery-Breast; Rhinoplasty; **Hospital:** St John's Hlth Ctr, Santa Monica; **Address:** 120 S Spalding Drive, Ste 222, Beverly Hills, CA 90212; **Phone:** 310-273-5995; **Board Cert:** Plastic Surgery 1993; **Med School:** Univ Miss 1984; **Resid:** Surgery, UC Irvine Med Ctr 1989; Plastic Surgery, UC Irvine Med Ctr 1991

Fodor, Peter B MD [PlS] - **Spec Exp:** Cosmetic Surgery; Liposuction & Body Contouring; **Hospital:** Olympia Med Ctr, Century City Hosp; **Address:** 2080 Century Park E, Ste 710, Century City, CA 90067; **Phone:** 310-203-9818; **Board Cert:** Plastic Surgery 1977; **Med School:** Univ Wisc 1966; **Resid:** Surgery, Columbia-Presby Med Ctr 1968; Plastic Surgery, St Luke's Hosp 1976; **Fac Appt:** Assoc Clin Prof S, UCLA

Garner, Warren L MD [PlS] - **Spec Exp:** Burns-Reconstructive Plastic Surgery; Wound Healing/Care; Skin Healing; **Hospital:** LAC & USC Med Ctr, USC Univ Hosp; **Address:** 1510 San Pablo St, Ste 415, Los Angeles, CA 90033; **Phone:** 323-442-7920; **Board Cert:** Plastic Surgery 1991; Surgical Critical Care 2001; **Med School:** Univ Kans 1978; **Resid:** Surgery, Ohio State Univ Hosp 1985; Plastic Surgery, Wash Univ Hosp 1989; **Fellow:** Critical Care Medicine, Ohio State Univ Hosp 1986; **Fac Appt:** Assoc Prof PlS, USC Sch Med

Gruss, Joseph MD [PlS] - **Spec Exp:** Maxillofacial & Craniofacial Surgery; Facial Trauma/Fractures; Cleft Palate/Lip; Pediatric Plastic Surgery; **Hospital:** Chldns Hosp and Regl Med Ctr - Seattle, Harborview Med Ctr; **Address:** Childrens Hosp & Regional Med Ctr, 4800 Sand Point Way NE, Box 5371, Seattle, WA 98105-3901; **Phone:** 206-987-2039; **Med School:** South Africa 1969; **Resid:** Plastic Surgery, Toronto Western Hosp 1976; Plastic Surgery, Hosp for Sick Children 1976; **Fellow:** Surgical Oncology, Princess Margaret Hosp 1977; Head and Neck Surgery, Princess Margaret Hosp 1977; **Fac Appt:** Prof PlS, Univ Wash

Hansen, Juliana MD [PlS] - **Spec Exp:** Breast Reconstruction; Cancer Reconstruction; **Hospital:** OR Hlth & Sci Univ; **Address:** 3303 SW Bond Ave, MC CH5P, Portland, OR 97239; **Phone:** 503-494-6687; **Board Cert:** Plastic Surgery 2008; **Med School:** Univ Wash 1988; **Resid:** Surgery, UCSF Med Ctr 1994; Plastic Surgery, UCSF Med Ctr 1996

Hardesty, Robert MD [PlS] - **Spec Exp:** Cosmetic Surgery-Face & Body; Cosmetic & Reconstructive Surgery; Body Contouring; Cosmetic Surgery-Breast; **Hospital:** Riverside Comm Hosp, Loma Linda Univ Med Ctr; **Address:** 4646 Brockton Ave, Ste 302, Riverside, CA 92506; **Phone:** 951-686-7600; **Board Cert:** Plastic Surgery 1989; **Med School:** Loma Linda Univ 1978; **Resid:** Surgery, Loma Linda Univ Med Ctr 1983; Plastic Surgery, Univ Pittsburgh 1986; **Fellow:** Pediatric Plastic Surgery, Washington Univ Chldns Hosp 1987; **Fac Appt:** Clin Prof PlS, Loma Linda Univ

Hoefflin, Steven M MD [PlS] - **Spec Exp:** Cosmetic Surgery-Face; Reconstructive Surgery; **Hospital:** St John's Hlth Ctr, Santa Monica; **Address:** 1530 Arizona Ave, Santa Monica, CA 90404-1234; **Phone:** 310-451-4733; **Board Cert:** Plastic Surgery 1978; **Med School:** UCLA 1972; **Resid:** Surgery, UCLA Med Ctr 1974; Plastic Reconstructive Surgery, UCLA Med Ctr 1977; **Fac Appt:** Assoc Clin Prof PlS, UCLA

Hoffman, William Y MD [PlS] - **Spec Exp:** Facial Plastic Surgery; Rhinoplasty; Liposuction & Body Contouring; Pediatric Plastic Surgery; **Hospital:** UCSF Med Ctr, CA Pacific Med Ctr - Pacific Campus; **Address:** UC San Francisco, Plastic Surgery, 350 Parnassus Ave, Ste 509, Box 0932, San Francisco, CA 94117; **Phone:** 415-476-9236; **Board Cert:** Plastic Surgery 1987; **Med School:** Univ Rochester 1977; **Resid:** Surgery, UCSF Med Ctr 1983; Plastic Surgery, UCSF Med Ctr 1985; **Fellow:** Craniofacial Surgery, NYU Med Ctr 1986; **Fac Appt:** Prof PlS, UCSF

Horowitz, Jed H MD [PlS] - **Spec Exp:** Cosmetic Surgery-Breast; Cosmetic Surgery-Face; Transumbilical Breast Augmentation(TUBA); **Hospital:** Hoag Meml Hosp Presby, Orange Coast Memorial Med Ctr; **Address:** 7677 Center Ave, Ste 401, Huntington Beach, CA 92647-3098; **Phone:** 714-902-1100; **Board Cert:** Plastic Surgery 1986; **Med School:** SUNY Buffalo 1977; **Resid:** Surgery, Grady Meml Hosp 1983; **Fellow:** Plastic Surgery, Univ Virginia 1985; **Fac Appt:** Asst Clin Prof PlS, USC Sch Med

Isik, Ferda Frank MD [PlS] - **Spec Exp:** Cosmetic Surgery-Face & Body; Breast Reconstruction; **Hospital:** Swedish Med Ctr - Seattle; **Address:** The Polyclinic, 1145 Broadway, Seattle, WA 98122; **Phone:** 206-860-4566; **Board Cert:** Surgery 2001; Plastic Surgery 2007; **Med School:** Mount Sinai Sch Med 1985; **Resid:** Surgery, Boston Univ Hosps 1990; Plastic Surgery, Univ Wash Affil Hosp 1995; **Fellow:** Pathology, NIH / Univ Wash 1992

Jewell, Mark L MD [PlS] - **Spec Exp:** Liposuction & Body Contouring; Cosmetic Surgery-Face; Breast Reconstruction; Cosmetic Surgery-Breast; **Hospital:** Sacred Heart Med Ctr; **Address:** 10 Coburg Rd, Ste 300, Eugene, OR 97401; **Phone:** 541-683-3234; **Board Cert:** Plastic Surgery 1981; **Med School:** Univ Kans 1973; **Resid:** Surgery, LAC-Harbor Med Ctr 1976; Plastic Surgery, Erlanger Hosp 1979; **Fellow:** Burn Surgery, LAC-USC Med Ctr 1977; **Fac Appt:** Asst Clin Prof PlS, Oregon Hlth & Sci Univ

Jones, Neil F MD [PlS] - **Spec Exp:** Hand Reconstruction-Pediatric; Nerve Disorders/Surgery; Tendon Surgery; Hand Surgery; **Hospital:** UC Irvine Med Ctr; **Address:** 101 The City Drive S, Route 94, Pavilion III, Los Angeles, CA 90095; **Phone:** 714-456-7012; **Board Cert:** Plastic Surgery 1985; **Med School:** England, UK 1974; **Resid:** Surgery, Radcliffe Infirmary 1979; Plastic Surgery, Univ Mich Med Ctr 1981; **Fellow:** Plastic Surgery, St Bartholomew's Hosp 1982; Hand & Microvascular Surgery, Mass Gen Hosp/Harvard 1983; **Fac Appt:** Prof PlS, UC Irvine

Kawamoto Jr, Henry K MD/DDS [PlS] - **Spec Exp:** Cosmetic Surgery; Craniofacial Surgery; Maxillofacial Surgery; **Hospital:** UCLA Ronald Reagan Med Ctr, St John's Hlth Ctr, Santa Monica; **Address:** 1301 20th St, Ste 460, Santa Monica, CA 90404; **Phone:** 310-829-0391; **Board Cert:** Surgery 1972; Plastic Surgery 1976; **Med School:** USC Sch Med 1964; **Resid:** Surgery, Columbia-Presby Med Ctr 1971; Plastic Surgery, NYU Med Ctr 1973; **Fellow:** Craniofacial Surgery, Dr Paul Tessier 1974; **Fac Appt:** Clin Prof S, UCLA

Koplin, Lawrence M MD [PlS] - **Spec Exp:** Cosmetic Surgery-Face; **Hospital:** Cedars-Sinai Med Ctr; **Address:** 465 N Roxbury Drive, Ste 800, Beverly Hills, CA 90210; **Phone:** 310-277-3223; **Board Cert:** Plastic Surgery 1985; **Med School:** Baylor Coll Med 1976; **Resid:** Surgery, Kaiser Fdn Hosp 1981; Plastic Surgery, St Joseph Hosp 1983

Leaf, Norman MD [PlS] - **Spec Exp:** Cosmetic Surgery-Face; Cosmetic Surgery-Breast; **Hospital:** Cedars-Sinai Med Ctr, UCLA Ronald Reagan Med Ctr; **Address:** 436 N Bedford, Ste 104, Beverly Hills, CA 90210-4310; **Phone:** 310-274-8001; **Board Cert:** Surgery 1973; Plastic Surgery 1974; **Med School:** Univ Chicago-Pritzker Sch Med 1966; **Resid:** Surgery, Univ Chicago Hosps 1972; Plastic Surgery, Univ Chicago Hosps 1973; **Fellow:** Research, Univ Chicago Hosp-US Pub Hlth Svc-NIH 1969; **Fac Appt:** Asst Clin Prof PlS, UCLA

Lesavoy, Malcolm A MD [PlS] - **Spec Exp:** Reconstructive Surgery; Cosmetic Surgery; Hand Surgery; **Hospital:** UCLA Ronald Reagan Med Ctr; **Address:** 16311 Ventura Blvd, Ste 555, Encino, CA 91436-4314; **Phone:** 818-986-8270; **Board Cert:** Plastic Surgery 1977; **Med School:** Ros Franklin Univ/Chicago Med Sch 1969; **Resid:** Surgery, Univ Chicago Hosps 1974; Plastic Surgery, Univ Miami Hosp/Clinics 1976; **Fac Appt:** Clin Prof PlS, UCLA

Markowitz, Bernard Lloyd MD [PlS] - **Spec Exp:** Cosmetic Surgery-Face; Craniofacial Surgery/Reconstruction; **Hospital:** UCLA Ronald Reagan Med Ctr, Cedars-Sinai Med Ctr; **Address:** 9675 Brighton Way, Ste 350, Beverly Hills, CA 90210; **Phone:** 310-205-5557; **Board Cert:** Plastic Surgery 1989; **Med School:** NYU Sch Med 1979; **Resid:** Surgery, NYU Med Ctr 1984; Plastic Surgery, NYU Med Ctr 1986; **Fellow:** Maxillofacial Surgery, Johns Hopkins Hosp 1987; Microvascular Surgery, Johns Hopkins Hosp 1987; **Fac Appt:** Clin Prof PlS, UCLA

Marten, Timothy Ja MD [PlS] - **Spec Exp:** Cosmetic Surgery-Face; Facial Rejuvenation; **Hospital:** CA Pacific Med Ctr, St Mary's Med Ctr - San Fran; **Address:** Marten Clinic of Plastic Surgery, 450 Sutter St, Ste 2222, San Francisco, CA 94108-4207; **Phone:** 415-677-9937; **Board Cert:** Plastic Surgery 1993; **Med School:** UC Davis 1982; **Resid:** Surgery, Kaiser Fdn Hosp 1987; Plastic Surgery, Univ Illinois Chicago Hosp 1989; **Fellow:** Cosmetic Plastic Surgery, Connell Aesthetic Network 1990; Cosmetic Plastic Surgery, Baker, Gordon, & Stuzin

Miller, Timothy A MD [PlS] - **Spec Exp:** Cosmetic Surgery-Face; Eyelid Cancer & Reconstruction; Skin Cancer; Nasal Reconstruction; **Hospital:** UCLA Ronald Reagan Med Ctr; **Address:** 200 UCLA Medical Plaza, Ste 465, Los Angeles, CA 90095-8344; **Phone:** 310-825-5644; **Board Cert:** Surgery 1971; Plastic Surgery 1973; **Med School:** UCLA 1963; **Resid:** Surgery, Johns Hopkins Hosp 1967; Thoracic Surgery, UCLA Med Ctr 1969; **Fellow:** Plastic Surgery, Univ Pittsburgh 1971; **Fac Appt:** Prof S, UCLA

Nichter, Larry S MD [PlS] - **Spec Exp:** Breast Reconstruction & Augmentation; Cosmetic Surgery-Face; Liposuction & Body Contouring; Hand Surgery; **Hospital:** Hoag Meml Hosp Presby, Orange Coast Memorial Med Ctr; **Address:** 7677 Center Ave, Ste 401, Huntington Beach, CA 92647-3098; **Phone:** 714-902-1100; **Board Cert:** Plastic Surgery 1986; **Med School:** Boston Univ 1978; **Resid:** Surgery, UCLA Medical Ctr 1982; Plastic Surgery, Univ Virginia Med Ctr 1985; **Fellow:** Hand & Microvascular Surgery, Univ Virginia 1983; Craniofacial Surgery, Univ Virginia 1985; **Fac Appt:** Clin Prof PlS, Univ SC Sch Med

Paul, Malcolm D MD [PlS] - **Spec Exp:** Cosmetic Surgery-Face; Cosmetic Surgery-Breast; Liposuction & Body Contouring; **Hospital:** Hoag Meml Hosp Presby; **Address:** 1401 Avocado Ave, Ste 810, Newport Beach, CA 92660-8708; **Phone:** 949-760-5047; **Board Cert:** Plastic Surgery 1976; **Med School:** Univ MD Sch Med 1969; **Resid:** Surgery, Geo Wash Med Ctr 1973; Plastic Surgery, Geo Wash Med Ctr 1975; **Fac Appt:** Clin Prof S, UC Irvine

Rand, Richard Pierce MD [PlS] - **Spec Exp:** Cosmetic Surgery-Face; Cosmetic Surgery-Breast; Abdominoplasty; **Hospital:** Overlake Hosp Med Ctr; **Address:** 1135 116th Ave NE, Ste 630, Bellevue, WA 98004-4623; **Phone:** 425-688-8828; **Board Cert:** Surgery 1998; Plastic Surgery 1991; **Med School:** Univ Mich Med Sch 1981; **Resid:** Surgery, Tufts-New England Med Ctr 1986; Plastic Surgery, Emory Univ Hosp 1989; **Fellow:** Craniofacial Surgery, Univ Miami 1989; **Fac Appt:** Assoc Prof S, Univ Wash

Reinisch, John F MD [PlS] - **Spec Exp:** Ear Reconstruction/Microtia; Cleft Palate/Lip; Craniofacial Surgery/Reconstruction; **Hospital:** Cedars-Sinai Med Ctr; **Address:** 250 N Robertson Blvd, Ste 506, Beverly Hills, CA 90211; **Phone:** 310-385-6090; **Board Cert:** Plastic Surgery 1980; **Med School:** Harvard Med Sch 1970; **Resid:** Surgery, Univ Mich Med Ctr 1975; Plastic Surgery, Univ Virginia Hosp 1978; **Fac Appt:** Prof S, USC Sch Med

Plastic Surgery

Ristow, Brunno MD [PlS] - **Spec Exp:** Cosmetic Surgery-Face; Facial Plastic & Reconstructive Surgery; Rhinoplasty; Nasal Reconstruction; **Hospital:** CA Pacific Med Ctr - Pacific Campus; **Address:** 2100 Webster St, Ste 501, San Francisco, CA 94115-2381; **Phone:** 415-202-1507; **Board Cert:** Plastic Surgery 1975; **Med School:** Brazil 1966; **Resid:** Surgery, NY Hosp-Cornell Med Ctr 1971; Plastic Surgery, NYU Med Ctr 1973; **Fellow:** Plastic Surgery, NYU Med Ctr 1968

Romano, James John MD [PlS] - **Spec Exp:** Cosmetic Surgery; Cosmetic Surgery-Breast; Rhinoplasty; **Hospital:** CA Pacific Med Ctr - CA Campus, Seton Med Ctr; **Address:** 126 Post St, Ste 618, San Francisco, CA 94108; **Phone:** 415-981-3911; **Board Cert:** Plastic Surgery 1990; **Med School:** Eastern VA Med Sch 1980; **Resid:** Surgery, Georgetown Univ Hosp 1985; Plastic Surgery, Johns Hopkins Hosp 1988; **Fac Appt:** Asst Prof PlS, USC Sch Med

Rosenberg, Howard L MD [PlS] - **Spec Exp:** Cosmetic Surgery-Breast; Cosmetic Surgery-Face; Liposuction; **Hospital:** El Camino Hosp; **Address:** 2204 Grant Rd, Ste 201, Mountain View, CA 94040; **Phone:** 650-961-2652; **Board Cert:** Surgery 1975; Plastic Surgery 1977; **Med School:** Johns Hopkins Univ 1969; **Resid:** Surgery, UCLA Med Ctr 1974; Plastic Surgery, Stanford Univ Med Ctr 1976; **Fac Appt:** Asst Clin Prof PlS, Stanford Univ

Sherman, Randolph MD [PlS] - **Spec Exp:** Facial Paralysis; Breast Reconstruction; Limb Surgery/Reconstruction; **Hospital:** Cedars-Sinai Med Ctr; **Address:** 8635 W 3rd St, Ste 770W, Los Angeles, CA 90048; **Phone:** 310-423-2129; **Board Cert:** Surgery 2004; Plastic Surgery 1986; Hand Surgery 2000; **Med School:** Univ MO-Columbia Sch Med 1977; **Resid:** Surgery, UCSF Hosps 1981; Surgery, State Univ of New York 1983; **Fellow:** Plastic Surgery, USC Med Ctr 1985; **Fac Appt:** Prof S, USC Sch Med

Singer, Robert MD [PlS] - **Spec Exp:** Cosmetic Surgery-Face; Cosmetic Surgery-Breast; Liposuction & Body Contouring; **Hospital:** Scripps Meml Hosp - La Jolla; **Address:** 9834 Genesee Ave, Ste 100, La Jolla, CA 92037-1214; **Phone:** 858-455-0290; **Board Cert:** Plastic Surgery 1977; **Med School:** SUNY Buffalo 1967; **Resid:** Surgery, Stanford Med Ctr 1969; Plastic Surgery, Vanderbilt Univ Hosp 1976; **Fellow:** Neurological Surgery, Rigs Hosp-Kommunes Hosp 1976

Stevenson, Thomas R MD [PlS] - ; **Address:** UC Davis Med Grp Surgical, 3301 C Rd, Ste 1100, Sacramento, CA 95816-4300; **Phone:** 916-734-4323; **Board Cert:** Surgery 1979; Plastic Surgery 1983; Hand Surgery 1994; **Med School:** Univ Kans 1972; **Resid:** Surgery, Univ VA Hosp 1978; Plastic Surgery, Emory Univ 1982; **Fac Appt:** Prof PlS, UC Davis

Urata, Mark M MD/DDS [PlS] - **Spec Exp:** Craniofacial Surgery-Pediatric; Craniofacial Surgery; **Hospital:** Chldns Hosp - Los Angeles; **Address:** CHLA, Plastic Surgery #96, Los Angeles, CA 90027-6062; **Phone:** 323-361-2154; **Board Cert:** Plastic Surgery 2005; **Med School:** USC Sch Med 1996; **Resid:** Oral & Maxillofacial Surgery, USC Med Ctr 1993; Plastic Surgery, USC Med Ctr 2002; **Fellow:** Craniofacial Surgery, LAC-USC Med Ctr 2003; **Fac Appt:** Prof PlS, USC-Keck School of Medicine

Wells, James H MD [PlS] - **Spec Exp:** Cleft Palate/Lip; Breast Surgery; **Hospital:** Long Beach Meml Med Ctr; **Address:** 2880 Atlantic Ave, Ste 209, Long Beach, CA 90806; **Phone:** 562-595-6543; **Board Cert:** Plastic Surgery 1978; **Med School:** Univ Tex Med Br, Galveston 1966; **Resid:** Surgery, Ochsner Fdn Hosp 1971; Plastic Surgery, Univ Virginia Hosp 1975

Cleveland Clinic

Plastic Surgery

Cleveland Clinic Department of Plastic Surgery, part of the Dermatology and Plastic Surgery Institute, offers a full array of subspecialized care for adult and pediatric patients.

Among the department's major advancements is the successful completion in 2008 of the first near-total face transplant in the United States.

The department has also focused on minimally invasive techniques in facial cosmetic surgery. This includes alternatives to face and necklift surgery, short-scar facelifts and minimally invasive facelift techniques. Cleveland Clinic plastic surgeons offer numerous methods of breast reconstruction that can be performed either at the time of mastectomy or as a secondary procedure. These techniques include breast implants and expanders; pedicled transverse rectus abdominis myocutaneous (TRAM) flaps (using abdominal skin and muscle); and free-tissue transfers such as deep inferior epigastric perforator (DIEP) flap. The DIEP flap minimizes injury to the abdominal wall while providing an ideal breast reconstruction using the patient's own tissue.

In addition to standard body contouring techniques including abdominoplasty and a wide variety of liposuction techniques, the department is particularly interested in plastic surgery after significant weight loss.

The department also includes a team of surgeons adept at handling all types of traumatic, congenital and work-related hand, peripheral nerve and upper-extremity problems.

Pediatric surgery and craniofacial surgery are strong specialties in this department.

For more information about the Cleveland Clinic Department of Plastic Surgery, to schedule a second opinion or to learn about assistance for out-of-town patients, call 800.890.2467 or visit clevelandclinic.org/plasticstopdocs.

Cleveland Clinic plastic surgeons offer expert diagnostic and management options including:

- Facial cosmetic surgery
- Reconstructive breast surgery
- Reconstruction after cancer
- Cosmetic breast surgery
- Body Contouring
- Liposuction
- Hand surgery
- Pediatric surgery and craniofacial surgery
- Microsurgery
- Complex wound repair

Cleveland Clinic Department of Plastic Surgery
9500 Euclid Avenue / AC311 | Cleveland OH 44195

NY Eye & Ear Infirmary

Continuum Health Partners, Inc.

THE NEW YORK EYE AND EAR INFIRMARY

310 East 14th Street
New York, New York 10003
Tel. 212.979.4000   Fax. 212.228.0664
http://www.nyee.edu

PROVIDING EXCEPTIONAL CARE

The Department of Plastic & Reconstructive Surgery is one of the region's most comprehensive centers for surgery which restores the body and spirit. More than 1,500 procedures a year are performed here, and 50 of the most noted board-certified plastic surgeons located throughout New York City and tri-state area comprise the attending medical staff.

IN A HIGHLY SPECIALIZED SETTING

As a specialty hospital, the Infirmary is uniquely qualified to handle the most complicated cases. It serves as a nationwide referral center with a commitment to teaching, research, and high-technology based patient care. Highly experienced staff using state-of-the-art instrumentation have made the Infirmary's 17 operating rooms a national benchmark in efficiency. In addition, private premium patient accommodations are available to assure that the hospital experience is as comfortable and convenient as possible.

FOR PATIENTS OF ALL AGES

Cutting edge technologies at New York Eye and Ear are continually improving peoples' lives. The latest version of a skin tightening Fraxel Re:pair laser enables many patients to avoid a surgical face and eyelid plastic operation. The Post Cancer Breast Reconstruction Institute performs the latest deep perforator microvascular flap reconstructions, and microvascular plastic surgeons aid in other post trauma and cancer reconstruction.

Childhood problems, such as cleft lip and palate and ear deformities also fall under the care of our surgeons.

The hospital has a Post Graduate Cosmetic Surgery Program which offers a year of intensive cosmetic surgery training to surgeons who have completed a formal plastic surgery residency. The program is the largest and most sought-after in the US and also provides a source for affordable cosmetic surgery for the community.

Innovative cosmetic surgery procedures such as endoscopic and other minimally invasive operations are offered. The Center for Nasal Plastic specializes in closed (no scar) nasal plastic techniques as well as repair of previous nasal surgeries, the secondary nasal plasty. Liposuction using the latest instrumentation and fat grafting by the latest technology is also available as are the latest variants of the abdominoplasty (tummy tuck) operation.

Plastic Surgery Clinical Services

Facial plasty

Eyelid plastic operations

Nasal plastic operations

Breast augmentation
Breast reduction procedures and suspension

Breast reconstruction using patient's own tissue
(DIEP, S-GAP, I-GAP and SIEA flap procedures)

Liposuction

Abdominoplasty

Facial resurfacing and dermabrasion

Fraxel laser

Botox

About The New York Eye and Ear Infirmary

Founded in 1820, it is the nation's oldest, continuously operating specialty hospital Throughout its history, the Infirmary has led clinical advances and research in vision, hearing, speech and restoration of the physical appearance.

**Physician Referral
1.800.449.HOPE (4673)**

Preventive & Occupational Medicine

A preventive medicine specialist focuses on the health of individuals and defined populations in order to protect, promote and maintain health and well-being, and to prevent disease, disability and premature death. A preventive medicine physician may be a specialist in general preventive medicine, public health, occupational medicine, or aerospace medicine. This specialist works with large population groups as well as with individual patients to promote health and understand the risks of disease, injury, disability, and death, seeking to modify and eliminate these risks.

Training Required: Three years

OCCUPATIONAL MEDICINE

Mid Atlantic

Gochfeld, Michael MD/PhD [OM] - **Spec Exp:** Environmental Medicine; Chemical Exposure; Mercury Toxic Exposure; **Hospital:** Robert Wood Johnson Univ Hosp - New Brunswick; **Address:** Enviro & Occupational Health - EOHSI, 170 Frelinghuysen Rd, Ste 200, Piscataway, NJ 08854; **Phone:** 732-445-0123 x627; **Board Cert:** Occupational Medicine 1983; **Med School:** Albert Einstein Coll Med 1965; **Resid:** Behavioral Medicine, Rockefeller Univ 1977; **Fac Appt:** Prof OM, UMDNJ-RW Johnson Med Sch

Landrigan, Philip MD [OM] - **Spec Exp:** Environmental Health in Children; **Hospital:** Mount Sinai Med Ctr (page 64); **Address:** Dept of Comm & Prev Med, One Gustave L Levy Pl, Box 1057, New York, NY 10029-6500; **Phone:** 212-824-7018; **Board Cert:** Pediatrics 1973; Public Health & Genl Preventive Med 1979; Occupational Medicine 1983; **Med School:** Harvard Med Sch 1967; **Resid:** Internal Medicine, Metro Genl Hosp 1968; Pediatrics, Chldns Hosp 1970; **Fellow:** Epidemiology, Ctrs for Disease Control 1973; Occupational Medicine, Univ London 1977; **Fac Appt:** Prof Ped, Mount Sinai Sch Med

West Coast and Pacific

Cullen, Mark R MD [OM] - **Spec Exp:** Mesothelioma; **Hospital:** Stanford Univ Med Ctr; **Address:** Stanford Gen'l Internal Med, 251 Campus Drive, MSOBx338, Stanford, CA 94306; **Phone:** 650-721-6209; **Board Cert:** Internal Medicine 1979; Occupational Medicine 1986; **Med School:** Yale Univ 1976; **Resid:** Internal Medicine, Yale-New Haven Hosp 1979; **Fac Appt:** Prof Med, Stanford Univ

Harber, Philip I MD [OM] - **Spec Exp:** Occupational Medicine; Environmental Medicine; **Hospital:** UCLA Ronald Reagan Med Ctr; **Address:** UCLA Med Ctr, Dept Occupational Med, 10880 Wilshire Blvd, Ste 1800, Los Angeles, CA 90024; **Phone:** 310-794-8144; **Board Cert:** Internal Medicine 1979; Pulmonary Disease 1980; Occupational Medicine 1982; **Med School:** Univ Pennsylvania 1972; **Resid:** Internal Medicine, Georgetown Univ Med Ctr 1978; Occupational Medicine, Johns Hopkins Hosp 1980; **Fellow:** Pulmonary Disease, Johns Hopkins Hosp 1980; **Fac Appt:** Assoc Prof Med, UCLA

PREVENTIVE MEDICINE

Mid Atlantic

Cahill, John MD [PrM] - **Spec Exp:** Tropical Diseases; Travel Medicine; Parasitic Infections; International Health; **Hospital:** St Luke's - Roosevelt Hosp Ctr - Roosevelt Div (page 57); **Address:** 425 W 59th St, Ste 8A, New York, NY 10019; **Phone:** 212-492-5500; **Board Cert:** Emergency Medicine 2001; **Med School:** Mount Sinai Sch Med 1996; **Resid:** Emergency Medicine, Rhode Island Hosp 1997; Emergency Medicine, Rhode Island Hosp 2000; **Fellow:** Tropical Medicine, Royal Coll Surgeons 1998; **Fac Appt:** Asst Clin Prof Med, Columbia P&S

Cahill, Kevin M MD [PrM] - **Spec Exp:** Tropical Diseases; International Health; Parasitic Infections; **Hospital:** Lenox Hill Hosp (page 62); **Address:** 850 5th Ave, New York, NY 10021; **Phone:** 212-434-2477; **Board Cert:** Public Health & Genl Preventive Med 1970; **Med School:** Cornell Univ-Weill Med Coll 1961; **Resid:** Internal Medicine, US Navy Med Res Unit 1965; Public Health & Genl Preventive Med, US Navy Med Res Unit 1965; **Fac Appt:** Clin Prof Med, NYU Sch Med

Hoffman, Robert S MD [PrM] - **Spec Exp:** Poison Control; Disaster Preparedness; **Hospital:** NYU Langone Med Ctr (page 67), Bellevue Hosp Ctr; **Address:** NY Poison Control Ctr, 455 1st Ave, rm 123, New York, NY 10016; **Phone:** 212-340-4494; **Board Cert:** Internal Medicine 1987; Emergency Medicine 2005; Medical Toxicology 1999; **Med School:** NYU Sch Med 1984; **Resid:** Internal Medicine, NYU Med Ctr 1987; **Fellow:** Medical Toxicology, NYU Med Ctr 1989; **Fac Appt:** Asst Clin Prof EM, NYU Sch Med

Lane, Dorothy S MD [PrM] - **Spec Exp:** Women's Health; Cancer Prevention; Health Promotion & Disease Prevention; **Hospital:** Stony Brook Univ Med Ctr; **Address:** Stony Brook Univ Sch Med, HSC L2, rm 142, Stony Brook, NY 11794-8222; **Phone:** 631-444-2094; **Board Cert:** Public Health & Genl Preventive Med 1970; **Med School:** Columbia P&S 1965; **Resid:** Public Health & Genl Preventive Med, NY Health Dept 1968; **Fac Appt:** Prof PrM, SUNY Stony Brook

Pearson, Thomas A MD/PhD [PrM] - **Spec Exp:** Preventive Cardiology; Cholesterol/Lipid Disorders; **Hospital:** Univ of Rochester Strong Meml Hosp; **Address:** 601 Elmwood Ave, Box 644, Rochester, NY 14642; **Phone:** 585-341-7100; **Board Cert:** Internal Medicine 1983; Preventive Medicine 1986; **Med School:** Johns Hopkins Univ 1976; **Resid:** Preventive Medicine, Johns Hopkins Hosp 1979; Internal Medicine, Johns Hopkins Hosp 1980; **Fellow:** Cardiovascular Disease, Johns Hopkins Hosp 1983; **Fac Appt:** Prof PrM, Univ Rochester

Weiss, Stanley H MD [PrM] - **Spec Exp:** Cancer Epidemiology & Control; AIDS Related Infections; Disaster Preparedness; Infections in Cancer Patients; **Hospital:** UMDNJ-Univ Hosp-Newark; **Address:** NJ Medical School-UMDNJ, 30 Bergen St, ADMC16, Ste 1614, Newark, NJ 07107-3000; **Phone:** 973-972-4623; **Board Cert:** Internal Medicine 1981; Medical Oncology 1985; **Med School:** Harvard Med Sch 1978; **Resid:** Internal Medicine, Montefiore Med Ctr 1981; **Fellow:** Medical Oncology, National Cancer Inst 1985; Epidemiology, National Cancer Inst 1987; **Fac Appt:** Prof PrM, UMDNJ-NJ Med Sch, Newark

THE MOUNT SINAI MEDICAL CENTER
OCCUPATIONAL AND ENVIRONMENTAL MEDICINE

One Gustave L. Levy Place
Fifth Avenue and 100th Street
New York, NY 10029-6574
Physician Referral: 1-800-MD-SINAI (637-4624)
www.mountsinai.org

THE IRVING J. SELIKOFF CLINICAL CENTER FOR OCCUPATIONAL AND ENVIRONMENTAL MEDICINE is an internationally respected diagnostic and treatment center. The mission of the Center is to prevent occupational disease in the workplace and reduce morbidity and mortality associated with work. To achieve this goal, we utilize a preventive medicine model that includes three integrated components:

Clinical Care – Our services include the diagnosis, treatment, and management of occupational diseases and work-related musculoskeletal disorders for current and retired workers. We offer disability assessment and rehabilitation services to facilitate a safe return to work and appropriate accommodations. Our social workers provide counseling regarding the financial, social, and psychological aspects of occupational disease.

Disease Prevention Services – Our team educates patients, health care providers, workers, unions, employers, and communities on the signs and symptoms of occupational disease. We provide comprehensive industrial hygiene and ergonomic services to evaluate exposures and recommend effective preventive measures. We also provide technical assistance and consultation services for employers, unions, and public health agencies.

Surveillance and Data Management – We study the pattern and prevalence of occupational disease and identify new links between workplace exposure and disease.

IMPROVING PUBLIC HEALTH

To promote disease prevention, the Center treats each newly identified case of occupational disease as a potential sentinel health event—that is, as a signal that there may be similar cases of disease in the patient's coworkers. This approach, coupled with our efforts to reduce workplace hazards, places the Center's impact well beyond individual patient evaluations. To help achieve our goal of improving public health by preventing occupational and environmental disease, we work closely with labor unions, employers, government and service organizations, health care providers, and community organizations.

The Clinical Center has satellite sites in Westchester County and Queens, where staff physicians see patients several days a week. Services available at the Irving J. Selikoff Center for Occupational and Environmental Medicine provide educational programs, guidance, and epidemiologic services to improve the health of workers.

PEDIATRIC ENVIRONMENTAL HEALTH SPECIALTY UNIT

We provide consultation and medical care for children with toxic environmental exposures and with diseases of suspected environmental origin. This unit serves New York, New Jersey, Puerto Rico, and the Virgin Islands.

WORLD TRADE CENTER (WTC) MEDICAL MONITORING AND TREATMENT PROGRAM
This federally funded program is available to workers and volunteers who participated in the rescue, recovery, and clean-up efforts following the 9/11 attacks. Services include:

• Medical evaluations for possible WTC-related health conditions

• Treatment at no cost for WTC workers covered under federally funded programs

• Mental health services

• Social work services to assist with Workers' Compensation and related benefits

• Patient education regarding WTC-related and other occupational health concerns

Psychiatry

A psychiatrist specializes in the prevention, diagnosis and treatment of mental, addictive and emotional disorders such as schizophrenia and other psychotic disorders, mood disorders, anxiety disorders, substance-related disorders, sexual and gender identity disorders and adjustment disorders. The psychiatrist is able to understand the biologic, psychologic and social components of illness, and therefore is uniquely prepared to treat the whole person. A psychiatrist is qualified to order diagnostic laboratory tests and to prescribe medications, evaluate and treat psychologic and interpersonal problems and to intervene with families who are coping with stress, crises and other problems in living.

Training Required: Four years

Certification in one of the following subspecialties requires additional training and examination.

Addiction Psychiatry: A psychiatrist who focuses on the evaluation and treatment of individuals with alcohol, drug, or other substance-related disorders and of individuals with the dual diagnosis of substance-related and other psychiatric disorders.

Child and Adolescent Psychiatry: A psychiatrist with additional training in the diagnosis and treatment of developmental, behavioral, emotional and mental disorders of childhood and adolescence.

Geriatric Psychiatry: A psychiatrist with expertise in the prevention, evaluation, diagnosis and treatment of mental and emotional disorders in the elderly. The geriatric psychiatrist seeks to improve the psychiatric care of the elderly both in health and in disease.

PSYCHIATRY

New England

Block, Susan D MD [Psyc] - **Spec Exp:** Psychiatry in Cancer; Palliative Care; **Hospital:** Dana-Farber Cancer Inst, Brigham & Women's Hosp; **Address:** Dana Farber Cancer Inst, 44 Binney St, SW 411, Boston, MA 02115; **Phone:** 617-632-5788; **Board Cert:** Psychiatry 1984; Internal Medicine 1981; Hospice & Palliative Medicine 2003; **Med School:** Case West Res Univ 1977; **Resid:** Internal Medicine, Beth Israel Hosp 1980; Psychiatry, Beth Israel Hosp 1982; **Fac Appt:** Prof Psyc, Harvard Med Sch

Ellison, James M MD [Psyc] - **Spec Exp:** Geriatric Psychiatry; **Hospital:** McLean Hosp; **Address:** McLean Hospital, 115 Mill St, Belmont, MA 02478; **Phone:** 617-855-2532; **Board Cert:** Psychiatry 1984; Geriatric Psychiatry 2007; **Med School:** UCSF 1978; **Resid:** Psychiatry, Mass Genl Hosp 1982; **Fac Appt:** Assoc Prof Psyc, Harvard Med Sch

Friedman, Matthew J MD/PhD [Psyc] - **Spec Exp:** Post Traumatic Stress Disorder; Psychopharmacology; Anxiety & Mood Disorders; **Hospital:** VA Aff Med Ctr - White River Junction, Dartmouth - Hitchcock Med Ctr; **Address:** National Center for PTSD, VA Medical Ctr, 215 N Main St, White River Junction, VT 05009; **Phone:** 802-296-5132; **Board Cert:** Psychiatry 1976; **Med School:** Univ KY Coll Med 1976; **Resid:** Psychiatry, Mass Genl Hosp 1972; Psychiatry, Dartmouth Hitchcock Med Ctr 1973; **Fac Appt:** Prof Psyc, Dartmouth Med Sch

Goff, Donald C MD [Psyc] - **Spec Exp:** Schizophrenia; Psychopharmacology; **Hospital:** Mass Genl Hosp; **Address:** Freedom Trail Clin, 25 Stainford St, Boston, MA 02114; **Phone:** 617-912-7899; **Board Cert:** Psychiatry 1986; **Med School:** UCLA 1980; **Resid:** Psychiatry, Mass Genl Hosp 1984; **Fellow:** Psychopharmacology, Tufts-New England Med Ctr 1985; **Fac Appt:** Assoc Prof Psyc, Tufts Univ

Greenberg, Donna B MD [Psyc] - **Spec Exp:** Psychiatry in Cancer; **Hospital:** Mass Genl Hosp; **Address:** Mass General Hospital, Warren 605, 55 Fruit St, Boston, MA 02114-2696; **Phone:** 617-724-8400; **Board Cert:** Internal Medicine 1978; Psychiatry 1990; **Med School:** Univ Rochester 1975; **Resid:** Internal Medicine, Boston City Hosp 1978; Psychiatry, Mass Genl Hosp 1989; **Fellow:** Psychiatry, Mass Genl Hosp 1979; **Fac Appt:** Assoc Prof Psyc, Harvard Med Sch

Gunderson, John G MD [Psyc] - **Spec Exp:** Personality Disorders; Personality Disorders-Borderline; Psychotherapy; **Hospital:** McLean Hosp; **Address:** McLean Hospital, 115 Mill St, Belmont, MA 02478-9106; **Phone:** 617-855-2293; **Board Cert:** Psychiatry 1974; **Med School:** Harvard Med Sch 1967; **Resid:** Psychiatry, Mass Mental Hlth Ctr 1971; **Fac Appt:** Prof Psyc, Harvard Med Sch

Herman, John B MD [Psyc] - **Spec Exp:** Depression; Anxiety Disorders; **Hospital:** Mass Genl Hosp; **Address:** Mass Genl Hosp, Dept Psychiatry, 55 Fruit St, Bulfinch 351, Boston, MA 02114-3139; **Phone:** 617-726-2993; **Board Cert:** Psychiatry 1987; **Med School:** Univ Wisc 1980; **Resid:** Psychiatry, Mass Genl Hosp 1984; **Fac Appt:** Asst Prof Psyc, Harvard Med Sch

Jacobson, Alan M MD [Psyc] - **Spec Exp:** Depression in Diabetes; **Hospital:** Beth Israel Deaconess Med Ctr - Boston; **Address:** Joslin Diabetes Ctr/Joslin Clin, One Joslin Pl, Boston, MA 02215; **Phone:** 617-732-2594; **Board Cert:** Psychiatry 1975; **Med School:** Univ Chicago-Pritzker Sch Med 1969; **Resid:** Psychiatry, Mass Genl Hosp 1973; **Fac Appt:** Prof Psyc, Harvard Med Sch

Jenike, Michael A MD [Psyc] - **Spec Exp:** Obsessive-Compulsive Disorder; Geriatric Psychiatry; **Hospital:** Mass Genl Hosp; **Address:** Obsessive Compulsive Disorders Unit, 185 Cambridge St, Ste 2200, Boston, MA 02114; **Phone:** 617-726-6766; **Board Cert:** Psychiatry 1984; **Med School:** Univ Okla Coll Med 1978; **Resid:** Psychiatry, Mass Genl Hosp 1982; **Fellow:** Psychiatry, Harvard Med Sch; Psychiatry, Mass Genl Hosp; **Fac Appt:** Prof Psyc, Harvard Med Sch

McGlashan, Thomas H MD [Psyc] - **Spec Exp:** Schizophrenia-Early Detection/Treatment; Personality Disorders; Schizophrenia-Clinical Trials; Personality Disorders-Clinical Trials; **Hospital:** Connecticut Mental Hlth Ctr, Yale-New Haven Hosp; **Address:** Yale Univ Sch Med, Dept Psychiatry, 301 Cedar St, New Haven, CT 06519; **Phone:** 203-737-2077; **Board Cert:** Psychiatry 1973; **Med School:** Univ Pennsylvania 1967; **Resid:** Psychiatry, Mass Mental Hlth Ctr 1971; **Fac Appt:** Prof Psyc, Yale Univ

Phillips, Katharine A MD [Psyc] - **Spec Exp:** Body Dysmorphic Disorder (BDD); Obsessive-Compulsive Disorder; **Hospital:** Butler Hosp; **Address:** Butler Hosp, The Body Image Prgm, 345 Blackstone Blvd, Providence, RI 02906; **Phone:** 401-455-6490; **Board Cert:** Psychiatry 1992; **Med School:** Dartmouth Med Sch 1987; **Resid:** Psychiatry, McLean Hosp 1991; **Fac Appt:** Prof Psyc, Brown Univ

Price, Lawrence H MD [Psyc] - **Spec Exp:** Anxiety & Mood Disorders; Depression; Bipolar/Mood Disorders; Obsessive-Compulsive Disorder; **Hospital:** Butler Hosp, Kent Hosp; **Address:** Butler Hospital, Dept Psychiatry, 345 Blackstone Blvd, Providence, RI 02906; **Phone:** 401-455-6533; **Board Cert:** Psychiatry 1983; **Med School:** Univ Mich Med Sch 1978; **Resid:** Psychiatry, Yale-New Haven Hosp 1982; **Fellow:** Psychiatry, Yale-New Haven Hosp 1983; **Fac Appt:** Prof Psyc, Brown Univ

Rasmussen, Steven A MD [Psyc] - **Spec Exp:** Obsessive-Compulsive Disorder; **Hospital:** Butler Hosp; **Address:** Butler Hosp, 345 Blackstone Blvd, Providence, RI 02906; **Phone:** 401-455-6209; **Board Cert:** Psychiatry 1983; **Med School:** Brown Univ 1977; **Resid:** Psychiatry, Yale Univ 1981; **Fac Appt:** Assoc Prof Psyc, Brown Univ

Rauch, Paula K MD [Psyc] - **Spec Exp:** Psychiatry in Childhood Cancer; Children/Families with Severe Illness; Parent Guidance in Parental Cancer; **Hospital:** Mass Genl Hosp; **Address:** Mass General Hosp, Dept Child Psychiatry, 32 Fruit St, Yawkey 6, Boston, MA 02114; **Phone:** 617-724-5600; **Board Cert:** Psychiatry 1990; Child & Adolescent Psychiatry 1991; **Med School:** Univ Cincinnati 1981; **Resid:** Psychiatry, Mass Genl Hosp 1984; **Fac Appt:** Asst Prof Psyc, Harvard Med Sch

Rosenbaum, Jerrold F MD [Psyc] - **Spec Exp:** Anxiety & Mood Disorders; **Hospital:** Mass Genl Hosp; **Address:** 55 Fruit St, Bulfinch 351, Boston, MA 02114; **Phone:** 617-726-3482; **Board Cert:** Psychiatry 1978; **Med School:** Yale Univ 1973; **Resid:** Psychiatry, Mass Genl Hosp 1977; **Fac Appt:** Prof Psyc, Harvard Med Sch

Salzman, Carl MD [Psyc] - **Spec Exp:** Psychopharmacology; Geriatric Psychiatry; Psychotherapy; **Hospital:** MA Mental Hlth Ctr, Beth Israel Deaconess Med Ctr - Boston; **Address:** Havard Medical School, Dept Psychiatry, 25 Shattuck St, Boston, MA 02115; **Phone:** 617-998-5006; **Board Cert:** Psychiatry 1970; **Med School:** SUNY Upstate Med Univ 1963; **Resid:** Psychiatry, Mass Mental Hlth Ctr 1967; Psychiatry, Natl Inst Mental Hlth 1969; **Fac Appt:** Prof Psyc, Harvard Med Sch

Shapiro, Edward R MD [Psyc] - **Spec Exp:** Psychoanalysis; **Hospital:** Austen Riggs Ctr; **Address:** Austen Riggs Ctr, 25 Main St, PO Box 962, Stockbridge, MA 01262; **Phone:** 413-298-5511; **Board Cert:** Psychiatry 1974; **Med School:** Harvard Med Sch 1968; **Resid:** Psychiatry, Mass Mental Hlth Ctr 1972; **Fellow:** Natl Inst Mental Hlth 1974; **Fac Appt:** Assoc Clin Prof Psyc, Harvard Med Sch

Psychiatry

Vanderkolk, Bessel MD [Psyc] - **Spec Exp:** Post Traumatic Stress Disorder; Child Abuse; **Hospital:** Boston Med Ctr, Arbour Hospital - Boston; **Address:** 16 Braddock Park, Boston, MA 02116-5804; **Phone:** 617-247-1720; **Board Cert:** Psychiatry 1976; **Med School:** Univ Chicago-Pritzker Sch Med 1970; **Resid:** Psychiatry, Harvard Med Sch 1974; **Fac Appt:** Prof Psyc, Boston Univ

Mid Atlantic

Akhtar, Salman MD [Psyc] - **Spec Exp:** Psychoanalysis; **Hospital:** Thomas Jefferson Univ Hosp; **Address:** Jefferson Med College, Dept Psychiatry, 833 Chestnut St, Ste 210, Philadelphia, PA 19107; **Phone:** 215-955-2547; **Board Cert:** Psychiatry 1977; **Med School:** India 1968; **Resid:** Psychiatry, UMDNJ Med Ctr 1974; Psychiatry, Univ Virginia Med Ctr 1976; **Fellow:** Psychoanalysis, Philadelphia Psych Inst 1986

Appelbaum, Paul S MD [Psyc] - **Spec Exp:** Forensic Psychiatry; Depression; Anxiety & Mood Disorders; **Hospital:** NY-Presby Hosp/Columbia (page 66); **Address:** NY State Psychiatric Inst, 1051 Riverside Drive, rm 6714, Box 122, New York, NY 10032; **Phone:** 212-543-4184; **Board Cert:** Psychiatry 1981; Forensic Psychiatry 2004; **Med School:** Harvard Med Sch 1976; **Resid:** Psychiatry, Mass Mental Health Ctr 1980; **Fac Appt:** Prof Psyc, Columbia P&S

Basch, Samuel MD [Psyc] - **Spec Exp:** Psychopharmacology; Psychiatry in Physical Illness; Psychiatry in Cancer; Psychoanalysis; **Hospital:** Mount Sinai Med Ctr (page 64); **Address:** 10 E 85th St, Ste 1B, New York, NY 10028-0412; **Phone:** 212-427-0344; **Board Cert:** Psychiatry 1970; **Med School:** Hahnemann Univ 1961; **Resid:** Psychiatry, Mount Sinai Hosp 1965; **Fellow:** Psychoanalysis, Columbia Presby Hosp 1976; **Fac Appt:** Clin Prof Psyc, Mount Sinai Sch Med

Boronow, John Joseph MD [Psyc] - **Spec Exp:** Psychotic Disorders; Schizophrenia; **Hospital:** Sheppard Pratt Hlth Sys; **Address:** 6501 N Charles St, rm TJ-113, Towson, MD 21284; **Phone:** 410-938-4306; **Board Cert:** Psychiatry 1983; **Med School:** Yale Univ 1977; **Resid:** Psychiatry, New York Hosp 1981; **Fellow:** Psychopharmacology, Natl Inst Mntl Hlth 1983; **Fac Appt:** Assoc Clin Prof Psyc, Univ MD Sch Med

Brandt, Harry A MD [Psyc] - **Spec Exp:** Eating Disorders; **Hospital:** St Joseph Med Ctr, Sheppard Pratt Hlth Sys; **Address:** Ctr Eating Disorders, 6535 N Charles St, Ste 300, Towson, MD 21204; **Phone:** 410-938-5252; **Board Cert:** Psychiatry 1989; **Med School:** Univ MD Sch Med 1983; **Resid:** Psychiatry, Univ Maryland Hosp 1986; **Fellow:** Biological Psychiatry, Natl Inst Mental Hlth 1988; **Fac Appt:** Assoc Clin Prof Psyc, Univ MD Sch Med

Breitbart, William MD [Psyc] - **Spec Exp:** Psychiatry in Cancer; AIDS Related Cancers; Pain-Cancer; Palliative Care; **Hospital:** Meml Sloan-Kettering Cancer Ctr; **Address:** 1275 York Avenue, New York, NY 10065; **Phone:** 646-888-0100; **Board Cert:** Internal Medicine 1982; Psychiatry 1986; Psychosomatic Medicine 2005; **Med School:** Albert Einstein Coll Med 1978; **Resid:** Internal Medicine, Bronx Muni Hosp Ctr 1982; Psychiatry, Bronx Muni Hosp Ctr 1984; **Fellow:** Psychiatric Oncology, Meml Sloan Kettering Cancer Ctr 1986; **Fac Appt:** Prof Psyc, Cornell Univ-Weill Med Coll

Brodkin, Edward S MD [Psyc] - **Spec Exp:** Autism; Asperger's Syndrome; **Hospital:** Hosp Univ Penn - UPHS (page 60), Pennsylvania Hosp (page 60); **Address:** Univ Penn Sch Med, Translational Rsch Lab, 125 S 31st St, rm 2220, Philadelphia, PA 19104-3403; **Phone:** 215-746-0118; **Board Cert:** Psychiatry 2006; **Med School:** Harvard Med Sch 1992; **Resid:** Psychiatry, Yale-New Haven Hosp 1996; **Fellow:** Neurological Biology, Yale Univ Sch Med 1998; Genetics, Princeton Univ 2002; **Fac Appt:** Asst Prof Psyc, Univ Pennsylvania

Bronheim, Harold MD [Psyc] - **Spec Exp:** Psychiatry in Body Image Awareness; Relationship Problems; Psychiatry in Physical Illness; Liaison Psychiatry; **Hospital:** Mount Sinai Med Ctr (page 64); **Address:** 1155 Park Ave, New York, NY 10128-1209; **Phone:** 212-996-5777; **Board Cert:** Psychiatry 1985; Internal Medicine 1986; Psychosomatic Medicine 2005; Geriatric Psychiatry 2001; **Med School:** SUNY Downstate 1980; **Resid:** Psychiatry, Mount Sinai Hosp 1984; **Fellow:** Internal Medicine, Beth Israel Hosp 1985; **Fac Appt:** Clin Prof Psyc, Mount Sinai Sch Med

Buysse, Daniel J MD [Psyc] - **Spec Exp:** Sleep Disorders; **Hospital:** UPMC Presby, Pittsburgh; **Address:** 3811 O'Hara St, rm E-1127, Pittsburgh, PA 15213; **Phone:** 412-246-6413; **Board Cert:** Psychiatry 1988; Sleep Medicine 2007; **Med School:** Univ Mich Med Sch 1983; **Resid:** Psychiatry, Western Psych Inst 1987; **Fellow:** Sleep Medicine, Univ of Pittsburgh; **Fac Appt:** Asst Prof Psyc, Univ Pittsburgh

Cohen, Mitchell Joseph MD [Psyc] - **Spec Exp:** Pain-Chronic; Psychiatry in Physical Illness; Anxiety Disorders; **Hospital:** Thomas Jefferson Univ Hosp; **Address:** 833 Chestnut St E, Ste 210B, Philadelphia, PA 19107; **Phone:** 215-955-6592; **Board Cert:** Psychiatry 1989; Pain Medicine 2002; **Med School:** Med Coll PA 1984; **Resid:** Psychiatry, Johns Hopkins Hosp 1988; **Fac Appt:** Prof Psyc, Thomas Jefferson Univ

DePaulo Jr, J Raymond MD [Psyc] - **Spec Exp:** Bipolar/Mood Disorders; Depression; **Hospital:** Johns Hopkins Hosp (page 61); **Address:** Johns Hopkins Hosp, Dept Psychiatry, 600 N Wolfe St, Meyer 4-113, Baltimore, MD 21287-7413; **Phone:** 410-955-3130; **Board Cert:** Psychiatry 1977; **Med School:** Johns Hopkins Univ 1972; **Resid:** Psychiatry, Johns Hopkins Hosp 1977; **Fac Appt:** Prof Psyc, Johns Hopkins Univ

Doghramji, Karl MD [Psyc] - **Spec Exp:** Sleep Disorders/Apnea; Narcolepsy; **Hospital:** Thomas Jefferson Univ Hosp; **Address:** 1015 Walnut St, Curtis Bldg Fl 3 - rm 319, Philadelphia, PA 19107; **Phone:** 215-955-6175; **Board Cert:** Psychiatry 1986; **Med School:** Thomas Jefferson Univ 1980; **Resid:** Psychiatry, Thomas Jefferson Univ Hosp 1984; **Fellow:** Sleep Medicine, Montefiore Med Ctr; **Fac Appt:** Prof Psyc, Thomas Jefferson Univ

Eaton Jr, James S MD [Psyc] - **Spec Exp:** Anxiety Disorders; Sexual Identity Issues; Depression; Diagnostic Second Opinions; **Hospital:** Georgetown Univ Hosp, G Washington Univ Hosp; **Address:** 4214 50th St NW, Washington, DC 20016; **Phone:** 202-333-5796; **Board Cert:** Psychiatry 1976; **Med School:** Tulane Univ 1962; **Resid:** Internal Medicine, Tulane Univ Med Ctr 1966; Psychiatry, Tulane Univ Med Ctr 1968; **Fellow:** Psychoanalysis, Tulane Univ Med Ctr 1973; **Fac Appt:** Clin Prof Psyc, Georgetown Univ

Eth, Spencer MD [Psyc] - **Spec Exp:** Forensic Psychiatry; Post Traumatic Stress Disorder; **Hospital:** St Vincent Cath Med Ctrs - Manhattan; **Address:** 144 W 12th St, rm 174, New York, NY 10011-8202; **Phone:** 212-604-8196; **Board Cert:** Child & Adolescent Psychiatry 1982; Geriatric Psychiatry 2000; Forensic Psychiatry 2005; **Med School:** UCLA 1976; **Resid:** Psychiatry, NY Cornell Med Ctr 1979; **Fellow:** Child & Adolescent Psychiatry, Cedars-Sinai Med Ctr 1981; **Fac Appt:** Prof Psyc, NY Med Coll

Fallon, Brian A MD [Psyc] - **Spec Exp:** Lyme Disease-Neuro Complications; Psychosomatic Disorders; Obsessive-Compulsive Disorder; Psychiatry in Physical Illness; **Hospital:** NY-Presby Hosp/Columbia (page 66); **Address:** NYS Psychiatric Institute, 1051 Riverside Drive, Room 3724, Unit/Box 69, New York, NY 10032; **Phone:** 212-543-5487; **Board Cert:** Psychiatry 1991; **Med School:** Columbia P&S 1985; **Resid:** Psychiatry, NYS Psychiatric Inst 1989; **Fellow:** Psychiatric Research, NYS Psychiatric Inst 1992; Psychodynamic Psychotherapy, Columbia Univ Psychoanalytic Inst 1990; **Fac Appt:** Asst Clin Prof Psyc, Columbia P&S

First, Michael B MD [Psyc] - **Spec Exp:** Psychotherapy; Psychopharmacology; Forensic Psychiatry; **Hospital:** NY-Presby Hosp/Columbia (page 66); **Address:** NY State Psychiatric Inst, Unit 60, 1051 Riverside Drive, New York, NY 10032; **Phone:** 212-543-5531; **Board Cert:** Psychiatry 1989; **Med School:** Univ Pittsburgh 1983; **Resid:** Psychiatry, NY State Psych Inst 1987; **Fellow:** Psychiatric Research, NY State Psych Inst 1988; **Fac Appt:** Clin Prof Psyc, Columbia P&S

Fyer, Abby J MD [Psyc] - **Spec Exp:** Anxiety Disorders; Panic Disorder; **Hospital:** NY State Psychiatric Inst; **Address:** 1051 Riverside Dr, Box 82, New York, NY 10032; **Phone:** 212-543-5372; **Board Cert:** Psychiatry 1980; **Med School:** NYU Sch Med 1973; **Resid:** Psychiatry, Montefiore Med Ctr 1978; **Fac Appt:** Prof Psyc, Columbia P&S

Ganguli, Rohan MD [Psyc] - **Spec Exp:** Schizophrenia; **Hospital:** Western Psych Inst & Clin - UPMC; **Address:** Western Psychiatric Inst & Clinic, 3811 O'Hara St, Pittsburgh, PA 15213; **Phone:** 412-246-5006; **Board Cert:** Psychiatry 1980; **Med School:** India 1973; **Resid:** Psychiatry, Memorial Univ 1978; Psychiatry, Univ Pittsburgh Med Ctr 1978; **Fac Appt:** Prof Psyc, Univ Pittsburgh

Guarda, Angela S MD [Psyc] - **Spec Exp:** Eating Disorders; **Hospital:** Johns Hopkins Hosp (page 61); **Address:** Johns Hopkins Hosp, Eating Disorder Program, 600 N Wolfe St, Baltimore, MD 21287; **Phone:** 410-614-4624; **Board Cert:** Psychiatry 2006; **Med School:** Univ MD Sch Med 1991; **Resid:** Psychiatry, Johns Hopkins Hosp 1995; **Fac Appt:** Assoc Prof Psyc, Johns Hopkins Univ

Haskett, Roger F MD [Psyc] - **Spec Exp:** Depression; Mood Disorders; Anxiety Disorders; **Hospital:** Western Psych Inst & Clin - UPMC; **Address:** Western Psychiatric Inst, 3811 O'Hara St, Pittsburgh, PA 15213; **Phone:** 412-586-9207; **Board Cert:** Psychiatry 1984; **Med School:** Australia 1968; **Resid:** Psychiatry, Royal Melbourne Hosp 1977; **Fellow:** Psychiatric Research, Uiv Michigan 1979; **Fac Appt:** Prof Psyc, Univ Pittsburgh

Hollander, Eric MD [Psyc] - **Spec Exp:** Obsessive-Compulsive Disorder; Anxiety Disorders; Autism; **Hospital:** Montefiore Med Ctr - Div. Moses; **Address:** 300 Central Park West, Ste 1C, New York, NY 10024-1513; **Phone:** 212-873-4051; **Board Cert:** Psychiatry 1987; **Med School:** SUNY Hlth Sci Ctr 1982; **Resid:** Internal Medicine, Mount Sinai Hosp 1983; Psychiatry, Mount Sinai Hosp 1986; **Fellow:** Psychiatry, Columbia-Presby Med Ctr 1988; **Fac Appt:** Prof Psyc, Mount Sinai Sch Med

Karasu, T Byram MD [Psyc] - **Spec Exp:** Depression; Personality Disorders; Psychotherapy; **Hospital:** Montefiore Med Ctr - Div. Moses; **Address:** 2 E 88th St, New York, NY 10128-0555; **Phone:** 212-426-5208; **Board Cert:** Psychiatry 1972; **Med School:** Turkey 1959; **Resid:** Psychiatry, Yale-New Haven Hosp 1968; **Fellow:** Psychiatry, Yale-New Haven Hosp 1969; **Fac Appt:** Prof Psyc, Albert Einstein Coll Med

Kavey, Neil B MD [Psyc] - **Spec Exp:** Narcolepsy; Sleep Disorders/Apnea; **Hospital:** NY-Presby Hosp/Columbia (page 66); **Address:** Columbia Presby Med Ctr, Sleep Disorders Ctr, 161 Ft Washington Ave Fl 3 - rm 342, New York, NY 10032; **Phone:** 212-305-1860; **Board Cert:** Psychiatry 1976; Sleep Medicine 2003; **Med School:** Columbia P&S 1969; **Resid:** Psychiatry, Columbia Presby Med Ctr 1973; **Fac Appt:** Clin Prof Psyc, Columbia P&S

Klagsbrun, Samuel C MD [Psyc] - **Spec Exp:** Psychiatry in Cancer; Psychiatry in Terminal Illness; **Hospital:** Four Winds Hosp; **Address:** Four Winds Hospital, 800 Cross River Rd, Katonah, NY 10536; **Phone:** 914-763-8151 x2222; **Board Cert:** Psychiatry 1977; **Med School:** Ros Franklin Univ/Chicago Med Sch 1962; **Resid:** Psychiatry, Yale-New Haven Hosp 1966; **Fac Appt:** Clin Prof Psyc, Albert Einstein Coll Med

Kunkel, Elisabeth J MD [Psyc] - **Spec Exp:** Psychiatry in Cancer; Psychiatry in Physical Illness; **Hospital:** Thomas Jefferson Univ Hosp, Methodist Hosp; **Address:** Thomas Jefferson Univ, 1020 Samson St, Thompson Bldg, Ste 1652, Philadelphia, PA 19107; **Phone:** 215-955-9545; **Board Cert:** Psychiatry 1989; Addiction Psychiatry 1998; Psychosomatic Medicine 2005; **Med School:** McGill Univ 1983; **Resid:** Psychiatry, NYU Med Ctr 1987; **Fellow:** Liaison Psychiatry, Meml Sloan Kettering Cancer Ctr 1989; Consultation Psychiatry, Meml Sloan Kettering Cancer Ctr 1989; **Fac Appt:** Prof Psyc, Jefferson Med Coll

Kupfer, David J MD [Psyc] - **Spec Exp:** Bipolar/Mood Disorders; **Hospital:** Western Psych Inst & Clin - UPMC; **Address:** Western Psychiatric Inst & Clinic, 3811 O'Hara St, Pittsburgh, PA 15213-2593; **Phone:** 412-246-6777; **Board Cert:** Psychiatry 1978; **Med School:** Yale Univ 1965; **Resid:** Psychiatry, Yale-New Haven Hosp 1970; Psychiatry, Natl Inst Mental Hlth 1969; **Fellow:** Psychiatry, Yale-New Haven Hosp 1967; **Fac Appt:** Prof Psyc, Univ Pittsburgh

Lawson, William B MD [Psyc] - **Spec Exp:** Bipolar/Mood Disorders; Addiction/Substance Abuse; Dual Diagnosis; **Hospital:** Howard Univ Hosp; **Address:** Howard Univ Hosp, Dept Psychiatry, 2041 Georgia Ave NW, Ste 5B01, Washington, DC 20060; **Phone:** 202-865-6611; **Board Cert:** Psychiatry 1984; Addiction Psychiatry 2006; **Med School:** Univ Chicago-Pritzker Sch Med 1978; **Resid:** Psychiatry, Stanford Univ Med Ctr 1981; Psychiatry, Natl Inst Mental Hlth 1982; **Fellow:** Neuropsychiatry, Natl Inst Mental Hlth 1984; **Fac Appt:** Prof Psyc, Howard Univ

Loewenstein, Richard MD [Psyc] - **Spec Exp:** Trauma Psychiatry; Dissociative Disorders; Child Abuse; Post Traumatic Stress Disorder; **Hospital:** Sheppard Pratt Hlth Sys; **Address:** 6501 N Charles St, Ste A305, Box 6815, Baltimore, MD 21204; **Phone:** 410-938-5070; **Board Cert:** Psychiatry 1980; **Med School:** Yale Univ 1975; **Resid:** Psychiatry, Yale Affil Hosps 1979; **Fellow:** Psychiatry, NIH,NIMH-Biol Psych Br 1982; **Fac Appt:** Assoc Clin Prof Psyc, Univ MD Sch Med

Manevitz, Alan MD [Psyc] - **Spec Exp:** Marital/Family/Sex Therapy; Fibromyalgia Syndrome (FMS); Post Traumatic Stress Disorder; ADD/ADHD; **Hospital:** NY-Presby Hosp/Weill Cornell (page 66), Lenox Hill Hosp (page 62); **Address:** 60 Sutton Place South, Ste 1CN, New York, NY 10022; **Phone:** 212-751-5072; **Board Cert:** Psychiatry 1987; **Med School:** Columbia P&S 1980; **Resid:** Psychiatry, NY Hosp 1984; **Fellow:** Psychopharmacology, NY Hosp 1985; **Fac Appt:** Assoc Clin Prof Psyc, Cornell Univ-Weill Med Coll

Mann, J John MD/PhD [Psyc] - **Spec Exp:** Mood Disorders; Clinical Trials; **Hospital:** NY-Presby Hosp/Columbia (page 66); **Address:** NYS Psychiatric Institute, 1051 Riverside Drive, Box 42, New York, NY 10032; **Phone:** 212-543-5571; **Board Cert:** Psychiatry 1980; **Med School:** Australia 1978; **Resid:** Psychiatry, Royal Melbourne Hosp 1976; **Fac Appt:** Prof Psyc, Columbia P&S

Marin, Deborah B MD [Psyc] - **Spec Exp:** Alzheimer's Disease; **Hospital:** Mount Sinai Med Ctr (page 64); **Address:** Mount Sinai Hospital, One Gustave L Levy Pl, Box 1068, New York, NY 10029; **Phone:** 212-241-7139; **Board Cert:** Psychiatry 1990; **Med School:** Mount Sinai Sch Med 1984; **Resid:** Psychiatry, Mount Sinai Hosp 1988; **Fellow:** Psychiatry, New York Hosp-Cornell Med Ctr 1991; **Fac Appt:** Prof Psyc, Mount Sinai Sch Med

McCann, Merle C MD [Psyc] - **Hospital:** Sheppard Pratt Hlth Sys; **Address:** Sheppard & Enoch Pratt Hosp, 6501 N Charles St,, rm PJ-111, Baltimore, MD 21204; **Phone:** 410-938-3000; **Board Cert:** Psychiatry 1986; **Med School:** Med Coll VA 1981; **Resid:** Psychiatry, Geo Wash Univ Hosp 1985; **Fac Appt:** Asst Clin Prof Psyc, Univ MD Sch Med

Oquendo, Maria A MD [Psyc] - **Spec Exp:** Bipolar/Mood Disorders-Consult; Depression-Consult; Suicidal Behavior-Consult; Cross Cultural Psychiatry; **Hospital:** NY State Psychiatric Inst; **Address:** 300 W 72nd St, Ste 1F, New York, NY 10023-2661; **Phone:** 212-721-2805; **Board Cert:** Psychiatry 1989; **Med School:** Columbia P&S 1984; **Resid:** Psychiatry, Payne Whitney Clinic 1988; **Fac Appt:** Clin Prof Psyc, Columbia P&S

Psychiatry

Roose, Steven MD [Psyc] - **Spec Exp:** Depression in the Elderly; **Hospital:** NY-Presby Hosp/Columbia (page 66); **Address:** NY State Psychiatric Institute, 1051 Riverside Drive, New York, NY 10032; **Phone:** 212-831-8644; **Board Cert:** Psychiatry 1979; **Med School:** Mount Sinai Sch Med 1974; **Resid:** Psychiatry, NY Psychiatric Inst 1978; **Fellow:** Research, Columbia-Presby Med Ctr 1981; **Fac Appt:** Clin Prof Psyc, Columbia P&S

Rosenthal, Richard N MD [Psyc] - **Spec Exp:** Anxiety & Mood Disorders; Addiction/Substance Abuse; **Hospital:** St Luke's - Roosevelt Hosp Ctr - Roosevelt Div (page 57), Beth Israel Med Ctr - Petrie Division (page 57); **Address:** 1090 Amerstdam Ave Fl 16 - Ste G, New York, NY 10025; **Phone:** 212-523-5366; **Board Cert:** Psychiatry 1985; Addiction Psychiatry 2003; **Med School:** SUNY Hlth Sci Ctr 1980; **Resid:** Psychiatry, Mount Sinai Hosp 1984; **Fac Appt:** Prof Psyc, Columbia P&S

Rosse, Richard B MD [Psyc] - **Hospital:** VA Med Ctr - Washington; **Address:** Mental Health Dept (116A), 50 Irving St NW, Washington, DC 20422-0001; **Phone:** 202-745-8156; **Board Cert:** Psychiatry 1986; **Med School:** Univ MD Sch Med 1980; **Resid:** Psychiatry, Georgetown Univ Med Ctr 1984; **Fac Appt:** Prof Psyc, Howard Univ

Roth, Andrew J MD [Psyc] - **Spec Exp:** Psychiatry of Prostate Cancer; Bereavement/Traumatic Grief; **Hospital:** Meml Sloan-Kettering Cancer Ctr; **Address:** 641 Lexington Ave Fl 7, New York, NY 10022; **Phone:** 646-888-0024; **Board Cert:** Psychiatry 1993; Geriatric Psychiatry 2005; Psychosomatic Medicine 2005; **Med School:** NY Med Coll 1988; **Resid:** Psychiatry, Mt Sinai Med Ctr 1992; **Fellow:** Liaison Psychiatry, Meml Sloan-Kettering Canc Ctr 1994

Sadock, Virginia MD [Psyc] - **Spec Exp:** Psychotherapy; Sexual Dysfunction; Anxiety & Depression; Marital/Family/Sex Therapy; **Hospital:** NYU Langone Med Ctr (page 67); **Address:** 4 E 89th St, Ste 1E, New York, NY 10128; **Phone:** 212-427-0885; **Board Cert:** Psychiatry 1975; **Med School:** NY Med Coll 1970; **Resid:** Psychiatry, Metropolitan Hosp 1973; **Fac Appt:** Clin Prof Psyc, NYU Sch Med

Samberg, Eslee MD [Psyc] - **Spec Exp:** Psychoanalysis; **Hospital:** NY-Presby Hosp/Weill Cornell (page 66); **Address:** 2211 Broadway, Ste 1H, New York, NY 10024-6263; **Phone:** 212-874-7725; **Board Cert:** Psychiatry 1983; **Med School:** Cornell Univ-Weill Med Coll 1978; **Resid:** Psychiatry, NY Hosp-Cornell Med Ctr 1982; **Fac Appt:** Assoc Clin Prof Psyc, Cornell Univ-Weill Med Coll

Scott, C Paul MD [Psyc] - **Spec Exp:** Anxiety & Mood Disorders; Psychoanalysis; **Hospital:** UPMC Presby, Pittsburgh; **Address:** 401 Shady Ave, Ste C202, Pittsburgh, PA 15206; **Phone:** 412-661-2354; **Board Cert:** Psychiatry 1976; **Med School:** Case West Res Univ 1968; **Resid:** Internal Medicine, Univ Cleveland Hosps 1970; Psychiatry, Western Psych Inst 1974; **Fellow:** Psychoanalysis, Western Psych Inst 1982; **Fac Appt:** Clin Prof Psyc, Univ Pittsburgh

Shear, M Katherine MD [Psyc] - **Spec Exp:** Panic Disorder; Anxiety Disorders; Bereavement/Traumatic Grief; Phobias; **Hospital:** NY-Presby Hosp/Columbia (page 66); **Address:** 1255 Amsterdam Ave, New York, NY 10027; **Phone:** 412-897-7449; **Board Cert:** Internal Medicine 1975; Psychiatry 1981; **Med School:** Tufts Univ 1972; **Resid:** Internal Medicine, Mt Sinai Hosp 1976; Psychiatry, Payne Whitney Clin 1979; **Fellow:** Psychosomatic Medicine, Montefiore Hosp 1980; **Fac Appt:** Prof Psyc, Colombia

Stone, Michael H MD [Psyc] - **Spec Exp:** Personality Disorders; Psychoanalysis; Forensic Psychiatry; **Hospital:** NY-Presby Hosp/Columbia (page 66); **Address:** 225 Central Park West, Ste 114, New York, NY 10024-6027; **Phone:** 212-758-2000; **Board Cert:** Psychiatry 1971; **Med School:** Cornell Univ-Weill Med Coll 1958; **Resid:** Internal Medicine, Bellevue Hosp 1961; Psychiatry, NYS Psych Inst 1966; **Fellow:** Hematology, Meml Sloan Kettering Cancer Ctr 1962; Medical Oncology, Meml Sloan Kettering Cancer Ctr 1963; **Fac Appt:** Clin Prof Psyc, Columbia P&S

Sussman, Norman MD [Psyc] - **Spec Exp:** Psychopharmacology; Anxiety & Mood Disorders; Bipolar/Mood Disorders; **Hospital:** NYU Langone Med Ctr (page 67); **Address:** 150 E 58th St, Fl 27, New York, NY 10155; **Phone:** 212-588-9722; **Board Cert:** Psychiatry 1980; **Med School:** NY Med Coll 1975; **Resid:** Psychiatry, Metropolitan Hosp Ctr 1977; Psychiatry, Westchester Co Med Ctr 1978; **Fac Appt:** Clin Prof Psyc, NYU Sch Med

Thase, Michael E MD [Psyc] - **Spec Exp:** Anxiety & Mood Disorders; Psychopharmacology; Depression; **Hospital:** Hosp Univ Penn - UPHS (page 60); **Address:** Univ Penn, Dept Psychiatry, 3535 Market St, Ste 670, Piladelphia, PA 19104; **Phone:** 215-746-6680; **Board Cert:** Psychiatry 1984; **Med School:** Ohio State Univ 1979; **Resid:** Psychiatry, Western Psych Inst 1983; **Fellow:** Research, Univ Pittsburgh Sch Med 1984; **Fac Appt:** Prof Psyc, Univ Pennsylvania

Wait, Susan B MD [Psyc] - **Spec Exp:** Post Traumatic Stress Disorder; Dissociative Disorders; Anxiety & Mood Disorders; Dialectical Behavioral Therapy; **Hospital:** Sheppard Pratt Hlth Sys; **Address:** Sheppard Pratt Hlth System, 6501 N Charles St, Baltimore, MD 21285; **Phone:** 410-938-5076; **Board Cert:** Psychiatry 1993; **Med School:** Med Coll PA Hahnemann 1987; **Resid:** Psychiatry, Sheppard Pratt Hosp 1991; **Fac Appt:** Assoc Clin Prof Psyc, Univ MD Sch Med

Walsh, B Timothy MD [Psyc] - **Spec Exp:** Eating Disorders; **Hospital:** NY State Psychiatric Inst, NY-Presby Hosp/Columbia (page 66); **Address:** NY State Psychiatric Inst-Unit 98, 1051 Riverside Dr, New York, NY 10032-2695; **Phone:** 212-543-5739; **Board Cert:** Psychiatry 1978; **Med School:** Harvard Med Sch 1972; **Resid:** Internal Medicine, Dartmouth Affil Hosps 1973; Psychiatry, Bronx Muni Hosp Ctr 1977; **Fac Appt:** Prof Psyc, Columbia P&S

Southeast

Blazer II, Dan G MD/PhD [Psyc] - **Spec Exp:** Geriatric Psychiatry; Mood Disorders; **Hospital:** Duke Univ Med Ctr; **Address:** Duke Univ Med Ctr, Dept Psychiatary, 3521 Hospital S, Box 3003, Durham, NC 27710-3003; **Phone:** 919-684-4128; **Board Cert:** Psychiatry 1977; Geriatric Psychiatry 2000; **Med School:** Univ Tenn Coll Med, Memphis 1969; **Resid:** Psychiatry, Duke Univ Med Ctr 1975; **Fellow:** Liaison Psychiatry, Montefiore Hosp 1976; **Fac Appt:** Prof Psyc, Duke Univ

Canterbury II, Randolph J MD [Psyc] - **Spec Exp:** Panic Disorder; Depression; Substance Abuse; **Hospital:** Univ Virginia Med Ctr; **Address:** Univ Virginia Dept Psychiatry, Div Outpatient Psychiatry, Box 800623, Charlottesville, VA 22908-0623; **Phone:** 434-243-5719; **Board Cert:** Internal Medicine 1983; Psychiatry 1985; Psychosomatic Medicine 2005; **Med School:** W VA Univ 1979; **Resid:** Internal Medicine, Univ Va Hosp 1983; Psychiatry, Univ Va Hosp 1985; **Fac Appt:** Prof Psyc, Univ VA Sch Med

Dell, Diana L MD [Psyc] - **Spec Exp:** Postpartum Depression; Menstrual Disorders (PMS); Psychiatry in Pregnancy; Women's Health-Mental & Reproductive; **Hospital:** Duke Univ Med Ctr; **Address:** Duke University Medical Ctr, Box 3263, Durham, NC 27710; **Phone:** 919-668-2570; **Board Cert:** Psychiatry 2001; Obstetrics & Gynecology 1998; **Med School:** Louisiana State U, New Orleans 1982; **Resid:** Obstetrics & Gynecology, Charity Hosp 1986; Psychiatry, Univ N Carolina Hosps 1998; **Fellow:** Psychosomatic Medicine, Univ Toronto Affil Hosp 1999; **Fac Appt:** Prof Psyc, Duke Univ

Giustra Jr, Lawrence J MD [Psyc] - **Spec Exp:** Psychotherapy; Marital/Family/Sex Therapy; Depression; **Hospital:** Emory Univ Hosp; **Address:** 1945 Cliff Valley Way NE, Ste 202, Atlanta, GA 30329; **Phone:** 404-325-2139; **Board Cert:** Psychiatry 1982; **Med School:** Johns Hopkins Univ 1976; **Resid:** Psychiatry, Mass General Hosp 1980; **Fac Appt:** Asst Prof Psyc, Emory Univ

Psychiatry

Klapheke, Martin M MD [Psyc] - **Spec Exp:** Transplantation Psychiatry; Psychoanalysis; **Hospital:** Univ of Louisville Hosp; **Address:** 2010 Cherokee Pkwy, Ste 3, Louisville, KY 40204; **Phone:** 502-456-1770; **Board Cert:** Psychiatry 1985; **Med School:** Univ KY Coll Med 1979; **Resid:** Psychiatry, Mayo Grad Sch Med 1982; **Fellow:** Child & Adolescent Psychiatry, Mayo Grad Sch Med 1984; Psychoanalysis, Topeka Inst Psychoanalysis 1994; **Fac Appt:** Clin Prof Psyc, Univ Louisville Sch Med

Levy, Steven T MD [Psyc] - **Spec Exp:** Depression; Anxiety & Mood Disorders; Bipolar/Mood Disorders; **Hospital:** Emory Univ Hosp; **Address:** Emory Univ Dept Psychiatry, 2004 Ridgewood Drive, Ste 300, Atlanta, GA 30322; **Phone:** 404-727-5886; **Board Cert:** Psychiatry 1976; **Med School:** Duke Univ 1969; **Resid:** Psychiatry, Yale-New Haven Hosp 1973; **Fac Appt:** Prof Psyc, Emory Univ

McCall, William V MD [Psyc] - **Spec Exp:** Sleep Disorders; Electroconvulsive Therapy (ECT); Depression; **Hospital:** Wake Forest Univ Baptist Med Ctr (page 72); **Address:** Wake Forest Univ Dept Psychiatry, Medical Center Blvd, Winston-Salem, NC 27157; **Phone:** 336-716-2911; **Board Cert:** Psychiatry 1990; Geriatric Psychiatry 2005; Sleep Medicine 2007; **Med School:** Duke Univ 1984; **Resid:** Psychiatry, Duke Univ Med Ctr 1987; **Fellow:** Sleep Medicine, Duke Univ Med Ctr 1988; **Fac Appt:** Prof Psyc, Wake Forest Univ

Powers, Pauline MD [Psyc] - **Spec Exp:** Eating Disorders; **Hospital:** Tampa Genl Hosp; **Address:** 1001 Macdill Ave, Tampa, FL 33629; **Phone:** 813-253-3094; **Board Cert:** Psychiatry 1977; **Med School:** Univ Iowa Coll Med 1971; **Resid:** Psychiatry, Univ Iowa Med Ctr 1974; Psychiatry, Univ Calif-Davis Med Ctr 1975; **Fac Appt:** Prof Psyc, Univ S Fla Coll Med

Weiner, Richard D MD/PhD [Psyc] - **Spec Exp:** Bipolar/Mood Disorders; Electroconvulsive Therapy (ECT); Depression; Schizophrenia; **Hospital:** Duke Univ Med Ctr, VA Med Ctr - Durham; **Address:** Duke Univ Medical Ctr, Dept Psychiatry, Box 3309, Durham, NC 27710; **Phone:** 919-681-8742; **Board Cert:** Psychiatry 1979; Clinical Neurophysiology 2003; **Med School:** Duke Univ 1973; **Resid:** Psychiatry, Duke Univ Med Ctr 1976; **Fellow:** Electroencephalography, Duke Univ Med Ctr 1977; **Fac Appt:** Prof Psyc, Duke Univ

Weisler, Richard H MD [Psyc] - **Spec Exp:** Depression; Bipolar/Mood Disorders; **Hospital:** Duke Univ Med Ctr, Univ NC Hosps; **Address:** 700 Spring Forest Rd, Ste 125, Raleigh, NC 27609; **Phone:** 919-872-5900; **Board Cert:** Psychiatry 1982; **Med School:** Univ NC Sch Med 1977; **Resid:** Psychiatry, Duke Univ Med Ctr 1982; **Fac Appt:** Assoc Prof Psyc, Duke Univ

Midwest

Andersen, Arnold MD [Psyc] - **Spec Exp:** Eating Disorders; **Hospital:** Univ Iowa Hosp & Clinics; **Address:** Univ Iowa, Dept Psychiatry, 200 Hawkins Drive, rm 2880-JPP, Iowa City, IA 52242; **Phone:** 319-356-1354; **Board Cert:** Psychiatry 1980; **Med School:** Cornell Univ-Weill Med Coll 1968; **Resid:** Psychiatry, NY Hosp 1970; Psychiatry, Johns Hopkins Hosp 1976; **Fellow:** Psychiatry, Natl Inst Mental Hlth 1975; **Fac Appt:** Prof Psyc, Univ Iowa Coll Med

Black, Kevin J MD [Psyc] - **Spec Exp:** Neuro-Psychiatry; **Hospital:** Barnes-Jewish Hosp; **Address:** 660 S Euclid Ave, CB 8134, St Louis, MO 63110; **Phone:** 314-362-1819; **Board Cert:** Psychiatry 2005; **Med School:** Duke Univ 1990; **Resid:** Psychiatry, Barnes Hosp-Washington Univ 1994; **Fellow:** Movement Disorders, Barnes Hosp-Washington Univ 1996; **Fac Appt:** Assoc Prof Psyc, Washington Univ, St Louis

Calabrese, Joseph R MD [Psyc] - **Spec Exp:** Bipolar/Mood Disorders; **Hospital:** Univ Hosps Case Med Ctr; **Address:** Case Western Reserve Univ, 10524 Euclid Ave Fl 12, Cleveland, OH 44106; **Phone:** 216-844-2865; **Board Cert:** Psychiatry 1989; **Med School:** Ohio State Univ 1980; **Resid:** Psychiatry, Cleveland Clinic 1984; **Fellow:** Biological Psychiatry, Natl Inst Mental Hlth 1986; **Fac Appt:** Prof Psyc, Case West Res Univ

Cloninger, C Robert MD [Psyc] - **Spec Exp:** Personality Disorders; **Hospital:** Barnes-Jewish Hosp; **Address:** Wash Univ Sch Med, Dept Psyc, 660 S Euclid Ave, Box 8134, St Louis, MO 63110; **Phone:** 314-362-7005; **Board Cert:** Psychiatry 1975; **Med School:** Washington Univ, St Louis 1970; **Resid:** Psychiatry, Barnes Hosp 1973; Psychiatry, Renard Hosp-Wash Univ 1973; **Fac Appt:** Prof Psyc, Washington Univ, St Louis

Crow, Scott J MD [Psyc] - **Spec Exp:** Eating Disorders; Obesity; **Hospital:** Univ Minn Med Ctr, Fairview - Univ Campus; **Address:** Univ Minn, Dept Psychiatry, 2450 Riverside Ave, F282/2A West, Minneapolis, MN 55454; **Phone:** 612-273-9807; **Board Cert:** Psychiatry 1994; **Med School:** Univ Minn 1988; **Resid:** Psychiatry, Univ Minn Hosp 1992; **Fellow:** Psychiatry, Univ Minn Hosp 1992; **Fac Appt:** Prof Psyc, Univ Minn

Gelenberg, Alan MD [Psyc] - **Spec Exp:** Psychopharmacology; Mood Disorders; Depression; **Hospital:** Rogers Meml Hosp.; **Address:** Healthcare Tech Sys, 7617 Mineral Point Rd, Ste 300, Madison, WI 53717; **Phone:** 608-827-2454; **Board Cert:** Psychiatry 1975; **Med School:** Univ Pennsylvania 1969; **Resid:** Psychiatry, Mass Genl Hosp 1973; **Fac Appt:** Clin Prof Psyc, Med Coll Wisc

Greden, John F MD [Psyc] - **Spec Exp:** Anxiety & Mood Disorders; Depression; **Hospital:** Univ Michigan Hlth Sys; **Address:** Univ Michigan Comp Depression Ctr, Rachel Upjohn Bldg, 4250 Plymouth Rd, Ann Arbor, MI 48109-2700; **Phone:** 734-763-9629; **Board Cert:** Psychiatry 1975; **Med School:** Univ Minn 1967; **Resid:** Psychiatry, Univ Minn Med Ctr 1969; Psychiatry, Walter Reed AMC 1972; **Fac Appt:** Prof Psyc, Univ Mich Med Sch

Janicak, Philip G MD [Psyc] - **Spec Exp:** Psychopharmacology; Mood Disorders; Psychotic Disorders; **Hospital:** Rush Univ Med Ctr; **Address:** Rush Univ Med Ctr, Dept Psych, 1720 W Polk St, M Field Bldg, rm 107, Chicago, IL 60612-4328; **Phone:** 312-942-7287; **Board Cert:** Psychiatry 1978; **Med School:** Loyola Univ-Stritch Sch Med 1973; **Resid:** Psychiatry, McGaw Hosp/Loyola Med Ctr 1976; **Fac Appt:** Prof Psyc, Rush Med Coll

Levine, Stephen B MD [Psyc] - **Spec Exp:** Sexual Dysfunction; Relationship Problems; Sexual Identity Issues; **Hospital:** Univ Hosps Case Med Ctr; **Address:** 23230 Chagrin Blvd, Ste 350, Beachwood, OH 44122-5446; **Phone:** 216-831-2900; **Board Cert:** Psychiatry 1976; **Med School:** Case West Res Univ 1967; **Resid:** Psychiatry, Univ Hosps Cleveland 1973; **Fac Appt:** Clin Prof Psyc, Case West Res Univ

Locala, Joseph MD [Psyc] - **Spec Exp:** Psychiatry in Transplant Patients; Psychiatry in Physical Illness; Anxiety & Mood Disorders; Neuro-Psychiatry; **Hospital:** Univ Hosps Case Med Ctr; **Address:** WO Walker Ctr, 10524 Euclid Ave Fl 13, Cleveland, OH 44106; **Phone:** 216-844-2400; **Board Cert:** Psychiatry 2006; Psychosomatic Medicine 2006; **Med School:** Temple Univ 1990; **Resid:** Psychiatry, Medical Ctr Hosp 1994; **Fellow:** Cleveland Clinic 1995; **Fac Appt:** Assoc Prof Psyc, Case West Res Univ

McCallum, Kimberli E MD [Psyc] - **Spec Exp:** Eating Disorders; **Hospital:** Rochelle Comm Hosp; **Address:** McCallum Place, 231 W Lockwood Ave, Ste 201, St. Louis, MO 63119; **Phone:** 314-968-1900; **Board Cert:** Psychiatry 1993; Child & Adolescent Psychiatry 1994; **Med School:** Yale Univ 1986; **Resid:** Psychiatry, UCLA Neuropsyc Inst 1991; **Fellow:** Child Psychiatry, Washington Univ 1993; **Fac Appt:** Assoc Clin Prof Psyc, Washington Univ, St Louis

Psychiatry

Nurnberger Jr, John I MD/PhD [Psyc] - **Spec Exp:** Bipolar/Mood Disorders; Depression; **Hospital:** Indiana Univ Hosp, Wishard Hlth Srvs; **Address:** Institute Psychiatric Research-IUMC, 791 Union Dr, Indianapolis, IN 46202-4887; **Phone:** 317-274-8382; **Board Cert:** Psychiatry 1981; **Med School:** Indiana Univ 1975; **Resid:** Psychiatry, Columbia-Presby Med Ctr 1978; **Fac Appt:** Prof Psyc, Indiana Univ

Riba, Michelle B MD [Psyc] - **Spec Exp:** Psychiatry in Cancer; **Hospital:** Univ Michigan Hlth Sys; **Address:** Univ Mich Med Ctr, Dept Psychiatry, 1500 E Medical Center Dr, MCHC, rm F6236, Ann Arbor, MI 48109-0295; **Phone:** 734-764-6879; **Board Cert:** Psychiatry 1991; Psychosomatic Medicine 2005; **Med School:** Univ Conn 1985; **Resid:** Psychiatry, Univ Connecticut 1988; **Fac Appt:** Clin Prof Psyc, Univ Mich Med Sch

Strakowski, Stephen M MD [Psyc] - **Spec Exp:** Bipolar/Mood Disorders; Psychotic Disorders; Dual Diagnosis; Addiction/Substance Abuse; **Hospital:** Univ Hosp - Cincinnati, Cincinnati Chldns Hosp Med Ctr; **Address:** Univ Cincinnati Coll Med, Dept Psychiatry, 231 Albert Sabin Way, Cincinnati, OH 45267-0559; **Phone:** 513-558-4274; **Board Cert:** Psychiatry 1993; **Med School:** Vanderbilt Univ 1988; **Resid:** Psychiatry, McLean Hosp-Harvard Med Sch 1992; **Fac Appt:** Prof Psyc, Univ Cincinnati

Wooten, Virgil D MD [Psyc] - **Spec Exp:** Sleep Disorders; **Hospital:** Bethesda North Hosp, Good Samaritan Hosp - Cincinnati; **Address:** Bethesda Sleep Ctr, 10475 Montgomery Rd, Ste 1D, Cincinnati, OH 45242; **Phone:** 513-865-1690; **Board Cert:** Psychiatry 1985; Sleep Medicine 2007; **Med School:** Univ Ark 1980; **Resid:** Psychiatry, Univ Hosp-VA Hosp 1984; **Fellow:** Sleep Medicine, Univ Hosp 1985

Zorumski, Charles F MD [Psyc] - **Spec Exp:** Neuro-Psychiatry; Psychopharmacology; **Hospital:** Barnes-Jewish Hosp; **Address:** 660 S Euclid Ave, CB 8134, St Louis, MO 63110-1010; **Phone:** 314-747-2680; **Board Cert:** Psychiatry 1984; **Med School:** St Louis Univ 1978; **Resid:** Psychiatry, Barnes-Jewish Hosp 1982; **Fac Appt:** Prof Psyc, Washington Univ, St Louis

Great Plains and Mountains

Freedman, Robert MD [Psyc] - **Spec Exp:** Schizophrenia; **Hospital:** Univ Colorado Hosp; **Address:** Univ Colorado, Dept Psychiatry, 13001 E 17th Ave, Box E2351, Aurora, CO 80045; **Phone:** 303-724-4940; **Board Cert:** Psychiatry 1980; **Med School:** Harvard Med Sch 1972; **Resid:** Psychiatry, Univ Chicago Hosps & Clins 1978; **Fellow:** Neuropharmacology, NIMH-Neuropharm Lab / St Elizabeth's Hosp; **Fac Appt:** Prof Psyc, Univ Colorado

Greiner, Carl B MD [Psyc] - **Spec Exp:** Psychiatry in Cancer; Psychiatry in Physical Illness; Palliative Care; Post Traumatic Stress Disorder; **Hospital:** Nebraska Med Ctr; **Address:** UNMC, dept Psychiatry, 985575 Nebraska Medical Ctr, Omaha, NE 68198-5575; **Phone:** 402-552-6002; **Board Cert:** Psychiatry 1984; Forensic Psychiatry 1999; **Med School:** Univ Cincinnati 1978; **Resid:** Psychiatry, Univ Cincinnati Med Ctr 1982; **Fac Appt:** Prof Psyc, Univ Nebr Coll Med

Hoffman, Daniel A MD [Psyc] - **Spec Exp:** ADD/ADHD; **Hospital:** Rose Med Ctr; **Address:** Neuro-Therapy Clin, Orchard Falls Bldg, 7800 E Orchard Rd, Ste 340, Greenwood Village, CO 80111; **Phone:** 303-741-4800; **Board Cert:** Psychiatry 1981; **Med School:** Wayne State Univ 1974; **Resid:** Psychiatry, Univ Colo Hlth Sci Ctr 1977; **Fac Appt:** Asst Clin Prof Psyc, Univ Colorado

McIntosh, J Michael MD [Psyc] - **Spec Exp:** Depression; Schizophrenia; Anxiety Disorders; Bipolar/Mood Disorders; **Hospital:** Univ Utah Hosps and Clins; **Address:** 30 N 1900 East, rm 5R110, Salt Lake City, UT 84108; **Phone:** 801-581-7951; **Board Cert:** Psychiatry 1994; **Med School:** UCLA 1987; **Resid:** Psychiatry, Univ Colo Hlth Sci Ctr 1991; Psychiatry, Univ Utah Hosps 1992; **Fac Appt:** Clin Prof Psyc, Univ Utah

Mitchell, James E MD [Psyc] - **Spec Exp:** Eating Disorders; **Hospital:** MeritCare Hosp; **Address:** NeuroPsychiatric Research Inst, 120 S 8th St Fl 2, Fargo, ND 58103; **Phone:** 701-293-1335; **Board Cert:** Psychiatry 1979; **Med School:** Northwestern Univ 1972; **Resid:** Psychiatry, Fairview-Univ Med Ctr 1976; **Fac Appt:** Prof Psyc, Univ ND Sch Med

Moench, Louis A MD [Psyc] - **Hospital:** LDS Hosp; **Address:** 333 South 9th East, Salt Lake City, UT 84102; **Phone:** 801-535-8398; **Board Cert:** Psychiatry 1978; Forensic Psychiatry 2004; **Med School:** Univ Utah 1970; **Resid:** Psychiatry, Hosp U Penn 1976; **Fellow:** Forensic Psychiatry, Hosp U Penn 1976; **Fac Appt:** Clin Prof Psyc, Univ Utah

Weiner, Kenneth L MD [Psyc] - **Spec Exp:** Eating Disorders; **Hospital:** Univ Colorado Hosp; **Address:** 1830 Franklin St, Ste 500, Denver, CO 80218; **Phone:** 303-220-1655; **Board Cert:** Psychiatry 1983; **Med School:** Tufts Univ 1977; **Resid:** Psychiatry, Univ Colorado Hlth Sci Ctr 1981; **Fac Appt:** Asst Clin Prof Psyc, Univ Colorado

Wilson, Daniel R MD/PhD [Psyc] - **Spec Exp:** Psychopharmacology; Forensic Psychiatry; **Hospital:** Creighton Univ Med Ctr; **Address:** 3528 Dodge St, Omaha, NE 68131; **Phone:** 402-345-8828; **Board Cert:** Psychiatry 1989; Forensic Psychiatry 1998; **Med School:** Univ Iowa Coll Med 1983; **Resid:** Psychiatry, McLean Hosp 1987; **Fellow:** Geriatric Psychiatry, McLean Hosp 1987; Genetics, Cambridge Univ 1993; **Fac Appt:** Prof Psyc, Creighton Univ

Southwest

Avery, Eric N MD [Psyc] - **Spec Exp:** Depression; Dementia; Arts in the Healing Process; AIDS/HIV Liaison Psychiatry; **Hospital:** UT Med Br Hosp at Galveston; **Address:** Dept Psychiatry, 301 University Blvd, Galveston, TX 77555-0193; **Phone:** 409-747-9667; **Board Cert:** Psychiatry 2003; **Med School:** Univ Tex Med Br, Galveston 1974; **Resid:** Psychiatry, NY State Psych Inst 1978; **Fellow:** Liaison Psychiatry for AIDS/HIV, NY State Psych Inst 1994; **Fac Appt:** Asst Prof Psyc, Univ Tex Med Br, Galveston

Baile, Walter F MD [Psyc] - **Spec Exp:** Psychiatry in Cancer; **Hospital:** UT MD Anderson Cancer Ctr; **Address:** Brain & Spine Inst, MD Anderson, Main Bldg Fl 7, 1515 Holcombe Blvd, Texas, TX 77030; **Phone:** 713-563-1484; **Board Cert:** Psychiatry 1980; **Med School:** Italy 1973; **Resid:** Psychiatry, Johns Hopkins Hosp 1976; **Fellow:** Behavioral Medicine, Natl Inst Aging 1978; **Fac Appt:** Prof Psyc, Univ Tex, Houston

Bowden, Charles L MD [Psyc] - **Spec Exp:** Bipolar/Mood Disorders; **Hospital:** Univ Hlth Syst-San Antonio; **Address:** Univ Tex Hlth Sci Ctr, Dept Psychiatry, 7526 Louis Pasteur, San Antonio, TX 78229-3900; **Phone:** 210-567-5555; **Board Cert:** Psychiatry 1970; **Med School:** Baylor Coll Med 1964; **Resid:** Psychiatry, NY State Psyc Inst/Columbia-Presby Med Ctr 1968; **Fac Appt:** Prof Psyc, Univ Tex, San Antonio

Davidson, Joyce E MD [Psyc] - **Spec Exp:** Obsessive-Compulsive Disorder; Bipolar/Mood Disorders; Schizophrenia; **Hospital:** Menninger Clinic; **Address:** 2801 Gessner Drive, Houston, TX 77080; **Phone:** 713-275-5419; **Board Cert:** Psychiatry 1988; **Med School:** Univ MO-Kansas City 1979; **Resid:** Psychiatry, Karl Menninger Sch Psyc 1982; **Fellow:** Child & Adolescent Psychiatry, Karl Menninger Sch Psyc 1984

Psychiatry

Gabbard, Glen O MD [Psyc] - **Spec Exp:** Personality Disorders-Borderline; Cognitive Psychotherapy; Psychoanalysis; **Hospital:** Baylor Univ Medical Ctr; **Address:** 6655 Travis, Ste 500, Houston, TX 77030; **Phone:** 713-798-6397; **Board Cert:** Psychiatry 1979; **Med School:** Rush Med Coll 1975; **Resid:** Psychiatry, Menninger Sch Psyc 1978; **Fellow:** Psychoanalysis, Topeka Inst Psychoanalysis 1984; **Fac Appt:** Clin Prof Psyc, Univ Kans

Haque, Waheedul MD [Psyc] - **Spec Exp:** Depression; Panic Disorder; **Hospital:** UT Med Br Hosp at Galveston; **Address:** Dept Psychiatry, 301 University Blvd, Route 0190, Galveston, TX 77555; **Phone:** 409-747-9722; **Board Cert:** Psychiatry 1970; **Med School:** India 1962; **Resid:** Psychiatry, Barnes Jewish Med Ctr 1969; **Fac Appt:** Prof Psyc, Univ Tex Med Br, Galveston

Hirschfeld, Robert M A MD [Psyc] - **Spec Exp:** Bipolar/Mood Disorders; Schizophrenia; Depression; Suicide; **Hospital:** UT Med Br Hosp at Galveston; **Address:** Dept Psychiatry, 301 University Blvd, Route 0188, Galveston, TX 77555-0188; **Phone:** 409-747-9722; **Board Cert:** Psychiatry 1975; **Med School:** Univ Mich Med Sch 1968; **Resid:** Psychiatry, Stanford Univ Med Ctr 1972; **Fac Appt:** Prof Psyc, Univ Tex Med Br, Galveston

Mohl, Paul C MD [Psyc] - **Spec Exp:** Psychopharmacology; Psychotherapy; **Hospital:** UT Southwestern Med Ctr at Dallas; **Address:** 5323 Harry Hines Blvd, Dallas, TX 75390-9070; **Phone:** 214-648-7312; **Board Cert:** Psychiatry 1977; **Med School:** Duke Univ 1971; **Resid:** Psychiatry, Duke Univ Hosp 1974; **Fac Appt:** Prof Psyc, Univ Tex SW, Dallas

Valentine, Alan D MD [Psyc] - **Spec Exp:** Psychiatry in Cancer; Palliative Care; **Hospital:** UT MD Anderson Cancer Ctr; **Address:** MD Anderson Cancer Center, Dept Psychiatry Unit 453, PO Box 301402, Houston, TX 77230-1402; **Phone:** 713-745-3344; **Board Cert:** Psychiatry 1992; Geriatric Psychiatry 2006; Psychosomatic Medicine 2005; **Med School:** Univ Tex, Houston 1986; **Resid:** Psychiatry, Univ Texas Affil Hosps; **Fac Appt:** Assoc Prof Psyc, Univ Tex, Houston

Weiner, Myron MD [Psyc] - **Spec Exp:** Psychiatry-Geriatric; Alzheimer's Disease; **Hospital:** UT Southwestern Med Ctr at Dallas; **Address:** Univ Texas SW Med Ctr, 5323 Harry Hines Blvd, Dallas, TX 75390-9129; **Phone:** 214-648-9353; **Board Cert:** Psychiatry 1966; Geriatric Psychiatry 2001; **Med School:** Tulane Univ 1957; **Resid:** Psychiatry, Parkland Hosp 1963; **Fellow:** Geriatric Psychiatry, Mt Sinai Med Ctr 1985; **Fac Appt:** Prof Psyc, Univ Tex SW, Dallas

West Coast and Pacific

Blumenfield, Michael MD [Psyc] - **Spec Exp:** Psychotherapy; Psychopharmacology; Psychosomatic Disorders; Disaster Psychiatry; **Address:** 5901 Nita Ave, Woodland Hills, CA 91367; **Phone:** 818-564-4207; **Board Cert:** Psychiatry 1970; Psychosomatic Medicine 2005; **Med School:** SUNY Downstate 1964; **Resid:** Psychiatry, Kings County Hosp 1968; **Fellow:** Psychosomatic Medicine, Kings County Hosp 1971; **Fac Appt:** Prof Emeritus Psyc, NY Med Coll

Burt, Vivien K MD/PhD [Psyc] - **Spec Exp:** Women's Health-Mental Health; Impulse-Control Disorders; Psychiatry in Pregnancy; Postpartum Depression; **Hospital:** UCLA Neuropsychiatric Hosp; **Address:** 300 UCLA Medical Plaza, Ste 2337, Los Angeles, CA 90095; **Phone:** 310-562-4942; **Board Cert:** Psychiatry 1990; **Med School:** McGill Univ 1984; **Resid:** Psychiatry, UCLA-Neurpsyc Inst 1988; **Fac Appt:** Assoc Prof Psyc, UCLA

Bystritsky, Alexander MD/PhD [Psyc] - **Spec Exp:** Obsessive-Compulsive Disorder; Anxiety Disorders; Psychopharmacology; **Hospital:** UCLA Neuropsychiatric Hosp; **Address:** 300 UCLA Med Plaza, Ste 2200, Box 956968, Los Angeles, CA 90095-6968; **Phone:** 310-206-5133; **Board Cert:** Psychiatry 1988; **Med School:** Russia 1977; **Resid:** Psychiatry, NYU Med Ctr 1985; **Fellow:** Psychiatry, UCLA 1987; **Fac Appt:** Prof Psyc, UCLA

Eisendrath, Stuart J MD [Psyc] - **Spec Exp:** Depression; Munchausen Syndrome; Cognitive Psychotherapy; **Hospital:** UCSF Med Ctr, Las Encinas Hosp; **Address:** UCSF Med Ctr, 401 Parnassus Ave, Box 0984, San Francisco, CA 94143-0984; **Phone:** 415-476-7868; **Board Cert:** Psychiatry 1980; Psychosomatic Medicine 2008; **Med School:** Med Coll Wisc 1974; **Resid:** Psychiatry, Langley Porter Neuropsych Inst 1978; **Fellow:** Liaison Psychiatry, Langley Porter Neuropsych Inst 1979; **Fac Appt:** Prof Psyc, UCSF

Fann, Jesse R MD [Psyc] - **Spec Exp:** Psychiatry in Physical Illness; Psychiatry in Cancer; Neuro-Psychiatry; **Hospital:** Univ Wash Med Ctr, Harborview Med Ctr; **Address:** Univ Washington Med Ctr, Psychiatry-Box 356560, 1959 NE Pacific St, Seattle, WA 98195-6560; **Phone:** 206-685-4280; **Board Cert:** Psychiatry 2005; **Med School:** Northwestern Univ 1989; **Resid:** Psychiatry, Univ Washington Med Ctr 1993; **Fellow:** Liaison Psychiatry, Univ Washington Med Ctr 1995; Epidemiology, Univ Washington 1996; **Fac Appt:** Assoc Prof Psyc, Univ Wash

Friedman, Barry MD [Psyc] - **Spec Exp:** Psychopharmacology; Psychoanalysis; **Address:** 435 N Bedford Dr, Ste 112, Beverly Hills, CA 90210; **Phone:** 310-274-4372; **Board Cert:** Psychiatry 1974; **Med School:** UCSF 1965; **Resid:** Psychiatry, UCLA Med Ctr 1971; **Fellow:** Psychoanalysis, Los Angeles Psychoanalytic Inst 1992; **Fac Appt:** Assoc Clin Prof Psyc, UCLA

Gitlin, Michael Jay MD [Psyc] - **Spec Exp:** Mood Disorders; **Hospital:** UCLA Neuropsychiatric Hosp; **Address:** UCLA NPI-Mood Disorders Clin, 300 Med Plaza, Ste 2200, Los Angeles, CA 90095-6968; **Phone:** 310-206-3654; **Board Cert:** Psychiatry 1981; **Med School:** Univ Pennsylvania 1975; **Resid:** Psychiatry, UCLA Med Ctr 1979; **Fac Appt:** Prof Psyc, UCLA

Guilleminault, Christian MD [Psyc] - **Spec Exp:** Sleep Disorders/Apnea; **Hospital:** Stanford Univ Med Ctr; **Address:** 401 Quarry Rd, Ste 3301A, Stanford, CA 94305; **Phone:** 650-723-6601; **Med School:** France 1968; **Fac Appt:** Prof Psyc, Stanford Univ

Keepers, George MD [Psyc] - **Spec Exp:** Neuro-Psychiatry; ADD/ADHD; **Hospital:** OR Hlth & Sci Univ; **Address:** 3181 SW Sam Jackson Park Rd, MC UHN80, Portland, OR 97239; **Phone:** 503-494-8144; **Board Cert:** Psychiatry 1984; **Med School:** Baylor Coll Med 1977; **Resid:** Psychiatry, Oregon Hlth Sci Univ 1981; **Fac Appt:** Prof Psyc, Oregon Hlth & Sci Univ

Kerrihard, Thomas MD [Psyc] - **Spec Exp:** Psychiatry in Physical Illness; Psychiatry in Cancer; **Hospital:** Cedars-Sinai Med Ctr; **Address:** Cedars Sinai Medical Ctr, Dept Psychiatry, 8700 Beverly Blvd, Ste AC1004, Los Angeles, CA 90048; **Phone:** 310-423-8030; **Board Cert:** Psychiatry 1999; Pain Medicine 2005; **Med School:** Harvard Med Sch 1994; **Resid:** Psychiatry, Mass Genl Hosp 1998; **Fellow:** Liaison Psychiatry, Meml Sloan Kettering Cancer Ctr 1999

Leuchter, Andrew F MD [Psyc] - **Spec Exp:** Depression; **Hospital:** UCLA Neuropsychiatric Hosp; **Address:** 760 Westwood Pl, rm 37-452, Los Angeles, CA 90024; **Phone:** 310-825-0207; **Board Cert:** Psychiatry 1986; Geriatric Psychiatry 2001; **Med School:** Baylor Coll Med 1980; **Resid:** Psychiatry, UCLA-Neuro Psyc Inst & Hosp 1984; **Fellow:** Geriatric Psychiatry, UCLA Med Ctr 1986; **Fac Appt:** Prof Psyc, UCLA

Liberman, Robert Paul MD [Psyc] - **Spec Exp:** Schizophrenia; Psychotic Disorders; Psychiatric Rehabilitation; **Hospital:** UCLA Neuropsychiatric Hosp; **Address:** UCLA Neuropsychiatric Institute, 760 Westwood Plaza, Los Angeles, CA 90095; **Phone:** 310-206-1616; **Board Cert:** Psychiatry 1969; **Med School:** Johns Hopkins Univ 1963; **Resid:** Psychiatry, Mass Mntl Hlth Ctr 1968; **Fellow:** Pharmacology, UCSF Med Ctr 1961; Research, Harvard Med Sch 1968; **Fac Appt:** Prof Psyc, UCLA

Psychiatry

Marder, Stephen R MD [Psyc] - **Spec Exp:** Schizophrenia; Psychopharmacology; **Hospital:** VA Med Ctr - W Los Angeles, UCLA Ronald Reagan Med Ctr; **Address:** West Los Angeles VA - Gr LA Hlth Svcs, 11301 Wilshire Blvd, Bldg MIRECC 210A, Los Angeles, CA 90073; **Phone:** 310-268-3647; **Board Cert:** Psychiatry 1977; **Med School:** SUNY Buffalo 1971; **Resid:** Psychiatry, LAC-USC Med Ctr 1975; **Fac Appt:** Prof Psyc, UCLA

Marmar, Charles MD [Psyc] - **Spec Exp:** Post Traumatic Stress Disorder; Bereavement/Traumatic Grief; **Hospital:** VA Med Ctr - San Francisco; **Address:** 4150 Clement St Bldg 8 - rm 320-1, Mental Hlth Svc 116A, San Francisco, CA 94941; **Phone:** 415-221-4810 x3436; **Board Cert:** Psychiatry 1982; **Med School:** Univ Manitoba 1970; **Resid:** Psychiatry, Univ Toronto Hosp 1976; **Fellow:** Anxiety Disorder, Langley Porter Inst-UCSF 1978; **Fac Appt:** Prof Psyc, UCSF

Nelson, James Craig MD [Psyc] - **Spec Exp:** Geriatric Psychiatry; Psychopharmacology; Mood Disorders; **Hospital:** UCSF Med Ctr; **Address:** UCSF-Langley Porter Psychiatric Inst, 401 Parnassus Ave, Box 0984, San Francisco, CA 94143-0984; **Phone:** 415-476-7500; **Board Cert:** Psychiatry 1974; Geriatric Psychiatry 2002; **Med School:** Univ Wisc 1968; **Resid:** Psychiatry, Yale-New Haven Hosp 1970; Psychiatry, Yale-New Haven Hosp 1974; **Fac Appt:** Prof Psyc, UCSF

Neppe, Vernon M MD/PhD [Psyc] - **Spec Exp:** Behavioral Neurology; Neuro-Psychiatry; Psychopharmacology; Forensic Psychiatry; **Hospital:** Overlake Hosp Med Ctr, Northwest Hosp; **Address:** Pacific Neuropsychiatric Inst, 6300 Ninth Ave NE, Ste 353, Seattle, WA 98115; **Phone:** 206-527-6289; **Board Cert:** Psychiatry 1988; Geriatric Psychiatry 2001; Behavioral Neurology & Neuropsychiatry 2006; **Med School:** South Africa 1973; **Resid:** Neurology, Univ Witwatersrand 1979; Psychiatry, Univ Witwatersrand 1980; **Fellow:** Psychopharmacology, Cornell Med Ctr 1983; Neuropsychiatry, Cornell Med Ctr 1983

Norman, Kim P MD [Psyc] - **Spec Exp:** Eating Disorders/Obesity; Personality Disorders; Dual Diagnosis; **Hospital:** UCSF Med Ctr; **Address:** UCSF-Langley Porter Psyc Inst, 401 Parnassus Ave, rm 250, Box A-221, San Francisco, CA 94143; **Phone:** 415-476-7402; **Board Cert:** Psychiatry 1983; **Med School:** Albert Einstein Coll Med 1977; **Resid:** Psychiatry, Langley Porter Psyc Inst 1981; **Fac Appt:** Clin Prof Psyc, UCSF

Pi, Edmond H MD [Psyc] - **Spec Exp:** Psychopharmacology; Cross Cultural Psychiatry; Anxiety Disorders; **Hospital:** LAC & USC Med Ctr; **Address:** LAC USC Healthcare Network, 1200 N State St, rm 10-621, Los Angeles, CA 90033; **Phone:** 323-226-7975; **Board Cert:** Psychiatry 1980; Psychosomatic Medicine 2008; **Med School:** South Korea 1972; **Resid:** Psychiatry, SUNY-Stony Brook Affil Hosp 1977; Psychiatry, Univ Kentucky Hosp-Chandler Med Ctr 1978; **Fac Appt:** Prof Psyc, USC Sch Med

Pynoos, Robert S MD [Psyc] - **Spec Exp:** Post Traumatic Stress Clinical Trials; **Hospital:** UCLA Neuropsychiatric Hosp; **Address:** Natl Ctr for Chld Traumatic Stress-UCLA, 11150 W Olympic Blvd, Ste 650, Los Angeles, CA 90064; **Phone:** 310-235-2633; **Board Cert:** Psychiatry 1980; **Med School:** Columbia P&S 1972; **Resid:** Pediatrics, Mt Sinai Hosp; Psychiatry, NY Presby-Cornell Med Ctr; **Fac Appt:** Prof Psyc, UCLA

Raskind, Murray MD [Psyc] - **Spec Exp:** Geriatric Psychiatry; Alzheimer's Disease; Post Traumatic Stress Disorder; **Hospital:** VA Puget Sound Hlth Care Sys, Univ Wash Med Ctr; **Address:** VA Puget Sound Health Care System, Mental Hlth Svc 116, 1660 S Columbia Way, Seattle, WA 98108; **Phone:** 206-768-5375; **Board Cert:** Psychiatry 1976; Geriatric Psychiatry 2001; **Med School:** Columbia P&S 1968; **Resid:** Internal Medicine, Harlem Hosp Ctr 1970; Psychiatry, Univ Wash Affil Hosps 1973; **Fac Appt:** Prof Psyc, Univ Wash

Reus, Victor I MD [Psyc] - **Spec Exp:** Psychopharmacology; Bipolar/Mood Disorders; Behavioral Disorders; **Hospital:** UCSF Med Ctr; **Address:** 401 Parnassus Ave, San Francisco, CA 94143-0984; **Phone:** 415-476-7478; **Board Cert:** Psychiatry 1977; Geriatric Psychiatry 2000; **Med School:** Univ MD Sch Med 1973; **Resid:** Psychiatry, Univ Wisc Med Ctr 1976; **Fellow:** Biological Psychiatry, Natl Inst Mntl Hlth 1978; **Fac Appt:** Prof Psyc, UCSF

Roy-Byrne, Peter P MD [Psyc] - **Spec Exp:** Anxiety & Mood Disorders; Panic Disorder; Bipolar/Mood Disorders; Post Traumatic Stress Disorder; **Hospital:** Harborview Med Ctr, Univ Wash Med Ctr; **Address:** 325 9th Ave, Box 359911, Seattle, WA 98104; **Phone:** 206-341-4200; **Board Cert:** Psychiatry 1983; **Med School:** Tufts Univ 1978; **Resid:** Psychiatry, UCLA Neuropsych Inst 1982; **Fellow:** Biological Psychiatry, Natl Inst Hlth - NIMH 1984; **Fac Appt:** Prof Psyc, Univ Wash

Saxena, Sanjaya MD [Psyc] - **Spec Exp:** Obsessive-Compulsive Disorder; **Hospital:** UCSD Med Ctr; **Address:** La Jolla Professional Building, 8950 Via La Jolla Drive, La Jolla, CA 92037; **Phone:** 858-534-6200; **Board Cert:** Psychiatry 2006; **Med School:** Univ Minn 1990; **Resid:** Psychiatry, UCLA Neuropsychiatric Hosp 1994; **Fellow:** Neuroimaging, Charles A. Dana Fdn 1996; **Fac Appt:** Asst Prof Psyc, UCSD

Schatzberg, Alan F MD [Psyc] - **Spec Exp:** Psychopharmacology; Anxiety & Mood Disorders; Depression; **Hospital:** Stanford Univ Med Ctr; **Address:** Stanford Univ, Dept Psychiatry, 401 Quarry Rd, Ste 3301A, Stanford, CA 94305-5717; **Phone:** 650-723-6811; **Board Cert:** Psychiatry 1975; **Med School:** NYU Sch Med 1968; **Resid:** Psychiatry, Mass Mental Hlth Ctr 1972; **Fellow:** Psychiatry, Mass Mental Hlth Ctr/Harvard 1972; **Fac Appt:** Prof Psyc, Stanford Univ

Spiegel, David MD [Psyc] - **Spec Exp:** Hypnosis; Psychiatry in Cancer; Post Traumatic Stress Disorder; **Hospital:** Stanford Univ Med Ctr; **Address:** Stanford Univ Sch Medicine, Dept Psychiatry & Behavioral Sciences, 401 Quarry Rd, rm 2325, Stanford, CA 94305-5718; **Phone:** 650-723-6421; **Board Cert:** Psychiatry 1976; **Med School:** Harvard Med Sch 1971; **Resid:** Psychiatry, Mass Mental Hlth Ctr 1974; Psychiatry, Cambridge Hosp-Harvard Med Sch 1974; **Fellow:** Community Psychiatry, Harvard Med Sch 1974; **Fac Appt:** Prof Psyc, Stanford Univ

Stein, Murray B MD [Psyc] - **Spec Exp:** Anxiety Disorders; Panic Disorder; Post Traumatic Stress Disorder; **Hospital:** UCSD Med Ctr, VA San Diego Hlthcre Sys; **Address:** UCSD Dept Psychiatry, 8939 Villa La Jolla Drive, Ste 200, La Jolla, CA 92037; **Phone:** 858-534-6400; **Board Cert:** Psychiatry 1989; **Med School:** Univ Manitoba 1983; **Resid:** Psychiatry, Univ Toronto Hosp 1986; Psychiatry, Natl Inst Mental Hlth-NIH 1987; **Fellow:** Anxiety Disorder, Natl Inst Mental Hlth-NIH 1990; **Fac Appt:** Prof Psyc, UCSD

Strouse, Thomas B MD [Psyc] - **Spec Exp:** Psychiatry in Cancer; Pain-Cancer; Psychiatry in Physical Illness; Psychopharmacology; **Hospital:** UCLA Ronald Reagan Med Ctr, Cedars-Sinai Med Ctr; **Address:** Resnick Neuropsychiatric Hosp at UCLA, 150 Medical Plaza, Ste 4230B, Los Angeles, CA 90025; **Phone:** 310-267-9159; **Board Cert:** Psychiatry 1993; Pain Medicine 2000; **Med School:** Case West Res Univ 1987; **Resid:** Psychiatry, UCLA Med Ctr 1991; **Fac Appt:** Clin Prof Psyc, UCLA

Weinstock, Robert MD [Psyc] - **Spec Exp:** Adolescent Psychiatry; Addiction/Substance Abuse; **Hospital:** Cedars-Sinai Med Ctr; **Address:** 1823 Sawtelle Blvd, Los Angeles, CA 90025; **Phone:** 310-477-9933; **Board Cert:** Psychiatry 1975; Forensic Psychiatry 2004; **Med School:** NYU Sch Med 1966; **Resid:** Psychiatry, McLean Hosp 1970; McLean Hosp 1972; **Fellow:** Psychiatric Research, Boston Univ 1974; **Fac Appt:** Clin Prof Psyc, UCLA

Psychiatry

Zerbe, Kathryn J MD [Psyc] - **Spec Exp:** Eating Disorders; Women's Health-Mental Health; Psychoanalysis; **Hospital:** OR Hlth & Sci Univ; **Address:** 3181 SW Sam Jackson Park Rd, MC OP02, Portland, OR 97239; **Phone:** 503-295-9909; **Board Cert:** Psychiatry 1984; **Med School:** Temple Univ 1978; **Resid:** Psychiatry, Menninger Clin 1982; Psychoanalysis, Topeka Inst for Psychoanalysis 1992; **Fac Appt:** Prof Psyc, Oregon Hlth & Sci Univ

Zisook, Sidney MD [Psyc] - **Spec Exp:** Bereavement/Traumatic Grief; Depression; Suicide; **Hospital:** VA San Diego Hlthcre Sys, UCSD Med Ctr; **Address:** UCSD, Dept Psychiatry, 9500 Gilman Drive, MS 9116A, La Jolla, CA 92093; **Phone:** 858-534-4040; **Board Cert:** Psychiatry 1975; **Med School:** Loyola Univ-Stritch Sch Med 1969; **Resid:** Psychiatry, Mass Genl Hosp 1973; **Fellow:** Psychiatry, Harvard 1973; **Fac Appt:** Prof Psyc, UCSD

ADDICTION PSYCHIATRY

New England

Schottenfeld, Richard MD [AdP] - **Spec Exp:** Drug Abuse-Consultation; Alcohol Abuse-Consultation; **Hospital:** Yale-New Haven Hosp, Connecticut Mental Hlth Ctr; **Address:** Connecticut Mental Health Ctr, 34 Park St, rm S-204, New Haven, CT 06519; **Phone:** 203-974-7349; **Board Cert:** Psychiatry 1984; **Med School:** Yale Univ 1976; **Resid:** Psychiatry, Yale Psych Inst 1982; **Fellow:** Epidemiology, Yale Univ 1984; **Fac Appt:** Assoc Prof Psyc, Yale Univ

Ziedonis, Douglas M MD [AdP] - **Spec Exp:** Tobacco Abuse; **Hospital:** UMass Memorial Med Ctr; **Address:** Univ Mass Medical School, Dept Psychiatry, 55 Lake Ave N, Worcester, MA 01655; **Phone:** 508-856-3066; **Board Cert:** Psychiatry 1994; Addiction Psychiatry 2006; **Med School:** Penn State Univ-Hershey Med Ctr 1985; **Resid:** Psychiatry, UCLA Med Ctr 1989; **Fellow:** Addiction Psychiatry, UCLA Med Ctr 1990; **Fac Appt:** Prof Psyc, Univ Mass Sch Med

Mid Atlantic

Frances, Richard J MD [AdP] - **Spec Exp:** Addiction/Substance Abuse; Anxiety & Mood Disorders; Forensic Psychiatry; **Hospital:** Silver Hill Hosp, NYU Langone Med Ctr (page 67); **Address:** 510 E 86th St, Ste 1D, New York, NY 10028; **Phone:** 212-861-0570; **Board Cert:** Psychiatry 1976; Addiction Psychiatry 2002; **Med School:** NYU Sch Med 1971; **Resid:** Psychiatry, Bronx Meml Hosp 1974; **Fellow:** Psychoanalysis, NY Psychoanalitic Inst 1984; **Fac Appt:** Clin Prof Psyc, NYU Sch Med

Galanter, Marc MD [AdP] - **Spec Exp:** Alcohol Abuse; Drug Abuse; **Hospital:** NYU Langone Med Ctr (page 67), Bellevue Hosp Ctr; **Address:** 285 Central Park West, New York, NY 10024-3006; **Phone:** 212-877-4093; **Board Cert:** Psychiatry 1974; Addiction Psychiatry 2002; **Med School:** Albert Einstein Coll Med 1967; **Resid:** Psychiatry, Bronx Muni Hosp-Einstein 1971; **Fac Appt:** Prof Psyc, NYU Sch Med

Kampman, Kyle M MD [AdP] - **Spec Exp:** Addiction/Substance Abuse; Cocaine Addiction; Opiate Addiction; **Hospital:** Hosp Univ Penn - UPHS (page 60); **Address:** Charles O'Brien Treatment Ctr, 3900 Chesnut St, Philadelphia, PA 19104; **Phone:** 215-222-3815; **Board Cert:** Psychiatry 2004; Addiction Psychiatry 2006; **Med School:** Tulane Univ 1985; **Resid:** Psychiatry, Univ Penn 1993; **Fellow:** Substance Abuse, Univ Penn 1994; **Fac Appt:** Assoc Prof Psyc, Univ Pennsylvania

Kleber, Herbert MD [AdP] - **Spec Exp:** Opiate Addiction; Cocaine Addiction; Drug Abuse; **Hospital:** NY-Presby Hosp/Columbia (page 66), NY State Psychiatric Inst; **Address:** NY State Psychiatric Inst, 1051 Riverside Drive, Room 3713, Unit 66, New York, NY 10032-1007; **Phone:** 212-543-5570; **Med School:** Jefferson Med Coll 1960; **Resid:** Psychiatry, Yale-New Haven Hosp 1964; **Fac Appt:** Prof Psyc, Columbia P&S

Serota, Ronald D MD [AdP] - **Spec Exp:** Addiction/Substance Abuse; **Hospital:** Thomas Jefferson Univ Hosp; **Address:** 833 Chestnut St, Ste 210, Philadelphia, PA 19107; **Phone:** 215-955-2542; **Board Cert:** Internal Medicine 1974; Psychiatry 1990; Addiction Psychiatry 1998; **Med School:** Thomas Jefferson Univ 1968; **Resid:** Internal Medicine, Mt Zion Hosp 1972; Psychiatry, Thomas Jefferson Univ Hosp 1981; **Fac Appt:** Asst Prof Psyc, Thomas Jefferson Univ

Strain, Eric C MD [AdP] - **Spec Exp:** Addiction/Substance Abuse; Dual Diagnosis; Opiate Addiction; **Hospital:** Johns Hopkins Bayview Med Ctr (page 61); **Address:** 4940 Eastern Ave, Baltimore, MD 21224; **Phone:** 410-550-0016; **Board Cert:** Psychiatry 1989; Addiction Psychiatry 2002; **Med School:** Ohio State Univ 1984; **Resid:** Psychiatry, Johns Hopkins Hosp 1988; **Fellow:** Addiction Psychiatry, Johns Hopkins Hosp 1990; **Fac Appt:** Prof Psyc, Johns Hopkins Univ

Southeast

Abou-Khalil, Bassel MD [AdP] - **Spec Exp:** Epilepsy; **Hospital:** Vanderbilt Univ Med Ctr; **Address:** Vanderbilt Univ-Dept Neurology, 1161 21st Ave, rm A-0118 MCN, Nashville, TN 37232-2551; **Phone:** 615-936-0060; **Board Cert:** Neurology 1986; Clinical Neurophysiology 2002; **Med School:** Amer Univ Beirut 1978; **Resid:** Neurology, Strong Meml Hosp 1980; Neurology, Univ Mich Hosps 1982; **Fellow:** Epilepsy, Univ Mich Hosps 1985; Electroencephalography, Univ Mich Hosps 1985; **Fac Appt:** Prof N, Vanderbilt Univ

Anton, Raymond F MD [AdP] - **Spec Exp:** Alcohol Abuse; Clinical Trials; **Hospital:** MUSC Med Ctr; **Address:** MUSC Dept Psychiatry, 67 President St, Box 250861, Charleston, SC 29425; **Phone:** 843-792-1226; **Board Cert:** Psychiatry 1982; **Med School:** UMDNJ-Rutgers Med Sch 1976; **Resid:** Psychiatry, Yale-New Haven Hosp/CT Mental Health Ctr 1980; **Fac Appt:** Prof Psyc, Med Univ SC

Brady, Kathleen T MD/PhD [AdP] - **Spec Exp:** Addiction/Substance Abuse; Dual Diagnosis; **Hospital:** MUSC Med Ctr; **Address:** MUSC Inst of Psychiatry, 67 President St, Box 250861, Charleston, SC 29425; **Phone:** 843-792-5205; **Board Cert:** Psychiatry 1992; Addiction Psychiatry 2002; **Med School:** Med Univ SC 1985; **Resid:** Psychiatry, Med Univ SC 1989; **Fellow:** Addiction Psychiatry, Med Univ SC 1989; **Fac Appt:** Prof Psyc, Med Univ SC

Midwest

Stine, Susan M MD/PhD [AdP] - **Spec Exp:** Addiction/Substance Abuse; Opiate Addiction; **Hospital:** Detroit Med Ctr, VA Med Ctr; **Address:** Wayne State Univ Sch Med, Dept Psychiatry, 2761 E Jefferson Ave, Detroit, MI 48207; **Phone:** 313-993-9879; **Board Cert:** Psychiatry 1993; Addiction Psychiatry 2002; **Med School:** Univ Miami Sch Med 1983; **Resid:** Psychiatry, Yale-New Haven Hosp 1987; **Fac Appt:** Assoc Prof Psyc, Wayne State Univ

Addiction Psychiatry

Great Plains and Mountains

Howell, Elizabeth F MD [AdP] - **Spec Exp:** Opiate Addiction; Alcohol Abuse; Addiction/Substance Abuse; Pain Management; **Hospital:** Univ Utah Hosps and Clins; **Address:** Univ Utah Neuropsychiatric Inst, 501 Chipeta Way, Salt Lake City, UT 84108; **Phone:** 801-585-1575; **Board Cert:** Psychiatry 1985; Addiction Psychiatry 2003; Addiction Medicine 1998; **Med School:** Med Univ SC 1980; **Resid:** Psychiatry, Med Univ South Carolina 1984; **Fellow:** Psychiatric Research, Med Univ South Carolina 1985; **Fac Appt:** Assoc Clin Prof Psyc, Univ Utah

Southwest

Kosten, Thomas MD [AdP] - **Spec Exp:** Cocaine Addiction; Alcohol Abuse; Psychopharmacology; Opiate Addiction; **Hospital:** DeBakey VA Med Ctr-Houston, UT MD Anderson Cancer Ctr; **Address:** Michael DeBakey VA Medical Ctr, 2002 Holcombe Blvd, Research - Building 110, Houston, TX 77030; **Phone:** 713-794-7032; **Board Cert:** Psychiatry 1984; Addiction Psychiatry 2002; **Med School:** Cornell Univ-Weill Med Coll 1977; **Resid:** Psychiatry, Yale-New Haven Hosp 1981; **Fellow:** Epidemiology, Yale-New Haven Hosp 1983; **Fac Appt:** Prof Psyc, Baylor Coll Med

West Coast and Pacific

Schuckit, Marc A MD [AdP] - **Spec Exp:** Alcohol Abuse; Psychopharmacology; **Hospital:** VA San Diego Hlthcre Sys, UCSD Med Ctr; **Address:** VA San Diego Healthcare System, Dept Psychiatry (116A), 3350 La Jolla Village Drive, San Diego, CA 92161-2002; **Phone:** 858-552-8585 x7978; **Board Cert:** Psychiatry 1974; **Med School:** Washington Univ, St Louis 1968; **Resid:** Psychiatry, Washington Univ Affil Hosp 1971; Psychiatry, UCSD Med Ctr 1972; **Fac Appt:** Prof Psyc, UCSD

Walker, R Dale MD [AdP] - **Spec Exp:** Alcohol Abuse-Consultation; Drug Abuse-Consultation; Substance Abuse-Consultation; **Hospital:** OR Hlth & Sci Univ; **Address:** Oregon Hlth & Sci Univ, 3181 SW Sam Jackson Pk Rd, MC GH151, Portland, OR 97239; **Phone:** 503-494-3703; **Board Cert:** Psychiatry 1982; **Med School:** Univ Okla Coll Med 1972; **Resid:** Psychiatry, Univ Oklahoma Med Ctr 1973; Psychiatry, UCSD Med Ctr 1977; **Fellow:** Public Health & Genl Preventive Med, Andriga Stampur; **Fac Appt:** Prof Psyc, Oregon Hlth & Sci Univ

CHILD & ADOLESCENT PSYCHIATRY

New England

Biederman, Joseph MD [ChAP] - **Spec Exp:** ADD/ADHD; Anxiety & Mood Disorders; Psychopharmacology; **Hospital:** Mass Genl Hosp; **Address:** 55 Fruit St Yawkey Bldg - rm 6900, Boston, MA 02114; **Phone:** 617-726-1743; **Board Cert:** Psychiatry 1983; Child & Adolescent Psychiatry 1984; **Med School:** Argentina 1971; **Resid:** Psychiatry, Hadassah Univ Hosp 1977; Psychiatry, Mass Genl Hosp 1981; **Fellow:** Child Psychiatry, Childrens Hosp 1979; **Fac Appt:** Prof Psyc, Harvard Med Sch

Fritz, Gregory K MD [ChAP] - **Spec Exp:** Asthma; Psychosomatic Disorders; **Hospital:** Rhode Island Hosp; **Address:** RI Hosp, Child & Family Psychiatry, 1 Hoppin St Fl 2, Providence, RI 02903; **Phone:** 401-444-7573; **Board Cert:** Psychiatry 1977; Child & Adolescent Psychiatry 1978; **Med School:** Tufts Univ 1971; **Resid:** Psychiatry, San Mateo Co Hosp 1974; Child Psychiatry, Stanford Univ Med Ctr 1977; **Fac Appt:** Prof Psyc, Brown Univ

Herzog, David B MD [ChAP] - **Spec Exp:** Eating Disorders; Somatic Disorders-Adolescent; **Hospital:** Mass Genl Hosp; **Address:** 2 Longfellow Place, Ste 200, Boston, MA 02114; **Phone:** 617-724-0799; **Board Cert:** Pediatrics 1980; Psychiatry 1982; Child & Adolescent Psychiatry 1986; **Med School:** Mexico 1973; **Resid:** Pediatrics, Univ Wisc 1975; Pediatrics, Boston City Hosp 1976; **Fellow:** Child & Adolescent Psychiatry, Chldns Hosp 1978; Psychiatry, Mass Genl Hosp 1980; **Fac Appt:** Prof Psyc, Harvard Med Sch

Hudziak, James MD [ChAP] - **Spec Exp:** ADD/ADHD; Obsessive-Compulsive Disorder; Psychopharmacology; **Hospital:** Fletcher Allen Health Care- Med Ctr Campus; **Address:** Univ Vermont Med Sch, Dept Psychiatry, 1 S Prospect Dr, MCHS-Arnold 6-UHC Campus, Burlington, VT 05401; **Phone:** 802-656-1084; **Board Cert:** Psychiatry 2005; Child & Adolescent Psychiatry 2005; **Med School:** Univ Minn 1988; **Resid:** Psychiatry, St Louis Chldns Hosp 1991; **Fac Appt:** Assoc Prof Psyc, Univ VT Coll Med

King, Robert A MD [ChAP] - **Spec Exp:** Tourette's Syndrome; Obsessive-Compulsive Disorder; Psychoanalysis; **Hospital:** Yale-New Haven Hosp, Greenwich Hosp; **Address:** Yale Child Study Ctr, 230 S Frontage Rd, Box 207900, New Haven, CT 06510; **Phone:** 203-785-5880; **Board Cert:** Psychiatry 1974; Child & Adolescent Psychiatry 1981; **Med School:** Harvard Med Sch 1968; **Resid:** Pediatrics, Chldns Hosp 1969; Psychiatry, Mass Mental Hlth Ctr 1971; **Fellow:** Child Psychiatry, Chldns Hosp 1972; Child Psychiatry, Chldns Hosp Natl Med Ctr 1974; **Fac Appt:** Prof ChAP, Yale Univ

Leckman, James F MD [ChAP] - **Spec Exp:** Tourette's Syndrome; Obsessive-Compulsive Disorder; Autism; **Hospital:** Yale-New Haven Hosp; **Address:** Yale Child Study Ctr, 230 S Frontage Rd, Box 207900, New Haven, CT 06520-7900; **Phone:** 203-785-7971; **Board Cert:** Psychiatry 1980; Child & Adolescent Psychiatry 1982; **Med School:** Univ New Mexico 1973; **Resid:** Psychiatry, Yale Univ 1979; Child Psychiatry, Yale Chld Stdy Ctr 1980; **Fellow:** Psychiatry, Natl Inst Mental Hlth 1976; **Fac Appt:** Prof Psyc, Yale Univ

Spencer, Thomas MD [ChAP] - **Spec Exp:** ADD/ADHD; **Hospital:** Mass Genl Hosp; **Address:** Mass General Hospital, 55 Fruit St, Ste YAW 6A, Boston, MA 02114; **Phone:** 617-724-5600; **Board Cert:** Psychiatry 1984; Child & Adolescent Psychiatry 1992; **Med School:** Univ Wisc 1978; **Resid:** Psychiatry, New England Med Ctr 1984; **Fellow:** Child & Adolescent Psychiatry, Mass Genl Hosp 1992; **Fac Appt:** Assoc Prof Psyc, Harvard Med Sch

Volkmar, Fred R MD [ChAP] - **Spec Exp:** Autism; Asperger's Syndrome; Developmental Disorders; Mental Retardation; **Hospital:** Yale-New Haven Hosp; **Address:** Yale Child Study Ctr, 230 S Frontage Rd, Box 207900, Rm NIHB 200, New Haven, CT 06520-7900; **Phone:** 203-785-5759; **Board Cert:** Psychiatry 1981; Child & Adolescent Psychiatry 1988; **Med School:** Stanford Univ 1976; **Resid:** Psychiatry, Stanford Univ 1980; Child Psychiatry, Yale Child Study Ctr 1982; **Fac Appt:** Prof Psyc, Yale Univ

Wilens, Timothy MD [ChAP] - **Spec Exp:** ADD/ADHD; Bipolar/Mood Disorders; Addiction/Substance Abuse; **Hospital:** Mass Genl Hosp; **Address:** Mass Genl Hosp, Dept Psyc, 55 Fruit St Yawkey Bldg - Ste 6A, Boston, MA 02114; **Phone:** 617-724-5600; **Board Cert:** Psychiatry 1990; Child & Adolescent Psychiatry 1991; Addiction Psychiatry 2004; **Med School:** Univ Mich Med Sch 1985; **Resid:** Internal Medicine, Henry Ford Hosp 1986; Psychiatry, Mass Genl Hosp 1988; **Fellow:** Child & Adolescent Psychiatry, Mass Genl Hosp 1990; **Fac Appt:** Assoc Prof Psyc, Harvard Med Sch

Child & Adolescent Psychiatry

Mid Atlantic

Abright, Arthur R MD [ChAP] - **Spec Exp:** Bipolar/Mood Disorders; ADD/ADHD; Post Traumatic Stress Disorder; Anxiety Disorders; **Hospital:** St Vincent Cath Med Ctrs - Manhattan; **Address:** 144 W 12th St, New York, NY 10011-8202; **Phone:** 212-604-8213; **Board Cert:** Psychiatry 1978; Child & Adolescent Psychiatry 1981; **Med School:** Univ Tex SW, Dallas 1973; **Resid:** Psychiatry, St Vincent's Hosp 1974; Psychiatry, NY Hosp-Cornell Med Ctr 1977; **Fellow:** Child & Adolescent Psychiatry, NY Hosp-Cornell Med Ctr 1979; **Fac Appt:** Clin Prof Psyc, NY Med Coll

Bird, Hector MD [ChAP] - **Spec Exp:** ADD/ADHD; Anxiety & Depression; Personality Disorders; **Hospital:** NY-Presby Hosp/Columbia (page 66); **Address:** 300 W 72nd St, Ste 1F, New York, NY 10023-2004; **Phone:** 212-874-5311; **Board Cert:** Psychiatry 1975; Child & Adolescent Psychiatry 1977; **Med School:** Yale Univ 1965; **Resid:** Psychiatry, NY State Psych Inst 1971; NY State Psych Inst 1972; **Fellow:** Psychoanalysis, WA White Institute 1977; **Fac Appt:** Prof Emeritus Psyc, Columbia P&S

Bogrov, Michael MD [ChAP] - **Spec Exp:** ADD/ADHD; Mood Disorders; **Hospital:** Sheppard Pratt Hlth Sys, Johns Hopkins Hosp (page 61); **Address:** 6501 N Charles St, P.O. Box 6815, Towson, MD 21204-6815; **Phone:** 410-938-4913; **Board Cert:** Psychiatry 1993; Child & Adolescent Psychiatry 1994; **Med School:** Emory Univ 1987; **Resid:** Psychiatry, Univ Maryland 1990; Critical Care Obstetrics, Johns Hopkins Hosp 1992; **Fac Appt:** Asst Prof Psyc, Johns Hopkins Univ

Brent, David A MD [ChAP] - **Spec Exp:** Suicide; **Hospital:** Western Psych Inst & Clin - UPMC; **Address:** Western Psych Inst & Clin, 3811 O'Hara St, Ste 315 BFT, Pittsburgh, PA 15213-2593; **Phone:** 412-246-5596; **Board Cert:** Pediatrics 1981; Psychiatry 1982; Child & Adolescent Psychiatry 1983; **Med School:** Jefferson Med Coll 1974; **Resid:** Psychiatry, Western Psych Inst 1982; **Fellow:** Psychiatry, Univ Colorado Med Ctr 1976; **Fac Appt:** Prof Psyc, Univ Pittsburgh

Bukstein, Oscar G MD [ChAP] - **Spec Exp:** ADD/ADHD; Substance Abuse; Clinical Trials; **Hospital:** Western Psych Inst & Clin - UPMC; **Address:** Western Psychiatric Inst & Clinic, 3811 O'Hara St, Pittsburgh, PA 15213; **Phone:** 412-246-5114; **Board Cert:** Psychiatry 1990; Child & Adolescent Psychiatry 1991; Addiction Psychiatry 2003; **Med School:** Univ Tex Med Br, Galveston 1983; **Resid:** Child Psychiatry, Western Psych Inst 1988; **Fellow:** Psychiatric Research, Western Psych Inst 1988; **Fac Appt:** Prof Psyc, Univ Pittsburgh

Coffey, Barbara J MD [ChAP] - **Spec Exp:** Tourette's Syndrome; ADD/ADHD; Obsessive-Compulsive Disorder; **Hospital:** NYU Langone Med Ctr (page 67); **Address:** NYU Child Study Ctr, 577 1st Ave, New York, NY 10016; **Phone:** 212-263-3926; **Board Cert:** Psychiatry 1981; Child & Adolescent Psychiatry 1986; **Med School:** Tufts Univ 1975; **Resid:** Psychiatry, Boston Univ Med Ctr 1978; **Fellow:** Child & Adolescent Psychiatry, Tufts Univ 1980; **Fac Appt:** Assoc Prof Psyc, NYU Sch Med

Foley, Carmel MD [ChAP] - **Spec Exp:** Mood Disorders; **Hospital:** Schneider Chldn's Hosp; **Address:** Schneider Chldns Hosp, 269-01 76th Ave Fl 4, New Hyde Park, NY 11040; **Phone:** 718-470-3550; **Board Cert:** Psychiatry 1979; Child & Adolescent Psychiatry 1981; Forensic Psychiatry 1999; **Med School:** Ireland 1972; **Resid:** Psychiatry, St Patrick's Hosp 1976; Psychiatry, Lafayette Clinic 1977; **Fellow:** Child & Adolescent Psychiatry, Lafayette Clinic 1979; **Fac Appt:** Assoc Prof Psyc, Albert Einstein Coll Med

Fornari, Victor MD [ChAP] - **Spec Exp:** Eating Disorders; Trauma Psychiatry; Post Traumatic Stress Disorder; **Hospital:** Zucker Hillside Hosp; **Address:** Zucker Hillside Hospital, Ambulatory Care Pavilion Lower Level, 75-59 263rd St, Glen Oaks, NY 11004; **Phone:** 718-470-3510; **Board Cert:** Psychiatry 1984; Child & Adolescent Psychiatry 1985; **Med School:** SUNY Downstate 1979; **Resid:** Psychiatry, Hosp Univ Penn 1982; **Fellow:** Child & Adolescent Psychiatry, LIJ Med Ctr 1984; **Fac Appt:** Prof Psyc, NYU Sch Med

Greenspan, Stanley I MD [ChAP] - **Spec Exp:** Autism; Infant/Toddler Psychiatry; **Hospital:** G Washington Univ Hosp; **Address:** 7201 Glenbrook Rd, Bethesda, MD 20814; **Phone:** 301-657-2348; **Board Cert:** Psychiatry 1972; **Med School:** Yale Univ 1966; **Resid:** Psychiatry, Columbia-Presby Psych Inst 1969; **Fellow:** Child & Adolescent Psychiatry, Childrens Hosp Natl Med Ctr 1971; **Fac Appt:** Clin Prof Psyc, Geo Wash Univ

Hertzig, Margaret MD [ChAP] - **Spec Exp:** Developmental Disorders; ADD/ADHD; **Hospital:** NY-Presby Hosp/Weill Cornell (page 66); **Address:** 525 E 68th St, Box 140, New York, NY 10021-4870; **Phone:** 212-746-5712; **Board Cert:** Psychiatry 1968; Child & Adolescent Psychiatry 1975; **Med School:** NYU Sch Med 1960; **Resid:** Pediatrics, Jewish Hosp 1962; Psychiatry, Bellevue Psych Hosp 1964; **Fellow:** Psychiatric Research, NYU Sch Med 1966; **Fac Appt:** Prof Psyc, Cornell Univ-Weill Med Coll

Hirsch, Glenn S MD [ChAP] - **Spec Exp:** Anxiety & Mood Disorders; Tourette's Syndrome; Bipolar/Mood Disorders; ADD/ADHD; **Hospital:** NYU Langone Med Ctr (page 67), Bellevue Hosp Ctr; **Address:** NYU Child Study Center, 577 First Ave, New York, NY 10016; **Phone:** 212-263-8704; **Board Cert:** Psychiatry 1984; Child & Adolescent Psychiatry 1985; **Med School:** Albert Einstein Coll Med 1979; **Resid:** Psychiatry, New York Hosp-Cornell 1982; **Fellow:** Child & Adolescent Psychiatry, Columbia-Presby Med Ctr 1984; **Fac Appt:** Asst Prof Psyc, NYU Sch Med

Pomeroy, John C MD [ChAP] - **Spec Exp:** Autism; Mental Retardation; Developmental Disorders; **Hospital:** Stony Brook Univ Med Ctr; **Address:** The Cody Center for Autism, 5 Medical Drive, Port Jefferson Stn, NY 11776; **Phone:** 631-632-3070; **Board Cert:** Psychiatry 1984; Child & Adolescent Psychiatry 1988; **Med School:** England, UK 1973; **Resid:** Psychiatry, St Mary's Hosp 1979; **Fellow:** Child & Adolescent Psychiatry, Univ Iowa Hosps 1981; **Fac Appt:** Assoc Prof Psyc, SUNY Stony Brook

Pruitt, David B MD [ChAP] - **Hospital:** Univ of MD Med Ctr; **Address:** Univ Maryland, Div Child & Adolescent Psychiatry, 701 W Pratt St, Ste 429, Baltimore, MD 21201; **Phone:** 410-328-3522; **Board Cert:** Psychiatry 1979; Child & Adolescent Psychiatry 1981; **Med School:** Univ Tex, Houston 1974; **Resid:** Psychiatry, Hosp Univ Penn 1978; Child Psychiatry, Child Guidance Ctr 1979; **Fac Appt:** Prof Psyc, Univ MD Sch Med

Rapoport, Judith MD [ChAP] - **Spec Exp:** Schizophrenia; Obsessive-Compulsive Disorder; **Hospital:** Natl Inst of Hlth - Clin Ctr; **Address:** 3010 44th Place NW, Washington, DC 20016; **Phone:** 202-966-7355; **Board Cert:** Psychiatry 1969; Child & Adolescent Psychiatry 1969; **Med School:** Harvard Med Sch 1959; **Resid:** Psychiatry, Mass Mental Hlth Ctr 1961; Psychiatry, St Elizabeth Hosp 1962; **Fellow:** Psychiatry, Karolinska Inst 1964; Child & Adolescent Psychiatry, Childns Hosp 1966

Riddle, Mark A MD [ChAP] - **Spec Exp:** Psychopharmacology; Anxiety Disorders; Mood Disorders; **Hospital:** Johns Hopkins Hosp (page 61); **Address:** 600 N Wolfe St, CMSC-346, Baltimore, MD 21287-3325; **Phone:** 410-955-2320; **Board Cert:** Psychiatry 1982; Child & Adolescent Psychiatry 1986; **Med School:** Indiana Univ 1977; **Resid:** Psychiatry, Yale-New Haven Hosp 1981; **Fellow:** Child & Adolescent Psychiatry, Yale Child Study Ctr 1983; **Fac Appt:** Prof Psyc, Johns Hopkins Univ

Rostain, Anthony L MD [ChAP] - **Spec Exp:** ADD/ADHD; Autism; Tourette's Syndrome; Asperger's Syndrome; **Hospital:** Chldns Hosp of Philadelphia, The, Penn Presby Med Ctr - UPHS (page 60); **Address:** Hosp Univ Penn, Dept Psychiatry, 3535 Market St Fl 2, Philadelphia, PA 19104; **Phone:** 215-746-7210; **Board Cert:** Pediatrics 1985; Psychiatry 1988; Child & Adolescent Psychiatry 1989; **Med School:** NYU Sch Med 1980; **Resid:** Pediatrics, Children's Hosp 1983; Psychiatry, Hosp Univ Penn 1987; **Fellow:** Child Psychiatry, Philadelphia Child Guidance Clin 1988; **Fac Appt:** Assoc Prof Psyc, Univ Pennsylvania

Child & Adolescent Psychiatry

Turecki, Stanley K MD [ChAP] - **Spec Exp:** Temperamentally Difficult Child; ADD/ADHD; Parenting Issues; **Hospital:** Lenox Hill Hosp (page 62), Beth Israel Med Ctr - Petrie Division (page 57); **Address:** 136 E 64th St, Ste 1B, New York, NY 10021-2137; **Phone:** 212-355-2535; **Board Cert:** Psychiatry 1978; Child & Adolescent Psychiatry 1981; **Med School:** South Africa 1961; **Resid:** Psychiatry, Tara Hospital 1969; Psychiatry, Mt Sinai Hosp 1971

Walkup, John MD [ChAP] - **Spec Exp:** Anxiety Disorders; **Hospital:** Johns Hopkins Hosp (page 61); **Address:** Johns Hopkins Hosp, Dept Child Psyc, 600 N Wolfe St, CMSC 314, Baltimore, MD 21287; **Phone:** 410-955-5823; **Board Cert:** Psychiatry 1987; Child & Adolescent Psychiatry 1992; **Med School:** Univ Minn 1982; **Resid:** Psychiatry, Yale Univ Med Sch 1985; Yale Chld Study Ctr 1988; **Fac Appt:** Asst Prof Psyc, Johns Hopkins Univ

Weller, Elizabeth B MD [ChAP] - **Spec Exp:** Anxiety & Mood Disorders; Bipolar/Mood Disorders; Depression; Bereavement/Traumatic Grief; **Hospital:** Chldns Hosp of Philadelphia, The; **Address:** Children's Hosp of Philadelphia, Mood & Anxiety Ctr, 34th & Civic Center Blvd, Philadelphia, PA 19104; **Phone:** 215-590-7555; **Board Cert:** Psychiatry 1981; Child & Adolescent Psychiatry 1982; **Med School:** Lebanon 1975; **Resid:** Psychiatry, Renard Hosp-Wash Univ 1978; **Fellow:** Child & Adolescent Psychiatry, Univ Kansas Med Ctr 1979; **Fac Appt:** Prof Psyc

Southeast

Deas, Deborah V MD [ChAP] - **Spec Exp:** Addiction/Substance Abuse; Dual Diagnosis; Substance Abuse in ADHD Patients; **Hospital:** MUSC Med Ctr; **Address:** MUSC, Ctr for Drug & Alcohol Programs, 67 President St, Charleston, SC 29425; **Phone:** 843-792-5214; **Board Cert:** Psychiatry 2005; Child & Adolescent Psychiatry 2007; **Med School:** Med Univ SC 1989; **Resid:** Psychiatry, MUSC Med Ctr 1992; **Fellow:** Child & Adolescent Psychiatry, MUSC Med Ctr 1994; Addiction Psychiatry, MUSC/Natl Inst Alcohol Abuse & Alcoholism 1994; **Fac Appt:** Prof Psyc, Med Univ SC

Heston, Jerry D MD [ChAP] - **Spec Exp:** ADD/ADHD; Depression; Asperger's Syndrome; **Hospital:** Le Bonheur Chldns Med Ctr, St Jude Children's Research Hosp; **Address:** Child & Adolescent Psychiatric Assocs, 1135 Cully Rd, Ste 100, Cordova, TN 38106; **Phone:** 901-752-1980; **Board Cert:** Psychiatry 1988; Pediatrics 2004; Child & Adolescent Psychiatry 1989; **Med School:** Univ S Fla Coll Med 1981; **Resid:** Pediatrics, LeBonheur Chldns Hosp 1984; Psychiatry, Univ Tennessee Affil Hosp 1986; **Fellow:** Child & Adolescent Psychiatry, Univ Tennessee Affil Hosp 1988; **Fac Appt:** Clin Prof Psyc, Univ Tenn Coll Med, Memphis

Sexson, Sandra G B MD [ChAP] - **Spec Exp:** Psychiatry in Transplant Patients; Death & Dying; **Hospital:** Med Coll of GA Hosp and Clin (MCG Health Inc); **Address:** Medical College Georgia, 997 St Sebastian Way, Augusta, GA 30912; **Phone:** 706-721-6699; **Board Cert:** Psychiatry 1980; Child & Adolescent Psychiatry 2004; **Med School:** Univ Miss 1971; **Resid:** Psychiatry, Tex Hlth Sci Ctr 1974; Child Psychiatry, Washington Univ Affil Hosp 1978; **Fac Appt:** Prof Psyc, Med Coll GA

Wright, Harry H MD [ChAP] - **Spec Exp:** Infant/Toddler Psychiatry; Autism & Developmental Disorders; Anxiety Disorders; **Hospital:** William S Hall Psyc Inst, Richland Mem Hosp; **Address:** 3555 Harden St Ext, Ste 301, Columbia, SC 29203-6894; **Phone:** 803-434-4250; **Board Cert:** Psychiatry 1982; Child & Adolescent Psychiatry 1984; **Med School:** Univ Pennsylvania 1976; **Resid:** Psychiatry, Wm S Hall Psyc Inst 1979; **Fellow:** Child & Adolescent Psychiatry, Wm S Hall Psyc Inst-Univ S Carolina 1981; **Fac Appt:** Prof Psyc, Univ SC Sch Med

Midwest

Alessi, Norman E MD [ChAP] - **Spec Exp:** Mood Disorders; Autism; Cognitive Psychotherapy; ADD/ADHD; **Hospital:** Univ Michigan Hlth Sys; **Address:** 825 Victors Way, Ste 310, Ann Arbor, MI 48108-2830; **Phone:** 734-222-6222; **Board Cert:** Psychiatry 1982; Child & Adolescent Psychiatry 1985; **Med School:** Emory Univ 1976; **Resid:** Psychiatry, Univ Mich Med Ctr 1980; Child Psychiatry, Univ Mich Med Ctr 1981; **Fellow:** Child & Adolescent Psychiatry, Univ Mich Med Ctr 1983; **Fac Appt:** Prof Emeritus Psyc, Univ Mich Med Sch

Boxer, Gary H MD [ChAP] - **Spec Exp:** ADD/ADHD; Parenting Issues; Mood Disorders; **Hospital:** St Louis Chldns Hosp, Barnes-Jewish Hosp; **Address:** St Louis Chldns Hosp, Dept Psychiatry, 24 S Kingshighway Blvd, St Louis, MO 63108; **Phone:** 314-286-1740; **Board Cert:** Psychiatry 1986; Child & Adolescent Psychiatry 1988; **Med School:** Univ Colorado 1980; **Resid:** Psychiatry, Univ Michigan Med Ctr 1983; **Fellow:** Child Psychiatry, Univ Colorado 1985; **Fac Appt:** Assoc Prof Psyc, Washington Univ, St Louis

Campo, John V MD [ChAP] - **Spec Exp:** Psychosomatic Disorders; Psychiatry in Physical Illness; **Hospital:** Nationwide Chldn's Hosp, Ohio St Univ Med Ctr; **Address:** Columbus Chldn's Hosp, 700 Childrens Drive, Timken Hall H2K, Columbus, OH 43205; **Phone:** 614-722-2291; **Board Cert:** Pediatrics 1986; Psychiatry 1989; Child & Adolescent Psychiatry 1993; **Med School:** Univ Pennsylvania 1982; **Resid:** Pediatrics, Childrens Hosp 1985; Psychiatry, West Psych Inst Clin 1989

Dulcan, Mina K MD [ChAP] - **Spec Exp:** ADD/ADHD; **Hospital:** Children's Mem Hosp; **Address:** Chldns Meml Hosp, Dept Psyc, 2300 Children's Plaza, Box 10, Chicago, IL 60614; **Phone:** 773-880-4811; **Board Cert:** Psychiatry 1978; Child & Adolescent Psychiatry 1979; **Med School:** Penn State Univ-Hershey Med Ctr 1974; **Resid:** Psychiatry, Western Psych Inst/Clinic 1977; **Fellow:** Child Psychiatry, Western Psych Inst 1978; **Fac Appt:** Prof Psyc, Northwestern Univ

Leventhal, Bennett MD [ChAP] - **Spec Exp:** Autism; ADD/ADHD; Psychopharmacology; **Hospital:** Univ of IL Med Ctr at Chicago; **Address:** Univ Illinois, Dept Psychiatry, 1747 W Roosevelt Rd, MC 747, Chicago, IL 60608; **Phone:** 312-355-3026; **Board Cert:** Psychiatry 1979; Child & Adolescent Psychiatry 1980; **Med School:** Louisiana State U, New Orleans 1974; **Resid:** Psychiatry, Duke Univ Med Ctr 1978; **Fellow:** Child & Adolescent Psychiatry, Duke Univ Med Ctr 1977; **Fac Appt:** Prof Psyc, Univ IL Coll Med

Luby, Joan L MD [ChAP] - **Spec Exp:** Mood Disorders; **Hospital:** Barnes-Jewish Hosp; **Address:** Wash Univ Sch Med, Dept Psychiatry, 660 S Euclid Ave, Box 8134, St Louis, MO 63110; **Phone:** 314-286-2730; **Board Cert:** Psychiatry 1993; Child & Adolescent Psychiatry 1993; **Med School:** Wayne State Univ 1985; **Resid:** Psychiatry, Stanford Univ Sch Med 1988; **Fellow:** Child & Adolescent Psychiatry, Stanford Univ Sch Med 1990; **Fac Appt:** Assoc Prof Psyc, Washington Univ, St Louis

Martini, D Richard MD [ChAP] - **Spec Exp:** Psychiatry in Physical Illness; Post Traumatic Stress Disorder; ADD/ADHD; Brain Injury; **Hospital:** Children's Mem Hosp; **Address:** Children's Meml Hospital, Psychiatry, 2300 Children's Plaza, Box 10, Chicago, IL 60614-3394; **Phone:** 773-880-4825; **Board Cert:** Psychiatry 1987; Child & Adolescent Psychiatry 1990; **Med School:** Univ Nebr Coll Med 1982; **Resid:** Psychiatry, Univ Pittsburgh Med Ctr 1985; Child Psychiatry, Univ Pittsburgh Med Ctr 1987; **Fac Appt:** Assoc Prof Psyc, Northwestern Univ

McDougle, Christopher J MD [ChAP] - **Spec Exp:** Autism & Developmental Disorders; Obsessive-Compulsive Disorder; Tourette's Syndrome; **Hospital:** Riley Hosp for Children, Methodist Hosp - Indianapolis; **Address:** 1111 W 10th St, Psychiatry Bldg - rm A-305, Indianapolis, IN 46202-4800; **Phone:** 317-274-8162; **Board Cert:** Psychiatry 1992; Child & Adolescent Psychiatry 2006; **Med School:** Indiana Univ 1986; **Resid:** Psychiatry, Yale Univ 1990; **Fellow:** Child & Adolescent Psychiatry, Yale Child Study Ctr 1995; **Fac Appt:** Prof Psyc, Indiana Univ

Child & Adolescent Psychiatry

Slomowitz, Marcia MD [ChAP] - **Spec Exp:** ADD/ADHD; Bipolar/Mood Disorders; Anxiety & Depression; **Hospital:** Northwestern Meml Hosp; **Address:** 333 N Michigan Ave, Ste 1125, Chicago, IL 60601; **Phone:** 312-726-1083; **Board Cert:** Psychiatry 1982; Child & Adolescent Psychiatry 1983; **Med School:** Univ Wisc 1977; **Resid:** Psychiatry, Univ Cincinnati Affil Hosp 1980; **Fellow:** Child & Adolescent Psychiatry, Univ Cincinnati Affil Hosp 1982; **Fac Appt:** Asst Prof Psyc, Northwestern Univ

Great Plains and Mountains

Hagman, Jennifer O MD [ChAP] - **Spec Exp:** Eating Disorders; Depression; Anxiety Disorders; **Hospital:** Chldn's Hosp - Aurora, The; **Address:** Chldns Hosp, Dept Psychiatry, 13123 E 16th Ave, Aurora, CO 80045; **Phone:** 720-777-2539; **Board Cert:** Psychiatry 1992; Child & Adolescent Psychiatry 1992; **Med School:** Univ Kans 1986; **Resid:** Psychiatry, UC Irvine Med Ctr 1990; **Fellow:** Child & Adolescent Psychiatry, UC Irvine Med Ctr 1991; **Fac Appt:** Assoc Prof Psyc, Univ Colorado

Wamboldt, Marianne Z MD [ChAP] - **Hospital:** Chldn's Hosp - Aurora, The; **Address:** Children's Hosp, Dept Psychiatry, 13123 E 16th Ave, Box B130, Aurora, CO 80045; **Phone:** 720-777-6096; **Board Cert:** Psychiatry 1986; Child & Adolescent Psychiatry 1991; **Med School:** Univ Wisc 1982; **Resid:** Psychiatry, Univ Wisconsin 1986

Southwest

Bleiberg, Efrain MD [ChAP] - **Spec Exp:** Trauma Psychiatry; Personality Disorders; **Hospital:** Menninger Clinic; **Address:** Menninger Hosp & Clinic, 2801 Gessner Drive, Box 809045, Houston, TX 77280-9045; **Phone:** 713-275-5213; **Board Cert:** Psychiatry 1985; Child & Adolescent Psychiatry 1986; **Med School:** Mexico 1976; **Resid:** Psychiatry, Menninger Fdn 1980; **Fellow:** Child & Adolescent Psychiatry, Menninger Fdn 1981

Emslie, Graham J MD [ChAP] - **Spec Exp:** Depression; **Hospital:** Chldns Med Ctr of Dallas; **Address:** UT SW Med Ctr at Dallas, 5323 Harry Hines Blvd, Dallas, TX 75390-8589; **Phone:** 214-456-5921; **Board Cert:** Psychiatry 1981; **Med School:** Scotland, UK 1974; **Resid:** Psychiatry, Univ Rochester 1978; Child Psychiatry, Stanford Med Ctr 1981; **Fac Appt:** Prof Psyc, Univ Tex SW, Dallas

Sargent III, Albert J MD [ChAP] - **Spec Exp:** Eating Disorders; Suicide; Family Therapy; Trauma Psychiatry; **Hospital:** Ben Taub Genl Hosp, Texas Chldns Hosp; **Address:** Baylor Coll Med, Dept Psychiatry, One Baylor Plaza, Houston, TX 77030-3411; **Phone:** 713-798-7889; **Board Cert:** Pediatrics 1979; Psychiatry 1988; Child & Adolescent Psychiatry 1989; **Med School:** Univ Rochester 1973; **Resid:** Pediatrics, Univ Wisc Hosp 1977; Phila Child Guidance Ctr 1980; **Fellow:** Ambulatory Pediatrics, Univ Wisc Hosp 1976; **Fac Appt:** Prof Psyc, Baylor Coll Med

Zeanah Jr, Charles H MD [ChAP] - **Spec Exp:** Attachment Disorders; Abuse/Neglect; Adoption-International; **Hospital:** Tulane Univ Hosp & Clin; **Address:** Tulane Univ Sch Med, Dept Psych & Neurology, 1440 Canal St, TB-52, New Orleans, LA 70112-2715; **Phone:** 504-988-5402; **Board Cert:** Psychiatry 1983; Child & Adolescent Psychiatry 1983; **Med School:** Tulane Univ 1977; **Resid:** Psychiatry, Duke Univ Med Ctr 1980; Stanford Univ Med Ctr 1982; **Fellow:** Research, Stanford Univ Med ctr 1984; **Fac Appt:** Prof Psyc, Tulane Univ

West Coast and Pacific

King, Bryan H MD [ChAP] - **Spec Exp:** Mental Retardation; Autism; Self-Injurious Behavior (SIB); **Hospital:** Chldns Hosp and Regl Med Ctr - Seattle; **Address:** Chldns Hosp & Regl Med Ctr, Dept Psych, 4800 Sand Point Way NE, MS W3636, Seattle, WA 98105; **Phone:** 206-987-4080; **Board Cert:** Psychiatry 1991; Child & Adolescent Psychiatry 2004; **Med School:** Med Coll Wisc 1983; **Resid:** Psychiatry, UCLA Neuropsych Inst 1987; **Fellow:** Child & Adolescent Psychiatry, UCLA Neuropsych Inst 1990; **Fac Appt:** Prof Psyc, Univ Wash

McCracken, James T MD [ChAP] - **Spec Exp:** Obsessive-Compulsive Disorder; Tourette's Syndrome; **Hospital:** UCLA Neuropsychiatric Hosp; **Address:** UCLA Neuropsychiatric Inst, 760 Westwood Plaza, Ste 48-270, Los Angeles, CA 90027; **Phone:** 310-825-0470; **Board Cert:** Psychiatry 1986; Child & Adolescent Psychiatry 1988; **Med School:** Baylor Coll Med 1980; **Resid:** Psychiatry, Duke Univ Med Ctr 1984; **Fellow:** Child & Adolescent Psychiatry, UCLA Neuropsych Inst 1985; **Fac Appt:** Prof Psyc, UCLA

McKelvey, Robert S MD [ChAP] - **Spec Exp:** Suicide; Depression; Cross Cultural Psychiatry; **Hospital:** Doernbecher Chldns Hosp/OHSU; **Address:** Oregon Hlth Sci Univ, 3181 SW Sam Jackson Park Rd, MC DC7P, Portland, OR 97239; **Phone:** 503-418-5775; **Board Cert:** Psychiatry 1980; Child & Adolescent Psychiatry 1982; **Med School:** Dartmouth Med Sch 1974; **Resid:** Psychiatry, Cambridge Hosp 1977; **Fellow:** Child Psychiatry, McLean Hosp 1979; **Fac Appt:** Prof Psyc, Oregon Hlth & Sci Univ

Ponton, Lynn Elisabeth MD [ChAP] - **Spec Exp:** Behavioral Disorders; Eating Disorders; **Hospital:** UCSF Med Ctr; **Address:** 201 Edgewood Ave, San Francisco, CA 94117; **Phone:** 415-664-3039; **Board Cert:** Psychiatry 1985; Child & Adolescent Psychiatry 1985; **Med School:** Univ Wisc 1978; **Resid:** Psychiatry, Hosp Univ Penn 1980; Psychiatry, UCSF Med Ctr 1981; **Fellow:** Child & Adolescent Psychiatry, UCSF Med Ctr 1983; **Fac Appt:** Prof Psyc, UCSF

Russell, Andrew T MD [ChAP] - **Spec Exp:** ADD/ADHD; Schizophrenia; Developmental Disorders; **Hospital:** UCLA Neuropsychiatric Hosp; **Address:** SEMEL Inst at UCLA, 760 Westwood Plaza, Los Angeles, CA 90024; **Phone:** 310-825-0389; **Board Cert:** Psychiatry 1980; Child & Adolescent Psychiatry 2004; **Med School:** Univ Colorado 1970; **Resid:** Psychiatry, UCLA Med Ctr 1973; **Fellow:** Child & Adolescent Psychiatry, UCLA Med Ctr 1977; **Fac Appt:** Prof Psyc, UCLA

Steiner, Hans MD [ChAP] - **Spec Exp:** Aggression Disorders; Eating Disorders; Trauma Psychiatry; **Hospital:** Stanford Univ Med Ctr, Lucile Packard Chldn's Hosp; **Address:** Division Child Psych & Child Devlp, 401 Quarry Rd, Ste MC 5719, Stanford, CA 94305-5719; **Phone:** 650-723-5511; **Board Cert:** Psychiatry 1979; Child & Adolescent Psychiatry 1981; **Med School:** Austria 1972; **Resid:** Psychiatry, SUNY Syracuse Med Ctr 1976; **Fellow:** Child & Adolescent Psychiatry, Univ Mich Hosps 1978; **Fac Appt:** Prof Psyc, Stanford Univ

Terr, Lenore MD [ChAP] - **Spec Exp:** Trauma Psychiatry; **Hospital:** UCSF Med Ctr; **Address:** 450 Sutter St, Ste 1336, San Francisco, CA 94108-4204; **Phone:** 415-433-7800; **Board Cert:** Psychiatry 1968; Child & Adolescent Psychiatry 1969; **Med School:** Univ Mich Med Sch 1961; **Resid:** Psychiatry, Univ Mich Med Ctr 1964; **Fellow:** Child & Adolescent Psychiatry, Univ Mich 1966; **Fac Appt:** Clin Prof Psyc, UCSF

GERIATRIC PSYCHIATRY

Mid Atlantic

Greenwald, Blaine MD [GerPsy] - **Spec Exp:** Depression; Dementia; **Hospital:** Zucker Hillside Hosp, N Shore Univ Hosp; **Address:** 75-59 263rd St, Div Geriatric Psychiatry, Glen Oaks, NY 11004; **Phone:** 718-470-8159; **Board Cert:** Psychiatry 1983; Geriatric Psychiatry 2000; **Med School:** NY Med Coll 1978; **Resid:** Psychiatry, Mt Sinai Hosp 1982; **Fellow:** Geriatric Psychiatry, Mt Sinai Hosp/Bronx VA Hosp 1983; **Fac Appt:** Assoc Prof Psyc, Albert Einstein Coll Med

Kennedy, Gary MD [GerPsy] - **Spec Exp:** Alzheimer's Disease; Dementia; Depression; **Hospital:** Montefiore Med Ctr - Div. Moses; **Address:** Dept Psyc & Behav Science, Montefiore Medical Center, 111 E 210th St, Bronx, NY 10467; **Phone:** 718-920-4236; **Board Cert:** Psychiatry 1980; Geriatric Psychiatry 2000; Psychosomatic Medicine 2005; **Med School:** Univ Tex, San Antonio 1975; **Resid:** Psychiatry, VA Hosp-Univ Texas 1979; **Fellow:** Geriatric Psychiatry, Montefiore Med Ctr 1984; **Fac Appt:** Prof Psyc, Albert Einstein Coll Med

Lyketsos, Constantine G MD [GerPsy] - **Spec Exp:** Alzheimer's Disease; Neuro-Psychiatry; Depression; **Hospital:** Johns Hopkins Bayview Med Ctr (page 61); **Address:** JHU Bayview Med Ctr, 5300 Alpha Commons Drive Fl 4th, Baltimore, MD 21224; **Phone:** 410-550-0062; **Board Cert:** Psychiatry 1994; Psychosomatic Medicine 2005; **Med School:** Washington Univ, St Louis 1988; **Resid:** Psychiatry, Johns Hopkins Hosp 1992; **Fellow:** Neuropsychiatry, Johns Hopkins Hosp 1994; **Fac Appt:** Prof Psyc, Johns Hopkins Univ

Reisberg, Barry MD [GerPsy] - **Spec Exp:** Alzheimer's Disease; Dementia; Depression; **Hospital:** NYU Langone Med Ctr (page 67); **Address:** Aging & Dementia Rsch Ctr - NYU, 550 First Ave, THN 316, New York, NY 10016; **Phone:** 212-263-8550; **Board Cert:** Psychiatry 1976; Geriatric Psychiatry 2000; **Med School:** NY Med Coll 1972; **Resid:** Psychiatry, Metropolitan Hosp 1975; **Fellow:** Psychiatric Research, Univ London 1975; **Fac Appt:** Prof Psyc, NYU Sch Med

Rosen, Jules MD [GerPsy] - **Spec Exp:** Alzheimer's Disease; Dementia; **Hospital:** Western Psych Inst & Clin - UPMC, UPMC Presby, Pittsburgh; **Address:** Western Psych Inst & Clin, 3811 O'Hara St, Pittsburgh, PA 15213; **Phone:** 412-246-5900; **Board Cert:** Psychiatry 1984; Geriatric Psychiatry 2003; **Med School:** Univ Cincinnati 1978; **Resid:** Psychiatry, Univ Mich Med Ctr 1982; **Fac Appt:** Prof Psyc, Univ Pittsburgh

Rovner, Barry W MD [GerPsy] - **Spec Exp:** Alzheimer's Disease; Behavioral Problems & Dementia; **Hospital:** Thomas Jefferson Univ Hosp; **Address:** Jefferson Hosp Neuroscience, 900 Walnut St Fl 4, Philadelphia, PA 19107; **Phone:** 215-503-1254; **Board Cert:** Psychiatry 1985; Geriatric Psychiatry 2000; **Med School:** Jefferson Med Coll 1980; **Resid:** Psychiatry, Johns Hopkins Hosp 1984; **Fac Appt:** Assoc Prof Psyc, Jefferson Med Coll

Streim, Joel E MD [GerPsy] - **Spec Exp:** Psychiatry in Physical Illness; Psychiatric Barriers to Physical Rehab; Alzheimer's Disease; **Hospital:** Hosp Univ Penn - UPHS (page 60), VA Med Ctr; **Address:** Univ Penn, Dept Geriatric Psychiatry, 3535 Market St Fl 3, Philadelphia, PA 19104; **Phone:** 215-615-3086; **Board Cert:** Psychiatry 1988; Geriatric Psychiatry 2000; **Med School:** Univ Rochester 1978; **Resid:** Psychiatry, Univ Wisconsin 1985; **Fellow:** Liaison Psychiatry, Univ Rochester/Strong Mem 1981; Geriatric Psychiatry, VA Med Ctr 1988; **Fac Appt:** Prof Psyc, Univ Pennsylvania

Southeast

Holroyd, Suzanne MD [GerPsy] - **Spec Exp:** Dementia; Psychoses-Late Onset; Mood Disorders; **Hospital:** Univ Virginia Med Ctr; **Address:** Univ of Virginia Health Sys, Dept Psych, Box 800623, Chalottesville, VA 22908; **Phone:** 434-924-2241; **Board Cert:** Psychiatry 1992; Geriatric Psychiatry 2004; **Med School:** Univ VA Sch Med 1986; **Resid:** Psychiatry, Johns Hopkins Hosp 1990; **Fellow:** Geriatric Psychiatry, Johns Hopkins Hosp 1991; **Fac Appt:** Prof Psyc, Univ VA Sch Med

Stein, Elliott M MD [GerPsy] - **Spec Exp:** Anxiety & Depression; Memory Disorders; Dementia; Stress Management; **Hospital:** Mount Sinai Med Ctr - Miami; **Address:** Mount Sinai Med Ctr, 4308 Alton Rd, Ste 910, Miami Beach, FL 33140; **Phone:** 305-534-3636; **Board Cert:** Psychiatry 1979; Geriatric Psychiatry 2001; **Med School:** Univ Miami Sch Med 1973; **Resid:** Psychiatry, Herrick Meml Hosp 1976; **Fac Appt:** Assoc Clin Prof Psyc, Univ Miami Sch Med

Tune, Larry E MD [GerPsy] - **Spec Exp:** Alzheimer's Disease; Dementia; Psychopharmacology; Psychoses-Late Onset; **Hospital:** Wesley Woods Ger Hosp; **Address:** Wesley Woods Ctr, Dept Psychiatry, 1841 Clifton Rd NE, Atlanta, GA 30329; **Phone:** 404-728-4969; **Board Cert:** Psychiatry 1991; Geriatric Psychiatry 2004; **Med School:** Univ VA Sch Med 1975; **Resid:** Psychiatry, Johns Hopkins Hosp 1979; Neurology, Johns Hopkins Hosp 1983; **Fellow:** Psychopharmacology, Johns Hopkins Univ 1981; **Fac Appt:** Prof Psyc, Emory Univ

Midwest

Grossberg, George MD [GerPsy] - **Spec Exp:** Alzheimer's Disease; Depression; Behavioral Problems & Dementia; **Hospital:** St Louis Univ Hosp; **Address:** St Louis Univ Sch Med, Dept Psychiatry, 1438 S Grand Blvd, St Louis, MO 63104; **Phone:** 314-977-4850; **Board Cert:** Psychiatry 1982; Geriatric Psychiatry 2001; **Med School:** St Louis Univ 1975; **Resid:** Psychiatry, St Louis Univ Med Ctr 1979; **Fac Appt:** Prof Psyc, St Louis Univ

Mellow, Alan M MD/PhD [GerPsy] - **Spec Exp:** Dementia; Depression; **Hospital:** Univ Michigan Hlth Sys; **Address:** Univ Mich, Dept Geriatric Psyc, 1500 E Med Ctr Drive, rm 1127, Box 0920, Ann Arbor, MI 48109; **Phone:** 734-222-4350; **Board Cert:** Psychiatry 1988; Geriatric Psychiatry 2002; **Med School:** Northwestern Univ 1981; **Resid:** Internal Medicine, Univ Chicago Hosp 1982; Psychiatry, McLean Hosp-Harvard 1985; **Fellow:** Psychiatry, Natl Inst Mental Hlth 1988; **Fac Appt:** Prof Psyc, Univ Mich Med Sch

Great Plains and Mountains

Burke, William J MD [GerPsy] - **Spec Exp:** Depression; Dementia; Alzheimer's Disease; Panic Disorder; **Hospital:** Nebraska Med Ctr; **Address:** Nebraska Medical Ctr, Dept Psychiatry, 985580 Nebraska Medical Ctr, Omaha, NE 68198-5580; **Phone:** 402-552-6062; **Board Cert:** Psychiatry 1986; Geriatric Psychiatry 2001; **Med School:** Univ Nebr Coll Med 1980; **Resid:** Internal Medicine, Univ Nebraska Med Ctr 1981; Psychiatry, Wash Univ Barnes Hosp 1984; **Fac Appt:** Prof Psyc, Univ Nebr Coll Med

Geriatric Psychiatry

West Coast and Pacific

Borson, Soo MD [GerPsy] - **Spec Exp:** Alzheimer's Disease; Psychiatry in Physical Illness; Dementia; Memory Disorders; **Hospital:** Univ Wash Med Ctr; **Address:** Univ Washington Hlth Sciences Ctr, 4225 Roosevelt Way NE, Ste 306, Seattle, WA 98105; **Phone:** 206-598-7792; **Board Cert:** Psychiatry 1985; Geriatric Psychiatry 2000; **Med School:** Stanford Univ 1969; **Resid:** Psychiatry, Univ Wash 1979; **Fellow:** Geriatric Psychiatry, Univ Wash 1981; **Fac Appt:** Prof Psyc, Univ Wash

Kramer, Barry A MD [GerPsy] - **Spec Exp:** Electroconvulsive Therapy (ECT); Depression; **Hospital:** Cedars-Sinai Med Ctr, Kaiser Permanente LA Med Ctr; **Address:** PO Box 5792, Beverly Hills, CA 90209; **Phone:** 310-423-4014; **Board Cert:** Psychiatry 1978; Geriatric Psychiatry 2001; **Med School:** Hahnemann Univ 1974; **Resid:** Psychiatry, Montefiore Hosp Med Ctr 1977; **Fellow:** Geriatric Psychiatry, UCLA-USC Long Term Gero Ctr 1986

Small, Gary W MD [GerPsy] - **Spec Exp:** Dementia; Alzheimer's Disease; Memory Disorders; Vascular Dementia; **Hospital:** UCLA Ronald Reagan Med Ctr; **Address:** UCLA, Neuropsych Inst, 760 Westwood Plaza, 88-201 NPI, Los Angeles, CA 90095; **Phone:** 310-825-0291; **Board Cert:** Psychiatry 1983; Geriatric Psychiatry 2001; **Med School:** USC Sch Med 1977; **Resid:** Psychiatry, Mass Genl Hosp 1981; **Fellow:** Psychiatry, UCLA Med Ctr 1983; **Fac Appt:** Prof Psyc, UCLA

Veith, Richard C MD [GerPsy] - **Spec Exp:** Depression in Cardiovascular Disease; **Hospital:** Univ Wash Med Ctr; **Address:** Univ Washington Health Sciences Ctr, BB 1644, Box 356560, 1959 NE Pacific St, Seattle, WA 98195; **Phone:** 206-543-3752; **Board Cert:** Psychiatry 1979; Geriatric Psychiatry 2000; **Med School:** Univ Wash 1973; **Resid:** Psychiatry, Univ Wash Med Ctr 1977; **Fac Appt:** Prof Psyc, Univ Wash

Cleveland Clinic

Psychiatry and Psychology

The Cleveland Clinic Department of Psychiatry and Psychology offers the full range of mental health and behavioral services for children, adolescents and adults. Our highly trained staff, offering expert clinical evaluation and treatment, includes psychiatrists, psychologists, clinical nurse specialists, social workers, counselors and therapists. In addition to evaluating and treating patients, our staff educates trainees, professionals and the public on the latest developments in psychiatry and the behavioral sciences.

The Department of Psychiatry and Psychology includes Adult Psychiatry, Child and Adolescent Psychiatry, Chemical Dependency, General Psychology, Habit Management, Neuropsychology, Psychosomatic Medicine and Psychiatric Occupational Therapy.

The department is part of the Cleveland Clinic Neurological Institute, a fully integrated entity with a disease-specific focus, combining all physicians and other healthcare providers in neurology, neurosurgery, neuroradiology, the behavioral sciences and nursing who treat children and adults with neurological and neurobehavioral disorders. Our staff of more than 250 specialists sees one of the largest and most diverse patient populations in the country. Because of our clinical expertise, academic achievement and innovative research, the Cleveland Clinic Neurological Institute has earned an international reputation for excellence.

Our staff treats a wide range of symptoms and problems involving personal or family crises. Among the types of problems for which children and adults seek our professional help:

- Attention Deficit Disorder
- Disruptive Behavior
- Mood and Anxiety Disorders
- Schizophrenia
- Sleeping Problems
- Stress
- Substance Abuse
- Work/Life/Family Problems

Our staff provides individualized assessments, medication management and counseling for individuals, couples, groups and families. The department offers care through outpatient, urgent care and routine visits, as well as inpatient treatment programs.

Our staff also serves as consultants for patients admitted to Cleveland Clinic medical and surgical units, and are key team members in the treatment of many conditions including epilepsy, movement disorders, organ transplantation, morbid obesity, chronic pain, headaches and cancer. Through the Psychiatric Neuromodulation Center, we offer both traditional and novel treatments to patients with psychiatric disorders resistant to common therapies.

For more information about the Cleveland Clinic Department of Psychiatry and Psychology, to schedule a second opinion or to learn about assistance for out-of-town patients, call 800.890.2467 or visit www.clevelandclinic.org/psychtopdocs.

Department of Psychiatry and Psychology
9500 Euclid Avenue / AC311 | Cleveland OH 44195

MOUNT SINAI
SCHOOL OF
MEDICINE

THE MOUNT SINAI MEDICAL CENTER
PSYCHIATRY

One Gustave L. Levy Place
Fifth Avenue and 100th Street
New York, NY 10029-6574
Physician Referral: 1-800-MD-SINAI (637-4624)
www.mountsinai.org

THE DEPARTMENT OF PSYCHIATRY at Mount Sinai strives to rapidly bring tomorrow's breakthrough treatments from clinical neuroscience research to clinical care today.

We serve infants, children, adolescents, adults, and seniors, offering mental health evaluation and treatment for autism, attention-deficit hyperactivity disorder, behavioral disorders, trauma responses in children, schizophrenia, Alzheimer's disease, mood and anxiety disorders, obsessive-compulsive disorder (OCD), substance abuse, post-traumatic stress disorder (PTSD), eating disorders, reproductive psychiatry, and personality disorders.

Clinical Services – The Department of Psychiatry is organized around key Centers of Excellence that link academic thought leaders to clinicians throughout the department in a diagnosis-based system. We offer a full range of diagnostic and treatment services, including psychotherapy, psychopharmacology, emergency services, electroconvulsive therapy, neuropsychological testing, and management of difficult clinical cases. We are engaged in Mount Sinai's World Trade Center Worker Medical Monitoring and Treatment Program.

Specialty Programs – The Seaver and New York Autism Center of Excellence offers a comprehensive assessment and treatment program that provides the finest patient care informed by the latest research. Our expert clinical staff are experienced in autism spectrum disorders, specializing in personalized and evidence-based treatment for very young children and high-functioning adults, as well as those individuals considered most difficult to assess and treat. Given the host of medical conditions associated with autism, the Center works closely with outstanding physicians from other specialties at Mount Sinai.

Our Center for Eating and Weight Disorders serves adults and children, offering innovative, proven-effective treatment for anorexia nervosa, bulimia nervosa, binge eating disorder, and obesity.

The Mood and Anxiety Disorders Program offers the latest integrative treatment strategies for patients who suffer from major depression, bipolar disorder, PTSD, panic attacks, generalized anxiety disorder, and social phobia.

The Obsessive Compulsive Disorders Center provides state-of-the-art diagnostic evaluation and treatment for OCD and related conditions. We offer intensive cognitive behavioral therapy on an outpatient basis for children, adolescents, and adults. We also specialize in biological interventions for patients who have not responded to conventional therapies.

TRANSLATING KNOWLEDGE INTO NEW SOLUTIONS
Mount Sinai is at the forefront of unlocking the interactions between biological processes and the myriad states of the human mind. At our Conte Center for the Neuroscience of Mental Disorders we are studying schizophrenia—pursuing breakthrough insights into the underlying neurobiology of the disease, and applying cutting-edge technology to convert those insights into new patient treatments. Among our other major research programs in psychiatry are the Alzheimer's Disease Research Center, which conducts both basic science and clinical research, and The Seaver and New York Autism Center of Excellence, which is dedicated to unraveling the biological causes of this disorder and to developing innovative treatment strategies. In shedding important new light on mental illness, psychiatrists at Mount Sinai are frequently able to offer the treatments of tomorrow—therapies that will not be widely available for years.

PSYCHIATRY

About the Department of Psychiatry:

The Department of Psychiatry is dedicated to improving the health and well-being of its patient population by delivering peerless psychiatric services and care. The Department is home to some of the nation's most respected clinical psychiatrists and psychologists, with specialties in psychoanalysis, psychopharmacology, behavioral therapy, child psychiatry, geriatric psychiatry, neuropsychiatry and positron emission tomography, a nuclear medicine imaging technique that produces a three-dimensional image of brain functions.

We specialize in the following areas:

INPATIENT SERVICES

The Inpatient Service Unit combines comprehensive diagnostic assessment and treatment including psychopharmacology, neuropsychology, psychotherapies and electroconvulsive therapy, a treatment in which seizures are electrically induced in anesthetized patients for therapeutic effect.

PSYCHOANALYTICS

The Psychoanalytic Institute at NYU Langone Medical Center offers low-fee programs in adult and child/adolescent psychodynamic psychotherapy (psychology focused on revealing the unconscious content of a client's psyche). The Institute offers patients the ability to relieve their emotional difficulties and problems through self-exploration under the guidance of a highly trained professional. Treatment is provided by psychiatrists, psychologists and clinical social workers under the supervision of senior faculty members.

OUTPATIENT PSYCHIATRY

The Outpatient Psychiatry Program at Tisch Hospital provides expert yet affordable treatment to individuals suffering from a broad range of mental disorders and emotional problems, including anxiety, depression, insomnia, manic-depression, reproductive psychiatry, attention-deficit hyperactivity disorder and schizophrenia. Our multidisciplinary team of licensed psychiatrists, psychologists and social workers offer the most up-to-date and scientifically validated treatments such as psychotherapy, medication, or the combination of the two.

MEMORY IMPAIRMENT

The Pearl Barlow Center for Memory Evaluation and Treatment specializes in treating patients with memory impairments caused by neurological, psychological and physical ailments, as well as memory issues resulting from medication side effects, anxiety, depression and the effects of normal aging, including illnesses such as Alzheimer's disease. This multidisciplinary medical approach integrated with the most advanced research capabilities is the most comprehensive and first of its kind in the treatment of memory disorders in New York City.

HUMAN SEXUALITY

The Human Sexuality Treatment Program provides a comprehensive examination of a full range of sexual disorders, including erectile disorder, premature ejaculation, male orgasmic disorder, female orgasmic and arousal disorders, vaginismus, dyspareunia, lack of desire, the unconsummated marriage and sexual incompatibility between partners. Experienced, skilled clinicians carry out treatment in complete confidence and in the best tradition of the doctor-patient relationship.

BEHAVIORAL HEALTH

About the Behavioral Health Program, Department of Psychiatry:

The Behavioral Health Program at NYU Langone Medical Center offers the most up-to-date treatments available for a wide range of disorders including: stress/anxiety, schizophrenia, depression, shyness, insomnia, low self esteem, women's issues, sexual difficulties, panic attacks and phobias, manic-depression, obsessions and compulsions and attention deficit/hyperactivity disorder. The Program serves its patients through a variety of approaches including career counseling, assertiveness training, martial/couples counseling and individual, group or family therapy.

We specialize in the following areas:

HUMAN SEXUALITY

The Human Sexuality Treatment Program provides a comprehensive examination of a full range of sexual disorders, including erectile disorder, premature ejaculation, male orgasmic disorder, female orgasmic and arousal disorders, vaginismus, dyspareunia, lack of desire, the unconsummated marriage and sexual incompatibility between partners. Experienced, skilled clinicians carry out treatment in complete confidence and ensure that couples and individuals who seek treatment receive individualized care appropriate to their concerns.

INPATIENT SERVICES

A 22-bed inpatient unit services an adult population including a Young Adult Program. The service combines comprehensive diagnostic assessment and treatment including psychopharmacology, neuropsychology, psychotherapies and electroconvulsive therapy, a treatment in which seizures are electrically induced in anesthetized patients for therapeutic effect. A multidisciplinary team approach provides a continuum of behavioral and therapeutic modalities.

OUTPATIENT PSYCHIATRY

The Outpatient Psychiatry Program at Tisch Hospital provides expert yet affordable treatment to individuals suffering from a broad range of mental disorders and emotional problems including anxiety, depression, insomnia, manic-depression, reproductive psychiatry, attention-deficit hyperactivity disorder and schizophrenia. Our multidisciplinary team of licensed psychiatrists, psychologists and social workers offer the most up-to-date and scientifically validated treatments such as psychotherapy, medication, or the combination of the two. For those who prefer it, direct treatment with a member of the faculty is also available as an option.

SCIENTIFIC INNOVATION

At NYU Langone Medical Center, scientific innovation goes hand in hand with patient care. Our physician-scientists continue to lead the way in psychopharmacology and continue to test new treatments for depression and bipolar disorder, with potentially life-altering results for the millions who suffer from these debilitating illnesses.

SLEEP DISORDERS

The Sleep Disorders Consultation and Treatment Service provides a thorough evaluation of a full range of sleep problems including insomnia, nightmares, narcolepsy, sleepwalking, and restless legs syndrome. Both behavioral and medication treatments are available.

NYU Child Study Center

NYU LANGONE MEDICAL CENTER

577 First Avenue
New York, NY 10016
212-263-6622
www.aboutourkids.org

NYU CHILD STUDY CENTER

About the Child Study Center, Department of Child and Adolescent Psychiatry:

The Child Study Center at NYU Langone Medical Center is dedicated to increasing the awareness of child and adolescent psychiatric and learning disorders and improving the prevention, identification and treatment of these disorders. For over a decade, the Child Study Center has been providing hope and care to children and their families. Its expert clinicians treat thousands of children from around the globe by providing diagnostic consultations and a wide variety of medication and evidence-based psychotherapeutic treatments for all conditions, in addition to the areas highlighted below. Through its website, www.AboutOurKids.org, and professional education programs, parents are provided with the tools and knowledge needed to promote children's mental health. The Department was also designated as the only New York State Center of Excellence in Mental Health.

We specialize in the following areas:

ANXIETY AND MOOD DISORDERS

The Anita Saltz Institute for Anxiety and Mood Disorders at NYU Langone Medical Center offers the most current and effective treatment for children, adolescents, and young adults, including thorough evaluation. Our psychopharmacologists are experts in understanding the issues of treating children with bipolar disorder and our researchers are studying treatments for children with severe temper outbursts and adolescent depression. We offer several programs including The Selective Mutism Service, providing specialized care for children who cannot speak in public; Dialectical Behavior Therapy (DBT) for adolescents with self-destructive behaviors; and Cognitive Behavior Therapy (CBT) for anxiety and mood disorders, including obsessive-compulsive disorder.

ATTENTION DEFICIT HYPERACTIVITY AND BEHAVIOR DISORDERS

The Institute for Attention Deficit Hyperactivity and Behavior Disorders focuses on the treatment of ADHD. Our Parent-Child Interaction Therapy Program (PCIT) is a state-of-the-art treatment for behavioral problems in young children and is the largest program of its kind in the northeast. The Institute is also developing new treatments for preschool children with ADHD and for children with severe organizational difficulties. We also offer a summer-long program for school-age children with ADHD.

AUTISM, ASPERGER'S SYNDROME AND COMMUNICATION DISORDERS

The Autism Spectrum programs at the Child Study Center provide extensive evaluations for toddlers and preschoolers having social and communication difficulties. Our Early Social Interaction treatment is a home-based intervention for children identified with symptoms of autism. Our specialists are also experienced at supporting the needs of teens and young adults who have been diagnosed with Asperger.

LEARNING DISORDERS

The Institute for Learning and Academic Achievement evaluates children with suspected learning weaknesses or poor academic achievement using a multidisciplinary team-based approach. We provide a carefully crafted, personalized set of recommendations that gives parent-, educator-, and child-friendly integrated strategies for improvement to help children achieve their academic potential.

TICS AND TOURETTE'S DISORDER

The Tics and Tourette's Clinical and Research programs are dedicated to the evaluation and treatment of individuals with tics, Tourette's disorder and related problems. Comprehensive evaluation and state-of-the-art treatment is provided including Habit Reversal Therapy (HRT) as well as opportunities for participation in research studies that include new treatments.

NYU **Langone Medical Center**

550 First Avenue (at 31St Street)
New York, NY 10016
Physician Referral:
(888)7-NYU-MED (888-769-8633)
www.med.nyu.edu

PSYCHIATRY

About the Department of Psychiatry:

The Department of Psychiatry is dedicated to improving the health and well-being of its patient population by delivering peerless psychiatric services and care. The Department is home to some of the nation's most respected clinical psychiatrists and psychologists, with specialties in psychoanalysis, psychopharmacology, behavioral therapy, child psychiatry, geriatric psychiatry, neuropsychiatry and positron emission tomography, a nuclear medicine imaging technique that produces a three-dimensional image of brain functions.

We specialize in the following areas:

INPATIENT SERVICES
The Inpatient Service Unit combines comprehensive diagnostic assessment and treatment including psychopharmacology, neuropsychology, psychotherapies and electroconvulsive therapy, a treatment in which seizures are electrically induced in anesthetized patients for therapeutic effect.

PSYCHOANALYTICS
The Psychoanalytic Institute at NYU Langone Medical Center offers low-fee programs in adult and child/adolescent psychodynamic psychotherapy (psychology focused on revealing the unconscious content of a client's psyche). The Institute offers patients the ability to relieve their emotional difficulties and problems through self-exploration under the guidance of a highly trained professional. Treatment is provided by psychiatrists, psychologists and clinical social workers under the supervision of senior faculty members.

OUTPATIENT PSYCHIATRY
The Outpatient Psychiatry Program at Tisch Hospital provides expert yet affordable treatment to individuals suffering from a broad range of mental disorders and emotional problems, including anxiety, depression, insomnia, manic-depression, reproductive psychiatry, attention-deficit hyperactivity disorder and schizophrenia. Our multidisciplinary team of licensed psychiatrists, psychologists and social workers offer the most up-to-date and scientifically validated treatments such as psychotherapy, medication, or the combination of the two.

MEMORY IMPAIRMENT
The Pearl Barlow Center for Memory Evaluation and Treatment specializes in treating patients with memory impairments caused by neurological, psychological and physical ailments, as well as memory issues resulting from medication side effects, anxiety, depression and the effects of normal aging, including illnesses such as Alzheimer's disease. This multidisciplinary medical approach integrated with the most advanced research capabilities is the most comprehensive and first of its kind in the treatment of memory disorders in New York City.

HUMAN SEXUALITY
The Human Sexuality Treatment Program provides a comprehensive examination of a full range of sexual disorders, including erectile disorder, premature ejaculation, male orgasmic disorder, female orgasmic and arousal disorders, vaginismus, dyspareunia, lack of desire, the unconsummated marriage and sexual incompatibility between partners. Experienced, skilled clinicians carry out treatment in complete confidence and in the best tradition of the doctor-patient relationship.

Pulmonary Disease
a subspecialty of Internal Medicine

An internist who treats diseases of the lungs and airways. The pulmonologist diagnoses and treats cancer, pneumonia, pleurisy, asthma, occupational diseases, bronchitis, sleep disorders, emphysema and other complex disorders of the lungs.

Training Required: Three years in internal medicine *plus* additional training and examination for certification in pulmonary disease.

PULMONARY DISEASE

New England

Beamis, John MD [Pul] - **Spec Exp:** Interventional Pulmonology; Bronchoscopy; **Hospital:** Lahey Clin; **Address:** Lahey Clinic, 41 Mall Rd, Burlington, MA 01805; **Phone:** 781-744-3240; **Board Cert:** Internal Medicine 1974; Pulmonary Disease 1978; Critical Care Medicine 1999; **Med School:** Univ VT Coll Med 1970; **Resid:** Internal Medicine, New Eng Deacones Hosp 1973; **Fellow:** Pulmonary Disease, New Eng Deacones Hosp 1974; Pulmonary Disease, Naval Hosp 1977; **Fac Appt:** Assoc Prof Med, Tufts Univ

Berk, John L MD [Pul] - **Spec Exp:** Interstitial Lung Disease; Amyloidosis; Pulmonary Fibrosis; **Hospital:** Boston Med Ctr; **Address:** The Pulmonary Ctr, 72 E Concord St, Ste R-3, Boston, MA 02118-2371; **Phone:** 617-638-4848; **Board Cert:** Critical Care Medicine 2002; Internal Medicine 1986; Pulmonary Disease 2000; **Med School:** Case West Res Univ 1983; **Resid:** Internal Medicine, Univ Hosp/VAMC 1986; **Fellow:** Pulmonary Critical Care Medicine, Boston Univ Med Ctr 1991; **Fac Appt:** Assoc Prof Med, Boston Univ

Braman, Sidney S MD [Pul] - **Spec Exp:** Asthma; Chronic Obstructive Lung Disease (COPD); **Hospital:** Rhode Island Hosp; **Address:** Rhode Island Hosp, Div Pulmonology, 593 Eddy St, APC Bldg Fl 7, Providence, RI 02903; **Phone:** 401-444-3567; **Board Cert:** Internal Medicine 1971; Pulmonary Disease 1972; **Med School:** Temple Univ 1967; **Resid:** Internal Medicine, Philadelphia Genl Hosp 1969; **Fellow:** Pulmonary Disease, Hosp Univ Penn 1970; Pulmonary Disease, Walter Reed AMC 1971; **Fac Appt:** Prof Med, Brown Univ

Celli, Bartolome MD [Pul] - **Spec Exp:** Chronic Obstructive Lung Disease (COPD); Mechanical Ventilation; Respiratory Failure; **Hospital:** Caritas St Elizabeth's Med Ctr; **Address:** St Elizabeth's Med Ctr, Dept Pulmonary Disease, 736 Cambridge St, Boston, MA 02135; **Phone:** 617-789-2545; **Board Cert:** Internal Medicine 1975; Pulmonary Disease 1978; **Med School:** Venezuela 1971; **Resid:** Internal Medicine, St Vincent Hosp 1973; Internal Medicine, Boston City Hosp 1976; **Fellow:** Pulmonary Disease, Boston Univ Med Ctr 1977; **Fac Appt:** Prof Med, Tufts Univ

Christiani, David MD [Pul] - **Spec Exp:** Occupational Lung Disease; **Hospital:** Mass Genl Hosp, MA Respiratory Hosp; **Address:** Mass Genl Hosp, Pulmonary Assocs, 55 Fruit St Cox 201B Bldg, Boston, MA 02114; **Phone:** 617-726-1721; **Board Cert:** Internal Medicine 1979; Occupational Medicine 1984; Pulmonary Disease 1988; **Med School:** Tufts Univ 1976; **Resid:** Internal Medicine, Boston City Hosp 1979; Occupational Medicine, Harvard Sch Public Hlth 1981; **Fellow:** Pulmonary Disease, Mass Genl Hosp 1987; **Fac Appt:** Prof Med, Harvard Med Sch

Enelow, Richard Ian MD [Pul] - **Spec Exp:** Interstitial Lung Disease; Lung Disease; **Hospital:** Dartmouth - Hitchcock Med Ctr; **Address:** Chief of Pulmonary & Critical Care, Dartmouth-Hitchcock Medical Ctr, 1 Medical Center Drive, Lebanon, NH 03756; **Phone:** 603-650-5383; **Board Cert:** Internal Medicine 1986; Pulmonary Disease 2002; **Med School:** Boston Univ 1983; **Resid:** Internal Medicine, New England Deaconess Med Ctr 1986; **Fellow:** Pulmonary Disease, Univ VA Hlth Scis Ctr 1992; **Fac Appt:** Prof Med, Dartmouth Med Sch

Ernst, Armin MD [Pul] - **Spec Exp:** Interventional Pulmonology; Tracheal Stenosis; Airway Disorders; Emphysema; **Hospital:** Beth Israel Deaconess Med Ctr - Boston; **Address:** Beth Israel Deaconess Med Ctr, 185 Pilgrim Rd, Deaconess Bldg - Ste 201, Boston, MA 02215; **Phone:** 617-632-8252; **Board Cert:** Internal Medicine 2003; Pulmonary Disease 2006; Critical Care Medicine 2007; **Med School:** Germany 1988; **Resid:** Internal Medicine, Thoraxklinik-Univ Heidelberg; Internal Medicine, Univ Tex Hlth Sci Ctr 1993; **Fellow:** Pulmonary Critical Care Medicine, Deaconess Med Ctr/Brigham & Women's 1996; Interventional Pulmonology, Thoraxklinik-Univ Heidelberg; **Fac Appt:** Assoc Prof Med, Harvard Med Sch

Fanta, Christopher MD [Pul] - **Spec Exp:** Asthma; Chronic Obstructive Lung Disease (COPD); Bronchiectasis; **Hospital:** Brigham & Women's Hosp, Faulkner Hosp; **Address:** 75 Francis St, Boston, MA 02115; **Phone:** 617-732-6770; **Board Cert:** Internal Medicine 1978; Pulmonary Disease 1980; **Med School:** Harvard Med Sch 1975; **Resid:** Internal Medicine, Peter Bent Brigham Hosp 1978; **Fellow:** Pulmonary Disease, Peter Bent Brigham Hosp 1980; **Fac Appt:** Assoc Prof Med, Harvard Med Sch

Friedman, Lloyd Neal MD [Pul] - **Spec Exp:** Tuberculosis; **Hospital:** Milford Hosp, Yale-New Haven Hosp; **Address:** Milford Hospital, 300 Seaside Ave, Milford, CT 06460; **Phone:** 203-876-4288; **Board Cert:** Internal Medicine 1983; Pulmonary Disease 1988; Critical Care Medicine 1999; **Med School:** Yale Univ 1979; **Resid:** Internal Medicine, Beth Israel Med Ctr 1980; Internal Medicine, Oregon Hlth Scis Univ 1983; **Fellow:** Pulmonary Intensive Care, Yale-New Haven Hosp 1988; **Fac Appt:** Clin Prof Med, Yale Univ

Irwin, Richard S MD [Pul] - **Spec Exp:** Cough; Asthma; Chronic Obstructive Lung Disease (COPD); Critical Care; **Hospital:** UMass Meml - Univ Campus; **Address:** 55 Lake Ave N, Worcester, MA 01655-0002; **Phone:** 508-856-1919; **Board Cert:** Internal Medicine 1972; Pulmonary Disease 1974; Critical Care Medicine 2007; **Med School:** Tufts Univ 1968; **Resid:** Internal Medicine, Tufts-New England Med Ctr 1970; **Fellow:** Pulmonary Disease, Columbia-Presby Hosp 1972; **Fac Appt:** Prof Med, Univ Mass Sch Med

Mahler, Donald A MD [Pul] - **Spec Exp:** Chronic Obstructive Lung Disease (COPD); Asthma; Breathing Disorders; **Hospital:** Dartmouth - Hitchcock Med Ctr; **Address:** Dartmouth-Hitchcock Med Ctr, Div Pulmonary Med, One Medical Center Drive, Lebanon, NH 03756-0001; **Phone:** 603-650-5533; **Board Cert:** Internal Medicine 1978; Pulmonary Disease 1980; **Med School:** Loyola Univ-Stritch Sch Med 1972; **Resid:** Internal Medicine, Dartmouth-Hitchcock Med Ctr 1977; **Fellow:** Pulmonary Disease, Yale-New Haven Hosp 1980; **Fac Appt:** Prof Med, Dartmouth Med Sch

Metersky, Mark L MD [Pul] - **Spec Exp:** Pulmonary Infections; Asthma; Bronchiectasis; **Hospital:** Univ of Conn Hlth Ctr, John Dempsey Hosp; **Address:** Univ Conn Hlth Ctr, 263 Farmington Ave, Farmington, CT 06030-1321; **Phone:** 860-679-3343; **Board Cert:** Internal Medicine 1988; Pulmonary Disease 2003; Critical Care Medicine 2003; **Med School:** NYU Sch Med 1985; **Resid:** Internal Medicine, Boston City Hosp 1988; **Fellow:** Pulmonary Critical Care Medicine, UCSD Med Ctr 1992; **Fac Appt:** Prof Med, Univ Conn

Millman, Richard P MD [Pul] - **Spec Exp:** Sleep Disorders/Apnea; **Hospital:** Rhode Island Hosp, Miriam Hosp; **Address:** RI Hosp, Div Pulm, Crit Care & Sleep Med, 593 Eddy St, APC 701, Providence, RI 02903-4923; **Phone:** 401-444-2670; **Board Cert:** Internal Medicine 1979; Pulmonary Disease 1982; Critical Care Medicine 1999; **Med School:** Univ Pennsylvania 1976; **Resid:** Internal Medicine, Univ Mich Hosp 1979; **Fellow:** Pulmonary Disease, Univ Penn 1981; **Fac Appt:** Prof Med, Brown Univ

Pulmonary Disease

Nardell, Edward MD [Pul] - **Spec Exp:** Tuberculosis; **Hospital:** Brigham & Women's Hosp; **Address:** Center for Health and Human Rights, 651 Huntington Ave, Boston, MA 02120; **Phone:** 617-432-6937; **Board Cert:** Internal Medicine 1975; Pulmonary Disease 1982; **Med School:** Hahnemann Univ 1972; **Resid:** Internal Medicine, Hahnemann Univ Hosp 1975; **Fellow:** Pulmonary Disease, Mass Genl Hosp 1977; **Fac Appt:** Assoc Prof Med, Harvard Med Sch

Parsons, Polly E MD [Pul] - **Spec Exp:** Critical Care; Lung Injury-Acute; **Hospital:** Fletcher Allen Health Care- Med Ctr Campus; **Address:** Fletcher Allen Health Care, 111 Colchester Ave, Fletcher 311, Burlington, VT 05401; **Phone:** 802-847-6177; **Board Cert:** Internal Medicine 1981; Pulmonary Disease 1986; Critical Care Medicine 2005; **Med School:** Univ Ariz Coll Med 1978; **Resid:** Internal Medicine, Univ Colorado Hosp 1981; **Fellow:** Pulmonary Disease, Univ Colorado Hosp 1985; **Fac Appt:** Prof Med, Univ VT Coll Med

Redlich, Carrie MD [Pul] - **Spec Exp:** Occupational Lung Disease; **Hospital:** Yale-New Haven Hosp; **Address:** Yale Occupational & Environmental Med, 135 College St Fl 3 - Ste 392, New Haven, CT 06510; **Phone:** 203-785-4197; **Board Cert:** Internal Medicine 1986; Occupational Medicine 1990; Pulmonary Disease 2002; **Med School:** Yale Univ 1982; **Resid:** Internal Medicine, Yale-New Haven Hosp 1986; Occupational Medicine, Yale-New Haven Hosp 1987; **Fellow:** Pulmonary Disease, Univ Washington 1989; **Fac Appt:** Assoc Prof Med, Yale Univ

Rochester, Carolyn L MD [Pul] - **Spec Exp:** Chronic Obstructive Lung Disease (COPD); **Hospital:** VA Conn Hlthcre Sys, Yale-New Haven Hosp; **Address:** Yale Univ Sch Med, Pulm & Crit Care Sect, 300 Cedar St, Box 208057, New Haven, CT 06520-8057; **Phone:** 203-785-3207; **Board Cert:** Internal Medicine 1986; Pulmonary Disease 2002; Critical Care Medicine 2006; **Med School:** Columbia P&S 1983; **Resid:** Internal Medicine, Columbia Presby Med Ctr 1986; **Fellow:** Pulmonary Disease, Columbia Presby Med Ctr 1988; **Fac Appt:** Asst Prof Med, Yale Univ

White, David P MD [Pul] - **Spec Exp:** Sleep Disorders/Apnea; **Hospital:** Brigham & Women's Hosp; **Address:** Brigham & Women's Hosp, Division of Sleep Med, 75 Francis St, Boston, MA 02115; **Phone:** 617-732-5778; **Board Cert:** Internal Medicine 1978; Pulmonary Disease 1982; Sleep Medicine 2007; **Med School:** Emory Univ 1975; **Resid:** Internal Medicine, Univ Colo Med Ctr 1978; **Fellow:** Pulmonary Disease, Univ Colo Med Ctr 1982; **Fac Appt:** Prof Med, Harvard Med Sch

Mid Atlantic

Arcasoy, Selim M MD [Pul] - **Spec Exp:** Transplant Medicine-Lung; Chronic Obstructive Lung Disease (COPD); Interstitial Lung Disease; Pulmonary Embolism; **Hospital:** NY-Presby Hosp/Columbia (page 66); **Address:** Ctr for Advanced Lung Dis/Transp, 622 W 168th St PH Bldg Fl 14E - rm 104, New York, NY 10032-3720; **Phone:** 212-305-6589; **Board Cert:** Internal Medicine 2003; Pulmonary Disease 2006; Critical Care Medicine 2007; **Med School:** Turkey 1990; **Resid:** Internal Medicine, SUNY Downstate Med Ctr 1994; **Fellow:** Pulmonary Critical Care Medicine, Univ Pittsburgh Med Ctr 1998; **Fac Appt:** Prof Med, Columbia P&S

Bascom, Rebecca MD [Pul] - **Spec Exp:** Environmental Medicine; Chemical Exposure; **Hospital:** Penn State Milton S Hershey Med Ctr; **Address:** Hershey Med Ctr, PO Box 850, MC HO41, Hershey, PA 17033-0850; **Phone:** 717-531-6525; **Board Cert:** Internal Medicine 1982; Occupational Medicine 1987; Pulmonary Disease 1988; Critical Care Medicine 1998; **Med School:** Oregon Hlth & Sci Univ 1979; **Resid:** Internal Medicine, Johns Hopkins Hosp 1982; Occupational Medicine, Johns Hopkins 1985; **Fellow:** Pulmonary Disease, Johns Hopkins 1985; **Fac Appt:** Prof Med, Penn State Univ-Hershey Med Ctr

Criner, Gerard J MD [Pul] - **Spec Exp:** Chronic Obstructive Lung Disease (COPD); Pulmonary Fibrosis; Pulmonary Hypertension; Critical Care; **Hospital:** Temple Univ Hosp; **Address:** Temple Univ Hosp, Pulmonary Med, 3401 N Broad St Fl 7, Philadelphia, PA 19140; **Phone:** 215-707-5555; **Board Cert:** Internal Medicine 1982; Critical Care Medicine 2007; Pulmonary Disease 1986; **Med School:** Temple Univ 1979; **Resid:** Internal Medicine, Temple Univ Hosp 1983; **Fellow:** Pulmonary Disease, Boston Univ 1986; **Fac Appt:** Prof Med, Temple Univ

Deitz, Joel L MD [Pul] - **Spec Exp:** Respiratory Failure; Chronic Obstructive Lung Disease (COPD); Cough; **Hospital:** Penn Presby Med Ctr - UPHS (page 60), Hosp Univ Penn - UPHS (page 60); **Address:** Penn-Presby Med Ctr, Pulmonology, 51 N 39th St, Philadelphia Heart Inst Fl 1 Rear, Philadelphia, PA 19104; **Phone:** 215-662-8766; **Board Cert:** Internal Medicine 1980; Pulmonary Disease 1984; Critical Care Medicine 2007; **Med School:** Tufts Univ 1977; **Resid:** Internal Medicine, Med Coll Va Med Ctr 1980; **Fellow:** Pulmonary Disease, Duke Univ Med Ctr 1984; **Fac Appt:** Assoc Clin Prof Med, Univ Pennsylvania

Greenberg, Harly MD [Pul] - **Spec Exp:** Sleep Disorders/Apnea; Lung Disease; Critical Care; **Hospital:** Long Island Jewish Med Ctr, N Shore Univ Hosp; **Address:** North Shore LIJ Sleep Disorders Ctr, 410 Lakeville Rd, Ste 105, New Hyde Park, NY 11040; **Phone:** 516-465-3899; **Board Cert:** Internal Medicine 1985; Pulmonary Disease 1988; **Med School:** NYU Sch Med 1982; **Resid:** Internal Medicine, North Shore Univ Hosp 1985; **Fellow:** Pulmonary Disease, NYU-Bellevue Hosp Ctr 1987; **Fac Appt:** Assoc Prof Med, Albert Einstein Coll Med

Hansen-Flaschen, John MD [Pul] - **Spec Exp:** Interstitial Lung Disease; Diagnostic Problems; Chronic Obstructive Lung Disease (COPD); **Hospital:** Hosp Univ Penn - UPHS (page 60); **Address:** Hosp Univ Penn, Div Pulm, Allergy and Crit Care, 3400 Spruce St Radvin Bldg Fl 3 - Ste F, Philadelphia, PA 19104; **Phone:** 215-662-3202; **Board Cert:** Pulmonary Disease 1982; Critical Care Medicine 1988; Internal Medicine 1979; **Med School:** NYU Sch Med 1976; **Resid:** Internal Medicine, Hosp Univ Penn 1979; **Fellow:** Pulmonary Disease, Hosp Univ Penn 1981; Critical Care Medicine, Hosp Univ Penn 1982; **Fac Appt:** Prof Med, Univ Pennsylvania

Kamholz, Stephan MD [Pul] - **Spec Exp:** Pulmonary Disease-Second Opinion Only; **Hospital:** N Shore Univ Hosp, Long Island Jewish Med Ctr; **Address:** 300 Community Drive, Dept Medicine, 4DSU, Manhasset, NY 11030; **Phone:** 516-562-2078; **Board Cert:** Internal Medicine 1987; Pulmonary Disease 1978; Critical Care Medicine 2009; **Med School:** NY Med Coll 1972; **Resid:** Internal Medicine, Montefiore Med Ctr 1975; **Fellow:** Pulmonary Disease, Montefiore Med Ctr 1977; **Fac Appt:** Prof Med, NYU Sch Med

King, Earl D MD [Pul] - **Spec Exp:** Lung Cancer; Critical Care; **Hospital:** Fox Chase Cancer Ctr (page 58); **Address:** Fox Chase Cancer Center, 333 Cottman Ave, Philadelphia, PA 19111; **Phone:** 215-728-5703; **Board Cert:** Internal Medicine 1990; Pulmonary Disease 2002; Critical Care Medicine 2003; **Med School:** Penn State Univ-Hershey Med Ctr 1986; **Resid:** Internal Medicine, Temple Univ Med Ctr 1989; **Fellow:** Pulmonary Disease, Johns Hopkins Hosp 1993; Sleep Medicine, Johns Hopkins Hosp 1993

Kotloff, Robert M MD [Pul] - **Spec Exp:** Transplant Medicine-Lung; Lung Disease-Complex; Interstitial Lung Disease; **Hospital:** Hosp Univ Penn - UPHS (page 60); **Address:** Hospital University of Pensylvania, Penn Lung Ctr, 3400 Spruce St, 838W Gates, Philadelphia, PA 19104; **Phone:** 215-662-3202; **Board Cert:** Internal Medicine 1986; Pulmonary Disease 1990; Critical Care Medicine 1991; **Med School:** Yale Univ 1983; **Resid:** Internal Medicine, Temple Univ Hosp 1986; **Fellow:** Pulmonary Disease, Hosp Univ Penn 1990; **Fac Appt:** Assoc Prof Med, Univ Pennsylvania

Pulmonary Disease

Libby, Daniel M MD [Pul] - **Spec Exp:** Asthma; Lung Cancer; Interstitial Lung Disease; Chronic Obstructive Lung Disease (COPD); **Hospital:** NY-Presby Hosp/Weill Cornell (page 66); **Address:** 635 Madison Ave, Ste 1101, New York, NY 10021; **Phone:** 212-628-6611; **Board Cert:** Internal Medicine 1977; Pulmonary Disease 1980; **Med School:** Baylor Coll Med 1974; **Resid:** Internal Medicine, NY Hosp 1977; **Fellow:** Pulmonary Disease, NY Hosp 1979; **Fac Appt:** Clin Prof Med, Cornell Univ-Weill Med Coll

Maxfield, Roger MD [Pul] - **Spec Exp:** Emphysema & Asthma; Occupational Lung Disease; Lung Cancer; Bronchoscopy; **Hospital:** NY-Presby Hosp/Columbia (page 66); **Address:** Columbia Presbyterian Eastside, 16 E 60th St, Ste 320, New York, NY 10022-1002; **Phone:** 212-326-8415; **Board Cert:** Internal Medicine 1980; Pulmonary Disease 1986; **Med School:** Brown Univ 1977; **Resid:** Internal Medicine, Georgetown Univ Hosp 1980; **Fellow:** Pulmonary Disease, Bellevue-NYU Med Ctr 1985; **Fac Appt:** Clin Prof Med, Columbia P&S

Nash, Thomas MD [Pul] - **Spec Exp:** Asthma; Cough; Pneumonia; **Hospital:** NY-Presby Hosp/Weill Cornell (page 66); **Address:** 310 E 72nd St, New York, NY 10021-4726; **Phone:** 212-734-6612; **Board Cert:** Internal Medicine 1981; Infectious Disease 1984; Pulmonary Disease 1988; **Med School:** NYU Sch Med 1978; **Resid:** Internal Medicine, New York Hosp-Cornell 1981; **Fellow:** Infectious Disease, New York Hosp-Cornell 1985; Pulmonary Disease, Meml Sloan Kettering Cancer Ctr 1985; **Fac Appt:** Assoc Clin Prof Med, NYU Sch Med

Nelson, Judith E MD [Pul] - **Spec Exp:** Palliative Care; Critical Care; **Hospital:** Mount Sinai Med Ctr (page 64); **Address:** Mt Sinai Medical Ctr, One Gustave Levy Pl, Box 1232, New York, NY 10029; **Phone:** 212-241-2587; **Board Cert:** Internal Medicine 1989; Pulmonary Disease 2002; Critical Care Medicine 2003; Hospice & Palliative Medicine 2005; **Med School:** NYU Sch Med 1986; **Resid:** Internal Medicine, Mt Sinai Med Ctr 1989; **Fellow:** Pulmonary Critical Care Medicine, Mt Sinai Med Ctr 1992; **Fac Appt:** Assoc Prof Med, Mount Sinai Sch Med

Niederman, Michael S MD [Pul] - **Spec Exp:** Infections-Respiratory; Emphysema; Respiratory Failure; Pneumonia; **Hospital:** Winthrop - Univ Hosp; **Address:** 222 Station Plaza N, Ste 400, Mineola, NY 11501-3893; **Phone:** 516-663-2834; **Board Cert:** Internal Medicine 1980; Pulmonary Disease 1983; Critical Care Medicine 2007; **Med School:** Boston Univ 1977; **Resid:** Internal Medicine, Northwestern Univ Med Ctr 1980; **Fellow:** Pulmonary Disease, Yale-New Haven Hosp 1983; **Fac Appt:** Prof Med, SUNY Stony Brook

Pack, Allan MD/PhD [Pul] - **Spec Exp:** Sleep Disorders/Apnea; **Hospital:** Hosp Univ Penn - UPHS (page 60); **Address:** Penn Sleep Center, 3624 Market St, Ste 201, Philadelphia, PA 19104; **Phone:** 215-615-3669; **Med School:** Scotland, UK 1967; **Resid:** Internal Medicine, Univ Glasgow Med Ctr 1972; **Fellow:** Pulmonary Disease, Univ Glasgow Med Ctr 1975; **Fac Appt:** Prof Med, Univ Pennsylvania

Palevsky, Harold I MD [Pul] - **Spec Exp:** Pulmonary Hypertension; Pulmonary Vascular Disease; Thromboembolic Disorders; Pulmonary Embolism; **Hospital:** Penn Presby Med Ctr - UPHS (page 60), Hosp Univ Penn - UPHS (page 60); **Address:** Penn Presbyterian Medical Ctr, 39th & Market Sts, Philadelphia Heart Inst Fl 1 Rear, Philadelphia, PA 19104; **Phone:** 215-662-8717; **Board Cert:** Internal Medicine 2007; Pulmonary Disease 2007; Critical Care Medicine 2007; **Med School:** Med Coll VA 1978; **Resid:** Internal Medicine, Hosp Univ Penn 1981; **Fellow:** Pulmonary Critical Care Medicine, Hosp Univ Penn 1984; **Fac Appt:** Prof Med, Univ Pennsylvania

Reilly Jr, John Joseph MD [Pul] - **Spec Exp:** Transplant Medicine-Lung; Emphysema; Chronic Obstructive Lung Disease (COPD); **Hospital:** UPMC Presby, Pittsburgh; **Address:** 1220 Scaife Hall, 3550 Terrace St, Pittsburgh, PA 15261; **Phone:** 412-648-9091; **Board Cert:** Internal Medicine 1984; Pulmonary Disease 1986; **Med School:** Harvard Med Sch 1981; **Resid:** Internal Medicine, Brigham & Women's Hosp 1984; **Fellow:** Pulmonary Disease, Brigham & Women's Hosp 1987; **Fac Appt:** Assoc Prof Med, Harvard Med Sch

Rossman, Milton D MD [Pul] - **Spec Exp:** Beryllium-induced Lung Disease; Sarcoidosis; Interstitial Lung Disease; **Hospital:** Hosp Univ Penn - UPHS (page 60); **Address:** Hosp of Univ Penn, 3400 Spruce St, 834W Gates Bldg, Philadelphia, PA 19104-4283; **Phone:** 215-662-6413; **Board Cert:** Internal Medicine 1975; Pulmonary Disease 1978; **Med School:** Jefferson Med Coll 1970; **Resid:** Internal Medicine, Univ Hosps 1975; **Fellow:** Pulmonary Disease, Hosp Univ Penn 1977; **Fac Appt:** Prof Med, Univ Pennsylvania

Schluger, Neil MD [Pul] - **Spec Exp:** Tuberculosis; Pulmonary Infections; Chronic Obstructive Lung Disease (COPD); **Hospital:** NY-Presby Hosp/Columbia (page 66); **Address:** Div Pulm, Allergy & Crit Care Med, 630 W 168th St, PH-8 East, Rm 101, New York, NY 10032; **Phone:** 212-305-1544; **Board Cert:** Internal Medicine 1988; Pulmonary Disease 2003; **Med School:** Univ Pennsylvania 1985; **Resid:** Internal Medicine, St Lukes Hosp 1989; **Fellow:** Pulmonary Critical Care Medicine, NY Hosp-Cornell 1992; **Fac Appt:** Prof Med, Columbia P&S

Schwab, Richard MD [Pul] - **Spec Exp:** Sleep Disorders/Apnea; **Hospital:** Hosp Univ Penn - UPHS (page 60); **Address:** Penn Sleep Center, 3624 Market St Fl 2 - Ste 201, Philadelphia, PA 19104; **Phone:** 215-662-7772; **Board Cert:** Internal Medicine 1986; Pulmonary Disease 2000; Critical Care Medicine 2000; **Med School:** Univ Pennsylvania 1983; **Resid:** Internal Medicine, Hosp Univ Penn 1986; **Fellow:** Pulmonary Critical Care Medicine, Hosp Univ Penn 1991; **Fac Appt:** Asst Prof Med, Univ Pennsylvania

Steiger, David MD [Pul] - **Spec Exp:** Rheumatologic Diseases of the Lung; Thromboembolic Disorders; Pulmonary Hypertension; Critical Care; **Hospital:** Hosp For Joint Diseases (page 67), NYU Langone Med Ctr (page 67); **Address:** 305 2nd Ave, Ste 16, New York, NY 10003; **Phone:** 212-598-6091; **Board Cert:** Internal Medicine 1987; Pulmonary Disease 2002; Critical Care Medicine 2005; **Med School:** England, UK 1981; **Resid:** Internal Medicine, St Thomas's Hosp 1984; Internal Medicine, St Lukes Hosp 1989; **Fellow:** Pulmonary Disease, UCSF Med Ctr 1994; **Fac Appt:** Asst Prof Med, NYU Sch Med

Steinberg, Harry MD [Pul] - **Spec Exp:** Asthma; Emphysema; Lung Cancer; **Hospital:** Long Island Jewish Med Ctr, N Shore Univ Hosp; **Address:** LI Jewish Med Ctr, Dept Med, 270-05 76th Ave, New Hyde Park, NY 11040-1433; **Phone:** 516-465-5400; **Med School:** Temple Univ 1966; **Resid:** Internal Medicine, LI Jewish Med Ctr 1969; Pulmonary Critical Care Medicine, LI Jewish Med Ctr 1970; **Fellow:** Pulmonary Disease, Hosp Univ Penn 1974; **Fac Appt:** Clin Prof Med, Albert Einstein Coll Med

Sterman, Daniel H MD [Pul] - **Spec Exp:** Interventional Pulmonology; Lung Cancer; Mesothelioma; Gene Therapy; **Hospital:** Hosp Univ Penn - UPHS (page 60); **Address:** Univ Penn Div Pul, Allergy & Crit Care, 833 W Gates Bldg, 3400 Spruce St, Philadelphia, PA 19104-4283; **Phone:** 215-662-6413; **Board Cert:** Internal Medicine 1992; Pulmonary Disease 1996; Critical Care Medicine 1997; **Med School:** Cornell Univ-Weill Med Coll 1989; **Resid:** Internal Medicine, Hosp Univ Penn 1992; **Fellow:** Pulmonary Critical Care Medicine, Univ Penn 1997; **Fac Appt:** Assoc Prof Med, Univ Pennsylvania

Stover-Pepe, Diane E MD [Pul] - **Spec Exp:** Interstitial Lung Disease; Pulmonary Infections; Pulmonary Disease/Immunocompromised; **Hospital:** Meml Sloan-Kettering Cancer Ctr; **Address:** 1275 York Avenue, New York, NY 10065; **Phone:** 800-525-2225; **Board Cert:** Internal Medicine 1975; Pulmonary Disease 1978; **Med School:** Albert Einstein Coll Med 1970; **Resid:** Internal Medicine, Harlem Hosp Ctr 1972; Internal Medicine, NY Hosp-Cornell Med Ctr 1975; **Fellow:** Pulmonary Disease, Montefiore Med Ctr 1977; **Fac Appt:** Prof Med, Cornell Univ-Weill Med Coll

Pulmonary Disease

Strollo, Patrick J MD [Pul] - **Spec Exp:** Sleep Disorders/Apnea; Respiratory Failure; **Hospital:** UPMC Montefiore, UPMC Presby, Pittsburgh; **Address:** Montefiore Univ Hospital, 3459 5th Ave, Ste S639.11, Pittsburgh, PA 15213; **Phone:** 412-692-2880; **Board Cert:** Internal Medicine 1984; Pulmonary Disease 1988; Sleep Medicine 2007; **Med School:** Uniformed Srvs Univ, Bethesda 1981; **Resid:** Internal Medicine, Wilford Hall Med Ctr 1984; **Fellow:** Pulmonary Disease, Wilford Hall Med Ctr 1987; **Fac Appt:** Assoc Prof Med, Univ Pittsburgh

Teirstein, Alvin S MD [Pul] - **Spec Exp:** Sarcoidosis; Interstitial Lung Disease; Occupational Lung Disease; Lung Cancer; **Hospital:** Mount Sinai Med Ctr (page 64), VA Med Ctr - Bronx; **Address:** Mount Sinai Med Ctr, 1 Gustave Levy Pl, Box 1232, New York, NY 10029; **Phone:** 212-241-5656; **Board Cert:** Internal Medicine 1961; Pulmonary Disease 1969; **Med School:** SUNY Downstate 1953; **Resid:** Internal Medicine, Mt Sinai Med Ctr 1957; **Fellow:** Pulmonary Disease, Mt Sinai Med Ctr 1954; Pulmonary Disease, VA Med Ctr 1956; **Fac Appt:** Prof Med, Mount Sinai Sch Med

Terry, Peter Browne MD [Pul] - **Hospital:** Johns Hopkins Hosp (page 61); **Address:** 1830 E Monument St Fl 5, Baltimore, MD 21205; **Phone:** 410-955-3467; **Board Cert:** Internal Medicine 1973; Pulmonary Disease 1976; **Med School:** St Louis Univ 1968; **Resid:** Internal Medicine, Univ Conn Hlth Ctr 1970; Internal Medicine, Johns Hopkins Hosp 1973; **Fellow:** Pulmonary Disease, Johns Hopkins Hosp 1974; Pulmonary Disease, Mayo Clinic 1975; **Fac Appt:** Prof Med, Johns Hopkins Univ

Thomashow, Byron MD [Pul] - **Spec Exp:** Emphysema; Asthma; Respiratory Failure; Chronic Obstructive Lung Disease (COPD); **Hospital:** NY-Presby Hosp/Columbia (page 66); **Address:** 161 Fort Washington Ave, rm 311, New York, NY 10032; **Phone:** 212-305-5261; **Board Cert:** Internal Medicine 1977; Pulmonary Disease 1980; **Med School:** Columbia P&S 1974; **Resid:** Internal Medicine, Roosevelt Hosp 1977; Pulmonary Disease, Roosevelt Hosp 1978; **Fellow:** Pulmonary Disease, Harlem Hosp Ctr 1979; **Fac Appt:** Clin Prof Med, Columbia P&S

Tino, Gregory MD [Pul] - **Spec Exp:** Emphysema-Lung Volume Reduction; Interstitial Lung Disease; Bronchiectasis; Chronic Obstructive Lung Disease (COPD); **Hospital:** Hosp Univ Penn - UPHS (page 60); **Address:** Hosp Univ Penn, Div Pulmonary & Critical Care, 3400 Spruce St Radvin Bldg Fl 3 - Ste F, Philadelphia, PA 19104; **Phone:** 215-349-5303; **Board Cert:** Internal Medicine 1989; **Med School:** Mount Sinai Sch Med 1986; **Resid:** Internal Medicine, Hosp Univ Penn 1989; **Fellow:** Pulmonary Disease, Hosp Univ Penn 1992; **Fac Appt:** Assoc Prof Med, Univ Pennsylvania

Unger, Michael MD [Pul] - **Spec Exp:** Lung Cancer; Bronchoscopy; Cancer Prevention; Interventional Pulmonology; **Hospital:** Fox Chase Cancer Ctr (page 58); **Address:** Fox Chase Cancer Center, 7701 Burholme Ave, Philadelphia, PA 19111; **Phone:** 215-728-6900; **Board Cert:** Internal Medicine 1977; Pulmonary Disease 1978; **Med School:** France 1971; **Resid:** Internal Medicine, Mt Sinai Hosp 1974; **Fellow:** Pulmonary Disease, NY Hosp-Cornell 1976; **Fac Appt:** Clin Prof Med, Thomas Jefferson Univ

Wenzel, Sally E MD [Pul] - **Spec Exp:** Asthma; Bronchiolitis Obliterans; Allergy; Inflammatory Pulmonary Diseases; **Hospital:** UPMC Montefiore; **Address:** UPMC Montefiore, 3601 Fifth Ave, Falk Medical Bldg Fl 4, Pittsburgh, PA 15213; **Phone:** 412-692-2139; **Board Cert:** Internal Medicine 1984; Pulmonary Disease 1986; **Med School:** Univ Fla Coll Med 1981; **Resid:** Internal Medicine, NC Baptist Hosp 1984; **Fellow:** Pulmonary Disease, Med Coll VA Hosp 1986; **Fac Appt:** Prof Med, Univ Colorado

White, Dorothy MD [Pul] - **Spec Exp:** Lung Cancer; Lung Disease(Drug-Induced); Lung Disease(Immunocompromised); **Hospital:** Meml Sloan-Kettering Cancer Ctr; **Address:** 1275 York Avenue, New York, NY 10065; **Phone:** 800-525-2225; **Board Cert:** Internal Medicine 1980; Pulmonary Disease 1984; **Med School:** SUNY Hlth Sci Ctr 1977; **Resid:** Internal Medicine, New York Hosp 1980; Internal Medicine, Meml Sloan Kettering Cancer Ctr 1981; **Fellow:** Pulmonary Disease, Yale-New Haven Hosp 1984; **Fac Appt:** Prof Med, Cornell Univ-Weill Med Coll

Southeast

Alberts, W Michael MD [Pul] - **Spec Exp:** Lung Cancer; **Hospital:** H Lee Moffitt Cancer Ctr & Research Inst; **Address:** H Lee Moffitt Cancer Ctr, Thoracic Onc, 12902 Magnolia Drive, Tampa, FL 33612; **Phone:** 813-979-3067; **Board Cert:** Internal Medicine 1980; Pulmonary Disease 1982; **Med School:** Univ IL Coll Med 1977; **Resid:** Internal Medicine, Ohio State Univ Hosp 1980; **Fellow:** Pulmonary Critical Care Medicine, UCSD Med Ctr 1983; **Fac Appt:** Prof Med, Univ S Fla Coll Med

Antony, Veena B MD [Pul] - **Spec Exp:** Pleural Disease; **Hospital:** Shands at Univ of FL; **Address:** Shands at the Univ of Florida, 1600 SW Archer Rd, Box 100225, Gainesville, FL 32610-0225; **Phone:** 352-265-0139; **Board Cert:** Internal Medicine 1979; Pulmonary Disease 1982; **Med School:** India 1974; **Resid:** Internal Medicine, Kingsbrook Jewish Med Ctr; **Fellow:** Pulmonary Disease, Univ Co Hlth Sci Ctr; Pulmonary Disease, Natl Jewish Hosp-Asthma Ctr

Brooks, Stuart M MD [Pul] - **Spec Exp:** Occupational Lung Disease; Asthma; Lung Injuries-Inhalation Induced; **Hospital:** Tampa Genl Hosp, H Lee Moffitt Cancer Ctr & Research Inst; **Address:** 1000 Chillum Ct, Safety Harbor, FL 34695; **Phone:** 813-389-6000; **Board Cert:** Internal Medicine 1977; Pulmonary Disease 1969; Occupational Medicine 1987; **Med School:** Univ Cincinnati 1962; **Resid:** Internal Medicine, Boston City Hosp 1967; **Fellow:** Pulmonary Disease, Boston City Hosp 1969; **Fac Appt:** Prof Med, Univ S Fla Coll Med

Campbell Jr, G Douglas MD [Pul] - **Spec Exp:** Infectious Disease-Lung; **Hospital:** Univ Mississippi Med Ctr, VA Med Ctr; **Address:** Univ Mississippi Med Ctr, Div Pulmonology, 2500 N State St, Jackson, MS 39216-4505; **Phone:** 601-984-5650; **Board Cert:** Internal Medicine 1979; Pulmonary Disease 1986; **Med School:** Univ Miss 1976; **Resid:** Internal Medicine, Univ Miss Hosp 1979; **Fellow:** Pulmonary Disease, Univ Tex Hlth Sci Ctr 1983; Infectious Disease, Univ Calgary HSC 1985; **Fac Appt:** Prof Med, Univ Miss

Christman, Brian W MD [Pul] - **Spec Exp:** Chronic Obstructive Lung Disease (COPD); Sepsis; Critical Care; Respiratory Distress Syndrome (ARDS); **Hospital:** VA Med Ctr - Nashville, Vanderbilt Univ Med Ctr; **Address:** VA Tennessee Valley Hlth Care System, 1310 24th Ave S, MC 111, Nashville, TN 37212; **Phone:** 615-327-4751 x5349; **Board Cert:** Internal Medicine 1984; Pulmonary Disease 1986; Critical Care Medicine 1999; **Med School:** Univ Okla Coll Med 1981; **Resid:** Internal Medicine, Vanderbilt Univ Med Ctr 1984; **Fellow:** Pulmonary Disease, Vanderbilt Univ Med Ctr 1987; **Fac Appt:** Prof Med, Vanderbilt Univ

Cooper, John Allen D MD [Pul] - **Spec Exp:** Drug Induced Lung Disease; Chronic Obstructive Lung Disease (COPD); **Hospital:** Univ of Ala Hosp at Birmingham, VA Med Ctr; **Address:** 422 Tinsley Harrison Tower, 1900 University Blvd, Birmingham, AL 35294; **Phone:** 205-975-6770; **Board Cert:** Internal Medicine 1981; Pulmonary Disease 1984; **Med School:** Duke Univ 1978; **Resid:** Internal Medicine, Univ Virginia Hosp 1981; **Fellow:** Pulmonary Disease, Yale Univ 1985; **Fac Appt:** Prof Med, Univ Alabama

Pulmonary Disease

Cooper, William R MD [Pul] - **Spec Exp:** Critical Care; Asthma; Chronic Obstructive Lung Disease (COPD); **Hospital:** Sentara VA Beach Genl Hosp; **Address:** 1008 First Colonial Rd, Ste 103, Virginia Beach, VA 23454-3071; **Phone:** 757-481-2515; **Board Cert:** Internal Medicine 1972; Pulmonary Disease 1974; Critical Care Medicine 1999; **Med School:** Univ VA Sch Med 1969; **Resid:** Internal Medicine, Cleveland Metro Genl Hosp 1971; Pulmonary Disease, Univ Va Hosp 1973; **Fellow:** Pulmonary Disease, Mt Sinai Med Ctr 1974

Doherty, Dennis E MD [Pul] - **Spec Exp:** Asthma; Chronic Obstructive Lung Disease (COPD); Interstitial Lung Disease; **Hospital:** Univ of Kentucky Chandler Hosp, VA Med Ctr - Lexington; **Address:** Univ Kentucky Med Ctr, Div Pulm & Crit Care, 740 S Limestone, rm L-543, Lexington, KY 40536; **Phone:** 859-323-5045; **Board Cert:** Internal Medicine 1985; Pulmonary Disease 1988; **Med School:** Ohio State Univ 1980; **Resid:** Internal Medicine, Ohio State Univ Hosp 1983; **Fellow:** Pulmonary Disease, Univ Colorado Hlth Sci Ctr 1986; **Fac Appt:** Prof Med, Univ KY Coll Med

Donohue, James Francis MD [Pul] - **Spec Exp:** Asthma; Chronic Obstructive Lung Disease (COPD); Sarcoidosis; **Hospital:** Univ NC Hosps; **Address:** Univ NC, Div Pulmonary Disease, 4125 Bio-informatics Bldg CB 7020, Chapel Hill, NC 27599-7020; **Phone:** 919-966-2531; **Board Cert:** Internal Medicine 1975; Pulmonary Disease 1976; **Med School:** UMDNJ-NJ Med Sch, Newark 1969; **Resid:** Internal Medicine, UMDNJ-Newark 1971; Internal Medicine, NC Meml Hosp 1974; **Fellow:** Pulmonary Disease, Univ North Carolina 1976; **Fac Appt:** Prof Med, Univ NC Sch Med

Dunlap, Nancy E MD/PhD [Pul] - **Spec Exp:** Tubercolosis; **Hospital:** Univ of Ala Hosp at Birmingham; **Address:** 2000 6th Ave S Fl 3/Admin, Birmingham, AL 35233; **Phone:** 205-801-7900; **Board Cert:** Internal Medicine 1984; Pulmonary Disease 1988; Critical Care Medicine 1999; **Med School:** Duke Univ 1981; **Resid:** Internal Medicine, Univ Alabama Med Ctr 1984; **Fellow:** Pulmonary Disease, Univ Alabama 1987; **Fac Appt:** Prof Med, Univ Alabama

Fulkerson Jr, William J MD [Pul] - **Spec Exp:** Respiratory Failure; Thromboembolic Disorders; **Hospital:** Duke Univ Med Ctr; **Address:** Duke Univ Med Ctr, Trent Drive, Box 3121, Durham, NC 27710; **Phone:** 919-684-1860; **Board Cert:** Internal Medicine 1981; Pulmonary Disease 1984; **Med School:** Univ NC Sch Med 1977; **Resid:** Internal Medicine, Vanderbilt Univ Hosp 1980; **Fellow:** Pulmonary Disease, Vanderbilt Univ Hosp 1983; **Fac Appt:** Prof Med, Duke Univ

Garver Jr, Robert MD [Pul] - **Spec Exp:** Lung Cancer; Lung Disease; **Hospital:** Univ of Ala Hosp at Birmingham; **Address:** 1900 University Blvd, THT 215, Birmingham, AL 35294; **Phone:** 205-934-7556; **Board Cert:** Internal Medicine 1984; Pulmonary Disease 1986; **Med School:** Johns Hopkins Univ 1981; **Resid:** Internal Medicine, Johns Hopkins Hosp 1984; **Fellow:** Pulmonary Disease, NHLBI 1985; **Fac Appt:** Prof Med, Univ Alabama

Goldman, Allan L MD [Pul] - **Spec Exp:** Occupational Lung Disease; Airway Disorders; Lung Cancer; **Hospital:** Tampa Genl Hosp, James A Haley VA Hosp; **Address:** USF Coll Med, Dept Internal Medicine, 12901 Bruce B Downs Blvd, Box MDC19, Tampa, FL 33612-4742; **Phone:** 813-974-2271; **Board Cert:** Internal Medicine 1972; Pulmonary Disease 1972; **Med School:** Univ Minn 1968; **Resid:** Internal Medicine, Brooke Army Hosp 1970; **Fellow:** Pulmonary Disease, Walter Reed Army Hosp 1972; **Fac Appt:** Prof Med, Univ S Fla Coll Med

Harman, Eloise M MD [Pul] - **Spec Exp:** Critical Care; Diagnostic Problems; Mechanical Ventilation; **Hospital:** Shands at Univ of FL; **Address:** Shands at Univ of Florida, 1600 SW Archer Rd, Box 100225, Gainesville, FL 32610-0225; **Phone:** 352-392-2666; **Board Cert:** Internal Medicine 1973; Pulmonary Disease 1976; Critical Care Medicine 2007; **Med School:** Johns Hopkins Univ 1970; **Resid:** Internal Medicine, Johns Hopkins Hosp 1972; **Fellow:** Pulmonary Disease, NY Hosp-Cornell Med Ctr 1974; **Fac Appt:** Prof Med, Univ Fla Coll Med

Haynes Jr, Johnson MD [Pul] - **Spec Exp:** Sickle Cell Disease-Lung; Chronic Obstructive Lung Disease (COPD); **Hospital:** Univ of S AL Med Ctr; **Address:** USA Comprehensive Sickle Cell Ctr, 2451 Fillingim St, MCSB 1530, Mobile, AL 36617; **Phone:** 251-471-7847; **Board Cert:** Internal Medicine 1983; Pulmonary Disease 1986; **Med School:** Univ S Ala Coll Med 1980; **Resid:** Internal Medicine, Univ S Alabama Med Ctr 1983; **Fellow:** Pulmonary Disease, Univ S Alabama Med Ctr 1986; **Fac Appt:** Prof Med, Univ S Ala Coll Med

Henke, David C MD [Pul] - **Spec Exp:** Asthma; Chronic Obstructive Lung Disease (COPD); Vasculitis; **Hospital:** Univ NC Hosps; **Address:** Univ NC Med Sch, Div Pulm Dis & Crit Care Med, 130 Mason Farm Rd, Box 7020, Chapel Hill, NC 27599-7020; **Phone:** 919-966-6838; **Board Cert:** Internal Medicine 1980; Dermatology 1983; Pulmonary Disease 1988; **Med School:** Univ NC Sch Med 1977; **Resid:** Internal Medicine, NC Memorial Hosp 1980; Dermatology, NC Meml NIEHS 1984; **Fellow:** Pulmonary Disease, NC Memorial Hosp 1986; **Fac Appt:** Assoc Prof Med, Univ NC Sch Med

Johnson, Bruce Ellsworth MD [Pul] - **Spec Exp:** Sleep Disorders/Apnea; **Hospital:** Sentara VA Beach Genl Hosp; **Address:** 1008 First Colonial Rd, Virginia Beach, VA 23454-3002; **Phone:** 757-481-2515; **Board Cert:** Internal Medicine 1981; Pulmonary Disease 1986; Critical Care Medicine 2001; **Med School:** Med Coll GA 1978; **Resid:** Internal Medicine, Univ VA Med Ctr 1981; **Fellow:** Pulmonary Disease, Univ VA Med Ctr 1983

Light, Richard W MD [Pul] - **Spec Exp:** Pleural Disease; **Hospital:** Vanderbilt Univ Med Ctr; **Address:** Vanderbilt Univ Med Ctr-Pulmonary Medicine, 1161 21st Ave S, T1218 MCN, Nashville, TN 37232-2650; **Phone:** 615-322-3412; **Board Cert:** Internal Medicine 1972; Pulmonary Disease 1974; **Med School:** Johns Hopkins Univ 1968; **Resid:** Internal Medicine, Johns Hopkins Hosp 1970; **Fellow:** Pulmonary Disease, Johns Hopkins Hosp 1972; **Fac Appt:** Prof Med, Vanderbilt Univ

LoRusso, Thomas J MD [Pul] - **Spec Exp:** Critical Care; Sleep Disorders/Apnea; **Hospital:** Inova Fairfax Hosp; **Address:** 1800 Town Ctr Drive, Ste 419, Reston, VA 20190; **Phone:** 703-620-3926; **Board Cert:** Internal Medicine 2001; Pulmonary Disease 2002; Critical Care Medicine 2003; **Med School:** SUNY Upstate Med Univ 1987; **Resid:** Internal Medicine, Univ Hosp-SUNY 1990; **Fellow:** Pulmonary Disease, Cedars Sinai Med Ctr 1993

Loyd, James E MD [Pul] - **Spec Exp:** Pulmonary Fibrosis; Interstitial Lung Disease; Transplant Medicine-Lung; Pulmonary Hypertension; **Hospital:** Vanderbilt Univ Med Ctr; **Address:** Vanderbilt Univ Med Ctr, Div Pulmonary Med, 1161 21st Ave S, rm T-1218 MCN, Nashville, TN 37232-2650; **Phone:** 615-322-4752; **Board Cert:** Internal Medicine 1978; Pulmonary Disease 1984; **Med School:** W VA Univ 1973; **Resid:** Internal Medicine, Vanderbilt Univ Hosp 1976; **Fellow:** Pulmonary Disease, Vanderbilt Univ Hosp 1978; **Fac Appt:** Prof Med, Vanderbilt Univ

Sahn, Steven A MD [Pul] - **Spec Exp:** Pleural Disease; Interstitial Lung Disease; Chronic Obstructive Lung Disease (COPD); Pulmonary Fibrosis; **Hospital:** MUSC Med Ctr, Charleston Mem Hosp; **Address:** MUSC, Div Pulm & Crit Care Med, 96 Jonathan Lucas St, Box 250630, Charleston, SC 29425-8900; **Phone:** 843-792-3167; **Board Cert:** Internal Medicine 1974; Pulmonary Disease 1974; **Med School:** Univ Louisville Sch Med 1968; **Resid:** Internal Medicine, Univ Iowa Hosp 1971; **Fellow:** Pulmonary Disease, Univ CO Hlth Sci Ctr 1973; **Fac Appt:** Prof Med, Med Univ SC

Staton Jr, Gerald W MD [Pul] - **Spec Exp:** Interstitial Lung Disease; Chronic Obstructive Lung Disease (COPD); Pulmonary Fibrosis; Sarcoidosis; **Hospital:** Wesley Woods Ger Hosp, Emory Univ Hosp Midtown; **Address:** 550 Peachtree St NE Fl 6, Atlanta, GA 30308; **Phone:** 404-686-2505; **Board Cert:** Internal Medicine 1978; Pulmonary Disease 1982; Critical Care Medicine 2007; **Med School:** Med Coll GA 1976; **Resid:** Internal Medicine, Stanford Univ Med Ctr 1979; **Fellow:** Pulmonary Disease, Mass Genl Hosp 1981; **Fac Appt:** Prof Med, Emory Univ

Pulmonary Disease

Tapson, Victor MD [Pul] - **Spec Exp:** Pulmonary Hypertension; Chronic Obstructive Lung Disease (COPD); Emphysema; **Hospital:** Duke Univ Med Ctr; **Address:** Duke Univ Med Ctr, Dept Pulm Critical Care Med, Box 102351, Durham, NC 27710; **Phone:** 919-684-6237; **Board Cert:** Internal Medicine 1986; Pulmonary Disease 2000; **Med School:** Hahnemann Univ 1982; **Resid:** Internal Medicine, Duke Univ Med Ctr 1986; **Fellow:** Pulmonary Disease, Boston Univ 1989; **Fac Appt:** Prof Med, Duke Univ

Vaughey, Ellen MD [Pul] - **Spec Exp:** Critical Care; Sleep Disorders/Apnea; **Hospital:** Inova Fairfax Hosp, Virginia Hosp Ctr - Arlington; **Address:** 3289 Woodburn Rd, Ste 350, Annandale, VA 22003; **Phone:** 703-641-8616; **Board Cert:** Internal Medicine 2001; Pulmonary Disease 2002; Critical Care Medicine 2003; **Med School:** Georgetown Univ 1987; **Resid:** Internal Medicine, Thomas Jefferson Univ Hosp 1990; **Fellow:** Pulmonary Disease, Roger Williams Hosp-Brown Univ 1993

Voelkel, Norbert F MD [Pul] - **Spec Exp:** Pulmonary Hypertension; Asthma; Emphysema; **Hospital:** Med Coll of VA Hosp; **Address:** Med Coll of VA Hosp, Box 980456, Richmond, VA 23298; **Phone:** 804-628-9614; **Med School:** Germany 1972; **Resid:** Internal Medicine, Univ Hamburg 1977; **Fellow:** Research, Univ Colorado 1978; Pulmonary Disease, Univ Colorado 1981; **Fac Appt:** Prof Med, Univ Colorado

Wanner, Adam MD [Pul] - **Spec Exp:** Asthma; **Hospital:** Jackson Meml Hosp (page 70), Univ of Miami Hosp (page 71); **Address:** Univ Miami Sch Med, Div Pulm & Crit Care, Box 016960 (R-47), Miami, FL 33101; **Phone:** 305-243-3045; **Board Cert:** Internal Medicine 1973; Pulmonary Disease 1974; **Med School:** Switzerland 1966; **Resid:** Internal Medicine, Kantonsspital Aarau 1970; **Fellow:** Pulmonary Disease, Mt Sinai Med Ctr 1972; **Fac Appt:** Prof Med, Univ Miami Sch Med

Wheeler, Arthur P MD [Pul] - **Spec Exp:** Critical Care; Sepsis; Respiratory Distress Syndrome (ARDS); **Hospital:** Vanderbilt Univ Med Ctr; **Address:** Vanderbilt Univ Medical Ctr, 1161 21st Ave S, rm T-1217 MCN, Nashville, TN 37232-2650; **Phone:** 615-322-3412; **Board Cert:** Internal Medicine 1985; Pulmonary Disease 1988; Critical Care Medicine 1999; **Med School:** Univ MD Sch Med 1982; **Resid:** Internal Medicine, Vanderbilt Univ Med Ctr 1985; **Fellow:** Pulmonary Disease, Vanderbilt Univ Med Ctr 1986; **Fac Appt:** Assoc Prof Med, Vanderbilt Univ

Young Jr, K Randall MD [Pul] - **Spec Exp:** Transplant Medicine-Lung; Cystic Fibrosis; **Hospital:** Univ of Ala Hosp at Birmingham; **Address:** 422 Tinsley Harrison Tower, 1900 University Blvd, Birmingham, AL 35294; **Phone:** 205-934-5400; **Board Cert:** Internal Medicine 1982; Pulmonary Disease 1986; Allergy & Immunology 1987; **Med School:** Jefferson Med Coll 1978; **Resid:** Internal Medicine, Yale-New Haven Hosp 1982; Pulmonary Critical Care Medicine, Yale-New Haven Hosp 1985; **Fellow:** Allergy & Immunology, Nat Inst Hlth 1988; **Fac Appt:** Prof Med, Univ Alabama

Midwest

Balk, Robert A MD [Pul] - **Spec Exp:** Asthma; Cystic Fibrosis; Respiratory Failure; Lung Injury/ARDS; **Hospital:** Rush Univ Med Ctr; **Address:** 1725 W Harrison St, Ste 054, Chicago, IL 60612; **Phone:** 312-942-6744; **Board Cert:** Internal Medicine 1981; Pulmonary Disease 1986; Critical Care Medicine 2008; **Med School:** Univ MO-Kansas City 1978; **Resid:** Internal Medicine, Univ MO-Kansas City Affil Hosps 1981; **Fellow:** Pulmonary Critical Care Medicine, Univ Ark Hosp 1983; **Fac Appt:** Prof Med, Rush Med Coll

Fahey, Patrick J MD [Pul] - **Hospital:** Loyola Univ Med Ctr, Hines VA Hosp; **Address:** Loyola Univ Med Ctr, 2160 1st Ave Bldg 54 - rm 131A, Maywood, IL 60153-3304; **Phone:** 708-216-3300; **Board Cert:** Internal Medicine 1976; Pulmonary Disease 1978; **Med School:** Univ Wisc 1973; **Resid:** Internal Medicine, St Elizabeth's Hosp 1976; **Fellow:** Pulmonary Disease, Strong Meml Hosp 1980; **Fac Appt:** Prof Med, Loyola Univ-Stritch Sch Med

Fletcher, Eugene MD [Pul] - **Spec Exp:** Chronic Obstructive Lung Disease (COPD); Sleep Disorders/Apnea; **Hospital:** Floyd Meml Hosp & Hlth Svcs; **Address:** 428 Vincennes St, New Albany, IN 47150; **Phone:** 812-948-5841; **Board Cert:** Internal Medicine 1974; Pulmonary Disease 1980; **Med School:** Temple Univ 1971; **Resid:** Internal Medicine, Univ Colo Affil Hosp 1973; Internal Medicine, Fitzsimons Army Med Ctr 1974; **Fellow:** Pulmonary Disease, Univ Okla Hlth Scis Ctr 1974

Garrity Jr, Edward MD [Pul] - **Spec Exp:** Transplant Medicine-Lung; Pulmonary Vascular Disease; Asthma; Cystic Fibrosis; **Hospital:** Univ of Chicago Med Ctr; **Address:** Lung Transplant Program, 5841 S Maryland Ave, MC 0999, Chicago, IL 60637; **Phone:** 773-834-1119; **Board Cert:** Internal Medicine 2003; Pulmonary Disease 1998; Critical Care Medicine 1998; **Med School:** Loyola Univ-Stritch Sch Med 1976; **Resid:** Internal Medicine, Loyola Univ Med Ctr 1979; **Fellow:** Pulmonary Disease, Univ Chicago Hosps 1983; **Fac Appt:** Prof Med, Univ Chicago-Pritzker Sch Med

Grum, Cyril M MD [Pul] - **Spec Exp:** Asthma; Cystic Fibrosis; **Hospital:** Univ Michigan Hlth Sys; **Address:** Univ Mich, Div Pulm & Crit Care Med, 1500 E Med Ctr Drive, rm 3110, Taubman Ctr-3rd flr reception C, Ann Arbor, MI 48109-0368; **Phone:** 734-647-9342; **Board Cert:** Internal Medicine 1980; Pulmonary Disease 1982; **Med School:** Med Coll Wisc 1977; **Resid:** Internal Medicine, Cleveland Clin; **Fellow:** Pulmonary Disease, Univ Mich Hosps; **Fac Appt:** Asst Prof Med, Univ Mich Med Sch

Hall, Jesse MD [Pul] - **Spec Exp:** Respiratory Failure; Critical Care; Sleep Disorders/Apnea; **Hospital:** Univ of Chicago Med Ctr; **Address:** 5841 S Maryland Ave, MC 6026, Chicago, IL 60637; **Phone:** 773-702-1454; **Board Cert:** Internal Medicine 1980; Critical Care Medicine 1998; **Med School:** Univ Chicago-Pritzker Sch Med 1977; **Resid:** Internal Medicine, Univ Chicago Hosps 1982; **Fac Appt:** Prof Med, Univ Chicago-Pritzker Sch Med

Hertz, Marshall I MD [Pul] - **Spec Exp:** Transplant Medicine-Lung; Transplant Medicine-Heart & Lung; Pulmonary Hypertension; **Hospital:** Univ Minn Med Ctr, Fairview - Univ Campus; **Address:** Pulmonary, Allergy & Critical Care Med, 420 Delaware St SE, MMC 276, Minneapolis, MN 55455; **Phone:** 612-624-0999; **Board Cert:** Internal Medicine 1981; Pulmonary Disease 1984; **Med School:** Univ Mich Med Sch 1978; **Resid:** Internal Medicine, Univ Minn Med Ctr 1982; **Fellow:** Pulmonary Critical Care Medicine, Univ Minn Med Ctr 1984; **Fac Appt:** Prof Med, Univ Minn

Hunninghake, Gary MD [Pul] - **Spec Exp:** Sarcoidosis; Interstitial Lung Disease; **Hospital:** Univ Iowa Hosp & Clinics; **Address:** Univ Iowa, Div Pulmonary Disease, 200 Hawkins Drive W319DGH, Iowa City, IA 52242-1081; **Phone:** 319-356-4187; **Board Cert:** Internal Medicine 1975; Pulmonary Disease 1980; Allergy & Immunology 1977; **Med School:** Univ Kans 1972; **Resid:** Internal Medicine, Univ Kansas Med Ctr 1974; Pulmonary Disease, Natl Inst Hlth 1976; **Fac Appt:** Prof Med, Univ Iowa Coll Med

Hyers, Thomas M MD [Pul] - **Spec Exp:** Thromboembolic Disorders; Chronic Obstructive Lung Disease (COPD); Occupational Medicine; **Hospital:** St Clare Hlth Ctr; **Address:** CARE Clinical Research, 522 N New Ballas Rd, Ste 350, St Louis, MO 63122; **Phone:** 314-699-9383; **Board Cert:** Internal Medicine 1974; Pulmonary Disease 1980; Critical Care Medicine 1999; **Med School:** Duke Univ 1968; **Resid:** Internal Medicine, Univ Wash Med Ctr 1975; Pulmonary Disease, Univ Colorado Hosp 1977; **Fellow:** Pulmonary Disease, Natl Inst Hlth 1972; **Fac Appt:** Clin Prof Med, St Louis Univ

Jett, James R MD [Pul] - **Spec Exp:** Lung Cancer; Mesothelioma; Thymoma; **Hospital:** Mayo Med Ctr & Clin - Rochester; **Address:** Mayo Clinic, Thoracic Diseases, 200 First St SW, Rochester, MN 55905; **Phone:** 507-284-5398; **Board Cert:** Internal Medicine 1976; Pulmonary Disease 1978; **Med School:** Univ MO-Columbia Sch Med 1973; **Resid:** Internal Medicine, Mayo Clinic 1976; **Fellow:** Pulmonary Disease, Mayo Clinic 1978; **Fac Appt:** Prof Med, Mayo Med Sch

Pulmonary Disease

Kaye, Mitchell MD [Pul] - **Spec Exp:** Chronic Obstructive Lung Disease (COPD); Asthma; **Hospital:** Abbott - Northwestern Hosp; **Address:** Minn Lung Ctr, 920 E 28th St, Ste 700, Minneapolis, MN 55407; **Phone:** 612-863-3750; **Board Cert:** Internal Medicine 1987; Pulmonary Disease 2000; Critical Care Medicine 2001; **Med School:** Univ Minn 1984; **Resid:** Internal Medicine, Univ Ill Hosps & Clins 1987; **Fellow:** Pulmonary Disease, Northwestern Univ Med Sch 1989

Kovitz, Kevin L MD [Pul] - **Spec Exp:** Interventional Pulmonology; **Hospital:** Central DuPage Hosp, Alexian Brothers Med Ctr; **Address:** Chicago Chest Ctr/Suburban Lung Assocs, 800 Biesterfield Rd, Ste 510, Elk Grove Village, IL 60007; **Phone:** 847-981-3660; **Board Cert:** Internal Medicine 1988; Pulmonary Disease 2002; Critical Care Medicine 2005; **Med School:** Israel 1985; **Resid:** Internal Medicine, Univ Maryland Hosps 1988; **Fellow:** Pulmonary Disease, Johns Hopkins Hosp 1992; Interventional Pulmonology, Sainte Marguerite Hosp 1993

Krowka, Michael J MD [Pul] - **Spec Exp:** Hepatopulmonary Syndrome; Pulmonary Hypertension; Chronic Obstructive Lung Disease (COPD); **Hospital:** Mayo Med Ctr & Clin - Rochester; **Address:** Mayo Clinic, Div Pulm & Crit Care Med, 200 First St SW, Rochester, MN 55905; **Phone:** 507-284-3764; **Board Cert:** Internal Medicine 1983; Pulmonary Disease 1986; **Med School:** Univ Nevada 1980; **Resid:** Internal Medicine, Evanston Hosp 1983; **Fellow:** Pulmonary Disease, Mayo Clinic 1986; **Fac Appt:** Prof Med, Mayo Med Sch

Lefrak, Stephen MD [Pul] - **Spec Exp:** Emphysema-Lung Volume Reduction; Critical Care; **Hospital:** Barnes-Jewish Hosp; **Address:** Wash Univ Sch Med, Div Pulm & Crit Care Med, 660 S Euclid Ave, Box 8052, St Louis, MO 63110; **Phone:** 314-362-6044; **Board Cert:** Internal Medicine 1972; Pulmonary Disease 1972; **Med School:** SUNY Downstate 1965; **Resid:** Internal Medicine, Boston Univ Hosp 1968; Pulmonary Disease, Kings Co Hosp Ctr 1969; **Fellow:** Cardiopulmonary Disease, Columbia-Presby Hosp 1970; **Fac Appt:** Prof Med, Washington Univ, St Louis

Lem, Vincent M MD [Pul] - **Spec Exp:** Asthma; **Hospital:** St Luke's Hosp of Kansas City; **Address:** 4321 Washington St, Ste 6000, Kansas City, MO 64111; **Phone:** 816-756-2255; **Board Cert:** Internal Medicine 1982; Pulmonary Disease 1984; Critical Care Medicine 2004; **Med School:** Univ Kans 1978; **Resid:** Internal Medicine, St Luke's Hosp 1982; **Fellow:** Pulmonary Disease, Univ Texas Hlth Sci Ctr 1984; **Fac Appt:** Assoc Clin Prof Med, Univ MO-Kansas City

Marini, John Joseph MD [Pul] - **Spec Exp:** Critical Care; Mechanical Ventilation; Chronic Obstructive Lung Disease (COPD); **Hospital:** Regions Hosp - St Paul; **Address:** 401 Phelon Blvd, St Paul, MN 55130; **Phone:** 952-967-7616; **Board Cert:** Internal Medicine 2003; Pulmonary Disease 2003; Critical Care Medicine 2002; **Med School:** Johns Hopkins Univ 1973; **Resid:** Internal Medicine, Univ Washington Med Ctr 1976; **Fellow:** Pulmonary Disease, Univ Washington Med Ctr 1978; **Fac Appt:** Prof Med, Univ Minn

Martinez, Fernando J MD [Pul] - **Spec Exp:** Lung Disease; Critical Care; **Hospital:** Univ Michigan Hlth Sys; **Address:** 1500 E Med Ctr Dr, Taubman Ctr-3916, 3rd flr-Reception C, Ann Arbor, MI 48109-0360; **Phone:** 734-763-7668; **Board Cert:** Internal Medicine 1986; Pulmonary Disease 1988; Critical Care Medicine 2000; **Med School:** Univ Fla Coll Med 1983; **Resid:** Internal Medicine, Beth Israel Hosp 1986; **Fellow:** Pulmonary Disease, Boston Univ 1989; **Fac Appt:** Prof Med, Univ Mich Med Sch

McLennan, Geoffrey MD/PhD [Pul] - **Spec Exp:** Lung Cancer; Emphysema; Chronic Obstructive Lung Disease (COPD); Bronchoscopy; **Hospital:** Univ Iowa Hosp & Clinics; **Address:** Univ Iowa Hosp, 200 Hawkins Drive, Ste 4900JPP, Iowa City, IA 52242; **Phone:** 319-353-8201; **Med School:** Australia 1970; **Resid:** Internal Medicine, Royal Adelaide Medical Sch; **Fellow:** Pulmonary Disease, Queen Elizabeth Hosp; **Fac Appt:** Prof Med, Univ Iowa Coll Med

Popovich Jr, John MD [Pul] - **Spec Exp:** Lung Disease; Pulmonary Embolism; Interstitial Lung Disease; Critical Care; **Hospital:** Henry Ford Hosp; **Address:** Henry Ford Hosp, Dept Int Med, 2799 W Grand Blvd, Detroit, MI 48202; **Phone:** 313-916-1828; **Board Cert:** Internal Medicine 1978; Pulmonary Disease 1980; **Med School:** Univ Mich Med Sch 1975; **Resid:** Internal Medicine, Henry Ford Hosp 1978; **Fellow:** Pulmonary Disease, Henry Ford Hosp 1980; **Fac Appt:** Prof Med, Wayne State Univ

Prakash, Udaya MD [Pul] - **Spec Exp:** Bronchoscopy; **Hospital:** Mayo Med Ctr & Clin - Rochester; **Address:** Mayo Clin, Div Pulm & Crit Care Med, 200 First St SW, Rochester, MN 55905; **Phone:** 507-284-4162; **Board Cert:** Internal Medicine 1987; Pulmonary Disease 1976; **Med School:** India 1969; **Resid:** Internal Medicine, Mayo Clin 1973; **Fellow:** Pulmonary Disease, Mayo Clin 1976; **Fac Appt:** Prof Med, Mayo Med Sch

Rosenbluth, Daniel B MD [Pul] - **Spec Exp:** Cystic Fibrosis; **Hospital:** Barnes-Jewish Hosp; **Address:** Washington Univ Sch Med, 660 S Euclid, Box 8052, St Louis, MO 63110; **Phone:** 314-454-8762; **Board Cert:** Pulmonary Disease 2004; Critical Care Medicine 2005; Internal Medicine 2002; **Med School:** Mount Sinai Sch Med 1989; **Resid:** Internal Medicine, Northwestern Meml Hosp 1992; **Fellow:** Pulmonary Critical Care Medicine, Barnes Hosp 1995; **Fac Appt:** Prof Med, Washington Univ, St Louis

Shore, Bernard L MD [Pul] - **Spec Exp:** Lung Disease; Palliative Care; Pain Management; **Hospital:** Barnes-Jewish Hosp; **Address:** 1110 Highland Plaza Drive E, Ste 375, St Louis, MO 63110; **Phone:** 314-367-3113; **Board Cert:** Internal Medicine 1980; Pulmonary Disease 1982; **Med School:** Washington Univ, St Louis 1977; **Resid:** Internal Medicine, Barnes Hosp 1980; **Fellow:** Pulmonary Disease, Wash Univ Med Ctr 1982; **Fac Appt:** Assoc Clin Prof Med, Washington Univ, St Louis

Silver, Michael R MD [Pul] - **Spec Exp:** Chronic Obstructive Lung Disease (COPD); Lung Cancer; Asthma; **Hospital:** Rush Univ Med Ctr, Rush Oak Park Hosp; **Address:** Rush Univ Med Ctr, Professional Office Bldg 3, 1725 W Harrison St, Ste 054, Chicago, IL 60612; **Phone:** 312-942-6744; **Board Cert:** Internal Medicine 1984; Pulmonary Disease 1988; Critical Care Medicine 1999; **Med School:** Albany Med Coll 1981; **Resid:** Internal Medicine, Rush-Presby-St Luke's Med Ctr 1985; **Fellow:** Pulmonary Critical Care Medicine, Rush-Presby-St Luke's Med Ctr 1987; **Fac Appt:** Assoc Prof Med, Rush Med Coll

Simon, Richard H MD [Pul] - **Spec Exp:** Cystic Fibrosis; **Hospital:** Univ Michigan Hlth Sys; **Address:** Univ Michigan Div Pulmonary Medicine, 1500 E Med Ctr Drive, Taubman Ctr-3rd flr Reception C, Ann Arbor, MI 48109; **Phone:** 734-647-9342; **Board Cert:** Internal Medicine 1976; Pulmonary Disease 1980; **Med School:** Duke Univ 1972; **Resid:** Internal Medicine, UCSF Med Ctr 1975; Internal Medicine, Univ Colorado Affil Hosps 1976; **Fellow:** Pulmonary Disease, Univ Colorado 1981; **Fac Appt:** Prof Med, Univ Mich Med Sch

Stoller, James MD [Pul] - **Spec Exp:** Emphysema/Alpha-1 Antitrypsin Deficiency; **Hospital:** Cleveland Clin Fdn (page 56); **Address:** Cleveland Clinic, Dept Education, 9500 Euclid Ave, Desk NA22, Cleveland, OH 44195; **Phone:** 216-444-1960; **Board Cert:** Internal Medicine 1982; Pulmonary Disease 1984; Critical Care Medicine 2007; **Med School:** Yale Univ 1979; **Resid:** Internal Medicine, Peter Bent Brigham Hosp 1982; **Fellow:** Pulmonary Disease, Brigham & Women's Hosp 1983; Critical Care Medicine, Mass Genl Hosp 1985; **Fac Appt:** Prof Med, Cleveland Cl Coll Med/Case West Res

Pulmonary Disease

Tobin, Martin MD [Pul] - **Spec Exp:** Mechanical Ventilation; Chronic Obstructive Lung Disease (COPD); **Hospital:** Loyola Univ Med Ctr, Hines VA Hosp; **Address:** Hines VA Hosp (111N), Fifth Ave and Roosevelt Rd, Bldg 1 - rm E438, Hines, IL 60141; **Phone:** 708-202-2705; **Board Cert:** Internal Medicine 1983; Pulmonary Disease 1984; **Med School:** Ireland 1975; **Resid:** Internal Medicine, Trinity Coll Hosps 1979; Pulmonary Disease, Kings Coll Hosp 1980; **Fellow:** Pulmonary Critical Care Medicine, Mt Sinai Hosp 1983; Pulmonary Critical Care Medicine, Univ Pittsburgh 1983; **Fac Appt:** Prof Med, Loyola Univ-Stritch Sch Med

Trulock, Elbert MD [Pul] - **Spec Exp:** Transplant Medicine-Lung; Emphysema-Lung Volume Reduction; Pulmonary Hypertension; Cystic Fibrosis; **Hospital:** Barnes-Jewish Hosp; **Address:** Wash Univ Sch Med, Dept Pulm, 660 S Euclid Ave, Box 8052, St Louis, MO 63110; **Phone:** 314-454-8766; **Board Cert:** Internal Medicine 1981; Pulmonary Disease 1984; **Med School:** Emory Univ 1978; **Resid:** Internal Medicine, Barnes Hosp 1981; **Fellow:** Pulmonary Disease, Wash Univ Med Ctr 1983; **Fac Appt:** Prof Med, Washington Univ, St Louis

Wiedemann, Herbert P MD [Pul] - **Spec Exp:** Respiratory Distress Syndrome (ARDS); Asthma; Emphysema; **Hospital:** Cleveland Clin Fdn (page 56); **Address:** Cleveland Clinic-Pulmonary & Allergy, 9500 Euclid Ave, Desk A90, Cleveland, OH 44195; **Phone:** 216-444-8335; **Board Cert:** Internal Medicine 1980; Pulmonary Disease 1984; **Med School:** Cornell Univ 1977; **Resid:** Internal Medicine, Univ Wash Hosps 1980; Internal Medicine, Harborview Hosp 1981; **Fellow:** Pulmonary Disease, Yale Univ 1984

Wunderink, Richard G MD [Pul] - **Spec Exp:** Infectious Disease-Lung; Pneumonia; Sepsis; **Hospital:** Northwestern Meml Hosp; **Address:** 675 N St Clair Galter Bldg - rm 18-250, Chicago, IL 60611; **Phone:** 312-695-1800; **Board Cert:** Internal Medicine 1983; Pulmonary Disease 1986; Critical Care Medicine 2008; **Med School:** Indiana Univ 1980; **Resid:** Internal Medicine, Butterworth Hosp 1983; **Fellow:** Pulmonary Disease, Henry Ford Hosp 1985; **Fac Appt:** Prof Med, Northwestern Univ

Great Plains and Mountains

Brown, Kevin K MD [Pul] - **Spec Exp:** Pulmonary Fibrosis; Interstitial Lung Disease; Autoimmune Lung Disease; **Hospital:** Natl Jewish Med & Rsch Ctr, Univ Colorado Hosp; **Address:** Natl Jewish Health, 1400 Jackson St, Denver, CO 80206-2762; **Phone:** 303-398-1621; **Board Cert:** Internal Medicine 1989; Pulmonary Disease 2005; **Med School:** Univ Minn 1984; **Resid:** Internal Medicine, Providence Med Ctr 1989; **Fellow:** Pulmonary Disease, Maine Med Ctr 1992; Pulmonary Disease, Univ Colo Hlth Scis Ctr 1994; **Fac Appt:** Assoc Prof Med, Univ Colorado

Elliott, C Gregory MD [Pul] - **Spec Exp:** Pulmonary Hypertension; Thromboembolic Disorders; **Hospital:** Intermountain Med Ctr, LDS Hosp; **Address:** Intermountain Med Ctr, Dept Medicine, 5121 S Cottonwood St, Ste 307, Murray, UT 84157; **Phone:** 801-507-3373; **Board Cert:** Internal Medicine 1976; Pulmonary Disease 1978; **Med School:** Univ MD Sch Med 1973; **Resid:** Internal Medicine, Univ Maryland Hosp 1976; **Fellow:** Pulmonary Disease, Univ Utah 1978; **Fac Appt:** Prof Med, Univ Utah

Iseman, Michael MD [Pul] - **Spec Exp:** Tuberculosis; Mycobacterial Infections; **Hospital:** Natl Jewish Med & Rsch Ctr; **Address:** Natl Jewish Med & Rsch Ctr, 1400 Jackson St, rm J223, Denver, CO 80206; **Phone:** 303-398-1667; **Board Cert:** Internal Medicine 1972; Pulmonary Disease 1976; **Med School:** Columbia P&S 1965; **Resid:** Internal Medicine, Bellevue Hosp 1967; Internal Medicine, Harlem Hosp 1970; **Fellow:** Pulmonary Disease, Harlem Hosp 1972; **Fac Appt:** Prof Med, Univ Colorado

Kaplan, James MD [Pul] - **Spec Exp:** Critical Care; Sleep Disorders/Apnea; **Hospital:** Overland Pk Regl Med Ctr, Providence Med Ctr; **Address:** 10550 Quivira, Ste 335, Overland Park, KS 66215-2304; **Phone:** 913-599-3800; **Board Cert:** Internal Medicine 1987; Pulmonary Disease 2000; Critical Care Medicine 2003; **Med School:** Univ MO-Kansas City 1984; **Resid:** Internal Medicine, Barnes Hosp 1987; **Fellow:** Pulmonary Disease, Barnes Hosp-Wash Univ 1987

Make, Barry J MD [Pul] - **Spec Exp:** Chronic Obstructive Lung Disease (COPD); Emphysema; Asthma; **Hospital:** Natl Jewish Med & Rsch Ctr, Rose Med Ctr; **Address:** Natl Jewish Health, 1400 Jackson St, rm K729, Denver, CO 80206-2762; **Phone:** 303-398-1720; **Board Cert:** Internal Medicine 1973; **Med School:** Jefferson Med Coll 1970; **Resid:** Internal Medicine, Univ Michigan Med Ctr 1973; **Fellow:** Pulmonary Disease, West Virginia Med Ctr 1974; Pulmonary Disease, Boston Univ Med Ctr 1976; **Fac Appt:** Prof Med, Univ Colorado

Martin, Richard J MD [Pul] - **Spec Exp:** Asthma; Vocal Cord Disorders; Chronic Obstructive Lung Disease (COPD); **Hospital:** Natl Jewish Med & Rsch Ctr, Univ Colorado Hosp; **Address:** 1400 Jackson St, Denver, CO 80206-2762; **Phone:** 303-398-1847; **Board Cert:** Internal Medicine 1976; Pulmonary Disease 1978; **Med School:** Univ Mich Med Sch 1971; **Resid:** Internal Medicine, Tulane Univ Affil Hosp 1976; **Fellow:** Pulmonary Disease, Univ Oklahoma 1978; **Fac Appt:** Prof Med, Univ Colorado

Rennard, Stephen I MD [Pul] - **Spec Exp:** Chronic Obstructive Lung Disease (COPD); Emphysema; **Hospital:** Nebraska Med Ctr; **Address:** 985910 Nebraska Med Ctr, Omaha, NE 68198-5910; **Phone:** 402-559-7313; **Board Cert:** Internal Medicine 1978; Pulmonary Disease 1982; **Med School:** Baylor Coll Med 1975; **Resid:** Internal Medicine, Barnes Hosp-Washington Univ 1977; **Fac Appt:** Prof Med, Univ Nebr Coll Med

Rose, Cecile MD [Pul] - **Spec Exp:** Occupational Lung Disease; Sarcoidosis; Pneumoconiosis; Asbestos-related Lung Disease; **Hospital:** Natl Jewish Med & Rsch Ctr, Univ Colorado Hosp; **Address:** 1400 Jackson St, rm G-211, Denver, CO 80206-2761; **Phone:** 303-398-1867; **Board Cert:** Internal Medicine 1983; Pulmonary Disease 1986; Occupational Medicine 1987; **Med School:** Univ IL Coll Med 1980; **Resid:** Internal Medicine, Med Coll Virginia Hosp 1983; **Fellow:** Pulmonary Disease, Med Coll Virginia Hosp 1985; **Fac Appt:** Assoc Prof Med, Univ Colorado

Schwarz, Marvin I MD [Pul] - **Spec Exp:** Interstitial Lung Disease; Pulmonary Vascular Disease; Lung Hemorrhage; **Hospital:** Univ Colorado Hosp, Natl Jewish Med & Rsch Ctr; **Address:** Div Pulmonary Science & Critical Care, 12700 E 19th Ave, C-272 Ave, Aurora, CO 80045; **Phone:** 303-724-4075; **Board Cert:** Internal Medicine 1970; Pulmonary Disease 1971; **Med School:** Tulane Univ 1964; **Resid:** Internal Medicine, Charity Hosp 1967; **Fellow:** Pulmonary Disease, Charity Hosp/Tulane Univ 1969; **Fac Appt:** Prof Med, Univ Colorado

Southwest

Arroliga, Alejandro C MD [Pul] - **Spec Exp:** Pulmonary Hypertension; Respiratory Distress Syndrome (ARDS); Critical Care; **Hospital:** Scott & White Mem Hosp; **Address:** 2401 S 31st St, Temple, TX 76508; **Phone:** 254-724-9887; **Board Cert:** Internal Medicine 2000; Pulmonary Disease 2000; Critical Care Medicine 2003; **Med School:** Mexico 1984; **Resid:** Internal Medicine, Coney Island Hosp 1990; **Fellow:** Pulmonary Critical Care Medicine, Yale-New Haven Hosp 1993; **Fac Appt:** Prof Med, Cleveland Cl Coll Med/Case West Res

Pulmonary Disease

Guidry, George Gary MD [Pul] - **Spec Exp:** Chronic Obstructive Lung Disease (COPD); Asthma; Pneumonia; Lung Cancer; **Hospital:** Lafayette Genl Med Ctr, Our Lady of Lourdes Reg Med Ctr - Lafayette; **Address:** 155 Hospital Drive, Ste 206, Lafayette, LA 70503-2852; **Phone:** 337-234-3204; **Board Cert:** Internal Medicine 1988; Pulmonary Disease 1999; **Med School:** Louisiana State U, New Orleans 1985; **Resid:** Internal Medicine, LSU Med Ctr 1988; **Fellow:** Pulmonary Disease, LSU Med Ctr 1991; **Fac Appt:** Assoc Clin Prof Med, Louisiana State U, New Orleans

Levin, David C MD [Pul] - **Spec Exp:** Asthma; Chronic Obstructive Lung Disease (COPD); **Hospital:** OU Med Ctr, VA Med Ctr - Oklahoma City; **Address:** OU Physicians Building, 825 NE 10th St, Ste 2500, Oklahoma City, OK 73104; **Phone:** 405-271-7001; **Board Cert:** Internal Medicine 1973; Pulmonary Disease 1976; **Med School:** Case West Res Univ 1970; **Resid:** Internal Medicine, Univ Colorado Affil Hosp 1974; **Fellow:** Pulmonary Disease, Univ Colorado 1975; **Fac Appt:** Prof Med, Univ Okla Coll Med

Perret, Philip S MD [Pul] - **Spec Exp:** Chronic Obstructive Lung Disease (COPD); **Hospital:** Our Lady of Lourdes Reg Med Ctr - Lafayette; **Address:** 614 W St Mary Blvd, Lafayette, LA 70506; **Phone:** 337-232-6435; **Board Cert:** Internal Medicine 1978; Pulmonary Disease 1980; **Med School:** Emory Univ 1974; **Resid:** Internal Medicine, Emory Univ Hosp 1977; **Fellow:** Pulmonary Disease, Emory Univ Hosp 1979

Shannon, John J MD [Pul] - **Spec Exp:** Asthma; Chronic Lung Disease; **Hospital:** Parkland Hlth & Hosp Sys; **Address:** Parkland Hlth & Hosp Ctr, 5201 Harry Hines Blvd, Dallas, TX 75235; **Phone:** 214-590-8000; **Board Cert:** Internal Medicine 1989; Pulmonary Disease 2004; Critical Care Medicine 2005; **Med School:** Rush Med Coll 1986; **Resid:** Internal Medicine, Parkland Meml Hosp-UTSW 1989; **Fellow:** Pulmonary Critical Care Medicine, Univ Mich Hosp 1995; **Fac Appt:** Asst Prof Med, Rush Med Coll

Shellito, Judd E MD [Pul] - **Spec Exp:** Pulmonary Infections; Occupational Lung Disease; **Hospital:** L Boggs Med Ctr; **Address:** 2820 Napoleon Ave, Ste 890, New Orleans, LA 70115; **Phone:** 504-895-5748; **Board Cert:** Internal Medicine 1977; Pulmonary Disease 1980; **Med School:** Tulane Univ 1974; **Resid:** Internal Medicine, Evanston Hosp 1978; **Fellow:** Pulmonary Critical Care Medicine, Univ New Mexico Hosp 1980; **Fac Appt:** Prof Med, Louisiana State U, New Orleans

Summer, Warren MD [Pul] - **Spec Exp:** Chronic Obstructive Lung Disease (COPD); Asthma; Respiratory Distress Syndrome (ARDS); **Hospital:** L Boggs Med Ctr; **Address:** 2820 Napoleon Ave, Ste 890, New Orleans, LA 70115; **Phone:** 504-895-5748; **Board Cert:** Internal Medicine 1972; Pulmonary Disease 1972; **Med School:** Georgetown Univ 1965; **Resid:** Internal Medicine, Maimonides Med Ctr 1968; **Fellow:** Pulmonary Disease, Georgetown Univ Hosp 1969; **Fac Appt:** Prof Med, Louisiana State U, New Orleans

Weissler, Jonathan C MD [Pul] - **Spec Exp:** Interstitial Lung Disease; Asthma; **Hospital:** UT Southwestern Med Ctr at Dallas, Parkland Hlth & Hosp Sys; **Address:** 5323 Harry Hines Blvd, Dallas, TX 75390-9034; **Phone:** 214-645-1825; **Board Cert:** Internal Medicine 1982; Pulmonary Disease 1984; Critical Care Medicine 2007; **Med School:** NYU Sch Med 1979; **Resid:** Internal Medicine, Univ Texas Hlth Sci Ctr 1982; **Fellow:** Pulmonary Disease, Univ Texas Hlth Sci Ctr 1985; **Fac Appt:** Prof Med, Univ Tex SW, Dallas

West Coast and Pacific

Albertson, Timothy MD/PhD [Pul] - **Spec Exp:** Critical Care; Transplant Medicine-Lung; **Hospital:** UC Davis Med Ctr; **Address:** UC Davis, Div Pulm Crit Care, 4150 V St, Ste 3400, Patient Support Svcs Bldg, Sacramento, CA 95817-9002; **Phone:** 916-734-3564; **Board Cert:** Pulmonary Disease 1984; Critical Care Medicine 2007; Emergency Medicine 2007; Medical Toxicology 2005; **Med School:** UC Davis 1977; **Resid:** Internal Medicine, Univ Arizona 1980; Internal Medicine, UC Davis Med Ctr 1981; **Fellow:** Pulmonary Critical Care Medicine, UC Davis Med Ctr 1983; **Fac Appt:** Prof Med, UC Davis

Auger, William R MD [Pul] - **Spec Exp:** Thromboembolic Disorders; Pulmonary Hypertension; **Hospital:** UCSD Med Ctr; **Address:** Thorton Hosp, UCSD, 9300 Campus Pt Dr, La Jolla, CA 92037; **Phone:** 858-657-7140; **Board Cert:** Internal Medicine 1986; Pulmonary Disease 1988; **Med School:** Univ Rochester 1982; **Resid:** Internal Medicine, Strong Meml Hosp 1985; **Fellow:** Critical Care Medicine, Ellis Hosp 1986; Pulmonary Disease, UCSD Med Ctr 1989; **Fac Appt:** Clin Prof Med, UCSD

Balmes, John Randolph MD [Pul] - **Spec Exp:** Beryllium-induced Lung Disease; **Hospital:** San Francisco Genl Hosp, UCSF Med Ctr; **Address:** UCSF, Div Occup & Envr Med, Campus Box 0843, San Francisco, CA 94143-0843; **Phone:** 415-206-8314; **Board Cert:** Internal Medicine 1979; Pulmonary Disease 1984; **Med School:** Mount Sinai Sch Med 1976; **Resid:** Internal Medicine, Mount Sinai Hosp 1979; **Fellow:** Pulmonary Disease, Yale-New Haven Hosp 1981; **Fac Appt:** Prof Med, UCSF

Bellamy, Paul E MD [Pul] - **Spec Exp:** Critical Care; **Hospital:** Kaiser Permanente Woodland Hills Med Ctr; **Address:** Kaiser Woodland Hills Med Ctr, Pulm Div, 5601 De Soto Ave, Med Office Twr, Fl 4, Woodland Hills, CA 91367; **Phone:** 818-719-3530; **Board Cert:** Internal Medicine 1978; Pulmonary Disease 1980; Critical Care Medicine 2007; **Med School:** SUNY Buffalo 1975; **Resid:** Internal Medicine, Univ Hosps-Case West Res 1978; **Fellow:** Pulmonary Disease, UCLA Med Ctr 1980; **Fac Appt:** Clin Prof Med, UCLA

Boushey Jr, Homer A MD [Pul] - **Spec Exp:** Asthma; **Hospital:** UCSF Med Ctr; **Address:** UCSF Med Ctr, Dept Med, 400 Parnassus Ave, Box 0359, San Francisco, CA 94143; **Phone:** 415-353-2961; **Board Cert:** Internal Medicine 1972; Pulmonary Disease 1974; **Med School:** UCSF 1968; **Resid:** Internal Medicine, UCSF Med Ctr 1970; Internal Medicine, Beth Israel Hosp 1971; **Fellow:** Pulmonary Disease, Oxford Univ 1972; Pulmonary Disease, UCSF Hosp 1973; **Fac Appt:** Prof Med, UCSF

Catanzaro, Antonino MD [Pul] - **Spec Exp:** Tuberculosis; Coccidioidomycosis; Mycobacterial Infections; **Hospital:** UCSD Med Ctr; **Address:** 200 W Arbor Drive, MC 8374, San Diego, CA 92103; **Phone:** 619-543-5550; **Board Cert:** Internal Medicine 1972; Pulmonary Disease 1976; **Med School:** SUNY Buffalo 1965; **Resid:** Internal Medicine, Georgetown Univ Hosp 1970; **Fellow:** Pulmonary Critical Care Medicine, UCSD Med Ctr 1972; Research, Scripps Clin Rsch Fdn 1972; **Fac Appt:** Prof Med, UCSD

Heffner, John E MD [Pul] - **Spec Exp:** Critical Care; Respiratory Failure; **Hospital:** Providence Portland Med Ctr; **Address:** 5050 NE Hoyt St, Ste 540, Portland, OR 97220; **Phone:** 503-215-6258; **Board Cert:** Internal Medicine 1977; Pulmonary Disease 1982; Critical Care Medicine 2005; **Med School:** UCLA 1974; **Resid:** Internal Medicine, Univ Colo Med Ctr 1978; **Fac Appt:** Prof Med, Med Univ SC

Pulmonary Disease

Hopewell, Philip C MD [Pul] - **Spec Exp:** AIDS/HIV; Tuberculosis; Infectious Disease-Lung; **Hospital:** San Francisco Genl Hosp; **Address:** UCSF, Div Occup & Envr Med, Campus Box 0841, San Francisco, CA 94110; **Phone:** 415-206-8314; **Board Cert:** Internal Medicine 1973; Pulmonary Disease 1974; **Med School:** W VA Univ 1965; **Resid:** Internal Medicine, UCSF Med Ctr 1971; **Fellow:** Pulmonary Disease, UCSF Med Ctr 1973; **Fac Appt:** Prof Med, UCSF

Huang, Laurence MD [Pul] - **Spec Exp:** AIDS/HIV; Pneumocystis Carinii Pneumonia (PCP); **Hospital:** San Francisco Genl Hosp; **Address:** UCSF Positive Health Program-SFGH, 995 Potrero Ave, Bldg 80-Ward 84, San Francisco, CA 94110; **Phone:** 415-206-2400; **Board Cert:** Internal Medicine 2003; Pulmonary Disease 2006; Critical Care Medicine 2007; **Med School:** Columbia P&S 1989; **Resid:** Internal Medicine, Columbia-Presby Hosp 1992; Pulmonary Critical Care Medicine, UCSF Med Ctr 1995; **Fac Appt:** Assoc Clin Prof Med, UCSF

Hudson, Leonard MD [Pul] - **Spec Exp:** Critical Care; Lung Injury-Acute; Respiratory Failure; **Hospital:** Harborview Med Ctr; **Address:** Harborview Medical Ctr, 325 9th Ave, Box 359762, Seattle, WA 98104; **Phone:** 206-744-3123; **Board Cert:** Internal Medicine 1973; Pulmonary Disease 1974; **Med School:** Univ Wash 1964; **Resid:** Internal Medicine, NY Hosp 1966; Internal Medicine, Univ Wash Hosps 1969; **Fellow:** Pulmonary Disease, Univ Colo Med Ctr 1971; **Fac Appt:** Prof Med, Univ Wash

Jacoby, David MD [Pul] - **Hospital:** OR Hlth & Sci Univ; **Address:** 3181 SW Sam Jackson Park Rd, MC UHN67, Dept Pulmonary/Crit Care, Portland, OR 97239; **Phone:** 503-494-6158; **Board Cert:** Internal Medicine 1983; Pulmonary Disease 1986; **Med School:** NY Med Coll 1980; **Resid:** Internal Medicine, Temple Univ Hosp 1983; **Fellow:** Pulmonary Critical Care Medicine, UCSF Hosp 1987; **Fac Appt:** Prof Med, Oregon Hlth & Sci Univ

King Jr, Talmadge E MD [Pul] - **Spec Exp:** Interstitial Lung Disease; Sarcoidosis; Asthma; **Hospital:** UCSF Med Ctr; **Address:** 505 Parnassus Ave, Ste 5H22, San Francisco, CA 94143-0120; **Phone:** 415-476-0909; **Board Cert:** Internal Medicine 1977; Pulmonary Disease 1982; **Med School:** Harvard Med Sch 1974; **Resid:** Internal Medicine, Grady-Emory Univ Affil Hosp 1977; **Fellow:** Pulmonary Critical Care Medicine, Univ Colo Hlth Sci Ctr 1979; **Fac Appt:** Prof Med, UCSF

Lynch, Joseph P MD [Pul] - **Spec Exp:** Transplant Medicine-Lung; Interstitial Lung Disease; Pulmonary Fibrosis; **Hospital:** UCLA Ronald Reagan Med Ctr; **Address:** UCLA - Div Pulmonary Med, 10833 Le Conte Ave, CHS Bldg - rm 37-131, Los Angeles, CA 90095-1690; **Phone:** 310-825-8599; **Board Cert:** Internal Medicine 1976; Pulmonary Disease 1980; **Med School:** Harvard Med Sch 1973; **Resid:** Internal Medicine, Univ Mich Med Ctr 1976; **Fellow:** Pulmonary Disease, Univ Mich Med Ctr 1978; **Fac Appt:** Prof Med, UCLA

Martin, Thomas R MD [Pul] - **Spec Exp:** Respiratory Distress Syndrome (ARDS); Critical Care; **Hospital:** VA Puget Sound Hlth Care Sys; **Address:** Seattle VA Hosp - Pulmonary Rsch 151L, 1660 S Columbian Way, Seattle, WA 98108; **Phone:** 206-764-2507; **Board Cert:** Internal Medicine 1976; Pulmonary Disease 1980; **Med School:** Univ Pennsylvania 1973; **Resid:** Internal Medicine, Univ Washington Med Ctr 1977; **Fellow:** Pulmonary Disease, Univ Washington 1980; **Fac Appt:** Prof Med, Univ Wash

Mosenifar, Zab MD [Pul] - **Spec Exp:** Chronic Obstructive Lung Disease (COPD); Interstitial Lung Disease; Asthma; Pulmonary Hypertension; **Hospital:** Cedars-Sinai Med Ctr; **Address:** Cedars-Sinai Med Ctr, Div Pulmonary Med, 8700 Beverly Blvd, rm 6732 South Twr, Los Angeles, CA 90048-1804; **Phone:** 310-423-4685; **Board Cert:** Internal Medicine 1978; Pulmonary Disease 1980; **Med School:** Iran 1973; **Resid:** Internal Medicine, Thomas Jefferson Univ Hosp; Internal Medicine, UCLA Med Ctr; **Fellow:** Pulmonary Disease, UCLA Med Ctr; **Fac Appt:** Prof Med, UCLA

Patterson, James R MD [Pul] - **Spec Exp:** Sleep Disorders/Apnea; **Hospital:** Providence Portland Med Ctr; **Address:** 1111 NE 99th Ave, Ste 200, Portland, OR 97220; **Phone:** 503-963-3030; **Board Cert:** Internal Medicine 1972; Pulmonary Disease 2001; **Med School:** Columbia P&S 1968; **Resid:** Internal Medicine, Columbia-Presby Med Ctr 1970; **Fellow:** Pulmonary Disease, Fitzsimons Army Med Ctr 1973; **Fac Appt:** Clin Prof Med, Oregon Hlth & Sci Univ

Raghu, Ganesh MD [Pul] - **Spec Exp:** Interstitial Lung Disease; Pulmonary Fibrosis; Sarcoidosis; Transplant-Lung; **Hospital:** Univ Wash Med Ctr; **Address:** 1959 NE Pacific St, Box 356166, Seattle, WA 98195; **Phone:** 206-598-4615; **Board Cert:** Internal Medicine 1982; **Med School:** India 1974; **Resid:** Internal Medicine, Univ Rochester-Strong Meml Hosp 1978; Internal Medicine, SUNY Buffalo Med Ctr 1981; **Fellow:** Pulmonary Critical Care Medicine, Univ Washington 1984; **Fac Appt:** Prof Med, Univ Wash

Rizk, Norman W MD [Pul] - **Spec Exp:** Critical Care; Asthma; **Hospital:** Stanford Univ Med Ctr; **Address:** 300 Pasteur Drive, Ste H3142, Stanford, CA 94305-5236; **Phone:** 650-725-7061; **Board Cert:** Internal Medicine 1979; Pulmonary Disease 1984; Critical Care Medicine 1996; **Med School:** Yale Univ 1976; **Resid:** Internal Medicine, San Fran Genl Hosp 1980; **Fellow:** Pulmonary Disease, Moffitt Hosp-UCSF 1983; **Fac Appt:** Prof Med, Stanford Univ

Rubin, Lewis J MD [Pul] - **Spec Exp:** Pulmonary Hypertension; Pulmonary Vascular Disease; **Hospital:** UCSD Med Ctr; **Address:** UCSD Med Ctr, Pulmonary & Critical Care, 9300 Campus Point Drive, MC 7381, La Jolla, CA 92037-7381; **Phone:** 858-657-8700; **Board Cert:** Internal Medicine 1978; Pulmonary Disease 1980; **Med School:** Albert Einstein Coll Med 1975; **Resid:** Internal Medicine, Duke Univ Med Ctr 1978; **Fellow:** Pulmonary Disease, Duke Univ Med Ctr 1979; **Fac Appt:** Prof Med, UCSD

Sharma, Om Prakash MD [Pul] - **Spec Exp:** Sarcoidosis; Interstitial Lung Disease; Hypersensitivity Pneumonitis; **Hospital:** LAC & USC Med Ctr, USC Univ Hosp; **Address:** 1200 N State St GNH Bldg - rm 11900, Los Angeles, CA 90033; **Phone:** 323-226-7923; **Board Cert:** Internal Medicine 1987; **Med School:** India 1959; **Resid:** Internal Medicine, Norwalk Hosp 1963; Internal Medicine, Montefiore Med Ctr 1965; **Fellow:** Pulmonary Disease, Montefiore Med Ctr 1966; Research, Royal Coll Physicians 1969; **Fac Appt:** Prof Med, USC Sch Med

Tharratt, Robert S MD [Pul] - **Spec Exp:** Disaster Preparedness; Critical Care; Toxicology; **Hospital:** UC Davis Med Ctr; **Address:** UC Davis Med Ctr, Div Pulm Crit Care, 4150 V St, Ste 3400-Pt Support Services Bldg, Sacramento, CA 95817-2214; **Phone:** 916-734-3564; **Board Cert:** Pulmonary Disease 1988; Critical Care Medicine 1999; Medical Toxicology 2004; Emergency Medicine 2007; **Med School:** UCLA 1983; **Resid:** Internal Medicine, UC Davis Med Ctr 1986; **Fellow:** Pulmonary Critical Care Medicine, UC Davis Med Ctr 1989; **Fac Appt:** Prof Med, UC Davis

Wallace, Jeanne M MD [Pul] - **Spec Exp:** Pulmonary Infections; Sleep Disorders/Apnea; Asthma; **Hospital:** Olive View Med Ctr; **Address:** Olive View UCLA Med Ctr, 14445 Olive View Dr, Sylmar, CA 91342-1437; **Phone:** 818-364-3205; **Board Cert:** Internal Medicine 1977; Pulmonary Disease 1980; Sleep Medicine 2007; **Med School:** UCLA 1974; **Resid:** Internal Medicine, UCSF Med Ctr 1977; **Fellow:** Pulmonary Disease, UCSD Med Ctr 1980; **Fac Appt:** Assoc Prof Med, UCLA

Cleveland Clinic

Pulmonary, Allergy and Critical Care Medicine

Individuals with all types of acute or chronic lung diseases, as well as sleep disordered breathing (sleep apnea) can access specialty care at Cleveland Clinic. In 2008, physicians in the Department of Pulmonary, Allergy and Critical Care Medicine provided over 78,000 outpatient visits and cared for more than 1,500 hospital admissions.

Lung Transplantation

Cleveland Clinic's Lung Transplant Program is the largest in Ohio and among the largest in the United States. In 2009 our program is on track to have a record setting year with over 100 transplants. The average wait time for a lung transplantation at Cleveland Clinic is significantly lower than the national average.

Sarcoidosis Center of Excellence

In January 2003, Cleveland Clinic was awarded a $2 million grant from the Department of Health and Human Services to establish a Sarcoidosis Center of Excellence. The only such center in Northeastern Ohio, the center aims to raise awareness of pulmonary sarcoidosis, improve the quality of sarcoidosis care and minimize the degree to which it can affect quality of life.

Areas of Expertise

Acute respiratory distress syndrome (ARDS), Allergy rhinitis, Allergies (drug and food; latex), Aspirin desensitization, Asthma, Beryllium-induced lung disease, Chronic obstructive pulmonary disease (COPD), Including alpha-1 antitrypsin deficiency, Interstitial lung disease, Interventional bronchology, Lung cancer, Lymphangioleiomyomatosis (LAM), Pulmonary alveolar proteinosis (PAP), Pulmonary vascular disease, Sarcoidosis, Sepsis, Sleep-disordered breathing, Urticaria, Weaning from mechanical ventilation

For more information about the Cleveland Clinic Department of Pulmonary, Allergy and Critical Care Medicine, to schedule a second opinion or to learn about assistance for out-of-town patients, call 800.890.2467 or visit www. clevelandclinic.org/pulmonarytopdocs.

Department of Pulmonology, Allergy and Critical Care Medicine
9500 Euclid Avenue / AC311 | Cleveland OH 44195

**MOUNT SINAI
SCHOOL OF
MEDICINE**

THE MOUNT SINAI MEDICAL CENTER
PULMONARY MEDICINE
One Gustave L. Levy Place
Fifth Avenue and 100th Street
New York, NY 10029-6574
Physician Referral: 1-800-MD-SINAI (637-4624)
www.mountsinai.org

The mission of Mount Sinai's **DIVISION OF PULMONARY, CRITICAL CARE, AND SLEEP MEDICINE** is to offer state-of-the-art clinical care to patients with all forms of lung disease and critical illness, cutting-edge research that will translate into improved patient care and outcomes, and hands-on training of future leaders in the field.

To achieve this goal, every faculty member is charged with the success of a specific program. Mount Sinai's Sarcoidosis Service, the largest of its kind in the world, is a Center of Excellence for sarcoidosis research. It is the only site in the United States that performs the diagnostic Kveim-Siltzbach skin test for sarcoidosis, which eliminates the need for more invasive, uncomfortable, and expensive procedures.

Through its Pulmonary Physiology Laboratory, Mount Sinai has been instrumental in establishing normal values for various pulmonary function tests and is currently conducting clinical studies of new tests for obesity, sarcoidosis, asthma, and lung cancer. Pulmonary specialists at Mount Sinai are investigating asthma and emphysema, lung cancer, collagen vascular diseases, pulmonary infections, and occupational lung diseases. Mount Sinai has the largest screening program for workers and anyone in the general population exposed to polluted air at the World Trade Center catastrophe site. Our critical care physicians are experts in treating liver disease and acute and chronic respiratory failure, using the most modern forms of delivery of intensive care and providing compassionate end-of-life care.

Our programs and services include:

- **The Asthma Program** uses a multidisciplinary team approach, focusing on patient education and skill-building to foster self-management;

- **The Chronic Obstructive Pulmonary Disease Program** offers a coordinated approach of exercise, treatment, and education that improves quality of life and clinical outlook, for one of the nation's most underdiagnosed conditions;

- **The Critical Care Medicine Program** features state-of-the-art medical intensive care and respiratory care units;

- **The Interventional Pulmonary Service** performs cutting-edge diagnostic and therapeutic procedures for patients with advanced pulmonary diseases;

- **The Lung Transplant Program,** which treats patients with advanced lung disease, has progressed despite optimal medical therapy;

- **The Occupational Lung Disorders Program** specializes in the diagnosis and management of occupational lung disorders, such as occupational asthma and bronchitis, asbestosis, silicosis, and heavy metal lung injury;

- **The Pulmonary Fibrosis/Interstitial Lung Disease Program** treats patients with chronic inflammatory and scarring disorders of the lungs, including collagen vascular-associated pulmonary diseases;

- **The Pulmonary Physiology Laboratory**, which has recently doubled in capacity, performs the full range of physiological testing for lung disease;

- **The Pulmonary Rehabilitation Program** provides occupational, physical, and cardiopulmonary rehabilitation programs for patients with disabling lung disorders, as well as pre- and post-operative consultation and therapy;

- **The Thoracic Oncology Service** provides multidisciplinary medical care for lung cancer, as a joint effort with the Department of Cardiothoracic Surgery; and,

- **The Sarcoidosis Service,** which has passed its 20,000 enrollee count, offers standard care as well as the opportunity to participate in new clinical trials to 60 new enrollees per week.

**MOUNT SINAI
SCHOOL OF
MEDICINE**

**THE MOUNT SINAI MEDICAL CENTER
SLEEP MEDICINE**
One Gustave L. Levy Place
Fifth Avenue and 100th Street
New York, NY 10029-6574
Physician Referral: 1-800-MD-SINAI (637-4624)
www.mountsinai.org

Mount Sinai's **CENTER FOR SLEEP MEDICINE** is a comprehensive, full-service program that has recently expanded and that specializes in the compassionate and personalized care of individuals with sleep disorders.

We use state-of-the-art equipment to diagnose and treat all aspects of sleep pathology, including breathing-related disorders, insomnia, restless leg syndrome, periodic limb movements, and narcolepsy. An initial consultation includes a clinical history and physical examination. In some cases, the diagnosis and treatment plan can be completed in a single visit. In other cases, the evaluation requires a sleep study—typically over one or two nights—or other tests. Overnight tests are completed by 7 am, so it is usually not necessary to miss a day of work. In rare instances, daytime studies are also recommended.

Services available at the Comprehensive Center for Sleep Medicine include:

- Consultations with board-certified sleep specialists.

- Overnight sleep testing and daytime testing provided by experienced physicians and technicians. During a sleep study, the patient is monitored by painless, noninvasive technology called polysomnography that records breathing, heart rate, brain waves, oxygen levels, and eye and leg movement.

- Treatment for a sleep disorder that may include a device to aid the patient's breathing while sleeping called Continuous Positive Airway Pressure or Bilevel Positive Airway Pressure, medication, or light therapy, as well as neuropsychiatric interventions. If indicated, consultations with other specialists are available to aid in diagnosis and therapy.

- Mechanical, behavioral, surgical, dental, and pharmacological therapies. Consultations can also be arranged with pulmonologists; ear, nose, and throat surgeons; bariatric surgeons; dentists; and psychiatrists.

MOUNT SINAI SPECIALIZES IN TREATING OBSTRUCTIVE SLEEP APNEA
Approximately 20 million Americans suffer from obstructive sleep apnea, which occurs when muscles of the back of the mouth and the throat relax during sleep, causing a complete (apnea) or partial (hypopnea) blockage of the airway. Apneic episodes lead to frequent awakenings and lowering of the oxygen level, causing the heart to work harder. When untreated, this disorder can lead to hypertension, heart failure, and stroke, as well as bouts of daytime sleepiness that increase the risk of motor vehicle and industrial accidents. Sleepiness is often misperceived as a natural consequence of aging. If you are overweight and snore, you may have sleep apnea or another sleep disorder.

NYU Langone Medical Center

550 First Avenue (at 31St Street)
New York, NY 10016
Physician Referral:
(888)7-NYU-MED (888-769-8633)
www.med.nyu.edu

PULMONOLOGY

About the Division of Pulmonary and Critical Care Medicine:

The NYU Langone Medical Center Pulmonary and Critical Care Medicine Division has a full continuum of services available for diagnosis, treatment and the research of both the inpatient and ambulatory patient. The Division grew out of the renowned Chest Service at Bellevue Hospital Center, an affiliate of NYU Langone Medical Center, which for more than a century has been a world leader in the delivery of state-of-the-art pulmonary care. Available services include a state-of-the-art Pulmonary Function Laboratory, a specialized inpatient pulmonary unit with a dedicated respiratory care unit, a specialized medical critical care unit staffed with dedicated pulmonary/critical care physicians and a multidisciplinary interventional bronchoscopy program integrated with thoracic radiology. Since 1990, research support for the Division has grown from zero to a dozen National Institute of Health and Centers for Disease Control and Prevention grant programs.

We specialize in the following areas:

ASTHMA
The Bellevue Asthma Clinic at Bellevue Hospital Center, an affiliate of NYU Langone Medical Center, offers an active research program dealing exclusively with particulate matter pollution and asthma. In addition, there is an ongoing gene banking program to study disease modifying genes in asthma and community-based studies of the health effects of the World Trade Center destruction.

CHEST SERVICES
The Division of Pulmonary and Critical Care Medicine at NYU Langone Medical Center provides clinical chest services at its affiliate hospital, Bellevue Hospital Center, which cares for patients with tuberculosis, lung cancer, asthma, and interstitial fibrosis. The inpatient service has also expanded to meet the needs of a growing population of patients with tuberculosis and AIDS. Current research is on bacterial pneumonia in HIV-1+ individuals.

INTERVENTIONAL BRONCHOSCOPY
The Interventional Bronchoscopy Program offered at Tisch Hospital at NYU Langone Medical Center employs leading-edge techniques to diagnose and treat tumors and inflammatory conditions of the lung.

NYU LUNG CANCER BIOMARKER CENTER
High-risk smokers can participate in a CT-scan lung cancer screening research program identifying molecular and protein biomarkers in blood and sputum.

SLEEP DISORDERS
The Sleep Disorders Center at NYU Langone Medical Center offers clinical and research services for physicians and patients in the diagnosis and treatment of severe or prolonged difficulties regarding sleep. The Center is also equipped for limited home or in-hospital monitoring for patient screening and follow up.

Radiation Oncology

a subspecialty of Radiology

A radiation oncologist deals with the therapeutic applications of radiant energy and its modifiers and the study and management of disease, especially malignant tumors.

Training Required: Four years in radiology *plus* additional training and examination.

RADIATION ONCOLOGY

New England

Choi, Noah C MD [RadRO] - **Spec Exp:** Lung Cancer; Esophageal Cancer; Mesothelioma; **Hospital:** Mass Genl Hosp; **Address:** Mass Genl Hosp, Dept Rad Oncology, 100 Blossom St, Cox 307, Boston, MA 02114; **Phone:** 617-726-6050; **Board Cert:** Therapeutic Radiology 1970; **Med School:** South Korea 1963; **Resid:** Radiation Oncology, Princess Margaret Hosp 1970; **Fac Appt:** Prof RadRO, Harvard Med Sch

D'Amico, Anthony V MD/PhD [RadRO] - **Spec Exp:** Prostate Cancer; Brachytherapy; **Hospital:** Dana-Farber Cancer Inst, Brigham & Women's Hosp; **Address:** Brigham & Women's Hosp, Dept Rad Onc, 75 Francis St, Ste L2, Boston, MA 02115; **Phone:** 617-732-7936; **Board Cert:** Radiation Oncology 1999; **Med School:** Univ Pennsylvania 1990; **Resid:** Radiation Oncology, Hosp Univ Penn 1994; **Fac Appt:** Prof RadRO, Harvard Med Sch

DeLaney, Thomas Francis MD [RadRO] - **Spec Exp:** Sarcoma; Proton Beam Therapy; **Hospital:** Mass Genl Hosp; **Address:** Francis H. Burr Proton Therapy Ctr, 30 Fruit St, Bosont, MA 02114; **Phone:** 617-726-6876; **Board Cert:** Therapeutic Radiology 1986; Radiation Oncology 1999; **Med School:** Harvard Med Sch 1982; **Resid:** Therapeutic Radiology, Mass Genl Hosp 1986; **Fac Appt:** Assoc Prof RadRO, Harvard Med Sch

Harris, Jay R MD [RadRO] - **Spec Exp:** Breast Cancer; **Hospital:** Brigham & Women's Hosp, Dana-Farber Cancer Inst; **Address:** Dana Farber Cancer Inst, 44 Binney St, rm D1622, Boston, MA 02115; **Phone:** 617-632-2291; **Board Cert:** Therapeutic Radiology 1999; **Med School:** Stanford Univ 1970; **Resid:** Radiation Oncology, Joint Ctr Rad Ther 1976; **Fellow:** Radiation Therapy, Harvard Med Sch 1977; **Fac Appt:** Prof RadRO, Harvard Med Sch

Kaplan, Irving D MD [RadRO] - **Spec Exp:** Prostate Cancer; Brachytherapy; **Hospital:** Beth Israel Deaconess Med Ctr - Boston; **Address:** Beth Israel Deaconess Med Ctr, Dept Radiation Oncology, 330 Brookline Ave, Boston, MA 02215; **Phone:** 617-667-2345; **Board Cert:** Radiation Oncology 1989; **Med School:** Stanford Univ 1985; **Resid:** Radiation Oncology, Stanford Univ Med Ctr 1989; **Fac Appt:** Asst Prof RadRO, Harvard Med Sch

Knisely, Jonathan MD [RadRO] - **Spec Exp:** Brain Tumors; Stereotactic Radiosurgery; Gastrointestinal Cancer; **Hospital:** Yale-New Haven Hosp; **Address:** Dept Therapeutic Radiology, 15 York St, Hunter Bldg-HRT 133, New Haven, CT 06520-8040; **Phone:** 203-785-2960; **Board Cert:** Internal Medicine 1989; Radiation Oncology 1993; **Med School:** Univ Pennsylvania 1986; **Resid:** Internal Medicine, Michael Reese Hosp 1989; Radiation Oncology, Univ Toronto Med Ctr 1992; **Fac Appt:** Assoc Prof RadRO, Yale Univ

Loeffler, Jay S MD [RadRO] - **Spec Exp:** Stereotactic Radiosurgery; Brain Tumors-Benign; Meningioma; Acoustic Neuroma; **Hospital:** Mass Genl Hosp; **Address:** Mass General Hosp, Radiation Oncology, 100 Blossom St, Boston, MA 02114; **Phone:** 617-724-1548; **Board Cert:** Therapeutic Radiology 1986; **Med School:** Brown Univ 1982; **Resid:** Radiation Oncology, Harvard Joint Ctr for Rad Ther 1986; **Fellow:** Cancer Biology, Harvard Sch Pub Hlth 1985; **Fac Appt:** Prof RadRO, Harvard Med Sch

Mauch, Peter M MD [RadRO] - **Spec Exp:** Lymphoma; Hodgkin's Disease; **Hospital:** Dana-Farber Cancer Inst; **Address:** Dana Farber Cancer Inst, 75 Francis St, Ste RadOnc L2, Boston, MA 02115; **Phone:** 617-632-4116; **Board Cert:** Therapeutic Radiology 1978; **Med School:** St Louis Univ 1974; **Resid:** Radiation Therapy, Harvard Joint Ctr 1978; **Fac Appt:** Prof, Harvard Med Sch

Peschel, Richard E MD [RadRO] - **Spec Exp:** Prostate Cancer; **Hospital:** Yale-New Haven Hosp, Bridgeport Hosp; **Address:** Yale-New Haven Hosp, Dept Therapeutic Radiology, 15 York St, rm HRT 142, New Haven, CT 06510; **Phone:** 203-785-2958; **Board Cert:** Therapeutic Radiology 1982; **Med School:** Yale Univ 1977; **Resid:** Radiation Oncology, Yale-New Haven Hosp 1981; **Fac Appt:** Prof RadRO, Yale Univ

Recht, Abram MD [RadRO] - **Spec Exp:** Breast Cancer; Gastrointestinal Cancer; Gynecologic Cancer; **Hospital:** Beth Israel Deaconess Med Ctr - Boston; **Address:** Beth Israel Deaconess Med Ctr, 330 Brookline Ave, Boston, MA 02215; **Phone:** 617-667-2345; **Board Cert:** Therapeutic Radiology 1984; **Med School:** Johns Hopkins Univ 1980; **Resid:** Radiation Oncology, Joint Ctr Radiation Therapy 1984; **Fac Appt:** Assoc Prof RadRO, Harvard Med Sch

Roberts, Kenneth MD [RadRO] - **Spec Exp:** Pediatric Cancers; Lymphoma; Hodgkin's Disease; **Hospital:** Yale-New Haven Hosp, Backus Hosp, Norwich; **Address:** Yale Univ School of Medicine, Dept Radiation Therapy, 15 York St, New Haven, CT 06520-8040; **Phone:** 203-785-2957; **Board Cert:** Internal Medicine 1987; Medical Oncology 1989; Radiation Oncology 1995; **Med School:** Duke Univ 1984; **Resid:** Internal Medicine, Ohio State Univ Hosps 1987; Radiation Oncology, Duke Univ Med Ctr 1992; **Fellow:** Hematology & Oncology, Duke Univ Med Ctr 1989; **Fac Appt:** Assoc Prof Rad, Yale Univ

Shipley, William U MD [RadRO] - **Spec Exp:** Bladder Cancer; Prostate Cancer; **Hospital:** Mass Genl Hosp; **Address:** Mass Genl Hosp, Dept Rad Oncology, 100 Blossom St, Cox Bldg, rm 347, Boston, MA 02114; **Phone:** 617-726-8146; **Board Cert:** Therapeutic Radiology 1975; **Med School:** Harvard Med Sch 1966; **Resid:** Surgery, Mass Genl Hosp 1971; Radiation Therapy, Harvard Joint Ctr Rad Therapy 1973; **Fellow:** Radiation Therapy, Royal Marsden Hosp 1974; **Fac Appt:** Prof RadRO, Harvard Med Sch

Taghian, Alphonse G MD/PhD [RadRO] - **Spec Exp:** Breast Cancer; **Hospital:** Mass Genl Hosp; **Address:** MGH Dept Radiation Oncology, 100 Blossom St, COX 3, Boston, MA 02114; **Phone:** 617-726-6050; **Board Cert:** Radiation Oncology 2006; **Med School:** Egypt 1980; **Resid:** Radiation Oncology, Vautrin Cancer Ctr 1987; Radiation Oncology, Inst Gustave Roussy 1989; **Fellow:** Radiation Oncology, Mass Genl Hosp 1993; **Fac Appt:** Assoc Prof RadRO, Harvard Med Sch

Tarbell, Nancy MD [RadRO] - **Spec Exp:** Brain Tumors-Pediatric; Proton Beam Therapy; **Hospital:** Mass Genl Hosp; **Address:** Massachusetts Genl Hosp, Proton Ctr, Boston, MA 02114; **Phone:** 617-724-1836; **Board Cert:** Therapeutic Radiology 1983; **Med School:** SUNY Upstate Med Univ 1979; **Resid:** Radiation Therapy, Harvard Med School 1983; **Fac Appt:** Prof RadRO, Harvard Med Sch

Wazer, David E MD [RadRO] - **Spec Exp:** Breast Cancer; Melanoma; **Hospital:** Rhode Island Hosp, Tufts Med Ctr; **Address:** 593 Eddy St, Providence, RI 02903; **Phone:** 401-444-8311; **Board Cert:** Radiation Oncology 1988; **Med School:** NYU Sch Med 1982; **Resid:** Radiation Oncology, Tufts New Eng Med Ctr 1988; **Fellow:** Neurological Chemistry, NYU Med Ctr 1984; **Fac Appt:** Prof RadRO, Tufts Univ

Wilson, Lynn D MD [RadRO] - **Spec Exp:** Lymphoma, Cutaneous T Cell (CTCL); Lymphoma, Cutaneous B Cell (CBCL); Lung Cancer; Head & Neck Cancer; **Hospital:** Yale-New Haven Hosp; **Address:** Yale Univ Sch Med, Dept Therapeutic Rad, PO Box 208040, New Haven, CT 06520-8040; **Phone:** 203-688-1861; **Board Cert:** Radiation Oncology 2004; **Med School:** Geo Wash Univ 1990; **Resid:** Therapeutic Radiology, Yale-New Haven Hosp 1994; **Fac Appt:** Prof RadRO, Yale Univ

Radiation Oncology

Zietman, Anthony L MD [RadRO] - **Spec Exp:** Prostate Cancer; Urologic Cancer; Proton Beam Therapy; **Hospital:** Mass Genl Hosp; **Address:** Mass Genl Hosp, 100 Blossom St Cox Bldg, rm 3, Boston, MA 02114; **Phone:** 617-724-4000; **Board Cert:** Radiation Oncology 1994; **Med School:** England, UK 1983; **Resid:** Internal Medicine, St Stephens & Westminster Hosp 1986; Radiation Oncology, Mass Genl Hosp 1989; **Fellow:** Radiation Oncology, Middlesex/Mt Vernon Hosps 1991; **Fac Appt:** Prof RadRO, Harvard Med Sch

Mid Atlantic

Berg, Christine D MD [RadRO] - **Spec Exp:** Breast Cancer-Early Detection; Breast Cancer-High Risk Women; **Hospital:** Natl Inst of Hlth - Clin Ctr; **Address:** 6130 Executive Blvd, Bethesda, MD 20892-7346; **Phone:** 301-496-8544; **Board Cert:** Internal Medicine 1980; Medical Oncology 1983; Therapeutic Radiology 1986; Radiation Oncology 1999; **Med School:** Northwestern Univ 1977; **Resid:** Internal Medicine, Northwestern Meml Hosp 1981; Radiation Oncology, Georgetown Univ Hosp 1986; **Fellow:** Medical Oncology, Natl Cancer Inst-NIH 1984

Bogart, Jeffrey A MD [RadRO] - **Spec Exp:** Lung Cancer; Thoracic Cancers; Clinical Trials; **Hospital:** Univ Hosp - SUNY Upstate; **Address:** SUNY Upstate Medical Ctr, Dept Radiation Oncology, 750 E Adams St, Syracuse, NY 13210; **Phone:** 315-464-5276; **Med School:** SUNY Upstate Med Univ 1989; **Resid:** Radiation Oncology, SUNY Hlth Sci Ctr 1993

Constine, Louis Sanders MD [RadRO] - **Spec Exp:** Pediatric Cancers; Lymphoma; Cancer Survivors-Late Effects of Therapy; Sarcoma; **Hospital:** Univ of Rochester Strong Meml Hosp; **Address:** 601 Elmwood Ave, Box 647, Rochester, NY 14642; **Phone:** 585-275-5622; **Board Cert:** Pediatrics 1978; Therapeutic Radiology 1981; Pediatric Hematology-Oncology 1978; **Med School:** Johns Hopkins Univ 1973; **Resid:** Pediatrics, Moffitt Hosp-UCSF Med Ctr 1975; Pediatrics, Stanford Hosp Med Ctr 1976; **Fellow:** Therapeutic Radiology, Stanford Hosp Med Ctr 1981; Pediatric Hematology-Oncology, Univ Wash/Chldns Ortho Hosp 1978; **Fac Appt:** Prof RadRO, Univ Rochester

DeWeese, Theodore L MD [RadRO] - **Spec Exp:** Urologic Cancer; Prostate Cancer; Testicular Cancer; **Hospital:** Johns Hopkins Hosp (page 61); **Address:** Johns Hopkins Hosp, Weinberg Bldg, 401 N Broadway, rm 1363, Baltimore, MD 21231; **Phone:** 410-955-8893; **Board Cert:** Radiation Oncology 1995; **Med School:** Univ Colorado 1990; **Resid:** Radiation Oncology, Johns Hopkins Hosp 1994; **Fellow:** Urologic Oncology, Johns Hopkins Hosp 1995; **Fac Appt:** Prof RadRO, Johns Hopkins Univ

Dicker, Adam P MD/PhD [RadRO] - **Spec Exp:** Prostate Cancer; **Hospital:** Thomas Jefferson Univ Hosp; **Address:** Bodine Cancer Treatment Ctr, 111 South 11th St, Philadelphia, PA 19107-5097; **Phone:** 215-955-6527; **Board Cert:** Radiation Oncology 2000; **Med School:** Cornell Univ-Weill Med Coll 1992; **Resid:** Surgery, Lenox Hill Hosp 1994; Radiation Oncology, Meml Sloan Kettering Cancer Ctr 1997; **Fac Appt:** Assoc Prof RadRO, Thomas Jefferson Univ

Donahue, Bernadine R MD [RadRO] - **Spec Exp:** Brain Tumors; Gastrointestinal Cancer; Pediatric Cancers; Solid Tumors; **Hospital:** Maimonides Med Ctr (page 63); **Address:** Maimonides Med Ctr, Dept Radiation Oncology, 6300 8th Ave, Lower Level, Brooklyn, NY 11220; **Phone:** 718-765-2700; **Board Cert:** Internal Medicine 1987; Radiation Oncology 1991; **Med School:** Boston Univ 1984; **Resid:** Internal Medicine, Boston Univ Med Ctr 1987; **Fellow:** Radiation Oncology, NYU Med Ctr 1990

Dritschilo, Anatoly MD [RadRO] - **Spec Exp:** Prostate Cancer; **Hospital:** Georgetown Univ Hosp; **Address:** Georgetown Univ Hosp, Dept Radiation Medicine, LL-Bliss, 3800 Reservoir Rd NW, Washington, DC 20007; **Phone:** 202-687-2144; **Board Cert:** Therapeutic Radiology 1977; **Med School:** UMDNJ-NJ Med Sch, Newark 1973; **Resid:** Radiation Therapy, Harvard Joint Rad Ther Ctr 1977; **Fac Appt:** Prof Med, Georgetown Univ

Ennis, Ronald D MD [RadRO] - **Spec Exp:** Prostate Cancer; Brachytherapy; Gynecologic Cancer; **Hospital:** St Luke's - Roosevelt Hosp Ctr - Roosevelt Div (page 57), Beth Israel Med Ctr - Petrie Division (page 57); **Address:** St Luke's Roosevelt Hosp, Dept Rad Oncol, 1000 10th Ave, Lower Level, New York, NY 10019; **Phone:** 212-523-7165; **Board Cert:** Radiation Oncology 2005; **Med School:** Yale Univ 1990; **Resid:** Therapeutic Radiology, Yale-New Haven Hosp 1994

Flickinger, John C MD [RadRO] - **Spec Exp:** Neuro-Oncology; Brain & Spinal Tumors; **Hospital:** UPMC Presby, Pittsburgh; **Address:** UPMC Cancer Ctr, Radiation Oncology, 5230 Centre Ave, Pittsburgh, PA 15213; **Phone:** 412-647-3600; **Board Cert:** Therapeutic Radiology 1985; **Med School:** Univ Chicago-Pritzker Sch Med 1981; **Resid:** Radiation Therapy, Mass Genl Hosp 1985; **Fac Appt:** Prof RadRO, Univ Pittsburgh

Formenti, Silvia C MD [RadRO] - **Spec Exp:** Breast Cancer; Chemo-Radiation Combined Therapy; **Hospital:** NYU Langone Med Ctr (page 67); **Address:** NYU Med Ctr, Dept Radiation Oncology, 160 E 34th St, New York, NY 10016; **Phone:** 212-263-2601; **Board Cert:** Radiation Oncology 1991; **Med School:** Italy 1980; **Resid:** Internal Medicine, San Carlo Borromeo Hosp 1983; Medical Oncology, Univ of Pavia Med Ctr 1985; **Fellow:** Radiation Oncology, USC Med Ctr 1990; **Fac Appt:** Asst Prof RadRO, NYU Sch Med

Freedman, Gary M MD [RadRO] - **Spec Exp:** Breast Cancer; **Hospital:** Fox Chase Cancer Ctr (page 58), Jeanes Hosp; **Address:** Fox Chase Cancer Ctr-Radiation Onc Dept, 333 Cottman Ave, Philadelphia, PA 19111; **Phone:** 215-728-3815; **Board Cert:** Radiation Oncology 2000; **Med School:** Temple Univ 1993; **Resid:** Radiation Oncology, Fox Chase Cancer Ctr 1998

Gejerman, Glen MD [RadRO] - **Spec Exp:** Prostate Cancer; Intensity Modulated Radiotherapy (IMRT); Breast Cancer; Brachytherapy; **Hospital:** Hackensack Univ Med Ctr; **Address:** Hackensack Univ Med Ctr, Radiation Onc, 30 Prospect Ave, Hackensack, NJ 07601; **Phone:** 201-996-2464; **Board Cert:** Radiation Oncology 2006; **Med School:** UMDNJ-NJ Med Sch, Newark 1990; **Resid:** Radiation Oncology, Montefiore Med Ctr 1995; **Fac Appt:** Asst Clin Prof RadRO, Albert Einstein Coll Med

Glassburn, John R MD [RadRO] - **Spec Exp:** Gynecologic Cancer; Prostate Cancer; Breast Cancer; **Hospital:** Pennsylvania Hosp (page 60), Hosp Univ Penn - UPHS (page 60); **Address:** Pennsylvania Hosp, Dept Radiation Oncology, 800 Spruce St, Philadelphia, PA 19107; **Phone:** 215-829-3873; **Board Cert:** Therapeutic Radiology 1973; **Med School:** Hahnemann Univ 1966; **Resid:** Radiation Oncology, Hahnemann Hosp 1972; **Fac Appt:** Clin Prof RadRO, Univ Pennsylvania

Glatstein, Eli MD [RadRO] - **Spec Exp:** Lymphoma; Lung Cancer; Photodynamic Therapy; Sarcoma; **Hospital:** Hosp Univ Penn - UPHS (page 60); **Address:** Hosp Univ Penn, Dept Rad Oncology, 3400 Spruce St, Donner Bldg Fl 2, Philadelphia, PA 19104; **Phone:** 215-662-3383; **Board Cert:** Therapeutic Radiology 1972; **Med School:** Stanford Univ 1964; **Resid:** Radiation Therapy, Stanford Med Ctr 1970; **Fellow:** Radiological Biology, Hammersmith Hosp 1972; **Fac Appt:** Prof RadRO, Univ Pennsylvania

Goodman, Robert L MD [RadRO] - **Spec Exp:** Breast Cancer; Lymphoma; Prostate Cancer; Brain Tumors; **Hospital:** St Barnabas Med Ctr; **Address:** St Barnabas Med Ctr, Dept Rad Oncology, 94 Old Short Hills Rd, Livingston, NJ 07039; **Phone:** 973-322-5133; **Board Cert:** Internal Medicine 1971; Therapeutic Radiology 1974; Medical Oncology 1975; **Med School:** Columbia P&S 1966; **Resid:** Internal Medicine, Beth Israel Hosp 1970; Radiation Therapy, Harvard Joint Ctr Rad Therapy 1974; **Fellow:** Hematology, NY-Presby Hosp 1969

Radiation Oncology

Greenberger, Joel S MD [RadRO] - **Spec Exp:** Lung Cancer; Esophageal Cancer; **Hospital:** UPMC Presby, Pittsburgh; **Address:** UPMC Cancer Ctr, Radiation Oncology, 5230 Centre Ave, Pittsburgh, PA 15232; **Phone:** 412-647-3600; **Board Cert:** Therapeutic Radiology 1977; **Med School:** Harvard Med Sch 1971; **Resid:** Radiation Therapy, Mass General Hosp 1977; **Fac Appt:** Prof RadRO, Univ Pittsburgh

Haffty, Bruce MD [RadRO] - **Spec Exp:** Breast Cancer; Head & Neck Cancer; Lung Cancer; **Hospital:** Robert Wood Johnson Univ Hosp - New Brunswick, Robert Wood Johnson Univ Hosp Hamilton; **Address:** The Cancer Institute of New Jersey, 195 Little Albany St, rm 2038, New Brunswick, NJ 08903; **Phone:** 732-253-3939; **Board Cert:** Radiation Oncology 1988; **Med School:** Yale Univ 1984; **Resid:** Radiation Oncology, Yale-New Haven Hosp 1988; **Fac Appt:** Prof RadRO, Robert W Johnson Med Sch

Hahn, Stephen M MD [RadRO] - **Spec Exp:** Lung Cancer; Prostate Cancer; Sarcoma; Photodynamic Therapy; **Hospital:** Hosp Univ Penn - UPHS (page 60), Penn Presby Med Ctr - UPHS (page 60); **Address:** Hosp of the Univ of Penn, 3400 Spruce St 2 Donner Bldg, Philadelphia, PA 19104; **Phone:** 215-662-7296; **Board Cert:** Radiation Oncology 2004; Internal Medicine 1987; Medical Oncology 2001; **Med School:** Temple Univ 1984; **Resid:** Internal Medicine, UCSF Med Ctr 1988; Medical Oncology, Natl Inst Hlth 1991; **Fellow:** Radiation Oncology, Natl Inst Hlth 1994; **Fac Appt:** Prof RadRO, Univ Pennsylvania

Harrison, Louis B MD [RadRO] - **Spec Exp:** Brachytherapy; Head & Neck Cancer; Radiation Therapy-Intraoperative; **Hospital:** Beth Israel Med Ctr - Petrie Division (page 57), St Luke's - Roosevelt Hosp Ctr - Roosevelt Div (page 57); **Address:** Beth Israel Med Ctr, Dept Rad Onc, 10 Union Square East, Ste 4G, New York, NY 10003-3314; **Phone:** 212-844-8087; **Board Cert:** Therapeutic Radiology 1986; **Med School:** SUNY Downstate 1982; **Resid:** Therapeutic Radiology, Yale-New Haven Hosp 1986; **Fac Appt:** Prof RadRO, Albert Einstein Coll Med

Horwitz, Eric MD [RadRO] - **Spec Exp:** Prostate Cancer; Intensity Modulated Radiotherapy (IMRT); Brachytherapy; **Hospital:** Fox Chase Cancer Ctr (page 58); **Address:** Fox Chase Cancer Ctr, Dept Radiation Oncology, 333 Cottman Ave, Philadelphia, PA 19111; **Phone:** 215-728-2995; **Board Cert:** Radiation Oncology 1999; **Med School:** Albany Med Coll 1992; **Resid:** Radiation Oncology, William Beaumont Hosp 1997

Isaacson, Steven R MD [RadRO] - **Spec Exp:** Brain Tumors; Neuro-Oncology; Stereotactic Radiosurgery; Arteriovenous Malformations; **Hospital:** NY-Presby Hosp/Columbia (page 66); **Address:** Columbia Presby Med Ctr, Dept Radiation Oncology, 622 W 168th St BHN Bldg - rm B-11, New York, NY 10032-3720; **Phone:** 212-305-2611; **Board Cert:** Radiation Oncology 1988; Otolaryngology 1978; **Med School:** Jefferson Med Coll 1973; **Resid:** Otolaryngology, Hosp Univ Penn 1978; Radiation Oncology, SUNY Hlth Sci Ctr 1988; **Fac Appt:** Clin Prof RadRO, Columbia P&S

Kleinberg, Lawrence MD [RadRO] - **Spec Exp:** Brain & Spinal Cord Tumors; Brain Tumors-Metastatic; Stereotactic Radiosurgery; Esophageal Cancer; **Hospital:** Johns Hopkins Hosp (page 61); **Address:** Johns Hopkins Oncology Ctr Weinberg Bldg, 401 N Broadway, Ste 1440, Baltimore, MD 21231; **Phone:** 410-614-2597; **Board Cert:** Radiation Oncology 1994; **Med School:** Yale Univ 1989; **Resid:** Radiation Oncology, Meml Sloan-Kettering Canc Ctr 1993; **Fac Appt:** Assoc Prof RadRO, Johns Hopkins Univ

Kuettel, Michael MD/PhD [RadRO] - **Spec Exp:** Prostate Cancer; **Hospital:** Roswell Park Cancer Inst; **Address:** Roswell Park Cancer Inst, Radiation Med, Elm and Carlton St, Buffalo, NY 14263; **Phone:** 716-845-1562; **Board Cert:** Radiation Oncology 1992; **Med School:** Northwestern Univ-Feinberg Sch Med 1985; **Resid:** Internal Medicine, Northwestern Hosp 1986; Radiation Oncology, Johns Hopkins Hosp 1990; **Fac Appt:** Prof RadRO, SUNY Buffalo

Lepanto, Philip B MD [RadRO] - **Hospital:** St Mary's Med Ctr - Huntington, Cabell Huntington Hosp; **Address:** St Mary's Med Ctr, Dept Radiation Oncology, 2900 First Ave, Huntington, WV 25702; **Phone:** 304-526-1143; **Board Cert:** Therapeutic Radiology 1975; **Med School:** Univ Louisville Sch Med 1970; **Resid:** Diagnostic Radiology, Graduate Hosp 1972; Radiation Therapy, Hosp Univ Penn 1975; **Fac Appt:** Clin Prof Rad, Marshall Univ

Machtay, Mitchell MD [RadRO] - **Spec Exp:** Head & Neck Cancer; Skin Cancer; Skull Base Tumors; **Hospital:** Thomas Jefferson Univ Hosp; **Address:** Bodine Ctr for Cancer Treatment, Dept Rad Onc, 111 S 11 St, Bodine Ctr, Philadelphia, PA 19107-5097; **Phone:** 215-955-6706; **Board Cert:** Radiation Oncology 1994; **Med School:** NYU Sch Med 1989; **Resid:** Radiation Oncology, Hosp Univ Penn 1993; **Fac Appt:** Assoc Prof RadRO, Jefferson Med Coll

McCormick, Beryl MD [RadRO] - **Spec Exp:** Breast Cancer; Eye Tumors/Cancer; **Hospital:** Meml Sloan-Kettering Cancer Ctr, NY-Presby Hosp/Weill Cornell (page 66); **Address:** 1275 York Avenue, New York, NY 10065; **Phone:** 800-525-2225; **Board Cert:** Therapeutic Radiology 1977; **Med School:** UMDNJ-NJ Med Sch, Newark 1973; **Resid:** Therapeutic Radiology, Meml Sloan Kettering Cancer Ctr 1977; **Fac Appt:** Prof RadRO, Cornell Univ-Weill Med Coll

Nicolaou, Nicos MD [RadRO] - **Spec Exp:** Lymphoma; Hodgkin's Disease; **Hospital:** Fox Chase Cancer Ctr (page 58); **Address:** 333 Cottman Avenue, Philadelphia, PA 19111-2497; **Phone:** 215-728-3058; **Board Cert:** Radiation Oncology 1999; **Med School:** Canada 1984; **Resid:** Radiation Oncology, British Columbia Cancer Agency 1989; **Fellow:** Radiation Oncology, Fox Chase Cancer Ctr 1990

Nori, Dattatreyudu MD [RadRO] - **Spec Exp:** Prostate Cancer; Brachytherapy; **Hospital:** NY-Presby Hosp/Weill Cornell (page 66), NY Hosp Queens; **Address:** 525 E 68th St, Box 575, New York, NY 10021-4870; **Phone:** 212-746-3679; **Board Cert:** Therapeutic Radiology 1979; **Med School:** India 1970; **Resid:** Radiation Oncology, Meml Sloan Kettering Cancer Ctr 1975; **Fellow:** Radiation Oncology, Meml Sloan Kettering Cancer Ctr 1978; **Fac Appt:** Prof RadRO, Cornell Univ-Weill Med Coll

Porrazzo, Michael S MD [RadRO] - **Spec Exp:** Prostate Cancer; Central Nervous System Cancer; Breast Cancer; Stereotactic Radiosurgery; **Hospital:** Washington Hosp Ctr; **Address:** Wash Hosp Ctr-Dept. Radiation Onc, 110 Irving St NW, Rm CG-107, Washington, DC 20010; **Phone:** 202-877-3925; **Board Cert:** Radiation Oncology 1990; **Med School:** Meharry Med Coll 1985; **Resid:** Radiation Oncology, Univ Hosp Brooklyn-SUNY Hlth 1989

Regine, William F MD [RadRO] - **Spec Exp:** Stereotactic Radiosurgery; Brain & Spinal Tumors; Gastrointestinal Cancer; **Hospital:** Univ of MD Med Ctr; **Address:** Univ MD Med System-Greenbaum Cancer Ctr, 22 S Green St Guldelsky Bldg, Baltimore, MD 21201; **Phone:** 410-328-6080; **Board Cert:** Radiation Oncology 1992; **Med School:** SUNY Upstate Med Univ 1987; **Resid:** Radiation Oncology, Thomas Jefferson Univ Hosp 1991; **Fellow:** Radiation Oncology, Thomas Jefferson Univ Hosp 1992; **Fac Appt:** Prof RadRO, Univ MD Sch Med

Rotman, Marvin MD [RadRO] - **Spec Exp:** Bladder Cancer; Gynecologic Cancer; Breast Cancer; Prostate Cancer; **Hospital:** SUNY Downstate Med Ctr, Long Island Coll Hosp (page 57); **Address:** 450 Clarkson Ave, Box 1211, Brooklyn, NY 11203-2056; **Phone:** 718-270-2181; **Board Cert:** Diagnostic Radiology 1966; Radiation Oncology 1999; **Med School:** Jefferson Med Coll 1958; **Resid:** Internal Medicine, Albert Einstein Med Ctr 1960; Radiation Oncology, Montefiore Hosp Med Ctr 1965; **Fac Appt:** Prof RadRO, SUNY Downstate

Radiation Oncology

Schiff, Peter B MD/PhD [RadRO] - **Spec Exp:** Prostate Cancer; Gynecologic Cancer; Breast Cancer; **Hospital:** NYU Langone Med Ctr (page 67); **Address:** NYU Clinical Cancer Ctr, 160 E 34th St Fl 1, New York, NY 10016; **Phone:** 212-731-5003; **Board Cert:** Radiation Oncology 1990; **Med School:** Albert Einstein Coll Med 1984; **Resid:** Radiation Oncology, Meml Sloan Kettering Cancer Ctr 1988; **Fac Appt:** Prof RadRO, NYU Sch Med

Solin, Lawrence J MD [RadRO] - **Spec Exp:** Breast Cancer; Head & Neck Cancer; **Hospital:** Albert Einstein Med Ctr; **Address:** Albert Einstein Medical Ctr, Dept Radiation Oncology, 5501 Old York Rd, Philadelphia, PA 19141; **Phone:** 215-456-6280; **Board Cert:** Radiation Oncology 1999; Therapeutic Radiology 1984; **Med School:** Brown Univ 1978; **Resid:** Surgery, Thos Jefferson Univ Hosp 1981; Radiation Oncology, Thos Jefferson Univ Hosp 1984; **Fac Appt:** Prof RadRO, Univ Pennsylvania

Stock, Richard MD [RadRO] - **Spec Exp:** Prostate Cancer; **Hospital:** Mount Sinai Med Ctr (page 64); **Address:** Dept Radiation Oncology, Box 1236, New York, NY 10029; **Phone:** 212-241-7502; **Board Cert:** Radiation Oncology 1993; **Med School:** Mount Sinai Sch Med 1988; **Resid:** Radiation Oncology, Meml Sloan Kettering Cancer Ctr 1992; **Fac Appt:** Prof RadRO, Mount Sinai Sch Med

Streeter Jr, Oscar E MD [RadRO] - **Spec Exp:** Lung Cancer; Head & Neck Cancer; **Hospital:** Howard Univ Hosp; **Address:** Howard Univ Hosp, Dept Radiation Onc, 2041 Georgia Ave NW, Washington, DC 20060; **Phone:** 202-865-6100; **Board Cert:** Radiation Oncology 1989; **Med School:** Howard Univ 1982; **Resid:** Radiation Oncology, Howard Univ 1986; **Fac Appt:** Assoc Prof RadRO, USC Sch Med

Weiss, Marisa C MD [RadRO] - **Spec Exp:** Breast Cancer; **Hospital:** Lankenau Hosp; **Address:** Lankenau Hospital, Dept Rad Oncology, 100 Lancaster Ave, Wynnewood, PA 19096; **Phone:** 610-645-2433; **Board Cert:** Radiation Oncology 1988; **Med School:** Univ Pennsylvania 1984; **Resid:** Radiation Oncology, Hosp Univ Penn 1988; **Fellow:** Radiological Biology, Hosp Univ Penn 1990

Werner-Wasik, Maria MD [RadRO] - **Spec Exp:** Brain Tumors; Lung Cancer; Melanoma; Breast Cancer; **Hospital:** Thomas Jefferson Univ Hosp; **Address:** Bodine Ctr, Ste G-301, 111 S 11 St, Philadelphia, PA 19107; **Phone:** 215-955-6702; **Board Cert:** Radiation Oncology 1994; **Med School:** Poland 1979; **Resid:** Internal Medicine, Framingham Union Hosp 1990; Radiation Oncology, Tufts/New England Med Ctr 1993; **Fellow:** Radiation Oncology, Hosp Univ Penn 1994; **Fac Appt:** Assoc Prof RadRO, Thomas Jefferson Univ

Wharam Jr, Moody D MD [RadRO] - **Spec Exp:** Pediatric Cancers; Brain Tumors; Sarcoma-Soft Tissue; **Hospital:** Johns Hopkins Hosp (page 61); **Address:** Kimmel Cancer Ctr, Dept Rad Oncology, 401 N Broadway St, Ste 1440, Baltimore, MD 21231-1146; **Phone:** 410-955-7313; **Board Cert:** Therapeutic Radiology 1974; **Med School:** Univ VA Sch Med 1969; **Resid:** Radiation Oncology, UCSF Med Ctr 1973; **Fac Appt:** Prof RadRO, Johns Hopkins Univ

Yahalom, Joachim MD [RadRO] - **Spec Exp:** Lymphoma; Hodgkin's Disease; Multiple Myeloma; **Hospital:** Meml Sloan-Kettering Cancer Ctr; **Address:** 1275 York Ave, SM03, Dept Radiation Onc, New York, NY 10065; **Phone:** 212-639-5999; **Board Cert:** Radiation Oncology 1988; **Med School:** Israel 1976; **Resid:** Internal Medicine, Hadassah Hosp 1979; Radiation Oncology, Hadassah Hosp 1984; **Fellow:** Radiation Oncology, Meml Sloan Kettering Canc Ctr 1986; **Fac Appt:** Prof RadRO, Cornell Univ-Weill Med Coll

Zelefsky, Michael J MD [RadRO] - **Spec Exp:** Prostate Cancer; Brachytherapy; Head & Neck Cancer; **Hospital:** Meml Sloan-Kettering Cancer Ctr; **Address:** 1275 York Avenue, New York, NY 10065; **Phone:** 800-525-2225; **Board Cert:** Radiation Oncology 1991; **Med School:** Albert Einstein Coll Med 1986; **Resid:** Radiation Oncology, Meml Sloan Kettering Cancer Ctr 1990; **Fac Appt:** Prof RadRO, Cornell Univ-Weill Med Coll

Southeast

Anscher, Mitchell S MD [RadRO] - **Spec Exp:** Prostate Cancer; Brachytherapy; **Hospital:** Med Coll of VA Hosp, Henrico Doctors Hosp; **Address:** Virginia Commonwealth Univ, Department of Radiation Oncology, Box 980058, Richmond, VA 23298-0058; **Phone:** 804-828-7238; **Board Cert:** Internal Medicine 1984; Radiation Oncology 1987; **Med School:** Med Coll VA 1981; **Resid:** Internal Medicine, St Marys Hosp 1984; Radiation Oncology, Duke Univ Med Ctr 1987; **Fac Appt:** Prof RadRO, Va Commonwealth Univ Sch Med

Blackstock, Arthur William MD [RadRO] - **Spec Exp:** Lung Cancer; Gastrointestinal Cancer; Clinical Trials; **Hospital:** Wake Forest Univ Baptist Med Ctr (page 72); **Address:** Wake Forest Univ Medical Ctr, Dept Radiation Oncology, Medical Center Blvd, Winston-Salem, NC 27157; **Phone:** 336-713-3600; **Board Cert:** Radiation Oncology 2006; **Med School:** E Carolina Univ 1989; **Resid:** Radiation Oncology, Univ NC Hosps 1994; **Fac Appt:** Prof RadRO, Wake Forest Univ

Bonner, James Alan MD [RadRO] - **Spec Exp:** Head & Neck Cancer; Lung Cancer; **Hospital:** Univ of Ala Hosp at Birmingham; **Address:** 1824 6th Ave S, WTI, rm 105, Birmingham, AL 35294; **Phone:** 205-934-2761; **Board Cert:** Radiation Oncology 1990; **Med School:** Wayne State Univ 1985; **Resid:** Radiation Oncology, Univ Michigan Med Ctr 1989; **Fac Appt:** Prof RadRO, Univ Alabama

Brizel, David M MD [RadRO] - **Spec Exp:** Head & Neck Cancer; Sarcoma; **Hospital:** Duke Univ Med Ctr; **Address:** Duke Univ Med Ctr, Dept Rad Onc, Box 3085, Durham, NC 27710-0001; **Phone:** 919-668-5637; **Board Cert:** Radiation Oncology 1987; **Med School:** Northwestern Univ 1983; **Resid:** Radiation Oncology, Harvard Joint Ctr Radiation Ther 1987; **Fac Appt:** Prof RadRO, Duke Univ

Chakravarthy, Anuradha MD [RadRO] - **Spec Exp:** Breast Cancer; Gastrointestinal Cancer; **Hospital:** Vanderbilt Univ Med Ctr; **Address:** Vanderbilt Univ Med Ctr, Dept Rad Onc, 1301 22nd Ave S, Preston Research Bldg, Ste 1003, Nashville, TN 37232; **Phone:** 615-322-2555; **Board Cert:** Radiation Oncology 1994; Internal Medicine 1986; Medical Oncology 1989; **Med School:** Geo Wash Univ 1983; **Resid:** Internal Medicine, Mayo Clinic 1986; Medical Oncology, Univ MD Cancer Ctr 1989; **Fellow:** Radiation Oncology, Johns Hopkins Hosp; **Fac Appt:** Asst Prof RadRO, Vanderbilt Univ

Crocker, Ian R MD [RadRO] - **Spec Exp:** Brain Tumors; Eye Tumors/Cancer; Vascular Brachytherapy; **Hospital:** Emory Univ Hosp, Emory Univ Hosp Midtown; **Address:** The Emory Clinic, Dept Radiation Onc, 1365 Clifton Rd NE, CT-104, Atlanta, GA 30322; **Phone:** 404-778-3473; **Board Cert:** Therapeutic Radiology 1999; Internal Medicine 1980; **Med School:** Univ Saskatchewan 1976; **Resid:** Internal Medicine, Univ Hosp-Univ West Ontario 1980; **Fellow:** Radiation Oncology, Princess Margaret Hosp-Univ Toronto 1983; **Fac Appt:** Prof RadRO, Emory Univ

Halle, Jan MD [RadRO] - **Spec Exp:** Breast Cancer; Lung Cancer; **Hospital:** Univ NC Hosps; **Address:** Univ North Carolina Sch Med, Dept Rad Onc, 101 Manning Drive, CB 7512, Gravely Bldg, Chapel Hill, NC 27599; **Phone:** 919-966-7700; **Board Cert:** Therapeutic Radiology 1982; **Med School:** Tufts Univ 1975; **Resid:** Radiation Oncology, North Carolina Meml Hosp 1981; **Fac Appt:** Assoc Prof RadRO, Univ NC Sch Med

Radiation Oncology

Jose, Baby Oliapuram MD [RadRO] - **Spec Exp:** Head & Neck Cancer; Lung Cancer; Gynecologic Cancer; Prostate Cancer; **Hospital:** Univ of Louisville Hosp, Floyd Meml Hosp & Hlth Svcs; **Address:** James G. Brown Cancer Center, 529 S Jackson St Fl 4, Louisville, KY 40202; **Phone:** 502-562-4759; **Board Cert:** Therapeutic Radiology 1978; **Med School:** India 1971; **Resid:** Surgery, CMC Hosp 1974; Radiation Oncology, CMC Hosp 1976; **Fellow:** Radiation Oncology, Brown Univ-RI Hosp 1979; **Fac Appt:** Prof RadRO, Univ Louisville Sch Med

Kiel, Krystyna D MD [RadRO] - **Spec Exp:** Breast Cancer; Sarcoma; Gastrointestinal Cancer; Colon & Rectal Cancer; **Hospital:** Meml Hlth Univ Med Ctr - Savannah; **Address:** Savannah Radiation Cancer Care, 4700 Waters Ave, Dept Radiation Onc, Savanna, GA 31404; **Phone:** 912-350-8490; **Board Cert:** Therapeutic Radiology 1983; Radiation Oncology 2000; **Med School:** Univ Mass Sch Med 1977; **Resid:** Radiation Oncology, Mass Genl Hosp 1982

Kun, Larry E MD [RadRO] - **Spec Exp:** Brain Tumors; Pediatric Cancers; **Hospital:** St Jude Children's Research Hosp, Le Bonheur Chldns Med Ctr; **Address:** St Jude Chldns Research Hosp-Dept Rad Onc, 262 Danny Thomas Pl, MS 220, Memphis, TN 38105; **Phone:** 901-495-3565; **Board Cert:** Therapeutic Radiology 1973; **Med School:** Jefferson Med Coll 1968; **Resid:** Therapeutic Radiology, Penrose Cancer Hosp 1972; **Fellow:** Radiation Oncology, Natl Cancer Inst 1974; Radiation Oncology, Rotterdam Radiotherapy Inst 1975; **Fac Appt:** Prof, Univ Tenn Coll Med, Memphis

Landry, Jerome C MD [RadRO] - **Spec Exp:** Gastrointestinal Cancer; Sarcoma-Soft Tissue; **Hospital:** Emory Univ Hosp, Grady Hlth Sys; **Address:** Emory Dept Rad Oncology, 1365 Clifton Rd NE, Ste A-1304, Atlanta, GA 30322; **Phone:** 404-778-3473; **Board Cert:** Radiation Oncology 1988; **Med School:** Harvard Med Sch 1983; **Resid:** Radiation Oncology, Mass Genl Hosp 1987; **Fac Appt:** Prof RadRO, Emory Univ

Larner, James M MD [RadRO] - **Spec Exp:** Neuro-Oncology; Brain Tumors; **Hospital:** Univ Virginia Med Ctr; **Address:** Univ Virginia Medical Ctr, Dept Radiation Oncology, PO Box 800383, Charlottesville, VA 22908; **Phone:** 434-924-5191; **Board Cert:** Internal Medicine 1983; Medical Oncology 1987; Hematology 1988; Radiation Oncology 1989; **Med School:** Univ VA Sch Med 1980; **Resid:** Internal Medicine, Thos Jefferson Univ Hosp 1983; Radiation Oncology, Montefiore-Einstein Med Ctr 1989; **Fellow:** Hematology & Oncology, Thos Jefferson Univ Hosp 1986; **Fac Appt:** Assoc Prof Med, Univ VA Sch Med

Lee, W Robert MD [RadRO] - **Spec Exp:** Prostate Cancer; Brachytherapy; Intensity Modulated Radiotherapy (IMRT); **Hospital:** Duke Univ Med Ctr; **Address:** Duke Univ Med Ctr, Div Radiation Oncology, Box 3085, Durham, NC 27710; **Phone:** 919-668-5640; **Board Cert:** Radiation Oncology 1994; **Med School:** Univ VA Sch Med 1989; **Resid:** Radiation Oncology, Univ Florida 1993; **Fac Appt:** Prof RadRO, Duke Univ

Lewin, Alan A MD [RadRO] - **Spec Exp:** Breast Cancer; Lung Cancer; Brain & Spinal Cord Tumors; **Hospital:** Baptist Hosp of Miami; **Address:** Baptist Hosp Miami, Dept Radiation Oncology, 8900 N Kendall Drive, Miami, FL 33176-2118; **Phone:** 786-596-6566; **Board Cert:** Therapeutic Radiology 1982; Internal Medicine 1976; Hematology 1978; Medical Oncology 1981; **Med School:** Geo Wash Univ 1973; **Resid:** Internal Medicine, Mt Sinai Hosp 1976; **Fellow:** Hematology & Oncology, Beth Israel Med Ctr 1978; Radiation Oncology, Joint Ctr Radiation Therapy 1980; **Fac Appt:** Clin Prof RadRO, Univ Miami Sch Med

Marcus Jr, Robert B MD [RadRO] - **Spec Exp:** Pediatric Cancers; Sarcoma; Bone Cancer; Brain/CNS Tumors; **Hospital:** Shands Jacksonville; **Address:** Univ Florida Proton Therapy Inst, 2015 N Jefferson St NE, Jacksonville, FL 32206; **Phone:** 904-588-1800; **Board Cert:** Therapeutic Radiology 1980; **Med School:** Univ Fla Coll Med 1975; **Resid:** Radiation Oncology, Shands Hosp 1979; **Fac Appt:** Prof RadRO, Univ Fla Coll Med

Markoe, Arnold M MD [RadRO] - **Spec Exp:** Eye Tumors/Cancer; Orbital Tumors/Cancer; Central Nervous System Cancer; Lymphoma; **Hospital:** Univ of Miami Hosp & Clins/Sylvester Comp Canc Ctr (page 70), Jackson Meml Hosp (page 70); **Address:** Univ of Miami Sylvester Comp Cancer Ctr, 1475 NW 12th Ave, Dept Radiation Onc-D31, Miami, FL 33136; **Phone:** 305-243-4319; **Board Cert:** Therapeutic Radiology 1983; **Med School:** Hahnemann Univ 1977; **Resid:** Radiation Oncology, Hahnemann Hosp 1981; **Fac Appt:** Prof RadRO, Univ Miami Sch Med

Marks, Lawrence MD [RadRO] - **Spec Exp:** Breast Cancer; Lung Cancer; **Hospital:** Univ NC Hosps; **Address:** UNC Dept Rad Onc, Campus Box 7512, Chapel Hill, NC 27599-7512; **Phone:** 919-966-0400; **Board Cert:** Radiation Oncology 1989; **Med School:** Univ Rochester 1985; **Resid:** Radiation Oncology, Mass Genl Hosp 1989; **Fac Appt:** Prof RadRO, Univ NC Sch Med

McGarry, Ronald C MD/PhD [RadRO] - **Spec Exp:** Lung Cancer; Lymphoma; Clinical Trials; Stereotactic Radiosurgery; **Hospital:** Univ of Kentucky Chandler Hosp; **Address:** Chandler Medical Ctr, Radiation Medicine, 800 Rose St, rm C1, Lexington, KY 40536; **Phone:** 859-323-6486; **Board Cert:** Radiation Oncology 1999; **Med School:** Canada 1992; **Resid:** Radiation Oncology, Univ W Ontario Regl Cancer Ctr 1997; **Fac Appt:** Prof RadRO, Univ KY Coll Med

Mendenhall, Nancy P MD [RadRO] - **Spec Exp:** Breast Cancer; Lymphoma; Hodgkin's Disease; **Hospital:** Shands at Univ of FL; **Address:** Univ Florida, Dept Radiation Oncology, Box 100385, Gainesville, FL 32610-0385; **Phone:** 352-265-0287; **Board Cert:** Therapeutic Radiology 1985; **Med School:** Univ Fla Coll Med 1980; **Resid:** Diagnostic Radiology, Shands-Univ of Florida 1984; **Fac Appt:** Prof RadRO, Univ Fla Coll Med

Mendenhall, William M MD [RadRO] - **Spec Exp:** Head & Neck Cancer; Stereotactic Radiosurgery; Colon Cancer; **Hospital:** Shands at Univ of FL; **Address:** Univ Florida, Dept Radiation Oncology, Box 100385, Gainesville, FL 32610-0385; **Phone:** 352-265-0287; **Board Cert:** Therapeutic Radiology 1983; **Med School:** Univ S Fla Coll Med 1978; **Resid:** Radiation Oncology, Univ Fla 1983; **Fac Appt:** Prof RadRO, Univ Fla Coll Med

Merchant, Thomas E DO [RadRO] - **Spec Exp:** Brain Tumors-Pediatric; **Hospital:** St Jude Children's Research Hosp; **Address:** St Jude Children's Research Hosp, 262 Danny Thomas Pl, MS 220, Memphis, TN 38105; **Phone:** 901-495-3604; **Board Cert:** Radiation Oncology 2004; **Med School:** Chicago Coll Osteo Med 1989; **Resid:** Radiation Oncology, Meml Sloan Kettering Cancer Ctr 1994

Meredith, Ruby F MD [RadRO] - **Spec Exp:** Multiple Myeloma; Breast Cancer; Radionuclide Therapy; Bone Tumors-Metastatic; **Hospital:** Univ of Ala Hosp at Birmingham; **Address:** Univ Alabama Hosps-Radiation Oncology, 619 19th St S, Birmingham, AL 35233; **Phone:** 205-934-2763; **Board Cert:** Radiation Oncology 1987; **Med School:** Ohio State Univ 1983; **Resid:** Radiation Oncology, Med College Va Hosps 1987; **Fac Appt:** Prof RadRO, Univ Alabama

Pollack, Alan MD/PhD [RadRO] - **Spec Exp:** Prostate Cancer; Genitourinary Cancer; Sarcoma; **Hospital:** Univ of Miami Hosp & Clins/Sylvester Comp Canc Ctr (page 70); **Address:** 1475 NW 12th Ave, Miami, FL 33136; **Phone:** 305-243-4200; **Board Cert:** Radiation Oncology 1993; **Med School:** Univ Miami Sch Med 1987; **Resid:** Radiation Oncology, MD Anderson Cancer Ctr 1992; **Fac Appt:** Prof RadRO, Univ Miami Sch Med

Prosnitz, Leonard MD [RadRO] - **Spec Exp:** Lymphoma; Breast Cancer; Hyperthermia Treatment of Cancer; Sarcoma; **Hospital:** Duke Univ Med Ctr; **Address:** Duke Univ Med Ctr, Dept Rad Onc, Box 3085, Durham, NC 27710; **Phone:** 919-668-5637; **Board Cert:** Therapeutic Radiology 1970; **Med School:** SUNY Downstate 1961; **Resid:** Internal Medicine, Dartmouth Affil Hosps 1963; Radiation Oncology, Yale-New Haven Hosp 1969; **Fellow:** Hematology & Oncology, Yale-New Haven Hosp 1967; **Fac Appt:** Prof RadRO, Duke Univ

Radiation Oncology

Randall, Marcus MD [RadRO] - **Spec Exp:** Gynecologic Cancer; Stereotactic Radiosurgery; **Hospital:** Univ of Kentucky Chandler Hosp; **Address:** Univ Kentucky Medical Ctr, 800 Rose St, rm C11-14D, Office of Radiation Med, Lexington, KY 40536-0001; **Phone:** 859-323-6487; **Board Cert:** Therapeutic Radiology 1986; **Med School:** Univ NC Sch Med 1982; **Resid:** Radiation Oncology, Univ Va Med Ctr 1986; **Fellow:** Radiation Oncology, Univ Va Med Ctr 1986; **Fac Appt:** Prof RadRO, Univ KY Coll Med

Rich, Tyvin Andrew MD [RadRO] - **Spec Exp:** Colon & Rectal Cancer; Chemo-Radiation Combined Therapy; Esophageal Cancer; Gallbladder & Biliary Cancer; **Hospital:** Univ Virginia Med Ctr; **Address:** Univ Va Hlth Sys, Dept Rad Onc, Box 800383, Charlottesville, VA 22908-0383; **Phone:** 434-924-5191; **Board Cert:** Radiation Oncology 1978; **Med School:** Univ VA Sch Med 1973; **Resid:** Mass Genl Hosp 1978; **Fellow:** Radiation Oncology, Mt Vernon Hosp/Gray Lab 1978; **Fac Appt:** Prof RadRO, Univ VA Sch Med

Rosenman, Julian MD/PhD [RadRO] - **Spec Exp:** Lung Cancer; Breast Cancer; Prostate Cancer; **Hospital:** Univ NC Hosps; **Address:** Univ North Carolina, Dept Rad Onc, 101 Manning Drive, CB 7512, Gravely Bldg, Chapel Hill, NC 27599-7512; **Phone:** 919-966-7700; **Board Cert:** Therapeutic Radiology 1981; **Med School:** Univ Tex SW, Dallas 1977; **Resid:** Therapeutic Radiology, Mass Genl Hosp 1981; **Fac Appt:** Prof RadRO, Univ NC Sch Med

Sailer, Scott MD [RadRO] - **Spec Exp:** Head & Neck Cancer; Genitourinary Cancer; Pediatric Cancers; Pediatric Radiology; **Hospital:** WakeMed Cary, WakeMed New Bern; **Address:** 300 Ashville Ave, Ste 110, Cary, NC 27518; **Phone:** 919-854-4588; **Board Cert:** Radiation Oncology 1988; **Med School:** Harvard Med Sch 1984; **Resid:** Radiation Therapy, Mass Genl Hosp 1988

Shaw, Edward G MD [RadRO] - **Spec Exp:** Stereotactic Radiosurgery; Brain Tumors; **Hospital:** Wake Forest Univ Baptist Med Ctr (page 72); **Address:** Wake Forest Med Ctr, Dept Rad Onc, Medical Center Blvd, Comp Cancer Ctr, Winston-Salem, NC 27157-1029; **Phone:** 336-713-6506; **Board Cert:** Radiation Oncology 1987; **Med School:** Rush Med Coll 1983; **Resid:** Radiation Oncology, Mayo Grad Sch Med 1987; **Fac Appt:** Prof RadRO, Wake Forest Univ

Tepper, Joel E MD [RadRO] - **Spec Exp:** Gastrointestinal Cancer; Sarcoma; Rectal Cancer; **Hospital:** Univ NC Hosps; **Address:** North Carolina Clin Cancer Ctr, Dept Rad Onc - CB#7512, Chapel Hill, NC 27599-7512; **Phone:** 919-966-0400; **Board Cert:** Therapeutic Radiology 1976; **Med School:** Washington Univ, St Louis 1972; **Resid:** Therapeutic Radiology, Mass Genl Hosp 1976; **Fellow:** Therapeutic Radiology, Mass Genl Hosp 1977; **Fac Appt:** Prof RadRO, Univ NC Sch Med

Toonkel, Leonard M MD [RadRO] - **Spec Exp:** Prostate Cancer; Breast Cancer; Brachytherapy; **Hospital:** Mount Sinai Med Ctr - Miami; **Address:** Dept Radiation Oncology, 4300 Alton Rd, Miami Beach, FL 33140; **Phone:** 305-535-3400; **Board Cert:** Therapeutic Radiology 1979; **Med School:** Univ Miami Sch Med 1975; **Resid:** Radiation Therapy, Jackson Meml Hosp 1977; Diagnostic Radiology, MD Anderson Hosp 1978; **Fellow:** Radiation Oncology, MD Anderson Hosp 1979; **Fac Appt:** Assoc Clin Prof Rad, Univ Miami Sch Med

Vijayakumar, Srinivasan MD [RadRO] - **Spec Exp:** Brachytherapy; Prostate Cancer; **Hospital:** Univ Mississippi Med Ctr; **Address:** 2500 N State St, Jackson, MS 39216; **Phone:** 601-815-2005; **Board Cert:** Therapeutic Radiology 1986; **Med School:** India 1978; **Resid:** Radiation Oncology, Madras Univ Med Ctr 1981; Radiation Oncology, Michael Reese Hosp 1984; **Fellow:** Brachytherapy, Univ Chicago Hosps 1985; **Fac Appt:** Prof RadRO, Univ Miss

Willett, Christopher MD [RadRO] - **Spec Exp:** Gastrointestinal Cancer; Clinical Trials; **Hospital:** Duke Univ Med Ctr; **Address:** Duke Univ Med Ctr, PO Box 3085, Durham, NC 27710; **Phone:** 919-668-5640; **Board Cert:** Therapeutic Radiology 1985; **Med School:** Tufts Univ 1981; **Resid:** Radiation Oncology, Mass Genl Hosp 1986; **Fac Appt:** Prof RadRO, Duke Univ

Wolfson, Aaron H MD [RadRO] - **Spec Exp:** Bone Tumors; Sarcoma-Soft Tissue; **Hospital:** Univ of Miami Hosp & Clins/Sylvester Comp Canc Ctr (page 70); **Address:** Univ of Miami Sylvester Comp Cancer Ctr, 1475 NW 12th Ave, Box D31, Miami, FL 33101; **Phone:** 305-243-4319; **Board Cert:** Radiation Oncology 1999; **Med School:** Univ Fla Coll Med 1982; **Resid:** Radiation Oncology, Med Coll of Virginia 1989; **Fac Appt:** Prof RadRO, Univ Miami Sch Med

Midwest

Abrams, Ross A MD [RadRO] - **Spec Exp:** Gastrointestinal Cancer; Lymphoma; **Hospital:** Rush Univ Med Ctr; **Address:** Women's Center for Radiation Therapy, 500 S Paulina, Ground Floor Atrium, Chicago, IL 60612; **Phone:** 312-942-5751; **Board Cert:** Internal Medicine 1976; Medical Oncology 1979; Hematology 1982; Radiation Oncology 1987; **Med School:** Univ Pennsylvania 1973; **Resid:** Internal Medicine, Pennsylvania Hosp 1975; Hematology & Oncology, Hosp Univ Penn 1976; **Fellow:** Hematology & Oncology, Natl Cancer Inst 1978; Radiation Oncology, Med Coll Wisconsin 1987; **Fac Appt:** Prof RadRO, Rush Med Coll

Awan, Azhar M MD [RadRO] - **Spec Exp:** Brain Tumors; Prostate Cancer; Breast Cancer; **Hospital:** Univ of IL Med Ctr at Chicago; **Address:** La Grange Meml Hosp, Outpatient Care Ctr, Chicago, IL 60612; **Phone:** 312-996-3630; **Board Cert:** Radiation Oncology 1985; **Med School:** Loyola Univ-Stritch Sch Med 1981; **Resid:** Radiation Oncology, Rush Presby/St Luke's Med Ctr 1985; **Fac Appt:** Assoc Prof RadRO, Univ Chicago-Pritzker Sch Med

Ben-Josef, Edgar MD [RadRO] - **Spec Exp:** Bone Cancer; Gastrointestinal Cancer; Pancreatic Cancer; Intensity Modulated Radiotherapy (IMRT); **Hospital:** Univ Michigan Hlth Sys; **Address:** Univ of Mich Hosp, 1500 E Medical Ctr Drive, rm UH B2C490, Ann Arbor, MI 48109-0010; **Phone:** 734-936-8207; **Board Cert:** Radiation Oncology 1994; **Med School:** Israel 1986; **Resid:** Radiation Oncology, Wayne State Univ Hosp 1994; **Fellow:** Cancer Biology, Wayne State Univ Hosp 1995; **Fac Appt:** Assoc Prof RadRO, Univ Mich Med Sch

Bradley, Jeffrey D MD [RadRO] - **Spec Exp:** Lung Cancer; Esophageal Cancer; Thoracic Cancers; Clinical Trials; **Hospital:** Barnes-Jewish Hosp; **Address:** Siteman Cancer Ctr, 4921 Parkview Pl Fl LL, St Louis, MO 63110; **Phone:** 314-747-7236; **Board Cert:** Radiation Oncology 1998; **Med School:** Univ Ark 1993; **Resid:** Radiation Oncology, Univ Chicago 1998; **Fac Appt:** Assoc Prof RadRO, Washington Univ, St Louis

Buatti, John M MD [RadRO] - **Spec Exp:** Central Nervous System Cancer; **Hospital:** Univ Iowa Hosp & Clinics; **Address:** 200 Hawkins Drive, rm 01626, Iowa City, IA 52242; **Phone:** 319-356-2699; **Board Cert:** Radiation Oncology 1994; **Med School:** Georgetown Univ 1986; **Resid:** Internal Medicine, Georgetown Univ 1989; **Fellow:** Radiation Oncology, Univ Arizona 1993; **Fac Appt:** Prof RadRO, Univ Iowa Coll Med

Charboneau, J William MD [RadRO] - **Spec Exp:** Radiofrequency Tumor Ablation; Liver Cancer; Thyroid Cancer; **Hospital:** Mayo Med Ctr & Clin - Rochester; **Address:** Mayo Clinic Dept of Radiology, 200 First St SW, Rochester, MN 55905-0002; **Phone:** 507-284-2097; **Board Cert:** Diagnostic Radiology 1980; **Med School:** Univ Wisc 1976; **Resid:** Diagnostic Radiology, Mayo Clinic 1980; **Fac Appt:** Prof, Mayo Med Sch

Ciezki, Jay P MD [RadRO] - **Spec Exp:** Brachytherapy; Prostate Cancer; Genitourinary Cancer; **Hospital:** Cleveland Clin Fdn (page 56); **Address:** Cleveland Clinic Fdn, 9500 Euclid Ave, MC T28, Cleveland, OH 44195; **Phone:** 216-445-9465; **Board Cert:** Radiation Oncology 2005; **Med School:** Med Coll Wisc 1991; **Resid:** Radiation Oncology, Cleveland Clinic 1995; **Fellow:** Brachytherapy, Cleveland Clinic 1996

Emami, Bahman MD [RadRO] - **Spec Exp:** Head & Neck Cancer; Lung Cancer; **Hospital:** Loyola Univ Med Ctr, Hines VA Hosp; **Address:** Loyola Univ Med Ctr, Dept Rad Onc, 2160 S First Ave Bldg 105 - rm 2932, Maywood, IL 60153-3328; **Phone:** 708-216-2729; **Board Cert:** Therapeutic Radiology 1976; **Med School:** Iran 1968; **Resid:** Radiation Therapy, St Vincents Hosp 1973; Radiation Therapy, New England Med Ctr 1977; **Fac Appt:** Prof RadRO, Loyola Univ-Stritch Sch Med

Forman, Jeffrey D MD [RadRO] - **Spec Exp:** Neutron Therapy for Advanced Cancer; Genitourinary Cancer; Prostate Cancer; **Address:** 70 Fulton St, Pontiac, MI 48341; **Phone:** 248-338-0300; **Board Cert:** Radiation Oncology 1986; **Med School:** NYU Sch Med 1982; **Resid:** Radiation Oncology, Johns Hopkins Hosp 1986; **Fellow:** Therapeutic Radiology, Johns Hopkins Hosp 1987; **Fac Appt:** Prof RadRO, Wayne State Univ

Grigsby, Perry W MD [RadRO] - **Spec Exp:** Gynecologic Cancer; Thyroid Cancer; **Hospital:** Barnes-Jewish Hosp, St Louis Chldns Hosp; **Address:** Washington Univ School Med, Dept Rad Onc, 4921 Parkview Pl, Box 8224, St Louis, MO 63110; **Phone:** 314-747-7236; **Board Cert:** Radiation Oncology 1987; **Med School:** Univ KY Coll Med 1982; **Resid:** Radiation Oncology, Barnes Jewish Hosp 1985; **Fac Appt:** Prof, Washington Univ, St Louis

Halpern, Howard MD/PhD [RadRO] - **Spec Exp:** Breast Cancer; Esophageal Cancer; Gynecologic Cancer; **Hospital:** Univ of Chicago Med Ctr, Univ of IL Med Ctr at Chicago; **Address:** 1801 W Taylor St, rm C400, MC-933, Chicago, IL 60612; **Phone:** 773-702-0817; **Board Cert:** Therapeutic Radiology 1984; **Med School:** Univ Miami Sch Med 1980; **Resid:** Therapeutic Radiology, Jnt Ctr Rad Ther Harvard 1984; **Fellow:** Therapeutic Radiology, Jnt Ctr Rad Ther Harvard 1985; **Fac Appt:** Prof Rad, Univ Chicago-Pritzker Sch Med

Haraf, Daniel J MD [RadRO] - **Spec Exp:** Head & Neck Cancer; Lung Cancer; Prostate Cancer; **Hospital:** Univ of Chicago Med Ctr; **Address:** Univ Chicago Hosps, Dept Rad Oncology, 5758 S Maryland, MS 9006, Chicago, IL 60637; **Phone:** 773-702-6870; **Board Cert:** Internal Medicine 1985; Radiation Oncology 1990; **Med School:** Ros Franklin Univ/Chicago Med Sch 1982; **Resid:** Internal Medicine, Michael Reese Hosp 1985; **Fellow:** Radiation Oncology, Michael Reese Hosp 1988; **Fac Appt:** Prof RadRO, Univ Chicago-Pritzker Sch Med

Harari, Paul M MD [RadRO] - **Spec Exp:** Head & Neck Cancer; **Hospital:** Univ WI Hosp & Clins; **Address:** Dept of Human Oncology, 600 Highland Ave, Ste K4/336, Madison, WI 53792; **Phone:** 608-263-5009; **Board Cert:** Radiation Oncology 1990; **Med School:** Univ VA Sch Med 1984; **Resid:** Radiation Oncology, Univ Arizona Med Ctr 1990; **Fac Appt:** Prof RadRO, Univ Wisc

Hayman, James A MD [RadRO] - **Spec Exp:** Breast Cancer; Stomach Cancer; Lung Cancer; Brain Tumors; **Hospital:** Univ Michigan Hlth Sys; **Address:** Univ Michigan Hosp, 1500 E Medical Ctr Drive, rm UH B2C490, Ann Arbor, MI 48109-0010; **Phone:** 734-647-9956; **Board Cert:** Radiation Oncology 2004; **Med School:** Univ Chicago-Pritzker Sch Med 1991; **Resid:** Radiation Therapy, Joint Ctr for Radiation Therapy 1996; **Fac Appt:** Assoc Prof RadRO, Univ Mich Med Sch

Kim, Jae Ho MD [RadRO] - **Spec Exp:** Brain Tumors; Spinal Cord Tumors; Breast Cancer; Lymphoma; **Hospital:** Henry Ford Hosp; **Address:** Radiation Oncology, 2799 W Grand Blvd, Detroit, MI 48202; **Phone:** 313-916-1029; **Board Cert:** Therapeutic Radiology 1973; **Med School:** Korea 1959; **Resid:** Therapeutic Radiology, Meml-Sloan-Kettering 1972; **Fellow:** Diagnostic Radiology, Meml-Sloan-Kettering 1968; **Fac Appt:** Prof RadRO, Wayne State Univ

Konski, Andre MD [RadRO] - **Spec Exp:** Esophageal Cancer; Rectal Cancer; Pancreatic Cancer; Gastrointestinal Cancer; **Hospital:** Karmanos Cancer Inst; **Address:** Dept Radiation Oncology, 4100 John R, Detroit, MI 48201; **Phone:** 313-745-2560; **Board Cert:** Radiation Oncology 2000; **Med School:** NY Med Coll 1984; **Resid:** Radiation Oncology, Stong Meml/Genesee Hosps 1988; **Fac Appt:** Prof RadRO, Wayne State Univ

Lawrence, Theodore S MD/PhD [RadRO] - **Spec Exp:** Gastrointestinal Cancer; Liver Cancer; Pancreatic Cancer; **Hospital:** Univ Michigan Hlth Sys; **Address:** Univ of Mich Hosp, Dept Rad Onc, 1500 E Med Ctr Dr, SPC5010, Box 5010, UH-B2-C502, Ann Arbor, MI 48109-5010; **Phone:** 734-936-4300; **Board Cert:** Internal Medicine 1983; Medical Oncology 1985; Radiation Oncology 1987; **Med School:** Cornell Univ-Weill Med Coll 1980; **Resid:** Internal Medicine, Stanford Univ Hosp 1983; Radiation Oncology, Natl Cancer Inst 1987; **Fellow:** Medical Oncology, Natl Cancer Inst 1986; **Fac Appt:** Prof RadRO, Univ Mich Med Sch

Lee, Chung K MD [RadRO] - **Spec Exp:** Head & Neck Cancer; Breast Cancer; Lymphoma; Gastrointestinal Cancer; **Hospital:** Univ Minn Med Ctr, Fairview - Univ Campus; **Address:** Dept of Radiation Oncology, 420 Delaware St SE, MMC 400, Minneapolis, MN 55455; **Phone:** 612-273-6700; **Board Cert:** Therapeutic Radiology 1976; **Med School:** Korea 1965; **Resid:** Therapeutic Radiology, Univ of Minn Hosp 1976; Diagnostic Radiology, Yonsei Univ Hosp 1971; **Fac Appt:** Prof, Univ Minn

Macklis, Roger M MD [RadRO] - **Spec Exp:** Radioimmunotherapy of Cancer; Breast Cancer; Lymphoma; **Hospital:** Cleveland Clin Fdn (page 56); **Address:** Cleveland Cin Fdn, Dept Rad Onc, 9500 Euclid Ave, Desk T28, Cleveland, OH 44195; **Phone:** 216-444-5576; **Board Cert:** Radiation Oncology 1989; **Med School:** Harvard Med Sch 1983; **Resid:** Radiation Oncology, Joint Ctr Radiotherapy Inst 1987; **Fellow:** Research, Dana Farber Cancer Inst 1987; **Fac Appt:** Prof RadRO, Case West Res Univ

Martenson Jr, James A MD [RadRO] - **Spec Exp:** Mucositis; Esophageal Cancer; **Hospital:** Mayo Med Ctr & Clin - Rochester; **Address:** Mayo Clinic, Dept Rad/Onc, 200 First St SW, Rochester, MN 55905; **Phone:** 507-284-4561; **Board Cert:** Therapeutic Radiology 1985; **Med School:** Univ Wash 1981; **Resid:** Radiation Oncology, Mayo Clinic 1985; **Fac Appt:** Assoc Prof, Mayo Med Sch

Mehta, Minesh P MD [RadRO] - **Spec Exp:** Brain Tumors; Lung Cancer; Pediatric Cancers; **Hospital:** Univ WI Hosp & Clins; **Address:** Univ Wisconsin, Dept Rad Oncology, 600 Highland Ave, K4B-100, Madison, WI 53792; **Phone:** 608-263-8500; **Board Cert:** Radiation Oncology 1988; **Med School:** Zambia 1981; **Resid:** Internal Medicine, Ndola Central Hosp 1983; Radiation Oncology, Univ WI Hosps 1988; **Fac Appt:** Prof RadRO, Univ Wisc

Michalski, Jeff M MD [RadRO] - **Spec Exp:** Prostate Cancer; Sarcoma; Pediatric Cancers; **Hospital:** Barnes-Jewish Hosp, St Louis Chldns Hosp; **Address:** Washington Univ Sch Med, Dept Rad Oncology, 4921 Parkview Place, Lower Level, Box 8224, St Louis, MO 63110; **Phone:** 314-747-7236; **Board Cert:** Radiation Oncology 1991; **Med School:** Med Coll Wisc 1986; **Resid:** Radiation Oncology, Columbia Presby Med Ctr 1988; Radiation Oncology, Mallinckrodt Inst of Radiology 1990; **Fellow:** Radiation Oncology, Mallinckrodt Inst of Radiology 1991; **Fac Appt:** Assoc Prof RadRO, Washington Univ, St Louis

Minsky, Bruce MD [RadRO] - **Spec Exp:** Gastrointestinal Cancer; Esophageal Cancer; Colon & Rectal Cancer; Pancreatic Cancer; **Hospital:** Univ of Chicago Med Ctr; **Address:** Univ Chicago Hosp, 5841 S Maryland Ave, MC 2004, Chicago, IL 60637; **Phone:** 773-834-1180; **Board Cert:** Radiation Oncology 1987; **Med School:** Univ Mass Sch Med 1982; **Resid:** Radiation Oncology, Harvard Jt Ctr Rad Ther 1986; **Fac Appt:** Prof RadRO, Univ Chicago-Pritzker Sch Med

Mittal, Bharat B MD [RadRO] - **Spec Exp:** Head & Neck Cancer; Lymphoma; Skin Cancer; **Hospital:** Northwestern Meml Hosp; **Address:** 251 E Huron St, Bldg LC-178, Chicago, IL 60611; **Phone:** 312-926-2520; **Board Cert:** Radiation Oncology 1981; **Med School:** India 1975; **Resid:** Internal Medicine, Christian Med Coll 1976; Radiation Oncology, Northwestern Meml Hosp 1980; **Fellow:** Radiation Oncology, Mallinckrodt Inst 1981; **Fac Appt:** Prof RadRO, Northwestern Univ

Radiation Oncology

Movsas, Benjamin MD [RadRO] - **Spec Exp:** Lung Cancer; Brain Tumors; Prostate Cancer; Stereotactic Radiosurgery; **Hospital:** Henry Ford Hosp; **Address:** Henry Ford Health Sys, Rad Oncology, 2799 W Grand Blvd, Detroit, MI 48202-2608; **Phone:** 313-916-5188; **Board Cert:** Radiation Oncology 1999; **Med School:** Washington Univ, St Louis 1990; **Resid:** Radiation Oncology, National Cancer Inst 1995

Myerson, Robert J MD [RadRO] - **Spec Exp:** Gastrointestinal Cancer; Breast Cancer; Hyperthermia Treatment of Cancer; **Hospital:** Barnes-Jewish Hosp; **Address:** Ctr for Advanced Med-Siteman Cancer Ctr, 4921 Parkview Pl, Box 9038635, St Louis, MO 63110; **Phone:** 314-747-7236; **Board Cert:** Therapeutic Radiology 1985; **Med School:** Univ Miami Sch Med 1980; **Resid:** Radiation Therapy, Hosp Univ Penn 1984; **Fac Appt:** Prof RadRO, Washington Univ, St Louis

Pierce, Lori J MD [RadRO] - **Spec Exp:** Breast Cancer; **Hospital:** Univ Michigan Hlth Sys; **Address:** Univ Hosp, Dept Rad Onc, 1500 E Med Ctr, rm B2C440, Box 5010, Ann Arbor, MI 48109-5099; **Phone:** 734-936-4300; **Board Cert:** Radiation Oncology 1989; **Med School:** Duke Univ 1985; **Resid:** Radiation Oncology, Hosp Univ Penn 1989; **Fac Appt:** Prof RadRO, Univ Mich Med Sch

Schomberg, Paula J MD [RadRO] - **Spec Exp:** Brain Tumors; Pediatric Cancers; **Hospital:** Mayo Med Ctr & Clin - Rochester; **Address:** Mayo Clinic - Charlton Bldg, Desk R, 200 1st St SW, Rochester, MN 55905; **Phone:** 507-284-3551; **Board Cert:** Therapeutic Radiology 1984; **Med School:** Med Coll Wisc 1979; **Resid:** Radiation Therapy, Mayo Clinic 1983; **Fac Appt:** Prof RadRO, Mayo Med Sch

Small Jr, William MD [RadRO] - **Spec Exp:** Gynecologic Cancer; Gastrointestinal Cancer; Breast Cancer; Pancreatic Cancer; **Hospital:** Northwestern Meml Hosp; **Address:** Northwestern Meml Hosp, Rad Oncology, 250 E Huron St Galter Bldg - Ste L178, Chicago, IL 60611; **Phone:** 312-472-3650; **Board Cert:** Radiation Oncology 2004; **Med School:** Northwestern Univ 1990; **Resid:** Radiation Oncology, Northwestern Univ 1994; **Fac Appt:** Prof RadRO, Northwestern Univ

Suh, John H MD [RadRO] - **Spec Exp:** Brain Tumors-Adult & Pediatric; Stereotactic Radiosurgery; Stereotactic Body Radiation Therapy; **Hospital:** Cleveland Clin Fdn (page 56); **Address:** Cleveland Clinic, Dept Rad/Onc, 9500 Euclid Ave, Desk T28, Cleveland, OH 44195-0001; **Phone:** 216-444-5574; **Board Cert:** Radiation Oncology 2000; **Med School:** Univ Miami Sch Med 1990; **Resid:** Radiation Oncology, Cleveland Clinic 1994; **Fellow:** Radiation Oncology, Cleveland Clinic 1995

Taylor, Marie E MD [RadRO] - **Spec Exp:** Breast Cancer; **Hospital:** Barnes-Jewish Hosp, Barnes-Jewish West County Hosp; **Address:** Center for Advanced Med-Siteman Cancer Ctr, 4921 Parkview Pl, Box 8224, St Louis, MO 63110; **Phone:** 314-747-7236; **Board Cert:** Radiation Oncology 1987; **Med School:** Univ Wash 1982; **Resid:** Radiation Oncology, Univ Wash Med Ctr 1986

Thornton Jr, Allan F MD [RadRO] - **Spec Exp:** Proton Beam Therapy; **Address:** Midwest Proton Radiotherapy Inst, 2425 N Milo B Sampson Lane, Bloomington, IN 47408; **Phone:** 812-349-5074; **Board Cert:** Radiation Oncology 1999; **Med School:** Univ VA Sch Med 1981; **Resid:** Radiation Oncology, Princess Margaret Hosp 1986

Vicini, Frank A MD [RadRO] - **Spec Exp:** Breast Cancer; Prostate Cancer; Brachytherapy; **Hospital:** William Beaumont Hosp; **Address:** William Beaumont Hospital, 3601 W 13 Mile Rd, Royal Oak, MI 48073; **Phone:** 248-551-1219; **Board Cert:** Radiation Oncology 1999; **Med School:** Wayne State Univ 1985; **Resid:** Radiation Oncology, William Beaumont Hosp 1989; **Fellow:** Radiation Oncology, Harvard Med Sch/Joint Ctr for Rad Ther 1990; **Fac Appt:** Clin Prof RadRO, Univ Mich Med Sch

Videtic, Gregory M MD [RadRO] - **Spec Exp:** Lung Cancer; Mesothelioma; Esophageal Cancer; Thymoma; **Hospital:** Cleveland Clin Fdn (page 56); **Address:** Cleveland Clinic, Radiation Oncology, 9500 Euclid Ave, MC T28, Cleveland, OH 44195; **Phone:** 216-444-9797; **Board Cert:** Radiation Oncology 1998; **Med School:** McGill Univ 1986; **Resid:** Radiation Oncology, Dalhousie Univ 1988; Radiation Oncology, London Regl Cancer Ctr 1997; **Fellow:** Radiation Oncology, Wayne State Univ 1998; **Fac Appt:** Assoc Prof Rad, Cleveland Cl Coll Med/Case West Res

Weichselbaum, Ralph R MD [RadRO] - **Spec Exp:** Gene Targeted Radiotherapy; Head & Neck Cancer; Esophageal Cancer; **Hospital:** Univ of Chicago Med Ctr; **Address:** Univ Chicago, Dept Rad Onc, 5758 S Maryland Ave, MC-9006-DCAM-1D, Chicago, IL 60637; **Phone:** 773-702-0817; **Board Cert:** Therapeutic Radiology 1975; **Med School:** Univ IL Coll Med 1971; **Resid:** Therapeutic Radiology, Harvard Jt Ctr Rad Therapy 1975; **Fellow:** Diagnostic Radiology, Harvard Med Sch 1976; **Fac Appt:** Prof Rad, Univ Chicago-Pritzker Sch Med

Wilson, J Frank MD [RadRO] - **Spec Exp:** Breast Cancer; Skin Cancer; **Hospital:** Froedtert Meml Lutheran Hosp; **Address:** Dept Radiation Oncology, 9200 W Wisconsin Ave, Milwaukee, WI 53226; **Phone:** 414-805-4400; **Board Cert:** Therapeutic Radiology 1971; **Med School:** Univ MO-Columbia Sch Med 1965; **Resid:** Radiation Therapy, Penrose Cancer Hosp 1969; **Fellow:** Radiation Therapy, Natl Cancer Inst/NIH 1971; **Fac Appt:** Prof RadRO, Med Coll Wisc

Great Plains and Mountains

Gaffney, David K MD/PhD [RadRO] - **Spec Exp:** Breast Cancer; Gynecologic Cancer; **Hospital:** Univ Utah Hosps and Clins; **Address:** Huntsman Cancer Hosp, Dept Rad Oncology, 1950 Circle of Hope, rm 1440, Salt Lake City, UT 84112-5560; **Phone:** 801-581-2396; **Board Cert:** Radiation Oncology 2007; **Med School:** Med Coll Wisc 1992; **Resid:** Radiation Oncology, Univ Utah Hosps 1996; **Fac Appt:** Assoc Prof, Univ Utah

Rabinovitch, Rachel A MD [RadRO] - **Spec Exp:** Breast Cancer; Lymphoma; **Hospital:** Univ Colorado Hosp; **Address:** Anschutz Cancer Pavilion, Dept Rad Oncology, 1665 Aurora Court, Ste 1032, MS F-706, Aurora, CO 80045; **Phone:** 720-848-0156; **Board Cert:** Radiation Oncology 1994; **Med School:** Albert Einstein Coll Med 1989; **Resid:** Radiation Oncology, Meml Sloan Kettering Cancer Ctr 1993; **Fac Appt:** Assoc Prof RadRO, Univ Colorado

Shrieve, Dennis C MD [RadRO] - **Spec Exp:** Brain Tumors-Adult & Pediatric; Genitourinary Cancer; Gastrointestinal Cancer; **Hospital:** Univ Utah Hosps and Clins, Primary Children's Med Ctr; **Address:** Huntsman Cancer Inst, Dept Rad Oncology, 1950 Circle of Hope, rm 1440, Salt Lake City, UT 84112; **Phone:** 801-581-2396; **Board Cert:** Radiation Oncology 1993; **Med School:** Univ Miami Sch Med 1989; **Resid:** Radiation Oncology, UCSF Med Ctr; **Fac Appt:** Prof RadRO, Univ Utah

Smalley, Stephen R MD [RadRO] - **Spec Exp:** Colon Cancer; Gastrointestinal Cancer; **Hospital:** Olathe Med Ctr; **Address:** Olathe Med Ctr, 20375 W 151st St, Doctors Bldg - Ste 180, Olathe, KS 66061-4575; **Phone:** 913-768-7200; **Board Cert:** Internal Medicine 1982; Radiation Oncology 1987; Medical Oncology 1985; **Med School:** Univ MO-Kansas City 1979; **Resid:** Internal Medicine, Mayo Clinic 1982; Radiation Oncology, Mayo Clinic 1986; **Fellow:** Medical Oncology, Mayo Clinic 1984; **Fac Appt:** Prof RadRO, Univ Kans

Radiation Oncology

Southwest

Ang, Kie-Kian MD/PhD [RadRO] - **Spec Exp:** Head & Neck Cancer; **Hospital:** UT MD Anderson Cancer Ctr; **Address:** UT MD Anderson Cancer Ctr, 1515 Holcombe Blvd, Box 97, Houston, TX 77030; **Phone:** 713-563-8400; **Board Cert:** Radiation Oncology 1987; **Med School:** Belgium 1975; **Resid:** Radiation Oncology, Univ Hosp Louvian 1980; **Fac Appt:** Prof, Univ Tex, Houston

Buchholz, Thomas A MD [RadRO] - **Spec Exp:** Breast Cancer; **Hospital:** UT MD Anderson Cancer Ctr; **Address:** Univ Texas MD Anderson Cancer Ctr, 1515 Holcombe Blvd, Unit 97, Houston, TX 77030-4000; **Phone:** 713-794-4892; **Board Cert:** Radiation Oncology 1993; **Med School:** Tufts Univ 1988; **Resid:** Radiation Oncology, Univ Washington Med Ctr 1993; **Fellow:** Research, Univ Washington Med Ctr 1994; **Fac Appt:** Prof RadRO, Univ Tex, Houston

Choy, Hak MD [RadRO] - **Spec Exp:** Lung Cancer; **Hospital:** UT Southwestern Med Ctr at Dallas; **Address:** UT SW Med Ctr - Dallas, Dept Rad-Onc, 5801 Forest Park Rd, Dallas, TX 75390-9183; **Phone:** 214-645-7600; **Board Cert:** Radiation Oncology 1993; **Med School:** Univ Tex Med Br, Galveston 1987; **Resid:** Radiation Oncology, Ohio State Univ Hosp 1989; Radiation Oncology, Univ Texas Hlth Sci Ctr 1991; **Fac Appt:** Prof RadRO, Univ Tex SW, Dallas

Cox, James D MD [RadRO] - **Spec Exp:** Lung Cancer; Esophageal Cancer; Thymoma; Thoracic Cancers; **Hospital:** UT MD Anderson Cancer Ctr; **Address:** Univ Tex MD Anderson Cancer Ctr, 1515 Holcombe Blvd, Unit 97, Houston, TX 77030; **Phone:** 713-563-2316; **Board Cert:** Radiation Oncology 1999; **Med School:** Univ Rochester 1965; **Resid:** Diagnostic Radiology, Penrose Cancer Hosp 1969; **Fellow:** Therapeutic Radiology, Inst Gustave-Roussy 1970; **Fac Appt:** Prof RadRO, Univ Tex, Houston

Eifel, Patricia J MD [RadRO] - **Spec Exp:** Cervical Cancer; Uterine Cancer; Vulvar Disease/Cancer; Vaginal Cancer; **Hospital:** UT MD Anderson Cancer Ctr; **Address:** MD Anderson Cancer Ctr, Dept Rad Onc, 1515 Holcombe Blvd, Unit 1202, Houston, TX 77030-4009; **Phone:** 713-563-6830; **Board Cert:** Therapeutic Radiology 1983; **Med School:** Stanford Univ 1977; **Resid:** Radiation Oncology, Stanford Univ Med Ctr 1981; **Fellow:** Therapeutic Radiology, Stanford Univ Med Ctr 1982

Grado, Gordon L MD [RadRO] - **Spec Exp:** Prostate Cancer; Brachytherapy; **Hospital:** Scottsdale Hlthcare - Shea, Univ Minn Med Ctr, Fairview - Univ Campus; **Address:** 2926 N Civic Center Plaza, Scottsdale, AZ 85251; **Phone:** 480-614-6300; **Board Cert:** Therapeutic Radiology 1981; Radiation Oncology 1999; **Med School:** Southern IL Univ 1977; **Resid:** Therapeutic Radiology, Mayo Clinic 1981; **Fac Appt:** Assoc Prof RadRO, Univ Minn

Gunderson, Leonard MD [RadRO] - **Spec Exp:** Gastrointestinal Cancer; Brachytherapy; Sarcoma; **Hospital:** Mayo Clinic - Scottsdale; **Address:** Mayo Clinic, Dept Radiation Onc, 5777 E Mayo Blvd, Phoenix, AZ 85054; **Phone:** 480-342-1262; **Board Cert:** Therapeutic Radiology 1975; **Med School:** Univ KY Coll Med 1969; **Resid:** Radiation Oncology, Latter Day Saints Hosp 1974; **Fac Appt:** Prof RadRO, Mayo Med Sch

Herman, Terence S MD [RadRO] - **Spec Exp:** Breast Cancer; Sarcoma; Brain Tumors; **Hospital:** OU Med Ctr; **Address:** Oklahoma Univ Health Sci Ctr, 825 NE 10th St, OUPB 1430, Oklahoma City, OK 73104-5417; **Phone:** 405-271-5641; **Board Cert:** Internal Medicine 1975; Medical Oncology 1977; Therapeutic Radiology 1985; **Med School:** Univ Conn 1972; **Resid:** Internal Medicine, Univ Arizona Med Ctr 1975; Radiation Oncology, Stanford Univ Med Ctr 1985; **Fellow:** Medical Oncology, Univ Arizona 1977; **Fac Appt:** Prof RadRO, Univ Okla Coll Med

Jhingran, Anuja MD [RadRO] - **Spec Exp:** Gynecologic Cancer; Brachytherapy; **Hospital:** UT MD Anderson Cancer Ctr; **Address:** MD Anderson Cancer Ctr, 1515 Holcombe Ave, Box 1202, Houston, TX 77030; **Phone:** 713-563-6900; **Board Cert:** Radiation Oncology 1993; **Med School:** Texas Tech Univ 1988; **Resid:** Radiation Oncology, Baylor College Med 1993; **Fac Appt:** Assoc Prof RadRO, Univ Tex, Houston

Komaki, Ritsuko U MD [RadRO] - **Spec Exp:** Lung Cancer; Thymoma; Esophageal Cancer; **Hospital:** UT MD Anderson Cancer Ctr; **Address:** UT-MD Anderson Cancer Ctr, Dept Rad Onc, 1515 Holcombe Blvd, Unit 97, Houston, TX 77030; **Phone:** 713-563-2300; **Board Cert:** Therapeutic Radiology 1977; Radiation Oncology 2001; **Med School:** Japan 1969; **Resid:** Radiation Oncology, Med Coll Wisc 1978; **Fac Appt:** Prof RadRO, Univ Tex, Houston

Kuske, Robert R MD [RadRO] - **Spec Exp:** Breast Cancer; **Hospital:** Scottsdale Hlthcare - Shea; **Address:** 9055 E Del Camino Drive, Ste 200, Scottsdale, AZ 85258; **Phone:** 480-922-4600; **Board Cert:** Therapeutic Radiology 1985; **Med School:** Univ Cincinnati 1980; **Resid:** Radiation Oncology, Univ Cincinnati Med Ctr 1984

Lee, Andrew K MD [RadRO] - **Spec Exp:** Prostate Cancer; Proton Beam Therapy; Genitourinary Cancer; **Hospital:** UT MD Anderson Cancer Ctr; **Address:** MD Anderson Cancer Ctr, 1515 Holcombe Blvd, Unit 1202, Houston, TX 77030; **Phone:** 713-563-2443; **Board Cert:** Radiation Oncology 2001; **Med School:** Univ Minn 1996; **Resid:** Radiation Oncology, Joint Ctr for Radiation Therapy/Harvard 2001; **Fac Appt:** Assoc Prof RadRO, Univ Tex, Houston

Medbery, Clinton A MD [RadRO] - **Spec Exp:** Breast Cancer; Prostate Cancer; Brachytherapy; Stereotactic Radiosurgery; **Hospital:** St Anthony Hosp -Oklahoma City; **Address:** Southwest Radiation Oncology, 1011 N Dewey Ave, Ste 101, Oklahoma City, OK 73101; **Phone:** 405-272-7311; **Board Cert:** Internal Medicine 1980; Medical Oncology 1983; Radiation Oncology 1987; **Med School:** Med Univ SC 1976; **Resid:** Internal Medicine, Naval Hosp 1980; Radiation Oncology, Natl Cancer Inst 1987; **Fellow:** Medical Oncology, Naval Hosp 1982

Schild, Steven E MD [RadRO] - **Spec Exp:** Lung Cancer; Brain Tumors; Gastrointestinal Cancer; Clinical Trials; **Hospital:** Mayo Clinic - Scottsdale; **Address:** Mayo Clinic, Dept Radiation Oncology, 13400 E Shea Blvd, Scottsdale, AZ 85259; **Phone:** 480-342-1262; **Board Cert:** Radiation Oncology 1989; **Med School:** Creighton Univ 1985; **Resid:** Radiation Oncology, Mayo Clinic 1989; **Fac Appt:** Prof RadRO, Mayo Med Sch

Senzer, Neil N MD [RadRO] - **Spec Exp:** Clinical Trials; Gene Targeted Radiotherapy; Gene Therapy; **Hospital:** Med City Dallas Hosp, Baylor Univ Medical Ctr; **Address:** Mary Crowley Cancer Research Ctr, 7777 Forest Ln C Bldg - Ste 707, Dallas, TX 75230; **Phone:** 214-370-1870; **Board Cert:** Pediatrics 1976; Pediatric Hematology-Oncology 1978; Therapeutic Radiology 1985; **Med School:** SUNY Buffalo 1971; **Resid:** Pediatrics, Johns Hopkins Hosp 1974; Radiation Oncology, St Barnabas Med Ctr 1985; **Fellow:** Pediatric Hematology-Oncology, St Jude Chldns Rsch Hosp 1978

Shina, Donald C MD [RadRO] - **Spec Exp:** Breast Cancer; **Hospital:** St Vincent Hosp - Santa Fe; **Address:** Santa Fe Cancer Ctr at St Vincent Hosp, 455 Saint Michael's Drive, Santa Fe, NM 87505; **Phone:** 505-820-5233; **Board Cert:** Internal Medicine 1977; Medical Oncology 1979; Therapeutic Radiology 1981; **Med School:** Case West Res Univ 1974; **Resid:** Internal Medicine, Univ Hosps 1977; **Fellow:** Radiation Oncology, Univ Hosps 1980; Medical Oncology, Univ Hosps 1980

Stea, Baldassarre MD/PhD [RadRO] - **Spec Exp:** Brain Tumors; Stereotactic Radiosurgery; Pediatric Cancers; **Hospital:** Univ Med Ctr - Tucson, Tucson Med Ctr; **Address:** Univ Hlth Scis Ctr, Dept Rad Onc, 1501 N Campbell Ave, Tucson, AZ 85724-0001; **Phone:** 520-626-6724; **Board Cert:** Radiation Oncology 1987; **Med School:** Geo Wash Univ 1983; **Resid:** Radiation Oncology, Natl Cancer Inst 1987; **Fac Appt:** Prof RadRO, Univ Ariz Coll Med

Radiation Oncology

Woo, Shiao Y MD [RadRO] - **Spec Exp:** Brain Tumors-Adult & Pediatric; Proton Beam Therapy; Stereotactic Radiosurgery; Pediatric Cancers; **Hospital:** UT MD Anderson Cancer Ctr, Texas Chldns Hosp; **Address:** UT-MD Anderson Cancer Ctr, 1515 Holcombe, Box 1150, Unit 97, Houston, TX 77030; **Phone:** 713-563-2324; **Board Cert:** Radiation Oncology 1988; Pediatrics 1980; **Med School:** Malaysia 1972; **Resid:** Pediatrics, Georgetown Univ Hosp 1978; **Fellow:** Pediatric Hematology-Oncology, Georgetown Univ Hosp 1980; Radiation Oncology, Georgetown Univ Hosp 1988; **Fac Appt:** Prof RadRO, Baylor Coll Med

West Coast and Pacific

Bahn, Duke K MD [RadRO] - **Spec Exp:** Prostate Cancer-Cryosurgery; Ultrasound; **Hospital:** Comm Meml Hosp - Ventura; **Address:** Prostate Inst of America, 168 N Brent St, Ste 402, Ventura, CA 93003; **Phone:** 805-585-3082; **Board Cert:** Diagnostic Radiology 1978; **Med School:** Korea 1970; **Resid:** Diagnostic Radiology, Wayne State Univ Med Ctr 1978

Donaldson, Sarah S MD [RadRO] - **Spec Exp:** Pediatric Cancers; Hodgkin's Disease; **Hospital:** Stanford Univ Med Ctr; **Address:** 875 Blake Wilbur Drive, CC Bldg Fl G - rm 226, MC 5847, Stanford, CA 94305-5847; **Phone:** 650-723-6195; **Board Cert:** Therapeutic Radiology 1974; **Med School:** Harvard Med Sch 1968; **Resid:** Radiation Oncology, Stanford Univ Med Ctr 1972; **Fellow:** Pediatric Hematology-Oncology, Inst Gustave-Roussy 1973; Pediatric Hematology-Oncology, MD Anderson Cancer Ctr 1971; **Fac Appt:** Prof RadRO, Stanford Univ

Douglas, James G MD [RadRO] - **Spec Exp:** Pediatric Cancers; Head & Neck Cancer; Brain Tumors; **Hospital:** Univ Wash Med Ctr, Chldns Hosp and Regl Med Ctr - Seattle; **Address:** Univ Washington Med Ctr, Dept Radiation Onc, 1959 NE Pacific St, Box 356043, Seattle, WA 98195-6043; **Phone:** 206-598-4100; **Board Cert:** Pediatrics 1986; Radiation Oncology 2007; **Med School:** Case West Res Univ 1980; **Resid:** Pediatrics, Children's Hosp Med Ctr 1983; Radiation Oncology, Univ Washington Med Ctr 1996; **Fellow:** Pediatric Hematology-Oncology, Natl Inst Hlth 1986; **Fac Appt:** Assoc Prof RadRO, Univ Wash

Fowble, Barbara MD [RadRO] - **Spec Exp:** Breast Cancer; **Hospital:** UCSF Med Ctr; **Address:** 1600 Divisiadero St, Ste H1031, 7701 Burholme Ave, San Francisco, CA 94143-1708; **Phone:** 415-353-9819; **Board Cert:** Therapeutic Radiology 1976; **Med School:** Jefferson Med Coll 1972; **Resid:** Therapeutic Radiology, Bellevue Hosp Ctr-NYU 1975; Therapeutic Radiology, Hahnemann 1976; **Fellow:** Radiation Therapy, Jefferson Hosp 1977; **Fac Appt:** Prof RadRO, UCSF

Halberg, Francine MD [RadRO] - **Spec Exp:** Breast Cancer; **Hospital:** Marin Genl Hosp, UCSF Med Ctr; **Address:** Marin Cancer Inst-Dept of Rad.Oncology, 1350 S Eliseo Drive, Ste 100, Greenbrae, CA 94904; **Phone:** 415-925-7326; **Board Cert:** Internal Medicine 1981; Therapeutic Radiology 1984; **Med School:** Cornell Univ-Weill Med Coll 1978; **Resid:** Internal Medicine, USPHS Hosp 1981; **Fellow:** Radiation Oncology, Stanford Univ Med Ctr 1984; **Fac Appt:** Assoc Prof RadRO, UCSF

Hancock, Steven MD [RadRO] - **Spec Exp:** Prostate Cancer; Breast Cancer; Cancer Survivors-Late Effects of Therapy; **Hospital:** Stanford Univ Med Ctr; **Address:** Stanford Cancer Center-Dept Rad Onc, 875 Blake Wilbur Drive, MC 5847, Stanford, CA 94305; **Phone:** 650-723-6440; **Board Cert:** Internal Medicine 1980; Therapeutic Radiology 1982; **Med School:** Stanford Univ 1976; **Resid:** Radiation Therapy, Stanford Univ Med Ctr 1981; Internal Medicine, Stanford Univ Med Ctr 1979; **Fac Appt:** Prof RadRO, Stanford Univ

Hoppe, Richard T MD [RadRO] - **Spec Exp:** Lymphoma; Hodgkin's Disease; **Hospital:** Stanford Univ Med Ctr; **Address:** Stanford Cancer Ctr, Dept Rad Onc, 875 Blake Wilbur, MC 5847, Stanford, CA 94305-5847; **Phone:** 650-723-5510; **Board Cert:** Therapeutic Radiology 1976; **Med School:** Cornell Univ-Weill Med Coll 1971; **Resid:** Radiation Therapy, Stanford Univ Med Ctr 1976; **Fac Appt:** Prof, Stanford Univ

Koh, Wui-Jin MD [RadRO] - **Spec Exp:** Gynecologic Cancer; Brachytherapy; Clinical Trials; **Hospital:** Univ Wash Med Ctr; **Address:** Univ Washington Med Ctr, Dept of Radiation Oncology, Box 356043, Seattle, WA 98195; **Phone:** 206-598-4121; **Board Cert:** Radiation Oncology 1988; **Med School:** Loma Linda Univ 1984; **Resid:** Radiation Oncology, Univ Washington Med Ctr 1988; **Fellow:** Tumor Imaging, Univ Washington Med Ctr 1988; **Fac Appt:** Prof RadRO, Univ Wash

Laramore, George E MD/PhD [RadRO] - **Spec Exp:** Neutron Therapy for Advanced Cancer; Salivary Gland Tumors; Head & Neck Cancer; Skin Cancer; **Hospital:** Univ Wash Med Ctr; **Address:** Univ Washington Med Ctr, Dept Rad Onc Box 356043, Seattle, WA 98195; **Phone:** 206-598-4110; **Board Cert:** Therapeutic Radiology 1980; Radiation Oncology 2000; **Med School:** Univ Miami Sch Med 1976; **Resid:** Radiation Oncology, Univ Washington 1980; **Fac Appt:** Prof RadRO, Univ Wash

Larson, David A MD/PhD [RadRO] - **Spec Exp:** Neuro-Oncology; Brain Tumors; Stereotactic Radiosurgery; **Hospital:** UCSF Med Ctr; **Address:** UCSF Med Ctr, Dept Rad Onc, 505 Parnassus Ave, rm L-75, San Francisco, CA 94143-0226; **Phone:** 415-353-8900; **Board Cert:** Therapeutic Radiology 1986; **Med School:** Univ Miami Sch Med 1981; **Resid:** Radiation Therapy, Joint Ctr RadTherapy 1985; **Fac Appt:** Prof RadRO, UCSF

Le, Quynh-Thu Xuan MD [RadRO] - **Spec Exp:** Head & Neck Cancer; Lung Cancer; Thoracic Cancers; Clinical Trials; **Hospital:** Stanford Univ Med Ctr; **Address:** Stanford Univ, Dept Rad Oncology, 875 Blake Wilbur Drive, MC 5847, Ground Flr, Stanford, CA 94305; **Phone:** 650-498-5032; **Board Cert:** Radiation Oncology 1998; **Med School:** UCSF 1993; **Resid:** Radiation Oncology, UCSF Med Ctr 1997; **Fac Appt:** Prof RadRO, Stanford Univ

Mundt, Arno J MD [RadRO] - **Spec Exp:** Gynecologic Cancer; Intensity Modulated Radiotherapy (IMRT); **Hospital:** UCSD Med Ctr; **Address:** Moores UCSD Cancer Ctr, Radiation Oncology Dept, 3855 Health Sciences Drive, MC 0843, La Jolla, CA 92093-0843; **Phone:** 858-822-6046; **Board Cert:** Radiation Oncology 1994; **Med School:** Univ Mich Med Sch 1987; **Resid:** Physical Medicine & Rehabilitation, George Washington Univ Hosp 1990; Radiation Oncology, Univ Chicago Hosps 1993; **Fellow:** Physical Medicine & Rehabilitation, Univ Chicago Hosps 1994; **Fac Appt:** Assoc Prof RadRO, Univ Chicago-Pritzker Sch Med

Park, Catherine C MD [RadRO] - **Spec Exp:** Breast Cancer; Lymphoma; **Hospital:** UCSF Med Ctr; **Address:** 1600 Divisadero St, Ste H1031, Box 1708, San Francisco, CA 94115; **Phone:** 415-353-7175; **Board Cert:** Radiation Oncology 2000; **Med School:** UCLA 1995; **Resid:** Radiation Oncology, Mass Genl Hosp 2000; **Fac Appt:** Assoc Prof RadRO, UCSF

Pezner, Richard D MD [RadRO] - **Spec Exp:** Sarcoma-Soft Tissue; Breast Cancer; Stereotactic Radiosurgery; **Hospital:** City of Hope Natl Med Ctr & Beckman Rsch; **Address:** City of Hope Med Ctr-Div Radiation Onc, 1500 E Duarte Rd, Duarte, CA 91010-3000; **Phone:** 626-301-8247; **Board Cert:** Therapeutic Radiology 1979; **Med School:** Northwestern Univ 1975; **Resid:** Radiation Oncology, Oregon Health Sci Ctr 1979; **Fac Appt:** Clin Prof RadRO, UC Irvine

Quivey, Jeanne M MD [RadRO] - **Spec Exp:** Head & Neck Cancer; Breast Cancer; Eye Tumors/Cancer; Intensity Modulated Radiotherapy (IMRT); **Hospital:** UCSF Med Ctr; **Address:** UCSF Med Ctr @ Mt Zion, Radiation Oncology Dept, 1600 Divisadero St, Ste H1031, San Francisco, CA 94115-3010; **Phone:** 415-353-7175; **Board Cert:** Therapeutic Radiology 1974; **Med School:** UCSF 1970; **Resid:** Radiation Therapy, UCSF Med Ctr 1974; **Fac Appt:** Prof RadRO, UCSF

Radiation Oncology

Roach III, Mack MD [RadRO] - **Spec Exp:** Prostate Cancer; Genitourinary Cancer; Lung Cancer; **Hospital:** UCSF - Mt Zion Med Ctr, UCSF Med Ctr; **Address:** UCSF Radiation Oncology, 1600 Divisadero St, Ste H1031, San Francisco, CA 94143-1708; **Phone:** 415-353-7181; **Board Cert:** Internal Medicine 1984; Medical Oncology 1985; Radiation Oncology 1987; **Med School:** Stanford Univ 1979; **Resid:** Internal Medicine, ML King Genl Hosp 1981; Radiation Oncology, Stanford Univ Med Ctr 1987; **Fellow:** Medical Oncology, UCSF Med Ctr 1983; **Fac Appt:** Prof RadRO, UCSF

Rose, Christopher M MD [RadRO] - **Spec Exp:** Prostate Cancer; Breast Cancer; Intensity Modulated Radiotherapy (IMRT); **Hospital:** Providence St Joseph Med Ctr; **Address:** Valley Radiotherapy Assocs, The Ctr for Radiation Therapy, 9229 Wilshire Blvd, Beverly Hills, CA 90210; **Phone:** 310-205-5777; **Board Cert:** Radiation Oncology 1999; **Med School:** Harvard Med Sch 1974; **Resid:** Internal Medicine, Beth Israel Deaconess 1976; Radiation Oncology, Joint Ctr Rad Therapy 1979; **Fellow:** Cancer Research, British Inst Cancer Rsch 1979; **Fac Appt:** Assoc Clin Prof RadRO, UCLA

Rossi, Carl John MD [RadRO] - **Spec Exp:** Prostate Cancer; Proton Beam Therapy; **Hospital:** Loma Linda Univ Med Ctr; **Address:** Loma Linda Univ Med Ctr, 11234 Anderson St, rm B124, Loma Linda, CA 92354; **Phone:** 909-558-4280; **Board Cert:** Radiation Oncology 1994; **Med School:** Loyola Univ-Stritch Sch Med 1988; **Resid:** Radiation Oncology, Loma Linda Univ Med Ctr 1992; **Fac Appt:** Asst Prof RadRO, Loma Linda Univ

Russell, Kenneth J MD [RadRO] - **Spec Exp:** Prostate Cancer; Lymphoma; Genitourinary Cancer; **Hospital:** Univ Wash Med Ctr; **Address:** Seattle Cancer Care Alliance, G1101, 825 Eastlake Ave E, Seattle, WA 98109; **Phone:** 206-288-7318; **Board Cert:** Therapeutic Radiology 1984; **Med School:** Harvard Med Sch 1979; **Resid:** Radiation Therapy, Stanford Univ Med Ctr 1983; **Fellow:** Radiological Biology, Stanford Univ Med Ctr 1985; **Fac Appt:** Prof Rad, Univ Wash

Sandler, Howard M MD [RadRO] - **Spec Exp:** Prostate Cancer; Genitourinary Cancer; Brain Tumors; **Hospital:** Cedars-Sinai Med Ctr; **Address:** S Oschin Comprehensive Cancer Inst, Cedars-Sinai Med Ctr, 8700 Beverly Blvd, Los Angeles, CA 90048; **Phone:** 310-423-4234; **Board Cert:** Radiation Oncology 1989; **Med School:** Univ Conn 1985; **Resid:** Radiation Oncology, Hosp Univ Penn 1989

Seung, Steven K MD/PhD [RadRO] - **Spec Exp:** Stereotactic Radiosurgery; Brain Tumors; Esophageal Cancer; Lung Cancer; **Hospital:** Providence Portland Med Ctr; **Address:** 4805 NE Glisan St, Garden Level, Portland, OR 97213; **Phone:** 503-215-6029; **Board Cert:** Radiation Oncology 1999; **Med School:** Univ Chicago-Pritzker Sch Med 1994; **Resid:** Radiation Oncology, UCSF Med Ctr 1998

Thomas, Charles R MD [RadRO] - **Hospital:** OR Hlth & Sci Univ; **Address:** 3181 SW Sam Jackson Park Rd, MC KPV4, Portland, OR 97239; **Phone:** 503-494-8756; **Board Cert:** Internal Medicine 1989; Radiation Oncology 1999; **Med School:** Univ IL Coll Med 1985; **Resid:** Internal Medicine, Baylor Coll Med 1988; Radiation Oncology, Univ Wash Med Ctr 1997; **Fellow:** Medical Oncology, Rush Univ Med Ctr 1999; **Fac Appt:** Prof RadRO, Oregon Hlth & Sci Univ

Tripuraneni, Prabhakar MD [RadRO] - **Spec Exp:** Prostate Cancer; Head & Neck Cancer; Lymphoma; **Hospital:** Scripps Green Hosp, Scripps Meml Hosp - La Jolla; **Address:** Scripps Clinic, Div Radiation Oncology, 10666 N Torrey Pines Rd, MSB 1, La Jolla, CA 92037; **Phone:** 858-554-2000; **Board Cert:** Therapeutic Radiology 1983; **Med School:** India 1976; **Resid:** Radiation Oncology, Univ Alberta 1981; Radiation Oncology, UCSF Med Ctr 1983; **Fac Appt:** Clin Prof RadRO, UCSD

Wara, William M MD [RadRO] - **Spec Exp:** Brain & Spinal Tumors; Sarcoma; Pediatric Cancers; **Hospital:** Kaiser Permanente S San Francisco Med Ctr; **Address:** Cancer Treatment Ctr, 220 Oyster Pt Blvd, San Francisco, CA 94080; **Phone:** 650-827-6500; **Board Cert:** Therapeutic Radiology 1974; **Med School:** UC Irvine 1969; **Resid:** Therapeutic Radiology, UCSF Medical Ctr 1973; **Fac Appt:** Prof RadRO, UCSF

Wong, Jeffrey Y C MD [RadRO] - **Spec Exp:** Radioimmunotherapy of Cancer; Prostate Cancer; Intensity Modulated Radiotherapy (IMRT); Multiple Myeloma; **Hospital:** City of Hope Natl Med Ctr & Beckman Rsch; **Address:** City of Hope Med Ctr-Dept Radiation Onc, 1500 E Duarte Rd, Duarte, CA 91768-3012; **Phone:** 626-359-8111 x62969; **Board Cert:** Therapeutic Radiology 1985; **Med School:** Johns Hopkins Univ 1981; **Resid:** Radiation Oncology, UCSF Med Ctr 1985; **Fac Appt:** Clin Prof RadRO, UC Irvine

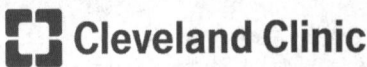 **Cleveland Clinic**

Radiation Oncology

The Department of Radiation Oncology at the Cleveland Clinic Taussig Cancer Institute is one of the busiest and most technologically advanced clinical radiotherapy programs in the country. Our specialists provide care at six facilities in Northeast Ohio and one in Florida.

Technology: Cleveland Clinic offers a full range of advanced technology equipment, including 13 linear accelerators, fully integrated CT simulators, and various image guided treatment technologies. Using multiple imaging modalities including PET/CT, SPECT/CT, and MRI, we offer patients accurately targeted treatment, and our state-of-the-art computer technologies provide precise external beam radiation. The department is equipped with a combined X-ray and optical imaging tracking system (Novalis, BrainLAB); kilo-voltage (KV) and Mega-voltage (MV) cone-beam computerized tomography (CT); electromagnetic emission detectors (Calypso system); and ultrasound imaging (CLARITY) to provide optimal cancer treatment.

> **How do you measure quality?**
> Visit clevelandclinic.org/quality for information on the criteria most often used to measure quality in health care; data on how Cleveland Clinic compares with other health care centers; patient satisfaction data; and quality measures for numerous specific diseases and conditions, including cancer.

Innovation: Cleveland Clinic Radiation Oncology was also one of the first programs to implement intensity-modulated radiation therapy (IMRT), image-guided radiation therapy (IGRT) and radioimmunotherapy (RIT). Cleveland Clinic has one of the most active brachytherapy programs in the U.S. In addition to intracavitary and intraluminal treatments, Cleveland Clinic has developed many novel approaches to brachytherapy, especially with prostate cancer.

Patient Services: Cleveland Clinic offers free round-trip transportation for patients who have difficulty getting to daily treatments from their homes. Our free wellness program, Reflections, offers a variety of complementary and aesthetic therapies, which allow patients the opportunity to be pampered, to regain a sense of control and to take some time for themselves. The treatments include healing therapies such as Reiki, reflexology, guided imagery, facials, makeovers and massotherapy.

Research: Cleveland Clinic is active in a number of in-house pharmaceutical and cooperative group trials. We are one of the leading enrollers in national studies and in combining novel agents such as radiation sensitizers with radiation therapy. In addition, the Department of Radiation Oncology houses one of the largest prostate cancer databases (>10,000 patients) in the nation.

For more information about the Cleveland Clinic Department of Radiation Oncology, to schedule a second opinion or to learn about assistance for out-of-town patients, call 800.890.2467 or visit www.clevelandclinic.org/radonctopdocs.

Department of Radiation Oncology | 9500 Euclid Avenue / AC311 | Cleveland OH 44195

NYU CANCER INSTITUTE

About the Cancer Institute:

The NYU Cancer Institute is an NCI-designated cancer center and provides personalized patient care that is both compassionate and state of the art. The doctors and researchers work together to develop innovative therapies for patients. The Institute is world-renowned for excellence in cancer-focused research, personalized care, education and community outreach. Its mission is to discover the origins of human cancer and to use that knowledge to eradicate the personal and societal burden of cancer in our community, the nation and the world. The center and its multidisciplinary team of experts provide access to the latest treatment options and clinical trials along with a variety of programs in cancer prevention, screening, diagnostics, genetic counseling and supportive services.

We specialize in the following areas:

PATIENT-FOCUSED SETTING

The NYU Clinical Cancer Center is the principal outpatient facility of The Cancer Institute and serves as home to our patients and their caregivers. The center and its multidisciplinary team of experts provide access to the latest treatment options and clinical trials along with a variety of programs in cancer prevention, screening, diagnostics, genetic counseling and supportive services. In addition the NYUCI emphasizes the importance of a holistic approach to management services in complementary medicine, psychosocial support, survivorship and palliative care.

RENOWNED EXPERTISE

The NYU Cancer Institute brings together experts from a variety of disciplines to create collaborative research endeavors and clinical care teams. The Institute offers a full continuum of personalized care, from prevention through diagnosis, treatment and post-treatment support. The compassion and expertise of our team members helps patients better manage the symptoms of their diseases as well as meet their special needs. Additionally, we have created special emphasis programs in diseases such as breast cancer, melanoma, GI cancer, prostate cancer, hematologic malignancies and lung cancer among others, as well as, translational programs in cancer healthcare disparities, molecularly-targeted therapy, and the cell signaling pathways involved in cancer.

A TRANSLATIONAL APPROACH

NYU Langone Medical Center scientists and other researchers excel in uncovering how cancer develops at the molecular level, and how we can harness that knowledge to reduce the risk of cancer and treat the disease. The Medical Center constantly seeks to create new opportunities for collaboration between investigators within our own institution, those located elsewhere in the NYU network of campuses, and researchers at other institutions.

THE STEPHEN D. HASSENFELD CHILDREN'S CENTER FOR CANCER AND BLOOD DISORDERS

The center is a leading pediatric outpatient facility for the treatment of childhood cancers and blood diseases. Its unique interdisciplinary and family-centered approach combines the most advanced medical treatments with psychosocial and emotional support services for young patients and their families.

FIGHTING **CANCER** JUST GOT **EASIER.**

Leksell® Gamma Knife Perfexion™

IN THE FIGHT AGAINST CANCER, NEW TECHNOLOGY REPRESENTS NEW HOPE.

So it is with genuine excitement that we announce the acquisition of two "next generation" tools that allow for treatment of tumors, from head to toe.

The Stereotactic Radiosurgery (SRS) Team at Wake Forest University Baptist Medical Center now offers **Leksell® Gamma Knife Perfexion™** and the **Axesse™** linear accelerator — the fastest, most accurate stereotactic radiosurgery/radiotherapy treatments available. For our patients, that means a faster return to daily life, with virtually no discomfort and no hospital stay.

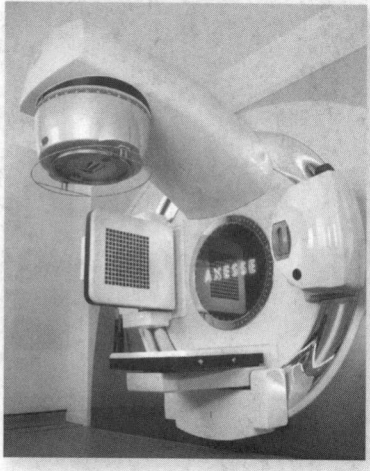
Axesse™ linear accelerator

We are honored to be named the nation's first Leksell Center for Radiosurgery training site for these exciting treatments. Our SRS team is one of the most experienced in the United States. We were first in North Carolina to offer non-invasive Gamma Knife, the "gold standard" treatment for selected benign and malignant brain tumors and vascular malformations. Today our Gamma Knife Center is among the busiest in the country.

Gamma Knife Perfexion hones an outstanding technology to an even higher level, now providing unequaled accuracy to spare healthy tissue and improving our ability to treat challenging skull and upper neck tumors.

Axesse Stereotactic Body Radiotherapy takes the linear accelerator to new heights of accuracy in targeting tumors virtually anywhere in the body. This technological advance vastly improves the patient experience by eliminating the need for repositioning after movement of any kind and **requiring just one to five treatment sessions.**

Conditions for which gamma Knife Perfexion is recommended: benign/malignant brain tumors (primary, metastatic); meningiomas; acoustic neuromas; ateriovenous malformations; trigeminal neuralgia; cervical, paranasal sinus and pharyngolaryngeal lesions.

Conditions for which Axesse Stereotactic Body Radiation is recommended: curative intent therapies for Stage I and recurrent lung cancers, spinal cord cancers, prostate cancer and recurrent head and neck cancers; metastatic cancers of the lung, spine, liver, bone, adrenal glands and oligometastatic cancer; curative intent image-guided therapies for head and neck cancer, locally advanced lung cancer, esophageal and stomach cancers, recurrent gynecological cancers and retroperitoneal sarcomas.

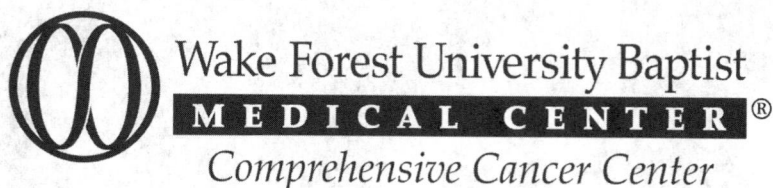

Wake Forest University Baptist
MEDICAL CENTER ®
Comprehensive Cancer Center

Our team looks forward to working with patients and their physicians to provide the most effective SRS therapies. For information call **336-716-5969** or toll-free **866-713-3228** or visit our **website wfubmc.edu/SRS.**

Radiology

A radiologist utilizes radiologic methodologies to diagnose and treat disease. Physicians practicing in the field of radiology most often specialize in radiology, diagnostic radiology, radiation oncology or radiological physics.

Diagnostic Radiology: A radiologist who utilizes X-ray, radionuclides, ultrasound and electromagnetic radiation to diagnose and treat disease.

Training Required: Four years

Radiation Oncology: A radiologist who deals with the therapeutic applications of radiant energy and its modifiers and the study and management of disease, especially malignant tumors.

Certification in one of the following subspecialties requires additional training and examination.

Neuroradiology: A radiologist who diagnoses and treats diseases utilizing imaging procedures as they relate to the brain, spine and spinal cord, head, neck and organs of special sense in adults and children.

Pediatric Radiology: A radiologist who is proficient in all forms of diagnostic imaging as it pertains to the treatment of diseases in the newborn, infant, child and adolescent. This specialist has knowledge of both imaging and interventional procedures related to the care and management of diseases of children. A pediatric radiologist must be highly knowledgeable of all organ systems as they relate to growth and development, congenital malformations, diseases peculiar to infants and children and diseases that begin in childhood but cause substantial residual impairment in adulthood.

Vascular and Interventional Radiology: A radiologist who diagnoses and treats diseases by various radiologic imaging modalities. These include fluoroscopy, digital radiography, computed tomography, sonography and magnetic resonance imaging.

DIAGNOSTIC RADIOLOGY

New England

Benson, Carol MD [DR] - **Spec Exp:** Obstetric Ultrasound; Thyroid Ultrasound; Fetal Surgical Imaging; **Hospital:** Brigham & Women's Hosp; **Address:** Brigham & Women's Hospital, Dept Radiology, 75 Francis St, Boston, MA 02115; **Phone:** 617-732-6280; **Board Cert:** Diagnostic Radiology 1984; **Med School:** Univ Pennsylvania 1980; **Resid:** Diagnostic Radiology, New York Hosp-Cornell 1984; **Fellow:** Ultrasound, Brigham & Womens Hosp 1985; **Fac Appt:** Prof Rad, Harvard Med Sch

Black, William C MD [DR] - **Spec Exp:** Chest Radiology; Lung Cancer; CT Chest Scan; **Hospital:** Dartmouth - Hitchcock Med Ctr; **Address:** Dartmouth Hitchcock Med Ctr, Dept Radiology, 1 Medical Center Drive, Lebanon, NH 03756; **Phone:** 603-650-7443; **Board Cert:** Diagnostic Radiology 1983; **Med School:** Med Coll VA 1979; **Resid:** Diagnostic Radiology, Univ Virginia Hosp 1983; **Fellow:** Ultrasound/CT, Univ Virginia Hosp 1984; **Fac Appt:** Prof Rad, Dartmouth Med Sch

Doubilet, Peter MD [DR] - **Spec Exp:** Ultrasound; Obstetric Ultrasound; **Hospital:** Brigham & Women's Hosp; **Address:** Brigham & Women's Hosp, Dept Radiology, 75 Francis St, Boston, MA 02115; **Phone:** 617-732-6251; **Board Cert:** Diagnostic Radiology 1981; **Med School:** Columbia P&S 1977; **Resid:** Diagnostic Radiology, Brigham Women's Hosp 1981; **Fac Appt:** Prof Rad, Harvard Med Sch

Kopans, Daniel B MD [DR] - **Spec Exp:** Breast Imaging; Breast Cancer; **Hospital:** Mass Genl Hosp; **Address:** Mass Genl Hosp, Avon Comprehensive Breast Ctr, 15 Parkman St, WAC 240, Boston, MA 02114-3117; **Phone:** 617-726-3093; **Board Cert:** Diagnostic Radiology 1977; **Med School:** Harvard Med Sch 1973; **Resid:** Diagnostic Radiology, Mass Genl Hosp 1977; **Fac Appt:** Prof Rad, Harvard Med Sch

McCarthy, Shirley M MD/PhD [DR] - **Spec Exp:** Gynecologic Cancer; Pelvic Imaging; **Hospital:** Yale-New Haven Hosp; **Address:** Yale-New Haven Hosp, 333 Cedar St, Ste TE2, New Haven, CT 06520-3206; **Phone:** 203-785-2384; **Board Cert:** Diagnostic Radiology 1983; **Med School:** Yale Univ 1979; **Resid:** Diagnostic Radiology, Yale-New Haven Hosp 1983; **Fellow:** Cross Sectional Imaging, UCSF Med Ctr 1984; **Fac Appt:** Prof Rad, Yale Univ

Palmer, William E MD [DR] - **Spec Exp:** Musculoskeletal Imaging; Pain-Vertebral Collapse/Osteoporosis; Sports Related Injuries; **Hospital:** Mass Genl Hosp; **Address:** 15 Parkman St, Wang Bldg, rm 515, Boston, MA 02114; **Phone:** 617-726-7717; **Board Cert:** Internal Medicine 1987; Diagnostic Radiology 1991; **Med School:** Yale Univ 1984; **Resid:** Internal Medicine, Hosp Univ Penn 1987; Diagnostic Radiology, Mass Genl Hosp 1991; **Fac Appt:** Assoc Prof Rad, Harvard Med Sch

Weinreb, Jeffrey C MD [DR] - **Spec Exp:** MRI; Breast Cancer; Abdominal Imaging; CT Scan; **Hospital:** Yale-New Haven Hosp; **Address:** Yale Univ Sch Medicine, Dept Radiology, 333 Cedar St, rm MRC147, Box 208042, New Haven, CT 06520-8042; **Phone:** 203-785-5913; **Board Cert:** Diagnostic Radiology 1983; **Med School:** Mount Sinai Sch Med 1978; **Resid:** Diagnostic Radiology, LI Jewish Med Ctr 1982; **Fellow:** Ultrasound/CT, Hosp Univ Penn 1983; **Fac Appt:** Prof Rad, Yale Univ

Diagnostic Radiology

Mid Atlantic

Adler, Ronald S MD/PhD [DR] - **Spec Exp:** Musculoskeletal Imaging; Ultrasound; Power Doppler Imaging; **Hospital:** Hosp For Special Surgery (page 59), NY-Presby Hosp/Weill Cornell (page 66); **Address:** Hospital for Special Surgery, 535 E 70th St, New York, NY 10021; **Phone:** 212-606-1635; **Board Cert:** Diagnostic Radiology 1988; **Med School:** Wayne State Univ 1984; **Resid:** Diagnostic Radiology, Univ Mich Med Ctr 1988; **Fellow:** Ultrasound/CT/MRI, Univ Mich Med Ctr 1989; **Fac Appt:** Prof Rad, Cornell Univ-Weill Med Coll

Austin, John H M MD [DR] - **Spec Exp:** Lung Cancer; Thoracic Radiology; **Hospital:** NY-Presby Hosp/Columbia (page 66); **Address:** Columbia Presby Hosp, Dept Radiology, 622 W 168th St, HP 3-305, New York, NY 10032-3784; **Phone:** 212-305-2986; **Board Cert:** Diagnostic Radiology 1970; **Med School:** Yale Univ 1965; **Resid:** Diagnostic Radiology, UCSF Med Ctr 1968; **Fellow:** Diagnostic Radiology, UCSF Med Ctr 1970; **Fac Appt:** Prof Rad, Columbia P&S

Berg, Wendie A MD/PhD [DR] - **Spec Exp:** Breast Imaging; Breast Cancer; **Hospital:** Johns Hopkins Hosp (page 61); **Address:** Johns Hopkins, Greenspring Station Breast Ctr, 10755 Falls Rd, Ste 440, Lutherville, MD 21093; **Phone:** 410-583-2700; **Board Cert:** Diagnostic Radiology 1992; **Med School:** Johns Hopkins Univ 1987; **Resid:** Diagnostic Radiology, Johns Hopkins Hosp 1992; **Fellow:** Abdominal Imaging, Johns Hopkins Univ 1992

Bluemke, David A MD/PhD [DR] - **Spec Exp:** Cardiac Imaging; MRI; **Hospital:** Natl Inst of Hlth - Clin Ctr; **Address:** 9000 Rockville Pike, Bldg 10 - Ste 1C351, Betheseda, MD 20892; **Phone:** 301-402-1854; **Board Cert:** Diagnostic Radiology 1993; **Med School:** Univ Chicago-Pritzker Sch Med 1989; **Resid:** Diagnostic Radiology, Johns Hopkins Hosp 1993; **Fellow:** Diagnostic Imaging, Johns Hopkins Hosp 1994; **Fac Appt:** Prof Rad, Johns Hopkins Univ

Brem, Rachel F MD [DR] - **Spec Exp:** Breast Imaging; Breast Cancer; **Hospital:** G Washington Univ Hosp; **Address:** GW Medical Faculty Assocs, 2150 Pennsylvania Ave NW, DC Level, Washington, DC 20037; **Phone:** 202-741-3036; **Board Cert:** Diagnostic Radiology 1990; **Med School:** Columbia P&S 1984; **Resid:** Diagnostic Radiology, Johns Hopkins Hosp 1989; **Fellow:** Mammography, Johns Hopkins Hosp 1990; **Fac Appt:** Prof Rad, Geo Wash Univ

Cohen, Burton A MD [DR] - **Spec Exp:** CT Scan; MRI; Ovarian Cancer Ultrasound Diagnosis; PET Imaging; **Hospital:** Mount Sinai Med Ctr (page 64); **Address:** 165 E 84th St, New York, NY 10028; **Phone:** 212-535-9770; **Board Cert:** Diagnostic Radiology 1979; **Med School:** NY Med Coll 1975; **Resid:** Diagnostic Radiology, Mt Sinai Hosp 1979; **Fac Appt:** Assoc Clin Prof Rad, Mount Sinai Sch Med

Coleman, Beverly G MD [DR] - **Spec Exp:** Ultrasound; **Hospital:** Hosp Univ Penn - UPHS (page 60); **Address:** Univ Penn Radiology, Ground Dulles, 3400 Spruce St, Philadelphia, PA 19104; **Phone:** 215-662-3046; **Board Cert:** Diagnostic Radiology 1978; **Med School:** Harvard Med Sch 1974; **Resid:** Diagnostic Radiology, Univ Penn Hosp 1975; Diagnostic Radiology, Univ Mich Hosp 1977; **Fellow:** Ultrasound, Univ Penn Hosp 1979; **Fac Appt:** Prof Rad, Univ Pennsylvania

Conant, Emily F MD [DR] - **Spec Exp:** Breast Cancer; Breast Imaging; **Hospital:** Hosp Univ Penn - UPHS (page 60); **Address:** Dept Radiology (Breast Imaging), 3400 Spruce St, 1 Silverstein, Philadelphia, PA 19104; **Phone:** 215-662-4032; **Board Cert:** Diagnostic Radiology 1989; **Med School:** Univ Pennsylvania 1983; **Resid:** Diagnostic Radiology, Hosp Univ Penn 1986; **Fellow:** Breast Imaging, Hosp Univ Penn 1989; **Fac Appt:** Prof Rad, Univ Pennsylvania

Dalinka, Murray MD [DR] - **Spec Exp:** Bone Disorders-Metabolic; Musculoskeletal Imaging; MRI; **Hospital:** Hosp Univ Penn - UPHS (page 60); **Address:** Dept Radiology, 3400 Spruce St, Philadelphia, PA 19104; **Phone:** 215-662-3019; **Board Cert:** Diagnostic Radiology 1969; **Med School:** Univ Mich Med Sch 1964; **Resid:** Diagnostic Radiology, Montefiore Med Ctr 1968; **Fac Appt:** Prof Rad, Univ Pennsylvania

Dershaw, D David MD [DR] - **Spec Exp:** Breast Imaging; Breast Cancer; Mammography; **Hospital:** Meml Sloan-Kettering Cancer Ctr; **Address:** 1275 York Avenue, New York, NY 10065; **Phone:** 800-525-2225; **Board Cert:** Diagnostic Radiology 1978; **Med School:** Jefferson Med Coll 1974; **Resid:** Diagnostic Radiology, New York Hosp 1978; **Fellow:** Ultrasound, Thos Jefferson Univ Hosp 1979; **Fac Appt:** Prof Rad, Cornell Univ-Weill Med Coll

Edelstein, Barbara A MD [DR] - **Spec Exp:** Breast Cancer; Women's Imaging; **Address:** 1045 Park Ave, New York, NY 10028; **Phone:** 212-860-7700; **Board Cert:** Diagnostic Radiology 1983; **Med School:** NY Med Coll 1977; **Resid:** Diagnostic Radiology, Montefiore Hosp 1982

Evers, Kathryn A MD [DR] - **Spec Exp:** Breast Cancer; Mammography; MRI-Breast; **Hospital:** Fox Chase Cancer Ctr (page 58); **Address:** Fox Chase Cancer Ctr, Diagnostic Imaging, 333 Cottman Ave, Philadelphia, PA 19111; **Phone:** 215-728-4316; **Board Cert:** Diagnostic Radiology 1980; **Med School:** NYU Sch Med 1975; **Resid:** Diagnostic Radiology, Hosp Univ Penn 1980; **Fellow:** Diagnostic Radiology, Hosp Univ Penn 1981; **Fac Appt:** Assoc Clin Prof Rad, Temple Univ

Fishman, Elliot MD [DR] - **Spec Exp:** CT Body Scan; Abdominal Imaging; Cardiac Imaging; Cancer Imaging; **Hospital:** Johns Hopkins Hosp (page 61); **Address:** Johns Hopkins Hosp, Dept Radiology, 601 N Caroline St, JHOC 3254, Baltimore, MD 21287-0006; **Phone:** 410-955-5173; **Board Cert:** Diagnostic Radiology 1981; **Med School:** Univ MD Sch Med 1977; **Resid:** Diagnostic Radiology, Sinai Hosp 1980; **Fellow:** Computerized Tomography, Johns Hopkins Hosp 1981; **Fac Appt:** Prof Rad, Johns Hopkins Univ

Fuhrman, Carl R MD [DR] - **Spec Exp:** Thoracic Imaging; **Hospital:** UPMC Presby, Pittsburgh; **Address:** UPMC-Dept Radiology, 200 Lothrop St, Ste E177 PUH, Pittsburgh, PA 15213; **Phone:** 412-647-7288; **Board Cert:** Diagnostic Radiology 1983; **Med School:** Univ Pittsburgh 1979; **Resid:** Diagnostic Radiology, Presby Univ Hosp 1983; **Fac Appt:** Prof Rad, Univ Pittsburgh

Gefter, Warren B MD [DR] - **Spec Exp:** Thoracic Imaging; **Hospital:** Hosp Univ Penn - UPHS (page 60); **Address:** Hospital Univ of Pennsylvania, 1 Silverstein, 3400 Spruce St, Philadelphia, PA 19104; **Phone:** 215-662-6724; **Board Cert:** Diagnostic Radiology 1978; **Med School:** Univ Pennsylvania 1974; **Resid:** Diagnostic Radiology, Hosp Univ Penn 1978; **Fac Appt:** Prof Rad, Univ Pennsylvania

Hann, Lucy MD [DR] - **Spec Exp:** Liver & Biliary Cancer Ultrasound; Ovarian Cancer Ultrasound Diagnosis; Thyroid Ultrasound; **Hospital:** Meml Sloan-Kettering Cancer Ctr; **Address:** 1275 York Avenue, New York, NY 10065; **Phone:** 800-525-2225; **Board Cert:** Diagnostic Radiology 1977; **Med School:** Harvard Med Sch 1971; **Resid:** Diagnostic Radiology, Hosp Univ Penn 1974; Diagnostic Radiology, Mass Genl Hosp 1977; **Fellow:** Body Imaging, Mass Genl Hosp 1978; **Fac Appt:** Prof Rad, Cornell Univ-Weill Med Coll

Henschke, Claudia L MD/PhD [DR] - **Spec Exp:** Lung Cancer; Lung Disease; Thoracic Radiology; **Hospital:** NY-Presby Hosp/Weill Cornell (page 66); **Address:** NY Weill Medical College, Dept Radiology, 525 E 68th St, Box 586, New York, NY 10021; **Phone:** 212-746-1325; **Board Cert:** Diagnostic Radiology 1981; **Med School:** Howard Univ 1977; **Resid:** Diagnostic Radiology, Brigham & Womens Hosp 1983; **Fac Appt:** Prof Rad, Cornell Univ-Weill Med Coll

Diagnostic Radiology

Holliday, Roy MD [DR] - **Spec Exp:** Head & Neck Radiology; **Hospital:** New York Eye & Ear Infirm (page 65), Beth Israel Med Ctr - Petrie Division (page 57); **Address:** 310 E 14th St, New York, NY 10003; **Phone:** 212-979-4397; **Board Cert:** Diagnostic Radiology 1986; **Med School:** NYU Sch Med 1982; **Resid:** Diagnostic Radiology, NYU Med Ctr 1986; **Fellow:** Neurological Radiology, NYU Med Ctr 1987; **Fac Appt:** Clin Prof Rad, NYU Sch Med

Hricak, Hedvig MD/PhD [DR] - **Spec Exp:** Prostate Cancer-MR Spectroscopy (MRSI); Breast Imaging; Breast Cancer; **Hospital:** Meml Sloan-Kettering Cancer Ctr; **Address:** 1275 York Avenue, New York, NY 10065; **Phone:** 800-525-2225; **Board Cert:** Diagnostic Radiology 1978; **Med School:** Yugoslavia 1970; **Resid:** Diagnostic Radiology, St Joseph Mercy Hosp 1977; **Fellow:** Ultrasound/CT, Henry Ford Hosp 1978; **Fac Appt:** Prof Rad, Cornell Univ-Weill Med Coll

Jaramillo, Diego MD [DR] - **Spec Exp:** Pediatric Radiology; **Hospital:** Chldns Hosp of Philadelphia, The; **Address:** Dept Radiology, 34th & Civic Center Blvd, rm 3NW-17, Philadelphia, PA 19104; **Phone:** 267-425-7110; **Board Cert:** Diagnostic Radiology 1987; Pediatric Radiology 2005; **Med School:** Colombia 1981; **Resid:** Diagnostic Radiology, Univ Texas 1987; **Fellow:** Pediatric Radiology, Children's Hosp 1989; **Fac Appt:** Prof Rad, Univ Pennsylvania

Kanal, Emanuel MD [DR] - **Spec Exp:** Neuroradiology; MRI; **Hospital:** UPMC Presby, Pittsburgh; **Address:** Univ Pittsburgh Med Ctr, Dept Radiology, 200 Lothrop St, rm D132, Pittsburgh, PA 15213-2582; **Phone:** 412-647-3540; **Board Cert:** Diagnostic Radiology 1985; **Med School:** Univ Pittsburgh 1981; **Resid:** Diagnostic Radiology, Univ Pittsburgh Med Ctr 1985; **Fellow:** Magnetic Resonance Imaging, Pittsburgh NMR Inst 1986; Neurological Radiology, Univ Pittsburgh Med Ctr 1993; **Fac Appt:** Prof Rad, Univ Pittsburgh

Kurtz, Alfred B MD [DR] - **Spec Exp:** Obstetric Ultrasound; **Hospital:** Thomas Jefferson Univ Hosp; **Address:** Thomas Jefferson Univ Hosp, Radiology, 111 S 11th St, Ste 3350A-B, Philadelphia, PA 19107; **Phone:** 215-955-6343; **Board Cert:** Diagnostic Radiology 1977; **Med School:** Stanford Univ 1972; **Resid:** Internal Medicine, Montefiore Med Ctr 1974; Diagnostic Radiology, Montefiore Med Ctr 1977; **Fellow:** Ultrasound, Thomas Jefferson Univ Hosp 1978; **Fac Appt:** Prof Rad, Jefferson Med Coll

Levy, Angela D MD [DR] - **Spec Exp:** Abdominal Imaging; **Hospital:** Unif Serv Univ of the Hlth Sci, Armed Forces Inst of Path; **Address:** Uniformed Services Univ of the Hlth Scis, Dept Radiology, 4301 Jones Bridge Rd, rm C1071, Bethesda, MD 20814; **Phone:** 301-295-3145; **Board Cert:** Diagnostic Radiology 1993; **Med School:** Uniformed Srvs Univ, Bethesda 1988; **Resid:** Diagnostic Radiology, Walter Reed Army Hosp 1992; **Fac Appt:** Assoc Prof Rad, Uniformed Srvs Univ, Bethesda

Megibow, Alec J MD [DR] - **Spec Exp:** Abdominal Imaging; Gastrointestinal Imaging; CT Body Scan; **Hospital:** NYU Langone Med Ctr (page 67); **Address:** 550 1st Ave, HHC 232, New York, NY 10016; **Phone:** 212-263-5222; **Board Cert:** Diagnostic Radiology 1978; **Med School:** SUNY Upstate Med Univ 1974; **Resid:** Diagnostic Radiology, Bellevue/NYU Med Ctr 1978; **Fac Appt:** Prof Rad, NYU Sch Med

Mirvis, Stuart E MD [DR] - **Spec Exp:** Trauma Radiology; **Hospital:** Univ of MD Med Ctr; **Address:** Univ Maryland Med Ctr, Dept Radiology, 22 S Greene St, Baltimore, MD 21201; **Phone:** 410-328-8845; **Board Cert:** Diagnostic Radiology 1984; **Med School:** Johns Hopkins Univ 1979; **Resid:** Diagnostic Radiology, Univ Maryland Med Ctr 1984; **Fellow:** Trauma Radiology, Univ Maryland Med Ctr 1985; **Fac Appt:** Prof Rad, Univ MD Sch Med

Mitnick, Julie MD [DR] - **Spec Exp:** Mammography; Breast Cancer; **Address:** 650 1st Ave, New York, NY 10016; **Phone:** 212-686-4440; **Board Cert:** Diagnostic Radiology 1977; **Med School:** NYU Sch Med 1973; **Resid:** Diagnostic Radiology, NYU Med Ctr 1977; **Fellow:** Pediatric Radiology, NYU Med Ctr 1978; **Fac Appt:** Assoc Clin Prof Rad, NYU Sch Med

Norton, Karen MD [DR] - **Spec Exp:** Pediatric Radiology; **Hospital:** Newark Beth Israel Med Ctr; **Address:** 201 Lyons Ave, Newark, NJ 07112; **Phone:** 973-926-6635; **Board Cert:** Diagnostic Radiology 1984; Pediatric Radiology 2005; **Med School:** Mount Sinai Sch Med 1980; **Resid:** Pediatrics, NYU Med Ctr 1981; Diagnostic Radiology, Mount Sinai Hosp 1984; **Fellow:** Pediatric Radiology, Mount Sinai Hosp 1985

Panicek, David M MD [DR] - **Spec Exp:** Bone Cancer; Soft Tissue Tumors; Musculoskeletal Tumor Imaging; **Hospital:** Meml Sloan-Kettering Cancer Ctr; **Address:** 1275 York Avenue, New York, NY 10065; **Phone:** 800-525-2225; **Board Cert:** Diagnostic Radiology 1984; **Med School:** Cornell Univ-Weill Med Coll 1980; **Resid:** Diagnostic Radiology, NY Hosp-Cornell Med Ctr 1984; **Fac Appt:** Prof Rad, Cornell Univ-Weill Med Coll

Parsons, Rosaleen B MD [DR] - **Spec Exp:** CT Body Scan; Gynecologic Cancer; Prostate Cancer; Interventional Radiology; **Hospital:** Fox Chase Cancer Ctr (page 58); **Address:** Fox Chase Cancer Ctr, Dept of Diagnostic Imaging, 333 Cottman Ave, Philadelphia, PA 19111; **Phone:** 215-728-3024; **Board Cert:** Diagnostic Radiology 1991; **Med School:** Med Coll PA Hahnemann 1986; **Resid:** Diagnostic Radiology, Med Coll Penn Affil Hosp 1991; **Fac Appt:** Prof Rad, Temple Univ

Potter, Hollis J MD [DR] - **Spec Exp:** Musculoskeletal Imaging; Cartilage Damage; Arthroplasty Imaging; **Hospital:** Hosp For Special Surgery (page 59); **Address:** Hosp for Special Surgery, MRI-basement, 535 E 70th St, New York, NY 10021-4892; **Phone:** 212-606-1882; **Board Cert:** Diagnostic Radiology 1990; **Med School:** NY Med Coll 1985; **Resid:** Diagnostic Radiology, North Shore Univ Hosp 1990; **Fellow:** Diagnostic Radiology, Hosp Special Surgery 1991; **Fac Appt:** Prof Rad, Cornell Univ-Weill Med Coll

Rao, Vijay M MD [DR] - **Spec Exp:** Head & Neck Tumors Imaging; TMJ Imaging; Ear Nose & Throat Imaging; **Hospital:** Thomas Jefferson Univ Hosp; **Address:** 132 S 10th St, 1087, Main Bldg, Philadelphia, PA 19107-4824; **Phone:** 215-955-4804; **Board Cert:** Diagnostic Radiology 1978; Neuroradiology 1997; **Med School:** India 1973; **Resid:** Diagnostic Radiology, Thomas Jefferson Univ Hosp 1978; **Fac Appt:** Prof Rad, Thomas Jefferson Univ

Reinus, William R MD [DR] - **Spec Exp:** Musculoskeletal Imaging; **Hospital:** Temple Univ Hosp; **Address:** Temple Univ Hospital, Dept Radiology, 3401 N Broad St, Philadelphia, PA 19140; **Phone:** 215-707-4264; **Board Cert:** Diagnostic Radiology 1983; **Med School:** NYU Sch Med 1979; **Resid:** Radiology, Mallinkradt Inst Rad 1983; **Fellow:** Musculoskeletal Imaging, Mallinkradt Inst Rad 1984; **Fac Appt:** Assoc Prof Rad, Temple Univ

Roth, Susan G MD [DR] - **Spec Exp:** Breast Imaging; Breast Cancer; **Hospital:** Hosp Univ Penn - UPHS (page 60); **Address:** Hosp Univ Penn, Dept Radiology, 3400 Physics Ctr Blvd Fl Ground, Philadelphia, PA 19104; **Phone:** 215-614-0124; **Board Cert:** Diagnostic Radiology 1989; **Med School:** Univ Pennsylvania 1986; **Resid:** Diagnostic Radiology, Johns Hopkins Hosp 1989; **Fac Appt:** Prof Rad, Univ Pennsylvania

Teal, James S MD [DR] - **Spec Exp:** Interventional Radiology; **Hospital:** Howard Univ Hosp; **Address:** Howard Univ Hosp, Dept Radiology, 2041 Georgia Ave NW, Washington, DC 20060-0001; **Phone:** 202-865-1571; **Board Cert:** Diagnostic Radiology 1970; **Med School:** Univ Tex Med Br, Galveston 1964; **Resid:** Diagnostic Radiology, Mt Zion Hosp 1969; **Fellow:** Neuroradiology, LAC-USC Med Ctr 1970; **Fac Appt:** Prof Rad, Howard Univ

White, Charles S MD [DR] - **Spec Exp:** Thoracic Imaging; **Hospital:** Univ of MD Med Ctr; **Address:** Univ Maryland Med Ctr, Dept Radiology, 22 S Greene St, Baltimore, MD 21201; **Phone:** 410-328-3477; **Board Cert:** Diagnostic Radiology 1991; Internal Medicine 1987; **Med School:** SUNY Buffalo 1984; **Resid:** Internal Medicine, Columbia-Presby Hosp 1987; Diagnostic Radiology, Columbia-Presby Hosp 1991; **Fellow:** Thoracic Radiology, Columbia-Presby Med Ctr; **Fac Appt:** Prof, Univ MD Sch Med

Diagnostic Radiology

Yankelevitz, David MD [DR] - **Spec Exp:** Lung Cancer; Thoracic Radiology; **Hospital:** NY-Presby Hosp/Weill Cornell (page 66); **Address:** 520 E 70th St, Weill Cornell Starr Bldg, New York, NY 10021; **Phone:** 212-746-9729; **Board Cert:** Diagnostic Radiology 1987; Nuclear Medicine 1987; **Med School:** SUNY Hlth Sci Ctr 1981; **Resid:** Diagnostic Radiology, Long Island Coll Hosp 1984; Nuclear Medicine, NY-Cornell Med Ctr 1987; **Fellow:** Diagnostic Radiology, NY-Cornell Med Ctr 1987; **Fac Appt:** Prof Rad, Cornell Univ-Weill Med Coll

Southeast

Abbitt, Patricia L MD [DR] - **Spec Exp:** Ultrasound; Interventional Radiology; Breast Imaging; Breast Cancer; **Hospital:** Shands at Univ of FL; **Address:** Shands Healthcare, Dept Radiology, 1600 SW Archer Rd, PO Box 100374, Gainesville, FL 32610; **Phone:** 352-265-0291; **Board Cert:** Diagnostic Radiology 1986; **Med School:** Tufts Univ 1981; **Resid:** Diagnostic Radiology, Univ VA Med Ctr 1986; **Fellow:** Breast Imaging, Univ VA Med Ctr 1987; **Fac Appt:** Prof Rad, Univ Fla Coll Med

Berland, Lincoln L MD [DR] - **Spec Exp:** Abdominal Imaging; Gastrointestinal Imaging; **Hospital:** Univ of Ala Hosp at Birmingham; **Address:** UAB Diagnositic Radiology, N348 Jefferson Tower Bldg, 619 19th St S, Birmingham, AL 35249-6830; **Phone:** 205-934-7978; **Board Cert:** Diagnostic Radiology 1980; **Med School:** Washington Univ, St Louis 1975; **Resid:** Diagnostic Radiology, Med Coll Wisconsin Hosps 1979; **Fellow:** Ultrasound/CT, Med Coll Wisconsin Hosps 1980; **Fac Appt:** Prof Rad, Univ Alabama

Cardenosa, Gilda MD [DR] - **Spec Exp:** Breast Imaging; **Hospital:** Med Coll of VA Hosp; **Address:** VCU Med Ctr at Stony Point, Dept Radiology, 9000 Stony Point Pkwy, Richmond, VA 23235; **Phone:** 804-560-8906 x7862; **Board Cert:** Diagnostic Radiology 1989; **Med School:** Columbia P&S 1984; **Resid:** Diagnostic Radiology, Mass Genl Hosp 1989; **Fac Appt:** Prof Rad, Med Coll VA

Cohen, Harris L MD [DR] - **Spec Exp:** Pediatric Radiology; Fetal Ultrasound/Obstetrical Imaging; Obstetric Ultrasound; **Hospital:** Le Bonheur Chldns Med Ctr; **Address:** Le Bonheur Children's Hospital, Dept Radiology, Ground FL, 50 N Dunlap St, Memphis, TN 38103-2807; **Phone:** 901-287-5901; **Board Cert:** Diagnostic Radiology 1980; Pediatric Radiology 2005; **Med School:** SUNY Downstate 1976; **Resid:** Diagnostic Radiology, Univ Hosp 1980; **Fellow:** Pediatric Radiology, Chldns Hosp 1981; **Fac Appt:** Prof Rad, Univ Tenn Coll Med, Memphis

Elster, Allen D MD [DR] - **Spec Exp:** MRI; Neuroradiology; Brain Tumors; Spinal Tumors; **Hospital:** Wake Forest Univ Baptist Med Ctr (page 72); **Address:** Wake Forest Univ Baptist Med Ctr, 1 Medical Center Blvd, Dept Radiology, Winston Salem, NC 27157-1088; **Phone:** 336-716-7095; **Board Cert:** Diagnostic Radiology 1987; Neuroradiology 2005; **Med School:** Baylor Coll Med 1980; **Resid:** Surgery, Mass Genl Hosp 1983; Diagnostic Radiology, Univ Texas 1986; **Fellow:** Neuroradiology, Bowman Gray Sch Med 1987; **Fac Appt:** Prof Rad, Wake Forest Univ

Mancuso, Anthony A MD [DR] - **Spec Exp:** Head & Neck Radiology; Neuroradiology; **Hospital:** Shands at Univ of FL; **Address:** Shands Hosp, Univ Florida, Dept Rad, Dept Radiology, 1600 SW Archer Rd, Gainesville, FL 32610; **Phone:** 352-265-0296; **Board Cert:** Diagnostic Radiology 1978; **Med School:** Univ Miami Sch Med 1973; **Resid:** Diagnostic Radiology, UCLA Med Ctr 1977; **Fellow:** Neuroradiology, UCLA Med Ctr 1978; **Fac Appt:** Prof Rad, Univ Fla Coll Med

Partain, Clarence L MD/PhD [DR] - **Spec Exp:** MRI; Nuclear Radiology; Chest Radiology; **Hospital:** Vanderbilt Univ Med Ctr; **Address:** Vanderbilt Univ Med Ctr, Dept Radiology, 1161 21st Ave S, rm RR1223 MCN, Nashville, TN 37232-2675; **Phone:** 615-343-3588; **Board Cert:** Nuclear Medicine 1979; Diagnostic Radiology 1980; Nuclear Radiology 1981; **Med School:** Washington Univ, St Louis 1975; **Resid:** Diagnostic Radiology, Univ North Carolina 1979; Nuclear Medicine, Univ North Carolina 1979; **Fac Appt:** Prof, Vanderbilt Univ

Patz, Edward F MD [DR] - **Spec Exp:** Thoracic Radiology; PET Imaging; Lung Cancer; **Hospital:** Duke Univ Med Ctr; **Address:** Duke Univ Med Ctr, Dept Radiology, Box 3808, Durham, NC 27710; **Phone:** 919-684-7367; **Board Cert:** Diagnostic Radiology 1990; **Med School:** Univ MD Sch Med 1985; **Resid:** Diagnostic Radiology, Brigham & Womens Hosp 1990; **Fellow:** Thoracic Radiology, Brigham & Womens Hosp 1990; **Fac Appt:** Prof, Duke Univ

White, Richard D MD [DR] - **Spec Exp:** Cardiovascular Imaging; **Hospital:** Shands Jacksonville; **Address:** Univ Fla Radiology at Shands, 655 W 8th St Fl 2, Box C-90, Jacksonville, FL 32209; **Phone:** 904-244-4224; **Board Cert:** Diagnostic Radiology 1986; **Med School:** Duke Univ 1981; **Resid:** Diagnostic Radiology, UCSF Med Ctr 1985; **Fellow:** Cardiovascular Radiology, UCSF Med Ctr 1987; **Fac Appt:** Prof, Univ Fla Coll Med

Yoon, Sydney S MD [DR] - **Spec Exp:** MRI; CT Body Scan; Uterine Fibroid Embolization; Interventional Radiology; **Address:** Sand Lake Imaging, 9350 Turkey Lake Rd, Orlando, FL 32819; **Phone:** 407-363-2772; **Board Cert:** Internal Medicine 1989; Diagnostic Radiology 1993; Vascular & Interventional Radiology 1998; Neuroradiology 2006; **Med School:** Univ Chicago-Pritzker Sch Med 1986; **Resid:** Internal Medicine, Johns Hopkins Hosp 1989; Diagnostic Radiology, UCLA Med Ctr 1993; **Fellow:** Neuroradiology, Columbia Presby Med Ctr 1995; Vascular & Interventional Radiology, UCLA Med Ctr 1997

Zagoria, Ronald J MD [DR] - **Spec Exp:** Abdominal Imaging; Genitourinary Radiology; Interventional Radiology; MRI; **Hospital:** Wake Forest Univ Baptist Med Ctr (page 72); **Address:** Wake Forest Univ Bapt Med Ct, One Medical Center Blvd, MRI Bldg Fl 3, Winston-Salem, NC 27157; **Phone:** 336-716-2471; **Board Cert:** Diagnostic Radiology 1987; Vascular & Interventional Radiology 2004; **Med School:** Univ MD Sch Med 1983; **Resid:** Radiology, Bowman Gray Med Ctr 1987; **Fellow:** Abdominal Imaging, Bowman Gray Med Ctr 1987; **Fac Appt:** Prof Rad, Wake Forest Univ

Midwest

Edelman, Robert R MD [DR] - **Spec Exp:** MRI; Cardiac CT Angiography; **Hospital:** NorthShore Univ HlthSys; **Address:** Evanston Hosp, Dept Radiology, 2650 Ridge Ave, rm 5108, Evanston, IL 60201; **Phone:** 847-570-2475; **Board Cert:** Diagnostic Radiology 1984; **Med School:** Boston Univ 1980; **Resid:** Diagnostic Radiology, Beth Israel Deaconess Med Ctr 1984; **Fac Appt:** Prof Rad, Northwestern Univ

Fidler, Jeff L MD [DR] - **Spec Exp:** Gastrointestinal Imaging; CT Colonography; MRI; **Hospital:** Mayo Med Ctr & Clin - Rochester; **Address:** Mayo Clin-Rochester, 200 1st St SW, rm #W4, Rochester, MN 55905-0002; **Phone:** 507-284-2511; **Board Cert:** Diagnostic Radiology 1993; **Med School:** Univ Nebr Coll Med 1988; **Resid:** Radiology, Duke Univ Med Ctr; **Fellow:** Diagnostic Radiology, Duke Univ Med Ctr; **Fac Appt:** Assoc Prof Rad, Mayo Med Sch

Flamm, Scott D MD [DR] - **Spec Exp:** Cardiac MRI; Cardiovascular Imaging; Congenital Heart Disease; **Hospital:** Cleveland Clin Fdn (page 56); **Address:** Cleveland Clinic, 9500 Euclid Ave, MC J1-4, Cleveland, OH 44195; **Phone:** 216-444-2740; **Board Cert:** Diagnostic Radiology 1993; **Med School:** Geo Wash Univ 1988; **Resid:** Diagnostic Radiology, UCLA Med Ctr 1992; **Fellow:** Cardiovascular Disease, UCSF Med Ctr 1994; **Fac Appt:** Assoc Prof Rad, Case West Res Univ

Goodman, Lawrence R MD [DR] - **Spec Exp:** Thoracic Imaging; Pulmonary Embolism; Lung Disease; **Hospital:** Froedtert Meml Lutheran Hosp; **Address:** Dept Radiology, 9200 W Wisconsin Ave, Milwaukee, WI 53226; **Phone:** 414-805-3120; **Board Cert:** Diagnostic Radiology 1973; **Med School:** SUNY Downstate 1968; **Resid:** Diagnostic Radiology, Boston Univ/City Hosp 1972; **Fellow:** Thoracic Radiology, UCSF Med Ctr 1973; **Fac Appt:** Prof Rad, Med Coll Wisc

Diagnostic Radiology

Helvie, Mark A MD [DR] - **Spec Exp:** Breast Imaging; Breast Cancer; Mammography; **Hospital:** Univ Michigan Hlth Sys; **Address:** 2910N Taubman Univ Michigan Health Ctr, 1500 E Medical Ctr Drive, Ann Arbor, MI 48109-0326; **Phone:** 734-936-4367; **Board Cert:** Internal Medicine 1983; Diagnostic Radiology 1986; **Med School:** Univ NC Sch Med 1980; **Resid:** Internal Medicine, Univ Michigan Hosps 1983; Diagnostic Radiology, Univ Michigan Hosps 1986; **Fellow:** Breast Imaging, Univ Michigan Hosps 1987; **Fac Appt:** Prof, Univ Mich Med Sch

Jackson, Valerie P MD [DR] - **Spec Exp:** Breast Imaging; **Hospital:** Indiana Univ Hosp, Wishard Hlth Srvs; **Address:** Indiana Univ Hosp, Dept Radiology, 550 N University Blvd, #0663, Indianapolis, IN 46202; **Phone:** 317-274-1866; **Board Cert:** Diagnostic Radiology 1982; **Med School:** Indiana Univ 1978; **Resid:** Diagnostic Radiology, Indiana Univ Med Ctr 1982; **Fac Appt:** Prof Rad, Indiana Univ

Monsees, Barbara MD [DR] - **Spec Exp:** Mammography; Breast Cancer; **Hospital:** Barnes-Jewish Hosp; **Address:** Ctr for Advanced Med, Campus Box 8131, 510 S Kingshighway Blvd, St Louis, MO 63110; **Phone:** 314-454-7500; **Board Cert:** Diagnostic Radiology 1980; **Med School:** Washington Univ, St Louis 1975; **Resid:** Pediatrics, St Louis Chldns Hosp 1977; Diagnostic Radiology, Mallinckrodt Inst Radiology 1980; **Fac Appt:** Prof, Washington Univ, St Louis

Sagel, Stuart S MD [DR] - **Spec Exp:** Lung Cancer; Occupational Lung Disease; Pulmonary Embolism; **Hospital:** Barnes-Jewish Hosp; **Address:** Mallinckrodt Inst Rad-Barnes Hosp, 510 S Kingshighway Blvd, Box 8131, St Louis, MO 63110-1016; **Phone:** 314-362-2927; **Board Cert:** Diagnostic Radiology 1970; **Med School:** Temple Univ 1965; **Resid:** Diagnostic Radiology, Yale New Haven Hosp 1968; Diagnostic Radiology, UCSF Med Ctr 1970; **Fac Appt:** Prof Rad, Washington Univ, St Louis

Sivit, Carlos MD [DR] - **Spec Exp:** Pediatric Radiology; Abdominal Imaging; Trauma Radiology; **Hospital:** Rainbow Babies & Chldns Hosp; **Address:** Dept Radiology, 11100 Euclid Ave, Cleveland, OH 44106-1736; **Phone:** 216-844-1172; **Board Cert:** Pediatrics 1987; Diagnostic Radiology 1987; **Med School:** Univ VA Sch Med 1981; **Resid:** Pediatrics, Vanderbilt Univ Hosp 1984; Diagnostic Radiology, George Washington Univ Hosp 1987; **Fellow:** Pediatric Radiology, Chldns Natl Med Ctr 1989; **Fac Appt:** Prof Rad, Case West Res Univ

Strife, Janet L MD [DR] - **Spec Exp:** Pediatric Radiology; Cardiac Imaging; **Hospital:** Cincinnati Chldns Hosp Med Ctr; **Address:** Children's Hospital, Dept Radiology, 3333 Burnet Ave, MC 5031, Cincinnati, OH 45229; **Phone:** 513-636-7535; **Board Cert:** Diagnostic Radiology 1974; Pediatric Radiology 2004; **Med School:** UMDNJ-NJ Med Sch, Newark 1968; **Resid:** Diagnostic Radiology, Univ Cincinnati Med Ctr 1971; Diagnostic Radiology, Johns Hopkins Hosp 1973; **Fellow:** Pediatrics, Johns Hopkins Hosp; **Fac Appt:** Prof, Univ Cincinnati

Swensen, Stephen J MD [DR] - **Spec Exp:** Lung Cancer; Lung Disease; **Hospital:** Mayo Med Ctr & Clin - Rochester; **Address:** Mayo Clinic - Diagnostic Radiology, 200 1st St SW, Rochester, MN 55905; **Phone:** 507-284-8550; **Board Cert:** Diagnostic Radiology 1986; **Med School:** Univ Wisc 1981; **Resid:** Diagnostic Radiology, Mayo Clinic 1986; **Fellow:** Pulmonary Radiology, Brigham & Womens Hosp 1987; **Fac Appt:** Prof Rad, Mayo Med Sch

Wells, Robert G MD [DR] - **Spec Exp:** Pediatric Radiology; **Hospital:** Chldns Hosp - Wisconsin; **Address:** Pediatric Diagnostic Imaging, 8522 W Capitol Drive, Milwaukee, WI 53222; **Phone:** 414-529-3100; **Board Cert:** Diagnostic Radiology 1984; Pediatric Radiology 2004; Vascular & Interventional Radiology 2004; **Med School:** Med Coll Wisc 1980; **Resid:** Diagnostic Radiology, St Luke's Hosp 1984; **Fellow:** Pediatric Radiology, Milwaukee Chldn's Hosp 1985; **Fac Appt:** Assoc Prof Rad, Med Coll Wisc

Great Plains and Mountains

Dodd III, Gerald Dewey MD [DR] - **Hospital:** Univ Colorado Hosp; **Address:** 12401 E 17th Ave, MS L954, Aurora, CO 80045; **Phone:** 720-848-6608; **Board Cert:** Diagnostic Radiology 1987; **Med School:** Univ Tex, Houston 1983; **Resid:** Diagnostic Radiology, Univ Hosp 1987; **Fellow:** Abdominal Imaging & Angio-Interventional, Univ Hosp 1988; **Fac Appt:** Prof, Univ Tex, San Antonio

Southwest

Erasmus, Jeremy J MD [DR] - **Spec Exp:** Lung Cancer; CT Body Scan; PET Imaging; **Hospital:** UT MD Anderson Cancer Ctr; **Address:** MD Anderson Cancer Ctr, Dept of Rad, 1515 Holcombe Blvd, Unit 0371, Houston, TX 77030; **Phone:** 713-792-5878; **Board Cert:** Diagnostic Radiology 1993; **Med School:** South Africa 1982; **Resid:** Diagnostic Radiology, Queens Univ 1993; **Fac Appt:** Prof Rad, Univ Tex, Houston

Harolds, Jay A MD [DR] - **Hospital:** OU Med Ctr; **Address:** Garrison Tower, Ste 4G 4250, Oklahoma City, OK 73104; **Phone:** 405-271-5125; **Board Cert:** Diagnostic Radiology 1975; Nuclear Radiology 1979; Nuclear Medicine 1980; **Med School:** SUNY Buffalo 1971; **Resid:** Diagnostic Radiology, Georgetown Univ Hosps 1975; Nuclear Medicine, Vanderbilt Univ Hosps 1980

Huynh, Phan Tuong MD [DR] - **Spec Exp:** Mammography; Breast Cancer; **Hospital:** St Luke's Episcopal Hosp-Houston; **Address:** 6624 Fannin St, St Luke's Tower, Womens Ctr Fl 10, Houston, TX 77030; **Phone:** 832-355-8130; **Board Cert:** Diagnostic Radiology 1994; **Med School:** Univ VA Sch Med 1989; **Resid:** Diagnostic Radiology, Univ Virginia Med Ctr 1994; **Fellow:** Mammography, Univ Virginia 1995; **Fac Appt:** Assoc Clin Prof Rad, Baylor Coll Med

Otto, Pamela MD [DR] - **Spec Exp:** Breast Imaging; Breast Cancer; **Hospital:** Univ Hlth Syst-San Antonio, Audie L Murphy Meml Vets Hosp; **Address:** 7703 Floyd Curl Drive, MC 7800, San Antonio, TX 78229-3900; **Phone:** 210-567-3448; **Board Cert:** Diagnostic Radiology 1993; **Med School:** Univ MO-Columbia Sch Med 1988; **Resid:** Diagnostic Radiology, Univ Texas Hlth Sci Ctr 1993; **Fellow:** Breast Imaging, Univ Texas Hlth Sci Ctr 1993; **Fac Appt:** Assoc Prof Rad, Univ Tex, San Antonio

West Coast and Pacific

Bassett, Lawrence W MD [DR] - **Spec Exp:** Breast Imaging; **Hospital:** UCLA Ronald Reagan Med Ctr; **Address:** 200 UCLA Med Plaza, rm 165-47, Los Angeles, CA 90095; **Phone:** 310-206-9608; **Board Cert:** Diagnostic Radiology 1975; **Med School:** UC Irvine 1968; **Resid:** Diagnostic Radiology, UCLA Med Ctr 1972; **Fac Appt:** Prof, UCLA

Coakley, Fergus V MD [DR] - **Spec Exp:** Abdominal Imaging; **Hospital:** UCSF Med Ctr; **Address:** UCSF Medical Ctr, 505 Parnassus Ave Fl 3 - rm M372, San Francisco, CA 94143; **Phone:** 415-353-1821; **Board Cert:** Diagnostic Radiology 2001; **Med School:** Ireland 1988

Federle, Michael P MD [DR] - **Spec Exp:** Abdominal Imaging; Gastrointestinal Imaging; **Hospital:** Stanford Univ Med Ctr; **Address:** 300 Pasteur Drive, SO92, MC 5105, Stanford, CA 94305; **Phone:** 650-650-2268; **Board Cert:** Diagnostic Radiology 1978; **Med School:** Georgetown Univ 1974; **Resid:** Diagnostic Radiology, Univ Cincinnati Hosp 1978; **Fellow:** Body Imaging, UCSF Med Ctr 1979; **Fac Appt:** Prof Rad, Stanford Univ

Diagnostic Radiology

Feig, Stephen A MD [DR] - **Spec Exp:** Breast Imaging; Breast Cancer; **Hospital:** UC Irvine Med Ctr; **Address:** UCI Medical Ctr, 101 City Drive South Route 140, Orange, CA 92868-3298; **Phone:** 714-456-6905; **Board Cert:** Diagnostic Radiology 1972; **Med School:** NYU Sch Med 1967; **Resid:** Radiology, Bronx Muni Hosp-Einstein 1971; **Fac Appt:** Prof Rad, UC Irvine

Filly, Roy A MD [DR] - **Spec Exp:** Obstetric Ultrasound; **Hospital:** UCSF Med Ctr; **Address:** UCSF Med Ctr, Dept Diagnostic Radiology, 505 Parnassus Ave, Box 0628, San Francisco, CA 94143-0628; **Phone:** 415-353-1628; **Board Cert:** Diagnostic Radiology 1974; **Med School:** Ohio State Univ 1970; **Resid:** Diagnostic Radiology, Stanford Univ Med Ctr 1974; **Fac Appt:** Prof Rad, UCSF

Gilsanz, Vicente MD [DR] - **Spec Exp:** Pediatric Radiology; Bone Disorders-Metabolic; **Hospital:** Chldns Hosp - Los Angeles; **Address:** Children's Hospital, LA, 4650 Sunset Blvd, MS 81, Los Angeles, CA 90027; **Phone:** 323-361-4571; **Board Cert:** Internal Medicine 1973; Diagnostic Radiology 1976; Pediatric Radiology 2004; **Med School:** Spain 1969; **Resid:** Internal Medicine, Mayo Clin 1973; Diagnostic Radiology, Mt Sinai Hosp 1976; **Fellow:** Pediatric Radiology, Chldns Hosp 1978; **Fac Appt:** Prof Rad, USC Sch Med

Lehman, Constance D MD/PhD [DR] - **Spec Exp:** Breast Imaging; **Hospital:** Univ Wash Med Ctr; **Address:** Seattle Cancer Care Alliance, 825 Eastlake Ave E, rm G2600, Seattle, WA 98109-1023; **Phone:** 206-288-2046; **Board Cert:** Diagnostic Radiology 1995; **Med School:** Yale Univ 1990; **Resid:** Diagnostic Radiology, Univ Wash Med Ctr 1995; **Fellow:** Diagnostic Radiology, Univ Wash Med Ctr 1996; **Fac Appt:** Prof Rad, Univ Wash

Pathria, Mini N MD [DR] - **Spec Exp:** Musculoskeletal Imaging; **Hospital:** UCSD Med Ctr; **Address:** UCSD Med Ctr, Dept Radiology, 200 W Arbor Drive, San Diego, CA 92103-8756; **Phone:** 858-543-5982; **Board Cert:** Diagnostic Radiology 1986; **Med School:** McMaster Univ 1982; **Resid:** Diagnostic Radiology, Mcmaster Univ 1983; **Fellow:** Skeletal Radiology, UCSD Med Ctr 1987; **Fac Appt:** Clin Prof Rad, UCSD

Rubin, Geoffrey D MD [DR] - **Spec Exp:** Cardiovascular Imaging; Cardiac Imaging; Thoracic Imaging; **Hospital:** Stanford Univ Med Ctr; **Address:** Stanford Univ Med Ctr, 300 Pasteur Drive, rm S 072, MC 5105, Stanford, CA 94305; **Phone:** 650-723-7647; **Board Cert:** Diagnostic Radiology 1992; **Med School:** UCSD 1987; **Resid:** Diagnostic Radiology, Stanford Univ Med Ctr 1992; **Fellow:** Body Imaging, Stanford Univ Med Ctr 1993; **Fac Appt:** Prof Rad, Stanford Univ

Thurmond, Amy S MD [DR] - **Spec Exp:** Women's Imaging; Infertility-Fallopian Tube Intervention; Gynecologic Imaging; **Hospital:** OR Hlth & Sci Univ; **Address:** 8950 SW Nimbus Ave, Beaverton, OR 97008; **Phone:** 503-643-7226; **Board Cert:** Diagnostic Radiology 1987; **Med School:** UCLA 1982; **Resid:** Cardiovascular Disease, St Vincent Hosp Med Ctr 1984; Diagnostic Radiology, Oreg Hlth Scis Univ 1987; **Fellow:** Interventional Radiology, Oreg Hlth Scis Univ 1988; **Fac Appt:** Assoc Prof Rad, Oregon Hlth & Sci Univ

Wood, Beverly MD/PhD [DR] - **Spec Exp:** Pediatric Radiology; **Hospital:** LAC & USC Med Ctr, Loma Linda Chldns Hosp; **Address:** Loma Linda Univ Chldns Hosp, Div Pediatric Radiology, 11234 Anderson St, rm 2835, Loma Linda, CA 92354; **Phone:** 909-558-4281; **Board Cert:** Diagnostic Radiology 1972; Pediatric Radiology 2003; **Med School:** Univ Rochester 1965; **Resid:** Diagnostic Radiology, Strong Meml Hosp 1971; **Fellow:** Pediatric Radiology, Strong Meml Hosp 1972; **Fac Appt:** Prof Rad, USC Sch Med

NEURORADIOLOGY

New England

Curtin, Hugh D MD [NRad] - **Spec Exp:** Head & Neck Radiology; **Hospital:** Mass Eye & Ear Infirmary; **Address:** Mass Eye & Ear Infirmary, Dept Radiology, 243 Charles St, Ground Level, Boston, MA 02114; **Phone:** 617-573-3563 x4; **Board Cert:** Diagnostic Radiology 1976; Neuroradiology 1999; **Med School:** SUNY Upstate Med Univ 1972; **Resid:** Diagnostic Radiology, Presby Univ Hosp 1976; **Fellow:** Neuroradiology, Foundation Rothschild; **Fac Appt:** Prof Rad, Harvard Med Sch

Hackney, David B MD [NRad] - **Hospital:** Beth Israel Deaconess Med Ctr - Boston; **Address:** BIDMC, Dept Radiology, 330 Brookline Ave, Boston, MA 02215; **Phone:** 617-754-2009; **Board Cert:** Diagnostic Radiology 1984; Neuroradiology 2005; **Med School:** Cornell Univ 1980; **Resid:** Diagnostic Radiology, UCSD Med Ctr 1983; **Fellow:** Neurological Radiology, Mass Genl Hosp 1985; **Fac Appt:** Prof Rad, Harvard Med Sch

Hirsch, Joshua A MD [NRad] - **Spec Exp:** Interventional Neuroradiology; Endovascular Surgery; Minimally Invasive Spinal Surgery; Osteoporosis Spine-Vertebroplasty; **Hospital:** Mass Genl Hosp; **Address:** Mass Genl Hospital, Interventional Neuroradiology, 55 Fruit St Gray Bldg - rm 241, Boston, MA 02114; **Phone:** 617-726-1767; **Board Cert:** Diagnostic Radiology 1996; **Med School:** Univ Pennsylvania 1991; **Resid:** Diagnostic Radiology, Hosp Univ Penn 1996; **Fellow:** Neuroradiology, Hosp Univ Penn 1995; Interventional Neuroradiology, Lahey Clinic 1998; **Fac Appt:** Asst Prof Rad, Harvard Med Sch

Norbash, Alexander M MD [NRad] - **Spec Exp:** Interventional Neuroradiology; Aneurysm-Cerebral; Osteoporosis Spine-Kyphoplasty; **Hospital:** Boston Med Ctr; **Address:** BMC, Dept Radiology, 820 Harrison Ave, Boston, MA 02118; **Phone:** 617-638-6610; **Board Cert:** Diagnostic Radiology 1991; Neuroradiology 2004; **Med School:** Univ MO-Kansas City 1986; **Resid:** Diagnostic Radiology, St Francis Hosp 1990; Diagnostic Radiology, Presby Univ Hosp 1991; **Fellow:** Neurological Radiology, Stanford Univ Hosp 1993; Interventional Radiology, Stanford Univ Hosp 1994; **Fac Appt:** Prof Rad, Boston Univ

Mid Atlantic

Berenstein, Alejandro MD [NRad] - **Spec Exp:** Interventional Neuroradiology; Aneurysm-Cerebral; Endovascular Surgery; **Hospital:** St Luke's - Roosevelt Hosp Ctr - Roosevelt Div (page 57); **Address:** Hyman-Newman Inst Neurolgy & Neuro Surg, 1000 10th Ave, rm GG16, New York, NY 10019; **Phone:** 212-636-3400; **Board Cert:** Diagnostic Radiology 1976; **Med School:** Mexico 1970; **Resid:** Diagnostic Radiology, Mt Sinai Med Ctr 1976; **Fellow:** Neuroradiology, NYU Med Ctr 1978; **Fac Appt:** Prof Rad, NYU Sch Med

Drayer, Burton P MD [NRad] - **Spec Exp:** Stroke; Parkinson's Disease/Aging Brain; MRI & CT of Brain & Spine; **Hospital:** Mount Sinai Med Ctr (page 64); **Address:** 1 Gustave Levy Pl, Box 1234, New York, NY 10029; **Phone:** 212-241-6403; **Board Cert:** Neurology 1976; Diagnostic Radiology 1978; Neuroradiology 2006; **Med School:** Ros Franklin Univ/Chicago Med Sch 1971; **Resid:** Neurology, Univ Vt Med Ctr 1975; Diagnostic Radiology, Univ Pitt Hlth Ctr 1978; **Fellow:** Neuroradiology, Univ Pitt Hlth Ctr 1978; **Fac Appt:** Prof Rad, Mount Sinai Sch Med

Neuroradiology

Flanders, Adam E MD [NRad] - **Spec Exp:** Spinal Trauma; Head Injury; **Hospital:** Thomas Jefferson Univ Hosp; **Address:** 132 10th St, 1072 Main Bldg, Philadelphia, PA 19107; **Phone:** 215-955-2430; **Board Cert:** Diagnostic Radiology 1987; Neuroradiology 1996; **Med School:** Rush Med Coll 1983; **Resid:** Diagnostic Radiology, Univ Illinois Hosps 1987; **Fellow:** Neuroradiology, Thos Jefferson Univ Hosp; **Fac Appt:** Prof Rad, Thomas Jefferson Univ

Grossman, Robert I MD [NRad] - **Spec Exp:** Multiple Sclerosis Imaging; Brain Injury; MRI; **Hospital:** NYU Langone Med Ctr (page 67), Bellevue Hosp Ctr; **Address:** NYU Med Ctr, Dept Radiology, 530 First Ave, HCC15, New York, NY 10016; **Phone:** 212-263-3269; **Board Cert:** Diagnostic Radiology 1979; Neuroradiology 2005; **Med School:** Univ Pennsylvania 1973; **Resid:** Neurological Surgery, Hosp Univ Penn 1976; Diagnostic Radiology, Hosp Univ Penn 1979; **Fellow:** Neuroradiology, Mass Genl Hosp 1981; **Fac Appt:** Prof Rad, NYU Sch Med

Hurst, Robert W MD [NRad] - **Spec Exp:** Interventional Neuroradiology; Aneurysm; Carotid Artery Stent Placement; Intracranial Angioplasty & Stent; **Hospital:** Hosp Univ Penn - UPHS (page 60); **Address:** Dept Radiology/Neuroradiology, HUP, 3400 Spruce St, Silverstein 1, 219 Dullis Bldg, Philadelphia, PA 19104; **Phone:** 215-662-3572; **Board Cert:** Neurology 1986; Diagnostic Radiology 1989; Neuroradiology 2005; **Med School:** Univ Tex, Houston 1981; **Resid:** Neurology, Univ Virginia Hosp 1985; Diagnostic Radiology, Univ Virginia Hosp 1989; **Fellow:** Neurological Radiology, Hosp Univ Penn 1990; Interventional Radiology, NYU Med Ctr 1991; **Fac Appt:** Prof Rad, Univ Pennsylvania

Khandji, Alexander G MD [NRad] - **Spec Exp:** Pituitary Disorders; Spine Imaging & Intervention; MRI; Brain Tumors; **Hospital:** NY-Presby Hosp/Columbia (page 66); **Address:** 177 Ft Washington Ave, Ste 4-156, New York, NY 10032-3173; **Phone:** 212-305-7669; **Board Cert:** Diagnostic Radiology 1985; Neuroradiology 2006; **Med School:** SUNY Downstate 1980; **Resid:** Surgery, MS Hershey Med Ctr 1982; Diagnostic Radiology, Columbia-Presby Med Ctr 1985; **Fellow:** Neuroradiology, Columbia-Presby Med Ctr 1987; **Fac Appt:** Clin Prof Rad, Columbia P&S

Litt, Andrew W MD [NRad] - **Spec Exp:** Vascular Lesions of the CNS; Cerebrovascular Disease; Stroke; **Hospital:** NYU Langone Med Ctr (page 67); **Address:** NYU Med Ctr, Dept Radiology, 560 1st Ave, IRM 232, New York, NY 10016-6402; **Phone:** 212-263-8121; **Board Cert:** Diagnostic Radiology 1988; Neuroradiology 2005; **Med School:** NYU Sch Med 1983; **Resid:** Diagnostic Radiology, NYU Med Ctr 1987; **Fellow:** Neuroradiology, NYU Med Ctr 1988; **Fac Appt:** Prof Rad, NYU Sch Med

Loevner, Laurie A MD [NRad] - **Spec Exp:** Head & Neck Cancer; Thyroid Cancer; Brain Tumor Imaging; Spinal Tumor Imaging; **Hospital:** Hosp Univ Penn - UPHS (page 60), Pennsylvania Hosp (page 60); **Address:** Univ Penn Med Ctr-Dept Rad, 3400 Spruce St, Philadelphia, PA 19104; **Phone:** 215-662-3020; **Board Cert:** Diagnostic Radiology 1993; Neuroradiology 2006; **Med School:** Univ Pennsylvania 1988; **Resid:** Diagnostic Radiology, Univ Michigan Hosps 1993; **Fellow:** Neuroradiology, Hosp Univ Penn 1995; **Fac Appt:** Prof Rad, Univ Pennsylvania

Pile-Spellman, John MD [NRad] - **Spec Exp:** Interventional Neuroradiology; Cerebrovascular Disease; Aneurysm; Arteriovenous Malformations; **Hospital:** NY-Presby Hosp/Columbia (page 66); **Address:** 177 Fort Washington Ave, MHB 8SK, New York, NY 10032-3713; **Phone:** 212-305-6515; **Board Cert:** Diagnostic Radiology 1984; **Med School:** Tufts Univ 1978; **Resid:** Neurological Surgery, New England Med Ctr 1981; Neurological Radiology, Mass Genl Hosp 1984; **Fellow:** Interventional Neuroradiology, NYU Med Ctr 1986; **Fac Appt:** Prof Rad, Columbia P&S

Tenner, Michael MD [NRad] - **Spec Exp:** Stroke; Aneurysm-Cerebral; Arteriovenous Malformations; Carotid Artery Stent Placement; **Hospital:** Westchester Med Ctr; **Address:** NY Med Coll, Dept Radiology, Route 100, Valhalla, NY 10595; **Phone:** 914-493-8158; **Board Cert:** Diagnostic Radiology 1967; Neuroradiology 2007; **Med School:** Univ MD Sch Med 1960; **Resid:** Diagnostic Radiology, Univ Maryland Hosp 1962; Diagnostic Radiology, Univ Maryland Hosp 1966; **Fellow:** Neuroradiology, Neurological Inst-Columbia Presby 1968; **Fac Appt:** Prof Rad, NY Med Coll

Vezina, L Gilbert MD [NRad] - **Spec Exp:** Pediatric Neuroradiology; Brain Tumors; Neurofibromatosis; **Hospital:** Chldns Natl Med Ctr; **Address:** Chldns Natl Med Ctr, Dept Radiology, 111 Michigan Ave NW, Washington, DC 20010-2970; **Phone:** 202-476-3651; **Board Cert:** Diagnostic Radiology 1987; Neuroradiology 1998; **Med School:** McGill Univ 1983; **Resid:** Diagnostic Radiology, Mass Genl Hosp 1987; **Fellow:** Neurological Radiology, Mass Genl Hosp 1989; Pediatric Neuroradiology, Chldns Natl Med Ctr 1991; **Fac Appt:** Prof, Geo Wash Univ

Yousem, David M MD [NRad] - **Hospital:** Johns Hopkins Hosp (page 61); **Address:** Johns Hopkins Hosp, Div Neuroradiology, 600 N Wolfe St Phipps Bldg - rm B-100, Baltimore, MD 21287; **Phone:** 410-955-2353; **Board Cert:** Diagnostic Radiology 1987; Neuroradiology 2005; **Med School:** Univ Mich Med Sch 1983; **Resid:** Diagnostic Radiology, Johns Hopkins Hosp 1987; **Fellow:** Neuroradiology, Hosp Univ Penn 1990; **Fac Appt:** Prof Rad, Johns Hopkins Univ

Zimmerman, Robert A MD [NRad] - **Spec Exp:** Pediatric Neuroradiology; **Hospital:** Chldns Hosp of Philadelphia, The; **Address:** Childrens Hosp Philadelphia, Radiology, 34th St & Civic Center Blvd, Philadelphia, PA 19104; **Phone:** 215-590-2569; **Board Cert:** Diagnostic Radiology 1970; Neuroradiology 2005; **Med School:** Georgetown Univ 1964; **Resid:** Diagnostic Radiology, Hosp Univ Penn 1969; **Fac Appt:** Prof Rad, Univ Pennsylvania

Zinreich, S James MD [NRad] - **Spec Exp:** Head & Neck Radiology; **Hospital:** Johns Hopkins Hosp (page 61); **Address:** Johns Hopkins Hospital, 600 N Wolfe St Phipps Bldg - rm B-100, Baltimore, MD 21287; **Phone:** 410-614-3020; **Board Cert:** Diagnostic Radiology 1982; Neuroradiology 2006; **Med School:** Belgium 1976; **Resid:** Diagnostic Radiology, Sinai Hosp; **Fac Appt:** Prof Oto, Johns Hopkins Univ

Southeast

Dion, Jacques E MD [NRad] - **Spec Exp:** Interventional Neuroradiology; Aneurysm-Cerebral; Intracranial Angioplasty & Stent; **Hospital:** Emory Univ Hosp; **Address:** Emory Univ Hosp, Dept Neuroradiology, 1364 Clifton Rd NE, rm A121, Atlanta, GA 30322; **Phone:** 404-712-4991; **Board Cert:** Diagnostic Radiology 1982; Neuroradiology 1998; **Med School:** Univ Ottawa 1978; **Resid:** Diagnostic Radiology, Harbor-UCLA Med Ctr 1981; Diagnostic Radiology, Notre Dame Hosp 1983; **Fellow:** Neuroradiology, Univ Hospital 1985; **Fac Appt:** Prof Rad, Emory Univ

Jensen, Mary E MD [NRad] - **Spec Exp:** Interventional Neuroradiology; Osteoporosis Spine-Vertebroplasty; Aneurysm-Cerebral; **Hospital:** Univ Virginia Med Ctr; **Address:** Univ of Virginia Med Ctr, Dept Radiology, Box 800170, Charlottsville, VA 22908; **Phone:** 434-924-9719; **Board Cert:** Diagnostic Radiology 1987; **Med School:** Med Coll VA 1982; **Resid:** Diagnostic Radiology, Univ Virginia Med Ctr 1991; **Fellow:** Interventional Neuroradiology, UCLA Med Ctr 1992; **Fac Appt:** Assoc Prof, Univ VA Sch Med

Joseph, Gregory J MD [NRad] - **Spec Exp:** Stroke; Aneurysm-Cerebral; Intracranial Angioplasty & Stent; **Hospital:** Presby Hosp - Charlotte; **Address:** Presbyterian Hosp, Dept Radiology, 200 Hawthorne Ln, Charlotte, NC 28204; **Phone:** 704-384-9654; **Board Cert:** Diagnostic Radiology 1989; **Med School:** Georgetown Univ 1984; **Resid:** Diagnostic Radiology, Georgetown Univ Hosp 1989; Vascular & Interventional Radiology, Emory Univ Hosp 1990; **Fellow:** Neuroradiology, Emory Univ Hosp 1991

Neuroradiology

Morris, P Pearse MD [NRad] - Spec Exp: Interventional Neuroradiology; Endovascular Neurosurgery; Aneurysm-Cerebral; Arteriovenous Malformations; **Hospital:** Wake Forest Univ Baptist Med Ctr (page 72); **Address:** Wake Forest Univ Bapt Med Ctr, One Medical Center Blvd, MRI Bldg, Fl 3, Winston-Salem, NC 27157; **Phone:** 336-716-7849; **Board Cert:** Psychiatry 1989; Diagnostic Radiology 1994; Neuroradiology 2007; **Med School:** Ireland 1983; **Resid:** Psychiatry, Johns Hopkins Hosp 1987; Diagnostic Radiology, Mass Genl Hosp 1994; **Fellow:** Geriatric Psychiatry, Cornell Univ 1988; Neuroradiology, Mass Genl Hosp 1995; **Fac Appt:** Prof Rad, Wake Forest Univ

Murtagh, F Reed MD [NRad] - Spec Exp: Neuro-Oncology; Brain Tumor Imaging; Spinal Tumor Imaging; Memory Disorders; **Hospital:** H Lee Moffitt Cancer Ctr & Research Inst; **Address:** Univ Diagnostic Institute-USF, 3301 Alumni Drive, Tampa, FL 33612; **Phone:** 813-975-0725; **Board Cert:** Diagnostic Radiology 1978; Neuroradiology 2004; **Med School:** Temple Univ 1971; **Resid:** Diagnostic Radiology, Jackson Meml Hosp 1978; **Fellow:** Neurological Radiology, Univ Miami 1979; **Fac Appt:** Prof Rad, Univ S Fla Coll Med

Provenzale, James M MD [NRad] - Spec Exp: Brain Tumor Imaging; Multiple Sclerosis Imaging; Brain Imaging-Pediatric; **Hospital:** Duke Univ Med Ctr; **Address:** Duke University Medical Ctr, Dept Radiology, Box 3808, Durham, NC 27710; **Phone:** 919-684-7218; **Board Cert:** Neurology 1988; Diagnostic Radiology 1991; Neuroradiology 2001; **Med School:** Albany Med Coll 1983; **Resid:** Neurology, NC Memorial Hosp 1987; Diagnostic Radiology, Mass Genl Hosp 1991; **Fellow:** Neuroradiology, Mass Genl Hosp 1992; **Fac Appt:** Prof, Duke Univ

Quencer, Robert MD [NRad] - Spec Exp: Spinal Cord Injury; **Hospital:** Univ of Miami Hosp & Clins/Sylvester Comp Canc Ctr (page 70); **Address:** Univ Miami, Dept Radiology, 1150 NW 14th St, Ste 511, M828, Miami, FL 33136-2116; **Phone:** 305-243-4701; **Board Cert:** Diagnostic Radiology 1972; Neuroradiology 2006; **Med School:** SUNY Upstate Med Univ 1967; **Resid:** Diagnostic Radiology, Columbia-Presbyterian Med Ctr 1971; **Fellow:** Neuroradiology, Neurological Inst 1972; **Fac Appt:** Prof, Univ Miami Sch Med

Midwest

Ball Jr, William S MD [NRad] - Spec Exp: Pediatric Neuroradiology; **Hospital:** Cincinnati Chldns Hosp Med Ctr; **Address:** Cincinnati Chldns Hosp, Dept Neuroradiology, 3333 Burnet Ave, ML 5031, Cincinnati, OH 45229-3039; **Phone:** 513-636-8574; **Board Cert:** Diagnostic Radiology 1982; Pediatrics 1982; Neuroradiology 1999; **Med School:** Tulane Univ 1974; **Resid:** Pediatrics, Oschner Fdn Hosp 1977; Diagnostic Radiology, Univ New Mexico 1978; **Fellow:** Pediatric Radiology, Chldns Hosp Med Ctr 1981; Neuroradiology, Univ New Mexico Med Ctr 1979; **Fac Appt:** Prof, Univ Cincinnati

Cross III, DeWitte T MD [NRad] - Spec Exp: Interventional Neuroradiology; Aneurysm-Cerebral; Stroke; **Hospital:** Barnes-Jewish Hosp, St Louis Chldns Hosp; **Address:** Wash Univ, Dept Radiology, 510 S Kingshighway Blvd, Box 8131, St Louis, MO 63110-1016; **Phone:** 314-362-5580; **Board Cert:** Diagnostic Radiology 1985; Neuroradiology 2006; **Med School:** Univ Alabama 1980; **Resid:** Diagnostic Radiology, Naval Hosp 1985; **Fellow:** Neuroradiology, NY Med Coll 1988; Neuroradiology, Columbia Univ 1989; **Fac Appt:** Assoc Prof Rad, Washington Univ, St Louis

Grobelny, Thomas MD [NRad] - Spec Exp: Interventional Neuroradiology; Aneurysm-Cerebral; Stroke; Arteriovenous Malformations; **Hospital:** Neuro & Ortho Hosp of Chicago, Adv Christ Med Ctr; **Address:** 4501 N Winchester Ave Fl 2, Chicago, IL 60640; **Phone:** 800-446-1234; **Board Cert:** Diagnostic Radiology 1996; Neuroradiology 1998; **Med School:** Poland 1986; **Resid:** Diagnostic Radiology, Harlem Hospital 1995; **Fellow:** Neurocritical Care, Thos Jefferson Univ Hosp 1998; Interventional Neuroradiology, UCLA Med Ctr 1989

Haughton III, Victor M MD [NRad] - **Spec Exp:** Spinal Imaging; **Hospital:** Univ WI Hosp & Clins; **Address:** Univ WI Hosps & Clins, Dept Radiology, 600 Highland Ave, MC 3252, Madison, WI 53792; **Phone:** 608-263-9179; **Board Cert:** Diagnostic Radiology 1974; **Med School:** Yale Univ 1967; **Resid:** Diagnostic Radiology, Peter Bent Brigham Hosp 1973; **Fellow:** Neurological Radiology, Peter Bent Brigham Hosp 1974; **Fac Appt:** Prof Rad, Univ Wisc

Kallmes, David F MD [NRad] - **Spec Exp:** Aneurysm-Cerebral; Stroke; Osteoporosis Spine-Vertebroplasty; **Hospital:** Mayo Med Ctr & Clin - Rochester; **Address:** Mayo Clinic, Old Marion Hall, 200 First St SW, Rochester, MN 55905; **Phone:** 507-266-3350; **Board Cert:** Diagnostic Radiology 1994; Neuroradiology 1998; **Med School:** Univ Mass Sch Med 1989; **Resid:** Diagnostic Radiology, Duke Univ Med Ctr 1993; **Fellow:** Neuroradiology, Univ Virginia Med Ctr 1995; **Fac Appt:** Assoc Prof Rad, Mayo Med Sch

Koeller, Kelly K MD [NRad] - **Spec Exp:** Brain Tumor Imaging; Head & Neck Tumors Imaging; Spinal Tumor Imaging; **Hospital:** Mayo Med Ctr & Clin - Rochester; **Address:** Mayo Clinic, 200 First St SW Charlton Bldg - rm 2-290, Rochester, MN 55905; **Phone:** 507-266-3412; **Board Cert:** Diagnostic Radiology 1990; Neuroradiology 2004; **Med School:** Univ Tenn Coll Med, Memphis 1982; **Resid:** Diagnostic Radiology, Naval Hosp 1990; **Fellow:** Neuroradiology, UCSF Med Ctr 1992

Masaryk, Thomas MD [NRad] - **Spec Exp:** Cerebrovascular Disease; Aneurysm-Cerebral; Vascular Lesions of the CNS; Carotid Artery Stent Placement; **Hospital:** Cleveland Clin Fdn (page 56); **Address:** Dept Radiology, 9500 Euclid Desk Ave P34, Cleveland, OH 44195; **Phone:** 216-444-6653; **Board Cert:** Diagnostic Radiology 1985; Neuroradiology 2005; **Med School:** Med Coll OH 1981; **Resid:** Diagnostic Radiology, Cleveland Clinic 1984; **Fellow:** Neurological Radiology, Cleveland Clinic 1985

Modic, Michael MD [NRad] - **Spec Exp:** MRI; Spinal Imaging; **Hospital:** Cleveland Clin Fdn (page 56); **Address:** 9500 Euclid Ave Desk, Cleveland, OH 44195; **Phone:** 216-444-9308; **Board Cert:** Diagnostic Radiology 1979; Neuroradiology 2003; **Med School:** Case West Res Univ 1975; **Resid:** Diagnostic Radiology, Cleveland Clin Fdn 1978; **Fellow:** Neuroradiology, Cleveland Clin Fdn 1979; **Fac Appt:** Prof Rad, Cleveland Cl Coll Med/Case West Res

Moran, Christopher J MD [NRad] - **Spec Exp:** Aneurysm-Cerebral; Cerebrovascular Disease/Stroke; Carotid Artery Stent Placement; Interventional Neuroradiology; **Hospital:** Barnes-Jewish Hosp; **Address:** Mallinckrodt Inst Radiology, Wash Univ Sch Med, Campus Box 8131, 510 S Kings Highway Blvd, St Louis, MO 63110; **Phone:** 314-362-5949; **Board Cert:** Diagnostic Radiology 1978; Neuroradiology 2004; **Med School:** St Louis Univ 1974; **Resid:** Diagnostic Radiology, Mallinckrodt Inst Rad/Wash U 1978; **Fellow:** Neuroradiology, Mallinckrodt Inst Rad/Wash U 1979; **Fac Appt:** Prof Rad, Washington Univ, St Louis

Mukherji, Suresh K MD [NRad] - **Spec Exp:** Head & Neck Radiology; Head & Neck Tumors Imaging; **Hospital:** Univ Michigan Hlth Sys; **Address:** Univ of Michigan-Dept Radiology, 1500 E Medical Ctr Drive, UH-B2A209B, Ann Arbor, MI 48109-0030; **Phone:** 734-936-8865; **Board Cert:** Diagnostic Radiology 1992; Neuroradiology 2006; **Med School:** Georgetown Univ 1987; **Resid:** Diagnostic Radiology, Brigham & Women's Hosp 1992; **Fellow:** Neuroradiology, Univ Florida 1994; **Fac Appt:** Prof Oto, Univ Mich Med Sch

Rowley, Howard A MD [NRad] - **Spec Exp:** Epilepsy; Cerebrovascular Disease/Stroke; **Hospital:** Univ WI Hosp & Clins; **Address:** Dept Neuroradiology, 600 Highland Ave, MC 3252, Madison, WI 53792; **Phone:** 608-265-8310; **Board Cert:** Neurology 1991; Diagnostic Radiology 1993; Neuroradiology 2007; **Med School:** Washington Univ, St Louis 1985; **Resid:** Neurology, UCSF Med Ctr 1989; Diagnostic Radiology, UCSF Med Ctr 1991; **Fellow:** Neurological Radiology, UCSF Med Ctr 1991; **Fac Appt:** Prof Rad, Univ Wisc

Neuroradiology

Great Plains and Mountains

Osborn, Anne G MD [NRad] - **Spec Exp:** Spinal Imaging; Brain Imaging; Head & Neck Radiology; **Hospital:** Univ Utah Hosps and Clins; **Address:** Dept Radiology, 30 N 1900 E, rm 1A71, Salt Lake City, UT 84132-2140; **Phone:** 801-581-7553; **Board Cert:** Diagnostic Radiology 1974; Neuroradiology 2004; **Med School:** Stanford Univ 1970; **Resid:** Diagnostic Radiology, Stanford Univ Hosp 1974; **Fellow:** Diagnostic Radiology, Univ Utah Hosp 1977; **Fac Appt:** Prof, Univ Utah

Southwest

Hunter, Jill V MD [NRad] - **Spec Exp:** Pediatric Neuroradiology; Brain Injury-Pediatric; **Hospital:** Texas Chldns Hosp; **Address:** 6621 Fannin, West Twr, Ste B120, MC 2-252, Houston, TX 77030; **Phone:** 832-822-5324; **Board Cert:** Diagnostic Radiology 1997; Neuroradiology 1998; **Med School:** England, UK 1975; **Resid:** Diagnostic Radiology, Baylor Coll Med 1978; **Fellow:** Neuroradiology, Queen Square Hosp 1992; **Fac Appt:** Assoc Prof Rad, Baylor Coll Med

Mawad, Michel E MD [NRad] - **Spec Exp:** Interventional Neuroradiology; **Hospital:** St Luke's Episcopal Hosp-Houston; **Address:** BCM Neurovascular, 6720 Bertner Ave, MC 4267, Houston, TX 77030; **Phone:** 713-798-2200; **Board Cert:** Diagnostic Radiology 1980; Neuroradiology 2006; **Med School:** Lebanon 1976; **Resid:** Diagnostic Radiology, St Luke's-Roosevelt Hosp 1979; **Fellow:** Neurological Radiology, Columbia-Presby Med Ctr 1980; **Fac Appt:** Prof, Baylor Coll Med

West Coast and Pacific

Atlas, Scott W MD [NRad] - **Spec Exp:** Stroke; MRI; Brain Tumors; **Hospital:** Stanford Univ Med Ctr; **Address:** Stanford Univ Med Ctr, Dept Rad, 300 Pasteur Drive, rm S-047, Stanford, CA 94304-2204; **Phone:** 650-498-7152; **Board Cert:** Diagnostic Radiology 1985; Neuroradiology 2005; **Med School:** Univ Chicago-Pritzker Sch Med 1981; **Resid:** Diagnostic Radiology, Northwestern Univ Med Ctr 1985; **Fellow:** Neuroradiology, Hosp Univ Pennsylvania 1987; **Fac Appt:** Prof, Stanford Univ

Barkovich, Anthony J MD [NRad] - **Spec Exp:** Pediatric Neuroradiology; MRI; Brain Development Abnormalities; **Hospital:** UCSF Med Ctr; **Address:** UCSF Med Ctr, Dept Neuroradiology, 505 Parnassus Ave, rm L371, Box 0628, San Francisco, CA 94143-0628; **Phone:** 415-353-1668; **Board Cert:** Diagnostic Radiology 1984; Neuroradiology 2006; **Med School:** Geo Wash Univ 1980; **Resid:** Diagnostic Radiology, Letterman AMC 1984; **Fellow:** Neuroradiology, Walter Reed AMC 1986; **Fac Appt:** Prof Rad, UCSF

Barnes, Patrick D MD [NRad] - **Spec Exp:** Pediatric Neuroradiology; Brain Injury-Pediatric; Brain Development Abnormalities; Fetal Neuroradiology; **Hospital:** Lucile Packard Chldn's Hosp; **Address:** Lucile Packard Chldns Hosp, Pediatric Neuroradiology, 725 Welch Rd, Palo Alto, CA 94304; **Phone:** 650-497-8376; **Board Cert:** Diagnostic Radiology 1977; Neuroradiology 2008; **Med School:** Univ Okla Coll Med 1973; **Resid:** Diagnostic Radiology, Univ Okla Coll Med 1976; **Fellow:** Pediatric Neuroradiology, Chldns Hosp/Harvard Med Sch 1977; **Fac Appt:** Assoc Prof, Stanford Univ

Cha, Soonmee MD [NRad] - **Spec Exp:** Brain Tumors; **Hospital:** UCSF Med Ctr; **Address:** 505 Parnassus Ave, Ste L-358, Neuroradiology Section, San Francisco, CA 94143-0628; **Phone:** 415-353-8913; **Board Cert:** Diagnostic Radiology 1996; Neuroradiology 1998; **Med School:** Georgetown Univ 1991; **Resid:** Diagnostic Radiology, North Shore Univ Hosp 1996; **Fellow:** Neuroradiology, NYU Med Ctr 1998; **Fac Appt:** Assoc Prof Rad, UCSF

Dillon, William P MD [NRad] - **Spec Exp:** Brain Tumors; **Hospital:** UCSF Med Ctr; **Address:** 505 Parnassus Ave, rm L 371, San Francisco, CA 94143-0628; **Phone:** 415-353-1668; **Board Cert:** Diagnostic Radiology 1982; Neuroradiology 2006; **Med School:** Loyola Univ-Stritch Sch Med 1978; **Resid:** Diagnostic Radiology, Univ Utah Hosp 1982; **Fellow:** Neuroradiology, UCSF Med Ctr 1983; **Fac Appt:** Prof, UCSF

Hesselink, John R MD [NRad] - **Spec Exp:** MRI & CT of Brain & Spine; Stroke; Brain Tumor Imaging; **Hospital:** UCSD Med Ctr; **Address:** UCSD Med Ctr, Div Neuroradiology, 200 W Arbor Drive, San Diego, CA 92013; **Phone:** 619-543-3736; **Board Cert:** Diagnostic Radiology 1975; Neuroradiology 2005; **Med School:** Univ Wisc 1971; **Resid:** Diagnostic Radiology, Univ Wisconsin-Madison 1975; **Fellow:** Neuroradiology, Mass Genl Hosp- Harvard Univ 1979; **Fac Appt:** Prof Rad, UCSD

Higashida, Randall T MD [NRad] - **Spec Exp:** Aneurysm-Cerebral; Stroke; Intracranial Angioplasty & Stent; **Hospital:** UCSF Med Ctr; **Address:** UCSF Med Ctr, Dept Interven Neurorad, 505 Parnassus Ave, rm L352, San Francisco, CA 94143-0628; **Phone:** 415-353-1863; **Board Cert:** Diagnostic Radiology 1984; **Med School:** Tulane Univ 1980; **Resid:** Diagnostic Radiology, UCLA Med Ctr 1984; **Fellow:** Neuroradiology, UCLA Med Ctr 1985; **Fac Appt:** Clin Prof, UCSF

Jarvik, Jeffrey G MD [NRad] - **Hospital:** Univ Wash Med Ctr; **Address:** Univ Washington, Dept of Radiology, 1959 NE Pacific St, Box 357115, Seattle, WA 98195; **Phone:** 206-598-6200; **Board Cert:** Diagnostic Radiology 1992; Neuroradiology 2005; **Med School:** UCSD 1987; **Resid:** Diagnostic Radiology, Hosp Univ Penn 1992; **Fellow:** Neuroradiology, Hosp Univ Penn 1993; **Fac Appt:** Prof Rad, Univ Wash

Larsen, Donald William MD [NRad] - **Spec Exp:** Interventional Neuroradiology; Stroke; Stroke Prevention; Aneurysm-Cerebral; **Hospital:** USC Univ Hosp; **Address:** 1520 San Pablo Rd, Ste 3800, Los Angeles, CA 90033; **Phone:** 323-447-5720; **Board Cert:** Diagnostic Radiology 1990; **Med School:** Ros Franklin Univ/Chicago Med Sch 1985; **Resid:** Diagnostic Radiology, USC Med Ctr 1990; **Fellow:** Vascular & Interventional Radiology, USC Med Ctr 1991; Neuroradiology, USF Med Ctr 1995; **Fac Appt:** Assoc Prof Rad, USC-Keck School of Medicine

Norman, David MD [NRad] - **Hospital:** UCSF Med Ctr; **Address:** UCSF Med Ctr, Dept Neuroradiology, 505 Parnassus Ave, rm L358, Box 0628, San Francisco, CA 94143-0628; **Phone:** 415-353-1668; **Board Cert:** Diagnostic Radiology 1972; Neuroradiology 2006; **Med School:** Univ Pennsylvania 1967; **Resid:** Diagnostic Radiology, Columbia-Presby Hosp 1971; **Fellow:** Neuroradiology, UCSF Med Ctr 1975; **Fac Appt:** Prof, UCSF

Teitelbaum, George P MD [NRad] - **Spec Exp:** Interventional Neuroradiology; Aneurysm-Cerebral; Carotid Artery Stent Placement; Vascular Lesions of the CNS; **Hospital:** St Joseph Hosp, Providence St Joseph Med Ctr; **Address:** 501 S Buena Vista St, Burbank, CA 91505; **Phone:** 818-847-4835; **Board Cert:** Diagnostic Radiology 1984; Neuroradiology 2008; **Med School:** UCSD 1980; **Resid:** Diagnostic Radiology, UC Irvine Med Ctr 1984; Interventional Radiology, George Washington 1985; **Fellow:** Magnetic Resonance Imaging, Huntington Med Research Inst 1988; Interventional Radiology, UCSF Med Ctr 1994; **Fac Appt:** Prof NS, USC-Keck School of Medicine

Vinuela, Fernando MD [NRad] - **Spec Exp:** Stroke; Intracranial Angioplasty & Stent; Aneurysm-Cerebral; **Hospital:** UCLA Ronald Reagan Med Ctr; **Address:** 757 West Wood Plaza, rm 2129, Los Angeles, CA 90095-7437; **Phone:** 310-267-8765; **Board Cert:** Diagnostic Radiology 1979; **Med School:** Uruguay 1970; **Resid:** Diagnostic Radiology, Westminster Hosp 1975; Diagnostic Radiology, Victoria Hosp 1977; **Fellow:** Neuroradiology, Univ Hosp 1979; **Fac Appt:** Prof, UCLA

VASCULAR & INTERVENTIONAL RADIOLOGY

New England

Aruny, John E MD [VIR] - **Spec Exp:** Thrombolytic Therapy; Dialysis Access; Vascular Disease; Vein Disorders; **Hospital:** Yale-New Haven Hosp; **Address:** Yale Univ School of Medicine, 333 Cedar St, New Haven, CT 06520; **Phone:** 203-785-7026; **Board Cert:** Diag Rad with Spec Comp in Nuc Rad 1989; **Med School:** Mexico 1983; **Resid:** Diagnostic Radiology, Westch Co Med Ctr 1989; **Fellow:** Interventional Radiology, Brigham & Women's Hosp 1992; **Fac Appt:** Assoc Prof Rad, Yale Univ

Hallisey, Michael J MD [VIR] - **Spec Exp:** Uterine Fibroid Embolization; Liver Cancer/Chemoembolization; **Hospital:** Hartford Hosp; **Address:** 399 Farmington Ave, Farmington, CT 06032; **Phone:** 860-246-6589; **Board Cert:** Diagnostic Radiology 1991; Vascular & Interventional Radiology 1998; **Med School:** Univ Conn 1986; **Resid:** Diagnostic Radiology, Hospital of St Raphael 1991

Murphy, Timothy P MD [VIR] - **Spec Exp:** Uterine Fibroid Embolization; Aneurysm-Aortic; Hypertension-Renovascular; **Hospital:** Rhode Island Hosp; **Address:** Rhode Island Hosp, Dept Diagnostic Imaging, 593 Eddy Street Fl 3rd, Providence, RI 02903-4970; **Phone:** 401-444-5194; **Board Cert:** Diagnostic Radiology 1992; Vascular & Interventional Radiology 2005; **Med School:** Boston Univ 1987; **Resid:** Diagnostic Radiology, Rhode Island Hosp 1992; **Fellow:** Vascular & Interventional Radiology, Rhode Island Hosp 1993; **Fac Appt:** Prof Rad, Brown Univ

White, Robert I MD [VIR] - **Spec Exp:** Uterine Fibroid Embolization; Pelvic Congestion Syndrome; Varicocele Embolization; Vascular Malformations; **Hospital:** Yale-New Haven Hosp; **Address:** Yale Univ Sch Med, Vasc & Interventional Rad, PO Box 208042, New Haven, CT 06520-8042; **Phone:** 203-737-5395; **Board Cert:** Diagnostic Radiology 1970; **Med School:** Baylor Coll Med 1963; **Resid:** Internal Medicine, Johns Hopkins Hosp 1967; Diagnostic Radiology, Johns Hopkins Hosp 1969; **Fellow:** Cardiovascular Disease, Johns Hopkins Hosp 1958; Cardiovascular Radiology, Univ Minn Med Ctr 1971; **Fac Appt:** Prof Rad, Yale Univ

Mid Atlantic

Brown, Daniel B MD [VIR] - **Spec Exp:** Liver Cancer/Chemoembolization; **Hospital:** Thomas Jefferson Univ Hosp; **Address:** Thos Jefferson Univ Hospital, Dept Radiology, 132 S 10th St, Philadelphia, PA 19107; **Phone:** 215-955-7976; **Board Cert:** Diagnostic Radiology 1997; Vascular & Interventional Radiology 2001; **Med School:** Hahnemann Univ 1993; **Resid:** Diagnostic Radiology, Bryn Mawr Hosp 1997; **Fellow:** Vascular & Interventional Radiology, Penn State 1999; **Fac Appt:** Assoc Prof Rad, Thomas Jefferson Univ

Denny, Donald F MD [VIR] - **Spec Exp:** Dialysis Access; Uterine Fibroids; **Hospital:** Univ Med Ctr - Princeton; **Address:** Princeton Radiology Assocs, 3674 Route 27, Kendall Park, NJ 08824; **Phone:** 609-497-4310; **Board Cert:** Diagnostic Radiology 1982; Vascular & Interventional Radiology 2005; **Med School:** Hahnemann Univ 1978; **Resid:** Diagnostic Radiology, Yale-New Haven Hosp 1982; **Fellow:** Diagnostic Radiology, Brigham & Womens Hosp 1983; **Fac Appt:** Assoc Clin Prof Rad, Yale Univ

Geschwind, Jean-Francois H MD [VIR] - **Spec Exp:** Liver Cancer/Chemoembolization; Cancer Chemoembolization; Cancer Radiotherapy; **Hospital:** Johns Hopkins Hosp (page 61); **Address:** Interventional Radiology, 600 N Wolfe St Blalock Bldg - rm 545, Baltimore, MD 21287; **Phone:** 410-955-6358; **Board Cert:** Diagnostic Radiology 1998; **Med School:** Boston Univ 1991; **Resid:** Diagnostic Radiology, UCSF Med Ctr 1996; **Fellow:** Interventional Radiology, Johns Hopkins Hosp 1998; **Fac Appt:** Assoc Prof, Johns Hopkins Univ

Haskal, Ziv MD [VIR] - **Spec Exp:** Uterine Fibroid Embolization; Vascular Malformations; Liver Cancer/Chemoembolization; **Hospital:** Univ of MD Med Ctr; **Address:** 22 S Greene St, rm G2K14, Baltimore, MD 21201; **Phone:** 410-328-7467; **Board Cert:** Diagnostic Radiology 1991; Vascular & Interventional Radiology 1999; **Med School:** Boston Univ 1986; **Resid:** Diagnostic Radiology, UCSF Med Ctr 1991; **Fellow:** Vascular & Interventional Radiology, UCSF Med Ctr 1992; **Fac Appt:** Prof Rad, Univ MD Sch Med

McLean, Gordon K MD [VIR] - **Spec Exp:** Uterine Fibroid Embolization; Angioplasty & Stent Placement; **Hospital:** Western Penn Hosp; **Address:** Western Pennsylvania Hosp, Dept Radiology, 4800 Friendship Ave, Pittsburgh, PA 15224-1722; **Phone:** 412-578-7412; **Board Cert:** Diagnostic Radiology 1979; Vascular & Interventional Radiology 2005; **Med School:** Dartmouth Med Sch 1975; **Resid:** Diagnostic Radiology, Hosp Univ Penn 1979; **Fellow:** Angiography, Hosp Univ Penn 1980; **Fac Appt:** Prof, Univ Pennsylvania

Shlansky-Goldberg, Richard MD [VIR] - **Spec Exp:** Uterine Fibroid Embolization; Varicocele Embolization; Pelvic Congestion Syndrome; **Hospital:** Hosp Univ Penn - UPHS (page 60); **Address:** Dept Radiology, 3400 Spruce St, 1 Silverstein Bldg, Philadelphia, PA 19104; **Phone:** 215-615-3541; **Board Cert:** Diagnostic Radiology 1989; Vascular & Interventional Radiology 2007; **Med School:** Univ Rochester 1984; **Resid:** Diagnostic Radiology, Thomas Jefferson Univ Hosp 1989; **Fellow:** Interventional Radiology, Hosp U Penn 1991; **Fac Appt:** Assoc Prof Rad, Univ Pennsylvania

Soulen, Michael C MD [VIR] - **Spec Exp:** Liver Cancer/Chemoembolization; Kidney Cancer; Radiofrequency Tumor Ablation; **Hospital:** Hosp Univ Penn - UPHS (page 60); **Address:** Hosp U Penn, Interventional Radiology, 3400 Spruce St, Philadelphia, PA 19104; **Phone:** 215-662-6839; **Board Cert:** Diagnostic Radiology 1989; Vascular & Interventional Radiology 1995; **Med School:** Univ Pennsylvania 1984; **Resid:** Diagnostic Radiology, Johns Hopkins Med Inst 1989; **Fellow:** Vascular & Interventional Radiology, Thomas Jefferson Univ Hosp 1991; **Fac Appt:** Prof Rad, Univ Pennsylvania

Trerotola, Scott O MD [VIR] - **Spec Exp:** Uterine Fibroid Embolization; Hereditary Hemorrhagic Telangiectasia; Varicocele Embolization; **Hospital:** Hosp Univ Penn - UPHS (page 60), Penn Presby Med Ctr - UPHS (page 60); **Address:** Hosp Univ Penn, Div Interventional Rad, 3400 Spruce St, 1 Silverstein, Philadelphia, PA 19104; **Phone:** 215-615-3540; **Board Cert:** Diagnostic Radiology 1991; Vascular & Interventional Radiology 2005; **Med School:** Univ Pennsylvania 1986; **Resid:** Diagnostic Radiology, Johns Hopkins Hosp 1991; **Fellow:** Vascular & Interventional Radiology, Johns Hopkins Hosp 1992; **Fac Appt:** Prof Rad, Univ Pennsylvania

Wood, Bradford J MD [VIR] - **Spec Exp:** Radiofrequency Tumor Ablation; Liver Cancer; Kidney Cancer; Gene Therapy Delivery Systems; **Hospital:** Natl Inst of Hlth - Clin Ctr; **Address:** National Inst Health, Bldg 10, 9000 Rockville Pike, msc 1182, Bethesda, MD 20892; **Phone:** 301-594-4511; **Board Cert:** Diagnostic Radiology 1996; Vascular & Interventional Radiology 2000; **Med School:** Univ VA Sch Med 1991; **Resid:** Diagnostic Radiology, Georgetown Univ Med Ctr 1996; **Fellow:** Abdominal/Interventional Radiology, Mass General Hosp 1997; **Fac Appt:** Asst Clin Prof Rad, Georgetown Univ

Vascular & Interventional Radiology

Southeast

Benenati, James F MD [VIR] - **Spec Exp:** Uterine Fibroid Embolization; Aneurysm-Abdominal Aortic; Peripheral Vascular Disease; **Hospital:** Baptist Hosp of Miami; **Address:** 8900 N Kendall Drive Fl 3, MC BCBI, Miami, FL 33176; **Phone:** 786-596-5990; **Board Cert:** Diagnostic Radiology 1988; Vascular & Interventional Radiology 2005; **Med School:** Univ S Fla Coll Med 1984; **Resid:** Diagnostic Radiology, Indiana Univ Hosp 1988; **Fellow:** Vascular & Interventional Radiology, Johns Hopkins Hosp 1989; **Fac Appt:** Prof Rad, Univ S Fla Coll Med

Bettmann, Michael A MD [VIR] - **Spec Exp:** Uterine Fibroid Embolization; Chemoembolization & Tumor Ablation; Carotid Artery Stent Placement; **Hospital:** Wake Forest Univ Baptist Med Ctr (page 72), Iredell Meml Hlthcare Sys; **Address:** Wake Forest Univ Sch Md-Radiology, Medical Center Blvd, Winston-Salem, NC 27157; **Phone:** 336-716-2463; **Board Cert:** Diagnostic Radiology 1975; Vascular & Interventional Radiology 2005; **Med School:** Albert Einstein Coll Med 1969; **Resid:** Diagnostic Radiology, Beth Israel Med Ctr-Harvard 1975; **Fellow:** Cardiovascular Radiology, Peter Bent Brigham Hosp-Harvard 1977; **Fac Appt:** Prof Rad, Wake Forest Univ

Hawkins Jr, Irvin MD [VIR] - **Hospital:** Shands at Univ of FL; **Address:** Univ Florida Dept Radiology, PO Box 100374, Gainesville, FL 32610-0374; **Phone:** 352-265-0291; **Board Cert:** Diagnostic Radiology 1969; **Med School:** Univ MD Sch Med 1962; **Resid:** Diagnostic Radiology, Ohio State Univ 1968; **Fellow:** Cardiovascular Radiology, Shands Tchg Hosps 1970; **Fac Appt:** Prof Rad, Univ Fla Coll Med

Katzen, Barry T MD [VIR] - **Spec Exp:** Peripheral Vascular Disease; Aneurysm-Aortic; Carotid Artery Disease; **Hospital:** Baptist Hosp of Miami; **Address:** Baptist Cardiac & Vascular Inst, 8900 N Kendall Drive, Miami, FL 33176-2118; **Phone:** 786-596-5990; **Board Cert:** Diagnostic Radiology 1974; Vascular & Interventional Radiology 2004; **Med School:** Univ Miami Sch Med 1970; **Resid:** Diagnostic Radiology, New York Hosp-Cornell Med Ctr 1974

Lewis, Curtis A MD [VIR] - **Spec Exp:** Interventional Radiology; Vein Disorders; **Hospital:** Grady Hlth Sys, Emory Univ Hosp; **Address:** Grady Meml Hosp, Dept Radiology, 80 Jesse Hill Jr Drive, 1B Admin Suite, Box 26298, Atlanta, GA 30303; **Phone:** 404-616-6753; **Board Cert:** Diagnostic Radiology 1991; Vascular & Interventional Radiology 2007; **Med School:** Emory Univ 1986; **Resid:** Diagnostic Radiology, Emory Univ Affil Hosps 1991; **Fellow:** Interventional Radiology, Emory Univ Affil Hosps 1992; **Fac Appt:** Asst Prof Rad, Emory Univ

Mauro, Matthew MD [VIR] - **Spec Exp:** Cancer Chemoembolization; Cancer Radiotherapy; Gastrointestinal Cancer; **Hospital:** Univ NC Hosps; **Address:** University NC Hosps, Dept Radiology, CB 7510, 2006 Old Clinic Bldg, Chapel Hill, NC 27514; **Phone:** 919-966-4238; **Board Cert:** Diagnostic Radiology 1981; Vascular & Interventional Radiology 2003; **Med School:** Cornell Univ-Weill Med Coll 1977; **Resid:** Diagnostic Radiology, Univ NC Hosps 1981; **Fellow:** Interventional Radiology, Mallinckrodt Inst 1982; **Fac Appt:** Prof Rad, Univ NC Sch Med

Midwest

Cho, Kyung J MD [VIR] - **Spec Exp:** Chemoembolization & Tumor Ablation; Vascular Malformations; Peripheral Vascular Disease; **Hospital:** Univ Michigan Hlth Sys; **Address:** Univ Michigan Med Ctr, Dept Radiology, 1500 E Med Ctr Drive, CVC 5582, Ann Arbor, MI 48109-5868; **Phone:** 734-936-4466; **Board Cert:** Diagnostic Radiology 1974; Vascular & Interventional Radiology 2005; **Med School:** Korea 1966; **Resid:** Diagnostic Radiology, Wayne Med Ctr 1973; **Fellow:** Cardiovascular Radiology, Univ Michigan 1975; **Fac Appt:** Prof Rad, Univ Mich Med Sch

Darcy, Michael MD [VIR] - **Spec Exp:** Portal Hypertension; Chemoembolization & Tumor Ablation; **Hospital:** Barnes-Jewish Hosp; **Address:** Washington Univ, Mallinckrodt Inst Radiology, 510 S Kingshighway Blvd, St Louis, MO 63110; **Phone:** 314-362-2900; **Board Cert:** Diagnostic Radiology 1985; Vascular & Interventional Radiology 2004; **Med School:** Ohio State Univ 1979; **Resid:** Surgery, Univ Minn Hosps 1982; Diagnostic Radiology, Univ Minn Hosps 1985; **Fellow:** Interventional Radiology, Univ Minn Hosps 1987; **Fac Appt:** Prof Rad, Washington Univ, St Louis

Johnson, Matthew S MD [VIR] - **Spec Exp:** Liver Tumors; Uterine Fibroid Embolization; Portal Hypertension; Varicocele Embolization; **Hospital:** Indiana Univ Hosp, Methodist Hosp - Indianapolis; **Address:** Indiana Univ Hosp, Interventional Radiology, 550 N University Blvd, rm 0276, Indianapolis, IN 46202-5253; **Phone:** 317-274-1840; **Board Cert:** Diagnostic Radiology 1992; Vascular & Interventional Radiology 2006; **Med School:** Univ Mich Med Sch 1986; **Resid:** Surgery, Loyola Univ Med Ctr 1988; Diagnostic Radiology, Loyola Univ Med Ctr 1992; **Fellow:** Interventional Radiology, Johns Hopkins Univ Hosp 1994; **Fac Appt:** Prof Rad, Indiana Univ

Ketcham, Douglas B MD [VIR] - **Spec Exp:** Uterine Fibroid Embolization; Varicocele Embolization; Osteoporosis Spine-Vertebroplasty; **Hospital:** United Hosp, Regions Hosp - St Paul; **Address:** 250 Thompson St, Affil United Hosp-Downtown Clin, St Paul, MN 55102; **Phone:** 651-297-6504; **Board Cert:** Diagnostic Radiology 1972; Vascular & Interventional Radiology 2005; **Med School:** Univ Wisc 1965; **Resid:** Diagnostic Radiology, Univ Minn Hosp 1971; **Fellow:** Neuroradiology, Univ Minn Hosp 1972

Nemcek, Albert A MD [VIR] - **Spec Exp:** Uterine Fibroid Embolization; Vascular Disease; **Hospital:** Northwestern Meml Hosp; **Address:** Feinberg Pavillion, 4-710T, 251 E Huron St, Chicago, IL 60611; **Phone:** 312-926-5302; **Board Cert:** Diagnostic Radiology 1986; Vascular & Interventional Radiology 2005; **Med School:** UCSD 1982; **Resid:** Diagnostic Radiology, UCSD Med Ctr 1986; **Fellow:** Interventional Radiology, Northwestern Meml Hosp 1987; **Fac Appt:** Assoc Prof Rad, Northwestern Univ

Rilling, William S MD [VIR] - **Spec Exp:** Liver Cancer/Chemoembolization; Arteriovenous Malformations; Uterine Fibroid Embolization; **Hospital:** Froedtert Meml Lutheran Hosp; **Address:** Froedtert Hosp, Dept Radiology, 9200 W Wisconsin Ave, Milwaukee, WI 53226; **Phone:** 414-805-3028; **Board Cert:** Diagnostic Radiology 1995; Vascular & Interventional Radiology 2007; **Med School:** Univ Wisc 1990; **Resid:** Diagnostic Radiology, Univ Wisc Affil Hosps 1995; **Fellow:** Vascular & Interventional Radiology, Northwestern Meml Hosp 1996; **Fac Appt:** Assoc Prof Rad, Univ Wisc

Salem, Riad MD [VIR] - **Spec Exp:** Cancer Radiotherapy; Cancer Chemoembolization; Liver Cancer/Chemoembolization; **Hospital:** Northwestern Meml Hosp; **Address:** Northwestern Univ Med Sch, Dept Radiology, 676 N St Clair St, Ste 800, Chicago, IL 60611; **Phone:** 312-695-5753; **Board Cert:** Diagnostic Radiology 1997; Vascular & Interventional Radiology 1999; **Med School:** McGill Univ 1993; **Resid:** Diagnostic Radiology, Geo Washington Univ Hosp 1997; **Fellow:** Interventional Radiology, Chldns Hosp 1998; Interventional Radiology, Hosp Univ Penn 1998; **Fac Appt:** Asst Prof Rad, Northwestern Univ

Smith, Steven J MD [VIR] - **Spec Exp:** Angioplasty-Peripheral; Uterine Fibroid Embolization; Varicocele Embolization; Pelvic Congestion Syndrome; **Hospital:** La Grange Meml Hosp, Hinsdale Hosp; **Address:** 333 Chestnut St, Hinsdale, IL 60521; **Phone:** 630-856-7460; **Board Cert:** Diagnostic Radiology 1983; Vascular & Interventional Radiology 2006; **Med School:** Wayne State Univ 1979; **Resid:** Diagnostic Radiology, Henry Ford Hosp 1983; **Fellow:** Vascular & Interventional Radiology, Northwestern Meml Hosp 1984; **Fac Appt:** Assoc Clin Prof Rad, Northwestern Univ

Vascular & Interventional Radiology

Vogelzang, Robert MD [VIR] - **Spec Exp:** Uterine Fibroid Embolization; Varicocele Embolization; Vascular Malformations; **Hospital:** Northwestern Meml Hosp; **Address:** Dept Radiology, 251 E Huron, Chicago, IL 60611; **Phone:** 312-926-5113; **Board Cert:** Diagnostic Radiology 1981; Vascular & Interventional Radiology 2005; **Med School:** Ros Franklin Univ/Chicago Med Sch 1977; **Resid:** Diagnostic Radiology, Northwestern Meml Hosp 1982; **Fellow:** Interventional Radiology, Northwestern Meml Hosp; **Fac Appt:** Prof Rad, Northwestern Univ

Great Plains and Mountains

Durham, Janette D MD [VIR] - **Spec Exp:** Uterine Fibroid Embolization; Peripheral Vascular Disease; **Hospital:** Univ Colorado Hosp; **Address:** Univ Hosp, Dept Radiology, 4200 E Ninth Ave, Box A030, Denver, CO 80262; **Phone:** 720-848-7630; **Board Cert:** Diagnostic Radiology 1987; Vascular & Interventional Radiology 2006; **Med School:** Indiana Univ 1983; **Resid:** Diagnostic Radiology, Indiana Univ Hosp 1987; **Fellow:** Vascular & Interventional Radiology, Mass General Hosp 1988; **Fac Appt:** Assoc Prof, Univ Colorado

Kumpe, David A MD [VIR] - **Spec Exp:** Aneurysm-Cerebral; Stroke; Arterial & Venous Stents; Interventional Neuroradiology; **Hospital:** Univ Colorado Hosp; **Address:** Univ Hosp, Dept Radiology, Leprino Bldg - rm 527, 12401 E 17th Ave, L954, PO Box 6511, Aurora, CO 80045; **Phone:** 720-848-6572; **Board Cert:** Diagnostic Radiology 1972; Vascular & Interventional Radiology 2005; **Med School:** Harvard Med Sch 1967; **Resid:** Diagnostic Radiology, Mass Genl Hosp 1971; **Fellow:** Neurological Radiology, Kantonsspital 1976; Angiography, Kantonsspital 1976; **Fac Appt:** Prof Rad, Univ Colorado

Yakes, Wayne MD [VIR] - **Spec Exp:** Vascular Malformations; Interventional Neuroradiology; **Hospital:** Swedish Med Ctr - Englewood; **Address:** CNI, Vasc Malformation Ctr, 501 E Hampden Ave, Ste 4600, Englewood, CO 80113; **Phone:** 303-788-4280; **Board Cert:** Diagnostic Radiology 1983; Vascular & Interventional Radiology 1998; Neuroradiology 1999; **Med School:** Creighton Univ 1979; **Resid:** Diagnostic Radiology, Fitzsimons Med Ctr 1983; **Fellow:** Angiography, Walter Reed Med Ctr 1984; Interventional Neuroradiology, Baptist Hosp 1992; **Fac Appt:** Clin Prof, Univ Colorado

Southwest

Kay, Dennis MD [VIR] - **Hospital:** Ochsner Fdn Hosp; **Address:** Ochsner Clin, Dept Interventional Radiology, 1514 Jefferson Hwy, New Orleans, LA 70121-2429; **Phone:** 504-842-3470; **Board Cert:** Diagnostic Radiology 1986; Vascular & Interventional Radiology 2004; **Med School:** Tulane Univ 1981; **Resid:** Diagnostic Radiology, Ochsner Fdn Hosp 1985; **Fellow:** Vascular & Interventional Radiology, Beth Israel Hosp 1986; **Fac Appt:** Assoc Clin Prof, Tulane Univ

West Coast and Pacific

Gomes, Antoinette S MD [VIR] - **Spec Exp:** Cardiovascular Interventional Radiology; Vascular Malformations; Chemoembolization & Tumor Ablation; **Hospital:** UCLA Ronald Reagan Med Ctr, Santa Clara Vly Med Ctr; **Address:** Dept Radiological Sciences, Ronald Reagan UCLA Med Ctr, 757 Westwood Plaza, Ste 2125, Los Angeles, CA 90095; **Phone:** 310-267-8769; **Board Cert:** Diagnostic Radiology 1975; Vascular & Interventional Radiology 2004; **Med School:** Med Coll PA Hahnemann 1969; **Resid:** Internal Medicine, LAC-USC Med Ctr 1972; Diagnostic Radiology, Stanford Univ Med Ctr 1975; **Fellow:** Cardiovascular Radiology, UCLA Med Ctr 1976; Cardiovascular Radiology, Univ Minn 1978; **Fac Appt:** Prof Rad, UCLA

Goodwin, Scott C MD [VIR] - **Spec Exp:** Uterine Fibroid Embolization; Liver Cancer/Chemoembolization; **Hospital:** UC Irvine Med Ctr; **Address:** 101 S City Drive, MC 5005, Route 140, Orange, CA 92868; **Phone:** 714-456-5033; **Board Cert:** Diagnostic Radiology 1989; Vascular & Interventional Radiology 2007; **Med School:** Harvard Med Sch 1984; **Resid:** Diagnostic Radiology, UCLA Medical Ctr 1988; **Fellow:** Vascular & Interventional Radiology, UCLA Medical Ctr 1989; **Fac Appt:** Prof, UCLA

Hovsepian, David M MD [VIR] - **Spec Exp:** Uterine Fibroid Embolization; Aneurysm-Aortic; Vascular Malformations-Pediatric; **Hospital:** Stanford Univ Med Ctr; **Address:** Interventional Radiology, 300 Pasteur Drive, rm H3649, Stanford, CA 94305-5642; **Phone:** 650-498-6022; **Board Cert:** Diagnostic Radiology 1991; Vascular & Interventional Radiology 2006; **Med School:** Columbia P&S 1986; **Resid:** Diagnostic Radiology, Columbia Presby Hosp 1991; **Fellow:** Interventional Radiology, Thomas Jefferson Univ Hosp 1993; **Fac Appt:** Prof Rad, Stanford Univ

Kaufman, John A MD [VIR] - **Spec Exp:** Uterine Fibroid Embolization; Angioplasty & Stent Placement; **Hospital:** Dotter Institute - OHSU; **Address:** Dotter Interven Inst-OHSU Hosps & Clins, 3181 SW Sam Jackson Park Rd, MC L605, Portland, OR 97239; **Phone:** 503-494-7660; **Board Cert:** Diagnostic Radiology 1990; Vascular & Interventional Radiology 2005; **Med School:** Boston Univ 1982; **Resid:** Diagnostic Radiology, Boston Univ Med Ctr 1990; **Fellow:** Vascular & Interventional Radiology, Boston Univ Med Ctr 1991; **Fac Appt:** Prof Rad, Oregon Hlth & Sci Univ

Keller, Frederick S MD [VIR] - **Spec Exp:** Uterine Fibroid Embolization; Arterial & Venous Stents; Urinary Tract Interventions; **Hospital:** OR Hlth & Sci Univ; **Address:** Dotter Interventional Inst, L-605, 3181 SW Sam Jackson Park Rd, Portland, OR 97239; **Phone:** 503-494-7660; **Board Cert:** Diagnostic Radiology 1977; Vascular & Interventional Radiology 2003; **Med School:** Univ Pennsylvania 1968; **Resid:** Diagnostic Radiology, Univ Oreg Hlth Scis Ctr 1977; **Fac Appt:** Prof, Oregon Hlth & Sci Univ

McGahan, John P MD [VIR] - **Spec Exp:** Radiofrequency Tumor Ablation; Liver Cancer; Kidney Cancer; **Hospital:** UC Davis Med Ctr; **Address:** UC Davis Medical Ctr, Dept Radiology, 4860 Y St, Ste 3100, Sacramento, CA 95817; **Phone:** 916-734-3606; **Board Cert:** Diagnostic Radiology 1979; **Med School:** Oregon Hlth & Sci Univ 1974; **Resid:** Surgery, UC Davis Med Ctr 1976; Diagnostic Radiology, UC Davis Med Ctr 1979; **Fac Appt:** Prof Rad, UC Davis

Valji, Karim MD [VIR] - **Spec Exp:** Dialysis Access; **Hospital:** Univ Wash Med Ctr; **Address:** Univ of WA Med Ctr-Dept Rad, 1959 NE Pacific St, Box 357115, Seattle, WA 98195; **Phone:** 206-543-3320; **Board Cert:** Diagnostic Radiology 1989; Vascular & Interventional Radiology 1998; **Med School:** Harvard Med Sch 1982; **Resid:** Internal Medicine, UCSF Med Ctr 1984; Diagnostic Radiology, UCSD Med Ctr 1988; **Fellow:** Angiography, UCSD Med Ctr 1989; **Fac Appt:** Prof, Univ SD Sch Med

MOUNT SINAI
SCHOOL OF
MEDICINE

THE MOUNT SINAI MEDICAL CENTER
RADIOLOGY

One Gustave L. Levy Place
Fifth Avenue and 100th Street
New York, NY 10029-6574
Physician Referral: 1-800-MD-SINAI (637-4624)
www.mountsinai.org

THE DEPARTMENT OF RADIOLOGY at Mount Sinai offers patients one of the world's most comprehensive and sophisticated arrays of diagnostic and interventional radiology services. The Department uses filmless digital technology that spans magnetic resonance imaging (MRI), multi-slice computed tomography (CT), positron emission tomography CT (PET-CT), single photon emission computed tomography CT (SPECT-CT), advanced ultrasound, conventional radiography, digital mammography, and state-of-the-art Picture Archiving Communication System (PACS) technology.

Comprehensive Diagnostic Services – Mount Sinai provides the entire range of diagnostic radiology services in a patient-friendly environment. Its nationally renowned radiologic physicians specialize in every area of disease diagnosis, as well as disease prevention and innovative therapeutic approaches. The combination of state-of-the-art imaging equipment with the finest imaging physicians makes Mount Sinai Radiology the "place to go" for all your imaging needs.

Early Detection Programs – We are committed to special screening approaches for early disease detection. We provide radiological screenings for colon, breast, and lung cancer and atherosclerosis. The early detection programs use a variety of imaging techniques, such as CT and MRI for atherosclerosis, CT for colon cancer, PET for oncology, and digital mammography, MRI, ultrasound, and computer-aided diagnosis for breast cancer.

Minimally Invasive Procedures – Radiology at Mount Sinai has moved beyond diagnosis to the most sophisticated therapeutic interventions. Interventional radiologists at Mount Sinai perform biopsies, vascular therapies, and uterine artery embolization for fibroids—an alternative to hysterectomy—as well as treatments for aneurysms, atherosclerosis, and many types of cancer. In addition, advanced CT and MR angiography techniques are widely utilized to diagnose vascular diseases in a minimally invasive yet highly accurate manner.

Oncology Imaging – Radiologists work closely with surgeons, oncologists, and other caregivers to optimize the diagnosis and treatment of patients with head and neck, liver, lung, breast, and gastrointestinal cancers.

DEVELOPING NEW DIAGNOSTIC TOOLS

Radiology at Mount Sinai is an active center of imaging research and development. Mount Sinai physicians and scientists developed a special form of MRI to diagnose heart disease and atherosclerosis noninvasively and thereby identify patients at greatest risk for stroke and heart attack. We actively collaborate with other disciplines to develop and refine imaging tools that will make prevention and diagnosis increasingly effective. That is the case, for example, in neuroscience, where the imaging innovations impact our understanding of neurodegenerative conditions such as Parkinson's disease, multiple sclerosis, stroke, brain tumors, and various psychiatric disorders; cardiovascular disease, where studies are under way to predict the risk associated with atherosclerotic plaques and assess new therapies for aortic and cerebral artery aneurysms; and liver disease, where radiologists, transplant surgeons, and hepatologists collaborate closely to develop optimal therapeutic strategies.

NYU Langone Medical Center

550 First Avenue (at 31St Street)
New York, NY 10016
Physician Referral:
(888)7-NYU-MED (888-769-8633)
www.med.nyu.edu

RADIOLOGY

About the Radiology Department:

The Radiology Department at NYU Langone Medical Center is committed to transforming the field of radiology to improve the lives of people. The Department understands that the field of radiology is changing and is determined to lead, define, and make these changes by integrating clinical and research activities leading to better diagnosis and less invasive treatment, as well as developing breakthrough technologies such as multichannel CT, parallel imaging in MR, and PET-CT.

The Radiology Department at NYU Langone Medical Center is in a unique position to take the lead in developing new algorithms and defining the role of an academic radiology department in this new environment. The staff consists of over 100 subspecialized academic radiologists, many of whom are acknowledged leaders and innovators in their fields; over 20 full-time basic scientists and several postdoctoral fellows; and approximately 70 residents and fellows. We have state-of-the-art equipment as well as the Center for Biomedical Imaging, a research facility specializing in high field and ultra high field MR including a 7T magnet.

We specialize in the following areas:

NYU Radiology offers an extensive range of diagnostic services in MRI, CT, ultrasound, PET/CT, X-ray, and interventional radiology and nuclear medicine. Subspecialized radiologists provide diagnostic interpretation in abdominal, biomedical, breast, cardiac, chest, emergency, general, musculoskeletal, neuroradiology, neuro interventional, nuclear medicine, pediatric, vascular interventional and women's imaging.

OUR STATE-OF-THE- ART EQUIPMENT INCLUDES:
- Siemens Dual Source CT— Somatom® Definition Flash™
- Siemens MAGNETOM® Verio—3T, 70 cm Open Bore and Tim™
  (Total imaging matrix) together in one powerful system
- 1.5 Tesla and 3 Tesla scanners
- 7 Tesla full-body research scanner
- High resolution/high sensitivity PET/CT
- State-of-the-art SPECT CT and SPECT gamma cameras
- Digital radiography, fluoroscopy, and mammography

OUR SPECIALTY PROCEDURES INCLUDE:
- Coronary artery disease and virtual colonoscopy screening programs
- Stereotactic biopsy capability
- Minimally invasive techniques including radiofrequency ablation and chemoembolization
- Radioimmunotherapy
- Bone densitometry

ADDITIONAL BENEFITS/SERVICES:
- American College of Radiology accredited
- Dedicated Image Processing Laboratory/3-D
- Pre- and post-consultation
- Ability to view patients' exam status, reports, and images online
- Appointment availability - we can accommodate same day appointments in most cases
- Timely delivery of reports and images
- Multilingual – our staff speaks multiple languages, and we provide on-site translation services
- Accepted insurance – we participate with an extensive list of insurances

RADIOLOGY

About the Radiology Department:

The Radiology Department at NYU Langone Medical Center is committed to transforming the field of radiology to improve the lives of people. The Department understands that the field of radiology is changing and is determined to lead, define, and make these changes by integrating clinical and research activities leading to better diagnosis and less invasive treatment, as well as developing breakthrough technologies such as multichannel CT, parallel imaging in MR, and PET-CT.

The Radiology Department at NYU Langone Medical Center is in a unique position to take the lead in developing new algorithms and defining the role of an academic radiology department in this new environment. The staff consists of over 100 subspecialized academic radiologists, many of whom are acknowledged leaders and innovators in their fields; over 20 full-time basic scientists and several postdoctoral fellows; and approximately 70 residents and fellows. We have state-of-the-art equipment as well as the Center for Biomedical Imaging, a research facility specializing in high field and ultra high field MR including a 7T magnet.

We specialize in the following areas:

NYU Radiology offers an extensive range of diagnostic services in MRI, CT, ultrasound, PET/CT, X-ray, and interventional radiology and nuclear medicine. Subspecialized radiologists provide diagnostic interpretation in abdominal, biomedical, breast, cardiac, chest, emergency, general, musculoskeletal, neuroradiology, neuro interventional, nuclear medicine, pediatric, vascular interventional and women's imaging.

OUR STATE-OF-THE- ART EQUIPMENT INCLUDES:
- Siemens Dual Source CT— Somatom® Definition Flash™
- Siemens MAGNETOM® Verio—3T, 70 cm Open Bore and Tim™
  (Total imaging matrix) together in one powerful system
- 1.5 Tesla and 3 Tesla scanners
- 7 Tesla full-body research scanner
- High resolution/high sensitivity PET/CT
- State-of-the-art SPECT CT and SPECT gamma cameras
- Digital radiography, fluoroscopy, and mammography

OUR SPECIALTY PROCEDURES INCLUDE:
- Coronary artery disease and virtual colonoscopy screening programs
- Stereotactic biopsy capability
- Minimally invasive techniques including radiofrequency ablation and chemoembolization
- Radioimmunotherapy
- Bone densitometry

ADDITIONAL BENEFITS/SERVICES:
- American College of Radiology accredited
- Dedicated Image Processing Laboratory/3-D
- Pre- and post-consultation
- Ability to view patients' exam status, reports, and images online
- Appointment availability - we can accommodate same day appointments in most cases
- Timely delivery of reports and images
- Multilingual – our staff speaks multiple languages, and we provide on-site translation services
- Accepted insurance – we participate with an extensive list of insurances

Reproductive Endocrinology

a subspecialty of Obstetrics & Gynecology

An obstetrician/gynecologist who is capable of managing complex problems relating to reproductive endocrinology and infertility.

Training Required: Four years *plus* two years in clinical practice before certification in obstetrics and gynecology is complete *plus* additional training and examination in reproductive endocrinology.

REPRODUCTIVE ENDOCRINOLOGY

New England

Carson, Sandra A MD [RE] - **Spec Exp:** Infertility-IVF; Laparoscopic Surgery; Endometriosis; Sexual Dysfunction; **Hospital:** Women & Infants Hosp of RI; **Address:** Women & Infants Hosp of RI, 101 Dudley St Fl 1, Providence, RI 02905; **Phone:** 401-274-1122 x8167; **Board Cert:** Obstetrics & Gynecology 2005; Reproductive Endocrinology 2005; **Med School:** Northwestern Univ 1977; **Resid:** Obstetrics & Gynecology, Prentice Womens Hosp 1981; **Fellow:** Reproductive Endocrinology, Michael Reese Hosp 1983; **Fac Appt:** Prof ObG, Brown Univ

Crowley, William F MD [RE] - **Spec Exp:** Pituitary Disorders; Kallmann's Syndrome; Fertility Preservation in Cancer; **Hospital:** Mass Genl Hosp; **Address:** Mass Genl Hosp, Reproductive Sci Ctr, 55 Fruit St, Bartlett Hall-Ext 5, Boston, MA 02114; **Phone:** 617-726-5390; **Board Cert:** Internal Medicine 1974; Endocrinology 1977; **Med School:** Tufts Univ 1969; **Resid:** Internal Medicine, Mass Genl Hosp 1971; Internal Medicine, Mass Genl Hosp 1974; **Fellow:** Endocrinology, Mass Genl Hosp 1976; **Fac Appt:** Prof Med, Harvard Med Sch

Ginsburg, Elizabeth MD [RE] - **Spec Exp:** Infertility-IVF; Fertility Preservation in Cancer; **Hospital:** Brigham & Women's Hosp, Dana-Farber Cancer Inst; **Address:** Brigham & Womens Hosp, Reproductive Med, 75 Francis St, Ste 3300, Boston, MA 02115; **Phone:** 617-732-4222; **Board Cert:** Obstetrics & Gynecology 2007; Reproductive Endocrinology 2007; **Med School:** Mount Sinai Sch Med 1985; **Resid:** Obstetrics & Gynecology, Brigham & Womens Hosp 1989; **Fellow:** Reproductive Endocrinology, Brigham & Womens Hosp 1991

Hill III, Joseph A MD [RE] - **Spec Exp:** Miscarriage-Recurrent; Infertility-Female; Gynecology; **Hospital:** Portsmouth Regl Hosp, Winchester Hosp; **Address:** Fertility Ctr of New England, 875 Greenland Rd C Bldg, Unit 1, Portsmouth, NH 03801; **Phone:** 781-942-7000 x601; **Board Cert:** Obstetrics & Gynecology 2007; Reproductive Endocrinology 2007; **Med School:** Med Coll GA 1981; **Resid:** Obstetrics & Gynecology, Med Coll Ga 1985; **Fellow:** Reproductive Endocrinology, Brigham-Womens Hosp/Harvard 1987; Reproductive Immunology, Brigham-Womens Hosp/Harvard 1988; **Fac Appt:** Prof ObG, Harvard Med Sch

Hornstein, Mark D MD [RE] - **Spec Exp:** Infertility-IVF; Endometriosis; Laparoscopic Surgery; Hysteroscopic Surgery; **Hospital:** Brigham & Women's Hosp, Newton - Wellesley Hosp; **Address:** Brigham & Women's Hosp, 75 Francis St, Boston, MA 02115; **Phone:** 617-732-4648; **Board Cert:** Obstetrics & Gynecology 2008; Reproductive Endocrinology 2008; **Med School:** Univ Cincinnati 1982; **Resid:** Obstetrics & Gynecology, Brigham & Women's Hosp 1986; **Fellow:** Reproductive Endocrinology, Brigham & Women's Hosp 1988; **Fac Appt:** Assoc Prof ObG, Harvard Med Sch

Isaacson, Keith B MD [RE] - **Spec Exp:** Infertility; Endometriosis; Minimally Invasive Surgery; **Hospital:** Newton - Wellesley Hosp, Mass Genl Hosp; **Address:** 2014 Washington St Fl 2 West, Newton, MA 02462; **Phone:** 617-243-5205; **Board Cert:** Obstetrics & Gynecology 2007; Reproductive Endocrinology 2007; **Med School:** Med Coll GA 1983; **Resid:** Obstetrics & Gynecology, Ochsner Fdn Hosp 1987; **Fellow:** Reproductive Endocrinology, Hosp Univ Penn 1989; **Fac Appt:** Assoc Prof ObG, Harvard Med Sch

Luciano, Anthony A MD [RE] - **Spec Exp:** Infertility; Endometriosis; Menopause Problems; Osteoporosis; **Hospital:** Hosp of Central CT at New Britain, Hartford Hosp; **Address:** Center for Fertility & Womens Health, 100 Grand St, Ste E3, New Britain, CT 06050; **Phone:** 860-224-5467; **Board Cert:** Obstetrics & Gynecology 1980; Reproductive Endocrinology 1981; **Med School:** Univ Conn 1973; **Resid:** Obstetrics & Gynecology, Univ Conn Hosp 1977; **Fellow:** Reproductive Endocrinology, Univ Conn Hosp 1979; **Fac Appt:** Prof ObG, Univ Conn

Manganiello, Paul D MD [RE] - **Spec Exp:** Infertility; Menopause Problems; **Hospital:** Dartmouth - Hitchcock Med Ctr; **Address:** Dartmouth-Hitchcock Med Ctr, Dept Ob/Gyn, One Medical Center Drive, Lebanon, NH 03756; **Phone:** 603-653-9240; **Board Cert:** Obstetrics & Gynecology 1980; Reproductive Endocrinology 1984; **Med School:** Jefferson Med Coll 1973; **Resid:** Obstetrics & Gynecology, Thomas Jefferson Univ Hosp 1977; **Fellow:** Reproductive Endocrinology, Med Coll Ga Hosp 1979; **Fac Appt:** Assoc Prof ObG, Dartmouth Med Sch

Patrizio, Pasquale MD [RE] - **Spec Exp:** Infertility-IVF; Fertility Preservation in Cancer; **Hospital:** Yale-New Haven Hosp; **Address:** Yale Fertility Ctr, Dept OB/GYN, 150 Sargent Drive, New Haven, CT 06511; **Phone:** 203-785-4708; **Board Cert:** Obstetrics & Gynecology 2007; Reproductive Endocrinology 2007; **Med School:** Italy 1983; **Resid:** Obstetrics & Gynecology, Univ Naples 1987; Reproductive Endocrinology, Univ Pisa 1990; **Fellow:** Infertility, UC Irvine 1995; **Fac Appt:** Prof ObG, Yale Univ

Toth, Thomas L MD [RE] - **Spec Exp:** Infertility-IVF; **Hospital:** Mass Genl Hosp, Newton - Wellesley Hosp; **Address:** Mass General Hospital, Dept Reproductive Endocrinology, 55 Fruit St, Boston, MA 02114-2621; **Phone:** 617-726-8868; **Board Cert:** Obstetrics & Gynecology 2007; Reproductive Endocrinology/Infertility 2007; **Med School:** Univ MO-Kansas City 1986; **Resid:** Obstetrics & Gynecology, Mass Genl Hosp/Brigham & Womens Hosp 1990; **Fellow:** Reproductive Endocrinology, E Virginia Med Sch Hosps 1992; **Fac Appt:** Assoc Prof ObG, Harvard Med Sch

Yeh, John J MD [RE] - **Spec Exp:** Infertility; Polycystic Ovarian Syndrome; Menstrual Disorders; **Hospital:** Beth Israel Deaconess Med Ctr - Boston; **Address:** BIDMC, Dept Ob/Gyn, 330 Brookline Ave, KS 03182, Boston, MA 02115; **Phone:** 617-667-2286; **Board Cert:** Obstetrics & Gynecology 2008; Reproductive Endocrinology 2007; **Med School:** UCSD 1983; **Resid:** Obstetrics & Gynecology, Beth Israel Hosp 1987; **Fellow:** Reproductive Endocrinology, Brigham & Womens Hosp 1989; **Fac Appt:** Prof ObG, Harvard Med Sch

Zinaman, Michael J MD [RE] - **Spec Exp:** Endometriosis; Infertility; Uterine Fibroids; **Hospital:** Caritas St Elizabeth's Med Ctr; **Address:** Caritas St Elizabeth's Med Ctr SMC5, 736 Cambridge St, Boston, MA 02135; **Phone:** 617-562-7018; **Board Cert:** Obstetrics & Gynecology 1996; Reproductive Endocrinology 1996; **Med School:** SUNY Downstate 1981; **Resid:** Obstetrics & Gynecology, Univ Chicago Hosps 1985; **Fellow:** Reproductive Endocrinology, Georgetown Univ 1987

Mid Atlantic

Bieber, Eric J MD [RE] - **Spec Exp:** Uterine Fibroids; Infertility; Endometriosis; **Hospital:** Geisinger Med Ctr; **Address:** 100 N Academy, MC 29-20, Danville, PA 17821; **Phone:** 570-271-7906; **Board Cert:** Obstetrics & Gynecology 2007; Reproductive Endocrinology 2007; **Med School:** Loyola Univ-Stritch Sch Med 1986; **Resid:** Obstetrics & Gynecology, Rush Presby-St Lukes Med Ctr 1990; **Fellow:** Reproductive Endocrinology, Univ Chicago 1993

Copperman, Alan B MD [RE] - **Spec Exp:** Infertility-IVF; Endometriosis; Laparoscopic Surgery; Hysteroscopic Surgery; **Hospital:** Mount Sinai Med Ctr (page 64); **Address:** 635 Madison Ave Fl 10, New York, NY 10022; **Phone:** 212-756-5777; **Board Cert:** Obstetrics & Gynecology 2007; Reproductive Endocrinology 2007; **Med School:** NY Med Coll 1989; **Resid:** Obstetrics & Gynecology, Yale-New Haven Hosp 1993; **Fellow:** Reproductive Endocrinology, Mt Sinai Med Ctr 1995; **Fac Appt:** Clin Prof ObG, Mount Sinai Sch Med

Reproductive Endocrinology

Coutifaris, Christos MD/PhD [RE] - **Spec Exp:** Infertility-IVF; Fertility Preservation in Cancer; Polycystic Ovarian Syndrome; **Hospital:** Hosp Univ Penn - UPHS (page 60); **Address:** Penn Fertility Care, 3701 Market St Fl 8 - Ste 800, Philadelphia, PA 19104; **Phone:** 215-662-6100; **Board Cert:** Obstetrics & Gynecology 2006; Reproductive Endocrinology 2006; **Med School:** Univ Pennsylvania 1982; **Resid:** Obstetrics & Gynecology, Hosp Univ Penn 1986; **Fellow:** Reproductive Endocrinology, Hosp Univ Penn 1987; **Fac Appt:** Prof ObG, Univ Pennsylvania

Damewood, Marian D MD [RE] - **Spec Exp:** Infertility-IVF; **Hospital:** York Hosp, Hosp Univ Penn - UPHS (page 60); **Address:** York Hosp, Dept Ob/Gyn, 1001 S George St, York, PA 17405; **Phone:** 717-851-2349; **Board Cert:** Obstetrics & Gynecology 1985; Reproductive Endocrinology 1987; **Med School:** Johns Hopkins Univ 1978; **Resid:** Obstetrics & Gynecology, Johns Hopkins Hosp 1982; **Fellow:** Reproductive Endocrinology, Johns Hopkins Hosp 1984; **Fac Appt:** Clin Prof ObG, Univ Pennsylvania

Grazi, Richard MD [RE] - **Spec Exp:** Infertility-IVF; Preimplantation Genetic Diagnosis; Fertility Preservation in Cancer; **Hospital:** Maimonides Med Ctr (page 63), Richmond Univ Med Ctr; **Address:** 1355 84th St, Brooklyn, NY 11228-3030; **Phone:** 718-283-8600; **Board Cert:** Obstetrics & Gynecology 2006; Reproductive Endocrinology 2006; **Med School:** SUNY Buffalo 1981; **Resid:** Obstetrics & Gynecology, NYU Med Ctr 1985; **Fellow:** Reproductive Endocrinology, UMDNJ Med Ctr 1987; **Fac Appt:** Assoc Clin Prof ObG, Mount Sinai Sch Med

Grifo, James A MD/PhD [RE] - **Spec Exp:** Infertility-IVF; Prenatal Genetic Diagnosis; Hysteroscopic Surgery; Laparoscopic Surgery; **Hospital:** NYU Langone Med Ctr (page 67); **Address:** 660 1st Ave Fl 5, New York, NY 10016; **Phone:** 212-263-7978; **Board Cert:** Obstetrics & Gynecology 2007; Reproductive Endocrinology 2007; **Med School:** Case West Res Univ 1984; **Resid:** Obstetrics & Gynecology, NY Hosp-Cornell Med Ctr 1988; **Fellow:** Reproductive Endocrinology, Yale-New Haven Hosp 1990; **Fac Appt:** Prof ObG, NYU Sch Med

Grunfeld, Lawrence MD [RE] - **Spec Exp:** Infertility-IVF; Hysteroscopic Surgery; Laparoscopic Surgery; **Hospital:** Mount Sinai Med Ctr (page 64), Lenox Hill Hosp (page 62); **Address:** 635 Madison Ave Fl 10, New York, NY 10022-1009; **Phone:** 212-756-5777; **Board Cert:** Obstetrics & Gynecology 2007; Reproductive Endocrinology 2007; **Med School:** Mount Sinai Sch Med 1979; **Resid:** Obstetrics & Gynecology, Montefiore Med Ctr 1984; **Fellow:** Reproductive Endocrinology, Montefiore Med Ctr 1987; **Fac Appt:** Assoc Clin Prof ObG, Mount Sinai Sch Med

Legro, Richard S MD [RE] - **Spec Exp:** Polycystic Ovarian Syndrome; Menstrual Disorders; Ovarian Failure; Infertility-IVF; **Hospital:** Penn State Milton S Hershey Med Ctr; **Address:** Hershey Med Ctr, 500 University Drive, PO Box 850, MC H103, Hershey, PA 17033; **Phone:** 717-531-8478; **Board Cert:** Obstetrics & Gynecology 2007; Reproductive Endocrinology 2007; **Med School:** Mount Sinai Sch Med 1987; **Resid:** Obstetrics & Gynecology, Magee Womens Hosp 1991; **Fellow:** Reproductive Endocrinology, USC Women's Hosp 1993; **Fac Appt:** Prof ObG, Penn State Univ-Hershey Med Ctr

Licciardi, Frederick L MD [RE] - **Spec Exp:** Infertility-IVF; Infertility; Fertility Preservation in Cancer; **Hospital:** NYU Langone Med Ctr (page 67); **Address:** NYU Medical Ctr, 660 First Ave, 5th Fl, New York, NY 10016; **Phone:** 212-263-7754; **Board Cert:** Obstetrics & Gynecology 2007; Reproductive Endocrinology 2007; **Med School:** UMDNJ-Rutgers Med Sch 1986; **Resid:** Obstetrics & Gynecology, St Barnabas Med Ctr 1990; **Fellow:** Reproductive Endocrinology, NY Hosp-Cornell Med Ctr 1992; **Fac Appt:** Assoc Prof ObG, NYU Sch Med

McClamrock, Howard D MD [RE] - **Spec Exp:** Infertility-IVF; Prenatal Genetic Diagnosis; **Hospital:** Univ of MD Med Ctr, St Joseph Med Ctr; **Address:** Univ Maryland, Dept OB/GYN, 405 W Redwood St Fl 3, Baltimore, MD 21201; **Phone:** 410-328-2304; **Board Cert:** Obstetrics & Gynecology 1998; Reproductive Endocrinology 1998; **Med School:** Univ NC Sch Med 1981; **Resid:** Obstetrics & Gynecology, Univ Maryland Hosp 1986; **Fellow:** Reproductive Endocrinology, Univ Maryland Hosp 1988; **Fac Appt:** Assoc Prof ObG, Univ MD Sch Med

McGovern, Peter G MD [RE] - **Spec Exp:** Infertility-IVF; Fertility Preservation in Cancer; **Hospital:** UMDNJ-Univ Hosp-Newark, Hackensack Univ Med Ctr; **Address:** University Reproductive Assocs, 214 Terrace Ave, Hasbrouck Heights, NJ 07604; **Phone:** 201-288-6330; **Board Cert:** Obstetrics & Gynecology 2008; Reproductive Endocrinology/Infertility 2008; **Med School:** NYU Sch Med 1986; **Resid:** Obstetrics & Gynecology, NYU-Bellevue Hosp Ctr 1990; **Fellow:** Reproductive Endocrinology, UMDNJ-Newark 1992; **Fac Appt:** Assoc Prof ObG, UMDNJ-NJ Med Sch, Newark

Mukherjee, Tanmoy MD [RE] - **Spec Exp:** Infertility-IVF; Endometriosis; Uterine Fibroids; **Hospital:** Mount Sinai Med Ctr (page 64); **Address:** 635 Madison Ave Fl 10, New York, NY 10022; **Phone:** 212-756-5777; **Board Cert:** Obstetrics & Gynecology 2007; Reproductive Endocrinology 2007; **Med School:** Albert Einstein Coll Med 1990; **Resid:** Obstetrics & Gynecology, Montefiore Med Ctr 1994; **Fellow:** Reproductive Endocrinology, Mt Sinai Hosp 1996

Noyes, Nicole MD [RE] - **Spec Exp:** Infertility-IVF; Fertility Preservation in Cancer; Reproductive Surgery; **Hospital:** NYU Langone Med Ctr (page 67); **Address:** NYU Med Ctr, 660 First Ave, 5th FL, New York, NY 10016; **Phone:** 212-263-7981; **Board Cert:** Obstetrics & Gynecology 2007; Reproductive Endocrinology 2007; **Med School:** Univ VT Coll Med 1986; **Resid:** Obstetrics & Gynecology, NY Hosp-Cornell Med Ctr 1990; **Fellow:** Reproductive Endocrinology, NY Hosp-Cornell Med Ctr 1992; **Fac Appt:** Assoc Prof ObG, NYU Sch Med

Pfeifer, Samantha MD [RE] - **Spec Exp:** Infertility-Female; Endometriosis; Laparoscopic Surgery; Robotic Surgery; **Hospital:** Hosp Univ Penn - UPHS (page 60); **Address:** Penn Health for Women, 250 King of Prussia Rd, Radnor, PA 19087; **Phone:** 610-902-2500; **Board Cert:** Obstetrics & Gynecology 2007; Reproductive Endocrinology 2007; **Med School:** Univ Pennsylvania 1986; **Resid:** Obstetrics & Gynecology, Hosp Univ Penn 1990; **Fellow:** Reproductive Endocrinology, Hosp Univ Penn 1993; **Fac Appt:** Assoc Prof ObG, Univ Pennsylvania

Rosenwaks, Zev MD [RE] - **Spec Exp:** Infertility-IVF; Genetic Disorders; Fertility Preservation in Cancer; **Hospital:** NY-Presby Hosp/Weill Cornell (page 66); **Address:** Ctr For Reproductive Medicine & Infertility, 1305 York Ave Fl 6, New York, NY 10021-4872; **Phone:** 646-962-3743; **Board Cert:** Obstetrics & Gynecology 1978; Reproductive Endocrinology 1981; **Med School:** SUNY Downstate 1972; **Resid:** Obstetrics & Gynecology, LI Jewish Med Ctr 1976; **Fellow:** Reproductive Endocrinology, Johns Hopkins Hosp 1978; **Fac Appt:** Prof ObG, Cornell Univ-Weill Med Coll

Sanfilippo, Joseph S MD [RE] - **Spec Exp:** Adolescent Gynecology; Infertility; Minimally Invasive Surgery; Menopause Problems; **Hospital:** Magee-Womens Hosp - UPMC; **Address:** Ctr for Fertility & Repro Endo-Magee Hosp, 300 Halket St, Ste 2309, Pittsburgh, PA 15213; **Phone:** 412-641-1204; **Board Cert:** Obstetrics & Gynecology 2008; Reproductive Endocrinology 2008; **Med School:** Ros Franklin Univ/Chicago Med Sch 1973; **Resid:** Obstetrics & Gynecology, SUNY Upstate 1977; **Fellow:** Reproductive Endocrinology, Univ of Louisville 1979; **Fac Appt:** Prof ObG, Univ Pittsburgh

Sauer, Mark MD [RE] - **Spec Exp:** Infertility-IVF; **Hospital:** NY-Presby Hosp/Columbia (page 66); **Address:** 1790 Broadway Fl 2, New York, NY 10019; **Phone:** 646-756-8282; **Board Cert:** Obstetrics & Gynecology 2009; Reproductive Endocrinology 2009; **Med School:** Univ IL Coll Med 1980; **Resid:** Obstetrics & Gynecology, Univ Illinois Med Ctr 1984; **Fellow:** Reproductive Endocrinology, Harbor-UCLA Med Ctr 1986; **Fac Appt:** Prof ObG, Columbia P&S

Reproductive Endocrinology

Seifer, David B MD [RE] - **Spec Exp:** Infertility-IVF; Infertility-Advanced Maternal Age; Fertility Preservation in Cancer; **Hospital:** Maimonides Med Ctr (page 63), Richmond Univ Med Ctr; **Address:** 1355 84th St, Brooklyn, NY 11228; **Phone:** 718-283-8600; **Board Cert:** Obstetrics & Gynecology 1998; Reproductive Endocrinology/Infertility 1998; **Med School:** Univ IL Coll Med 1981; **Resid:** Obstetrics & Gynecology, Stanford Univ Hosp 1985; **Fellow:** Reproductive Endocrinology, Yale-New Haven Hosp 1991; **Fac Appt:** Prof ObG, Mount Sinai Sch Med

Simon, James A MD [RE] - **Spec Exp:** Infertility; Menopause Problems; Osteoporosis; **Hospital:** G Washington Univ Hosp, Sibley Mem Hosp; **Address:** 1850 M St NW, Ste 450, Washington, DC 20036; **Phone:** 202-293-1000; **Board Cert:** Obstetrics & Gynecology 1998; Reproductive Endocrinology 1998; **Med School:** Rush Med Coll 1978; **Resid:** Obstetrics & Gynecology, George Washington Univ Hosp 1982; **Fellow:** Reproductive Endocrinology, Harbor-UCLA Medical Ctr 1985; **Fac Appt:** Clin Prof ObG, Geo Wash Univ

Sondheimer, Steven MD [RE] - **Spec Exp:** Infertility; **Hospital:** Hosp Univ Penn - UPHS (page 60); **Address:** Penn Fertility Care, 3701 Market St Fl 8, Philadelphia, PA 19104; **Phone:** 215-662-6100; **Board Cert:** Obstetrics & Gynecology 2005; Reproductive Endocrinology 2005; **Med School:** Univ Pennsylvania 1974; **Resid:** Obstetrics & Gynecology, Hosp Univ Penn 1978; **Fellow:** Endocrinology, Hosp Univ Penn 1980; **Fac Appt:** Prof ObG, Univ Pennsylvania

Stangel, John MD [RE] - **Spec Exp:** Infertility-IVF; Endometriosis; Pregnancy Loss; **Hospital:** Northern Westchester Hosp, Phelps Meml Hosp Ctr; **Address:** 70 Maple Ave, Rye, NY 10580-1568; **Phone:** 914-967-6800; **Board Cert:** Obstetrics & Gynecology 1976; Reproductive Endocrinology 1981; **Med School:** NY Med Coll 1969; **Resid:** Obstetrics & Gynecology, Mount Sinai Med Ctr 1974; **Fellow:** Reproductive Endocrinology, Metropolitan Hosp Ctr 1976

Tureck, Richard W MD [RE] - **Spec Exp:** Reproductive Surgery; Infertility; **Hospital:** Hosp Univ Penn - UPHS (page 60); **Address:** Penn Fertility Care, 3701 Market St Fl 8 - Ste 800, Philadelphia, PA 19104; **Phone:** 215-662-6100; **Board Cert:** Obstetrics & Gynecology 1982; **Med School:** Cornell Univ-Weill Med Coll 1975; **Resid:** Obstetrics & Gynecology, Roosevelt Hosp/Columbia Presby Med Ctr 1979; **Fellow:** Reproductive Endocrinology, Hosp Univ Penn 1981; **Fac Appt:** Prof ObG, Univ Pennsylvania

Wallach, Edward E MD [RE] - **Spec Exp:** Uterine Fibroids; Infertility-IVF; **Hospital:** Johns Hopkins Hosp (page 61), Johns Hopkins Bayview Med Ctr (page 61); **Address:** Johns Hopkins at Greenspring Station, 2330 W Joppa Rd, Ste 301, Lutherville, MD 21093; **Phone:** 410-583-2751; **Board Cert:** Obstetrics & Gynecology 1979; Reproductive Endocrinology 1975; **Med School:** Cornell Univ-Weill Med Coll 1958; **Resid:** Obstetrics & Gynecology, Kings Co Hosp 1963; **Fellow:** Reproductive Endocrinology, Worcester Fdn Exper Biol 1962; **Fac Appt:** Prof ObG, Johns Hopkins Univ

Weiss, Gerson MD [RE] - **Spec Exp:** Infertility; Menopause Problems; **Hospital:** Hackensack Univ Med Ctr, UMDNJ-Univ Hosp-Newark; **Address:** 214 Terrace Ave, Hasbrouck Heights, NJ 07604-1815; **Phone:** 201-288-6330; **Board Cert:** Obstetrics & Gynecology 1993; Reproductive Endocrinology 1974; **Med School:** NYU Sch Med 1964; **Resid:** Obstetrics & Gynecology, Bellevue Hosp Ctr 1969; **Fellow:** Reproductive Endocrinology, Univ Pittsburgh 1973; **Fac Appt:** Prof ObG, UMDNJ-NJ Med Sch, Newark

Zacur, Howard A MD/PhD [RE] - **Spec Exp:** Prolactin Disorders; Uterine Fibroids; Hormonal Disorders; **Hospital:** Johns Hopkins Hosp (page 61); **Address:** Johns Hopkins at Green Spring Station, 10753 Falls Rd, Pavilion 2, Ste 335, Lutherville, MD 21093; **Phone:** 410-616-7140; **Board Cert:** Obstetrics & Gynecology 1994; Reproductive Endocrinology 1984; **Med School:** Univ Miami Sch Med 1973; **Resid:** Obstetrics & Gynecology, Johns Hopkins Hosp 1980; **Fellow:** Reproductive Endocrinology, Johns Hopkins Hosp 1982; **Fac Appt:** Prof ObG, Johns Hopkins Univ

Southeast

Berga, Sarah L MD [RE] - **Spec Exp:** Infertility-IVF; Hormonal Disorders; Menstrual Disorders; Polycystic Ovarian Syndrome; **Hospital:** Emory Univ Hosp, Emory Univ Hosp Midtown; **Address:** Dept Gynecology & Obstetrics, 1639 Pierce Drive, rm 4208-WMB, Atlanta, GA 30322; **Phone:** 404-778-3401; **Board Cert:** Obstetrics & Gynecology 2008; Reproductive Endocrinology 2008; **Med School:** Univ VA Sch Med 1980; **Resid:** Obstetrics & Gynecology, Mass Genl Hosp 1984; **Fellow:** Reproductive Endocrinology, UCSD Med Ctr 1986; **Fac Appt:** Prof ObG, Emory Univ

Blackwell, Richard E MD/PhD [RE] - **Spec Exp:** Infertility-Female; Women's Health; **Hospital:** Univ of Ala Hosp at Birmingham, St Vincent's Hosp - Birmingham; **Address:** 618 S 20th St, Birmingham, AL 35294; **Phone:** 205-934-6090; **Board Cert:** Obstetrics & Gynecology 1982; Reproductive Endocrinology 1987; **Med School:** Baylor Coll Med 1975; **Resid:** Obstetrics & Gynecology, Univ Alabama Hosp 1979; **Fellow:** Reproductive Endocrinology, Univ Alabama Hosp 1981; Reproductive Endocrinology, Sack Inst 1982; **Fac Appt:** Prof ObG, Univ Alabama

Broderick, Gregory MD [RE] - **Spec Exp:** Erectile Dysfunction; Voiding Dysfunction; Peyronie's Disease; **Hospital:** Mayo - Jacksonville; **Address:** Mayo Clinic, Dept Urology, 4500 San Pablo Rd, Jacksonville, FL 32224; **Phone:** 904-953-7330; **Board Cert:** Urology 2002; **Med School:** UCSF 1983; **Resid:** Surgery, UCSF Med Ctr 1985; Urology, UCSF Med Ctr 1988; **Fellow:** Neurourology, UC Davis Med Ctr 1990; **Fac Appt:** Prof U, Mayo Med Sch

Cowan, Bryan D MD [RE] - **Spec Exp:** Infertility-IVF; Uterine Fibroids; **Hospital:** Univ Mississippi Med Ctr; **Address:** University Hosp & Clinics, Dept Ob/Gyn, 2500 N State St, Jackson, MS 39216; **Phone:** 601-984-5300; **Board Cert:** Obstetrics & Gynecology 2007; Reproductive Endocrinology 2007; **Med School:** Univ Colorado 1975; **Resid:** Obstetrics & Gynecology, Portsmouth Naval Hosp 1979; **Fellow:** Reproductive Endocrinology, WRAH/NIH 1981; **Fac Appt:** Prof ObG, Univ Miss

DeVane, Gary W MD [RE] - **Spec Exp:** Infertility-IVF; Miscarriage-Recurrent; Endometriosis; Vaginal/Uterine Abnormalities; **Hospital:** Florida Hosp - Orlando, Arnold Palmer Hosp for Chldn; **Address:** 3435 Pinehurst Ave, Orlando, FL 32804-4049; **Phone:** 407-740-0909; **Board Cert:** Obstetrics & Gynecology 1977; Reproductive Endocrinology 1982; **Med School:** Baylor Coll Med 1971; **Resid:** Obstetrics & Gynecology, UCSD Hosp 1975; **Fellow:** Reproductive Endocrinology, Univ Texas SW Hosp 1980

Fritz, Marc A MD [RE] - **Spec Exp:** Infertility; Menopause Problems; Menstrual Disorders; **Hospital:** Univ NC Hosps; **Address:** Univ NC Sch Med, Dept Ob/Gyn, CB 7570, 4001 Old Clinic, Chapel Hill, NC 27599-7570; **Phone:** 919-966-5283; **Board Cert:** Obstetrics & Gynecology 1996; Reproductive Endocrinology 1996; **Med School:** Tulane Univ 1977; **Resid:** Obstetrics & Gynecology, Wright State Univ 1981; **Fellow:** Reproductive Endocrinology, Oregon Hlth Sci Univ 1983; **Fac Appt:** Prof ObG, Univ NC Sch Med

Goodman, Neil F MD [RE] - **Spec Exp:** Polycystic Ovarian Syndrome; Hormonal Disorders; Infertility; **Hospital:** Baptist Hosp of Miami, South Miami Hosp; **Address:** 9150 SW 87th Ave, Ste 210, Miami, FL 33176-2313; **Phone:** 305-595-6855; **Board Cert:** Internal Medicine 1973; Endocrinology, Diabetes & Metabolism 1975; **Med School:** Columbia P&S 1970; **Resid:** Internal Medicine, Beth Israel Hosp 1972; **Fellow:** Endocrinology, Mass Genl Hosp 1974; **Fac Appt:** Clin Prof Med, Univ Miami Sch Med

Reproductive Endocrinology

Hammond, Charles B MD [RE] - **Spec Exp:** Menopause Problems; Trophoblastic Disease; **Hospital:** Duke Univ Med Ctr; **Address:** Duke Univ Med Ctr, Box 3853, Durham, NC 27710-0001; **Phone:** 919-684-3008; **Board Cert:** Obstetrics & Gynecology 1972; Reproductive Endocrinology 1974; **Med School:** Duke Univ 1961; **Resid:** Obstetrics & Gynecology, Duke Med Ctr 1963; Obstetrics & Gynecology, Duke Med Ctr 1968; **Fellow:** Gynecology, Duke Med Ctr 1964; Reproductive Endocrinology, Natl Inst Hlth 1966; **Fac Appt:** Prof ObG, Duke Univ

Keefe, David Lawrence MD [RE] - **Spec Exp:** Infertility-IVF; Infertility-Advanced Maternal Age; **Hospital:** Univ of S FL - Tampa; **Address:** 2 Tampa Genl Cir, Tampa, FL 33606; **Phone:** 813-259-8500; **Board Cert:** Obstetrics & Gynecology 2007; Reproductive Endocrinology 2007; **Med School:** Georgetown Univ 1980; **Resid:** Psychiatry, Harvard Psych Srv/Camb Hosp 1983; Obstetrics & Gynecology, Yale New Haven Hosp 1989; **Fellow:** Psychiatry, Univ Chicago Hosp & Clins 1985; Reproductive Endocrinology, Yale New Haven Hosp 1991; **Fac Appt:** Prof ObG, Univ S Fla Coll Med

Kutteh, William H MD/PhD [RE] - **Spec Exp:** Miscarriage-Recurrent; Infertility; **Hospital:** Baptist Memorial Hospital - Memphis, Methodist LeBonheur Germantown Hosp; **Address:** 80 Humphrey's Ctr, Ste 307, Memphis, TN 38120-2363; **Phone:** 901-747-2229; **Board Cert:** Obstetrics & Gynecology 2007; Reproductive Endocrinology/Infertility 2007; **Med School:** Wake Forest Univ 1985; **Resid:** Obstetrics & Gynecology, UAB Med Ctr 1989; **Fellow:** Reproductive Endocrinology, Univ Tennessee Affil Hosp 1991; **Fac Appt:** Prof Med, Univ Tenn Coll Med, Memphis

Murphy, Ana A MD [RE] - **Spec Exp:** Infertility; Endometriosis; Pelvic Surgery; **Hospital:** Med Coll of GA Hosp and Clin (MCG Health Inc); **Address:** Med Coll Ga - Dept Ob/Gyn, BA-7313, 1120 15th St, Agusta, GA 30912; **Phone:** 706-722-4434; **Board Cert:** Obstetrics & Gynecology 2007; Reproductive Endocrinology 2007; **Med School:** Univ Mich Med Sch 1980; **Resid:** Obstetrics & Gynecology, Johns Hopkins Univ 1984; **Fellow:** Reproductive Endocrinology, Johns Hopkins Univ 1986; **Fac Appt:** Prof ObG, Med Coll GA

Ory, Steven J MD [RE] - **Spec Exp:** Infertility; Hormonal Disorders; Endometriosis; **Hospital:** Northwest Med Ctr, Meml Regl Hosp; **Address:** 2960 N State Road 7, Ste 300, Margate, FL 33063-5737; **Phone:** 954-247-6200; **Board Cert:** Obstetrics & Gynecology 2007; Reproductive Endocrinology 2007; **Med School:** Baylor Coll Med 1976; **Resid:** Obstetrics & Gynecology, Mayo Clinic 1980; **Fellow:** Reproductive Endocrinology, Duke Univ 1982; **Fac Appt:** Assoc Clin Prof ObG, Univ Miami Sch Med

Session, Donna R MD [RE] - **Spec Exp:** Ultrasound Guided Surgery; Infertility-Female; **Hospital:** Emory Univ Hosp, Emory Univ Hosp Midtown; **Address:** Emory Reproductive Endocrinology, 550 Peachtree St, Ste 1800 MOT, Atlanta, GA 30308; **Phone:** 404-778-3401; **Board Cert:** Obstetrics & Gynecology 2004; Reproductive Endocrinology 2004; **Med School:** Eastern VA Med Sch 1986; **Resid:** Obstetrics & Gynecology, Winthrop Hosp 1990; **Fellow:** Reproductive Endocrinology, Columbia-Presby Med Ctr 1993; **Fac Appt:** Assoc Prof ObG, Emory Univ

Steinkampf, Michael MD [RE] - **Spec Exp:** Infertility; **Hospital:** Brookwood Med Ctr; **Address:** 2700 Highway 280, Ste 370 East, East Birmingham, AL 35223; **Phone:** 205-874-0000; **Board Cert:** Obstetrics & Gynecology 1997; Reproductive Endocrinology 1997; **Med School:** Louisiana State U, New Orleans 1981; **Resid:** Obstetrics & Gynecology, Parkland Meml Hosp 1985; **Fellow:** Reproductive Endocrinology, Univ Texas SW Med Ctr 1987; **Fac Appt:** Prof ObG, Univ Alabama

Walmer, David K MD/PhD [RE] - **Spec Exp:** Infertility; Miscarriage-Recurrent; DES-Exposed Females; Endometriosis; **Hospital:** Duke Univ Med Ctr; **Address:** Duke Fertility Center, 5704 Fayetteville Rd, Durham, NC 27713; **Phone:** 919-572-4673; **Board Cert:** Obstetrics & Gynecology 2007; Reproductive Endocrinology 2007; **Med School:** Univ NC Sch Med 1982; **Resid:** Obstetrics & Gynecology, Univ Texas Health Sci Ctr 1987; **Fellow:** Reproductive Endocrinology, Duke Univ Med Ctr 1989; **Fac Appt:** Assoc Prof ObG, Duke Univ

Midwest

Barnes, Randall B MD [RE] - **Spec Exp:** Infertility-IVF; Polycystic Ovarian Syndrome; Miscar-riage-Recurrent; **Hospital:** Northwestern Meml Hosp; **Address:** 675 N St Clair St Fl 14 - Ste 200, Chicago, IL 60611; **Phone:** 312-695-7269; **Board Cert:** Obstetrics & Gynecology 2007; Reproduc-tive Endocrinology 2007; **Med School:** Johns Hopkins Univ 1979; **Resid:** Obstetrics & Gynecology, LAC-USC Med Ctr 1983; **Fellow:** Reproductive Endocrinology, LAC-USC Med Ctr 1985; **Fac Appt:** Assoc Prof ObG, Northwestern Univ

Christman, Gregory MD [RE] - **Spec Exp:** Infertility-IVF; Uterine Fibroids; **Hospital:** Univ Michigan Hlth Sys; **Address:** 475 Market Pl, Ste B, Ann Arbor, MI 48108; **Phone:** 734-763-4323; **Board Cert:** Obstetrics & Gynecology 2002; Reproductive Endocrinology 2002; **Med School:** Univ Wisc 1983; **Resid:** Obstetrics & Gynecology, Univ Wisconsin Med Sch 1987; **Fellow:** Reproductive Endocrinology, Univ North Carolina 1992; **Fac Appt:** Assoc Prof ObG, Univ Mich Med Sch

Diamond, Michael P MD [RE] - **Spec Exp:** Infertility-IVF; Infertility-Female; Polycystic Ovarian Syndrome; Hysteroscopic Surgery; **Hospital:** Hutzel Hosp - Detroit, Harper Univ Hosp; **Address:** Univ Ctr for Women's Medicine, 26400 W 12 Mile Rd, Southfield, MI 48034; **Phone:** 248-352-8200; **Board Cert:** Obstetrics & Gynecology 2007; Reproductive Endocrinology 2007; **Med School:** Vanderbilt Univ 1981; **Resid:** Obstetrics & Gynecology, Vanderbilt Univ Med Ctr 1985; **Fellow:** Reproductive Endocrinology, Yale-New Haven Hosp 1987; Univ Penn 1996; **Fac Appt:** Prof ObG, Wayne State Univ

Dodds, William G MD [RE] - **Spec Exp:** Infertility; Endometriosis; Infertility-IVF; **Hospital:** Spectrum Hlth Butterworth Campus, Bronson Meth Hosp; **Address:** 3230 Eagle Park Drive NE, Grand Rapids, MI 49525; **Phone:** 616-988-2229; **Board Cert:** Obstetrics & Gynecology 2007; Reproduc-tive Endocrinology 2007; **Med School:** Ohio State Univ 1982; **Resid:** Obstetrics & Gynecology, Ohio State Univ Med Ctr 1986; **Fellow:** Reproductive Endocrinology, Ohio State Univ 1988; **Fac Appt:** Assoc Prof ObG, Univ Mich Med Sch

Dumesic, Daniel Anthony MD [RE] - **Spec Exp:** Infertility-Female; Hormonal Disorders; En-dometriosis; **Address:** Reproductive Med & Infertility Assocs, 2101 Woodwinds Drive, Ste 100, Woodbury, MN 55125; **Phone:** 651-222-6050; **Board Cert:** Obstetrics & Gynecology 1995; Re-productive Endocrinology 1995; **Med School:** Univ Wisc 1978; **Resid:** Obstetrics & Gynecology, UCSF Med Ctr 1982; **Fellow:** Reproductive Endocrinology, UCSF Med Ctr 1987

Falcone, Tommaso MD [RE] - **Spec Exp:** Minimally Invasive Surgery; Infertility-IVF; Endometrio-sis; **Hospital:** Cleveland Clin Fdn (page 56); **Address:** Cleveland Clin, Dept Ob/Gyn, 9500 Euclid Ave, Desk A81, Cleveland, OH 44195-0001; **Phone:** 216-444-1758; **Board Cert:** Obstetrics & Gy-necology 1998; Reproductive Endocrinology 1998; **Med School:** McGill Univ 1981; **Resid:** Obstet-rics & Gynecology, McGill Univ 1986; **Fellow:** Reproductive Endocrinology, McGill Univ 1989

Haney, Arthur F MD [RE] - **Spec Exp:** Infertility-Female; DES-Exposed Females; **Hospital:** Univ of Chicago Med Ctr; **Address:** 5841 S Maryland Ave, MC 2050, Chicago, IL 60637; **Phone:** 773-702-6127; **Board Cert:** Obstetrics & Gynecology 2007; Reproductive Endocrinology 2007; **Med School:** Univ Ariz Coll Med 1972; **Resid:** Obstetrics & Gynecology, Duke Univ Med Ctr 1976; **Fellow:** Reproductive Endocrinology, Duke Univ Med Ctr 1978; **Fac Appt:** Prof ObG, Univ Chicago-Pritzker Sch Med

Jacobs, Laurence A MD [RE] - **Spec Exp:** Infertility-IVF; Polycystic Ovarian Syndrome; En-dometriosis; **Hospital:** Adv Luth Genl Hosp, Northwest Comm Hosp; **Address:** 135 N Arlington Hts Rd, Ste 195, Buffalo Grove, IL 60089; **Phone:** 847-215-8899; **Board Cert:** Obstetrics & Gynecol-ogy 1981; **Med School:** Northwestern Univ 1975; **Resid:** Obstetrics & Gynecology, Northwestern Meml Hosp 1979; **Fellow:** Reproductive Endocrinology, Mayo Clinic 1988; **Fac Appt:** Assoc Prof ObG, Northwestern Univ

Reproductive Endocrinology

Kazer, Ralph MD [RE] - **Spec Exp:** Polycystic Ovarian Syndrome; Infertility-IVF; **Hospital:** Northwestern Meml Hosp; **Address:** Northwestern Meml Hospital, 675 N St Clair St Fl 14 - Ste 200, Chicago, IL 60611; **Phone:** 312-695-7269; **Board Cert:** Obstetrics & Gynecology 2007; Reproductive Endocrinology 2007; **Med School:** Tufts Univ 1979; **Resid:** Obstetrics & Gynecology, Tufts Univ Med Ctr 1983; **Fellow:** Reproductive Endocrinology, UC San Diego Med Ctr 1986; **Fac Appt:** Assoc Prof ObG, Northwestern Univ

Milad, Magdy P MD [RE] - **Spec Exp:** Reproductive Surgery; Infertility; Uterine Fibroids; **Hospital:** Northwestern Meml Hosp, Children's Mem Hosp; **Address:** Northwestern Med Fac Fdn, 675 North St Clair, Fl 14 - Ste 200, Chicago, IL 60611-5975; **Phone:** 312-695-7269; **Board Cert:** Obstetrics & Gynecology 2007; Reproductive Endocrinology 2007; **Med School:** Wayne State Univ 1987; **Resid:** Obstetrics & Gynecology, William Beaumont Hosp 1991; **Fellow:** Reproductive Endocrinology, Mayo Clinic 1993; **Fac Appt:** Prof ObG, Northwestern Univ

Miller, Charles E MD [RE] - **Spec Exp:** Infertility-IVF; Minimally Invasive Surgery; Endometriosis; Uterine Fibroids; **Hospital:** Edward Hosp, Adv Luth Genl Hosp; **Address:** 120 Osler Drive, Ste 100, Naperville, IL 60540; **Phone:** 630-428-2229; **Board Cert:** Obstetrics & Gynecology 1984; **Med School:** Northwestern Univ 1977; **Resid:** Obstetrics & Gynecology, Univ Texas SW Med Ctr 1980; **Fellow:** Reproductive Endocrinology, Hosp Univ Penn 1983; **Fac Appt:** Assoc Clin Prof ObG, Univ Chicago-Pritzker Sch Med

Molo, Mary W MD [RE] - **Spec Exp:** Infertility-IVF; Uterine Fibroids; Fertility Preservation in Cancer; **Hospital:** Rush Univ Med Ctr; **Address:** 1725 W Harrison St, Ste 408 East, Chicago, IL 60612; **Phone:** 312-997-2229; **Board Cert:** Obstetrics & Gynecology 2007; Reproductive Endocrinology 2007; **Med School:** Southern IL Univ 1982; **Resid:** Obstetrics & Gynecology, Southern Illinois Affil Hosps 1984; Obstetrics & Gynecology, Rush Presby St Lukes Hosp 1987; **Fellow:** Reproductive Endocrinology, Rush Presby St Lukes Hosp 1989; **Fac Appt:** Asst Prof ObG, Rush Med Coll

Nagel, Theodore C MD [RE] - **Spec Exp:** Infertility-IVF; Hysteroscopic Surgery; Vaginal/Uterine Abnormalities; Laparoscopic Surgery; **Hospital:** Univ Minn Med Ctr, Fairview - Riverside Campus; **Address:** Reproductive Med Ctr, Univ Minnesota, 606 24th Ave S, Ste 500, Minnneapolis, MN 55454; **Phone:** 612-627-4564; **Board Cert:** Internal Medicine 1970; Endocrinology 1975; Obstetrics & Gynecology 1981; Reproductive Endocrinology 1983; **Med School:** Cornell Univ-Weill Med Coll 1963; **Resid:** Internal Medicine, Bellevue Hosp Ctr 1968; Obstetrics & Gynecology, Univ Minn Hosps 1977; **Fellow:** Endocrinology, Diabetes & Metabolism, Northwestern Univ Med Sch 1972; Reproductive Endocrinology, Univ Minnesota 1980; **Fac Appt:** Assoc Clin Prof ObG, Univ Minn

Odem, Randall R MD [RE] - **Spec Exp:** Infertility; Reproductive Surgery; Miscarriage-Recurrent; Hysteroscopic Surgery; **Hospital:** Barnes-Jewish Hosp; **Address:** 4444 Forest Park Ave, Ste 3100, St Louis, MO 63108-2212; **Phone:** 314-286-2421; **Board Cert:** Obstetrics & Gynecology 2007; Reproductive Endocrinology 2007; **Med School:** Univ Iowa Coll Med 1981; **Resid:** Obstetrics & Gynecology, Univ Illinois Hosps 1985; **Fellow:** Reproductive Endocrinology, Wash Univ Sch Med Affil Hosp 1987; **Fac Appt:** Prof ObG, Washington Univ, St Louis

Ratts, Valerie S MD [RE] - **Spec Exp:** Polycystic Ovarian Syndrome; Uterine Fibroids; Infertility-IVF; **Hospital:** Barnes-Jewish Hosp; **Address:** Washington Univ, Ctr for Reproductive Med/Infertility, 4444 Forest Park Ave, Ste 3100, St Louis, MO 63108; **Phone:** 314-286-2400; **Board Cert:** Obstetrics & Gynecology 2007; Reproductive Endocrinology 2007; **Med School:** Johns Hopkins Univ 1987; **Resid:** Obstetrics & Gynecology, Johns Hopkins Hosp 1991; **Fellow:** Reproductive Endocrinology, Johns Hopkins Hosp 1993; **Fac Appt:** Assoc Prof ObG, Washington Univ, St Louis

Smith, Yolanda R MD [RE] - **Spec Exp:** Infertility; Polycystic Ovarian Syndrome; **Hospital:** Univ Michigan Hlth Sys; **Address:** Women's Hosp, 1500 E Med Ctr Drive, rm L4100, Box 0276, Ann Arbor, MI 48109-0276; **Phone:** 734-763-4323; **Board Cert:** Obstetrics & Gynecology 2007; Reproductive Endocrinology 2007; **Med School:** Wake Forest Univ 1989; **Resid:** Obstetrics & Gynecology, Univ Mich Hosp 1993; **Fellow:** Reproductive Endocrinology, Johns Hopkins Hosp 1995; **Fac Appt:** Assoc Prof ObG, Univ Mich Med Sch

Great Plains and Mountains

Richardson, Marilyn MD [RE] - **Spec Exp:** Menopause Problems; Infertility; Polycystic Ovarian Syndrome; **Hospital:** Univ of Kansas Hosp; **Address:** 12616 W 62nd Terr, Ste 111, Shawnee, KS 66216; **Phone:** 913-631-0277; **Board Cert:** Obstetrics & Gynecology 2007; **Med School:** Univ Kans 1979; **Resid:** Obstetrics & Gynecology, Truman Med Ctr 1983; **Fellow:** Reproductive Endocrinology, Univ Texas Hlth Scis Ctr 1985; **Fac Appt:** Asst Clin Prof ObG, Univ Kans

Schlaff, William D MD [RE] - **Spec Exp:** Infertility; Endometriosis; Vaginal/Uterine Abnormalities; **Hospital:** Univ Colorado Hosp; **Address:** Dept of OB & Gyn, 1635 Aurora Ct, MS F701, Aurora, CO 80045; **Phone:** 720-848-1690; **Board Cert:** Obstetrics & Gynecology 2008; Reproductive Endocrinology 2008; **Med School:** Univ Mich Med Sch 1977; **Resid:** Obstetrics & Gynecology, Univ Mich Hosps 1981; **Fellow:** Reproductive Endocrinology, Johns Hopkins Med Ctr 1985; **Fac Appt:** Prof ObG, Univ Colorado

Surrey, Eric S MD [RE] - **Spec Exp:** Infertility-IVF; Endometriosis; **Hospital:** Swedish Med Ctr - Englewood, Sky Ridge Med Ctr; **Address:** 10290 RidgeGate Circle, Lone Tree, CO 80124; **Phone:** 303-788-8300; **Board Cert:** Obstetrics & Gynecology 1998; Reproductive Endocrinology 1998; **Med School:** Univ Pennsylvania 1981; **Resid:** Obstetrics & Gynecology, UCLA Med Ctr 1986; **Fellow:** Reproductive Endocrinology, UCLA Med Ctr 1988

Southwest

Dickey, Richard P MD/PhD [RE] - **Spec Exp:** Infertility-IVF; **Hospital:** Tulane-Lakeside Hosp; **Address:** The Fertility Institute, 800 N Causeway Blvd, Ste 2C, Mandeville, LA 70448; **Phone:** 985-892-7621; **Board Cert:** Obstetrics & Gynecology 1967; Reproductive Endocrinology/Infertility 1976; **Med School:** Case West Res Univ 1960; **Resid:** Obstetrics & Gynecology, Ohio State Univ Hosp 1965; **Fellow:** Reproductive Endocrinology, Ohio State Univ Hosp 1966; **Fac Appt:** Clin Prof ObG, Louisiana State U, New Orleans

Schenken, Robert S MD [RE] - **Spec Exp:** Infertility-Female; Endometriosis; **Hospital:** Univ Hlth Syst-San Antonio, Baptist Hlth Sys; **Address:** Dept OB/GYN, 7703 Floyd Curl Dr, MSC 7836, San Antonio, TX 78229-3900; **Phone:** 210-567-4950; **Board Cert:** Obstetrics & Gynecology 1995; Reproductive Endocrinology 1995; **Med School:** Baylor Coll Med 1977; **Resid:** Obstetrics & Gynecology, Bexar Co Hosp 1981; **Fellow:** Reproductive Endocrinology, Natl Inst Hlth 1982; Reproductive Endocrinology, Univ Tex Hlth Sci Ctr 1983; **Fac Appt:** Prof ObG, Univ Tex, San Antonio

West Coast and Pacific

Adamson, G David MD [RE] - **Spec Exp:** Infertility-Female; Endometriosis; Infertility-IVF; **Hospital:** Good Samaritan Hosp - San Jose, Stanford Univ Med Ctr; **Address:** 540 University Ave, Ste 200, Palo Alto, CA 94301; **Phone:** 650-322-1900; **Board Cert:** Obstetrics & Gynecology 1980; Reproductive Endocrinology 1982; **Med School:** Univ Toronto 1973; **Resid:** Obstetrics & Gynecology, Toronto Genl Hosp 1977; **Fellow:** Obstetrics & Gynecology, Toronto Genl Hosp 1978; Reproductive Endocrinology, Stanford Univ Hosp 1980; **Fac Appt:** Clin Prof ObG, Stanford Univ

Reproductive Endocrinology

Agarwal, Sanjay K MD [RE] - **Spec Exp:** Infertility-IVF; Endometriosis; **Hospital:** UCSD Med Ctr; **Address:** Univ California-San Diego Medical Ctr, 9500 Gilman Drive, MC 0633, La Jolla, CA 92093-0633; **Phone:** 858-657-8745; **Board Cert:** Obstetrics & Gynecology 2007; Reproductive Endocrinology/Infertility 2007; **Med School:** England, UK 1987; **Resid:** Obstetrics & Gynecology, Duke Univ Med Ctr 1997; **Fellow:** Reproductive Endocrinology, UCLA Med Ctr 2000; **Fac Appt:** Prof ObG, UCSD

Azziz, Ricardo MD [RE] - **Spec Exp:** Infertility-Female; Reproductive Surgery; Polycystic Ovarian Syndrome; **Hospital:** Cedars-Sinai Med Ctr; **Address:** Cedars Sinai-Ctr Fertility & Reproductive Med, 8700 Beverly Blvd, Ste 3611, Los Angeles, CA 90048; **Phone:** 310-423-9964; **Board Cert:** Obstetrics & Gynecology 2007; Reproductive Endocrinology 2007; **Med School:** Penn State Univ-Hershey Med Ctr 1981; **Resid:** Obstetrics & Gynecology, Georgetown Univ Hosp 1985; **Fellow:** Reproductive Endocrinology, Johns Hopkins Hosp 1987; **Fac Appt:** Prof ObG, UCLA

Chang, R Jeffrey MD [RE] - **Spec Exp:** Polycystic Ovarian Syndrome; Hormonal Disorders; **Hospital:** UCSD Med Ctr; **Address:** Univ California-San Diego Medical Ctr, 9500 Gilman Drive, MC 0633, La Jolla, CA 92093-0633; **Phone:** 858-657-8745; **Board Cert:** Obstetrics & Gynecology 2002; Reproductive Endocrinology/Infertility 2002; **Med School:** Oregon Hlth & Sci Univ 1969; **Resid:** Obstetrics & Gynecology, Harbor Genl Hosp-UCLA 1974; **Fellow:** Reproductive Endocrinology, Harbor Genl Hosp-UCLA 1975; Reproductive Endocrinology, UCSF Med Ctr 1977; **Fac Appt:** Prof ObG, UCSD

Marrs, Richard P MD [RE] - **Spec Exp:** Infertility-Female; Endometriosis; Uterine Fibroids; **Hospital:** Santa Monica - UCLA Med Ctr & Ortho Hosp; **Address:** 11818 Wilshire Blvd, Ste 300, Los Angeles, CA 90025; **Phone:** 310-828-4008; **Board Cert:** Obstetrics & Gynecology 1980; Reproductive Endocrinology 1983; **Med School:** Univ Tex Med Br, Galveston 1974; **Resid:** Obstetrics & Gynecology, Univ Tex Hosps 1977; **Fellow:** Reproductive Endocrinology, USC Med Ctr 1979

Paulson, Richard J MD [RE] - **Spec Exp:** Infertility-IVF; Infertility-Advanced Maternal Age; **Hospital:** LAC & USC Med Ctr, Good Samaritan Hosp - LA; **Address:** USC Fertility, 1127 Wilshire Blvd, Ste 1400, Los Angeles, CA 90017; **Phone:** 213-975-9990; **Board Cert:** Obstetrics & Gynecology 2007; Reproductive Endocrinology 2007; **Med School:** UCLA 1980; **Resid:** Obstetrics & Gynecology, Harbor-UCLA Med Ctr 1984; **Fellow:** Reproductive Endocrinology, LAC-USC Med Ctr 1986; **Fac Appt:** Prof ObG, USC Sch Med

Soules, Michael R MD [RE] - **Spec Exp:** Infertility-Female; Infertility-IVF; **Hospital:** Northwest Hosp; **Address:** 1505 Westlake Ave N, Ste 400, Seattle, WA 98109; **Phone:** 206-301-5000; **Board Cert:** Obstetrics & Gynecology 2002; Reproductive Endocrinology 2002; **Med School:** UCLA 1972; **Resid:** Obstetrics & Gynecology, Univ Colorado Med Ctr 1976; **Fellow:** Reproductive Endocrinology, Duke Univ Hosp 1978; **Fac Appt:** Prof ObG, Univ Wash

Winer, Sharon A MD [RE] - **Spec Exp:** Hormonal Disorders; Infertility-Female; Vaginitis; Gynecology; **Hospital:** Cedars-Sinai Med Ctr, USC Univ Hosp; **Address:** 9400 Brighton Way, Ste 206, Beverly Hills, CA 90210-4709; **Phone:** 310-274-9100; **Board Cert:** Obstetrics & Gynecology 2007; Reproductive Endocrinology 2007; **Med School:** USC Sch Med 1978; **Resid:** Obstetrics & Gynecology, LAC-USC Med Ctr 1982; **Fellow:** Microsurgery, Hammersmith Hosp 1983; Reproductive Endocrinology, LAC-USC Med Ctr 1985; **Fac Appt:** Clin Prof ObG, USC Sch Med

Yee, Billy MD [RE] - **Spec Exp:** Infertility-IVF; **Hospital:** Long Beach Meml Med Ctr, Little Co of Mary-Torrance Hosp; **Address:** 13950 Milton Ave, Ste 100, Westminster, CA 92683; **Phone:** 714-702-3001; **Board Cert:** Obstetrics & Gynecology 2007; Reproductive Endocrinology 2007; **Med School:** UC Davis 1978; **Resid:** Obstetrics & Gynecology, LAC-USC Med Ctr 1982; **Fellow:** Reproductive Endocrinology, LAC-USC Med Ctr 1985; **Fac Appt:** Assoc Clin Prof ObG, UC Irvine

Rheumatology

a subspecialty of Internal Medicine

An internist who treats diseases of joints, muscle, bones and tendons. This specialist diagnoses and treats arthritis, back pain, muscle strains, common athletic injuries and "collagen" diseases.

Training Required: Three years in internal medicine *plus* additional training and examination for certification in rheumatology.

RHEUMATOLOGY

New England

Albert, Daniel A MD [Rhu] - **Spec Exp:** Juvenile Arthritis; Rheumatology-Adult & Pediatric; **Hospital:** Dartmouth - Hitchcock Med Ctr; **Address:** Dartmouth-Hitchcock Med Ctr, Dept Rheumatology, One Medical Center Drive, Lebanon, NH 03756; **Phone:** 603-650-8622; **Board Cert:** Internal Medicine 1977; Rheumatology 1980; **Med School:** NYU Sch Med 1974; **Resid:** Internal Medicine, NC Meml Hosp 1977; **Fellow:** Rheumatology, UCSD 1981; **Fac Appt:** Prof Med, Univ Pennsylvania

Brenner, Michael B MD [Rhu] - **Spec Exp:** Gout; Rheumatoid Arthritis; Lupus/SLE; **Hospital:** Brigham & Women's Hosp; **Address:** Div Rheumatology Smith Bldg - rm 552, 1 Jimmy Fund Way, Boston, MA 02115; **Phone:** 617-525-1000; **Board Cert:** Internal Medicine 1978; Rheumatology 1982; **Med School:** Vanderbilt Univ 1975; **Resid:** Internal Medicine, Vanderbilt Univ Hosp 1979; **Fellow:** Rheumatology, UCLA Med Ctr 1981; **Fac Appt:** Prof Med, Harvard Med Sch

Coblyn, Jonathan S MD [Rhu] - **Spec Exp:** Rheumatoid Arthritis; Lupus/SLE; Vasculitis; Musculoskeletal Disorders; **Hospital:** Brigham & Women's Hosp, New England Bapt Hosp; **Address:** Brigham & Women's Hosp, Div Rheumatology, 75 Francis St, PBB-B3, Boston, MA 02115; **Phone:** 617-732-5347; **Board Cert:** Internal Medicine 1977; Rheumatology 1980; **Med School:** Johns Hopkins Univ 1974; **Resid:** Internal Medicine, Peter Bent Brigham Hosp 1976; Internal Medicine, Stanford Univ Hosps 1977; **Fellow:** Rheumatology, Peter Bent Brigham Hosp 1979; **Fac Appt:** Assoc Prof Med, Harvard Med Sch

Kay, Jonathan MD [Rhu] - **Spec Exp:** Rheumatoid Arthritis; Psoriatic Arthritis; Ankylosing Spondylitis; Nephrogenic Fibrosing Dermopathy; **Hospital:** UMass Meml - Meml Campus; **Address:** Rheumatology Ctr, Meml Campus, 119 Belmont St, Worcester, MA 01605; **Phone:** 508-334-6273; **Board Cert:** Internal Medicine 1986; Rheumatology 1988; **Med School:** UCSF 1983; **Resid:** Internal Medicine, Hosp Univ Penn 1986; **Fellow:** Rheumatology/Immunology, Brigham & Womens Hosp 1989; **Fac Appt:** Prof Med, Univ Mass Sch Med

Massarotti, Elena M MD [Rhu] - **Spec Exp:** Lupus/SLE; Rheumatoid Arthritis; Psoriatic Arthritis; Gout; **Hospital:** Brigham & Women's Hosp; **Address:** Brigham & Women's Hosp, Div Rheumatology, PBB-B3, 75 Francis St, Boston, MA 02115; **Phone:** 617-732-6523; **Board Cert:** Internal Medicine 1989; Rheumatology 2000; **Med School:** Tufts Univ 1984; **Resid:** Internal Medicine, Tufts-New England Med Ctr 1987; **Fellow:** Rheumatology, Tufts-New England Med Ctr 1989; **Fac Appt:** Assoc Prof Med, Tufts Univ

Merkel, Peter MD [Rhu] - **Spec Exp:** Vasculitis; Scleroderma; **Hospital:** Boston Med Ctr; **Address:** Boston Univ Vasculitis Ctr, 72 E Concord St, E 533, Boston, MA 02118; **Phone:** 617-414-2500; **Board Cert:** Internal Medicine 2000; Rheumatology 2000; **Med School:** Yale Univ 1988; **Resid:** Internal Medicine, Hosp Univ Penn 1991; **Fellow:** Rheumatology, Mass General Hosp 1994

Polisson, Richard P MD [Rhu] - **Spec Exp:** Rheumatoid Arthritis; Lupus/SLE; **Hospital:** Mass Genl Hosp; **Address:** 55 Fruit St Yawkey Bldg - Ste 2C, Boston, MA 02114; **Phone:** 617-726-7938; **Board Cert:** Internal Medicine 1979; Rheumatology 1984; **Med School:** Duke Univ 1976; **Resid:** Internal Medicine, Duke Univ Med Ctr 1978; Internal Medicine, Natl Inst Hlth/NCI 1980; **Fellow:** Rheumatology, Mass Genl Hosp 1982; **Fac Appt:** Assoc Prof Med, Harvard Med Sch

Schoen, Robert T MD [Rhu] - **Spec Exp:** Rheumatoid Arthritis; Lyme Disease; Osteoporosis; **Hospital:** Yale-New Haven Hosp; **Address:** 60 Temple St, Ste 6A, New Haven, CT 06510-2716; **Phone:** 203-789-2255; **Board Cert:** Internal Medicine 1979; Rheumatology 1982; **Med School:** Columbia P&S 1976; **Resid:** Internal Medicine, Yale New Haven Hosp 1979; **Fellow:** Rheumatology, Brigham & Womens Hosp 1981; **Fac Appt:** Clin Prof Med, Yale Univ

Seton, Margaret P MD [Rhu] - **Spec Exp:** Paget's Disease of Bone; **Hospital:** Mass Genl Hosp; **Address:** Rheumatology Assocs, 55 Fruit St, Yawkey 2C, Boston, MA 02114; **Phone:** 617-726-7938; **Board Cert:** Internal Medicine 1986; Rheumatology 2002; **Med School:** Med Coll VA 1980; **Resid:** Internal Medicine, Univ Hosp 1984; **Fellow:** Immunology, Mass Genl Hosp 1986; Rheumatology, Mass Genl Hosp 1991; **Fac Appt:** Asst Prof Med, Harvard Med Sch

Shadick, Nancy A MD [Rhu] - **Spec Exp:** Lyme Disease; Rheumatoid Arthritis; Osteoarthritis; **Hospital:** Brigham & Women's Hosp; **Address:** Brigham & Womens Hosp, Arthritis Ctr, Dept Rheumatology, 75 Francis St, Boston, MA 02115-6105; **Phone:** 617-732-5266; **Board Cert:** Internal Medicine 1989; Rheumatology 2002; **Med School:** NYU Sch Med 1986; **Resid:** Internal Medicine, Columbia-Presby Hosp 1989; **Fellow:** Rheumatology, Brigham & Womens Hosp 1992; **Fac Appt:** Asst Prof Med, Harvard Med Sch

Simms, Robert W MD [Rhu] - **Spec Exp:** Rheumatoid Arthritis; Scleroderma; Lyme Disease; **Hospital:** Boston Med Ctr; **Address:** Boston Univ Sch Med, Arthritis Ctr, 72 E Concord St, Evans-501, Boston, MA 02118; **Phone:** 617-638-4312; **Board Cert:** Internal Medicine 1985; Rheumatology 1988; **Med School:** Univ Rochester 1980; **Resid:** Internal Medicine, N Shore Hosp 1982; Internal Medicine, Brigham & Women's Hosp 1985; **Fellow:** Rheumatology, Boston Univ Med Ctr 1987; **Fac Appt:** Prof Med, Boston Univ

Tsokos, George MD [Rhu] - **Spec Exp:** Lupus/SLE; **Hospital:** Beth Israel Deaconess Med Ctr - Boston; **Address:** Beth Israel Deaconess Med Ctr, Dept Rheumatology, 110 Francis St, Ste 4B, Boston, MA 02215; **Phone:** 617-632-8658; **Board Cert:** Internal Medicine 1983; Diagnostic Lab Immunology 1986; Rheumatology 1984; **Med School:** Greece 1975; **Resid:** Internal Medicine, Natl Univ 1979; Immunology, NIH-NIADDK 1981; **Fellow:** Rheumatology, NIH-NIADDK 1983

Weinblatt, Michael E MD [Rhu] - **Spec Exp:** Rheumatoid Arthritis; **Hospital:** Brigham & Women's Hosp; **Address:** Brigham & Womens Hosp, Arthritis Ctr, 45 Francis St, Boston, MA 02115-6110; **Phone:** 617-732-5331; **Board Cert:** Internal Medicine 1978; Rheumatology 1980; **Med School:** Univ MD Sch Med 1975; **Resid:** Internal Medicine, Univ Maryland Hosp 1978; **Fellow:** Rheumatology, Peter Bent Brigham Hosp 1980; **Fac Appt:** Prof Med, Harvard Med Sch

Mid Atlantic

Belmont, H Michael MD [Rhu] - **Spec Exp:** Lupus/SLE; Rheumatoid Arthritis; Scleroderma; **Hospital:** Hosp For Joint Diseases (page 67), NYU Langone Med Ctr (page 67); **Address:** 305 2nd Ave, Ste 16, New York, NY 10003-2739; **Phone:** 212-598-6516; **Board Cert:** Internal Medicine 1983; Rheumatology 1986; **Med School:** Univ Pittsburgh 1980; **Resid:** Internal Medicine, Mt Sinai Hosp 1983; **Fellow:** Rheumatology, NYU/Bellevue Hosp 1985; **Fac Appt:** Assoc Prof Med, NYU Sch Med

Blume, Ralph S MD [Rhu] - **Spec Exp:** Vasculitis; Lupus/SLE; Rheumatoid Arthritis; **Hospital:** NY-Presby Hosp/Columbia (page 66); **Address:** 161 Fort Washington Ave, Ste 537, New York, NY 10032-3713; **Phone:** 212-305-5512; **Board Cert:** Internal Medicine 1972; Rheumatology 1974; **Med School:** Columbia P&S 1964; **Resid:** Internal Medicine, Columbia-Presby Med Ctr 1968; **Fellow:** Rheumatology, Columbia-Presby Med Ctr 1970; **Fac Appt:** Clin Prof Med, Columbia P&S

Rheumatology

Bunning, Robert D MD [Rhu] - **Spec Exp:** Exercise Physiology; Rheumatoid Arthritis; Muscu-loskeletal Disorders; **Hospital:** Natl Rehab Hosp; **Address:** National Rehab Hosp, 102 Irving St NW Fl 2 - rm 2141, Washington, DC 20010; **Phone:** 202-877-1660; **Board Cert:** Internal Medicine 1984; Rheumatology 1986; **Med School:** Univ Cincinnati 1979; **Resid:** Internal Medicine, Wash Hosp Ctr 1984; **Fellow:** Rheumatology, Wash Hosp Ctr 1983; **Fac Appt:** Asst Clin Prof Med, Geo Wash Univ

Buyon, Jill P MD [Rhu] - **Spec Exp:** Lupus/SLE in Pregnancy; Lupus/SLE in Menopause; **Hospi-tal:** Hosp For Joint Diseases (page 67), NYU Langone Med Ctr (page 67); **Address:** 246 E 20th St, New York, NY 10003; **Phone:** 646-356-9400; **Board Cert:** Internal Medicine 1981; Rheumatology 1984; **Med School:** Albert Einstein Coll Med 1978; **Resid:** Internal Medicine, Montefiore Med Ctr 1981; **Fellow:** Rheumatology, NYU Med Ctr 1983; **Fac Appt:** Prof Med, NYU Sch Med

Cupps, Thomas R MD [Rhu] - **Spec Exp:** Vasculitis; Hepatitis B-Immune Response; **Hospital:** Georgetown Univ Hosp; **Address:** 3800 Resevoir Rd NW, George Univ Hosp, Dept of Med, Pas-querilla Bldg, Ste 3004G, Washington, DC 20007; **Phone:** 202-444-6200; **Board Cert:** Internal Medicine 1978; Allergy & Immunology 1981; **Med School:** Stanford Univ 1975; **Resid:** Internal Medicine, Strong Meml Hosp 1978; **Fellow:** Allergy & Immunology, Natl Inst Allergy & Inf Dis 1980; **Fac Appt:** Assoc Prof Med, Georgetown Univ

Farber, Martin Stuart MD/PhD [Rhu] - **Hospital:** Sunnyview Hosp & Rehab Ctr, Ellis Hosp; **Address:** Sunnyview Hospital, 124 Rosa Rd, Schenectady, NY 12308-2198; **Phone:** 518-386-3644; **Board Cert:** Internal Medicine 1982; Rheumatology 1984; **Med School:** Albert Einstein Coll Med 1979; **Resid:** Internal Medicine, Boston City Hosp 1982; **Fellow:** Rheumatology, Boston Univ Sch Med 1984; **Fac Appt:** Asst Clin Prof Med, Albany Med Coll

Fields, Theodore R MD [Rhu] - **Spec Exp:** Gout; Rheumatoid Arthritis; Osteoarthritis; **Hospi-tal:** Hosp For Special Surgery (page 59), NY-Presby Hosp/Weill Cornell (page 66); **Address:** Hosp Special Surg-Faculty Practice, 535 E 70th St Fl 7 - Ste 719, New York, NY 10021-4872; **Phone:** 212-606-1286; **Board Cert:** Internal Medicine 1979; Rheumatology 1982; **Med School:** SUNY Down-state 1976; **Resid:** Internal Medicine, Nassau Co Med Ctr 1979; **Fellow:** Rheumatology, Univ Hosp 1982; **Fac Appt:** Assoc Clin Prof Med, Cornell Univ-Weill Med Coll

Ginzler, Ellen MD [Rhu] - **Spec Exp:** Lupus/SLE; **Hospital:** SUNY Downstate Med Ctr, Kings County Hosp Ctr; **Address:** SUNY Downstate, Dept Rheumatology, 450 Clarkson Ave, Box 42, Brook-lyn, NY 11203-0042; **Phone:** 718-270-1662; **Board Cert:** Internal Medicine 1972; Rheumatology 1974; **Med School:** Case West Res Univ 1969; **Resid:** Internal Medicine, Kings Co Hosp 1971; In-ternal Medicine, Bellevue Hosp 1972; **Fellow:** Rheumatology, Univ Hosp 1974; **Fac Appt:** Prof Med, SUNY Downstate

Gorevic, Peter D MD [Rhu] - **Spec Exp:** Autoimmune Disease; Amyloidosis/Joint Disease; Cryoglobulinemia; **Hospital:** Mount Sinai Med Ctr (page 64), Huntington Hosp; **Address:** Mount Sinai Medical Ctr, 1 Gustave L Levy Pl, New York, NY 10029; **Phone:** 212-241-1671; **Board Cert:** Allergy & Immunology 1977; Rheumatology 1976; Diagnostic Lab Immunology 1986; Internal Medi-cine 1973; **Med School:** NYU Sch Med 1970; **Resid:** Internal Medicine, NYU Med Ctr 1974; **Fel-low:** Rheumatology, NYU Med Ctr 1976; Allergy & Immunology, NYU Med Ctr 1977; **Fac Appt:** Prof Med, Mount Sinai Sch Med

Gourley, Mark F MD [Rhu] - **Spec Exp:** Autoimmune Disease; Lupus/SLE; **Hospital:** Natl Inst of Hlth - Clin Ctr; **Address:** Natl Inst Hlth, 10 Center Drive Bldg 10 - rm 10/6N216F, Bethesda, MD 20892-1616; **Phone:** 301-451-6269; **Board Cert:** Internal Medicine 1988; Rheumatology 2002; **Med School:** Tulane Univ 1985; **Resid:** Internal Medicine, Univ Wisconsin Hosps 1988; **Fellow:** Rheumatology, Natl Inst Hlth 1996

Hochberg, Marc C MD [Rhu] - **Spec Exp:** Osteoporosis; Osteoarthritis; Rheumatoid Arthritis; **Hospital:** Univ of MD Med Ctr, Taylor Manor Hosp; **Address:** Univ MD Sch Med, Div Rheum, 10 S Pine St, MSTF 8-34, Baltimore, MD 21201; **Phone:** 410-706-6474; **Board Cert:** Internal Medicine 1976; Rheumatology 1978; **Med School:** Johns Hopkins Univ 1973; **Resid:** Internal Medicine, Johns Hopkins Hosp 1975; **Fellow:** Rheumatology, Johns Hopkins Hosp 1977; **Fac Appt:** Prof Med, Univ MD Sch Med

Lahita, Robert G MD/PhD [Rhu] - **Spec Exp:** Lupus/SLE; Endocrinology & Joint Disorders; Immunodeficiency Disorders; **Hospital:** Newark Beth Israel Med Ctr, St Vincent Cath Med Ctrs - Manhattan; **Address:** 201 Lyons Ave, Newark, NJ 07112; **Phone:** 973-926-7472; **Board Cert:** Internal Medicine 2004; Rheumatology 2007; **Med School:** Jefferson Med Coll 1973; **Resid:** Internal Medicine, New York Hosp-Cornell 1976; **Fellow:** Rheumatology, Rockefeller Hosp 1978; **Fac Appt:** Prof Med, Mount Sinai Sch Med

Lockshin, Michael D MD [Rhu] - **Spec Exp:** Lupus/SLE in Women; Antiphospholipid Syndrome (APS); Pregnancy & Rheumatic Disease; Lupus/SLE in Pregnancy; **Hospital:** Hosp For Special Surgery (page 59), NY-Presby Hosp/Weill Cornell (page 66); **Address:** 535 E 70th St, rm 661, New York, NY 10021-4872; **Phone:** 212-606-1461; **Board Cert:** Internal Medicine 1969; Rheumatology 1972; **Med School:** Harvard Med Sch 1963; **Resid:** Internal Medicine, Bellevue Hosp 1968; **Fellow:** Rheumatology, Columbia-Presby Hosp 1970; **Fac Appt:** Prof Med, Cornell Univ-Weill Med Coll

Magid, Steven K MD [Rhu] - **Spec Exp:** Rheumatoid Arthritis; Osteoarthritis; Lyme Disease; Polymyalgia Rheumatica; **Hospital:** Hosp For Special Surgery (page 59), NY-Presby Hosp/Weill Cornell (page 66); **Address:** 535 E 70th St West Bldg Fl 7 - rm 778, New York, NY 10021; **Phone:** 212-606-1060; **Board Cert:** Internal Medicine 1979; Rheumatology 1984; **Med School:** Cornell Univ-Weill Med Coll 1976; **Resid:** Internal Medicine, New York Hosp 1979; **Fellow:** Rheumatology, Hosp For Special Surgery 1981; **Fac Appt:** Assoc Clin Prof Med, Cornell Univ-Weill Med Coll

Manzi, Susan MD [Rhu] - **Spec Exp:** Lupus/SLE; Lupus/SLE in Women; **Hospital:** UPMC Presby, Pittsburgh; **Address:** Lupus Center at Magee Womens Hosp, 300 Halket St, #5710, Pittsburgh, PA 15213; **Phone:** 412-641-7600; **Board Cert:** Internal Medicine 1988; Rheumatology 2000; **Med School:** Univ Pittsburgh 1985; **Resid:** Internal Medicine, Duke Univ Med Ctr 1988; **Fellow:** Rheumatology, Univ Pittsburgh 1991; **Fac Appt:** Assoc Prof Med, Univ Pittsburgh

Medsger Jr, Thomas A MD [Rhu] - **Spec Exp:** Scleroderma; Raynaud's Disease; Polymyositis; Dermatomyositis; **Hospital:** UPMC Presby, Pittsburgh; **Address:** Arthritis & Autoimmunity Ctr, 3601 Fifth Ave, Suite 2B Falk Med Bldg, Pittsburgh, PA 15213; **Phone:** 412-647-6700; **Board Cert:** Internal Medicine 1972; Rheumatology 1972; **Med School:** Univ Pennsylvania 1962; **Resid:** Internal Medicine, Univ Pittsburgh 1968; **Fellow:** Rheumatology, Univ Pittsburgh 1966; Rheumatology, Univ Tenn Coll Med 1969; **Fac Appt:** Prof Med, Univ Pittsburgh

Mitnick, Hal J MD [Rhu] - **Spec Exp:** Rheumatoid Arthritis; Psoriatic Arthritis; Osteoporosis; **Hospital:** NYU Langone Med Ctr (page 67); **Address:** 333 E 34th St, Ste 1C, New York, NY 10016-4977; **Phone:** 212-889-7217; **Board Cert:** Internal Medicine 1976; Rheumatology 1978; **Med School:** NYU Sch Med 1972; **Resid:** Internal Medicine, Bellevue Hosp 1976; **Fellow:** Rheumatology, NYU Med Ctr 1978; **Fac Appt:** Clin Prof Med, NYU Sch Med

Oddis, Chester V MD [Rhu] - **Spec Exp:** Polymyositis; Dermatomyositis; Connective Tissue Disorders; **Hospital:** UPMC Presby, Pittsburgh; **Address:** Univ Pittsburgh-Div Rheumatology, 3500 Terrace St, Suite 2B, Pittsburgh, PA 15261; **Phone:** 412-647-6700; **Board Cert:** Internal Medicine 1983; Rheumatology 1986; **Med School:** Penn State Univ-Hershey Med Ctr 1980; **Resid:** Internal Medicine, Hershey Med Ctr 1984; **Fellow:** Rheumatology, Univ Pittsburgh 1986; **Fac Appt:** Prof Med, Univ Pittsburgh

Rheumatology

Paget, Stephen MD [Rhu] - **Spec Exp:** Rheumatoid Arthritis; Lupus/SLE; **Hospital:** Hosp For Special Surgery (page 59); **Address:** 535 E 70th St, rm 721 West, New York, NY 10021; **Phone:** 212-606-1845; **Board Cert:** Internal Medicine 1974; Rheumatology 1976; **Med School:** SUNY Downstate 1971; **Resid:** Internal Medicine, Johns Hopkins Hosp 1973; **Fellow:** Rheumatology, Hosp Special Surg 1975; **Fac Appt:** Clin Prof Med, Cornell Univ-Weill Med Coll

Petri, Michelle A MD [Rhu] - **Spec Exp:** Lupus/SLE; Antiphospholipid Syndrome (APS); **Hospital:** Johns Hopkins Hosp (page 61); **Address:** Lupus Ctr, Div Rheumatology, 1830 E Monument St, Ste 7500, Baltimore, MD 21205-2100; **Phone:** 410-955-9114; **Board Cert:** Internal Medicine 1983; Allergy & Immunology 1985; Rheumatology 1986; **Med School:** Harvard Med Sch 1980; **Resid:** Internal Medicine, Mass Genl Hosp 1983; **Fellow:** Allergy & Immunology, UCSF Med Ctr 1985; Rheumatology, UCSF Med Ctr 1986; **Fac Appt:** Prof Med, Johns Hopkins Univ

Plotz, Paul MD [Rhu] - **Hospital:** Natl Inst of Hlth - Clin Ctr; **Address:** Bldg 50 - rm 1503, 50 South Drive, MC 8023, Bethesda, MD 20892-1820; **Phone:** 301-496-9904; **Board Cert:** Internal Medicine 1970; **Med School:** Harvard Med Sch 1963; **Resid:** Internal Medicine, Beth Israel Hosp 1965; **Fellow:** Rheumatology, Clin Ctr- NIH 1968

Rosen, Antony MD [Rhu] - **Spec Exp:** Arthritis; Vasculitis; Musculoskeletal Disorders; **Hospital:** Johns Hopkins Hosp (page 61); **Address:** Johns Hopkins School of Medicine, Mason Lord Bldg, Center Toweer, 5200 Eastern Ave, rm 412, Baltimore, MD 21224; **Phone:** 410-550-1894; **Board Cert:** Internal Medicine 2003; Rheumatology 1996; **Med School:** South Africa 1984; **Resid:** Internal Medicine, Johns Hopkins Hosp 1992; **Fellow:** Rheumatology, Johns Hopkins Hosp 1994; Immunological Biology, Rockefeller Inst 1990; **Fac Appt:** Prof Med, Johns Hopkins Univ

Rothenberg, Russell R MD [Rhu] - **Spec Exp:** Fibromyalgia; Lupus/SLE; Rheumatoid Arthritis; **Hospital:** G Washington Univ Hosp; **Address:** 10215 Fernwood Rd, Ste 401, Bethesda, MD 20817; **Phone:** 301-571-2273; **Board Cert:** Internal Medicine 1980; Rheumatology 1982; **Med School:** Albany Med Coll 1977; **Resid:** Internal Medicine, LIJ Med Ctr 1980; **Fellow:** Rheumatology, Mt Sinai Med Ctr 1982; **Fac Appt:** Assoc Prof Med, Geo Wash Univ

Solomon, Gary MD [Rhu] - **Spec Exp:** Psoriatic Arthritis; Rheumatoid Arthritis; Autoimmune Disease; **Hospital:** Hosp For Joint Diseases (page 67), NYU Langone Med Ctr (page 67); **Address:** Hosp Joint Diseases, Dept Rheumatology, 305 2nd Ave, Ste 16, New York, NY 10003-2747; **Phone:** 212-598-6516; **Board Cert:** Internal Medicine 1980; Rheumatology 1982; **Med School:** Mount Sinai Sch Med 1977; **Resid:** Internal Medicine, Mt Sinai Med Ctr 1980; **Fellow:** Rheumatology, Montefiore Med Ctr 1982; **Fac Appt:** Assoc Clin Prof Med, NYU Sch Med

Spiera, Harry MD [Rhu] - **Spec Exp:** Lupus/SLE; Scleroderma; Vasculitis; **Hospital:** Mount Sinai Med Ctr (page 64), NY-Presby Hosp/Weill Cornell (page 66); **Address:** 1088 Park Ave, New York, NY 10128-1132; **Phone:** 212-860-4000 x36; **Board Cert:** Internal Medicine 1965; Rheumatology 1972; **Med School:** NYU Sch Med 1958; **Resid:** Internal Medicine, VA Med Ctr 1960; Internal Medicine, Mt Sinai Hosp 1961; **Fellow:** Rheumatology, Columbia-Presby Med Ctr 1963; **Fac Appt:** Clin Prof Med, Mount Sinai Sch Med

Starz, Terence W MD [Rhu] - **Spec Exp:** Arthritis; **Hospital:** UPMC St Margaret; **Address:** Arthritis & Int Medicine Assocs-UPMC, 3500 Fifth Ave Hieber Bldg Fl 4, Pittsburgh, PA 15213; **Phone:** 412-682-2434; **Board Cert:** Internal Medicine 1975; Rheumatology 1978; **Med School:** Jefferson Med Coll 1971; **Resid:** Internal Medicine, Presby-Univ Hosp 1975; **Fellow:** Rheumatology, Presby-Univ Hosp 1977; **Fac Appt:** Clin Prof Med, Univ Pittsburgh

Steen, Virginia MD [Rhu] - **Spec Exp:** Scleroderma; Lupus/SLE; Polymyositis; **Hospital:** Georgetown Univ Hosp; **Address:** 3800 Reservoir Rd, 3004 PHC Bldg, Washington, DC 20007; **Phone:** 202-687-8233; **Board Cert:** Internal Medicine 1978; Rheumatology 1980; **Med School:** Univ Pittsburgh 1975; **Resid:** Internal Medicine, Hosp Univ Penn 1978; **Fellow:** Rheumatology, Presby Hosp 1980; **Fac Appt:** Prof Med, Georgetown Univ

Vivino, Frederick B MD [Rhu] - **Spec Exp:** Sjogren's Syndrome; **Hospital:** Penn Presby Med Ctr - UPHS (page 60); **Address:** Presbyterian Medical Ctr, 39th & Filberts Sts, PHI-2B, Philadelphia, PA 19104; **Phone:** 215-662-4333; **Board Cert:** Internal Medicine 1986; Rheumatology 1988; **Med School:** Temple Univ 1983; **Resid:** Internal Medicine, Hosp U Penn 1986; **Fellow:** Rheumatology, Hosp U Penn 1989; **Fac Appt:** Asst Clin Prof Med, Univ Pennsylvania

Weinstein, Arthur MD [Rhu] - **Spec Exp:** Lyme Disease; Lupus/SLE; **Hospital:** Washington Hosp Ctr, Georgetown Univ Hosp; **Address:** Washington Hosp Ctr, Div Rheumatology, 110 Irving St NW, rm 2A-66, Washington, DC 20010; **Phone:** 202-877-0333; **Board Cert:** Rheumatology 1976; Diagnostic Lab Immunology 1986; **Med School:** Univ Toronto 1967; **Resid:** Internal Medicine, Toronto Wellesley Hosp 1972; Rheumatology, Hammersmith Hosp 1971; **Fellow:** Rheumatology, Toronto Wellesley Hosp 1973; **Fac Appt:** Prof Med, Georgetown Univ

Wigley, Frederick M MD [Rhu] - **Spec Exp:** Scleroderma; Raynaud's Disease; **Hospital:** Johns Hopkins Bayview Med Ctr (page 61), Johns Hopkins Hosp (page 61); **Address:** 5501 Hopkins Bayview Cir, Ste 1B32, Baltimore, MD 21224; **Phone:** 410-550-7715; **Board Cert:** Internal Medicine 1975; Rheumatology 1980; **Med School:** Univ Fla Coll Med 1972; **Resid:** Internal Medicine, Johns Hopkins Hosp 1975; **Fellow:** Rheumatology, Johns Hopkins Hosp 1979; **Fac Appt:** Prof Med, Johns Hopkins Univ

Southeast

Allen, Nancy B MD [Rhu] - **Spec Exp:** Vasculitis; Wegener's Granulomatosis; Lupus/SLE; **Hospital:** Duke Univ Med Ctr; **Address:** Duke Univ Med Ctr, Box 3440, Durham, NC 27710; **Phone:** 919-668-7630; **Board Cert:** Internal Medicine 1981; Rheumatology 1984; **Med School:** Tufts Univ 1978; **Resid:** Internal Medicine, Duke Univ Med Ctr 1981; **Fellow:** Rheumatology, Duke Univ Med Ctr 1983; **Fac Appt:** Prof Med, Duke Univ

Chatham, Walter W MD [Rhu] - **Spec Exp:** Lupus/SLE; Connective Tissue Disorders; Rheumatoid Arthritis; **Hospital:** Univ of Ala Hosp at Birmingham; **Address:** UAB Med Ctr FOT Bldg - Ste 802, 1530 3rd Ave S, Birmingham, AL 35294-3408; **Phone:** 205-934-4212; **Board Cert:** Internal Medicine 1983; Rheumatology 1988; **Med School:** Vanderbilt Univ 1980; **Resid:** Internal Medicine, North Carolina Meml Hosp 1983; **Fellow:** Rheumatology, Univ Alabama Birmingham 1988; **Fac Appt:** Assoc Prof Med, Univ Alabama

Crofford, Leslie J MD [Rhu] - **Spec Exp:** Fibromyalgia; Rheumatoid Arthritis; Lupus/SLE; **Hospital:** Univ of Kentucky Chandler Hosp; **Address:** 740 S Limestone St, rm J509, Lexington, KY 40536-0284; **Phone:** 859-323-4939; **Board Cert:** Internal Medicine 1987; Rheumatology 2003; **Med School:** Univ Tenn Coll Med, Memphis 1984; **Resid:** Internal Medicine, Barnes/Wash Univ 1987; **Fellow:** Rheumatology, Natl Inst Hlth Clin Ctr 1992; **Fac Appt:** Prof Med, Univ KY Coll Med

Hadler, Nortin MD [Rhu] - **Spec Exp:** Occupational Musculoskeletal Disorders; Musculoskeletal Disorders; Spondylitis-Back Pain; **Hospital:** Univ NC Hosps; **Address:** Univ North Carolina, Dept Medicine, 3300 Thurston Building, Box 7280, Chapel Hill, NC 27599-7280; **Phone:** 919-966-0566; **Board Cert:** Rheumatology 1974; Allergy & Immunology 1975; Internal Medicine 1987; **Med School:** Harvard Med Sch 1968; **Resid:** Internal Medicine, Mass Genl Hosp 1973; **Fellow:** Rheumatology, Natl Inst Hlth 1972; Allergy & Immunology, Clin Res Ctr 1974; **Fac Appt:** Prof Med, Univ NC Sch Med

Rheumatology

Kimberly, Robert P MD [Rhu] - **Spec Exp:** Immunodeficiency Disorders; Lupus/SLE; Vasculitis; **Hospital:** Univ of Ala Hosp at Birmingham; **Address:** Univ of Alabama Hospital, 1825 University Blvd, SHEL 172B, Birmingham, AL 35294; **Phone:** 205-934-0245; **Board Cert:** Internal Medicine 1976; Rheumatology 1978; **Med School:** Harvard Med Sch 1973; **Resid:** Internal Medicine, Hosp U Penn 1975; **Fellow:** Rheumatology, NIH 1977; Rheumatology, NY Hosp=Cornell Med Ctr 1979; **Fac Appt:** Prof Med, Univ Alabama

Moore, Walter J MD [Rhu] - **Spec Exp:** Rheumatoid Arthritis; Lupus/SLE; **Hospital:** Med Coll of GA Hosp and Clin (MCG Health Inc); **Address:** Medical College of Georgia, 1120 15th St, rm BI 5083, Augusta, GA 30912; **Phone:** 706-721-2981; **Board Cert:** Internal Medicine 1980; Rheumatology 1984; **Med School:** Georgetown Univ 1977; **Resid:** Internal Medicine, Walter Reed AMC 1980; **Fellow:** Rheumatology, Walter Reed AMC 1983; **Fac Appt:** Assoc Prof Med, Med Coll GA

Sergent, John S MD [Rhu] - **Spec Exp:** Vasculitis; **Hospital:** Vanderbilt Univ Med Ctr; **Address:** Vanderbilt Univ Med Ctr - Dept Medicine, 1301 Medical Ctr Drive, Ste 250, Nashville, TN 37232-2358; **Phone:** 615-322-1900; **Board Cert:** Internal Medicine 1972; Rheumatology 1974; **Med School:** Vanderbilt Univ 1966; **Resid:** Internal Medicine, Johns Hopkins Hosp 1968; Internal Medicine, Vanderbilt Univ Hosp 1972; **Fellow:** Rheumatology, Hosp Special Surgery 1974; **Fac Appt:** Prof Med, Vanderbilt Univ

Silver, Richard M MD [Rhu] - **Spec Exp:** Scleroderma & Lung Disease; Pediatric Rheumatology; Connective Tissue Disorders; **Hospital:** MUSC Med Ctr; **Address:** MUSC Med Ctr, PO Box 250623, 96 Jonathan Lucas St, Ste 912, Charleston, SC 29425; **Phone:** 843-876-0500; **Board Cert:** Internal Medicine 1978; Rheumatology 1982; **Med School:** Vanderbilt Univ 1975; **Resid:** Internal Medicine, Univ NC Hosps 1978; **Fellow:** Rheumatology, UCSD Med Ctr 1981; **Fac Appt:** Prof Med, Med Univ SC

Sundy, John S MD/PhD [Rhu] - **Spec Exp:** Rheumatoid Arthritis; Gout; Lupus/SLE; Allergic Rhinitis; **Hospital:** Duke Univ Med Ctr, Durham Regional Hosp; **Address:** 4309 Med Park Drive, Ste 100, Duke Univ Med Ctr Box 3278, Durham, NC 27710; **Phone:** 919-668-2169; **Board Cert:** Rheumatology 1998; Allergy & Immunology 1999; Internal Medicine 2006; **Med School:** Hahnemann Univ 1991; **Resid:** Internal Medicine, Duke Univ Med Ctr 1993; **Fellow:** Rheumatology, Duke Univ Med Ctr 1996; Allergy & Immunology, Duke Univ Med Ctr 1998; **Fac Appt:** Asst Prof Med, Duke Univ

Wise, Christopher M MD [Rhu] - **Spec Exp:** Gout; Sjogren's Syndrome; Rheumatoid Arthritis; **Hospital:** Med Coll of VA Hosp; **Address:** Virginia Commonwealth Univ/MCV Campus, Box 980647, Richmond, VA 23298; **Phone:** 804-828-9341; **Board Cert:** Internal Medicine 1980; Rheumatology 1982; **Med School:** Univ NC Sch Med 1977; **Resid:** Internal Medicine, Med Coll Virginia Hosp 1980; **Fellow:** Rheumatology, Med Coll Virginia Hosp 1982; **Fac Appt:** Prof Med, Va Commonwealth Univ Sch Med

Midwest

Adams, Elaine MD [Rhu] - **Spec Exp:** Rheumatoid Arthritis; Lupus/SLE; Spondyloarthropathies; **Hospital:** Loyola Univ Med Ctr, Hines VA Hosp; **Address:** Loyola Univ Med Ctr, Dept Rheumatology, 2160 S 1st Ave, Bldg 54 - rm 121, Maywood, IL 60153-5590; **Phone:** 708-216-8563; **Board Cert:** Internal Medicine 1981; Rheumatology 1984; **Med School:** Loyola Univ-Stritch Sch Med 1978; **Resid:** Internal Medicine, Loyola Univ Med Ctr 1981; **Fellow:** Rheumatology, Univ Wisconsin Med Ctr 1983; **Fac Appt:** Prof Med, Loyola Univ-Stritch Sch Med

Brasington, Richard MD [Rhu] - **Hospital:** Barnes-Jewish Hosp; **Address:** 4921 Parkview Pl Fl 5 - Ste C, CB 8124, St Louis, MO 63110; **Phone:** 314-286-2635; **Board Cert:** Internal Medicine 1985; Rheumatology 1986; **Med School:** Duke Univ 1980; **Resid:** Internal Medicine, Univ Iowa Med Ctr 1982; Internal Medicine, Univ Iowa Med Ctr 1985; **Fellow:** Rheumatology, Univ Iowa 1986; **Fac Appt:** Assoc Prof Med, Washington Univ, St Louis

Chang, Rowland W MD [Rhu] - **Spec Exp:** Rheumatoid Arthritis; Arthritis; Ankylosing Spondylitis; **Hospital:** Rehab Inst of Chicago, Northwestern Meml Hosp; **Address:** Rehab Inst of Chicago Arthritis Ctr, 345 E Superior St Fl 9, Chicago, IL 60611-2654; **Phone:** 312-238-2784; **Board Cert:** Internal Medicine 1979; Rheumatology 1982; **Med School:** Tufts Univ 1976; **Resid:** Internal Medicine, Mt Auburn Hosp 1979; **Fellow:** Rheumatology, Hammersmith Hosp 1980; Rheumatology, Brigham & Womens Hosp 1982; **Fac Appt:** Prof Med, Northwestern Univ

Curran, James J MD [Rhu] - **Spec Exp:** Rheumatoid Arthritis; Lupus/SLE; Sjogren's Syndrome; Polymyositis; **Hospital:** Univ of Chicago Med Ctr; **Address:** 5841 S Maryland Ave, MC-0930, Chicago, IL 60637-1463; **Phone:** 773-702-1232; **Board Cert:** Internal Medicine 1980; Rheumatology 1982; **Med School:** Univ IL Coll Med 1976; **Resid:** Internal Medicine, Bethesda Naval Hosp 1980; **Fellow:** Rheumatology, Univ Chicago Hosps 1982; **Fac Appt:** Prof Med, Univ Chicago-Pritzker Sch Med

Fischbein, Lewis C MD [Rhu] - **Spec Exp:** Rheumatoid Arthritis; Lupus/SLE; Hypertension; Preventive Medicine; **Hospital:** Barnes-Jewish Hosp; **Address:** 4921 Parkview Pl, Ste 5G, St Louis, MO 63110; **Phone:** 314-747-1970; **Board Cert:** Internal Medicine 1977; Rheumatology 1980; **Med School:** Washington Univ, St Louis 1974; **Resid:** Internal Medicine, Barnes Jewish Hosp 1977; **Fellow:** Rheumatology, Barnes Jewish Hosp 1979; **Fac Appt:** Assoc Prof Med, Washington Univ, St Louis

Katz, Robert S MD [Rhu] - **Spec Exp:** Rheumatoid Arthritis; Lupus/SLE; Fibromyalgia; **Hospital:** Rush Univ Med Ctr, Northwestern Meml Hosp; **Address:** 1725 W Harrison St, Ste 1039, Chicago, IL 60612-3841; **Phone:** 312-942-2159; **Board Cert:** Internal Medicine 1975; Rheumatology 1976; **Med School:** Univ MD Sch Med 1970; **Resid:** Internal Medicine, Washington Univ Med Ctr 1972; **Fellow:** Rheumatology, Johns Hopkins Hosp 1976; **Fac Appt:** Assoc Prof Med, Rush Med Coll

Langford, Carol MD [Rhu] - **Spec Exp:** Vasculitis; **Hospital:** Cleveland Clin Fdn (page 56); **Address:** Cleveland Clinic, 9500 Euclid Ave, Ste A50, Cleveland, OH 44195; **Phone:** 216-445-6056; **Board Cert:** Internal Medicine 2000; Rheumatology 2000; **Med School:** UCLA 1987; **Resid:** Internal Medicine, Univ Mich 1990; **Fellow:** Rheumatology, Duke Univ Med Ctr 1991

Lawry, George V MD [Rhu] - **Hospital:** Univ Iowa Hosp & Clinics; **Address:** Univ Iowa Hosp & Clins, Dept Rheumatology, 200 Hawkins Drive, rm C31-GGH, Iowa City, IA 52242-1009; **Phone:** 319-356-1777; **Board Cert:** Internal Medicine 1978; Rheumatology 1982; **Med School:** Johns Hopkins Univ 1975; **Resid:** Internal Medicine, Mass Genl Hosp 1977; Internal Medicine, Stanford Hosp 1978; **Fellow:** Rheumatology, Wadsworth VA-UCLA Med Ctr 1981; **Fac Appt:** Clin Prof Med, Univ Iowa Coll Med

Luggen, Michael MD [Rhu] - **Hospital:** Univ Hosp - Cincinnati, Christ Hospital; **Address:** Christ Hosp Office Bldg, 2123 Auburn Ave, Ste 630, Cincinnati, OH 45219; **Phone:** 513-585-1970; **Board Cert:** Internal Medicine 1978; Rheumatology 1982; **Med School:** Columbia P&S 1974; **Resid:** Internal Medicine, Cinn Genl Hosp 1977; **Fellow:** Rheumatology, Univ Cincinnati 1982; **Fac Appt:** Prof Med, Univ Cincinnati

Rheumatology

Luthra, Harvinder Singh MD [Rhu] - **Spec Exp:** Rheumatoid Arthritis; Ankylosing Spondylitis; Relapsing Polychondritis; **Hospital:** St Mary's Hosp - Rochester, Rochester Methodist Hosp; **Address:** Mayo Clinic, 200 First St SW, Rochester, MN 55905-0002; **Phone:** 507-266-4439; **Board Cert:** Internal Medicine 1973; Rheumatology 2002; **Med School:** India 1967; **Resid:** Ophthalmology, Christian Med Coll; Internal Medicine, Mount Sinai Hosp 1972; **Fellow:** Rheumatology, Mayo Grad School Affil Hosp 1974; **Fac Appt:** Prof Med, Mayo Med Sch

McCune, W Joseph MD [Rhu] - **Spec Exp:** Lupus/SLE; Rheumatoid Arthritis; **Hospital:** Univ Michigan Hlth Sys; **Address:** Univ Mich, Dept Rheum, 1500 E Med Ctr, rm 3918 Taubman Ctr, Ann Arbor, MI 48109-0358; **Phone:** 734-647-5900; **Board Cert:** Internal Medicine 1978; Rheumatology 1982; **Med School:** Univ Cincinnati 1975; **Resid:** Internal Medicine, Univ Mich Hosps 1978; **Fellow:** Rheumatology, Brigham Womens Hosp 1981; **Fac Appt:** Prof Med, Univ Mich Med Sch

Michalska, Margaret MD [Rhu] - **Spec Exp:** Rheumatoid Arthritis; Connective Tissue Disorders; Osteoporosis; **Hospital:** Adv Illinois Masonic Med Ctr; **Address:** 3000 N Halsted St, MOC Bldg - Ste 409, Chicago, IL 60657; **Phone:** 773-296-7150; **Board Cert:** Internal Medicine 1988; Rheumatology 2000; **Med School:** Poland 1979; **Resid:** Internal Medicine, Hines VA Hosp 1988; **Fellow:** Biochemistry, Nortwestern Univ 1985; Rheumatology, Rush-Presby-St Lukes Med Ctr 1990; **Fac Appt:** Assoc Prof Med, Rush Med Coll

Moder, Kevin G MD [Rhu] - **Spec Exp:** Rheumatoid Arthritis; Lupus/SLE; **Hospital:** Mayo Med Ctr & Clin - Rochester; **Address:** Mayo Clin, Div Rheumatology, 200 First St SW, Rochester, MN 55905-0002; **Phone:** 507-284-4550; **Board Cert:** Internal Medicine 2000; Rheumatology 2000; **Med School:** Univ MO-Columbia Sch Med 1987; **Resid:** Internal Medicine, Mayo Clinic 1990; **Fellow:** Rheumatology, Mayo Clinic 1993; **Fac Appt:** Asst Prof Med, Mayo Med Sch

Pope, Richard M MD [Rhu] - **Spec Exp:** Rheumatoid Arthritis; Sjogren's Syndrome; Psoriatic Arthritis; **Hospital:** Northwestern Meml Hosp; **Address:** 675 N St Clair, Ste 14-100, Chicago, IL 60611-5966; **Phone:** 312-695-8628; **Board Cert:** Internal Medicine 1973; Rheumatology 1976; Clinical & Laboratory Immunology 1986; **Med School:** Loyola Univ-Stritch Sch Med 1970; **Resid:** Internal Medicine, Michael Reese Hosp 1972; **Fellow:** Rheumatology, Univ Wash Med Ctr 1974; **Fac Appt:** Prof Med, Northwestern Univ

Warner, Ann E MD [Rhu] - **Hospital:** St Luke's Hosp of Kansas City; **Address:** 4330 Wornall St, Ste 40, Kansas City, MO 64111-3210; **Phone:** 816-531-0930; **Board Cert:** Internal Medicine 1986; Rheumatology 1988; Allergy & Immunology 1999; **Med School:** Univ Kans 1983; **Resid:** Internal Medicine, St Luke's Hosp 1986; **Fellow:** Rheumatology, Univ Kansas Med Ctr 1989; **Fac Appt:** Asst Clin Prof Med, Univ MO-Kansas City

Great Plains and Mountains

Arend, William P MD [Rhu] - **Spec Exp:** Arthritis; Rheumatoid Arthritis; **Hospital:** Univ Colorado Hosp; **Address:** 1775 N Ursula St, Box 6511, MC b115, Univ of Colo, Dept of Rheumatology, Aurora, CO 80045; **Phone:** 720-848-1940; **Board Cert:** Internal Medicine 1971; Rheumatology 1980; **Med School:** Columbia P&S 1964; **Resid:** Internal Medicine, Univ Washington Hosp 1969; **Fellow:** Rheumatology, Univ Washington Hosp 1971; **Fac Appt:** Prof Med, Univ Colorado

O'Dell, James R MD [Rhu] - **Spec Exp:** Osteoarthritis; Rheumatoid Arthritis; **Hospital:** Nebraska Med Ctr; **Address:** 983025 Nebraska Med Ctr, Omaha, NE 68198-3025; **Phone:** 402-559-4015; **Board Cert:** Internal Medicine 1980; Rheumatology 1984; **Med School:** Univ Nebr Coll Med 1977; **Resid:** Internal Medicine, Univ Nebraska Med Ctr 1981; **Fellow:** Rheumatology, Univ Colorado 1984; **Fac Appt:** Prof Med, Univ Nebr Coll Med

West, Sterling MD [Rhu] - **Spec Exp:** Lupus/SLE; Vasculitis; Osteoporosis; **Hospital:** Univ Colorado Hosp; **Address:** Barbara Davis Ctr, 1775 N Ursula St, Box B115, 1635 aurora court, Aurora, CO 80045; **Phone:** 720-848-1940; **Board Cert:** Internal Medicine 1979; Rheumatology 2005; **Med School:** Emory Univ 1976; **Resid:** Internal Medicine, Fitzsimons Army Med Ctr 1979; **Fellow:** Rheumatology, Walter Reed Army Med Ctr 1981; **Fac Appt:** Prof Med, Univ Colorado

Southwest

Arnett Jr, Frank C MD [Rhu] - **Spec Exp:** Reiter's Syndrome; Spondylitis; Scleroderma; **Hospital:** Meml Hermann Hosp - Texas Med Ctr; **Address:** Hermann Prof Bldg, 6410 Fannin St, Ste 600, Houston, TX 77030-5302; **Phone:** 832-325-7191; **Board Cert:** Internal Medicine 1972; Rheumatology 1976; Clinical & Laboratory Immunology 1990; **Med School:** Univ Cincinnati 1968; **Resid:** Internal Medicine, Johns Hopkins Hosp 1970; **Fellow:** Rheumatology, Johns Hopkins Hosp 1972; **Fac Appt:** Prof Med, Univ Tex, Houston

Chang-Miller, April MD [Rhu] - **Spec Exp:** Connective Tissue Disorders; Spondyloarthropathies; **Hospital:** Mayo Clinic - Scottsdale; **Address:** Mayo Clinic, Div Rheumatology, 13400 E Shea Blvd, Scottsdale, AZ 85259; **Phone:** 480-301-4342; **Board Cert:** Internal Medicine 1986; Rheumatology 2000; **Med School:** Yale Univ 1983; **Resid:** Internal Medicine, Mayo Clinic 1985; **Fellow:** Rheumatology, Mayo Clinic 1989; Biochemical and Molecular Biology, Mayo Clinic 1990; **Fac Appt:** Asst Prof Med, Mayo Med Sch

Davis, William Eugene MD [Rhu] - **Spec Exp:** Lupus/SLE; Rheumatoid Arthritis; Gout; **Hospital:** Ochsner Fdn Hosp; **Address:** Ochsner Clinic, Rheum, 1514 Jefferson Hwy, CA5, New Orleans, LA 70121-2483; **Phone:** 504-842-3920; **Board Cert:** Internal Medicine 1987; Rheumatology 1988; **Med School:** Louisiana State U, New Orleans 1983; **Resid:** Internal Medicine, Ochsner Fdn Hosp 1986; **Fellow:** Rheumatology, Univ Michigan 1988

Lindsey, Stephen M MD [Rhu] - **Spec Exp:** Osteoporosis; Lupus/SLE; **Hospital:** Ochsner Baptist Med Ctr; **Address:** 9001 Summa Ave, Baton Rouge, LA 70809; **Phone:** 225-761-5481; **Board Cert:** Internal Medicine 1975; Rheumatology 1980; **Med School:** Louisiana State U, New Orleans 1972; **Resid:** Internal Medicine, Letterman AMC 1975; **Fellow:** Rheumatology, Walter Reed AMC 1979

Lipstate, James M MD [Rhu] - **Spec Exp:** Arthritis; Osteoporosis; **Hospital:** Our Lady of Lourdes Reg Med Ctr - Lafayette, Lafayette Genl Med Ctr; **Address:** 401 Audubon Blvd, Ste 102B, Lafayette, LA 70503; **Phone:** 337-237-7801; **Board Cert:** Internal Medicine 1983; Rheumatology 1986; **Med School:** Tulane Univ 1980; **Resid:** Internal Medicine, Univ Alabama Hosp 1983; **Fellow:** Rheumatology, Univ Alabama Hosp 1986; **Fac Appt:** Asst Clin Prof Med, Louisiana State U, New Orleans

Mayes, Maureen D MD [Rhu] - **Spec Exp:** Scleroderma; **Hospital:** Meml Hermann Hosp - Texas Med Ctr, LBJ General Hosp; **Address:** Univ Tex Hlth Sci Ctr, Div Rheum, 6410 Fannin St, Ste 600, Houston, TX 77030-1501; **Phone:** 832-325-7191; **Board Cert:** Internal Medicine 1980; Rheumatology 1982; **Med School:** Eastern VA Med Sch 1976; **Resid:** Internal Medicine, Cleveland Clinic Fnd 1979; **Fellow:** Rheumatology, Cleveland Clinic Fnd 1981; **Fac Appt:** Prof Med, Univ Tex, Houston

Sessoms, Sandra Lee MD [Rhu] - **Spec Exp:** Arthritis; Lupus/SLE; Autoimmune Disease; **Hospital:** Methodist Hosp - Houston, St Luke's Episcopal Hosp-Houston; **Address:** Meth Hosp, Div Rheum, 6550 Fannin St, Smith Twr, Ste 2500, Houston, TX 77030; **Phone:** 713-441-9000; **Board Cert:** Internal Medicine 1981; Rheumatology 1984; **Med School:** Baylor Coll Med 1978; **Resid:** Internal Medicine, Baylor Coll Med 1979; **Fellow:** Rheumatology, Baylor Coll Med 1983; **Fac Appt:** Assoc Prof Med, Baylor Coll Med

Rheumatology

West Coast and Pacific

Bobrove, Arthur M MD [Rhu] - **Spec Exp:** Psoriatic Arthritis; Ankylosing Spondylitis; Sjogren's Syndrome; **Hospital:** Stanford Univ Med Ctr; **Address:** 795 El Camino Real, Palo Alto, CA 94301-2302; **Phone:** 650-853-2972; **Board Cert:** Internal Medicine 1972; Rheumatology 1976; **Med School:** Temple Univ 1967; **Resid:** Internal Medicine, Univ Mich Hosp 1969; Internal Medicine, Univ Mich Hosp 1972; **Fellow:** Immunology, Stanford Univ Hosp 1974; **Fac Appt:** Clin Prof Med, Stanford Univ

Clements, Philip J MD [Rhu] - **Spec Exp:** Scleroderma; Raynaud's Disease; **Hospital:** UCLA Ronald Reagan Med Ctr; **Address:** UCLA Sch Med, Rehab 32-59, 1000 Veteran Ave, Los Angeles, CA 90095-1670; **Phone:** 310-825-8414; **Board Cert:** Internal Medicine 1972; Rheumatology 1974; **Med School:** Indiana Univ 1965; **Resid:** Internal Medicine, Cedars-Sinai Med Ctr 1971; **Fellow:** Rheumatology, UCLA Med Ctr 1974; **Fac Appt:** Prof Med, UCLA

Ehresmann, Glenn R MD [Rhu] - **Hospital:** USC Univ Hosp; **Address:** 1520 San Pablo St, Ste 1000, Los Angeles, CA 90033; **Phone:** 323-442-5100; **Board Cert:** Internal Medicine 1977; Rheumatology 1978; **Med School:** UC Irvine 1973; **Resid:** Internal Medicine, LAC-USC Med Ctr 1976; **Fellow:** Rheumatology, LAC-USC Med Ctr 1978; **Fac Appt:** Assoc Clin Prof Med, USC-Keck School of Medicine

Gershwin, Merrill E MD [Rhu] - **Spec Exp:** Allergy; Rheumatoid Arthritis; **Hospital:** UC Davis Med Ctr; **Address:** UC Davis Sch Med, Div Rheum, 451 E Health Sciences Drive, Ste 6510, Davis, CA 95616; **Phone:** 530-752-2884; **Board Cert:** Internal Medicine 1974; Rheumatology 1976; Allergy & Immunology 1979; **Med School:** Stanford Univ 1971; **Resid:** Internal Medicine, Tufts-New Eng Med Ctr 1972; Allergy & Immunology, Tufts-New Eng Med Ctr 1973; **Fellow:** Rheumatology, Natl Inst Hlth 1975; Allergy & Immunology, Natl Inst Hlth 1977; **Fac Appt:** Prof Med, UC Davis

Mease, Philip J MD [Rhu] - **Spec Exp:** Arthritis; Autoimmune Disease; Fibromyalgia; Lupus/SLE; **Hospital:** Swedish Med Ctr - Seattle, Swedish Med Ctr Providence Campus; **Address:** 1101 Madison St, Ste 1000, Seattle, WA 98104; **Phone:** 206-386-2000; **Board Cert:** Internal Medicine 1980; Rheumatology 1982; **Med School:** Stanford Univ 1977; **Resid:** Internal Medicine, Univ Wash Med Ctr 1981; **Fellow:** Rheumatology, Univ Wash Med Ctr 1982; **Fac Appt:** Clin Prof Med, Univ Wash

Wallace, Daniel J MD [Rhu] - **Spec Exp:** Lupus/SLE; Rheumatoid Arthritis; Scleroderma; **Hospital:** Cedars-Sinai Med Ctr, UCLA Ronald Reagan Med Ctr; **Address:** 8737 Beverly Blvd, Ste 302, Los Angeles, CA 90048-1828; **Phone:** 310-652-0920; **Board Cert:** Internal Medicine 1978; Rheumatology 1982; **Med School:** USC Sch Med 1974; **Resid:** Internal Medicine, Cedars-Sinai Med Ctr 1977; **Fellow:** Rheumatology, UCLA Med Ctr 1979; **Fac Appt:** Clin Prof Med, UCLA

Wener, Mark MD [Rhu] - **Spec Exp:** Lupus/SLE; Vasculitis; Immunodeficiency Disorders; Scleroderma; **Hospital:** Univ Wash Med Ctr; **Address:** Univ Washington Med Ctr, Div Rheumatology, 1959 NE Pacific St, Box 356166, Seattle, WA 98195; **Phone:** 206-598-4615; **Board Cert:** Internal Medicine 1978; Rheumatology 1980; Clinical & Laboratory Immunology 1986; **Med School:** Washington Univ, St Louis 1974; **Resid:** Internal Medicine, Univ Iowa Hosps 1978; **Fellow:** Rheumatology, Univ Iowa Hosp 1980; Immunology, Univ Wash 1981; **Fac Appt:** Prof Med, Univ Wash

Wofsy, David MD [Rhu] - **Spec Exp:** Lupus/SLE; **Hospital:** VA Med Ctr - San Francisco, UCSF Med Ctr; **Address:** 533 Parnassus Ave, Box 0633, San Francisco, CA 94143; **Phone:** 415-750-2104; **Board Cert:** Internal Medicine 1977; Rheumatology 1980; **Med School:** UCSD 1974; **Resid:** Internal Medicine, UCSF Hosps 1977; **Fellow:** Rheumatology, UCSF 1979; **Fac Appt:** Prof Med, UCSF

Cleveland Clinic

Rheumatic and Immunologic Diseases

Cleveland Clinic's Department of Rheumatic and Immunologic Diseases has a long-standing commitment to excellence and innovation in the research and care of patients with illnesses such as arthritis, osteoporosis and vasculitis. For the past several years, *U.S.News & World Report* has consistently ranked it among the nation's top five rheumatology programs.

Arthritis

Arthritis is a general term for more than 100 diseases involving inflammation in the joints, characterized by redness, warmth, swelling and pain. Some of the conditions most commonly treated at the Department of Rheumatic and Immunologic Diseases include rheumatoid arthritis and osteoarthritis.

Osteoporosis

Cleveland Clinic's Center for Osteoporosis and Metabolic Bone Diseases is devoted to the evaluation and treatment of patients with osteoporosis and other diseases that affect bones. The Center's goal is to evaluate patients at an early stage to prevent the complications and additional disease manifestations of osteoporosis.

Vasculitis

Cleveland Clinic's Center for Vasculitis Care and Research aims to ensure the best possible care for patients with vasculitis, discover the causes of these diseases and identify improved therapies. The department faculty has special expertise in vasculitis and has established extensive collaborations with other Cleveland Clinic departments to bring complementary skills to both service and research.

Autoimmune Disease

The Department of Rheumatic and Immunologic Diseases also provides expert care for a variety of illnesses for which arthritis may not be a major feature. These include conditions for which the body's immune defense system, in part, turns on itself and damages a person's own body. Examples of such "autoimmune" disorders include systemic lupus, scleroderma, myositis, polychondritis and vasculitis.

For more information about the Cleveland Clinic Department of Rheumatic and Immunologic Diseases, to schedule a second opinion, or to learn about assistance for out-of-town patients, call 800.890.2467 or visit www. clevelandclinic.org/arthritistopdocs.

Department of Rheumatic and Immunologic Diseases
9500 Euclid Avenue / AC311 | Cleveland OH 44195

NYU Hospital for Joint Diseases
NYU LANGONE MEDICAL CENTER

301 East 17th Street
(at Second Avenue)
New York, NY 10003
212-598-6000 FAX: 212-260-1203
www.nyuhjd.org

RHEUMATOLOGY

About the Division of Rheumatology, Department of Medicine:

The Division of Rheumatology at NYU Langone Medical Center is dedicated to the diagnosis and treatment of patients with rheumatic illnesses with a focus on autoimmune diseases. The Division has a long and illustrious track record in the study and treatment of rheumatic diseases and in the mentoring and training of leaders in the field of rheumatology. The specialty was recently recognized by *U.S. News and World Report* as among the most prestigious rheumatology programs in the country.

We specialize in the following areas:

ARTHRITIS AND AUTOIMMUNITY
Staffed by a select group of leading academic researchers and physicians, the Center for Arthritis and Autoimmunity at NYU Langone Medical Center offers a comprehensive program for the prevention, diagnosis and treatment of all rheumatologic conditions. Patients receive complete rheumatologic evaluations, orthopaedic and neurological consultative services, sophisticated diagnostic testing, physical therapy and complementary medicine.

BEHCET'S SYNDROME
In close collaboration with the American Bechet's Disease Association, the only North American Behcet's Center was established for research and the evaluation and treatment of patients with Behcet's syndrome, a disease that involves inflammation of the blood vessels.

BIOLOGICAL TREATMENT
Biological treatments for inflammatory arthritis and osteoporosis are administered within the Hospital for Joint Diseases' Infusion Center at NYU Langone Medical Center, a dedicated unit where each patient has a personalized LCD television and support of a hospital-based pharmacy.

LUPUS
The Lupus Center at NYU Langone Medical Center is devoted solely to the treatment and research of patients with this multifaceted disease. Patients are seen regularly by rheumatologists and have ready access to specialists in dermatology, nephrology, orthopaedics and neurology, all of whom have expertise in systemic lupus erythematosus, a chronic autoimmune connective tissue disease. The center also offers expertise in pregnancy and hormonal issues.

MEDICAL MILESTONES
While working in the Department of Microbiology at the NYU School of Medicine, two professors developed the monoclonal antibody that is the basis for the drug now known as Remicade®. The drug is a potent anti-inflammatory agent now used in the treatment of rheumatoid arthritis, Crohn's disease, ankylosing spondylitis, psoriatic arthritis and other inflammatory diseases.

OSTEOPOROSIS
Osteoporosis is a bone disease that leads to an increased risk of bone fractures. The Osteoporosis Center offers comprehensive care for the prevention, evaluation and treatment of osteoporosis, and includes state-of-the art bone densitometers used to measure bone density.

PSORIATIC ARTHRITIS
The Psoriatic Arthritis Center is a collaborative effort with the Department of Dermatology at NYU Langone Medical Center. Patients are seen at the department for two half-day sessions in the presence of both a rheumatologist and dermatologist with particular expertise in psoriatic arthritis.

RESEARCH
The Peter D. Seligman Center for Advanced Therapeutics focuses on developing improved treatments for rheumatic diseases and promotes new initiatives in clinical and translational investigations. Researchers conduct protocols using a wide variety of new medications for the treatment of rheumatoid arthritis,

Sports Medicine

a subspecialty of Internal Medicine, Family Practice, Pediatrics, Orthopaedics and Physical Medicine & Rehabilitation

A specialist trained to be responsible for continuous care in the field of sports medicine, not only for the enhancement of health and fitness, but also for the prevention of injury and illness. A sports medicine physician must have knowledge and experience in the promotion of wellness and the prevention of injury. Knowledge about special areas of medicine such as exercise physiology, biomechanics, nutrition, psychology, physical rehabilitation, epidemiology, physical evaluation, injuries (treatment and prevention and referral practice) and the role of exercise in promoting a healthy life style are essential to the practice of sports medicine. The sports medicine physician requires special education to provide the knowledge to improve the healthcare of the individual engaged in physical exercise (sports) whether as an individual or in team participation.

Training Required: Three years in internal medicine, family practice, or pediatrics or seven years in orthopaedics *plus* additional training and examination for certification in sports medicine.

For more information about the main specialties of these physicians, see **Internal Medicine, Family Practice, Pediatrics, Orthopaedics** section(s).

Sports Medicine

New England

Micheli, Lyle J MD [SM] - **Spec Exp:** Pediatric Sports Medicine; Dance/Ballet Injuries; **Hospital:** Children's Hospital - Boston, Beth Israel Deaconess Med Ctr - Boston; **Address:** Chldns Hosp, Div Sports Medicine, 319 Longwood Ave, Boston, MA 02115; **Phone:** 617-355-3501; **Board Cert:** Orthopaedic Surgery 1973; **Med School:** Harvard Med Sch 1966; **Resid:** Surgery, Univ Hosps 1968; Orthopaedic Surgery, Mass Genl Hosp/Chldns Hosp 1972; **Fellow:** Pediatric Orthopaedic Surgery, Orth Rsch Soc-Traveling Fell 1973; **Fac Appt:** Assoc Clin Prof OrS, Harvard Med Sch

Scheller, Arnold D MD [SM] - **Spec Exp:** Sports Injuries; Ankle Surgery; Shoulder Surgery; Knee Surgery; **Hospital:** New England Bapt Hosp; **Address:** Pro Sports Orthopaedics, 235 Cypres St, Ste 300, Brookline, MA 02445; **Phone:** 617-738-8642; **Board Cert:** Orthopaedic Surgery 1983; **Med School:** Rush Med Coll 1973; **Resid:** Orthopaedic Surgery, New England Hosp 1983; **Fac Appt:** Asst Clin Prof OrS, Tufts Univ

Schepsis, Anthony A MD [SM] - **Spec Exp:** Arthroscopic Surgery; Shoulder & Knee Surgery; Knee-Patella Problems; Cartilage Restoration; **Hospital:** Boston Med Ctr; **Address:** Boston Med Ctr, 720 Harrison Ave Ste 805, Boston, MA 02118-2334; **Phone:** 617-638-5633; **Board Cert:** Orthopaedic Surgery 1983; **Med School:** Boston Univ 1976; **Resid:** Orthopaedic Surgery, Boston University Med Ctr Hosp 1981; **Fellow:** Sports Medicine/Knee Surgery, Travelling Fellowship 1982; **Fac Appt:** Prof OrS, Boston Univ

Steiner, Mark E MD [SM] - **Spec Exp:** Shoulder Injuries; Knee Injuries; Arthroscopic Surgery; **Hospital:** New England Bapt Hosp; **Address:** 830 Boylston St, Ste 205, Chestnut Hill, MA 02467; **Phone:** 617-739-2003; **Board Cert:** Orthopaedic Surgery 2008; **Med School:** Columbia P&S 1978; **Resid:** Surgery, Mass General Hosp 1980; Orthopaedic Surgery, Mass General Hosp 1984; **Fellow:** Sports Medicine, U Oklahoma Med Ctr 1985

Mid Atlantic

Altchek, David MD [SM] - **Spec Exp:** Shoulder Surgery; Elbow Surgery; Knee Surgery; Arthroscopic Surgery; **Hospital:** Hosp For Special Surgery (page 59), NY-Presby Hosp/Weill Cornell (page 66); **Address:** Hospital for Special Surgery, 535 E 70th St, New York, NY 10021; **Phone:** 212-606-1909; **Board Cert:** Orthopaedic Surgery 2001; **Med School:** Cornell Univ-Weill Med Coll 1982; **Resid:** Orthopaedic Surgery, Hosp for Special Surg 1987; **Fellow:** Sports Medicine, Hosp for Special Surg 1988; **Fac Appt:** Assoc Prof OrS, Cornell Univ-Weill Med Coll

Bradley, James P MD [SM] - **Spec Exp:** Reconstructive Surgery; Shoulder Surgery; Knee Surgery; **Hospital:** UPMC St Margaret, UPMC Shadyside; **Address:** 200 Delafield Ave, Ste 4010, Pittsburgh, PA 15215; **Phone:** 412-784-5783; **Board Cert:** Orthopaedic Surgery 2001; **Med School:** Georgetown Univ 1982; **Resid:** Surgery, Univ Tennessee Affil Hosp 1984; Orthopaedic Surgery, Univ Hlth Ctr 1987; **Fellow:** Sports Medicine, Kerlan-Jobe Ortho Clinic 1988; **Fac Appt:** Assoc Prof OrS, Univ Pittsburgh

Burke, Charles J MD [SM] - **Spec Exp:** Knee Injuries; Shoulder Injuries; **Hospital:** UPMC St Margaret, UPMC Shadyside; **Address:** 200 Delafield Rd, 200 Medical Arts Bldg, Ste 4010, Pittsburgh, PA 15215; **Phone:** 412-784-5770; **Board Cert:** Orthopaedic Surgery 2009; **Med School:** Univ Cincinnati 1981; **Resid:** Therapeutic Radiology, Univ Mass Med Ctr 1983; Orthopaedic Surgery, Univ Pittsburgh Med Ctr 1986; **Fac Appt:** Asst Prof OrS, Univ Pittsburgh

Ciccotti, Michael G MD [SM] - **Spec Exp:** Knee Reconstruction; Elbow Reconstruction; Shoulder Reconstruction; Arthroscopic Surgery; **Hospital:** Thomas Jefferson Univ Hosp, Bryn Mawr Hosp; **Address:** Rothman Institute, 925 Chestnut St Fl 5, Philadelphia, PA 19107; **Phone:** 800-321-9999; **Board Cert:** Orthopaedic Surgery 2005; **Med School:** Georgetown Univ 1986; **Resid:** Orthopaedic Surgery, Thos Jefferson Univ Med Ctr 1991; **Fellow:** Sports Medicine, Kerlan-Jobe Clinic/USC 1992; **Fac Appt:** Assoc Prof OrS, Jefferson Med Coll

Harner, Christopher D MD [SM] - **Spec Exp:** Knee Injuries; **Hospital:** UPMC South Side; **Address:** UPMC Ctr for Sports Med, 3200 S Water St, Pittsburgh, PA 15203; **Phone:** 412-432-3661; **Board Cert:** Orthopaedic Surgery 2010; Orthopaedic Sports Medicine 2007; **Med School:** Univ Mich Med Sch 1981; **Resid:** Orthopaedic Surgery, Univ Pittsburgh 1986; **Fellow:** Sports Medicine/Knee Surgery, Salt Lake City Knee & Sport 1987; **Fac Appt:** Prof OrS, Univ Pittsburgh

Hershman, Elliott MD [SM] - **Spec Exp:** Knee Injuries; Knee Surgery; Arthroscopic Surgery; Ligament Reconstruction; **Hospital:** Lenox Hill Hosp (page 62); **Address:** 130 E 77th St Fl 7, New York, NY 10021-1851; **Phone:** 212-744-8114; **Board Cert:** Orthopaedic Surgery 2008; **Med School:** Univ Rochester 1979; **Resid:** Orthopaedic Surgery, Lenox Hill Hosp 1984; **Fellow:** Sports Medicine, Cleveland Clinic 1985; **Fac Appt:** Asst Clin Prof OrS, Mount Sinai Sch Med

Levine, William MD [SM] - **Spec Exp:** Arthroscopic Surgery; Shoulder & Elbow Surgery; Knee Injuries; **Hospital:** NY-Presby Hosp/Columbia (page 66); **Address:** 622 W 168th St Fl PH-11, New York, NY 10032; **Phone:** 212-305-0762; **Board Cert:** Orthopaedic Surgery 1999; **Med School:** Case West Res Univ 1990; **Resid:** Surgery, Beth Israel Hosp 1991; Orthopaedic Surgery, New Eng Med Ctr Hosps 1995; **Fellow:** Shoulder Surgery, Columbia-Presby Med Ctr 1996; Sports Medicine, Univ MD Med Ctr 1998; **Fac Appt:** Clin Prof OrS, Columbia P&S

Maharam, Lewis G MD [SM] - **Spec Exp:** Running Injuries; Primary Care Sports Medicine; Knee Injuries; Shoulder Injuries; **Hospital:** Hosp For Joint Diseases (page 67), NYU Langone Med Ctr (page 67); **Address:** 24 W 57th St, New York, NY 10019-3918; **Phone:** 212-765-5763; **Med School:** Emory Univ 1985; **Resid:** Internal Medicine, Danbury Hosp 1987; Internal Medicine, NY Infirm/Beekman Downtown 1989; **Fellow:** Sports Medicine, Pascack Valley Hosp 1990; **Fac Appt:** Asst Clin Prof OrS, NYU Sch Med

Metzl, Jordan D MD [SM] - **Spec Exp:** Primary Care Sports Medicine; Adolescent Sports Medicine; Running Injuries; **Hospital:** Hosp For Special Surgery (page 59); **Address:** Hospital for Special Surgery, Sports Med, 535 E 70 St, New York, NY 10021-4872; **Phone:** 212-606-1678; **Board Cert:** Sports Medicine 2001; **Med School:** Univ MO-Columbia Sch Med 1993; **Resid:** Pediatrics, New Eng Med Ctr 1996; **Fellow:** Sports Medicine, Vanderbilt Univ Med Ctr 1996; Sports Medicine, Hosp Special Surgery 1997; **Fac Appt:** Asst Prof Ped, Cornell Univ-Weill Med Coll

Nisonson, Barton MD [SM] - **Spec Exp:** Shoulder & Knee Surgery; **Hospital:** Lenox Hill Hosp (page 62); **Address:** 130 E 77th St, New York, NY 10021-1851; **Phone:** 212-570-9120; **Board Cert:** Orthopaedic Surgery 1974; **Med School:** Columbia P&S 1966; **Resid:** Surgery, Columbia-Presby Med Ctr 1968; Orthopaedic Surgery, Columbia-Presby Med Ctr 1973

Plancher, Kevin D MD [SM] - **Spec Exp:** Shoulder Surgery; Elbow Surgery; Cartilage Damage & Transplant; Shoulder Replacement; **Hospital:** Beth Israel Med Ctr - Petrie Division (page 57), Lenox Hill Hosp (page 62); **Address:** 1160 Park Ave, New York, NY 10128; **Phone:** 212-876-5200; **Board Cert:** Orthopaedic Surgery 2007; Hand Surgery 2008; **Med School:** Georgetown Univ 1986; **Resid:** Orthopaedic Surgery, Mass Genl Hosp/Brigham & Womens Hosp 1991; **Fellow:** Hand Surgery, Indiana Hand Ctr 1993; Sports Medicine, Steadman-Hawkins Clinic 1994; **Fac Appt:** Assoc Clin Prof OrS, Albert Einstein Coll Med

Sports Medicine

Rodeo, Scott A MD [SM] - **Spec Exp:** Knee Injuries; Cartilage Damage; **Hospital:** Hosp For Special Surgery (page 59); **Address:** Hospital for Special Surgery, 535 E 70th St, New York, NY 10021; **Phone:** 212-606-1513; **Board Cert:** Orthopaedic Surgery 1998; **Med School:** Cornell Univ-Weill Med Coll 1989; **Resid:** Orthopaedic Surgery, Hosp Special Surgery 1994; **Fellow:** Sports Medicine, Hosp Special Surgery 1996; **Fac Appt:** Assoc Clin Prof OrS, Cornell Univ-Weill Med Coll

Southeast

Andrews, James R MD [SM] - **Spec Exp:** Shoulder Surgery; Elbow Surgery; Knee Surgery; **Hospital:** St Vincent's Hosp - Birmingham; **Address:** 805 St Vincent's Drive, Ste 100, Birmingham, AL 35205; **Phone:** 205-939-3099; **Board Cert:** Orthopaedic Surgery 1974; **Med School:** Louisiana State U, New Orleans 1967; **Resid:** Orthopaedic Surgery, USPHS Hosp 1969; Orthopaedic Surgery, Touro Infirm-Tulane 1970; **Fellow:** Hand Surgery, VA Med Ctr; **Fac Appt:** Clin Prof OrS, Univ Alabama

Garth Jr, William P MD [SM] - **Spec Exp:** Knee Ligament Reconstruction; Shoulder Reconstruction; **Hospital:** Univ of Ala Hosp at Birmingham, Children's Hospital - Birmingham; **Address:** Univ Alabama Birmingham - Sports Medicine, Ste 402, Birmingham, AL 35233-1711; **Phone:** 205-934-1041; **Board Cert:** Orthopaedic Surgery 1980; Orthopaedic Sports Medicine 2007; **Med School:** Tulane Univ 1973; **Resid:** Surgery, Duke Univ Hosp 1975; Orthopaedic Surgery, Campbell Clinic 1979; **Fellow:** Sports Medicine, Sports Med Clinic 1984; **Fac Appt:** Prof OrS, Univ Alabama

Speer, Kevin MD [SM] - **Spec Exp:** Shoulder Surgery; **Hospital:** Duke Health Raleigh; **Address:** 3404 Wake Forest Rd, Ste 201, Raleigh, NC 27609; **Phone:** 919-256-1511; **Board Cert:** Orthopaedic Surgery 2005; **Med School:** Johns Hopkins Univ 1985; **Resid:** Orthopaedic Surgery, Duke Univ Med Ctr 1991; **Fellow:** Sports Medicine, Hosp Special Surgery 1992; **Fac Appt:** Assoc Prof OrS, Duke Univ

Midwest

Cole, Brian J MD [SM] - **Spec Exp:** Cartilage Damage; Shoulder & Elbow Surgery; Knee Injuries; **Hospital:** Rush Univ Med Ctr; **Address:** 1725 W Harrison St, Ste 1063, Chicago, IL 60612-3841; **Phone:** 312-432-2381; **Board Cert:** Orthopaedic Surgery 1999; **Med School:** Univ Chicago-Pritzker Sch Med 1990; **Resid:** Orthopaedic Surgery, Hosp for Special Surgery 1996; **Fellow:** Sports Medicine, Univ Pittsburgh Med Ctr 1997; **Fac Appt:** Prof OrS, Rush Med Coll

Dimeff, Robert J MD [SM] - **Spec Exp:** Primary Care Sports Medicine; Nutrition; **Hospital:** Cleveland Clin Fdn (page 56); **Address:** 5555 Transportation Blvd, Garfield Heights, OH 44125; **Phone:** 216-518-3470; **Board Cert:** Family Medicine 2003; Sports Medicine 2003; **Med School:** NE Ohio Univ 1985; **Resid:** Family Medicine, Presbyterian-St Lukes Med Ctr 1989; **Fellow:** Sports Medicine, Cleveland Clinic 1990; **Fac Appt:** Assoc Prof FMed, Ohio State Univ

Ho, Sherwin S MD [SM] - **Spec Exp:** Shoulder & Knee Surgery; Arthroscopic Surgery; Cartilage Damage; **Hospital:** Univ of Chicago Med Ctr; **Address:** Dept Surgery, 5841 S Maryland Ave, MS 3079, Chicago, IL 60637-3079; **Phone:** 773-702-5978; **Board Cert:** Orthopaedic Surgery 2005; **Med School:** Univ Hawaii JA Burns Sch Med 1985; **Resid:** Orthopaedic Surgery, Univ Hawaii Med Ctr 1991; **Fellow:** Sports Medicine, Univ Chicago Hosp 1992; **Fac Appt:** Assoc Prof OrS, Univ Chicago-Pritzker Sch Med

Miniaci, Anthony MD [SM] - **Spec Exp:** Shoulder Reconstruction; Shoulder Arthroscopic Surgery; Knee Reconstruction; Cartilage Damage; **Hospital:** Cleveland Clin Fdn (page 56); **Address:** Cleveland Clinic, Sports Hlth Ctr, 5555 Transportation Blvd, Garfield Heights, OH 44125; **Phone:** 216-518-3466; **Med School:** Univ Western Ontario 1982; **Resid:** Orthopaedic Surgery, Univ Western Ontario 1987; **Fellow:** Sports Medicine, Kerlan-Jobe Orthopaedic Clin 1989; Orthopaedic Research, Univ Calgary 1990; **Fac Appt:** Prof S, Case West Res Univ

Paletta, George A MD [SM] - **Spec Exp:** Ankle Surgery; Knee Surgery; **Address:** The Orthopaedic Ctr of St Louis, 14825 N Outer Forty Rd, Ste 200, Chesterfield, MO 63017; **Phone:** 314-336-2555; **Board Cert:** Orthopaedic Surgery 2009; **Med School:** Johns Hopkins Univ 1988; **Resid:** Orthopaedic Surgery, Cornell Univ Med Ctr 1994; **Fellow:** Sports Medicine, Cleveland Clin Fnd 1995; Pediatric Sports Medicine, Chldns Hosp Michigan; **Fac Appt:** Assoc Prof OrS, Washington Univ, St Louis

Great Plains and Mountains

Saint-Phard, Deborah MD [SM] - **Spec Exp:** Sports Medicine-Women; Spinal Rehabilitation; **Hospital:** Univ Colorado Hosp; **Address:** Univ Sports Med, 2000 S Colorado Blvd, Ste 4500, Denver, CO 80222; **Phone:** 720-848-8200; **Board Cert:** Physical Medicine & Rehabilitation 2007; Pain Medicine 2004; Sports Medicine 2008; **Med School:** Temple Univ 1992; **Resid:** Physical Medicine & Rehabilitation, Univ Colorado 1996; **Fellow:** Sports Medicine, Mayo Clin 1997; **Fac Appt:** Assoc Prof PMR, Univ Colorado

West Coast and Pacific

Fronek, Jan MD [SM] - **Spec Exp:** Knee Injuries; Shoulder Injuries; Arthroscopic Surgery; Rotator Cuff Surgery; **Hospital:** Scripps Green Hosp; **Address:** Scripps Clinic, 10666 N Torrey Pines Rd, MS B4, La Jolla, CA 92037; **Phone:** 858-554-9753; **Board Cert:** Orthopaedic Surgery 2008; **Med School:** Univ Rochester 1978; **Resid:** Orthopaedic Surgery, UCSD Med Ctr 1984; **Fellow:** Sports Medicine, Hosp Special Surgery 1985

Gambardella, Ralph A MD [SM] - **Spec Exp:** Cartilage Damage; Shoulder & Elbow Surgery; Knee Surgery; **Hospital:** Centinela Freeman Reg Med Ctr-Centinela, USC Univ Hosp; **Address:** Kerlan-Jobe Clinic, 6801 Park Terr, Ste 400, Los Angeles, CA 90045; **Phone:** 310-665-7200; **Board Cert:** Orthopaedic Surgery 1985; **Med School:** USC Sch Med 1977; **Resid:** Orthopaedic Surgery, USC Med Ctr 1982; **Fellow:** Sports Medicine, Southwestern Ortho Grp 1983; **Fac Appt:** Assoc Clin Prof S, USC Sch Med

Mirzayan, Raffy MD [SM] - **Spec Exp:** Fractures-Non Union; Cartilage Damage; Knee Injuries; **Hospital:** Kaiser Permanente Baldwin Pk Med Ctr; **Address:** Kaiser Permanente Med Ctr, Orthopaedics, 1011 Baldwin Park Blvd, Baldwin Park, CA 91706; **Phone:** 626-851-5256; **Board Cert:** Orthopaedic Surgery 2003; Sports Medicine 2007; **Med School:** USC Sch Med 1995; **Resid:** Orthopaedic Surgery, LAC/USC Med Ctr 2000; **Fellow:** Sports Medicine, Kerlan Jobe Ortho Clinic 2001

Schechter, David L MD [SM] - **Spec Exp:** Pain-Back; Sports Injuries; Muscle Pain-Stress Related; Sciatica; **Hospital:** Cedars-Sinai Med Ctr; **Address:** 8500 Wilshire Blvd, Ste 705, Beverly Hills, CA 90211; **Phone:** 310-657-1022; **Board Cert:** Family Medicine 2008; Sports Medicine 2003; **Med School:** NYU Sch Med 1984; **Resid:** Family Medicine, UCLA/Santa Monica Hosp 1987; **Fac Appt:** Assoc Clin Prof FMed, USC Sch Med

Cleveland Clinic

Sports Health

Cleveland Clinic Sports Health brings together top orthopaedic surgeons, primary care and chiropractic sports physicians, sports psychologists, physical therapists, athletic trainers, exercise physiologists, strength and conditioning specialists, physician's assistants and nurses to get athletes back in the game. Leaders in their specialties, our physicians diagnose, treat and rehabilitate injuries so athletes can perform at their best.

Our Cleveland Clinic Sports Health team treats athletes of all sports, ages and skill levels. We offer care that is focused, one-on-one and state-of-the-art. This involves conditioning to become stronger and faster, maximizing abilities, preventing and treating injuries, and improving future performance.

As one of the largest sports health practices in the nation, Cleveland Clinic Sports Health provides a host of services to many of the world's top professional and amateur athletes.

We've provided the physicians for Cleveland's professional teams for more than 25 years. Currently, we are the team physicians for the Cleveland Browns, Cleveland Cavaliers and Cleveland Indians. Our experienced staff has treated athletes from the AHL, EPL (English Premier League), NBA, NCAA, NFL, NHL, MLB, MLS, PBA, USA Boxing, USA Hockey, US Olympic teams and WNBA.

Our world-renowned team of physicians is trained in diagnosing and treating the unique problems of amateur to high-performance athletes. Our staff is involved in research every day to improve patient care and bring new treatments to the clinical setting.

For more information about the Cleveland Clinic Sports Health, to schedule a second opinion, or to learn about assistance for out-of-town patients, call 800.890.2467 or visit www.clevelandclinic.org/ sportstopdocs.

Sports Health
9500 Euclid Avenue / AC311 | Cleveland OH 44195

Cleveland Clinic Sports Health offers specialized programs that focus on injury evaluation and re-hab, injury prevention, and strength and conditioning tailored to your sport. These programs include:

- Golf Smart – a program designed for golfers of all ages and skill levels

- Jump Right – an eight-week program designed to teach proper jumping and landing mechanics to help reduce the risk of serious knee injury

- Run Smart – A program involving gait analysis, body composition test-ing, strength and flexibil-ity testing, VO2 analysis, injury assessment and conditioning

- Match Fit – A soccer performance program offering conditioning, injury assessment and prevention

- Throw Right – A special-ized program designed to meet the needs of baseball and fast-pitch softball players

- Strength and Condition-ing (Train Right): A specialized program that enhances your strength, speed, agility and overall performance

About the Hospital:

The Hospital for Joint Diseases (HJD) at NYU Langone Medical Center is one of the nation's leading orthopaedic, rheumatologic, and neurologic specialty hospitals dedicated to the prevention and treatment of neuromusculoskeletal diseases. The hospital offers one of the leading and most advanced orthopaedic programs in the region for musculoskeletal disorders and the largest pediatric orthopaedic program in New York City. HJD was recently recognized as the 9th best hospital in America for orthopaedics by *U.S. News and World Report*.

We specialize in the following areas:

NEUROLOGY

HJD provides a broad range of diagnostic and therapeutic services to patients with neurological disorders. Our outstanding clinical staff includes specialists in multiple sclerosis, pain management, spine and nerve pain, attention deficit disorder and cerebral palsy. Our Neurorehabilitation and Traumatic Brain Injury programs are centers of innovation and excellence for the treatment of neurobehavioral disorders. Additionally, the Initiative for Women with Disabilities is a center committed to providing high quality medical, gynecological and wellness programs promoting services for women with disabilities and chronic conditions in a fully accessible environment. We also provide multidisciplinary treatment to both children and adults with ADD at our Attention Deficit Disorder Center.

ORTHOPAEDIC SURGERY

HJD faculty includes world-renowned surgeons working to treat a wide variety of orthopaedic and rheumatologic conditions. Areas of specialty include trauma and fractures, adult reconstructive surgery, hip and knee replacement, spine surgery, sports medicine, hand and wrist disorders, musculoskeletal oncology, foot and ankle care, shoulder and elbow problems, minimally invasive surgery of hip, knee, shoulder and spine, robotic-assisted joint replacement and pediatric orthopaedics.

RADIOLOGY

HDJ provides complete inpatient and outpatient diagnostic orthopaedic radiology services, including MRI, computed tomography, ultrasonography and conventional radiography, as well as a multitude of musculoskeletal interventional procedures. Our neurointerventional specialist also performs the highly effective new vertebroplasty (a medical spinal repair procedure) for treatment of osteoporotic compression fractures. The faculty includes several internationally known musculoskeletal radiologists with expertise in all aspects of osteo-radiology.

RHEUMATOLOGY

HJD is devoted to the care of patients with clinical problems involving joints, soft tissues and the combined conditions of connective tissues. Conditions treated include rheumatoid arthritis, osteoarthritis, lupus, pediatric rheumatology and Lyme disease.

Surgery

A surgeon manages a broad spectrum of surgical conditions affecting almost any area of the body. The surgeon establishes the diagnosis and provides the preoperative, operative and postoperative care to surgical patients and is usually responsible for the comprehensive management of the trauma victim and the critically ill surgical patient.

The surgeon uses a variety of diagnostic techniques, including endoscopy, for observing internal structures and may use specialized instruments during operative procedures. A general surgeon is expected to be familiar with the salient features of other surgical specialties in order to recognize problems in those areas and to know when to refer a patient to another specialist.

Training Required: Five years

For a description of the subspecialty **Hand Surgery**, **Pediatric Surgery** and **Vascular Surgery** see the corresponding section(s).

SURGERY

New England

Ashley, Stanley W MD [S] - **Spec Exp:** Gastrointestinal Cancer & Surgery; **Hospital:** Brigham & Women's Hosp, Dana-Farber Cancer Inst; **Address:** Brigham & Women's Hosp, Dept Surgery, 75 Francis St, Boston, MA 02115; **Phone:** 617-732-6730; **Board Cert:** Surgery 2004; Surgical Critical Care 1999; **Med School:** Cornell Univ-Weill Med Coll 1981; **Resid:** Surgery, Barnes Jewish Med Ctr 1989; **Fac Appt:** Prof S, Harvard Med Sch

Becker, James M MD [S] - **Spec Exp:** Inflammatory Bowel Disease; Gastrointestinal Cancer; Gastrointestinal Surgery; **Hospital:** Boston Med Ctr, Qunicy Med Ctr; **Address:** Boston Med Ctr, Dept Surg, 88 E Newton St, rm C500, Boston, MA 02118-2393; **Phone:** 617-638-8600; **Board Cert:** Surgery 1999; **Med School:** Case West Res Univ 1975; **Resid:** Surgery, Univ Utah Med Ctr 1980; **Fellow:** Research, Mayo Clinic 1982; **Fac Appt:** Prof S, Boston Univ

Brooks, David C MD [S] - **Spec Exp:** Gastrointestinal Surgery; **Hospital:** Brigham & Women's Hosp; **Address:** Brigham & Women's Hospital, Dept Surgery, 75 Francis St, ASB II Fl 3, Boston, MA 02115; **Phone:** 617-732-6337; **Board Cert:** Surgery 2003; **Med School:** Brown Univ 1976; **Resid:** Surgery, Brigham & Women's Hosp 1983; **Fac Appt:** Assoc Prof S, Harvard Med Sch

Burke, Peter A MD [S] - **Spec Exp:** Trauma; Critical Care; **Hospital:** Boston Med Ctr; **Address:** Boston Medical Ctr, Dowling 2 South, 1 Boston Pl, Boston, MA 02118; **Phone:** 617-414-8056; **Board Cert:** Surgery 1999; Surgical Critical Care 2001; **Med School:** Tufts Univ 1983; **Resid:** Surgery, New England Deaconess Med Ctr 1990; **Fac Appt:** Assoc Prof S, Boston Univ

Callery, Mark P MD [S] - **Spec Exp:** Pancreatic Cancer; Liver Cancer; Laparoscopic Surgery; **Hospital:** Beth Israel Deaconess Med Ctr - Boston; **Address:** Beth Israel Deaconess Med Ctr, Dept Surgery, 330 Brookline Ave, Ste 928, Boston, MA 02215; **Phone:** 617-667-3798; **Board Cert:** Surgery 2004; **Med School:** Albany Med Coll 1985; **Resid:** Surgery, Albany Med Coll Hosp 1987; Surgery, Barnes Jewish Med Ctr 1992; **Fellow:** Research, Wash Univ Sch Med 1990; **Fac Appt:** Assoc Prof S, Harvard Med Sch

Cioffi, William G MD [S] - **Spec Exp:** Trauma; Cancer Surgery; **Hospital:** Rhode Island Hosp; **Address:** Rhode Island Hosp, Dept Surg, 2 Dudley St, Ste 470, Providence, RI 02905; **Phone:** 401-553-8348; **Board Cert:** Surgery 2007; Surgical Critical Care 1997; **Med School:** Univ VT Coll Med 1981; **Resid:** Surgery, Med Ctr Hosp 1986; **Fac Appt:** Prof S, Brown Univ

Cushing, Brad M MD [S] - **Spec Exp:** Trauma; Critical Care; **Hospital:** Maine Med Ctr; **Address:** Maine Medical Ctr Surgical Assocs, 887 Congress St, Ste 210, Portland, ME 04102-3113; **Phone:** 207-774-2381; **Board Cert:** Surgery 2005; Surgical Critical Care 2003; **Med School:** Univ Rochester 1980; **Resid:** Surgery, St Francis Hosp 1985; **Fellow:** Trauma/Critical Care, Iniv MD Med Ctr 1987; **Fac Appt:** Clin Prof S, Univ VT Coll Med

Eisenberg, Burton L MD [S] - **Spec Exp:** Breast Cancer; Melanoma; Sarcoma; **Hospital:** Dartmouth - Hitchcock Med Ctr; **Address:** DHMC, Dept General Surgery, One Medical Center Drive, Lebanon, NH 03756; **Phone:** 603-650-9479; **Board Cert:** Surgery 1999; **Med School:** Univ Tenn Coll Med, Memphis 1974; **Resid:** Surgery, Wilford Hall USAF Med Ctr 1979; **Fellow:** Surgical Oncology, Meml Sloan-Kettering Cancer Ctr 1981; **Fac Appt:** Prof S, Dartmouth Med Sch

Emhoff, Timothy A MD [S] - **Spec Exp:** Trauma; Critical Care; **Hospital:** UMass Meml - Univ Campus; **Address:** U Mass Memorial Medical Ctr, Dept Surgery, 55 Lake Ave N, Worcester, MA 01655; **Phone:** 508-856-1168; **Board Cert:** Surgery 2004; Surgical Critical Care 2007; **Med School:** Geo Wash Univ 1976; **Resid:** Surgery, Wilford Hall Army Med Ctr 1983; **Fellow:** Trauma/Critical Care, Baltimore Shock Trauma Ctr 1984; **Fac Appt:** Assoc Prof S, Univ Mass Sch Med

Emre, Sukru MD [S] - **Spec Exp:** Transplant-Liver-Adult & Pediatric; Hepatobiliary Surgery; Portal Hypertension; **Hospital:** Yale-New Haven Hosp; **Address:** 333 Cedar St, rm FMB112, Yale, CT 06520; **Phone:** 203-785-2565; **Med School:** Turkey 1977; **Resid:** Surgery, Univ Istanbul 1982; **Fellow:** Hepatobiliary Surgery, Univ Istanbul 1988; Transplant Surgery, Mount Sinai Med Ctr 1994; **Fac Appt:** Prof S, Mount Sinai Sch Med

Gupta, Rajan MD [S] - **Spec Exp:** Trauma; Critical Care; **Hospital:** Dartmouth - Hitchcock Med Ctr; **Address:** Dartmouth Hitchcock Med Ctr, Dept Surgery, One Medical Center Drive, Lewbanon, NH 03756; **Phone:** 603-650-8022; **Board Cert:** Surgery 2001; Surgical Critical Care 2003; **Med School:** Boston Univ 1991; **Resid:** Surgery, Dartmouth-Hitchcock Med Ctr 1997; **Fellow:** Trauma/Critical Care, Hosp U Penn 1999; **Fac Appt:** Asst Prof S, Dartmouth Med Sch

Hebert, James C MD [S] - **Spec Exp:** Biliary Surgery; Colon & Rectal Surgery; **Hospital:** Fletcher Allen Health Care- Med Ctr Campus; **Address:** Fletcher Allen Hlth Care, 111 Colchester Ave, Burlington, VT 05401; **Phone:** 802-847-3344; **Board Cert:** Surgery 2000; **Med School:** Univ VT Coll Med 1977; **Resid:** Surgery, Med Ctr Hosp 1982; **Fac Appt:** Prof S, Univ VT Coll Med

Hughes, Kevin S MD [S] - **Spec Exp:** Breast Cancer; Ovarian Cancer; **Hospital:** Mass Genl Hosp; **Address:** Mass Genl Hosp, Dept Surgery, 55 Fruit St, Yawkey Center Fl 9 - Ste A, Boston, MA 02114; **Phone:** 617-724-4800; **Board Cert:** Surgery 2006; **Med School:** Dartmouth Med Sch 1979; **Resid:** Surgery, Mercy Hosp 1984; **Fellow:** Surgical Oncology, National Cancer Inst 1986; **Fac Appt:** Assoc Prof S, Harvard Med Sch

Iglehart, J Dirk MD [S] - **Spec Exp:** Breast Cancer; **Hospital:** Brigham & Women's Hosp, Dana-Farber Cancer Inst; **Address:** Dana-Farber Cancer Inst, 44 binney, Smith Bldg, Boston, MA 02115; **Phone:** 617-632-5178 x1; **Board Cert:** Surgery 2005; **Med School:** Harvard Med Sch 1975; **Resid:** Surgery, Duke Univ Med Ctr 1981; Thoracic Surgery, Duke Univ Med Ctr 1984; **Fac Appt:** Prof S, Harvard Med Sch

Jenkins, Roger L MD [S] - **Spec Exp:** Transplant-Liver; Liver & Biliary Cancer; Pancreatic Cancer; **Hospital:** Lahey Clin, Children's Hospital - Boston; **Address:** Lahey Clinic, Div Hepatobiliary Surgery, 41 Mall Rd, Burlington, MA 01805; **Phone:** 781-744-2500; **Board Cert:** Surgery 2005; **Med School:** Univ VT Coll Med 1977; **Resid:** Surgery, New Eng Deaconess Hosp 1982; **Fellow:** Cardiac Surgery, New Eng Deaconess Hosp 1983; Transplant Surgery, Univ Pittsburgh Hosp 1983; **Fac Appt:** Prof S, Tufts Univ

Kavanah, Maureen MD [S] - **Spec Exp:** Breast Cancer; Gynecologic Cancer; Melanoma; **Hospital:** Boston Med Ctr; **Address:** Boston Medical Ctr, 820 Harrison Ave, rm 5009, Bldg FGH, Boston, MA 02118; **Phone:** 617-638-8473; **Board Cert:** Surgery 1999; **Med School:** Tufts Univ 1975; **Resid:** Surgery, St Elizabeths Hosp 1979; **Fellow:** Surgical Oncology, Boston Univ Med Ctr 1981; **Fac Appt:** Assoc Prof S, Boston Univ

Krag, David N MD [S] - **Spec Exp:** Sentinel Node Surgery; Breast Cancer; Cancer Surgery; Melanoma; **Hospital:** Fletcher Allen Health Care- Med Ctr Campus; **Address:** Univ Vermont Coll Med, Dept Surgery, 89 Beaumont Ave, Given Bldg - E309C, Burlington, VT 05405; **Phone:** 802-656-5830; **Board Cert:** Surgery 2006; **Med School:** Loyola Univ-Stritch Sch Med 1980; **Resid:** Surgery, UC Davis Med Ctr 1983; **Fellow:** Surgical Oncology, UCLA Med Ctr 1984; **Fac Appt:** Assoc Prof S, Univ VT Coll Med

Lannin, Donald R MD [S] - **Spec Exp:** Breast Cancer; Breast Surgery; **Hospital:** Yale-New Haven Hosp; **Address:** Yale-New Haven Breast Ctr, 800 Howard Ave, Yale Physicians Bldg, Lower Level 38, New Haven, CT 06520-8062; **Phone:** 203-785-2328; **Board Cert:** Surgery 2002; **Med School:** Univ Minn 1974; **Resid:** Surgery, Univ Minnesota Med Ctr 1982; **Fac Appt:** Prof S, Yale Univ

Lipkowitz, George S MD [S] - **Spec Exp:** Transplant-Kidney; Dialysis Access; **Hospital:** Baystate Med Ctr, Mercy Med Ctr; **Address:** 208 Ashley Ave, West Springfield, MA 01089; **Phone:** 413-747-4170 x151; **Board Cert:** Surgery 2006; **Med School:** SUNY Downstate 1980; **Resid:** Surgery, SUNY Kings Co Hosp 1985; **Fellow:** Transplant Surgery, SUNY Hlth Scis Ctr 1986; **Fac Appt:** Assoc Prof S, Tufts Univ

Pomposelli, Frank B MD [S] - **Spec Exp:** Diabetic Leg/Foot; Aortic Surgery; Carotid Artery Disease; Endovascular Surgery; **Hospital:** Beth Israel Deaconess Med Ctr - Boston, New England Bapt Hosp; **Address:** Beth Israel Deac Med Ctr, 110 Francis St, Ste 5B, Boston, MA 02215-5566; **Phone:** 617-632-9847; **Board Cert:** Vascular Surgery 1998; **Med School:** Boston Univ 1979; **Resid:** Surgery, New England Deaconess Hosp 1986; **Fellow:** Peripheral Vascular Surgery, NYU Med Ctr 1987; **Fac Appt:** Assoc Prof S, Harvard Med Sch

Ponn, Teresa MD [S] - **Spec Exp:** Breast Cancer; **Hospital:** Elliot Hosp; **Address:** Elliot Breast Health Center, 275 Mammoth Rd, Ste 1, Manchester, NH 03109; **Phone:** 603-668-3067; **Board Cert:** Surgery 2000; **Med School:** Univ Fla Coll Med 1976; **Resid:** Surgery, Stanford Univ Med Ctr 1982

Ryan, Colleen M MD [S] - **Spec Exp:** Burn Care; Toxic Epidermal Neurolysis; Wound Healing/Care; **Hospital:** Mass Genl Hosp, Boston Shriners Hosp; **Address:** MGH Burn Assocs, 55 Fruit St GRB Bldg - Ste 1303, Boston, MA 02114-2621; **Phone:** 617-726-3712; **Board Cert:** Surgery 1999; Surgical Critical Care 2003; **Med School:** Georgetown Univ 1982; **Resid:** Surgery, NE Deaconess Hosp 1988; **Fellow:** Hepatology, Hammersmith Hosp 1986; Burn Surgery, Mass Genl Hosp 1989; **Fac Appt:** Assoc Prof S, Harvard Med Sch

Salem, Ronald R MD [S] - **Spec Exp:** Cancer Surgery; Liver & Biliary Surgery; Gastrointestinal Cancer; Liver Cancer; **Hospital:** Yale-New Haven Hosp; **Address:** Dept Surgery, 333 Cedar St, TMP 202, New Haven, CT 06520-8062; **Phone:** 203-785-3577; **Board Cert:** Surgery 2000; **Med School:** Zimbabwe 1978; **Resid:** Surgery, Hammersmith Hosp 1985; Surgery, New England Deaconess Hosp 1989; **Fac Appt:** Assoc Prof S, Yale Univ

Shikora, Scott A MD [S] - **Spec Exp:** Obesity/Bariatric Surgery; Laparoscopic Abdominal Surgery; **Hospital:** Tufts Med Ctr; **Address:** Tufts-New England Med Ctr, 800 Washington St, Box 900, Boston, MA 02111; **Phone:** 617-636-6093; **Board Cert:** Surgery 2001; **Med School:** Columbia P&S 1985; **Resid:** Surgery, New England Deaconess Hosp 1991; **Fellow:** Nutrition & Metabolism, New England Deaconess Hos 1989; **Fac Appt:** Prof S, Tufts Univ

Smith, Barbara Lynn MD/PhD [S] - **Spec Exp:** Breast Cancer; **Hospital:** Mass Genl Hosp; **Address:** Mass Genl Hosp, Dept Surgery, 55 Fruit St, Yawkey Center Fl 9 - Ste A, Boston, MA 02114; **Phone:** 617-724-4800; **Board Cert:** Surgery 2000; **Med School:** Harvard Med Sch 1983; **Resid:** Surgery, Brigham & Women's Hosp 1989; **Fac Appt:** Asst Prof S, Harvard Med Sch

Sutton, John E MD [S] - **Spec Exp:** Esophageal Cancer; Liver & Biliary Surgery; Pancreatic Cancer; **Hospital:** Dartmouth - Hitchcock Med Ctr; **Address:** One Medical Center Drive, Lebanon, NH 03756; **Phone:** 603-650-8022; **Board Cert:** Surgery 2001; Surgical Critical Care 2007; **Med School:** Georgetown Univ 1974; **Resid:** Surgery, Dartmouth-Hitchcock Med Ctr 1981; **Fellow:** Surgical Critical Care, Dartmouth-Hitchcock Med Ctr 1983; **Fac Appt:** Prof S, Dartmouth Med Sch

Tanabe, Kenneth K MD [S] - **Spec Exp:** Liver Cancer; Colon & Rectal Cancer; Melanoma; **Hospital:** Mass Genl Hosp, Newton - Wellesley Hosp; **Address:** Mass General Hosp, Div Surgical Oncology, 55 Fruit St, Yawkey 7.924, Boston, MA 02114; **Phone:** 617-724-3868; **Board Cert:** Surgery 2000; **Med School:** UCSD 1985; **Resid:** Surgery, New York Hosp-Cornell 1990; **Fellow:** Surgical Oncology, MD Anderson Cancer Ctr 1993; **Fac Appt:** Assoc Prof S, Harvard Med Sch

Udelsman, Robert MD [S] - **Spec Exp:** Parathyroid Cancer; Adrenal Tumors; Thyroid Cancer; **Hospital:** Yale-New Haven Hosp; **Address:** Yale School Medicine, Dept Surgery, 330 Cedar St, FMB 102, New Haven, CT 06511; **Phone:** 203-785-2697; **Board Cert:** Surgery 1999; **Med School:** Geo Wash Univ 1981; **Resid:** Surgery, Natl Inst Hlth 1986; Surgery, Johns Hopkins Hosp 1989; **Fellow:** Gastrointestinal Surgery, Johns Hopkins Hosp 1990; **Fac Appt:** Prof S, Yale Univ

Vlahakes, Gus J MD [S] - **Spec Exp:** Cardiac Surgery-Adult & Pediatric; Transplant-Heart; Maze Procedure for Atrial Fibrillation; **Hospital:** Mass Genl Hosp, Children's Hospital - Boston; **Address:** Mass General Hospital, 55 Fruit St, Ste COX 652, Boston, MA 02114-2621; **Phone:** 617-726-1861; **Board Cert:** Surgery 2002; Surgical Critical Care 2000; Thoracic Surgery 2005; **Med School:** Harvard Med Sch 1975; **Resid:** Surgery, Mass Genl Hosp 1983; Cardiothoracic Surgery, Mass Genl Hosp 1985; **Fellow:** Pediatric Cardiac Surgery, Chldns Hosp 1985; **Fac Appt:** Prof S, Harvard Med Sch

Ward, Barbara MD [S] - **Spec Exp:** Breast Cancer; Breast Disease; **Hospital:** Greenwich Hosp; **Address:** 77 Lafayette Pl, Ste 302, Greenwich, CT 06830-5426; **Phone:** 203-863-4250; **Board Cert:** Surgery 2002; **Med School:** Temple Univ 1983; **Resid:** Surgery, Yale-New Haven Hosp 1990; **Fellow:** Surgical Oncology, Natl Cancer Inst 1987; **Fac Appt:** Assoc Clin Prof S, Yale Univ

Warshaw, Andrew L MD [S] - **Spec Exp:** Pancreatic Cancer; Pancreatic Surgery; **Hospital:** Mass Genl Hosp; **Address:** Mass Genl Hosp, Dept Surg, 55 Fruit St, WHT 506, Boston, MA 02114-2696; **Phone:** 617-726-8254; **Board Cert:** Surgery 1971; **Med School:** Harvard Med Sch 1963; **Resid:** Surgery, Mass Genl Hosp 1971; **Fellow:** Internal Medicine, Mass Genl Hosp 1970; **Fac Appt:** Prof S, Harvard Med Sch

Winchell, Robert J MD [S] - **Spec Exp:** Critical Care; Trauma; Burn Care; **Hospital:** Maine Med Ctr; **Address:** Maine Medical Partners, 887 Congress St, Ste 210, Portland, ME 04102-3113; **Phone:** 207-774-2381; **Board Cert:** Surgery 1999; Surgical Critical Care 2001; **Med School:** Yale Univ 1984; **Resid:** Surgery, UCSD Med Ctr 1990; **Fellow:** Trauma/Critical Care, UCSD Med Ctr 1991; **Fac Appt:** Assoc Clin Prof S, Univ VT Coll Med

Zinner, Michael MD [S] - **Spec Exp:** Colon & Rectal Cancer; Gastrointestinal Surgery; Pancreatic Cancer; **Hospital:** Brigham & Women's Hosp, Dana-Farber Cancer Inst; **Address:** Brigham & Women's Hosp, Dept Surg, 75 Francis St, Twr 1, Ste 220, Boston, MA 02115; **Phone:** 617-732-8181; **Board Cert:** Surgery 2000; **Med School:** Univ Fla Coll Med 1971; **Resid:** Surgery, Johns Hopkins Hosp 1974; Surgery, Johns Hopkins Hosp 1979; **Fac Appt:** Prof S, Harvard Med Sch

Mid Atlantic

Alfonso, Antonio MD [S] - **Spec Exp:** Breast Cancer; Head & Neck Surgery; Thyroid Cancer; **Hospital:** Long Island Coll Hosp (page 57), SUNY Downstate Med Ctr; **Address:** Long Island Coll Hosp, 339 Hicks St, Brooklyn, NY 11201; **Phone:** 718-875-3244; **Board Cert:** Surgery 1973; **Med School:** Philippines 1968; **Resid:** Surgery, Temple Univ Hosp 1972; **Fellow:** Surgical Oncology, Meml Sloan Kettering Cancer Ctr 1974; **Fac Appt:** Prof S, SUNY Downstate

August, David MD [S] - **Spec Exp:** Pancreatic Cancer; Esophageal Cancer; Stomach Cancer; Sarcoma-Soft Tissue; **Hospital:** Robert Wood Johnson Univ Hosp - New Brunswick; **Address:** Canc Inst NJ, 195 Little Albany St, New Brunswick, NJ 08903-1914; **Phone:** 732-235-7701; **Board Cert:** Surgery 2005; **Med School:** Yale Univ 1980; **Resid:** Surgery, Yale-New Haven Hosp 1986; **Fellow:** Surgical Oncology, Natl Cancer Inst 1984; **Fac Appt:** Prof S, UMDNJ-RW Johnson Med Sch

Axelrod, Deborah MD [S] - **Spec Exp:** Breast Cancer; Breast Disease; **Hospital:** NYU Langone Med Ctr (page 67), St Vincent Cath Med Ctrs - Manhattan; **Address:** NYU Clinical Cancer Ctr, 160 E 34th St, New York, NY 10016; **Phone:** 212-731-5366; **Board Cert:** Surgery 1997; **Med School:** Israel 1982; **Resid:** Surgery, Beth Israel Med Ctr 1988; **Fellow:** Surgical Oncology, Meml Sloan Kettering Cancer Ctr 1986; **Fac Appt:** Assoc Prof S, NYU Sch Med

Balch, Charles M MD [S] - **Spec Exp:** Sentinel Node Surgery; Melanoma; Cancer Surgery; **Hospital:** Johns Hopkins Hosp (page 61); **Address:** 600 N Wolfe St Osler Bldg - Ste 624, Baltimore, MD 21287; **Phone:** 410-502-5977; **Board Cert:** Surgery 1997; **Med School:** Columbia P&S 1967; **Resid:** Surgery, Univ Alabama Med Ctr 1971; Surgery, Univ Alabama Med Ctr 1975; **Fellow:** Immunology, Scripps Clin-Rsch Fdn 1973; **Fac Appt:** Prof Surg & Onc, Johns Hopkins Univ

Ballantyne, Garth H MD [S] - **Spec Exp:** Laparoscopic Surgery; Gastroesophageal Reflux Disease (GERD); Colon Cancer; Obesity/Bariatric Surgery; **Hospital:** Hackensack Univ Med Ctr; **Address:** 20 Prospect Ave, Ste 901, Hackensack, NJ 07601-1974; **Phone:** 201-996-2959; **Board Cert:** Surgery 2006; Colon & Rectal Surgery 1985; **Med School:** Columbia P&S 1977; **Resid:** Surgery, UCLA Med Ctr 1980; Surgery, Northwestern Univ 1982; **Fellow:** Colon & Rectal Surgery, Mayo Clinic 1984; **Fac Appt:** Prof S, UMDNJ-NJ Med Sch, Newark

Barie, Philip MD [S] - **Spec Exp:** Trauma; Critical Care; Hernia; Sepsis; **Hospital:** NY-Presby Hosp/Weill Cornell (page 66), Hosp For Special Surgery (page 59); **Address:** Weill Med College-Cornell Univ, 525 E 68th St, Ste P713A, New York, NY 10021-4873; **Phone:** 212-746-5401; **Board Cert:** Surgery 2004; Surgical Critical Care 2005; **Med School:** Boston Univ 1977; **Resid:** Surgery, NY Hosp-Cornell Med Ctr 1984; **Fellow:** Trauma, Albany Med Coll 1981; **Fac Appt:** Prof S, Cornell Univ-Weill Med Coll

Bartlett, David L MD [S] - **Spec Exp:** Peritoneal Carcinomatosis; Pancreatic Cancer; Liver Cancer; Appendix Cancer; **Hospital:** UPMC Shadyside; **Address:** UPMC Cancer Ctr, 5150 Centre Ave Fl 4 - rm 415, Pittsburgh, PA 15232; **Phone:** 412-692-2852; **Board Cert:** Surgery 2004; **Med School:** Univ Tex, Houston 1987; **Resid:** Surgery, Hosp Univ Penn 1993; **Fellow:** Surgical Oncology, Meml Sloan-Kettering Cancer Ctr 1995; **Fac Appt:** Assoc Prof S, Univ Pittsburgh

Bartlett, Stephen Thomas MD [S] - **Spec Exp:** Transplant-Pancreas; Transplant-Kidney; **Hospital:** Univ of MD Med Ctr; **Address:** 22 S Greene St, rm N4E40, Baltimore, MD 21201; **Phone:** 410-328-8407; **Board Cert:** Surgery 2004; Vascular Surgery 2007; **Med School:** Univ Chicago-Pritzker Sch Med 1979; **Resid:** Surgery, Hosp Univ Penn 1985; **Fellow:** Vascular Surgery, Northwestern Univ Affil Hosp 1986; **Fac Appt:** Prof S, Univ MD Sch Med

Bessler, Marc MD [S] - **Spec Exp:** Obesity/Bariatric Surgery; Laparoscopic Surgery; Gastrointestinal Metabolic Surgery; **Hospital:** NY-Presby Hosp/Columbia (page 66); **Address:** NY Presby Med Ctr, Dept of Surgery, 161 Fort Washington Ave, rm 612, New York, NY 10032; **Phone:** 212-305-9506; **Board Cert:** Surgery 2007; **Med School:** NYU Sch Med 1989; **Resid:** Surgery, Columbia Presby Med Ctr 1995; **Fac Appt:** Assoc Prof S, Columbia P&S

Borgen, Patrick I MD [S] - **Spec Exp:** Breast Cancer; **Hospital:** Maimonides Med Ctr (page 63); **Address:** Maimonides Breast Ctr, 6300 8th Ave, Brooklyn, NY 11220; **Phone:** 718-765-2570; **Board Cert:** Surgery 2002; **Med School:** Louisiana State U, New Orleans 1984; **Resid:** Surgery, Ochsner Fdn Hosp 1989; **Fellow:** Surgical Oncology, Meml Sloan Kettering Canc Ctr 1990; **Fac Appt:** Prof S, Cornell Univ-Weill Med Coll

Brennan, Murray MD [S] - **Spec Exp:** Sarcoma; Pancreatic Cancer; Stomach Cancer; Endocrine Cancers; **Hospital:** Meml Sloan-Kettering Cancer Ctr; **Address:** 1275 York Avenue, New York, NY 10065; **Phone:** 800-525-2225; **Board Cert:** Surgery 1975; **Med School:** New Zealand 1964; **Resid:** Surgery, Univ Otago Hosp 1969; **Fellow:** Surgery, Harvard Med Sch 1972; Surgery, Peter Bent Brigham Hosp 1975; **Fac Appt:** Prof S, Cornell Univ-Weill Med Coll

Brody, Fred J MD [S] - **Spec Exp:** Gastrointestinal Surgery; Laparoscopic Surgery; Hernia; **Hospital:** G Washington Univ Hosp; **Address:** George Washington Univ Dept Surgery, 2150 Pennsylvania Ave NW, Ste 6B-412, Washington, DC 20037; **Phone:** 202-741-2587; **Board Cert:** Surgery 1998; **Med School:** Univ NC Sch Med 1991; **Resid:** Surgery, George Washington Univ Med Ctr 1997; **Fellow:** Laparoscopic Surgery, Duke Univ Med Ctr 1998; **Fac Appt:** Assoc Prof S, Geo Wash Univ

Bromberg, Jonathan S MD/PhD [S] - **Spec Exp:** Transplant-Kidney; Transplant-Pancreas; **Hospital:** Mount Sinai Med Ctr (page 64); **Address:** Mount Sinai Medical Ctr, One Gustave Levy Pl, Box 1104, New York, NY 10029-6500; **Phone:** 212-659-8086; **Board Cert:** Surgery 1997; **Med School:** Harvard Med Sch 1983; **Resid:** Surgery, Univ Washington Med Ctr 1988; **Fellow:** Transplant Surgery, Hosp U Penn 1990; **Fac Appt:** Prof S, Mount Sinai Sch Med

Brooks, Ari D MD [S] - **Spec Exp:** Breast Cancer; **Hospital:** Hahnemann Univ Hosp; **Address:** Drexel Surgical Assocs, 219 N Broad St Fl 8, Philadelphia, PA 19107; **Phone:** 215-762-2295; **Board Cert:** Surgery 2000; **Med School:** Hahnemann Univ 1992; **Resid:** Surgery, NYU Med Ctr 1999; **Fellow:** Surgical Oncology, Meml Sloan-Kettering Cancer Ctr 2001; **Fac Appt:** Assoc Prof S, Drexel Univ Coll Med

Cance, William G MD [S] - **Spec Exp:** Pancreatic Cancer; Colon & Rectal Cancer; Endocrine Cancers; **Hospital:** Roswell Park Cancer Inst; **Address:** Roswell Park Cancer Inst, Dept Surgery, Elm & Carlton Sts, Buffalo, NY 14263; **Phone:** 716-845-8204; **Board Cert:** Surgery 1998; **Med School:** Duke Univ 1982; **Resid:** Surgery, Barnes Jewish Hosp 1988; **Fellow:** Surgical Oncology, Meml Sloan Kettering Canc Ctr 1990; **Fac Appt:** Prof S, SUNY Buffalo

Carty, Sally E MD [S] - **Spec Exp:** Endocrine Tumors; Parathyroid Surgery; **Hospital:** UPMC Montefiore; **Address:** 3471 Fifth Ave, Ste 101, Pittsburgh, PA 15213; **Phone:** 412-647-0467; **Board Cert:** Surgery 1999; **Med School:** Penn State Univ-Hershey Med Ctr 1984; **Resid:** Surgery, Penn State Hershey Med Ctr 1989; **Fellow:** Surgical Oncology, Natl Cancer Inst 1991; **Fac Appt:** Prof S, Univ Pittsburgh

Chabot, John A MD [S] - **Spec Exp:** Liver & Biliary Surgery; Pancreatic Cancer; Pancreatic Surgery; Thyroid & Parathyroid Surgery; **Hospital:** NY-Presby Hosp/Columbia (page 66); **Address:** NY Presby-Columbia Medical Ctr, 161 Ft Washington Ave Fl 8 - Ste 819, New York, NY 10032; **Phone:** 212-305-9468; **Board Cert:** Surgery 2000; **Med School:** Dartmouth Med Sch 1983; **Resid:** Surgery, Columbia-Presby Med Ctr 1990; **Fac Appt:** Prof S, Columbia P&S

Choti, Michael A MD [S] - **Spec Exp:** Pancreatic Cancer; Liver Cancer-Metastatic; Carcinoid Tumors; **Hospital:** Johns Hopkins Hosp (page 61); **Address:** Johns Hopkins Hosp, 600 N Wolfe St Blalock Bldg - rm 665, Baltimore, MD 21287; **Phone:** 410-955-7113; **Board Cert:** Surgery 2002; **Med School:** Yale Univ 1983; **Resid:** Surgery, Hosp Univ Penn 1990; **Fellow:** Surgical Oncology, Meml Sloan-Kettering Canc Ctr 1992; **Fac Appt:** Prof S, Johns Hopkins Univ

Coit, Daniel G MD [S] - **Spec Exp:** Melanoma; Pancreatic Cancer; Stomach Cancer; **Hospital:** Meml Sloan-Kettering Cancer Ctr; **Address:** 1275 York Avenue, New York, NY 10065; **Phone:** 800-525-2225; **Board Cert:** Surgery 2004; **Med School:** Univ Cincinnati 1976; **Resid:** Internal Medicine, New Eng Deaconess Hosp 1978; Surgery, New Eng Deaconess Hosp 1983; **Fellow:** Surgical Oncology, Meml Sloan Kettering Canc Ctr 1985; **Fac Appt:** Prof S, Cornell Univ-Weill Med Coll

Conti, David J MD [S] - **Spec Exp:** Transplant-Kidney; **Hospital:** Albany Med Ctr; **Address:** Albany Medical Center, 47 New Scotland Ave, MC 61GE, Albany, NY 12208; **Phone:** 518-262-5614; **Board Cert:** Surgery 1998; **Med School:** Northwestern Univ 1981; **Resid:** Surgery, Northwestern Meml Hosp 1987; **Fellow:** Transplant Surgery, Mass Genl Hosp 1989; **Fac Appt:** Prof S, Albany Med Coll

Cornwell III, Edward E MD [S] - **Spec Exp:** Trauma; **Hospital:** Howard Univ Hosp; **Address:** Howard Univ Hospital, 2041 Georgia Ave NW, Ste 4B02, Washington, DC 20060; **Phone:** 202-865-1441; **Board Cert:** Surgery 2006; Surgical Critical Care 1998; **Med School:** Howard Univ 1982; **Resid:** Surgery, LAC-USC Med Ctr 1987; **Fellow:** Trauma, Emer/Med Svcs System 1989; **Fac Appt:** Assoc Prof S, Johns Hopkins Univ

Courcoulas, Anita P MD [S] - **Spec Exp:** Obesity/Bariatric Surgery; Minimally Invasive Surgery; **Hospital:** Magee-Womens Hosp - UPMC; **Address:** Magee-Women's Hospital, 3380 Boulevard of the Allies, Ste 390, Pittsburgh, PA 15213; **Phone:** 412-641-3632; **Board Cert:** Surgery 2005; **Med School:** Boston Univ 1988; **Resid:** Surgery, Univ Pittsburgh Med Ctr 1996; **Fac Appt:** Assoc Prof S, Univ Pittsburgh

Curcillo, Paul G MD [S] - **Spec Exp:** Laparoscopic Surgery; Hernia; Robotic Surgery; **Hospital:** Hahnemann Univ Hosp; **Address:** 219 N Broad St Fl 10, Philadelphia, PA 19107; **Phone:** 215-762-5577; **Board Cert:** Surgery 2007; **Med School:** Univ Pennsylvania 1989; **Resid:** Surgery, Thos Jefferson Univ Hosp 1995; **Fac Appt:** Assoc Prof S, Drexel Univ Coll Med

Dayton, Merril T MD [S] - **Spec Exp:** Gastrointestinal Surgery; Inflammatory Bowel Disease; **Hospital:** Buffalo General Hosp; **Address:** Buffalo General Hospital, Dept Surgery, 100 High St, Buffalo, NY 14203; **Phone:** 716-859-3911; **Board Cert:** Surgery 2004; **Med School:** Univ Utah 1976; **Resid:** Surgery, UCLA Med Ctr 1982; **Fellow:** Gastrointestinal Surgery, UCLA Med Ctr 1983; **Fac Appt:** Prof S, SUNY Buffalo

Deitch, Edwin A MD [S] - **Spec Exp:** Trauma; Burn Care; Critical Care; **Hospital:** UMDNJ-Univ Hosp-Newark; **Address:** 185 S Orange Ave, MSB, rm G506, Newark, NJ 07103; **Phone:** 973-972-5045; **Board Cert:** Surgery 1997; Surgical Critical Care 2006; **Med School:** Univ MD Sch Med 1973; **Resid:** Surgery, US Public Hlth Svc Hosp 1976; Surgery, US Public Hlth Svc Hosp 1978; **Fac Appt:** Prof S, UMDNJ-NJ Med Sch, Newark

Dempsey, Daniel MD [S] - **Spec Exp:** Gastrointestinal & Esophageal Surgery; Laparoscopic Surgery; Gastroesophageal Reflux Disease (GERD); **Hospital:** Temple Univ Hosp, Jeanes Hosp; **Address:** Temple Univ Hosp - Dept Surgery, 3401 N Broad St, 400 Parkinson Pavilion, Philadelphia, PA 19140; **Phone:** 215-707-5080; **Board Cert:** Surgery 2006; **Med School:** Univ Rochester 1979; **Resid:** Surgery, Hosp Univ Penn 1986; **Fac Appt:** Prof S, Temple Univ

Drebin, Jeffrey A MD/PhD [S] - **Spec Exp:** Pancreatic Cancer; Liver Cancer; Biliary Cancer; Gastrointestinal Cancer; **Hospital:** Hosp Univ Penn - UPHS (page 60); **Address:** Hosp Univ Penn, Dept Surgery, 3400 Spruce St, 4 Silverstein Pavilion, Philadelphia, PA 19104; **Phone:** 215-662-2165; **Board Cert:** Surgery 2004; **Med School:** Harvard Med Sch 1987; **Resid:** Surgery, Johns Hopkins Hosp 1994; **Fellow:** Surgical Oncology, Johns Hopkins Hosp 1995; **Fac Appt:** Prof S, Univ Pennsylvania

Edge, Stephen B MD [S] - **Spec Exp:** Breast Cancer; **Hospital:** Roswell Park Cancer Inst; **Address:** Roswell Park Cancer Inst, Dept Surg Onc, Elm & Carlton Streets, Buffalo, NY 14263; **Phone:** 716-845-3152; **Board Cert:** Surgery 2006; **Med School:** Case West Res Univ 1979; **Resid:** Surgery, Univ Hosp 1986; **Fellow:** Surgical Oncology, Natl Cancer Inst 1984; **Fac Appt:** Prof S, SUNY Buffalo

Edington, Howard D MD [S] - **Spec Exp:** Melanoma; Breast Reconstruction; Reconstructive Surgery; **Hospital:** Magee-Womens Hosp - UPMC; **Address:** Magee-Women's Hospital, Dept Surgery, 300 Halket St, rm 2502, Pittsburgh, PA 15213; **Phone:** 412-641-1342; **Board Cert:** Surgery 1998; Plastic Surgery 1993; **Med School:** Temple Univ 1983; **Resid:** Surgery, Univ Pittsburgh Med Ctr 1989; Plastic Surgery, Univ Pittsburgh Med Ctr 1990; **Fellow:** Hand Surgery, Univ Pittsburgh Med Ctr 1991; Surgical Oncology, National Cancer Inst 1993; **Fac Appt:** Assoc Prof S, Univ Pittsburgh

Edye, Michael MD [S] - **Spec Exp:** Laparoscopic Abdominal Surgery; Colon Cancer; Diverticulitis; Obesity/Bariatric Surgery; **Hospital:** Mount Sinai Med Ctr (page 64), Westchester Med Ctr; **Address:** 1060 Fifth Ave, New York, NY 10128; **Phone:** 212-241-0872; **Med School:** Australia 1977; **Resid:** Surgery, St Vincents Hosp 1980; Surgery, Royal N Shore Hosp 1984; **Fellow:** Laparoscopic Surgery, Univ Bordeaux 1992; **Fac Appt:** Assoc Clin Prof S, Mount Sinai Sch Med

Emond, Jean C MD [S] - **Spec Exp:** Transplant-Liver; Liver Cancer; Liver & Biliary Cancer; Hepatobiliary Surgery; **Hospital:** NY-Presby Hosp/Columbia (page 66), Holy Name Hosp; **Address:** 622 W 168th St, PH - Fl 14, New York, NY 10032; **Phone:** 212-305-9691; **Board Cert:** Surgery 2006; **Med School:** Univ Chicago-Pritzker Sch Med 1979; **Resid:** Surgery, Cook Cty Hosp 1984; **Fellow:** Surgery, Hopital P Brousse/Univ de Paris Sud 1985; Transplant Surgery, Univ Chicago Hosps 1987; **Fac Appt:** Prof S, Columbia P&S

Eng, Kenneth MD [S] - **Spec Exp:** Colon & Rectal Cancer & Surgery; Pancreatic Cancer; Inflammatory Bowel Disease; **Hospital:** NYU Langone Med Ctr (page 67); **Address:** 530 1st Ave, Ste 6B, New York, NY 10016-6402; **Phone:** 212-263-7301; **Board Cert:** Surgery 1982; **Med School:** NYU Sch Med 1967; **Resid:** Surgery, NYU Med Ctr 1972; **Fac Appt:** Prof S, NYU Sch Med

Estabrook, Alison MD [S] - **Spec Exp:** Breast Cancer; Breast Disease; Breast Cancer-High Risk Women; **Hospital:** St Luke's - Roosevelt Hosp Ctr - Roosevelt Div (page 57); **Address:** 425 W 59th St, Ste 7A, New York, NY 10019-1104; **Phone:** 212-523-7500; **Board Cert:** Surgery 2004; **Med School:** NYU Sch Med 1978; **Resid:** Surgery, Columbia Presby Med Ctr 1984; **Fellow:** Surgical Oncology, Columbia Presby Med Ctr 1982; **Fac Appt:** Prof S, Columbia P&S

Fahey III, Thomas J MD [S] - **Spec Exp:** Endocrine Surgery; Pheochromocytoma; Pancreatic Cancer; **Hospital:** NY-Presby Hosp/Weill Cornell (page 66); **Address:** NY Presby Cornell Med Ctr, Dept Surgery, 525 E 68 St, rm F2024, Box 249, New York, NY 10065; **Phone:** 212-746-5130; **Board Cert:** Surgery 2002; **Med School:** Cornell Univ-Weill Med Coll 1986; **Resid:** Surgery, New York Hosp 1992; **Fellow:** Endocrine Surgery, Royal North Shore Hosp 1993; **Fac Appt:** Prof S, Cornell Univ-Weill Med Coll

Fong, Yuman MD [S] - **Spec Exp:** Pancreatic Cancer; Liver & Biliary Cancer; Stomach Cancer; **Hospital:** Meml Sloan-Kettering Cancer Ctr, NY-Presby Hosp/Weill Cornell (page 66); **Address:** 1275 York Avenue, New York, NY 10065; **Phone:** 800-525-2225; **Board Cert:** Surgery 2002; **Med School:** Cornell Univ-Weill Med Coll 1984; **Resid:** Surgery, NY Hosp-Cornell Med Ctr 1992; **Fellow:** Surgical Oncology, Meml Sloan-Kettering Cancer Ctr 1994; **Fac Appt:** Prof S, Cornell Univ-Weill Med Coll

Fraker, Douglas L MD [S] - **Spec Exp:** Melanoma; Endocrine Tumors; Liver Cancer; Sarcoma; **Hospital:** Hosp Univ Penn - UPHS (page 60); **Address:** Hosp Univ Penn, Dept Surgery, 3400 Spruce St, 4 Silverstein Pavilion, Philadelphia, PA 19104; **Phone:** 215-662-7866; **Board Cert:** Surgery 2002; **Med School:** Harvard Med Sch 1983; **Resid:** Surgery, UCSF Med Ctr 1986; Surgery, UCSF Med Ctr 1991; **Fellow:** Surgical Oncology, National Cancer Inst 1989; **Fac Appt:** Prof S, Univ Pennsylvania

Surgery

Frazier, Thomas G MD [S] - **Spec Exp:** Breast Cancer; Breast Disease; **Hospital:** Bryn Mawr Hosp; **Address:** 101 S Bryn Mawr Ave, Ste 201, Bryn Mawr, PA 19010; **Phone:** 610-520-0700; **Board Cert:** Surgery 2004; **Med School:** Univ Pennsylvania 1968; **Resid:** Surgery, Hosp Univ Penn 1975; **Fellow:** Surgical Oncology, MD Anderson Cancer Ctr 1976; **Fac Appt:** Clin Prof S, Drexel Univ Coll Med

Gibbs, John F MD [S] - **Spec Exp:** Liver Cancer; Liver & Biliary Surgery; Pancreatic Cancer; **Hospital:** Roswell Park Cancer Inst; **Address:** Roswell Park Cancer Inst, Dept Surg Onc, Elm & Carlton Streets, Buffalo, NY 14263-0001; **Phone:** 716-845-5807; **Board Cert:** Surgery 2000; **Med School:** UCSD 1985; **Resid:** Surgery, Rush Presby-St Lukes Med Ctr 1990; **Fellow:** Transplant Surgery, Baylor Univ Med Ctr 1992; Surgical Oncology, Roswell Park Cancer Inst 1996; **Fac Appt:** Assoc Prof S, SUNY Buffalo

Hanna, Nader N MD [S] - **Spec Exp:** Pancreatic Cancer; Adrenal Tumors; Peritoneal Carcinomatosis; Sarcoma-Soft Tissue; **Hospital:** Univ of MD Med Ctr; **Address:** Univ MD Med Sys, 22 S Greene St, Ste S4B-12, Baltimore, MD 21201; **Phone:** 410-328-7320; **Board Cert:** Surgery 2005; **Med School:** Egypt 1985; **Resid:** Surgery, St. Elizabeth's Med Ctr-Tuft's Univ 1994; **Fellow:** Surgical Oncology, Univ Chicago 1997; Research, Univ Chicago; **Fac Appt:** Assoc Prof Surg & Onc, Univ MD Sch Med

Hoffman, John P MD [S] - **Spec Exp:** Pancreatic Cancer; Gastrointestinal Cancer; Hepatobiliary Surgery; Liver Cancer; **Hospital:** Fox Chase Cancer Ctr (page 58); **Address:** Fox Chase Cancer Ctr, 333 Cottman Ave, Philadelphia, PA 19111-2497; **Phone:** 215-728-3518; **Board Cert:** Surgery 1998; **Med School:** Case West Res Univ 1970; **Resid:** Surgery, Virginia Mason Hosp 1977; **Fellow:** Surgical Oncology, Meml Sloan Kettering Cancer Ctr 1980; **Fac Appt:** Prof S, Temple Univ

Jarnagin, William MD [S] - **Spec Exp:** Hepatobiliary Surgery; Liver Cancer; Pancreatic Cancer; **Hospital:** Meml Sloan-Kettering Cancer Ctr; **Address:** 1275 York Ave, New York, NY 10065; **Phone:** 212-639-7601; **Board Cert:** Surgery 2006; **Med School:** Rush Med Coll 1988; **Resid:** Surgery, Univ Calif San Francisco 1996; **Fellow:** Hepatopancreatobiliary Surgery, Meml Sloan-Kettering Cancer Ctr 1997

Johnson, Ronald R MD [S] - **Spec Exp:** Breast Cancer; **Hospital:** Magee-Womens Hosp - UPMC; **Address:** Magee-Womens Hosp - UPMC, 300 Halket St, Ste 2601, Pittsburgh, PA 15213; **Phone:** 412-641-1225; **Board Cert:** Surgery 1999; **Med School:** Univ Pittsburgh 1983; **Resid:** Surgery, Univ Pittsburgh Med Ctr 1989; **Fac Appt:** Asst Prof S, Univ Pittsburgh

Julian, Thomas B MD [S] - **Spec Exp:** Breast Cancer & Surgery; Clinical Trials; **Hospital:** Allegheny General Hosp; **Address:** Allegheny Cancer Center, 320 E North Ave Fl 5, Pittsburgh, PA 15212; **Phone:** 412-359-8229; **Board Cert:** Surgery 2001; **Med School:** Univ Pittsburgh 1976; **Resid:** Surgery, Univ Pittsburgh Med Ctr 1982; **Fac Appt:** Assoc Prof S, Drexel Univ Coll Med

Kapur, Sandip MD [S] - **Spec Exp:** Transplant-Kidney; Islet Cell Transplant; Hepatobiliary Surgery; Transplant-Pancreas; **Hospital:** NY-Presby Hosp/Weill Cornell (page 66); **Address:** 520 E 68th St, Ste F1919, New York, NY 10065; **Phone:** 212-746-5330; **Board Cert:** Surgery 2007; **Med School:** Cornell Univ-Weill Med Coll 1990; **Resid:** Surgery, Cornell Univ Med Ctr 1996; **Fellow:** Research, The Rogosin Inst 1994; Transplant Surgery, Thomas E Starzl Transplant Inst 1998; **Fac Appt:** Assoc Prof S, Cornell Univ-Weill Med Coll

Karpeh Jr, Martin S MD [S] - **Spec Exp:** Gastrointestinal Cancer; Esophageal Cancer; Colon & Rectal Cancer; **Hospital:** Beth Israel Med Ctr - Petrie Division (page 57); **Address:** Beth Israel Med Ctr, Philips Ambulatory Ctr, 10 Union Square E, Ste 4C, New York, NY 10003; **Phone:** 212-420-4041; **Board Cert:** Surgery 1998; **Med School:** Penn State Univ-Hershey Med Ctr 1983; **Resid:** Surgery, Hosp Univ Penn 1989; **Fellow:** Surgical Oncology, Meml Sloan Kettering Cancer Ctr 1991; **Fac Appt:** Prof S, Mount Sinai Sch Med

Kato, Tomoaki MD [S] - **Spec Exp:** Transplant-Liver; Transplant Surgery-Pediatric; Transplant-Multi Organ; Transplant-Auto Transplantation; **Hospital:** NY-Presby Hosp/Columbia (page 66); **Address:** Columbia Univ Med Ctr, PH Bldg - rm 14-105, 622 W 168 St, New York, NY 10032; **Phone:** 212-305-8936; **Med School:** Japan 1991; **Resid:** Surgery, Itami City Hospital 1995; **Fellow:** Transplant Surgery, Jackson Meml Hosp 1997; **Fac Appt:** Asst Prof S, Columbia P&S

Kaufman, Howard L MD [S] - **Spec Exp:** Cancer Surgery; Vaccine Therapy; Melanoma; Immunotherapy; **Hospital:** Mount Sinai Med Ctr (page 64); **Address:** Mount Sinai Med Ctr, Dept Surgery, 5 E 98th St, Box 1259, New York, NY 10029; **Phone:** 212-241-4757; **Board Cert:** Surgery 2007; **Med School:** Loyola Univ-Stritch Sch Med 1986; **Resid:** Surgery, Boston Univ Hosp 1995; **Fellow:** Surgical Oncology, Natl Cancer Inst 1996; **Fac Appt:** Prof S, Mount Sinai Sch Med

Lee, Kenneth K W MD [S] - **Spec Exp:** Pancreatic Cancer; Gastrointestinal Cancer & Surgery; **Hospital:** UPMC Presby, Pittsburgh, UPMC Shadyside; **Address:** UPMC Presbyterian, 200 Lothrop St, Ste 497, Scaife Hall, Pittsburgh, PA 15261; **Phone:** 412-647-0457; **Board Cert:** Surgery 1998; **Med School:** Univ Chicago-Pritzker Sch Med 1981; **Resid:** Surgery, Univ Chicago Hosps 1988; **Fac Appt:** Assoc Prof S, Univ Pittsburgh

Lentz, Christopher W MD [S] - **Spec Exp:** Burn Care; Trauma; Critical Care; Wound Healing/Care; **Hospital:** Univ of Rochester Strong Meml Hosp; **Address:** Univ Rochester, Surgery Dept, 601 Elmwood Ave, Box SURG, Rochester, NY 14642; **Phone:** 585-275-2876; **Board Cert:** Surgery 2006; Surgical Critical Care 2006; **Med School:** Wayne State Univ 1988; **Resid:** Surgery, Med Coll Wisc 1994; **Fellow:** Surgical Critical Care, Shriners Burns Inst 1991; Burn Surgery, Univ N Carolina Med Ctr 1996; **Fac Appt:** Assoc Prof S, Univ Rochester

Libutti, Steven K MD [S] - **Spec Exp:** Liver Cancer; Pancreatic Cancer; Endocrine Tumors; Gastrointestinal Cancer; **Hospital:** Montefiore Med Ctr - Div. Moses, Montefiore Med Ctr - Div. Weiler; **Address:** 3400 Bainbridge Ave Fl 4th, Bronx, NY 10467; **Phone:** 718-920-4231; **Board Cert:** Surgery 2004; **Med School:** Columbia P&S 1990; **Resid:** Surgery, Columbia Presby Med Ctr 1995; **Fellow:** Surgical Oncology, Natl Cancer Inst 1996; **Fac Appt:** Prof S, Albert Einstein Coll Med

Marsh Jr, James W MD [S] - **Spec Exp:** Transplant-Liver; Liver Cancer; Pancreatic Cancer; **Hospital:** UPMC Presby, Pittsburgh; **Address:** UPMC, Starzl Transplant Inst, 3459 Fifth Ave 7 South, Pittsburgh, PA 15213; **Phone:** 412-647-5800; **Board Cert:** Surgery 2003; **Med School:** Univ Ark 1979; **Resid:** Surgery, St Paul Hosp 1984; **Fellow:** Transplant Surgery, Mayo Clin 1985; Transplant Surgery, Univ Pittsburgh Hosps 1986; **Fac Appt:** Prof S, Univ Pittsburgh

Meyers, William C MD [S] - **Spec Exp:** Hernia; Liver & Biliary Surgery; **Hospital:** Hahnemann Univ Hosp; **Address:** 245 N 15th St, MS 413, Philadelphia, PA 19102; **Phone:** 215-762-1078; **Board Cert:** Surgery 2004; **Med School:** Columbia P&S 1975; **Resid:** Surgery, Duke U Med Ctr 1983; Surgery, Duke U Med Ctr 1982; **Fellow:** Gastroenterology, Duke U Med Ctr 1983; **Fac Appt:** Prof S, Drexel Univ Coll Med

Michelassi, Fabrizio MD [S] - **Spec Exp:** Gastrointestinal Cancer; Crohn's Disease; Ulcerative Colitis; Colon Cancer; **Hospital:** NY-Presby Hosp/Weill Cornell (page 66); **Address:** Weill Cornell Med College, Surg Dept, 525 E 68th St, rm F-739, New York, NY 10021; **Phone:** 212-746-6006; **Board Cert:** Surgery 2002; **Med School:** Italy 1975; **Resid:** Surgery, NYU Med Ctr 1981; **Fellow:** Research, Mass Genl Hosp 1983; **Fac Appt:** Prof S, Cornell Univ-Weill Med Coll

Montgomery, Robert A MD/PhD [S] - **Spec Exp:** Transplant-Kidney; **Hospital:** Johns Hopkins Hosp (page 61); **Address:** Johns Hopkins Hosp, Transplant Surgery, 720 Rutland Ave Ross Bldg - Ste 765, Baltimore, MD 21205; **Phone:** 410-614-8297; **Board Cert:** Surgery 2006; **Med School:** Univ Rochester 1987; **Resid:** Surgery, Johns Hopkins Hosp 1995; **Fellow:** Transplant Surgery, Johns Hopkins Hosp 1997; **Fac Appt:** Assoc Prof S, Johns Hopkins Univ

Morrow, Monica MD [S] - **Spec Exp:** Breast Cancer; **Hospital:** Meml Sloan-Kettering Cancer Ctr; **Address:** 1275 York Avenue, New York, NY 10065; **Phone:** 800-525-2225; **Board Cert:** Surgery 2001; **Med School:** Jefferson Med Coll 1976; **Resid:** Surgery, Med Ctr Hosp Vermont 1981; **Fellow:** Surgical Oncology, Meml Sloan Kettering Cancer Ctr 1983; **Fac Appt:** Prof S, Cornell Univ-Weill Med Coll

Nava-Villarreal, Hector MD [S] - **Spec Exp:** Esophageal Cancer; Stomach Cancer; Barrett's Esophagus; **Hospital:** Roswell Park Cancer Inst; **Address:** Roswell Park Cancer Inst, Elm & Carlton Sts, Buffalo, NY 14263; **Phone:** 716-845-5915; **Board Cert:** Surgery 2001; **Med School:** Mexico 1967; **Resid:** Surgery, Buffalo Genl Hosp 1974; **Fellow:** Surgical Oncology, Roswell Park Cancer Inst 1976; **Fac Appt:** Assoc Prof S, SUNY Buffalo

Nowak, Eugene MD [S] - **Spec Exp:** Breast Cancer; Hernia; Gastrointestinal Surgery; Sentinel Node Surgery; **Hospital:** NY-Presby Hosp/Weill Cornell (page 66); **Address:** 325 E 79th St, New York, NY 10021-0954; **Phone:** 212-517-6693; **Board Cert:** Surgery 2002; **Med School:** UMDNJ-NJ Med Sch, Newark 1975; **Resid:** Surgery, NY Hosp-Cornell Med Ctr 1980; **Fac Appt:** Assoc Prof S, Cornell Univ-Weill Med Coll

O'Hea, Brian J MD [S] - **Spec Exp:** Breast Cancer; Sentinel Node Surgery; **Hospital:** Stony Brook Univ Med Ctr; **Address:** SUNY Stony Brook, Dept Surgery, HSC T-18, Rm 060, Stony Brook, NY 11794-8191; **Phone:** 631-444-1795; **Board Cert:** Surgery 2002; **Med School:** Georgetown Univ 1986; **Resid:** Surgery, St Vincent's Hosp 1991; **Fellow:** Breast Disease, Meml Sloan-Kettering Cancer Ctr 1996; **Fac Appt:** Asst Prof S, SUNY Stony Brook

Olthoff, Kim M MD [S] - **Spec Exp:** Transplant-Liver-Adult & Pediatric; Liver & Biliary Surgery; Liver Cancer; **Hospital:** Hosp Univ Penn - UPHS (page 60), Chldns Hosp of Philadelphia, The; **Address:** Hosp Univ Penn - Dept Surgery, 3400 Spruce St Dulles Bldg Fl 2, Philadelphia, PA 19104; **Phone:** 215-662-6136; **Board Cert:** Surgery 2003; **Med School:** Univ Chicago-Pritzker Sch Med 1986; **Resid:** Surgery, UCLA Med Ctr 1990; **Fellow:** Transplant Surgery, UCLA Med Ctr; **Fac Appt:** Prof S, Univ Pennsylvania

Osborne, Michael P MD [S] - **Spec Exp:** Breast Cancer; Breast Cancer-High Risk Women; Breast Disease; **Hospital:** Beth Israel Med Ctr - Petrie Division (page 57); **Address:** Philip Ambulatory Care Ctr, 10 Union Square E, Ste 4E, New York, NY 10003; **Phone:** 212-844-8770; **Med School:** England, UK 1970; **Resid:** Surgery, Charing Cross Hosp 1977; Surgery, Royal Marsden Hosp 1980; **Fellow:** Surgical Oncology, Meml Sloan-Kettering Canc Ctr 1981; **Fac Appt:** Prof S, Cornell Univ-Weill Med Coll

Pachter, H Leon MD [S] - **Spec Exp:** Adrenal Surgery; Gastrointestinal Surgery; Pancreatic Cancer; Hernia; **Hospital:** NYU Langone Med Ctr (page 67), Bellevue Hosp Ctr; **Address:** 530 1st Ave, Ste 6C, New York, NY 10016; **Phone:** 212-263-7302; **Board Cert:** Surgery 2000; **Med School:** NYU Sch Med 1971; **Resid:** Surgery, NYU Med Ctr 1976; **Fac Appt:** Prof S, NYU Sch Med

Park, Adrian E MD [S] - **Spec Exp:** Minimally Invasive Surgery; Gastrointestinal Surgery; Laparoscopic Surgery; **Hospital:** Univ of MD Med Ctr; **Address:** Univ Maryland Dept Surgery, 22 S Greene St, S4B14, Baltimore, MD 21201; **Phone:** 410-328-7994; **Board Cert:** Surgery 2005; **Med School:** McMaster Univ 1987; **Resid:** Surgery, MC Master Univ 1992; **Fellow:** Laparoscopic Surgery, Hotel Dieu de Montreal 1993; **Fac Appt:** Prof S, Univ MD Sch Med

Paty, Philip B MD [S] - **Spec Exp:** Colon & Rectal Cancer; Pelvic Tumors; Appendix Cancer; **Hospital:** Meml Sloan-Kettering Cancer Ctr; **Address:** 1275 York Avenue, New York, NY 10065; **Phone:** 800-525-2225; **Board Cert:** Surgery 2001; **Med School:** Stanford Univ 1983; **Resid:** Surgery, UCSF Med Ctr 1990; **Fellow:** Surgical Oncology, Meml Sloan Kettering Cancer Ctr 1992; **Fac Appt:** Prof S, Cornell Univ-Weill Med Coll

Peitzman, Andrew B MD [S] - **Spec Exp:** Trauma; **Hospital:** UPMC Presby, Pittsburgh, UPMC Shadyside; **Address:** Presbyterian Univ Hosp, Dept Surg - F 1281, 200 Lothrop St, Pittsburgh, PA 15213; **Phone:** 412-647-0635; **Board Cert:** Surgery 2004; Surgical Critical Care 1997; **Med School:** Univ Pittsburgh 1976; **Resid:** Surgery, Univ Pittsburgh Med Ctr 1979; Surgery, Univ Pittsburgh Med Ctr 1984; **Fellow:** Surgery, NY Hosp-Cornell Univ 1981; **Fac Appt:** Prof S, Univ Pittsburgh

Peters, Jeffrey H MD [S] - **Spec Exp:** Esophageal Surgery; Gastroesophageal Reflux Disease (GERD); **Hospital:** Univ of Rochester Strong Meml Hosp; **Address:** 601 Elmwood Ave, Box SURG, Rochester, NY 14642-8410; **Phone:** 585-275-2725; **Board Cert:** Surgery 2007; **Med School:** Ohio State Univ 1981; **Resid:** Surgery, Johns Hopkins Hosp 1988; **Fellow:** Allergy & Immunology, Johns Hopkins Hosp 1985; Esophageal Surgery, Creighton Univ; **Fac Appt:** Prof S, Univ Rochester

Petrelli, Nicholas J MD [S] - **Spec Exp:** Cancer Surgery; Gastrointestinal Cancer; Colon & Rectal Cancer; **Hospital:** Christiana Care Hlth Svs; **Address:** Helen F Graham Cancer Ctr, 4701 Ogletown-Stanton Rd, Ste 1213, Newark, DE 19713; **Phone:** 302-623-4550; **Board Cert:** Surgery 1997; **Med School:** Tulane Univ 1973; **Resid:** Surgery, St Mary's Hosp-Med Ctr 1978; **Fellow:** Surgical Oncology, Roswell Park Cancer Inst 1980; **Fac Appt:** Prof S, Thomas Jefferson Univ

Pomp, Alfons MD [S] - **Spec Exp:** Obesity/Bariatric Surgery; Laparoscopic Abdominal Surgery; Hernia; **Hospital:** NY-Presby Hosp/Weill Cornell (page 66); **Address:** Weill Cornell College of Medicine, 525 E 68th St, Box 294, New York, NY 10021; **Phone:** 212-746-5294; **Board Cert:** Surgery 1999; **Med School:** Univ Sherbrooke 1980; **Resid:** Surgery, Univ Montreal Med Ctr 1985; **Fellow:** Nutrition, Rhode Island Hosp 1988; **Fac Appt:** Prof S, Cornell Univ-Weill Med Coll

Ramanathan, Ramesh Chandran MD [S] - **Spec Exp:** Obesity/Bariatric Surgery; Minimally Invasive Surgery; Colon Cancer; Clinical Trials; **Hospital:** Magee-Womens Hosp - UPMC, UPMC Presby, Pittsburgh; **Address:** 3380 Boulevard of the Allies, Ste 390, Pittsburgh, PA 15213; **Phone:** 412-641-3668; **Board Cert:** Surgery 2004; **Med School:** India 1988; **Resid:** Surgery, Univ Pitt Med Ctr 2003; **Fellow:** Surgical Oncology, Univ Pitt Med Ctr 1999; Minimally Invasive Surgery, Univ Pitt Med Ctr 2000; **Fac Appt:** Asst Prof S, Univ Pittsburgh

Reich, David MD [S] - **Spec Exp:** Transplant-Liver; Hepatobiliary Surgery; Liver Cancer; **Hospital:** Hahnemann Univ Hosp; **Address:** 216 N Broad St Fl 5, Philadelphia, PA 19102; **Phone:** 215-762-8153; **Board Cert:** Surgery 2003; **Med School:** McGill Univ 1989; **Resid:** Surgery, Beth Israel Med Ctr 1994; **Fellow:** Hepatobiliary Surgery, Mt Sinai Med Ctr 1996

Reiner, Mark MD [S] - **Spec Exp:** Laparoscopic Surgery; Hernia; Esophageal Surgery; Pancreatic Surgery; **Hospital:** Mount Sinai Med Ctr (page 64); **Address:** 1010 5th Ave, New York, NY 10028-0130; **Phone:** 212-879-6677; **Board Cert:** Surgery 2001; **Med School:** SUNY Downstate 1974; **Resid:** Surgery, Mt Sinai Hosp 1979; **Fac Appt:** Clin Prof S, Mount Sinai Sch Med

Ridge, John Andrew MD/PhD [S] - **Spec Exp:** Head & Neck Cancer & Surgery; Thyroid Cancer & Surgery; Laryngeal Cancer; **Hospital:** Fox Chase Cancer Ctr (page 58); **Address:** Fox Chase Cancer Ctr, Dept Surgical Oncology, 333 Cottman Ave, Philadelphia, PA 19111; **Phone:** 215-728-3517; **Board Cert:** Surgery 2006; **Med School:** Stanford Univ 1981; **Resid:** Surgery, Univ Colorado Med Ctr 1987; **Fellow:** Surgical Oncology, Meml Sloan-Kettering Cancer Ctr 1989

Roh, Mark S MD [S] - **Spec Exp:** Liver Cancer; Cancer Surgery; **Hospital:** Allegheny General Hosp; **Address:** Allegheny General Hospital, Dept Surgery, 320 E North Ave, Pittsburgh, PA 15212; **Phone:** 412-359-6738; **Board Cert:** Surgery 2006; **Med School:** Ohio State Univ 1979; **Resid:** Surgery, Univ Pittsburgh Med Ctr 1982; Surgery, Univ Pittsburgh Med Ctr 1986; **Fellow:** Surgical Oncology, Meml Sloan-Kettering Cancer Ctr 1984; Surgical Oncology, Meml Sloan-Kettering Cancer Ctr 1987; **Fac Appt:** Prof S, Drexel Univ Coll Med

Rosato, Ernest F MD [S] - **Spec Exp:** Gastrointestinal Cancer & Surgery; Esophageal Cancer; Pancreatic Cancer; **Hospital:** Hosp Univ Penn - UPHS (page 60); **Address:** Hosp Univ Penn, Dept Surg, 3400 Spruce St, 4 Silverstein, Philadelphia, PA 19104; **Phone:** 215-662-2033; **Board Cert:** Surgery 1969; **Med School:** Univ Pennsylvania 1962; **Resid:** Surgery, Hosp Univ Penn 1968; **Fac Appt:** Prof S, Univ Pennsylvania

Rosenberg, Steven A MD [S] - **Spec Exp:** Melanoma; Kidney Cancer; **Hospital:** Natl Inst of Hlth - Clin Ctr; **Address:** National Cancer Institute, 9000 Rockville Pike CRC Bldg, rm 3W-3940, Bethesda, MD 20892; **Phone:** 301-496-4164; **Board Cert:** Surgery 1975; **Med School:** Johns Hopkins Univ 1964; **Resid:** Surgery, Peter Bent Brigham Hosp 1974

Roses, Daniel F MD [S] - **Spec Exp:** Breast Cancer; Melanoma; Thyroid Cancer; Parathyroid Surgery; **Hospital:** NYU Langone Med Ctr (page 67); **Address:** 530 First Ave, Ste 6B, New York, NY 10016-6402; **Phone:** 212-263-7329; **Board Cert:** Surgery 1975; **Med School:** NYU Sch Med 1969; **Resid:** Surgery, NYU-Bellevue Hosp 1974; **Fellow:** Surgical Oncology, NYU-Bellevue Hosp 1978; **Fac Appt:** Prof Surg & Onc, NYU Sch Med

Rubino, Francesco MD [S] - **Spec Exp:** Gastrointestinal Metabolic Surgery; Diabetes Surgery-Rubino's Procedure; Obesity/Bariatric Surgery; **Hospital:** NY-Presby Hosp/Weill Cornell (page 66); **Address:** NY Presbyterian Hosp/Weill Cornell, 525 E 68th St, rm P714, New York, NY 10065; **Phone:** 212-746-5925; **Med School:** Italy 1994; **Resid:** Surgery, Catholic Univ/Policlinico Gemelli; **Fellow:** Laparoscopic Surgery, European Inst of Telesurgery; Research, Catholic Univ; **Fac Appt:** Asst Prof S, Cornell Univ-Weill Med Coll

Salky, Barry A MD [S] - **Spec Exp:** Laparoscopic Abdominal Surgery; Gastroesophageal Reflux Disease (GERD); Colon Cancer; Ulcerative Colitis; **Hospital:** Mount Sinai Med Ctr (page 64); **Address:** Mt Sinai Medical Center, Div of Laparoscopic Surgery, 5 E 98th St, Box 1259, New York, NY 10029; **Phone:** 212-241-6156; **Board Cert:** Surgery 1998; **Med School:** Univ Tenn Coll Med, Memphis 1970; **Resid:** Surgery, Mount Sinai Hosp 1973; Surgery, Mount Sinai Hosp 1978; **Fac Appt:** Prof S, Mount Sinai Sch Med

Scantlebury, Velma P MD [S] - **Spec Exp:** Transplant-Kidney; Kidney Disease; **Hospital:** Christiana Care Hlth Svs; **Address:** 4735 Ogletown-Stanton Rd, Med Arts Pavilion II, Ste 2224, Newark, DE 19713; **Phone:** 302-623-3866; **Board Cert:** Surgery 2001; **Med School:** Columbia P&S 1981; **Resid:** Surgery, Harlem Hosp 1986; **Fellow:** Transplant Surgery, Univ Pittsburgh Med Ctr 1988

Schnabel, Freya MD [S] - **Spec Exp:** Breast Cancer; Breast Cancer-High Risk Women; **Hospital:** NYU Langone Med Ctr (page 67); **Address:** 160 E 34th St Fl 3, New York, NY 10016; **Phone:** 212-731-5367; **Board Cert:** Surgery 1998; **Med School:** NYU Sch Med 1982; **Resid:** Surgery, NYU Med Ctr 1987; **Fellow:** Research, SUNY Hlth Sci Ctr 1988; **Fac Appt:** Prof S, NYU Sch Med

Schraut, Wolfgang H MD [S] - **Spec Exp:** Inflammatory Bowel Disease; Gastrointestinal Surgery; Colon & Rectal Cancer & Surgery; Laparoscopic Surgery; **Hospital:** UPMC Presby, Pittsburgh, Magee-Womens Hosp - UPMC; **Address:** Univ Pittsburgh Med Ctr, Dept Surgery, 200 Lothrop St, Ste 497, Scaife Hall, Pittsburgh, PA 15261; **Phone:** 412-647-0457; **Board Cert:** Surgery 1999; **Med School:** Germany 1970; **Resid:** Surgery, Univ Chicago Hosps 1978; **Fac Appt:** Prof S, Univ Pittsburgh

Schulick, Richard D MD [S] - **Spec Exp:** Liver Cancer; Biliary Cancer; Pancreatic Cancer; Adrenal Tumors; **Hospital:** Johns Hopkins Hosp (page 61); **Address:** Johns Hopkins Hosp-Dept Surgery, 600 N Wolfe St, Blalock 685, Baltimore, MD 21287; **Phone:** 410-614-9879; **Board Cert:** Surgery 2007; **Med School:** Johns Hopkins Univ 1989; **Resid:** Surgery, Johns Hopkins Hosp 1994; **Fellow:** Clinical Pharmacology, NIH 1995; Thyroid Oncology, Maml Sloan Kettering Cancer Ctr 1996; **Fac Appt:** Prof Surg & Onc, Johns Hopkins Univ

America's Top Doctors® 9th Edition

Shah, Jatin P MD/PhD [S] - **Spec Exp:** Head & Neck Cancer & Surgery; Thyroid Cancer & Surgery; Skull Base Tumors; Salivary Gland Tumors & Surgery; **Hospital:** Meml Sloan-Kettering Cancer Ctr; **Address:** 1275 York Avenue, New York, NY 10065; **Phone:** 800-525-2225; **Board Cert:** Surgery 1975; **Med School:** India 1964; **Resid:** Surgery, SSG Hosp 1967; Surgery, NY Eye & Ear Infirm 1974; **Fellow:** Head & Neck Surgical Oncology, Meml Sloan-Kettering Hosp 1972; **Fac Appt:** Prof S, Cornell Univ-Weill Med Coll

Shapiro, Ron MD [S] - **Spec Exp:** Transplant-Kidney; Transplant-Pancreas; Islet Cell Transplant; **Hospital:** UPMC Presby, Pittsburgh, Chldns Hosp of Pittsburgh - UPMC; **Address:** Starzl Transplantation Inst, UPMC Montefiore - 7 South, 3459 Fifth Ave, Pittsburgh, PA 15213-2582; **Phone:** 412-647-5800; **Board Cert:** Surgery 2005; **Med School:** Stanford Univ 1980; **Resid:** Surgery, Mt Sinai Hosp 1986; **Fellow:** Transplant Surgery, Univ Pittsburgh 1988; **Fac Appt:** Prof S, Univ Pittsburgh

Sigurdson, Elin R MD [S] - **Spec Exp:** Breast Cancer; Colon & Rectal Cancer; Melanoma; Gastrointestinal Cancer; **Hospital:** Fox Chase Cancer Ctr (page 58); **Address:** 333 Cottman Ave, Philadelphia, PA 19111-2412; **Phone:** 215-728-3519; **Board Cert:** Surgery 2006; **Med School:** Canada 1980; **Resid:** Surgery, Univ Toronto Med Ctr 1984; **Fellow:** Surgical Oncology, Meml Sloan-Kettering Cancer Ctr 1987; **Fac Appt:** Assoc Prof S

Singer, Samuel MD [S] - **Spec Exp:** Sarcoma-Soft Tissue; **Hospital:** Meml Sloan-Kettering Cancer Ctr; **Address:** 1275 York Avenue, New York, NY 10065; **Phone:** 800-525-2225; **Board Cert:** Surgery 1998; **Med School:** Harvard Med Sch 1982; **Resid:** Surgery, Brigham & Women's Hosp 1988; **Fellow:** Surgical Oncology, Dana Farber Cancer Inst 1990; **Fac Appt:** Assoc Prof S, Cornell Univ-Weill Med Coll

Skinner, Kristin A MD [S] - **Spec Exp:** Breast Cancer; Gastrointestinal Cancer; Melanoma; **Hospital:** Univ of Rochester Strong Meml Hosp; **Address:** Univ Rochester Med Ctr, 601 Elmwood Ave, Box SURG, Rochester, NY 14642; **Phone:** 585-276-3332; **Board Cert:** Surgery 2005; **Med School:** Johns Hopkins Univ 1988; **Resid:** Surgery, UCLA Med Ctr 1995; **Fellow:** Surgical Oncology, UCLA Med Ctr 1994; **Fac Appt:** Assoc Prof S, Univ Rochester

Sugarbaker, Paul H MD [S] - **Spec Exp:** Appendix Cancer; Peritoneal Carcinomatosis; Cystadenocarcinoma; Ovarian Cancer; **Hospital:** Washington Hosp Ctr; **Address:** Washington Hosp Ctr, 106 Irving St NW, Ste 3900N, Washington, DC 20010; **Phone:** 202-877-3908; **Board Cert:** Surgery 1973; **Med School:** Cornell Univ-Weill Med Coll 1967; **Resid:** Surgery, Peter Bent Brigham Hosp 1973; **Fellow:** Surgical Oncology, Mass Genl Hosp 1976; **Fac Appt:** Prof S, Univ Wash

Sundaram, Magesh MD [S] - **Spec Exp:** Gastrointestinal Cancer & Surgery; Pancreatic Cancer; Stomach Cancer; Liver & Biliary Cancer; **Hospital:** WV Univ Hosp - Ruby Memorial; **Address:** WV Univ Hosp-Dept Surgery, P.O. BOX 9238, 6309 HSC, Morgantown, WV 26506; **Phone:** 304-293-7095; **Board Cert:** Surgery 2006; **Med School:** Univ MD Sch Med 1990; **Resid:** Surgery, Delaware Med Ctr 1995; **Fellow:** Surgical Oncology, Jackson Meml Hosp 1997; **Fac Appt:** Assoc Prof Surg & Onc, W VA Univ

Swistel, Alexander J MD [S] - **Spec Exp:** Breast Cancer; Breast Disease; Sentinel Node Surgery; **Hospital:** NY-Presby Hosp/Weill Cornell (page 66), St Luke's - Roosevelt Hosp Ctr - Roosevelt Div (page 57); **Address:** 425 E 61st St Fl 10, New York, NY 10021; **Phone:** 212-821-0602; **Board Cert:** Surgery 2005; **Med School:** Brown Univ 1975; **Resid:** Surgery, St Luke's Roosevelt Hosp Ctr 1981; **Fellow:** Surgical Oncology, Meml Sloan Kettering Canc Ctr 1983; **Fac Appt:** Asst Prof S, Cornell Univ-Weill Med Coll

Tafra, Lorraine MD [S] - **Spec Exp:** Breast Cancer; **Hospital:** Anne Arundel Med Ctr; **Address:** 2002 Medical Parkway, Ste 120, Annapolis, MD 21401; **Phone:** 443-481-5300; **Board Cert:** Surgery 2005; **Med School:** Case West Res Univ 1986; **Resid:** Surgery, Rhode Island Hosp 1988; Surgery, Hosp Univ Penn 1992; **Fellow:** Surgical Oncology, John Wayne Cancer Inst 1994

Tartter, Paul MD [S] - **Spec Exp:** Breast Cancer; Breast Cancer in Elderly; Sentinel Node Surgery; **Hospital:** St Luke's - Roosevelt Hosp Ctr - Roosevelt Div (page 57), Mount Sinai Med Ctr (page 64); **Address:** 425 W 59th St, Ste 7A, New York, NY 10019-1104; **Phone:** 212-523-7500; **Board Cert:** Surgery 2003; **Med School:** Brown Univ 1977; **Resid:** Surgery, Mt Sinai Hosp 1982; **Fac Appt:** Assoc Prof S, Columbia P&S

Teperman, Lewis W MD [S] - **Spec Exp:** Transplant-Liver; Transplant-Kidney; Liver Tumors; **Hospital:** NYU Langone Med Ctr (page 67); **Address:** 403 E 34th St Fl 3, Transplant Assocs, New York, NY 10016; **Phone:** 212-263-8134; **Board Cert:** Surgery 1997; **Med School:** Mount Sinai Sch Med 1981; **Resid:** Surgery, Columbia Presby Med Ctr 1984; Surgery, LI Jewish Med Ctr 1986; **Fellow:** Transplant Surgery, Univ Pittsburgh 1988; **Fac Appt:** Assoc Prof S, NYU Sch Med

Tsangaris, Theodore N MD [S] - **Spec Exp:** Breast Cancer; **Hospital:** Johns Hopkins Hosp (page 61); **Address:** Johns Hopkins Hospital, 600 N Wolfe St, Carnegie 686, Baltimore, MD 21287; **Phone:** 410-955-2615; **Board Cert:** Surgery 2005; **Med School:** Geo Wash Univ 1983; **Resid:** Surgery, Geo Washington Univ Med Ctr 1989; **Fellow:** Surgical Oncology, Baylor Univ Med Ctr 1990; **Fac Appt:** Assoc Prof S, Johns Hopkins Univ

Willey, Shawna C MD [S] - **Spec Exp:** Breast Cancer; Clinical Trials; **Hospital:** Georgetown Univ Hosp; **Address:** 3800 Reservoir Rd NW, PHC Bldg Fl 4, Washington, DC 20007; **Phone:** 202-444-0241; **Board Cert:** Surgery 1998; **Med School:** Univ Iowa Coll Med 1982; **Resid:** Surgery, George Washington Univ Med Ctr 1988; **Fac Appt:** Asst Prof S, Georgetown Univ

Yang, James C MD [S] - **Spec Exp:** Kidney Cancer; Kidney Cancer Clinical Trials; Clinical Trials; Immunotherapy; **Hospital:** Natl Inst of Hlth - Clin Ctr; **Address:** National Cancer Institute, 9000 Rockville Pike CRC Bldg - rm 3-5952, Bethesda, MD 20892; **Phone:** 301-496-1574; **Board Cert:** Surgery 2005; **Med School:** UCSD 1978; **Resid:** Surgery, UCSD Med Ctr 1984; **Fellow:** Surgical Oncology, Natl Cancer Inst 1986

Yeo, Charles J MD [S] - **Spec Exp:** Pancreatic Cancer; Biliary Cancer; **Hospital:** Thomas Jefferson Univ Hosp; **Address:** 1015 Walnut St, Ste 620, Philadelphia, PA 19107; **Phone:** 215-955-9402; **Board Cert:** Surgery 2005; **Med School:** Johns Hopkins Univ 1979; **Resid:** Surgery, Johns Hopkins Hosp 1985; **Fellow:** Research, SUNY Downstate 1982; **Fac Appt:** Prof S, Thomas Jefferson Univ

Yurt, Roger W MD [S] - **Spec Exp:** Burn Care; Wound Healing/Care; Hyperbaric Medicine; **Hospital:** NY-Presby Hosp/Weill Cornell (page 66); **Address:** 525 E 68th St, rm L706, New York, NY 10021-4885; **Phone:** 212-746-5410; **Board Cert:** Surgery 1999; **Med School:** Univ Miami Sch Med 1972; **Resid:** Surgery, Parkland Meml Hosp 1974; Surgery, New York Hosp-Cornell Med Ctr 1980; **Fellow:** Internal Medicine, Brigham & Womens Hosp 1978; **Fac Appt:** Prof S, Cornell Univ-Weill Med Coll

Southeast

Adams, Reid B MD [S] - **Spec Exp:** Hepatobiliary Surgery; Liver Cancer; Pancreatic & Biliary Surgery; **Hospital:** Univ Virginia Med Ctr; **Address:** UVA Health System, Dept Surgery, PO Box 800709, Charlottesville, VA 22908; **Phone:** 434-924-2839; **Board Cert:** Surgery 2003; **Med School:** Univ VA Sch Med 1987; **Resid:** Surgery, Univ Va Hlth Sci Ctr 1994; **Fellow:** Hepatopancreatobiliary Surgery, Univ Toronto Med Ctr 1995; **Fac Appt:** Assoc Prof S, Univ VA Sch Med

Albertson, David A MD [S] - **Spec Exp:** Endocrine Surgery; **Hospital:** Wake Forest Univ Baptist Med Ctr (page 72); **Address:** Wake Forest Univ Sch Med, Dept Surgery, Medical Center Blvd, Winston-Salem, NC 27157-1095; **Phone:** 336-716-0664; **Board Cert:** Surgery 2007; **Med School:** Univ VA Sch Med 1972; **Resid:** Surgery, NC Bapt Hosp 1977; **Fellow:** Endocrine Surgery, Boston Univ 1978; **Fac Appt:** Assoc Prof S, Wake Forest Univ

Bear, Harry D MD/PhD [S] - **Spec Exp:** Breast Cancer; Melanoma; Gastrointestinal Cancer; **Hospital:** Med Coll of VA Hosp; **Address:** Med Coll Virginia - VCU, PO Box 980011, Richmond, VA 23298; **Phone:** 804-828-9325; **Board Cert:** Surgery 2003; **Med School:** Med Coll VA 1975; **Resid:** Surgery, Brigham & Women's Hosp 1983; **Fellow:** Surgical Oncology, Med Coll Virgina 1984; **Fac Appt:** Prof Surg & Onc, Med Coll VA

Beauchamp, Robert D MD [S] - **Spec Exp:** Breast Cancer; Colon & Rectal Cancer; Pancreatic Cancer; **Hospital:** Vanderbilt Univ Med Ctr; **Address:** Medical Center North, rm D4316, 1161 21st Ave S, Nashville, TN 37232; **Phone:** 615-322-2363; **Board Cert:** Surgery 2007; **Med School:** Univ Tex Med Br, Galveston 1982; **Resid:** Surgery, Univ Tex Med Br 1987; **Fellow:** Cellular Molecular Biology, Vanderbilt Univ 1989; **Fac Appt:** Prof S, Vanderbilt Univ

Behrns, Kevin E MD [S] - **Spec Exp:** Pancreatic Cancer; Gastrointestinal Cancer & Surgery; **Hospital:** Shands at Univ of FL; **Address:** Shands Healthcare at Univ Florida, PO Box 100286, Gainesville, FL 32610-0286; **Phone:** 352-265-0761; **Board Cert:** Surgery 2005; **Med School:** Mayo Med Sch 1988; **Resid:** Surgery, Mayo Clinic 1995; **Fac Appt:** Prof S, Univ Fla Coll Med

Bland, Kirby MD [S] - **Spec Exp:** Breast Cancer; Colon Cancer; Thyroid & Parathyroid Cancer & Surgery; **Hospital:** Univ of Ala Hosp at Birmingham; **Address:** UAB, Dept Surgery, 1530 3rd Ave S, BDB 502, Birmingham, AL 35294-0002; **Phone:** 205-975-2193; **Board Cert:** Surgery 2000; **Med School:** Univ Alabama 1968; **Resid:** Surgery, Univ Fla Hosp 1970; Surgery, Univ Fla Hosp 1976; **Fellow:** Surgical Oncology, MD Anderson Cancer Ctr 1977; **Fac Appt:** Prof S, Univ Alabama

Britt, L D MD [S] - **Spec Exp:** Trauma; Head Injury; **Hospital:** Sentara Norfolk Genl Hosp; **Address:** Eastern Virginia Med Sch, Dept Surgery, 825 Fairfax Ave, Ste 610, Norfolk, VA 23507; **Phone:** 757-446-8950; **Board Cert:** Surgery 2003; Surgical Critical Care 2006; **Med School:** Harvard Med Sch 1977; **Resid:** Surgery, Barnes Hosp-Wash Univ 1979; Surgery, Univ Illinois Chicago Med Ctr 1984; **Fellow:** Trauma, Md Inst Emer Med Serv Sys 1986; **Fac Appt:** Prof S, Eastern VA Med Sch

Buchman, Timothy G MD/PhD [S] - **Spec Exp:** Critical Care; Pilonidal Disease; Wound Healing/Care; Sepsis; **Hospital:** Emory Univ Hosp; **Address:** Director, Emory Ctr for Crtical Care, 1364 Clifton Rd NE, Ste F524, Atlanta, GA 30322; **Phone:** 404-712-2609; **Board Cert:** Surgery 2004; Surgical Critical Care 2005; **Med School:** Univ Chicago-Pritzker Sch Med 1980; **Resid:** Surgery, Johns Hopkins Hosp 1985; **Fellow:** Trauma, Maryland Inst for Emergency Med 1987; **Fac Appt:** Prof S, Emory Univ

Calvo, Benjamin MD [S] - **Spec Exp:** Colon Cancer; Endocrine Cancers; Breast Cancer; **Hospital:** Univ NC Hosps; **Address:** Dept Surg CB 7213, Chapel Hill, NC 27599; **Phone:** 919-966-5221; **Board Cert:** Surgery 1999; **Med School:** Univ MD Sch Med 1981; **Resid:** Surgery, G Washington Univ Hosp 1988; Surgery, Natl Inst Hlth 1991; **Fellow:** Surgery, Meml Sloan Kettering Cancer Ctr 1993; **Fac Appt:** Assoc Prof S, Univ NC Sch Med

Chari, Ravi S MD [S] - **Spec Exp:** Liver Cancer; Biliary Cancer; Transplant-Liver; **Hospital:** Centennial Med Ctr, Vanderbilt Univ Med Ctr; **Address:** Centennial Med Ctr, 2300 Patterson St, Nashville, TN 37203; **Phone:** 615-936-2573; **Board Cert:** Surgery 2005; **Med School:** Canada 1989; **Resid:** Surgery, Duke Univ Med Ctr 1996; **Fellow:** Transplant Surgery, Univ Toronto-Toronto Hosp 1998; **Fac Appt:** Prof S, Vanderbilt Univ

Cole, David J MD [S] - **Spec Exp:** Breast Brachytherapy; Gastrointestinal Cancer; Vaccine Therapy; Gene Therapy; **Hospital:** MUSC Med Ctr; **Address:** 96 Jonathan Lucas St, PO BOX 250613, Charleston, SC 29425; **Phone:** 843-792-4638; **Board Cert:** Surgery 2000; **Med School:** Cornell Univ-Weill Med Coll 1986; **Resid:** Surgery, Emory Univ Affil Hosp 1991; **Fellow:** Surgical Oncology, Natl Cancer Institute 1994; **Fac Appt:** Prof S, Med Univ SC

Dilawari, Raza A MD [S] - **Spec Exp:** Liver & Biliary Cancer; Melanoma; Skin Cancer; Breast Cancer; **Hospital:** Methodist Univ Hosp - Memphis, St Francis Hosp - Memphis; **Address:** Methodist Univ Hosp, 1325 Eastmoreland Ave, Ste 410, Memphis, TN 38104; **Phone:** 901-725-1921; **Board Cert:** Surgery 1975; **Med School:** Pakistan 1968; **Resid:** Surgery, SUNY-Upstate Med Ctr 1974; **Fellow:** Surgical Oncology, Roswell Park Meml Hosp 1976; **Fac Appt:** Prof S, Univ Tenn Coll Med, Memphis

Eason, James MD [S] - **Spec Exp:** Transplant-Kidney; Transplant-Pancreas & Liver; Liver Cancer; **Hospital:** Methodist Univ Hosp - Memphis; **Address:** Transplant Inst, 1265 Union Ave, rm S1011, Memphis, TN 38104; **Phone:** 866-805-7710; **Board Cert:** Surgery 2002; **Med School:** Univ Tenn Coll Med, Memphis 1987; **Resid:** Surgery, Wilford Hall USAF Med Ctr 1992; **Fellow:** Transplant Surgery, Mass Genl Hosp 1994; **Fac Appt:** Prof S, Univ Tenn Coll Med, Memphis

Eckhoff, Devin E MD [S] - **Spec Exp:** Transplant-Liver; Hepatobiliary Surgery; Transplant-Kidney; Hepatitis C; **Hospital:** Univ of Ala Hosp at Birmingham; **Address:** University of Alabama School of Medicine, 701 S 19th St LHRB Bldg - rm 710, Birmingham, AL 35294-0007; **Phone:** 205-975-7622; **Board Cert:** Surgery 2000; Surgical Critical Care 2001; **Med School:** Univ Minn 1986; **Resid:** Surgery, Univ Wisconsin Med Ctr 1992; **Fellow:** Transplant Surgery, Univ Wisconsin Med Ctr 1994; **Fac Appt:** Prof S, Univ Alabama

Feliciano, David V MD [S] - **Spec Exp:** Vascular Surgery; Trauma; **Hospital:** Grady Hlth Sys; **Address:** Emory Univ Dept Surgery, 69 Jesse Hill Jr Dr SE, rm 304, Atlanta, GA 30303; **Phone:** 404-616-5456; **Board Cert:** Surgery 1998; Surgical Critical Care 1998; **Med School:** Georgetown Univ 1970; **Resid:** Surgery, Mayo Clinic 1977; **Fellow:** Cardiovascular Surgery, Texas Med Ctr/Baylor 1978; **Fac Appt:** Prof S, Emory Univ

Flynn, Michael B MD [S] - **Spec Exp:** Head & Neck Cancer; Head & Neck Surgery; **Hospital:** Univ of Louisville Hosp, Norton Hosp; **Address:** 401 E Chestnut St, Ste 710, Louisville, KY 40202; **Phone:** 502-583-8303; **Board Cert:** Surgery 1972; **Med School:** Ireland 1962; **Resid:** Surgery, Univ Maryland Hosp 1969; **Fellow:** Surgical Oncology, MD Anderson Hosp 1971; **Fac Appt:** Prof S, Univ Louisville Sch Med

Gabram, Sheryl G A MD [S] - **Spec Exp:** Breast Cancer; Breast Cancer-High Risk Women; Breast Disease; **Hospital:** Emory Univ Hosp, Grady Hlth Sys; **Address:** Winship Cancer Institute, 1365 Clifton Rd NE C Bldg Fl 2, Atlanta, GA 30322; **Phone:** 404-778-1230; **Board Cert:** Surgery 2006; **Med School:** Georgetown Univ 1982; **Resid:** Surgery, Washington Hosp Ctr 1987; **Fellow:** Trauma, Hartford Hosp 1988; **Fac Appt:** Prof S, Emory Univ

Gagner, Michel MD [S] - **Spec Exp:** Obesity/Bariatric Surgery; Adrenal Surgery; Pancreatic Surgery; Diabetes Surgery-Rubino's Procedure; **Hospital:** Mount Sinai Med Ctr - Miami; **Address:** 4775 Collins Ave, Ste 2003, aMiami Beach, FL 33140; **Phone:** 305-336-5704; **Board Cert:** Surgery 2003; **Med School:** Canada 1982; **Resid:** Surgery, Royal Victoria Hosp/McGill 1988; **Fellow:** Hepatobiliary Surgery, Hosp Paul-Brousse 1989; Hepatobiliary Surgery, Lahey Clinic 1990; **Fac Appt:** Prof S, FIU Coll Med

Goldstein, Richard E MD/PhD [S] - **Spec Exp:** Endocrine Tumors; Thyroid Cancer & Surgery; Parathyroid Cancer; Parathyroid Surgery; **Hospital:** Univ of Louisville Hosp; **Address:** University Surgical Assocs, 401 E Chestnut St, Ste 710, Louisville, KY 40202; **Phone:** 502-583-8303; **Board Cert:** Surgery 1999; **Med School:** Jefferson Med Coll 1982; **Resid:** Surgery, Vanderbilt Univ Hosp 1990; **Fac Appt:** Prof S, Univ Louisville Sch Med

Greene, Frederick L MD [S] - **Spec Exp:** Gastrointestinal Surgery; Gastrointestinal Cancer; Hernia; **Hospital:** Carolinas Med Ctr; **Address:** Carolinas Medical Ctr, 1025 Morehead Medical Drive, Ste 275, Charlotte, NC 28203; **Phone:** 704-355-1813; **Board Cert:** Surgery 1998; **Med School:** Univ VA Sch Med 1970; **Resid:** Surgery, Yale-New Haven Hosp 1976; **Fellow:** Surgical Oncology, Yale-New Haven Hosp 1973; **Fac Appt:** Prof S, Univ NC Sch Med

Hanks, John B MD [S] - **Spec Exp:** Endocrine Cancers; Breast Cancer; Thyroid Cancer & Surgery; Endocrine Surgery; **Hospital:** Univ Virginia Med Ctr; **Address:** Univ VA Hlth Sys, Dept Surgery, PO Box 800709, Charlottesville, VA 22908-0709; **Phone:** 434-924-0376; **Board Cert:** Surgery 2001; **Med School:** Univ Rochester 1973; **Resid:** Surgery, Duke Univ Med Ctr 1982; **Fac Appt:** Prof S, Univ VA Sch Med

Herrmann, Virginia M MD [S] - **Spec Exp:** Breast Cancer; Nutrition & Cancer Prevention/Control; **Hospital:** Hilton Head Reg Med Ctr, MUSC Med Ctr; **Address:** Hilton Head Reg Med Ctr, 25 Hospital Center Drive, Ste 300, Hilton Head Isl, SC 29926; **Phone:** 843-682-7377; **Board Cert:** Surgery 2000; **Med School:** St Louis Univ 1974; **Resid:** Surgery, St Louis Univ Hosps 1979; **Fellow:** Surgery, Brigham & Women's Hosp 1980; **Fac Appt:** Prof S, Med Univ SC

Heslin, Martin J MD [S] - **Spec Exp:** Gastrointestinal Cancer; Pancreatic Cancer; Biliary Cancer; Sarcoma-Soft Tissue; **Hospital:** Univ of Ala Hosp at Birmingham; **Address:** Univ Alabama, 1922 7th Ave S, Ste 321, Birmingham, AL 35294-0016; **Phone:** 205-934-3064; **Board Cert:** Surgery 2006; **Med School:** SUNY Upstate Med Univ 1987; **Resid:** Surgery, NYU Med Ctr 1994; Surgery, Meml Sloan-Kettering Canc Ctr 1991; **Fellow:** Surgical Oncology, Meml Sloan-Kettering Cancer Ctr 1996; **Fac Appt:** Prof S, Univ Alabama

Howard, Richard J MD [S] - **Spec Exp:** Endocrine Surgery; Transplant-Kidney; Gastrointestinal Surgery; **Hospital:** Shands at Univ of FL; **Address:** Univ Florida Dept Surgery, 1600 SW Archer Rd, Ste 6142, Gainesville, FL 32610; **Phone:** 352-265-0606; **Board Cert:** Surgery 2004; **Med School:** Yale Univ 1966; **Resid:** Surgery, Univ Minn Hosp 1975; **Fac Appt:** Prof S, Univ Fla Coll Med

Howerton, Russell M MD [S] - **Spec Exp:** Hepatobiliary Surgery; Pancreatic Surgery; Colon & Rectal Surgery; Laparoscopic Surgery; **Hospital:** Wake Forest Univ Baptist Med Ctr (page 72); **Address:** Dept of Genl Surgery, Medical Ctr Blvd, Winston-Salem, NC 27157; **Phone:** 336-716-0664; **Board Cert:** Surgery 1998; **Med School:** Vanderbilt Univ 1983; **Resid:** Surgery, Tufts/New England Med Ctr 1989; **Fellow:** Hepatobiliary Surgery, Hammersmith Hosp 1992; **Fac Appt:** Assoc Prof S, Wake Forest Univ

Kelley, Mark C MD [S] - **Spec Exp:** Breast Cancer; Melanoma; **Hospital:** Vanderbilt Univ Med Ctr; **Address:** Div Surgical Oncology, 2220 Pierce Ave, 597 Preston Rsch Bldg, Nashville, TN 37232; **Phone:** 615-322-2391; **Board Cert:** Surgery 2005; **Med School:** Univ Fla Coll Med 1989; **Resid:** Surgery, Univ Fla-Shands Hosp 1995; **Fellow:** Surgical Oncology, John Wayne Cancer Inst-St Johns Hosp 1997; **Fac Appt:** Asst Prof Surg & Onc, Vanderbilt Univ

Knechtle, Stuart J MD [S] - **Spec Exp:** Transplant-Liver; Transplant-Kidney; Transplant Immunology; Hepatobiliary Surgery; **Hospital:** Emory Univ Hosp; **Address:** Emory Div Transplant Surgery, 1364 Clifton Rd, WMB-5105, Atlanta, GA 30322; **Phone:** 404-712-5676; **Board Cert:** Surgery 1998; **Med School:** Cornell Univ 1982; **Resid:** Surgery, Duke Univ Med Ctr 1989; **Fellow:** Transplant Surgery, Univ Wisconsin Hosp 1991; **Fac Appt:** Prof S, Emory Univ

Surgery

Koruda, Mark J MD [S] - **Spec Exp:** Gastrointestinal Surgery; Minimally Invasive Surgery; Inflammatory Bowel Disease; **Hospital:** Univ NC Hosps; **Address:** Div Gastorintestinal Surgery, 4035 Burnett-Womack Bldg, Campus Box 7081, Chapel Hill, NC 27599-7081; **Phone:** 919-966-8436; **Board Cert:** Surgery 1999; **Med School:** Yale Univ 1981; **Resid:** Surgery, Hosp Univ Penn 1988; **Fac Appt:** Prof S, Univ NC Sch Med

Larsen, Christian P MD/PhD [S] - **Spec Exp:** Islet Cell Transplant; Transplant-Pancreas; Transplant-Kidney; **Hospital:** Emory Univ Hosp; **Address:** Emory Transplant Center, Emory Univ Hosp, 1364 Clifton Rd NE, Box 7, Atlanta, GA 30322; **Phone:** 404-727-0717; **Board Cert:** Surgery 2001; **Med School:** Emory Univ 1984; **Resid:** Surgery, Emory Univ Hosp 1988; **Fellow:** Surgical Research, Oxford Univ 1990; Transplant Surgery, Emory Univ Hosp 1993; **Fac Appt:** Prof S, Emory Univ

Levi, Joe U MD [S] - **Spec Exp:** Pancreatic Cancer; Liver Disease; Liver Tumors; Biliary Surgery; **Hospital:** Jackson Meml Hosp (page 70), Univ of Miami Hosp & Clins/Sylvester Comp Canc Ctr (page 70); **Address:** 1475 NW 12th Ave, Ste 3524, Miami, FL 33136; **Phone:** 305-243-4211; **Board Cert:** Surgery 1975; **Med School:** Univ Fla Coll Med 1967; **Resid:** Surgery, Johns Hopkins Hosp 1969; Surgery, Jackson Meml Hosp 1974; **Fac Appt:** Prof S, Univ Miami Sch Med

Levine, Edward A MD [S] - **Spec Exp:** Breast Cancer; Esophageal Cancer; Peritoneal Carcinomatosis; **Hospital:** Wake Forest Univ Baptist Med Ctr (page 72); **Address:** Wake Forest Univ Baptist Med Ctr, Dept Surgery, Medical Center Blvd, Winston-Salem, NC 27157; **Phone:** 336-716-4276; **Board Cert:** Surgery 1999; **Med School:** Ros Franklin Univ/Chicago Med Sch 1985; **Resid:** Surgery, Michael Reese Hosp 1990; **Fellow:** Surgical Oncology, Univ Illinois 1992; **Fac Appt:** Prof S, Wake Forest Univ

Lind, David Scott MD [S] - **Spec Exp:** Breast Cancer; Melanoma; Sarcoma; **Hospital:** Med Coll of GA Hosp and Clin (MCG Health Inc); **Address:** MCG Health-Comp Cancer Center, Div Surgical Oncology, 1120 15th St, Augusta, GA 30912; **Phone:** 706-721-6744; **Board Cert:** Surgery 2000; **Med School:** Eastern VA Med Sch 1984; **Resid:** Surgery, Univ Texas Affil Hosp 1989; **Fellow:** Medical Oncology, Med Coll Virginia 1992; **Fac Appt:** Prof Surg & Onc, Med Coll GA

Livingstone, Alan S MD [S] - **Spec Exp:** Liver & Biliary Cancer; Stomach Cancer; Esophageal Cancer; Pancreatic Cancer; **Hospital:** Jackson Meml Hosp (page 70), Univ of Miami Hosp & Clins/Sylvester Comp Canc Ctr (page 70); **Address:** Sylvester Comp Cancer Ctr, Dept Surgery (310T), 1475 NW 12th Ave, rm 3550, Miami, FL 33136-1002; **Phone:** 305-243-4902; **Board Cert:** Surgery 2007; **Med School:** McGill Univ 1971; **Resid:** Surgery, Montreal Genl Hosp 1976; Surgery, Jackson Meml Hosp 1975; **Fac Appt:** Prof S, Univ Miami Sch Med

Luterman, Arnold MD [S] - **Spec Exp:** Burn Care; Wound Healing/Care; Critical Care; **Hospital:** Univ of S AL Med Ctr; **Address:** Univ of S Alabama Med Ctr, Mastin Bldg, 2451 Fillingim St, rm 701, Mobile, AL 36617; **Phone:** 251-415-1475; **Board Cert:** Surgery 2006; **Med School:** McGill Univ 1970; **Resid:** Surgery, Sinai Hospital 1973; Surgery, Jewish Gen Hosp. McGill U 1976; **Fellow:** Burn Surgery, Univ Washington Medical Ctr 1976; **Fac Appt:** Prof S, Univ S Ala Coll Med

Lyerly, H Kim MD [S] - **Spec Exp:** Breast Cancer; Immunotherapy; **Hospital:** Duke Univ Med Ctr, Durham Regional Hosp; **Address:** Duke Comprehensive Cancer Center, DUMC Box 2714, Durham, NC 27710; **Phone:** 919-684-5613; **Board Cert:** Surgery 2001; **Med School:** UCLA 1983; **Resid:** Surgery, Duke Univ Med Ctr 1990; **Fac Appt:** Prof S, Duke Univ

MacDonald Jr, Kenneth G MD [S] - **Spec Exp:** Gastrointestinal Surgery; Obesity/Bariatric Surgery; Pancreatic Surgery; **Hospital:** Pitt Cty Mem Hosp - Univ Med Ctr East Carolina, Nash Genl Hosp; **Address:** Southern Surgical Assocs, 2455 Emerald Pl, Greenville, NC 27834; **Phone:** 252-758-2224; **Board Cert:** Surgery 1998; **Med School:** W VA Univ 1981; **Resid:** Surgery, NC Baptist Hosp 1984; Surgery, Univ Med Ctr E Carolina 1987; **Fac Appt:** Prof S, E Carolina Univ

MacFadyen Jr, Bruce V MD [S] - **Spec Exp:** Laparoscopic Surgery; Gastrointestinal Surgery; Endoscopy; **Hospital:** Med Coll of GA Hosp and Clin (MCG Health Inc); **Address:** Medical College GA, Dept Surgery, 1120 15th St, Ste 4076, Augusta, GA 30912; **Phone:** 706-721-4651; **Board Cert:** Surgery 1975; **Med School:** Hahnemann Univ 1968; **Resid:** Surgery, Hosp Univ Penn 1972; Surgery, Hermann Hosp 1974; **Fellow:** MD Anderson Cancer Ctr 1978; **Fac Appt:** Prof S, Med Coll GA

McGrath, Patrick C MD [S] - **Spec Exp:** Breast Cancer; Cancer Surgery; **Hospital:** Univ of Kentucky Chandler Hosp; **Address:** Univ Kentucky Med Ctr, Dept Genl Surgery, 800 Rose St, rm C224, Lexington, KY 40536-0293; **Phone:** 859-323-6346 x233; **Med School:** Univ IL Coll Med 1980; **Resid:** Surgery, Med Coll Virginia Hosp 1986; **Fellow:** Surgical Oncology, Med Coll Virginia Hosp 1988; **Fac Appt:** Prof S, Univ KY Coll Med

McMasters, Kelly M MD [S] - **Spec Exp:** Melanoma; Breast Cancer; Liver Cancer; **Hospital:** Univ of Louisville Hosp; **Address:** 401 S Chestnut St, Ste 710, Louisville, KY 40202; **Phone:** 502-583-8303; **Board Cert:** Surgery 2005; **Med School:** UMDNJ-RW Johnson Med Sch 1989; **Resid:** Surgery, Univ Louisville Sch Med 1994; **Fellow:** Surgical Oncology, Texas-MD Anderson Cancer Ctr 1995; **Fac Appt:** Prof S, Univ Louisville Sch Med

Meyer, Anthony A MD [S] - **Spec Exp:** Trauma/Critical Care; Burn Care; **Hospital:** Univ NC Hosps; **Address:** Univ NC-Sch Med, Dept Surgery, 4041 Burnett-Womack Bldg, CB7050, Chapel HIll, NC 27599-7050; **Phone:** 919-966-4321; **Board Cert:** Surgery 2001; Surgical Critical Care 2005; **Med School:** Univ Chicago-Pritzker Sch Med 1977; **Resid:** Surgery, UCSF Med Ctr 1982; **Fac Appt:** Prof S, Univ NC Sch Med

Neifeld, James P MD [S] - **Spec Exp:** Melanoma; Head & Neck Cancer; Gastrointestinal Cancer; **Hospital:** Med Coll of VA Hosp; **Address:** Medical College Virginia Hosp, PO Box 980645, Richmond, VA 23298-0645; **Phone:** 804-828-9324; **Board Cert:** Surgery 2009; **Med School:** Med Coll VA 1972; **Resid:** Surgery, Med Coll Va Hosps 1978; **Fac Appt:** Prof S, Va Commonwealth Univ Sch Med

Newell, Kenneth A MD/PhD [S] - **Spec Exp:** Transplant-Kidney; Transplant-Pancreas; **Hospital:** Emory Univ Hosp; **Address:** Emory Transplant Ctr, 101 Woodruff Cir, rm 5105 WMB, Atlanta, GA 30322; **Phone:** 404-727-2489; **Board Cert:** Surgery 2009; **Med School:** Univ Mich Med Sch 1984; **Resid:** Surgery, Loyola Univ Med Ctr 1989; **Fellow:** Transplant Surgery, Univ Chicago 1994; **Fac Appt:** Prof S, Emory Univ

Pappas, Theodore N MD [S] - **Spec Exp:** Pancreatic Surgery; Laparoscopic Surgery; **Hospital:** Duke Univ Med Ctr; **Address:** Duke Univ Med Ctr, Dept Surgery, DUMC Box 3479, Durham, NC 27710-0001; **Phone:** 919-681-3442; **Board Cert:** Surgery 1997; **Med School:** Ohio State Univ 1981; **Resid:** Surgery, Brigham & Womens Hosp 1988; **Fellow:** Research, Wadworth VA Med Ctr 1985; **Fac Appt:** Prof S, Duke Univ

Pinson, C Wright MD [S] - **Spec Exp:** Transplant-Liver; Liver & Biliary Cancer; Pancreatic Cancer; Liver & Biliary Surgery; **Hospital:** Vanderbilt Univ Med Ctr; **Address:** Vanderbilt Univ Med Ctr, TVC 3810A, 1301 Med Center Drive, Nashville, TN 37232-5545; **Phone:** 615-343-9324; **Board Cert:** Surgery 2007; Surgical Critical Care 2007; **Med School:** Vanderbilt Univ 1980; **Resid:** Surgery, Oregon Health Sci Ctr 1986; **Fellow:** Gastrointestinal Surgery, Lahey Clinic 1987; Transplant Surgery, Deaconess Hosp 1988; **Fac Appt:** Prof S, Vanderbilt Univ

Rosemurgy, Alexander S MD [S] - **Spec Exp:** Pancreatic Cancer; Gastrointestinal Surgery; Minimally Invasive Surgery; **Hospital:** Tampa Genl Hosp; **Address:** Digestive Disorders Ctr, Tampa General Hospital, 2 Columbia Drive, rm F145, Tampa, FL 33601; **Phone:** 813-844-7393; **Board Cert:** Surgery 2005; **Med School:** Univ Mich Med Sch 1979; **Resid:** Surgery, Univ Chicago Hosps 1984; **Fac Appt:** Prof S, Univ S Fla Coll Med

Surgery

Salo, Jonathan C MD [S] - **Spec Exp:** Gastrointestinal Cancer; Esophageal Cancer; **Hospital:** Carolinas Med Ctr; **Address:** Blumenthal Cancer Center, 1025 Morehead Medical Drive, Ste 600, Charlotte, NC 28204; **Phone:** 704-355-2884; **Board Cert:** Surgery 2005; **Med School:** UCSF 1981; **Resid:** Surgery, UCSF Med Ctr 1993; **Fellow:** Surgical Oncology, Natl Cancer Inst 1991; Surgical Oncology, Meml Sloan-Kettering Cancer Ctr 1998; **Fac Appt:** Asst Prof S, Univ NC Sch Med

Schirmer, Bruce D MD [S] - **Spec Exp:** Laparoscopic Surgery; Gastrointestinal Surgery; Pancreatic Surgery; Liver Surgery; **Hospital:** Univ Virginia Med Ctr; **Address:** Univ VA Hlth Sys, Dept Surgery, PO Box 800709, Charlottesville, VA 22908; **Phone:** 434-924-2104; **Board Cert:** Surgery 2005; **Med School:** Duke Univ 1978; **Resid:** Surgery, Duke Univ Med Ctr 1985; **Fac Appt:** Prof S, Univ VA Sch Med

Sharp, Kenneth MD [S] - **Spec Exp:** Gastrointestinal Surgery; Esophageal Disorders; Laparoscopic Surgery; Pancreatic Surgery; **Hospital:** Vanderbilt Univ Med Ctr; **Address:** Vanderbilt Univ Med Ctr, Div Gen Surgery, D-5203 Medical Center North, Nashville, TN 37232-2577; **Phone:** 615-322-0259; **Board Cert:** Surgery 2003; **Med School:** Johns Hopkins Univ 1977; **Resid:** Surgery, Johns Hopkins Univ Med Ctr 1984; **Fellow:** Hepatobiliary Surgery, Loch Raven VA Hosp 1981; Surgery, John Radcliffe Hosp 1982; **Fac Appt:** Prof S, Vanderbilt Univ

Shen, Perry MD [S] - **Spec Exp:** Liver & Biliary Cancer; Pancreatic Cancer; Gastrointestinal Cancer; Melanoma; **Hospital:** Wake Forest Univ Baptist Med Ctr (page 72); **Address:** Wake Forest Univ Baptist Med Ctr, Dept Surgery, Medical Center Blvd, Winston-Salem, NC 27157; **Phone:** 336-716-4276; **Board Cert:** Surgery 1999; **Med School:** USC Sch Med 1992; **Resid:** Surgery, LAC-USC Med Ctr 1998; **Fellow:** Surgical Oncology, John Wayne Cancer Inst 2000; **Fac Appt:** Assoc Prof S, Wake Forest Univ

Slingluff Jr, Craig L MD [S] - **Spec Exp:** Melanoma; Immunotherapy; **Hospital:** Univ Virginia Med Ctr; **Address:** UVA Health System, Dept Surgery, PO Box 800709, Charlottesville, VA 22908; **Phone:** 434-924-1730; **Board Cert:** Surgery 2002; **Med School:** Univ VA Sch Med 1984; **Resid:** Surgery, Duke Univ Med Ctr 1991; **Fellow:** Surgical Research, Duke Univ Med Ctr 1992; **Fac Appt:** Prof S, Univ VA Sch Med

Sondak, Vernon K MD [S] - **Spec Exp:** Cancer Surgery; Melanoma; Sarcoma; **Hospital:** H Lee Moffitt Cancer Ctr & Research Inst; **Address:** H Lee Moffitt Cancer Ctr, Cutaneous Program, 12902 Magnolia Drive, Tampa, FL 33612; **Phone:** 813-745-1968; **Board Cert:** Surgery 1996; **Med School:** Boston Univ 1980; **Resid:** Surgery, UCLA Med Ctr 1987; **Fellow:** Surgical Oncology, UCLA Med Ctr 1984; **Fac Appt:** Prof S, Univ S Fla Coll Med

Stratta, Robert J MD [S] - **Spec Exp:** Transplant-Pancreas; Transplant-Kidney; Gastrointestinal Surgery; **Hospital:** Wake Forest Univ Baptist Med Ctr (page 72); **Address:** Wake Forest Univ Baptist Med Ctr, Dept Surgery, Medical Center Blvd, Winston-Salem, NC 27157-1095; **Phone:** 336-716-6371; **Board Cert:** Surgery 2006; **Med School:** Univ Chicago-Pritzker Sch Med 1980; **Resid:** Surgery, Univ Utah Med Ctr 1986; **Fellow:** Transplant Surgery, Univ Wisc Hosps & Clins 1988; **Fac Appt:** Prof S, Wake Forest Univ

Sweeney, John F MD [S] - **Spec Exp:** Obesity/Bariatric Surgery; Laparoscopic Surgery; Gastroesophageal Reflux Disease (GERD); Minimally Invasive Surgery; **Hospital:** Emory Univ Hosp; **Address:** Emory Univ Dept Surgery, 1364 Clifton Rd NE, rm B206, Atlanta, GA 30322; **Phone:** 404-778-3712; **Board Cert:** Surgery 2004; **Med School:** Rush Med Coll 1988; **Resid:** Surgery, Univ South Florida Med Ctr 1995; **Fellow:** Surgical Research, Univ South Florida 1993; **Fac Appt:** Prof S, Emory Univ

Tyler, Douglas S MD [S] - **Spec Exp:** Pancreatic Cancer; Colon & Rectal Cancer; Rectal Cancer/Sphincter Preservation; Melanoma; **Hospital:** Duke Univ Med Ctr; **Address:** Duke University Med Ctr, Box 3118, Durham, NC 27710; **Phone:** 919-684-6858; **Board Cert:** Surgery 2000; **Med School:** Dartmouth Med Sch 1985; **Resid:** Surgery, Duke Univ Med Ctr 1992; **Fellow:** Surgical Oncology, MD Anderson Cancer Ctr 1994; **Fac Appt:** Prof S, Duke Univ

Tzakis, Andreas G MD [S] - **Spec Exp:** Transplant-Liver; Transplant-Bowel; **Hospital:** Jackson Meml Hosp (page 70); **Address:** Miami Transplant Institute, 1801 NW 9th Ave, Ste 310, Miami, FL 33136; **Phone:** 305-355-5748; **Board Cert:** Surgery 2003; **Med School:** Greece 1974; **Resid:** Surgery, Mt Sinai Hosp 1979; Surgery, SUNY Stony Brook 1983; **Fellow:** Transplant Surgery, Univ Pittsburgh 1985; **Fac Appt:** Prof S, Univ Miami Sch Med

Urist, Marshall M MD [S] - **Spec Exp:** Cancer Surgery; Breast Cancer; Melanoma; **Hospital:** Univ of Ala Hosp at Birmingham; **Address:** Univ Alabama Sch Med, Dept Surgery, 1922 7th Ave S, Kracke Bldg, Ste 321, Birmingham, AL 35294; **Phone:** 205-934-3065; **Board Cert:** Surgery 2000; **Med School:** Univ Chicago-Pritzker Sch Med 1971; **Resid:** Surgery, Johns Hopkins Hosp 1978; **Fellow:** Surgical Oncology, UCLA Med Ctr 1976; **Fac Appt:** Prof S, Univ Alabama

White Jr, Richard L MD [S] - **Spec Exp:** Breast Cancer; Melanoma; Sarcoma; Immunotherapy; **Hospital:** Carolinas Med Ctr; **Address:** Carolinas Medical Center, 1000 Blythe Blvd, Box 32861, Charlotte, NC 28203; **Phone:** 704-355-2884; **Board Cert:** Surgery 2002; **Med School:** Columbia P&S 1986; **Resid:** Surgery, Georgetown Univ Hosp 1992; **Fellow:** Surgical Oncology, NIH-Natl Cancer Inst 1995; **Fac Appt:** Assoc Clin Prof S, Univ NC Sch Med

Whitworth, Pat W MD [S] - **Spec Exp:** Breast Cancer; **Hospital:** Baptist Hosp - Nashville, Centennial Med Ctr; **Address:** 300 20th Ave N, Ste 401, Nashville, TN 37203; **Phone:** 615-620-5535; **Board Cert:** Surgery 1999; **Med School:** Univ Tenn Coll Med, Memphis 1983; **Resid:** Surgery, Univ Louisville Med Ctr 1988; **Fellow:** Surgical Oncology, MD Anderson Cancer Ctr 1991; **Fac Appt:** Assoc Clin Prof S, Vanderbilt Univ

Willis, Irvin MD [S] - **Spec Exp:** Pancreatic Surgery; Cancer Surgery; Laparoscopic Surgery; **Hospital:** Mount Sinai Med Ctr - Miami; **Address:** 4302 Alton Rd, Ste 630, Miami Beach, FL 33140-2876; **Phone:** 305-534-6050; **Board Cert:** Surgery 1970; **Med School:** Univ Cincinnati 1964; **Resid:** Surgery, Univ Miami-Jackson Meml 1969

Wood, William C MD [S] - **Spec Exp:** Breast Cancer; **Hospital:** Emory Univ Hosp; **Address:** Emory Univ Hosp, Dept Surgery, 1364 Clifton Rd NE, Ste B206, Atlanta, GA 30322; **Phone:** 404-778-4720; **Board Cert:** Surgery 1974; **Med School:** Harvard Med Sch 1966; **Resid:** Surgery, Mass Genl Hosp 1968; Surgery, Mass Genl Hosp 1974; **Fac Appt:** Prof S, Emory Univ

Yeatman, Timothy J MD [S] - **Spec Exp:** Liver Cancer; **Hospital:** H Lee Moffitt Cancer Ctr & Research Inst; **Address:** H Lee Moffitt Cancer Ctr, 12902 Magnolia Drive, Tampa, FL 33612-9497; **Phone:** 813-979-7292; **Board Cert:** Surgery 2000; **Med School:** Emory Univ 1984; **Resid:** Surgery, Univ Florida 1990; **Fellow:** Surgical Oncology, MD Anderson Cancer Ctr 1992; **Fac Appt:** Prof S, Univ S Fla Coll Med

Midwest

Abecassis, Michael MD [S] - **Spec Exp:** Transplant-Liver; Transplant-Kidney; Pancreatic & Biliary Surgery; Liver Cancer; **Hospital:** Northwestern Meml Hosp; **Address:** Northwestern Medical Faculty Fdn, 675 N St Clair St, Galter Pavilion, Ste 17-200, Chicago, IL 60611; **Phone:** 312-695-8900; **Board Cert:** Surgery 1998; **Med School:** Univ Toronto 1983; **Resid:** Surgery, Toronto Genl Hosp 1989; **Fellow:** Hepatopancreatobiliary Surgery, Toronto Genl Hosp 1990; Transplant Surgery, Univ Iowa Hosp 1991; **Fac Appt:** Prof S, Northwestern Univ-Feinberg Sch Med

Surgery

Angelos, Peter MD/PhD [S] - **Spec Exp:** Endocrine Tumors; Pheochromocytoma; Thyroid Surgery; Parathyroid Surgery; **Hospital:** Univ of Chicago Med Ctr; **Address:** 5841 S Maryland Ave, MC 4052, Chicago, IL 60637; **Phone:** 773-702-4429; **Board Cert:** Surgery 2004; **Med School:** Boston Univ 1989; **Resid:** Surgery, Northwestern Univ 1995; **Fellow:** Medical Ethics, Univ of Chicago Hosps 1992; Endocrine Surgery, Univ of Michigan Med Sch 1996; **Fac Appt:** Prof S, Univ Chicago-Pritzker Sch Med

Aranha, Gerard V MD [S] - **Spec Exp:** Pancreatic & Biliary Surgery; Stomach Cancer; Esophageal Cancer; **Hospital:** Loyola Univ Med Ctr, Hines VA Hosp; **Address:** Loyola Univ Med Ctr, Dept Surg, 2160 S First Ave Bldg 110 - rm 3236, Maywood, IL 60153-3328; **Phone:** 708-327-3430; **Board Cert:** Surgery 2006; **Med School:** India 1969; **Resid:** Surgery, Loyola Univ Med Ctr 1975; **Fellow:** Surgical Oncology, Univ Minn Hosp 1977; **Fac Appt:** Prof S, Loyola Univ-Stritch Sch Med

Averbook, Bruce J MD [S] - **Spec Exp:** Melanoma; Clinical Trials; **Hospital:** MetroHealth Med Ctr; **Address:** Metrohealth Medical Ctr, Surgical Oncology, 2500 Metrohealth Drive, rm C2110, Cleveland, OH 44109; **Phone:** 216-778-4795; **Board Cert:** Surgery 2000; **Med School:** Geo Wash Univ 1983; **Resid:** Surgery, UC Irvine Med Ctr 1990; **Fellow:** Surgical Oncology, NCI, NIH Surg Br 1993; **Fac Appt:** Assoc Prof S, Case West Res Univ

Benedetti, Enrico MD [S] - **Spec Exp:** Transplant-Liver; Transplant-Pancreas; Transplant-Kidney; Transplant-Bowel; **Hospital:** Univ of IL Med Ctr at Chicago, Adv Luth Genl Hosp; **Address:** Univ Illinois, Dept Surgery/Transplant, 840 S Wood St, rm 402, Chicago, IL 60612; **Phone:** 312-996-6771; **Board Cert:** Surgery 2003; **Med School:** Italy 1985; **Resid:** Surgery, Univ IL at Chicago Med Ctr 1993; **Fellow:** Transplant Surgery, Univ Minn Med Ctr 1994; **Fac Appt:** Prof S, Univ IL Coll Med

Brems, John J MD [S] - **Spec Exp:** Pancreatic Cancer; Liver Cancer; Transplant-Liver; Liver & Biliary Surgery; **Hospital:** Loyola Univ Med Ctr; **Address:** 2160 S 1st Ave, MC-EMS-3268, Maywood, IL 60153-3328; **Phone:** 708-327-2539; **Board Cert:** Surgery 2004; Surgical Critical Care 2000; **Med School:** St Louis Univ 1981; **Resid:** Surgery, St Louis Univ 1986; **Fellow:** Transplant Surgery, UCLA Med Ctr 1987; **Fac Appt:** Prof S, Loyola Univ-Stritch Sch Med

Brunt, L Michael MD [S] - **Spec Exp:** Minimally Invasive Surgery; Adrenal Tumors; Hernia; **Hospital:** Barnes-Jewish Hosp; **Address:** Washington Univ Sch Medicine, Dept Surg, 660 S Euclid Ave, Box 8109, St Louis, MO 63110; **Phone:** 314-454-7194; **Board Cert:** Surgery 2006; **Med School:** Johns Hopkins Univ 1980; **Resid:** Surgery, Barnes Jewish Hosp 1987; **Fellow:** Surgery, Barnes Jewish Hosp 1984; **Fac Appt:** Prof S, Washington Univ, St Louis

Chand, Bipan MD [S] - **Spec Exp:** Obesity/Bariatric Surgery; Gastrointestinal Metabolic Surgery; Gastroesophageal Reflux Disease (GERD); Barrett's Esophagus; **Hospital:** Cleveland Clin Fdn (page 56); **Address:** Cleveland Clinic, 9500 Euclid Ave, MC 61, Cleveland, OH 44195; **Phone:** 216-444-6668; **Board Cert:** Surgery 2003; **Med School:** Univ MO-Kansas City 1996; **Resid:** Surgery, Cleveland Clinic 2002; **Fellow:** Laparoscopic Surgery, Cleveland Clinic 2003

Chang, Alfred E MD [S] - **Spec Exp:** Breast Cancer; Gastrointestinal Cancer; Melanoma; Sarcoma; **Hospital:** Univ Michigan Hlth Sys; **Address:** Univ Mich Comp Cancer Ctr, 1500 E Med Ctr Dr 3302 CGC, Ann Arbor, MI 48109-5932; **Phone:** 734-936-6000; **Board Cert:** Surgery 2001; **Med School:** Harvard Med Sch 1974; **Resid:** Surgery, Duke Univ Med Ctr 1976; Surgery, Hosp Univ Penn 1982; **Fellow:** Surgical Oncology, Natl Cancer Inst 1979; **Fac Appt:** Prof S, Univ Mich Med Sch

Chapman, William C MD [S] - **Spec Exp:** Transplant-Liver-Adult & Pediatric; Liver Cancer; Liver & Biliary Surgery; **Hospital:** Barnes-Jewish Hosp, St Louis Chldns Hosp; **Address:** Washington Univ Sch Med, 660 S Euclid Ave, Box 8109, St Louis, MO 63110; **Phone:** 314-362-7792; **Board Cert:** Surgery 2001; Surgical Critical Care 2001; **Med School:** Med Univ SC 1984; **Resid:** Surgery, Vanderbilt Univ Med Ctr 1991; **Fellow:** Hepatobiliary Surgery, Kings College Hosp 1992; **Fac Appt:** Prof S, Washington Univ, St Louis

Cronin II, David C MD/PhD [S] - **Spec Exp:** Transplant-Liver; Transplant Surgery-Pediatric; Liver & Biliary Surgery; Pancreatic Surgery; **Hospital:** Froedtert Meml Lutheran Hosp; **Address:** Div Transplant Surgery, 9200 W Wisconsin Ave, Ste 5700, Milwaukee, WI 53226; **Phone:** 414-955-6920; **Board Cert:** Surgery 2005; **Med School:** Mount Sinai Sch Med 1987; **Resid:** Surgery, Univ Chicago Hosps 1995; **Fellow:** Transplant Surgery, Univ Chicago Hosps 1997; Medical Ethics, Univ Chicago Hosps 2002; **Fac Appt:** Assoc Prof S, Univ Wisc

Crowe Jr, Joseph P MD [S] - **Spec Exp:** Breast Cancer; Tumor Surgery; **Hospital:** Cleveland Clin Fdn (page 56); **Address:** Cleveland Clinic Fdn, Dept Surg, 9500 Euclid Ave, Desk A10, Cleveland, OH 44195; **Phone:** 216-444-3024; **Board Cert:** Surgery 2004; **Med School:** Case West Res Univ 1978; **Resid:** Surgery, Univ Hosp-Case West Reserve 1983; **Fellow:** Surgical Oncology, Meml Sloan Kettering Cancer Ctr 1985

Deziel, Daniel J MD [S] - **Spec Exp:** Hepatobiliary Surgery; Pancreatic Surgery; Laparoscopic Surgery; **Hospital:** Rush Univ Med Ctr; **Address:** 1725 W Harrison, Ste 810, Chicago, IL 60612-3828; **Phone:** 312-942-6500; **Board Cert:** Surgery 2003; **Med School:** Univ Minn 1979; **Resid:** Surgery, Rush-Presby-St Luke's Med Ctr 1984; **Fellow:** Gastrointestinal Surgery, Lahey Clinic 1985; **Fac Appt:** Prof S, Rush Med Coll

Doherty, Gerard M MD [S] - **Spec Exp:** Endocrine Surgery; Adrenal Surgery; Laparoscopic Surgery; Thyroid Surgery; **Hospital:** Univ Michigan Hlth Sys; **Address:** Taubman Hlth Care Ctr, 1500 E Med Ctr Drive, rm 2920, Ann Arbor, MI 48109-5331; **Phone:** 734-615-4741; **Board Cert:** Surgery 2003; **Med School:** Yale Univ 1986; **Resid:** Surgery, UCSF Med Ctr 1993; **Fellow:** Medical Oncology, Natl Cancer Inst 1991; **Fac Appt:** Prof S, Univ Mich Med Sch

Donohue, John H MD [S] - **Spec Exp:** Gastrointestinal Cancer; Breast Cancer; Stomach Cancer; **Hospital:** Mayo Med Ctr & Clin - Rochester; **Address:** Mayo Clinic, Dept General Surgery, 200 First St SW, Rochester, MN 55905; **Phone:** 507-284-0362; **Board Cert:** Surgery 2005; **Med School:** Harvard Med Sch 1978; **Resid:** Surgery, UCSF Med Ctr 1981; Surgery, UCSF Med Ctr 1985; **Fellow:** Surgery, Natl Inst Hlth 1983; Surgical Oncology, Meml Sloan-Kettering Canc Ctr 1987; **Fac Appt:** Prof S, Mayo Med Sch

Eberlein, Timothy J MD [S] - **Spec Exp:** Breast Cancer; Melanoma; Immunotherapy; **Hospital:** Barnes-Jewish Hosp, St Louis Chldns Hosp; **Address:** Wash Univ School Med, Dept Surgery, 660 S Euclid Ave, Box 8109, St Louis, MO 63110-1093; **Phone:** 314-362-8020; **Board Cert:** Surgery 2006; **Med School:** Univ Pittsburgh 1977; **Resid:** Surgery, Peter Bent Brigham Hosp 1979; Surgery, Brigham-Womens Hosp 1985; **Fellow:** Allergy & Immunology, Natl Inst Hlth 1982; **Fac Appt:** Prof S, Washington Univ, St Louis

Edwards, Michael J MD [S] - **Spec Exp:** Breast Cancer; Melanoma; **Hospital:** Univ Hosp - Cincinnati; **Address:** 234 Goodman St, ML 0772, Cincinnati, OH 45219; **Phone:** 513-584-8900; **Board Cert:** Surgery 2005; **Med School:** Emory Univ 1981; **Resid:** Surgery, Univ Louisville Hosp 1986; **Fellow:** Surgical Oncology, MD Anderson Cancer Ctr 1987; **Fac Appt:** Prof S, Univ Ark

Ellison, E Christopher MD [S] - **Spec Exp:** Biliary Surgery; Biliary Cancer; Pancreatic Cancer; **Hospital:** Ohio St Univ Med Ctr; **Address:** 1654 Upham Drive, Ste 327 Means Hall, Columbus, OH 43210-1236; **Phone:** 614-293-9722; **Board Cert:** Surgery 2001; **Med School:** Univ Wisc 1975; **Resid:** Surgery, Ohio State Univ 1981; **Fac Appt:** Prof S, Ohio State Univ

Surgery

Evans, Douglas B MD [S] - **Spec Exp:** Pancreatic Cancer; Thyroid Cancer; Endocrine Cancers; **Hospital:** Froedtert Meml Lutheran Hosp, Clement J Zablocki VA Med Ctr; **Address:** Medical Coll Wisconsin, Dept Surgery, 9200 W Wisconsin Ave, Ste 3510, Milwaukee, WI 53226-6533; **Phone:** 414-805-5706; **Board Cert:** Surgery 1996; **Med School:** Boston Univ 1983; **Resid:** Surgery, Dartmouth-Hitchcock Med Ctr 1988; **Fellow:** Surgical Oncology, MD Anderson Cancer Ctr 1990; **Fac Appt:** Prof S, Med Coll Wisc

Farley, David R MD [S] - **Spec Exp:** Endocrine Surgery; Hepatobiliary Surgery; Laparoscopic Surgery; Hernia; **Hospital:** Mayo Med Ctr & Clin - Rochester; **Address:** Mayo Clin, 200 First St SW, Mayo West 12, Rochester, MN 55905; **Phone:** 507-284-2644; **Board Cert:** Surgery 2002; **Med School:** Univ Wisc 1988; **Resid:** Surgery, Mayo Clin 1994; **Fellow:** Endocrinology, Mayo Clin 1995; **Fac Appt:** Assoc Prof S, Mayo Med Sch

Farrar, William B MD [S] - **Spec Exp:** Breast Cancer; Thyroid Cancer; **Hospital:** Arthur G James Cancer Hosp & Research Inst, Ohio St Univ Med Ctr; **Address:** 410 W 10th Ave, N924 Doan Hall, Columbus, OH 43210-1240; **Phone:** 614-293-8890; **Board Cert:** Surgery 2000; **Med School:** Univ VA Sch Med 1975; **Resid:** Surgery, Ohio State Univ Hosps 1980; **Fellow:** Surgical Oncology, Meml Sloan-Kettering Cancer Ctr 1982; **Fac Appt:** Prof S, Ohio State Univ

Frantzides, Constantine T MD/PhD [S] - **Spec Exp:** Minimally Invasive Surgery; Laparoscopic Surgery; Obesity/Bariatric Surgery; Laparoscopic Abdominal Surgery; **Hospital:** Evanston/Northshore Univ Hlth Syst, St Francis Hosp - Evanston; **Address:** Chicago Inst Minimally Invasive Surgery, 64 Old Orchard Ctr, Ste 409, Skokie, IL 60076; **Phone:** 847-676-2200; **Med School:** Greece 1976; **Resid:** Surgery, Athens Univ Affil Hosp 1982; **Fellow:** Surgery, Med Coll Wisc 1985; **Fac Appt:** Prof S, Northwestern Univ-Feinberg Sch Med

Fung, John J MD/PhD [S] - **Spec Exp:** Transplant-Liver; Transplant-Kidney; Liver & Biliary Cancer; **Hospital:** Cleveland Clin Fdn (page 56), Euclid Hosp; **Address:** Cleveland Clinic, Dept Surgery, 9500 Euclid Ave, Desk A80, Cleveland, OH 44195-0001; **Phone:** 216-444-3776; **Board Cert:** Surgery 2008; **Med School:** Univ Chicago-Pritzker Sch Med 1982; **Resid:** Surgery, Strong Memorial Hosp 1988; **Fellow:** Transplant Surgery, Univ Pittsburgh 1986; **Fac Appt:** Prof S, Cleveland Cl Coll Med/Case West Res

Gamelli, Richard L MD [S] - **Spec Exp:** Burn Care; Trauma/Critical Care; **Hospital:** Loyola Univ Med Ctr; **Address:** 2160 S First Ave Bldg 103 - rm 1075, Maywood, IL 60153; **Phone:** 708-216-4444; **Board Cert:** Surgery 1999; **Med School:** Univ VT Coll Med 1974; **Resid:** Surgery, Vermont Med Ctr Hosp 1979; **Fac Appt:** Prof S, Loyola Univ-Stritch Sch Med

Goulet Jr, Robert J MD [S] - **Spec Exp:** Breast Cancer; Breast Surgery; **Hospital:** Indiana Univ Hosp; **Address:** Indiana Cancer Pavilion, 535 Barnhill Drive, Ste 253, Indianapolis, IN 46202-5112; **Phone:** 317-274-9800; **Board Cert:** Surgery 2006; **Med School:** SUNY Downstate 1979; **Resid:** Surgery, SUNY-Downstate Med Ctr 1986; **Fellow:** Surgical Research, SUNY-Downstate Med Ctr 1983; **Fac Appt:** Assoc Prof S, Indiana Univ

Grant, Clive S MD [S] - **Spec Exp:** Thyroid & Parathyroid Cancer & Surgery; Adrenal Tumors; Breast Cancer; **Hospital:** Mayo Med Ctr & Clin - Rochester; **Address:** Mayo Clinic, Dept Surgery, 200 First St SW, Rochester, MN 55905-0001; **Phone:** 507-284-2644; **Board Cert:** Surgery 2001; **Med School:** Univ Colorado 1975; **Resid:** Surgery, Mayo Clinic 1980; **Fac Appt:** Prof S, Mayo Med Sch

Gruber, Scott A MD/PhD [S] - **Spec Exp:** Transplant-Kidney; Transplant-Pancreas; **Hospital:** Harper Univ Hosp, Chldns Hosp of Michigan; **Address:** Harper Professional Bldg, 3990 John R, Ste 400, Detroit, MI 48201; **Phone:** 313-745-7319; **Board Cert:** Surgery 2001; **Med School:** SUNY Downstate 1983; **Resid:** Surgery, Univ Minnesota Med Ctr 1986; **Fellow:** Surgery, Univ Minnesota Med Ctr 1989; Transplant Surgery, Univ Minnesota Med Ctr 1993; **Fac Appt:** Prof S, Wayne State Univ

Hansen, Nora M MD [S] - **Spec Exp:** Sentinel Node Surgery; Breast Cancer-High Risk Women; Breast Cancer Risk Assessment; **Hospital:** Northwestern Meml Hosp; **Address:** Lynn Sage Breast Surgery Ctr, 250 E Superior St Fl 4 - Ste 420, Chicago, IL 60611; **Phone:** 312-472-4720; **Board Cert:** Surgery 2006; **Med School:** NY Med Coll 1988; **Resid:** Surgery, Univ Chicago Hosps 1995; **Fellow:** Surgical Oncology, Univ Chicago Hosps 1996; **Fac Appt:** Assoc Prof S, Northwestern Univ

Hering, Bernhard J MD [S] - **Spec Exp:** Islet Cell Transplant; Diabetes; **Hospital:** Univ Minn Med Ctr, Fairview - Univ Campus; **Address:** University of Minnesotta, Dept Surgery, MMC 195, 420 Delaware St SE, Minneapolis, MN 55455; **Phone:** 612-626-5697; **Med School:** Germany 1983; **Resid:** Research, Islet Transplant lab, Justus Liebig Univ 1986; Internal Medicine, Justus Liebig Univ 1995; **Fellow:** Endocrinology, Justus Liebig Univ 1996; **Fac Appt:** Prof S, Univ Minn

Hinshaw, Daniel B MD [S] - **Spec Exp:** Palliative Care; **Hospital:** VA Med Ctr - Ann Arbor, Univ Michigan Hlth Sys; **Address:** VA Medical Ctr, 2215 Fuller Rd, rm 530, MS 112, Ann Arbor, MI 48105; **Phone:** 734-769-7100 x5939; **Board Cert:** Surgery 2003; **Med School:** Loma Linda Univ 1978; **Resid:** Surgery, Loma Linda U Med Ctr 1983; **Fellow:** Immunology, Scripps Clinic Rsch Fdn 1985; Cleveland Clinic 2001; **Fac Appt:** Clin Prof S, Univ Mich Med Sch

Howe, James MD [S] - **Spec Exp:** Endocrine Surgery; Gastrointestinal Cancer; Colon & Rectal Cancer; **Hospital:** Univ Iowa Hosp & Clinics; **Address:** Univ Iowa, Dept Surgery, 200 Hawkins Drive, 4645 JCP, Iowa City, IA 52242-1086; **Phone:** 319-356-1727; **Board Cert:** Surgery 2006; **Med School:** Univ VT Coll Med 1987; **Resid:** Surgery, Barnes Hosp-Wash Univ 1994; **Fellow:** Research, Wash Univ-NCI 1991; Surgical Oncology, Meml Sloan Kettering Cancer Ctr 1996; **Fac Appt:** Prof S, Univ Iowa Coll Med

Ikramuddin, Sayeed MD [S] - **Spec Exp:** Minimally Invasive Surgery; Obesity/Bariatric Surgery; **Hospital:** Univ Minn Med Ctr, Fairview - Univ Campus, Univ Minn Med Ctr, Fairview - Riverside Campus; **Address:** 420 Delaware St SE, Mayo, MC 290, Minneapolis, MN 55455; **Phone:** 612-625-8446; **Board Cert:** Surgery 2007; **Med School:** Albany Med Coll 1990; **Resid:** Surgery, SUNY Hlth Sciences Ctr 1992; Surgery, SUNY Hlth Sciences Ctr 1996; **Fellow:** Research, SUNY Hlth Sciences Ctr 1993; Laparoscopic Surgery, Ohio State Univ Affil Hosp 1997; **Fac Appt:** Assoc Prof S, Univ Minn

Kagan, Richard J MD [S] - **Spec Exp:** Burn Care; **Hospital:** Cincinnati Shriners Hosp, Univ Hosp - Cincinnati; **Address:** Cincinnati Shriners Hosp, 3229 Burnet Ave, Cincinnati, OH 45229; **Phone:** 513-872-6210; **Board Cert:** Surgery 2007; **Med School:** St Louis Univ 1974; **Resid:** Surgery, Univ IL Hosp 1980; **Fac Appt:** Prof S, Univ Cincinnati

Kim, Julian A MD [S] - **Spec Exp:** Melanoma; Breast Cancer; Gastrointestinal Cancer; Immunotherapy; **Hospital:** Univ Hosps Case Med Ctr; **Address:** Univ Hosps of Cleveland, LKS 5047, 11100 Euclid Ave, Cleveland, OH 44106-1716; **Phone:** 216-844-8247; **Board Cert:** Surgery 2002; **Med School:** Med Univ Ohio at Toledo 1986; **Resid:** Surgery, Univ Maryland Hosps 1991; **Fellow:** Surgical Oncology, Arthur James Cancer Hosp & Rsch Inst 1993; Immunotherapy, Ohio State Univ Comp Cancer Ctr 1994; **Fac Appt:** Assoc Prof S, Case West Res Univ

Surgery

Lillemoe, Keith D MD [S] - **Spec Exp:** Pancreatic Cancer; Colon Cancer; Pancreatic & Biliary Surgery; Gastrointestinal Cancer; **Hospital:** Indiana Univ Hosp; **Address:** Indiana Univ, Dept Surgery, 545 Barnhill Drive, EH 203, Indianapolis, IN 46202-5112; **Phone:** 317-274-5707; **Board Cert:** Surgery 2007; **Med School:** Johns Hopkins Univ 1978; **Resid:** Surgery, Johns Hopkins Hosp 1985; **Fac Appt:** Prof S, Indiana Univ

Mamounas, Eleftherios P MD [S] - **Spec Exp:** Breast Cancer; **Hospital:** Aultman Hosp; **Address:** Aultman Cancer Ctr, 2600 6th St SW, Main 1, Clinical Trials Dept, Canton, OH 44710; **Phone:** 330-363-6281; **Board Cert:** Surgery 1999; **Med School:** Greece 1983; **Resid:** Surgery, McKeesport Hosp 1989; **Fellow:** Clinical Oncology, Univ Pittsburgh 1991; Surgical Oncology, Roswell Park Cancer Inst 1992; **Fac Appt:** Prof S, NE Ohio Univ

Matas, Arthur J MD [S] - **Spec Exp:** Transplant-Kidney; **Hospital:** Univ Minn Med Ctr, Fairview - Univ Campus; **Address:** Univ Minn Med Ctr-Dept Surgery, 420 Delaware St SE, MMC 328, Minneapolis, MN 55455; **Phone:** 612-625-6460; **Board Cert:** Surgery 2000; **Med School:** Univ Manitoba 1972; **Resid:** Surgery, Univ Minnesota Hosps 1979; **Fellow:** Transplant Surgery, Univ Minnesota Hosps 1980; **Fac Appt:** Prof S, Univ Minn

Matthews, Jeffrey MD [S] - **Spec Exp:** Gastrointestinal Surgery; Pancreatic Surgery; Liver & Biliary Surgery; **Hospital:** Univ of Chicago Med Ctr; **Address:** 5841 S Maryland Ave, MC 5029, Chicago, IL 60637; **Phone:** 773-702-0881; **Board Cert:** Surgery 2001; **Med School:** Harvard Med Sch 1985; **Resid:** Surgery, Beth Israel Hosp 1990; **Fellow:** Hepatobiliary Surgery, Univ Bern 1989; **Fac Appt:** Prof S, Univ Chicago-Pritzker Sch Med

McHenry, Christopher R MD [S] - **Spec Exp:** Adrenal Surgery; Thyroid Surgery; Parathyroid Surgery; **Hospital:** MetroHealth Med Ctr; **Address:** MetroHealth Medical Ctr, Dept Surgery, 2500 Metro Health Drive, Cleveland, OH 44109-1998; **Phone:** 216-778-4753; **Board Cert:** Surgery 1997; **Med School:** NE Ohio Univ 1984; **Resid:** Surgery, Loyola Univ Med Ctr 1989; **Fellow:** Endocrinology, Univ Toronto Med Ctr 1990; Head and Neck Surgery, Univ Toronto Med Ctr 1990; **Fac Appt:** Prof S, Case West Res Univ

Melvin, W Scott MD [S] - **Spec Exp:** Liver & Biliary Surgery; Pancreatic Cancer; Laparoscopic Surgery; **Hospital:** Ohio St Univ Med Ctr; **Address:** 410 W 10th Ave, Ste N729 Doan, Columbus, OH 43210; **Phone:** 614-293-4499; **Board Cert:** Surgery 2002; **Med School:** Med Coll OH 1987; **Resid:** Surgery, Univ Maryland 1992; **Fellow:** Gastrointestinal Surgery, Grant Med Ctr 1993; **Fac Appt:** Prof S, Ohio State Univ

Merrick III, Hollis W MD [S] - **Spec Exp:** Cancer Surgery; **Hospital:** Univ of Toledo Med Ctr; **Address:** 3065 Arlington Ave, Toledo, OH 43614-2570; **Phone:** 419-383-3759; **Board Cert:** Surgery 1997; **Med School:** McGill Univ 1964; **Resid:** Surgery, Royal Victoria Hosp 1972; **Fac Appt:** Prof S, Med Coll OH

Millis, J Michael MD [S] - **Spec Exp:** Transplant-Liver-Adult & Pediatric; Liver Cancer; Transplant-Pancreas; Critical Care; **Hospital:** Univ of Chicago Med Ctr; **Address:** Univ Chicago, Dept Surgery, 5841 S Maryland Ave, MC 5027, Chicago, IL 60637; **Phone:** 773-702-6319; **Board Cert:** Surgery 2001; Surgical Critical Care 2001; **Med School:** Univ Tenn Coll Med, Memphis 1985; **Resid:** Surgery, UCLA Med Ctr 1992; **Fellow:** Transplant Surgery, UCLA Med Ctr 1994; **Fac Appt:** Prof S, Univ Chicago-Pritzker Sch Med

Moley, Jeffrey F MD [S] - **Spec Exp:** Thyroid Cancer & Surgery; Endocrine Cancers; Melanoma; **Hospital:** Barnes-Jewish Hosp; **Address:** Washington Univ School Med, Dept Surgery, 660 S Euclid Ave, Box 8109, St Louis, MO 63110; **Phone:** 314-362-2280; **Board Cert:** Surgery 2005; **Med School:** Columbia P&S 1980; **Resid:** Surgery, Yale-New Haven Hosp 1985; **Fellow:** Surgical Oncology, National Cancer Inst 1987; **Fac Appt:** Prof S, Washington Univ, St Louis

Nagorney, David M MD [S] - **Spec Exp:** Pancreatic Cancer; Hepatobiliary Surgery; Gastrointestinal Cancer; **Hospital:** Mayo Med Ctr & Clin - Rochester; **Address:** Mayo Clin, Dept Surgery, 200 1st St SW, Mayo E12, Rochester, MN 55905; **Phone:** 507-284-2644; **Board Cert:** Surgery 2001; **Med School:** Univ Kans 1975; **Resid:** Surgery, Mayo Clin 1982; **Fellow:** Hepatobiliary Surgery, Hammersmith Hosp 1985; **Fac Appt:** Prof S, Mayo Med Sch

Nathanson, S David MD [S] - **Spec Exp:** Breast Cancer; Breast Cancer Risk Assessment; Melanoma; Sarcoma; **Hospital:** Henry Ford Hosp; **Address:** 2799 W Grand Blvd, Detroit, MI 48202; **Phone:** 313-916-2917; **Board Cert:** Surgery 2002; **Med School:** South Africa 1966; **Resid:** Surgery, Univ Witwaterstrand 1974; Surgical Oncology, UCLA Med Ctr 1980; **Fellow:** Surgery, UC Davis 1982; **Fac Appt:** Prof S, Case West Res Univ

Newman, Lisa A MD [S] - **Spec Exp:** Breast Cancer; **Hospital:** Univ Michigan Hlth Sys; **Address:** Univ Michigan Cancer Center, 1500 E Medical Center Drive, rm 3308-CGC, Ann Arbor, MI 48109-5932; **Phone:** 734-936-8771; **Board Cert:** Surgery 2001; **Med School:** SUNY Downstate 1985; **Resid:** Surgery, Downstate Med Ctr 1990; **Fac Appt:** Assoc Prof S, Univ Mich Med Sch

Oberholzer, Jose MD [S] - **Spec Exp:** Diabetes; Transplant-Pancreas; Islet Cell Transplant; Hepatobilliary Surgery; **Hospital:** Univ of IL Med Ctr at Chicago, Adv Luth Genl Hosp; **Address:** Univ Illinois Med Ctr at Chicago, Div Transplantation, 840 S Wood St, Ste 402, MC 958, Chicago, IL 60612; **Phone:** 312-996-6771; **Med School:** Switzerland 1992; **Resid:** Surgery, Triemli Hosp 1996; Surgery, Univ Geneva Hosp 1998; **Fellow:** Transplant Surgery, Univ Geneva Hosp 2002; Hepatopancreatobiliary Surgery, Univ Alberta Hosp 2003; **Fac Appt:** Assoc Prof S, Univ IL Coll Med

Onders, Raymond P MD [S] - **Spec Exp:** Laparoscopic Surgery; Diaphragm Pacing via Laparoscopy; Gastrointestinal Cancer; **Hospital:** Univ Hosps Case Med Ctr; **Address:** University Hosps Cleveland, 11100 Euclid Ave, LKS 5047, Cleveland, OH 44106; **Phone:** 216-844-5797; **Board Cert:** Surgery 2001; **Med School:** NE Ohio Univ 1988; **Resid:** Surgery, Case Western Reserve Univ 1993; **Fac Appt:** Asst Prof S, Case West Res Univ

Ponsky, Jeffrey L MD [S] - **Spec Exp:** Minimally Invasive Surgery; Gastrointestinal Surgery; Endoscopy; **Hospital:** Univ Hosps Case Med Ctr; **Address:** Univ Hosps Cleveland, Dept Surgery, 11100 Euclid Ave, Cleveland, OH 44106; **Phone:** 216-844-3209; **Board Cert:** Surgery 2007; **Med School:** Case West Res Univ 1971; **Resid:** Surgery, Univ Hosps 1976; **Fac Appt:** Prof S, Case West Res Univ

Posner, Mitchell C MD [S] - **Spec Exp:** Pancreatic Cancer; Gastrointestinal Cancer; Esophageal Cancer; **Hospital:** Univ of Chicago Med Ctr; **Address:** Univ Chicago Hospitals, 5841 S Maryland Ave, Ste G209, MC 9045, Chicago, IL 60637-1447; **Phone:** 773-834-0156; **Board Cert:** Surgery 2006; **Med School:** SUNY Buffalo 1981; **Resid:** Surgery, Univ Colorado Med Ctr 1986; **Fellow:** Surgical Oncology, Meml Sloan Kettering Cancer Ctr 1988; **Fac Appt:** Prof S, Univ Chicago-Pritzker Sch Med

Prinz, Richard A MD [S] - **Spec Exp:** Adrenal Surgery; Thyroid & Parathyroid Surgery; Pancreatic & Biliary Surgery; Laparoscopic Surgery; **Hospital:** Rush Univ Med Ctr, Rush Oak Park Hosp; **Address:** 1725 W Harrison, Ste 818, Chicago, IL 60612-3841; **Phone:** 312-942-6511; **Board Cert:** Surgery 2007; **Med School:** Loyola Univ-Stritch Sch Med 1972; **Resid:** Surgery, Barnes Hosp 1974; Surgery, Loyola Univ Hosp 1977; **Fellow:** Endocrine Surgery, Hammersmith Hosp 1980; **Fac Appt:** Prof S, Rush Med Coll

Rikkers, Layton F MD [S] - **Spec Exp:** Liver & Biliary Surgery; Pancreatic Cancer; Liver & Biliary Cancer; **Hospital:** Univ WI Hosp & Clins; **Address:** 600 Highland Ave, rm K4/761, Madison, WI 53705-2275; **Phone:** 608-263-1383; **Board Cert:** Surgery 2007; **Med School:** Stanford Univ 1970; **Resid:** Surgery, Univ Utah Hosp 1973; Surgery, Univ Utah Hosp 1976; **Fellow:** Hepatology, Royal Free Hosp 1974; **Fac Appt:** Prof S, Univ Wisc

Surgery

Rosen, Charles B MD [S] - **Spec Exp:** Transplant-Liver; Transplant-Bile Duct; **Hospital:** Mayo Med Ctr & Clin - Rochester; **Address:** Dept Surg-Div Transplantation, 200 First St SW, Charlton 10A, Rochester, MN 55905-0001; **Phone:** 507-266-6640; **Board Cert:** Surgery 1999; **Med School:** Mayo Med Sch 1984; **Resid:** Surgery, Mayo Clin 1989; **Fellow:** Transplant Surgery, Mayo Clin 1991; **Fac Appt:** Assoc Prof S, Mayo Med Sch

Saha, Sukamal MD [S] - **Spec Exp:** Sentinel Node Surgery; Colon Cancer; Head & Neck Cancer & Surgery; **Hospital:** McLaren Reg Med Ctr, Genesys Reg Med Ctr - St Joseph Campus; **Address:** 3500 Calkins Rd, Ste A, Flint, MI 48532; **Phone:** 810-230-9600 x500; **Board Cert:** Surgery 2000; **Med School:** India 1977; **Resid:** Surgery, Hahnemann Univ Hosp 1985; Surgery, Easton Hosp 1987; **Fellow:** Surgical Oncology, Tulane Univ Med Ctr 1989; Head and Neck Surgery, Roswell Park Meml Hosp; **Fac Appt:** Asst Prof S, Mich State Univ

Sarr, Michael G MD [S] - **Spec Exp:** Pancreatic Cancer; Gastrointestinal Cancer; Obesity/Bariatric Surgery; Gastrointestinal Motility Disorders; **Hospital:** Mayo Med Ctr & Clin - Rochester; **Address:** Mayo Clinic, Dept Surg, Desk West 12A, Rochester, MN 55905; **Phone:** 507-284-2863; **Board Cert:** Surgery 2001; **Med School:** Johns Hopkins Univ 1976; **Resid:** Surgery, Johns Hopkins Hosp 1982; **Fellow:** Surgery, Mayo Clinic 1984; Surgery, Johns Hopkins Hosp 1985; **Fac Appt:** Prof S, Mayo Med Sch

Schauer, Philip MD [S] - **Spec Exp:** Obesity/Bariatric Surgery; Minimally Invasive Surgery; **Hospital:** Cleveland Clin Fdn (page 56); **Address:** Cleveland Clinic, 9500 Euclid Ave, MC M61, Cleveland, OH 44195; **Phone:** 216-444-4794; **Board Cert:** Surgery 2004; **Med School:** Baylor Coll Med 1986; **Resid:** Surgery, Univ Texas Med Ctr 1991; **Fellow:** Laparoscopic Surgery, Duke Univ Med Ctr 1992; **Fac Appt:** Prof S, Cleveland Cl Coll Med/Case West Res

Schulak, James A MD [S] - **Spec Exp:** Transplant-Kidney-Adult & Pediatric; Transplant-Pancreas & Liver; Pancreatic Surgery; **Hospital:** Univ Hosps Case Med Ctr; **Address:** Univ Hosps of Cleveland, Dept Surgery, 11100 Euclid Ave, MS 5047, Cleveland, OH 44106-5407; **Phone:** 216-844-0307; **Board Cert:** Surgery 2000; **Med School:** Univ Chicago-Pritzker Sch Med 1974; **Resid:** Surgery, Univ Chicago Hosp 1980; **Fellow:** Transplant Surgery, Univ Chicago Hosp 1981; **Fac Appt:** Prof S, Case West Res Univ

Schwartzentruber, Douglas J MD [S] - **Spec Exp:** Cancer Surgery; Melanoma; Kidney Cancer; Cancer Surgery; **Hospital:** Goshen Genl Hosp; **Address:** Cancer Ctr at Goshen Health System, 200 High Park Ave, Goshen, IN 46526; **Phone:** 574-535-2888; **Board Cert:** Surgery 1997; **Med School:** Indiana Univ 1982; **Resid:** Surgery, Indiana Univ Med Ctr 1987; **Fellow:** Surgical Oncology, Natl Cancer Inst 1990; **Fac Appt:** Assoc Clin Prof S, Indiana Univ

Scott-Conner, Carol E H MD/PhD [S] - **Spec Exp:** Breast Cancer; Cancer Surgery; Laparoscopic Surgery; **Hospital:** Univ Iowa Hosp & Clinics, VA Med Ctr - Iowa City; **Address:** Univ Iowa, Dept Surg, 200 Hawkins Drive, 4622-JCP, Iowa City, IA 52242-1086; **Phone:** 319-356-0330; **Board Cert:** Surgery 2000; Surgical Critical Care 1998; **Med School:** NYU Sch Med 1976; **Resid:** Surgery, NYU Med Ctr 1981; **Fac Appt:** Prof S, Univ Iowa Coll Med

Shenk, Robert R MD [S] - **Spec Exp:** Breast Cancer; Melanoma; Pancreatic Cancer; Stomach Cancer; **Hospital:** Univ Hosps Case Med Ctr; **Address:** Univ Hosp Case Med Ctr, 11100 Euclid Ave, Dept General Surgery, Cleveland, OH 44106; **Phone:** 216-844-3026; **Board Cert:** Surgery 2004; **Med School:** Case West Res Univ 1978; **Resid:** Surgery, Univ Hosp 1985; Immunology, Natl Cancer Inst 1982; **Fellow:** Surgical Oncology, Anderson Hosp 1987; **Fac Appt:** Assoc Prof S, Case West Res Univ

Sielaff, Timothy D MD/PhD [S] - **Spec Exp:** Liver Cancer; Pancreatic Cancer; Gallbladder & Biliary Cancer; **Hospital:** Abbott - Northwestern Hosp; **Address:** Virginia Piper Cancer Inst, Liver and Pancreas Clinic, 800 E 28th St, Minneapolis, MN 55407; **Phone:** 612-863-7553; **Board Cert:** Surgery 1998; **Med School:** Med Coll VA 1989; **Resid:** Surgery, Univ Minn Hosps 1997; **Fellow:** Transplant Surgery, Univ Toronto Affil Hosp 1998; **Fac Appt:** Assoc Prof S, Univ Minn

Simeone, Diane M MD [S] - **Spec Exp:** Pancreatic Cancer; Cancer Surgery; **Hospital:** Univ Michigan Hlth Sys; **Address:** Univ Michigan Hlth Sys, 1500 E Med Ctr Drive, 2210B Taubman Center SPC 5343, Ann Arbor, MI 48109-5331; **Phone:** 734-936-5738; **Board Cert:** Surgery 2005; **Med School:** Duke Univ 1988; **Resid:** Surgery, Univ Mich Med Ctr 1995; **Fac Appt:** Prof S, Univ Mich Med Sch

Siperstein, Allan E MD [S] - **Spec Exp:** Laparoscopic Surgery; Endocrine Tumors; Thyroid & Parathyroid Cancer & Surgery; **Hospital:** Cleveland Clin Fdn (page 56); **Address:** Cleveland Clinic Fdn, Dept Genl Surg, 9500 Euclid Ave, Desk A80, Cleveland, OH 44195; **Phone:** 216-444-5664; **Board Cert:** Surgery 1997; **Med School:** Univ Tex SW, Dallas 1983; **Resid:** Surgery, UCSF Med Ctr 1990; **Fellow:** Research, UCSF Med Ctr 1988

Soper, Nathaniel MD [S] - **Spec Exp:** Laparoscopic Surgery; Gastroesophageal Reflux Disease (GERD); Biliary Surgery; **Hospital:** Northwestern Meml Hosp; **Address:** Northwestern Meml Hosp, Dept Surg, 251 E Huron St Galter Bldg - rm 3-150, Chicago, IL 60611; **Phone:** 312-926-4962; **Board Cert:** Surgery 2005; **Med School:** Univ Iowa Coll Med 1980; **Resid:** Surgery, Univ Utah Hosps 1986; **Fellow:** Digestive Dis, Mayo Clinic 1988; **Fac Appt:** Prof S, Northwestern Univ

Stahl, Donna L MD [S] - **Spec Exp:** Breast Cancer; Breast Surgery; **Hospital:** Jewish Hosp - Kenwood - Cincinnati; **Address:** 4750 E Galbraith Rd, Ste 112, Cincinnati, OH 45236; **Phone:** 513-686-3109; **Board Cert:** Surgery 2000; **Med School:** Univ Iowa Coll Med 1971; **Resid:** Surgery, Univ Cincinnati Hosps 1978

Staren, Edgar MD/PhD [S] - **Spec Exp:** Breast Cancer; Endocrine Cancers; Liver Cancer; **Hospital:** Midwest Reg Med Ctr; **Address:** Cancer Treatment Centers of America, 2610 Sheridan Rd, Zion, IL 60099; **Phone:** 847-731-5805; **Board Cert:** Surgery 2006; **Med School:** Loyola Univ-Stritch Sch Med 1982; **Resid:** Surgery, Rush-Presby-St Lukes Med Ctr 1987; **Fellow:** Surgical Oncology, Rush-Presby-St Lukes Med Ctr 1988

Sutherland, David E MD/PhD [S] - **Spec Exp:** Transplant-Pancreas; Transplant-Kidney; Immunotherapy; **Hospital:** Univ Minn Med Ctr, Fairview - Univ Campus; **Address:** 420 Delaware St SE, MMC 195, Univ Minn Med Ctr-Dept Surgery, Minneapolis, MN 55455-0341; **Phone:** 612-625-7600; **Board Cert:** Surgery 2007; **Med School:** Univ Minn 1966; **Resid:** Surgery, West Virginia Univ Hosp 1968; **Fellow:** Transplant Surgery, Univ Minn Hosps 1975; **Fac Appt:** Prof S, Univ Minn

Talamonti, Mark S MD [S] - **Spec Exp:** Pancreatic Cancer; Liver Cancer; Gastrointestinal Cancer & Surgery; Melanoma; **Hospital:** Evanston/Northshore Univ Hlth Syst, Highland Park/North Shore Univ Hlth Syst; **Address:** North Shore Univ Health System, 2560 Ridge Ave, Evanston, IL 60201; **Phone:** 847-570-1700; **Board Cert:** Surgery 1999; **Med School:** Northwestern Univ 1983; **Resid:** Surgery, Northwestern Meml Hosp 1989; **Fellow:** Surgical Oncology, MD Anderson Cancer Ctr 1991; **Fac Appt:** Prof S, Northwestern Univ

Thistlethwaite, J Richard MD/PhD [S] - **Spec Exp:** Transplant-Kidney; Transplant-Pancreas; Transplant-Liver; Transplant Surgery-Pediatric; **Hospital:** Univ of Chicago Med Ctr; **Address:** 5841 S Maryland Ave, rm J-517, MC 5026, Chicago, IL 60637; **Phone:** 773-834-3537; **Med School:** Duke Univ 1977; **Resid:** Surgery, Mass Genl Hosp 1983; **Fellow:** Surgical Oncology, Natl Inst Hlth 1981; Transplant Surgery, Mass Genl Hosp 1984; **Fac Appt:** Prof S, Univ Chicago-Pritzker Sch Med

Surgery

Tuttle, Todd M MD [S] - **Spec Exp:** Breast Cancer; Minimally Invasive Surgery; Cancer Surgery; **Hospital:** Univ Minn Med Ctr, Fairview - Univ Campus; **Address:** Univ Minn, Dept Surgery, 420 Delaware St SE, MMC 195, Minneapolis, MN 55455; **Phone:** 612-625-2991; **Board Cert:** Surgery 2004; **Med School:** Johns Hopkins Univ 1988; **Resid:** Surgery, Med Coll Virginia Hosps 1994; **Fellow:** Surgical Oncology, MD Anderson Cancer Ctr 1996; **Fac Appt:** Assoc Prof S

Vickers, Selwyn M MD [S] - **Spec Exp:** Pancreatic Cancer; Liver Tumors; Gastrointestinal Surgery; **Hospital:** Univ Minn Med Ctr, Fairview - Univ Campus; **Address:** University of Minnesota, 420 Delaware St SE, Phillips Wangensteen Bldg, MMC 88, Minneapolis, MN 55455; **Phone:** 612-625-5411; **Board Cert:** Surgery 2003; **Med School:** Johns Hopkins Univ 1986; **Resid:** Surgery, Johns Hopkins Hosp 1992; **Fac Appt:** Prof S, Johns Hopkins Univ

Wakefield, Thomas MD [S] - **Spec Exp:** Thrombotic Disorders; Bleeding/Coagulation Disorders; Pulmonary Embolism; **Hospital:** Univ Michigan Hlth Sys, VA Med Ctr - Ann Arbor; **Address:** Univ Mich, Dept Surg, Div Vasc Surg, 1500 E Med Ctr Drive, CVC5179 SPC5867, Ann Arbor, MI 48109; **Phone:** 734-936-5820; **Board Cert:** Surgery 2002; Vascular Surgery 2005; Surgical Critical Care 2000; **Med School:** Med Coll OH 1978; **Resid:** Surgery, Univ Mich Med Ctr 1984; **Fellow:** Peripheral Vascular Surgery, Univ Mich Med Ctr 1986; **Fac Appt:** Prof S, Univ Mich Med Sch

Walker, Alonzo P MD [S] - **Spec Exp:** Breast Cancer; **Hospital:** Froedtert Meml Lutheran Hosp; **Address:** Dept Surgery, 9200 W Wisconsin Ave, Milwaukee, WI 53226-3522; **Phone:** 414-805-5737; **Board Cert:** Surgery 2004; **Med School:** Univ Fla Coll Med 1976; **Resid:** Surgery, Univ Maryland Hosps 1983; **Fac Appt:** Prof S, Med Coll Wisc

Walsh, R Matthew MD [S] - **Spec Exp:** Pancreatic Cancer; Gastrointestinal Surgery; Hepatobiliary Surgery; **Hospital:** Cleveland Clin Fdn (page 56); **Address:** Cleveland Clin Dept Surgery, Desk A110, 9500 Euclid Ave, Cleveland, OH 44195; **Phone:** 216-445-7576; **Board Cert:** Surgery 1999; **Med School:** Med Coll Wisc 1985; **Resid:** Surgery, Loyola Univ Hosp 1990; **Fellow:** Endoscopy, Mass General Hosp 1991; Hepatopancreatobiliary Surgery, Cleveland Clinic; **Fac Appt:** Assoc Prof S, Cleveland Cl Coll Med/Case West Res

Weigel, Ronald J MD/PhD [S] - **Spec Exp:** Breast Cancer; Endocrine Surgery; **Hospital:** Univ Iowa Hosp & Clinics; **Address:** Univ Iowa Carver Coll Med-Dept Surgery, 200 Hawkins Drive, 1516 JCP, Iowa City, IA 52242-1086; **Phone:** 319-356-4200; **Board Cert:** Surgery 2001; **Med School:** Yale Univ 1986; **Resid:** Surgery, Duke Univ Med Ctr 1992; **Fellow:** Immunology, Duke Univ Med Ctr; **Fac Appt:** Prof S, Univ Iowa Coll Med

Wiebke, Eric A MD [S] - **Spec Exp:** Gastrointestinal Cancer & Surgery; Laparoscopic Surgery; Gastrointestinal Motility Disorders; **Hospital:** Indiana Univ Hosp; **Address:** Indiana Univ Med Ctr-Emerson Hall 244, 545 Barnhill Drive, Indianapolis, IN 46202; **Phone:** 317-274-4990; **Board Cert:** Surgery 1998; Surgical Critical Care 2002; **Med School:** Vanderbilt Univ 1983; **Resid:** Surgery, Johns Hopkins Hosp 1989; **Fellow:** Surgical Oncology, Natl Cancer Inst/NIH 1987; **Fac Appt:** Prof S, Indiana Univ

Witt, Thomas R MD [S] - **Spec Exp:** Breast Cancer; Breast Disease; **Hospital:** Rush Univ Med Ctr, Glenbrook/NorthShore Univ Hlth Syst; **Address:** 1725 W Harrison St, Ste 409, Chicago, IL 60612-3828; **Phone:** 312-942-2302; **Board Cert:** Surgery 2000; **Med School:** Northwestern Univ 1975; **Resid:** Surgery, Rush Presby-St Lukes Med Ctr 1980; **Fellow:** Surgical Oncology, Meml Sloan Kettering Cancer Ctr 1982; **Fac Appt:** Assoc Prof S, Rush Med Coll

Great Plains and Mountains

Edney, James A MD [S] - **Spec Exp:** Breast Cancer; Thyroid & Parathyroid Cancer & Surgery; Cancer Surgery; **Hospital:** Nebraska Med Ctr; **Address:** Univ Nebraska Med Ctr, Dept Surgery, 984030 Nebraska Medical Ctr, Omaha, NE 68198-4030; **Phone:** 402-559-7272; **Board Cert:** Surgery 2000; **Med School:** Univ Nebr Coll Med 1975; **Resid:** Surgery, Univ Nebraska Med Ctr 1980; **Fellow:** Surgical Oncology, Univ Colorado Med Ctr 1981; **Fac Appt:** Prof S, Univ Nebr Coll Med

Finlayson, Christina A MD [S] - **Spec Exp:** Breast Cancer; Breast Disease; **Hospital:** Univ Colorado Hosp; **Address:** Univ Colorado Hlth Sci Ctr, Dept Surgery, GI Tumor C313 Academic Office 1, rm 6001, 12631 E 17th Ave, PO Box 6511, Auora, CO 80045; **Phone:** 720-848-1030; **Board Cert:** Surgery 2004; **Med School:** Univ Utah 1989; **Resid:** Surgery, Univ Colorado Hlth Sci Ctr 1994; **Fellow:** Surgical Oncology, Fox Chase Cancer Ctr 1996; **Fac Appt:** Assoc Prof S, Univ Colorado

Fitzgibbons Jr, Robert J MD [S] - **Spec Exp:** Hernia; Minimally Invasive Surgery; Gastrointestinal Surgery; **Hospital:** Creighton Univ Med Ctr, Archbishop Bergan Mercy Med Ctr; **Address:** Creighton Univ, Dept Surgery, 601 N 30th St, Ste 3700, Omaha, NE 68131-2100; **Phone:** 402-280-4503; **Board Cert:** Surgery 2002; **Med School:** Creighton Univ 1974; **Resid:** Surgery, Charity Hosp/LA State Univ 1979; **Fellow:** Surgery, Lahey Clin 1980; **Fac Appt:** Prof S, Creighton Univ

Loggie, Brian MD [S] - **Spec Exp:** Cancer Surgery; Mesothelioma; Solid Tumors; Melanoma; **Hospital:** Creighton Univ Med Ctr; **Address:** 601 N 30th St, Ste 2801, Omaha, NE 68131; **Phone:** 402-280-4100; **Board Cert:** Surgery 1998; **Med School:** McGill Univ 1979; **Resid:** Surgery, Montreal Genl Hosp 1986; **Fellow:** Surgical Oncology, Univ Illinois 1988; **Fac Appt:** Prof S, Creighton Univ

McIntyre Jr, Robert C MD [S] - **Spec Exp:** Endocrine Surgery; Trauma; Critical Care; **Hospital:** Univ Colorado Hosp, Chldn's Hosp - Aurora, The; **Address:** Univ Colorado at Denver & Hlth Sci Ctr, 12631 E 17th Ave, PO Box 6511, MS C313, Aurora, CO 80045; **Phone:** 303-724-2724; **Board Cert:** Surgery 2002; Surgical Critical Care 2003; **Med School:** Tulane Univ 1987; **Resid:** Surgery, Univ Colorado 1992; **Fac Appt:** Assoc Prof S, Univ Colorado

Mulvihill, Sean J MD [S] - **Spec Exp:** Gastrointestinal Surgery; Liver & Biliary Cancer; Pancreatic Cancer; **Hospital:** Univ Utah Hosps and Clins; **Address:** Univ Utah, Dept Surgery, 30 N 1900 E, rm 3B110, Salt Lake City, UT 84132; **Phone:** 801-581-7304; **Board Cert:** Surgery 1999; **Med School:** USC Sch Med 1981; **Resid:** Surgery, UCLA Med Ctr 1987; **Fac Appt:** Prof S, Univ Utah

Nelson, Edward W MD [S] - **Spec Exp:** Breast Cancer; **Hospital:** Univ Utah Hosps and Clins; **Address:** Univ Utah Med Ctr, Div Genl Surgery, 30 N 1900 E, rm 3B322, Salt Lake City, UT 84132; **Phone:** 801-581-7738; **Board Cert:** Surgery 2008; **Med School:** Univ Utah 1974; **Resid:** Surgery, Univ Utah Med Ctr 1979; **Fac Appt:** Prof S, Univ Utah

Pearlman, Nathan W MD [S] - **Spec Exp:** Gastrointestinal Cancer; Melanoma; Head & Neck Cancer; **Hospital:** Univ Colorado Hosp; **Address:** 12631 E 17th Ave, MS C-313, Aurora, CO 80045; **Phone:** 303-724-2728; **Board Cert:** Surgery 1974; **Med School:** Univ IL Coll Med 1966; **Resid:** Surgery, Univ Colorado Med Ctr 1973; **Fellow:** Surgical Oncology, Sloan-Kettering Cancer Ctr 1975; **Fac Appt:** Prof S, Univ Colorado

Petelin, Joseph B MD [S] - **Spec Exp:** Laparoscopic Abdominal Surgery; **Hospital:** Shawnee Mission Med Ctr; **Address:** 9119 W 74th St, Ste 255, Shawnee Mission, KS 66204; **Phone:** 913-432-5420; **Board Cert:** Surgery 2001; **Med School:** Univ Kans 1976; **Resid:** Surgery, Univ Kansas 1981; **Fac Appt:** Assoc Clin Prof S, Univ Kans

Surgery

Saffle, Jeffrey MD [S] - **Spec Exp:** Burn Care; Wound Healing/Care; **Hospital:** Univ Utah Hosps and Clins; **Address:** Dept Surgery, 30 N 1900 E, rm 3B306, Salt Lake City, UT 84132; **Phone:** 801-581-3595; **Board Cert:** Surgery 2002; Surgical Critical Care 2007; **Med School:** Univ Chicago-Pritzker Sch Med 1976; **Resid:** Surgery, Univ Utah Med Ctr 1982; **Fellow:** Burn Surgery, Univ Utah Med Ctr 1980; **Fac Appt:** Prof S, Univ Utah

Sasson, Aaron R MD [S] - **Spec Exp:** Gastrointestinal Cancer; Pancreatic Cancer; Liver Cancer; Neuroendocrine Tumors; **Hospital:** Nebraska Med Ctr; **Address:** Univ Nebraska Med Ctr, Box 984030, Omaha, NE 68198-0001; **Phone:** 402-559-8941; **Board Cert:** Surgery 2000; **Med School:** UMDNJ-NJ Med Sch, Newark 1993; **Resid:** Surgery, UCSD Med Ctr 1999; **Fellow:** Surgical Oncology, Fox Chase Cancer Ctr 2001; **Fac Appt:** Assoc Prof S, Univ Nebr Coll Med

Shaw Jr, Byers W MD [S] - **Spec Exp:** Transplant-Liver; Hepatobiliary Surgery; Liver Tumors; **Hospital:** Nebraska Med Ctr; **Address:** 983285 Nebraska Med Ctr, Omaha, NE 68198-3285; **Phone:** 402-559-5000; **Board Cert:** Surgery 2003; Surgical Critical Care 1996; **Med School:** Case West Res Univ 1976; **Resid:** Surgery, Univ Utah Med Ctr 1981; **Fellow:** Transplant Surgery, Univ Pittsburgh 1983; **Fac Appt:** Prof S, Univ Nebr Coll Med

Southwest

Ames, Frederick C MD [S] - **Spec Exp:** Breast Cancer; **Hospital:** UT MD Anderson Cancer Ctr; **Address:** MD Anderson Cancer Ctr, Dept Surgery, 1515 Holcombe Blvd, Unit 444, Houston, TX 77030-4009; **Phone:** 713-792-6929; **Board Cert:** Surgery 1975; **Med School:** Univ Tex Med Br, Galveston 1969; **Resid:** Surgery, Univ Texas Med Branch 1971; Surgery, St Joseph Hosp 1974; **Fellow:** Surgical Oncology, MD Anderson Cancer Ctr 1975; **Fac Appt:** Prof S, Univ Tex, Houston

Babiera, Gildy V MD [S] - **Spec Exp:** Breast Cancer; **Hospital:** UT MD Anderson Cancer Ctr; **Address:** MD Anderson Cancer Ctr, 1515 Holcombe Blvd., Unit 444, Houston, TX 77030-4009; **Phone:** 713-792-6937; **Board Cert:** Surgery 2007; **Med School:** NY Med Coll 1991; **Resid:** Surgery, NYU Med Ctr 1995; Surgery, NYU Med Ctr 1997; **Fellow:** Surgical Oncology, MD Anderson Cancer Ctr 1996; **Fac Appt:** Assoc Prof Surg & Onc, Univ Tex, Houston

Baker, Christopher C MD [S] - **Spec Exp:** Trauma/Critical Care; Colon & Rectal Surgery; Hernia; **Hospital:** LSU Interim Public Hosp; **Address:** LSUHSC Sch Med, Dept Surg, 1542 Tulane Ave, rm 741, New Orleans, LA 70112; **Phone:** 504-568-4751; **Board Cert:** Surgery 2002; Surgical Critical Care 2007; **Med School:** Harvard Med Sch 1974; **Resid:** Surgery, UCSF Med Ctr 1981; **Fellow:** Trauma, San Francisco Genl Hosp 1979; **Fac Appt:** Prof S, Louisiana State U, New Orleans

Beitsch, Peter D MD [S] - **Spec Exp:** Breast Cancer; **Hospital:** Med City Dallas Hosp, Presby Hosp of Dallas; **Address:** 7777 Forrest Ln C Bldg - Ste 760, Dallas, TX 75230; **Phone:** 972-566-8039; **Board Cert:** Surgery 2002; **Med School:** Univ Tex SW, Dallas 1986; **Resid:** Surgery, Univ TX SW Med Ctr 1993; **Fellow:** Surgical Oncology, MD Anderson Cancer Ctr 1990; Surgical Oncology, John Wayne Cancer Inst 1994

Bentley, Frederick R MD [S] - **Spec Exp:** Transplant Surgery; Transplant-Kidney; Transplant-Pancreas; Colon Cancer; **Hospital:** UAMS Med Ctr; **Address:** 4301 W Markham St, Slot 520, Little Rock, AR 72205; **Phone:** 501-526-7053; **Board Cert:** Surgery 2006; **Med School:** Louisiana State U, New Orleans 1977; **Resid:** Surgery, LSU Med Ctr 1983; **Fellow:** Research, Univ Minnesota Affil Hosp 1982; Transplant Surgery, Univ Minnesota Affil Hosp 1984; **Fac Appt:** Assoc Prof S, Univ Louisville Sch Med

Bolton, John MD [S] - **Spec Exp:** Cancer Surgery; Esophageal Cancer; Pancreatic Cancer; Liver Cancer; **Hospital:** Ochsner Fdn Hosp; **Address:** Ochsner Clin, Dept Surg, 1514 Jefferson Hwy, New Orleans, LA 70121; **Phone:** 504-842-4072; **Board Cert:** Surgery 2002; **Med School:** Louisiana State U, New Orleans 1976; **Resid:** Surgery, Charity Hosp 1981; **Fellow:** Hepatopancreatobiliary Surgery, Lahey Clinic 1980; Surgical Oncology, Meml Sloan Kettering Cancer Ctr 1982; **Fac Appt:** Asst Clin Prof S, Louisiana State U, New Orleans

Brunicardi, F Charles MD [S] - **Spec Exp:** Islet Cell Transplant; Pancreatic Cancer; Gastroesophageal Reflux Disease (GERD); **Hospital:** St Luke's Episcopal Hosp-Houston; **Address:** 6620 Main St, Ste 1475, Houston, TX 77030; **Phone:** 713-798-8070; **Board Cert:** Surgery 1998; **Med School:** UMDNJ-Rutgers Med Sch 1980; **Resid:** Surgery, SUNY Brooklyn Hlth Sci Ctr 1989; **Fellow:** Pancreatic Physiology, SUNY Brooklyn Hlth Sci Ctr 1986; **Fac Appt:** Prof S, Baylor Coll Med

Curley, Steven A MD [S] - **Spec Exp:** Colon & Rectal Cancer; Liver Cancer; Hepatobiliary Surgery; **Hospital:** UT MD Anderson Cancer Ctr; **Address:** MD Anderson Cancer Ctr, Dept Surg Oncology, Unit 444, PO Box 301402, Houston, TX 77230-1402; **Phone:** 713-792-6937; **Board Cert:** Surgery 1997; **Med School:** Univ Tex, Houston 1982; **Resid:** Surgery, Univ New Mexico Hosps 1988; **Fellow:** Surgical Oncology, MD Anderson Cancer Ctr 1990; **Fac Appt:** Prof S, Univ Tex, Houston

Demarest III, Gerald B MD [S] - **Spec Exp:** Trauma; Burn Care; **Hospital:** Univ NM Hlth & Sci Ctr; **Address:** Univ New Mexico Health Science Ctr, Dept Surgery, MSC 10-5610, 1 University New Mexico, Albuquerque, NM 83131-0001; **Phone:** 505-272-6441; **Board Cert:** Surgery 1999; Surgical Critical Care 2005; **Med School:** Columbia P&S 1973; **Resid:** Surgery, Univ Washington Med Ctr 1978; **Fellow:** Burn Surgery, Harborview Med Ctr 1979; Harborview Med Ctr 1980; **Fac Appt:** Assoc Prof S, Univ New Mexico

Dooley, William C MD [S] - **Spec Exp:** Breast Cancer; Tumors-Rare & Multiple; **Hospital:** OU Med Ctr, VA Med Ctr - Oklahoma City; **Address:** 825 NE 10th St, Ste 4500, Oklahoma City, OK 73104; **Phone:** 405-271-7867; **Board Cert:** Surgery 1997; **Med School:** Vanderbilt Univ 1982; **Resid:** Surgery, Johns Hopkins Hosp 1987; Surgical Oncology, Oxford Univ 1986; **Fellow:** Surgical Oncology, Johns Hopkins 1988; **Fac Appt:** Prof S, Univ Okla Coll Med

Ellis, Lee M MD [S] - **Spec Exp:** Liver Cancer; Colon & Rectal Cancer; Metastatic Cancer; Peritoneal Carcinomatosis; **Hospital:** UT MD Anderson Cancer Ctr; **Address:** MD Anderson Cancer Ctr, Dept Surgery, 1515 Holcombe Blvd, Box 444, Houston, TX 77030; **Phone:** 713-792-6937; **Board Cert:** Surgery 1999; **Med School:** Univ VA Sch Med 1983; **Resid:** Surgery, Univ Fla-Shands Hosp 1990; **Fellow:** Surgical Oncology, MD Anderson Cancer Ctr 1992; **Fac Appt:** Prof S, Univ Tex, Houston

Euhus, David M MD [S] - **Spec Exp:** Breast Cancer; **Hospital:** UT Southwestern Med Ctr at Dallas; **Address:** Univ Texas SW Med Ctr - Div Surg Oncology, 5323 Harry Hines Blvd, MC 9155, Dallas, TX 75390-9155; **Phone:** 214-648-6467; **Board Cert:** Surgery 2001; **Med School:** St Louis Univ 1984; **Resid:** Surgery, UCLA Med Ctr 1991; **Fellow:** Surgical Oncology, UCLA Med Ctr 1988; Breast Disease, Queens Med Ctr 1990; **Fac Appt:** Prof S, Univ Tex SW, Dallas

Feig, Barry W MD [S] - **Spec Exp:** Gastrointestinal Cancer; Sarcoma; Breast Cancer; **Hospital:** UT MD Anderson Cancer Ctr; **Address:** UT MD Anderson Cancer Ctr, Dept Surg Onc, Unit 444, PO Box 301402, Houston, TX 77230-1402; **Phone:** 713-792-6937; **Board Cert:** Surgery 1998; **Med School:** SUNY Upstate Med Univ 1984; **Resid:** Surgery, Northwestern Univ Med Ctr 1990; **Fellow:** Trauma, Univ Minnesota Affil Hosp 1991; Surgical Oncology, UT MD Anderson Cancer Ctr 1994; **Fac Appt:** Prof S, Univ Tex, Houston

Surgery

Fisher, William E MD [S] - **Spec Exp:** Pancreatic Cancer; **Hospital:** St Luke's Episcopal Hosp-Houston; **Address:** 6620 Main St, Ste 1475, Houston, TX 77030; **Phone:** 713-798-8070; **Board Cert:** Surgery 2006; **Med School:** Univ Cincinnati 1990; **Resid:** Surgery, Ohio State U Hosps 1996; **Fellow:** Cancer Research, Ohio State U Hosps 1998; **Fac Appt:** Asst Prof S, Baylor Coll Med

Franklin, Morris E MD [S] - **Spec Exp:** Laparoscopic Abdominal Surgery; Colon & Rectal Surgery; **Hospital:** Southeast Baptist Hosp, Baptist Med Ctr - San Antonio; **Address:** 4242 E Southcross Blvd, Ste 1, San Antonio, TX 78222; **Phone:** 210-333-7510; **Board Cert:** Surgery 1973; **Med School:** Univ Tex SW, Dallas 1967; **Resid:** Surgery, Bexar Co Hosp 1972; **Fac Appt:** Clin Prof S, Univ Tex, San Antonio

Grant, Michael D MD [S] - **Spec Exp:** Breast Cancer; Breast Surgery; **Hospital:** Baylor Univ Medical Ctr; **Address:** 3900 Junius, Ste 220, Baylor Medical Pavillion, Dallas, TX 75246; **Phone:** 214-826-7300; **Board Cert:** Surgery 2001; **Med School:** Univ Tex, Houston 1987; **Resid:** Surgery, Baylor Univ Med Ctr 1992; **Fellow:** Breast Cancer, Baylor Univ Med Ctr 1993

Gray, Richard J MD [S] - **Spec Exp:** Breast Cancer; Melanoma; **Hospital:** Mayo Clinic - Phoenix, Mayo Clinic - Scottsdale; **Address:** Mayo Clinic, 5777 E Mayo Blvd, Phoenix, AZ 85054; **Phone:** 480-342-2849; **Board Cert:** Surgery 2001; **Med School:** Mich State Univ 1995; **Resid:** Surgery, Mayo Clinic 2000; **Fellow:** Surgical Oncology, H Lee Moffitt Cancer Ctr 2001; **Fac Appt:** Assoc Prof S, Mayo Med Sch

Griswold, John A MD [S] - **Spec Exp:** Burn Care; **Hospital:** Univ Med Ctr-Lubbock; **Address:** Dept Surgery, 3601 4th St, MS 9905, Lubbock, TX 79430; **Phone:** 806-743-2373; **Board Cert:** Surgery 1999; Surgical Critical Care 2000; **Med School:** Creighton Univ 1981; **Resid:** Surgery, Texas Tech Univ Hlth Scis Ctr 1986; **Fellow:** Burn Surgery, Univ Washington 1988

Halff, Glenn A MD [S] - **Spec Exp:** Transplant-Liver; Liver Surgery; **Hospital:** Univ Hlth Syst-San Antonio, Christus Santa Rosa Children's Hosp; **Address:** University Transplant Center, 7703 Floyd Curl Drive, MC 785, San Antonio, TX 78229; **Phone:** 210-567-5777; **Board Cert:** Surgery 2007; Surgical Critical Care 2000; **Med School:** Univ Tex, Houston 1983; **Resid:** Surgery, NYU Med Ctr 1987; **Fellow:** Transplant Surgery, Univ Pittsburgh 1989; **Fac Appt:** Assoc Prof S, Univ Tex, San Antonio

Hunt, John L MD [S] - **Spec Exp:** Trauma; Burn Care; **Hospital:** UT Southwestern Med Ctr at Dallas; **Address:** Dept Surgery, 5323 Harry Hines Blvd, MC 9158, Dallas, TX 75390-9158; **Phone:** 214-648-2152; **Board Cert:** Surgery 1972; Surgical Critical Care 1996; **Med School:** Univ Cincinnati 1964; **Resid:** Surgery, Cincinnati Genl Hosp 1971; **Fac Appt:** Prof S, Univ Tex SW, Dallas

Hunt, Kelly K MD [S] - **Spec Exp:** Breast Cancer; Sarcoma-Soft Tissue; Gene Therapy; **Hospital:** UT MD Anderson Cancer Ctr; **Address:** MD Anderson Cancer Ctr, 1515 Holcombe Blvd, Box 444, Houston, TX 77030-4000; **Phone:** 713-792-7216; **Board Cert:** Surgery 2001; **Med School:** Univ Tenn Coll Med, Memphis 1986; **Resid:** Surgery, UCLA Med Ctr 1993; **Fellow:** Surgical Oncology, MD Anderson Cancer Ctr 1996; **Fac Appt:** Prof S, Univ Tex, Houston

Jackson, Gilchrist MD [S] - **Spec Exp:** Thyroid & Parathyroid Surgery; Head & Neck Cancer & Surgery; Endocrine Tumors; Gastrointestinal Cancer & Surgery; **Hospital:** St Luke's Episcopal Hosp-Houston, Woman's Hosp TX; **Address:** 2727 W Holcombe Blvd Fl 3 A, Houston, TX 77027; **Phone:** 713-442-1132; **Board Cert:** Surgery 1998; **Med School:** Univ Louisville Sch Med 1974; **Resid:** Surgery, Parkland Hosp 1979; **Fellow:** Surgical Oncology, MD Anderson Hosp 1980; **Fac Appt:** Assoc Clin Prof S, Baylor Coll Med

Kim, Lawrence Thomas MD [S] - **Spec Exp:** Endocrine Surgery; Thyroid Cancer; Parathyroid Disease; **Hospital:** UAMS Med Ctr; **Address:** 4301 W Markham, Slot# 721-2, Little Rock, AR 72205; **Phone:** 501-686-8211; **Board Cert:** Surgery 2005; **Med School:** Univ Tex SW, Dallas 1987; **Resid:** Surgery, South Western Med Ctr 1994; **Fellow:** Research, South Western Med Ctr 1991; Research, Natl Inst Health 1996; **Fac Appt:** Prof S, Univ Ark

Klimberg, Vicki S MD [S] - **Spec Exp:** Breast Cancer; Radiofrequency Tumor Ablation; Sentinel Node Surgery; **Hospital:** UAMS Med Ctr; **Address:** Univ Arkansas Medical Sciences, 4301 W Markham, MS 725, Little Rock, AR 72205-7199; **Phone:** 501-686-5669; **Board Cert:** Surgery 1999; **Med School:** Univ Fla Coll Med 1984; **Resid:** Surgery, Univ Fla Med Ctr 1989; **Fellow:** Clinical Oncology, Univ Fla 1990; Breast Disease, Univ Arkansas for Med Scis 1991; **Fac Appt:** Prof S, Univ Ark

Krouse, Robert S MD [S] - **Spec Exp:** Cancer Surgery; Gastrointestinal Cancer; Palliative Care; **Hospital:** VA Medical Center - Tucson; **Address:** Southern AZ VA Hosp Care System, Surg Care Line, 2-112, 3601 S 6th Ave, Tucson, AZ 85723; **Phone:** 520-792-1450 x6145; **Board Cert:** Surgery 2007; **Med School:** Hahnemann Univ 1991; **Resid:** Surgery, Univ Hawaii Integrated Surg Prog 1993; Immunotherapy, Natl Cancer Inst 1994; **Fellow:** Surgery, W Virginia Univ Sch Med 1997; Surgical Oncology, City of Hope Natl Med Ctr 2000; **Fac Appt:** Asst Prof S, Univ Ariz Coll Med

Kuhn, Joseph A MD [S] - **Spec Exp:** Liver Cancer; Peritoneal Carcinomatosis; Melanoma; Thyroid Cancer; **Hospital:** Baylor Univ Medical Ctr; **Address:** 7777 Forest Lane St, Ste C-410, Dallas, TX 75230; **Phone:** 214-823-5000; **Board Cert:** Surgery 1999; Surgical Critical Care 2003; **Med School:** Univ Tex Med Br, Galveston 1984; **Resid:** Surgery, Baylor Univ Med Ctr 1989; **Fellow:** Surgical Oncology, City Hosp Natl Med Ctr 1992

Lee, Jeffrey E MD [S] - **Spec Exp:** Melanoma; Pancreatic Cancer; Endocrine Tumors; **Hospital:** UT MD Anderson Cancer Ctr; **Address:** UT MD Anderson Cancer Ctr, 1400 Holcombe Blvd, Unit 444 Fl 12, Houston, TX 77030-4009; **Phone:** 713-792-7218; **Board Cert:** Surgery 1999; **Med School:** Stanford Univ 1984; **Resid:** Surgery, Stanford Univ Hosp 1987; Surgery, Stanford Univ Hosp 1991; **Fellow:** Immunology, Stanford Univ Sch Med 1989; Surgical Oncology, Univ Tex-MD Anderson Cancer Ctr 1993; **Fac Appt:** Prof S, Univ Tex, Houston

Leitch, A Marilyn MD [S] - **Spec Exp:** Breast Cancer & Surgery; Melanoma; Sarcoma; **Hospital:** UT Southwestern Med Ctr at Dallas; **Address:** UT Southwestern Med Ctr - Dept Surgery, 5323 Harry Hines Blvd, MC 9155, Dallas, TX 75390-9155; **Phone:** 214-648-3039; **Board Cert:** Surgery 2003; **Med School:** Univ Tex SW, Dallas 1978; **Resid:** Surgery, UCLA Med Ctr 1984; **Fellow:** Surgical Oncology, MD Anderson Cancer Ctr 1985; **Fac Appt:** Prof S, Univ Tex SW, Dallas

Li, Benjamin D L MD [S] - **Spec Exp:** Gastrointestinal Cancer; Sarcoma; Breast Cancer; **Hospital:** Louisiana State Univ Hosp, Willis Knighton Hlth Sys; **Address:** LSU Hlth Scis Ctr, Dept Surgery, 1501 Kings Hwy, Shreveport, LA 71130; **Phone:** 318-675-6100; **Board Cert:** Surgery 2002; **Med School:** Yale Univ 1986; **Resid:** Surgery, Northwestern Univ-McGraw Med Ctr 1992; **Fellow:** Surgical Oncology, Roswell Park Cancer Inst 1995; **Fac Appt:** Prof S, Louisiana State U, New Orleans

Livingston, Edward H MD [S] - **Spec Exp:** Gastrointestinal Surgery; Endocrine Surgery; Obesity/Bariatric Surgery; **Hospital:** UT Southwestern Med Ctr at Dallas; **Address:** Dept Surgery, 5323 Harry Hines Blvd, MC 9156, Dallas, TX 75390-9156; **Phone:** 214-648-7956; **Board Cert:** Surgery 2003; **Med School:** UCLA 1985; **Resid:** Surgery, UCLA Med Ctr 1992; **Fac Appt:** Prof S, Univ Tex SW, Dallas

Surgery

Mansfield, Paul F MD [S] - **Spec Exp:** Appendix Cancer; Stomach Cancer; Colon Cancer; Melanoma; **Hospital:** UT MD Anderson Cancer Ctr; **Address:** UT MD Anderson Cancer Ctr, 1515 Holcombe Blvd, rm 444, Houston, TX 77030; **Phone:** 713-794-5499; **Board Cert:** Surgery 2006; **Med School:** Jefferson Med Coll 1983; **Resid:** Surgery, Pennsylvania Hosp 1988; **Fellow:** Surgical Oncology, MD Anderson Cancer Ctr 1991; **Fac Appt:** Prof Surg & Onc, Univ Tex, Houston

Pisters, Peter MD [S] - **Spec Exp:** Pancreatic Cancer; Sarcoma-Soft Tissue; Gastrointestinal Cancer; **Hospital:** UT MD Anderson Cancer Ctr; **Address:** MD Anderson Cancer Ctr, PO Box 301402, Unit 444, Houston, TX 77230-1402; **Phone:** 713-792-6397; **Board Cert:** Surgery 2001; **Med School:** Univ Western Ontario 1985; **Resid:** Surgery, NYU/Bellevue Hosp 1992; **Fellow:** Surgical Research, Meml Sloan-Kettering Cancer Ctr 1989; Surgical Oncology, Meml Sloan-Kettering Cancer Ctr 1994; **Fac Appt:** Prof S, Univ Tex, Houston

Pockaj, Barbara A MD [S] - **Spec Exp:** Melanoma; Breast Cancer; Stomach Cancer; Clinical Trials; **Hospital:** Mayo Clinic - Scottsdale; **Address:** Mayo Clinic, Dept Surgery, 5779 E Mayo Blvd, Phoenix, AZ 85054; **Phone:** 480-342-1051; **Board Cert:** Surgery 2005; **Med School:** Vanderbilt Univ 1987; **Resid:** Surgery, Case Western Res Univ Affil Hosps 1995; **Fellow:** Surgical Oncology, Natl Inst Hlth 1992; **Fac Appt:** Assoc Prof S, Mayo Med Sch

Pollock, Raphael E MD/PhD [S] - **Spec Exp:** Sarcoma; **Hospital:** UT MD Anderson Cancer Ctr; **Address:** MD Anderson Cancer Ctr, Dept Surg Oncology, 1515 Holcombe Blvd, Unit 444, Houston, TX 77030; **Phone:** 713-792-6928; **Board Cert:** Surgery 2003; **Med School:** St Louis Univ 1977; **Resid:** Surgery, Univ Chicago 1979; Surgery, Rush Presby-St Lukes Hosp 1982; **Fellow:** Surgical Oncology, MD Anderson Cancer Ctr 1984; **Fac Appt:** Prof S, Univ Tex, Houston

Postier, Russell G MD [S] - **Spec Exp:** Pancreatic Cancer; Biliary Surgery; **Hospital:** OU Med Ctr; **Address:** OU Physicians, Dept Surgery, 825 NE 10th St, Ste 4500, Oklahoma City, OK 73104; **Phone:** 405-271-1400; **Board Cert:** Surgery 2000; **Med School:** Univ Okla Coll Med 1975; **Resid:** Surgery, Johns Hopkins Hosp 1981; **Fac Appt:** Prof S, Univ Okla Coll Med

Purdue, Gary F MD [S] - **Spec Exp:** Burn Care; **Hospital:** Parkland Hlth & Hosp Sys; **Address:** UT Southwestern Med Ctr, 5323 Harry Hines Blvd, MC 9158, Dept Surgery, Dallas, TX 75390-9158; **Phone:** 214-648-2041; **Board Cert:** Surgery 1999; Surgical Critical Care 2006; **Med School:** Jefferson Med Coll 1976; **Resid:** Surgery, Mercy Hosp 1981; **Fellow:** Burn Surgery, Parkland Meml Hosp 1982; **Fac Appt:** Prof S, Univ Tex SW, Dallas

Ross, Merrick I MD [S] - **Spec Exp:** Sentinel Node Surgery; Breast Cancer; Melanoma; **Hospital:** UT MD Anderson Cancer Ctr; **Address:** UT MD Anderson Cancer Ctr, Dept Surg Onc, PO Box 301402, Unit 444, Houston, TX 77230-1402; **Phone:** 713-792-6937; **Board Cert:** Surgery 2007; **Med School:** Univ IL Coll Med 1980; **Resid:** Surgery, Univ Illinois Hosp & Clin 1982; Surgery, Univ Illinois Hosp & Clin 1987; **Fellow:** Research, Scripps Clin & Rsch 1984; Surgical Oncology, Univ TX-MD Anderson Cancer Ctr 1989; **Fac Appt:** Prof S, Univ Tex, Houston

Schlinkert, Richard T MD [S] - **Spec Exp:** Endocrine Surgery; Laparoscopic Surgery; Gastrointestinal Surgery; Adrenal Surgery; **Hospital:** Mayo Clinic - Phoenix; **Address:** Mayo Clinic, Dept Surgery, 13400 E Shea Blvd, Scottsdale, AZ 85259-5404; **Phone:** 480-342-1051; **Board Cert:** Surgery 2006; **Med School:** Med Coll OH 1981; **Resid:** Surgery, Mayo Clinic 1986; **Fellow:** Hepatobiliary Surgery, Royal Infirmary 1987; **Fac Appt:** Prof S, Mayo Med Sch

Singletary, S Eva MD [S] - **Spec Exp:** Breast Cancer; **Hospital:** UT MD Anderson Cancer Ctr; **Address:** Univ Tex MD Anderson Cancer Ctr, 1515 Holcombe Blvd, Box 444, Houston, TX 77030-4009; **Phone:** 713-792-6937; **Board Cert:** Surgery 2003; **Med School:** Med Univ SC 1977; **Resid:** Surgery, Shands Hosp-Univ Florida 1983; **Fellow:** Surgery, UT MD Anderson Hosp 1985; **Fac Appt:** Prof S, Univ Tex, Houston

Skibber, John M MD [S] - **Spec Exp:** Rectal Cancer/Sphincter Preservation; Colon & Rectal Cancer-Familial Polyposis; **Hospital:** UT MD Anderson Cancer Ctr; **Address:** Unit 444 PO Box 301402, Houston, TX 77230-1402; **Phone:** 713-792-5165; **Board Cert:** Surgery 1998; **Med School:** Jefferson Med Coll 1981; **Resid:** Surgery, NYU Med Ctr 1989; **Fellow:** Surgical Oncology, Univ Texas-MD Anderson 1991; **Fac Appt:** Prof S, Univ Tex, Houston

Stewart, Ronald M MD [S] - **Spec Exp:** Trauma; **Hospital:** Univ Hlth Syst-San Antonio; **Address:** Univ Tex Hlth Sci Ctr, Dept Surg-Trauma, 7703 Floyd Curl Drive, MC 7740, San Antonio, TX 78229-3900; **Phone:** 210-567-3623; **Board Cert:** Surgery 2000; Surgical Critical Care 2002; **Med School:** Univ Tex, San Antonio 1985; **Resid:** Surgery, Univ Tex Hlth Sci Ctr 1991; **Fellow:** Trauma, Univ Tenn Coll Med 1993; **Fac Appt:** Assoc Prof S, Univ Tex, San Antonio

Stolier, Alan J MD [S] - **Spec Exp:** Breast Cancer; **Hospital:** Ochsner Baptist Med Ctr, Louisiana State Univ Hosp; **Address:** 2525 Severn Ave, Metairie, LA 70002; **Phone:** 504-832-4200; **Board Cert:** Surgery 2006; **Med School:** Louisiana State U, New Orleans 1970; **Resid:** Surgery, Charity Hosp 1974; **Fellow:** Surgical Oncology, MD Anderson Hosp 1976

Vauthey, Jean Nicholas MD [S] - **Spec Exp:** Hepatobiliary Surgery; Liver Cancer; Gallbladder & Biliary Cancer; **Hospital:** UT MD Anderson Cancer Ctr; **Address:** UT MD Anderson Cancer Ctr -Surg Oncology, 1515 Holcombe Blvd, Unit 444, Houston, TX 77030; **Phone:** 713-792-6937; **Board Cert:** Surgery 2000; **Med School:** Switzerland 1979; **Resid:** Surgery, Ochsner Med Fdn 1989; **Fellow:** Hepatobiliary Surgery, Med Fac Univ Bern 1991; Surgical Oncology, Meml Sloan-Kettering Cancer Ctr 1993; **Fac Appt:** Prof S, Univ Tex, Houston

Woltering, Eugene MD [S] - **Spec Exp:** Carcinoid Tumors; **Hospital:** Ochsner Fdn Hosp; **Address:** 200 W Esplanade, Ste 200, Kenner, LA 70062; **Phone:** 504-464-8500; **Board Cert:** Surgery 2002; **Med School:** Ohio State Univ 1975; **Resid:** Surgery, Vanderbilt Med Ctr 1982; Surgical Oncology, Natl Inst Hlth 1979; **Fellow:** Surgical Oncology, Ohio State Univ 1984; **Fac Appt:** Prof S, Louisiana State U, New Orleans

Wood, R Patrick MD [S] - **Spec Exp:** Liver Cancer; Liver Surgery; **Hospital:** St Luke's Episcopal Hosp-Houston; **Address:** 6624 Fannin St, Ste 1200, Houston, TX 77030; **Phone:** 713-795-8994; **Board Cert:** Surgery 2004; **Med School:** Univ Rochester 1979; **Resid:** Surgery, NYU/Bellevue Hosp Ctr 1984; **Fellow:** Transplant Surgery, Univ Pittsburgh 1985; **Fac Appt:** Clin Prof S, Univ Tex, Houston

Zannis, Victor J MD [S] - **Spec Exp:** Breast Cancer; **Hospital:** Phoenix Baptist Hosp & Med Ctr, J C Lincoln Hosp - North Mountain; **Address:** 2525 W Greenway Rd, Ste 130, Phoenix, AZ 85023; **Phone:** 602-942-8000; **Board Cert:** Surgery 2000; **Med School:** UCLA 1976; **Resid:** Surgery, Maricopa Med Ctr 1982

West Coast and Pacific

Anderson, Benjamin O MD [S] - **Spec Exp:** Breast Cancer & Surgery; **Hospital:** Univ Wash Med Ctr; **Address:** Univ Washington Dept Surgery, 1959 NE Pacific St, Box 356410, Seattle, WA 98195-6410; **Phone:** 206-288-6487; **Board Cert:** Surgery 2002; **Med School:** Albert Einstein Coll Med 1985; **Resid:** Surgery, Univ Colorado 1992; **Fellow:** Surgical Oncology, Meml Sloan Kettering Cancer Ctr 1994; **Fac Appt:** Prof S, Univ Wash

Ascher, Nancy L MD/PhD [S] - **Spec Exp:** Transplant-Liver; Transplant-Kidney; **Hospital:** UCSF Med Ctr; **Address:** 513 Parnassus Ave, Box 0104, San Francisco, CA 94143-0104; **Phone:** 415-476-1236; **Board Cert:** Surgery 2002; **Med School:** Univ Mich Med Sch 1974; **Resid:** Surgery, Univ Minn Hosp 1981; **Fellow:** Transplant Surgery, Univ Minn Hosp 1982; **Fac Appt:** Prof S, UCSF

Bilchik, Anton J MD/PhD [S] - **Spec Exp:** Gastrointestinal Cancer; Laparoscopic Surgery; **Hospital:** St John's Hlth Ctr, Santa Monica, Cedars-Sinai Med Ctr; **Address:** John Wayne Cancer Institute, 2336 Santa Monica Blvd, Ste 206, Santa Monica, CA 90404; **Phone:** 310-696-0716; **Board Cert:** Surgery 2004; **Med School:** South Africa 1985; **Resid:** Surgery, UCLA Med Ctr 1996; **Fellow:** John Wayne Cancer Inst. 1998; **Fac Appt:** Asst Clin Prof S, UCLA

Bouvet, Michael MD [S] - **Spec Exp:** Endocrine Surgery; Pancreatic Cancer; Biliary Cancer; **Hospital:** UCSD Med Ctr; **Address:** UCSD Moores Cancer Ctr, 3855 Health Science Ctr, La Jolla, CA 92093; **Phone:** 858-822-6191; **Board Cert:** Surgery 2004; **Med School:** Univ Wash 1989; **Resid:** Surgery, UCSD Med Ctr 1995; **Fellow:** Surgical Oncology, MD Anderson Cancer Ctr 1998; **Fac Appt:** Assoc Prof S, UCSD

Busuttil, Ronald W MD/PhD [S] - **Spec Exp:** Transplant-Liver; Liver Cancer; **Hospital:** UCLA Ronald Reagan Med Ctr; **Address:** UCLA Dept Surg, Transplant, 77-120 CHS Box 957054, Los Angeles, CA 90095-7054; **Phone:** 310-825-5318; **Board Cert:** Surgery 2007; **Med School:** Tulane Univ 1971; **Resid:** Surgery, UCLA Med Ctr 1976; **Fellow:** Surgery, UCLA Med Ctr 1975; **Fac Appt:** Prof S, UCLA

Butler, John A MD [S] - **Spec Exp:** Breast Cancer; Thyroid Cancer; Adrenal Tumors; Small Bowel Cancer; **Hospital:** UC Irvine Med Ctr; **Address:** UC-Irvine Medical Ctr, 101 City Drive S, Bldg 56 Office 252 Rt 81, Orange, CA 92868-3298; **Phone:** 714-456-8030; **Board Cert:** Surgery 2003; **Med School:** Loyola Univ-Stritch Sch Med 1976; **Resid:** Surgery, LAC-USC Med Ctr 1982; Surgery, Harbor-UCLA Med Ctr 1982; **Fellow:** Surgical Oncology, Meml Sloan-Kettering Cancer Ctr 1984; **Fac Appt:** Prof S, UC Irvine

Byrd, David MD [S] - **Spec Exp:** Tumor Surgery; Breast Cancer; Melanoma; **Hospital:** Univ Wash Med Ctr; **Address:** Univ Washington Med Ctr, Dept Surgical Specialites Center, 1959 NE Pacific St, Box 356165, Seattle, WA 98195; **Phone:** 206-598-4477; **Board Cert:** Surgery 1998; **Med School:** Tulane Univ 1982; **Resid:** Surgery, Univ Wash Med Ctr 1987; **Fellow:** Surgical Oncology, Univ Tex-MD Anderson Cancer Ctr 1992; **Fac Appt:** Assoc Prof S, Univ Wash

Chang, Helena MD [S] - **Spec Exp:** Breast Cancer; Cancer Surgery; **Hospital:** UCLA Ronald Reagan Med Ctr; **Address:** 200 Westwood Plaza Drive, Ste B265, Revlon Breast Clinic, Los Angeles, CA 90095-7028; **Phone:** 310-825-2144; **Board Cert:** Surgery 1997; **Med School:** Temple Univ 1981; **Resid:** Surgery, Episcopal Hosp 1986; **Fellow:** Cellular Molecular Biology, Temple Univ 1977; Surgical Oncology, Meml Sloan-Kettering Cancer Ctr 1988; **Fac Appt:** Prof S, UCLA

Clark, Orlo H MD [S] - **Spec Exp:** Thyroid Cancer & Surgery; Neuroendocrine Tumors; Parathyroid Cancer; **Hospital:** UCSF - Mt Zion Med Ctr, UCSF Med Ctr; **Address:** UCSF Mt Zion Med Ctr, 1600 Divisadero St Fl 3, Box 1674, San Francisco, CA 94115-1926; **Phone:** 415-353-7687; **Board Cert:** Surgery 1974; **Med School:** Cornell Univ-Weill Med Coll 1967; **Resid:** Surgery, UCSF Med Ctr 1970; Surgery, UCSF Med Ctr 1973; **Fellow:** Surgery, Royal Med Sch London 1971; **Fac Appt:** Prof S, UCSF

Colquhoun, Steven D MD [S] - **Spec Exp:** Liver Cancer; Transplant-Liver; Pancreatic Cancer; Hepatobiliary Surgery; **Hospital:** Cedars-Sinai Med Ctr; **Address:** Cedars-Sinai Med Center, 8635 W 3rd St, Ste 590-W, Los Angeles, CA 90048; **Phone:** 310-423-2641; **Board Cert:** Surgery 2003; Surgical Critical Care 2008; **Med School:** Loyola Univ-Stritch Sch Med 1984; **Resid:** Surgery, UCLA Med Ctr 1990; **Fellow:** Surgical Oncology, UCLA Med Ctr 1993; Transplant Surgery, UCLA Med Ctr 1994; **Fac Appt:** Assoc Clin Prof S, UCLA

Curet, Myriam J MD [S] - **Spec Exp:** Obesity/Bariatric Surgery; Robotic Surgery; Minimally Invasive Surgery; **Hospital:** Stanford Univ Med Ctr; **Address:** 300 Pasteur Drive, rm H3680, Stanford, CA 94305-5655; **Phone:** 650-736-1613; **Board Cert:** Surgery 2008; **Med School:** Harvard Med Sch 1982; **Resid:** Surgery, Univ Chicago Hosps 1989; **Fellow:** Univ New Mexico 1994; **Fac Appt:** Prof S, Stanford Univ

Dixon, Sherwood M MD [S] - **Spec Exp:** Wound Healing/Care; **Hospital:** Northern Nevada Med Ctr; **Address:** 1500 E 2nd St, Ste 206, Reno, NV 89502; **Phone:** 775-789-7000; **Board Cert:** Surgery 2000; **Med School:** Univ Alabama 1976; **Resid:** Surgery, UC Davis Med Ctr 1981; **Fellow:** Vascular Surgery, UCLA Ctr Hlth Scis 1982

Duh, Quan-Yang MD [S] - **Spec Exp:** Endocrine Surgery; Thyroid & Parathyroid Cancer & Surgery; Adrenal Tumors; Minimally Invasive Surgery; **Hospital:** UCSF Med Ctr, VA Med Ctr - San Francisco; **Address:** UCSF Medical Ctr, Box 1926, San Francisco, CA 94143-1926; **Phone:** 415-353-7687; **Board Cert:** Surgery 2007; **Med School:** UCSF 1981; **Resid:** Surgery, UCSF Med Ctr 1988; **Fellow:** Endocrine Surgery, UCSF Med Ctr 1987; **Fac Appt:** Prof S, UCSF

Easter, David W MD [S] - **Spec Exp:** Breast Cancer; Gastrointestinal Cancer; **Hospital:** UCSD Med Ctr; **Address:** UCSD Dept Surgery, 200 W Arbor Drive, MC 8401, San Diego, CA 92103-8401; **Phone:** 619-543-2826; **Board Cert:** Surgery 2000; **Med School:** Yale Univ 1983; **Resid:** Surgery, UCSD Med Ctr 1989; **Fellow:** Surgical Oncology, Ninewells, Dundee 1990; **Fac Appt:** Clin Prof S, UCSD

Eilber, Frederick R MD [S] - **Spec Exp:** Tumor Surgery; Sarcoma; **Hospital:** UCLA Ronald Reagan Med Ctr; **Address:** 200 UCLA Medical Plaza, Ste 120, Los Angeles, CA 90095-1718; **Phone:** 310-825-7086; **Board Cert:** Surgery 1973; **Med School:** Univ Mich Med Sch 1965; **Resid:** Surgery, Univ Maryland Hosp 1972; **Fellow:** Surgery, Univ Tex-MD Anderson Hosp 1973; **Fac Appt:** Prof S, UCLA

Ellenhorn, Joshua DI MD [S] - **Spec Exp:** Gastrointestinal Cancer; Pancreatic Cancer; Cancer Surgery; **Hospital:** City of Hope Natl Med Ctr & Beckman Rsch, Huntington Memorial Hosp; **Address:** City of Hope Med Ctr, 1500 E Duarte Rd, Duarte, CA 91010; **Phone:** 626-471-7100; **Board Cert:** Surgery 2000; **Med School:** Boston Univ 1984; **Resid:** Surgery, Univ Cincinnati Hosp 1991; **Fellow:** Surgical Oncology, Meml Sloan-Kettering Cancer Ctr 1993

Esquivel, Carlos O MD [S] - **Spec Exp:** Transplant-Liver; **Hospital:** Stanford Univ Med Ctr, Lucile Packard Chldn's Hosp; **Address:** 750 Welch Rd, Ste 319, Palo Alto, CA 94304; **Phone:** 650-498-5689; **Board Cert:** Surgery 2003; Surgical Critical Care 1999; **Med School:** Costa Rica 1975; **Resid:** Surgery, UC- Davis Med Ctr 1984; **Fellow:** Transplant Surgery, Univ Hlth Ctr Pittsburgh 1985; **Fac Appt:** Prof S, Stanford Univ

Esserman, Laura J MD [S] - **Spec Exp:** Breast Cancer; **Hospital:** UCSF - Mt Zion Med Ctr, UCSF Med Ctr; **Address:** UCSF-Helen Diller Family Comp Cancer Ctr, 1600 Divisadero St Fl 2, Box 1710, San Francisco, CA 94115; **Phone:** 415-353-7070; **Board Cert:** Surgery 2001; **Med School:** Stanford Univ 1983; **Resid:** Surgery, Stanford Univ Med Ctr 1991; **Fellow:** Oncology, Stanford Univ Med Ctr 1988; **Fac Appt:** Assoc Prof S, UCSF

Essner, Richard MD [S] - **Spec Exp:** Sentinel Node Surgery; Melanoma; Gastrointestinal Surgery; **Hospital:** St John's Hlth Ctr, Santa Monica, Century City Hosp; **Address:** John Wayne Cancer Inst, 2336 Santa Monica Blvd, Ste 206, Santa Monica, CA 90404-2302; **Phone:** 310-696-0716; **Board Cert:** Surgery 2002; **Med School:** Emory Univ 1985; **Resid:** Surgery, Univ NC Hosps 1992; **Fac Appt:** Asst Clin Prof S, USC Sch Med

Surgery

Giuliano, Armando E MD [S] - **Spec Exp:** Breast Cancer; Thyroid & Parathyroid Surgery; **Hospital:** St John's Hlth Ctr, Santa Monica, UCLA Ronald Reagan Med Ctr; **Address:** John Wayne Cancer Inst, 2200 Santa Monica Blvd, Santa Monica, CA 90404; **Phone:** 310-829-8089; **Board Cert:** Surgery 1999; **Med School:** Univ Chicago-Pritzker Sch Med 1973; **Resid:** Surgery, UCSF Med Ctr 1980; **Fellow:** Surgical Oncology, UCLA Med Ctr 1978; **Fac Appt:** Prof S, UCLA

Goodnight, James E MD [S] - **Spec Exp:** Melanoma; Breast Cancer; Bone & Soft Tissue Tumors; **Hospital:** UC Davis Med Ctr; **Address:** 4610 X St, Ste 3101, Sacramento, CA 95817; **Phone:** 916-703-5569; **Board Cert:** Surgery 2007; **Med School:** Baylor Coll Med 1968; **Resid:** Surgery, Univ Utah Hosp 1976; **Fellow:** Surgical Oncology, UCLA Med Ctr 1978; **Fac Appt:** Prof S, UC Davis

Goodson III, William H MD [S] - **Spec Exp:** Breast Cancer; Breast Disease; **Hospital:** CA Pacific Med Ctr - Pacific Campus, UCSF - Mt Zion Med Ctr; **Address:** 2100 Webster St, Ste 401, San Francisco, CA 94115-2378; **Phone:** 415-923-3925; **Board Cert:** Surgery 2006; **Med School:** Harvard Med Sch 1971; **Resid:** Surgery, Univ Hosps 1976; Surgery, Childrens Hosp 1977

Gower, Roland E MD [S] - **Spec Exp:** Breast Surgery; Biliary Surgery; Thyroid Surgery; **Hospital:** Providence Alaska Med Ctr, Alaska Regl Hosp; **Address:** 2841 De Barr Rd, Ste 41, Anchorage, AK 99508-2973; **Phone:** 907-279-3564; **Board Cert:** Surgery 1997; **Med School:** Vanderbilt Univ 1971; **Resid:** Surgery, Kansas Med Ctr 1975

Greenhalgh, David G MD [S] - **Spec Exp:** Burn Care; Nutrition; Wound Healing/Care; **Hospital:** Northern CA Shriners Hosp, UC Davis Med Ctr; **Address:** Shriners Hosp Chldn, 2425 Stockton Blvd, Sacramento, CA 95817; **Phone:** 916-453-2050; **Board Cert:** Surgery 2005; Surgical Critical Care 1998; **Med School:** SUNY Upstate Med Univ 1981; **Resid:** Surgery, MC Hosp of VT 1986; **Fellow:** Burn Surgery, Univ Wash Hosp 1989; **Fac Appt:** Prof S, UC Davis

Hemming, Alan W MD [S] - **Spec Exp:** Liver Cancer; Transplant-Liver; Hepatobiliary Surgery; Pancreatic Cancer; **Hospital:** UCSD Med Ctr; **Address:** UCSD Transplant Surgery, 200 W Arbor Drive, San Diego, CA 92103-8401; **Phone:** 619-543-5870; **Board Cert:** Surgery 2004; **Med School:** Univ British Columbia Fac Med 1987; **Resid:** Surgery, Univ British Columbia Med Ctr 1993; **Fellow:** Transplant Surgery, Univ Toronto/Hosp for Sick Children 1995; Hepatobiliary Surgery, Univ Toronto 1996; **Fac Appt:** Prof S, UCSD

Hoyt, David B MD [S] - **Spec Exp:** Trauma; Critical Care; Burn Care; **Hospital:** UC Irvine Med Ctr; **Address:** UC Irvine, Dept Surgery, 333 City Blvd West, City Twr, Ste 700, Orange, CA 92868; **Phone:** 714-456-6262; **Board Cert:** Surgery 2004; Surgical Critical Care 2007; **Med School:** Case West Res Univ 1976; **Resid:** Surgery, UCSD Med Ctr 1984; **Fellow:** Immunopathology, Scripps Clin 1982; **Fac Appt:** Prof S, UC Irvine

Hunter, John G MD [S] - **Spec Exp:** Gastrointestinal & Esophageal Surgery; Laparoscopic Abdominal Surgery; Gastroesophageal Reflux Disease (GERD); **Hospital:** OR Hlth & Sci Univ; **Address:** Digestive Hlth Ctr, 3303 SW Bond Ave, MC CH6D, Portland, OR 97239; **Phone:** 503-494-4373; **Board Cert:** Surgery 2006; **Med School:** Univ Pennsylvania 1981; **Resid:** Surgery, Univ Utah Med Ctr 1987; **Fellow:** Gastrointestinal Surgery, Mass Genl Hosp 1988; Endoscopy, Univ West Ontario 1989; **Fac Appt:** Assoc Prof S, Oregon Hlth & Sci Univ

Johnson, Denise L MD [S] - **Spec Exp:** Melanoma; Breast Cancer; **Hospital:** Stanford Univ Med Ctr; **Address:** Stanford Univ Med Ctr-Dept Surgery, 300 Pasteur Drive, Ste H3680, MC 5655, Stanford, CA 94305; **Phone:** 650-723-5672; **Board Cert:** Surgery 2001; **Med School:** Washington Univ, St Louis 1978; **Resid:** Surgery, Univ Illinois Med Ctr 1986; Immunology, Univ Texas SW Med Ctr 1982; **Fellow:** Surgical Oncology, City of Hope Med Ctr 1989; **Fac Appt:** Assoc Prof S, Stanford Univ

Karlan, Scott R MD [S] - **Spec Exp:** Breast Cancer & Surgery; **Hospital:** Cedars-Sinai Med Ctr; **Address:** 310 N San Vicente Blvd Fl 3, Los Angeles, CA 90048; **Phone:** 310-423-9331; **Board Cert:** Surgery 2005; **Med School:** Harvard Med Sch 1982; **Resid:** Surgery, Yale-New Haven Hosp 1987; **Fac Appt:** Clin Prof S, UCLA

Kaufman, Cary S MD [S] - **Spec Exp:** Breast Cancer; Breast Disease; **Hospital:** St Joseph Hosp - Bellingham; **Address:** 2940 Squalicum Pkwy, Ste 101, Bellingham, WA 98225; **Phone:** 360-671-9877; **Board Cert:** Surgery 2000; **Med School:** UCLA 1973; **Resid:** Surgery, Univ Wash Med Ctr 1975; Surgery, Harbor-UCLA Med Ctr 1979; **Fac Appt:** Asst Clin Prof S, Univ Wash

Klein, Andrew S MD [S] - **Spec Exp:** Transplant-Liver; Liver Cancer; Liver Failure; **Hospital:** Cedars-Sinai Med Ctr; **Address:** Liver & Transplant Ctr at Cedars-Sinai, 8635 W Third St, Ste 590W, Los Angeles, CA 90048; **Phone:** 310-423-2641; **Board Cert:** Surgery 2007; **Med School:** Johns Hopkins Univ 1979; **Resid:** Surgery, Johns Hopkins Hosp 1982; Surgery, Johns Hopkins Hosp 1986; **Fellow:** Transplant Surgery, UCLA-CHS 1988; **Fac Appt:** Clin Prof S, UCLA

Knudson, Mary Margaret MD [S] - **Spec Exp:** Breast Cancer; Trauma; **Hospital:** UCSF Med Ctr, San Francisco Genl Hosp; **Address:** 1001 Potrero Ave, Ste 3A, San Francisco, CA 94110; **Phone:** 415-206-4623; **Board Cert:** Surgery 2002; Surgical Critical Care 1998; **Med School:** Univ Mich Med Sch 1976; **Resid:** Surgery, Beth Israel Hosp 1979; Surgery, Univ Mich Med Ctr 1982; **Fellow:** Pediatric Surgery, Stanford Univ Hosps 1983; **Fac Appt:** Assoc Prof S, UCSF

Lowy, Andrew M MD [S] - **Spec Exp:** Pancreatic Cancer; Gastrointestinal Cancer; Peritoneal Carinomatosis; Clinical Trials; **Hospital:** UCSD Med Ctr; **Address:** Moores UCSD Cancer Ctr, 3855 Health Sciences Drive, MC 0987, La Jolla, CA 92093-0987; **Phone:** 858-822-2124; **Board Cert:** Surgery 2003; **Med School:** Cornell Univ-Weill Med Coll 1988; **Resid:** Surgery, NY-Cornell Med Ctr 1993; **Fellow:** Surgical Oncology, MD Anderson Cancer Ctr 1994; **Fac Appt:** Prof S, UCSD

Moossa, AR MD [S] - **Spec Exp:** Pancreatic Cancer; Gastrointestinal Cancer; Hepatobiliary Surgery; **Hospital:** UCSD Med Ctr; **Address:** 9300 Campus Point Drive, MC 7212, La Jolla, CA 92037; **Phone:** 858-657-6113; **Med School:** England, UK 1965; **Resid:** Surgery, Liverpool Univ Hosps 1970; **Fellow:** Surgical Oncology, Johns Hopkins Hosp 1972; **Fac Appt:** Prof S, UCSD

Morton, John Magana MD [S] - **Spec Exp:** Obesity/Bariatric Surgery; **Hospital:** Stanford Univ Med Ctr, Lucile Packard Chldn's Hosp; **Address:** Surgical Specialties, 300 Pasteur Drive, rm H3680, MC 5655, Stanford, CA 94305; **Phone:** 650-725-9777; **Board Cert:** Surgery 2002; **Med School:** Tulane Univ 1993; **Resid:** Surgery, Tulane Univ Hosp 1999; Surgery, Swedish Med Ctr 2001; **Fellow:** Laparoscopic Surgery, Univ N Carolina Affil Hosp 2003; **Fac Appt:** Assoc Prof S, Stanford Univ

Nakakura, Eric MD/PhD [S] - **Spec Exp:** Pancreatic Cancer; Liver Cancer; Gastrointestinal Cancer; Sarcoma; **Hospital:** UCSF Med Ctr; **Address:** 1600 Divisadero St Fl 4 - rm 4202, San Francisco, CA 94115; **Phone:** 415-353-9888; **Board Cert:** Surgery 2004; **Med School:** Stanford Univ 1995; **Resid:** Surgery, Johns Hopkins Hosp 2000; **Fellow:** Surgical Oncology, Johns Hopkins Hosp 2004; **Fac Appt:** Asst Prof S, UCSF

Nguyen, Ninh T MD [S] - **Spec Exp:** Laparoscopic Surgery; Obesity/Bariatric Surgery; Gastrointestinal Cancer & Surgery; **Hospital:** UC Irvine Med Ctr; **Address:** Div Gastrointestinal Surgery, 333 City Blvd W, Ste 850, Orange, CA 92868; **Phone:** 714-456-8598; **Board Cert:** Surgery 2006; **Med School:** Univ Tex, San Antonio 1990; **Resid:** Surgery, Mt Sinai Med Ctr 1995; **Fellow:** Surgical Oncology, Univ Pittsburgh Med Ctr 1997; Laparoscopic Surgery, Univ Pittsburgh Med Ctr 1998; **Fac Appt:** Assoc Prof S, UC Irvine

Nissen, Nicholas N MD [S] - **Spec Exp:** Liver Cancer; Transplant-Liver; Pancreatic Cancer; Minimally Invasive Surgery; **Hospital:** Cedars-Sinai Med Ctr; **Address:** Cedars-Sinai Medical Center, 8635 W 3rd St, Ste 590-W, Los Angeles, CA 90048; **Phone:** 310-423-2641; **Board Cert:** Surgery 1999; Surgical Critical Care 1999; **Med School:** Univ Minn 1991; **Resid:** Surgery, Loyola Univ Med Ctr 1998; **Fellow:** Surgical Critical Care, Univ Pittsburgh Med Ctr 1999; Hepatobiliary Surgery, UCLA Med Ctr 2001

Norton, Jeffrey A MD [S] - **Spec Exp:** Pancreatic Cancer; Gastrointestinal Cancer & Surgery; Endocrine Surgery; **Hospital:** Stanford Univ Med Ctr; **Address:** 875 Blake Wilbur Drive, Clinic F, Stanford, CA 94305; **Phone:** 650-723-5461; **Board Cert:** Surgery 2001; **Med School:** SUNY Upstate Med Univ 1973; **Resid:** Surgery, Duke Univ Med Ctr 1982; **Fellow:** Research, Natl Cancer Inst 1989; **Fac Appt:** Prof S, Stanford Univ

Paz, Isaac Benjamin MD [S] - **Spec Exp:** Breast Cancer; Esophageal Cancer; **Hospital:** City of Hope Natl Med Ctr & Beckman Rsch; **Address:** 209 S Fair Oaks Ave, South Pasadena, CA 91030; **Phone:** 626-256-4673 x67100; **Board Cert:** Surgery 2000; **Med School:** Chile 1981; **Resid:** Surgery, Univ Catolica de Chile 1985; Surgery, Univ Arizona 1990; **Fellow:** Surgical Oncology, City of Hope Med Ctr 1993

Pellegrini, Carlos MD [S] - **Spec Exp:** Esophageal Cancer; Esophageal Surgery; Barrett's Esophagus; Gastrointestinal Cancer & Surgery; **Hospital:** Univ Wash Med Ctr; **Address:** Univ Washington Medical Ctr, Dept Surgery, 1959 NE Pacific St, Box 356165, Seattle, WA 98195; **Phone:** 206-598-4477; **Board Cert:** Surgery 1998; **Med School:** Argentina 1971; **Resid:** Surgery, Granadero Hosp 1975; Surgery, Univ Chicago Hosps 1979; **Fac Appt:** Prof S, Univ Wash

Perkins, James D MD [S] - **Spec Exp:** Transplant-Pancreas; Transplant-Liver; Transplant-Kidney; **Hospital:** Univ Wash Med Ctr, Chldns Hosp and Regl Med Ctr - Seattle; **Address:** Univ Wash Med Ctr, Dept Surg, 1959 NE Pacific St, Box 356410, Seattle, WA 98195; **Phone:** 206-543-3825; **Board Cert:** Surgery 2004; **Med School:** Univ Ark 1979; **Resid:** Surgery, St Francis Regl Med Ctr 1984; **Fellow:** Transplant Surgery, Mayo Grad Sch 1985; **Fac Appt:** Prof S, Univ Wash

Peterson, Laura D MD [S] - **Spec Exp:** Breast Cancer; **Hospital:** Kapiolani Med Ctr for Women & Chldn; **Address:** Kapi'olani Womens Ctr, 1907 S Beretania St, Ste 501, Honolulu, HI 96826; **Phone:** 808-949-3444; **Board Cert:** Surgery 2004; **Med School:** UCSD 1998; **Resid:** Surgery, UCSD Med Ctr 2004

Phillips, Edward H MD [S] - **Spec Exp:** Laparoscopic Surgery; Obesity/Bariatric Surgery; **Hospital:** Cedars-Sinai Med Ctr; **Address:** 8635 W 3rd St, Ste 795, Los Angeles, CA 90048-6101; **Phone:** 310-423-8350; **Board Cert:** Surgery 1998; **Med School:** USC Sch Med 1973; **Resid:** Surgery, USC Medical Ctr 1978; Vascular Surgery, Los Angeles Co-USC Medical Ctr 1979; **Fac Appt:** Assoc Clin Prof S, USC Sch Med

Potenza, Bruce M MD [S] - **Spec Exp:** Burn Care; Critical Care; **Hospital:** UCSD Med Ctr; **Address:** UCSD Med Ctr, 200 W Arbor Drive, MC 8896, San Diego, CA 92103-8896; **Phone:** 619-543-6001; **Board Cert:** Surgery 2004; Internal Medicine 1988; Surgical Critical Care 2006; Critical Care Medicine 2006; **Med School:** Loyola Univ-Stritch Sch Med 1983; **Resid:** Internal Medicine, Good Samaritan Med Ctr 1987; Surgery, SUNY Syracuse Med Ctr 1993; **Fac Appt:** Clin Prof S, UCSD

Rassman, William R MD [S] - **Spec Exp:** Hair Restoration/Transplant; **Address:** 2080 Century Park East, rm 607, Los Angeles, CA 90067; **Phone:** 310-553-9113; **Board Cert:** Surgery 1975; **Med School:** Med Coll VA 1966; **Resid:** Surgery, New York Hos -Cornell 1969; Surgery, Dartmouth Med Ctr 1973

Reber, Howard A MD [S] - **Spec Exp:** Pancreatic Cancer; Pancreatic Surgery; Gastrointestinal Cancer; **Hospital:** UCLA Ronald Reagan Med Ctr; **Address:** UCLA General Surgery, Box 956904, Los Angeles, CA 90095-6904; **Phone:** 310-825-4976; **Board Cert:** Surgery 1971; **Med School:** Univ Pennsylvania 1964; **Resid:** Surgery, Hosp Univ Penn 1970; **Fac Appt:** Prof S, UCLA

Roberts, John P MD [S] - **Spec Exp:** Transplant-Liver; **Hospital:** UCSF Med Ctr, CA Pacific Med Ctr - Pacific Campus; **Address:** UCSF Medical Ctr, Div Transplant Surgery, 505 Parnassus Ave, rm M896, Box 0780, San Francisco, CA 94143-0780; **Phone:** 415-353-1888; **Board Cert:** Surgery 2006; **Med School:** UCSD 1980; **Resid:** Surgery, Univ Wash 1983; Surgery, Univ Wash 1987; **Fellow:** Surgery, Cornell-New York Hosp 1986; Transplant Surgery, Univ Minn Med Ctr 1988; **Fac Appt:** Prof S, UCSF

Rogers, Stanley J MD [S] - **Spec Exp:** Minimally Invasive Surgery; Gastrointestinal Surgery; Obesity/Bariatric Surgery; **Hospital:** San Francisco Genl Hosp, UCSF Med Ctr; **Address:** San Francisco General Hosp, Surgery, 1001 Potrero Ave, San Francisco, CA 94110; **Phone:** 415-206-6775; **Board Cert:** Surgery 2006; **Med School:** Univ Utah 1991; **Resid:** Surgery, UCSF Med Ctr 1997; **Fac Appt:** Assoc Prof S, UCSF

Satava, Richard M MD [S] - **Spec Exp:** Laparoscopic Abdominal Surgery; Gastrointestinal Surgery; **Hospital:** Univ Wash Med Ctr; **Address:** Univ Washington Med Ctr, Dept Surgery, 1959 NE Pacific St, Box 356410, Seattle, WA 98195; **Phone:** 206-685-0052; **Board Cert:** Surgery 2000; **Med School:** Hahnemann Univ 1968; **Resid:** Surgery, Mayo Clinic 1974; **Fellow:** Research, Mayo Clinic 1972

Selby, Robert R MD [S] - **Spec Exp:** Transplant-Liver; Transplant-Kidney; Transfusion Free Surgery; **Hospital:** USC Univ Hosp; **Address:** USC Univ Hosp, Organ Transplant, 1510 San Pablo St, Ste 200, Los Angeles, CA 90033-4612; **Phone:** 323-442-5908; **Board Cert:** Surgery 1999; Surgical Critical Care 2001; **Med School:** Univ MO-Columbia Sch Med 1979; **Resid:** Internal Medicine, Good Samaritan Hosp 1981; Surgery, Good Samaritan Hosp 1986; **Fellow:** Transplant Surgery, Presby Univ Hosp 1988; **Fac Appt:** Prof S, USC Sch Med

Sener, Stephen F MD [S] - **Spec Exp:** Breast Cancer; Lymphedema; Gastrointestinal Cancer & Surgery; Pancreatic Cancer; **Hospital:** USC Norris Cancer Hosp; **Address:** USC Norris Comprehensive Cancer Ctr, 1441 Eastlake Ave, Los Angeles, CA 90033; **Phone:** 323-865-3535; **Board Cert:** Surgery 2001; **Med School:** Northwestern Univ 1977; **Resid:** Surgery, Northwestern Univ 1982; **Fellow:** Surgery, Meml Sloan Kettering Cancer Ctr 1984; **Fac Appt:** Prof S, USC-Keck School of Medicine

Silverstein, Melvin J MD [S] - **Spec Exp:** Breast Cancer; **Hospital:** Hoag Meml Hosp Presby; **Address:** 1 Hoag Drive, Breast Care Ctr, Newport Beach, CA 92658; **Phone:** 949-764-8281; **Board Cert:** Surgery 1971; **Med School:** Albany Med Coll 1965; **Resid:** Surgery, Boston City Hosp-Tufts Univ 1970; **Fellow:** Surgical Oncology, UCLA Med Ctr 1975

Sinanan, Mika N MD [S] - **Spec Exp:** Gastrointestinal Surgery; Gastrointestinal Cancer; Liver & Biliary Cancer; Laparoscopic Surgery; **Hospital:** Univ Wash Med Ctr; **Address:** Univ Washington, Dept Surgery, 1959 NE Pacific St, Box 356165, Seattle, WA 98195-6410; **Phone:** 206-598-7915; **Board Cert:** Surgery 1998; **Med School:** Johns Hopkins Univ 1980; **Resid:** Surgery, Univ Washington Hosp 1988; **Fellow:** Gastrointestinal Surgery, Univ Brit Columbia Med Ctr 1986; **Fac Appt:** Prof S, Univ Wash

Sobel, Michael MD [S] - **Spec Exp:** Vein Disorders; **Hospital:** Univ Wash Med Ctr; **Address:** East Side Specialty Center, 1700 116th Ave NE, Bellevue, WA 98004; **Phone:** 425-646-7777; **Board Cert:** Surgery 2002; Vascular Surgery 1996; **Med School:** Albert Einstein Coll Med 1975; **Resid:** Surgery, Beth Israel Hosp 1982; **Fellow:** Vascular Surgery, NYU Med Ctr 1983; **Fac Appt:** Prof VascS, Univ Wash

Swanstrom, Lee L MD [S] - **Spec Exp:** Minimally Invasive Surgery; Esophageal Disorders; Endoscopy; Gastrointestinal Motility Disorders; **Hospital:** Providence Portland Med Ctr, Legacy Good Samaritan Hosp and Med Ctr; **Address:** 1040 NW 22nd Ave, Ste 560, Portland, OR 97210; **Phone:** 503-281-0561; **Board Cert:** Surgery 1997; **Med School:** Creighton Univ 1983; **Resid:** Surgery, Emanuel Hosp 1988; **Fac Appt:** Clin Prof S, Oregon Hlth & Sci Univ

Traverso, L William MD [S] - **Spec Exp:** Pancreatic Cancer; Laparoscopic Surgery; **Hospital:** Virginia Mason Med Ctr; **Address:** Virginia Mason Med Ctr, Dept Surg, 1100 9th Ave, Seattle, WA 98101; **Phone:** 206-223-8855; **Board Cert:** Surgery 1998; **Med School:** UCLA 1973; **Resid:** Surgery, UCLA Med Ctr 1978; **Fac Appt:** Clin Prof S, Univ Wash

Trisal, Vijay MD [S] - **Spec Exp:** Skin Cancer; **Hospital:** City of Hope Natl Med Ctr & Beckman Rsch; **Address:** 1500 E Duarte Rd, Duarte, CA 91010; **Phone:** 626-256-4673 x67100; **Board Cert:** Surgery 2003; **Med School:** India 1993; **Resid:** Surgery, Providence Hosp & Med Ctrs 2002; **Fellow:** Surgical Oncology, City of Hope Natl Med Ctr 2004

Vetto, John MD [S] - **Spec Exp:** Cancer Surgery; **Hospital:** OR Hlth & Sci Univ; **Address:** 3181 SW Sam Jackson Park Rd, MC L619, Portland, OR 97239; **Phone:** 503-494-5501; **Board Cert:** Surgery 2000; **Med School:** Oregon Hlth & Sci Univ 1982; **Resid:** Surgery, Brigham & Women's Hosp 1984; Surgery, UCLA Med Ctr 1989; **Fellow:** Surgical Oncology, Natl Cancer Inst 1986; Surgical Oncology, Meml Sloan Kettering Cancer Ctr 1991; **Fac Appt:** Assoc Prof S, Oregon Hlth & Sci Univ

Wagman, Lawrence D MD [S] - **Spec Exp:** Liver Cancer; Gastrointestinal Cancer; Breast Cancer; Liver Surgery; **Hospital:** St Joseph's Hosp - Orange, City of Hope Natl Med Ctr & Beckman Rsch; **Address:** Ctr for Cancer Prevention & Treatment, 1000 W La Veta Ave, Orange, CA 92868; **Phone:** 714-734-6215; **Board Cert:** Surgery 2004; **Med School:** Columbia P&S 1978; **Resid:** Surgery, Med Coll Virginia Hosp 1985; **Fellow:** Surgical Oncology, NIH/NCI 1982; **Fac Appt:** Assoc Clin Prof S, UCSD

Wallace, Anne Marie MD [S] - **Spec Exp:** Breast Cancer; Breast Reconstruction; Melanoma; **Hospital:** UCSD Med Ctr; **Address:** UCSD Moores Cancer Ctr, 3855 Health Sciences Drive #0987, La Jolla, CA 92093; **Phone:** 858-822-6193; **Board Cert:** Surgery 2001; Plastic Surgery 2005; **Med School:** Creighton Univ 1987; **Resid:** Surgery, Washington Hosp Ctr 1992; Plastic Surgery, UCSD Med Ctr 1994; **Fellow:** Surgical Breast Oncology, MD Anderson Cancer Ctr 1995; **Fac Appt:** Clin Prof S, UCSD

Warren, Robert Samuel MD [S] - **Spec Exp:** Liver Cancer; **Hospital:** UCSF Med Ctr; **Address:** UCSF Comprehensive Cancer Center, 1600 Divisadero St Fl 4, San Francisco, CA 94115; **Phone:** 415-353-9846; **Board Cert:** Surgery 1998; **Med School:** Univ Minn 1980; **Resid:** Surgery, Univ Minn Hosps 1988; **Fellow:** Surgical Oncology, Meml Sloan-Kettering Cancer Ctr 1986; **Fac Appt:** Prof S, UCSF

Yeung, Raymond S W MD [S] - **Spec Exp:** Liver & Biliary Cancer; Liver Cancer; Melanoma; Breast Cancer; **Hospital:** Univ Wash Med Ctr; **Address:** Univ of Washington, Dept Surgery, 1959 NE Pacific St, Box 356165, Seattle, WA 98195; **Phone:** 202-598-4477; **Board Cert:** Surgery 1999; **Med School:** Univ Toronto 1982; **Resid:** Surgery, University of Toronto 1987; **Fellow:** Surgical Oncology, Fox Chase Cancer Ctr 1992; **Fac Appt:** Prof S, Univ Wash

FOX CHASE
CANCER CENTER

333 Cottman Avenue
Philadelphia, PA 19111-2497
Phone: 1-888-FOX CHASE
www.fccc.edu

SURGICAL ONCOLOGY

The most experienced surgical oncologists have the best treatment outcomes. At Fox Chase, our surgeons are fellowship-trained, meaning they have one to three years of additional training in the highly complex techniques of cancer surgery. They focus entirely on cancer care, including a wide variety of options from minimally invasive approaches to complex plastic and reconstructive surgery.

Breast Cancer: We offer the most advanced diagnostic techniques, including digital mammography, stereotactic breast biopsy and sentinel lymph-node surgery. Treatment options include breast-preserving surgery with radiation therapy as well as skin-sparing mastectomy with cosmetic reconstructive surgery.

Gastrointestinal Cancers: Our gastrointestinal surgeons have extensive expertise with colorectal, pancreatic, gallbladder, liver and other bowel cancers and are the most experienced laparoscopic and robotic experts in the region. We also offer the most advanced endoscopic and minimally invasive techniques to avoid major surgery.

Genitourinary Cancers: Our urologic surgical oncologists have extensive expertise in the treatment of prostate, bladder, kidney, ureteral, adrenal, testicular and penile cancers. Our urologists emphasize organ preservation, quality of life and minimally invasive/robotic approaches to cancer surgery.

Gynecologic Cancers: Our gynecologic surgeons offer the most advanced laparoscopic and robotic techniques as well as complex open surgery for women with cancers of the uterus, ovary and cervix.

Head and Neck Cancers: The head and neck cancer center at Fox Chase provides patients with one-stop consultations with surgical, radiation and medical oncologists. Expertise includes otolaryngology, transoral laser surgery, plastic and microvascular reconstruction as well as robotic surgery.

Lung and Esophageal Cancers: Our thoracic surgeons offer a variety of minimally invasive techniques for patients with lung and esophageal cancers, including video-assisted thoracic surgery (VATS) and laparoscopic esophageal surgery. Fox Chase is one of only a few centers in the country offering these options.

Minimally Invasive Surgery

At Fox Chase, we offer the broadest range of minimally invasive treatment options for your cancer. Our highly skilled surgeons specialize in da Vinci robot-assisted surgery for more types of cancers than other hospitals across the country. This includes prostate, gynecologic, kidney, bladder, colon, lung, and head and neck cancers. In addition, Fox Chase is one of only a few places in the nation to offer advanced laparoscopic and minimally invasive techniques for patients with cancers of the liver, pancreas, bile ducts, and gallbladder.

For more about Fox Chase physicians and services, visit our web site, www.fccc.edu, or call 1-888-FOX CHASE.

PENN ROBOTIC SURGERY

For more than 200 years, Penn has expanded the frontiers of medicine. Today, surgeons at Penn Medicine are leading the way in robotic-assisted surgery.

Most Comprehensive Program in the United States

Penn is home to five daVinci® Surgical Systems making it one of the largest robotic-assisted surgical programs in the United States. The equipment has been used for some time in urologic/prostate procedures, cardiac surgery, gastrointestinal and gynecological operations.

In addition, Penn surgeons have pioneered new procedures in head and neck surgery using the robotic-assisted technology. Penn was the first medical center in the world with an approved study to perform this surgery and many patients have benefited from transoral robotic surgery (TORS).

Benefits of Robotic Surgery

The advantages of robotic-assisted surgery include a tremendous enhancement in the surgeon's control of the instruments and the ability to perform more intricate procedures.

For patients, the benefits of robotic-assisted surgery may include:

- Less post-operative pain
- Less risk of infection
- Less anesthesia
- Less blood loss
- Shorter hospital stay
- Faster and more complete recovery
- Quicker return to normal daily activities

Experience Makes the Difference

Because of its many benefits, robotic-assisted surgery has gained increased popularity among the medical community in recent years. But technology is only as good as the hands that control it. Robotic technology is meant to be operated by skilled and experienced surgeons. The robotic surgery program at Penn is staffed by surgeons who far exceed the recommended level of experience required for its use.

Penn is also one of the largest, state-of-the-art surgical training centers in the country and the only training center on the East Coast for the new surgical system.

As the medical community embraces robotic-assisted surgery, our researchers, nurses, and surgeons remain at the forefront of this field by relentlessly advancing the application of this technology as well as educating the next generation of surgeons who will use it. The result is that Penn is the first place surgeons turn to learn the technology of tomorrow and the first place you should turn for answers.

Robotic Surgery Available at Penn:

- Cancer: Head and Neck, Throat, Mouth and Tongue, Prostate, Kidney, Heart, Uterus, Cervix

- Gastrointestinal: Bariatric LAP BAND®, Anti-reflux, Motility Disorders

- Gynecology: Pelvic Floor Reconstruction, Hysterectomy, Fibroid Removal, Myomectomy, Tubal Anastomosis

- Heart: Coronary Bypass, Mitral Valve Repair, Atrial Septal Defect Closure, Tumor Resection

- Urology: Prostatectomy, Nephrectomy, Pelvic Reconstruction

**MOUNT SINAI
SCHOOL OF
MEDICINE**

THE MOUNT SINAI MEDICAL CENTER
DEPARTMENT OF SURGERY
One Gustave L. Levy Place
Fifth Avenue and 100th Street
New York, NY 10029-6574
Physician Referral: 1-800-MD-SINAI (637-4624)
www.mountsinai.org/surgery

THE DEPARTMENT OF SURGERY at Mount Sinai continues to be at the forefront of minimally invasive surgery. Mount Sinai surgeons build upon the legacy of those who have gone before, caring for the very sickest of patients while developing new therapies and training tomorrow's physicians to save and enhance lives. Patients today are experiencing less pain, shorter hospital stays, and faster recovery times than was ever imaginable just 20 years ago.

Bariatric Surgery – The latest minimally invasive techniques are used to perform laparoscopic gastric bypass, lap band placement, duodenal switch, and sleeve gastrectomy. In addition, a full inter-disciplinary team follows all aspects of pre- and post-operative care.

Colon and Rectal Surgery – Leaders in the treatment of gastrointestinal disorders, our surgeons care for a wide range of diseases, including: inflammatory bowel disease (Crohn's disease and ulcerative colitis), diverticulitis, and colon and rectal cancers. We offer many important procedures not commonly available.

General Surgery – Treatment is individualized based on the patient's condition, with options from advanced laparoscopic procedures to complex operations.

Laparoscopic and Minimally Invasive Surgery – Mount Sinai surgeons include the world's most respected and innovative surgeons, who perform more laparoscopic procedures than surgeons at any other hospital in New York.

Pediatric Surgery – Surgeries involving children can be met with even more apprehension than those for adults. Fortunately, Mount Sinai surgeons offer a full range of pediatric surgical procedures in a family-focused, child-sensitive environment.

Plastic and Reconstructive Surgery – Surgical care from aesthetic to complex reconstruction is offered for benign and malignant disease, as well as for deformities that are either congenital or acquired. The aim is to restore function and correct deformities caused by birth defects, aging, accident, or illness.

Surgical Oncology – Patients are seen promptly and are cared for by a team of medical and surgical experts, enabling them to benefit from the opinions of dozens of nationally renowned doctors.

Vascular Surgery – A recognized world leader in the development of new techniques for the treatment of aortic aneurysms, Mount Sinai continues to perform extensive research to advance the field of vascular surgery. A wide array of advanced patient services are available, ensuring that conditions are managed successfully.

TOP-RANKING MINIMALLY INVASIVE SURGEONS

In surveys of leading minimally invasive surgeons in a variety of specialties, Mount Sinai's physicians are consistently at the top of the list in surgery of the colon and rectum, liver and bile ducts, thyroid, hernia, chest, and blood vessels. Compared with traditional open surgery, minimally invasive procedures result in less tissue trauma, less scarring, and shorter postoperative recovery time. Although the techniques vary from procedure to procedure and among different surgical subspecialties, minimally invasive surgical procedures typically employ video cameras and lens systems to provide anatomic visualization within a region of the body.

MOUNT SINAI
SCHOOL OF
MEDICINE

**THE MOUNT SINAI MEDICAL CENTER
TRANSPLANTATION**
One Gustave L. Levy Place
Fifth Avenue and 100th Street
New York, NY 10029-6574
Physician Referral: 1-800-MD-SINAI (637-4624)
www.mountsinai.org

Scientific breakthroughs, technological advances, and improved clinical therapies make it possible to save more lives through organ transplantation than ever before. The Mount Sinai Medical Center's **RECANATI MILLER/TRANSPLANTATION INSTITUTE (RMTI)** has been a world leader in these advances. The RMTI brings together clinical programs in adult and pediatric liver, kidney, pancreas, and intestinal transplantation. It is one of the largest transplant centers in the US and one of the longest running transplant programs in the Northeast. The RMTI performs more than 350 procedures annually.

History of Achievement – Mount Sinai surgeons were the first in New York State to perform many transplant procedures, including combined liver and kidney transplantation, pediatric liver transplantation, living adult- and pediatric-donor liver transplantation, and split liver transplantation. Our surgeons have successfully performed more than 3,000 liver transplants and 2,000 kidney transplants.

Tradition of Excellence – Mount Sinai is one of the few hospitals in the country that offers comprehensive, multi-organ transplant services for both children and adults. The RMTI houses the adult and pediatric liver, kidney, pancreas, and intestine programs. Heart and lung transplant programs are also offered within the Department of Cardiothoracic Surgery and the Cardiovascular Institute. Because of this collaboration, our physicians are able to accept the sickest and most complex patients. However, despite the severity of our cases, patient and graft survival rates still exceed national standards.

Innovative Programs

- HIV/Protocol Study – In 2001, the RMTI was one of the only National Institutes of Health-sponsored transplant centers to participate in a national study on transplantation for patients with HIV.

- Living Donor Program – Mount Sinai has an active living donor program. We participate in local and national paired exchange and donor chain initiatives.

- Desensitization Program – We treat many patients who, due to their high immunologic risk, were not previously eligible for transplantation.

- Multi-organ Transplantation Program – We have performed more combined kidney and liver pediatric transplants than any other program in the world. In addition, we have completed the most combined kidney/pancreas transplants in the Northeast.

CARDIAC SURGERY

About the Division of Cardiac Surgery:

The Division of Cardiac Surgery is a nationally recognized leader in advanced treatments and technologies for both adult and congenital heart disease. Our team's multidisciplinary approach to high quality patient-centered care and commitment to research are just a few of the many factors that set us apart. NYU Langone Medical Center is one of the tri-state area's largest cardiac surgery centers and our world renowned surgeons are true pioneers in minimally invasive heart surgery and mitral valve repair. We have performed over 4,750 minimally invasive heart surgery procedures since pioneering the technique in 1996 and offer over 30 years of experience in mitral valve repair. We also perform state-of-the-art surgical procedures for heart valve replacement and aortic aneurysm repair and specialize in high-risk and elderly patients.

We specialize in the following areas:

AORTIC ANEURYSM REPAIR
NYU Langone Medical Center was one of the first centers in the U.S. to adopt the minimally invasive approach to thoracic aneurysm repair. We have participated in numerous FDA clinical trials to determine the efficacy of endovascular repair. Our approach to endovascular repair includes a catheter-based intervention with insertion of a stent graft into the aorta to the site of the aneurysm. The Department of Cardiothoracic Surgery also treats hundreds of patients with aneurysms each year with traditional surgical techniques.

HIGH-RISK CARDIAC SURGERY
Our cardiac surgery team also specializes in the surgical care of high-risk patients. Surgical procedures for high-risk patients include, but are not limited to, coronary revascularization for severe left main disease, heart valve repair or replacement, surgical ventricular restoration, ventricular assist device implantations, and thoracic aortic dissection repair.

MINIMALLY INVASIVE CARDIAC SURGERY
Over 4,750 minimally invasive heart surgery procedures have been performed at NYU Langone Medical Center since 1996. Benefits include dramatic reduction in pain, lower risk of bleeding and infection and an accelerated recovery. Most patients are candidates for minimally invasive procedures which have become the preferred approach for the majority of our heart surgery patients, including mitral valve repair and replacement, aortic valve replacement and coronary artery bypass.

MITRAL VALVE REPAIR
Our heart surgeons introduced mitral valve repair into the U.S., and have refined the technique over the last 30 years. We have performed the most mitral valve repair procedures in the country, avoiding the need to replace the mitral valve, which would require future reoperations. The 3,500 mitral valve repair procedures performed at NYU Langone Medical Center since 1979 have demonstrated that repair is preferable over replacement and that surgery should be performed as early as possible when the risks of treatment are the lowest. We are a leader in the field of mitral valve repair, training visiting surgeons from around the world.

NYU Langone Medical Center

550 First Avenue (at 31St Street)
New York, NY 10016
Physician Referral:
(888)7-NYU-MED (888-769-8633)
www.med.nyu.edu

MINIMALLY INVASIVE SURGERY

About Minimally Invasive Surgery, Department of Surgery:

NYU Langone Medical Center has been at the forefront of minimally invasive surgery for more than 20 years, treating conditions from heart disease to prostate cancer; to obesity to fetal abnormalities in-utero. Minimally invasive procedures result in less discomfort, scarring and surgical trauma. Post-operative recovery is also significantly reduced, allowing patients to resume their normal activities much sooner than with traditional surgery.

We specialize in the following areas:

MINIMALLY INVASIVE CARDIAC SURGERY

Since 1996, the 4,750 minimally invasive heart surgery procedures performed here, including mitral valve repair and replacement, aortic valve replacement and coronary artery bypass, have demonstrated that they are safe and broadly applicable techniques for performing a wide range of complex heart procedures. Benefits include dramatic reduction in pain, lower risk of bleeding and infection and an accelerated recovery.

MINIMALLY INVASIVE THORACIC SURGERY

The Division of Thoracic Surgery at NYU Langone Medical Center offers a minimally invasive surgery program, incorporating both video-assisted and "open chest" techniques along with the newest methods for post-operative pain relief. The use of video-assisted equipment allows for a smaller incision resulting in greater comfort, a shorter recovery and decreased length of stay.

CRYOTHERAPY

For patients with early-stage kidney cancers, surgeons at NYU Langone Medical Center offer minimally invasive cryotherapy to treat tumors. Cryotherapy is also commonly used to treat patients with prostate cancer due to its ability to attack cancer cells without injuring any of the nearby structures.

GYNECOLOGIC SURGERY

The Pelvic Pain Center at the Medical Center offers minimally invasive gynecological procedures such as hysteroscopy (inspection of the uterine cavity), cystoscopy (endoscopy of the urinary bladder), vaginal rejuvenation surgery, endometriosis surgery and laparoscopic hysterectomy.

LAPAROSCOPIC SURGERY

Surgeons at NYU Langone Medical Center use minimally invasive surgery to manage kidney cancers, remove diseased adrenal glands, perform renal biopsies, remove renal cysts and perform innovative urinary reconstruction. Kidney donations can also be performed laparoscopically.

NEUROSURGICAL TECHNOLOGY

Using the Leksell Gamma Knife, neurosurgeons at NYU Langone Medical Center remove deep-seated tumors, vascular malformations and other sites of dysfunction with outstanding results. Aided by three-dimensional MRI technology, the Knife bombards its target with precise doses of radiation, while still preserving healthy tissue. NYU Langone Medical Center is one of the only two hospitals on the east coast to have this tool.

ROBOTIC SURGERY

We are the first hospital in New York City to use the minimally invasive da Vinci Si HD robotic surgical system which allows for a 40 percent higher definition view of the surgical field. The device also allows physicians to import and display medical test results from any computer or diagnostic medical device.

VARICOSE VEIN RESEARCH

Physicians at NYU Langone Medical Center pioneered two minimally invasive procedures that do not require surgical incisions to treat varicose veins: Endovascular closure uses radio heat waves to close down inadequate valves, while scope-based varicose vein treatment introduces a scope under the skin, allowing veins to be removed without an open incision.

NYU Langone Medical Center

550 First Avenue (at 31St Street)
New York, NY 10016
Physician Referral:
(888)7-NYU-MED (888-769-8633)
www.med.nyu.edu

THORACIC SURGERY

About the Division of Thoracic Surgery:

The Division of Thoracic Surgery at NYU Langone Medical Center offers the most advanced diagnosis and treatment options for patients with both benign and malignant lesions of the lung, esophagus, mediastinum and chest wall. All of the thoracic attending physicians at the Medical Center are experts in minimally invasive, video-assisted thoracic surgery and prefer this technique to minimize discomfort in all possible cases.

We specialize in the following areas:

AIRWAY STENTING

Patients experiencing trouble breathing may require airway stenting in order to maintain an open airway (windpipe). Treatment of primary and metastatic lung cancer often includes the use of hollow tubes (stents) to maintain an unobstructed airway. At NYU Langone Medical Center, stent placement is performed in the operating room by an experienced team that includes a surgeon, anesthesiologist and nursing staff. The procedure can be performed through either rigid or flexible bronchoscopy, using either temporary (plastic) or more permanent (metal) stents. Post-operative patients are carefully monitored by a multidisciplinary team to ensure their comfort and care.

MINIMALLY INVASIVE THORACIC SURGERY

The Division of Thoracic Surgery at NYU Langone Medical Center offers a minimally invasive surgery program, incorporating both video-assisted and "open chest" techniques along with the newest methods for post-operative pain relief. The use of video-assisted equipment allows for a smaller incision without spreading the rib spaces leading to greater patient comfort, a shorter recovery time and decreased length of stay for patients. Procedures offered include video-assisted thoracoscopy for biopsy with or without removal of a portion of the lungs as well as repair of hiatal hernias and minimally invasive esophagectomy.

PIONEERING TREATMENTS

The Division of Thoracic Surgery at NYU Langone Medical Center offers new, pioneering treatments including: early detection of airway malignancies, diagnosis and treatment strategies for endobronchial abnormalities, investigation of non-surgical techniques selectively used for destruction of lung cancer nodules and the use of stents (and replaceable stents) to relieve blockages of the windpipe and esophagus.

RESEARCH

The Medical Center is committed to state-of-the-art surgical management and developing novel treatment strategies using clinical trials. The Medical Center also uses the resources at the New York Thoracic Surgery Laboratory housed at Bellevue Hospital to search for genes and proteins in malignancies of the chest in order to detect them earlier or develop novel targeted therapies. Through studies like these, the Medical Center makes clinically relevant

NYU **Cardiac and Vascular Institute**
NYU LANGONE MEDICAL CENTER

550 First Avenue (at 31St Street)
New York, NY 10016
Physician Referral:
(888)7-NYU-MED (888-769-8633)
www.med.nyu.edu

VASCULAR SURGERY

About the Division of Vascular and Endovascular Surgery:

Staffed by one of the largest vascular surgery teams in the country, the Division of Vascular and Endovascular Surgery at the Cardiac and Vascular Institute at NYU Langone Medical Center offers expert patient care with an emphasis on minimally invasive therapies. Our physicians have extensive experience in performing the most up-to-date procedures including stents, angioplasty for carotid artery disease, aortic aneurysms and blockages in arteries throughout the body.

We specialize in the following areas:

AORTIC PATHOLOGY

NYU Langone Medical Center is among a select group of institutions worldwide that offer minimally invasive surgical solutions for complex aortic problems. Patients usually require no blood transfusions and are able to leave the hospital just one or two days after surgery. NYU Langone Medical Center is a leading center for treatment of aortic disease and is a training center for endovascular management of abdominal and thoracic aneurysms.

CAROTID ARTERY DISEASE

NYU Langone Medical Center remains a leader in both the screening for carotid disease (using ultrasound technologies) and the prevention of stroke for those being treated for carotid artery occlusive disease, known to predispose patients to stroke. Doctors at NYU Langone Medical Center assisted in pioneering carotid endarterectomy as an open surgical procedure, as well as playing a pivotal role in the development of the carotid stenting procedure. The Division of Vascular Surgery has remained on the cutting edge of clinical trials in carotid artery disease.

PERIPHERAL ARTERIAL DISEASE

The Division of Vascular and Endovascular Surgery at NYU Langone Medical Center has a wealth of experience in treating peripheral arterial disease (PAD) and specializes in new and innovative technologies such as laser and "silverhawk" atherectomy procedures as well as cryoplasty. Additionally, the Medical Center is one of the only centers in the tristate area with access to drug-eluting stents as part of clinical trial protocols. These stents are coated with special medicines that, over time, may prevent scar formation and re-occlusion of the stent.

VASCULAR SCREENINGS

Our doctors are committed to improving the public awareness and understanding of vascular disease through preventative screenings. The disease is among the leading causes of death in the U.S., yet is generally asymptomatic until a stroke or aneurysm rupture. Effective screenings performed include ultrasound scans of the aorta to identify aortic aneurysms, ultrasound scans of the carotid arteries to assess stroke risk and blood pressure measurements to identify the risk of peripheral arterial disease and heart disease.

VENOUS DISEASE

The Vein Center at NYU Langone Medical Center is considered an authority in the treatment of venous disease, treating patients with all forms of venous pathology ranging from venous insufficiency and varicose veins to occlusive disease and deep vein thrombosis.

Thoracic Surgery

A thoracic surgeon provides the operative, perioperative care and critical care of patients with pathologic conditions within the chest. Included is the surgical care of coronary artery disease, cancers of the lung, esophagus and chest wall, abnormalities of the trachea, abnormalities of the great vessels and heart valves, congenital anomalies, tumors of the mediastinum and diseases of the diaphragm. The management of the airway and injuries of the chest is within the scope of the specialty.

Thoracic surgeons have the knowledge, experience and technical skills to accurately diagnose, operate upon safely and effectively manage patients with thoracic diseases of the chest. This requires substantial knowledge of cardiorespiratory physiology and oncology, as well as capability in the use of heart assist devices, management of abnormal heart rhythms and drainage of the chest cavity, respiratory support systems, endoscopy and invasive and noninvasive diagnostic techniques.

Training Required: Seven to eight years

THORACIC SURGERY

New England

Akins, Cary W MD [TS] - **Spec Exp:** Heart Valve Surgery; Coronary Artery Surgery; Aneurysm-Thoracic Aortic; **Hospital:** Mass Genl Hosp; **Address:** Mass Genl Hosp, Dept Surgery, Cox 648, Boston, MA 02114; **Phone:** 617-726-8218; **Board Cert:** Thoracic Surgery 2005; **Med School:** Harvard Med Sch 1970; **Resid:** Cardiovascular Surgery, Mass Genl Hosp 1975; **Fac Appt:** Clin Prof S, Harvard Med Sch

Bolman III, Ralph Morton MD [TS] - **Spec Exp:** Heart Failure & Ventricular Containment; Ventricular Assist Device (LVAD); Mitral Valve Surgery; Aneurysm; **Hospital:** Brigham & Women's Hosp; **Address:** Brigham & Womens Hosp, Dept Cardiac Surg, 75 Francis St, rm CA211, Boston, MA 02115; **Phone:** 617-732-7678; **Board Cert:** Thoracic Surgery 2004; **Med School:** St Louis Univ 1973; **Resid:** Surgery, Duke Univ Med Ctr 1980; **Fellow:** Thoracic Surgery, Univ Minn Hosp 1982; **Fac Appt:** Prof S, Harvard Med Sch

Bueno, Raphael MD [TS] - **Spec Exp:** Lung Cancer; **Hospital:** Brigham & Women's Hosp, Dana-Farber Cancer Inst; **Address:** Brigham and Women's Hospital, 75 Francis St, Division of Thoracic Surgery Clin, Boston, MA 02115; **Phone:** 617-732-6824; **Board Cert:** Thoracic Surgery 2006; Surgery 2002; Surgical Critical Care 2003; **Med School:** Harvard Med Sch 1985; **Resid:** Surgery, Brigham & Women's Hosp 1992; **Fellow:** Surgical Critical Care, Brigham & Women's Hosp 1993; Cardiothoracic Surgery, Mass Genl Hosp 1997; **Fac Appt:** Assoc Prof S, Harvard Med Sch

DeCamp Jr, Malcolm M MD [TS] - **Spec Exp:** Lung Surgery; Esophageal Surgery; emphysema-Lung Volume Reduction; **Hospital:** Beth Israel Deaconess Med Ctr - Boston; **Address:** BIDMC-185 Pilgrim Rd, Deaconess Bldg - Ste 201, Boston, MA 02215; **Phone:** 617-632-8252; **Board Cert:** Surgery 2001; Thoracic Surgery 2003; **Med School:** Univ Louisville Sch Med 1983; **Resid:** Surgery, Brighams & Womens Hosp 1986; Surgery, Brighams & Womens Hosp 1990; **Fellow:** Cardiac Surgery, Brighams & Womens Hosp 1993; **Fac Appt:** Assoc Prof S, Harvard Med Sch

Elefteriades, John MD [TS] - **Spec Exp:** Aneurysm-Thoracic Aortic; Transplant-Heart; Ventricular Assist Device (LVAD); **Hospital:** Yale-New Haven Hosp; **Address:** Yale Sch of Medicine, Dept Cardiothoracic Surgery, PO Box 208039, New Haven, CT 06520; **Phone:** 203-785-2705; **Board Cert:** Thoracic Surgery 2004; **Med School:** Yale Univ 1976; **Resid:** Surgery, Yale-New Haven Hosp 1981; Cardiothoracic Surgery, Yale-New Haven Hosp 1983; **Fellow:** Cardiothoracic Surgery, Yale-New Haven Hosp 1983; **Fac Appt:** Prof S, Yale Univ

Gaissert, Henning A MD [TS] - **Spec Exp:** Esophageal Cancer; Tracheal Surgery; Lung Cancer; **Hospital:** Mass Genl Hosp; **Address:** Division of Thoracic Surgery, 55 Fruit St, BLK 1570, Boston, MA 02114; **Phone:** 617-726-5341; **Board Cert:** Surgery 2001; Thoracic Surgery 2004; **Med School:** Germany 1984; **Resid:** Surgery, Mass Genl Hosp 1989; Surgery, Barnes Jewish Hosp 1991; **Fellow:** Research, Harvard Med Sch 1993; Cardiothoracic Surgery, Barnes Jewish Hosp 1996; **Fac Appt:** Assoc Prof S, Harvard Med Sch

Hashim, Sabet W MD [TS] - **Spec Exp:** Mitral Valve Surgery; Heart Valve Surgery; Maze Procedure for Atrial Fibrillation; **Hospital:** Yale-New Haven Hosp, Hosp of St Raphael; **Address:** Yale Univ Cardiothoracic Surgery, 333 Cedar St, Boardman 2, New Haven, CT 06520; **Phone:** 203-785-6214; **Board Cert:** Thoracic Surgery 2001; **Med School:** Lebanon 1975; **Resid:** Surgery, St Lukes Roosevely Hosp 1979; Cardiothoracic Surgery, Yale-New Haven Hosp 1981

Kopf, Gary S MD [TS] - **Spec Exp:** Cardiac Surgery; Pediatric Cardiothoracic Surgery; Congenital Heart Disease; **Hospital:** Yale-New Haven Hosp; **Address:** Yale University School of Medicine, Dept of Surgery, Box 208039, New Haven, CT 06520-8039; **Phone:** 203-785-2702; **Board Cert:** Thoracic Surgery 2000; **Med School:** Harvard Med Sch 1970; **Resid:** Surgery, Peter Bent Brigham Hosp 1977; Cardiothoracic Surgery, Chldns Hosp Med Ctr 1980; **Fellow:** Cardiothoracic Surgery, Peter Bent Brigham Hosp 1980; **Fac Appt:** Prof S, Yale Univ

Mathisen, Douglas MD [TS] - **Spec Exp:** Tracheal Surgery; Lung Cancer; Esophageal Cancer; **Hospital:** Mass Genl Hosp, Newton - Wellesley Hosp; **Address:** Mass Genl Hosp, Dept Thor Surg, 55 Fruit St, Blake 1570, Boston, MA 02114; **Phone:** 617-726-6826; **Board Cert:** Thoracic Surgery 2002; **Med School:** Univ IL Coll Med 1974; **Resid:** Surgery, Mass Genl Hosp 1981; Thoracic Surgery, Mass Genl Hosp 1982; **Fellow:** Surgical Oncology, Natl Cancer Inst 1979; **Fac Appt:** Prof S, Harvard Med Sch

Nugent, William C MD [TS] - **Spec Exp:** Thoracic Cancers; Hyperhidrosis-Palmar; **Hospital:** Dartmouth - Hitchcock Med Ctr; **Address:** Dartmouth-Hitchcock Med Ctr, Dept Cardiothoracic Surgery, 1 Medical Center Drive, Lebanon, NH 03756-1000; **Phone:** 603-650-8572; **Board Cert:** Thoracic Surgery 2002; **Med School:** Albany Med Coll 1975; **Resid:** Surgery, Beth Israel Hosp 1980; Thoracic Surgery, Univ Michigan Med Ctr 1983; **Fellow:** Cardiothoracic Surgery, Mass Genl Hosp 1981; **Fac Appt:** Prof S, Dartmouth Med Sch

Sellke, Frank W MD [TS] - **Spec Exp:** Heart Valve Surgery; Angiogenesis; Coronary Artery Surgery; Aortic Surgery; **Hospital:** Rhode Island Hosp, Miriam Hosp; **Address:** Rhode Island Hosp, 2 Dudley St, MOC 500, Providence, RI 02905; **Phone:** 401-444-2732; **Board Cert:** Surgery 2005; Thoracic Surgery 1999; **Med School:** Indiana Univ 1981; **Resid:** Surgery, Akron City Hosp 1987; Cardiothoracic Surgery, Univ Iowa Hosps & Clinics 1990; **Fac Appt:** Prof S, Brown Univ

Singh, Arun K MD [TS] - **Spec Exp:** Cardiac Surgery; **Hospital:** Rhode Island Hosp; **Address:** University Cardiovascular Surgical, 2 Dudley St, Ste 470, Providence, RI 02905-3248; **Phone:** 401-274-7546; **Board Cert:** Surgery 1973; Thoracic Surgery 1975; **Med School:** India 1967; **Resid:** Surgery, Columbia Presby Med Ctr 1972; Cardiothoracic Surgery, Rhode Island Hosp 1974; **Fellow:** Cardiac Surgery, Hosp Sick Chldn 1975; **Fac Appt:** Clin Prof S, Brown Univ

Sugarbaker, David J MD [TS] - **Spec Exp:** Mesothelioma; Transplant-Lung; Esophageal Cancer; **Hospital:** Brigham & Women's Hosp, Dana-Farber Cancer Inst; **Address:** Brigham & Women's Hosp, 75 Francis St, Division of Thoracic Surgery, Boston, MA 02115-6110; **Phone:** 617-732-6824; **Board Cert:** Thoracic Surgery 1999; **Med School:** Cornell Univ-Weill Med Coll 1979; **Resid:** Surgery, Brigham & Women's Hosp 1982; Surgery, Brigham & Women's Hosp 1986; **Fellow:** Thoracic Surgery, Toronto Genl Hosp 1988; **Fac Appt:** Prof S, Harvard Med Sch

Swanson, Scott J MD [TS] - **Spec Exp:** Lung Cancer; Video Assisted Thoracic Surgery (VATS); Esophageal Cancer; **Hospital:** Brigham & Women's Hosp, Dana-Farber Cancer Inst; **Address:** Div Thoracic Surgery, Brigham & Women's Hosp, 75 Francis St, Boston, MA 02115; **Phone:** 617-525-7532; **Board Cert:** Surgery 2003; Thoracic Surgery 2006; **Med School:** Harvard Med Sch 1985; **Resid:** Surgery, Brigham & Womens Hosp 1990; **Fellow:** Cardiothoracic Surgery, Brigham & Womens Hosp 1994

Vander Salm, Thomas MD [TS] - **Spec Exp:** Heart Valve Surgery-Mitral; Cardiovascular Surgery; **Hospital:** N Shore Med Ctr - Salem Hosp; **Address:** Salem Hosp, Div Cardiac Surgery, 81 Highland Ave, Salem, MA 01970; **Phone:** 978-354-2500; **Board Cert:** Surgery 1974; Thoracic Surgery 2006; **Med School:** Johns Hopkins Univ 1966; **Resid:** Surgery, Mass Genl Hosp 1968; Thoracic Surgery, Johns Hopkins Hosp 1969; **Fac Appt:** Prof S, Univ Mass Sch Med

Thoracic Surgery

Wain, John MD [TS] - **Spec Exp:** Transplant-Lung; Lung Cancer; Esophageal Cancer; **Hospital:** Mass Genl Hosp; **Address:** Mass Genl Hosp, Dept Thoracic Surg, 55 Fruit St, Blake 1570, Boston, MA 02114; **Phone:** 617-726-5200; **Board Cert:** Thoracic Surgery 2000; **Med School:** Jefferson Med Coll 1980; **Resid:** Surgery, Mass Genl Hosp 1985; **Fellow:** Cardiothoracic Surgery, Mass Genl Hosp 1988; **Fac Appt:** Asst Prof TS, Harvard Med Sch

Wright, Cameron D MD [TS] - **Spec Exp:** Lung Cancer; Esophageal Cancer; Tracheal Surgery; **Hospital:** Mass Genl Hosp; **Address:** Mass Genl Hosp, Div Thoracic Surg, 55 Fruit St, Blake 1570, Boston, MA 02114-2696; **Phone:** 617-726-5801; **Board Cert:** Surgery 2006; Thoracic Surgery 2007; **Med School:** Univ Mich Med Sch 1980; **Resid:** Surgery, Mass Genl Hosp 1986; Thoracic Surgery, Mass Genl Hosp 1988; **Fac Appt:** Assoc Prof S, Harvard Med Sch

Mid Atlantic

Acker, Michael A MD [TS] - **Spec Exp:** Transplant-Heart; Ventricular Assist Device (LVAD); Coronary Artery Surgery; Heart Valve Surgery; **Hospital:** Hosp Univ Penn - UPHS (page 60); **Address:** 3400 Spruce St, 6 Silverstein Pavillion, Philadelphia, PA 19104-4227; **Phone:** 215-349-8305; **Board Cert:** Surgery 2001; Thoracic Surgery 2001; **Med School:** Brown Univ 1981; **Resid:** Surgery, Hosp Univ Penn 1988; Cardiothoracic Surgery, Johns Hopkins Hosp 1991; **Fac Appt:** Assoc Prof S, Univ Pennsylvania

Adams, David H MD [TS] - **Spec Exp:** Mitral Valve Surgery; Heart Valve Surgery; Minimally Invasive Cardiac Surgery; Coronary Artery Surgery; **Hospital:** Mount Sinai Med Ctr (page 64); **Address:** Mt Sinai Hosp, Cardiac & Thoracic Surg, 1190 Fifth Ave, Box 1028, New York, NY 10029; **Phone:** 212-659-6820; **Board Cert:** Thoracic Surgery 2003; **Med School:** Duke Univ 1983; **Resid:** Surgery, Brigham & Women's Hosp 1988; Thoracic Surgery, Brigham & Women's Hosp 1990; **Fac Appt:** Prof TS, Mount Sinai Sch Med

Altorki, Nasser MD [TS] - **Spec Exp:** Esophageal Cancer; Lung Cancer; Thoracic Cancers; Vaccine Therapy; **Hospital:** NY-Presby Hosp/Weill Cornell (page 66); **Address:** 525 E 68th St, New York, NY 10021-4870; **Phone:** 212-746-5156; **Board Cert:** Surgery 2006; Thoracic Surgery 1998; **Med School:** Egypt 1978; **Resid:** Surgery, Univ Chicago Hosps 1985; **Fellow:** Cardiothoracic Surgery, Univ Chicago Hosps 1987; **Fac Appt:** Prof S, Cornell Univ-Weill Med Coll

Argenziano, Michael MD [TS] - **Spec Exp:** Robotic Cardiac Surgery; Coronary Artery Surgery; Maze Procedure for Atrial Fibrillation; **Hospital:** NY-Presby Hosp/Columbia (page 66); **Address:** Columbia Presby Med Ctr, Milstein Bldg, 177 Fort Washington Ave, rm 7-435, New York, NY 10032; **Phone:** 212-305-5888; **Board Cert:** Surgery 1999; Thoracic Surgery 2002; **Med School:** Columbia P&S 1992; **Resid:** Surgery, Columbia Presby Med Ctr 1998; **Fellow:** Cardiothoracic Surgery, Columbia Presby Med Ctr 1999; **Fac Appt:** Asst Prof S, Columbia P&S

Bains, Manjit MD [TS] - **Spec Exp:** Cardiothoracic Surgery; Esophageal Cancer; Lung Cancer; **Hospital:** Meml Sloan-Kettering Cancer Ctr; **Address:** 1275 York Avenue, New York, NY 10065; **Phone:** 800-525-2225; **Board Cert:** Surgery 1971; Thoracic Surgery 1972; **Med School:** India 1963; **Resid:** Surgery, Rochester Genl Hosp 1970; **Fellow:** Thoracic Surgery, Sloan Kettering Cancer Ctr 1972; **Fac Appt:** Clin Prof S, Cornell Univ-Weill Med Coll

Battafarano, Richard J MD [TS] - **Spec Exp:** Lung Cancer; Barrett's Esophagus; Esophageal Surgery; Mesothelioma; **Hospital:** Barnes-Jewish Hosp; **Address:** Univ MD Med Ctr, Greenebaum Cancer Ctr-Dept Thoracic Surgery, 22 S Greeene St, Baltimore, MD 21210; **Phone:** 410-328-6366; **Board Cert:** Surgery 1998; Thoracic Surgery 2000; **Med School:** Hahnemann Univ 1988; **Resid:** Surgery, Univ Minn Hosp & Clin 1997; **Fellow:** Thoracic Surgery, Meml Sloan Kettering Cancer Ctr 1999; **Fac Appt:** Assoc Prof S, Univ MD Sch Med

Bavaria, Joseph E MD [TS] - **Spec Exp:** Aortic Surgery; Transplant-Lung; Heart Valve Surgery; **Hospital:** Hosp Univ Penn - UPHS (page 60); **Address:** Hosp Univ Pennsylvania, 3400 Spruce St, 6 Silverstein, Philadelphia, PA 19104; **Phone:** 215-662-2017; **Board Cert:** Thoracic Surgery 2001; **Med School:** Tulane Univ 1983; **Resid:** Surgery, Hosp Univ Penn 1990; Cardiothoracic Surgery, Hosp Univ Penn/Children's Hosp 1992; **Fac Appt:** Prof S, Univ Pennsylvania

Bridges, Charles R MD [TS] - **Spec Exp:** Minimally Invasive Cardiac Surgery; Maze Procedure for Atrial Fibrillation; Aneurysm-Aortic; Heart Valve Surgery; **Hospital:** Pennsylvania Hosp (page 60), Hosp Univ Penn - UPHS (page 60); **Address:** 230 W Washington Square Fl 3, Farm Journal Bldg, Philadelphia, PA 19107; **Phone:** 215-829-8713; **Board Cert:** Surgery 2003; Thoracic Surgery 2004; **Med School:** Harvard Med Sch 1981; **Resid:** Internal Medicine, Brigham & Women's Hosp 1984; Surgery, Hosp U Penn 1991; **Fellow:** Cardiothoracic Surgery, Hosp U Penn 1993; **Fac Appt:** Assoc Prof S, Univ Pennsylvania

Conte Jr, John V MD [TS] - **Spec Exp:** Transplant-Heart; Transplant-Lung; Cardiac Surgery-Adult; Coronary Artery Surgery; **Hospital:** Johns Hopkins Hosp (page 61); **Address:** 600 N Wolfe St, Blalock 618, Baltimore, MD 21287-4618; **Phone:** 410-955-1753; **Board Cert:** Thoracic Surgery 2007; **Med School:** Georgetown Univ 1986; **Resid:** Surgery, Georgetown Univ Med Ctr 1992; Stanford Univ Med Ctr 1995

Cooper, Joel D MD [TS] - **Spec Exp:** Transplant-Lung; Emphysema-Lung Volume Reduction; Lung Surgery; **Hospital:** Hosp Univ Penn - UPHS (page 60); **Address:** Hosp Univ Penn, 3400 Spruce St, 4 Silverstein, Philadelphia, PA 19104; **Phone:** 215-662-2022; **Board Cert:** Surgery 1971; Thoracic Surgery 1972; **Med School:** Harvard Med Sch 1964; **Resid:** Surgery, Mass Genl Hosp 1968; Thoracic Surgery, Frenchay Hosp; **Fellow:** Research, Hammersmith Hosp; Thoracic Surgery, Mass Genl Hosp; **Fac Appt:** Prof S, Univ Pennsylvania

Demmy, Todd L MD [TS] - **Spec Exp:** Lung Cancer; Thoracic Cancers; Esophageal Cancer; Minimally Invasive Thoracic Surgery; **Hospital:** Roswell Park Cancer Inst, Buffalo General Hosp; **Address:** Roswell Park Cancer Inst, Dept Thoracic Surgery, Elm & Carlton Sts, Buffalo, NY 14263; **Phone:** 716-845-5873; **Board Cert:** Surgery 2008; Thoracic Surgery 2000; Surgical Critical Care 2001; **Med School:** Jefferson Med Coll 1983; **Resid:** Surgery, Baylor Univ Medical Ctr 1988; Thoracic Surgery, Allegheny Genl Hosp 1991; **Fac Appt:** Assoc Prof S, SUNY Buffalo

DeRose Jr, Joseph J MD [TS] - **Spec Exp:** Robotic Cardiac Surgery; Minimally Invasive Cardiac Surgery; **Hospital:** Montefiore Med Ctr - Div. Weiler, Montefiore Med Ctr - Div. Moses; **Address:** Montefiore-Weiler Medical Ctr, Dept Cardiothoracic Surgery, 1575 Blondell Ave, Ste 125, Bronx, NY 10461; **Phone:** 718-405-8371; **Board Cert:** Surgery 2000; Thoracic Surgery 2002; **Med School:** Columbia P&S 1993; **Resid:** Surgery, Columbia Presby Med Ctr 1995; **Fellow:** Cardiothoracic Surgery, Columbia Presby Med Ctr 1999; **Fac Appt:** Assoc Prof TS, Albert Einstein Coll Med

Diehl, James T MD [TS] - **Spec Exp:** Cardiac Surgery-Adult; Aortic Surgery; Heart Valve Surgery-Aortic; Heart Valve Surgery-Mitral; **Hospital:** Thomas Jefferson Univ Hosp, Albert Einstein Med Ctr; **Address:** 1025 Walnut St, Ste 607, Philadelphia, PA 19107; **Phone:** 215-955-6996; **Board Cert:** Thoracic Surgery 2004; **Med School:** Albert Einstein Coll Med 1978; **Resid:** Surgery, Cleveland Clinic 1984; Cardiothoracic Surgery, Univ Toronto Med Ctr 1986; **Fac Appt:** Prof S, Thomas Jefferson Univ

Friedberg, Joseph MD [TS] - **Spec Exp:** Lung Cancer; Mesothelioma; Photodynamic Therapy; Thoracic Cancers; **Hospital:** Penn Presby Med Ctr - UPHS (page 60), Hosp Univ Penn - UPHS (page 60); **Address:** Penn-Presbyterian Medical Ctr, 51 N 39th St, rm W250, Philadelphia, PA 19104; **Phone:** 215-662-9195; **Board Cert:** Surgery 2006; Thoracic Surgery 2006; **Med School:** Harvard Med Sch 1986; **Resid:** Surgery, Mass General Hosp 1994; **Fellow:** Cardiothoracic Surgery, Brigham & Womens Hosp 1996

Thoracic Surgery

Furukawa, Satoshi MD [TS] - **Spec Exp:** Transplant-Heart & Lung; Cardiac Surgery-High Risk; Heart Valve Surgery; Minimally Invasive Cardiac Surgery; **Hospital:** Temple Univ Hosp; **Address:** 3401 N Broad St, Ste 300, Philadelphia, PA 19140; **Phone:** 215-707-3601; **Board Cert:** Surgery 2003; Thoracic Surgery 2005; **Med School:** Univ Pennsylvania 1984; **Resid:** Surgery, Hosp Univ Penn 1991; Thoracic Surgery, Hosp Univ Penn 1993; **Fac Appt:** Prof TS, Temple Univ

Galloway, Aubrey MD [TS] - **Spec Exp:** Minimally Invasive Heart Valve Surgery; Coronary Artery Surgery; Aneurysm-Thoracic Aortic; **Hospital:** NYU Langone Med Ctr (page 67), Bellevue Hosp Ctr; **Address:** 530 1st Ave, Ste 9V, New York, NY 10016-6402; **Phone:** 212-263-7185; **Board Cert:** Thoracic Surgery 2006; **Med School:** Tulane Univ 1978; **Resid:** Surgery, Univ Colo Hlth Sci Ctr 1983; Cardiovascular Surgery, NYU Med Ctr 1985; **Fellow:** Research, Boston Chldns Hosp 1981; Cardiothoracic Surgery, NYU Med Ctr 1985; **Fac Appt:** Prof TS, NYU Sch Med

Gharagozloo, Farid MD [TS] - **Spec Exp:** Video Assisted Thoracic Surgery (VATS); Lung Cancer; **Hospital:** G Washington Univ Hosp, Harbor Hosp Ctr; **Address:** 2175 K St NW, Ste 300, Washington, DC 20037; **Phone:** 202-775-8600; **Board Cert:** Thoracic Surgery 2001; **Med School:** Johns Hopkins Univ 1983; **Resid:** Surgery, Mayo Clinic 1989; Research, Harvard Med Sch 1986; **Fellow:** Cardiothoracic Surgery, Mayo Clinic 1992; **Fac Appt:** Prof S, Geo Wash Univ

Ginsburg, Mark MD [TS] - **Spec Exp:** Lung Cancer; Transplant-Lung; Emphysema-Lung Volume Reduction; **Hospital:** NY-Presby Hosp/Columbia (page 66), Good Samaritan Hosp - Suffern; **Address:** 161 Ft Washington Ave Fl 3 - rm 301, New York, NY 10032; **Phone:** 212-305-3408; **Board Cert:** Surgery 2006; Thoracic Surgery 2005; **Med School:** Tufts Univ 1980; **Resid:** Surgery, Strong Meml Hosp 1985; **Fellow:** Thoracic Surgery, Strong Meml Hosp 1987; **Fac Appt:** Asst Clin Prof S, Columbia P&S

Girardi, Leonard N MD [TS] - **Spec Exp:** Aneurysm-Aortic; Cardiac Surgery; Marfan's Syndrome; Cardiothoracic Surgery; **Hospital:** NY-Presby Hosp/Weill Cornell (page 66); **Address:** 525 E 68th St, M404, New York, NY 10021; **Phone:** 212-746-5194; **Board Cert:** Surgery 2005; Thoracic Surgery 2007; **Med School:** Cornell Univ-Weill Med Coll 1989; **Resid:** Surgery, NY Presby-Cornell Med Ctr 1994; **Fellow:** Cardiothoracic Surgery, NY Presby Hosp 1996; Cardiothoracic Surgery, Baylor Coll Med 1997; **Fac Appt:** Assoc Prof TS, Cornell Univ-Weill Med Coll

Graver, L Michael MD [TS] - **Spec Exp:** Heart Valve Surgery-Aortic; Coronary Artery Surgery; Atrial Fibrillation; **Hospital:** Long Island Jewish Med Ctr, N Shore Univ Hosp; **Address:** 270-05 76th Ave, New Hyde Park, NY 11040-1433; **Phone:** 718-470-7460; **Board Cert:** Surgery 2003; Thoracic Surgery 2004; **Med School:** Albany Med Coll 1977; **Resid:** Surgery, St Luke's-Roosevelt Hosp Ctr 1982; Cardiovascular Surgery, Deaconness Hosp 1983; **Fellow:** Cardiovascular Pathology, NY Hosp-Cornell Med Ctr 1985; **Fac Appt:** Prof TS, Albert Einstein Coll Med

Griepp, Randall B MD [TS] - **Spec Exp:** Aneurysm-Abdominal Aortic; Aneurysm-Thoracic Aortic; **Hospital:** Mount Sinai Med Ctr (page 64); **Address:** Mt Sinai Med Ctr, Dept Cardiothoracic Surg, 1190 5th Ave, New York, NY 10029; **Phone:** 212-659-9495; **Board Cert:** Thoracic Surgery 2007; **Med School:** Stanford Univ 1967; **Resid:** Surgery, Stanford Univ Hosp 1973; **Fellow:** Cardiothoracic Surgery, Stanford Univ Hosp 1972; **Fac Appt:** Prof TS, Mount Sinai Sch Med

Griffith, Bartley MD [TS] - **Spec Exp:** Transplant-Heart & Lung; Heart Valve Surgery; Aneurysm-Aortic; **Hospital:** Univ of MD Med Ctr; **Address:** Univ Maryland, Div Cardiac Surg, N4W94, 22 S Greene St, Baltimore, MD 21201; **Phone:** 410-328-3822; **Board Cert:** Thoracic Surgery 2001; **Med School:** Jefferson Med Coll 1974; **Resid:** Surgery, Univ Hlth Ctr Hosps 1979; Thoracic Surgery, Univ Hlth Ctr Hosps 1981; **Fellow:** Research, Univ Hlth Ctr Hosps 1978; **Fac Appt:** Prof S, Univ MD Sch Med

Grossi, Eugene A MD [TS] - **Spec Exp:** Minimally Invasive Cardiac Surgery; Mitral Valve Surgery; Cardiac Tumors, Myxomas; **Hospital:** NYU Langone Med Ctr (page 67); **Address:** NYU Med Ctr, 530 1st Ave, Ste 9V, New York, NY 10016-6402; **Phone:** 212-263-7452; **Board Cert:** Thoracic Surgery 2002; **Med School:** Columbia P&S 1981; **Resid:** Surgery, NYU Med Ctr 1987; Thoracic Surgery, NYU Med Ctr 1991; **Fac Appt:** Assoc Prof S, NYU Sch Med

Hargrove III, W Clark MD [TS] - **Spec Exp:** Mitral Valve Robotic Surgery; Heart Valve Surgery; Minimally Invasive Cardiac Surgery; **Hospital:** Penn Presby Med Ctr - UPHS (page 60); **Address:** Philadelphia Heart Inst, 51 N 39th St, Ste 2D, Philadelphia, PA 19104; **Phone:** 215-662-9595; **Board Cert:** Thoracic Surgery 2004; **Med School:** Wake Forest Univ 1973; **Resid:** Surgery, Hosp U Penn 1979; Cardiothoracic Surgery, Hosp U Penn 1984; **Fellow:** Vascular Surgery, Hosp U Penn 1981; **Fac Appt:** Clin Prof S, Univ Pennsylvania

Heitmiller, Richard F MD [TS] - **Spec Exp:** Esophageal Surgery; Esophageal Cancer; Lung Cancer; **Hospital:** Union Meml Hosp-Baltimore; **Address:** 3333 N Calvert St, Ste 610, Baltimore, MD 21218; **Phone:** 410-554-2063; **Board Cert:** Surgery 1997; Thoracic Surgery 1999; **Med School:** Johns Hopkins Univ 1979; **Resid:** Surgery, Mass Genl Hosp 1985; **Fellow:** Thoracic Surgery, Mass Genl Hosp 1987; **Fac Appt:** Assoc Prof Surg & Onc, Johns Hopkins Univ

Horvath, Keith MD [TS] - **Spec Exp:** Minimally Invasive Cardiac Surgery; Heart Valve Surgery; Heart Laser Revascularization; **Hospital:** Suburban Hosp, Johns Hopkins Hosp (page 61); **Address:** Suburban Hospital, 8600 Old Georgetown Rd, Bethesda, MD 20814; **Phone:** 301-896-7610; **Board Cert:** Thoracic Surgery 2005; **Med School:** Univ Chicago-Pritzker Sch Med 1987; **Resid:** Surgery, Brigham & Women's Hosp 1994; Brigham & Women's Hosp 1996; **Fellow:** Research, Mass Genl Hosp 1991; **Fac Appt:** Assoc Prof S, Northwestern Univ

Isom, O Wayne MD [TS] - **Spec Exp:** Cardiac Surgery; Coronary Artery Surgery; Heart Valve Surgery; **Hospital:** NY-Presby Hosp/Weill Cornell (page 66), NY Hosp Queens; **Address:** 525 E 68th St, rm M-404, New York, NY 10065; **Phone:** 212-746-5151; **Board Cert:** Surgery 1971; Thoracic Surgery 1972; **Med School:** Univ Tex, Houston 1965; **Resid:** Surgery, Parkland Meml Hosp 1970; **Fellow:** Thoracic Surgery, NYU Med Ctr 1972; **Fac Appt:** Prof TS, Cornell Univ-Weill Med Coll

Jonas, Richard A MD [TS] - **Spec Exp:** Pediatric Cardiothoracic Surgery; Congenital Heart Surgery; **Hospital:** Chldns Natl Med Ctr, Georgetown Univ Hosp; **Address:** 111 Michigan Ave NW, Washington, DC 20010; **Phone:** 202-476-2811; **Med School:** Australia 1974; **Resid:** Surgery, Royal Melbourne Hosp 1979; Thoracic Surgery, Green Lane Hosp 1982; **Fellow:** Thoracic Surgery, Brigham & Women's Hosp 1984; **Fac Appt:** Prof S, Geo Wash Univ

Kanda, Louis T MD [TS] - **Spec Exp:** Heart Valve Surgery; **Hospital:** Washington Hosp Ctr; **Address:** 110 Irving St NW, Ste 1041, Washington, DC 20010; **Phone:** 202-877-5039; **Board Cert:** Thoracic Surgery 2002; **Med School:** Geo Wash Univ 1970; **Resid:** Surgery, Washington Hosp Ctr 1975; **Fellow:** Cardiothoracic Surgery, Cleveland Clin Fdn 1980; **Fac Appt:** Asst Prof S, Howard Univ

Katz, Nevin M MD [TS] - **Spec Exp:** Critical Care; **Hospital:** G Washington Univ Hosp; **Address:** 2175 K St NW, Ste 300, Washington, DC 20037; **Phone:** 202-775-8600; **Board Cert:** Thoracic Surgery 2000; **Med School:** Case West Res Univ 1971; **Resid:** Surgery, Mass Genl Hosp 1976; Cardiothoracic Surgery, Univ Alabama Hosp 1980; **Fellow:** Cardiovascular Surgery, Univ Alabama 1978; **Fac Appt:** Clin Prof S, Geo Wash Univ

Thoracic Surgery

Keenan, Robert J MD [TS] - **Spec Exp:** Lung Cancer; Esophageal Cancer; Mediastinal Tumors; Emphysema-Lung Volume Reduction; **Hospital:** Allegheny General Hosp, Westmoreland Hosp; **Address:** Allegheny Genl Hosp, 14th Fl, 320 E North Ave, Pittsburgh, PA 15212; **Phone:** 412-359-6137; **Board Cert:** Surgery 2000; **Med School:** Canada 1984; **Resid:** Surgery, Univ Toronto Med Ctr 1989; **Fellow:** Thoracic Surgery, Univ Pittsburgh Med Ctr 1990; Thoracic Surgery, Univ Toronto Med Ctr 1991; **Fac Appt:** Prof TS, Drexel Univ Coll Med

Keller, Steven M MD [TS] - **Spec Exp:** Lung Cancer; Esophageal Cancer; Hyperhidrosis-Palmar; **Hospital:** Montefiore Med Ctr - Div. Moses, Montefiore Med Ctr - Div. Weiler; **Address:** Montefiore-Moses Medical Ctr, 3400 Bainbridge Ave Fl 5 - Ste A, Bronx, NY 10467-2404; **Phone:** 718-920-7580; **Board Cert:** Thoracic Surgery 2008; **Med School:** Albany Med Coll 1977; **Resid:** Surgery, Mount Sinai Hosp 1985; Thoracic Surgery, Mem Sloan Kettering Cancer Ctr 1987; **Fellow:** Surgical Oncology, NIH/National Cancer Inst 1983; **Fac Appt:** Prof TS, Albert Einstein Coll Med

Kiev, Jonathan MD [TS] - **Spec Exp:** Chest Wall Tumors; Esophageal Cancer; Lung Cancer; **Hospital:** Anne Arundel Med Ctr; **Address:** Annapolis Thoracic Surgery, 2001 Medical Pkwy, Donner Pavilion, 2nd Fl, Annapolis, MD 21401; **Phone:** 443-481-3300; **Board Cert:** Surgery 2005; Thoracic Surgery 2002; **Med School:** Tulane Univ 1989; **Resid:** Surgery, Hahnemann Univ Hosp 1996; Cardiothoracic Surgery, Loma Linda Univ 2000; **Fellow:** Thoracic Surgery, Univ Pittsburgh 2001; Thoracic Surgery, Mayo Clinic 2001

Kormos, Robert MD [TS] - **Spec Exp:** Transplant-Heart; Artificial Heart Devices; **Hospital:** UPMC Presby, Pittsburgh; **Address:** UPMC Presbyterian Hosp, 200 Lothrop St, Ste C700, Pittsburgh, PA 15213; **Phone:** 412-648-6259; **Med School:** Univ Western Ontario 1976; **Resid:** Surgery, Toronto Western Hosp 1978; Cardiothoracic Surgery, Toronto Genl Hosp/Hosp for Sick Chldn 1982; **Fellow:** Transplant Surgery, Univ Pittsburgh Med Ctr 1987; **Fac Appt:** Prof S, Univ Pittsburgh

Krasna, Mark MD [TS] - **Spec Exp:** Esophageal Cancer; Lung Cancer; Mesothelioma; **Hospital:** St Joseph Med Ctr, Univ of MD Med Ctr; **Address:** 7501 Osler Drive Odea Bldg - Ste 204, Towson, MD 21204; **Phone:** 410-427-2220; **Board Cert:** Thoracic Surgery 2000; **Med School:** Israel 1982; **Resid:** Surgery, CMDNJ-Rutgers Med Sch 1988; **Fellow:** Cardiothoracic Surgery, New England Deaconess-Harvard 1990; **Fac Appt:** Prof S, Univ MD Sch Med

Krellenstein, Daniel J MD [TS] - **Spec Exp:** Lung Cancer; Minimally Invasive Thoracic Surgery; Asbestos-related Lung Disease; **Hospital:** Mount Sinai Med Ctr (page 64), Lenox Hill Hosp (page 62); **Address:** 16 E 98th St, Ste 1F, New York, NY 10029-6545; **Phone:** 212-423-9311; **Board Cert:** Surgery 1974; Thoracic Surgery 2006; **Med School:** SUNY Buffalo 1964; **Resid:** Surgery, SUNY Downstate Med Ctr 1972; **Fac Appt:** Assoc Clin Prof TS, Mount Sinai Sch Med

Krieger, Karl H MD [TS] - **Spec Exp:** Heart Valve Surgery; Coronary Artery Surgery; Cardiac Surgery-Adult; **Hospital:** NY-Presby Hosp/Weill Cornell (page 66), NY Hosp Queens; **Address:** Cardiothoracic Surgery Dept, 525 E 68th St, Ste M404, New York, NY 10021-4873; **Phone:** 212-746-5152; **Board Cert:** Thoracic Surgery 2004; **Med School:** Johns Hopkins Univ 1975; **Resid:** Surgery, Johns Hopkins 1976; Bellevue Hosp 1979; **Fellow:** Thoracic Surgery, NYU Med Ctr 1981; **Fac Appt:** Prof S, Cornell Univ-Weill Med Coll

Lang, Samuel MD [TS] - **Spec Exp:** Minimally Invasive Cardiac Surgery; Heart Valve Surgery; **Hospital:** NY Hosp Queens; **Address:** 46-45 Main St, Cardiac Surgery -WA100, Flushing, NY 11355; **Phone:** 718-670-2439; **Board Cert:** Thoracic Surgery 2006; **Med School:** Univ Alabama 1978; **Resid:** Surgery, UCLA Med Ctr 1982; Thoracic Surgery, NYU Med Ctr 1983; **Fellow:** Cardiothoracic Surgery, UCLA Med Ctr 1985; Pediatric Cardiac Surgery, Hosp for Sick Chldn 1986

Lansman, Steven MD/PhD [TS] - **Spec Exp:** Coronary Artery Surgery; Heart Valve Surgery; Ventricular Assist Device (LVAD); Transplant-Heart; **Hospital:** Westchester Med Ctr; **Address:** Westchester Medical Ctr, 95 Grasslands Rd, Macy Pavilion, rm 114W, Valhalla, NY 10595; **Phone:** 914-493-8793; **Board Cert:** Thoracic Surgery 2004; **Med School:** SUNY Hlth Sci Ctr 1977; **Resid:** Surgery, Montefiore Med Ctr 1982; **Fellow:** Thoracic Surgery, Univ Hosp 1984; **Fac Appt:** Prof S, NY Med Coll

Loulmet, Didier MD [TS] - **Spec Exp:** Heart Valve Surgery; Robotic Cardiac Surgery; Minimally Invasive Cardiac Surgery; **Hospital:** NYU Langone Med Ctr (page 67); **Address:** NYU Medical Ctr, Cardiothoracic Surgery, 550 1st Ave, Ste 9V, New York, NY 10016; **Phone:** 212-263-2329; **Med School:** France 1984; **Resid:** Cardiothoracic Surgery, Paris Univ Hosp 1990; Cardiothoracic Surgery, Brigham & Women's Hosp 1991; **Fellow:** Pediatric Cardiac Surgery, Chldn's Hosp, Harvard Univ 1992

Magovern Jr, George J MD [TS] - **Spec Exp:** Cardiothoracic Surgery; Ventricular Assist Device (LVAD); **Hospital:** Allegheny General Hosp; **Address:** Cardiovascular Surgery Ctr, CVI-1, 320 E North Ave, NW Wing-Snyder Pavilion, Pittsburgh, PA 15212; **Phone:** 412-359-8820; **Board Cert:** Thoracic Surgery 2005; **Med School:** Univ Pittsburgh 1978; **Resid:** Surgery, Johns Hopkins Hosp 1981; Cardiovascular Surgery, Johns Hopkins Hosp 1985; **Fac Appt:** Prof S, Drexel Univ Coll Med

Marshall, Margaret Blair MD [TS] - **Spec Exp:** Lung Cancer; Esophageal Cancer; Thymoma; Chest Wall Tumors; **Hospital:** Georgetown Univ Hosp, Sibley Mem Hosp; **Address:** Georgetown Univ Hosp, 3800 Reservoir Rd NW, 4PHC, Washington, DC 20007; **Phone:** 202-444-5045; **Board Cert:** Surgery 2000; Thoracic Surgery 2002; **Med School:** Georgetown Univ 1991; **Resid:** Surgery, Georgetown Univ Med Ctr 1995; Cardiothoracic Surgery, Hosp Univ Penn 2001; **Fellow:** Research, Chldn's Hosp 1998; **Fac Appt:** Assoc Prof S, Georgetown Univ

McGrath, Lynn B MD [TS] - **Spec Exp:** Cardiac Surgery-Adult & Pediatric; Congenital Heart Disease; Coronary Artery Surgery; Heart Valve Surgery; **Hospital:** Deborah Hrt & Lung Ctr; **Address:** Deborah Heart & Lung Ctr, Dept Surgery, 200 Trenton Rd, Brown Mills, NJ 08015; **Phone:** 609-893-6611; **Board Cert:** Thoracic Surgery 2002; **Med School:** Canada 1974; **Resid:** Surgery, Peter Bent Brigham Hosp 1981; Cardiothoracic Surgery, Univ Ala Med Ctr 1983; **Fellow:** Congenital Heart Surgery, Univ Ala Med Ctr 1984; **Fac Appt:** Assoc Prof S, Robert W Johnson Med Sch

Morris, Rohinton J MD [TS] - **Spec Exp:** Transplant-Heart; Ventricular Assist Device (LVAD); Coronary Artery Surgery; **Hospital:** Penn Presby Med Ctr - UPHS (page 60), Hosp Univ Penn - UPHS (page 60); **Address:** Philadelphia Heart Inst, 51 N 39th St, Ste 2D, Philadelphia, PA 19104-4227; **Phone:** 215-349-8419; **Board Cert:** Thoracic Surgery 2003; **Med School:** Hahnemann Univ 1984; **Resid:** Surgery, Hahnemann Univ Hosp 1989; Thoracic Surgery, Hahnemann Univ Hosp 1992; **Fac Appt:** Assoc Clin Prof TS, Univ Pennsylvania

Naka, Yoshifumi MD/PhD [TS] - **Spec Exp:** Transplant-Heart & Lung; Ventricular Assist Device (LVAD); Heart Failure & Ventricular Containment; Mitral Valve Surgery; **Hospital:** NY-Presby Hosp/Columbia (page 66); **Address:** 177 Fort Washington Ave, MHB 7-435, New York, NY 10032; **Phone:** 212-305-0828; **Med School:** Japan 1984; **Resid:** Surgery, Osaka Police Hosp 1991; **Fellow:** Cardiovascular Surgery, Osaka Police Hosp 1993; Cardiothoracic Surgery, Columbia Univ 1998; **Fac Appt:** Asst Prof S, Columbia P&S

Oz, Mehmet C MD [TS] - **Spec Exp:** Transplant-Heart; Heart Valve Surgery; Minimally Invasive Cardiac Surgery; **Hospital:** NY-Presby Hosp/Columbia (page 66); **Address:** NY Presby Hosp, Dept Cardiothoracic Surg, 177 Ft Washington Ave, MHB- Rm 7, GN435, New York, NY 10032; **Phone:** 212-305-4434; **Board Cert:** Thoracic Surgery 2003; **Med School:** Univ Pennsylvania 1986; **Resid:** Surgery, Columbia Presby Med Ctr 1991; **Fellow:** Cardiothoracic Surgery, Columbia Presby Med Ctr 1993; **Fac Appt:** Prof S, Columbia P&S

Thoracic Surgery

Pass, Harvey MD [TS] - **Spec Exp:** Lung Cancer; Mesothelioma; Clinical Trials; **Hospital:** NYU Langone Med Ctr (page 67); **Address:** NYU Cancer Ctr, 160 E 34th St Fl 8, New York, NY 10016; **Phone:** 212-731-5414; **Board Cert:** Thoracic Surgery 2001; **Med School:** Duke Univ 1973; **Resid:** Surgery, Duke Univ Med Ctr 1975; Surgery, Univ Miss Med Ctr 1980; **Fellow:** Cardiothoracic Surgery, MUSC Med Ctr 1982; **Fac Appt:** Prof S, NYU Sch Med

Pierson III, Richard N MD [TS] - **Spec Exp:** Transplant-Lung; Lung Cancer; Transplant-Heart; **Hospital:** Univ of MD Med Ctr; **Address:** Univ Md Med Ctr, Dept Cardiothoracic Surg, 22 S Greene St, rm N4W94, Baltimore, MD 21201; **Phone:** 410-328-5842; **Board Cert:** Surgery 2000; Thoracic Surgery 2002; **Med School:** Columbia P&S 1983; **Resid:** Surgery, Univ Mich Med Ctr 1990; **Fellow:** Cardiothoracic Surgery, Mass General Hosp 1992; **Fac Appt:** Assoc Prof TS, Univ MD Sch Med

Pochettino, Alberto MD [TS] - **Spec Exp:** Aneurysm-Thoracic Aortic; Transplant-Lung; Left Ventricular Assist Device (LVAD); Heart Valve Surgery; **Hospital:** Hosp Univ Penn - UPHS (page 60), Penn Presby Med Ctr - UPHS (page 60); **Address:** Dept Thoracic Surgery, 3400 Spruce St, 6 Silverstein Pavillion, Philadelphia, PA 19104; **Phone:** 215-662-2957; **Board Cert:** Surgery 2005; Thoracic Surgery 2005; **Med School:** Northwestern Univ 1987; **Resid:** Surgery, SUNY-Upstate Med Ctr 1992; Thoracic Surgery, Hosp Univ Penn 1994; **Fac Appt:** Assoc Prof TS, Univ Pennsylvania

Rosengart, Todd MD [TS] - **Spec Exp:** Transfusion Free Surgery; Gene Therapy-Cardiac Angiogenesis; Minimally Invasive Surgery; Cardiac Surgery; **Hospital:** Stony Brook Univ Med Ctr; **Address:** Stonybrook Univ Hosp, Health Sci Ctr, Cardiothoracic Surgery, HSC-T19, rm 080, Stonybrook, NY 11794-0001; **Phone:** 631-444-7875; **Board Cert:** Surgery 1999; Thoracic Surgery 2002; **Med School:** Northwestern Univ 1983; **Resid:** Surgery, NYU Med Ctr 1985; Surgery, NYU Med Ctr 1989; **Fellow:** Thoracic Surgery, Natl Inst Hlth 1987; Cardiothoracic Surgery, NY-Cornell Med Ctr 1991; **Fac Appt:** Prof S, SUNY Stony Brook

Samuels, Louis MD [TS] - **Spec Exp:** Transplant-Heart; Artificial Heart Devices; Ventricular Assist Device (LVAD); **Hospital:** Lankenau Hosp; **Address:** 100 Lancaster Ave, 280 Lankenau Medical Science Bldg, Wynnwood, PA 19096; **Phone:** 610-896-9255; **Board Cert:** Surgery 1994; Thoracic Surgery 1996; **Med School:** Hahnemann Univ 1987; **Resid:** Surgery, Hahnemann Hosp 1992; Thoracic Surgery, Hahnemann Hosp 1995; **Fac Appt:** Prof S, Hahnemann Univ

Scott, Walter J MD [TS] - **Spec Exp:** Lung Cancer; Esophageal Cancer; Mediastinal Tumors; Minimally Invasive Surgery; **Hospital:** Fox Chase Cancer Ctr (page 58); **Address:** Fox Chase Cancer Ctr, 333 Cottman Ave, rm C308, Philadelphia, PA 19111; **Phone:** 215-214-1427; **Board Cert:** Thoracic Surgery 1998; **Med School:** Univ Chicago-Pritzker Sch Med 1981; **Resid:** Surgery, Univ Chicago Med Ctr 1987; **Fellow:** Cardiothoracic Surgery, Univ Chicago Med Ctr 1989; **Fac Appt:** Assoc Prof TS, Temple Univ

Smith, Craig R MD [TS] - **Spec Exp:** Mitral Valve Surgery; Transplant-Heart; Minimally Invasive Cardiac Surgery; Robotic Cardiac Surgery; **Hospital:** NY-Presby Hosp/Columbia (page 66); **Address:** Columbia Presbyterian Med Ctr, 177 Fort Washington Ave, Ste 7-435, New York, NY 10032; **Phone:** 212-305-8312; **Board Cert:** Thoracic Surgery 2004; **Med School:** Case West Res Univ 1977; **Resid:** Surgery, Strong Meml Hosp 1982; **Fellow:** Cardiothoracic Surgery, Columbia Presby Med Ctr 1984; **Fac Appt:** Prof S, Columbia P&S

Sonett, Joshua R MD [TS] - **Spec Exp:** Minimally Invasive Thoracic Surgery; Transplant-Lung; Thoracic Cancers; Emphysema-Lung Volume Reduction; **Hospital:** NY-Presby Hosp/Columbia (page 66); **Address:** 161 Fort Washington Ave, Ste 301, New York, NY 10032; **Phone:** 212-305-8086; **Board Cert:** Surgery 1994; Thoracic Surgery 1997; **Med School:** E Carolina Univ 1988; **Resid:** Surgery, Univ Mass Med Ctr 1993; **Fellow:** Cardiothoracic Surgery, Univ Pittsburgh Med Ctr 1994; Thoracic Surgery, Meml Sloan Kettering Cancer Ctr; **Fac Appt:** Assoc Prof S, Columbia P&S

Strong III, Michael D MD [TS] - **Spec Exp:** Coronary Artery Surgery; Heart Valve Surgery; Thoracic Aortic Surgery; **Hospital:** Hahnemann Univ Hosp; **Address:** Div Cardiothoracic Surgery, 245 N 15th St, 744 N Tower, Philadelphia, PA 19102; **Phone:** 215-762-7802; **Board Cert:** Surgery 1974; Thoracic Surgery 2006; **Med School:** Jefferson Med Coll 1966; **Resid:** Surgery, Jefferson Hosp 1973; Thoracic Surgery, Temple Univ Hosp 1975; **Fac Appt:** Assoc Prof TS, Drexel Univ Coll Med

Tortolani, Anthony J MD [TS] - **Spec Exp:** Transfusion Free Surgery; Heart Valve Surgery; Coronary Artery Surgery; **Hospital:** NY-Presby Hosp/Weill Cornell (page 66), New York Methodist Hosp; **Address:** NY Presby Hosp, Dept Cardiothoracic Surg, 525 E 68th St, rm M-404, New York, NY 10021-4870; **Phone:** 212-746-5155; **Board Cert:** Surgery 1975; Thoracic Surgery 1999; **Med School:** Geo Wash Univ 1969; **Resid:** Surgery, N Shore Univ Hosp 1974; **Fellow:** Cardiothoracic Surgery, NYU Med Ctr 1978; **Fac Appt:** Clin Prof S, Cornell Univ-Weill Med Coll

Tranbaugh, Robert MD [TS] - **Spec Exp:** Coronary Artery Surgery; Heart Valve Surgery; Aneurysm-Thoracic Aortic; **Hospital:** Beth Israel Med Ctr - Petrie Division (page 57); **Address:** 317 E 17th St Fl 11, New York, NY 10003; **Phone:** 212-420-2584; **Board Cert:** Thoracic Surgery 2004; **Med School:** Univ Pennsylvania 1976; **Resid:** Surgery, UCSF Med Ctr 1983; Cardiothoracic Surgery, UCSF Med Ctr 1985; **Fac Appt:** Assoc Prof TS, Albert Einstein Coll Med

Watson, Thomas J MD [TS] - **Spec Exp:** Esophageal Cancer; Gastroesophageal Reflux Disease (GERD); Lung Cancer; **Hospital:** Univ of Rochester Strong Meml Hosp, Highland Hosp of Rochester; **Address:** 601 Elmwood Ave, Box SURG, Rochester, NY 14642; **Phone:** 585-275-1509; **Board Cert:** Thoracic Surgery 2007; Surgery 2003; **Med School:** Univ SC Sch Med 1988; **Resid:** Surgery, LAC-USC Med Ctr 1993; Cardiothoracic Surgery, LAC-USC Med Ctr 1996; **Fellow:** Esophageal Surgery, LAC-USC Med Ctr 1994; **Fac Appt:** Assoc Prof S, Univ Rochester

Weksler, Benny MD [TS] - **Spec Exp:** Thoracic Cancers; Cancer Surgery; Esophageal Cancer; Minimally Invasive Thoracic Surgery; **Hospital:** Thomas Jefferson Univ Hosp; **Address:** 1025 Walnut St, 607 College, Philadelphia, PA 19107; **Phone:** 215-955-6996; **Board Cert:** Surgery 2007; Thoracic Surgery 2007; **Med School:** Brazil 1987; **Resid:** Surgery, NY Med Coll/ Lincoln Med Ctr 1991; Surgery, NY Med Coll/Lincoln Med Ctr 1995; **Fellow:** Cardiothoracic Surgery, Meml Sloan Kettering Cancer Ctr 1997; Minimally Invasive Surgery, Univ Pittsburgh Med Ctr 2008; **Fac Appt:** Assoc Prof S, Thomas Jefferson Univ

Woo, Y Joseph MD [TS] - **Spec Exp:** Minimally Invasive Cardiac Surgery; Robotic Cardiac Surgery; Aneurysm-Abdominal & Thoracic Aortic; Mitral Valve Robotic Surgery; **Hospital:** Hosp Univ Penn - UPHS (page 60); **Address:** Penn Cardiac Care, 6 Silverstein Bldg, 3400 Spruce St, Philadelphia, PA 19104; **Phone:** 215-662-2956; **Board Cert:** Surgery 2000; Thoracic Surgery 2002; **Med School:** Univ Pennsylvania 1992; **Resid:** Surgery, Hosp Univ Penn 1998; Thoracic Surgery, Hosp Univ Penn 2001; **Fac Appt:** Asst Prof S, Univ Pennsylvania

Yang, Stephen C MD [TS] - **Spec Exp:** Mesothelioma; Lung Cancer; Esophageal Cancer; **Hospital:** Johns Hopkins Hosp (page 61), Johns Hopkins Bayview Med Ctr (page 61); **Address:** Johns Hopkins Hosp, 600 N Wolfe St Blalock Bldg - rm 240, Baltimore, MD 21287-5674; **Phone:** 410-614-3891; **Board Cert:** Surgery 2003; Thoracic Surgery 2005; **Med School:** Med Coll VA 1984; **Resid:** Surgery, Univ Tex Hlth Sci Ctr 1990; **Fellow:** Thoracic Surgery, MD Anderson Cancer Ctr 1992; Cardiothoracic Surgery, Med Coll Virginia 1994; **Fac Appt:** Assoc Prof TS, Johns Hopkins Univ

Thoracic Surgery

Southeast

Bichell, David P MD [TS] - **Spec Exp:** Cardiac Surgery-Neonatal; Cardiac Surgery-Pediatric; Congenital Heart Surgery; Minimally Invasive Cardiac Surgery; **Hospital:** Vanderbilt Children's Hosp, Vanderbilt Univ Med Ctr; **Address:** Vanderbilt Childrens Hosp, Div Pediatric Cardiac Surgery, 2200 Childrens Way, 5247 DOT, Nashville, TN 37232-9292; **Phone:** 615-343-6525; **Board Cert:** Thoracic Surgery 2006; **Med School:** Columbia P&S 1987; **Resid:** Surgery, Barnes Jewish Hosp 1994; Cardiothoracic Surgery, Brigham & Womens Hosp/Chldns Hosp 1996; **Fellow:** Cardiac Surgery, Brigham & Womens Hosp 1997; **Fac Appt:** Prof TS, Vanderbilt Univ

Brunsting III, Louis A MD [TS] - **Spec Exp:** Robotic Cardiac Surgery; **Hospital:** Centennial Med Ctr, Baptist Hosp - Nashville; **Address:** Cardiothoracic Surgery Associates, 2400 Patterson St, Ste 223, Nashville, TN 37203; **Phone:** 615-329-1122; **Board Cert:** Thoracic Surgery 2001; **Med School:** UCSD 1983; **Resid:** Surgery, Univ Rochester 1985; Surgery, Univ Rochester 1989; **Fellow:** Surgery, Duke Univ 1987; Thoracic Surgery, Duke Univ 1991

Cerfolio, Robert J MD [TS] - **Spec Exp:** Lung Cancer; Tracheal Surgery; Chest Wall Tumors; Esophageal Cancer; **Hospital:** Univ of Ala Hosp at Birmingham; **Address:** 703 19th St S, Ste 739, Zigler Rsch Bldg, Birmingham, AL 35294-0007; **Phone:** 205-934-5937; **Board Cert:** Surgery 2003; Thoracic Surgery 2006; **Med School:** Univ Rochester 1988; **Resid:** Surgery, Cornell-NY Hosp 1990; Surgery, Mayo Clinic 1993; **Fellow:** Cardiothoracic Surgery, Mayo Clinic 1996; **Fac Appt:** Prof TS, Univ Alabama

Chitwood Jr, W Randolph MD [TS] - **Spec Exp:** Robotic Cardiac Surgery; Minimally Invasive Cardiac Surgery; Heart Valve Surgery; Mitral Valve Surgery; **Hospital:** Pitt Cty Mem Hosp - Univ Med Ctr East Carolina; **Address:** E Carolina Heart Inst @ ECU, 115 Heart Drive, rm 3153, Greenville, NC 27834; **Phone:** 252-744-4536; **Board Cert:** Thoracic Surgery 2005; **Med School:** Univ VA Sch Med 1974; **Resid:** Surgery, Duke Univ Med Ctr 1983; **Fellow:** Cardiovascular Surgery, Duke Univ Med Ctr 1984; **Fac Appt:** Prof S, E Carolina Univ

Christian, Karla G MD [TS] - **Spec Exp:** Congenital Heart Surgery; Transplant-Heart-Adult & Pediatric; Cardiac Surgery-Adult & Pediatric; **Hospital:** Vanderbilt Children's Hosp, Vanderbilt Univ Med Ctr; **Address:** Vanderbilt Chldns Hosp, Cardiac Surgery, 2200 Childrens Way, 5247 DOT, Nashville, TN 37232-9292; **Phone:** 615-343-6525; **Board Cert:** Surgery 2001; Thoracic Surgery 2003; **Med School:** Univ Wash 1985; **Resid:** Surgery, Univ Washington Med Ctr 1987; Surgery, Vanderbilt Univ Med Ctr 1991; **Fellow:** Cardiothoracic Surgery, Vanderbilt Univ Med Ctr 1994; **Fac Appt:** Assoc Prof S, Vanderbilt Univ

D'Amico, Thomas MD [TS] - **Spec Exp:** Lung Cancer; Esophageal Cancer; **Hospital:** Duke Univ Med Ctr; **Address:** Duke Univ Med Ctr, Dept Thoracic Surg, Box 3496, Durham, NC 27710; **Phone:** 919-684-4891; **Board Cert:** Surgery 2004; Thoracic Surgery 2006; **Med School:** Columbia P&S 1987; **Resid:** Surgery, Duke Univ Med Ctr 1989; Cardiothoracic Surgery, Duke Univ Med Ctr 1996; **Fellow:** Thoracic Oncology, Meml Sloan Kettering Cancer Ctr; **Fac Appt:** Assoc Prof S, Duke Univ

Drinkwater Jr, Davis C MD [TS] - **Spec Exp:** Transplant-Heart & Lung; Cardiac Surgery-Adult & Pediatric; **Hospital:** Centennial Med Ctr, Vanderbilt Children's Hosp; **Address:** 2400 Patterson St, Ste 400, Nashville, TN 37203; **Phone:** 615-342-5812; **Board Cert:** Thoracic Surgery 2005; **Med School:** Univ VT Coll Med 1976; **Resid:** Surgery, McGill Univ 1981; Cardiothoracic Surgery, McGill Univ 1983; **Fellow:** Cardiothoracic Surgery, Childrens Hosp 1984; **Fac Appt:** Clin Prof TS, Vanderbilt Univ

Glassford Jr, David M MD [TS] - **Spec Exp:** Cardiothoracic Surgery; **Hospital:** Saint Thomas Hosp - Nashville; **Address:** Cardiovascular Surgery Assocs, 4230 Harding Rd, Ste 202, Nashville, TN 37205; **Phone:** 615-385-4781; **Board Cert:** Surgery 1998; Surgical Critical Care 1999; Thoracic Surgery 2007; **Med School:** Univ Tex Med Br, Galveston 1970; **Resid:** Surgery, Univ Texas Med Br 1975; Thoracic Surgery, Ochsner Clinic 1977; **Fac Appt:** Asst Clin Prof TS, Vanderbilt Univ

Guyton, Robert A MD [TS] - **Spec Exp:** Coronary Artery Surgery; Minimally Invasive Cardiac Surgery; Heart Valve Surgery; Heart Valve-Percutaneous; **Hospital:** Emory Univ Hosp Midtown, Emory Univ Hosp; **Address:** Crawford Long Hospital of Emory Univ, 550 Peachtree St, MOT Fl 6, Atlanta, GA 30308; **Phone:** 404-686-2513; **Board Cert:** Thoracic Surgery 2000; **Med School:** Harvard Med Sch 1971; **Resid:** Surgery, Mass Genl Hosp 1975; **Fellow:** Thoracic Surgery, National Heart Lung Inst 1975; **Fac Appt:** Prof TS, Emory Univ

Harpole Jr, David H MD [TS] - **Spec Exp:** Lung Cancer; Mesothelioma; Esophageal Cancer; **Hospital:** Duke Univ Med Ctr; **Address:** Duke Univ Med Ctr-Thoracic Surgery, 2424 Erwin Rd, Ste 403 - rm 4071, Durham, NC 27705; **Phone:** 919-668-8413; **Board Cert:** Surgery 2002; Thoracic Surgery 2003; **Med School:** Univ VA Sch Med 1984; **Resid:** Surgery, Duke Univ Med Ctr 1991; **Fellow:** Thoracic Surgery, Duke Univ Med Ctr 1993; **Fac Appt:** Prof S, Duke Univ

Heidary, Dariush H MD [TS] - **Spec Exp:** Cardiothoracic Surgery; Cardiovascular Surgery; **Hospital:** Meml Hlth Univ Med Ctr - Savannah, St Joseph's-Candler Hosp; **Address:** Memorial Hlth Univ Med Ctr, 4700 Waters Ave, Ste 403, Savannah, GA 31404-6220; **Phone:** 912-354-7188; **Board Cert:** Thoracic Surgery 2007; **Med School:** Iran 1967; **Resid:** Surgery, Albert Einstein Med Ctr 1974; Cardiothoracic Surgery, Albert Einstein Med Ctr 1975; **Fellow:** Cardiothoracic Surgery, Med Coll Georgia 1977

Jones, David R MD [TS] - **Spec Exp:** Lung Cancer; Esophageal Cancer; Minimally Invasive Thoracic Surgery; **Hospital:** Univ Virginia Med Ctr; **Address:** Department of Surgery, Box 800679, Charlottesville, VA 22901; **Phone:** 434-243-6443; **Board Cert:** Surgery 2005; Thoracic Surgery 2007; **Med School:** W VA Univ 1989; **Resid:** Surgery, West Va Univ 1995; **Fellow:** Thoracic Surgery, Univ North Carolina 1998; **Fac Appt:** Assoc Prof S, Univ VA Sch Med

Kanter, Kirk R MD [TS] - **Spec Exp:** Pediatric Cardiac Surgery; Transplant-Heart-Pediatric; Transplant-Lung-Pediatric; **Hospital:** Chldns Hlthcare Atlanta @ Egleston, Emory Univ Hosp; **Address:** Childrens Hlthcare Atlanta at Egleston, Pediatric Cardiothoracic Surgery, 1405 Clifton Rd NE Fl 2, Atlanta, GA 30322; **Phone:** 404-785-6300; **Board Cert:** Thoracic Surgery 1996; **Med School:** Albany Med Coll 1976; **Resid:** Surgery, Johns Hopkins Hosp 1982; Thoracic Surgery, Johns Hopkins Hosp 1984; **Fellow:** Pediatric Cardiac Surgery, Brompton/Harefield Hosps 1985; **Fac Appt:** Prof S, Emory Univ

Kiernan, Paul D MD [TS] - **Spec Exp:** Lung Cancer; Esophageal Cancer; Mediastinal Tumors; **Hospital:** Inova Fairfax Hosp, Inova Alexandria Hosp; **Address:** 2921 Telestar Court, Falls Church, VA 22042; **Phone:** 703-280-5858; **Board Cert:** Thoracic Surgery 2002; **Med School:** Georgetown Univ 1974; **Resid:** Surgery, Mayo Clinic 1979; Cardiothoracic Surgery, Mayo Clinic 1981; **Fellow:** Vascular Surgery, Mayo Clinic 1982; **Fac Appt:** Assoc Clin Prof S, Georgetown Univ

Kirklin, James K MD [TS] - **Spec Exp:** Transplant-Heart-Adult & Pediatric; Cardiac Surgery-Adult & Pediatric; Transplant-Heart & Lung; **Hospital:** Univ of Ala Hosp at Birmingham; **Address:** Univ Alabama Med Ctr, THT 760, 1900 University Blvd, Birmingham, AL 35294; **Phone:** 205-934-3368; **Board Cert:** Thoracic Surgery 2000; **Med School:** Harvard Med Sch 1973; **Resid:** Surgery, Mass Genl Hosp 1977; Cardiothoracic Surgery, Mass Genl Hosp 1979; **Fellow:** Cardiothoracic Surgery, Chidren's Hosp Med Ctr 1979; **Fac Appt:** Prof S, Univ Alabama

Thoracic Surgery

Kron, Irving L MD [TS] - **Spec Exp:** Coronary Artery Surgery; Transplant-Heart; **Hospital:** Univ Virginia Med Ctr; **Address:** Univ VA Hlth Sys, Div Cardiovascular Surg, PO Box 800679, Charlottesville, VA 22908; **Phone:** 434-924-2158; **Board Cert:** Surgery 1999; Thoracic Surgery 2001; Vascular Surgery 2006; **Med School:** Med Coll Wisc 1975; **Resid:** Surgery, Maine Med Ctr 1980; **Fellow:** Cardiothoracic Surgery, Univ Virginia Med Ctr 1982; **Fac Appt:** Prof S, Univ VA Sch Med

Martin, Tomas D MD [TS] - **Spec Exp:** Cardiothoracic Surgery; Aortic Surgery; Aneurysm-Abdominal Aortic; **Hospital:** Shands at Univ of FL; **Address:** Dept of Surgery, 1600 SW Archer Rd, Box 100129, Gainesville, FL 32610-0129; **Phone:** 352-273-5505; **Board Cert:** Thoracic Surgery 1999; **Med School:** Univ Tex, Houston 1981; **Resid:** Surgery, Baylor Coll Med 1986; Vascular Surgery, Baylor Coll Med 1987; **Fellow:** Cardiothoracic Surgery, Shands/Univ Florida 1989; **Fac Appt:** Assoc Prof S, Univ Fla Coll Med

Miller, Daniel L MD [TS] - **Spec Exp:** Esophageal Cancer; Lung Cancer; Mesothelioma; Emphysema-Lung Volume Reduction; **Hospital:** Emory Univ Hosp; **Address:** The Emory Clinic, 1365A Clifton Rd NE, Ste 2219, Atlanta, GA 30322; **Phone:** 404-778-3755; **Board Cert:** Thoracic Surgery 2005; Surgery 2001; **Med School:** Univ KY Coll Med 1985; **Resid:** Surgery, Georgetown Univ Hosp 1991; **Fellow:** Cardiothoracic Surgery, Mayo Clinic 1994; **Fac Appt:** Assoc Prof S, Emory Univ

Miller, Joseph I MD [TS] - **Spec Exp:** Lung Cancer; **Hospital:** Emory Univ Hosp, Emory Univ Hosp Midtown; **Address:** 550 Peachtree St NE, MOT-6th Fl, Atlanta, GA 30308; **Phone:** 404-686-2515; **Board Cert:** Surgery 1973; Thoracic Surgery 1975; **Med School:** Emory Univ 1965; **Resid:** Surgery, Mayo Clin 1972; Thoracic Surgery, Emory Univ Hosp 1974; **Fac Appt:** Prof S, Emory Univ

Mullett, Timothy W MD [TS] - **Spec Exp:** Lung Cancer; Transplant-Heart & Lung; Cardiac Surgery-Adult & Pediatric; Esophageal Surgery; **Hospital:** Univ of Kentucky Chandler Hosp; **Address:** 800 Rose St Fl 4th, Lexington, KY 40536; **Phone:** 859-323-1691; **Board Cert:** Thoracic Surgery 1997; Surgery 2005; **Med School:** Univ Fla Coll Med 1987; **Resid:** Surgery, Shands/Univ of FL 1993; **Fellow:** Pediatric Surgery, Shands/Univ of FL 1994; Cardiothoracic Surgery, Shands/Univ of FL 1995; **Fac Appt:** Assoc Prof S, Univ KY Coll Med

Murphy, Douglas A MD [TS] - **Spec Exp:** Mitral Valve Robotic Surgery; Minimally Invasive Heart Surgery; **Hospital:** St Joseph's Hosp - Atlanta; **Address:** 5665 Peachtree Dunwoody Rd NE, Ste 150, Atlanta, GA 30342; **Phone:** 404-252-6104; **Board Cert:** Internal Medicine 1978; Thoracic Surgery 2004; **Med School:** Univ Pennsylvania 1975; **Resid:** Internal Medicine, Mass Genl Hosp 1977; Surgery, Mass Genl Hosp 1981; **Fellow:** Thoracic Surgery, Emory Univ Affil Hosp 1983

Nesbitt, Jonathan C MD [TS] - **Spec Exp:** Lung Cancer; Esophageal Cancer; Chest Diseases-Benign; **Hospital:** Vanderbilt Univ Med Ctr, Saint Thomas Hosp - Nashville; **Address:** The Vanderbilt Clinic, 609 Oxford House, 1313 21st Ave S, Nashville, TN 37232-4682; **Phone:** 615-322-0064; **Board Cert:** Surgery 1998; Thoracic Surgery 1998; **Med School:** Georgetown Univ 1981; **Resid:** Surgery, Vanderbilt Univ Med Ctr 1987; Thoracic Surgery, Albany Med Ctr 1989; **Fac Appt:** Asst Clin Prof S, Vanderbilt Univ

Ninan, Mathews MD [TS] - **Spec Exp:** Lung Cancer; Transplant-Lung; Esophageal Cancer; **Hospital:** Baptist Memorial Hospital - Memphis, Methodist Univ Hosp - Memphis; **Address:** 7945 Wolf River Blvd, Ste 280, Germantown, TN 38138; **Phone:** 901-347-8270; **Med School:** India 1988; **Resid:** Surgery, Univ London Affil Hosp 1994; **Fellow:** Cardiothoracic Surgery, Univ Pittsburgh Affil Hosp 1998; **Fac Appt:** Assoc Prof TS, Vanderbilt Univ

Oaks, Timothy E MD [TS] - **Spec Exp:** Transplant-Heart; Cardiovascular Surgery-Complex; Lung Cancer; **Hospital:** Wake Forest Univ Baptist Med Ctr (page 72); **Address:** Wake Forest Baptist Med Ctr, Dept Cardiothoracic Surgery, Medical Center Blvd, Winston-Salem, NC 27157; **Phone:** 336-716-9800; **Board Cert:** Thoracic Surgery 2001; **Med School:** Penn State Univ Coll Med 1984; **Resid:** Surgery, Penn State-Hershey Med Ctr 1990; **Fellow:** Cardiothoracic Surgery, Penn State-Hershey Med Ctr 1992; Cardiothoracic Surgery, Papworth Hosp 1993; **Fac Appt:** Assoc Prof TS, Wake Forest Univ

Putnam Jr, Joe B MD [TS] - **Spec Exp:** Lung Cancer; Esophageal Cancer; Sarcoma-Soft Tissue; **Hospital:** Vanderbilt Univ Med Ctr, VA Med Ctr - Nashville; **Address:** Vanderbilt Univ Med Ctr - Thoracic Surgery, 609 Oxford House, 1313 21st Ave S, Nashville, TN 37232-4682; **Phone:** 615-343-9202; **Board Cert:** Thoracic Surgery 2007; **Med School:** Univ NC Sch Med 1979; **Resid:** Surgery, Univ Rochester 1986; Thoracic Surgery, Univ Mich Med Ctr 1988; **Fellow:** Surgical Oncology, NCI/NIH-Surg Branch 1984; **Fac Appt:** Prof TS, Vanderbilt Univ

Quintessenza, James A MD [TS] - **Spec Exp:** Transplant-Heart; Coronary Artery Surgery; Cardiovascular Surgery; **Hospital:** All Children's Hosp; **Address:** 625 6th Ave S, Ste 475, St Petersburg, FL 33701; **Phone:** 727-822-6666; **Board Cert:** Thoracic Surgery 2007; **Med School:** Univ Fla Coll Med 1981; **Resid:** Surgery, Univ Florida Hosps 1986; **Fellow:** Thoracic Surgery, UCSD Medical Ctr 1988; **Fac Appt:** Assoc Clin Prof S, Univ S Fla Coll Med

Reed, Carolyn E MD [TS] - **Spec Exp:** Esophageal Cancer; Lung Cancer; **Hospital:** MUSC Med Ctr; **Address:** Med Univ S Carolina, 25 Courtenay Drive, Ste 7018, Charleston, SC 29425; **Phone:** 843-876-4845; **Board Cert:** Thoracic Surgery 2006; **Med School:** Univ Rochester 1977; **Resid:** Surgery, NY Hosp 1982; Thoracic Surgery, NY Hosp 1985; **Fellow:** Surgical Oncology, Meml Sloan Kettering Cancer Ctr 1983; **Fac Appt:** Prof S, Med Univ SC

Robinson, Lary A MD [TS] - **Spec Exp:** Lung Cancer; Mesothelioma; **Hospital:** H Lee Moffitt Cancer Ctr & Research Inst, Tampa Genl Hosp; **Address:** H Lee Moffitt Cancer Ctr, Div Thoracic Oncology, 12902 Magnolia Drive, Tampa, FL 33612-9497; **Phone:** 813-745-7282; **Board Cert:** Thoracic Surgery 2003; Surgery 2002; Surgical Critical Care 2000; **Med School:** Washington Univ, St Louis 1972; **Resid:** Surgery, Duke Univ Med Ctr 1974; Thoracic Surgery, Duke Univ Med Ctr 1981; **Fellow:** Cardiothoracic Surgery, St Thomas Hosp 1982; Cardiothoracic Surgery, Duke Univ Med Ctr 1983; **Fac Appt:** Prof S, Univ S Fla Coll Med

Slaughter, Mark S MD [TS] - **Spec Exp:** Ventricular Assist Device (LVAD); Mitral Valve Surgery; Transplant-Heart; **Hospital:** Jewish Hosp HlthCre Svcs Inc; **Address:** 201 Abraham Flexner Way, Ste 1200, Louisville, KY 40202; **Phone:** 502-583-8383; **Board Cert:** Surgery 2002; Thoracic Surgery 1995; **Med School:** Indiana Univ 1987; **Resid:** Surgery, Northwestern Meml Hosp 1992; **Fellow:** Thoracic Surgery, Univ Minnesota 1994

Smith, Peter K MD [TS] - **Spec Exp:** Coronary Artery Surgery; Heart Valve Surgery; **Hospital:** Duke Univ Med Ctr, VA Med Ctr - Durham; **Address:** Duke Univ Med Ctr, Cardiothoracic Surg, Box 3442, Durham, NC 27710; **Phone:** 919-684-2890; **Board Cert:** Thoracic Surgery 2007; **Med School:** Duke Univ 1977; **Resid:** Surgery, Duke Univ Med Ctr 1984; Thoracic Surgery, Duke Univ Med Ctr 1987; **Fac Appt:** Prof S, Duke Univ

Srivastava, Sudhir P MD [TS] - **Spec Exp:** Robotic Cardiac Surgery; **Hospital:** St Joseph's Hosp - Atlanta; **Address:** Peachtree Cardiovascular/Thoracic Surgeons, 5665 Peachtree Dunwoody Rd, Ste 150, Atlanta, GA 30342; **Phone:** 404-252-6104; **Board Cert:** Thoracic Surgery 1999; **Med School:** India 1970; **Resid:** Vascular Surgery, Vancouver Genl Hosp 1977; Thoracic Surgery, Vancouver Genl Hosp 1978; **Fellow:** Surgery, Vancouver Genl Hosp 1979

Thoracic Surgery

Staples, Edward D MD [TS] - **Spec Exp:** Transplant-Heart & Lung; Ventricular Assist Device (LVAD); **Hospital:** Shands at Univ of FL, Malcolm Randall VA Med Ctr; **Address:** Shands-Dept Cardiothoracic Surg, 1600 SW Archer Rd, rm NG-33, Gainesville, FL 32610; **Phone:** 352-273-5507; **Board Cert:** Thoracic Surgery 2004; Surgical Critical Care 2002; **Med School:** Univ S Fla Coll Med 1977; **Resid:** Surgery, Med Coll Va 1979; Surgery, Univ Hosp 1982; **Fellow:** Cardiothoracic Surgery, Univ Florida 1984; **Fac Appt:** Assoc Prof S, Univ Fla Coll Med

Stowe, Cary MD [TS] - **Spec Exp:** Aortic Surgery; **Hospital:** Indian River Med Ctr; **Address:** 1040 37th Pl, Ste 101, Vero Beach, FL 32960; **Phone:** 772-563-4580; **Board Cert:** Thoracic Surgery 1999; **Med School:** Univ Alabama 1978; **Resid:** Surgery, Barnes Hosp 1982; **Fellow:** Vascular Surgery, Baylor Coll Med 1983; Cardiothoracic Surgery, Emory Univ Sch Med 1994

Tedder, Mark MD [TS] - **Spec Exp:** Transplant-Heart; Cardiac Surgery; Artificial Heart Devices; **Hospital:** Saint Thomas Hosp - Nashville; **Address:** 4230 Harding Rd, Ste 202, Nashville, TN 37205; **Phone:** 615-385-4781; **Board Cert:** Thoracic Surgery 1998; **Med School:** Duke Univ 1988; **Resid:** Surgery, Duke Univ Med Ctr 1995; Cardiothoracic Surgery, Duke Univ Med Ctr 1997

Weiman, Darryl S MD [TS] - **Spec Exp:** Cardiothoracic Surgery; Lung Cancer; **Hospital:** Methodist Univ Hosp - Memphis, VA Med Ctr - Memphis; **Address:** 956 Court Ave, Memphis, TN 38163; **Phone:** 901-448-5912; **Board Cert:** Thoracic Surgery 2000; Surgery 2002; **Med School:** St Louis Univ 1978; **Resid:** Surgery, Univ Chicago Pritzker Sch Med 1983; Thoracic Surgery, Univ Chicago Pritzker Sch Med 1984; **Fellow:** Cardiothoracic Surgery, Long Island Jewish Hosp 1991; **Fac Appt:** Prof S, Univ Tenn Coll Med, Memphis

Zwischenberger, Joseph B MD [TS] - **Spec Exp:** Thoracic Cancers; Lung Cancer; Esophageal Cancer; Respiratory Failure; **Hospital:** Univ of Kentucky Chandler Hosp; **Address:** MN264 A B Chandler Med Ctr, 800 Rose St, Lexington, KY 40536; **Phone:** 859-323-6013; **Board Cert:** Surgery 2002; Thoracic Surgery 2005; Surgical Critical Care 1996; **Med School:** Univ KY Coll Med 1977; **Resid:** Surgery, Univ Michigan Hosp 1984; Cardiothoracic Surgery, Univ Michigan Hosp 1985; **Fellow:** Cardiac Surgery, Natl Inst Hlth 1981; **Fac Appt:** Prof S, Univ KY Coll Med

Midwest

Alexander Jr, John C MD [TS] - **Spec Exp:** Minimally Invasive Cardiac Surgery; Robotic Cardiac Surgery; Mitral Valve Surgery; Arrhythmias; **Hospital:** Evanston/Northshore Univ Hlth Syst; **Address:** Evanston Hosp, Cardiothoracic Surgery, 2650 Ridge Ave Walgreens Bldg - Ste 3507, Evanston, IL 60201; **Phone:** 847-570-2868; **Board Cert:** Thoracic Surgery 2001; **Med School:** Duke Univ 1972; **Resid:** Surgery, Duke Univ Med Ctr 1979; **Fellow:** Cardiothoracic Surgery, Duke Univ Med Ctr 1980; **Fac Appt:** Prof S, Northwestern Univ-Feinberg Sch Med

Bakhos, Mamdouh MD [TS] - **Spec Exp:** Mitral Valve Surgery; Minimally Invasive Cardiac Surgery; Transplant-Heart & Lung; Cardiovascular Surgery; **Hospital:** Loyola Univ Med Ctr, Adv Good Samaritan Hosp; **Address:** Loyola Univ, Dept Cardiothoracic Surgery, 2160 S First Ave, Bldg 110 - rm 6240, Maywood, IL 60153; **Phone:** 708-327-2503; **Board Cert:** Thoracic Surgery 2007; **Med School:** Syria 1971; **Resid:** Surgery, Huron Road Hosp 1976; **Fellow:** Thoracic Surgery, Loyola Univ Med Ctr 1978; **Fac Appt:** Prof TS, Loyola Univ-Stritch Sch Med

Brown, John W MD [TS] - **Spec Exp:** Cardiac Surgery-Neonatal & Pediatric; Transplant-Heart; Heart Valve Surgery; Congenital Heart Disease; **Hospital:** Riley Hosp for Children, Methodist Hosp - Indianapolis; **Address:** 545 Barnhill Drive, EH215, Indianapolis, IN 46202-5112; **Phone:** 317-274-7150; **Board Cert:** Thoracic Surgery 2007; **Med School:** Indiana Univ 1970; **Resid:** Surgery, Univ Mich Med Ctr 1976; Cardiothoracic Surgery, Univ Mich Med Ctr 1978; **Fellow:** Cardiovascular Surgery, Natl Heart Lung-Blood Inst 1974; **Fac Appt:** Prof S, Indiana Univ

Damiano Jr, Ralph J MD [TS] - **Spec Exp:** Minimally Invasive Cardiac Surgery; Robotic Cardiac Surgery; Endoscopic Coronary Bypass Surgery; **Hospital:** Barnes-Jewish Hosp; **Address:** 660 S Euclid Ave, Campus Box 8234, St Louis, MO 63110; **Phone:** 314-362-7327; **Board Cert:** Thoracic Surgery 2002; **Med School:** Duke Univ 1980; **Resid:** Surgery, Duke Univ Med Ctr 1988; **Fellow:** Cardiothoracic Surgery, Duke Univ Med Ctr 1989; **Fac Appt:** Prof S, Washington Univ, St Louis

Deschamps, Claude MD [TS] - **Spec Exp:** Gastroesophageal Reflux Disease (GERD); Esophageal Cancer; Lung Cancer; **Hospital:** St Mary's Hosp - Rochester; **Address:** Mayo Clinic, Div Thoracic Surgery, 200 First St SW, Rochester, MN 55905; **Phone:** 507-284-8462; **Board Cert:** Surgery 2004; **Med School:** Univ Montreal 1979; **Resid:** Surgery, Univ Montreal Hosps 1984; Thoracic Surgery, Univ Montreal Hosps 1985; **Fellow:** Thoracic Surgery, Mayo Clinic 1987; **Fac Appt:** Prof S, Mayo Med Sch

Durham, Samuel J MD [TS] - **Spec Exp:** Cardiothoracic Surgery; **Hospital:** Univ of Toledo Med Ctr; **Address:** Univ of Toledo Med Ctr, Dowling Hall, 3065 Arlington Ave, Ste 2261, Toledo, OH 43614; **Phone:** 419-383-5150; **Board Cert:** Surgery 2001; Thoracic Surgery 2003; **Med School:** Harvard Med Sch 1983; **Resid:** Surgery, Univ Pittsburgh Med Ctr 1987; Thoracic Surgery, Univ Pittsburgh Med Ctr 1988; **Fellow:** Pediatric Surgery, Chlidren's Hosp 1993; **Fac Appt:** Prof S, Ohio State Univ

Ferguson, Mark K MD [TS] - **Spec Exp:** Barrett's Esophagus; Esophageal Cancer; Lung Cancer; **Hospital:** Univ of Chicago Med Ctr; **Address:** 5841 S Maryland Ave, MC 5035, Univ Chicago Hosps, Chicago, IL 60637-1470; **Phone:** 773-702-3551; **Board Cert:** Thoracic Surgery 2003; **Med School:** Univ Chicago-Pritzker Sch Med 1977; **Resid:** Surgery, Univ Chicago Hosps 1982; **Fellow:** Cardiothoracic Surgery, Univ Chicago Hosps 1984; **Fac Appt:** Prof S, Univ Chicago-Pritzker Sch Med

Howington, John A MD [TS] - **Spec Exp:** Lung Cancer; Esophageal Cancer; Thymoma; Minimally Invasive Thoracic Surgery; **Hospital:** NorthShore Univ HlthSys, Highland Park/North Shore Univ Hlth Syst; **Address:** Evanston Northwestern Hosp, 2650 Ridge Ave, Walgreen Bldg - Ste 3507, Evanston, IL 60201; **Phone:** 847-570-2868; **Board Cert:** Thoracic Surgery 2006; Surgery 2004; **Med School:** Univ Tenn Coll Med, Memphis 1989; **Resid:** Surgery, Truman Med Ctr/U Missouri 1994; Cardiothoracic Surgery, Vanderbilt Univ Med Ctr 1997; **Fac Appt:** Assoc Prof S, Northwestern Univ

Huddleston, Charles B MD [TS] - **Spec Exp:** Transplant-Lung-Pediatric; Transplant-Heart-Pediatric; **Hospital:** St Louis Chldns Hosp, Barnes-Jewish Hosp; **Address:** St Louis Children's Hospital, One Children's Pl, Ste 5 South 50, St Louis, MO 63110; **Phone:** 314-454-6165; **Board Cert:** Thoracic Surgery 2007; **Med School:** Vanderbilt Univ 1978; **Resid:** Surgery, Vanderbilt Univ Hosp 1986; Cardiothoracic Surgery, Vanderbilt Univ Hosp 1988; **Fellow:** Pediatric Cardiothoracic Surgery, Hosp for Sick Chldn 1989; **Fac Appt:** Prof S, Washington Univ, St Louis

Iannettoni, Mark D MD [TS] - **Spec Exp:** Transplant-Lung; Lung Cancer; Esophageal Surgery; **Hospital:** Univ Iowa Hosp & Clinics; **Address:** Univ Iowa Hosp & Clinics, 200 Hawkins Drive, rm SE514GH, Iowa City, IA 52242; **Phone:** 319-356-1133; **Board Cert:** Surgery 2002; Thoracic Surgery 2002; **Med School:** SUNY Upstate Med Univ 1985; **Resid:** Surgery, SUNY Upstate Med Ctr 1991; Thoracic Surgery, Univ Mich Med Ctr 1993; **Fellow:** Thoracic Surgery, Univ Mich Med Sch 1994

Jeevanandam, Valluvan MD [TS] - **Spec Exp:** Minimally Invasive Heart Valve Surgery; Transplant-Heart; Artificial Heart Devices; **Hospital:** Univ of Chicago Med Ctr; **Address:** 5841 S Maryland Ave, MC 5040, Chicago, IL 60637-1483; **Phone:** 773-702-2500; **Board Cert:** Thoracic Surgery 2002; **Med School:** Columbia P&S 1984; **Resid:** Surgery, Columbia-Presby Med Ctr 1989; **Fellow:** Cardiothoracic Surgery, Columbia-Presby Med Ctr 1991; **Fac Appt:** Prof S, Univ Chicago-Pritzker Sch Med

Thoracic Surgery

Little, Alex G MD [TS] - **Hospital:** Wright State Univ, Miami Valley Hosp; **Address:** 30 E Apple St, Ste 5253, Dayton, OH 45409; **Phone:** 937-208-2552; **Board Cert:** Surgery 1998; Thoracic Surgery 2000; **Med School:** Johns Hopkins Univ 1974; **Resid:** Surgery, Univ Chicago Hosp 1979; Thoracic Surgery, Univ Chicago Hosp 1981; **Fellow:** Research, Univ Chicago Hosp 1977; **Fac Appt:** Prof TS, Wright State Univ

Love, Robert B MD [TS] - **Spec Exp:** Transplant-Heart & Lung; Lung Cancer; Esophageal Cancer; Heart Valve Surgery; **Hospital:** Loyola Univ Med Ctr; **Address:** Loyola Univ Med Ctr, 2160 S First Ave Bldg 110 - rm 6243, Maywood, IL 60153; **Phone:** 708-327-2488; **Board Cert:** Surgery 2007; Thoracic Surgery 2000; Surgical Critical Care 2001; **Med School:** Rush Med Coll 1982; **Resid:** Surgery, Univ of Wisconsin Hosp 1988; Thoracic Surgery, Gloucestershire Royal Hosp 1989; **Fellow:** Cardiothoracic Surgery, Univ of Wisconsin Hosp 1991; **Fac Appt:** Prof TS, Loyola Univ-Stritch Sch Med

Lytle, Bruce W MD [TS] - **Spec Exp:** Heart Valve Surgery; Coronary Artery Surgery; Aortic Surgery; **Hospital:** Cleveland Clin Fdn (page 56); **Address:** Cleveland Clinic, Dept Thoracic Surgery, 9500 Euclid Ave, J1-227, Cleveland, OH 44195; **Phone:** 216-444-6962; **Board Cert:** Thoracic Surgery 2007; **Med School:** Harvard Med Sch 1971; **Resid:** Surgery, Mass Genl Hsop 1975; Surgery, Shotley Bridge Hosp 1976; **Fellow:** Thoracic Surgery, Mass Genl Hosp 1979; **Fac Appt:** Prof TS, Cleveland Cl Coll Med/Case West Res

Maddaus, Michael A MD [TS] - **Spec Exp:** Esophageal Cancer; Lung Cancer; Minimally Invasive Thoracic Surgery; **Hospital:** Univ Minn Med Ctr, Fairview - Univ Campus, Abbott - Northwestern Hosp; **Address:** Div General Thoracic Surgery, 420 Delaware St SE, MMC 207, Minneapolis, MN 55455; **Phone:** 612-624-9461; **Board Cert:** Surgery 2000; Thoracic Surgery 2003; **Med School:** Univ Minn 1982; **Resid:** Surgery, Univ Minn Affil Hosp 1990; Thoracic Surgery, Univ Toronto Affil Hosp 1991; **Fellow:** Cardiac Surgery, St Michael's Hosp/Hosp Sick Chldn 1992; Thoracic Oncology, Meml Sloan Kettering Cancer Ctr 1992; **Fac Appt:** Prof S, Univ Minn

McCarthy, Patrick M MD [TS] - **Spec Exp:** Heart Valve Surgery; Coronary Artery Surgery; Ventricular Assist Device (LVAD); **Hospital:** Northwestern Meml Hosp; **Address:** Bluhm Cardiovascular Inst, 675 N St Clair St, Galter 19-100, Chicago, IL 60611-2968; **Phone:** 312-695-6984; **Board Cert:** Thoracic Surgery 1998; **Med School:** Loyola Univ-Stritch Sch Med 1980; **Resid:** Surgery, Mayo Clinic 1985; Thoracic Surgery, Mayo Clinic 1988; **Fellow:** Cardiopulmonary Transplant Surgery, Stanford Univ 1989; **Fac Appt:** Prof S, Northwestern Univ

Merrill, Walter H MD [TS] - **Spec Exp:** Cardiothoracic Surgery; Cardiac Surgery-Adult & Pediatric; Transplant-Heart; **Hospital:** Univ Hosp - Cincinnati, VA Med Ctr; **Address:** Univ Cincinnati, Sect Cardiothoracic Surg, 231 Albert Sabin Way, ML 0558, Cincinnati, OH 45267-0001; **Phone:** 513-584-3278; **Board Cert:** Surgery 2000; Thoracic Surgery 2001; Surgical Critical Care 1999; **Med School:** Johns Hopkins Univ 1974; **Resid:** Thoracic Surgery, Natl Inst Hlth 1978; Thoracic Surgery, Johns Hopkins Hosp 1982; **Fellow:** Pediatric Surgery, Hosp for Sick Chldn 1983; **Fac Appt:** Prof S, Univ Cincinnati

Meyers, Bryan MD [TS] - **Spec Exp:** Lung Cancer; Esophageal Cancer; Transplant-Lung; Emphysema-Lung Volume Reduction; **Hospital:** Barnes-Jewish Hosp, Barnes-Jewish West County Hosp; **Address:** 4921 Parkview Pl, Ste 8B, St Louis, MO 63110; **Phone:** 314-362-8598; **Board Cert:** Surgery 1998; Thoracic Surgery 1999; **Med School:** Univ Chicago-Pritzker Sch Med 1986; **Resid:** Surgery, Mass Genl Hosp 1996; **Fellow:** Cardiothoracic Surgery, Barnes Hosp-Wash Univ 1998; **Fac Appt:** Assoc Prof S, Washington Univ, St Louis

Naunheim, Keith S MD [TS] - **Spec Exp:** Lung Cancer; Esophageal Cancer; Chest Wall Tumors; Video Assisted Thoracic Surgery (VATS); **Hospital:** St Louis Univ Hosp, SSM St Mary's Hlth Ctr - St Louis; **Address:** St Louis Univ Med Ctr, Dept Surgery, 3635 Vista Ave, St Louis, MO 63110-0250; **Phone:** 314-577-8360; **Board Cert:** Thoracic Surgery 2004; **Med School:** Univ Chicago-Pritzker Sch Med 1978; **Resid:** Surgery, Univ Chicago Hosp 1983; **Fellow:** Cardiothoracic Surgery, Univ Chicago Hosp 1985; **Fac Appt:** Prof S, St Louis Univ

Orringer, Mark B MD [TS] - **Spec Exp:** Esophageal Cancer; Lung Cancer; Mediastinal Tumors; Lung Cancer; **Hospital:** Univ Michigan Hlth Sys; **Address:** Univ Mich, Taubman Ctr, 1500 E Med Ctr Drive, rm TC 2120, Box 0344, Ann Arbor, MI 48109-0344; **Phone:** 734-936-4975; **Board Cert:** Surgery 1973; Thoracic Surgery 1974; **Med School:** Univ Pittsburgh 1967; **Resid:** Thoracic Surgery, Johns Hopkins Hosp 1973; **Fac Appt:** Prof S, Univ Mich Med Sch

Pagani, Francis D MD/PhD [TS] - **Spec Exp:** Transplant-Heart; Coronary Artery Surgery; Left Ventricular Assist Device (LVAD); **Hospital:** Univ Michigan Hlth Sys; **Address:** Univ Mich Med Ctr, 5144 Cardiovascular Ctr, 1500 E Med Ctr Drive, SPC 5864, Ann Arbor, MI 48109-5864; **Phone:** 734-647-2894; **Board Cert:** Surgery 2002; Thoracic Surgery 2004; **Med School:** Georgetown Univ 1986; **Resid:** Surgery, Georgetown Univ Med Ctr 1993; Thoracic Surgery, Univ Mich Hosp 1995; **Fellow:** Research, Univ Mass Med Ctr 1990; **Fac Appt:** Prof S, Univ Mich Med Sch

Patterson, G Alexander MD [TS] - **Spec Exp:** Lung Cancer; Esophageal Cancer; Transplant-Lung; Transplant-Heart & Lung; **Hospital:** Barnes-Jewish Hosp; **Address:** 660 S Euclid Ave, Box 8234, St Louis, MO 63110; **Phone:** 314-362-6025; **Board Cert:** Surgery 1978; Thoracic Surgery 1981; Vascular Surgery 1982; **Med School:** Canada 1974; **Resid:** Surgery, Queens Univ Med Ctr 1978; Vascular Surgery, Univ Toronto Med Ctr 1979; **Fellow:** Research, Toronto Genl Hosp 1981; Surgical Critical Care, Johns Hopkins Hosp 1982; **Fac Appt:** Prof S, Washington Univ, St Louis

Raman, Jai MD/PhD [TS] - **Spec Exp:** Robotic Cardiac Surgery; Heart Failure & Ventricular Containment; Transplant-Heart; Atrial Fibrillation; **Hospital:** Univ of Chicago Med Ctr; **Address:** 5841 S Maryland Ave, MC 5040, Chicago, IL 60637; **Phone:** 773-702-2500; **Med School:** India 1990; **Resid:** Cardiothoracic Surgery, St Vincent's Hosp 1991; Cardiothoracic Surgery, Austin Hospital 1995; **Fellow:** Thoracic Surgery, Austin Hosp 1994; Pediatric Cardiac Surgery, Royal Children's Hosp 1996; **Fac Appt:** Assoc Prof S, Univ Chicago-Pritzker Sch Med

Rice, Thomas W MD [TS] - **Spec Exp:** Esophageal Surgery; Minimally Invasive Thoracic Surgery; Lung Cancer; **Hospital:** Cleveland Clin Fdn (page 56); **Address:** Cleveland Clinic, 9500 Euclid Ave, Desk J4-1, Cleveland, OH 44195; **Phone:** 216-444-1921; **Board Cert:** Surgery 2004; Thoracic Surgery 2005; **Med School:** Univ Toronto 1978; **Resid:** Surgery, Univ Toronto Med Ctr 1983; Thoracic Surgery, Univ Toronto Med Ctr 1986; **Fellow:** Pulmonary Disease, UCSF Med Ctr 1984; **Fac Appt:** Prof S, Cleveland Cl Coll Med/Case West Res

Schaff, Hartzell MD [TS] - **Spec Exp:** Heart Valve Surgery; Congenital Heart Disease; Maze Procedure for Atrial Fibrillation; **Hospital:** St Mary's Hosp - Rochester; **Address:** Mayo Clin, Div Cardiovasc Surg, 200 First St SW, Rochester, MN 55905-0001; **Phone:** 507-255-7068; **Board Cert:** Thoracic Surgery 2000; **Med School:** Univ Okla Coll Med 1973; **Resid:** Surgery, Johns Hopkins Hosp 1978; Thoracic Surgery, Johns Hopkins Hosp 1980; **Fellow:** Surgery, Johns Hopkins Hosp 1976; **Fac Appt:** Prof S, Mayo Med Sch

Smedira, Nicholas MD [TS] - **Spec Exp:** Transplant-Heart; Transplant-Lung; Ventricular Assist Device (LVAD); Aortic Surgery; **Hospital:** Cleveland Clin Fdn (page 56); **Address:** Cleveland Clin, Dept Cardiothoracic Surg, 9500 Euclid Ave, Desk J4-1, Cleveland, OH 44195; **Phone:** 216-445-7052; **Board Cert:** Thoracic Surgery 2003; **Med School:** Univ Rochester 1984; **Resid:** Surgery, UCSF Med Ctr 1991; Thoracic Surgery, UCSF Med Ctr 1994; **Fellow:** Cardiothoracic Surgery, UCSF Med Ctr 1994

Smith, John Michael MD [TS] - **Spec Exp:** Mitral Valve Robotic Surgery; **Hospital:** Good Samaritan Hosp - Cincinnati; **Address:** 4030 Smith Rd, Ste 300, Cincinnati, OH 45209; **Phone:** 513-421-3494; **Board Cert:** Surgery 2003; Thoracic Surgery 2006; **Med School:** Univ Louisville Sch Med 1989; **Resid:** Surgery, Good Samaritan Hosp 1994; **Fellow:** Cardiothoracic Surgery, Yale Univ Hosp 1996

Stuart, Richard MD [TS] - **Spec Exp:** Cardiac Surgery; Thoracic Surgery; Robotic Cardiac Surgery; **Hospital:** St Luke's Hosp of Kansas City, N Kansas City Hosp; **Address:** 4320 Wornall Rd Bldg 2 - Ste 50, Kansas City, MO 64111; **Phone:** 816-931-3312; **Board Cert:** Thoracic Surgery 1999; Surgical Critical Care 2003; **Med School:** Johns Hopkins Univ 1981; **Resid:** Surgery, Johns Hopkins Hosp 1986; **Fellow:** Cardiothoracic Surgery, Johns Hopkins Hosp 1989; **Fac Appt:** Clin Prof TS, Univ MO-Kansas City

Sundt III, Thoralf MD [TS] - **Spec Exp:** Heart Valve Surgery; Aneurysm-Thoracic Aortic; Pulmonary Embolism; Coronary Artery Surgery; **Hospital:** Mayo Med Ctr & Clin - Rochester, St Mary's Hosp - Rochester; **Address:** Mayo Clinic, 200 First St SW, Rochester, MN 55905-0002; **Phone:** 507-255-7064; **Board Cert:** Surgery 2000; Thoracic Surgery 2004; **Med School:** Johns Hopkins Univ 1984; **Resid:** Surgery, Mass Genl Hosp 1991; Cardiothoracic Surgery, Wash Univ Sch Med 1993; **Fellow:** Cardiothoracic Surgery, Harefield Hosp 1994; **Fac Appt:** Prof S, Mayo Med Sch

Svensson, Lars G MD/PhD [TS] - **Spec Exp:** Aortic Surgery; Heart Valve Surgery; Heart Valve-Percutaneous; Marfan's Syndrome; **Hospital:** Cleveland Clin Fdn (page 56); **Address:** Cleveland Clinic, Main Campus, 9500 Euclid Ave, MC J4-1, Cleveland, OH 44195; **Phone:** 216-445-4813; **Med School:** South Africa 1978; **Resid:** Cardiothoracic Surgery, Johannesburg Hosp; **Fellow:** Cardiothoracic Surgery, Cleveland Clinic; **Fac Appt:** Prof S, Case West Res Univ

Turrentine, Mark W MD [TS] - **Spec Exp:** Cardiac Surgery-Pediatric; Transplant-Heart; Transplant-Lung; Congenital Heart Disease; **Hospital:** Riley Hosp for Children, Methodist Hosp - Indianapolis; **Address:** 545 Barnhill Dr, Emerson Hall, Ste 215, Indianapolis, IN 46202; **Phone:** 317-274-1121; **Board Cert:** Thoracic Surgery 2002; **Med School:** Univ Kans 1983; **Resid:** Surgery, Univ Kansas Med Ctr 1988; Cardiothoracic Surgery, Indiana Univ Med Ctr 1991; **Fellow:** Cardiothoracic Surgery, Texas Heart Inst 1986; Transplant Surgery, Indiana Univ Med Ctr 1989; **Fac Appt:** Prof S, Indiana Univ

Ungerleider, Ross M MD [TS] - **Spec Exp:** Congenital Heart Disease; Cardiac Surgery; Pediatric Cardiac Surgery; **Hospital:** Rainbow Babies & Chldns Hosp; **Address:** 11100 Euclid Ave, MS RBC6021, Cleveland, OH 44106; **Phone:** 216-844-3058; **Board Cert:** Thoracic Surgery 2007; **Med School:** Rush Med Coll 1977; **Resid:** Surgery, Duke Univ Med Ctr 1987; **Fellow:** Cardiothoracic Surgery, Duke Univ Med Ctr 1989; Pediatric Cardiac Surgery, UCSF Med Ctr; **Fac Appt:** Prof S, Oregon Hlth & Sci Univ

Vigneswaran, Wickii MD [TS] - **Spec Exp:** Transplant-Heart & Lung; Lung Cancer; Mesothelioma; Hyperhidrosis-Palmar; **Hospital:** Univ of Chicago Med Ctr; **Address:** Univ Chicago Hospitals, Lung Transplant Div, 5841 S Maryland Ave, MC 5040, Chicago, IL 60637; **Phone:** 773-795-1267; **Med School:** Sri Lanka 1978; **Resid:** Surgery, Royal College of Surgeons 1983; Cardiothoracic Surgery, Royal College of Surgeons 1990; **Fellow:** Cardiothoracic Transplant Surg, Mayo Clinic 1994; **Fac Appt:** Prof S, Univ Chicago-Pritzker Sch Med

Great Plains and Mountains

Bull, David A MD [TS] - **Spec Exp:** Cardiothoracic Surgery; Esophageal Cancer; **Hospital:** Univ Utah Hosps and Clins; **Address:** Univ Utah, Dept Cardiothoracic Surgery, 30 N 1900 East, rm 3C127, Salt Lake City, UT 84132; **Phone:** 801-581-5311; **Board Cert:** Thoracic Surgery 2004; Vascular Surgery 2003; Surgery 1999; Surgical Critical Care 1999; **Med School:** UCSF 1985; **Resid:** Surgery, UCSF Medical Ctr 1987; Surgery, Univ Arizona Hosps 1990; **Fellow:** Vascular Surgery, Univ Arizona Hosps 1992; Cardiothoracic Surgery, Univ Arizona Hosps 1994; **Fac Appt:** Assoc Prof TS, Univ Utah

Campbell, David N MD [TS] - **Spec Exp:** Pediatric Cardiothoracic Surgery; Transplant-Heart-Pediatric; Transplant-Lung; Congenital Heart Surgery; **Hospital:** Chldn's Hosp - Aurora, The, Univ Colorado Hosp; **Address:** 13123 E 16th Ave, Ste B-200, Denver, CO 80218; **Phone:** 720-777-6624; **Board Cert:** Surgery 1999; Thoracic Surgery 2000; Surgical Critical Care 2000; **Med School:** Rush Med Coll 1974; **Resid:** Surgery, Univ Colo Med Ctr 1980; Cardiothoracic Surgery, Univ Colo Med Ctr 1979; **Fellow:** Cardiovascular Surgery, Boston Chldns Hosp 1980; **Fac Appt:** Prof S, Univ Colorado

Fullerton, David A MD [TS] - **Spec Exp:** Maze Procedure for Atrial Fibrillation; Ross Procedure for Aortic Valve Disease; Mitral Valve Surgery; Transplant-Heart & Lung; **Hospital:** Univ Colorado Hosp, VA Med Ctr; **Address:** Univ of Colorado, Cardiothoracic Surgery, 12631 E 17th Ave, L15, rm 6602, MS C310, PO Box 6511, Aurora, CO 80045; **Phone:** 303-724-2798; **Board Cert:** Surgery 2007; Surgical Critical Care 2001; Thoracic Surgery 2001; **Med School:** Univ MO-Columbia Sch Med 1981; **Resid:** Surgery, Univ Wash Med Ctr 1987; Thoracic Surgery, Univ Colorado Hosp 1990; **Fac Appt:** Prof S, Univ Colorado

Karwande, Shreekanth V MD [TS] - **Spec Exp:** Thoracic Cancers; Lung Cancer; Cardiac Surgery; **Hospital:** St Mark's Hosp - Salt Lake City; **Address:** St Mark's Hosp, 1160 E 3900 St, Ste 3500, Salt Lake City, UT 84124; **Phone:** 801-743-4750; **Board Cert:** Thoracic Surgery 2003; **Med School:** India 1973; **Resid:** Surgery, Erie Co Med Ctr 1981; Cardiothoracic Surgery, NY Hosp 1985; **Fellow:** Cardiothoracic Surgery, Meml Sloan Kettering Cancer Ctr

Mitchell, John D MD [TS] - **Spec Exp:** Lung Cancer; Esophageal Surgery; Transplant-Lung; Hyperhidrosis-Palmar; **Hospital:** Univ Colorado Hosp, VA Med Ctr; **Address:** Univ CO Hosp, Dept Cardiothoracic Surgery, 4200 E Ninth Ave, Ste C 310, Denver, CO 80262; **Phone:** 303-724-2800; **Board Cert:** Surgery 2005; Thoracic Surgery 2007; **Med School:** Univ Mich Med Sch 1987; **Resid:** Surgery, Mass Genl Hosp 1994; Cardiothoracic Surgery, Mass Genl Hosp 1996; **Fac Appt:** Assoc Prof TS, Univ Colorado

Mitchell, Max B MD [TS] - **Spec Exp:** Congenital Heart Surgery; Heart Valve Surgery; Pediatric Cardiac Surgery; Transplant-Lung; **Hospital:** Chldn's Hosp - Aurora, The, Univ Colorado Hosp; **Address:** 13123 E 16th Ave, Ste B200, Denver, CO 80045; **Phone:** 720-777-6624; **Board Cert:** Surgery 2004; Thoracic Surgery 1999; **Med School:** Geo Wash Univ 1988; **Resid:** Surgery, Univ Colorado Hlth Sci Ctr 1995; Cardiovascular Surgery, Univ Colorado Hlth Sci Ctr 1998; **Fellow:** Pediatric Cardiac Surgery, Royal Childrens Hosp 1999; **Fac Appt:** Assoc Prof S, Univ Colorado

Southwest

Aklog, Lishan MD [TS] - **Spec Exp:** Mitral Valve Surgery; Minimally Invasive Cardiac Surgery; Coronary Artery Surgery; Heart Failure; **Hospital:** St Joseph's Hosp & Med Ctr - Phoenix; **Address:** Heart and Lung Inst, St Joseph's Hosp Med Ctr, 500 W Thomas Rd, Ste 500, Phoenix, AZ 85013-4224; **Phone:** 602-406-4000; **Board Cert:** Thoracic Surgery 2000; **Med School:** Harvard Med Sch 1989; **Resid:** Surgery, Brigham & Women's Hosp 1996; **Fellow:** Cardiothoracic Surgery, Brigham & Women's Hosp 1998; Cardiac Surgery, Harefield Hosp 1999

Thoracic Surgery

Calhoon, John H MD [TS] - **Spec Exp:** Transplant-Heart & Lung; Congenital Heart Surgery; Cardiac Surgery-Adult & Pediatric; **Hospital:** Univ Hlth Syst-San Antonio, Christus Santa Rosa Children's Hosp; **Address:** UTHSCSA, Dept Thoracic Surg, 7703 Floyd Curl Drive, MC 7841, San Antonio, TX 78229-3901; **Phone:** 210-567-6863; **Board Cert:** Surgery 2004; Thoracic Surgery 2007; **Med School:** Baylor Coll Med 1981; **Resid:** Surgery, Univ Hosp/Univ Texas HSC 1986; Univ Hosp/Univ Texas HSC 1988; **Fellow:** Pediatric Cardiac Surgery, Chldns Hosp/Harvard 1989; **Fac Appt:** Prof TS, Univ Tex, San Antonio

Copeland III, Jack G MD [TS] - **Spec Exp:** Transplant-Heart; Transplant-Heart & Lung; Artificial Heart Devices; **Hospital:** Univ Med Ctr - Tucson, VA Medical Center - Tucson; **Address:** Univ Ariz Hlth Sci Ctr, 1501 N Campbell Ave, rm 4402, Box 245071, Tucson, AZ 85724-5071; **Phone:** 520-626-6339; **Board Cert:** Thoracic Surgery 1997; **Med School:** Stanford Univ 1969; **Resid:** Surgery, UCSD Med Ctr 1971; Cardiovascular Surgery, Natl Inst Hlth 1973; **Fellow:** Cardiothoracic Surgery, Stanford Univ 1977; **Fac Appt:** Prof TS, Univ Ariz Coll Med

Coselli, Joseph S MD [TS] - **Spec Exp:** Aneurysm-Abdominal & Thoracic Aortic; Marfan's Syndrome; Aortic Surgery; **Hospital:** St Luke's Episcopal Hosp-Houston; **Address:** 6770 Bertner St, Ste C350, Houston, TX 77030; **Phone:** 832-355-9910; **Board Cert:** Thoracic Surgery 2004; **Med School:** Univ Tex Med Br, Galveston 1977; **Resid:** Surgery, Baylor Coll Med 1982; Thoracic Surgery, Baylor Coll Med 1984; **Fac Appt:** Assoc Prof S, Baylor Coll Med

Diethrich, Edward B MD [TS] - **Spec Exp:** Vascular Surgery; Endovascular Surgery; Cardiovascular Surgery; **Hospital:** Arizona Heart Hosp; **Address:** Arizona Heart Inst, 2632 N 20th St, Phoenix, AZ 85006-1339; **Phone:** 602-266-2200; **Board Cert:** Thoracic Surgery 1967; Surgery 1966; **Med School:** Univ Mich Med Sch 1960; **Resid:** Surgery, St Joseph Mercy Hosp 1964; **Fellow:** Cardiothoracic Surgery, Baylor Coll Med 1966; **Fac Appt:** Prof TS, Univ Ariz Coll Med

Echeverri, Luis G MD [TS] - **Spec Exp:** Cardiac Surgery; Aortic Surgery; Transplant-Heart; **Hospital:** St Luke's Episcopal Hosp-Houston; **Address:** 7737 SW Freeway, Ste 201, Houston, TX 77074; **Phone:** 713-776-3402; **Board Cert:** Surgery 2007; Thoracic Surgery 2002; **Med School:** Colombia 1982; **Resid:** Surgery, Univ Texas Med Ctr 1996; Cardiothoracic Surgery, Univ Arizona 2001; **Fellow:** Transplant Surgery, Univ Pittsburgh 1993; Cardiovascular Surgery, Texas Heart Inst 1998

Forbess, Joseph M MD [TS] - **Spec Exp:** Pediatric Cardiothoracic Surgery; Heart Valve Surgery-Pediatric; **Hospital:** Chldns Med Ctr of Dallas, UT Southwestern Med Ctr at Dallas; **Address:** Univ Texas SW Med Ctr, Div Ped Cardiothor Surg, 1935 Medical District Drive, Ste C-3211, Dallas, TX 75235; **Phone:** 214-456-5000; **Board Cert:** Surgery 2000; Thoracic Surgery 1998; **Med School:** Harvard Med Sch 1990; **Resid:** Surgery, Duke Univ Med Ctr 1997; Cardiothoracic Surgery, Duke Univ Med Ctr 1999; **Fellow:** Cardiac Surgery, Childrens Hosp 1994; **Fac Appt:** Assoc Prof TS, Univ Tex SW, Dallas

Fraser, Charles D MD [TS] - **Spec Exp:** Pediatric Cardiothoracic Surgery; Congenital Heart Surgery; **Hospital:** Texas Chldns Hosp; **Address:** Texas Chldns Hosp-Heart Ctr, 6621 Fannin St, MC 19-345H, Houston, TX 77030-2399; **Phone:** 832-826-2030; **Board Cert:** Surgery 2000; Thoracic Surgery 2002; **Med School:** Univ Tex Med Br, Galveston 1984; **Resid:** Surgery, Johns Hopkins Hosp 1990; Cardiovascular Surgery, Johns Hopkins Hosp 1993; **Fac Appt:** Prof S, Baylor Coll Med

Frazier, Oscar Howard MD [TS] - **Spec Exp:** Transplant-Heart; Lung Surgery; Artificial Heart Devices; **Hospital:** St Luke's Episcopal Hosp-Houston; **Address:** Surgical Assocs - Texas Heart Institute, PO Box 20345, MC 2-114A, Houston, TX 77030; **Phone:** 832-355-4900; **Board Cert:** Surgery 1975; Thoracic Surgery 2005; **Med School:** Baylor Coll Med 1967; **Resid:** Surgery, Baylor Affil Hosp 1974; Thoracic Surgery, Texas Heart Inst 1976; **Fac Appt:** Prof S, Univ Tex, Houston

Harrell Jr, James E MD [TS] - **Spec Exp:** Transplant-Heart; Cardiac Surgery-Pediatric; **Hospital:** Covenant Children's Hosp; **Address:** 3606 21st St, Ste 103, Lubbock, TX 79410; **Phone:** 806-725-4425; **Board Cert:** Surgery 2006; Thoracic Surgery 2006; **Med School:** Baylor Coll Med 1978; **Resid:** Surgery, Univ Tex Hlth Scis Ctr 1984; Thoracic Surgery, Baylor Coll Med 1986; **Fellow:** Cardiovascular Surgery, Hosp Sick Chldn 1987

Lanza, Louis MD [TS] - **Spec Exp:** Lung Cancer; Cardiac Surgery; **Hospital:** Mayo Clinic - Scottsdale; **Address:** Mayo Clinic Hosp, 5779 E Mayo Blvd MCSB Bldg Fl 1, Phoenix, AZ 85054; **Phone:** 480-342-2270; **Board Cert:** Thoracic Surgery 2002; **Med School:** Loyola Univ-Stritch Sch Med 1981; **Resid:** Surgery, Univ Michigan Med Ctr 1988; Cardiovascular Surgery, Texas Heart Inst 1991; **Fellow:** Surgical Oncology, Natl Cancer Inst 1986; Thoracic Oncology, MD Anderson Cancer Ctr 1989

Ott, David A MD [TS] - **Spec Exp:** Heart Valve Surgery; Coronary Artery Surgery; Aneurysm-Abdominal Aortic; **Hospital:** St Luke's Episcopal Hosp-Houston; **Address:** 1101 Bates St, Ste P-514, Houston, TX 77030-2607; **Phone:** 832-355-4900; **Board Cert:** Thoracic Surgery 1997; **Med School:** Baylor Coll Med 1972; **Resid:** Surgery, Baylor Coll Med 1976; Cardiothoracic Surgery, Tex Heart Inst 1978; **Fac Appt:** Clin Prof S, Baylor Coll Med

Reardon, Michael J MD [TS] - **Spec Exp:** Cardiac Tumors/Cancer; Heart Valve Surgery-Aortic; **Hospital:** Methodist Hosp - Houston, UT MD Anderson Cancer Ctr; **Address:** 6560 Fannin St, Ste 1401, Houston, TX 77030; **Phone:** 713-441-5200; **Board Cert:** Thoracic Surgery 2006; **Med School:** Baylor Coll Med 1978; **Resid:** Surgery, Baylor Affil Hosps 1983; Thoracic Surgery, Texas Heart Inst 1985; **Fac Appt:** Clin Prof S, Baylor Coll Med

Ring, W Steves MD [TS] - **Spec Exp:** Cardiac Surgery-Adult & Pediatric; Transplant-Heart & Lung; Congenital Heart Surgery; Coronary Revascularization; **Hospital:** UT Southwestern Med Ctr at Dallas, Chldns Med Ctr of Dallas; **Address:** 5323 Harry Hines Blvd, MC 8879, Dallas, TX 75390-8879; **Phone:** 214-645-7706; **Board Cert:** Surgery 1999; Thoracic Surgery 2004; **Med School:** Harvard Med Sch 1971; **Resid:** Surgery, Duke Univ Med Ctr 1977; Surgery, Univ Minn Hosps 1980; **Fellow:** Thoracic Surgery, Univ Minn Hosps 1982; **Fac Appt:** Prof TS, Univ Tex SW, Dallas

Roth, Jack MD [TS] - **Spec Exp:** Esophageal Cancer; Lung Cancer; Gene Therapy; **Hospital:** UT MD Anderson Cancer Ctr; **Address:** Dept Thoracic & Cardiovasc Surg Unit 445, 1515 Holcombe Blvd, Houston, TX 77030-4000; **Phone:** 713-792-7664; **Board Cert:** Thoracic Surgery 2002; **Med School:** Johns Hopkins Univ 1971; **Resid:** Surgery, Johns Hopkins Hosp 1973; Thoracic Surgery, UCLA Ctr Hlth Sci 1979; **Fellow:** Surgical Oncology, UCLA 1975; **Fac Appt:** Prof TS, Univ Tex, Houston

Safi, Hazim J MD [TS] - **Spec Exp:** Aneurysm-Abdominal Aortic; **Hospital:** Meml Hermann Hosp - Texas Med Ctr; **Address:** UT, Dept Cardiothoracic & Vascular Surg, 6400 Fannin St, Ste 2850, Houston, TX 77030; **Phone:** 713-500-5304; **Board Cert:** Thoracic Surgery 2007; Vascular Surgery 2005; **Med School:** Iraq 1970; **Resid:** Surgery, Baylor Coll Med 1980; Radiation Oncology, Baylor Coll Med 1981; **Fellow:** Thoracic Surgery, Baylor Coll Med 1983; **Fac Appt:** Assoc Prof S, Univ Tex, Houston

Smythe, W Roy MD [TS] - **Spec Exp:** Lung Cancer; Mesothelioma; **Hospital:** Scott & White Mem Hosp; **Address:** 2401 S 31st St, Temple, TX 76508; **Phone:** 254-724-2334; **Board Cert:** Surgery 1998; Thoracic Surgery 2000; **Med School:** Texas A&M Univ 1989; **Resid:** Surgery, Hosp Univ Penn 1996; **Fellow:** Cardiothoracic Surgery, Hosp Univ Penn 1998; Surgical Oncology, Am Cancer Soc 1996; **Fac Appt:** Asst Prof S, Univ Tex, Houston

Thoracic Surgery

Swisher, Stephen G MD [TS] - **Spec Exp:** Esophageal Cancer; Lung Cancer; Mesothelioma; Thoracic Cancers; **Hospital:** UT MD Anderson Cancer Ctr; **Address:** Dept of Thoracic & Cardiovasc Surg, 1515 Holcombe Blvd, Unit 445, Houston, TX 77030; **Phone:** 713-792-8659; **Board Cert:** Surgery 2002; Thoracic Surgery 2006; **Med School:** UCSD 1986; **Resid:** Surgery, UCLA Med Ctr 1993; **Fellow:** Surgical Oncology, UCLA Med Ctr 1990; Cardiothoracic Surgery, MD Anderson Canc Ctr 1996; **Fac Appt:** Prof TS, Univ Tex, Houston

Turner, William F MD [TS] - **Spec Exp:** Coronary Artery Surgery; Cardiac Surgery; **Hospital:** E TX Med Ctr-Tyler, Trinity Mother Frances Hosp; **Address:** 1100 E Lake St, Ste 210, Tyler, TX 75701; **Phone:** 903-593-0900; **Board Cert:** Surgery 1997; Thoracic Surgery 1998; **Med School:** Baylor Coll Med 1981; **Resid:** Surgery, Baylor Coll Med 1987; Thoracic Surgery, Baylor Coll Med 1989

West Coast and Pacific

Bailey, Leonard L MD [TS] - **Spec Exp:** Cardiac Surgery-Pediatric; Congenital Heart Surgery; Transplant-Heart-Pediatric; **Hospital:** Loma Linda Chldns Hosp, Loma Linda Univ Med Ctr; **Address:** 11234 Anderson St, rm 1617, Loma Linda, CA 92354; **Phone:** 909-558-4200; **Board Cert:** Surgery 1975; Thoracic Surgery 2006; **Med School:** Loma Linda Univ 1969; **Resid:** Surgery, Loma Linda Univ Med Ctr 1973; Thoracic Surgery, Loma Linda Univ Med Ctr 1974; **Fellow:** Cardiovascular Surgery, Hosp Sick Chldn 1975; **Fac Appt:** Prof S, Loma Linda Univ

Cameron, Robert B MD [TS] - **Spec Exp:** Lung Cancer; Mesothelioma; **Hospital:** UCLA Ronald Reagan Med Ctr; **Address:** UCLA Medical Ctr-Dept of Thoracic Surg, 10833 Le Conte Ave, Los Angeles, CA 90095; **Phone:** 310-794-7333; **Board Cert:** Surgery 2002; Thoracic Surgery 2005; **Med School:** UCLA 1984; **Resid:** Surgery, UCLA Hosp & Clinic 1992; **Fellow:** Surgical Oncology, National Inst Health 1989; Cardiothoracic Surgery, NY Hosp/Cornell 1994

Cohen, Robbin G MD [TS] - **Spec Exp:** Minimally Invasive Surgery; Heart Valve Surgery; Thoracic Aortic Surgery; **Hospital:** USC Univ Hosp, Huntington Memorial Hosp; **Address:** 1520 San Pueblo St, Ste 4300, Los Angeles, CA 90033; **Phone:** 323-442-5850; **Board Cert:** Thoracic Surgery 1999; **Med School:** Univ Colorado 1980; **Resid:** Surgery, Stanford Univ Med Ctr 1986; **Fellow:** Cardiothoracic Surgery, Stanford Univ Med Ctr 1989; **Fac Appt:** Assoc Prof TS, USC Sch Med

Dang, Michael H MD [TS] - **Spec Exp:** Cardiac Surgery; Peripheral Vascular Disease; Transplant-Heart; **Hospital:** Queen's Med Ctr - Honolulu; **Address:** Queens Heart Physicians Practice, 550 S Beretania St, Ste 300, Honolulu, HI 96813; **Phone:** 808-545-8900; **Board Cert:** Thoracic Surgery 2002; **Med School:** Univ Colorado 1968; **Resid:** Surgery, Baylor Univ Med Ctr 1976; Thoracic Surgery, Baylor Univ Med Ctr 1978

De Meester, Tom R MD [TS] - **Spec Exp:** Stomach Cancer; Esophageal Cancer; Lung Cancer; Tracheal Surgery; **Hospital:** USC Univ Hosp; **Address:** 1510 San Pablo St, Ste 514, Los Angeles, CA 90033; **Phone:** 323-442-5925; **Board Cert:** Surgery 1971; Thoracic Surgery 1971; **Med School:** Univ Mich Med Sch 1963; **Resid:** Surgery, Johns Hopkins Hosp 1966; **Fellow:** Thoracic Surgery, Johns Hopkins Hosp 1968; **Fac Appt:** Prof S, USC Sch Med

DeFilippi, Vincent J MD [TS] - **Spec Exp:** Minimally Invasive Cardiac Surgery; Mitral Valve Surgery; Maze Procedure for Atrial Fibrillation; Robotic Cardiac Surgery; **Hospital:** Salinas Valley Meml Hlthcare Systs, Stanford Univ Med Ctr; **Address:** Stanford Univ at Salinas Valley, Cardiac Surgery Program, 212 San Jose St, Ste 301, Salinas, CA 93901; **Phone:** 831-759-3289; **Board Cert:** Thoracic Surgery 2005; **Med School:** Columbia P&S 1988; **Resid:** Surgery, Univ Chicago Hosps 1994; **Fellow:** Cardiothoracic Surgery, New York Hosp/Meml Sloan Kettering Cancer Ctr 1995; **Fac Appt:** Assoc Clin Prof TS, Stanford Univ

Fontana, Gregory MD [TS] - **Spec Exp:** Minimally Invasive Surgery; Cardiac Surgery-Pediatric; Mitral Valve Surgery; Coronary Artery Surgery; **Hospital:** Cedars-Sinai Med Ctr; **Address:** 8700 Beverly Blvd, North Twr, rm 6215, Los Angeles, CA 90048-1804; **Phone:** 310-423-1874; **Board Cert:** Thoracic Surgery 2004; **Med School:** UCLA 1984; **Resid:** Surgery, Duke Univ Med Ctr 1990; Thoracic Surgery, Duke Univ Med Ctr 1993; **Fellow:** Pediatric Cardiac Surgery, UCLA Med Ctr; Pediatric Cardiac Surgery, Chldns Hosp; **Fac Appt:** Assoc Clin Prof S, UCLA

Grannis Jr, Frederic W MD [TS] - **Spec Exp:** Lung Cancer; Tobacco Abuse; Thoracic Cancers; Palliative Care; **Hospital:** City of Hope Natl Med Ctr & Beckman Rsch, Methodist Hosp - Southern California; **Address:** Thor Surg-City of Hope Natl Med Ctr, 1500 E Duarte Rd, Duarte, CA 91010; **Phone:** 626-359-8111 x62669; **Board Cert:** Surgery 1975; Thoracic Surgery 2000; **Med School:** NY Med Coll 1969; **Resid:** Surgery, Mayo Clinic 1974; Thoracic Surgery, Mayo Clinic 1977; **Fac Appt:** Assoc Prof TS, UCSD

Gundry, Steven MD [TS] - **Spec Exp:** Cardiac Surgery-Adult & Pediatric; Cardiac Surgery-High Risk; Nutrition in Heart Disease; **Hospital:** Desert Regl Med Ctr; **Address:** International Heart & Lung Inst, 555 Tachevah Drive, 3W - Ste 103, Palm Springs, CA 92262; **Phone:** 760-323-5553; **Board Cert:** Thoracic Surgery 2005; **Med School:** Med Coll GA 1977; **Resid:** Surgery, Univ Michigan Hosps 1983; Thoracic Surgery, Univ Michigan Hosps 1985; **Fellow:** Pediatric Cardiac Surgery, Hosp-Sick Chldn 1986; **Fac Appt:** Clin Prof S, Loma Linda Univ

Handy Jr, John R MD [TS] - **Spec Exp:** Lung Cancer; Esophageal Cancer; Mesothelioma; Chest Wall Tumors; **Hospital:** Providence Portland Med Ctr; **Address:** Oregon Clinic-Cardiothoracic Surgery, 1111 NE 99th Ave, Ste 201, Portland, OR 97220; **Phone:** 503-963-3030; **Board Cert:** Thoracic Surgery 2001; Surgery 1999; **Med School:** Duke Univ 1983; **Resid:** Surgery, Brown Univ Hosp 1990; **Fellow:** Cardiothoracic Surgery, MUSC Med Ctr 1993

Hanley, Frank L MD [TS] - **Spec Exp:** Pediatric Thoracic Surgery; **Hospital:** Lucile Packard Chldn's Hosp, Chldns Hosp - Oakland; **Address:** 300 Pasteur Drive, FALK CVRB, Stanford, CA 94305-5407; **Phone:** 650-723-0190; **Board Cert:** Thoracic Surgery 2002; **Med School:** Tufts Univ 1978; **Resid:** Surgery, UCSF Med Ctr 1981; Cardiothoracic Surgery, UCSF Med Ctr 1988; **Fellow:** Research, UCSF Sch Med 1984; **Fac Appt:** Prof S, UCSF

Harken, Alden H MD [TS] - **Spec Exp:** Arrhythmias; Cardiac Surgery; Coronary Artery Disease; **Hospital:** UCSF Med Ctr, Alameda County Med Ctr-Highland Campus; **Address:** Univ Cal San Francisco, 1411 E 31st St, Oakland, CA 94602; **Phone:** 510-437-4091; **Board Cert:** Surgery 1990; Thoracic Surgery 2006; **Med School:** Case West Res Univ 1967; **Resid:** Surgery, Peter Bent Brigham Hosp 1970; Thoracic Surgery, Peter Bent Brigham Hosp 1973; **Fellow:** Cardiovascular Surgery, Boston Chldns Hosp 1971; **Fac Appt:** Prof S, Univ Colorado

Jablons, David M MD [TS] - **Spec Exp:** Lung Cancer; Mesothelioma; Esophageal Surgery; **Hospital:** UCSF - Mt Zion Med Ctr; **Address:** UCSF Thoracic Surgery, 1600 Divisadero St Fl 4, San Francisco, CA 94115; **Phone:** 415-885-3882; **Board Cert:** Thoracic Surgery 2002; **Med School:** Albany Med Coll 1984; **Resid:** Surgery, New Eng Med Ctr-Tufts Univ 1986; Surgery, New Eng Med Ctr-Tufts Univ 1991; **Fellow:** Surgical Oncology, Natl Cancer Inst-NIH 1989; Cardiothoracic Surgery, New York Hosp-Cornell 1993; **Fac Appt:** Prof S, UCSF

Jamieson, Stuart W MD [TS] - **Spec Exp:** Pulmonary Embolism; Transplant-Heart & Lung; **Hospital:** UCSD Med Ctr; **Address:** UCSD Med Ctr, Div CTS, 200 W Arbor Drive, MC 8892, San Diego, CA 92103; **Phone:** 619-543-7777; **Med School:** England, UK 1971; **Resid:** Surgery 1975; **Fellow:** Cardiothoracic Surgery 1977; Cardiothoracic Surgery, Stanford Univ/American Heart Assoc 1980; **Fac Appt:** Prof S, UCSD

Thoracic Surgery

Kernstine, Kemp H MD/PhD [TS] - **Spec Exp:** Lung Cancer; Esophageal Cancer; Tracheal Surgery; Esophageal Surgery; **Hospital:** City of Hope Natl Med Ctr & Beckman Rsch; **Address:** City of Hope Comprehensive Cancer Ctr, 1500 E Duarte Rd, Duarte, CA 91010; **Phone:** 626-359-8111 x68845; **Board Cert:** Thoracic Surgery 2004; Surgery 2001; **Med School:** Duke Univ 1982; **Resid:** Surgery, Univ Minn Med Ctr 1988; **Fellow:** Cardiothoracic Surgery, Brigham & Women's Hosp 1994; **Fac Appt:** Prof S, Univ Iowa Coll Med

Laks, Hillel MD [TS] - **Spec Exp:** Congenital Heart Disease; Transplant-Heart; **Hospital:** UCLA Ronald Reagan Med Ctr; **Address:** UCLA Med Ctr, 10833 Le Conte Ave, rm 62-215 CHS, Los Angeles, CA 90095-1741; **Phone:** 310-206-1837; **Board Cert:** Surgery 1975; Thoracic Surgery 2006; **Med School:** Africa 1965; **Resid:** Surgery, Peter Bent Brigham Hosp 1969; Thoracic Surgery, Peter Bent Brigham Hosp 1973; **Fac Appt:** Prof S, UCLA

Lamberti Jr, John J MD [TS] - **Spec Exp:** Pediatric Cardiac Surgery; Heart Valve Surgery; Congenital Heart Surgery; **Hospital:** Rady Children's Hosp - San Diego, UCSD Med Ctr; **Address:** Rady Chldns Hosp, 3030 Children's Way, Ste 202, San Diego, CA 92123-4227; **Phone:** 858-966-8030; **Board Cert:** Surgery 1973; Thoracic Surgery 1975; **Med School:** Univ Pittsburgh 1967; **Resid:** Surgery, Peter Bent Brigham Hosp 1972; Thoracic Surgery, Peter Bent Brigham Hosp 1973; **Fellow:** Pediatric Cardiac Surgery, Chldns Hosp 1974; **Fac Appt:** Prof S, UCSD

Merrick, Scot H MD [TS] - **Spec Exp:** Cardiac Surgery-Adult; Heart Valve Surgery; Coronary Revascularization; **Hospital:** UCSF Med Ctr; **Address:** UCSF Med Ctr, Div Cardiothoracic Surg, 500 Parnassus Ave, San Francisco, CA 94143-0118; **Phone:** 415-353-1606; **Board Cert:** Thoracic Surgery 1997; **Med School:** Univ Wash 1980; **Resid:** Surgery, UCSF Med Ctr 1985; **Fellow:** Cardiothoracic Surgery, UCSF Med Ctr 1987; **Fac Appt:** Assoc Prof S, UCSF

Miller, David Craig MD [TS] - **Spec Exp:** Thoracic Aortic Surgery; Heart Valve Surgery; Endovascular Stent Grafts; **Hospital:** Stanford Univ Med Ctr; **Address:** Stanford Univ Sch Medicine, Div Cardiothoracic Surgery, 300 Pasteur Drive Falk Rsch Bldg, Stanford, CA 94305-5407; **Phone:** 650-725-3826; **Board Cert:** Thoracic Surgery 1998; **Med School:** Stanford Univ 1972; **Resid:** Thoracic Surgery, Standford Univ Med Ctr 1978; **Fac Appt:** Prof TS, Stanford Univ

Reitz, Bruce A MD [TS] - **Spec Exp:** Transplant-Heart & Lung; Heart Valve Surgery; Congenital Heart Surgery; Coronary Artery Surgery; **Hospital:** Stanford Univ Med Ctr, El Camino Hosp; **Address:** Stanford Univ Sch Med, Dept Cardiothoracic Surgery, 300 Pasteur Drive, Falk CVRB ULN, Stanford, CA 94305-5407; **Phone:** 650-725-4497; **Board Cert:** Thoracic Surgery 1999; **Med School:** Yale Univ 1970; **Resid:** Cardiovascular Surgery, Stanford Univ Hosp 1972; Thoracic Surgery, Stanford Univ Hosp 1978; **Fellow:** Cardiac Surgery, Natl Heart Inst 1974; **Fac Appt:** Prof TS, Stanford Univ

Robbins, Robert C MD [TS] - **Spec Exp:** Transplant-Heart; Transplant-Lung; **Hospital:** Stanford Univ Med Ctr, El Camino Hosp; **Address:** Cardiovascular Rsch Bldg, Fl 2, 300 Pasteur Drive, Stanford, CA 94305-5407; **Phone:** 650-725-3828; **Board Cert:** Thoracic Surgery 2002; Surgery 2002; **Med School:** Univ Miss 1983; **Resid:** Surgery, Univ Miss Med Ctr 1988; **Fellow:** Thoracic Surgery, Stanford Univ Med Ctr 1991; **Fac Appt:** Prof TS, Stanford Univ

Shemin, Richard MD [TS] - **Spec Exp:** Minimally Invasive Cardiac Surgery; Heart Valve Surgery; Aneurysm-Thoracic Aortic; **Hospital:** UCLA Ronald Reagan Med Ctr; **Address:** UCLA-David Geffen Sch Med, Le Conte Ave, rm 62182, Los Angeles, CA 90095; **Phone:** 310-206-8232; **Board Cert:** Thoracic Surgery 2002; **Med School:** Boston Univ 1974; **Resid:** Surgery, PB Brigham Hosp 1980; NYU Med Ctr 1982; **Fellow:** Cardiac Surgery, Natl Inst Hlth 1978; **Fac Appt:** Prof TS, UCLA-David Geffen Sch Med

Shrager, Joseph B MD [TS] - **Spec Exp:** Lung Cancer; Thymoma; Mediastinal Tumors; Emphysema-Lung Volume Reduction; **Hospital:** Stanford Univ Med Ctr, VA Hlth Care Sys - Palo Alto; **Address:** Stanford Univ Medical Ctr, Falk Bldg, 300 Pasteur Drive Fl 2 - rm CV207, Stanford, CA 94305-5407; **Phone:** 650-721-2086; **Board Cert:** Thoracic Surgery 1999; **Med School:** Harvard Med Sch 1988; **Resid:** Surgery, Hosp Univ Penn 1995; Thoracic Surgery, Mass Genl Hosp 1997; **Fac Appt:** Prof TS, Stanford Univ

Starnes, Vaughn A MD [TS] - **Spec Exp:** Transplant-Heart & Lung; Heart Valve Surgery; Ross Procedure for Aortic Valve Disease; Robotic Cardiac Surgery; **Hospital:** USC Univ Hosp, Huntington Memorial Hosp; **Address:** USC Cardiothoracic Surgery, 1520 San Pablo St, Ste 4300, Los Angeles, CA 90033; **Phone:** 323-442-5849; **Board Cert:** Thoracic Surgery 2007; **Med School:** Univ NC Sch Med 1977; **Resid:** Surgery, Vanderbilt Univ Hosp 1984; Cardiovascular Surgery, Stanford Unv Hosp 1986; **Fellow:** Cardiothoracic Transplant Surg, Stanford Unv Hosp 1987; Pediatric Cardiac Surgery, Univ NC Hosp; **Fac Appt:** Prof TS, USC Sch Med

Thistlethwaite, Patricia A MD/PhD [TS] - **Spec Exp:** Cardiac Surgery; Lung Cancer; **Hospital:** UCSD Med Ctr; **Address:** UCSD Med Ctr, Div CTS, 200 W Arbor Drive, MC 8892, San Diego, CA 92103; **Phone:** 619-543-7777; **Board Cert:** Surgery 2005; Thoracic Surgery 2007; **Med School:** Harvard Med Sch 1989; **Resid:** Surgery, Mass Genl Hosp 1994; **Fellow:** Cardiothoracic Surgery, Univ Pittsburgh 1997; **Fac Appt:** Assoc Prof S, UCSD

Trento, Alfredo MD [TS] - **Spec Exp:** Transplant-Heart; Cardiac Surgery; Pediatric Cardiac Surgery; Coronary Artery Surgery; **Hospital:** Cedars-Sinai Med Ctr; **Address:** Cedars-Sinai Med Ctr, Dept Thoracic Surg, 8700 Beverly Blvd, North Tower - rm 6215, Los Angeles, CA 90048; **Phone:** 310-423-3851; **Board Cert:** Thoracic Surgery 2005; **Med School:** Italy 1975; **Resid:** Surgery, Univ Mass Med Ctr 1982; Thoracic Surgery, Univ Pittsburgh Med Ctr 1985; **Fellow:** Cardiothoracic Surgery, Univ Mass Med Ctr 1982; **Fac Appt:** Prof S, UCLA

Vallieres, Eric MD [TS] - **Spec Exp:** Lung Cancer; Mesothelioma; Mediastinal Tumors; Thoracic Cancers; **Hospital:** Swedish Med Ctr - Seattle; **Address:** 1101 Madison St, Ste 850, Seattle, WA 98104; **Phone:** 206-215-6800; **Board Cert:** Surgery 1988; Thoracic Surgery 1990; **Med School:** Canada 1982; **Resid:** Surgery, Univ Toronto Affil Hosp 1988; Thoracic Surgery, Univ Toronto Affil Hosp 1989; **Fellow:** Cardiovascular Surgery, Univ Montreal 1990

Verrier, Edward D MD [TS] - **Spec Exp:** Coronary Artery Surgery; Heart Valve Surgery; **Hospital:** Univ Wash Med Ctr, Northwest Hosp; **Address:** University Washington Medical Ctr, 1959 NE Pacific St, Ste AA115, Box 356310, Seattle, WA 98195-6310; **Phone:** 206-598-3636; **Board Cert:** Thoracic Surgery 2003; **Med School:** Tufts Univ 1974; **Resid:** Surgery, UCSF Med Ctr 1982; Thoracic Surgery, UCSF Med Ctr 1984; **Fellow:** Cardiac Surgery, UCSF Med Ctr 1980; **Fac Appt:** Prof TS, Univ Wash

Wells, Winfield J MD [TS] - **Spec Exp:** Tracheal Surgery-Pediatric; Congenital Heart Surgery; **Hospital:** Chldns Hosp - Los Angeles; **Address:** Chlds Hosp, Div Cardiothoracic Surgery, 4650 W Sunset Blvd, MS 66, Los Angeles, CA 90027; **Phone:** 323-361-4148; **Board Cert:** Thoracic Surgery 2007; **Med School:** USC Sch Med 1970; **Resid:** Surgery, Columbia-Presby Med Ctr 1976; **Fac Appt:** Assoc Prof S, USC Sch Med

Whyte, Richard MD [TS] - **Spec Exp:** Lung Cancer; Esophageal Cancer; Chest Wall Tumors; **Hospital:** Stanford Univ Med Ctr; **Address:** Stanford Univ Sch Med, Div Thor Surg, 300 Pasteur Dr, Bldg CVRB - rm 205, Stanford, CA 94305-5407; **Phone:** 650-723-6649; **Board Cert:** Surgery 2001; Thoracic Surgery 2003; **Med School:** Univ Pittsburgh 1983; **Resid:** Surgery, Mass Genl Hosp 1990; Thoracic Surgery, Univ Michigan Hosp 1992; **Fac Appt:** Prof TS, Stanford Univ

Thoracic Surgery

Wood, Douglas E MD [TS] - **Spec Exp:** Lung Cancer; Esophageal Cancer; Tracheal Surgery; Mesothelioma; **Hospital:** Univ Wash Med Ctr, Northwest Hosp; **Address:** Univ Washington, Div Cardiothoracic Surg, 1959 NE Pacific St, AA Bldg - rm 115, Box 356310, Seattle, WA 98195-6310; **Phone:** 206-685-3228; **Board Cert:** Surgery 1999; Thoracic Surgery 2001; **Med School:** Harvard Med Sch 1983; **Resid:** Surgery, Mass Genl Hosp 1989; Thoracic Surgery, Mass Genl Hosp 1991; **Fellow:** Surgical Critical Care, Mass Genl Hosp 1991; **Fac Appt:** Prof S, Univ Wash

Mount Sinai

MOUNT SINAI SCHOOL OF MEDICINE

THE MOUNT SINAI MEDICAL CENTER
THORACIC SURGERY
One Gustave L. Levy Place
Fifth Avenue and 100th Street
New York, NY 10029-6574
Physician Referral: 1-800-MD-SINAI (637-4624)
www.mountsinai.org

THORACIC SURGERY at Mount Sinai is world renowned for its state-of-the-art surgery, multidisciplinary team approach to treatment, and commitment to compassionate patient care. Protocol-driven therapy ensures that Mount Sinai patients are given access to many clinical trials.

Our team of dedicated thoracic surgeons are experts in the treatment of all primary cancers of the chest, lung, esophagus, mediastinum, and airway, and all metastatic tumors of the chest. We also diagnose and treat patients who are affected by benign esophageal disorders such as gastroesophageal reflux disease, achalasia, and motility disorders.

Mount Sinai is a leader in the development and implementation of the latest technologies and treatment options for disorders of the lung and esophagus, including:

- Video-assisted thoracic surgery (VATS)
- VATS lobectomy
- VATS thymectomy
- VATS sympathectomy for patients with excessive sweating of the hands
- Minimally invasive esophagectomy
- Robotic surgery
- Endobronchial ultrasound—a new noninvasive method for staging lung cancers
- Stent and laser treatment of the airway and esophagus
- Radiofrequency ablation of lung tumors
- Stereotactic radiosurgery of the lung
- Navigational bronchoscopy—a new, innovative, noninvasive method via bronchoscopy to perform biopsies on small lung lesions, including those in subpleural locations
- Lung volume reduction surgery

TAKING CARE OF ONE PATIENT AT A TIME
At Mount Sinai we believe in personalized care. Each patient benefits from a team approach that includes thoracic surgeons, anesthesiologists, medical oncologists, radiation oncologists, and oncology-dedicated nurses. Coordinating information among team members to ensure seamless delivery of care is a top priority.

Transplant Program – Our transplant program is one of two accredited programs in the New York metropolitan area dedicated to lung transplantation for a wide variety of conditions. Patients enrolled in this program receive a multidisciplinary team approach to their condition.

Translational Research – Mount Sinai's scientists are conducting state-of-the-art translational thoracic research, including genomic analysis of tumors to better understand and predict behavior in order to develop more directed, personalized therapeutic approaches to treatment.

Screening and Diagnosis – Mount Sinai offers comprehensive screening and diagnostic tests, including CT scans for early detection, advanced endoscopic techniques to detect early lesions and recurrence, PET scans, and innovative MRI technology with ultrasensitive resolution. Our developing program for the screening and detection of esophageal cancer is the first of its kind in New York City.

NYU **Langone Medical Center**

550 First Avenue (at 31St Street)
New York, NY 10016
Physician Referral:
(888)7-NYU-MED (888-769-8633)
www.med.nyu.edu

THORACIC SURGERY

About the Division of Thoracic Surgery:

The Division of Thoracic Surgery at NYU Langone Medical Center offers the most advanced diagnosis and treatment options for patients with both benign and malignant lesions of the lung, esophagus, mediastinum and chest wall. All of the thoracic attending physicians at the Medical Center are experts in minimally invasive, video-assisted thoracic surgery and prefer this technique to minimize discomfort in all possible cases.

We specialize in the following areas:

AIRWAY STENTING

Patients experiencing trouble breathing may require airway stenting in order to maintain an open airway (windpipe). Treatment of primary and metastatic lung cancer often includes the use of hollow tubes (stents) to maintain an unobstructed airway. At NYU Langone Medical Center, stent placement is performed in the operating room by an experienced team that includes a surgeon, anesthesiologist and nursing staff. The procedure can be performed through either rigid or flexible bronchoscopy, using either temporary (plastic) or more permanent (metal) stents. Post-operative patients are carefully monitored by a multidisciplinary team to ensure their comfort and care.

MINIMALLY INVASIVE THORACIC SURGERY

The Division of Thoracic Surgery at NYU Langone Medical Center offers a minimally invasive surgery program, incorporating both video-assisted and "open chest" techniques along with the newest methods for post-operative pain relief. The use of video-assisted equipment allows for a smaller incision without spreading the rib spaces leading to greater patient comfort, a shorter recovery time and decreased length of stay for patients. Procedures offered include video-assisted thoracoscopy for biopsy with or without removal of a portion of the lungs as well as repair of hiatal hernias and minimally invasive esophagectomy.

PIONEERING TREATMENTS

The Division of Thoracic Surgery at NYU Langone Medical Center offers new, pioneering treatments including: early detection of airway malignancies, diagnosis and treatment strategies for endobronchial abnormalities, investigation of non-surgical techniques selectively used for destruction of lung cancer nodules and the use of stents (and replaceable stents) to relieve blockages of the windpipe and esophagus.

RESEARCH

The Medical Center is committed to state-of-the-art surgical management and developing novel treatment strategies using clinical trials. The Medical Center also uses the resources at the New York Thoracic Surgery Laboratory housed at Bellevue Hospital to search for genes and proteins in malignancies of the chest in order to detect them earlier or develop novel targeted therapies. Through studies like these, the Medical Center makes clinically relevant

Urology

A urologist manages benign and malignant medical and surgical disorders of the genitourinary system and the adrenal gland. This specialist has comprehensive knowledge of, and skills in, endoscopic, percutaneous and open surgery of congenital and acquired conditions of the urinary and reproductive systems and their contiguous structures.

Training Required: Five years

UROLOGY

New England

Albertsen, Peter Christian MD [U] - **Spec Exp:** Prostate Cancer; **Hospital:** Univ of Conn Hlth Ctr, John Dempsey Hosp; **Address:** 263 Farmington Ave Fl 2 - Ste 223, Farmington, CT 06030; **Phone:** 860-679-4100; **Board Cert:** Urology 2004; **Med School:** Columbia P&S 1978; **Resid:** Surgery, New England Deaconess Hosp 1980; Urology, Johns Hopkins Hospital 1984; **Fellow:** Preventive Medicine, Univ WI Affil Hosp 1990; **Fac Appt:** Prof U, Univ Conn

Caldamone, Anthony A MD [U] - **Spec Exp:** Pediatric Urology; **Hospital:** Rhode Island Hosp; **Address:** 2 Dudley St, Ste 185, Providence, RI 02905; **Phone:** 401-421-0710; **Board Cert:** Urology 1983; Pediatric Urology 2008; **Med School:** Brown Univ 1975; **Resid:** Urology, Strong Meml Hosp 1981; **Fellow:** Pediatric Urology, Childrens Hosp 1982; **Fac Appt:** Prof U, Brown Univ

Colberg, John W MD [U] - **Spec Exp:** Prostate Cancer; Bladder Cancer; Kidney Cancer; Testicular Cancer; **Hospital:** Yale-New Haven Hosp; **Address:** Yale Urology Group, 800 Howard Ave Fl 3, New Haven, CT 06520-8062; **Phone:** 203-785-2815; **Board Cert:** Urology 2001; **Med School:** Washington Univ, St Louis 1985; **Resid:** Surgery, Yale-New Haven Hosp 1987; Urology, Yale-New Haven Hosp 1990; **Fac Appt:** Assoc Prof U, Yale Univ

Foster Jr, Harris E MD [U] - **Spec Exp:** Urology-Female; Urodynamics; Neurogenic Bladder; Voiding Dysfunction; **Hospital:** Yale-New Haven Hosp; **Address:** Yale Urology Group, 800 Howard Ave Fl 3, New Haven, CT 06520-8062; **Phone:** 203-785-2815; **Board Cert:** Urology 2003; **Med School:** Univ Miami Sch Med 1987; **Resid:** Surgery, Univ Michigan Med Ctr 1989; Urology, Univ Michigan Med Ctr 1992; **Fac Appt:** Prof U, Yale Univ

Gomery, Pablo MD [U] - **Spec Exp:** Neuro-Urology; Erectile Dysfunction; Voiding Dysfunction; Infertility-Male; **Hospital:** Mass Genl Hosp, Spaulding Rehab Hosp; **Address:** Mass Genl Hosp-Dept Urology, 55 Fruit St, GRB 1102, Boston, MA 02114; **Phone:** 617-726-8482; **Board Cert:** Urology 2000; **Med School:** Albert Einstein Coll Med 1974; **Resid:** Surgery, New England Deaconess Hosp 1977; Urology, Mass General Hosp 1980

Heney, Niall M MD [U] - **Spec Exp:** Urologic Cancer; **Hospital:** Mass Genl Hosp; **Address:** Mass Genl Hosp, Dept Urol, 55 Fruit St Fl 5th, 528 rm, Boston, MA 02114; **Phone:** 617-726-3011; **Board Cert:** Urology 1977; **Med School:** Ireland 1965; **Resid:** Urology, Regional Hosp 1972; Urology, Mass Genl Hosp 1976; **Fac Appt:** Prof U, Harvard Med Sch

Janeiro Jr, John J MD [U] - **Spec Exp:** Urologic Cancer; Kidney Stones; Vasectomy Reversal; **Hospital:** Southern NH Med Ctr, St Joseph Hosp; **Address:** Urology Center Southern New Hampshire, 17 Riverside St, Ste 201, Nashua, NH 03062; **Phone:** 603-883-1550; **Board Cert:** Urology 2008; **Med School:** Univ Mass Sch Med 1982; **Resid:** Urology, Lahey Clinic 1987; **Fellow:** Pediatric Urology, Childrens Hosp 1989

Libertino, John A MD [U] - **Spec Exp:** Kidney Cancer; Prostate Cancer; Adrenal Tumors; **Hospital:** Lahey Clin; **Address:** Lahey Clinic, Dept Urology, 41 Mall Rd, Burlington, MA 01805-0001; **Phone:** 781-744-2750; **Board Cert:** Urology 1973; **Med School:** Georgetown Univ 1965; **Resid:** Urology, Univ Rochester-Strong Meml Hosp 1967; Urology, Yale-New Haven Hosp 1970; **Fellow:** Surgery, Yale-New Haven Hosp 1968; **Fac Appt:** Assoc Clin Prof S, Harvard Med Sch

Loughlin, Kevin R MD [U] - **Spec Exp:** Prostate Cancer; Bladder Cancer; Penile Cancer; Incontinence-Female; **Hospital:** Brigham & Women's Hosp, Dana-Farber Cancer Inst; **Address:** Brigham & Women's Hosp, Div Urology, 45 Francis St, ASBII-3, Boston, MA 02115; **Phone:** 617-732-6325; **Board Cert:** Urology 2004; **Med School:** NY Med Coll 1975; **Resid:** Pediatrics, New York Hosp-Cornell 1978; Surgery, Bellevue Hosp Ctr-NYU 1979; **Fellow:** Urology, Brigham & Women's Hosp 1983; Urologic Oncology, Meml Sloan Kettering Cancer Ctr 1983; **Fac Appt:** Prof S, Harvard Med Sch

McDougal, W Scott MD [U] - **Spec Exp:** Penile Cancer; Prostate Cancer; Bladder Cancer; Urologic Cancer; **Hospital:** Mass Genl Hosp; **Address:** Mass Genl Hosp, 55 Fruit St, Bldg GRB - rm 1102, Boston, MA 02114; **Phone:** 617-726-3010; **Board Cert:** Surgery 1975; Urology 1978; **Med School:** Cornell Univ-Weill Med Coll 1968; **Resid:** Surgery, Univ Hosps Cleveland 1975; Urology, Univ Hosps Cleveland 1975; **Fellow:** Physiology, Yale Med Sch 1972; **Fac Appt:** Prof U, Harvard Med Sch

McGovern, Francis MD [U] - **Spec Exp:** Prostate Cancer; **Hospital:** Mass Genl Hosp; **Address:** One Hawthorne Pl, Ste 109, Boston, MA 02114; **Phone:** 617-726-3560; **Board Cert:** Urology 1999; **Med School:** Case West Res Univ 1983; **Resid:** Urology, Mass Genl Hosp 1989

O'Leary, Michael P MD [U] - **Spec Exp:** Sexual Dysfunction; Kidney Stones; Prostate Disease; **Hospital:** Brigham & Women's Hosp, Dana-Farber Cancer Inst; **Address:** Brigham & Women's Hosp, Div Urology, 45 Francis St, ASBII-3, Boston, MA 02155; **Phone:** 617-732-6325; **Board Cert:** Urology 2000; **Med School:** Geo Wash Univ 1980; **Resid:** Urology, Tufts New Eng Med Ctr 1982; Urology, Mass Genl Hosp 1986; **Fellow:** Urology, UCSF Med Ctr 1989; **Fac Appt:** Assoc Prof S, Harvard Med Sch

Oates, Robert D MD [U] - **Spec Exp:** Infertility-Male; Vasectomy Reversal; Reproductive Genetics; **Hospital:** Boston Med Ctr; **Address:** Boston Univ Med Ctr, Dept Urology, 720 Harrison Ave, Ste 606, Boston, MA 02118-2334; **Phone:** 617-638-8485; **Board Cert:** Urology 2000; **Med School:** Boston Univ 1982; **Resid:** Surgery, Boston Univ Hosp 1984; Urology, Boston Univ Hosp 1987; **Fellow:** Reproductive Medicine, Baylor Coll Med 1988; **Fac Appt:** Prof U, Boston Univ

Richie, Jerome MD [U] - **Spec Exp:** Prostate Cancer; Testicular Cancer; Kidney Cancer; **Hospital:** Brigham & Women's Hosp, Dana-Farber Cancer Inst; **Address:** Brigham & Womens Hosp, 75 Francis St, Ste ASB2, Boston, MA 02115; **Phone:** 617-732-6325; **Board Cert:** Urology 1992; **Med School:** Univ Tex Med Br, Galveston 1969; **Resid:** Surgery, UCLA Med Ctr 1971; Urology, UCLA Med Ctr 1975; **Fac Appt:** Prof U, Harvard Med Sch

Sanda, Martin G MD [U] - **Spec Exp:** Prostate Cancer; Bladder Cancer; Kidney Cancer; Urologic Cancer; **Hospital:** Beth Israel Deaconess Med Ctr - Boston; **Address:** Beth Israel Deaconess Medical Ctr, 330 Brookline Ave, Rabb 440, Boston, MA 02115; **Phone:** 617-735-2100; **Board Cert:** Urology 2007; **Med School:** Columbia P&S 1987; **Resid:** Surgery, Med Coll Virginia 1989; Urology, Johns Hopkins Hosp 1994; **Fellow:** Surgical Oncology, Natl Cancer Inst 1991; **Fac Appt:** Assoc Prof U, Harvard Med Sch

Sigman, Mark MD [U] - **Spec Exp:** Infertility-Male; Vasectomy Reversal; **Hospital:** Rhode Island Hosp; **Address:** 2 Dudley St, Ste 175, Providence, RI 02905-3247; **Phone:** 401-421-0710; **Board Cert:** Urology 2000; **Med School:** Univ Conn 1981; **Resid:** Urology, Univ VA 1987; Surgery, Univ VA 1983; **Fellow:** Male Reproduction, Baylor Coll Med 1989; **Fac Appt:** Assoc Prof U, Brown Univ

Urology

Weiss, Robert M MD [U] - **Spec Exp:** Pediatric Urology; Testicular Cancer; Penile Cancer; Bladder Cancer; **Hospital:** Yale-New Haven Hosp; **Address:** Yale Univ Sch Med, Dept Urology, 800 Howard Ave, Box 208041, New Haven, CT 06520-8041; **Phone:** 203-785-2815; **Board Cert:** Urology 1970; **Med School:** SUNY Downstate 1960; **Resid:** Surgery, Beth Israel Hosp 1962; Urology, Columbia Presby Hosp 1967; **Fellow:** Pharmacology, Columbia Presby Hosp 1965; **Fac Appt:** Prof U, Yale Univ

Mid Atlantic

Alexander, Richard B MD [U] - **Spec Exp:** Prostate Disease; Prostate Cancer; **Hospital:** Univ of MD Med Ctr; **Address:** 29 SE Greene St, Ste 500, Baltimore, MD 21201; **Phone:** 410-328-5109; **Board Cert:** Urology 1999; **Med School:** Johns Hopkins Univ 1981; **Resid:** Surgery, Vanderbilt Univ Affl Hosps 1983; Urology, Johns Hopkins Hosp 1988; **Fellow:** Cancer Immunology, Natl Cancer Inst 1989; **Fac Appt:** Prof U, Univ MD Sch Med

Bagley, Demetrius H MD [U] - **Spec Exp:** Endourology; Kidney Stones; Kidney Cancer; Ureter & Renal Pelvis Cancer; **Hospital:** Thomas Jefferson Univ Hosp; **Address:** 833 Chestnut St E, Ste 703, Philadelphia, PA 19107; **Phone:** 215-955-1000; **Board Cert:** Urology 1981; **Med School:** Johns Hopkins Univ 1970; **Resid:** Surgery, Yale-New Haven Hosp 1972; Urology, Yale-New Haven Hosp 1979; **Fellow:** Surgery, NCI-USPHS 1975; **Fac Appt:** Prof U, Thomas Jefferson Univ

Bar-Chama, Natan MD [U] - **Spec Exp:** Infertility-Male; Erectile Dysfunction; Varicocele Microsurgery; Vasectomy Reversal; **Hospital:** Mount Sinai Med Ctr (page 64); **Address:** 5 E 98th St, Box 1272, New York, NY 10029-6501; **Phone:** 212-241-4812; **Board Cert:** Urology 2006; **Med School:** Albert Einstein Coll Med 1987; **Resid:** Urology, Montefiore Med Ctr 1993; **Fellow:** Male Infertility, Baylor Coll Med 1994; **Fac Appt:** Assoc Prof U, Mount Sinai Sch Med

Belman, A Barry MD [U] - **Spec Exp:** Pediatric Urology; Hypospadias; **Hospital:** Chldns Natl Med Ctr; **Address:** Chldns Natl Med Ctr, 111 Michigan Ave NW, Washington, DC 20010-2978; **Phone:** 202-476-5042; **Board Cert:** Urology 1973; Pediatric Urology 2008; **Med School:** Northwestern Univ 1964; **Resid:** Urology, Northwestern Univ Med Ctr 1970; **Fac Appt:** Prof U, Geo Wash Univ

Benson, Mitchell C MD [U] - **Spec Exp:** Prostate Cancer/Robotic Surgery; Bladder Cancer; Kidney Cancer; Continent Urinary Diversions; **Hospital:** NY-Presby Hosp/Columbia (page 66); **Address:** NY Presby Hosp-Columbia, Dept Urology, 161 Ft Washington Ave Fl 11 - rm 1102, New York, NY 10032-3713; **Phone:** 212-305-5201; **Board Cert:** Urology 1984; **Med School:** Columbia P&S 1977; **Resid:** Surgery, Mount Sinai Med Ctr 1979; Urology, Columbia-Presby Hosp 1982; **Fellow:** Oncology, Johns Hopkins Hosp 1984; **Fac Appt:** Prof U, Columbia P&S

Blaivas, Jerry G MD [U] - **Spec Exp:** Uro-Gynecology; Urology-Female; Neurogenic Bladder; Incontinence after Prostate Cancer; **Hospital:** NY-Presby Hosp/Weill Cornell (page 66), Lenox Hill Hosp (page 62); **Address:** 445 E 77th St, New York, NY 10021; **Phone:** 212-772-3900; **Board Cert:** Urology 1978; **Med School:** Tufts Univ 1964; **Resid:** Surgery, Boston Med Ctr 1971; Urology, New England Med Ctr 1976; **Fac Appt:** Clin Prof U, Cornell Univ-Weill Med Coll

Burnett II, Arthur L MD [U] - **Spec Exp:** Prostate Cancer; Erectile Dysfunction; **Hospital:** Johns Hopkins Hosp (page 61); **Address:** 600 N Wolfe St, Marburg Bldg, Ste 407, Baltimore, MD 21287; **Phone:** 410-614-3986; **Board Cert:** Urology 2007; **Med School:** Johns Hopkins Univ 1988; **Resid:** Surgery, Johns Hopkins Hosp 1990; Urology, Johns Hopkins Hosp 1994; **Fac Appt:** Prof U, Johns Hopkins Univ

Canning, Douglas MD [U] - **Spec Exp:** Pediatric Urology; Hypospadias; **Hospital:** Chldns Hosp of Philadelphia, The; **Address:** Childrens Hosp, Div Urology, 34th St & Civic Center Blvd, Wood Bldg, 3rd Fl, Philadelphia, PA 19104; **Phone:** 215-590-2754; **Board Cert:** Urology 2000; **Med School:** Dartmouth Med Sch 1982; **Resid:** Urology, Naval Hosp 1987; **Fellow:** Pediatric Urology, Johns Hopkins Hosp 1988; **Fac Appt:** Assoc Prof U, Univ Pennsylvania

Carter, H Ballentine MD [U] - **Spec Exp:** Prostate Cancer; **Hospital:** Johns Hopkins Hosp (page 61); **Address:** Brady Urological Inst, Johns Hopkins Hosp, 600 N Wolfe St Marburg Bldg - rm 145, Baltimore, MD 21287-2101; **Phone:** 410-955-0833; **Board Cert:** Urology 1999; **Med School:** Med Univ SC 1981; **Resid:** Surgery, New York Hosp 1983; Urology, New York Hosp 1987; **Fellow:** Research, Johns Hopkins Hosp 1989; **Fac Appt:** Prof U, Johns Hopkins Univ

Docimo, Steven G MD [U] - **Spec Exp:** Pediatric Urology; Minimally Invasive Surgery; Bladder Reconstruction; Voiding Dysfunction; **Hospital:** Chldns Hosp of Pittsburgh - UPMC; **Address:** Executive Suites Children's Hosp of Pittsburgh, Children's Hosp Drive, Pittsburgh, PA 15201; **Phone:** 412-692-7932; **Board Cert:** Urology 2000; Pediatric Urology 2008; **Med School:** Johns Hopkins Univ 1984; **Resid:** Surgery, Georgetown Univ Med Ctr 1986; Urology, Brigham & Womens Hosp 1990; **Fellow:** Pediatric Urology, Johns Hopkins 1994; Research, Childrens Hosp 1988; **Fac Appt:** Prof U, Univ Pittsburgh

Droller, Michael J MD [U] - **Spec Exp:** Urologic Cancer; Bladder Cancer; Prostate Cancer; Kidney Cancer; **Hospital:** Mount Sinai Med Ctr (page 64); **Address:** 5 E 98th St Fl 6, Box 1272, New York, NY 10029-6501; **Phone:** 212-241-3868; **Board Cert:** Urology 2001; **Med School:** Harvard Med Sch 1968; **Resid:** Surgery, Peter Bent Brigham Hosp 1970; Urology, Stanford Univ Med Ctr 1976; **Fellow:** Immunology, Univ Stockholm 1977; **Fac Appt:** Prof U, Mount Sinai Sch Med

Fisch, Harry MD [U] - **Spec Exp:** Infertility-Male; Microsurgery; Vasectomy Reversal; **Hospital:** NY-Presby Hosp/Columbia (page 66), Lenox Hill Hosp (page 62); **Address:** 944 Park Ave, Ste 1C, New York, NY 10028; **Phone:** 212-879-0800; **Board Cert:** Urology 1999; **Med School:** Mount Sinai Sch Med 1983; **Resid:** Surgery, Montefiore Med Ctr 1985; Urology, Montefiore Med Ctr 1989; **Fac Appt:** Prof U, Columbia P&S

Gearhart, John P MD [U] - **Spec Exp:** Pediatric Urology; **Hospital:** Johns Hopkins Hosp (page 61); **Address:** Johns Hopkins Hospital, Brady Urological Institute, 600 N Wolfe St Marburg Bldg - Ste 146, Baltimore, MD 21287-2101; **Phone:** 410-955-5358; **Board Cert:** Urology 1982; **Med School:** Univ Louisville Sch Med 1975; **Resid:** Urology, Med Coll Georgia Hosp 1980; **Fellow:** Pediatric Urology, Alder Hey Chldns Hosp 1981; Pediatric Urology, Johns Hopkins Hosp 1985; **Fac Appt:** Prof U, Johns Hopkins Univ

Glassberg, Kenneth MD [U] - **Spec Exp:** Pediatric Urology; Genital Reconstruction; Varicocele In Adolescents; **Hospital:** NYPresby-Morgan Stanley Children's Hosp (page 66); **Address:** Morgan Stanley Chlds Hosp of NY-Presby, 3959 Broadway, BHN 1118, New York, NY 10032; **Phone:** 212-305-9918; **Board Cert:** Urology 1977; **Med School:** SUNY Downstate 1968; **Resid:** Surgery, Montefiore Hosp Med Ctr 1972; Urology, Univ Hosp 1975; **Fellow:** Pediatric Urology, Adler Hey Chldns Hosp 1976; Pediatric Urology, Hosp For Sick Chldn 1976; **Fac Appt:** Prof U, Columbia P&S

Goldstein, Marc MD [U] - **Spec Exp:** Infertility-Male; Vasectomy Reversal; Varicocele Microsurgery; Erectile Dysfunction; **Hospital:** NY-Presby Hosp/Weill Cornell (page 66); **Address:** Cornell Inst for Reproductive Med, 525 E 68th St, Box 580, New York, NY 10021-4870; **Phone:** 212-746-5470; **Board Cert:** Urology 1982; **Med School:** SUNY Downstate 1972; **Resid:** Surgery, Columbia-Presby Med Ctr 1974; Urology, SUNY Downstate Med Ctr 1980; **Fellow:** Microsurgery, Rockefeller Univ 1982; **Fac Appt:** Prof U, Cornell Univ-Weill Med Coll

Urology

Gomella, Leonard G MD [U] - **Spec Exp:** Prostate Cancer; Minimally Invasive Urologic Surgery; Urologic Cancer; **Hospital:** Thomas Jefferson Univ Hosp; **Address:** Thomas Jefferson Univ, 1015 Walnut St Fl 11 - Ste 1112, Philadelphia, PA 19107-5001; **Phone:** 215-955-1000; **Board Cert:** Urology 1998; **Med School:** Univ KY Coll Med 1980; **Resid:** Surgery, Univ Kentucky Med Ctr 1982; Urology, Univ Kentucky Med Ctr 1986; **Fellow:** Urologic Oncology, Natl Cancer Inst 1988; **Fac Appt:** Prof U, Jefferson Med Coll

Grasso, Michael MD [U] - **Spec Exp:** Urologic Cancer; Laparoscopic Surgery; Kidney Stones; Testicular Cancer; **Hospital:** St Vincent Cath Med Ctrs - Manhattan; **Address:** 170 W 12th St, Dept Urology - Cronin 205, New York, NY 10011; **Phone:** 212-604-1270; **Board Cert:** Urology 2002; **Med School:** Jefferson Med Coll 1986; **Resid:** Surgery, Jefferson Univ Hosp 1988; Urology, Jefferson Univ Hosp 1992; **Fac Appt:** Prof U, NY Med Coll

Greenberg, Richard E MD [U] - **Spec Exp:** Prostate Cancer; Bladder Cancer; Kidney Cancer; Prostate Cancer/Robotic Surgery; **Hospital:** Fox Chase Cancer Ctr (page 58), Abington Mem Hosp; **Address:** Fox Chase Cancer Ctr, Div Urol-Dept Surg, 333 Cottman Ave, Ste H3 - rm H3-116, Philadelphia, PA 19111; **Phone:** 215-728-5341; **Board Cert:** Urology 2005; **Med School:** Cornell Univ-Weill Med Coll 1976; **Resid:** Surgery, New York Hosp 1979; Urology, New York Hosp 1983; **Fac Appt:** Prof U, Temple Univ

Gribetz, Michael MD [U] - **Spec Exp:** Prostate Disease; Urology-Female; Sexual Dysfunction; Kidney Stones; **Hospital:** Mount Sinai Med Ctr (page 64); **Address:** 1155 Park Ave, New York, NY 10128-1209; **Phone:** 212-831-1300; **Board Cert:** Urology 1980; **Med School:** Albert Einstein Coll Med 1973; **Resid:** Surgery, Montefiore Med Ctr 1975; Urology, Mt Sinai Hosp 1978; **Fac Appt:** Asst Clin Prof U, Mount Sinai Sch Med

Hall, Simon J MD [U] - **Spec Exp:** Urologic Cancer; Minimally Invasive Urologic Surgery; Continent Urinary Diversions; Prostate Cancer; **Hospital:** Mount Sinai Med Ctr (page 64); **Address:** Mount Sinai Medical Ctr, 5 98th St, Box 1272, New York, NY 10029; **Phone:** 212-241-4812; **Board Cert:** Urology 2009; **Med School:** Columbia P&S 1988; **Resid:** Surgery, Mt Sinai Med Ctr 1990; Urology, Boston Univ 1994; **Fellow:** Urology, Baylor Coll Med 1996; **Fac Appt:** Assoc Prof U, Mount Sinai Sch Med

Hensle, Terry MD [U] - **Spec Exp:** Pediatric Urology; Hypospadias; Urinary Reconstruction; Wilms' Tumor; **Hospital:** NYPresby-Morgan Stanley Children's Hosp (page 66), Hackensack Univ Med Ctr; **Address:** Morgan Stanley Chldns Hosp of NY-Presby, 3959 Broadway, Ste 219N, New York, NY 10032; **Phone:** 212-305-8510; **Board Cert:** Urology 1978; **Med School:** Cornell Univ-Weill Med Coll 1968; **Resid:** Surgery, Boston City Hosp 1973; Urology, Mass Genl Hosp 1976; **Fellow:** Pediatric Urology, Mass Genl Hosp 1977; Pediatric Urology, Great Ormond St Hosp 1978; **Fac Appt:** Prof U, Columbia P&S

Herr, Harry W MD [U] - **Spec Exp:** Bladder Cancer; Prostate Cancer; Testicular Cancer; **Hospital:** Meml Sloan-Kettering Cancer Ctr, NY-Presby Hosp/Weill Cornell (page 66); **Address:** 1275 York Avenue, New York, NY 10065; **Phone:** 800-525-2225; **Board Cert:** Urology 1976; **Med School:** UCSF 1969; **Resid:** Urology, UC Irvine Med Ctr 1974; **Fellow:** Urology, Meml Sloan Kettering Cancer Ctr 1976; **Fac Appt:** Assoc Prof S, Cornell Univ-Weill Med Coll

Hrebinko Jr, Ronald L MD [U] - **Spec Exp:** Urologic Cancer; Kidney Cancer; Bladder Cancer; Testicular Cancer; **Hospital:** UPMC Presby, Pittsburgh; **Address:** Univ Pittsburgh Dept of Urology, Shadyside Medical Bldg, Ste 209, 5200 Centre Ave, Pittsburgh, PA 15232; **Phone:** 412-605-3022; **Board Cert:** Urology 2004; **Med School:** Univ Pittsburgh 1986; **Resid:** Urology, Univ Pittsburgh Med Ctr 1992; **Fellow:** Urologic Oncology, Roswell Park Cancer Ctr 1993; **Fac Appt:** Assoc Prof U, Univ Pittsburgh

Huben, Robert P MD [U] - **Spec Exp:** Prostate Cancer; Kidney Cancer; Urologic Cancer; **Hospital:** Roswell Park Cancer Inst; **Address:** Roswell Park Cancer Inst, Dept Urology, Elm & Carlton Sts, Buffalo, NY 14263-0001; **Phone:** 716-845-3389; **Board Cert:** Urology 1983; **Med School:** Cornell Univ-Weill Med Coll 1976; **Resid:** Urology, East Virginia Med Ctr 1981; **Fellow:** Urologic Oncology, Roswell Park Meml Inst 1982

Jackman, Stephen V MD [U] - **Spec Exp:** Prostate Cancer/Robotic Surgery; Laparoscopic Surgery; Kidney Stones; **Hospital:** UPMC Shadyside, UPMC Presby, Pittsburgh; **Address:** UPMC, Kaufman Bldg, 3471 Fifth Ave, Ste 700, Pittsburgh, PA 15213; **Phone:** 412-692-4095; **Board Cert:** Urology 2002; **Med School:** Yale Univ 1994; **Resid:** Urology, Johns Hopkins Hosp 1999; **Fac Appt:** Assoc Prof U, Univ Pittsburgh

Jarow, Jonathan P MD [U] - **Spec Exp:** Infertility-Male; Prostate Cancer; Erectile Dysfunction; Incontinence after Prostate Cancer; **Hospital:** Johns Hopkins Hosp (page 61); **Address:** Johns Hopkins Outpatient Ctr-Urology, 601 N Caroline St, Fl 4, Baltimore, MD 21287; **Phone:** 410-955-3617; **Board Cert:** Urology 2007; **Med School:** Northwestern Univ 1980; **Resid:** Surgery, Johns Hopkins Hosp 1982; Urology, Johns Hopkins Hosp 1986; **Fellow:** Andrology, Baylor Univ 1989; **Fac Appt:** Assoc Prof U, Johns Hopkins Univ

Kaplan, Steven A MD [U] - **Spec Exp:** Urodynamics; Voiding Dysfunction; Incontinence after Prostate Cancer; Incontinence; **Hospital:** NY-Presby Hosp/Weill Cornell (page 66); **Address:** NY Presbyterian-Weill Cornell Med Ctr, 525 E 68th St, rm F9West, New York, NY 10021-4870; **Phone:** 212-746-4811; **Board Cert:** Urology 2001; **Med School:** Mount Sinai Sch Med 1982; **Resid:** Surgery, Mount Sinai Hosp 1984; Urology, Columbia Presby Med Ctr 1988; **Fellow:** Urology, Columbia Presby Med Ctr 1990; **Fac Appt:** Prof U, Cornell Univ-Weill Med Coll

Katz, Aaron E MD [U] - **Spec Exp:** Prostate Cancer-Cryosurgery; Kidney Cancer-Cryosurgery; Complementary Medicine; Nutrition & Cancer Prevention; **Hospital:** NY-Presby Hosp/Columbia (page 66); **Address:** NY Presby Med Ctr, Herbert Irving Pav, 161 Ft Washington Ave Fl 11, New York, NY 10032; **Phone:** 212-305-6408; **Board Cert:** Urology 2006; **Med School:** NY Med Coll 1986; **Resid:** Urology, Maimonides Med Ctr 1992; **Fellow:** Urologic Oncology, Columbia Presby Med Ctr 1993; **Fac Appt:** Assoc Clin Prof U, Columbia P&S

Kavoussi, Louis R MD [U] - **Spec Exp:** Laparoscopic Surgery; Kidney Stones; Urologic Cancer; Prostate Cancer; **Hospital:** Long Island Jewish Med Ctr, N Shore Univ Hosp; **Address:** 450 Lakeville Rd, Ste M-41, New Hyde Park, NY 11040; **Phone:** 516-734-8558; **Board Cert:** Urology 1999; **Med School:** SUNY Buffalo 1983; **Resid:** Surgery, Barnes Jewish Hosp 1985; Urology, Barnes Jewish Hosp 1989; **Fac Appt:** Prof U, NYU Sch Med

Kirschenbaum, Alexander M MD [U] - **Spec Exp:** Prostate Cancer; Bladder Cancer; Kidney Cancer; **Hospital:** Mount Sinai Med Ctr (page 64); **Address:** 58A E 79th St, New York, NY 10021; **Phone:** 646-422-0926; **Board Cert:** Urology 2006; **Med School:** Mount Sinai Sch Med 1980; **Resid:** Surgery, Mt Sinai Hosp 1982; Urology, Mt Sinai Hosp 1985; **Fellow:** Urologic Oncology, Mt Sinai Hosp 1987; **Fac Appt:** Assoc Prof U, Mount Sinai Sch Med

Lanteri, Vincent J MD [U] - **Spec Exp:** Prostate Cancer/Robotic Surgery; Urologic Cancer; Minimally Invasive Urologic Surgery; **Hospital:** Hackensack Univ Med Ctr, Monmouth Med Ctr; **Address:** 255 W Spring Valley Ave, Ste 101, Maywood, NJ 07607; **Phone:** 201-487-8866; **Board Cert:** Urology 1982; **Med School:** Mexico 1974; **Resid:** Surgery, UMDNJ Med Ctr 1977; Urology, UMDNJ Med Ctr 1980; **Fellow:** Urologic Oncology, Roswell Park Cancer Inst 1981

Lepor, Herbert MD [U] - **Spec Exp:** Prostate Cancer; **Hospital:** NYU Langone Med Ctr (page 67); **Address:** 150 E 32nd St Fl 2, New York, NY 10016; **Phone:** 646-825-6327; **Board Cert:** Urology 2006; **Med School:** Johns Hopkins Univ 1975; **Resid:** Urology, Johns Hopkins Hosp 1986; **Fac Appt:** Prof U, NYU Sch Med

Urology

Linsenmeyer, Todd A MD [U] - **Spec Exp:** Infertility-Male in Spinal Cord Injury; Voiding Dysfunction/Spinal Cord Injury; Urodynamics in Spinal Cord Injury; **Hospital:** Kessler Inst for Rehab - W Orange; **Address:** Kessler Inst Rehab, 1199 Pleasant Valley Way, West Orange, NJ 07052; **Phone:** 973-731-3900 x2274; **Board Cert:** Urology 2005; Physical Medicine & Rehabilitation 1990; Spinal Cord Injury Medicine 2002; **Med School:** Univ Hawaii JA Burns Sch Med 1979; **Resid:** Urology, Tripler AMC 1984; **Fellow:** Physical Medicine & Rehabilitation, Stanford Univ Hosp 1989; **Fac Appt:** Assoc Prof S, UMDNJ-NJ Med Sch, Newark

Lowe, Franklin MD [U] - **Spec Exp:** Prostate Disease; Complementary Medicine; Prostate Cancer; **Hospital:** St Luke's - Roosevelt Hosp Ctr - Roosevelt Div (page 57), NY-Presby Hosp/Columbia (page 66); **Address:** 425 W 59th St, Ste 3A, New York, NY 10019-1104; **Phone:** 212-523-7790; **Board Cert:** Urology 2006; **Med School:** Columbia P&S 1979; **Resid:** Surgery, Johns Hopkins Hosp 1981; Urology, Johns Hopkins Hosp 1984; **Fac Appt:** Clin Prof U, Columbia P&S

Malkowicz, S Bruce MD [U] - **Spec Exp:** Prostate Cancer; Bladder Cancer; Kidney Cancer; Gene Therapy; **Hospital:** Hosp Univ Penn - UPHS (page 60); **Address:** Hosp Univ Penn, Dept Urology, 3400 Spruce St, 9 Penn Tower, Philadelphia, PA 19104; **Phone:** 215-662-2891; **Board Cert:** Urology 2000; **Med School:** Univ Pennsylvania 1981; **Resid:** Surgery, Hosp Univ Penn 1983; Urology, Hosp Univ Penn 1987; **Fellow:** Urologic Oncology, USC Med Ctr 1998; Urologic Oncology, Hosp Univ Penn/Wistar Inst 1990; **Fac Appt:** Assoc Prof U, Univ Pennsylvania

McCullough, Andrew R MD [U] - **Spec Exp:** Erectile Dysfunction; Infertility-Male; Prostate Cancer; **Hospital:** NYU Langone Med Ctr (page 67); **Address:** NYU Med Ctr, Dept Urology, 150 E 32nd St Fl 2, New York, NY 10016; **Phone:** 646-825-6311; **Board Cert:** Urology 2005; **Med School:** Univ MD Sch Med 1978; **Resid:** Urology, Johns Hopkins Hosp 1983; **Fellow:** Urologic Oncology, Johns Hopkins Hosp 1984; **Fac Appt:** Assoc Prof U, NYU Sch Med

Mohler, James L MD [U] - **Spec Exp:** Prostate Cancer; **Hospital:** Roswell Park Cancer Inst; **Address:** Roswell Park Cancer Institute, Elm and Carlton Streets, Buffalo, NY 14263; **Phone:** 716-845-3159; **Board Cert:** Urology 2007; **Med School:** Med Coll GA 1980; **Resid:** Surgery, Univ Kentucky Med Ctr 1982; Urology, Univ Kentucky Med Ctr 1985; **Fellow:** Urologic Oncology, Johns Hopkins Hosp 1987; **Fac Appt:** Prof U, SUNY Buffalo

Mostwin, Jacek L MD/PhD [U] - **Spec Exp:** Prostate Cancer; **Hospital:** Johns Hopkins Hosp (page 61); **Address:** Johns Hopkins Hosp, 600 N Wolfe St Park 207 Bldg, Baltimore, MD 21287; **Phone:** 410-955-4461; **Board Cert:** Urology 2007; **Med School:** Univ MD Sch Med 1975; **Resid:** Surgery, Univ Michigan Med Ctr 1978; Urology, Johns Hopkins Hosp 1983; **Fac Appt:** Prof U, Johns Hopkins Univ

Mulhall, John P MD [U] - **Spec Exp:** Erectile Dysfunction; Peyronie's Disease; Penile Prostheses; Infertility-Male; **Hospital:** Meml Sloan-Kettering Cancer Ctr; **Address:** Prostate Ctr at Meml Sloan Kettering, 353 E 68th St Fl 5, New York, NY 10021; **Phone:** 646-422-4359; **Board Cert:** Urology 1999; **Med School:** Ireland 1985; **Resid:** Urology, Univ Conn Health Ctr 1995; **Fellow:** Urology, Boston Univ Med Ctr 1996; **Fac Appt:** Assoc Prof U, Cornell Univ-Weill Med Coll

Nagler, Harris M MD [U] - **Spec Exp:** Vasectomy Reversal; Infertility-Male; Varicocele Microsurgery; Erectile Dysfunction; **Hospital:** Beth Israel Med Ctr - Petrie Division (page 57); **Address:** Beth Israel Med Ctr, Dept Urology, 10 Union Square E, Ste 3A, New York, NY 10003-3314; **Phone:** 212-844-8700; **Board Cert:** Urology 1982; **Med School:** Temple Univ 1975; **Resid:** Urology, Columbia Presby Med Ctr 1980; **Fellow:** Reproductive Medicine, Columbia Presby Med Ctr 1981; **Fac Appt:** Prof U, Albert Einstein Coll Med

Naslund, Michael MD [U] - **Spec Exp:** Prostate Cancer; Prostate Disease; **Hospital:** Univ of MD Med Ctr; **Address:** Maryland Prostate Ctr, 419 W Redwood St, Ste 320, Baltimore, MD 21201; **Phone:** 410-328-0800; **Board Cert:** Urology 2008; **Med School:** Johns Hopkins Univ 1981; **Resid:** Surgery, Johns Hopkins Hosp 1983; Urology, Johns Hopkins Hosp 1987; **Fac Appt:** Prof U, Univ MD Sch Med

Nelson, Joel B MD [U] - **Spec Exp:** Prostate Cancer; **Hospital:** UPMC Shadyside; **Address:** UPMC Shadyside Med Ctr, 5200 Centre Ave, Ste 209, Pittsburgh, PA 15232-1312; **Phone:** 412-605-3013; **Board Cert:** Urology 2008; **Med School:** Northwestern Univ 1988; **Resid:** Surgery, Northwestern Meml Hosp 1990; Urology, Northwestern Meml Hosp 1994; **Fellow:** Urology, Johns Hopkins Hosp; **Fac Appt:** Prof U, Univ Pittsburgh

Nitti, Victor MD [U] - **Spec Exp:** Urology-Female; Incontinence-Male & Female; Urodynamics; Voiding Dysfunction; **Hospital:** NYU Langone Med Ctr (page 67); **Address:** 150 E 32nd St, Ste 200, New York, NY 10016; **Phone:** 646-825-6324; **Board Cert:** Urology 2002; **Med School:** UMDNJ-NJ Med Sch, Newark 1985; **Resid:** Surgery, Univ Hosp 1987; Urology, Univ Hosp 1991; **Fellow:** Urology, UCLA Med Ctr 1992; **Fac Appt:** Assoc Prof U, NYU Sch Med

Partin, Alan W MD/PhD [U] - **Spec Exp:** Prostate Cancer; Prostate Disease; **Hospital:** Johns Hopkins Hosp (page 61); **Address:** Johns Hopkins Hosp, 600 N Wolfe St Marburg Bldg - rm 134, Baltimore, MD 21287; **Phone:** 410-614-4876; **Board Cert:** Urology 2007; **Med School:** Johns Hopkins Univ 1989; **Resid:** Surgery, Johns Hopkins Hosp 1991; Urology, Johns Hopkins Hosp 1996; **Fac Appt:** Prof U, Johns Hopkins Univ

Poppas, Dix P MD [U] - **Spec Exp:** Genital Reconstruction-Pediatric; Robotic Surgery-Pediatric; Minimally Invasive Surgery-Pediatric; **Hospital:** NY-Presby Hosp/Weill Cornell (page 66); **Address:** Inst for Pediatric Urology, NY Presby Hosp-Weill Cornell, 525 E 68th St, Box 94, New York, NY 10021-4870; **Phone:** 212-746-5337; **Board Cert:** Urology 1999; Pediatric Urology 2008; **Med School:** Eastern VA Med Sch 1988; **Resid:** Urology, NY Hosp-Cornell Med Ctr 1994; **Fellow:** Pediatric Urology, Chldns Hosp Harvard Med Sch 1996; **Fac Appt:** Prof U, Cornell Univ-Weill Med Coll

Rushton Jr, H Gil MD [U] - **Spec Exp:** Pediatric Urology; Fetal Urology; Hypospadias; **Hospital:** Chldns Natl Med Ctr; **Address:** Dept Urology, 111 Michigan Ave NW, Washington, DC 20010; **Phone:** 202-476-5042; **Board Cert:** Urology 2004; **Med School:** Univ SC Sch Med 1978; **Resid:** Urology, Univ SC Med Ctr 1983; **Fellow:** Pediatric Urology, Hosp Sick Chldn 1984; Pediatric Urology, Emory Chldns Hosp 1986; **Fac Appt:** Prof U, Geo Wash Univ

Samadi, David B MD [U] - **Spec Exp:** Prostate Cancer/Robotic Surgery; Kidney Cancer; Bladder Cancer; Urologic Cancer; **Hospital:** Mount Sinai Med Ctr (page 64), N Genl Hosp; **Address:** 625 Madison Ave Fl 2, New York, NY 10029; **Phone:** 212-241-8779; **Board Cert:** Urology 2004; **Med School:** SUNY Stony Brook 1994; **Resid:** Surgery, Montefiore Med Ctr 2000; Urology, Montefiore Med Ctr 2002; **Fellow:** Urologic Oncology, Meml Sloan Kettering Cancer Ctr 2003; Laparoscopic Surgery, Henri Mondor Hosp; **Fac Appt:** Assoc Prof U, Mount Sinai Sch Med

Sawczuk, Ihor S MD [U] - **Spec Exp:** Kidney Cancer; Bladder Cancer; Prostate Cancer/Robotic Surgery; Bladder Reconstruction; **Hospital:** Hackensack Univ Med Ctr, NY-Presby Hosp/Columbia (page 66); **Address:** Hackensack Univ Med Ctr, 360 Essex St, Ste 403, Hackensack, NJ 07601; **Phone:** 201-336-8090; **Board Cert:** Urology 2005; **Med School:** Med Coll PA Hahnemann 1979; **Resid:** Surgery, St Vincents Hosp 1981; Urology, Columbia-Presby Med Ctr 1984; **Fellow:** Urologic Oncology, Columbia-Presby Med Ctr 1986; **Fac Appt:** Prof U, Columbia P&S

Urology

Scardino, Peter T MD [U] - **Spec Exp:** Prostate Cancer; Bladder Cancer; Urologic Cancer; Urinary Reconstruction; **Hospital:** Meml Sloan-Kettering Cancer Ctr; **Address:** 1275 York Avenue, New York, NY 10065; **Phone:** 646-422-4329; **Board Cert:** Urology 1981; **Med School:** Duke Univ 1971; **Resid:** Surgery, Mass Genl Hosp 1973; Urology, UCLA Med Ctr 1979; **Fellow:** Urology, Natl Cancer Inst 1976; **Fac Appt:** Prof U, Cornell Univ-Weill Med Coll

Scherr, Douglas S MD [U] - **Spec Exp:** Prostate Cancer/Robotic Surgery; Bladder Cancer; Robotic Surgery; Testicular Cancer; **Hospital:** NY-Presby Hosp/Weill Cornell (page 66); **Address:** NY Cornell Medical Ctr, Dept Urology, 525 E 68th St Starr 900, New York, NY 10021; **Phone:** 212-746-5788; **Board Cert:** Urology 2003; **Med School:** Geo Wash Univ 1994; **Resid:** Urology, NY Hosp-Cornell Med Ctr 1999; **Fellow:** Urologic Oncology, Meml Sloan-Kettering Canc Ctr 2002; **Fac Appt:** Assoc Prof U, Cornell Univ-Weill Med Coll

Schlegel, Peter N MD [U] - **Spec Exp:** Prostate Cancer; Infertility-Male; **Hospital:** NY-Presby Hosp/Weill Cornell (page 66); **Address:** 525 E 68th St, Starr 900, New York, NY 10021-4870; **Phone:** 212-746-5491; **Board Cert:** Urology 2001; **Med School:** Univ Mass Sch Med 1983; **Resid:** Surgery, Johns Hopkins Hosp 1985; Urology, Johns Hopkins Hosp 1989; **Fellow:** Medical Oncology, Johns Hopkins Hosp 1987; Male Reproduction, NY Hosp-Cornell Med Ctr 1991; **Fac Appt:** Prof U, Cornell Univ-Weill Med Coll

Schoenberg, Mark P MD [U] - **Spec Exp:** Bladder Cancer; Urinary Reconstruction; **Hospital:** Johns Hopkins Hosp (page 61); **Address:** Johns Hopkins Hospital, 150 Marburg Bldg, 600 N Wolfe St, Baltimore, MD 21287-2101; **Phone:** 410-502-3803; **Board Cert:** Urology 2005; **Med School:** Univ Tex, Houston 1986; **Resid:** Surgery, Hosp U Penn 1988; Urologic Surgery, Hosp U Penn 1992; **Fellow:** Urologic Oncology, Brady Inst/Johns Hopkins 1994; **Fac Appt:** Prof U, Johns Hopkins Univ

Sheinfeld, Joel MD [U] - **Spec Exp:** Testicular Cancer; Bladder Cancer; Fertility Preservation in Cancer; **Hospital:** Meml Sloan-Kettering Cancer Ctr; **Address:** 1275 York Avenue, New York, NY 10065; **Phone:** 800-525-2225; **Board Cert:** Urology 2000; **Med School:** Univ Fla Coll Med 1981; **Resid:** Urology, Strong Meml Hosp 1986; **Fellow:** Urologic Oncology, Meml Sloan Kettering Cancer Ctr 1989; **Fac Appt:** Assoc Prof U, Cornell Univ-Weill Med Coll

Shenot, Patrick J MD [U] - **Spec Exp:** Voiding Dysfunction/Spinal Cord Injury; Voiding Dysfunction; Genitourinary Disorders; Incontinence; **Hospital:** Thomas Jefferson Univ Hosp, Magee Rehab Hosp; **Address:** 833 Chestnut St, Ste 703, Philadelphia, PA 19107; **Phone:** 215-955-1000; **Board Cert:** Urology 2000; **Med School:** SUNY Stony Brook 1991; **Resid:** Surgery, Thos Jefferson Univ Hosp 1993; Urology, Thos Jefferson Univ Hosp 1997; **Fac Appt:** Asst Prof U, Thomas Jefferson Univ

Snyder III, Howard M MD [U] - **Spec Exp:** Pediatric Urology; Genital Reconstruction; Reconstructive Urologic Surgery; **Hospital:** Chldns Hosp of Philadelphia, The; **Address:** Chldrns Hosp, Dept Ped Urology, 34th St & Civic Ctr Blvd, Wood Bldg, Fl 3, Philadelphia, PA 19104; **Phone:** 215-590-2767; **Board Cert:** Surgery 1995; Urology 1982; Pediatric Surgery 1995; **Med School:** Harvard Med Sch 1969; **Resid:** Surgery, Peter Bent Brigham Hosp 1973; Pediatric Surgery, Boston Chldns Hosp Med Ctr 1974; **Fellow:** Urology, Peter Bent Brigham Hosp 1980; **Fac Appt:** Prof U, Univ Pennsylvania

Sosa, R Ernest MD [U] - **Spec Exp:** Kidney Stones; Laparoscopic Surgery; Adrenal Surgery; **Hospital:** NY-Presby Hosp/Weill Cornell (page 66), Lenox Hill Hosp (page 62); **Address:** 880 5th Ave, New York, NY 10021; **Phone:** 212-570-6800; **Board Cert:** Urology 2006; **Med School:** Cornell Univ-Weill Med Coll 1978; **Resid:** Surgery, NY Hosp-Cornell 1980; Urology, NY Hosp-Cornell 1984; **Fellow:** Renal Physiology, NY Hosp-Cornell 1986; **Fac Appt:** Assoc Clin Prof U, Cornell Univ-Weill Med Coll

Taneja, Samir S MD [U] - **Spec Exp:** Kidney Cancer; Prostate Cancer; Bladder Cancer; **Hospital:** NYU Langone Med Ctr (page 67); **Address:** NYU Urology Assocs, 150 E 32nd St Fl 2, New York, NY 10016-6024; **Phone:** 646-825-6321; **Board Cert:** Urology 1999; **Med School:** Northwestern Univ 1990; **Resid:** Urology, UCLA Med Ctr 1996; **Fellow:** Urologic Oncology, NYU Med Ctr 1998; **Fac Appt:** Assoc Prof U, NYU Sch Med

Tewari, Ashutosh MD [U] - **Spec Exp:** Prostate Cancer/Robotic Surgery; **Hospital:** NY-Presby Hosp/Weill Cornell (page 66); **Address:** Weill Cornell Brady Urologic Health Ct, 525 E 68th St, Starr 916, New York, NY 10065; **Phone:** 212-746-5638; **Board Cert:** Urology 2006; **Med School:** India 1984; **Resid:** Surgery, GSVM Medical College 1990; Urology, Henry Ford Hosp 2003; **Fellow:** Transplant Surgery, Liverpool Univ Med Ctr 1993; Urologic Oncology, Shands Healthcare 1995; **Fac Appt:** Assoc Prof U, Cornell Univ-Weill Med Coll

Uzzo, Robert MD [U] - **Spec Exp:** Bladder Cancer; Prostate Cancer; Robotic Surgery; Minimally Invasive Urologic Surgery; **Hospital:** Fox Chase Cancer Ctr (page 58); **Address:** 333 Cottman Ave, rm H3116, Philadelphia, PA 19111; **Phone:** 215-728-3501; **Board Cert:** Urology 2001; **Med School:** Cornell Univ-Weill Med Coll 1991; **Resid:** Surgery, New York Hosp-Cornell Med Ctr 1993; Urology, New York Hosp-Cornell Med Ctr 1997; **Fellow:** Urologic Oncology, Cleveland Clinic 1999; Renal Transplant, Cleveland Clinic 2000; **Fac Appt:** Assoc Prof S, Temple Univ

Van Arsdalen, Keith N MD [U] - **Spec Exp:** Infertility-Male; Varicocele Microsurgery; Urologic Cancer; Vasectomy Reversal; **Hospital:** Hosp Univ Penn - UPHS (page 60), Chldns Hosp of Philadelphia, The; **Address:** Hosp Univ Penn, Div Urology, 3400 Spruce St, 9 Penn Tower, Philadelphia, PA 19104-4283; **Phone:** 215-662-2891; **Board Cert:** Urology 1984; **Med School:** Med Coll VA 1977; **Resid:** Surgery, Univ Maryland Hosp 1979; Urology, Med Coll Virginia 1982; **Fellow:** Urodynamics, Hosp Univ Penn 1983; **Fac Appt:** Prof U, Univ Pennsylvania

Vapnek, Jonathan M MD [U] - **Spec Exp:** Incontinence; Urology-Female; Neurogenic Bladder; Urodynamics; **Hospital:** Mount Sinai Med Ctr (page 64); **Address:** 229 E 79th St, New York, NY 10021; **Phone:** 212-717-9500; **Board Cert:** Urology 2005; **Med School:** UCSD 1986; **Resid:** Surgery, UCSD Med Ctr 1988; Urology, UCSF Med Ctr 1992; **Fellow:** Neurourology, UC Davis Med Ctr 1993; **Fac Appt:** Assoc Clin Prof U, Mount Sinai Sch Med

Vaughan, Edwin D MD [U] - **Spec Exp:** Urologic Cancer; Adrenal Tumors; Prostate Disease; **Hospital:** NY-Presby Hosp/Weill Cornell (page 66); **Address:** New York Presby Hosp, Dept Urology, 525 E 68th St, Starr 900, Box 94, New York, NY 10021-4870; **Phone:** 212-746-5480; **Board Cert:** Urology 1986; **Med School:** Univ VA Sch Med 1965; **Resid:** Surgery, Vanderbilt Univ Med Ctr 1967; Urology, Univ Virginia Hosp 1971; **Fellow:** Internal Medicine, Columbia Univ 1973; **Fac Appt:** Prof U, Cornell Univ-Weill Med Coll

Walsh, Patrick MD [U] - **Spec Exp:** Prostate Cancer; **Hospital:** Johns Hopkins Hosp (page 61); **Address:** Brady Urological Inst, 600 N Wolfe St, Park 224, Baltimore, MD 21287-2101; **Phone:** 410-955-6100; **Board Cert:** Urology 1975; **Med School:** Case West Res Univ 1964; **Resid:** Surgery, Peter Bent Brigham Hosp/Childrens Hosp 1967; Urology, UCLA Med Ctr 1971; **Fellow:** Endocrinology, Harbor Genl Hosp 1970; **Fac Appt:** Prof U, Johns Hopkins Univ

Wein, Alan J MD [U] - **Spec Exp:** Neuro-Urology; Prostate Cancer; Testicular Cancer; Bladder Cancer; **Hospital:** Hosp Univ Penn - UPHS (page 60), Pennsylvania Hosp (page 60); **Address:** Univ Penn Hlth System, Div Urology, 34th & Civic Center Blvd, 9 Penn Tower, Philadelphia, PA 19104-4283; **Phone:** 215-662-6755; **Board Cert:** Urology 1995; **Med School:** Univ Pennsylvania 1966; **Resid:** Surgery, Hosp Univ Penn 1968; Urology, Hosp Univ Penn 1972; **Fellow:** Urology, Hosp Univ Penn 1969; **Fac Appt:** Prof U, Univ Pennsylvania

Urology

Weiss, Robert E MD [U] - **Spec Exp:** Bladder Cancer; Kidney Cancer; Testicular Cancer; **Hospital:** Robert Wood Johnson Univ Hosp - New Brunswick, Univ Med Ctr - Princeton; **Address:** 1 Robert Wood Johnson Pl Ste MB588, New Brunswick, NJ 08901-1928; **Phone:** 732-235-7775; **Board Cert:** Urology 2004; **Med School:** NYU Sch Med 1985; **Resid:** Surgery, Mount Sinai Med Ctr 1987; Urology, Mount Sinai Med Ctr 1991; **Fellow:** Urologic Oncology, Meml Sloan Kettering Cancer Ctr 1994; **Fac Appt:** Assoc Prof U, UMDNJ-RW Johnson Med Sch

Yu, George W MD [U] - **Spec Exp:** Nutrition & Disease Prevention/Control; Nutrition & Cancer Prevention/Control; **Hospital:** G Washington Univ Hosp, Anne Arundel Med Ctr; **Address:** 122 Defense Hwy, Ste 224, Annapolis, MD 21401; **Phone:** 410-897-0540; **Board Cert:** Urology 1981; **Med School:** Tufts Univ 1973; **Resid:** Surgery, Brigham & Women's Hosp 1976; Urology, Johns Hopkins Hosp 1981; **Fac Appt:** Prof U, Geo Wash Univ

Southeast

Albala, David M MD [U] - **Spec Exp:** Prostate Cancer/Robotic Surgery; Kidney Stones; Laparoscopic Surgery; **Hospital:** Duke Univ Med Ctr, VA Med Ctr - Durham; **Address:** Duke Univ Med Ctr, Green Zone, Box 3457, Durham, NC 27710; **Phone:** 919-668-6401; **Board Cert:** Urology 2002; **Med School:** Mich State Univ 1983; **Resid:** Surgery, Dartmouth-Hitchcock Med Ctr 1985; Urology, Dartmouth-Hitchcock Med Ctr 1990; **Fellow:** Endourology, Wash Univ Med Ctr 1991; **Fac Appt:** Prof U, Duke Univ

Assimos, Dean G MD [U] - **Spec Exp:** Kidney Stones; Reconstructive Urologic Surgery; **Hospital:** Wake Forest Univ Baptist Med Ctr (page 72); **Address:** Wake Forest, Dept Urology, 140 Charlois Blvd, Winston-Salem, NC 27103; **Phone:** 336-716-4131; **Board Cert:** Urology 2003; **Med School:** Loyola Univ-Stritch Sch Med 1977; **Resid:** Surgery, Northwestern Univ Hosp 1979; Urology, Northwestern Univ Hosp 1983; **Fellow:** Urology, Bowman Gray Sch Med 1984; **Fac Appt:** Prof S, Wake Forest Univ

Atala, Anthony MD [U] - **Spec Exp:** Pediatric Urology; Reconstructive Surgery; Hernia; Microsurgery; **Hospital:** Wake Forest Univ Baptist Med Ctr (page 72); **Address:** Wake Forest Univ-Baptist, MC, Dept Urology, Medical Center Blvd, Winston-Salem, NC 27157-1094; **Phone:** 336-716-4131; **Board Cert:** Urology 2004; Pediatric Urology 2008; **Med School:** Univ Louisville Sch Med 1985; **Resid:** Surgery, Univ Louisville Hosp 1987; Urology, Univ Louisville Hosp 1990; **Fellow:** Research, Childrens Hosp/Harvard 1991; Pediatric Urology, Childrens Hosp/Harvard 1992; **Fac Appt:** Prof U, Wake Forest Univ

Beall, Michael E MD [U] - **Spec Exp:** Prostate Cancer; Testicular Cancer; Vasectomy Reversal; **Hospital:** Inova Fairfax Hosp, Reston Hosp Ctr; **Address:** 8503 Arlington Blvd, Ste 310, Fairfax, VA 22031; **Phone:** 703-208-4200; **Board Cert:** Urology 1979; **Med School:** Geo Wash Univ 1972; **Resid:** Urology, Geo Wash Univ Hosp 1977; **Fac Appt:** Assoc Clin Prof U, Geo Wash Univ

Brock III, John W MD [U] - **Spec Exp:** Pediatric Urology; Reconstructive Surgery; **Hospital:** Vanderbilt Children's Hosp; **Address:** Vanderbilt Chldns Hosp, Div Ped Urology, 2200 Childrens Way, 4102 DOT, Nashville, TN 37232-9820; **Phone:** 615-936-1060; **Board Cert:** Urology 2004; Pediatric Urology 2008; **Med School:** Med Coll GA 1978; **Resid:** Urology, Vanderbilt Univ Med Ctr 1983; **Fac Appt:** Prof U, Vanderbilt Univ

Carson III, Culley C MD [U] - **Spec Exp:** Erectile Dysfunction; Kidney Stones; Peyronie's Disease; **Hospital:** Univ NC Hosps; **Address:** Univ North Carolina, Dept Urol, 2113 Physicians Office Bldg, Chapel Hill, NC 27599-7235; **Phone:** 919-966-2571; **Board Cert:** Urology 1980; **Med School:** Geo Wash Univ 1971; **Resid:** Surgery, Dartmouth-Hitchcock Med Ctr 1973; Urology, Mayo Clinic 1978; **Fac Appt:** Prof U, Univ NC Sch Med

Chang, Sam S MD [U] - **Spec Exp:** Urologic Cancer; Prostate Cancer; Prostate Cancer-HIFU Therapy; High Intensity Focused Ultrasound(HIFU); **Hospital:** Vanderbilt Univ Med Ctr; **Address:** Vanderbilt University Med Ctr, A-1302 MCN, Nashville, TN 37232-2765; **Phone:** 615-322-2880; **Board Cert:** Urology 2002; **Med School:** Vanderbilt Univ 1992; **Resid:** Surgery, Vanderbilt Univ 1998; **Fellow:** Urologic Oncology, Meml Sloan Kettering Cancer Ctr 1999; **Fac Appt:** Assoc Prof U, Vanderbilt Univ

Cookson, Michael MD [U] - **Spec Exp:** Bladder Cancer; Testicular Cancer; Prostate Cancer; **Hospital:** Vanderbilt Univ Med Ctr, Saint Thomas Hosp - Nashville; **Address:** Vanderbilt Univ Med Ctr, Urol Surg A1302 MCN, Nashville, TN 37232-0001; **Phone:** 615-322-2101; **Board Cert:** Urology 2006; **Med School:** Univ Okla Coll Med 1988; **Resid:** Urology, Univ Tex San Antonio-Univ Hosp 1994; **Fellow:** Urologic Oncology, Meml Sloan-Kettering Cancer Ctr 1996; **Fac Appt:** Prof U, Vanderbilt Univ

El-Galley, Rizk MD [U] - **Spec Exp:** Urologic Cancer; Laparoscopic Surgery; Bladder Cancer; Hydrocele; **Hospital:** Univ of Ala Hosp at Birmingham; **Address:** UAB Hosp FOT-1105, 1530 3rd Ave S, Birmingham, AL 35294-3411; **Phone:** 205-996-8765; **Board Cert:** Urology 2003; **Med School:** Egypt 1983; **Resid:** Urology, Emory Univ Hosp 1999; **Fac Appt:** Asst Prof U, Univ Alabama

Fraser, Lionel B MD [U] - **Spec Exp:** Prostate Cancer; Incontinence after Prostate Cancer; Erectile Dysfunction; **Hospital:** Baptist Hosp - Jackson; **Address:** Metropolitan Urology, St Dominics West Med Tower, 971 Lakeland Drive, Ste 360, Jackson, MS 39216; **Phone:** 601-982-0982; **Board Cert:** Urology 2005; **Med School:** Univ Mich Med Sch 1977; **Resid:** Surgery, New England Deaconness Hosp 1979; **Fellow:** Urology, Brigham & Womens Hosp 1983

Harty, James MD [U] - **Spec Exp:** Urologic Cancer; **Hospital:** Norton Hosp, Jewish Hosp HlthCre Svcs Inc; **Address:** Allied Urology, 250 E Liberty St, Ste 500, Louisville, KY 40202; **Phone:** 502-584-0651; **Board Cert:** Urology 1979; **Med School:** Ireland 1969; **Resid:** Surgery, Johns Hopkins Hosp 1973; Urology, Johns Hopkins Hosp 1977; **Fac Appt:** Prof S, Univ Louisville Sch Med

Hemal, Ashok K MD [U] - **Spec Exp:** Urologic Cancer; Robotic Surgery; Reconstructive Urologic Surgery; Laparoscopic Surgery; **Hospital:** Wake Forest Univ Baptist Med Ctr (page 72); **Address:** Wake Forest Sch Med, Dept Urology, 140 Charlois Blvd, Winston-Salem, NC 27103; **Phone:** 336-716-4131; **Med School:** India 1981; **Resid:** Surgery, G R Med College 1985; Urology, Post Grad Inst Med Ed & Rsch 1988; **Fellow:** Robotic Surgery, Henry Ford Hosp; **Fac Appt:** Prof U, Wake Forest Univ

Irby III, Pierce B MD [U] - **Spec Exp:** Kidney Stones; Minimally Invasive Surgery; Vasectomy & Vasectomy Reversal; **Hospital:** Carolinas Med Ctr, Presby Hosp - Charlotte; **Address:** McKay Urology, 1023 Edgehill Rd S, Charlotte, NC 28207; **Phone:** 704-355-8686; **Board Cert:** Urology 2003; **Med School:** Uniformed Srvs Univ, Bethesda 1983; **Resid:** Urology, Letterman Army Med Ctr 1990; **Fellow:** Endourology, UCSF Med Ctr 1992; **Fac Appt:** Asst Clin Prof U, Univ NC Sch Med

Jordan, Gerald H MD [U] - **Spec Exp:** Incontinence; Urinary Reconstruction; Prostate Cancer; **Hospital:** Sentara Norfolk Genl Hosp; **Address:** 400 W Brambleton Ave, Ste 100, Norfolk, VA 23510; **Phone:** 757-457-5100; **Board Cert:** Urology 2008; **Med School:** Univ Tex, San Antonio 1977; **Resid:** Urology, Naval Reg Med Ctr 1978; **Fellow:** Reconstructive Surgery, Eastern Va Med Sch 1984; **Fac Appt:** Prof U, Eastern VA Med Sch

Joseph, David B MD [U] - **Spec Exp:** Pediatric Urology; Urodynamics; Neuro-Urology; **Hospital:** Children's Hospital - Birmingham, Univ of Ala Hosp at Birmingham; **Address:** Childrens Hospital, Dept Urology, 1600 7th Ave S, Ste ACC-318, Birmingham, AL 35233; **Phone:** 205-939-9840; **Board Cert:** Urology 2005; Pediatric Urology 2008; **Med School:** Univ Wisc 1980; **Resid:** Urology, Univ Wisconsin Med Ctr 1985; **Fellow:** Pediatric Urology, Boston Childrens Hosp 1986; **Fac Appt:** Prof U, Univ Alabama

Urology

Keane, Thomas E MD [U] - **Spec Exp:** Urologic Cancer; Genitourinary Cancer; Prostate Cancer; Clinical Trials; **Hospital:** MUSC Med Ctr; **Address:** MUSC-Urology Dept, 96 Jonathan Lucas St, Ste CSB644, Charleston, SC 29425; **Phone:** 843-792-1666; **Board Cert:** Urology 2003; **Med School:** Ireland 1981; **Resid:** Urology, St Vincents Hosp 1986; Urology, N Tees Gen Hosp 1988; **Fellow:** Urology, Duke Univ Med Ctr 1993; **Fac Appt:** Prof U, Univ SC Sch Med

Kennelly, Michael J MD [U] - **Spec Exp:** Incontinence; Voiding Dysfunction; Pelvic Organ Prolapse Repair; Neurogenic Bladder; **Hospital:** Carolinas Med Ctr, Presby Hosp - Charlotte; **Address:** 1023 Edgehill Rd S, Charlotte, NC 28207; **Phone:** 704-355-8686; **Board Cert:** Urology 2005; **Med School:** Univ Cincinnati 1989; **Resid:** Urology, Univ Mich Med Ctr 1994; **Fellow:** Neurology, Univ Tex Hlth Sci Ctr 1995; **Fac Appt:** Clin Prof U, Univ NC Sch Med

Kim, Edward D MD [U] - **Spec Exp:** Infertility-Male; Prostate Cancer; Bladder Cancer; **Hospital:** Univ of Tennessee Mem Hosp; **Address:** University Urology, 1928 Alcoa Hwy, Med Office B Bldg - Ste 222, Knoxville, TN 37920; **Phone:** 865-305-9254; **Board Cert:** Urology 2007; **Med School:** Northwestern Univ 1989; **Resid:** Urology, Northwestern Meml Hosp 1995; **Fellow:** Baylor Coll Med 1996; **Fac Appt:** Assoc Prof U, Univ Tenn Coll Med, Memphis

Lloyd, L Keith MD [U] - **Spec Exp:** Erectile Dysfunction; Incontinence; Interstitial Cystitis; Neurogenic Bladder; **Hospital:** Univ of Ala Hosp at Birmingham; **Address:** FOT 1120, 510 20th St S, Birmingham, AL 35294-3411; **Phone:** 205-975-0088; **Board Cert:** Urology 1976; **Med School:** Tulane Univ 1966; **Resid:** Urology, Tulane Univ Hosp 1974; **Fac Appt:** Prof U, Univ Alabama

Lockhart, Jorge L MD [U] - **Spec Exp:** Voiding Dysfunction; Bladder Cancer; Incontinence; Urinary Reconstruction; **Hospital:** Tampa Genl Hosp, H Lee Moffitt Cancer Ctr & Research Inst; **Address:** USF College of Medicine, Div Urology, 2 Tampa General Circle Fl 7, Tampa, FL 33606; **Phone:** 813-259-8702; **Board Cert:** Urology 1980; **Med School:** Uruguay 1973; **Resid:** Urology, Duke Univ Med Ctr 1977; **Fellow:** Urodynamics, Duke Univ Med Ctr 1978; **Fac Appt:** Prof S, Univ S Fla Coll Med

Lynne, Charles M MD [U] - **Spec Exp:** Infertility-Male in Spinal Cord Injury; Voiding Dysfunction/Spinal Cord Injury; Urodynamics; **Hospital:** Jackson Meml Hosp (page 70), Univ of Miami Hosp (page 71); **Address:** Univ Miami, Dept Urology 814, PO Box 016960, Miami, FL 33101; **Phone:** 305-243-6590; **Board Cert:** Urology 1974; **Med School:** Univ Miami Sch Med 1964; **Resid:** Urology, Univ Miami Affil Hosps 1971; **Fac Appt:** Prof U, Univ Miami Sch Med

Marshall, Fray F MD [U] - **Spec Exp:** Prostate Cancer; **Hospital:** Emory Univ Hosp; **Address:** Emory Urology, 1365 Clifton Rd NE B Bldg - Ste 1400, Atlanta, GA 30322; **Phone:** 404-778-4898; **Board Cert:** Urology 1977; **Med School:** Univ VA Sch Med 1969; **Resid:** Surgery, Univ Mich Hosps 1972; Urology, Mass Genl Hosp 1975; **Fac Appt:** Prof U, Emory Univ

McConnell, John D MD [U] - **Spec Exp:** Prostate Cancer; **Hospital:** Wake Forest Univ Baptist Med Ctr (page 72); **Address:** Wake Forest Univ Baptist Med Ctr, Medical Center Blvd, Winston-Salem, NC 27157; **Phone:** 336-716-3408; **Board Cert:** Urology 2004; **Med School:** Loyola Univ-Stritch Sch Med 1978; **Resid:** Surgery, Parkland Hosp 1980; Urology, Parkland Hosp 1984; **Fac Appt:** Prof U, Wake Forest Univ

Milam, Douglas F MD [U] - **Spec Exp:** Urodynamics; Voiding Dysfunction; **Hospital:** Vanderbilt Univ Med Ctr; **Address:** Vanderbilt Univ-Dept Urology, 1301 Medical Center Drive, Ste 3823, Nashville, TN 37232; **Phone:** 615-322-2880; **Board Cert:** Urology 2003; **Med School:** W VA Univ 1986; **Resid:** Surgery, Univ Utah Hosps 1988; Urology, Univ Utah Hosps 1991; **Fac Appt:** Assoc Prof U, Vanderbilt Univ

Moul, Judd W MD [U] - **Spec Exp:** Prostate Cancer; Testicular Cancer; Minimally Invasive Urologic Surgery; Clinical Trials; **Hospital:** Duke Univ Med Ctr, VA Med Ctr - Durham; **Address:** Duke Univ Med Ctr, Div Urologic Surgery, Box 3707, Durham, NC 27710; **Phone:** 919-668-8180; **Board Cert:** Urology 2007; **Med School:** Jefferson Med Coll 1982; **Resid:** Urology, Walter Reed Army Med Ctr 1987; **Fellow:** Urologic Oncology, Duke Univ Med Ctr 1989; **Fac Appt:** Prof S, Duke Univ

Patel, Vipul R MD [U] - **Spec Exp:** Prostate Cancer/Robotic Surgery; Kidney Cancer; **Hospital:** Florida Hosp Celebration Hlth; **Address:** 410 Celebration Pl, Ste 200, Celebration, FL 34747; **Phone:** 407-303-4673; **Board Cert:** Urology 2004; **Med School:** Baylor Coll Med 1995; **Resid:** Urology, Univ Miami; **Fellow:** Urologic Laparoscopic Surgery-Endourology, Univ Miami

Patterson, Anthony L MD [U] - **Spec Exp:** Laparoscopic Surgery; Kidney Stones; **Hospital:** Univ of Tennessee Mem Hosp; **Address:** UT Medical Group, 7945 Wolf River Blvd, Ste 350, Germantown, TN 38138-1733; **Phone:** 901-347-8350; **Board Cert:** Urology 2007; **Med School:** Univ Tenn Coll Med, Memphis 1982; **Resid:** Surgery, Univ Tenn Med Ctr 1984; Urology, Univ Tenn Med Ctr 1987; **Fac Appt:** Assoc Prof U, Univ Tenn Coll Med, Memphis

Pope IV, John C MD [U] - **Spec Exp:** Pediatric Urology; Kidney Stones; **Hospital:** Vanderbilt Children's Hosp; **Address:** 2200 Children's Way, Ste 4102, Nashville, TN 37232-9820; **Phone:** 615-936-1060; **Board Cert:** Urology 1999; Pediatric Urology 2008; **Med School:** Univ Tenn Coll Med, Memphis 1989; **Resid:** Surgery, Vanderbilt Univ Med Ctr 1991; Urology, Vanderbilt Univ Med Ctr 1995; **Fellow:** Pediatric Urology, Indiana Univ Med Ctr 1997; **Fac Appt:** Assoc Prof U, Vanderbilt Univ

Pow-Sang, Julio M MD [U] - **Spec Exp:** Prostate Cancer; **Hospital:** H Lee Moffitt Cancer Ctr & Research Inst; **Address:** H Lee Moffitt Cancer Ctr, GU Clinic, 12902 Magnolia Drive, Tampa, FL 33612-9416; **Phone:** 813-972-8418; **Board Cert:** Urology 1999; **Med School:** Mexico 1978; **Resid:** Surgery, Univ Miami Sch Med 1983; Urology, Univ Miami Sch Med 1986; **Fellow:** Urologic Oncology, Univ Fla Coll Med 1987; **Fac Appt:** Prof S, Univ S Fla Coll Med

Preminger, Glenn M MD [U] - **Spec Exp:** Kidney Stones; **Hospital:** Duke Univ Med Ctr; **Address:** Duke Univ Med Ctr, Div Urologic Surgery, rm 1587, Box 3167, White Zone Duke S, Durham, NC 27710; **Phone:** 919-681-5506; **Board Cert:** Urology 2003; **Med School:** NY Med Coll 1977; **Resid:** Surgery, N Carolina Meml Hosp 1979; Urology, N Carolina Meml Hosp 1983; **Fellow:** Urology, Univ Texas SW Med Ctr 1985; **Fac Appt:** Prof U, Duke Univ

Robertson, Cary N MD [U] - **Spec Exp:** Prostate Cancer; Kidney Cancer; High Intensity Focused Ultrasound(HIFU); Testicular Cancer; **Hospital:** Duke Univ Med Ctr; **Address:** Duke Univ Med Ctr, Trent Drive, Box 3833, Durham, NC 27710; **Phone:** 919-681-6768; **Board Cert:** Urology 2006; **Med School:** Tulane Univ 1977; **Resid:** Urology, Duke Univ Med Ctr 1985; **Fellow:** Urologic Oncology, Natl Inst Hlth 1987; **Fac Appt:** Assoc Prof U, Duke Univ

Rowland, Randall MD [U] - **Spec Exp:** Urologic Cancer; **Hospital:** Univ of Kentucky Chandler Hosp; **Address:** Univ Kentucky Med Ctr, Div Urology, 800 Rose St, rm MS283, Lexington, KY 40536-0001; **Phone:** 859-323-6677; **Board Cert:** Urology 1980; **Med School:** Northwestern Univ 1972; **Resid:** Urology, Northwestern Meml Hosp 1978; **Fellow:** Urology, Northwestern Meml Hosp 1977; **Fac Appt:** Prof U, Univ KY Coll Med

Sanders, William H MD [U] - **Spec Exp:** Prostate Cancer; Kidney Stones; Kidney Cancer; **Hospital:** St Joseph's Hosp - Atlanta, Northside Hosp; **Address:** 980 Johnson Ferry Rd, Ste 490, Atlanta, GA 30342-1767; **Phone:** 404-257-0133; **Board Cert:** Urology 2006; **Med School:** Emory Univ 1988; **Resid:** Urology, Yale-New Haven Hosp 1993

Urology

Shaban, Stephen F MD [U] - **Spec Exp:** Infertility-Male; **Hospital:** Rex HlthCare, WakeMed New Bern; **Address:** 2800 Blue Ridge Rd, Ste 405, Raleigh, NC 27607; **Phone:** 919-790-5500; **Board Cert:** Urology 2004; **Med School:** Mount Sinai Sch Med 1982; **Resid:** Urology, Univ S Fla 1987; **Fellow:** Male Reproduction, Baylor Coll Med 1988; **Fac Appt:** Prof U, Univ NC Sch Med

Smith, Joseph A MD [U] - **Spec Exp:** Prostate Cancer/Robotic Surgery; Bladder Cancer; Kidney Cancer; **Hospital:** Vanderbilt Univ Med Ctr; **Address:** Vanderbilt Univ Med Ctr, Dept Urology, A-1302 MCN, Nashville, TN 37232-2765; **Phone:** 615-343-0234; **Board Cert:** Urology 2000; **Med School:** Univ Tenn Coll Med, Memphis 1974; **Resid:** Surgery, Parkland Meml Hosp 1976; Urology, Univ Utah 1979; **Fellow:** Urologic Oncology, Meml Sloan Kettering Cancer Ctr 1980; **Fac Appt:** Prof U, Vanderbilt Univ

Soloway, Mark S MD [U] - **Spec Exp:** Bladder Cancer; Kidney Cancer; Prostate Cancer; Urologic Pathology; **Hospital:** Jackson Meml Hosp (page 70), Univ of Miami Hosp & Clins/Sylvester Comp Canc Ctr (page 70); **Address:** 1150 NW 14th St, Ste 309, Miami, FL 33136; **Phone:** 305-243-6596; **Board Cert:** Urology 1977; **Med School:** Case West Res Univ 1968; **Resid:** Surgery, Univ Hosps 1970; Urology, Univ Hosps 1975; **Fellow:** Surgery, Natl Cancer Inst 1972; **Fac Appt:** Prof U, Univ Miami Sch Med

Steers, William D MD [U] - **Spec Exp:** Incontinence; Erectile Dysfunction; Prostate Cancer/Robotic Surgery; **Hospital:** Univ Virginia Med Ctr; **Address:** UVA Hlth System, Dept Urology, PO Box 800422, Charlottesville, VA 22908-0422; **Phone:** 434-924-9107; **Board Cert:** Urology 1999; **Med School:** Med Coll OH 1980; **Resid:** Urology, Univ Tex Hlth Sci Ctr 1986; **Fellow:** Neurology, Univ Pittsburgh Med Ctr 1988; **Fac Appt:** Prof U, Univ VA Sch Med

Strup, Stephen E MD [U] - **Spec Exp:** Urologic Cancer; Minimally Invasive Urologic Surgery; Robotic Surgery; **Hospital:** Univ of Kentucky Chandler Hosp; **Address:** MS-283 Chandler Medical Ctr, 800 Rose St, Lexington, KY 40536; **Phone:** 859-323-6679; **Board Cert:** Urology 2007; **Med School:** Indiana Univ 1988; **Resid:** Urology, Thomas Jefferson Univ Hosp 1994; **Fellow:** Urologic Oncology, National Cancer Inst 1996; **Fac Appt:** Prof S, Univ KY Coll Med

Teigland, Chris M MD [U] - **Spec Exp:** Prostate Cancer/Robotic Surgery; Kidney Cancer; Laparoscopic Surgery; **Hospital:** Carolinas Med Ctr; **Address:** Mckay Urology, 1023 Edgehill Rd S, Charlotte, NC 28207; **Phone:** 704-355-8686; **Board Cert:** Urology 2007; **Med School:** Duke Univ 1980; **Resid:** Surgery, Univ Utah Affil Hosps 1982; Urology, Univ Texas SW Med Ctr 1987; **Fac Appt:** Clin Prof S, Univ NC Sch Med

Terris, Martha K MD [U] - **Spec Exp:** Prostate Cancer; Brachytherapy; Urologic Cancer; Bladder Cancer; **Hospital:** VA Medical Ctr - Augusta, Med Coll of GA Hosp and Clin (MCG Health Inc); **Address:** Charlie Norwood VA Medical Center, 1 Freedom Way, Augusta, GA 30904; **Phone:** 706-733-0188; **Board Cert:** Urology 2007; **Med School:** Univ Miss 1986; **Resid:** Surgery, Duke Univ Med Ctr 1988; Urology, Stanford Univ Med Ctr 1995; **Fellow:** Ultrasound, Stanford Univ 1991; **Fac Appt:** Prof S, Med Coll GA

Theodorescu, Dan MD/PhD [U] - **Spec Exp:** Prostate Cancer; Clinical Trials; Bladder Cancer; Kidney Cancer; **Hospital:** Univ Virginia Med Ctr; **Address:** UVA Health System, Dept Urology, PO Box 800422, Charlottesville, VA 22908; **Phone:** 434-924-0042; **Board Cert:** Urology 2007; **Med School:** Canada 1986; **Resid:** Urology, Univ Toronto Med Ctr 1993; **Fellow:** Urologic Oncology, Meml Sloan Kettering Cancer Ctr 1995; **Fac Appt:** Prof U, Univ VA Sch Med

Webster, George D MD [U] - **Spec Exp:** Reconstructive Urologic Surgery; Urology-Female; Urodynamics; **Hospital:** Duke Univ Med Ctr; **Address:** Dept Urolology, Box 3146, Durham, NC 27710; **Phone:** 919-684-2516; **Board Cert:** Urology 1981; **Med School:** England, UK 1968; **Resid:** Surgery, Harare Hosp 1972; Urology, Inst Urology 1974; **Fellow:** Urology, Duke Univ Med Ctr 1978; **Fac Appt:** Prof U, Duke Univ

Winfield, Howard N MD [U] - **Spec Exp:** Kidney Stones; Laparoscopic Surgery; Robotic Surgery; **Hospital:** DCH Reg Med Ctr; **Address:** W Alabama Urology Assoc, DCH Med Towers, Suite 908, 701 Univ Blvd E, Tuscaloosa, AL 35401; **Phone:** 205-344-9393; **Board Cert:** Urology 2008; **Med School:** McGill Univ 1978; **Resid:** Urology, McGill Univ Tchg Hosp 1984; **Fellow:** Urology, Washington Univ 1985; Urology, UCLA 1986; **Fac Appt:** Prof U, Univ Iowa Coll Med

Midwest

Andriole, Gerald L MD [U] - **Spec Exp:** Urologic Cancer; Prostate Cancer; Laparoscopic Surgery; **Hospital:** Barnes-Jewish Hosp; **Address:** 4960 Children's Place, Campus Box 8242, St Louis, MO 63110; **Phone:** 314-362-8212; **Board Cert:** Urology 2003; **Med School:** Jefferson Med Coll 1978; **Resid:** Surgery, Strong Meml Hosp 1980; Urology, Brigham & Womens Hosp 1983; **Fellow:** Urologic Oncology, NCI/NIH 1985; **Fac Appt:** Prof U, Washington Univ, St Louis

Bahnson, Robert MD [U] - **Spec Exp:** Prostate Cancer; Bladder Cancer; Continent Urinary Diversions; **Hospital:** Ohio St Univ Med Ctr, Arthur G James Cancer Hosp & Research Inst; **Address:** 456 West 10th Avenue, Dept of Urology, 4960 Cramblett Med Ctr, Columbus, OH 43210-1228; **Phone:** 614-293-3646; **Board Cert:** Urology 2006; **Med School:** Tufts Univ 1979; **Resid:** Surgery, Northwestern Univ 1981; Urology, Northwestern Univ 1985; **Fellow:** Urology, Northwestern Univ 1984; Research, Univ Pittsburgh 1991; **Fac Appt:** Prof U, Ohio State Univ

Bloom, David A MD [U] - **Spec Exp:** Pediatric Urology; Voiding Dysfunction; Genitourinary Reconstruction; Spina Bifida; **Hospital:** Univ Michigan Hlth Sys; **Address:** Univ Mich, Dept Ped Urology, 1500 E Med Ctr Dr, 3875 Taubman Ctr, Ann Arbor, MI 48109-5330; **Phone:** 734-232-4943; **Board Cert:** Urology 1982; Pediatric Urology 2008; **Med School:** SUNY Buffalo 1971; **Resid:** Surgery, UCLA Med Ctr 1976; Urology, UCLA Med Ctr 1980; **Fellow:** Pediatric Urology, Inst Urol-St Peters Hosp 1978; **Fac Appt:** Prof U, Univ Mich Med Sch

Brendler, Charles B MD [U] - **Spec Exp:** Prostate Cancer; **Hospital:** Evanston/Northshore Univ Hlth Syst; **Address:** Evanston/Northshore Univ Hosp, 2650 Ridge Ave Walgreen Bldg - Ste 2507, Evanston, IL 60201; **Phone:** 847-657-5730; **Board Cert:** Urology 1981; **Med School:** Univ VA Sch Med 1974; **Resid:** Surgery, Duke Univ Med Ctr 1976; Urology, Duke Univ Med Ctr 1979; **Fellow:** Urologic Oncology, Univ Hosp Wales 1980; Urologic Oncology, Johns Hopkins Hosp 1982; **Fac Appt:** Prof U, Northwestern Univ-Feinberg Sch Med

Bushman, Wade MD [U] - **Spec Exp:** Neuro-Urology; Urodynamics; Urology-Female; **Hospital:** Univ WI Hosp & Clins; **Address:** Dept Urology, 600 Highland Ave, C52, Madison, WI 53792-3236; **Phone:** 608-263-4757; **Board Cert:** Urology 2006; **Med School:** Univ Chicago-Pritzker Sch Med 1986; **Resid:** Urology, Univ VA Med Ctr 1992; **Fac Appt:** Assoc Prof U, Univ Wisc

Campbell, Steven C MD/PhD [U] - **Spec Exp:** Kidney Cancer; Prostate Cancer; Bladder Cancer; **Hospital:** Cleveland Clin Fdn (page 56); **Address:** Cleveland Clinic, Glickman Urological Inst, 9500 Euclid Ave, MS Q10-1, Cleveland, OH 44195; **Phone:** 216-444-5595; **Board Cert:** Urology 1999; **Med School:** Univ Chicago-Pritzker Sch Med 1989; **Resid:** Urology, Cleveland Clinic 1995; **Fellow:** Urology, Meml Sloan Kettering Cancer Ctr 1996; **Fac Appt:** Prof S, Cleveland Cl Coll Med/Case West Res

Catalona, William J MD [U] - **Spec Exp:** Prostate Cancer; Prostate Disease; **Hospital:** Northwestern Meml Hosp; **Address:** Northwestern Med Faculty Foundation, 675 N St Clair St, Ste 20-150, Chicago, IL 60611; **Phone:** 312-695-6126; **Board Cert:** Urology 1978; **Med School:** Yale Univ 1968; **Resid:** Surgery, UCSF Med Ctr 1970; Urology, Johns Hopkins Hosp 1976; **Fellow:** Surgical Oncology, Natl Cancer Inst 1972; **Fac Appt:** Prof U, Northwestern Univ

Urology

Chancellor, Michael B MD [U] - **Spec Exp:** Incontinence-Female; Urology-Female; Neuro-Urology; **Hospital:** William Beaumont Hosp; **Address:** William Beaumont Hospital, Urology, 3535 W 13 Mile Rd, Ste 438, Royal Oak, MI 48073; **Phone:** 248-551-3519; **Board Cert:** Urology 2000; **Med School:** Med Coll Wisc 1983; **Resid:** Surgery, Univ Michigan 1985; Urology, Univ Michigan 1988; **Fellow:** Neurourology, Columbia-Presby Med Ctr 1990; **Fac Appt:** Prof U, Univ Mich Med Sch

Coplen, Douglas E MD [U] - **Spec Exp:** Pediatric Urology; Urologic Cancer-Pediatric; Testicular Cancer-Pediatric; Fetal Urology; **Hospital:** St Louis Chldns Hosp; **Address:** St Louis Children's Hosp, 4990 Children's Pl, Northwest Tower, Ste 1120, St Louis, MO 63110; **Phone:** 314-454-6034; **Board Cert:** Urology 2005; Pediatric Urology 2008; **Med School:** Indiana Univ 1985; **Resid:** Urology, Barnes Jewish Hosp 1992; **Fellow:** Pediatric Urology, Childrens Hosp 1994; **Fac Appt:** Asst Prof S, Washington Univ, St Louis

Donovan Jr, James F MD [U] - **Spec Exp:** Prostate Cancer/Robotic Surgery; Infertility-Male; Erectile Dysfunction; Kidney Cancer; **Hospital:** Univ Hosp - Cincinnati, Christ Hospital; **Address:** Univ Cincinnati Med Ctr, Medical Arts Bldg, 222 Piedmont Ave, Ste 7000, Cincinnati, OH 45219; **Phone:** 513-475-8787; **Board Cert:** Surgery 1997; Urology 1999; **Med School:** Northwestern Univ 1978; **Resid:** Surgery, Northwestern Meml Hosp 1982; Urology, Northwestern Meml Hosp 1986; **Fellow:** Male Infertility, Baylor Coll Med 1986; **Fac Appt:** Prof U, Univ Cincinnati

Elder, Jack S MD [U] - **Spec Exp:** Pediatric Urology; Hypospadias; Urinary Reconstruction; Robotic Surgery; **Hospital:** Henry Ford Hosp, Chldns Hosp of Michigan; **Address:** Henry Ford Hosp, 2799 W Grand Blvd Fl K-9, Detroit, MI 48202; **Phone:** 313-916-2626; **Board Cert:** Urology 1984; **Med School:** Univ Okla Coll Med 1976; **Resid:** Surgery, Yale-New Haven Hosp 1978; Urology, Johns Hopkins Hosp 1982; **Fellow:** Pediatric Urology, Johns Hopkins Hosp 1982; Pediatric Urology, Chldns Hosp 1986; **Fac Appt:** Prof U, Case West Res Univ

Firlit, Casimir MD/PhD [U] - **Spec Exp:** Pediatric Urology; Genitourinary Reconstruction; Transplant-Kidney-Pediatric; **Hospital:** Cardinal Glennon Mem Children's Hosp; **Address:** Cardinal Glennon Chlds Hosp, 1465 S Grand Blvd Fl 5, Glennon Hall, St Louis, MO 63104; **Phone:** 314-577-5334; **Board Cert:** Urology 1975; **Med School:** Loyola Univ-Stritch Sch Med 1965; **Resid:** Surgery, Hines VA Hosp 1970; Urology, Hines VA Hosp 1973; **Fellow:** Pediatric Urology, Chldns Meml Hosp 1974; **Fac Appt:** Prof U, Univ MO-Columbia Sch Med

Flanigan, Robert C MD [U] - **Spec Exp:** Prostate Cancer; Bladder Cancer; Kidney Cancer; **Hospital:** Loyola Univ Med Ctr; **Address:** Loyola Univ Med-Fahey Bldg 54, 2160 S First Ave, rm 267, Maywood, IL 60153; **Phone:** 708-216-5100; **Board Cert:** Surgery 1998; Urology 2001; **Med School:** Case West Res Univ 1972; **Resid:** Surgery, Case West Univ Med Ctr 1978; Urology, Case West Univ Med Ctr 1978; **Fac Appt:** Prof U, Loyola Univ-Stritch Sch Med

Foster, Richard S MD [U] - **Spec Exp:** Testicular Cancer; Reconstructive Surgery; **Hospital:** Indiana Univ Hosp; **Address:** 535 N Barnhill Drive, Ste 420, Indianapolis, IN 46202; **Phone:** 317-274-3458; **Board Cert:** Urology 2008; **Med School:** Indiana Univ 1980; **Resid:** Urology, Indiana Univ Hosp 1986; **Fac Appt:** Prof U, Indiana Univ

Gluckman, Gordon R MD [U] - **Spec Exp:** Prostate Cancer; Kidney Cancer; Minimally Invasive Urologic Surgery; **Hospital:** Adv Luth Genl Hosp, Resurrection Med Ctr; **Address:** 900 Grand Rd, Ste 120, Des Plaines, IL 60016; **Phone:** 847-823-3185; **Board Cert:** Urology 2006; **Med School:** Northwestern Univ 1989; **Resid:** Surgery, UCSF Med Ctr 1991; Urology, UCSF Med Ctr 1995

Gujral, Saroj MD [U] - **Spec Exp:** Urologic Cancer; Urology-Female; **Hospital:** Albert Lea Med Ctr-Mayo Hlth Sys; **Address:** 404 W Fountain St, Albert Lea, MN 56007; **Phone:** 507-379-2130; **Board Cert:** Urology 1979; **Med School:** India 1970; **Resid:** Urology, Suburban Hosp 1978; Urology, Dalhousie Univ Med Ctrs

Kaouk, Jihad MD [U] - **Spec Exp:** Minimally Invasive Urologic Surgery; Robotic Surgery; Kidney Cancer; Bladder Cancer; **Hospital:** Cleveland Clin Fdn (page 56); **Address:** Cleveland Clinic main campus, 9500 Euclid Ave, MC Q10-1, Cleveland, OH 44195; **Phone:** 216-444-2976; **Med School:** Lebanon 1993; **Resid:** Urology, Amer Univ of Beirut Med Ctr; Surgery, Amer Univ of Beitut Med Ctr; **Fellow:** Minimally Invasive Surgery, Cleveland Clinic; Research, Cleveland Clinic; **Fac Appt:** Assoc Prof S, Cleveland Cl Coll Med/Case West Res

Kass, Evan MD [U] - **Spec Exp:** Pediatric Urology; **Hospital:** William Beaumont Hosp; **Address:** 2221 Livernois, Ste 103, Troy, MI 48083; **Phone:** 248-519-0305; **Board Cert:** Urology 1978; **Med School:** SUNY Downstate 1968; **Resid:** Urology, Univ Mich Hosp 1976; **Fellow:** Pediatric Urology, Hosp for Sick Chldn 1978; **Fac Appt:** Assoc Prof U, Wayne State Univ

Kibel, Adam S MD [U] - **Spec Exp:** Prostate Cancer; Bladder Cancer; Kidney Cancer; Minimally Invasive Surgery; **Hospital:** Barnes-Jewish Hosp; **Address:** Director Urologic Oncology, Washington Univ School of Medicine, 4960 Children's Place, Box 8242, St Louis, MO 63105-1000; **Phone:** 314-362-8295; **Board Cert:** Urology 2001; **Med School:** Cornell Univ-Weill Med Coll 1991; **Resid:** Urology, Brigham & Women's Hosp 1996; **Fellow:** Urologic Oncology, Johns Hopkins Hosp 1999; **Fac Appt:** Prof U, Washington Univ, St Louis

Klein, Eric A MD [U] - **Spec Exp:** Prostate Cancer; Testicular Cancer; Urologic Cancer; **Hospital:** Cleveland Clin Fdn (page 56); **Address:** Cleveland Clinic Fdn, Dept Urol, Sect Urol-Onc, 9500 Euclid Ave, Desk A100, Cleveland, OH 44195-0001; **Phone:** 216-444-5591; **Board Cert:** Urology 2008; **Med School:** Univ Pittsburgh 1981; **Resid:** Urology, Cleveland Clinic Fdn 1986; **Fellow:** Urologic Oncology, Meml Sloan Kettering Canc Ctr 1989; **Fac Appt:** Prof S, Cleveland Cl Coll Med/Case West Res

Klutke, Carl G MD [U] - **Spec Exp:** Urology-Female; Incontinence; Urodynamics; **Hospital:** Barnes-Jewish Hosp; **Address:** 1040 N Mason Rd, Ste 122, St Louis, MO 63141; **Phone:** 314-996-8060; **Board Cert:** Urology 2000; **Med School:** Univ Mich Med Sch 1983; **Resid:** Surgery, Henry Ford Hosp 1985; Urology, Henry Ford Hosp 1988; **Fellow:** Female Urology, UCLA Med Ctr 1989; **Fac Appt:** Assoc Prof S, Washington Univ, St Louis

Koff, Stephen A MD [U] - **Spec Exp:** Pediatric Urology; **Hospital:** Nationwide Chldn's Hosp; **Address:** Chldns Hosp, Dept Urology, 555 S 18th St, Ste 6D, Columbus, OH 43205; **Phone:** 614-722-3114; **Board Cert:** Urology 1978; **Med School:** Duke Univ 1969; **Resid:** Internal Medicine, New York Hosp 1971; Urology, Univ Mich Med Ctr 1975; **Fellow:** Pediatric Urology, Alder Hey Chldns Hosp 1977; **Fac Appt:** Prof U, Ohio State Univ

Kozlowski, James M MD [U] - **Spec Exp:** Prostate Cancer; Continent Urinary Diversions; Laparoscopic Surgery; **Hospital:** Northwestern Meml Hosp, Jesse A Brown VA Med Ctr; **Address:** 675 N St Clair St, Galter Bldg Fl 20 - Ste 150, Chicago, IL 60611; **Phone:** 312-695-8146; **Board Cert:** Surgery 2004; Urology 1983; **Med School:** Northwestern Univ 1975; **Resid:** Surgery, Northwestern Univ-McGaw 1979; Urology, Northwestern Univ-McGaw 1981; **Fellow:** Research, NCI-Frederick Cancer Rsch 1984; **Fac Appt:** Assoc Prof U, Northwestern Univ

Lee, Cheryl T MD [U] - **Spec Exp:** Urologic Cancer; Bladder Cancer; **Hospital:** Univ Michigan Hlth Sys; **Address:** Univ of Michigan Cancer Ctr, 1500 E Medical Ctr Drive, Reception D LB1-229, Ann Arbor, MI 48109-5913; **Phone:** 734-647-8903; **Board Cert:** Urology 2002; **Med School:** Albany Med Coll 1991; **Resid:** Urology, Albany Med Ctr; **Fellow:** Urologic Oncology, Meml Sloan Kettering Cancer Ctr 2000; **Fac Appt:** Assoc Prof U, Univ Mich Med Sch

Urology

Levine, Laurence Adan MD [U] - **Spec Exp:** Erectile Dysfunction; Infertility-Male; Peyronie's Disease; Prostate Cancer; **Hospital:** Rush Univ Med Ctr; **Address:** 1725 W Harrison St, Ste 352, Chicago, IL 60612; **Phone:** 312-563-5000; **Board Cert:** Urology 2009; **Med School:** Univ Colorado 1980; **Resid:** Surgery, Tufts-New Eng Med Ctr 1982; Urology, Brigham & Women's Hosp 1987; **Fac Appt:** Prof U, Rush Med Coll

McGuire, Edward J MD [U] - **Spec Exp:** Incontinence; Urology-Female; Neurogenic Bladder; **Hospital:** Univ Michigan Hlth Sys; **Address:** Univ Mich Med Ctr, Dept Urology, 1500 E Med Ctr Drive, rm 3875-TC, Ann Arbor, MI 48109-5330; **Phone:** 734-936-7030; **Board Cert:** Urology 1975; **Med School:** Wayne State Univ 1965; **Resid:** Surgery, Yale-New Haven Hosp 1969; Urology, Yale-New Haven Hosp 1972; **Fac Appt:** Prof U, Univ Mich Med Sch

McVary, Kevin MD [U] - **Spec Exp:** Prostate Cancer; Erectile Dysfunction; Prostate Disease; **Hospital:** Northwestern Meml Hosp; **Address:** 675 N St Clair St, Galter Bldg Fl 20 - Ste 150, Chicago, IL 60611-4813; **Phone:** 312-695-8146; **Board Cert:** Urology 2000; **Med School:** Northwestern Univ 1983; **Resid:** Surgery, Northwestern Meml Hosp 1985; Urology, Northwestern Meml Hosp 1988; **Fellow:** Research, Northwestern Meml Hosp; **Fac Appt:** Prof U, Northwestern Univ

Menon, Mani MD [U] - **Spec Exp:** Prostate Cancer/Robotic Surgery; Transplant-Kidney; Urologic Cancer; **Hospital:** Henry Ford Hosp; **Address:** Henry Ford Hosp - Vattikuti Urology Inst, 2799 W Grand Bvd, Clinic Bldg - #K-9, Detroit, MI 48202; **Phone:** 888-881-1117; **Board Cert:** Urology 1982; **Med School:** India 1969; **Resid:** Urology, Bryn Mawr Hosp 1974; Urology, Johns Hopkins Hosp 1980; **Fellow:** Transplant Surgery, Johns Hopkins Univ 1977; **Fac Appt:** Prof S, Univ Mass Sch Med

Mesrobian, Hrair-George O MD [U] - **Spec Exp:** Pediatric Urology; **Hospital:** Chldns Hosp - Wisconsin; **Address:** 999 N 92nd St, Ste 330, Milwaukee, WI 53226; **Phone:** 414-266-3794; **Board Cert:** Urology 2005; Pediatric Urology 2008; **Med School:** Lebanon 1978; **Resid:** Surgery, SUNY Upstate Med Ctr 1980; Urology, UCSF Med Ctr 1983; **Fellow:** Pediatric Urology, Mayo Clinic 1984; **Fac Appt:** Prof U, Med Coll Wisc

Mitchell, Michael E MD [U] - **Spec Exp:** Genitourinary Congenital Abnormality; Pediatric Urology; Bladder Reconstruction; **Hospital:** Chldns Hosp - Wisconsin; **Address:** Children's Hospital of Wisconsin, 999 N 92nd St, Ste 330, Milwaukee, WI 53226; **Phone:** 414-266-3794; **Board Cert:** Urology 2000; **Med School:** Harvard Med Sch 1969; **Resid:** Surgery, Peter Bent Brigham Hosp 1974; Urology, Mass Genl Hosp 1977; **Fellow:** Pediatric Urology, Mass Genl Hosp 1978; **Fac Appt:** Prof U, Univ Wisc

Montague, Drogo K MD [U] - **Spec Exp:** Erectile Dysfunction; Genitourinary Prosthetics; Incontinence; **Hospital:** Cleveland Clin Fdn (page 56); **Address:** Urological Inst, 9500 Euclid Ave, Q10-1, Cleveland, OH 44195-5041; **Phone:** 216-444-5590; **Board Cert:** Urology 1995; **Med School:** Univ Mich Med Sch 1968; **Resid:** Surgery, Cleveland Clinic 1970; Urology, Cleveland Clinic 1973; **Fac Appt:** Prof U, Cleveland Cl Coll Med/Case West Res

Montie, James MD [U] - **Spec Exp:** Bladder Cancer; Prostate Cancer; Genitourinary Cancer; **Hospital:** Univ Michigan Hlth Sys; **Address:** UMH Cancer Ctr, Team 3, Reception D, Level B1-229, 1500 E Med Ctr Drive, Ann Arbor, MI 48109-5913; **Phone:** 734-647-8903; **Board Cert:** Urology 1978; **Med School:** Univ Mich Med Sch 1971; **Resid:** Urology, Cleveland Clinic Fdn 1976; **Fellow:** Urologic Oncology, Meml Sloan-Kettering Cancer Ctr 1979; **Fac Appt:** Prof U, Univ Mich Med Sch

America's Top Doctors® 9th Edition

Myers, Robert P MD [U] - **Spec Exp:** Prostate Cancer; **Hospital:** Mayo Med Ctr & Clin - Rochester, Rochester Methodist Hosp; **Address:** Mayo Clinic, Dept Urology, 200 First St SW, Rochester, MN 55905; **Phone:** 507-284-3077; **Board Cert:** Urology 1976; **Med School:** Columbia P&S 1967; **Resid:** Urology, Mayo Clinic 1972; **Fac Appt:** Prof U, Mayo Med Sch

Nehra, Ajay MD [U] - **Spec Exp:** Erectile Dysfunction; **Hospital:** Mayo Med Ctr & Clin - Rochester; **Address:** 200 First St SW, Rochester, MN 55905; **Phone:** 507-266-4446; **Board Cert:** Urology 2006; **Med School:** India 1982; **Resid:** Surgery, Boston Univ Sch Med 1987; Urology, Maimonides Med Ctr 1993; **Fellow:** Female Urology, Boston Univ Sch Med 1989; Male Infertility, Boston Univ Sch Med 1995; **Fac Appt:** Prof U, Mayo Med Sch

O'Donnell, Michael A MD [U] - **Spec Exp:** Bladder Cancer; Immunotherapy; Urologic Cancer; **Hospital:** Univ Iowa Hosp & Clinics; **Address:** Univ Iowa Hosp & Clins, Dept Urology, 200 Hawkins Drive, 3RCP, Iowa City, IA 52242-1089; **Phone:** 319-384-6040; **Board Cert:** Urology 2005; **Med School:** Duke Univ 1984; **Resid:** Surgery, Brigham & Womens Hosp 1987; Urology, Brigham & Womens Hosp 1991; **Fellow:** Urology, Brigham & Womens Hosp 1993; **Fac Appt:** Prof U, Univ Iowa Coll Med

Ohl, Dana MD [U] - **Spec Exp:** Infertility-Male; Erectile Dysfunction; **Hospital:** Univ Michigan Hlth Sys; **Address:** Univ Mich Med Ctr, Dept Urology, 1500 E Med Ctr Drive, rm 3875-TC, Ann Arbor, MI 48109-5330; **Phone:** 734-936-7030; **Board Cert:** Urology 2008; **Med School:** Univ Mich Med Sch 1982; **Resid:** Urology, Univ Mich Hosps 1987; **Fac Appt:** Prof U, Univ Mich Med Sch

Rink, Richard C MD [U] - **Spec Exp:** Pediatric Urology; Reconstructive Urologic Surgery; Genital Reconstruction; Neurogenic Bladder; **Hospital:** Riley Hosp for Children, Indiana Univ Hosp; **Address:** Indiana Univ Med Ctr, 702 Barnhill Drive, Ste 4230, Indianapolis, IN 46202-5128; **Phone:** 317-274-7472; **Board Cert:** Urology 2004; Pediatric Urology 2008; **Med School:** Indiana Univ 1978; **Resid:** Surgery, Emory Univ Med Ctr 1980; Urology, Indiana Univ Med Ctr 1984; **Fellow:** Pediatric Urology, Chldns Hosp-Harvard 1985; **Fac Appt:** Prof U, Indiana Univ

Ross, Lawrence S MD [U] - **Spec Exp:** Infertility-Male; Erectile Dysfunction; Prostate Disease; **Hospital:** Univ of IL Med Ctr at Chicago; **Address:** Univ Ctr fo Urology, 60 E Delaware Pl, Ste 1420, Chicago, IL 60611; **Phone:** 312-440-5127; **Board Cert:** Urology 1974; **Med School:** Univ Chicago-Pritzker Sch Med 1965; **Resid:** Urology, Michael Reese Hosp 1970; **Fac Appt:** Prof U, Univ IL Coll Med

Sandlow, Jay I MD [U] - **Spec Exp:** Infertility-Male; Varicocele Microsurgery; Vasectomy & Vasectomy Reversal; **Hospital:** Froedtert Meml Lutheran Hosp; **Address:** Med Coll of WI, Urology Dept, 9200 W Wisconsin Ave, Milwaukee, WI 53226-3522; **Phone:** 414-805-0805; **Board Cert:** Urology 2005; **Med School:** Rush Med Coll 1987; **Resid:** Surgery, Univ Iowa Hosps 1993; **Fellow:** Infertility, Univ Iowa Hosps 1995; **Fac Appt:** Assoc Prof U, Med Coll Wisc

Schaeffer, Anthony MD [U] - **Spec Exp:** Interstitial Cystitis; Incontinence after Prostate Cancer; Urology-Female; **Hospital:** Northwestern Meml Hosp; **Address:** 675 N St Clair, Galter Bldg Fl 20 - Ste 150, Chicago, IL 60611; **Phone:** 312-695-8146; **Board Cert:** Urology 1978; **Med School:** Northwestern Univ 1968; **Resid:** Surgery, Northwestern Meml Hosp 1970; Urology, Stanford Med Ctr 1976; **Fac Appt:** Prof U, Northwestern Univ

See, William A MD [U] - **Spec Exp:** Prostate Cancer; Bladder Cancer; Testicular Cancer; **Hospital:** Froedtert Meml Lutheran Hosp; **Address:** Med Coll Wisconsin, Dept Urology, 9200 W Wisconsin Ave, Milwaukee, WI 53226; **Phone:** 414-805-0805; **Board Cert:** Urology 2008; **Med School:** Univ Chicago-Pritzker Sch Med 1982; **Resid:** Urology, Univ Washington 1988; **Fellow:** Research, Natl Kidney Fdn/Univ Wash 1986; Research, Amer Fdn for Urol Dis/Univ Iowa 1990; **Fac Appt:** Prof U, Med Coll Wisc

Urology

Seftel, Allen D MD [U] - **Spec Exp:** Sexual Dysfunction; Infertility-Male; Prostate Disease; **Hospital:** Univ Hosps Case Med Ctr; **Address:** Univ Hosp-Cleveland, 11100 Euclid Ave, Ste 4550, Office # 4564, Cleveland, OH 44106-1736; **Phone:** 216-844-3009; **Board Cert:** Urology 2003; **Med School:** SUNY Downstate 1984; **Resid:** Urology, SUNY Downstate Med Ctr 1987; Urology, Univ Hosps-Case West Res 1990; **Fellow:** Reproductive Medicine, Boston Univ Med Ctr 1992; **Fac Appt:** Prof U, Case West Res Univ

Sheldon, Curtis A MD [U] - **Spec Exp:** Pediatric Urology; Genitourinary Reconstruction; Transplant-Kidney-Pediatric; **Hospital:** Cincinnati Chldns Hosp Med Ctr; **Address:** Childrens Hosp, Div Pediatric Urology, 3333 Burnet Ave, MC 5037, Cincinnati, OH 45229; **Phone:** 513-636-4975; **Board Cert:** Urology 1993; Pediatric Urology 2008; **Med School:** UCSD 1976; **Resid:** Urology, Univ Minnesota Affil Hosp 1981; Surgery, Univ Minnesota Affil Hosp 1983; **Fellow:** Pediatric Surgery, Chldns Hosp Med Ctr 1985; Pediatric Urology, Hosp for Sick Chldn 1986; **Fac Appt:** Prof S, Univ Cincinnati

Silber, Sherman J MD [U] - **Spec Exp:** Infertility-Male; Vasectomy Reversal; Infertility-IVF; Transplant-Ovarian Tissue; **Hospital:** St Luke's Hosp - Chesterfield, MO; **Address:** 224 S Woods Mill Rd, Ste 730, St Louis, MO 63017-3451; **Phone:** 314-576-1400; **Board Cert:** Urology 1977; **Med School:** Univ Mich Med Sch 1966; **Resid:** Internal Medicine, PH Service Comm Corps 1969; Urology, Univ Michigan 1973; **Fellow:** Microsurgery, Univ Melbourne 1974

Steinberg, Gary D MD [U] - **Spec Exp:** Bladder Cancer; Kidney Cancer; Prostate Cancer; **Hospital:** Univ of Chicago Med Ctr; **Address:** 5841 S Maryland Ave, rm J653, MC 6038, Chicago, IL 60637-1447; **Phone:** 773-702-3080; **Board Cert:** Urology 2003; **Med School:** Univ Chicago-Pritzker Sch Med 1985; **Resid:** Surgery, Johns Hopkins Hosp 1987; Urology, Brady Urol Inst/Johns Hopkins 1991; **Fellow:** Oncology, Johns Hopkins Hosp 1989; **Fac Appt:** Prof U, Univ Chicago-Pritzker Sch Med

Williams, Richard D MD [U] - **Spec Exp:** Kidney Cancer; Bladder Cancer; Prostate Cancer; **Hospital:** Univ Iowa Hosp & Clinics; **Address:** Univ Iowa Hosp, Dept Urology, 200 Hawkins Dr, rm 3251 RCP, Iowa City, IA 52242-1089; **Phone:** 319-356-0760; **Board Cert:** Urology 1979; **Med School:** Univ Kans 1970; **Resid:** Surgery, Univ Minn Hosp 1972; Urology, Univ Minn Hosp 1976; **Fellow:** Urologic Oncology, Univ Minn Hosp 1979; **Fac Appt:** Prof U, Univ Iowa Coll Med

Wood, David P MD [U] - **Spec Exp:** Genitourinary Cancer; Bladder Cancer; Prostate Cancer; Robotic Surgery; **Hospital:** Univ Michigan Hlth Sys; **Address:** UMH Cancer Ctr, Team 3, Reception D, Level B1-229, 1500 E Medical Center Drive, Ann Arbor, MI 48109-5913; **Phone:** 734-647-8903; **Board Cert:** Urology 2002; **Med School:** Univ Mich Med Sch 1983; **Resid:** Urology, Cleveland Clinic 1988; **Fellow:** Urologic Oncology, Meml Sloan-Kettering Cancer Ctr 1991; **Fac Appt:** Prof U, Univ Mich Med Sch

Zippe, Craig D MD [U] - **Spec Exp:** Prostate Cancer; Bladder Cancer; Incontinence after Prostate Cancer; **Hospital:** Univ Hosps Case Med Ctr; **Address:** 88 Center Rd, Ste 360, Bedford, OH 44146; **Phone:** 440-232-8955; **Board Cert:** Urology 2007; **Med School:** Rush Med Coll 1980; **Resid:** Urology, Columbia Presby Med Ctr 1989; **Fellow:** Urologic Oncology, Meml Sloan Kettering Cancer Ctr 1992

Great Plains and Mountains

Cartwright, Patrick C MD [U] - **Spec Exp:** Pediatric Urology; **Hospital:** Primary Children's Med Ctr, Univ Utah Hosps and Clins; **Address:** Pediatric Urology, 100 N Mario Capecchi Drive, Ste 2200, Salt Lake City, UT 84113-1100; **Phone:** 801-662-5555; **Board Cert:** Urology 2001; **Med School:** Univ Tex SW, Dallas 1984; **Resid:** Urology, Univ Utah Affil Hosp 1989; **Fellow:** Pediatric Urology, Chldns Hosp 1990; **Fac Appt:** Assoc Prof S, Univ Utah

Childs, Stacy J MD [U] - **Spec Exp:** Voiding Dysfunction; Erectile Dysfunction; Prostate Cancer; Bladder Cancer; **Hospital:** Yampa Valley Med Ctr, Memorial Hosp - Craig; **Address:** 501 Anglers Drive, Ste 202, Steamboat Springs, CO 80487-8841; **Phone:** 970-871-9710; **Board Cert:** Urology 1979; **Med School:** Louisiana State U, New Orleans 1972; **Resid:** Urology, Carraway Meth Med Ctr 1977; **Fac Appt:** Clin Prof U, Univ Colorado

Crawford, E David MD [U] - **Spec Exp:** Prostate Cancer; Testicular Cancer; Bladder Cancer; **Hospital:** Univ Colorado Hosp; **Address:** Urologic Oncology, MS F710, 1665 Aurora Ct, rm 1004, Box 6510, Aurora, CO 80045; **Phone:** 720-848-0170; **Board Cert:** Urology 1980; **Med School:** Univ Cincinnati 1973; **Resid:** Urology, Good Samaritan Hosp 1977; **Fellow:** Genitourinary Surgery, UCLA Med Ctr 1978; **Fac Appt:** Prof U, Univ Colorado

Davis, Bradley E MD [U] - **Spec Exp:** Urologic Cancer; Bladder Cancer; Reconstructive Surgery; Prostate Cancer; **Hospital:** Overland Pk Regl Med Ctr, St Luke's Hosp of Kansas City; **Address:** Urologic Surgical Associates, 10550 Quivira Rd, Ste 105, Overland Park, KS 66215; **Phone:** 913-438-3833; **Board Cert:** Urology 2004; **Med School:** Univ Kans 1986; **Resid:** Surgery, St Lukes Hosp 1991; Urology, Univ Kansas Med Ctr 1991; **Fellow:** Urologic Oncology, Meml Sloan-Kettering Cancer Ctr 1993; **Fac Appt:** Asst Clin Prof U, Univ Kans

Lugg, James A MD [U] - **Spec Exp:** Prostate Cancer; Laparoscopic Surgery; Incontinence after Prostate Cancer; **Hospital:** Cheyenne Regl Med Ctr, Univ Colorado Hosp; **Address:** 2301 House Ave, Ste 502, Cheyenne, WY 82001; **Phone:** 307-635-4131; **Board Cert:** Urology 2008; **Med School:** Northwestern Univ 1990; **Resid:** Urology, UCLA Med Ctr 1995; **Fac Appt:** Asst Prof U, Univ Colorado

Southwest

Appell, Rodney A MD [U] - **Spec Exp:** Voiding Dysfunction; Urology-Female; Uro-Gynecology; **Hospital:** Methodist Hosp - Houston; **Address:** 6400 Fannin St, Ste 2300, Houston, TX 77030; **Phone:** 713-366-7800; **Board Cert:** Urology 1981; **Med School:** Jefferson Med Coll 1973; **Resid:** Surgery, George Wash Univ Med Ctr 1975; **Fellow:** Urology, Yale Univ Sch Med 1979; **Fac Appt:** Prof U, Baylor Coll Med

Bans, Larry L MD [U] - **Spec Exp:** Prostate Cancer; Prostate Disease; **Hospital:** Banner Good Samaritan Regl Med Ctr - Phoenix; **Address:** Prostate Solutions of Arizona, 2525 E Arizona Biltmore Cir, Ste C236, Phoenix, AZ 85016; **Phone:** 602-426-9772; **Board Cert:** Urology 2004; **Med School:** Cornell Univ-Weill Med Coll 1978; **Resid:** Urology, Ind Univ Med Ctr 1983

Bardot, Stephen F MD [U] - **Spec Exp:** Urologic Cancer; Prostate Cancer; **Hospital:** Ochsner Fdn Hosp; **Address:** Ochsner Clinic, 1514 Jefferson Hwy Fl 4, Atrium 4 West, Dept of Urology, New Orleans, LA 70121-2483; **Phone:** 504-842-4083; **Board Cert:** Urology 2002; **Med School:** Univ Kans 1985; **Resid:** Surgery, St Luke's Hosp 1987; Urology, Kansas City Univ Med Ctr 1990; **Fellow:** Urologic Oncology, Cleveland Clinic 1991

Basler, Joseph W MD [U] - **Spec Exp:** Prostate Cancer; Urologic Cancer; Kidney Stones; **Hospital:** Audie L Murphy Meml Vets Hosp; **Address:** 7703 Floyd Curl Dr, MC-7845, San Antonio, TX 78229-3900; **Phone:** 210-567-5640; **Board Cert:** Urology 2001; **Med School:** Univ MO-Columbia Sch Med 1984; **Resid:** Surgery, Univ Missouri Affil Hosp 1986; Urology, Barnes Hosp/Wash Univ 1990; **Fac Appt:** Prof U, Univ Tex, San Antonio

Urology

Boone, Timothy B MD/PhD [U] - **Spec Exp:** Neuro-Urology; Urinary Reconstruction; Incontinence; **Hospital:** Methodist Hosp - Houston, St Luke's Episcopal Hosp-Houston; **Address:** Scurlock Tower, 6560 Fannin, Ste 2100, Houston, TX 77030-2769; **Phone:** 713-441-6455; **Board Cert:** Urology 2004; **Med School:** Univ Tex, Houston 1985; **Resid:** Surgery, Univ Tex SW Med Ctr 1987; Urology, Univ Tex SW Med Ctr 1991; **Fac Appt:** Prof U, Baylor Coll Med

Buch, Jeffrey Phillip MD [U] - **Spec Exp:** Vasectomy Reversal; Infertility-Male; Sexual Dysfunction; **Address:** Legacy Male Health Institute, 5516 Warren Pkwy, Ste 101, Frisco, TX 75034; **Phone:** 972-612-7131; **Board Cert:** Urology 2005; **Med School:** Univ Mich Med Sch 1980; **Resid:** Surgery, Albany Med Ctr 1982; Urology, Albany Med Ctr 1985; **Fellow:** Male Infertility, Baylor Coll Med 1987; Microsurgery, Baylor Coll Med 1987; **Fac Appt:** Assoc Clin Prof U, Univ Tex SW, Dallas

Culkin, Daniel J MD [U] - **Spec Exp:** Voiding Dysfunction; Interstitial Cystitis; Urologic Cancer; Laparoscopic Surgery; **Hospital:** OU Med Ctr, VA Med Ctr - Oklahoma City; **Address:** Oklahoma Univ Med Ctr, Div Urology, 920 Stanton L Young Blvd, Ste WP 3150, Oklahoma City, OK 73104; **Phone:** 405-271-8156; **Board Cert:** Urology 2006; **Med School:** Creighton Univ 1979; **Resid:** Surgery, Loyola Univ Med Ctr 1981; Urology, Loyola Univ Med Ctr 1983; **Fellow:** Neurourology, Loyola Univ Med Ctr 1984; **Fac Appt:** Prof U, Univ Okla Coll Med

Ellis, David S MD [U] - **Spec Exp:** Prostate Cancer-Cryosurgery; **Hospital:** Arlington Meml Hosp; **Address:** Urology Assocs of N Texas (UANT), Arlington-North, 1001 Waldrop Drive, Ste 708, Arlington, TX 76012; **Phone:** 817-465-0373; **Board Cert:** Urology 2000; **Med School:** Univ Tex, Houston 1982; **Resid:** Urology, Univ Texas Med Ctr 1988

Ewalt, David H MD [U] - **Spec Exp:** Pediatric Urology; Hypospadias; Urinary Reconstruction; Neurogenic Bladder; **Hospital:** Chldns Med Ctr of Dallas, Med City Dallas Hosp; **Address:** 8315 Walnut Hill Lane, Ste 205, Dallas, TX 75231; **Phone:** 214-750-0808; **Board Cert:** Urology 2003; Pediatric Urology 2008; **Med School:** Univ Tex SW, Dallas 1984; **Resid:** Urology, Univ Texas SW Affil Hosps 1990; **Fellow:** Pediatric Urology, Chldns Hosp 1992

Gonzales, Edmond T MD [U] - **Spec Exp:** Pediatric Urology; **Hospital:** Texas Chldns Hosp; **Address:** Clinical Care Center, Ste 660, 6701 Fannin St, Houston, TX 77030; **Phone:** 832-822-3160; **Board Cert:** Urology 1975; Pediatric Urology 2008; **Med School:** Tulane Univ 1965; **Resid:** Surgery, Duke Univ Med Ctr 1968; Urology, Duke Univ Med Ctr 1972; **Fellow:** Pediatric Urology, Childrens Hosp; **Fac Appt:** Prof U, Baylor Coll Med

Greene, Graham MD [U] - **Spec Exp:** Urologic Cancer; **Hospital:** UAMS Med Ctr, Arkansas Chldns Hosp; **Address:** 4301 W Markham, Slot 774, Little Rock, AR 72205; **Phone:** 501-296-1545; **Board Cert:** Urology 2007; **Med School:** Dalhousie Univ 1989; **Resid:** Urology, Victoria Genl 1994; **Fellow:** Urologic Oncology, M.D. Anderson Cancer Ctr 1997; **Fac Appt:** Assoc Prof U, Univ Ark

Grossman, H Barton MD [U] - **Spec Exp:** Bladder Cancer; Bladder Reconstruction; Urinary Reconstruction; **Hospital:** UT MD Anderson Cancer Ctr; **Address:** MD Anderson Cancer Ctr, Dept Urology, 1373, 1515 Holcombe Blvd, Houston, TX 77030; **Phone:** 713-792-3250; **Board Cert:** Urology 1979; **Med School:** Temple Univ 1972; **Resid:** Surgery, St Joseph Mercy Hosp 1974; Urology, Univ Michigan Med Ctr 1977; **Fellow:** Research, Meml Sloan Kettering Cancer Ctr 1979; **Fac Appt:** Prof U, Univ Tex, Houston

Hellstrom, Wayne J MD [U] - **Spec Exp:** Infertility-Male; Erectile Dysfunction; Peyronie's Disease; Penile Prostheses; **Hospital:** Tulane Univ Hosp & Clin; **Address:** 1430 Tulane Ave, SL42, New Orleans, LA 70112; **Phone:** 504-988-7308; **Board Cert:** Urology 2007; **Med School:** Canada 1981; **Resid:** Surgery, Montreal Genl/Royal Vistoria Hosp 1983; Urology, UCSF Med Ctr 1985; **Fellow:** Andrology, UC Davis Med Ctr 1988; **Fac Appt:** Prof U, Tulane Univ

Kadmon, Dov MD [U] - **Spec Exp:** Prostate Cancer; **Hospital:** St Luke's Episcopal Hosp-Houston, Methodist Hosp - Houston; **Address:** Baylor Dept Urology, 6620 Main St, Ste 1325, Houston, TX 77030; **Phone:** 713-798-4001; **Board Cert:** Urology 1984; **Med School:** Israel 1970; **Resid:** Surgery, Barnes Jewish Hosp 1977; Urology, Barnes Jewish Hosp 1980; **Fellow:** Urology, Barnes Jewish Hosp 1982; **Fac Appt:** Prof U, Baylor Coll Med

Lerner, Seth P MD [U] - **Spec Exp:** Bladder Cancer; Testicular Cancer; Urinary Reconstruction; **Hospital:** St Luke's Episcopal Hosp-Houston, Methodist Hosp - Houston; **Address:** 6620 Main St, Ste 1325, Houston, TX 77030; **Phone:** 713-798-6841; **Board Cert:** Urology 2002; **Med School:** Baylor Coll Med 1984; **Resid:** Surgery, Virginia Mason Hosp 1986; Urology, Baylor Coll Med 1990; **Fellow:** Urologic Oncology, LAC-USC Med Ctr 1992; **Fac Appt:** Prof U, Baylor Coll Med

Lipshultz, Larry MD [U] - **Spec Exp:** Infertility-Male; Microsurgery; Erectile Dysfunction; **Hospital:** St Luke's Episcopal Hosp-Houston, Methodist Hosp - Houston; **Address:** 6560 Fannin St, Scurlock Twr, Ste 2100, Houston, TX 77030-2706; **Phone:** 713-798-4001; **Board Cert:** Urology 1977; **Med School:** Univ Pennsylvania 1968; **Resid:** Urology, Hosp Univ Penn 1971; **Fellow:** Reproductive Medicine, Univ Tex Med Sch Affil Hosp 1971; **Fac Appt:** Prof U, Baylor Coll Med

Miles, Brian J MD [U] - **Spec Exp:** Prostate Cancer; Urologic Cancer; Gene Therapy; **Hospital:** Methodist Hosp - Houston, St Luke's Episcopal Hosp-Houston; **Address:** 6624 Fannin St, Ste 2280, Houston, TX 77030-2769; **Phone:** 713-799-8896; **Board Cert:** Urology 1984; **Med School:** Univ Mich Med Sch 1974; **Resid:** Urology, Walter Reed Army Med Ctr 1982; **Fac Appt:** Clin Prof U, Baylor Coll Med

Pisters, Louis L MD [U] - **Spec Exp:** Prostate Cancer; Bladder Cancer; Genitourinary Cancer; Prostate Cancer/Robotic Surgery; **Hospital:** UT MD Anderson Cancer Ctr; **Address:** MD Anderson Cancer Ctr, 1515 Holcombe Blvd, Unit 1373, Houston, TX 77030; **Phone:** 713-792-3250; **Board Cert:** Urology 2003; **Med School:** Univ Western Ontario 1986; **Resid:** Urology, Shands Hosp/UNIV Florida 1991; **Fellow:** Urologic Oncology, MD Anderson Cancer Ctr 1993; **Fac Appt:** Assoc Prof U, Univ Tex, Houston

Roehrborn, Claus MD [U] - **Spec Exp:** Prostate Disease; Prostate Cancer; **Hospital:** UT Southwestern Med Ctr at Dallas, Parkland Hlth & Hosp Sys; **Address:** Dept Urology, 5323 Harry Hines Blvd, J8-148, Dallas, TX 75390-9110; **Phone:** 214-645-8765; **Board Cert:** Urology 2004; **Med School:** Germany 1980; **Resid:** Surgery, W Germany Army Hosp 1982; Urology, UT SW Med Ctr 1989; **Fellow:** Urology, Am Fdn Urol Dis 1991; **Fac Appt:** Prof U, Univ Tex SW, Dallas

Sagalowsky, Arthur I MD [U] - **Spec Exp:** Urologic Cancer; Transplant-Kidney; Testicular Cancer; **Hospital:** UT Southwestern Med Ctr at Dallas; **Address:** UT SW Med Ctr, Dept Urology, 5323 Harry Hines Blvd, J8.114, Dallas, TX 75390-9110; **Phone:** 214-648-3976; **Board Cert:** Urology 1980; **Med School:** Indiana Univ 1973; **Resid:** Surgery, Indiana Univ Hosps 1975; Urology, Indiana Univ Hosps 1978; **Fellow:** Clinical Pharmacology, Univ Tex SW Med Ctr 1980; **Fac Appt:** Prof U, Univ Tex SW, Dallas

Slawin, Kevin Mark MD [U] - **Spec Exp:** Prostate Cancer; Prostate Cancer/Robotic Surgery; Prostate Disease; **Hospital:** Meml Hermann Hosp - Texas Med Ctr, Methodist Hosp - Houston; **Address:** Vanguard Urologic Inst, Memorial Hermann Medical Plaza, 6400 Fannin, Ste 2300, Houston, TX 77030; **Phone:** 713-366-7848; **Board Cert:** Urology 2005; **Med School:** Columbia P&S 1986; **Resid:** Surgery, Mt Sinai Med Ctr 1988; Urology, Columbia-Presby Hosp 1992; **Fellow:** Urologic Oncology, Am Fdn Urol Dis/Baylor Coll Med 1994; **Fac Appt:** Clin Prof U, Baylor Coll Med

Urology

Strand, William R MD [U] - **Spec Exp:** Pediatric Urology; Laparoscopic Surgery; Hypospadias; Reconstructive Surgery; **Hospital:** Chldns Med Ctr of Dallas; **Address:** 4001 W 15th St Bldg 3 - Ste 300, Plano, TX 75093; **Phone:** 214-750-0808 x5400; **Board Cert:** Urology 2001; Pediatric Urology 2008; **Med School:** Mayo Med Sch 1983; **Resid:** Surgery, Naval Med Ctr 1984; Urology, Natl Naval Med Ctr 1988; **Fellow:** Pediatric Urology, Chldns Med Ctr of Dallas; **Fac Appt:** Assoc Prof U, Univ Tex SW, Dallas

Swanson, David A MD [U] - **Spec Exp:** Kidney Cancer; Prostate Cancer; Testicular Cancer; **Hospital:** UT MD Anderson Cancer Ctr; **Address:** UT MD Anderson Canc Ctr, Dept Urol, 1515 Holcombe Blvd , Unit 1373, Houston, TX 77030-4009; **Phone:** 713-792-3250; **Board Cert:** Urology 1977; **Med School:** Univ Pennsylvania 1967; **Resid:** Surgery, Harbor Genl Hosp 1969; Urology, UC Davis Med Ctr 1975; **Fellow:** Urologic Oncology, Univ Tex-MD Anderson Hosp 1978

Thompson Jr, Ian M MD [U] - **Spec Exp:** Prostate Cancer; Prostate Disease; **Hospital:** Univ Hlth Syst-San Antonio; **Address:** Univ Tex Hlth Scis Ctr, Dept Urol, 7703 Floyd Curl Drive, rm 306L, MC 7845, San Antonio, TX 78229-3900; **Phone:** 210-567-5643; **Board Cert:** Urology 2005; **Med School:** Tulane Univ 1980; **Resid:** Urology, Brooke Army Med Ctr 1985; **Fellow:** Medical Oncology, Meml Sloan-Kettering Canc Ctr 1988; **Fac Appt:** Prof S, Univ Tex, San Antonio

Winters, Jack C MD [U] - **Spec Exp:** Voiding Dysfunction; Urology-Female; Urinary Reconstruction; **Hospital:** Ochsner Fdn Hosp; **Address:** Ochsner Clinic, Dept Urology, 1514 Jefferson Hwy Fl 4, New Orleans, LA 70121; **Phone:** 504-842-4083; **Board Cert:** Urology 2006; **Med School:** Louisiana State U, New Orleans 1988; **Resid:** Surgery, Ochsner Fdn Hosp 1990; Urology, Ochsner Fdn Hosp 1994; **Fellow:** Female Urology, Cleveland Clinic Fdn 1995

Woo, Howard H MD [U] - **Spec Exp:** Pain-Pelvic; Voiding Dysfunction; ncontinence; **Hospital:** Ochsner Fdn Hosp; **Address:** Ochsner Clinic Foundation, Dept Urology, 1516 Jefferson Hwy, New Orleans, LA 70121; **Phone:** 504-842-4084; **Board Cert:** Urology 2006; **Med School:** Med Coll Wisc 1989; **Resid:** Urology, Univ Colorado Hlth Sci Ctr 1995

West Coast and Pacific

Ahlering, Thomas E MD [U] - **Spec Exp:** Prostate Cancer/Robotic Surgery; **Hospital:** UC Irvine Med Ctr, VA Med Ctr - Long Beach, CA; **Address:** UC Irvine Med Ctr, 333 City Blvd W, Ste 2100, Orange, CA 92868; **Phone:** 714-456-6068; **Board Cert:** Urology 2005; **Med School:** St Louis Univ 1979; **Resid:** Urology, LAC-USC Med Ctr 1984; **Fellow:** Urologic Oncology, USC-Norris Comp Cancer Ctr 1986; **Fac Appt:** Prof U, UC Irvine

Amling, Christopher L MD [U] - **Spec Exp:** Prostate Cancer/Robotic Surgery; Kidney Cancer; Bladder Cancer; Testicular Cancer; **Hospital:** OR Hlth & Sci Univ; **Address:** 3303 SW Bond Ave, MC CC10U, Portland, OR 97239; **Phone:** 503-494-4779; **Board Cert:** Urology 1999; **Med School:** Oregon Hlth & Sci Univ 1985; **Resid:** Urology, Duke Univ Med Ctr 1996; **Fellow:** Urologic Oncology, Mayo Clinic 1997; **Fac Appt:** Prof U, Univ Alabama

Baskin, Laurence S MD [U] - **Spec Exp:** Pediatric Urology; Hypospadias; **Hospital:** UCSF Med Ctr, CA Pacific Med Ctr - Pacific Campus; **Address:** Urology Faculty Practice, 400 Parnassus Ave Fl 6th, Ste 610A, Box 0330, San Francisco, CA 94143-0330; **Phone:** 415-353-2200; **Board Cert:** Urology 2004; Pediatric Urology 2008; **Med School:** UCLA 1986; **Resid:** Urology, UCSF Med Ctr 1991; **Fellow:** Pediatric Urology, Childrens Hosp 1993; **Fac Appt:** Assoc Prof U, UCSF

Belldegrun, Arie S MD [U] - **Spec Exp:** Urologic Cancer; Gene Therapy; **Hospital:** UCLA Ronald Reagan Med Ctr; **Address:** UCLA-Geffen Sch Med, Dep Urology, 108-33 Leconte Ave, rm 66-118, Los Angeles, CA 90095; **Phone:** 310-206-1434; **Board Cert:** Urology 1999; **Med School:** Israel 1974; **Resid:** Urology, Brigham and Women's Hosp 1985; **Fellow:** Urologic Oncology, Natl Cancer Inst, NIH 1988; **Fac Appt:** Prof U, UCLA

Boyd, Stuart D MD [U] - **Spec Exp:** Incontinence; Erectile Dysfunction; Urologic Cancer; **Hospital:** USC Norris Cancer Hosp, USC Univ Hosp; **Address:** 1441 Eastlake Ave, Ste 7416, Los Angeles, CA 90089-9178; **Phone:** 323-865-3704; **Board Cert:** Urology 1984; **Med School:** UCLA 1975; **Resid:** Urology, UCLA Med Ctr 1982; **Fac Appt:** Prof U, USC Sch Med

Carroll, Peter R MD [U] - **Spec Exp:** Testicular Cancer; Prostate Cancer; Bladder Cancer; Bladder Reconstruction; **Hospital:** UCSF - Mt Zion Med Ctr; **Address:** UCSF Urologic Oncology Practice, Fl 3, Box 1711, 1600 Divisadero St, San Francisco, CA 94115-1711; **Phone:** 415-353-7171; **Board Cert:** Urology 2006; **Med School:** Georgetown Univ 1979; **Resid:** Surgery, UCSF Med Ctr 1984; **Fellow:** Urology, Meml Sloan Kettering Cancer Ctr 1986; **Fac Appt:** Prof U, UCSF

Clayman, Ralph V MD [U] - **Spec Exp:** Kidney Stones; Kidney Cancer; Laparoscopic Surgery; Robotic Surgery; **Hospital:** UC Irvine Med Ctr; **Address:** UCI Med Ctr, Dept Urology, 333 City Blvd W, Ste 2100, Orange, CA 92868; **Phone:** 714-456-3330; **Board Cert:** Urology 2007; **Med School:** UCSD 1973; **Resid:** Urology, Univ Minn Med Ctr 1979; **Fac Appt:** Prof U, UC Irvine

Daneshmand, Siamak MD [U] - **Spec Exp:** Bladder Cancer; Prostate Cancer; Kidney Cancer; Testicular Cancer; **Hospital:** OR Hlth & Sci Univ; **Address:** Division of Urology, 10th FL, Center for Health & Healing, 3303 SW Bond Ave, Ste CH10U, Portland, OR 97239; **Phone:** 503-346-1500; **Board Cert:** Urology 2006; **Med School:** UC Davis 1996; **Resid:** Surgery, UC Med Ctr 1998; Urology, UC Med Ctr 2002; **Fellow:** Urologic Oncology, UC Med Ctr 2004; **Fac Appt:** Assoc Prof S, Oregon Hlth & Sci Univ

Danoff, Dudley S MD [U] - **Spec Exp:** Prostate Cancer; Bladder Cancer; Erectile Dysfunction; **Hospital:** Cedars-Sinai Med Ctr; **Address:** 8635 W 3rd St, Ste 1 West, Los Angeles, CA 90048; **Phone:** 310-854-9898; **Board Cert:** Urology 1974; **Med School:** Yale Univ 1963; **Resid:** Urology, Yale-New Haven Hosp 1965; Urology, Columbia-Presby Med Ctr 1969

de Kernion, Jean B MD [U] - **Spec Exp:** Urologic Cancer; Kidney Cancer; Prostate Cancer; Prostate Disease; **Hospital:** UCLA Ronald Reagan Med Ctr; **Address:** UCLA-Geffen Sch Med, Dept Urology, rm 66-133CHS, Box 951738, Los Angeles, CA 90095-1738; **Phone:** 310-206-6453; **Board Cert:** Surgery 1973; Urology 1975; **Med School:** Louisiana State U, New Orleans 1965; **Resid:** Surgery, Univ Hosps-Case West Res 1967; Urology, Univ Hosps-Case West Res 1973; **Fellow:** Urologic Oncology, Natl Cancer Inst 1969; **Fac Appt:** Prof U, UCLA

Ellis, William J MD [U] - **Spec Exp:** Prostate Cancer; Prostate Disease; Kidney Cancer; **Hospital:** Univ Wash Med Ctr; **Address:** Univ Wash Med Ctr, Dept Urology, 1959 NE Pacific St, Box 356158, Seattle, WA 98195; **Phone:** 206-598-4294; **Board Cert:** Urology 2001; **Med School:** Johns Hopkins Univ 1985; **Resid:** Surgery, Northwestern Meml Hosp 1987; Urology, Northwestern Meml Hosp 1991; **Fac Appt:** Assoc Prof U, Univ Wash

Fuchs, Eugene F MD [U] - **Spec Exp:** Infertility-Male; Kidney Stones; Vasectomy Reversal; **Hospital:** OR Hlth & Sci Univ, Legacy Emanuel Hospitals; **Address:** 3303 SW Bond Ave Fl 10, Portland, OR 97239; **Phone:** 503-418-9032; **Board Cert:** Urology 1977; **Med School:** Univ VT Coll Med 1970; **Resid:** Urology, Univ Oregon Hosp 1975; **Fac Appt:** Prof U, Oregon Hlth & Sci Univ

Urology

Gill, Harcharan Singh MD [U] - **Spec Exp:** Urologic Cancer; Prostate Cancer; Prostate Disease; **Hospital:** Stanford Univ Med Ctr; **Address:** 875 Blake Wilbur Drive, rm 2216, Stanford, CA 94305-5826; **Phone:** 650-725-5544; **Board Cert:** Urology 2004; **Med School:** Kenya 1977; **Resid:** Urology, Inst of Urol; Urology, Univ Penn 1991; **Fellow:** Urology, Univ Penn 1986; **Fac Appt:** Prof U, Stanford Univ

Gill, Inderbir Singh MD [U] - **Spec Exp:** Prostate Cancer; Kidney Cancer; Urologic Cancer; Minimally Invasive Urologic Surgery; **Hospital:** USC Norris Cancer Hosp; **Address:** USC/Norris Cancer Ctr, Dept Urology, 1441 Eastlake Ave, Ste 7416, Los Angeles, CA 90089; **Phone:** 323-865-3700; **Board Cert:** Urology 2008; **Med School:** India 1980; **Resid:** Surgery, Dayanand Med Coll & Hosp; Urology, Univ Kentucky Hosp 1993; **Fac Appt:** Prof U, Univ SC Sch Med

Ginsberg, David A MD [U] - **Spec Exp:** Incontinence; Urinary Reconstruction; Neuro-Urology; Neurogenic Bladder; **Hospital:** USC Univ Hosp; **Address:** USC-Norris Cancer Ctr, 1441 Eastlake Ave, Ste 7416, Los Angeles, CA 90033; **Phone:** 323-865-3703; **Board Cert:** Urology 2008; **Med School:** USC Sch Med 1990; **Resid:** Surgery, LAC-USC Med Ctr 1992; Urology, LAc-USC Med Ctr 1996; **Fellow:** Reconstructive Surgery, UCLA Med Ctr 1997; **Fac Appt:** Assoc Clin Prof U, USC-Keck School of Medicine

Holden, Stuart MD [U] - **Spec Exp:** Kidney Cancer; **Hospital:** Cedars-Sinai Med Ctr; **Address:** 8635 W 3rd St, Ste 1 West, Los Angeles, CA 90048; **Phone:** 310-854-9898; **Board Cert:** Urology 1977; **Med School:** Cornell Univ-Weill Med Coll 1968; **Resid:** Surgery, NY Hosp-Cornell 1970; Urology, Emory Univ Hosp 1975; **Fellow:** Urology, Meml Sloan Kettering Cancer Ctr 1978

Kawachi, Mark H MD [U] - **Spec Exp:** Prostate Cancer/Robotic Surgery; Minimally Invasive Urologic Surgery; **Hospital:** City of Hope Natl Med Ctr & Beckman Rsch; **Address:** Div Urologic Oncology, 1500 E Duarte Rd, Duarte, CA 91010-3012; **Phone:** 626-359-8111 x62655; **Board Cert:** Urology 2004; **Med School:** USC Sch Med 1979; **Resid:** Urology, USC Med Ctr 1984

Koyle, Martin A MD [U] - **Spec Exp:** Pediatric Urology; Genitourinary Reconstruction; Transplant-Kidney-Pediatric; **Hospital:** Chldns Hosp and Regl Med Ctr - Seattle; **Address:** Pediatric Urology W-7729, 4800 Sand Point Way NE, W-7729, Seattle, WA 98105-0371; **Phone:** 206-987-5893; **Board Cert:** Urology 2004; Pediatric Urology 2008; **Med School:** Canada 1976; **Resid:** Surgery, Hlth Scis Ctr 1978; Urology, Brigham & Womens Hosp 1984; **Fellow:** Transplant Surgery, Pacific Med Ctr 1982; **Fac Appt:** Prof U, Univ Wash

Lange, Paul H MD [U] - **Spec Exp:** Prostate Cancer; **Hospital:** Univ Wash Med Ctr; **Address:** Univ Wash Med Ctr, Dept Urology, 1959 NE Pacific St, Box 356158, Seattle, WA 98195; **Phone:** 206-598-4294; **Board Cert:** Urology 2006; **Med School:** Washington Univ, St Louis 1967; **Resid:** Surgery, Duke Univ Med Ctr 1972; Urology, Univ Minn Med Ctr 1975; **Fellow:** Immunology, Univ Minn 1973; Research, Natl Inst Hlth 1970; **Fac Appt:** Prof U, Univ Wash

Lieskovsky, Gary MD [U] - **Spec Exp:** Prostate Cancer; **Hospital:** USC Norris Cancer Hosp, USC Univ Hosp; **Address:** 1441 Eastlake Ave, Ste 7416, Los Angeles, CA 90089-0112; **Phone:** 323-865-3702; **Board Cert:** Urology 1980; **Med School:** Canada 1973; **Resid:** Urology, Univ Alberta Hosp 1978; **Fellow:** Urology, UCLA Med Ctr 1980; **Fac Appt:** Prof U, USC Sch Med

Marsh, Christopher L MD [U] - **Spec Exp:** Transplant-Kidney; Transplant-Pancreas; Islet Cell Transplant; Adrenal Surgery; **Hospital:** Scripps Green Hosp; **Address:** Scripps Green Hospital, 10666 N Torrey Pines Rd, MC 200N, La Jolla, CA 92037; **Phone:** 858-554-4310; **Board Cert:** Urology 2006; **Med School:** Loma Linda Univ 1980; **Resid:** Urology, Loma Linda U Med Ctr 1986; **Fellow:** Transplant Surgery, Mayo Clinic 1987

McAninch, Jack W MD [U] - **Spec Exp:** Genitourinary Trauma; Genitourinary Reconstruction; **Hospital:** UCSF Med Ctr, San Francisco Genl Hosp; **Address:** San Francisco Genl Hosp, Dept Urology, 1001 Potrero Ave, Ste 3A20, San Francisco, CA 94110; **Phone:** 415-476-3372; **Board Cert:** Urology 1995; **Med School:** Univ Tex Med Br, Galveston 1964; **Resid:** Surgery, Darnall Army Hosp 1966; Urology, Letterman AMC 1969; **Fac Appt:** Prof U, UCSF

McClure, Robert D MD [U] - **Spec Exp:** Infertility-Male; **Hospital:** Virginia Mason Med Ctr; **Address:** Virginia Mason Med Ctr, 1100 9th Ave, MS C7-URO, Seattle, WA 98101; **Phone:** 206-223-6179; **Board Cert:** Urology 1979; **Med School:** Canada 1968; **Resid:** Urology, McGill Univ Hosp 1975; **Fellow:** Endocrinology, Univ Washington Med Ctr 1977

Payne, Christopher K MD [U] - **Spec Exp:** Interstitial Cystitis; Pelvic Organ Prolapse Repair; Incontinence; Neurogenic Bladder; **Hospital:** Stanford Univ Med Ctr; **Address:** Stanford Univ, Dept Urology, 300 Pasteur Drive, rm A-260, Stanford, CA 94305-5118; **Phone:** 650-723-3391; **Board Cert:** Urology 2004; **Med School:** Vanderbilt Univ 1986; **Resid:** Urology, Univ Penn 1992; **Fellow:** Urology, UCLA Med Ctr 1993; **Fac Appt:** Assoc Prof U, Stanford Univ

Penson, David F MD [U] - **Spec Exp:** Urologic Cancer; Prostate Disease; Bladder Cancer; Erectile Dysfunction; **Hospital:** USC Univ Hosp, Good Sam Hosp; **Address:** 1441 Eastlake Ave, Ste 7416, Los Angeles, CA 90089; **Phone:** 323-865-3716; **Board Cert:** Urology 2001; **Med School:** Boston Univ 1991; **Resid:** Urology, UCLA Med Ctr 1997; **Fellow:** Urologic Oncology, Yale-New Haven Hosp 1999; **Fac Appt:** Assoc Prof U, USC-Keck School of Medicine

Perkash, Inder MD [U] - **Spec Exp:** Neurogenic Bladder; Neuro-Urology; Spinal Cord Injury; Voiding Dysfunction/Spinal Cord Injury; **Hospital:** VA Hlth Care Sys - Palo Alto, Stanford Univ Med Ctr; **Address:** VA Med Ctr-Spinal Cord Injury Svc, Urology Dept-MC 112C, 3801 Miranda Ave, Palo Alto, CA 94304-1207; **Phone:** 650-849-1916; **Board Cert:** Physical Medicine & Rehabilitation 1977; Spinal Cord Injury Medicine 2001; **Med School:** India 1957; **Resid:** Urology, Hammersmith Hosp 1963; Physical Medicine & Rehabilitation, Baylor Affil Hosp 1973; **Fellow:** Urology, Stanford Univ Med Ctr 1965; **Fac Appt:** Prof U, Stanford Univ

Presti Jr, Joseph C MD [U] - **Spec Exp:** Prostate Cancer; Bladder Cancer; Kidney Cancer; **Hospital:** Stanford Univ Med Ctr; **Address:** Stanford Cancer Ctr, 875 Blake Wilbur Dr MC 5826, Stanford, CA 94305; **Phone:** 650-725-5544; **Board Cert:** Urology 2002; **Med School:** UC Irvine 1984; **Resid:** Surgery, UCSF Med Ctr 1986; Urology, UCSF Med Ctr 1989; **Fellow:** Urologic Oncology, Meml Sloan-Kettering Cancer Ctr 1992; **Fac Appt:** Prof U, Stanford Univ

Rajfer, Jacob MD [U] - **Spec Exp:** Erectile Dysfunction; Prostate Disease; Infertility-Male; **Hospital:** LAC - Harbor - UCLA Med Ctr, UCLA Ronald Reagan Med Ctr; **Address:** 21840 S Normandy Ave, Ste 600, Torrance, CA 90502; **Phone:** 310-222-5189; **Board Cert:** Urology 1980; **Med School:** Northwestern Univ 1972; **Resid:** Surgery, St Josephs Hosp 1974; Urology, Johns Hopkins Hosp 1978; **Fellow:** Research, Johns Hopkins Hosp 1976; **Fac Appt:** Prof U, UCLA

Raz, Shlomo MD [U] - **Spec Exp:** Incontinence-Female; Urology-Female; **Hospital:** UCLA Ronald Reagan Med Ctr; **Address:** 200 Medical Plaza, Ste 140, Los Angeles, CA 90095; **Phone:** 310-794-0206; **Board Cert:** Urology 1979; **Med School:** Uruguay 1962; **Resid:** Surgery, Hadassah Univ Hosp 1973; **Fellow:** Urology, UCLA Med Ctr 1975; **Fac Appt:** Prof U, UCLA

Sharlip, Ira D MD [U] - **Spec Exp:** Vasectomy Reversal; Erectile Dysfunction; Infertility-Male; **Hospital:** CA Pacific Med Ctr - Pacific Campus, UCSF Med Ctr; **Address:** 2100 Webster St, Ste 222, San Francisco, CA 94115-2376; **Phone:** 415-202-0250; **Board Cert:** Internal Medicine 1972; Urology 1977; **Med School:** Univ Pennsylvania 1965; **Resid:** Internal Medicine, Hosp Univ Penn 1967; Urology, UCSF Med Ctr 1975; **Fellow:** Urology, Middlesex Hosp 1976; **Fac Appt:** Clin Prof U, UCSF

Shortliffe, Linda M MD [U] - **Spec Exp:** Pediatric Urology; Hypospadias; Hydronephrosis; **Hospital:** Lucile Packard Chldn's Hosp, Stanford Univ Med Ctr; **Address:** 300 Pasteur Drive, rm S287, Stanford, CA 94305-5118; **Phone:** 650-724-7608; **Board Cert:** Urology 2002; Pediatric Urology 2008; **Med School:** Stanford Univ 1975; **Resid:** Surgery, Tufts-New England Med Ctr 1977; Urology, Stanford Univ Med Ctr 1981; **Fellow:** Pediatric Urology, Childrens Hosp 1987; **Fac Appt:** Prof U, Stanford Univ

Skinner, Eila C MD [U] - **Spec Exp:** Urologic Cancer; Genitourinary Disorders-Geriatric; Urinary Reconstruction; **Hospital:** USC Norris Cancer Hosp, USC Univ Hosp; **Address:** USC-Keck Sch Med, Dept Urology, 1441 Eastlake Ave, Ste 7416, Los Angeles, CA 90089; **Phone:** 323-865-3707; **Board Cert:** Urology 2001; **Med School:** USC Sch Med 1983; **Resid:** Urology, LAC-USC Med Ctr 1988; **Fellow:** Urologic Oncology, LAC-USC Med Ctr 1990; **Fac Appt:** Assoc Prof U, USC Sch Med

Stoller, Marshall L MD [U] - **Spec Exp:** Laparoscopic Surgery; Kidney Stones; **Hospital:** UCSF Med Ctr; **Address:** 400 Parnassus Ave Fl 6, San Francisco, CA 94143; **Phone:** 415-353-2200; **Board Cert:** Urology 1999; **Med School:** Baylor Coll Med 1981; **Resid:** Surgery, UCSF Med Ctr 1983; Urology, UCSF Med Ctr 1987; **Fellow:** Urology, Prince Henry Hosptial 1986; **Fac Appt:** Prof U, UCSF

Stone, Anthony R MD [U] - **Spec Exp:** Urology-Female; Voiding Dysfunction; **Hospital:** UC Davis Med Ctr; **Address:** 4860 Y St, Ste 3500, Sacramento, CA 95817-2214; **Phone:** 916-734-2222; **Board Cert:** Urology 2006; **Med School:** Scotland, UK 1972; **Resid:** Western Genl Hosp 1980; Urology, Cardiff Royal Infirm 1983; **Fellow:** Urodynamics, Duke Univ Med Ctr 1986; **Fac Appt:** Prof U, UC Davis

Turek, Paul J MD [U] - **Spec Exp:** Infertility-Male; Microsurgery; Fertility Preservation in Cancer; Erectile Dysfunction; **Address:** 55 Francisco St, Ste 300, San Francisco, CA 94133; **Phone:** 415-392-3200; **Board Cert:** Urology 2005; **Med School:** Stanford Univ 1987; **Resid:** Surgery, Hosp Univ Penn 1989; Urology, Hosp Univ Penn 1993; **Fellow:** Microsurgery, Baylor Coll Med 1994; **Fac Appt:** Prof U, UCSF

Wilson, Timothy G MD [U] - **Spec Exp:** Prostate Cancer/Robotic Surgery; Minimally Invasive Urologic Surgery; Urinary Reconstruction; **Hospital:** City of Hope Natl Med Ctr & Beckman Rsch; **Address:** Div Urologic Oncology, 1500 E Duarte Rd, Duarte, CA 91010; **Phone:** 626-359-8111 x62655; **Board Cert:** Urology 2001; **Med School:** Oregon Hlth & Sci Univ 1984; **Resid:** Urology, USC Med Ctr 1990; **Fellow:** Urologic Oncology, City Hosp Natl Med Ctr 1991; **Fac Appt:** Assoc Clin Prof U, USC Sch Med

Cleveland Clinic

Glickman Urological and Kidney Institute

One of the Best

With nearly 70 physicians and scientists, the Cleveland Clinic Glickman Urological and Kidney Institute's Department of Urology is is the largest and most comprehensive urological group in the world. Many procedures have been developed or perfected here and adopted around the world. These include laparoscopic urological surgery, single-port urological procedures, female incontinence procedures, kidney-sparing surgery for kidney cancer, kidney artery reconstruction and kidney transplantation. The Institute also offers innovative treatment for sexual dysfunction, male infertility and testicular and bladder cancer. The latest and most effective treatments are provided for every urological disorder in adults and children. Because of its clinical and academic achievements, the Glickman Urological and Kidney Institute has consistently received national and international recognition. *U.S.News & World Report* **ranks the Cleveland Clinic Glickman Urological and Kidney Institute one of the top two urology programs in the United States.**

A National Leader in Urology

The Glickman Urological and Kidney Institute provides the highest quality of care for adult and pediatric patients with routine or complex disorders. Successful results in the practice and science of urology have won the Institute international acclaim as one of the most progressive and accomplished urologic groups in the country.

Innovative Care

In the treatment of kidney cancer, the Cleveland Clinic Glickman Urological and Kidney Institute has made numerous pioneering contributions, including the development of "bench surgery," a technique designed to repair the kidney outside the body and then transplant it back into the patient. The Cleveland Clinic Glickman Urological & Kidney Institute is also a recognized leader in partial nephrectomies, or kidney-sparing surgery, for the treatment of kidney cancer. More than 1,000 laparoscopic, or minimally invasive kidney-sparing procedures, have been performed here, representing the largest experience in the world. Another treatment option pioneered at Cleveland Clinic for kidney cancer is cryoablation, a minimally invasive treatment that uses a freezing probe to destroy the cancerous portion of the kidney. An Institute urologist performed the world's first laparoscopic cryoablation.

Defining State of the Art

The Cleveland Clinic Glickman Urological and Kidney Institute has been instrumental in perfecting and refining many laparoscopic techniques that may offer patients improved outcomes. These techniques are now routinely used for many urological diseases and conditions including prostate cancer, kidney and bladder cancer, urinary incontinence and in removing and transplanting kidneys in live-donor transplants. As one of the first centers in the country to begin using the latest versions of robotic surgery systems for prostate cancer, the Cleveland Clinic Glickman Urological and Kidney Institute is leading the way in minimally invasive urologic surgery. In addition, the Institute is pioneering advancements in single-port surgery that include performing surgery through a single incision in the belly button.

For more information about Glickman Urological and Kidney Institute, to schedule a second opinion or learn about assistance for out-of-state patients, call 800.890.2467 or visit www.clevelandclinic.org/urologytopdocs.

Glickman Urological and Kidney Institute
9500 Euclid Avenue / AC311 | Cleveland OH 44195

MOUNT SINAI
SCHOOL OF
MEDICINE

THE MOUNT SINAI MEDICAL CENTER
UROLOGY

One Gustave L. Levy Place
Fifth Avenue and 100th Street
New York, NY 10029-6574
Physician Referral: 1-800-MD-SINAI (637-4624)
www.mountsinai.org

THE MILTON AND CARROLL PETRIE DEPARTMENT OF UROLOGY at The Mount Sinai Medical Center offers the latest technologic advances for the diagnosis and treatment of urologic diseases and conditions, while supporting a strong translational and clinical research program.

Prostate Cancer – The Department of Urology's Barbara and Maurice Deane Prostate Health and Research Center offers a full range of surgical and radiation treatments for the management of localized prostate cancer, including minimally invasive laparoscopic and robotic prostatectomy. For more advanced disease, options include hormonal therapy, new chemotherapy regimens, and a clinical trial with a new prostate cancer vaccine. Current gene therapy research also offers hope for the future.

Bladder Cancer – As recognized leaders in the assessment and treatment of all forms of bladder cancer, Mount Sinai oncologists employ knowledge of tumor markers and new diagnostic techniques and work with Department of Urology surgeons to determine the most effective treatment approaches. Robotic surgeons can perform cystectomies with a variety of diversions, resulting in minimal impact on quality of life.

Kidney Cancer – A majority of kidney tumors can be removed by Department of Urology surgeons via minimally invasive robotic surgical techniques, reducing pain and recovery time. Laparoscopic surgery may be utilized to remove all or a portion of a kidney. Other less-invasive modalities—such as freezing, or radiofrequency ablation—may be recommended to treat small kidney cancers while preserving maximum function.

Prostatic Enlargement (benign prostatic hyperplasia) – The Deane Center offers the latest technologies and treatments, including Holmium Laser Ablation and transurethral microwave dilation therapy, highly effective approaches to relieving urinary problems associated with an enlarged prostate, including urinary frequency, pain, burning, and retention. Many of these procedures are offered in an outpatient setting.

Urinary Dysfunction – Mount Sinai provides comprehensive resources for the evaluation and treatment, both medical and surgical, of urinary incontinence, neuro-urologic problems, and pelvic pain syndrome for both men and women. Many procedures can now be performed on an outpatient basis in a new, state-of-the-art facility within the Deane Center.

THE BARBARA AND MAURICE DEANE PROSTATE HEALTH AND RESEARCH CENTER offers a multidisciplinary approach for the assessment and treatment of all aspects of prostate disease, including cancer, benign enlargement, and inflammation. The Center strives to empower the patient and his family, as well as help them to better understand various prostate conditions so they can choose the most appropriate treatment and derive lasting benefits.

Mount Sinai offers a comprehensive **Minimally Invasive Urologic Surgery Program** and is a recognized leader in the greater New York area for performing complex robotic and laparoscopic procedures to treat urologic cancers. Areas of focus also include the treatment and management of stone disease and reconstructive procedures for various urologic cancers and anatomic abnormalities.

Urologic Stone Disease – Mount Sinai's expertise in kidney stone disease ranges from stone prevention to minimally invasive therapies with lasers, sonic energies, and extracorporeal shock wave lithotripsy.

Pediatric Conditions – Mount Sinai has a strong reputation in the area of pediatric urology, offering expertise in minimally invasive reconstructive procedures for both infants and children.

Male Infertility – Mount Sinai offers state-of-the-art approaches using medications and in vitro fertilization techniques that result in high success rates.

Sexuality-Related Health Concerns – For both men and women, sexuality-related issues are addressed with both medical and surgical approaches.

NYU Langone Medical Center

550 First Avenue (at 31St Street)
New York, NY 10016
Physician Referral:
(888)7-NYU-MED (888-769-8633)
www.med.nyu.edu

UROLOGY

About the Department of Urology:

Urologists at NYU Langone Medical Center continue to pioneer advances in the surgical and pharmacological treatments of urological disease. Committed to developing new technologies to treat even the most complex disorders more effectively and less invasively, patients experience less discomfort and a faster recovery. The Department was recently recognized as one of the top 20 urology programs in the country by U.S. News and World Report.

We specialize in the following areas:

BENIGN PROSTATIC DISEASES
NYU Langone Medical Center offers innovative medical and surgical therapies for benign prostatic diseases, a condition that increases the size of the prostate in middle-aged and elderly men, as well as prostatitis, the inflammation of the prostate gland.

UROLOGICAL DISEASES
Specialists at the Center of Excellence on Urological Diseases are focused on finding ways in which bladder-specific cancer markers, discovered here at NYU Langone Medical Center, can be used to assess how well bladder cancer treatments are working. Bladder cancer is the fourth most common cancer in men and eighth in women. NYU Langone Medical Center is at the forefront of science in this field.

FEMALE UROLOGY AND INCONTINENCE
The Department of Urology specializes in urological problems unique to women, including recurrent urinary tract infections, pelvic pain, prolapse and sexual dysfunction.

LATEST MINIMALLY INVASIVE TREATMENTS
The Department of Urology focuses on discovering and implementing innovative treatments for the most prevalent urological disorders, including prostate cancer. One such treatment is our High Intensity Focused Ultrasound (HIFU), a minimally invasive incision-less treatment using high energy sound waves to precisely destroy prostate cancer cells. Another example is our Photodynamic Therapy (PDT), which destroys cancer cells using laser light energy.

PEDIATRIC UROLOGY AND RECONSTRUCTIVE SURGERY
Pediatric urology focuses on disorders of children's urinary systems. Pediatric urologists provide care for both boys and girls ranging from birth to early adult age.

PROSTATE CANCER SURGERY
The Department of Urology features some of the most experienced open minimally invasive robotic and cryo prostate cancer surgeons in the northeast, offering the best possible outcomes for men with prostate cancer.

ROBOTIC UROLOGICAL SURGERY
NYU Langone Medical Center provides a comprehensive robotic urological surgery program, which includes surgery for prostate and kidney cancers, female incontinence and urinary tract reconstruction. Robotic urological surgery maximizes surgical precision, is less invasive, decreases incision size, maximizes surgical precision and minimizes discomfort and recovery time.

UROLOGIC ONCOLOGY
The Department of Urology at NYU Langone Medical Center aggressively treats and cures urological cancers while maintaining the highest quality of life for its patients. Because cancer treatment often requires a collaborative approach, urologists work closely with NYU Langone Medical Center's radiation oncologists to tailor individual treatments for each patient.

UHEALTH UROLOGY: TRUSTED BY PATIENTS, RECOGNIZED BY PEERS

A TEAM OF EXCELLENCE

Mark Soloway, M.D., one of a select group of urologists honored with the Gold Cystoscope award by the American Urological Association, leads the urology team at UHealth – University of Miami Health System. Under his direction, each year, several members of the urology team rank among the "Best Doctors" in national and regional listings. They are recognized, in part, because of their outstanding patient care, but also for their work with fellow doctors and research scientists with whom they collaborate to improve the understanding of urologic diseases and translate discoveries to patient care.

Based on listings provided by Best Doctors®, Castle Connolly Medical Ltd., and Florida Super Doctors.

SPECIALIZED CARE

UHealth's urology team provides novel treatment, including the pioneering use of Botox and interstim for the treatment of overactive bladder and the management of stress-related urinary incontinence for both men and women. UHealth boasts Miami's only female urologist, fellowship-trained in voiding dysfunction.

They also provide highly specialized surgical care – laparoscopic, robotic and open field – for partial nephrectomy, treatment of all aspects of bladder cancer, the construction of orthotopic neobladders following cystectomy, total prostatectomy, placement of artificial sphincters for urinary incontinence, radio frequency ablation for small renal tumors, ureteroscopic management of upper urinary tract tumors, surgical management and lithotripsy for renal and ureteral stones, and erectile dysfunction and infertility.

ON A MISSION

UHealth urology team seeks to enhance the quality of patients' lives by providing the highest quality, comprehensive treatment for all urologic conditions and to diagnose and prevent urologic disease. Through their innovative and groundbreaking research, our urologists work to advance medical science. As the only university-based urology team in the region, UHealth applies the latest clinical techniques – every day – for a wide range of urologic subspecialty care.

UHealth Urology Physicians

- Mark S. Soloway, M.D.
  Chairman
  Urologic Oncology

- Vincent Bird, M.D.
  Laparoscopic Surgery and Renal Stone Disease

- Richard Boxer, M.D.
  General Urology

- Angelo Gousse, M.D.
  Female Urology and Voiding Dysfunction

- Bruce Kava, M.D.
  Urologic Oncology and Erectile Dysfunction

- Yvonne Koch, M.D.
  Female Urology and Voiding Dysfunction

- Raymond Leveillee, M.D.
  Laparoscopic Surgery and Renal Stone Disease

- Charles Lynne, M.D.
  Neurology/Urodynamics and Male Infertility

- Murugesan Manoharan, M.D.
  Urologic Oncology

UHealth Urology Research

- Bal Lokeshwar, Ph.D
- Vinata Lokeshwar, Ph.D.

Vascular Surgery

a subspecialty of Surgery

A surgeon with expertise in the management of surgical disorders of the blood vessels, excluding the intercranial vessels or the heart.

Training Required: Five years in surgery *plus* additional training and examination.

VASCULAR SURGERY

New England

Belkin, Michael MD [VascS] - **Spec Exp:** Aneurysm; Arterial Bypass Surgery; Carotid Artery Surgery; **Hospital:** Brigham & Women's Hosp, Faulkner Hosp; **Address:** Brigham & Women's Hosp, Dept Vasc Surg, 75 Francis St, Boston, MA 02115; **Phone:** 857-307-1920; **Board Cert:** Surgery 1997; Vascular Surgery 1998; **Med School:** Univ Conn 1982; **Resid:** Surgery, Hartford Hosp 1987; **Fellow:** Vascular Surgery, Brigham & Women's Hosp 1989; **Fac Appt:** Assoc Prof S, Harvard Med Sch

Brewster, David C MD [VascS] - **Spec Exp:** Aneurysm-Abdominal Aortic; Endovascular Surgery; Angioplasty & Stent Placement; **Hospital:** Mass Genl Hosp, Newton - Wellesley Hosp; **Address:** Massachusetts General Hosp, 15 Parkman St, WAC 440, Boston, MA 02114; **Phone:** 617-726-3567; **Board Cert:** Surgery 1975; Vascular Surgery 2003; **Med School:** Columbia P&S 1967; **Resid:** Surgery, Mass Genl Hosp 1975; **Fellow:** Vascular Surgery, Mass Genl Hosp 1976; **Fac Appt:** Clin Prof S, Harvard Med Sch

Cambria, Richard P MD [VascS] - **Spec Exp:** Aneurysm-Abdominal Aortic; Cerebrovascular Disease; Renovascular Disease; Aortic Reconstruction; **Hospital:** Mass Genl Hosp; **Address:** Mass Genl Hosp, Dept Vascular Surgery, 15 Parkman St, WAC 440, Boston, MA 02114-3117; **Phone:** 617-726-8278; **Board Cert:** Vascular Surgery 2006; **Med School:** Columbia P&S 1977; **Resid:** Surgery, Mass Genl Hosp 1978; **Fellow:** Vascular Surgery, Mass Genl Hosp 1984; **Fac Appt:** Prof S, Harvard Med Sch

Cronenwett, Jack MD [VascS] - **Spec Exp:** Peripheral Vascular Surgery; Aneurysm-Abdominal Aortic; Carotid Artery Surgery; **Hospital:** Dartmouth - Hitchcock Med Ctr, Mary Hitchcock Mem Hosp; **Address:** Dartmouth-Hitchcock Med Ctr, Sect Vascular Surgery, One Medical Center Drive, Lebanon, NH 03756; **Phone:** 603-650-8670; **Board Cert:** Vascular Surgery 2003; **Med School:** Stanford Univ 1973; **Resid:** Surgery, Univ Mich Hosp 1979; **Fellow:** Vascular Surgery, Univ Tenn Hosp 1980; **Fac Appt:** Prof S, Dartmouth Med Sch

Gusberg, Richard J MD [VascS] - **Spec Exp:** Endovascular Surgery; Aneurysm-Aortic; Renovascular Disease; **Hospital:** Yale-New Haven Hosp, VA Conn Hlthcre Sys; **Address:** Yale Univ School of Med-Dept Surgery, 333 Cedar St, Box 208062, New Haven, CT 06520-8062; **Phone:** 203-785-6217; **Board Cert:** Surgery 1996; Vascular Surgery 1997; **Med School:** Columbia P&S 1970; **Resid:** Surgery, Columbia-Presby Med Ctr 1975; **Fellow:** Vascular Surgery, Columbia-Presby Med Ctr 1976; **Fac Appt:** Prof S, Yale Univ

Kwolek, Christopher J MD [VascS] - **Spec Exp:** Aneurysm-Abdominal & Thoracic Aortic; Endovascular Surgery; Carotid Artery Stent Placement; **Hospital:** Mass Genl Hosp, Newton - Wellesley Hosp; **Address:** 15 Parkman St, Wang Bldg Fl 4, Boston, MA 02114; **Phone:** 617-724-6101; **Board Cert:** Surgery 2003; Vascular Surgery 2006; **Med School:** UCSF 1987; **Resid:** Surgery, New England Deaconess Hosp 1993; Vascular Surgery, Mass Genl Hosp 1995; **Fellow:** Endovascular Surgery, Arizona Heart Inst 1999; **Fac Appt:** Assoc Prof VascS, Harvard Med Sch

LaMuraglia, Glenn M MD [VascS] - **Spec Exp:** Carotid Body Tumors; Aneurysm-Aortic; Endovascular Surgery; Vascular Disease; **Hospital:** Mass Genl Hosp; **Address:** Mass General Hospital, Vascular Surgery, 55 Fruit St, Boston, MA 02114; **Phone:** 617-726-6997; **Board Cert:** Surgery 2004; Vascular Surgery 2007; **Med School:** Harvard Med Sch 1979; **Resid:** Surgery, Mass General Hosp 1985; Vascular Surgery, Mass General Hosp 1986; **Fac Appt:** Assoc Prof S, Harvard Med Sch

Mackey, William C MD [VascS] - **Spec Exp:** Carotid Artery Surgery; Aneurysm-Abdominal Aortic; Lower Limb Arterial Disease; **Hospital:** Tufts Med Ctr; **Address:** 750 Washington St, Ste 1035, Boston, MA 02111-1526; **Phone:** 617-636-5927; **Board Cert:** Surgery 2002; Vascular Surgery 2004; Surgical Critical Care 2007; **Med School:** Duke Univ 1977; **Resid:** Surgery, New York Hosp 1982; **Fellow:** Vascular Surgery, Tufts-New Eng Med Ctr 1984; **Fac Appt:** Prof S, Tufts Univ

Sumpio, Bauer E MD/PhD [VascS] - **Spec Exp:** Diabetic Leg/Foot; Endovascular Surgery; **Hospital:** Yale-New Haven Hosp, VA Conn Hlthcre Sys; **Address:** Yale Univ School Medicine, Dept Surgery, 333 Cedar St, rm FMB137, Box 208062, New Haven, CT 06520; **Phone:** 203-785-6217; **Board Cert:** Vascular Surgery 1999; Surgery 2007; **Med School:** Cornell Univ-Weill Med Coll 1980; **Resid:** Surgery, Yale-New Haven Hosp 1986; **Fellow:** Vascular Surgery, Univ N Carolina Hosp 1987; **Fac Appt:** Prof S, Yale Univ

Mid Atlantic

Adelman, Mark MD [VascS] - **Spec Exp:** Carotid Artery Surgery; Aneurysm-Abdominal Aortic; Vein Disorders; Endovascular Surgery; **Hospital:** NYU Langone Med Ctr (page 67), Bellevue Hosp Ctr; **Address:** 530 1st Ave, Ste 6F, New York, NY 10016-6402; **Phone:** 212-263-7311; **Board Cert:** Surgery 1999; Vascular Surgery 2001; **Med School:** NYU Sch Med 1985; **Resid:** Surgery, NYU Med Ctr 1990; **Fellow:** Vascular Surgery, NYU Med Ctr 1991; **Fac Appt:** Prof VascS, NYU Sch Med

Ascher, Enrico MD [VascS] - **Spec Exp:** Endovascular Surgery; Carotid Artery Surgery; Limb Sparing Surgery; Aneurysm; **Hospital:** Maimonides Med Ctr (page 63), Mount Sinai Med Ctr (page 64); **Address:** Maimonides Med Ctr, Dept Vascular Surg, 4802 10th Ave Fl 4, Brooklyn, NY 11219-2844; **Phone:** 718-283-7957; **Board Cert:** Vascular Surgery 2004; **Med School:** Brazil 1974; **Resid:** Surgery, NY Med Coll 1981; **Fellow:** Vascular Surgery, Montefiore Hosp Med Ctr 1982; **Fac Appt:** Prof S, SUNY Downstate

Atnip, Robert G MD [VascS] - **Spec Exp:** Aneurysm-Abdominal Aortic; Peripheral Vascular Disease; Carotid Artery Disease; Endovascular Surgery; **Hospital:** Penn State Milton S Hershey Med Ctr; **Address:** Hershey Med Ctr Vascular Surgery, 500 University Dr, rm 4628, Hershey, PA 17033; **Phone:** 717-531-4554; **Board Cert:** Surgery 2005; Vascular Surgery 2007; Surgical Critical Care 2000; **Med School:** Univ Alabama 1978; **Resid:** Surgery, Mass Genl Hosp 1984; **Fellow:** Vascular Surgery, Mass Genl Hosp 1985; **Fac Appt:** Prof S, Penn State Univ-Hershey Med Ctr

Benvenisty, Alan I MD [VascS] - **Spec Exp:** Renovascular Disease; Aneurysm-Aortic; Endovascular Surgery; Minimally Invasive Vascular Surgery; **Hospital:** St Luke's - Roosevelt Hosp Ctr - St Luke's Hosp (page 57), St Luke's - Roosevelt Hosp Ctr - Roosevelt Div (page 57); **Address:** 1090 Amsterdam Ave Fl 12, New York, NY 10025; **Phone:** 212-523-4706; **Board Cert:** Surgery 2004; Vascular Surgery 1999; **Med School:** Columbia P&S 1978; **Resid:** Surgery, Columbia-Presby Med Ctr 1983; **Fellow:** Vascular Surgery, Columbia-Presby Med Ctr 1984; Transplant Surgery, Columbia-Presby Med Ctr 1984; **Fac Appt:** Clin Prof S, Columbia P&S

Brener, Bruce J MD [VascS] - **Spec Exp:** Endovascular Surgery; Minimally Invasive Vascular Surgery; Carotid Artery Surgery; Aneurysm-Aortic; **Hospital:** Newark Beth Israel Med Ctr, St Barnabas Med Ctr; **Address:** 200 South Orange Ave, Livingston, NJ 07039; **Phone:** 973-322-7233; **Board Cert:** Surgery 1972; Vascular Surgery 2005; **Med School:** Harvard Med Sch 1966; **Resid:** Surgery, Chldns Hosp Med Ctr 1968; Surgery, Peter Bent Brigham Hosp 1972; **Fellow:** Vascular Surgery, Mass Genl Hosp 1973; **Fac Appt:** Assoc Clin Prof S, Columbia P&S

Vascular Surgery

Calligaro, Keith D MD [VascS] - **Spec Exp:** Aneurysm-Abdominal & Thoracic Aortic; Carotid Artery Disease; Renal Artery Stenosis; **Hospital:** Pennsylvania Hosp (page 60); **Address:** 700 Spruce St, Ste 101, Philadelphia, PA 19106; **Phone:** 215-829-5000; **Board Cert:** Surgery 1997; Vascular Surgery 1999; **Med School:** UMDNJ-Rutgers Med Sch 1982; **Resid:** Surgery, St Barnabas Med Ctr 1984; Surgery, Univ Hlth Scis/Chicago Med Sch 1987; **Fellow:** Vascular Surgery, Montefiore Med Ctr 1989; **Fac Appt:** Clin Prof S, Univ Pennsylvania

Carpenter, Jeffrey P MD [VascS] - **Spec Exp:** Aneurysm-Abdominal & Thoracic Aortic; Carotid Artery Surgery; Peripheral Vascular Disease; **Hospital:** Cooper Univ Hosp; **Address:** 3 Cooper Plaza, Ste 411, Camden, NJ 08104; **Phone:** 856-325-6516; **Board Cert:** Surgery 2001; Vascular Surgery 2001; **Med School:** Yale Univ 1986; **Resid:** Surgery, Hosp Univ Penn 1991; **Fellow:** Vascular Surgery, Hosp Univ Penn 1992; **Fac Appt:** Prof S, Univ Pennsylvania

Criado, Frank J MD [VascS] - **Spec Exp:** Endovascular Surgery; Aneurysm-Abdominal & Thoracic Aortic; Carotid Artery Stent Placement; **Hospital:** Union Meml Hosp-Baltimore; **Address:** 3333 N Calvert St, Ste 570, Baltimore, MD 21218; **Phone:** 410-554-6400; **Board Cert:** Vascular Surgery 1997; **Med School:** Uruguay 1974; **Resid:** Surgery, Union Memorial Hosp 1980; Vascular Surgery, Union Memorial Hosp 1985; **Fellow:** Cardiovascular Surgery, Baylor Univ Med Ctr 1981

Darling III, R Clement MD [VascS] - **Spec Exp:** Aneurysm-Abdominal & Thoracic Aortic; Arterial Bypass Surgery; Carotid Artery Surgery; **Hospital:** Albany Med Ctr, St Peter's Hosp - Albany; **Address:** Albany Med Ctr, Vascular Inst, 43 New Scotland Ave, MC 157, Albany, NY 12208; **Phone:** 518-262-5640; **Board Cert:** Surgery 1999; Vascular Surgery 2002; **Med School:** Univ Cincinnati 1984; **Resid:** Surgery, Beth Israel Deaconess Hosp 1989; **Fellow:** Vascular Surgery, Albany Med Ctr 1991; **Fac Appt:** Prof S, Albany Med Coll

Dougherty, Matthew J MD [VascS] - **Spec Exp:** Endovascular Stent Grafts; Aneurysm; **Hospital:** Pennsylvania Hosp (page 60); **Address:** 700 Spruce St, Ste 101, Philadelphia, PA 19106; **Phone:** 215-829-5000; **Board Cert:** Vascular Surgery 2001; Surgery 1999; **Med School:** Harvard Med Sch 1984; **Resid:** Surgery, Mass Genl Hosp 1990; **Fellow:** Vascular Surgery, Mayo Clinic 1992; **Fac Appt:** Assoc Clin Prof S, Univ Pennsylvania

Fairman, Ronald M MD [VascS] - **Spec Exp:** Aneurysm-Aortic; Peripheral Vascular Disease; Carotid Artery Surgery; Aneurysm-Abdominal & Thoracic Aortic; **Hospital:** Hosp Univ Penn - UPHS (page 60); **Address:** Hosp Univ Penn, 4 Silverstein Pavilion, 3400 Spruce St, Philadelphia, PA 19104; **Phone:** 215-662-2050; **Board Cert:** Surgery 1996; Vascular Surgery 2000; **Med School:** Thomas Jefferson Univ 1977; **Resid:** Surgery, Hosp U Penn 1983; **Fellow:** Vascular Surgery, Hosp U Penn 1984; **Fac Appt:** Assoc Prof S, Univ Pennsylvania

Fantini, Gary A MD [VascS] - **Spec Exp:** Spinal Access Surgery; Thoracic Outlet Syndrome; **Hospital:** Hosp For Special Surgery (page 59), NY-Presby Hosp/Weill Cornell (page 66); **Address:** 635 Madison Ave Fl 7, New York, NY 10022; **Phone:** 212-317-4550; **Board Cert:** Surgery 2007; Vascular Surgery 2000; **Med School:** Albert Einstein Coll Med 1983; **Resid:** Surgery, NY Hosp-Cornell Med Ctr 1989; **Fellow:** Vascular Surgery, UCSF Med Ctr 1990; **Fac Appt:** Assoc Prof S, Cornell Univ-Weill Med Coll

Faries, Peter MD [VascS] - **Spec Exp:** Aneurysm-Abdominal Aortic; Peripheral Vascular Disease; Renovascular Disease; Carotid Artery Surgery; **Hospital:** Mount Sinai Med Ctr (page 64); **Address:** 5 E 98th St, Ste 415, New York, NY 10021; **Phone:** 212-415-5386; **Board Cert:** Surgery 1999; Vascular Surgery 2001; **Med School:** Univ Pennsylvania 1992; **Resid:** Surgery, Montefiore Med Ctr 1998; **Fellow:** Vascular Surgery, Beth Israel Deaconess Med Ctr 2000; **Fac Appt:** Prof S, Mount Sinai Sch Med

Freischlag, Julie A MD [VascS] - **Spec Exp:** Aneurysm-Aortic; Carotid Artery Disease; Thoracic Outlet Syndrome; **Hospital:** Johns Hopkins Hosp (page 61); **Address:** Johns Hopkins Hosp, Dept Surg, 720 Rutland Ave, Ross Bldg-759, Baltimore, MD 21205; **Phone:** 443-287-3497; **Board Cert:** Surgery 2005; Vascular Surgery 2005; **Med School:** Rush Med Coll 1980; **Resid:** Surgery, UCLA Medical Ctr 1986; **Fellow:** Vascular Surgery, UCLA Medical Ctr 1987; **Fac Appt:** Prof S, Johns Hopkins Univ

Golden, Michael A MD [VascS] - **Spec Exp:** Aneurysm; Endovascular Surgery; **Hospital:** Penn Presby Med Ctr - UPHS (page 60); **Address:** Penn Presbyterian, Vascular Surgery, 266 Wright Saunders Bldg, 39th & Market Sts, Philadelphia, PA 19104; **Phone:** 215-662-9660; **Board Cert:** Surgery 1989; Vascular Surgery 2001; **Med School:** Univ Pennsylvania 1981; **Resid:** Surgery, Brigham & Women's Hosp 1987; **Fellow:** Vascular Surgery, Brigham & Women's Hosp 1990; **Fac Appt:** Assoc Prof S, Univ Pennsylvania

Green, Richard M MD [VascS] - **Spec Exp:** Aneurysm-Abdominal Aortic; Carotid Artery Surgery; Percutaneous Vascular Interventions; **Hospital:** Lenox Hill Hosp (page 62); **Address:** 130 E 77th St Fl 13, New York, NY 10021; **Phone:** 212-434-3420; **Board Cert:** Vascular Surgery 2003; **Med School:** Univ Rochester 1970; **Resid:** Surgery, Strong Meml Hosp 1976

Harrington, Elizabeth MD [VascS] - **Spec Exp:** Carotid Artery Surgery; Aneurysm-Aortic; Arterial Bypass Surgery-Leg; **Hospital:** Mount Sinai Med Ctr (page 64); **Address:** 1225 Park Ave, Ste 1D, New York, NY 10128-1758; **Phone:** 212-876-7400; **Board Cert:** Surgery 1999; Vascular Surgery 2006; **Med School:** NY Med Coll 1975; **Resid:** Surgery, Mt Sinai Hosp 1980; **Fellow:** Vascular Surgery, Mt Sinai Hosp 1981; **Fac Appt:** Assoc Prof VascS, Mount Sinai Sch Med

Makaroun, Michel S MD [VascS] - **Spec Exp:** Endovascular Surgery; Aneurysm; Carotid Artery Disease; Peripheral Vascular Surgery; **Hospital:** UPMC Shadyside, UPMC Presby, Pittsburgh; **Address:** Presby-Univ Hosp, A-1011, 200 Lothrop St, Pittsburgh, PA 15213; **Phone:** 412-802-3028; **Board Cert:** Surgery 2004; Vascular Surgery 1998; **Med School:** Lebanon 1978; **Resid:** Surgery, American Univ Hosp 1980; Surgery, Univ Pittsburgh Med Ctr 1985; **Fac Appt:** Prof S, Univ Pittsburgh

Marin, Michael L MD [VascS] - **Spec Exp:** Aneurysm-Aortic; Carotid Artery Surgery; Limb Sparing Surgery; Endovascular Surgery; **Hospital:** Mount Sinai Med Ctr (page 64), N Genl Hosp; **Address:** Mount Sinai Medical Ctr, 5 E 98th St, Box 1273, New York, NY 10029; **Phone:** 212-241-5315; **Board Cert:** Surgery 1999; **Med School:** Mount Sinai Sch Med 1984; **Resid:** Surgery, Columbia-Presby Med Ctr 1990; **Fellow:** Transplant Surgery, Columbia-Presby Med Ctr 1988; Vascular Surgery, Montefiore Med Ctr 1992; **Fac Appt:** Prof S, Mount Sinai Sch Med

Neville Jr, Richard F MD [VascS] - **Spec Exp:** Endovascular Surgery; Wound Healing/Care; **Hospital:** Georgetown Univ Hosp; **Address:** 3800 Reservoir Rd NW, PHC Bldg Fl 4, Washington, DC 20007; **Phone:** 202-444-2255; **Board Cert:** Surgery 2000; Vascular Surgery 2002; **Med School:** Univ MD Sch Med 1983; **Resid:** Surgery, Georgetown Univ Hosp 1988; **Fellow:** Vascular Surgery, UMDNJ Affil Hosp 1991; **Fac Appt:** Assoc Prof S, Georgetown Univ

Perler, Bruce MD [VascS] - **Spec Exp:** Carotid Artery Surgery; Aneurysm; Arterial Bypass Surgery-Leg; **Hospital:** Johns Hopkins Hosp (page 61), Johns Hopkins Bayview Med Ctr (page 61); **Address:** Johns Hopkins Hosp-Surg, 600 N Wolfe St Bldg Harvey - Ste 611, Baltimore, MD 21287-8611; **Phone:** 410-955-2618; **Board Cert:** Vascular Surgery 1997; **Med School:** Duke Univ 1976; **Resid:** Surgery, Mass Genl Hosp 1981; **Fellow:** Vascular Surgery, Mass Genl Hosp 1982; **Fac Appt:** Prof S, Johns Hopkins Univ

Vascular Surgery

Ricotta, John MD [VascS] - **Spec Exp:** Aneurysm; Carotid Artery Surgery; Vein Disorders; **Hospital:** Washington Hosp Ctr; **Address:** Washington Hospital Ctr, Dept Surgery, 110 Irving St NW, rm G253, Washington, DC 20010; **Phone:** 202-877-8089; **Board Cert:** Surgery 2004; Vascular Surgery 2003; **Med School:** Johns Hopkins Univ 1973; **Resid:** Surgery, Johns Hopkins Hosp 1977; **Fellow:** Vascular Surgery, Johns Hopkins Hosp 1979; **Fac Appt:** Prof S

Riles, Thomas MD [VascS] - **Spec Exp:** Aneurysm-Abdominal Aortic; Carotid Artery Surgery; **Hospital:** NYU Langone Med Ctr (page 67); **Address:** NYU Med Ctr, Univ Vascular Assoc, 530 1st Ave, HCC-6D, New York, NY 10016; **Phone:** 212-263-6360; **Board Cert:** Vascular Surgery 2003; **Med School:** Baylor Coll Med 1969; **Resid:** Surgery, NYU Med Ctr 1976; **Fellow:** Vascular Surgery, NYU Med Ctr 1977; **Fac Appt:** Prof S, NYU Sch Med

Steed, David L MD [VascS] - **Spec Exp:** Wound Healing/Care; **Hospital:** UPMC Presby, Pittsburgh; **Address:** UPMC Presbyterian Hosp, 200 Lothrop St, Ste A-1011, Pittsburgh, PA 15213; **Phone:** 412-802-3024; **Board Cert:** Surgery 1999; Vascular Surgery 1997; **Med School:** Univ Pittsburgh 1973; **Resid:** Surgery, Univ Pittsburgh Med Ctr 1980; **Fellow:** Vascular Surgery, UCLA Med Ctr 1977; **Fac Appt:** Prof S, Univ Pittsburgh

Todd, George MD [VascS] - **Spec Exp:** Minimally Invasive Vascular Surgery; Aneurysm-Abdominal Aortic; Carotid Artery Surgery; **Hospital:** St Luke's - Roosevelt Hosp Ctr - Roosevelt Div (page 57); **Address:** St Luke's-Roosevelt Hosp Ctr, Dept Surg, 1000 10th Ave, rm 5G77, New York, NY 10019; **Phone:** 212-523-7481; **Board Cert:** Surgery 2000; **Med School:** Penn State Univ-Hershey Med Ctr 1974; **Resid:** Surgery, Columbia-Presby Med Ctr 1979; **Fellow:** Vascular Surgery, Columbia-Presby Med Ctr 1980; **Fac Appt:** Prof S, Columbia P&S

Southeast

Bandyk, Dennis F MD [VascS] - **Spec Exp:** Endovascular Stent Grafts; Lower Limb Arterial Disease; Thoracic Outlet Syndrome; **Hospital:** Tampa Genl Hosp, Univ of S FL - Tampa; **Address:** USF Physicians Group, 2 Tampa General Circle, Ste 7001, Tampa, FL 33606; **Phone:** 813-259-0921; **Board Cert:** Surgery 2001; Vascular Surgery 2000; **Med School:** Univ Mich Med Sch 1975; **Resid:** Surgery, Univ Wash Hosp 1980; **Fellow:** Vascular Surgery, Univ Wash Hosp 1981; **Fac Appt:** Prof S, Univ S Fla Coll Med

Chaikof, Elliot L MD/PhD [VascS] - **Spec Exp:** Aneurysm-Aortic; Carotid Artery Disease; Peripheral Vascular Disease; Endovascular Surgery; **Hospital:** Emory Univ Hosp, Chldns Hlthcare Atlanta @ Egleston; **Address:** Emory Vascular Surgery, 101 Woodruff Cir, Ste 5501 WMB, Atlanta, GA 30322; **Phone:** 404-778-5451; **Board Cert:** Surgery 2002; Vascular Surgery 2003; **Med School:** Johns Hopkins Univ 1982; **Resid:** Surgery, Mass Genl Hosp 1985; Surgery, Mass Genl Hosp 1991; **Fellow:** Vascular Surgery, Emory Univ Hosp 1992; **Fac Appt:** Prof S, Emory Univ

Cherry Jr, Kenneth J MD [VascS] - **Spec Exp:** Vascular Reconstruction; Aortic Graft Infections; **Hospital:** Univ Virginia Med Ctr; **Address:** Univ Virginia Health System, PO Box 800679, Charlottesville, VA 22908-0679; **Phone:** 434-243-7052; **Board Cert:** Vascular Surgery 2004; **Med School:** Univ VA Sch Med 1974; **Resid:** Surgery, Univ Virginia Hosp 1980; Vascular Surgery, UCSF Med Ctr 1981; **Fac Appt:** Prof S, Univ VA Sch Med

Flynn, Timothy C MD [VascS] - **Spec Exp:** Peripheral Vascular Disease; Aortic Graft Infections; **Hospital:** Shands at Univ of FL; **Address:** Shands Hlthcare Univ Florida, PO Box 100321, Gainesville, FL 32610-0286; **Phone:** 352-265-0152; **Board Cert:** Surgery 1999; Vascular Surgery 1994; Surgical Critical Care 1998; **Med School:** Baylor Coll Med 1974; **Resid:** Surgery, Univ Texas 1980; **Fac Appt:** Prof S, Univ Fla Coll Med

Hakaim, Albert G MD [VascS] - **Spec Exp:** Aneurysm-Abdominal Aortic; Endovascular Surgery; **Hospital:** Mayo - Jacksonville; **Address:** Mayo Clinic, Dept Vascular Surgery, 4500 San Pablo Rd, Ste 323N, Jacksonville, FL 32224; **Phone:** 904-953-2077; **Board Cert:** Surgery 2002; Vascular Surgery 2003; **Med School:** Ohio State Univ 1984; **Resid:** Surgery, Cleveland Clinic 1989; **Fellow:** Transplant Surgery, Boston Univ Hosp 1991; Vascular Surgery, Cleveland Clinic 1992; **Fac Appt:** Assoc Prof S, Mayo Med Sch

Hallett Jr, John W MD [VascS] - **Spec Exp:** Aneurysm-Abdominal Aortic; Carotid Artery Surgery; Thoracic Outlet Syndrome; **Hospital:** Roper Hosp; **Address:** Roper St Francis Heart & Vascular Ctr, 316 Calhoun St, Charleston, SC 29401; **Phone:** 843-720-5665; **Board Cert:** Surgery 1999; Vascular Surgery 2003; **Med School:** Duke Univ 1973; **Resid:** Surgery, Wilford Hall USAF Med Ctr 1978; **Fellow:** Vascular Surgery, Mass Genl Hosp-Harvard Med Sch 1979; **Fac Appt:** Assoc Clin Prof VascS, Med Univ SC

Hansen, Kimberley J MD [VascS] - **Spec Exp:** Aortic & Visceral Artery Surgery; Renovascular Disease; Carotid Artery Surgery; **Hospital:** Wake Forest Univ Baptist Med Ctr (page 72), Forsyth Med Ctr; **Address:** Dept Vascular & Endovascular Surgery, Wake Forest Univ Sch Med, Medical Center Blvd, Winston-Salem, NC 27157-1095; **Phone:** 336-716-4151; **Board Cert:** Vascular Surgery 1998; Surgery 2006; Surgical Critical Care 2001; **Med School:** Univ Alabama 1980; **Resid:** Surgery, NC Baptist Hosp/WFU Sch MEd 1986; **Fellow:** Vascular Surgery, Univ California 1987; **Fac Appt:** Prof S, Wake Forest Univ

McCann, Richard L MD [VascS] - **Spec Exp:** Endovascular Surgery; **Hospital:** Duke Univ Med Ctr; **Address:** Duke Univ Med Ctr, Box 2990, Durham, NC 27710; **Phone:** 919-684-2620; **Board Cert:** Surgery 2003; Vascular Surgery 2006; **Med School:** Cornell Univ-Weill Med Coll 1974; **Resid:** Surgery, Duke Univ Med Ctr 1983; **Fac Appt:** Prof S, Duke Univ

Mitchell, Marc E MD [VascS] - **Spec Exp:** Aneurysm-Aortic; Cartoid Artery Disease; Endovascular Surgery; Peripheral Vascular Disease; **Hospital:** Univ Mississippi Med Ctr; **Address:** Univ Mississippi Med Ctr, Dept Surgery, 2500 N State St, Jackson, MS 39216; **Phone:** 601-815-2005; **Board Cert:** Surgery 1999; Surgical Critical Care 2005; Vascular Surgery 2007; **Med School:** Georgetown Univ 1984; **Resid:** Surgery, UCSF Med Ctr 1986; Surgery, Univ Mississippi Med Ctr 1991; **Fellow:** Cardiac Surgery, NIH 1998; Vascular Surgery, Univ Penn 1997; **Fac Appt:** Prof S, Univ Miss

Rosenthal, David MD [VascS] - **Spec Exp:** Stroke; Aneurysm; Endovascular Surgery; **Hospital:** Atlanta Med Ctr, Piedmont Hosp; **Address:** Atlanta Vascular Specialists, 315 Boulevard NE, Ste 412, Atlanta, GA 30312; **Phone:** 404-524-0095; **Board Cert:** Vascular Surgery 2003; **Med School:** SUNY Downstate 1973; **Resid:** Surgery, Tufts-New Eng Med Ctr 1977; **Fellow:** Vascular Surgery, Tufts-New Eng Med Ctr 1978; **Fac Appt:** Clin Prof S, Med Coll GA

Seeger, James M MD [VascS] - **Spec Exp:** Lower Limb Arterial Disease; Aneurysm-Aortic; Kidney & Bowel Arterial Disease; **Hospital:** Shands at Univ of FL; **Address:** Univ Florida, Dept Vascular Surgery, 1600 SW Archer Rd, NG-45, PO Box 100286, Gainesville, FL 32610-0286; **Phone:** 352-273-5484; **Board Cert:** Surgery 2000; Vascular Surgery 1992; **Med School:** Med Coll GA 1973; **Resid:** Surgery, Univ Utah Med Ctr 1980; **Fellow:** Vascular Surgery, Eastern VA Med Sch 1981; **Fac Appt:** Prof S, Univ Fla Coll Med

Sivina, Manuel MD [VascS] - **Hospital:** Mount Sinai Med Ctr - Miami; **Address:** Mount Sinai Med Ctr, 4300 Alton Rd, Ste 2240, Miami Beach, FL 33140; **Phone:** 305-674-2760; **Board Cert:** Surgery 2000; **Med School:** Peru 1969; **Resid:** Surgery, Mt Sinai Med Ctr 1975; **Fellow:** Vascular Surgery, Mt Sinai Med Ctr 1976

Vascular Surgery

Midwest

Alexander, J Jeffrey MD [VascS] - **Hospital:** MetroHealth Med Ctr; **Address:** Metrohealth Med Ctr, Heart & Vascular Dept, 2500 Metrohealth Drive, Cleveland, OH 44109; **Phone:** 216-778-4811; **Board Cert:** Surgery 2002; Vascular Surgery 2006; **Med School:** Univ Pittsburgh 1978; **Resid:** Surgery, Univ Chicago Hosps 1983; **Fellow:** Vascular Surgery, Univ Chicago Hosps 1984; **Fac Appt:** Assoc Prof S, Case West Res Univ

Berguer, Ramon MD/PhD [VascS] - **Spec Exp:** Cerebrovascular Disease; Aortic & Visceral Artery Surgery; **Hospital:** Univ Michigan Hlth Sys; **Address:** Univ Michigan Hlth Sys, 1500 E Med Ctr Dr, SPC5867, Ann Arbor, MI 48109; **Phone:** 734-936-8247; **Board Cert:** Surgery 1970; Vascular Surgery 2003; **Med School:** Spain 1963; **Resid:** Surgery, Henry Ford Hosp 1969; **Fellow:** Vascular Surgery, Henry Ford Hosp 1970; Vascular Surgery, Kings College Hosp; **Fac Appt:** Prof S, Univ Mich Med Sch

Blebea, John MD [VascS] - **Spec Exp:** Endovascular Surgery; Radiofrequency Tumor Ablation; **Hospital:** Univ Hosps Case Med Ctr; **Address:** Univ Hosps, Dept Vascular Surgery, 11100 Euclid Ave, Cleveland, OH 44106-7060; **Phone:** 216-844-3013; **Board Cert:** Vascular Surgery 2000; Surgery 1998; **Med School:** Case West Res Univ 1982; **Resid:** Surgery, Georgetown Univ Hosp 1985; Vascular Surgery, UMDNJ 1986; **Fellow:** Vascular Surgery, Univ Rochester 1991; **Fac Appt:** Prof S, Case West Res Univ

Clair, Daniel G MD [VascS] - **Spec Exp:** Carotid Artery Surgery; Aneurysm-Abdominal & Thoracic Aortic; Peripheral Vascular Surgery; Endovascular Stent Grafts; **Hospital:** Cleveland Clin Fdn (page 56); **Address:** Cleveland Clinic, Dept Vascular Surgery, 9500 Euclid Ave, MC H32, Cleveland, OH 44195; **Phone:** 216-444-3857; **Board Cert:** Surgery 2003; Vascular Surgery 2004; **Med School:** Univ VA Sch Med 1986; **Resid:** Surgery, Brigham & Women's Hosp 1992; **Fellow:** Oncology, Brigham & Women's Hosp 1991; Vascular Surgery, Brigham & Women's Hosp 1994

Comerota, Anthony J MD [VascS] - **Spec Exp:** Carotid Artery Disease; Gene Therapy; Aneurysm-Aortic; Peripheral Vascular Disease; **Hospital:** Toledo Hosp; **Address:** Jobst Vascular Ctr, 2109 Hughes Drive, Ste 400, Toledo, OH 43606; **Phone:** 419-291-2088; **Board Cert:** Surgery 1999; Vascular Surgery 2003; **Med School:** Temple Univ 1974; **Resid:** Surgery, Temple Univ Hosp 1978; **Fellow:** Vascular Surgery, Good Samaritan Hosp 1981; **Fac Appt:** Clin Prof S, Univ Mich Med Sch

Dalsing, Michael C MD [VascS] - **Spec Exp:** Peripheral Vascular Surgery; Vein Disorders; Renovascular Disease; Carotid Artery Surgery; **Hospital:** Methodist Hosp - Indianapolis, Clarian West Med Ctr; **Address:** 1801 N Senate Blvd, MC 3500, Indianapolis, IN 46202; **Phone:** 317-962-0280; **Board Cert:** Surgery 2002; Vascular Surgery 2003; Surgical Critical Care 2001; **Med School:** Med Coll Wisc 1978; **Resid:** Surgery, Ind Univ Med Ctr 1983; **Fellow:** Vascular Surgery, Northwestern Univ Med Ctr 1984; **Fac Appt:** Prof S, Indiana Univ

Gloviczki, Peter MD [VascS] - **Spec Exp:** Aneurysm-Abdominal Aortic; Lower Limb Arterial Disease; Vein Disorders; **Hospital:** Mayo Med Ctr & Clin - Rochester; **Address:** Mayo Clin, Div Vasc Surg, 200 First St SW, Rochester, MN 55905-0001; **Phone:** 507-284-4652; **Board Cert:** Surgery 1998; Vascular Surgery 1998; **Med School:** Hungary 1972; **Resid:** Vascular Surgery, Semmelweis Med Sch 1980; Surgery, Mayo Clin 1987; **Fellow:** Vascular Surgery, Mayo Clin 1983; **Fac Appt:** Prof S, Mayo Med Sch

Greisler, Howard MD [VascS] - **Spec Exp:** Peripheral Vascular Surgery; Aneurysm; Carotid Artery Disease; **Hospital:** Hines VA Hosp, Loyola Univ Med Ctr; **Address:** VA Hospital, 5000 S 5th Ave Bldg 1 - rm C417, Hines, IL 60141; **Phone:** 708-216-8541; **Board Cert:** Vascular Surgery 2003; **Med School:** Penn State Univ-Hershey Med Ctr 1975; **Resid:** Surgery, Columbia Presby Med Ctr 1980; **Fellow:** Vascular Surgery, Columbia Presby Med Ctr 1981; **Fac Appt:** Prof S, Loyola Univ-Stritch Sch Med

Hodgson, Kim John MD [VascS] - **Spec Exp:** Aneurysm; Carotid Artery Surgery; Endovascular Surgery; **Hospital:** St John's Hosp - Springfield, Memorial Med Ctr-Springfield; **Address:** PO Box 19638, Springfield, IL 62794-9638; **Phone:** 217-545-5555; **Board Cert:** Vascular Surgery 2005; **Med School:** Univ Pennsylvania 1981; **Resid:** Surgery, Albany Med Ctr 1986; **Fellow:** Vascular Surgery, Southern Ill Univ 1987; **Fac Appt:** Prof VascS, Southern IL Univ

Kent, Kenneth C MD [VascS] - **Spec Exp:** Carotid Artery Surgery; Aneurysm-Abdominal Aortic; Lower Limb Arterial Disease; **Hospital:** Univ WI Hosp & Clins, Meriter Hosp; **Address:** Univ Wisconsin-Madison, Dept Surgery, H4/710D Clinical Sciences Ctr, 600 Highland Ave, Madison, WI 53792-7375; **Phone:** 608-265-8854; **Board Cert:** Surgery 2007; Vascular Surgery 2008; **Med School:** UCSF 1981; **Resid:** Surgery, UCSF Med Ctr 1986; **Fellow:** Vascular Surgery, Brigham & Women's Hosp 1988; **Fac Appt:** Prof S, Univ Wisc

McLafferty, Robert B MD [VascS] - **Spec Exp:** Minimally Invasive Vascular Surgery; Endovascular Stent Grafts; Carotid Artery Stent Placement; Aneurysm; **Hospital:** Memorial Med Ctr-Springfield, St John's Hosp - Springfield; **Address:** PO Box 19680, Springfield, IL 62794-9680; **Phone:** 217-545-5555; **Board Cert:** Surgery 2005; Vascular Surgery 2007; **Med School:** Univ VT Coll Med 1990; **Resid:** Surgery, Oregon Hlth Sci Ctr 1996; **Fellow:** Vascular Surgery, Oregon Hlth Sci Ctr 1998; **Fac Appt:** Prof VascS, Southern IL Univ

Pearce, William H MD [VascS] - **Spec Exp:** Aneurysm-Abdominal Aortic; Stroke; Peripheral Vascular Disease; **Hospital:** Northwestern Meml Hosp; **Address:** Galter Pavilion, 675 N St Clair St, Ste 19-100, Chicago, IL 60611-2647; **Phone:** 312-695-2714; **Board Cert:** Surgery 2001; Vascular Surgery 2003; Surgical Critical Care 1999; **Med School:** Univ Colorado 1975; **Resid:** Surgery, Univ Co Hlth Sci Ctr 1981; **Fellow:** Vascular Surgery, Northwestern Meml Hosp 1982; **Fac Appt:** Prof S, Northwestern Univ

Sanchez, Luis A MD [VascS] - **Spec Exp:** Aneurysm-Abdominal & Thoracic Aortic; Endovascular Stent Grafts; Peripheral Vascular Disease; **Hospital:** Barnes-Jewish Hosp, Barnes-Jewish West County Hosp; **Address:** Washington Univ School Medicine, 660 S Euclid Ave, Box 8109-Surgery, St Louis, MO 63110; **Phone:** 314-362-7408; **Board Cert:** Surgery 2004; Vascular Surgery 2003; **Med School:** Harvard Med Sch 1987; **Resid:** Surgery, Montefiore Med Ctr 1992; **Fellow:** Vascular Surgery, Montefiore Med Ctr 1994; **Fac Appt:** Prof VascS, Washington Univ, St Louis

Shepard, Alexander D MD [VascS] - **Spec Exp:** Aneurysm-Aortic; Aortic Reconstruction; Vascular Surgery-Secondary; **Hospital:** Henry Ford Hosp; **Address:** 2799 W Grand Blvd, Detroit, MI 48202-2608; **Phone:** 313-916-3155; **Board Cert:** Surgery 2001; Vascular Surgery 2005; **Med School:** Johns Hopkins Univ 1976; **Resid:** Surgery, Johns Hopkins Hosp 1982; **Fellow:** Vascular Surgery, New England Med Ctr 1985; **Fac Appt:** Prof S, Wayne State Univ

Sicard, Gregorio A MD [VascS] - **Spec Exp:** Aneurysm-Abdominal Aortic; **Hospital:** Barnes-Jewish Hosp; **Address:** Wash Univ Vascular Surgery, 660 S Euclid Ave, Box 8109, St Louis, MO 63110; **Phone:** 314-362-7841; **Board Cert:** Vascular Surgery 2002; **Med School:** Univ Puerto Rico 1972; **Resid:** Surgery, Barnes Hosp 1977; **Fellow:** Transplant Surgery, Wash Univ Hosp 1978; **Fac Appt:** Prof S, Washington Univ, St Louis

Vascular Surgery

Stanley, James C MD [VascS] - **Spec Exp:** Peripheral Vascular Surgery; Renovascular Disease; Aneurysm; **Hospital:** Univ Michigan Hlth Sys; **Address:** Univ Mich, Dept Vascular Surgery, 1500 E Med Ctr Drive, rm 5167CVC, Taubman Ctr, Ann Arbor, MI 48109-5867; **Phone:** 734-936-5786; **Board Cert:** Surgery 1973; Vascular Surgery 2001; **Med School:** Univ Mich Med Sch 1964; **Resid:** Surgery, Univ Mich Med Ctr 1972; **Fac Appt:** Prof S, Univ Mich Med Sch

Great Plains and Mountains

Annest, Stephen J MD [VascS] - **Spec Exp:** Thoracic Outlet Syndrome; **Hospital:** Presby - St Luke's Med Ctr, Exempla Saint Jos. Hosp. - Denver; **Address:** Vascular Inst of The Rockies, 1601 E 19th Ave, Ste 3950, Denver, CO 80218; **Phone:** 303-539-0736; **Board Cert:** Surgery 2000; Vascular Surgery 2005; **Med School:** Univ Wash 1975; **Resid:** Surgery, Albany Med Ctr 1981; **Fellow:** Trauma, Albany Med Ctr 1980; Vascular Surgery, Baylor Univ Med Ctr 1982; **Fac Appt:** Asst Clin Prof S, Hahnemann Univ

Cooper, Michael A MD [VascS] - **Hospital:** Rose Med Ctr; **Address:** Colorado Cardiovascular Surgical Assocs, 4600 E Hale Pkwy, Ste 460, Denver, CO 80218; **Phone:** 303-388-7265; **Board Cert:** Surgery 1998; Vascular Surgery 2001; **Med School:** Univ Nebr Coll Med 1984; **Resid:** Surgery, Univ Kansas Med Ctr 1989; **Fellow:** Vascular Surgery, LSU Med Ctr 1992

Howard, Thomas C MD [VascS] - **Spec Exp:** Aortic Surgery; Aneurysm-Aortic; Carotid Artery Surgery; Lower Limb Arterial Disease; **Hospital:** Nebraska Med Ctr, Immanuel Med Ctr; **Address:** Surgery Ctr of the Heartland, 4239 Farnam St, Ste 823, Omaha, NE 68131; **Phone:** 402-552-3015; **Board Cert:** Surgery 1975; Vascular Surgery 2002; **Med School:** Yale Univ 1969; **Resid:** Surgery, Yale-New Haven Hosp 1974; **Fac Appt:** Assoc Prof S, Univ Nebr Coll Med

Southwest

Clagett, George Patrick MD [VascS] - **Spec Exp:** Aneurysm-Abdominal Aortic; **Hospital:** UT Southwestern Med Ctr at Dallas, Parkland Hlth & Hosp Sys; **Address:** Univ Tex SW Med Ctr, 5909 Harry Hines Blvd, HA8.130, Dallas, TX 75390-9157; **Phone:** 214-645-0548; **Board Cert:** Surgery 1996; Vascular Surgery 2004; **Med School:** Univ VA Sch Med 1968; **Resid:** Surgery, Univ Mich Med Ctr 1972; Surgery, Univ Mich Med Ctr 1976; **Fellow:** Research, Beth Israel-Harvard 1974; Vascular Surgery, Walter Reed Army Med Ctr 1979; **Fac Appt:** Prof S, Univ Tex SW, Dallas

Eidt, John F MD [VascS] - **Spec Exp:** Aneurysm-Abdominal Aortic; Carotid Artery Stent Placement; Endovascular Surgery; Peripheral Vascular Disease; **Hospital:** UAMS Med Ctr; **Address:** 4301 W Markham St, Slot 520-2, Little Rock, AR 72205; **Phone:** 501-686-6176; **Board Cert:** Surgery 2004; Vascular Surgery 2006; **Med School:** Univ Tex SW, Dallas 1981; **Resid:** Surgery, Brigham-Womens Hosp 1986; **Fellow:** Vascular Surgery, Univ Tex SW Med Ctr 1988; **Fac Appt:** Prof S, Univ Ark

Fowl, Richard J MD [VascS] - **Spec Exp:** Aneurysm-Aortic; Carotid Artery Surgery; Arterial Bypass Surgery-Leg; **Hospital:** Mayo Clinic - Scottsdale; **Address:** Mayo Clinic, Dept Vascular Surgery, 5777 E Mayo Blvd, Phoenix, AZ 85054; **Phone:** 480-342-2868; **Board Cert:** Surgery 2002; Vascular Surgery 2004; **Med School:** Rush Med Coll 1978; **Resid:** Surgery, Med Coll Virginia 1980; Surgery, Univ Iowa Med Ctr 1983; **Fellow:** Vascular Surgery, Mayo Clinic 1985; **Fac Appt:** Prof S, Mayo Med Sch

Hollier, Larry H MD [VascS] - **Spec Exp:** Aortic Surgery; Carotid Artery Surgery; Endovascular Surgery; **Hospital:** West Jefferson Med Ctr, LSU Interim Public Hosp; **Address:** 433 Bolivar St, Ste 815, New Orleans, LA 70112; **Phone:** 504-568-4800; **Board Cert:** Surgery 2007; Vascular Surgery 2001; **Med School:** Louisiana State U, New Orleans 1968; **Resid:** Surgery, Charity Hosp 1973; **Fellow:** Vascular Surgery, Baylor Med Ctr 1974; **Fac Appt:** Prof S, Louisiana State U, New Orleans

Kougias, Panagiotis MD [VascS] - **Spec Exp:** Vascular Reconstruction; Carotid Artery Surgery; Stroke; Endovascular Surgery; **Hospital:** St Luke's Episcopal Hosp-Houston; **Address:** 1709 Dryden Rd, Ste 1500, Houston, TX 77030; **Phone:** 713-794-7892; **Board Cert:** Surgery 2005; Vascular Surgery 2007; **Med School:** Greece 1992; **Resid:** Surgery, East Tennessee State Univ 2004; **Fellow:** Vascular Surgery, Baylor Coll Med 2006; **Fac Appt:** Asst Prof VascS, Baylor Coll Med

Lumsden, Alan B MD [VascS] - **Spec Exp:** Aortic Stent Grafts; Minimally Invasive Surgery; Vein Disorders; **Hospital:** Methodist Hosp - Houston, St Luke's Episcopal Hosp-Houston; **Address:** 6550 Fannin St, Ste 1401, Scurlock Tower, Houston, TX 77030; **Phone:** 713-441-5200; **Board Cert:** Vascular Surgery 2002; **Med School:** Scotland, UK 1981; **Resid:** Surgery, Emory Univ Hosp 1987; **Fellow:** Vascular Surgery, Emory Univ Hosp 1989; **Fac Appt:** Prof VascS, Baylor Coll Med

Money, Samuel R MD [VascS] - **Spec Exp:** Aneurysm-Abdominal Aortic; Arterial Bypass Surgery-Leg; Endovascular Surgery; **Hospital:** Mayo Clinic - Scottsdale; **Address:** Mayo Clinic, Dept Surgery, 5777 E Mayo Blvd, Phoenix, AZ 85054; **Phone:** 480-342-2868; **Board Cert:** Surgery 2000; Vascular Surgery 2002; **Med School:** SUNY Downstate 1983; **Resid:** Surgery, Kings Co Med Ctr 1990; **Fellow:** Vascular Surgery, Ochsner Clinic 1993; **Fac Appt:** Prof S, Mayo Med Sch

West Coast and Pacific

Ahn, Sam S MD [VascS] - **Spec Exp:** Minimally Invasive Vascular Surgery; Endovascular Surgery; Thoracic Outlet Syndrome; Hyperhidrosis; **Hospital:** UCLA Ronald Reagan Med Ctr, St John's Hlth Ctr, Santa Monica; **Address:** 1082 Glendon Ave, Los Angeles, CA 90024; **Phone:** 310-209-2011; **Board Cert:** Surgery 2004; Vascular Surgery 1997; **Med School:** Univ Tex SW, Dallas 1978; **Resid:** Surgery, UCLA Med Ctr 1984; **Fellow:** Vascular Surgery, UCLA Med Ctr 1986; **Fac Appt:** Prof S, UCLA

Angle, Niren MD [VascS] - **Spec Exp:** Endovascular Surgery; Aneurysm-Abdominal & Thoracic Aortic; Cerebrovascular Disease; Carotid Artery Surgery; **Hospital:** UCSD Med Ctr; **Address:** UCSD Med Ctr, 200 W Arbor Drive, MC 8403, San Diego, CA 92103-8403; **Phone:** 619-543-6980; **Board Cert:** Surgery 2000; Vascular Surgery 2002; **Med School:** Loyola Univ-Stritch Sch Med 1992; **Resid:** Surgery, UCSD Med Ctr 1999; **Fellow:** Vascular Surgery, UCLA Ctr Hlth Scis 2001; **Fac Appt:** Assoc Prof S, UCSD

Dilley, Ralph B MD [VascS] - **Spec Exp:** Vascular Reconstruction; **Hospital:** Scripps Green Hosp; **Address:** Scripps Clinic-Torrey Pines, 10666 N Torrey Pines Rd, rm SW208, La Jolla, CA 92037; **Phone:** 858-554-8988; **Board Cert:** Surgery 1966; Thoracic Surgery 1966; Vascular Surgery 2002; **Med School:** Stanford Univ 1959; **Resid:** Surgery, UCLA Med Ctr 1965; Surgery, Johns Hopkins Hosp 1961; **Fellow:** Cardiovascular Surgery, UCSF Med Ctr 1970; **Fac Appt:** Clin Prof S, UCSD

Flanigan, D Preston MD [VascS] - **Spec Exp:** Carotid Artery Disease; Aneurysm; Vein Disorders; **Hospital:** St Joseph's Hosp - Orange; **Address:** 1140 W LaVeta Ave, Ste 850, Orange, CA 92868; **Phone:** 714-560-4450; **Board Cert:** Vascular Surgery 2002; **Med School:** Jefferson Med Coll 1972; **Resid:** Surgery, St Joseph-Mercy Hosp 1977; **Fellow:** Vascular Surgery, Northwest Med Ctr 1978; **Fac Appt:** Clin Prof S, UC Irvine

Vascular Sugery

Gewertz, Bruce MD [VascS] - **Spec Exp:** Carotid Artery Surgery; Peripheral Vascular Disease; Aneurysm-Aortic; Renovascular Disease; **Hospital:** Cedars-Sinai Med Ctr; **Address:** 8700 Beverly Blvd, N Tower, Ste 8215, Los Angeles, CA 90048; **Phone:** 310-423-5884; **Board Cert:** Vascular Surgery 2002; **Med School:** Jefferson Med Coll 1972; **Resid:** Surgery, Univ Mich Hosp 1977; **Fac Appt:** Prof S, UCLA

Pevec, William C MD [VascS] - **Spec Exp:** Vascular Disease; Angioplasty & Stent Placement; **Hospital:** UC Davis Med Ctr; **Address:** UC Davis Med Ctr, Dept Vascular Surgery, 4860 Y St, Ste 2100, Sacramento, CA 95817; **Phone:** 916-734-3524; **Board Cert:** Surgery 1999; Vascular Surgery 2001; **Med School:** Univ Cincinnati 1984; **Resid:** Surgery, U Pittsburgh Med Ctr 1990; **Fellow:** Vascular Surgery, Mass Genl Hosp 1992; **Fac Appt:** Assoc Prof VascS, UC Davis

White, Rodney Allen MD [VascS] - **Spec Exp:** Endovascular Surgery; Aneurysm; Carotid Artery Surgery; **Hospital:** LAC - Harbor - UCLA Med Ctr; **Address:** Harbor-UCLA Med Ctr, 1000 W Carson St, Box 11, Torrance, CA 90502; **Phone:** 310-222-2704; **Board Cert:** Surgery 1998; Vascular Surgery 2006; **Med School:** SUNY Upstate Med Univ 1974; **Resid:** Surgery, LAC-Harbor-UCLA Med Ctr 1979; **Fellow:** Vascular Surgery, LAC-Harbor-UCLA Med Ctr 1980; **Fac Appt:** Prof S, UCLA

Zarins, Christopher K MD [VascS] - **Spec Exp:** Carotid Artery Surgery; Aneurysm-Abdominal Aortic; Endovascular Surgery; **Hospital:** Stanford Univ Med Ctr, El Camino Hosp; **Address:** Stanford Univ Med Ctr, Div Vascular Surg, 300 Pasteur Drive, rm H-3600, Stanford, CA 94305; **Phone:** 650-725-5227; **Board Cert:** Surgery 1975; Vascular Surgery 2002; **Med School:** Johns Hopkins Univ 1968; **Resid:** Surgery, Univ Michigan Hosp 1974; **Fellow:** Surgery, Johns Hopkins Hosp 1972; **Fac Appt:** Prof S, Stanford Univ

Sponsored Page

Appendices

APPENDIX A:
Medical Boards

Introduction to ABMS and Osteopathic Specialties

The following pages contain descriptions of the "official" medical specialties, approved by the American Board of Medical Specialists (for M.D.s) or by the American Osteopathic Association (for D.O.s). These are important because they are the only specialties recognized by the official governing boards. There may be physicians who call themselves one kind of specialist or another, but they may not be certified by the "official" boards. There are, in fact, over 100 such "self-designated" boards, some simply groups of physicians interested in a given area of medicine with no qualifications for membership to other groups with very specific qualifications for membership.

It is important for the medical consumer to seek out physicians certified by the ABMS or AOA to assure their doctor has had the appropriate training and passed the board certification exam.

ABMS

The ABMS is an organization of ABMS Approved medical specialty boards. The mission of the ABMS is to maintain and improve the quality of medical care by assisting the Member Boards in their efforts to develop and utilize professional and educational standards for the evaluation and certification of physician specialists. The intent of certification of physicians is to provide assurance to the public that a physician specialist certified by a Member Board of the ABMS has successfully completed an approved educational program and evaluation process which includes an examination designed to assess the knowledge, skills, and experience required to provide quality patient care in that specialty. The ABMS serves to coordinate the activities of its Member Boards and to provide information to the public, the government, the profession and its Members concerning issues involving specialization and certification in medicine.

Following is a list of the addresses of the various medical specialty boards approved by the ABMS. Note that there are 24 board organizations for 25 medical specialties. Psychiatry and Neurology share the same board.

To find out if a physician is certified, consumers can call the individual boards which may charge a fee for the information, or they can contact the ABMS at (866) 275-2267 (no fee) or www.abms.org.

Appendix A: Medical Boards

American Board of Allergy and Immunology
510 Walnut Street, Suite 1701
Philadelphia, PA 19106-3699
(215) 592-9466, (866) 264-5568

General Certification in Allergy and Immunology. Certifications awarded since 1989 are valid for 10 years. For those certified prior to 1989 there is no recertification requirement.

American Board of Anesthesiology
4101 Lake Boone Trail
Raleigh, NC 27607-7506
(919) 881-2570

General Certification in Anesthesiology; with Special and Added Qualifications in Critical Care Medicine and Pain Management. Certifications awarded since 2000 are valid for 10 years.

American Board of Colon and Rectal Surgery
20600 Eureka Road, Suite 600
Taylor, MI 48180
(734) 282-9400

General Certification is in Colon and Rectal Surgery. Certifications awarded since 1990 are valid for 10 years.

American Board of Dermatology
Henry Ford Health System
Detroit, MI 48202-3450
(313) 874-1088

General Certification in Dermatology; with Special Qualifications in Clinical and Laboratory Dermatological Immunology, Dermatopathology, and Pediatric Dermatology. Certifications awarded since 1991 are valid for 10 years.

American Board of Emergency Medicine
3000 Coolidge Road
East Lansing, MI 48823-6319
(517) 332-4800

General Certification in Emergency Medicine; with Special and Added Qualifications in Medical Toxicology, Pediatric Emergency Medicine, Sports Medicine and Undersea and Hyperbaric Medicine. Certifications awarded since 1980 are valid for 10 years

American Board of Family Practice
2228 Young Drive
Lexington, KY 40505-4294
(859) 269-5626, (888) 995-5700

General Certification in Family Practice; with Added Qualifications in Adolescent
Medicine, Geriatric Medicine and Sports Medicine. Certifications awarded since 1970
are valid for 7 years.

American Board of Internal Medicine
510 Walnut Street, Suite 1700
Philadelphia, PA 19106-3699
(215) 446-3500, (800) 441-ABIM

General Certification in Internal Medicine; with Special Qualifications in Cardiovascular
Disease, Endocrinology, Diabetes and Metabolism, Gastroenterology, Hematology,
Infectious Disease, Medical Oncology, Nephrology, Pulmonary Disease, and
Rheumatology; and Added Qualifications in Adolescent Medicine, Clinical Cardiac
Electrophysiology, Critical Care Medicine, Geriatric Medicine, Interventional Cardiology,
Sleep Medicine, Sports Medicine and Transplant Hepatology. Certifications awarded
since 1990 are valid for 10 years.

American Board of Medical Genetics
9650 Rockville Pike
Bethesda, MD 20814-3998
(301) 634-7315

General Certification in Clinical Genetics (MD), PhD Medical Genetics, Clinical
Biochemical Genetics, Clinical Cytogenetics and Clinical Molecular Genetics; with
Added Qualifications in Molecular Genetic Pathology. Certifications awarded since 2002
are valid for 2 years.

American Board of Neurological Surgery
6550 Fannin Street, Suite 2139
Houston, TX 77030-2701
(713) 441-6015

General Certification in Neurological Surgery. Certifications awarded since 1999 are
valid for 10 years.

Appendix A: Medical Boards

American Board of Nuclear Medicine
4555 Forest Park Boulevard, Suite 119
St. Louis, MO 63108
(314) 367-2225

General Certification in Nuclear Medicine. Certifications awarded since 1992 are valid for 10 years.

American Board of Obstetrics and Gynecology
2915 Vine Street, Suite 300
Dallas, TX 75204
(214) 871-1619

General Certification in Obstetrics and Gynecology; with Special Qualifications in Gynecologic Oncology, Maternal and Fetal Medicine, Reproductive Endocrinology; and Added Qualifications in Critical Care Medicine. Certifications awarded since 1986 are valid for 6 years.

American Board of Ophthalmology
111 Presidential Boulevard, Suite 241
Bala Cynwyd, PA 19004-1075
(610) 664-1175

Certifications Awarded since 1992 are valid for 10 years. For those certified prior to 1992, there is no recertification requirement.

American Board of Orthopaedic Surgery
400 Silver Cedar Court
Chapel Hill, NC 27514
(919) 929-7103

General Certification in Orthopaedic Surgery; with Added Qualification in Hand Surgery; with Added Qualifications in Hand Surgery and Orthopaedic Sports Medicine. Certifications awarded since 1986 are valid for 10 years.

American Board of Otolaryngology
5615 Kirby Drive, Suite 600
Houston, TX 77005
(713) 850-0399

General Certification in Otolaryngology; with Added Qualifications in Neurotology, Pediatric Otolaryngology and Plastic Surgery within the Head and Neck. Certifications awarded since 2002 are valid for10 years.

American Board of Pathology
P.O. Box 25915
Tampa, FL 33622-5915
(813) 286-2444

General Certification in Anatomic and Clinical Pathology, Anatomic Pathology and Clinical Pathology; with Special Qualifications in Blood Banking/Transfusion Medicine, Chemical Pathology, Dermatopathology, Forensic Pathology, Hematology, Medical Microbiology, Molecular Genetic Pathology, Neuropathology and Pediatric Pathology; and Added Qualifications in Cytopathology. Certifications awarded since 1997 are valid for 10 years.

American Board of Pediatrics
111 Silver Cedar Court
Chapel Hill, NC 27514-1651
(919) 929-0461

General Certification in Pediatrics; with Special Qualifications in Adolescent Medicine, Developmental-Behavioral Pediatrics, Neonatal-Perinatal Medicine, Pediatric Cardiology, Pediatric Critical Care Medicine, Pediatric Emergency Medicine, Pediatric Endocrinology, Pediatric Gastroenterology, Pediatric Hematology-Oncology, Pediatric Infectious Diseases, Pediatric Nephrology, Pediatric Pulmonology, and Pediatric Rheumatology; and Added Qualifications in Medical Toxicology, Neurodevelopmental Disabilities, Pediatric Transplant Hepatology and Sports Medicine. Certifications awarded since 1988 valid for 7 years.

American Board of Physical Medicine and Rehabilitation
3015 Allegro Park Lane, S.W.
Rochester, MN 55902-4139
(507) 282-1776

General Certification in Physical Medicine and Rehabilitation; with Special Qualifications in Pain Medicine, Pediatric Rehabilitation Medicine, and Spinal Cord Injury Medicine. Certifications awarded since 1993 are valid for 10 years.

American Board of Plastic Surgery
Seven Penn Center, Suite 400
Philadelphia, PA 19103-2204
(215) 587-9322

General Certification in Plastic Surgery; with Added Qualifications in Hand Surgery. Certifications awarded since 1995 are valid for a 10-year period.

American Board of Preventive Medicine
330 South Wells Street, Suite 1018
Chicago, IL 60606-7106
(312) 939-ABPM [2276]

General Certification in Aerospace Medicine, Occupational Medicine and Public Health
and General Preventive Medicine; with Added Qualifications in Undersea and
Hyperbaric Medicine and Medical Toxicology. Certifications awarded since 1997 are
valid for 10 years.

American Board of Psychiatry and Neurology
500 Lake Cook Road, Suite 335
Deerfield, IL 60015-5349
(847) 945-7900

General Certification in Psychiatry, Neurology and Neurology with Special Qualification
in Child Neurology; with Special Qualifications in Child and Adolescent Psychiatry, Pain
Medicine and Sleep Medicine; and Added Qualifications in Addiction Psychiatry,
Clinical Neurophysiology, Forensic Psychiatry, Geriatric Psychiatry, Neurodevelopmental
Disabilities, Psychosomatic Medicine and Vascular Neurology . Certifications awarded
since 1994 are valid for 10 years.

American Board of Radiology
5441 E. Williams Boulevard, Suite 200
Tucson, AZ 85711
(520) 790-2900

General Certification in Diagnostic Radiology or Radiation Oncology; with Special
Competency in Nuclear Radiology; and Added Qualifications in Neuroradiology,
Pediatric Radiology and Vascular and Interventional Radiology. Radiological Physics is a
non-clinical certification. Certificates are valid for 10 years.

American Board of Surgery
1617 John F. Kennedy Boulevard, Suite 860
Philadelphia, PA 19103-1847
(215) 568-4000

General Certification in Surgery and Vascular Surgery; with Special Qualifications in
Pediatric Surgery and Surgery of the Hand; and Added Qualifications in Surgical Critical
Care. Certifications awarded since 1976 are valid for 10 years.

American Board of Thoracic Surgery
633 North St. Clair Street, Suite 2320
Chicago, IL 60611
(312 202-5900

General Certification in Thoracic Surgery. Certifications awarded since 1976 are valid for 10 years.

American Board of Urology
2216 Ivy Road, Suite 210
Charlottesville, VA 22903
(434) 979-0059

General Certification in Urology. Certifications awarded as of 1985 are valid for 10 years.

Osteopathic

The American Osteopathic Association (AOA) is a member association representing more than 56,000 osteopathic physicians (D.O.s). The AOA serves as the primary certifying body for D.O.s, and is the accrediting agency for all osetopathic medical colleges and health care facilities. The AOA's mission is to advance the philosophy and practice of osteopathic medicine by promoting excellence in education, research, and the delivery of quality, cost-effective healthcare within a distinct, unified profession. American Osteopathic Association 142 E Ontario Street Chicago, IL 60611.

Consumers may call the American Osteopathic Association at (800) 621-1773 or visit the website, www.osteopathic.org, for general certification information.

American Osteopathic Board of Anesthesiology

General certification in Anesthesiology; with Added Qualifications in Addiction Medicine, Critical Care Medicine, and Pain Management. Certifications awarded since 2004 are valid for 10 years. For those certified prior to 2004 there is no recertification requirement.

American Osteopathic Board of Dermatology

General certification in Dermatology; with Added Qualifications in Dermatopathology and MOHS-Micrographic Surgery. Certifications awarded since 2004 are valid for 10 years.

Appendix A: Medical Boards

American Osteopathic Board of Emergency Medicine

General certification in Emergency Medicine; with Added Qualifications in Emergency Medical Services, Medical Toxicology, and Sports Medicine. Certifications awarded since 1994 are valid for 10 years.

American Osteopathic Board of Family Physicians

General certification in Family Practice and Osteopathic Manipulative Treatment (OMT); with Added Qualifications in Geriatric Medicine and Sports Medicine. Certifications awarded since March 1,1997 are valid for 8 years.

American Osteopathic Board of Internal Medicine

General certification in Internal Medicine; with Special Qualifications in Allergy/Immunology, Cardiology, Endocrinology, Gastroenterology, Hematology, Infectious Disease, Nephrology, Oncology, Pulmonary Disease, Rheumatology; with Added Qualifications in Addiction Medicine, Critical Care Medicine, Clinical Cardiac Electrophysiology, Geriatric Medicine, Interventional Cardiology and Sports Medicine. Certifications awarded since 1993 are valid for 10 years.

American Osteopathic Board of Neurology and Psychiatry

General certification in Neurology and Psychiatry; with Special Qualifications in Child/Adolescent Psychiatry and Child/Adolescent Neurology; with Added Qualifications in Addiction Medicine, Neurophysiology, and Sports Medicine. Certifications awarded since 1995 are valid for 10 years.

American Osteopathic Board of Neuromusculoskeletal Medicine

(Formerly American Osteopathic Board of Special Proficiency in Osteopathic Manipulative Medicine)

General certification in Neuromusculoskeletal Medicine. Certifications awarded since 1995 are valid for 10 years. For those certified prior to 1995 there is no recertification requirement.

American Osteopathic Board of Nuclear Medicine

General certification in Nuclear Medicine. Certifications awarded since 1995 are valid for 10 years

American Osteopathic Board of Obstetrics and Gynecology

General certification in Obstetrics and Gynecology; with Special Qualifications in Gynecologic Oncology; Maternal and Fetal Medicine and Reproductive Endocrinology. Certifications awarded since June, 2002 are valid for 6 years.

American Osteopathic Board of Ophthalmology and Otolaryngology/Head and Neck Surgery

General certification in Ophthalmology, Otolaryngolgy, Facial Plastic Surgery and Otolaryngology/Facial Plastic Surgery; with Added Qualifications in Otolaryngic Allergy. Certifications awarded in Ophthalmology since 2000 are valid for 10 years. For those certified prior to 2000 there is no recertification requirement. Certifications awarded in Otolaryngology and/or Otolaryngology/Facial Plastic Surgery since 2002 are valid for 10 years.

American Osteopathic Board of Orthopaedic Surgery

General certification in Orthopaedic Surgery; with Added Qualifications in Hand Surgery. Certifications awarded since 1994 are valid for 10 years.

American Osteopathic Board of Pathology

General certification in Laboratory Medicine, Anatomic Pathology and Anatomic Pathology and Laboratory Medicine; with Special Qualifications in Forensic Pathology; and with Added Qualifications in Dermatopathology. Certifications awarded since 1995 are valid for 10 years.

American Osteopathic Board of Pediatrics

General certification in Pediatrics with Special Qualifications in Adolescent and Young Adult Medicine, Neonatology, Pediatric Allergy/Immunology and Pediatric Endocrinology; with Added Qualifications in Sports Medicine. Certifications awarded since 1995 are valid for 7 years.

American Osteopathic Board of Physical Medicine and Rehabilitation Medicine

General certification in Physical Medicine and Rehabilitation; with Added Qualifications in Sports Medicine. Certifications awarded since 2004 are valid for 10 years.

American Osteopathic Board of Preventive Medicine

General certification in Preventive Medicine/Aerospace Medicine, Preventive Medicine/Occupational-Environmental Medicine and Preventive Medicine/Public Health; with Added Qualifications in Occupational Medicine and Sports Medicine. Certifications awarded since 1994 are valid for 10 years.

American Osteopathic Board of Proctology

General certification in Proctology. Certifications awarded since 2004 are valid for 10 years.

Appendix A: Medical Boards

American Osteopathic Board of Radiology

General certification in Diagnostic Radiology and Radiation Oncology; with Added Qualifications in Body Imaging, Diagnostic Ultrasound, Neuroradiology, Pediatric Radiology and Vascular and Interventional Radiology. Certifications awarded since 2002 are valid for 10 years.

American Osteopathic Board of Surgery

General certification in Surgery, Neurological Surgery, Plastic and Reconstructive Surgery, Cardiothoracic Surgery, Urological Surgery and General Vascular Surgery; with Added Qualifications in Surgical Critical Care. Certifications awarded since 1997 are valid for 10 years.

Appendix B:
Self-Designated Medical Specialties

This list of self-designated medical specialty groups was obtained from the American Board of Medical Specialties. However, it is important to point out that these groups are not recognized by the ABMS, the governing board for the recognized twenty-four medical specialty boards (listed in Appendix A).

The organizations listed below range from highly organized groups that are attempting to formalize training and certification in their field to informal groups interested in a particular aspect of medicine.

If you wish to obtain information from any of these groups you will have to do some detective work. Because so many are informal, the location, phone and mailing addresses change frequently, depending upon the person who is functioning as secretary or administrator.

The best way to track down one of these groups is to consult the doctor listings to find a doctor who has expressed a special interest in that field, and call his or her office. You might also call a nearby academic health center in the area to see if they have a faculty or staff member known to be involved in that particular medical interest. If that fails, take the same approach with your community hospital.

A

Abdominal Surgeons
Acupuncture Medicine
Addiction Medicine
Addictionology
Adolescent Psychiatry
Aesthetic Plastic Surgery
Alcoholism and Other Drug
    Dependencies (AMSAODD)
Algology (Chronic Pain)
Alternative Medicine
Ambulatory Anesthesia
Ambulatory Foot Surgery
Anesthesia
Arthroscopic Surgery
Arthroscopy (Board of North America)

B

Bariatric Medicine
Bionic Psychology
Bloodless Medicine & Surgery

C

Chelation Therapy
Chemical Dependence
Clinical Chemistry
Clinical Ecology
Clinical Medicine and Surgery
Clinical Neurology
Clinical Neurophysiology
Clinical Neurosurgery
Clinical Nutrition
Clinical Orthopaedic Surgery
Clinical Pharmacology
Clinical Polysomnography
Clinical Psychiatry
Clinical Psychology
Clinical Toxicology
Cosmetic Plastic Surgery
Cosmetic Surgery
Council of Non-Board Certified Physicians
Critical Care in Medicine & Surgery

D

Disability Analysis
Disability Evaluating Physicians

E

Electrodiagnostic Medicine
Electroencephalography
Electromyography & Electrodiagnosis
Environmental Medicine
Epidemiology (College)
Eye Surgery

F

Facial Cosmetic Surgery
Facial Plastic & Reconstructive Surgery
Family Practice, Certification
Forensic Examiners
Forensic Psychiatry
Forensic Toxicology

H

Hand Surgery
Head, Facial & Neck Pain & TMJ Orthopaedics
Health Physics
Homeopathic Physicians
Homeotherapeutics
Hypnotic Anesthesiology, National Board for

I

Independent Medical Examiners
Industrial Medicine & Surgery
Insurance Medicine
International Cosmetic & Plastic
    Facial Reconstructive Standards
Interventional Radiology

L

Laser Surgery
Law in Medicine
Longevity Medicine/Surgery

M

Malpractice Physicians
Maxillofacial Surgeons
Medical Accreditation (American Federation for)
Medical Hypnosis
Medical Laboratory Immunology
Medical-Legal Analysis of Medicine & Surgery
Medical Legal & Workers
  Comp. Medicine & Surgery
Medical-Legal Consultants
Medical Management
Medical Microbiology
Medical Preventics (Academy)
Medical Psychotherapists
Medical Toxicology
Microbiology (Medical Microbiology)
Military Medicine
Mohs Micrographic Surgery &
  Cutaneous Oncology

N

Neuroimaging
Neurologic & Orthopaedic Dental
  Medicine and Surgery
Neurological & Orthopaedic Medicine
Neurological & Orthopaedic Surgery
Neurological Microsurgery
Neurology
Neuromuscular Thermography
Neuro-Orthopaedic Dental Medicine
Neuro-Orthopaedic Electrodiagnosis
Neuro-Orthopaedic Laser Surgery
Neuro-Orthopaedic Psychiatry
Neuro-Orthopaedic Thoracic Medicine
Neurorehabilitation
Nutrition

O

Orthopaedic Medicine
Orthopaedic Microneurosurgery
Otorhinolaryngology

P

Pain Management (American Academy of)
Pain Management Specialties
Pain Medicine
Palliative Medicine
Percutaneous Diskectomy
Plastic Esthetic Surgeons
Prison Medicine
Professional Disability Consultants Psychiatric
  Medicine
Psychiatry (American National Board of)
Psychoanalysis (American Examining
  Board in)
Psychological Medicine (International)

Q

Quality Assurance & Utilization Review

R

Radiology & Medical Imaging
Rheumatologic Surgery
Rheumatological & Reconstructive Medicine
Ringside Medicine & Surgery

S

Skin Specialists
Sleep Medicine (Polysomnography)
Spinal Cord Injury
Spinal Surgery
Sports Medicine
Sports Medicine/Surgery

T

Toxicology
Trauma Surgery
Traumatologic Medicine & Surgery
Tropical Medicine

U

Ultrasound Technology
Urologic Allied Health Professionals
Urological Surgery

W

Weight Reduction Medicine

APPENDIX C:
Hospital Listings

The following is an alphabetical listing of all hospitals that have at least one Castle Connolly Top Doctor in this guide. Institutions listed in **Bold** are profiled in this Guide in association with Castle Connolly's *Partnership for Excellence* program. The abbreviations as they appear in the listings are in italics below. Due to the many changes taking place in the hospital industry, the names on this list may have changed subsequent to publication of this guide.

Abbott - Northwestern Hospital		(612) 863-4000
Abbott - Northwestern Hosp		
800 E 28th St	Minneapolis, MN 55407	MIDWEST
Advocate Christ Medical Center		(708) 684-8000
Adv Christ Med Ctr		
4440 W 95th St	Oak Lawn, IL 60453	MIDWEST
Advocate Good Samaritan Hospital		(630) 275-5900
Adv Good Samaritan Hosp		
3815 Highland Ave	Downers Grove, IL 60515	MIDWEST
Advocate Illinois Masonic Medical Center		(773) 975-1600
Adv Illinois Masonic Med Ctr		
836 W Wellington Ave	Chicago, IL 60657-5147	MIDWEST
Advocate Lutheran General Hospital		(847) 723-2210
Adv Luth Genl Hosp		
1775 West Dempster St	Park Ridge, IL 60068	MIDWEST
Albany Medical Center		(518) 262-3125
Albany Med Ctr		
43 New Scotland Ave	Albany, NY 12208	MID ATLANTIC
Albert Einstein Medical Center		(215) 456-7890
Albert Einstein Med Ctr		
5501 Old York Rd	Philadelphia, PA 19141	MID ATLANTIC
Albert Lea Medical Center-Mayo Health System		(507) 373-2384
Albert Lea Med Ctr-Mayo Hlth Sys		
404 W Fountain St	Albert Lea, MN 56007	MIDWEST
Alexian Brothers Medical Center		(847) 437-5500
Alexian Brothers Med Ctr		
800 Biesterfield Rd	Elk Grove Village, IL 60007	MIDWEST

Alfred I duPont Hospital for Children   (302) 651-4000
Alfred I duPont Hosp for Children
1600 Rockland Rd   Wilmington, DE 19803   MID ATLANTIC

All Children's Hospital   (727) 767-7451
All Children's Hosp
801 Sixth Street South   St. Petersburg, FL 33701   SOUTHEAST

Allegheny General Hospital   (412) 359-3131
Allegheny General Hosp
320 E. North Avenue   Pittsburgh, PA 15212   MID ATLANTIC

Allenmore Hospital   (206) 552-5000
Allenmore Hosp
S 19th & Union, Box 11414   Tacoma, WA 98405   WEST COAST AND PACIFIC

Alta Bates Summit Medical Center-Alta Bates Campus   (510) 204-4444
Alta Bates Summit Med Ctr-Alta Bates Campus
2450 Ashby Avenue   Berkeley, CA 94705   WEST COAST AND PACIFIC

Anne Arundel Medical Center   (443) 481-1000
Anne Arundel Med Ctr
64 Franklin Street   Annapolis, MD 21401   MID ATLANTIC

Arizona Heart Hospital   (602) 532-1000
Arizona Heart Hosp
1930 Thomas Rd   Phoenix, AZ 85016   SOUTHWEST

Arkansas Children's Hospital   (501) 364-1100
Arkansas Chldns Hosp
800 Marshall St   Little Rock, AR 72202   SOUTHWEST

Arlington Memorial Hospital   (817) 548-6100
Arlington Meml Hosp
800 W Randol Mill Rd   Arlington, TX 76012-2503   SOUTHWEST

Arthur G. James Cancer Hospital & Research Institute   (614) 293-3300
Arthur G James Cancer Hosp & Research Inst
300 West 10th Avenue   Columbus, OH 43210   MIDWEST

Atlanta Medical Center   (404) 265-4000
Atlanta Med Ctr
303 Parkway Dr. NE   Atlanta, GA 30312   SOUTHEAST

Audie L Murphy Memorial Veterans Hospital   (210) 617-5300
Audie L Murphy Meml Vets Hosp
7400 Merton Minter Blvd   San Antonio, TX 78229   SOUTHWEST

Aultman Hospital (330) 452-9911
Aultman Hosp
2600 6th St SW   Canton, OH 44710-1799   MIDWEST

Austen Riggs Center (413) 298-5511
Austen Riggs Ctr
25 Main Street or PO Box 962   Stockbridge, MA 01262-0962   NEW ENGLAND

Aventura Hosp & Medical Center (305) 682-7000
Aventura Hosp & Med Ctr
20900 Biscayne Blvd   Aventura, FL 33180   SOUTHEAST

Banner Desert Medical Center (480) 512-3000
Banner Desert Med Ctr
1400 S Dobson Rd   Mesa, AZ 85202   SOUTHWEST

Banner Good Samaritan Regional Medical Center - Phoenix (602) 239-2000
Banner Good Samaritan Regl Med Ctr - Phoenix
1111 E McDowell Rd   Phoenix, AZ 85060   SOUTHWEST

Baptist Hospital - Jackson (601) 968-1000
Baptist Hosp - Jackson
1225 N State St   Jackson, MS 39202   SOUTHEAST

Baptist Hospital - Nashville (615) 284-5555
Baptist Hosp - Nashville
2000 Church St   Nashville, TN 37236   SOUTHEAST

Baptist Hospital of Miami (786) 596-1960
Baptist Hosp of Miami
8900 N Kendall Dr   Miami, FL 33176   SOUTHEAST

Baptist Medical Center - San Antonio (210) 297-7000
Baptist Med Ctr - San Antonio
111 Dallas St   San Antonio, TX 78205   SOUTHWEST

Baptist Memorial Hospital - Memphis (901) 226-5000
Baptist Memorial Hospital - Memphis
6019 Walnut Grove Rd   Memphis, TN 38120   SOUTHEAST

Barnes-Jewish Hospital (314) 362-5000
Barnes-Jewish Hosp
One Barnes-Jewish Hospital Plaza   St. Louis, MO 63110   MIDWEST

Barnes-Jewish West County Hospital (314) 996-8000
Barnes-Jewish West County Hosp
12634 Olive Blvd   St. Louis, MO 63141   MIDWEST

Bascom Palmer Eye Institute   (305) 326-6000
Bascom Palmer Eye Inst
900 NW 17 St   Miami, FL 33136   SOUTHEAST

Baylor University Medical Center   (214) 820-0111
Baylor Univ Medical Ctr
3500 Gaston Avenue   Dallas, TX 75246   SOUTHWEST

Baystate Medical Center   (413) 794-0000
Baystate Med Ctr
759 Chestnut Street   Springfield, MA 01199   NEW ENGLAND

Ben Taub General Hospital   (713) 873-2000
Ben Taub Genl Hosp
1504 Taub Loop   Houston, TX 77001   SOUTHWEST

Beth Israel Deaconess Medical Center - Boston   (617) 667-7000
Beth Israel Deaconess Med Ctr - Boston
330 Brookline Ave   Boston, MA 02215   NEW ENGLAND

Beth Israel Medical Center - Milton & Caroll Petrie Division   (212) 420-2000
Beth Israel Med Ctr - Petrie Division
First Avenue @ 16th Street   New York, NY 10003   MID ATLANTIC

Bethesda North Hospital   (513) 745-1111
Bethesda North Hosp
10500 Montgomery Rd   Cincinnati, OH 45242-4415   MIDWEST

Boca Raton Community Hospital   (561) 395-7100
Boca Raton Comm Hosp
800 Meadows Road   Boca Raton, FL 33486   SOUTHEAST

Boston Medical Center   (617) 638-8000
Boston Med Ctr
1 Boston Medical Center Pl   Boston, MA 02118   NEW ENGLAND

Boulder Community Hospital   (303) 440-2273
Boulder Community Hospital
1100 Balsam Ave, Box 9019   Boulder, CO 80301-9019   GREAT PLAINS AND MOUNTAINS

Boys Town National Research Hospital   (402) 498-6511
Boys Town Natl Rsch Hosp
555 N 30th St   Omaha, NE 68101   GREAT PLAINS AND MOUNTAINS

Brenner Children's Hospital   (336) 716-2011
Brenner Chldrn's Hosp
Medical Center Blvd   Winston-Salem, NC 27157-1015   SOUTHEAST

Brigham & Women's Hospital	(617) 732-5500
Brigham & Women's Hosp	
75 Francis St Boston, MA 02115	NEW ENGLAND

Brooklyn Hospital Center-Downtown	(718) 250-8000
Brooklyn Hosp Ctr-Downtown	
121 DeKalb Avenue Brooklyn, NY 11201	MID ATLANTIC

Brookwood Medical Center	(205) 877-1000
Brookwood Med Ctr	
2010 Brookwood Med Ctr Drive Birmingham, AL 35209-6804	SOUTHEAST

Broward General Medical Center	(954) 355-4400
Broward General Med Ctr	
1600 S Andrews Ave Fort Lauderdale, FL 33316	SOUTHEAST

Bryn Mawr Hospital	(610) 526-3000
Bryn Mawr Hosp	
130 S Bryn Mawr Ave Bryn Mawr, PA 19010-3143	MID ATLANTIC

Buffalo General Hospital	(716) 859-5600
Buffalo General Hosp	
100 High Street Buffalo, NY 14203	MID ATLANTIC

Burke Rehabilitation Hospital	(914) 597-2500
Burke Rehab Hosp	
785 Mamaroneck Avenue White Plains, NY 10605	MID ATLANTIC

Butler Hospital	(401) 455-6200
Butler Hosp	
345 Blackstone Blvd Providence, RI 02906	NEW ENGLAND

California Pacific Medical Center	(415) 600-6000
CA Pacific Med Ctr	
PO Box 7999 San Francisco, CA 94120	WEST COAST AND PACIFIC

California Pacific Medical Center - California Campus	(415) 600-6000
CA Pacific Med Ctr - CA Campus	
3700 California St San Francisco, CA 94114	WEST COAST AND PACIFIC

California Pacific Medical Center - Pacific Campus	(415) 600-6000
CA Pacific Med Ctr - Pacific Campus	
2333 Buchanan St San Francisco, CA 94115	WEST COAST AND PACIFIC

Carilion Roanoke Memorial Hospital	(540) 224-4966
Carilion Roanoke Meml Hosp	
1906 Belleview Ave Roanoke, VA 24014	SOUTHEAST

Caritas St Elizabeth's Medical Center   (617) 789-3000
Caritas St Elizabeth's Med Ctr
736 Cambridge St   Boston, MA 02135   NEW ENGLAND

Carolinas Medical Center   (704) 355-2000
Carolinas Med Ctr
1000 Blythe Blvd   Charlotte, NC 28203-5871   SOUTHEAST

Carolinas Medical Center-University   (704) 548-6000
Carolinas Med Ctr-Univ
PO Box 560727   Charlotte, NC 28256   SOUTHEAST

Cedars-Sinai Medical Center   (310) 423-3277
Cedars-Sinai Med Ctr
8700 Beverly Boulevard   Los Angeles, CA 90048   WEST COAST AND PACIFIC

Centennial Medical Center   (615) 342-1000
Centennial Med Ctr
2300 Patterson Street   Nashville, TN 37203   SOUTHEAST

Centinela Freeman Regional Medical Center-Centinela Campus   (310) 673-4660
Centinela Freeman Reg Med Ctr-Centinela
555 East Hardy Street   Inglewood, CA 90301   WEST COAST AND PACIFIC

Central Baptist Hospital   (859) 260-6592
Central Baptist Hosp
1740 Nicholasville Rd   Lexington, KY 40503-1499   SOUTHEAST

Central DuPage Hospital   (630) 933-1600
Central DuPage Hosp
25 N Winfield Rd   Winfield, IL 60190   MIDWEST

Chelsea Community Hospital   (734) 475-1311
Chelsea Comm Hosp
775 S Main St   Chelsea, MI 48118   MIDWEST

Cheyenne Regional Medical Center   (307) 634-2273
Cheyenne Regl Med Ctr
214 E 23rd St   Cheyenne, WY 82001   GREAT PLAINS AND MOUNTAINS

Children's Healthcare of Atlanta - Scottish Rite   (404) 250-5437
Chldns Hlthcare Atlanta - Scottish Rite
1001 Johnson Ferry Rd   Atlanta, GA 30342   SOUTHEAST

Children's Healthcare of Atlanta at Egleston   (404) 325-6000
Chldns Hlthcare Atlanta @ Egleston
1405 Clifton Rd NE   Atlanta, GA 30322   SOUTHEAST

Children's Hospital - Aurora, The   (720) 777-1234
Chldn's Hosp - Aurora, The
13123 E 16th Ave   Aurora, CO 80045   GREAT PLAINS AND MOUNTAINS

Children's Hospital - Austin   (512) 324-8832
Children's Hospital - Austin
609 W 15th St   Austin, TX 78701   SOUTHWEST

Children's Hospital - Boston   (617) 355-6000
Children's Hospital - Boston
300 Longwood Avenue   Boston, MA 02115   NEW ENGLAND

Children's Hospital - Los Angeles   (323) 660-2450
Chldns Hosp - Los Angeles
4650 Sunset Blvd   Los Angeles, CA 90027   WEST COAST AND PACIFIC

Children's Hospital - New Orleans   (504) 899-9511
Children's Hospital - New Orleans
200 Henry Clay Ave   New Orleans, LA 70118   SOUTHWEST

Children's Hospital - Oakland   (510) 428-3000
Chldns Hosp - Oakland
747 52nd St   Oakland, CA 94609   WEST COAST AND PACIFIC

Children's Hospital - Omaha   (402) 955-5400
Children's Hosp - Omaha
8200 Dodge St   Omaha, NE 68114   GREAT PLAINS AND MOUNTAINS

Children's Hospital and Clinics - Minneapolis   (612) 813-6111
Chldns Hosp and Clinics - Minneapolis
2525 Chicago Ave S   Minneapolis, MN 55404   MIDWEST

Children's Hospital and Regional Medical Center - Seattle   (206) 987-2000
Chldns Hosp and Regl Med Ctr - Seattle
4800 Sand Point Way NE   Seattle, WA 98145   WEST COAST AND PACIFIC

Children's Hospital at OU Medical Center   (405) 271-5437
Chldns Hosp OU Med Ctr
940 Northeast 13th St   Oklahoma City, OK 73104   SOUTHWEST

Children's Hospital Central California   (559) 353-3000
Chldns Hosp Central CA
9300 Valley Children's Pl   Madera, CA 93638   WEST COAST AND PACIFIC

Children's Hospital Medical Center - Akron   (330) 379-8200
Children's Hosp & Med Ctr- Akron
One Perkins Square   Akron, OH 44308   MIDWEST

Children's Hospital of Alabama - Birmingham	(205) 939-9100
Children's Hospital - Birmingham	
1600 7th Ave South Birmingham, AL 35233	SOUTHEAST
Children's Hospital of Michigan	(313) 745-5437
Chldns Hosp of Michigan	
3901 Beaubian Blvd Detroit, MI 48201	MIDWEST
Children's Hospital of Orange County	(714) 997-3000
Chldns Hosp Orange Co	
455 South Main Street Orange, CA 92868	WEST COAST AND PACIFIC
Children's Hospital of Philadelphia, The	(215) 590-1000
Chldns Hosp of Philadelphia, The	
34th St & Civic Center Blvd Philadelphia, PA 19104	MID ATLANTIC
Children's Hospital of Pittsburgh - UPMC	(412) 692-5325
Chldns Hosp of Pittsburgh - UPMC	
3705 Fifth Avenue Pittsburgh, PA 15213	MID ATLANTIC
Children's Hospital of the King's Daughters	(757) 668-7500
Chldns Hosp of King's Daughters	
601 Children's Ln Norfolk, VA 23507	SOUTHEAST
Children's Hospital of Wisconsin	(414) 266-2000
Chldns Hosp - Wisconsin	
9000 W Wisconsin Ave Milwaukee, WI 53201	MIDWEST
Children's Institute - Pittsburgh	(412) 420-2400
Children's Inst - Pittsburgh	
1405 Shady Avenue Pittsburgh, PA 15217	MID ATLANTIC
Children's Medical Center of Dallas	(214) 456-7000
Chldns Med Ctr of Dallas	
1935 Motor St Dallas, TX 75235	SOUTHWEST
Children's Memorial Hospital	(773) 880-4000
Children's Mem Hosp	
2300 Children's Plaza Chicago, IL 60614	MIDWEST
Children's Mercy Hospitals & Clinics	(816) 234-3000
Chldns Mercy Hosps & Clinics	
2401 Gilham Rd Kansas City, MO 64108	MIDWEST
Children's National Medical Center - DC	(202) 884-5000
Chldns Natl Med Ctr	
111 Michigan Ave NW Washington, DC 20010	MID ATLANTIC

Christ Hospital, The   (513) 585-2000
Christ Hospital
2139 Auburn Ave   Cincinnati, OH 45219   MIDWEST

Christiana Care Health Services   (302) 428-2229
Christiana Care Hlth Svs
501 W 14th St   Wilmington, DE 19899-1038   MID ATLANTIC

Christiana Hospital   (302) 733-1000
Christiana Hospital
4755 Ogletown-Stanton Rd   Newark, DE 19718-0001   MID ATLANTIC

Christus Santa Rosa Children's Hospital   (512) 228-2011
Christus Santa Rosa Children's Hosp
333 N Santa Rosa St   San Antonio, TX 78207   SOUTHWEST

Christus Santa Rosa Medical Center Hospital   (210) 705-6300
Christus Santa Rosa Med Ctr Hosp
2827 Babcock Rd   San Antonio, TX 78229-6098   SOUTHWEST

Cincinnati Children's Hospital Medical Center   (800) 344-2462
Cincinnati Chldns Hosp Med Ctr
3333 Burnet Ave   Cincinnati, OH 45229-3039   MIDWEST

Cincinnati Shriners Hospital   (513) 872-6000
Cincinnati Shriners Hosp
3229 Burnet Ave   Cincinnati, OH 45229-3095   MIDWEST

City of Hope National Medical Center & Beckman Research   (626) 359-8111
City of Hope Natl Med Ctr & Beckman Rsch
1500 E Duarte Rd   Duarte, CA 91010   WEST COAST AND PACIFIC

CJW Medical Center Johnston-Willis Campus   (804) 330-2000
CJW Med Ctr
1401 Johnston-Willis Dr   Richmond, VA 23235   SOUTHEAST

Clara Maass Medical Center   (973) 450-2000
Clara Maass Med Ctr
One Clara Maass Drive   Belleville, NJ 07109   MID ATLANTIC

Cleveland Clinic Florida - Weston   (954) 659-5000
Cleveland Clin - Weston
2950 Cleveland Clinic Blvd   Weston, FL 33331   SOUTHEAST

Cleveland Clinic Foundation   (800) 223-2273
Cleveland Clin Fdn
9500 Euclid Avenue   Cleveland, OH 44195   MIDWEST

Columbia Hospital - West Palm Beach	(561) 842-6141
Columbia Hosp - W Palm Beach	
2201 45th St West Palm Beach, FL 33407	SOUTHEAST

Community Memorial Hospital - Ventura	(805) 652-5011
Comm Meml Hosp - Ventura	
147 N Brent St Ventura, CA 93003	WEST COAST AND PACIFIC

Concord Hospital	(603) 225-2711
Concord Hospital	
250 Pleasant St Concord, NH 03301-2598	NEW ENGLAND

Connecticut Children's Medical Center	(860) 545-9000
CT Chldns Med Ctr	
282 Washington St Hartford, CT 06106	NEW ENGLAND

Connecticut Mental Health Center	(203) 789-7092
Connecticut Mental Hlth Ctr	
34 Park St New Haven, CT 06508-1842	NEW ENGLAND

Cook Children's Medical Center	(682) 885-4000
Cook Chldns Med Ctr	
801 7th Ave Fort Worth, TX 76104-2796	SOUTHWEST

Cooper University Hospital	(856) 342-2000
Cooper Univ Hosp	
1 Cooper Plaza Camden, NJ 08103-1489	MID ATLANTIC

Covenant Children's Hospital	(806) 725-1011
Covenant Children's Hosp	
3610 21st St Lubbock, TX 79410	SOUTHWEST

Covenant Medical Center	(319) 272-8000
Covenant Med Ctr	
3421 W 9th St Waterloo, IA 50702-5499	MIDWEST

Creighton University Medical Center	(402) 449-4000
Creighton Univ Med Ctr	
601 N 30th St Omaha, NE 68131-2197	GREAT PLAINS AND MOUNTAINS

Dana-Farber Cancer Institute	(617) 632-3000
Dana-Farber Cancer Inst	
44 Binney St Boston, MA 02115	NEW ENGLAND

Dartmouth - Hitchcock Medical Center	(603) 650-5000
Dartmouth - Hitchcock Med Ctr	
1 Medical Center Dr Lebanon, NH 03756-0002	NEW ENGLAND

DCH Regional Medical Center
DCH Reg Med Ctr
809 Univ Blvd E   Tuscaloosa, AL 35401-2029

(205) 759-7111

SOUTHEAST

Deborah Heart and Lung Center
Deborah Hrt & Lung Ctr
200 Trenton Rd   Brown Mills, NJ 08015-1705

(609) 893-6611

MID ATLANTIC

Denver Health Medical Center
Denver Health Med Ctr
777 Bannock St   Denver, CO 80204

(303) 436-6000

GREAT PLAINS AND MOUNTAINS

Desert Regional Medical Center
Desert Regl Med Ctr
1150 N Indian Canyon Dr   Palm Springs, CA 92262

(760) 323-6511

WEST COAST AND PACIFIC

Detroit Medical Center
Detroit Med Ctr
3663 Woodward Ave, Ste 200   Detroit, MI 48201-2403

(313) 578-3930

MIDWEST

DeVos Children's Hospital
DeVos Children's Hosp
1000 E Paris SE   Grand Rapids, MI 49546

(616) 957-0866

MIDWEST

Doctors' Hospital
Doctors' Hosp
5000 University Dr   Coral Gables, FL 33146

(305) 666-2111

SOUTHEAST

Doernbecher Children's Hospital/Oregon Health Science University
Doernbecher Chldns Hosp/OHSU
3181 SW Sam Jackson Park Rd   Portland, OR 97201-3098

(503) 494-8811

WEST COAST AND PACIFIC

Dotter Interventional Institute - OHSU
Dotter Institute - OHSU
3181 SW Sam Jackson Park Rd   Portland, OR 97201

(503) 494-7660

WEST COAST AND PACIFIC

Duke Health Raleigh Hospital
Duke Health Raleigh
3400 Wake Forest Rd   Raleigh, NC 27609

(919) 954-3000

SOUTHEAST

Duke University Medical Center
Duke Univ Med Ctr
DUMC, Box 3708   Durham, NC 27710

(919) 684-8111

SOUTHEAST

East Texas Medical Center-Tyler
E TX Med Ctr-Tyler
1000 S Beckham Ave   Tyler, TX 75701

(903) 597-0351

SOUTHWEST

Edward Hines Jr Veterans Affairs Hospital   (708) 202-8387
Hines VA Hosp
5th Ave & Roosevelt Rd, Box 5000 Hines, IL 60141   MIDWEST

Edward Hospital   (630) 355-0450
Edward Hosp
801 S Washington St   Naperville, IL 60540   MIDWEST

El Camino Hospital   (650) 940-7000
El Camino Hosp
2500 Grant Road   Mountain View, CA 94039   WEST COAST AND PACIFIC

Elliot Hospital   (603) 669-5300
Elliot Hosp
1 Elliot Way   Manchester, NH 03103   NEW ENGLAND

Emory University Hospital   (404) 712-2000
Emory Univ Hosp
1364 Clifton Rd NE   Atlanta, GA 30322   SOUTHEAST

Emory University Hospital Midtown   (404) 686-4411
Emory Univ Hosp Midtown
550 Peachtree St NE   Atlanta, GA 30365   SOUTHEAST

Englewood Hospital & Medical Center   (201) 894-3000
Englewood Hosp & Med Ctr
350 Engle Street   Englewood, NJ 07631   MID ATLANTIC

Evanston/Northshore University Health System   (847) 570-2000
Evanston/Northshore Univ Hlth Syst
2650 Ridge Ave   Evanston, IL 60201   MIDWEST

Fairview Southdale Hospital   (952) 924-5000
Fairview Southdale Hosp
6401 France Ave S   Edina, MN 55435-2199   MIDWEST

Fletcher Allen Health Care-Medical Center Campus   (802) 658-4310
Fletcher Allen Health Care- Med Ctr Campus
111 Colchester Ave   Burlington, VT 05401   NEW ENGLAND

Florida Hospital - Celebration Health   (407) 764-4000
Florida Hosp Celebration Hlth
400 Celebration Pl   Celebration, FL 34747   SOUTHEAST

Florida Hospital - Orlando   (407) 303-5600
Florida Hosp - Orlando
601 E Rollins St   Orlando, FL 32803   SOUTHEAST

Floyd Memorial Hospital & Health Services	(812) 944-7701
Floyd Meml Hosp & Hlth Svcs	
1850 State St New Albany, IN 47150-4997	MIDWEST

Forsyth Medical Center	(336) 718-5000
Forsyth Med Ctr	
3333 Silas Creek Pkwy Winston-Salem, NC 27103	SOUTHEAST

Four Winds Hospital	(914) 763-8151
Four Winds Hosp	
800 Cross River Road Katonah, NY 10536	MID ATLANTIC

Fox Chase Cancer Center	(215) 728-6900
Fox Chase Cancer Ctr	
333 Cottman Avenue Philadelphia, PA 19111	MID ATLANTIC

Franklin Square Hospital	(443) 777-7000
Franklin Square Hosp	
9000 Franklin Square Drive Baltimore, MD 21237	MID ATLANTIC

Froedtert Memorial Lutheran Hospital	(414) 805-6644
Froedtert Meml Lutheran Hosp	
9200 W Wisconsin Ave Milwaukee, WI 53226	MIDWEST

Gaston Memorial Hospital	(704) 834-2000
Gaston Meml Hosp	
2525 Court Dr Gastonia, NC 28054	SOUTHEAST

Geisinger Medical Center	(570) 271-6211
Geisinger Med Ctr	
100 N Academy Ave Danville, PA 17822	MID ATLANTIC

George Washington University Hospital	(202) 715-4000
G Washington Univ Hosp	
900 23rd St NW Washington, DC 20037	MID ATLANTIC

Georgetown University Hospital	(202) 444-2000
Georgetown Univ Hosp	
3800 Reservoir Rd NW Washington, DC 20007	MID ATLANTIC

Glenbrook/NorthShore University Health System	(847) 657-5800
Glenbrook/NorthShore Univ Hlth Syst	
2100 Pfingsten Rd Glenview, IL 60025	MIDWEST

Good Samaritan Hosp - Cincinnati	(513) 872-1400
Good Samaritan Hosp - Cincinnati	
375 Dixmyth Ave Cincinnati, OH 45220	MIDWEST

Good Samaritan Hospital	(410) 532-8000
Good Samaritan Hosp	
5601 Loch Raven Blvd Baltimore, MD 21208	MID ATLANTIC

Good Samaritan Hospital - Los Angeles	(213) 977-2121
Good Samaritan Hosp - LA	
1225 Wilshire Boulevard Los Angeles, CA 90017	WEST COAST AND PACIFIC

Good Samaritan Hospital - San Jose	(408) 559-2011
Good Samaritan Hosp - San Jose	
2425 Samaritan Drive San Jose, CA 95124	WEST COAST AND PACIFIC

Goshen General Hospital	(574) 533-2141
Goshen Genl Hosp	
200 High Park Ave Goshen, IN 46526	MIDWEST

Gottlieb Memorial Hospital	(708) 681-3200
Gottlieb Meml Hosp	
701 W North Ave Melrose Park, IL 60160	MIDWEST

Grady Health System	(404) 616-4307
Grady Hlth Sys	
80 Jesse Hill Jr Dr Atlanta, GA 30303	SOUTHEAST

Greater Baltimore Medical Center	(443) 849-2000
Greater Baltimore Med Ctr	
6701 N Charles St Baltimore, MD 21204	MID ATLANTIC

Greenwich Hospital	(203) 863-3000
Greenwich Hosp	
Five Perryridge Road Greenwich, CT 06830	NEW ENGLAND

H Lee Moffitt Cancer Center & Research Institute	(813) 972-4673
H Lee Moffitt Cancer Ctr & Research Inst	
12902 Magnolia Drive Tampa, FL 33612-9497	SOUTHEAST

Hackensack University Medical Center	(201) 996-2000
Hackensack Univ Med Ctr	
30 Prospect Avenue Hackensack, NJ 07601	MID ATLANTIC

Hahnemann University Hospital	(215) 762-7000
Hahnemann Univ Hosp	
Broad & Vine St Philadelphia, PA 19102	MID ATLANTIC

Hamot Medical Center	(814) 877-6000
Hamot Med Ctr	
201 State Street Erie, PA 16550-0001	MID ATLANTIC

Harborview Medical Center
Harborview Med Ctr
325 9th Ave, Box 359717   Seattle, WA 98104
(206) 731-3000
WEST COAST AND PACIFIC

Harlem Hospital Center
Harlem Hosp Ctr
506 Lenox Avenue   New York, NY 10037
(212) 939-1000
MID ATLANTIC

Harper University Hospital
Harper Univ Hosp
3990 John R St   Detroit, MI 48201-2097
(313) 745-8040
MIDWEST

Harrison Memorial Hospital
Harrison Meml Hosp
2520 Cherry Ave   Bremerton, WA 98310-4270
(360) 377-3911
WEST COAST AND PACIFIC

Hartford Hospital
Hartford Hosp
80 Seymour St, Box 5037   Hartford, CT 06102-5037
(860) 545-5000
NEW ENGLAND

Healthsouth Lakeshore Rehabilitation Hospital
Healthsouth Lakeshore Rehab Hosp
3800 Ridgeway   Birmingham, AL 35209
(205) 868-2000
SOUTHEAST

Hennepin County Medical Center
Hennepin Cnty Med Ctr
701 Park Ave S   Minneapolis, MN 55415
(612) 347-2121
MIDWEST

Henry Ford Hospital
Henry Ford Hosp
2799 W Grand Blvd   Detroit, MI 48202
(313) 916-2600
MIDWEST

Henry Mayo Newhall Memorial Hospital
Henry Mayo Newhall Memorial Hosp
23845 McBean Parkway   Valencia, CA 91355
(805) 253-8000
WEST COAST AND PACIFIC

Highland Park/North Shore University Health System
Highland Park/North Shore Univ Hlth Syst
718 Glenview Ave   Highland Park, IL 60035
(847) 432-8000
MIDWEST

Hillcrest Hospital Cleveland Clinic Health System
Hillcrest Hosp-Mayfield Hts
6780 Mayfield Rd   Mayfield Heights, OH 44124
(440) 449-4500
MIDWEST

Hilton Head Regional Medical Center
Hilton Head Reg Med Ctr
25 Hosp Ctr Blvd, PO Box 21117   Hartsville, SC 29925-1117
(843) 681-6122
SOUTHEAST

Hinsdale Hospital   (630) 856-9000
Hinsdale Hosp
120 N Oak St   Hinsdale, IL 60521   MIDWEST

Hoag Memorial Hospital Presbyterian   (949) 645-8600
Hoag Meml Hosp Presby
One Hoag Drive   Newport Beach, CA 92663   WEST COAST AND PACIFIC

Hollywood Presbyterian Medical Center   (213) 413-3000
Hollywood Presby Med Ctr
1300 N Vermont Ave   Los Angeles, CA 90027-6069   WEST COAST AND PACIFIC

Holy Cross Hospital - Fort Lauderdale   (954) 771-8000
Holy Cross Hosp - Fort Lauderdale
4725 N Federal Hwy   Fort Lauderdale, FL 33308   SOUTHEAST

Holy Cross Hospital - Silver Spring   (301) 754-7000
Holy Cross Hospital - Silver Spring
1500 Forest Glen Road   Silver Spring, MD 20910   MID ATLANTIC

Hospital for Joint Diseases   (212) 598-6000
Hosp For Joint Diseases
301 East 17th Street   New York, NY 10003   MID ATLANTIC

Hospital for Special Surgery   (212) 606-1000
Hosp For Special Surgery
535 East 70th Street   New York, NY 10021   MID ATLANTIC

Hospital of Central CT at New Britain   (860) 224-5011
Hosp of Central CT at New Britain
100 Grand St   New Britain, CT 06050   NEW ENGLAND

Hospital of St Raphael   (203) 789-3000
Hosp of St Raphael
1450 Chapel Street   New Haven, CT 06511   NEW ENGLAND

Hospital of the University of Pennsylvania - UPHS   (215) 662-4000
Hosp Univ Penn - UPHS
3400 Spruce Street   Philadelphia, PA 19104   MID ATLANTIC

Howard University Hospital   (202) 865-6100
Howard Univ Hosp
2041 Georgia Ave NW   Washington, DC 20060   MID ATLANTIC

Hunter Holmes McGuire Veterans Affairs Medical Center   (804) 675-5500
Hunter Holmes McGuire VA Med Ctr
1201 Broad Rock Boulevard   Richmond, VA 23249   SOUTHEAST

Hutzel Women's Hospital - Detroit		(313) 745-7555
Hutzel Hosp - Detroit		
3980 John R. Blvd	Detroit, MI 48201-2018	MIDWEST

Imperial Point Medical Center		(954) 776-8500
Imperial Point Med Ctr		
6401 N Federal Hwy	Fort Lauderdale, FL 33308	SOUTHEAST

Indian River Medical Center		(772) 567-4311
Indian River Med Ctr		
1000 36th St	Vero Beach, FL 32960	SOUTHEAST

Indiana University Hospital		(317) 274-5000
Indiana Univ Hosp		
550 N University Blvd	Indianapolis, IN 46202	MIDWEST

Ingalls Memorial Hospital		(708) 333-2300
Ingalls Meml Hosp		
1 Ingalls Dr	Harvey, IL 60426	MIDWEST

Inova Fair Oaks Hospital		(703) 391-3600
Inova Fair Oaks Hosp		
3600 Joseph Siewick Dr	Fairfax, VA 22033	SOUTHEAST

Inova Fairfax Hospital		(703) 698-1110
Inova Fairfax Hosp		
3300 Gallows Road	Falls Church, VA 22042	SOUTHEAST

Inova Fairfax Hospital for Children		(703) 204-6777
Inova Fairfax Hosp for Chldn		
3300 Gallows Rd	Fairfax, VA 22042	SOUTHEAST

Integris Baptist Medical Center - Oklahoma		(405) 949-3011
Integris Baptist Med Ctr - OK		
3300 NW Expressway	Oklahoma City, OK 73112-9028	SOUTHWEST

Intermountain Medical Center		(801) 507-7000
Intermountain Med Ctr		
5121 S Cottonwood St	Salt Lake City, UT 84107	GREAT PLAINS AND MOUNTAINS

Iowa Methodist Medical Center		(515) 241-6212
Iowa Methodist Med Ctr		
1200 Pleasant St	Des Moines, IA 50309	MIDWEST

Jackson Memorial Hospital		(305) 585-1111
Jackson Meml Hosp		
1611 NW 12th Ave	Miami, FL 33136	SOUTHEAST

Jackson North Medical Center   (305) 651-1100
Jackson N Med Ctr
160 NW 170 St   North Miami Beach, FL 33169   SOUTHEAST

Jewish Hospital - Kenwood - Cincinnati   (513) 686-3000
Jewish Hosp - Kenwood - Cincinnati
4777 E Galbraith Rd   Cincinnati, OH 45236-2891   MIDWEST

Jewish Hospital HealthCare Services, Inc.   (502) 587-4011
Jewish Hosp HlthCre Svcs Inc
200 Abraham Slexner Way   Louisville, KY 40202   SOUTHEAST

JFK Medical Center - Atlantis   (561) 642-3791
JFK Med Ctr - Atlantis
5301 S Congress Ave   Atlantis, FL 33462   SOUTHEAST

JFK Medical Center - Edison   (732) 321-7000
JFK Med Ctr - Edison
65 James Street   Edison, NJ 08818   MID ATLANTIC

John L McClellan VA Medical Center   (501) 257-1000
John L McClellan VA Med Ctr
4300 W 7th St   Little Rock, AR 72205   SOUTHWEST

John Sealy Hospital - UTMB   (409) 747-1935
UTMB - John Sealy Hospital
301 University Blvd   Galveston, TX 77555   SOUTHWEST

Johns Hopkins Bayview Medical Center   (410) 550-0100
Johns Hopkins Bayview Med Ctr
4940 Eastern Avenue   Baltimore, MD 21224   MID ATLANTIC

Johns Hopkins Hospital   (410) 955-5000
Johns Hopkins Hosp
600 N Wolfe St   Baltimore, MD 21287   MID ATLANTIC

Kaiser Permanente Baldwin Park Medical Center   (626) 851-1011
Kaiser Permanente Baldwin Pk Med Ctr
1011 Baldwin Park Blvd   Baldwin Park, CA 91706   WEST COAST AND PACIFIC

Kaiser Permanente Oakland Medical Center   (510) 752-1000
Kaiser Permanente Oakland Med Ctr
280 West MacArthur Boulevard   Oakland, CA 94611   WEST COAST AND PACIFIC

Kaiser Permanente Santa Clara Medical Center   (408) 236-6400
Kaiser Permanente Santa Clara Med Ctr
700 Lawrence Expy   Santa Clara, CA 95051   WEST COAST AND PACIFIC

Kaiser Permanente South San Francisco Medical Center   (650) 742-2000
Kaiser Permanente S San Francisco Med Ctr
1200 El Camino Real   South San Francisco, CA 94080   WEST COAST AND PACIFIC

Kaiser Permanente Woodland Hills Medical Center   (818) 719-2000
Kaiser Permanente Woodland Hills Med Ctr
5601 DeSoto Ave   Woodland Hills, CA 91365   WEST COAST AND PACIFIC

Kapiolani Medical Center for Women & Children   (808) 983-6000
Kapiolani Med Ctr for Women & Chldn
1319 Punahou St   Honolulu, HI 96826   WEST COAST AND PACIFIC

Karmanos Cancer Institute   (800) 527-6266
Karmanos Cancer Inst
4100 John R   Detroit, MI 48201   MIDWEST

Kenmore Mercy Hospital   (845) 331-3131
Kenmore Mercy Hosp
2950 Elmwood Ave   Kenmore, NY 14217   MID ATLANTIC

Kennedy Krieger Institute   (443) 923-9200
Kennedy Krieger Inst
707 N Broadway   Baltimore, MD 21205   MID ATLANTIC

Kessler Institute for Rehabilitation - West Orange   (973) 243-6800
Kessler Inst for Rehab - W Orange
1199 Pleasant Valley Way   West Orange, NJ 07052-1499   MID ATLANTIC

Kootenai Medical Center   (208) 666-2000
Kootenai Med Ctr
2003 Lincoln Way   Coeur d'Alene, ID 83814-2677   GREAT PLAINS AND MOUNTAINS

Kosair Children's Hospital   (502) 629-6000
Kosair Chldn's Hosp
231 E Chestnut St   Louisville, KY 40202   SOUTHEAST

La Grange Memorial Hospital   (708) 352-1200
La Grange Meml Hosp
5101 S Willow Springs Rd   La Grange, IL 60525   MIDWEST

LAC & USC Medical Center   (323) 226-2622
LAC & USC Med Ctr
1200 N State St   Los Angeles, CA 90033-4525   WEST COAST AND PACIFIC

LAC - Harbor - UCLA Medical Center   (310) 222-2345
LAC - Harbor - UCLA Med Ctr
1000 W Carson St   Torrance, CA 90509-2059   WEST COAST AND PACIFIC

Lafayette General Medical Center   (337) 289-7991
Lafayette Genl Med Ctr
1214 Coolidge Blvd   Lafayette, LA 70503   SOUTHWEST

Lahey Clinic   (781) 744-5100
Lahey Clin
41 Mall Road   Burlington, MA 01805   NEW ENGLAND

Lancaster General Hospital   (717) 290-5511
Lancaster Genl Hosp
555 N Duke St, PO Box 3555   Lancaster, PA 17604-3555   MID ATLANTIC

Lankenau Hospital   (610) 645-2000
Lankenau Hosp
100 Lancaster Ave   Wynnewood, PA 19096-3498   MID ATLANTIC

Laureate Psychiatric Clinic & Hospital   (918) 481-4000
Laureate Psyc Clinic & Hosp
6655 S Yale Ave, Box 470207   Tulsa, OK 74147   SOUTHWEST

LDS Hospital   (801) 408-1100
LDS Hosp
8th Ave & C St   Salt Lake City, UT 84143   GREAT PLAINS AND MOUNTAINS

Le Bonheur Children's Medical Center   (901) 572-3000
Le Bonheur Chldns Med Ctr
50 N Dunlap   Memphis, TN 38103-2893   SOUTHEAST

Lee Memorial Health Systems   (239) 334-5314
Lee Memorial Hlth Systems
2776 Cleveland Ave   Fort Myers, FL 33901   SOUTHEAST

Legacy Good Samaritan Hospital and Medical Center   (503) 413-7711
Legacy Good Samaritan Hosp and Med Ctr
1015 NW 22nd Ave   Portland, OR 97210-3025   WEST COAST AND PACIFIC

Lenox Hill Hospital   (212) 434-2000
Lenox Hill Hosp
100 East 77th Street   New York, NY 10021   MID ATLANTIC

Lenox Hill Hospital (Manhattan Eye, Ear & Throat Hosp)   (212) 838-9200
Lenox Hill Hosp (Manh Eye, Ear & Throat Hosp)
210 East 64th Street   New York, NY 10021   MID ATLANTIC

Lindy Boggs Medical Center   (504) 483-5000
L Boggs Med Ctr
301 N Jefferson Davis Pkwy   New Orleans, LA 70119   SOUTHWEST

Loma Linda Children's Hospital		(909) 558-8000
Loma Linda Chldns Hosp		
11234 Anderson St	Loma Linda, CA 92354	WEST COAST AND PACIFIC

Loma Linda University Medical Center		(909) 558-4000
Loma Linda Univ Med Ctr		
11234 Anderson St	Loma Linda, CA 92354	WEST COAST AND PACIFIC

Long Beach Memorial Medical Center		(562) 933-2000
Long Beach Meml Med Ctr		
2801 Atlantic Ave	Long Beach, CA 90801	WEST COAST AND PACIFIC

Long Island College Hospital		(718) 780-1000
Long Island Coll Hosp		
339 Hicks Street	Brooklyn, NY 11201	MID ATLANTIC

Long Island Jewish Medical Center		(516) 470-7000
Long Island Jewish Med Ctr		
270-05 76th Avenue	New Hyde Park, NY 11040	MID ATLANTIC

Los Alamitos Medical Center		(562) 598-1311
Los Alamitos Med Ctr		
3751 Katella Ave	Los Alamitos, CA 90720	WEST COAST AND PACIFIC

Louisiana State University Hospital		(318) 675-4239
Louisiana State Univ Hosp		
1501 Kings Hwy, PO Box 33932	Shreveport, LA 71130	SOUTHWEST

Loyola University Medical Center		(708) 216-9000
Loyola Univ Med Ctr		
2160 S 1st Ave	Maywood, IL 60153	MIDWEST

LSU Interim Public Hospital		(504) 903-3000
LSU Interim Public Hosp		
2021 Perdido St	New Orleans, LA 70112	SOUTHWEST

Lucile Packard Children's Hospital		(650) 497-8000
Lucile Packard Chldn's Hosp		
725 Welch Rd	Palo Alto, CA 94304	WEST COAST AND PACIFIC

Lutheran Medical Center - Cleveland		(216) 696-4300
Lutheran Med Ctr - Cleveland		
1730 W 25th St	Cleveland, OH 44113	MIDWEST

Magee Rehabilitation Hospital		(215) 587-3000
Magee Rehab Hosp		
1513 Race St	Philadelphia, PA 19102-1177	MID ATLANTIC

Magee-Womens Hospital - UPMC		(412) 641-1000
Magee-Womens Hosp - UPMC		
300 Halket Street	Pittsburgh, PA 15213	MID ATLANTIC

Maimonides Medical Center		(718) 283-6000
Maimonides Med Ctr		
4802 Tenth Avenue	Brooklyn, NY 11219	MID ATLANTIC

Maine Medical Center		(207) 871-0111
Maine Med Ctr		
22 Bramhall St	Portland, ME 04102	NEW ENGLAND

Marianjoy Rehabilitation Hospital		(630) 462-4000
Marianjoy Rehab Hosp		
26 W 171 Roosevelt Rd	Wheaton, IL 60187	MIDWEST

Marin General Hospital		(415) 925-7000
Marin Genl Hosp		
250 Bon Air Rd	Greenbrae, CA 94904	WEST COAST AND PACIFIC

Mary Shiels Hospital		(214) 443-3000
Mary Shiels Hosp		
3515 Howell St	Dallas, TX 75204	SOUTHWEST

Maryland General Hospital		(410) 225-8000
Maryland Genl Hosp		
827 Linden Ave	Baltimore, MD 21201	MID ATLANTIC

Massachusetts Eye and Ear Infirmary		(617) 523-7900
Mass Eye & Ear Infirmary		
243 Charles Street	Boston, MA 02114	NEW ENGLAND

Massachusetts General Hospital		(617) 726-2000
Mass Genl Hosp		
55 Fruit St	Boston, MA 02114	NEW ENGLAND

Massachusetts Mental Health Center		(617) 626-9300
MA Mental Hlth Ctr		
180 Morton St	Jamaica Plain, MA 02130	NEW ENGLAND

Mattel Children's Hospital at UCLA		(310) 825-9111
Mattel Chldns Hosp at UCLA		
10833 Le Conte Ave	Los Angeles, CA 90095-1752	WEST COAST AND PACIFIC

Mayo Clinic - Jacksonville, FL		(904) 953-2000
Mayo - Jacksonville		
4500 San Pablo Road	Jacksonville, FL 32224	SOUTHEAST

Mayo Clinic - Phoenix
Mayo Clinic - Phoenix
5777 E Mayo Blvd   Phoenix, AZ 85054

(480) 515-6296

SOUTHWEST

Mayo Clinic - Rochester, MN
Mayo Med Ctr & Clin - Rochester
200 First St SW   Rochester, MN 55905

(507) 284-2511

MIDWEST

Mayo Clinic - Scottsdale
Mayo Clinic - Scottsdale
13400 E Shea Blvd   Scottsdale, AZ 85259

(480) 301-8000

SOUTHWEST

McLaren Regional Medical Center
McLaren Reg Med Ctr
401 S. Ballenger Highway   Flint, MI 48532

(810) 342-2000

MIDWEST

McLean Hospital
McLean Hosp
115 Mill St   Belmont, MA 02478

(617) 855-2000

NEW ENGLAND

Medical Center of Central Georgia
Med Ctr of Central GA
777 Hemlock Street   Macon, GA 31201

(478) 633-1000

SOUTHEAST

Medical City Dallas Hospital
Med City Dallas Hosp
7777 Forest Ln   Dallas, TX 75230-2594

(972) 566-7000

SOUTHWEST

Medical College of Georgia Hospital & Clinic (MCG Health Inc)
Med Coll of GA Hosp and Clin (MCG Health Inc)
1120 15th Street   Augusta, GA 30912

(706) 721-6569

SOUTHEAST

Medical College of Virginia Hospitals
Med Coll of VA Hosp
1250 E Marshall St, Box 980510   Richmond, VA 23219

(804) 828-9000

SOUTHEAST

Medical University of South Carolina Children's Hospital
MUSC Chldns Hosp
169 Ashley Ave   Charleston, SC 29425

(843) 792-1414

SOUTHEAST

Medical University of South Carolina Medical Center
MUSC Med Ctr
169 Ashley Ave   Charleston, SC 29425

(843) 792-2300

SOUTHEAST

Memorial Health University Medical Center - Savannah
Meml Hlth Univ Med Ctr - Savannah
4700 Waters Ave   Savannah, GA 31404

(912) 350-8000

SOUTHEAST

Memorial Hermann Hospital - Texas Medical Center	(713) 704-4000
Meml Hermann Hosp - Texas Med Ctr	
6411 Fannin Houston, TX 77030	SOUTHWEST

Memorial Hermann Memorial City Hospital	(713) 242-3000
Meml Hermann Meml City Hosp	
921 Gessner Ave Houston, TX 77024-2412	SOUTHWEST

Memorial Medical Center-Springfield	(217) 788-3340
Memorial Med Ctr-Springfield	
701 N First St Springfield, IL 62781	MIDWEST

Memorial Regional Hospital	(954) 987-2000
Meml Regl Hosp	
3501 Johnson Street Hollywood, FL 33021	SOUTHEAST

Memorial Sloan-Kettering Cancer Center	(212) 639-2000
Meml Sloan-Kettering Cancer Ctr	
1275 York Avenue New York, NY 10021	MID ATLANTIC

Menninger Clinic	(800) 351-9058
Menninger Clinic	
PO Box 809045 Houston, TX 77280	SOUTHWEST

Mercy General Hospital - Sacramento	(916) 453-4545
Mercy General Hosp - Sacramento	
4001 J Street Sacramento, CA 95819	WEST COAST AND PACIFIC

Mercy Hospital	(305) 854-4400
Mercy Hosp	
3663 S Miami Ave Miami, FL 33133	SOUTHEAST

Mercy Hospital - Coon Rapids	(763) 236-6000
Mercy Hosp - Coon Rapids	
4050 Coon Rapids Blvd Coon Rapids, MN 55433-2522	MIDWEST

Mercy Hospital - Fairfield	(513) 870-7000
Mercy Hosp - Fairfield	
3000 Mack Rd Fairfield, OH 45014	MIDWEST

Mercy Medical Center	(410) 332-9000
Mercy Med Ctr	
301 St Paul Pl Baltimore, MD 21202	MID ATLANTIC

MeritCare Hospital	(701) 234-6000
MeritCare Hosp	
720 Fourth Street North Fargo, ND 58122	GREAT PLAINS AND MOUNTAINS

Methodist Hospital - Indianapolis	(317) 962-2000
Methodist Hosp - Indianapolis	
1701 N Senate Blvd Indianapolis, IN 46202	MIDWEST

Methodist Hospital Healthsystem - Minnesota	(952) 993-5000
Methodist Hosp - Minnesota	
6500 Excelsior Blvd Minneapolis, MN 55426-4700	MIDWEST

Methodist Hospital System	(713) 790-3311
Methodist Hosp - Houston	
6565 Fannin St Houston, TX 77030	SOUTHWEST

Methodist Hospital-Omaha	(402) 354-4000
Methodist Hosp - Omaha	
8303 Dodge St Omaha, NE 68114	GREAT PLAINS AND MOUNTAINS

Methodist Hospital-San Antonio	(210) 575-4000
Methodist Hosp-San Antonio	
7700 Floyd Curl Drive San Antonio, TX 78229	SOUTHWEST

Methodist Specialty & Transplant Hospital	(210) 575-8110
Methodist Spec & Transpl Hosp	
8026 Floyd Curl Dr San Antonio, TX 78229	SOUTHWEST

Methodist University Hospital - Memphis	(901) 516-7000
Methodist Univ Hosp - Memphis	
1265 Union Ave Memphis, TN 38104	SOUTHEAST

MetroHealth Medical Center	(216) 778-7800
MetroHealth Med Ctr	
2500 MetroHealth Drive Cleveland, OH 44109-1998	MIDWEST

Miami Children's Hospital	(305) 666-6511
Miami Children's Hosp	
3100 SW 62nd Ave Miami, FL 33155	SOUTHEAST

Michael E. DeBakey VA Medical Center	(713) 791-1414
DeBakey VA Med Ctr-Houston	
2002 Holcombe Blvd Houston, TX 77030-1414	SOUTHWEST

Michigan State University-Sparrow Hospital	(517) 364-1000
Mich State Univ-Sparrow Hos	
1215 E Michigan Ave, MS 0 Lansing, MI 48912	MIDWEST

Midwestern Regional Medical Center	(847) 872-4561
Midwest Reg Med Ctr	
2520 Elisha Ave Zion, IL 60099	MIDWEST

Milford Hospital
Milford Hosp
300 Seaside Ave   Milford, CT 06460
(203) 876-4000
NEW ENGLAND

Millard Fillmore Gates Circle Hospital
Millard Fillmore Gates Cir Hosp
3 Gates Cir   Buffalo, NY 14209
(716) 887-4600
MID ATLANTIC

Miriam Hospital
Miriam Hosp
164 Summit Avenue   Providence, RI 02906-2894
(401) 793-2500
NEW ENGLAND

Montefiore Medical Center - Henry and Lucy Moses Division
Montefiore Med Ctr - Div. Moses
111 East 210 Street   Bronx, NY 10467
(718) 920-4321
MID ATLANTIC

Montefiore Medical Center - Jack D. Weiler Division
Montefiore Med Ctr - Div. Weiler
1825 Eastchester Road   Bronx, NY 10461
(718) 904-2000
MID ATLANTIC

Montgomery Rehabilitation Hospital
Montgomery Rehab Hosp
8601 Stenton Ave   Wyndmoor, PA 19038
(215) 233-6200
MID ATLANTIC

Morristown Memorial Hospital
Morristown Mem Hosp
100 Madison Avenue   Morristown, NJ 07960
(973) 971-5000
MID ATLANTIC

MossRehab Hospital
MossRehab Hosp
60 E Township Line Rd   Elkins Park, PA 19027
(215) 663-6000
MID ATLANTIC

Mott Children's Hospital
Mott Chldns Hosp
1500 E Medical Center Dr   Ann Arbor, MI 48109
(734) 936-4000
MIDWEST

Mount Auburn Hospital
Mount Auburn Hosp
330 Mount Auburn St   Cambridge, MA 02238
(617) 492-3500
NEW ENGLAND

Mount Carmel West Hospital
Mt Carmel W Hosp
793 W State St   Columbus, OH 43085
(614) 234-5000
MIDWEST

Mount Clemens Regional Medical Center
Mount Clemens Regional Med Ctr
1000 Harrington Blvd   Mount Clemens, MI 48043
(586) 493-8000
MIDWEST

Mount Sinai Medical Center (212) 241-6500
Mount Sinai Med Ctr
One Gustave L. Levy Pl   New York, NY 10029   MID ATLANTIC

Mount Sinai Medical Center - Miami (305) 674-2121
Mount Sinai Med Ctr - Miami
4300 Alton Rd   Miami Beach, FL 33140   SOUTHEAST

National Institutes of Health - Clinical Center (301) 496-4000
Natl Inst of Hlth - Clin Ctr
10 Center Drive   Bethesda, MD 20892-0001   MID ATLANTIC

National Jewish Medical & Research Center (303) 388-4461
Natl Jewish Med & Rsch Ctr
1400 Jackson St   Denver, CO 80206-2762   GREAT PLAINS AND MOUNTAINS

National Naval Medical Center (301) 295-4611
Natl Naval Med Ctr
8901 Wisconsin Ave   Bethesda, MD 20889   MID ATLANTIC

National Rehabilitation Hospital (202) 877-1000
Natl Rehab Hosp
102 Irving St NW   Washington, DC 20010   MID ATLANTIC

Nationwide Children's Hospital (614) 722-2000
Nationwide Chldn's Hosp
700 Children's Drive   Columbus, OH 43205   MIDWEST

Nebraska Medical Center (402) 559-2000
Nebraska Med Ctr
42nd & Dewey St   Omaha, NE 68198   GREAT PLAINS AND MOUNTAINS

Nebraska Methodist Hospital (402) 354-4000
Nebraska Meth Hosp
8303 Dodge St   Omaha, NE 68114   GREAT PLAINS AND MOUNTAINS

Neurologic & Orthopedic Hosp of Chicago (800) 411-2466
Neuro & Ortho Hosp of Chicago
4501 N Winchester   Chicago, IL 60640   MIDWEST

New England Baptist Hospital (617) 754-5800
New England Bapt Hosp
125 Parker Hill Ave   Boston, MA 02120   NEW ENGLAND

New Hanover Regional Medical Center (910) 343-7000
New Hanover Reg Med Ctr
2131 S 17th St   Wilmington, NC 28401   SOUTHEAST

New York Eye & Ear Infirmary   (212) 979-4000
New York Eye & Ear Infirm
310 East 14th Street   New York, NY 10003   MID ATLANTIC

New York Hospital Queens   (718) 670-1231
NY Hosp Queens
56-45 Main Street   Flushing, NY 11355   MID ATLANTIC

New York Methodist Hospital   (718) 780-3000
New York Methodist Hosp
506 Sixth Street   Brooklyn, NY 11215   MID ATLANTIC

New York State Psychiatric Institute   (212) 543-5000
NY State Psychiatric Inst
1051 Riverside Dr   New York, NY 10032   MID ATLANTIC

Newark Beth Israel Medical Center   (973) 926-7000
Newark Beth Israel Med Ctr
201 Lyons Ave   Newark, NJ 07112   MID ATLANTIC

Newton - Wellesley Hospital   (617) 243-6000
Newton - Wellesley Hosp
2014 Washington St   Newton, MA 02462   NEW ENGLAND

NewYork-Presbyterian Hospital/Columbia   (212) 305-2500
NY-Presby Hosp/Columbia
622 W 168th St   New York, NY 10032   MID ATLANTIC

NewYork-Presbyterian Hospital/Weill Cornell   (212) 746-5454
NY-Presby Hosp/Weill Cornell
525 E 68th St   New York, NY 10021   MID ATLANTIC

NewYork-Presbyterian/Morgan Stanley Children's Hospital   (212) 305-2500
NYPresby-Morgan Stanley Children's Hosp
622 W 168th St   New York, NY 10032   MID ATLANTIC

North Florida Regional Medical Center   (352) 333-4000
North Florida Regl Med Ctr
6500 Newberry Rd   Gainesville, FL 32605   SOUTHEAST

North Oaks Medical Center   (985) 230-6601
North Oaks Med Ctr
15790 Paul Vega MD Dr   Hammond, LA 70403   SOUTHWEST

North Shore Medical Center - Salem Hospital   (978) 741-1215
N Shore Med Ctr - Salem Hosp
81 Highland Avenue   Salem, MA 01970   NEW ENGLAND

North Shore University Hospital — (516) 562-0100
N Shore Univ Hosp
300 Community Dr — Manhasset, NY 11030 — MID ATLANTIC

North Shore-LIJ Health System — (516) 465-2600
NS-LIJ Hlth Sys
125 Community Drive — Great Neck, NY — MID ATLANTIC

Northern California Shriners Hospital — (916) 453-2000
Northern CA Shriners Hosp
2425 Stockton Blvd — Sacramento, CA 95817 — WEST COAST AND PACIFIC

Northern Memorial Health Care, Robbinsdale — (763) 520-5200
Northern Meml Hlth Care
3300 Oakdale Ave N — Robbinsdale, MN 55422 — MIDWEST

Northern Nevada Medical Center — (775) 531-7000
Northern Nevada Med Ctr
2375 E Prater Way — Sparks, NV 89434-9644 — WEST COAST AND PACIFIC

Northern Westchester Hospital — (914) 666-1200
Northern Westchester Hosp
400 East Main Street — Mount Kisco, NY 10549 — MID ATLANTIC

NorthShore University HealthSystem — (847) 570-2000
NorthShore Univ HlthSys
1301 Central Ave — Evanston, IL 60201 — MIDWEST

Northside Hospital - Atlanta — (404) 851-8000
Northside Hosp
1000 Johnson Ferry Rd NE — Atlanta, GA 30342 — SOUTHEAST

Northwest Hospital — (206) 364-0500
Northwest Hosp
1550 N 115th St — Seattle, WA 98133-0806 — WEST COAST AND PACIFIC

Northwest Medical Center — (954) 974-0400
Northwest Med Ctr
2801 N State Rd 7 — Margate, FL 33063 — SOUTHEAST

Northwestern Memorial Hospital — (312) 926-2000
Northwestern Meml Hosp
251 E Huron St — Chicago, IL 60611 — MIDWEST

Norton Hospital — (502) 629-8000
Norton Hosp
200 E Chestnut St — Louisville, KY 40202 — SOUTHEAST

NYU Langone Medical Center   (212) 263-7300
NYU Langone Med Ctr
550 First Avenue   New York, NY 10016   MID ATLANTIC

NYU Rusk Institute   (212) 263-2606
NYU Rusk Inst
400 East 34th Street   New York, NY 10016   MID ATLANTIC

Ochsner Baptist Medical Center   (504) 899-9311
Ochsner Baptist Med Ctr
2700 Napoleon Ave   New Orleans, LA 70115   SOUTHWEST

Ochsner Foundation Hospital   (504) 842-3000
Ochsner Fdn Hosp
1516 Jefferson Hwy   New Orleans, LA 70121   SOUTHWEST

Ohio State University Medical Center   (614) 293-8000
Ohio St Univ Med Ctr
410 W 10th Avenue   Columbus, OH 43210   MIDWEST

Olathe Medical Center   (913) 791-4200
Olathe Med Ctr
20333 W 151st St   Olathe, KS 66061-5352   GREAT PLAINS AND MOUNTAINS

Olive View Medical Center   (818) 364-1555
Olive View Med Ctr
14445 Olive View Dr   Sylmar, CA 91342   WEST COAST AND PACIFIC

Olympia Medical Center   (310) 657-5900
Olympia Med Ctr
5900 W Olympic Blvd   Los Angeles, CA 90036   WEST COAST AND PACIFIC

Oregon Health & Science University   (503) 494-8311
OR Hlth & Sci Univ
3181 SW Sam Jackson Park Rd   Portland, OR 97239-3098   WEST COAST AND PACIFIC

Orlando Regional Medical Center   (407) 841-5111
Orlando Regl Med Ctr
1414 Kuhl Ave   Orlando, FL 32806   SOUTHEAST

Orthopedic Specialty Hospital, The (TOSH)   (801) 314-4100
Ortho Spec Hosp, The (TOSH)
5848 Fashion Blvd   Salt Lake City, UT 84107   GREAT PLAINS AND MOUNTAINS

OU Medical Center   (405) 271-4700
OU Med Ctr
1200 Everett Dr   Oklahoma City, OK 73104-5098   SOUTHWEST

Our Lady of Lourdes Regional Medical Center - Lafayette	(337) 289-2000	
Our Lady of Lourdes Reg Med Ctr - Lafayette		
611 St. Landry St	Lafayette, LA 70506-4697	SOUTHWEST
Our Lady of the Lake Regional Medical Center	(225) 765-6565	
Our Lady of the Lake Regl Med Ctr		
5000 Hennessy Blvd	Baton Rouge, LA 70808-4398	SOUTHWEST
Overlake Hospital Medical Center	(425) 688-5000	
Overlake Hosp Med Ctr		
1035 116th Ave NE	Bellevue, WA 98004-4687	WEST COAST AND PACIFIC
Overland Park Regional Medical Center	(913) 541-5000	
Overland Pk Regl Med Ctr		
10500 Quivira Rd	Overland Park, KS 66215	GREAT PLAINS AND MOUNTAINS
Palmetto Richland Memorial Hospital	(803) 434-7000	
Palmetto Richland Mem Hosp		
5 Richland Medical Park Drive	Columbia, SC 29203	SOUTHEAST
Park Plaza Hospital	(713) 527-5000	
Park Plaza Hosp		
1313 Herman Dr	Houston, TX 77004	SOUTHWEST
Parkinson's Institute/Movement Disorders Treament Center, The	(408) 734-2800	
Parkinson's Inst/Movement Disorders Trmt Ctr, The		
1170 Morse Ave	Sunnyvale, CA 94089-1605	WEST COAST AND PACIFIC
Parkland Health & Hospital System	(214) 590-8000	
Parkland Hlth & Hosp Sys		
5201 Harry Hines Blvd	Dallas, TX 75235	SOUTHWEST
Peninsula Medical Center	(650) 696-5400	
Peninsula Med Ctr		
1783 El Camino Real	Burlingame, CA 94010	WEST COAST AND PACIFIC
Penn Presbyterian Medical Center - UPHS	(215) 662-8000	
Penn Presby Med Ctr - UPHS		
51 N 39th St	Philadelphia, PA 19104	MID ATLANTIC
Penn State Milton S Hershey Medical Center	(717) 531-8521	
Penn State Milton S Hershey Med Ctr		
500 University Drive	Hershey, PA 17033-0850	MID ATLANTIC
Pennsylvania Hospital	(215) 829-3000	
Pennsylvania Hosp		
800 Spruce St, Ste 240	Philadelphia, PA 19107	MID ATLANTIC

Penrose Hospital   (719) 776-5000
Penrose Hosp
2222 N Nevada   Colorado Springs, CO 80907   GREAT PLAINS AND MOUNTAINS

Philadelphia Shriners Hospital   (215) 430-4000
Philadelphia Shriners Hosp
3351 N Broad St   Philadelphia, PA 19140   MID ATLANTIC

Phillips Eye Institute   (612) 775-8800
Phillips Eye Inst
2215 Park Ave S   Minneapolis, MN 55404   MIDWEST

Phoenix Baptist Hospital & Medical Center   (602) 249-0212
Phoenix Baptist Hosp & Med Ctr
2000 West Bethany Home Rd   Phoenix, AZ 85015-2184   SOUTHWEST

Phoenix Children's Hospital   (602) 546-1000
Phoenix Children's Hosp
1919 E Thomas Rd   Phoenix, AZ 85106   SOUTHWEST

Physicians Regional Medical Center   (239) 348-4000
Physicians Regl Med Ctr
6101 Pine Ridge Rd   Naples, FL 34119   SOUTHEAST

Piedmont Hospital   (404) 605-5000
Piedmont Hosp
1968 Peachtree Rd NW   Atlanta, GA 30309   SOUTHEAST

Pitt County Memorial Hospital - Univ Health System East Carolina   (252) 847-4100
Pitt Cty Mem Hosp - Univ Med Ctr East Carolina
2100 Stantonsburg Rd   Greenville, NC 27835-6028   SOUTHEAST

Portsmouth Regional Hospital   (603) 436-5110
Portsmouth Regl Hosp
333 Borthwick Ave   NH 03801-7002   NEW ENGLAND

Presbyterian - St Luke's Medical Center   (303) 839-6000
Presby - St Luke's Med Ctr
1719 E 19th Ave   Denver, CO 80218   GREAT PLAINS AND MOUNTAINS

Presbyterian Hospital - Charlotte   (704) 384-4000
Presby Hosp - Charlotte
200 Hawthorne Ln   Charlotte, NC 28204-2528   SOUTHEAST

Presbyterian Hospital of Dallas   (214) 345-6789
Presby Hosp of Dallas
8200 Walnut Hill Ln   Dallas, TX 75231   SOUTHWEST

Presbyterian Hospital of Plano
Presby Hosp of Plano
6200 West Parker Road   Plano, TX 75093

(972) 608-8000

SOUTHWEST

Primary Children's Medical Center
Primary Children's Med Ctr
100 N Medical Drive   Salt Lake City, UT 84113-1100

(801) 588-2000

GREAT PLAINS AND MOUNTAINS

Providence Alaska Medical Center
Providence Alaska Med Ctr
3200 Providence Dr   Anchorage, AK 99508-4615

(907) 562-2211

WEST COAST AND PACIFIC

Providence Centralia Hospital
Providence Centralia Hosp
914 Scheuber Rd   Centralia, WA 98531

(360) 736-2803

WEST COAST AND PACIFIC

Providence Hospital - Southfield
Providence Hosp - Southfield
16001 W Nine Mile Rd   Southfield, MI 48075

(248) 424-3000

MIDWEST

Providence Portland Medical Center
Providence Portland Med Ctr
4805 NE Glisan   Portland, OR 97213-2967

(503) 215-1111

WEST COAST AND PACIFIC

Providence Saint Joseph Medical Center
Providence St Joseph Med Ctr
501 S Buena Vista St   Burbank, CA 91505

(818) 843-5111

WEST COAST AND PACIFIC

Queen's Medical Center - Honolulu
Queen's Med Ctr - Honolulu
1301 Punchbowl Street   Honolulu, HI 96813

(808) 538-9011

WEST COAST AND PACIFIC

Rady Children's Hospital - San Diego
Rady Children's Hosp - San Diego
3020 Children's Way   San Diego, CA 92123

(858) 576-1700

WEST COAST AND PACIFIC

Rainbow Babies & Children's Hospital
Rainbow Babies & Chldns Hosp
11100 Euclid Ave   Cleveland, OH 44106

(216) 844-1000

MIDWEST

Rancho Los Amigos National Rehabilitation Center
Rancho Los Amigos Natl Rehab Ctr
7601 East Imperial Highway   Downey, CA 90242

(562) 401-7111

WEST COAST AND PACIFIC

Rapid City Regional Hospital
Rapid City Reg Hosp
353 Fairmount Blvd   Rapid City, SD 57701

(605) 719-1000

GREAT PLAINS AND MOUNTAINS

Regional Medical Center - Memphis   (901) 545-7100
Regional Med Ctr - Memphis
877 Jefferson Avenue   Memphis, TN 38103   SOUTHEAST

Regions Hospital - St Paul   (651) 254-3456
Regions Hosp - St Paul
640 Jackson Street   St Paul, MN 55101   MIDWEST

Rehabilitation Institute of Chicago   (312) 238-1000
Rehab Inst of Chicago
345 E. Superior Street   Chicago, IL 60611   MIDWEST

Rehabilitation Institute of St. Louis   (314) 658-3800
Rehab Inst St. Louis
4455 Duncan Ave   St. Louis, MO 63110   MIDWEST

Rex HealthCare   (919) 784-3100
Rex HlthCare
4420 Lake Boone Trail   Raleigh, NC 27607   SOUTHEAST

Rhode Island Hospital   (401) 444-4000
Rhode Island Hosp
593 Eddy Street   Providence, RI 02903-4923   NEW ENGLAND

Riddle Memorial Hospital   (610) 566-9400
Riddle Meml Hosp
1068 W Baltimore Pike   Media, PA 19063   MID ATLANTIC

Riley Hospital for Children   (317) 274-5000
Riley Hosp for Children
702 Barnhill Drive   Indianapolis, IN 46202   MIDWEST

Riverside Community Hospital   (951) 788-3000
Riverside Comm Hosp
4445 Magnolia Avenue   Riverside, CA 92502   WEST COAST AND PACIFIC

Riverview Medical Center   (732) 741-2700
Riverview Med Ctr
1 Riverview Plaza   Red Bank, NJ 07701   MID ATLANTIC

Robert Wood Johnson University Hospital - New Brunswick   (732) 828-3000
Robert Wood Johnson Univ Hosp - New Brunswick
1 Robert Wood Johnson Pl   New Brunswick, NJ 08901   MID ATLANTIC

Rochester General Hospital   (585) 922-4000
Rochester Genl Hosp
1425 Portland Avenue   Rochester, NY 14621   MID ATLANTIC

Rochester Methodist Hospital
Rochester Methodist Hosp
201 W Center St   Rochester, MN 55905-3003
(507) 284-2511
MIDWEST

Rockefeller University
Rockefeller Univ
1230 York Avenue   New York, NY 10021
(212) 327-8000
MID ATLANTIC

Roger Williams Hospital
Roger Williams Hosp
825 Chalkstone Avenue   Providence, RI 02908
(401) 456-2000
NEW ENGLAND

Rogers Memorial Hospital
Rogers Meml Hosp.
34700 Valley Rd   Oconomowoc, WI 53066-4599
(262) 646-4411
MIDWEST

Roper Hospital
Roper Hosp
316 Calhoun St   Charleston, SC 29401
(843) 724-2000
SOUTHEAST

Rose Medical Center
Rose Med Ctr
4567 E 9th Ave   Denver, CO 80220-3941
(303) 320-2121
GREAT PLAINS AND MOUNTAINS

Roswell Park Cancer Institute
Roswell Park Cancer Inst
Elm and Carlton Streets   Buffalo, NY 14263
(716) 845-5770
MID ATLANTIC

Rush Copley Medical Center
Rush Copley Med Ctr
2000 Ogden Ave   Aurora, IL 60504-4206
(630) 978-6200
MIDWEST

Rush University Medical Center
Rush Univ Med Ctr
1653 W Congress Pkwy   Chicago, IL 60612-3833
(312) 942-5000
MIDWEST

Sacred Heart Medical Center
Sacred Heart Med Ctr
1255 Hilyard St   Eugene, OR 97440-3700
(541) 686-7300
WEST COAST AND PACIFIC

Saint Francis Hospital - Memphis
St Francis Hosp - Memphis
5959 Park Ave   Memphis, TN 38119
(901) 765-1000
SOUTHEAST

Saint John's Health Center
St John's Hlth Ctr, Santa Monica
1328 22nd St   Santa Monica, CA 90404
(310) 829-5511
WEST COAST AND PACIFIC

Saint Thomas Hospital - Nashville	(615) 222-2111
Saint Thomas Hosp - Nashville	
4220 Harding Road Nashville, TN 37205	SOUTHEAST

Saint Vincent Catholic Medical Centers - St Vincent's Manhattan	(212) 604-7000
St Vincent Cath Med Ctrs - Manhattan	
170 West 12th Street New York, NY 10011	MID ATLANTIC

Salinas Valley Memorial Healthcare Systems	(831) 757-4333
Salinas Valley Meml Hlthcare Systs	
450 E Romie Ln Salinas, CA 93901	WEST COAST AND PACIFIC

Salt Lake Regional Medical Center	(801) 350-4111
Salt Lake Regional Med Ctr	
1050 E South Temple Salt Lake City, UT 84102	GREAT PLAINS AND MOUNTAINS

San Diego Hospice	(619) 688-1600
San Diego Hospice	
4311 3rd Ave0 San Diego, CA 92103-7499	WEST COAST AND PACIFIC

San Francisco General Hospital	(415) 206-8000
San Francisco Genl Hosp	
1001 Potrero Avenue San Francisco, CA 94110	WEST COAST AND PACIFIC

Sanford Health -South Dakota	(605) 333-1000
Sanford Health SD	
1100 S Euclid Ave, PO Box 5039 Sioux Falls, SD 57717	GREAT PLAINS AND MOUNTAINS

Santa Barbara Cottage Hospital	(805) 682-7111
Santa Barbara Cottage Hosp	
Pueblo at Bath St Santa Barbara, CA 93105	WEST COAST AND PACIFIC

Santa Clara Valley Medical Center	(408) 885-5000
Santa Clara Vly Med Ctr	
751 S Bascom Ave San Jose, CA 95128	WEST COAST AND PACIFIC

Santa Monica - UCLA Medical Center and Orthopaedic Hospital	(310) 319-4000
Santa Monica - UCLA Med Ctr & Ortho Hosp	
1250 16th St Santa Monica, CA 90404	WEST COAST AND PACIFIC

Sarasota Memorial Hospital	(941) 917-9000
Sarasota Meml Hosp	
1700 S Tamiami Trail Sarasota, FL 34239	SOUTHEAST

Schneider Children's Hospital	(718) 470-3000
Schneider Chldn's Hosp	
269-01 76th Ave New Hyde Park, NY 11040	MID ATLANTIC

Schwab Rehabilitation Hospital (773) 522-2010
Schwab Rehab Hosp
1401 S. California Boulevard   Chicago, IL 60608   MIDWEST

Scott & White Memorial Hospital (254) 724-2111
Scott & White Mem Hosp
2401 S 31st St   Temple, TX 76508-0001   SOUTHWEST

Scottsdale Healthcare - Osborn (480) 675-4000
Scottsdale Hlthcare - Osborn
7400 E Osborn Rd   Scottsdale, AZ 85251-6403   SOUTHWEST

Scottsdale Healthcare - Shea (480) 860-3000
Scottsdale Hlthcare - Shea
9000 E Shea Blvd   Scottsdale, AZ 85258-4514   SOUTHWEST

Scripps Green Hospital (858) 455-9100
Scripps Green Hosp
10666 N Torrey Pines Rd   La Jolla, CA 92037   WEST COAST AND PACIFIC

Scripps Memorial Hospital - La Jolla (858) 457-4123
Scripps Meml Hosp - La Jolla
9888 Genesee Ave   La Jolla, CA 92037   WEST COAST AND PACIFIC

Scripps Mercy Hospital & Medical Center (619) 294-8111
Scripps Mercy Hosp & Med Ctr
4077 Fifth Ave   San Diego, CA 92103   WEST COAST AND PACIFIC

Self Regional Healthcare (864) 227-4111
Self Regional Healthcare
1325 Spring St   Greenwood, SC 29646   SOUTHEAST

Sentara Leigh Hospital (757) 466-6000
Sentara Leigh Hosp
830 Kempsville Rd   Norfolk, VA 23502-3981   SOUTHEAST

Sentara Norfolk General Hospital (757) 668-3000
Sentara Norfolk Genl Hosp
600 Gresham Dr   Norfolk, VA 23507   SOUTHEAST

Sentara Virginia Beach General Hospital (757) 395-8000
Sentara VA Beach Genl Hosp
1060 First Colonial Rd   Virginia Beach, VA 23454   SOUTHEAST

Shady Grove Adventist Hospital (301) 279-6000
Shady Grove Adven Hosp
9901 Medical Center Drive   Rockville, MD 20850   MID ATLANTIC

Shands at University of Florida		(352) 265-0111
Shands at Univ of FL		
1600 SW Archer Rd	Gainesville, FL 32610	SOUTHEAST

Shands Jacksonville		(904) 244-0411
Shands Jacksonville		
655 W 8th St	Jacksonville, FL 32209	SOUTHEAST

Sharp Memorial Hospital		(858) 541-3400
Sharp Meml Hosp		
7901 Frost St	San Diego, CA 92123	WEST COAST AND PACIFIC

Shawnee Mission Medical Center		(913) 676-2000
Shawnee Mission Med Ctr		
9100 W 74th St	Shawnee Mission, KS 66204	GREAT PLAINS AND MOUNTAINS

Shepherd Center - Atlanta		(404) 352-2020
Shepherd Ctr - Atlanta		
2020 Peachtree Road NW	Atlanta, GA 30309	SOUTHEAST

Sheppard Pratt Health System		(410) 938-3000
Sheppard Pratt Hlth Sys		
6501 N Charles St	Baltimore, MD 21285-6815	MID ATLANTIC

Shriners Hospital for Children-Philadelphia		(215) 430-4000
Shriners Hosp for Chldn-Phila		
3551 N Broad St	Philadelphia, PA 19140	MID ATLANTIC

Sibley Memorial Hospital		(202) 537-4000
Sibley Mem Hosp		
5255 Loughboro Road NW	Washington, DC 20016	MID ATLANTIC

Silver Hill Hospital		(203) 966-3561
Silver Hill Hosp		
208 Valley Rd	New Canaan, CT 06840-3899	NEW ENGLAND

Sinai Hospital - Baltimore		(410) 601-9000
Sinai Hosp - Baltimore		
2401 W Belvedere Ave	Baltimore, MD 21215	MID ATLANTIC

Sinai-Grace Hospital - Detroit		(313) 966-3300
Sinai-Grace Hosp - Detroit		
6071 W. Outer Drive	Detroit, MI 48235	MIDWEST

South Miami Hospital		(305) 661-4611
South Miami Hosp		
6200 SW 73 St	South Miami, FL 33143	SOUTHEAST

Southeast Baptist Hospital		(210) 297-3000
Southeast Baptist Hosp		
4214 E Southcross Blvd	San Antonio, TX 78222	SOUTHWEST

Southern New Hampshire Medical Center		(603) 577-2000
Southern NH Med Ctr		
8 Prospect St	Nashua, NH 03061	NEW ENGLAND

Southwest Texas Methodist Hospital		(210) 575-4000
SW TX Meth Hosp		
7700 Floyd Curl Dr	San Antonio, TX 78229	SOUTHWEST

Spaulding Rehabilitation Hospital		(617) 720-6400
Spaulding Rehab Hosp		
125 Nashua Street	Boston, MA 02114	NEW ENGLAND

Spectrum Health - Blodgett Campus		(616) 774-7444
Spectrum Hlth Blodgett Campus		
1840 Wealthy St SE	Grand Rapids, MI 49506	MIDWEST

Spectrum Health Butterworth Campus		(616) 391-1774
Spectrum Hlth Butterworth Campus		
100 Michigan St NE	Grand Rapids, MI 49503	MIDWEST

SSM Cardinal Glennon Children's Hospital		(314) 577-5600
Cardinal Glennon Mem Children's Hosp		
1465 S Grand Blvd	St Louis, MO 63104	MIDWEST

St Alphonsus Regional Medical Center		(208) 367-2121
St Alphonsus Regl Med Ctr		
1055 N Curtis Rd	Boise, ID 83706-1370	GREAT PLAINS AND MOUNTAINS

St Anthony Hospital - Oklahoma City		(405) 272-7000
St Anthony Hosp -Oklahoma City		
1000 N Lee St	Oklahoma City, OK 73102	SOUTHWEST

St Anthony's Hospital - St Petersburg		(727) 893-6814
St Anthony's Hosp - St Petersburg		
1200 7th Avenue North	St Petersburg, FL 33705	SOUTHEAST

St Barnabas Medical Center		(973) 322-5000
St Barnabas Med Ctr		
94 Old Short Hills Rd	Livingston, NJ 07039-5672	MID ATLANTIC

St Christopher's Hospital for Children		(215) 427-5000
St Christopher's Hosp for Chldn		
Erie Ave at Front St	Philadelphia, PA 19134	MID ATLANTIC

St Clare Health Center — (636) 496-2000
St Clare Hlth Ctr
Bowles Ave & Hwy 141 — St Louis, MO 63122 — MIDWEST

St David's Medical Center — (512) 476-7111
St David's Med Ctr
919 E 32rd st — Austin, TX 78705 — SOUTHWEST

St Elizabeth Medical Center (South Unit) — (859) 344-2000
St Elizabeth Med Ctr (South Unit)
1 Medical Village Dr — Edgewood, KY 41017 — SOUTHEAST

St Francis Hospital & Medical Center — (860) 714-4000
St Francis Hosp & Med Ctr
114 Woodland St — Hartford, CT 06105 — NEW ENGLAND

St Francis Hospital - The Heart Center — (516) 562-6000
St Francis Hosp - The Heart Ctr
100 Port Washington Boulevard — Roslyn, NY 11576 — MID ATLANTIC

St Francis Medical Center — (318) 362-4000
St Francis Med Ctr
309 Jackson St — Monroe, LA 71210-7498 — SOUTHWEST

St John's Hospital - Springfield — (217) 544-6464
St John's Hosp - Springfield
800 E Carpenter St — Springfield, IL 62769 — MIDWEST

St John's Mercy Medical Center - St Louis — (314) 569-6000
St John's Mercy Med Ctr - St Louis
615 S New Ballas Rd — St Louis, MO 63141 — MIDWEST

St Joseph Hospital — (773) 665-3000
St Joseph Hosp
2900 N Lake Shore Drive — Chicago, IL 60657 — MIDWEST

St Joseph Hospital — (603) 882-3000
St Joseph Hosp
172 Kinsley St — Nashua, NH 03060 — NEW ENGLAND

St Joseph Hospital — (707) 445-8121
St Joseph Hosp
2700 Dolbeer St — Eureka, CA 95501 — WEST COAST AND PACIFIC

St Joseph Hospital — (360) 734-5400
St Joseph Hosp - Bellingham
2901 Squalicum Pkwy — Bellingham, WA 98225-1898 — WEST COAST AND PACIFIC

St Joseph Medical Center
St Joseph Med Ctr
7601 Osler Drive   Baltimore, MD 21208
(410) 337-1000
MID ATLANTIC

St Joseph Medical Center - Tacoma
St Joseph Med Ctr - Tacoma
1717 South J St   Tacoma, WA 98401
(253) 627-4101
WEST COAST AND PACIFIC

St Joseph Mercy Hospital - Ann Arbor
St Joseph Mercy Hosp - Ann Arbor
5301 E Huron River Dr, Box 992   Ann Arbor, MI 48106
(734) 712-3456
MIDWEST

St Joseph Mercy Oakland Hospital
St Joseph Mercy Oakland Hosp
44405 Woodward Ave   Pontiac, MI 48341
(248) 858-3000
MIDWEST

St Joseph's Children's Hospital
St Josephs Chldns Hosp
3001 W Dr MLK Jr Blvd   Tampa, FL 33607
(813) 554-8500
SOUTHEAST

St Joseph's Hospital & Medical Center - Phoenix
St Joseph's Hosp & Med Ctr - Phoenix
350 W Thomas Rd   Phoenix, AZ 85013-4496
(602) 406-3000
SOUTHWEST

St Joseph's Hospital - Atlanta
St Joseph's Hosp - Atlanta
5665 Peachtree Dunwoody Rd NE Atlanta, GA 30342
(404) 851-7001
SOUTHEAST

St Joseph's Hospital - Orange
St Joseph's Hosp - Orange
1100 West Stewart Drive   Orange, CA 92868
(714) 633-9111
WEST COAST AND PACIFIC

St Joseph's Hospital - Tampa
St Joseph's Hosp - Tampa
3001 W MLK Jr Blvd   Tampa, FL 33607
(813) 870-4000
SOUTHEAST

St Joseph's Hospital - Tucson
St Joseph's Hosp - Tucson
350 N Wilmot Rd   Tucson, AZ 85711
(520) 296-3211
SOUTHWEST

St Jude Children's Research Hospital
St Jude Children's Research Hosp
262 Danny Thomas Pl   Memphis, TN 38105
(901) 495-3300
SOUTHEAST

St Louis Children's Hospital
St Louis Chldns Hosp
One Children's Pl   St Louis, MO 63110
(314) 454-6000
MIDWEST

St Louis University Hospital   (314) 577-8000
St Louis Univ Hosp
3635 Vista at Grand Blvd   St Louis, MO 63110   MIDWEST

St Luke's - Roosevelt Hospital Center - Roosevelt Division   (212) 523-4000
St Luke's - Roosevelt Hosp Ctr - Roosevelt Div
1000 Tenth Avenue   New York, NY 10019   MID ATLANTIC

St Luke's - Roosevelt Hospital Center - St Luke's Hospital   (212) 523-4000
St Luke's - Roosevelt Hosp Ctr - St Luke's Hosp
1111 Amsterdam Ave   New York, NY 10025   MID ATLANTIC

St Luke's Episcopal Hospital-Houston   (832) 355-1000
St Luke's Episcopal Hosp-Houston
6720 Bertner Avenue   Houston, TX 77030   SOUTHWEST

St Luke's Hospital - Bethlehem   (610) 954-4000
St Luke's Hosp - Bethlehem
801 Ostrum Street   Bethlehem, PA 18015   MID ATLANTIC

St Luke's Hospital - Chesterfield, MO   (314) 434-1500
St Luke's Hosp - Chesterfield, MO
232 S Woods Mill Rd   Chesterfield, MO 63017   MIDWEST

St Luke's Hospital - Duluth   (218) 249-5555
St Luke's Hosp - Duluth
915 E 1st St   Duluth, MN 55805-2193   MIDWEST

St Luke's Hospital of Kansas City   (816) 932-2000
St Luke's Hosp of Kansas City
4401 Wornall Rd   Kansas City, MO 64111   MIDWEST

St Mark's Hospital - Salt Lake City   (801) 268-7111
St Mark's Hosp - Salt Lake City
1200 E. 3900 S   Salt Lake City, UT 84124   GREAT PLAINS AND MOUNTAINS

St Mary Medical Center - Long Beach   (562) 491-9000
St Mary Med Ctr - Long Beach
1050 Linden Ave   Long Beach, CA 90813   WEST COAST AND PACIFIC

St Mary's Hospital - Rochester, MN (Mayo Clinic)   (507) 255-5123
St Mary's Hosp - Rochester
1216 2nd St SW   Rochester, MN 55902   MIDWEST

St Mary's Medical Center - Huntington   (304) 526-1234
St Mary's Med Ctr - Huntington
2900 First Ave   Huntington, WV 25702-1272   MID ATLANTIC

St Mary's Medical Center - West Palm Beach (561) 844-6300
St Mary's Med Ctr - W Palm Bch
901 45th St   West Palm Beach, FL 33407   SOUTHEAST

St Patrick Hospital & Health Sciences Center (406) 543-7271
St Patrick Hospital - Missoula
500 W Broadway   Missoula, MT 59802   GREAT PLAINS AND MOUNTAINS

St Peter's University Hospital (732) 745-8600
St Peter's Univ Hosp
254 Easton Ave   New Brunswick, NJ 08901-1780   MID ATLANTIC

St Vincent Carmel Hospital (317) 573-7000
St Vincent Carmel Hosp
13500 N Meridian St   Carmel, IN 46032-1496   MIDWEST

St Vincent Hospital - Green Bay (920) 433-0111
St Vincent Hosp - Green Bay
835 S Van Buren St, Box 13508   Green Bay, WI 54307-3508   MIDWEST

St Vincent Hospital - Santa Fe (505) 983-3361
St Vincent Hosp - Santa Fe
455 St Michaels Dr   Santa Fe, NM 87504-2107   SOUTHWEST

St Vincent Indianapolis Hospital (317) 338-2345
St Vincent Indianapolis Hosp
2001 W 86th St   Indianapolis, IN 46260-1991   MIDWEST

St Vincent's Hospital - Birmingham (205) 939-7000
St Vincent's Hosp - Birmingham
810 St. Vincent's Dr, Box 12407   Birmingham, AL 35202-2407   SOUTHEAST

St Vincent's Medical Center - Jacksonville (904) 308-7300
St Vincent's Med Ctr - Jacksonville
1800 Barrs St   Jacksonville, FL 32204   SOUTHEAST

St Vincent's Medical Center - Los Angeles (213) 484-7111
St Vincent's Med Ctr - Los Angeles
2131 W 3rd St   Los Angeles, CA 90057   WEST COAST AND PACIFIC

St. Alexius Medical Center (701) 530-7000
St. Alexius Med Ctr - Bismarck
900 E Broadway Ave   Bismarck, ND 58501   GREAT PLAINS AND MOUNTAINS

St. John's Health East Hospital (651) 232-7000
St. John's Hosp
1575 Beam Ave   Maplewood, MN 55109   MIDWEST

St. Luke's Regional Medical Center   (208) 381-2222
St. Luke's Reg Med Ctr - Boise
190 E Bannock St   Boise, ID 83712   GREAT PLAINS AND MOUNTAINS

St. Vincent Infirmary Medical Center & Doctors Hospital   (501) 552-3000
St Vincent Med Ctr
2 St. Vincent Cir   Little Rock, AR 72205   SOUTHWEST

Stamford Hospital   (203) 325-7000
Stamford Hosp
30 Shelburne Rd, Box 9317   Stamford, CT 06902   NEW ENGLAND

Stanford University Medical Center   (650) 723-4000
Stanford Univ Med Ctr
300 Pasteur Dr   Stanford, CA 94305   WEST COAST AND PACIFIC

Stony Brook University Medical Center   (631) 689-8333
Stony Brook Univ Med Ctr
Nicolls Rd   Stony Brook, NY 11794-8410   MID ATLANTIC

Suburban Hospital   (301) 896-3100
Suburban Hosp
8600 Old Georgetown Rd   Bethesda, MD 20814   MID ATLANTIC

Sunnyview Hospital & Rehabilitation Center   (518) 382-4500
Sunnyview Hosp & Rehab Ctr
1270 Belmont Ave   Schenectady, NY 12308-2198   MID ATLANTIC

Sunrise Hospital & Medical Center/Sunrise Children's Hospital   (702) 731-8000
Sunrise Hosp & Med Ctr/Sunrise Chldn's Hosp
3186 Maryland Pkwy   Las Vegas, NV 89109-2306   WEST COAST AND PACIFIC

SUNY Downstate Medical Center   (718) 270-1000
SUNY Downstate Med Ctr
450 Clarkson Ave   Brooklyn, NY 11203   MID ATLANTIC

Swedish Covenant Hospital   (773) 878-8200
Swedish Covenant Hosp
5145 N California Ave   Chicago, IL 60625   MIDWEST

Swedish Medical Center - Englewood   (303) 788-5000
Swedish Med Ctr - Englewood
501 E Hamden Ave   Englewood, CO 80110-2795   GREAT PLAINS AND MOUNTAINS

Swedish Medical Center - Seattle   (206) 386-6000
Swedish Med Ctr - Seattle
747 Broadway   Seattle, WA 98122   WEST COAST AND PACIFIC

Tampa General Hospital   (813) 844-7000
Tampa Genl Hosp
PO BOX 1289   Tampa, FL 33601   SOUTHEAST

Tanner Medical Center - Carrollton   (770) 836-9666
Tanner Med Ctr
705 Dixie Street   Carrollton, GA 30117   SOUTHEAST

Temple University Hospital   (215) 707-2000
Temple Univ Hosp
3401 N Broad St   Philadelphia, PA 19140-5189   MID ATLANTIC

Texas Children's Hospital   (832) 824-1000
Texas Chldns Hosp
6621 Fannin St   Houston, TX 77030   SOUTHWEST

Texas Orthopedic Hospital   (713) 799-8600
Texas Ortho Hosp
7401 S Main   Houston, TX 77030   SOUTHWEST

Texas Scottish Rite Hospital for Children   (214) 559-5000
Texas Scottish Rite Hosp for Chldn
2222 Welborn St   Dallas, TX 75219   SOUTHWEST

Thomas Jefferson University Hospital   (215) 955-6000
Thomas Jefferson Univ Hosp
111 S 11th St   Philadelphia, PA 19107   MID ATLANTIC

TIRR   (713) 799-5000
TIRR
1333 Moursund   Houston, TX 77030   SOUTHWEST

Toledo Hospital   (419) 291-4000
Toledo Hosp
2142 N Cove Blvd   Toledo, OH 43606   MIDWEST

Tucson Medical Center   (520) 327-5461
Tucson Med Ctr
5301 E Grant Rd   Tucson, AZ 85712-2874   SOUTHWEST

Tufts Medical Center   (617) 636-5000
Tufts Med Ctr
750 Washington St   Boston, MA 02111   NEW ENGLAND

Tulane University Hospital & Clinic   (504) 588-5263
Tulane Univ Hosp & Clin
1415 Tulane Ave   New Orleans, LA 70112   SOUTHWEST

Tulane-Lakeside Hospital	(504) 780-8282
Tulane-Lakeside Hosp	
4700 I-10 Service Rd Metairie, LA 70001	SOUTHWEST
UAB Highlands Hospital	(205) 930-7000
UAB Highlands Hosp	
1201 11th Ave S Birmingham, AL 35205-5299	SOUTHEAST
UCLA Neuropsychiatric Hospital	(310) 825-9989
UCLA Neuropsychiatric Hosp	
760 Westwood Plaza Los Angeles, CA 90024	WEST COAST AND PACIFIC
UCLA Ronald Reagan Medical Center	(310) 825-9111
UCLA Ronald Reagan Med Ctr	
757 Westwood Plaza Los Angeles, CA 90095	WEST COAST AND PACIFIC
UCSD Medical Center	(619) 543-6222
UCSD Med Ctr	
200 W Arbor Dr San Diego, CA 92103	WEST COAST AND PACIFIC
UCSF - Mount Zion Medical Center	(415) 567-6600
UCSF - Mt Zion Med Ctr	
1600 Divisadero St San Francisco, CA 94115	WEST COAST AND PACIFIC
UCSF Medical Center	(415) 476-1000
UCSF Med Ctr	
500 Parnassus Ave San Francisco, CA 94143	WEST COAST AND PACIFIC
UMass Memorial - Memorial Campus	(508) 793-6611
UMass Meml - Meml Campus	
119 Belmont St Worcester, MA 01605	NEW ENGLAND
UMass Memorial - University Campus	(508) 856-0011
UMass Meml - Univ Campus	
55 Lake Ave N Worcester, MA 01655-0002	NEW ENGLAND
UMass Memorial Medical Center	(508) 334-1000
UMass Memorial Med Ctr	
55 Lake Ave N Worcester, MA 01655	NEW ENGLAND
UMDNJ-University Hospital-Newark	(973) 972-4300
UMDNJ-Univ Hosp-Newark	
150 Bergen St Newark, NJ 07103-2406	MID ATLANTIC
Uniformed Services University of the Health Sciences	(301) 295-9390
Unif Serv Univ of the Hlth Sci	
4301 Jones Bridge Rd Bethesda, MD 20814-4799	MID ATLANTIC

Union Memorial Hospital-Baltimore		(410) 554-2000
Union Meml Hosp-Baltimore		
201 E University Pkwy	Baltimore, MD 21218	MID ATLANTIC

United Hospital		(651) 241-8000
United Hosp		
333 N Smith Ave	St Paul, MN 55102	MIDWEST

University Community Hospital		(813) 971-6000
University Comm Hosp		
3100 E Fletcher Avenue	Tampa, FL 33613	SOUTHEAST

University Health System-San Antonio		(210) 358-4000
Univ Hlth Syst-San Antonio		
4502 Medical Dr	San Antonio, TX 78229	SOUTHWEST

University Hospital - Cincinnati		(513) 584-1000
Univ Hosp - Cincinnati		
234 Goodman St	Cincinnati, OH 45219	MIDWEST

University Hospital - SUNY Upstate Medical University		(315) 464-5540
Univ Hosp - SUNY Upstate		
750 E Adams Street	Syracuse, NY 13210	MID ATLANTIC

University Hospital of New Mexico		(505) 272-2111
Univ Hosp of New Mexico		
2211 Lomas Blvd NE	Albuquerque, NM 87106	SOUTHWEST

University Hospitals Case Medical Center		(216) 844-1000
Univ Hosps Case Med Ctr		
11100 Euclid Ave	Cleveland, OH 44106	MIDWEST

University Medical Center at Princeton		(609) 497-4000
Univ Med Ctr - Princeton		
253 Witherspoon St	Princeton, NJ 08540	MID ATLANTIC

University Medical Center of Southern Nevada - Las Vegas		(702) 383-2000
Univ Med Ctr - Las Vegas		
1800 W Charleston Blvd	Las Vegas, NV 89102	WEST COAST AND PACIFIC

University Medical Center- Tucson		(520) 694-0111
Univ Med Ctr - Tucson		
1501 N Campbell Ave	Tucson, AZ 85724-5128	SOUTHWEST

University Medical Center-Lubbock		(806) 775-8200
Univ Med Ctr-Lubbock		
602 Indiana Ave	Lubbock, TX 79408	SOUTHWEST

Appendix C

University New Mexico Health & Science Center   (505) 272-2111
Univ NM Hlth & Sci Ctr
2211 Lomas Blvd NE   Albuquerque, NM 87106   SOUTHWEST

University of Alabama Hospital at Birmingham   (205) 934-4011
Univ of Ala Hosp at Birmingham
619 South 19th Street   Birmingham, AL 35249-6544   SOUTHEAST

University of Arkansas for Medical Sciences Medical Center   (501) 686-7000
UAMS Med Ctr
4301 W Markham St   Little Rock, AR 72205   SOUTHWEST

University of California - Davis Medical Center   (916) 734-2011
UC Davis Med Ctr
2315 Stockton Blvd   Sacramento, CA 95817   WEST COAST AND PACIFIC

University of California - Irvine Medical Center   (714) 456-6011
UC Irvine Med Ctr
101 The City Dr   Orange, CA 92868   WEST COAST AND PACIFIC

University of Chicago Medical Center   (773) 702-1000
Univ of Chicago Med Ctr
5841 S Maryland Ave   Chicago, IL 60637   MIDWEST

University of Colorado Hospital   (730) 848-4011
Univ Colorado Hosp
12605 E 16th Ave   Aurora, CO 80045   GREAT PLAINS AND MOUNTAINS

University of Connecticut Health Center, John Dempsey Hospital   (860) 679-2100
Univ of Conn Hlth Ctr, John Dempsey Hosp
263 Farmington Ave   Farmington, CT 06030   NEW ENGLAND

University of Illinois at Chicago Eye & Ear Infirmary   (312) 996-6500
Univ of IL at Chicago Eye & Ear Infirm
1855 W Taylor St   Chicago, IL 60612   MIDWEST

University of Illinois Medical Center at Chicago   (312) 996-7000
Univ of IL Med Ctr at Chicago
1740 W Taylor St   Chicago, IL 60612   MIDWEST

University of Iowa Hospitals and Clinics   (319) 356-1616
Univ Iowa Hosp & Clinics
200 Hawkins Drive   Iowa City, IA 52242   MIDWEST

University of Kansas Hospital   (913) 588-5000
Univ of Kansas Hosp
3901 Rainbow Blvd   Kansas City, KS 66160   GREAT PLAINS AND MOUNTAINS

University of Kentucky Chandler Hospital		(800) 333-8874
Univ of Kentucky Chandler Hosp		
800 Rose Street	Lexington, KY 40536	SOUTHEAST
University of Louisville Hospital		(502) 562-3000
Univ of Louisville Hosp		
530 S Jackson St	Louisville, KY 40202	SOUTHEAST
University of Maryland Medical Center		(410) 328-8667
Univ of MD Med Ctr		
22 S Greene St	Baltimore, MD 21201	MID ATLANTIC
University of Miami Hosp & Clinics/Sylvester Comprehensive Cancer Cntr		(305) 243-1000
Univ of Miami Hosp & Clins/Sylvester Comp Canc Ctr		
1475 NW 12th Ave	Miami, FL 33136	SOUTHEAST
University of Miami Hospital		(305) 325-5511
Univ of Miami Hosp		
1400 NW 12 Ave	Miami, FL 33136	SOUTHEAST
University of Michigan Health System		(734) 936-4000
Univ Michigan Hlth Sys		
1500 E Medical Center Dr	Ann Arbor, MI 48109	MIDWEST
University of Minnesota Medical Center, Fairview - Riverside Campus		(612) 672-6000
Univ Minn Med Ctr, Fairview - Riverside Campus		
2450 Riverside Ave S	Minneapolis, MN 55454	MIDWEST
University of Minnesota Medical Center, Fairview - University Campus		(612) 273-3000
Univ Minn Med Ctr, Fairview - Univ Campus		
420 Delaware St SE	Minneapolis, MN 55455	MIDWEST
University of Mississippi Medical Center		(601) 984-1000
Univ Mississippi Med Ctr		
2500 N State St	Jackson, MS 39216	SOUTHEAST
University of Missouri Hospitals & Clinics		(573) 882-4141
Univ of Missouri Hosp & Clins		
1 Hospital Dr	Columbia, MO 65212	MIDWEST
University of North Carolina Hospitals		(919) 966-4131
Univ NC Hosps		
101 Manning Drive, Box 7600	Chapel Hill, NC 27514	SOUTHEAST
University of Rochester Strong Memorial Hospital		(585) 275-2121
Univ of Rochester Strong Meml Hosp		
601 Elmwood Ave	Rochester, NY 14642	MID ATLANTIC

University of South Alabama Medical Center	(251) 471-7000
Univ of S AL Med Ctr	
2451 Fillingim St Mobile, AL 36617	SOUTHEAST

University of South Florida - Tampa	(813) 974-2011
Univ of S FL - Tampa	
4202 E Fowler Ave Tampa, FL 33620	SOUTHEAST

University of Tennesee Memorial Hospital	(865) 544-9000
Univ of Tennesee Mem Hosp	
1924 Alcoa Hwy Knoxville, TN 37920	SOUTHEAST

University of Texas Health Center at Tyler	(903) 877-3451
UT Hlth Ctr at Tyler	
11937 US Hwy 271 Tyler, TX 75708	SOUTHWEST

University of Texas MD Anderson Cancer Center	(713) 792-2121
UT MD Anderson Cancer Ctr	
1515 Holcombe Blvd Houston, TX 77030-4095	SOUTHWEST

University of Texas Medical Branch Hospital at Galveston	(409) 772-1011
UT Med Br Hosp at Galveston	
301 University Blvd Galveston, TX 77555	SOUTHWEST

University of Toledo Medical Center	(419) 383-4000
Univ of Toledo Med Ctr	
3000 Arlington Ave Toledo, OH 43614	MIDWEST

University of Utah Hospitals and Clinics	(801) 581-2121
Univ Utah Hosps and Clins	
50 N Medical Dr Salt Lake City, UT 84132	GREAT PLAINS AND MOUNTAINS

University of Virginia Medical Center	(434) 924-0211
Univ Virginia Med Ctr	
1215 Lee Street Charlottesville, VA 22908-0001	SOUTHEAST

University of Washington Medical Center	(206) 598-3300
Univ Wash Med Ctr	
1959 NE Pacific St, Box 356355 Seattle, WA 98195	WEST COAST AND PACIFIC

University of Wisconsin Hospital & Clinics	(608) 263-6400
Univ WI Hosp & Clins	
600 Highland Avenue Madison, WI 53792	MIDWEST

UPMC Mercy	(412) 232-8111
UPMC Mercy, Pittsburgh	
1400 Locust Street Pittsburgh, PA 15213	MID ATLANTIC

UPMC Montefiore		(412) 647-2345
UPMC Montefiore		
200 Lothrop St	Pittsburgh, PA 15213	MID ATLANTIC

UPMC Passavant		(412) 367-6700
UPMC Passavant		
9100 Babcock Blvd	Pittsburgh, PA 15237	MID ATLANTIC

UPMC Presbyterian		(412) 647-2345
UPMC Presby, Pittsburgh		
200 Lothrop St	Pittsburgh, PA 15213	MID ATLANTIC

UPMC Shadyside		(412) 623-2121
UPMC Shadyside		
5230 Centre Ave	Pittsburgh, PA 15232	MID ATLANTIC

UPMC South Side		(412) 488-5550
UPMC South Side		
2000 Mary St	Pittsburgh, PA 15203	MID ATLANTIC

UPMC St Margaret		(412) 784-4000
UPMC St Margaret		
815 Freeport Rd	Pittsburgh, PA 15215-3301	MID ATLANTIC

USC Norris Cancer Hospital		(323) 865-3000
USC Norris Cancer Hosp		
1441 Eastlake Ave	Los Angeles, CA 90033	WEST COAST AND PACIFIC

USC University Hospital		(323) 442-8444
USC Univ Hosp		
1500 San Pablo St	Los Angeles, CA 90033	WEST COAST AND PACIFIC

UT Southwestern Medical Center at Dallas		(214) 648-3111
UT Southwestern Med Ctr at Dallas		
5323 Harry Hines Blvd	Dallas, TX 75390	SOUTHWEST

VA Connecticut Healthcare System		(203) 932-5711
VA Conn Hlthcre Sys		
950 Campbell Ave	West Haven, CT 06516	NEW ENGLAND

VA Health Care System - Palo Alto		(650) 493-5000
VA Hlth Care Sys - Palo Alto		
3801 Miranda Ave	Palo Alto, CA 94304	WEST COAST AND PACIFIC

VA Healthcare System North Texas-Dallas		(214) 742-8387
VA Healthcare Syst N TX-Dallas		
4500 S Lancaster Rd	Dallas, TX 75216	SOUTHWEST

VA Medical Center - Ann Arbor		(734) 769-7100
VA Med Ctr - Ann Arbor		
2215 Fuller Rd	Ann Arbor, MI 48105	MIDWEST

VA Medical Center - Atlanta		(404) 321-6111
VA Med Ctr - Atlanta		
1670 Clairmont Rd	Decatur, GA 30033	SOUTHEAST

VA Medical Center - Cleveland		(216) 791-3800
VA Med Ctr - Cleveland		
10701 East Blvd	Cleveland, OH 44106	MIDWEST

VA Medical Center - Durham		(919) 286-0411
VA Med Ctr - Durham		
508 Fulton St	Durham, NC 27705	SOUTHEAST

VA Medical Center - Memphis		(901) 523-8990
VA Med Ctr - Memphis		
1030 Jefferson Ave	Memphis, TN 38104	SOUTHEAST

VA Medical Center - Nashville		(615) 327-4751
VA Med Ctr - Nashville		
1310 24th Ave S	Nashville, TN 37212	SOUTHEAST

VA Medical Center - Portland		(503) 220-8262
VA Medical Center - Portland		
3710 SW US Veteran Hospital Rd	Portland, OR 97239	WEST COAST AND PACIFIC

VA Medical Center - San Francisco		(415) 221-4810
VA Med Ctr - San Francisco		
4150 Clement St	San Francisco, CA 94121	WEST COAST AND PACIFIC

VA Medical Center - Washington, DC		(202) 745-8000
VA Med Ctr - Washington		
50 Irving St NW	Washington, DC 20422	MID ATLANTIC

VA Medical Center - West Los Angeles		(310) 478-3711
VA Med Ctr - W Los Angeles		
11301 Wilshire Blvd	Los Angeles, CA 90073	WEST COAST AND PACIFIC

VA Puget Sound Health Care System		(206) 762-1010
VA Puget Sound Hlth Care Sys		
1660 S Columbian Way	Seattle, WA 98108	WEST COAST AND PACIFIC

VA San Diego Healthcare System		(858) 552-8585
VA San Diego Hlthcre Sys		
3350 La Jolla Village Drive	San Diego, CA 92161	WEST COAST AND PACIFIC

Vail Valley Medical Center		(970) 476-2451
Vail Valley Med Ctr		
181 W Meadow Dr	Vail, CO 81657-5058	GREAT PLAINS AND MOUNTAINS
Vanderbilt Children's Hospital		(615) 936-1000
Vanderbilt Children's Hosp		
2200 Children's Way	Nashville, TN 37232	SOUTHEAST
Vanderbilt University Medical Center		(615) 322-5000
Vanderbilt Univ Med Ctr		
1313 21st Avenue South	Nashville, TN 37232	SOUTHEAST
Veterans Affairs Medical Center - Albuquerque		(505) 265-1711
VA Med Ctr		
1501 San Pedro SE	Albuquerque, NM 87108	SOUTHWEST
Veterans Affairs Medical Center - Augusta		(706) 733-0188
VA Medical Ctr - Augusta		
One Freedom Way	Augusta, GA 30904	SOUTHEAST
Veterans Affairs Medical Center - Tucson		(520) 792-1450
VA Medical Center - Tucson		
3601 S 6th Avenue	Tucson, AZ 85723	SOUTHWEST
Veterans Affairs Medical Center - White River Junction		(802) 295-9363
VA Aff Med Ctr - White River Junction		
215 North Maine Street	White River Junction, VT 05009	NEW ENGLAND
Virginia Commonwealth University Medical Center		(904) 828-9000
VCU Med Ctr		
1250 E Marshall St, Box 980510	Richmond, VA 23298	SOUTHEAST
Virginia Hospital Center - Arlington		(703) 558-5000
Virginia Hosp Ctr - Arlington		
1701 N George Mason Dr	Arlington, VA 22205-3698	SOUTHEAST
Virginia Mason Medical Center		(206) 223-6600
Virginia Mason Med Ctr		
1100 Ninth Ave, Box 900	Seattle, WA 98111	WEST COAST AND PACIFIC
Wake Forest University Baptist Medical Center		(336) 716-2011
Wake Forest Univ Baptist Med Ctr		
Medical Center Blvd	Winston-Salem, NC 27157-1015	SOUTHEAST
WakeMed Cary Hospital		(919) 350-2300
WakeMed Cary		
1900 Kildaire Farm Rd	Cary, NC 27511-6616	SOUTHEAST

WakeMed New Bern Avenue Campus   (919) 350-8000
WakeMed New Bern
3000 New Bern Ave   Raleigh, NC 27610   SOUTHEAST

Walter Reed Army Medical Center   (202) 782-3501
W Reed Army Med Ctr
6900 Georgia Ave NW   Washington, DC 20307-5001   MID ATLANTIC

Washington Hospital Center   (202) 877-7000
Washington Hosp Ctr
110 Irving St NW   Washington, DC 20010   MID ATLANTIC

Washington University Medical Center   (314) 362-6828
Washington Univ Med Ctr
4444 Forest Park Ave   St Louis, MO 63108   MIDWEST

WellStar Windy Hill Hospital   (770) 644-1000
WellStar Windy Hill Hosp
2540 Windy Hill Road   Marietta, GA 30067   SOUTHEAST

Wesley Woods Geriatric Hospital   (404) 728-6200
Wesley Woods Ger Hosp
1821 Clifton Rd   Atlanta, GA 30329   SOUTHEAST

West Jefferson Medical Center   (504) 347-5511
West Jefferson Med Ctr
1101 Medical Ctr Blvd   Marrero, LA 70072   SOUTHWEST

West Virginia University Hospital - Ruby Memorial   (304) 598-4000
WV Univ Hosp - Ruby Memorial
1 Medical Center Drive   Morgantown, WV 26506   MID ATLANTIC

Westchester Medical Center   (914) 493-7000
Westchester Med Ctr
95 Grasslands Road   Valhalla, NY 10595   MID ATLANTIC

Western Maryland Hospital Center   (301) 745-4200
W MD Hosp Ctr
1500 Pennsylvania Ave   Hagerstown, MD 21742   MID ATLANTIC

Western Pennsylvania Hospital   (412) 578-5120
Western Penn Hosp
4800 Friendship Avenue   Pittsburgh, PA 15224   MID ATLANTIC

Western Psychiatric Institute and Clinic - UPMC   (412) 624-2100
Western Psych Inst & Clin - UPMC
3811 O'Hara St   Pittsburgh, PA 15213   MID ATLANTIC

Western Reserve Care System
Western Reserve Care Sys
345 Oak Hill Avenue   Youngstown, OH 44501
(330) 740-3223
MIDWEST

Wheaton Franciscan Healthcare-St Joseph
Wheaton Franciscan Hlthcare-St Joseph-Milwaukee
5000 W. Chambers Street   Milwaukee, WI 53210
(414) 447-2000
MIDWEST

William Beaumont Hospital
William Beaumont Hosp
3601 W 13 Mile Rd   Royal Oak, MI 48073
(248) 551-5000
MIDWEST

William S Hall Psychiatric Institute
William S Hall Psyc Inst
1800 Colonial Dr, Box 202   Columbia, SC 29202-6827
(803) 898-1693
SOUTHEAST

Wills Eye Hospital
Wills Eye Hosp
840 Walnut St   Philadelphia, PA 19107-5598
(215) 928-3000
MID ATLANTIC

Winthrop - University Hospital
Winthrop - Univ Hosp
259 1st St   Mineola, NY 11501
(516) 663-0333
MID ATLANTIC

Wolfson Children's Hospital
Wolfson Chldns Hosp
800 Prudential Dr   Jacksonville, FL 32207
(904) 202-8000
SOUTHEAST

Woman's Hospital of Texas
Woman's Hosp TX
7600 Fannin St   Houston, TX 77054
(713) 790-1234
SOUTHWEST

Women & Infants Hospital of Rhode Island
Women & Infants Hosp of RI
101 Dudley Street   Providence, RI 02905
(401) 274-1100
NEW ENGLAND

Women's & Children's Hospital-Los Angeles
Women's & Children's Hosp-LA
1240 North Mission Road   Los Angeles, CA 90033
(323) 226-3427
WEST COAST AND PACIFIC

Women's and Children's Hospital of Buffalo, The
Women's & Chldn's Hosp of Buffalo, The
219 Bryant St   Buffalo, NY 14222
(716) 878-7000
MID ATLANTIC

Wright State University
Wright State Univ
3640 Colonel Glenn Hwy   Dayton, OH 45435-0001
(937) 775-2550
MIDWEST

Yakima Valley Memorial Hospital   (509) 575-8000
Yakima Valley Mem Hosp
2811 Tieton Dr   Yakima, WA 98902-3799   WEST COAST AND PACIFIC

Yale-New Haven Hospital   (203) 688-4242
Yale-New Haven Hosp
20 York St   New Haven, CT 06510   NEW ENGLAND

Yampa Valley Medical Center   (970) 879-1322
Yampa Valley Med Ctr
1024 Central Park Dr   Steamboat Springs, CO 80487   GREAT PLAINS AND MOUNTAINS

York Hospital   (717) 851-3500
York Hosp
1001 S George St   York, PA 17405-7198   MID ATLANTIC

Zucker Hillside Hospital   (718) 470-8000
Zucker Hillside Hosp
75-59 263rd St   Glen Oaks, NY 11004   MID ATLANTIC

Appendix D:
Selected Resources

AMERICAN AMBULANCE ASSOCIATION (AAA)

The American Ambulance Association represents emergency and non-emergency medical transportation providers, advocating high quality pre-hospital care and keeping these providers aware of legislation and news that may affect them.

8201 Greensboro Drive, Ste 300
McLean, VA 22102

800-523-4447
703-610-9018
fax 703-610-9005
www.the-aaa.org/

AMERICA'S HEALTH INSURANCE PLANS (AHIP)

America's Health Insurance Plans is a national trade association representing nearly 1,300 member companies providing health benefits to more than 200 million Americans.

601 Pennsylvania Ave, NW
South Building Suite 500
Washington, DC 20004

202-778-3200
fax: 202-331-7487
www.ahip.org/

AMERICAN BOARD OF MEDICAL SPECIALTIES (ABMS)

The ABMS is the authoritative body for the recognition of medical specialties, coordinating 24 medical specialty boards (including 25 medical specialties) and providing information on the board certification of doctors.

1007 Church Street, Suite 404
Evanston, Illinois 60201-5913

847-491-9091 or 866-ASK-ABMS
fax 847-328-3596
www.abms.org

AMERICAN HOSPITAL ASSOCIATION (AHA)

A national health advocacy organization, the AHA represents hospitals and healthcare networks in legislative and regulatory matters. In 1973 the AHA adopted the Patient Bill of Rights to help patients understand their rights and responsibilities.

1 North Franklin
Chicago, IL 60606

800-424-4301 or 312-422-3000
fax 312-422-4796
www.aha.org/

325 7th St. NW
Washington, DC 20004

800-424-4301 or 202-638-1100
fax 202-626-2345

Appendix D

AMERICAN MEDICAL ASSOCIATION (AMA)
The AMA is an association that maintains information on physicians practicing throughout the nation. Healthcare consumers can use their database to check the location, licensing, education and specialty of many doctors in the United States.

515 North State Street
Chicago, IL 60610

800-621-8335
www.ama-assn.org/

CENTER FOR MEDICAL CONSUMERS
Provides volume and outcome data on certain medical procedures performed in New York state.

239 Thompson St.
New York, NY 10012

212-674-7105
fax 212-674-7100
medconsumers@earthlink.net
www.medicalconsumers.org

CENTERS FOR DISEASE CONTROL AND PREVENTION (CDC)
Part of the Department of Health and Human Services, the CDC's mission is to prevent and manage diseases and illnesses. Its Web site contains information on a range of illnesses and the research being pursued to manage them. It also provides free faxed reports on disease risk and prevention in various parts of the world.

Public Inquiries/MASO
Mailstop E11
1600 Clifton Road
Atlanta, GA 30333

1-800-311-3435

toll free number for international travelers 877 FYI-TRIP or 404-639-3534
fax information service for international travelers 888-232-3299
www.cdc.gov/netinfo.htm

THE CENTERWATCH CLINICAL TRIALS LISTING SERVICE
Profiles centers conducting clinical research by therapeutic area and geographic region, including more than 41,000 international industry and government-sponsored clinical trials and new FDA approved drug therapies, as well as 5,200 clinical trials that are actively recruiting patients.

100 N. Washington St
Ste 301
Boston, MA 02114

617-948-5100
fax 617-948-5101
www.centerwatch.com

HEALTH CARE CHOICES
Provides information on volume and outcomes of certain medical procedures performed in hospitals in various states throughout the country.

P.O. Box 21039
Columbus Circle Station
New York, NY 10023

212-724-9395
www.healthcarechoices.org
info@healthcarechoices.org

INTERNATIONAL ASSOCIATION FOR MEDICAL ASSISTANCE TO TRAVELLERS (IAMAT)

IAMAT is a non-profit organization that disseminates information on health and sanitary conditions worldwide. Membership is free but donations are appreciated. Members will receive a membership card making them eligible to access English speaking physicians all over the world. The organization also provides information on immunization requirements, malaria, and other tropical diseases, and sanitary and climactic conditions around the world. For information, send request in writing.

1623 Military Road #279
Niagra Falls, New York 14304-1745

716-754-4883
www.iamat.org

JOINT COMMISSION ON ACCREDITATION OF HEALTHCARE ORGANIZATIONS

The Joint Commission (JCAHO) is an independent, not-for-profit organization, which evaluates the quality and safety of care for nearly 17,000 health care organizations. To maintain and earn accreditation, organizations must have an extensive on-site review by a team of JCAHO health care professionals, at least once every three years. JCAHO is governed by a board that includes physicians, nurses, and consumers. JCAHO sets the standards by which health care quality is measured in America and around the world.

One Renaissance Boulevard
Oakbrook Terrace, IL 60181

630-792-5000
fax 630-792-5005
www.jcaho.org

MEDIC ALERT FOUNDATION

The Medic Alert Foundation (a non-profit organization) provides an "ID tag" engraved with personal medical facts, as well as a 24-hour emergency response center which can release additional personal medical details. Membership is $20/year (waived for the first year) and members need to purchase the "ID tag" which sells for as low as $35.

2323 Colorado Avenue
Turlock, CA 95382

888-633-4298
Fax 209-669-2450
www.medicalert.org

MEDLINE

One Medline Place
Mundelein, Illinois 60060

1-800-MEDLINE (800-633-5463)
fax 1-800-351-1512
www.medline.com

A medical database including millions of medical references and abstracts from thousands of scientific and medical journals.

THE NATIONAL CANCER INSTITUTE (NCI)

Part of the NIH, the NCI sponsors cancer clinical trials at more than 100 sites in the United States. Trials are carried out in major medical research centers, such as teaching hospitals, as well as in community hospitals, specialized medical clinics and even in doctors' offices.

Clinical Studies Support Center (CSSC)
6116 Executive Boulevard
Bethesda, MD 20892-8322

800-4-CANCER (800-422-6237)
www.nci.nih.gov
www.cancer.gov
cancergovstaff@mail.nih.gov

NATIONAL CENTER FOR COMPLEMENTARY AND ALTERNATIVE MEDICINE CLEARINGHOUSE (NCCAMC)

The NCCAMC facilitates the evaluation of alternative medical treatment modalities to help determine their effectiveness and bring alternative medicine into mainstream medicine. This agency does not provide referrals.

9000 Rockville Pike
Bethesda, MD 20892

888-644-6226
fax 866-464-3616
www.nccam.nih.gov
info@nccam.nih.gov

NATIONAL CONSUMERS LEAGUE (NCL)

NCL is a private, nonprofit consumer advocacy organization. NCL strives to investigate, educate, and advocate on a variety of issues including healthcare. Membership is $20 annually, but individuals can also write to the organization for a list of publications that non-members can purchase.

1701 K Street, NW, Suite 1200
Washington, DC 20006

202-835-3323
fax 202-835-0747
www.nclnet.org
info@nclnet.org

THE NATIONAL INSTITUTES OF HEALTH (NIH)

An organization operated by the U.S. government, the NIH operates its own hospital at which the care provided is usually related to clinical studies its researchers are undertaking. Information about the Warren G. Magnuson Clinical Center is also available.

Patient Recruitment Referral Center
9000 Rockville Pike
Bethesda, MD 20892

800-411-1222 or 301-496-4000
www.nih.gov
www.clinicaltrials.gov
nihinfo@od.nih.gov

NATIONAL INSURANCE INFORMATION INSTITUTE

The National Insurance Information Institute Helpline advises consumers on how to choose an insurance company or broker. It also offers an analysis of life insurance and assists in insurance complaints.

110 William St
New York, NY 10038

800-942-4242 or 212-346-5500
www.iii.org

THE PATIENT ADVOCATE FOUNDATION

A national non-profit organization that provides consultation, referrals and case management to patients to ensure that they are not denied access to healthcare, insurance coverage, employment and public assistance programs during an illness. In particular, the organization maintains comprehensive information on cancer treatment options that are available to consumers through a separate Web site: www.oncology.com.

700 Thimble Shoals Boulevard, Suite 200
Newport News, VA 23606

800-532-5274
fax 757-873-8999
www.patientadvocate.org/
help@patientadvocate.org

PEOPLE'S MEDICAL SOCIETY

The People's Medical Society, a nonprofit organization, is focused on educating the healthcare consumer about healthcare issues and medical rights. Their Web site provides information on useful books and publications as well as the latest healthcare developments.

P.O. Box 868
Allentown, PA 18105

610-770-1670
fax 610-770-0607
cbi@peoplesmed.org

PERSONS UNITED LIMITING SUBSTANDARDS AND ERRORS IN HEALTHCARE (P.U.L.S.E.)

A support group for the survivors of medical malpractice and substandard healthcare, this nonprofit group also advocates patient education and patient-doctor communication.

PO Box 353
3300 Park Avenue
Wantagh NY 11793-0353

800-96-pulse (800-967-8573) or
516-579-4711
fax: 516-520-8105
www.PULSEamerica.org
www.PULSEofNY.com
pulse516@aol.com

Colorado Office

719-250-1286
PULSECOLO@YAHOO.COM

PUBLIC CITIZEN'S HEALTH AND RESEARCH GROUP

A non-profit organization, the Public Citizen's Group acts as a watchdog agency by advocating accountability and the open use of doctors' disciplinary backgrounds.

1600 20th Street NW
Washington, D.C. 20009

202-588-1000
www.citizen.org/hrg/

VERITAS MEDICINE

An organization that allows individuals to perform confidential, personalized searches of their clinical trials database and to access information on new treatment and drug options. The text is submitted by Harvard-affiliated doctors.

11 Cambridge Center
Cambridge, Massachusetts 02142

617-234-1500 or
877-5-TRIALS (877-587-4257)
fax 617-234-1555
www.veritasmedicine.com
info@veritasmedicine.com

Indices

Subject Index

Prevention Trials 27

Primary Care 1, 4, 7, 8, 15, 18, 19, 31, 42, 43, 49

Private Insurance 29

Professional Reputation 13

Protocol 27, 28, 30

R

Recertification 12, 50

Referral 8, 18, 35, 53

Residency 10, 11, 16, 17, 37, 49, 50

S

Second Opinions 17

Selection Process 2

Self-Designated Medical Specialties 12

Side Effects 27, 32, 33

Special Resources 25, 26, 28, 30, 32, 34

Specialists 1, 3, 4, 5, 6, 7, 8, 9, 10, 12, 14, 15, 16, 18, 19, 21, 24, 37, 38, 41, 43, 49, 50, 51

Specialties 3, 5, 6, 9, 10, 11, 12, 14, 24, 41, 42, 43, 44, 45, 46, 47, 49, 50, 51, 53

Standard Therapies 25

Subspecialties 1, 5, 6, 10, 12, 13, 15, 41, 42, 49, 50, 53

T

Therapeutic Approaches 1, 6, 25

Treatment Plan 21, 30

Treatment Studies 25, 30

Trust 19

U

United States Department of Health 33

United States Medical Licensing Exam 9

V

W

Special Expertise Index

This index lists the areas that the physicians listed in the Guide have identified as their "special expertise." These are not medical specialties. They are specific elements of disease, procedures, techniques and treatments for which these physicians are best known and are referred patients.

Spec	Name	St	Pg

A

Abdominal Imaging

Spec	Name	St	Pg
DR	Berland, L	AL	904
DR	Coakley, F	CA	907
DR	Federle, M	CA	907
DR	Fishman, E	MD	901
DR	Levy, A	MD	902
DR	Megibow, A	NY	902
DR	Sivit, C	OH	906
DR	Weinreb, J	CT	899
DR	Zagoria, R	NC	905

Abdominal Wall Reconstruction

Spec	Name	St	Pg
PIS	Kuzon, W	MI	786
PIS	Stahl, R	CT	773

Abdominoplasty

Spec	Name	St	Pg
PIS	Bermant, M	VA	781
PIS	Eriksson, E	MA	772
PIS	Gallico, G	MA	772
PIS	Matarasso, A	NY	778
PIS	Pitman, G	NY	778
PIS	Rand, R	WA	795

Abuse/Neglect

Spec	Name	St	Pg
AM	Diaz, A	NY	76
ChAP	Zeanah, C	LA	828
Ger	Lachs, M	NY	247

Achalasia

Spec	Name	St	Pg
Ge	Lind, C	TN	227
Ge	Vaezi, M	TN	229

Acne

Spec	Name	St	Pg
D	Del Giudice, S	NH	178
D	Eichenfield, L	CA	193
D	James, W	PA	182
D	Lucky, A	OH	189
D	Shalita, A	NY	184

Acoustic Neuroma

Spec	Name	St	Pg
NS	Adler, J	CA	451
NS	Eisenberg, H	MD	431
NS	Giannotta, S	CA	453
NS	Golfinos, J	NY	431
NS	Grubb, R	MO	444

Spec	Name	St	Pg
NS	Gutin, P	NY	432
NS	Harsh, G	CA	453
NS	Martuza, R	MA	429
NS	Mayberg, M	WA	454
NS	Sisti, M	NY	435
NS	Stieg, P	NY	436
NS	Thompson, B	MI	447
Oto	Arriaga, M	PA	601
Oto	Beatty, C	MN	614
Oto	Brackmann, D	CA	624
Oto	De la Cruz, A	CA	625
Oto	Driscoll, C	MN	615
Oto	Feghali, J	NY	602
Oto	Jenkins, H	CO	621
Oto	Kveton, J	CT	599
Oto	Lambert, P	SC	610
Oto	Leonetti, J	IL	617
Oto	Linstrom, C	NY	605
Oto	Miyamoto, R	IN	617
Oto	Roland, J	NY	606
Oto	Shelton, C	UT	621
Oto	Telian, S	MI	619
Oto	Wackym, P	WI	619
Oto	Wazen, J	FL	613
Oto	Wiet, R	IL	620
RadRO	Loeffler, J	MA	870

Acromegaly

Spec	Name	St	Pg
EDM	Biller, B	MA	198
EDM	Klibanski, A	MA	199
EDM	Melmed, S	CA	212

Acupuncture

Spec	Name	St	Pg
PM	Ngeow, J	NY	635
PMR	Dillard, J	NY	759

Acute Coronary Syndromes

Spec	Name	St	Pg
Cv	Brindis, R	CA	112
Cv	Eagle, K	MI	105
Cv	Ohman, E	NC	103
IC	Gibson, C	MA	120
IC	Henry, T	MN	124
IC	Holmes, D	MN	124

ADD/ADHD

Spec	Name	St	Pg
ChAP	Abright, A	NY	824
ChAP	Alessi, N	MI	827
ChAP	Biederman, J	MA	822
ChAP	Bird, H	NY	824
ChAP	Bogrov, M	MD	824

Spec	Name	St	Pg
ChAP	Boxer, G	MO	827
ChAP	Bukstein, O	PA	824
ChAP	Coffey, B	NY	824
ChAP	Dulcan, M	IL	827
ChAP	Hertzig, M	NY	825
ChAP	Heston, J	TN	826
ChAP	Hirsch, G	NY	825
ChAP	Hudziak, J	VT	823
ChAP	Leventhal, B	IL	827
ChAP	Martini, D	IL	827
ChAP	Rostain, A	PA	825
ChAP	Russell, A	CA	829
ChAP	Slomowitz, M	IL	828
ChAP	Spencer, T	MA	823
ChAP	Turecki, S	NY	826
ChAP	Wilens, T	MA	823
N	Finkel, M	FL	477
Ped	Burgess, D	NJ	662
Ped	Hershorin, E	FL	663
Ped	Jacob, M	IL	664
Psyc	Hoffman, D	CO	814
Psyc	Keepers, G	OR	817
Psyc	Manevitz, A	NY	809

Addiction/Substance Abuse

Spec	Name	St	Pg
AdP	Brady, K	SC	821
AdP	Frances, R	NY	820
AdP	Howell, E	UT	822
AdP	Kampman, K	PA	820
AdP	Serota, R	PA	821
AdP	Stine, S	MI	821
AdP	Strain, E	MD	821
ChAP	Deas, D	SC	826
ChAP	Wilens, T	MA	823
IM	Selwyn, P	NY	389
Psyc	Lawson, W	DC	809
Psyc	Rosenthal, R	NY	810
Psyc	Strakowski, S	OH	814
Psyc	Weinstock, R	CA	819

Adolescent Behavior-High Risk

Spec	Name	St	Pg
AM	Ginsburg, K	PA	76
AM	Staggers, B	CA	78

Adolescent Gynecology

Spec	Name	St	Pg
AM	Diaz, A	NY	76
AM	Emans, S	MA	76
AM	Hergenroeder, A	TX	77
AM	Irwin, C	CA	77
AM	Kaplan, D	CO	77
AM	Kokotailo, P	WI	77

Special Expertise Index

Special Expertise Index

Special Expertise Index

Special Expertise Index

Spec	Name	St	Pg
Bone Densitometry			
NuM	Dillehay, G	IL	504
Bone Disorders			
Nep	Hruska, K	MO	421
Bone Disorders-Inherited			
CG	Weaver, D	IN	156
Bone Disorders-Metabolic			
DR	Dalinka, M	PA	901
DR	Gilsanz, V	CA	908
EDM	Bilezikian, J	NY	200
EDM	Bockman, R	NY	200
EDM	Clutter, W	MO	206
EDM	Dalkin, A	VA	204
EDM	Econs, M	IN	206
EDM	Khosla, S	MN	207
EDM	LeBoff, M	MA	199
EDM	Licata, A	OH	208
EDM	Siris, E	NY	203
EDM	Watts, N	OH	209
Ger	Lyles, K	NC	248
Nep	Ott, S	WA	424
OrS	Einhorn, T	MA	556
OrS	Kaplan, F	PA	565
OrS	Lane, J	NY	565
OrS	O'Keefe, R	NY	567
OrS	Rosier, R	NY	568
PEn	Friedman, N	NC	681
PEn	Gordon, C	MA	678
PEn	Levine, M	PA	679
Bone Infections			
Inf	Nahass, R	NJ	377
Inf	Slama, T	IN	381
OrS	Browner, B	CT	556
OrS	Schurman, D	CA	588
OrS	Swiontkowski, M	MN	581
OrS	Wilkins, R	CO	582
Bone Infections in Children			
OrS	Kocher, M	MA	557
Bone Marrow & Stem Cell Transplant			
Hem	Yeager, A	AZ	302
Onc	Ball, E	CA	354
Onc	Horning, S	CA	357
Onc	Maloney, D	WA	358
Onc	Stadtmauer, E	PA	323
PHO	Matthay, K	CA	710
Bone Marrow Failure Disorders			
Onc	Deeg, H	WA	355

Spec	Name	St	Pg
PHO	Corey, S	IL	702
PHO	Hord, J	OH	704
PHO	Lipton, J	NY	695
PHO	Wang, W	TN	701
Bone Marrow Pathology			
Path	Arber, D	CA	655
Path	Foucar, M	NM	653
Path	Knowles, D	NY	645
Path	Kurtin, P	MN	651
Path	Orazi, A	NY	646
Bone Marrow Transplant			
Hem	Barlogie, B	AR	300
Hem	Bigelow, C	MS	293
Hem	Brenner, M	TX	300
Hem	Champlin, R	TX	300
Hem	Cobos, E	TX	300
Hem	Copelan, E	OH	295
Hem	Di Persio, J	MO	295
Hem	Farag, S	IN	296
Hem	Files, J	MS	293
Hem	Forman, S	CA	302
Hem	Goldberg, J	NJ	290
Hem	Gordon, L	IL	296
Hem	Juckett, M	WI	297
Hem	Larson, R	IL	297
Hem	Laughlin, M	OH	297
Hem	Lazarus, H	OH	298
Hem	Linenberger, M	WA	303
Hem	Linker, C	CA	303
Hem	Litzow, M	MN	298
Hem	Mangan, K	PA	291
Hem	Maziarz, R	OR	303
Hem	McGlave, P	MN	298
Hem	Meehan, K	NH	288
Hem	Miller, K	MA	289
Hem	Munker, R	LA	301
Hem	Negrin, R	CA	303
Hem	Nimer, S	NY	291
Hem	Porter, D	PA	291
Hem	Rowley, S	NJ	292
Hem	Schuster, M	NY	292
Hem	Snyder, D	CA	304
Hem	Solberg, L	FL	294
Hem	Spitzer, T	MA	289
Hem	Stiff, P	IL	299
Hem	Tallman, M	IL	299
Hem	Uberti, J	MI	299
Hem	Winter, J	IL	299
Onc	Antin, J	MA	304
Onc	Appelbaum, F	WA	354
Onc	Armitage, J	NE	345
Onc	Bierman, P	NE	345
Onc	Bitran, J	IL	336
Onc	Bolwell, B	OH	336
Onc	Camoriano, J	AZ	349
Onc	Carabasi, M	PA	311
Onc	Chao, N	NC	327

Spec	Name	St	Pg
Onc	Claxton, D	PA	311
Onc	Fay, J	TX	349
Onc	Flinn, I	TN	327
Onc	Flomenberg, N	PA	314
Onc	Hurd, D	NC	329
Onc	Jillella, A	GA	329
Onc	Kalaycio, M	OH	340
Onc	Kaminski, M	MI	340
Onc	Livingston, R	AZ	350
Onc	Pohlman, B	OH	342
Onc	Press, O	WA	359
Onc	Shea, T	NC	333
Onc	Soiffer, R	MA	308
Onc	Vaughan, W	AL	335
Onc	Wade, J	WI	344
Onc	Wingard, J	FL	335
PA&I	Cowan, M	CA	668
PA&I	Kamani, N	DC	665
PHO	Abella, E	AZ	707
PHO	Andrews, R	WA	709
PHO	Arceci, R	MD	697
PHO	Bertolone, S	KY	697
PHO	Cairo, M	NY	692
PHO	Camitta, B	WI	702
PHO	Chen, A	MD	692
PHO	Civin, C	MD	692
PHO	Coccia, P	NE	707
PHO	Davies, S	OH	702
PHO	Ferrara, J	MI	703
PHO	Garvin, J	NY	693
PHO	Graham, M	AZ	708
PHO	Grupp, S	PA	693
PHO	Haut, P	IN	703
PHO	Hayashi, R	MO	703
PHO	Horn, B	CA	710
PHO	Kadota, R	CA	710
PHO	Kapoor, N	CA	710
PHO	Kurtzberg, J	NC	699
PHO	Kushner, B	NY	694
PHO	Lipton, J	NY	695
PHO	Nieder, M	FL	700
PHO	O'Reilly, R	NY	695
PHO	Rosenthal, J	CA	711
PHO	Sakamoto, K	CA	711
PHO	Sandler, E	FL	700
PHO	Weinstein, H	MA	691
Bone Pathology			
Path	Kahn, L	NY	645
Bone Tumors			
Onc	Demetri, G	MA	305
Onc	Forscher, C	CA	356
OrS	Conrad, E	WA	585
OrS	Eckardt, J	CA	586
OrS	Gebhardt, M	MA	557
OrS	Healey, J	NY	563
OrS	Hornicek, F	MA	557
OrS	Kenan, S	NY	565

Special Expertise Index

Special Expertise Index

Spec	Name	St	Pg
S	Babiera, G	TX	994
S	Bear, H	VA	977
S	Beauchamp, R	TN	977
S	Beitsch, P	TX	994
S	Bland, K	AL	977
S	Borgen, P	NY	966
S	Brooks, A	PA	967
S	Butler, J	CA	1000
S	Byrd, D	WA	1000
S	Calvo, B	NC	977
S	Chang, A	MI	984
S	Chang, H	CA	1000
S	Crowe, J	OH	985
S	Dilawari, R	TN	978
S	Donohue, J	MN	985
S	Dooley, W	OK	995
S	Easter, D	CA	1001
S	Eberlein, T	MO	985
S	Edge, S	NY	968
S	Edney, J	NE	993
S	Edwards, M	OH	985
S	Eisenberg, B	NH	962
S	Esserman, L	CA	1001
S	Estabrook, A	NY	969
S	Euhus, D	TX	995
S	Farrar, W	OH	986
S	Feig, B	TX	995
S	Finlayson, C	CO	993
S	Frazier, T	PA	970
S	Gabram, S	GA	978
S	Giuliano, A	CA	1002
S	Goodnight, J	CA	1002
S	Goodson, W	CA	1002
S	Goulet, R	IN	986
S	Grant, C	MN	986
S	Grant, M	TX	996
S	Gray, R	AZ	996
S	Hanks, J	VA	979
S	Herrmann, V	SC	979
S	Hughes, K	MA	963
S	Hunt, K	TX	996
S	Iglehart, J	MA	963
S	Johnson, D	CA	1002
S	Johnson, R	PA	970
S	Kaufman, C	WA	1003
S	Kavanah, M	MA	963
S	Kelley, M	TN	979
S	Kim, J	OH	987
S	Klimberg, V	AR	977
S	Knudson, M	CA	1003
S	Krag, D	VT	963
S	Lannin, D	CT	964
S	Levine, E	NC	980
S	Li, B	LA	997
S	Lind, D	GA	980
S	Lyerly, H	NC	980
S	Mamounas, E	OH	988
S	McGrath, P	KY	981
S	McMasters, K	KY	981
S	Morrow, M	NY	972

Spec	Name	St	Pg
S	Nathanson, S	MI	989
S	Nelson, E	UT	993
S	Newman, L	MI	989
S	Nowak, E	NY	972
S	O'Hea, B	NY	972
S	Osborne, M	NY	972
S	Paz, I	CA	1004
S	Peterson, L	HI	1004
S	Pockaj, B	AZ	998
S	Ponn, T	NH	964
S	Roses, D	NY	974
S	Ross, M	TX	998
S	Schnabel, F	NY	974
S	Scott-Conner, C	IA	990
S	Sener, S	CA	1005
S	Shenk, R	OH	990
S	Sigurdson, E	PA	975
S	Silverstein, M	CA	1005
S	Singletary, S	TX	998
S	Skinner, K	NY	975
S	Smith, B	MA	964
S	Stahl, D	OH	991
S	Staren, E	IL	991
S	Stolier, A	LA	999
S	Swistel, A	NY	975
S	Tafra, L	MD	975
S	Tartter, P	NY	976
S	Tsangaris, T	MD	976
S	Tuttle, T	MN	992
S	Urist, M	AL	983
S	Wagman, L	CA	1006
S	Walker, A	WI	992
S	Wallace, A	CA	1006
S	Ward, B	CT	965
S	Weigel, R	IA	992
S	White, R	NC	983
S	Whitworth, P	TN	983
S	Willey, S	DC	976
S	Witt, T	IL	992
S	Wood, W	GA	983
S	Yeung, R	WA	1006
S	Zannis, V	AZ	999

Breast Cancer & Surgery

Spec	Name	St	Pg
PlS	Fox, J	PA	776
S	Anderson, B	WA	999
S	Julian, T	PA	970
S	Karlan, S	CA	1003
S	Leitch, A	TX	997

Breast Cancer Genetics

Spec	Name	St	Pg
ObG	Shulman, L	IL	512
Onc	Buys, S	UT	346
Onc	Graham, M	NC	328
Onc	Olopade, O	IL	341

Breast Cancer in Elderly

Spec	Name	St	Pg
S	Tartter, P	NY	976

Breast Cancer Risk Assessment

Spec	Name	St	Pg
CG	Plon, S	TX	157
GO	Cain, J	RI	258
Onc	Buys, S	UT	346
Onc	Daly, M	PA	312
Onc	Fabian, C	KS	346
Onc	Isaacs, C	DC	317
Onc	Legare, R	RI	307
Onc	O'Regan, R	GA	332
Onc	Perez, E	FL	332
Onc	Stopeck, A	AZ	353
Path	Allred, D	MO	650
S	Hansen, N	IL	987
S	Nathanson, S	MI	989

Breast Cancer Vaccine Therapy

Spec	Name	St	Pg
Onc	Serody, J	NC	333

Breast Cancer-Early Detection

Spec	Name	St	Pg
RadRO	Berg, C	MD	872

Breast Cancer-High Risk Women

Spec	Name	St	Pg
RadRO	Berg, C	MD	872
S	Estabrook, A	NY	969
S	Gabram, S	GA	978
S	Hansen, N	IL	987
S	Osborne, M	NY	972
S	Schnabel, F	NY	974

Breast Cancer-Novel Therapies

Spec	Name	St	Pg
Onc	Fleming, G	IL	339
Onc	Rugo, H	CA	360

Breast Cosmetic & Reconstructive Surgery

Spec	Name	St	Pg
PlS	Ascherman, J	NY	774
PlS	Butler, C	TX	790
PlS	Sood, R	IN	788

Breast Disease

Spec	Name	St	Pg
S	Axelrod, D	NY	966
S	Estabrook, A	NY	969
S	Finlayson, C	CO	993
S	Frazier, T	PA	970
S	Gabram, S	GA	978
S	Goodson, W	CA	1002
S	Kaufman, C	WA	1003
S	Osborne, M	NY	972
S	Swistel, A	NY	975
S	Ward, B	CT	965
S	Witt, T	IL	992

Breast Imaging

Spec	Name	St	Pg
DR	Abbitt, P	FL	904
DR	Bassett, L	CA	907

Special Expertise Index

Special Expertise Index

Special Expertise Index

Special Expertise Index

Special Expertise Index

Spec	Name	St	Pg
PlS	Losee, J	PA	777
PlS	Markowitz, B	CA	795
PlS	Marsh, J	MO	787
PlS	Matthews, D	NC	783
PlS	Posnick, J	MD	778
PlS	Reinisch, J	CA	795
PlS	Spinelli, H	NY	779
PlS	Staffenberg, D	NY	779
PlS	Vander Kolk, C	MD	780
PlS	Vasconez, H	KY	784
PlS	Whitaker, L	PA	780
PlS	Wolfe, S	FL	784

Craniosynostosis

CG	Zackai, E	PA	154
NS	Bierbrauer, K	OH	442
NS	Dias, M	PA	431
NS	Jimenez, D	TX	449
NS	Shuer, L	CA	455
NS	Winston, K	CO	448

Creutzfeldt-Jakob Disease (CJD)

Path	Gambetti, P	OH	651

Critical Care

Inf	Maki, D	WI	381
Inf	Masur, H	MD	376
MF	Besinger, R	IL	398
MF	Gianopoulos, J	IL	398
N	Gress, D	VA	478
N	Suarez, J	TX	491
NP	Gross, I	CT	406
PCCM	Anand, K	TN	677
PCCM	Sarnaik, A	MI	677
PCCM	Thompson, A	PA	676
PM	Berde, C	MA	634
PPul	Kurachek, S	MN	728
PS	Bensard, D	CO	740
PS	Karrer, F	CO	740
PS	Nance, M	PA	735
PS	Reynolds, M	IL	739
PS	Shamberger, R	MA	733
Pul	Albertson, T	CA	861
Pul	Arroliga, A	TX	859
Pul	Bellamy, P	CA	861
Pul	Christman, B	TN	851
Pul	Cooper, W	VA	852
Pul	Criner, G	PA	847
Pul	Greenberg, H	NY	847
Pul	Hall, J	IL	855
Pul	Harman, E	FL	852
Pul	Heffner, J	OR	861
Pul	Hudson, L	WA	862
Pul	Irwin, R	MA	845
Pul	Kaplan, J	KS	859
Pul	King, E	PA	847
Pul	Lefrak, S	MO	856
Pul	LoRusso, T	VA	853

Spec	Name	St	Pg
Pul	Marini, J	MN	856
Pul	Martin, T	WA	862
Pul	Martinez, F	MI	856
Pul	Nelson, J	NY	848
Pul	Parsons, P	VT	846
Pul	Popovich, J	MI	857
Pul	Rizk, N	CA	863
Pul	Steiger, D	NY	849
Pul	Tharratt, R	CA	863
Pul	Vaughey, E	VA	854
Pul	Wheeler, A	TN	854
S	Barie, P	NY	966
S	Buchman, T	GA	977
S	Burke, P	MA	962
S	Cushing, B	ME	962
S	Deitch, E	NJ	968
S	Emhoff, T	MA	963
S	Gupta, R	NH	963
S	Hoyt, D	CA	1002
S	Lentz, C	NY	971
S	Luterman, A	AL	980
S	McIntyre, R	CO	993
S	Millis, J	IL	988
S	Potenza, B	CA	1004
S	Winchell, R	ME	965
TS	Katz, N	DC	1021

Crohn's Disease

CRS	Milsom, J	NY	166
CRS	Rafferty, J	OH	169
CRS	Welton, M	CA	173
CRS	Wolff, B	MN	170
Ge	Abreu, M	FL	225
Ge	Hanauer, S	IL	231
Ge	Isaacs, K	NC	227
Ge	Loftus, E	MN	232
Ge	Sandborn, W	MN	234
Ge	Siegel, C	NH	216
Ge	Targan, S	CA	241
Ge	Young, R	NE	236
PGe	Baldassano, R	PA	684
PGe	Dubinsky, M	CA	689
S	Michelassi, F	NY	971

Cross Cultural Psychiatry

ChAP	McKelvey, R	OR	829
Psyc	Oquendo, M	NY	809
Psyc	Pi, E	CA	818

Cryoglobulinemia

Rhu	Gorevic, P	NY	942

CT Body Scan

DR	Erasmus, J	TX	907
DR	Fishman, E	MD	901
DR	Megibow, A	NY	902
DR	Parsons, R	PA	903
DR	Yoon, S	FL	905

Spec	Name	St	Pg
	CT Chest Scan		
DR	Black, W	NH	899
	CT Colonography		
DR	Fidler, J	MN	905
	CT Scan		
DR	Cohen, B	NY	900
DR	Weinreb, J	CT	899
NuM	Freeman, L	NY	502
	Cushing's Syndrome		
EDM	Biller, B	MA	198
PEn	Levitsky, L	MA	678
	Cutaneous Lymphoma		
D	Belsito, D	KS	190
D	Bowen, G	UT	191
D	Duvic, M	TX	191
D	Edelson, R	CT	178
D	Kim, Y	CA	194
D	Kupper, T	MA	179
D	Lebwohl, M	NY	183
D	Lessin, S	PA	183
D	Lim, H	MI	189
D	McDonald, C	RI	179
D	Olsen, E	NC	187
D	Ramsay, D	NY	183
D	Rook, A	PA	184
D	Thiers, B	SC	188
D	Wood, G	WI	190
Hem	Kuzel, T	IL	297
Path	Le Boit, P	CA	657
	Cystadenocarcinoma		
S	Sugarbaker, P	DC	975
	Cystic Fibrosis		
PA&I	Fanous, Y	CA	669
PGe	Baker, R	NY	684
PPul	Accurso, F	CO	728
PPul	Borowitz, D	NY	725
PPul	Dozor, A	NY	725
PPul	Kattan, M	NY	725
PPul	Konstan, M	OH	728
PPul	Lapey, A	MA	725
PPul	Morgan, W	AZ	729
PPul	Murphy, T	NC	727
PPul	Orenstein, D	PA	726
PPul	Panitch, H	PA	726
PPul	Platzker, A	CA	729
PPul	Quittell, L	NY	726
PPul	Ramsey, B	WA	729
PPul	Rubin, B	NC	727
PPul	Stern, R	OH	728
PPul	Wall, M	OR	729

Special Expertise Index

Special Expertise Index

Special Expertise Index

Special Expertise Index

Special Expertise Index

Special Expertise Index

Special Expertise Index

America's Top Doctors® 9th Edition

Special Expertise Index

Spec	Name	St	Pg
Hepatobiliary Surgery			
S	Adams, R	VA	976
S	Colquhoun, S	CA	1000
S	Curley, S	TX	995
S	Deziel, D	IL	985
S	Eckhoff, D	AL	978
S	Emond, J	NY	969
S	Emre, S	CT	963
S	Farley, D	MN	986
S	Hemming, A	CA	1002
S	Hoffman, J	PA	970
S	Howerton, R	NC	979
S	Jarnagin, W	NY	970
S	Kapur, S	NY	970
S	Knechtle, S	GA	979
S	Moossa, A	CA	1003
S	Nagorney, D	MN	989
S	Reich, D	PA	973
S	Shaw, B	NE	994
S	Vauthey, J	TX	999
S	Walsh, R	OH	992
Hepatobilliary Surgery			
S	Oberholzer, J	IL	989
Hepatopulmonary Syndrome			
Pul	Krowka, M	MN	856
Pul	Krowka, M	MN	856
Hereditary Cancer			
CG	Grody, W	CA	158
CG	Ostrer, H	NY	153
CG	Plon, S	TX	157
CG	Shapiro, L	NY	154
CG	Sutphen, R	FL	155
CG	Weitzel, J	CA	159
CG	Whelan, A	MO	156
Onc	Markowitz, S	OH	341
Onc	Nissenblatt, M	NJ	319
Onc	Olopade, O	IL	341
Hereditary Hemorrhagic Telangiectasia			
CG	Pyeritz, R	PA	154
VIR	Trerotola, S	PA	917
Hernia			
PS	Aiken, J	WI	737
PS	Paidas, C	FL	736
PS	Velcek, F	NY	735
S	Baker, C	LA	994
S	Barie, P	NY	966
S	Brody, F	DC	967
S	Brunt, L	MO	984
S	Curcillo, P	PA	968
S	Farley, D	MN	986

Spec	Name	St	Pg
S	Fitzgibbons, R	NE	993
S	Greene, F	NC	979
S	Meyers, W	PA	971
S	Nowak, E	NY	972
S	Pachter, H	NY	972
S	Pomp, A	NY	973
S	Reiner, M	NY	973
U	Atala, A	NC	1058
Herpes Simplex			
PInf	Bryson, Y	CA	716
Herpetic Neuralgia (Shingles)			
PM	Audell, L	CA	639
PM	Raja, S	MD	635
PM	Rowbotham, M	CA	640
Heterotopic Ossification			
OrS	Keenan, M	PA	565
High Intensity Focused Ultrasound(HIFU)			
U	Chang, S	TN	1059
U	Robertson, C	NC	1061
Hip & Knee Reconstruction			
OrS	Einhorn, T	MA	556
OrS	McDonald, D	MO	579
OrS	Rosenberg, A	IL	580
Hip & Knee Replacement			
OrS	Blaha, J	MI	576
OrS	Bucholz, R	TX	583
OrS	Callaghan, J	IA	577
OrS	Copp, S	CA	585
OrS	Dorr, L	CA	585
OrS	Einhorn, T	MA	556
OrS	Finerman, G	CA	586
OrS	Goldberg, V	OH	577
OrS	Grant, H	OH	578
OrS	Johanson, N	PA	565
OrS	Luck, J	CA	586
OrS	Padgett, D	NY	567
OrS	Ready, J	MA	558
OrS	Reilly, D	MA	558
OrS	Rosenberg, A	IL	580
OrS	Salvati, E	NY	569
OrS	Schurman, D	CA	588
OrS	Stuchin, S	NY	570
OrS	Stulberg, S	IL	580
OrS	Thornhill, T	MA	558
OrS	Vail, T	CA	588
OrS	Wittig, J	NY	571
OrS	Wixson, R	IL	581
Hip & Knee Replacement in Bone			

Spec	Name	St	Pg
Tumors			
OrS	Healey, J	NY	563
OrS	Ready, J	MA	558
Hip Disorders & Dysplasia			
OrS	Aronson, J	AR	583
OrS	Weinstein, S	IA	581
Hip Disorders-Pediatric			
OrS	Roye, D	NY	568
OrS	Weinstein, S	IA	581
Hip Replacement			
OrS	Brick, G	MA	556
OrS	Bronson, M	NY	560
OrS	Buly, R	NY	560
OrS	Burke, D	MA	556
OrS	Di Cesare, P	CA	585
OrS	Gitelis, S	IL	577
OrS	Goldstein, W	IL	577
OrS	Hume, E	NJ	564
OrS	Jiranek, W	VA	573
OrS	Kenan, S	NY	565
OrS	Macaulay, W	NY	566
OrS	Muschler, G	OH	579
OrS	Ranawat, C	NY	568
OrS	Rothman, R	PA	568
OrS	Schmalzried, T	CA	587
OrS	Scott, R	MA	558
OrS	Sculco, T	NY	569
OrS	Trick, L	TX	584
OrS	Westrich, G	NY	570
OrS	Zuckerman, J	NY	571
Hip Replacement & Revision			
OrS	Cuckler, J	AL	572
OrS	Hungerford, M	MD	564
OrS	Krackow, K	NY	565
OrS	Mabrey, J	TX	583
Hip Replacement-Young Adults			
OrS	Pellicci, P	NY	567
Hip Resurfacing			
OrS	Di Cesare, P	CA	585
OrS	Pellicci, P	NY	567
OrS	Stuchin, S	NY	570
OrS	Vail, T	CA	588
Hip Surgery			
OrS	Crossett, L	PA	561
OrS	Garvin, K	NE	581
OrS	Hozack, W	PA	564
OrS	Salvati, E	NY	569
OrS	Weiner, R	FL	576

Special Expertise Index

Special Expertise Index

Special Expertise Index

Special Expertise Index

Special Expertise Index

Spec	Name	St	Pg
CRS	Stryker, S	IL	170
CRS	Thorson, A	NE	171
CRS	Wexner, S	FL	168
CRS	Whelan, R	NY	166
CRS	Wong, R	HI	173
GO	Azodi, M	CT	258
GO	Barakat, R	NY	260
GO	Barter, J	MD	260
GO	Burnett, A	AR	268
GO	Curtin, J	NY	261
GO	DeMars, L	NH	258
GO	Dottino, P	NY	261
GO	Fowler, J	OH	266
GO	Herzog, T	NY	261
GO	Horowitz, I	GA	264
GO	Morgan, M	PA	262
GO	Stern, J	CA	272
ObG	Brodman, M	NY	508
ObG	Cornella, J	AZ	513
ObG	Goldstein, M	NY	509
ObG	Hager, W	KY	510
ObG	Steege, J	NC	511
PS	Albanese, C	CA	741
PS	Nuchtern, J	TX	741
PS	Shlasko, E	NY	735
RE	Carson, S	RI	926
RE	Copperman, A	NY	927
RE	Grifo, J	NY	928
RE	Grunfeld, L	NY	928
RE	Hornstein, M	MA	926
RE	Nagel, T	MN	934
RE	Pfeifer, S	PA	929
S	Ballantyne, G	NJ	966
S	Bessler, M	NY	966
S	Bilchik, A	CA	1000
S	Brody, F	DC	967
S	Callery, M	MA	962
S	Curcillo, P	PA	968
S	Dempsey, D	PA	968
S	Deziel, D	IL	985
S	Doherty, G	MI	985
S	Farley, D	MN	986
S	Frantzides, C	IL	986
S	Howerton, R	NC	979
S	MacFadyen, B	GA	981
S	Melvin, W	OH	988
S	Nguyen, N	CA	1003
S	Onders, R	OH	989
S	Pappas, T	NC	981
S	Park, A	MD	972
S	Phillips, E	CA	1004
S	Prinz, R	IL	989
S	Reiner, M	NY	973
S	Schirmer, B	VA	982
S	Schlinkert, R	AZ	998
S	Schraut, W	PA	974
S	Scott-Conner, C	IA	990
S	Sharp, K	TN	982
S	Sinanan, M	WA	1005
S	Siperstein, A	OH	991

Spec	Name	St	Pg
S	Soper, N	IL	991
S	Sweeney, J	GA	982
S	Traverso, L	WA	1006
S	Wiebke, E	IN	992
S	Willis, I	FL	983
U	Albala, D	NC	1058
U	Andriole, G	MO	1063
U	Clayman, R	CA	1073
U	Culkin, D	OK	1070
U	El-Galley, R	AL	1059
U	Grasso, M	NY	1052
U	Hemal, A	NC	1059
U	Jackman, S	PA	1053
U	Kavoussi, L	NY	1053
U	Kozlowski, J	IL	1065
U	Lugg, J	WY	1069
U	Patterson, A	TN	1061
U	Sosa, R	NY	1056
U	Stoller, M	CA	1076
U	Strand, W	TX	1072
U	Teigland, C	NC	1062
U	Winfield, H	AL	1063

Laparoscopy & Thoracostomy

PS	Dolgin, S	NY	734
PS	Sato, T	WI	740

Laryngeal & Tracheal Disorders

Oto	Weissler, M	NC	613
Oto	Zalzal, G	DC	609

Laryngeal & Vocal Cord Surgery

Oto	Caldarelli, D	IL	615
Oto	Sulica, R	NY	608

Laryngeal & Voice Disorders

Oto	Fried, M	NY	602

Laryngeal Cancer

Onc	Pfister, D	NY	321
Oto	Courey, M	CA	624
Oto	Grillone, G	MA	599
Oto	Shapshay, S	NY	607
Oto	Shindo, M	OR	626
Oto	Weinstein, G	PA	608
Oto	Wolf, G	MI	620
Oto	Woo, P	NY	608
Oto	Zeitels, S	MA	600
S	Ridge, J	PA	973

Laryngeal Cancer-Organ Preservation

Oto	Rassekh, C	WV	606

Laryngeal Disorders

Oto	Bastian, R	IL	614
Oto	Berke, G	CA	624
Oto	Courey, M	CA	624
Oto	Flint, P	OR	625
Oto	Ford, C	WI	615
Oto	Grillone, G	MA	599
Oto	Koufman, J	NY	604
Oto	Sataloff, R	PA	607
Oto	Stasney, C	TX	624
Oto	Suen, J	AR	624
Oto	Woo, P	NY	608
Oto	Zeitels, S	MA	600
PO	April, M	NY	720
PO	Tunkel, D	MD	722

Laser Resurfacing

D	Grossman, M	NY	182

Laser Surgery

D	Burton, C	NC	185
D	Cook, J	NC	186
ObG	Bury, R	ND	512
Oph	Caster, A	CA	544
Oph	Gaasterland, D	MD	522
PlS	Morgan, R	VA	783

Laser Vision Surgery

Oph	Caster, A	CA	544
Oph	Dodick, J	NY	521
Oph	Gibralter, R	NY	522
Oph	Kornmehl, E	MA	518
Oph	Lane, S	MN	536
Oph	McCulley, J	TX	541
Oph	Stulting, R	GA	532
Oph	Wang, M	TN	532
Oph	Zaidman, G	NY	528

LASIK-Refractive Surgery

Oph	Boxer Wachler, B	CA	543
Oph	Caster, A	CA	544
Oph	Culbertson, W	FL	529
Oph	Durrie, D	KS	540
Oph	Feder, R	IL	534
Oph	Gorovoy, M	FL	530
Oph	Hersh, P	NJ	523
Oph	Holladay, J	TX	541
Oph	Mackool, R	NY	524
Oph	Maloney, R	CA	546
Oph	Manche, E	CA	546
Oph	Mandel, E	NY	525
Oph	Pepose, J	MO	537
Oph	Salz, J	CA	547
Oph	Serafano, D	CA	548
Oph	Waring, G	GA	533

Special Expertise Index

Special Expertise Index

M

Special Expertise Index

Spec	Name	St	Pg
Mercury Toxic Exposure			
OM	Gochfeld, M	NJ	800
Merkel Cell Carcinoma			
Onc	Cohen, S	NY	312
Onc	Johnson, B	MA	306
Onc	Kelsen, D	NY	317
Mesothelioma			
OM	Cullen, M	CA	800
Onc	Algazy, K	PA	309
Onc	Bonomi, P	IL	336
Onc	Dakhil, S	KS	346
Onc	Ilson, D	NY	317
Onc	Kalemkerian, G	MI	340
Onc	Kindler, H	IL	341
Onc	Langer, C	PA	318
Onc	Martins, R	WA	358
Onc	Robert-Vizcarrondo, F	AL	332
Onc	Ross, H	AZ	352
Onc	Ruckdeschel, J	MI	342
Onc	Salgia, R	IL	343
Onc	Shin, D	GA	333
Onc	Simon, G	PA	322
Onc	Verschraegen, C	NM	353
Onc	Vogelzang, N	NV	362
Path	Cagle, P	TX	653
Path	Moran, C	TX	654
Pul	Jett, J	MN	855
Pul	Sterman, D	PA	849
RadRO	Choi, N	MA	870
RadRO	Videtic, G	OH	885
S	Loggie, B	NE	993
TS	Battafarano, R	MD	1018
TS	Cameron, R	CA	1038
TS	Friedberg, J	PA	1019
TS	Handy, J	OR	1039
TS	Harpole, D	NC	1027
TS	Jablons, D	CA	1039
TS	Krasna, M	MD	1022
TS	Miller, D	GA	1028
TS	Pass, H	NY	1024
TS	Robinson, L	FL	1029
TS	Smythe, W	TX	1037
TS	Sugarbaker, D	MA	1017
TS	Swisher, S	TX	1038
TS	Vallieres, E	WA	1041
TS	Vigneswaran, W	IL	1034
TS	Wood, D	WA	1042
TS	Yang, S	MD	1025
Metabolic Disorders			
ChiN	Ashwal, S	CA	147
ChiN	De Vivo, D	NY	143
ChiN	Patterson, M	MN	146
EDM	Dobs, A	MD	201
IM	Rader, D	PA	389

Spec	Name	St	Pg
Metabolic Genetic Disorders			
CG	Bialer, M	NY	153
CG	Fernhoff, P	GA	154
Metabolic Syndrome			
EDM	Schwartz, S	PA	202
PEn	De Luca, F	PA	679
Metastatic Cancer			
S	Ellis, L	TX	995
Microdiscectomy			
NS	Chen, T	CA	452
NS	Haid, R	GA	438
NS	Maroon, J	PA	434
OrS	Boden, S	GA	572
Microscopic Colitis			
Ge	Loftus, E	MN	232
Microsurgery			
HS	Bishop, A	MN	280
HS	Culp, R	PA	277
HS	Fischer, T	IN	281
HS	Lubahn, J	PA	278
HS	Mih, A	IN	282
HS	Rayan, G	OK	283
HS	Stern, P	OH	282
NS	Barrow, D	GA	437
NS	Chen, C	NY	430
NS	Selman, W	OH	447
ObG	Bury, R	ND	512
Oto	Strome, S	MD	608
PlS	Andersen, J	CA	792
PlS	Brandt, K	MO	785
PlS	Cederna, P	MI	786
PlS	Dagum, A	NY	775
PlS	Fix, R	AL	781
PlS	Levin, L	PA	776
PlS	Low, D	PA	777
PlS	Mehrara, B	NY	778
PlS	Neumeister, M	IL	787
PlS	Sanger, J	WI	788
PlS	Siebert, J	NY	779
PlS	Siemionow, M	OH	788
PlS	Wilkins, E	MI	788
U	Atala, A	NC	1058
U	Fisch, H	NY	1051
U	Lipshultz, L	TX	1071
U	Turek, P	CA	1076
Microvascular Surgery			
Oto	Hayden, R	AZ	623
Oto	Wax, M	OR	627

Spec	Name	St	Pg
Middle Ear Disorders			
Oto	Miyamoto, R	IN	617
Oto	Tucci, D	NC	613
Migraine			
ChiN	Epstein, L	IL	146
ChiN	Maytal, J	NY	144
ChiN	Sankar, R	CA	148
N	Aurora, S	WA	491
N	Bernad, P	VA	476
N	Buchholz, D	MD	467
N	Charles, A	CA	492
N	Cutrer, F	MN	482
N	Dodick, D	AZ	489
N	Finkel, A	NC	477
N	Mohammad, Y	IL	484
N	Raskin, N	CA	494
N	Silberstein, S	PA	475
N	Swanson, J	MN	486
N	Wright, R	IL	487
PM	Loder, E	MA	634
PM	Robbins, L	IL	637
Migraine in Women			
N	Rubin, S	IL	486
Minimally Invasive Cardiac Surgery			
TS	Adams, D	NY	1018
TS	Aklog, L	AZ	1035
TS	Alexander, J	IL	1030
TS	Bakhos, M	IL	1030
TS	Bichell, D	TN	1026
TS	Bridges, C	PA	1019
TS	Chitwood, W	NC	1026
TS	Damiano, R	MO	1031
TS	DeFilippi, V	CA	1038
TS	DeRose, J	NY	1019
TS	Furukawa, S	PA	1020
TS	Grossi, E	NY	1021
TS	Guyton, R	GA	1027
TS	Hargrove, W	PA	1021
TS	Horvath, K	MD	1021
TS	Lang, S	NY	1022
TS	Loulmet, D	NY	1023
TS	Oz, M	NY	1023
TS	Shemin, R	CA	1040
TS	Smith, C	NY	1024
TS	Woo, Y	PA	1025
Minimally Invasive Heart Surgery			
TS	Murphy, D	GA	1028
Minimally Invasive Heart Valve Surgery			
TS	Galloway, A	NY	1020
TS	Jeevanandam, V	IL	1031

Special Expertise Index

Special Expertise Index

Special Expertise Index

America's Top Doctors® 9th Edition

Special Expertise Index

Special Expertise Index

Special Expertise Index

Special Expertise Index

Special Expertise Index

Special Expertise Index

Special Expertise Index

Spec	Name	St	Pg
GerPsy	Streim, J	PA	830
Psyc	Basch, S	NY	806
Psyc	Bronheim, H	NY	807
Psyc	Cohen, M	PA	807
Psyc	Fallon, B	NY	807
Psyc	Fann, J	WA	817
Psyc	Greiner, C	NE	814
Psyc	Kerrihard, T	CA	817
Psyc	Kunkel, E	PA	809
Psyc	Locala, J	OH	813
Psyc	Strouse, T	CA	819

Psychiatry in Pregnancy

Spec	Name	St	Pg
Psyc	Burt, V	CA	816
Psyc	Dell, D	NC	811

Psychiatry in Terminal Illness

Spec	Name	St	Pg
Psyc	Klagsbrun, S	NY	808

Psychiatry in Transplant Patients

Spec	Name	St	Pg
ChAP	Sexson, S	GA	826
Psyc	Locala, J	OH	813

Psychiatry of Prostate Cancer

Spec	Name	St	Pg
Psyc	Roth, A	NY	810

Psychiatry-Geriatric

Spec	Name	St	Pg
Psyc	Weiner, M	TX	816

Psychoanalysis

Spec	Name	St	Pg
ChAP	King, R	CT	823
Psyc	Akhtar, S	PA	806
Psyc	Basch, S	NY	806
Psyc	Friedman, B	CA	817
Psyc	Gabbard, G	TX	816
Psyc	Klapheke, M	KY	812
Psyc	Samberg, E	NY	810
Psyc	Scott, C	PA	810
Psyc	Shapiro, E	MA	805
Psyc	Stone, M	NY	810
Psyc	Zerbe, K	OR	820

Psychodermatology

Spec	Name	St	Pg
D	Koo, J	CA	194

Psychopharmacology

Spec	Name	St	Pg
AdP	Kosten, T	TX	822
AdP	Schuckit, M	CA	822
ChAP	Biederman, J	MA	822
ChAP	Hudziak, J	VT	823
ChAP	Leventhal, B	IL	827
ChAP	Riddle, M	MD	825
GerPsy	Tune, L	GA	831
PM	Robbins, L	IL	637
Psyc	Basch, S	NY	806

Spec	Name	St	Pg
Psyc	Blumenfield, M	CA	816
Psyc	Bystritsky, A	CA	816
Psyc	First, M	NY	808
Psyc	Friedman, B	CA	817
Psyc	Friedman, M	VT	804
Psyc	Gelenberg, A	WI	813
Psyc	Goff, D	MA	804
Psyc	Janicak, P	IL	813
Psyc	Marder, S	CA	818
Psyc	Mohl, P	TX	816
Psyc	Nelson, J	CA	818
Psyc	Neppe, V	WA	818
Psyc	Pi, E	CA	818
Psyc	Reus, V	CA	819
Psyc	Salzman, C	MA	805
Psyc	Schatzberg, A	CA	819
Psyc	Strouse, T	CA	819
Psyc	Sussman, N	NY	811
Psyc	Thase, M	PA	811
Psyc	Wilson, D	NE	815
Psyc	Zorumski, C	MO	814

Psychoses-Late Onset

Spec	Name	St	Pg
GerPsy	Holroyd, S	VA	831
GerPsy	Tune, L	GA	831

Psychosocial Support in Childhood Cancer

Spec	Name	St	Pg
PHO	Siegel, S	CA	711

Psychosomatic Disorders

Spec	Name	St	Pg
ChAP	Campo, J	OH	827
ChAP	Fritz, G	RI	822
Psyc	Blumenfield, M	CA	816
Psyc	Fallon, B	NY	807

Psychotherapy

Spec	Name	St	Pg
Psyc	Blumenfield, M	CA	816
Psyc	First, M	NY	808
Psyc	Giustra, L	GA	811
Psyc	Gunderson, J	MA	804
Psyc	Karasu, T	NY	808
Psyc	Mohl, P	TX	816
Psyc	Sadock, V	NY	810
Psyc	Salzman, C	MA	805

Psychotic Disorders

Spec	Name	St	Pg
Psyc	Boronow, J	MD	806
Psyc	Janicak, P	IL	813
Psyc	Liberman, R	CA	817
Psyc	Strakowski, S	OH	814

Pubertal Disorders

Spec	Name	St	Pg
PEn	Allen, D	WI	681
PEn	Alter, C	PA	679
PEn	Eugster, E	IN	682

Spec	Name	St	Pg
PEn	Foster, C	UT	683
PEn	Freemark, M	NC	681
PEn	Geffner, M	CA	683
PEn	Kappy, M	CO	683
PEn	Plotnick, L	MD	680
PEn	Rosenfield, R	IL	682

Pulmonary Complications-Cancer Therapy

PPul	Kim, Y	IN	728

Pulmonary Complications-Sickle Cell Dis

PPul	Kim, Y	IN	728

Pulmonary Disease-Second Opinion Only

Pul	Kamholz, S	NY	847

Pulmonary Disease/Immunocompromised

Pul	Stover-Pepe, D	NY	849

Pulmonary Embolism

DR	Goodman, L	WI	905
DR	Sagel, S	MO	906
Pul	Arcasoy, S	NY	846
Pul	Palevsky, H	PA	848
Pul	Popovich, J	MI	857
S	Wakefield, T	MI	992
TS	Jamieson, S	CA	1039
TS	Sundt, T	MN	1034

Pulmonary Fibrosis

Pul	Berk, J	MA	844
Pul	Brown, K	CO	858
Pul	Criner, G	PA	847
Pul	Loyd, J	TN	853
Pul	Lynch, J	CA	862
Pul	Raghu, G	WA	863
Pul	Sahn, S	SC	853
Pul	Staton, G	GA	853

Pulmonary Hypertension

Cv	Bashore, T	NC	100
Cv	Bourge, R	AL	101
Cv	Horn, E	NY	97
Cv	Poon, M	NY	98
Cv	Rich, S	IL	108
Cv	Wagoner, L	OH	109
NP	Steinhorn, R	IL	411
Pul	Arroliga, A	TX	859
Pul	Auger, W	CA	861
Pul	Criner, G	PA	847

Special Expertise Index

Special Expertise Index

America's Top Doctors® 9th Edition

Special Expertise Index

Special Expertise Index

Special Expertise Index

Special Expertise Index

Special Expertise Index

Special Expertise Index

Special Expertise Index

Special Expertise Index

Special Expertise Index

Special Expertise Index

Special Expertise Index

Alphabetical Listing of Doctors

Name	Specialty	Pg
A		
Abaza, Mona (CO)	Oto	620
Abbas, Fouad (MD)	GO	259
Abbitt, Patricia (FL)	DR	904
Abbott, Richard (CA)	Oph	543
Abbruzzese, James (TX)	Onc	347
Abcarian, Herand (IL)	CRS	168
Abecassis, Michael (IL)	S	983
Abella, Esteban (AZ)	PHO	707
Abou-Khalil, Bassel (TN)	AdP	821
Abrahamson, Martin (MA)	EDM	198
Abrahm, Janet (MA)	PM	634
Abram, Stephen (WI)	PM	636
Abrams, Charles (PA)	Hem	289
Abrams, Donald (CA)	Onc	354
Abrams, Gary (MI)	Oph	533
Abrams, Ross (IL)	RadRO	881
Abramson, David (NY)	Oph	519
Abrass, Itamar (WA)	Ger	251
Abreu, Maria (FL)	Ge	225
Abright, Arthur (NY)	ChAP	824
Abromowitch, Minnie (NE)	PHO	706
Abu-Rustum, Nadeem (NY)	GO	259
Abuhamad, Alfred (VA)	MF	397
Accurso, Frank (CO)	PPul	728
Achkar, Edgar (OH)	Ge	229
Acker, David (MA)	MF	394
Acker, Michael (PA)	TS	1018
Ackerman, Michael (MN)	PCd	673
Adams, David (NY)	TS	1018
Adams, David (FL)	N	476
Adams, Elaine (IL)	Rhu	946
Adams, Harold (IA)	N	481
Adams, James (TX)	NP	411
Adams, Reid (VA)	S	976
Adams, Robert (SC)	N	476
Adams-Graves, Patricia (TN)	Hem	293
Adamson, G David (CA)	RE	935

Name	Specialty	Pg
Adamson, Peter (PA)	PHO	691
Adelman, Mark (NY)	VascS	1083
Adelson, P David (AZ)	NS	449
Adelstein, David (OH)	Onc	335
Adkins, Terrance (AZ)	CRS	171
Adler, John (CA)	NS	451
Adler, Kenneth (NJ)	Onc	309
Adler, Ronald (NY)	DR	900
Adornato, Bruce (CA)	N	491
Adzick, N Scott (PA)	PS	733
Agarwal, Animesh (TX)	OrS	583
Agarwal, Sanjay (CA)	RE	936
Agarwala, Brojendra (IL)	PCd	673
Ahern, Geoffrey (AZ)	N	488
Ahlering, Thomas (CA)	U	1072
Ahlgren, James (DC)	Onc	309
Ahlskog, J Eric (MN)	N	481
Ahmad, Suhail (WA)	Nep	424
Ahmann, Frederick (AZ)	Onc	347
Ahn, Jung (NY)	PMR	758
Ahn, Sam (CA)	VascS	1091
Aiello, Lloyd (MA)	Oph	518
Aiken, John (WI)	PS	737
Ain, Kenneth (KY)	EDM	204
Aisner, Joseph (NJ)	Onc	309
Ajani, Jaffer (TX)	Onc	348
Akelman, Edward (RI)	HS	276
Akerley, Wallace (UT)	Onc	345
Akhtar, Salman (PA)	Psyc	806
Akins, Cary (MA)	TS	1016
Aklog, Lishan (AZ)	TS	1035
Al-Mefty, Ossama (AR)	NS	449
Alavi, Abass (PA)	NuM	502
Alazraki, Naomi (GA)	NuM	504
Albain, Kathy (IL)	Onc	336
Albala, David (NC)	U	1058
Albanese, Craig (CA)	PS	741
Albers, Gregory (CA)	N	491
Albert, Daniel (WI)	Oph	533

Alphabetical Listing of Doctors

Name	Specialty	Pg	Name	Specialty	Pg
Albert, Daniel (NH)	Rhu	940	Amato, Anthony (MA)	N	464
Albert, Michael (DC)	Ge	217	Ambinder, Richard (MD)	Onc	309
Albert, Todd (PA)	OrS	559	Ames, Frederick (TX)	S	994
Albertini, Mark (WI)	Onc	336	Amin, Mahul (CA)	Path	655
Alberts, David (AZ)	Onc	348	Amin, Sandeep (IL)	PM	636
Alberts, Mark (IL)	N	481	Aminoff, Michael (CA)	N	491
Alberts, W Michael (FL)	Pul	851	Amling, Christopher (OR)	U	1072
Albertsen, Peter (CT)	U	1048	Amonette, Rex (TN)	D	185
Albertson, David (NC)	S	977	An, Howard (IL)	OrS	576
Albertson, Timothy (CA)	Pul	861	Anand, Kanwaljeet (TN)	PCCM	677
Albright, A Leland (WI)	NS	441	Andersen, Arnold (IA)	Psyc	812
Albritton, Karen (MA)	PHO	690	Andersen, James (CA)	PlS	792
Aledo, Alexander (NY)	PHO	691	Anderson, Benjamin (WA)	S	999
Alessi, Norman (MI)	ChAP	827	Anderson, Corrie (WA)	PM	639
Alexander, Frederick (NJ)	PS	733	Anderson, Jeffrey (UT)	Cv	110
Alexander, J Jeffrey (OH)	VascS	1088	Anderson, Joseph (MI)	Onc	336
Alexander, John (IL)	TS	1030	Anderson, Karl (TX)	Ge	236
Alexander, Kenneth (IL)	PInf	714	Anderson, Kenneth (MA)	Hem	288
Alexander, Richard (MD)	U	1050	Anderson, Lesley (CA)	OrS	584
Alexander, Steven (CA)	PNep	719	Anderson, Mark (IA)	CE	117
Alfonso, Antonio (NY)	S	965	Anderson, Martin (CA)	AM	77
Alfonso, Eduardo (FL)	Oph	528	Anderson, Richard (MA)	D	178
Algazy, Kenneth (PA)	Onc	309	Anderson, Richard (UT)	Oph	540
Allen, David (WI)	PEn	681	Andiman, Warren (CT)	PInf	711
Allen, Jeffrey (NY)	ChiN	143	Andreoli, Sharon (IN)	PNep	718
Allen, Nancy (NC)	Rhu	945	Andrews, David (PA)	NS	429
Allen, Robert (SC)	PlS	781	Andrews, James (AL)	SM	956
Allon, Michael (AL)	Nep	418	Andrews, Robert (WA)	PHO	709
Allred, D Craig (MO)	Path	650	Andriole, Gerald (MO)	U	1063
Alster, Tina (DC)	D	180	Ang, Kie-Kian (TX)	RadRO	886
Altchek, David (NY)	SM	954	Angelos, Peter (IL)	S	984
Alter, Craig (PA)	PEn	679	Anghelescu, Doralina (TN)	PM	636
Alter, Gary (CA)	PlS	792	Angle, Niren (CA)	VascS	1091
Altman, Arnold (CT)	PHO	690	Anhalt, Grant (MD)	D	180
Altman, Leonard (WA)	A&I	87	Annest, Stephen (CO)	VascS	1090
Altorki, Nasser (NY)	TS	1018	Anscher, Mitchell (VA)	RadRO	877
Alvarez, Ronald (AL)	GO	263	Anthony, Lowell (LA)	Onc	348
Alvarez-Elcoro, Salvador (FL)	Inf	378	Antin, Joseph (MA)	Onc	304
Alward, Wallace (IA)	Oph	533	Anton, Raymond (SC)	AdP	821
Amar, Arun (CA)	NS	451	Antonia, Scott (FL)	Onc	325

Alphabetical Listing of Doctors

Name	Specialty	Pg	Name	Specialty	Pg
Antony, Veena (FL)	Pul	851	Arroliga, Alejandro (TX)	Pul	859
Anyane-Yeboa, Kwame (NY)	CG	152	Arslanian, Silva (PA)	PEn	679
Apatoff, Brian (NY)	N	466	Arteaga, Carlos (TN)	Onc	325
Apfelbaum, Ronald (UT)	NS	447	Arts, H Alexander (MI)	Oto	614
Appel, Gerald (NY)	Nep	417	Arun, Banu (TX)	Onc	348
Appelbaum, Frederick (WA)	Onc	354	Aruny, John (CT)	VIR	916
Appelbaum, Paul (NY)	Psyc	806	Ascher, Enrico (NY)	VascS	1083
Appell, Rodney (TX)	U	1069	Ascher, Nancy (CA)	S	999
Appelman, Henry (MI)	Path	650	Ascherman, Jeffrey (NY)	PlS	774
Applegate, Robert (NC)	IC	122	Aseff, John (DC)	PMR	758
April, Max (NY)	PO	720	Asher, Anthony (NC)	NS	437
Apuzzo, Michael (CA)	NS	451	Ashizawa, Tetsuo (FL)	N	476
Aranha, Gerard (IL)	S	984	Ashley, Stanley (MA)	S	962
Arber, Daniel (CA)	Path	655	Ashwal, Stephen (CA)	ChiN	147
Arcasoy, Selim (NY)	Pul	846	Assimos, Dean (NC)	U	1058
Arceci, Robert (MD)	PHO	692	Aston, Sherrell (NY)	PlS	774
Archer, Steven (MI)	Oph	533	Atala, Anthony (NC)	U	1058
Arend, William (CO)	Rhu	948	Athanasian, Edward (NY)	HS	276
Arensman, Robert (IL)	PS	737	Atkins, Michael (MA)	Onc	304
Argenta, Louis (NC)	PlS	781	Atkinson, John (MN)	NS	442
Argenziano, Michael (NY)	TS	1018	Atkinson, Robert (HI)	HS	283
Argiris, Athanassios (PA)	Onc	309	Atlas, Scott (CA)	NRad	914
Ariagno, Ronald (CA)	NP	412	Atmar, Robert (TX)	Inf	382
Arjmand, Ellis (OH)	PO	722	Atnip, Robert (PA)	VascS	1083
Arlen, Philip (MD)	Onc	310	Attas, Lewis (NJ)	Onc	310
Armitage, James (NE)	Onc	345	Attinger, Christopher (DC)	PlS	774
Armon, Carmel (MA)	N	464	Audell, Laura (CA)	PM	639
Armstrong, William (MI)	Cv	104	Auger, William (CA)	Pul	861
Arnason, Barry (IL)	N	481	Augsburger, James (OH)	Oph	534
Arndt, Carola (MN)	PHO	701	August, David (NJ)	S	966
Arndt, Kenneth (MA)	D	178	August, Phyllis (NY)	Nep	417
Arnett, Frank (TX)	Rhu	949	Aurora, Sheena (WA)	N	491
Arnold, Anthony (CA)	Oph	543	Austin, John (NY)	DR	900
Arnold, James (OH)	PO	723	Auwaerter, Paul (MD)	Inf	374
Arnold, Robert (PA)	IM	388	Averbook, Bruce (OH)	S	984
Aronchick, Craig (PA)	Ge	217	Avery, Eric (TX)	Psyc	815
Aronson, James (AR)	OrS	583	Aviv, Jonathan (NY)	Oto	601
Aronson, Peter (CT)	Nep	416	Avner, Ellis (WI)	PNep	718
Arpey, Christopher (IA)	D	188	Awan, Azhar (IL)	RadRO	881
Arriaga, Moises (PA)	Oto	601	Axelrod, Deborah (NY)	S	966

Alphabetical Listing of Doctors

Name	Specialty	Pg	Name	Specialty	Pg
Axelrod, Lloyd (MA)	EDM	198	Baker, Stephen (DC)	PlS	774
Axelrod, Rita (PA)	Onc	310	Baker, Susan (NY)	PGe	684
Azar, Dimitri (IL)	Oph	534	Bakhos, Mamdouh (IL)	TS	1030
Azodi, Masoud (CT)	GO	258	Bakken, Johan (MN)	Inf	380
Azziz, Ricardo (CA)	RE	936	Balady, Gary (MA)	Cv	92
			Balart, Luis (LA)	Ge	236
			Balch, Charles (MD)	S	966
B			Baldassano, Robert (PA)	PGe	684
			Balderston, Richard (PA)	OrS	559
Babiera, Gildy (TX)	S	994	Baldridge, Alan (PA)	PGe	684
Bach, Bernard (IL)	OrS	576	Balducci, Lodovico (FL)	Onc	325
Bach, John (NJ)	PMR	759	Bale, Allen (CT)	CG	152
Back, Anthony (WA)	Onc	354	Bale, James (UT)	ChiN	147
Bacon, Bruce (MO)	Ge	230	Balk, Robert (IL)	Pul	854
Badie, Behnam (CA)	NS	452	Balkany, Thomas (FL)	Oto	609
Baer, Maria (MD)	Hem	289	Ball, Douglas (MD)	EDM	200
Baerveldt, George (CA)	Oph	543	Ball, Edward (CA)	Onc	354
Bagg, Adam (PA)	Path	643	Ball, William (OH)	NRad	912
Bagley, Demetrius (PA)	U	1050	Balla, Andre (IL)	Path	650
Bahado-Singh, Ray (MI)	MF	398	Ballantyne, Garth (NJ)	S	966
Bahn, Duke (CA)	RadRO	888	Ballard, Pamela (DC)	PMR	759
Bahn, Rebecca (MN)	EDM	206	Ballon-Landa, Gonzalo (CA)	Inf	383
Bahna, Sami (LA)	PA&I	668	Balmes, John (CA)	Pul	861
Bahnson, Robert (OH)	U	1063	Baltimore, Robert (CT)	PInf	711
Baile, Walter (TX)	Psyc	815	Baltuch, Gordon (PA)	NS	429
Bailey, H Randolph (TX)	CRS	171	Bancalari, Eduardo (FL)	NP	408
Bailey, Leonard (CA)	TS	1038	Bandyk, Dennis (FL)	VascS	1086
Bailey, Steven (TX)	IC	125	Banks, Peter (NC)	Path	648
Bailin, Philip (OH)	D	188	Bans, Larry (AZ)	U	1069
Baim, Howard (IL)	Oto	614	Bar-Chama, Natan (NY)	U	1050
Bains, Manjit (NY)	TS	1018	Barakat, Richard (NY)	GO	260
Bairey-Merz, C Noel (CA)	Cv	112	Baratz, Mark (PA)	HS	277
Bakay, Roy (IL)	NS	442	Barber, Douglas (TX)	PMR	766
Baker, Carol (TX)	PInf	715	Bardot, Stephen (LA)	U	1069
Baker, Christopher (LA)	S	994	Barger, Geoffrey (MI)	N	482
Baker, Daniel (NY)	PlS	774	Barie, Philip (NY)	S	966
Baker, Emily (NH)	MF	394	Barkin, Jamie (FL)	Ge	225
Baker, James (MI)	A&I	85	Barkovich, Anthony (CA)	NRad	914
Baker, John (MI)	Oph	534	Barksdale, Edward (OH)	PS	737
Baker, Robert (NY)	PGe	684	Barlogie, Bart (AR)	Hem	300
Baker, Shan (MI)	Oto	614			

Alphabetical Listing of Doctors

Name	Specialty	Pg	Name	Specialty	Pg
Belmont, H Michael (NY)	Rhu	941	Bergey, Gregory (MD)	N	466
Belsito, Donald (KS)	D	190	Bergman, Donald (NY)	EDM	200
Belsky, Mark (MA)	HS	276	Bergman, Ira (PA)	ChiN	143
Belzberg, Allan (MD)	NS	430	Bergsagel, Peter Leif (AZ)	Onc	348
Ben-Josef, Edgar (MI)	RadRO	881	Berguer, Ramon (MI)	VascS	1088
Benedetti, Costantino (OH)	PM	637	Berk, John (MA)	Pul	844
Benedetti, Enrico (IL)	S	984	Berke, Gerald (CA)	Oto	624
Benedetti, Thomas (WA)	MF	401	Berkowitz, Carol (CA)	Ped	664
Benedetto, Pasquale (FL)	Onc	325	Berkowitz, Leonard (NY)	Inf	375
Benenati, James (FL)	VIR	918	Berkowitz, Richard (NY)	MF	395
Benenati, Susan (FL)	A&I	84	Berkowitz, Ross (MA)	GO	258
Benevenia, Joseph (NJ)	OrS	559	Berkson, Richard (CA)	EDM	211
Benjamin, Ivor (UT)	Cv	110	Berl, Tomas (CO)	Nep	422
Benjamin, Robert (TX)	Onc	348	Berland, Lincoln (AL)	DR	904
Benkov, Keith (NY)	PGe	685	Berlin, Cheston (PA)	Ped	662
Bennett, Richard (CA)	D	192	Berlin, Jordan (TN)	Onc	325
Bennett, William (OR)	Nep	424	Berman, Brian (OH)	Ped	663
Benninger, Michael (OH)	Oto	614	Berman, James (IL)	PGe	687
Bensard, Denis (CO)	PS	740	Berman, Michael (CA)	GO	270
Bensinger, William (WA)	Onc	354	Bermant, Michael (VA)	PlS	781
Benson, Al (IL)	Onc	336	Bermudez, Ovidio (OK)	AM	77
Benson, Carol (MA)	DR	899	Bernad, Peter (VA)	N	476
Benson, Mitchell (NY)	U	1050	Bernard, Stephen (NC)	Onc	326
Bentley, Frederick (AR)	S	994	Bernstein, Daniel (CA)	PCd	676
Bentz, Michael (WI)	PlS	785	Bernstein, David (OH)	PInf	714
Benvenisty, Alan (NY)	VascS	1083	Bernstein, David (OH)	A&I	85
Benzel, Edward (OH)	NS	442	Bernstein, Jonathan (OH)	A&I	85
Benzon, Honorio (IL)	PM	637	Bernstein, Richard (IL)	N	482
Berchuck, Andrew (NC)	GO	263	Bernstein, Robert (NY)	D	180
Berde, Charles (MA)	PM	634	Berrey, B Hudson (FL)	OrS	572
Berek, Jonathan (CA)	GO	270	Bertolone, Salvatore (KY)	PHO	697
Berenstein, Alejandro (NY)	NRad	909	Bertorini, Tulio (TN)	N	477
Berg, Christine (MD)	RadRO	872	Besinger, Richard (IL)	MF	398
Berg, Daniel (WA)	D	192	Bessler, Marc (NY)	S	966
Berg, Stacey (TX)	PHO	707	Bettmann, Michael (NC)	VIR	918
Berg, Wendie (MD)	DR	900	Betz, Randal (PA)	OrS	559
Berga, Sarah (GA)	RE	931	Beyer, Eric (IL)	PHO	701
Berger, Joseph (KY)	N	476	Bhan, Atul (MA)	Path	642
Berger, Melvin (OH)	A&I	85	Bhattacharyya, Neil (MA)	Oto	599
Berger, Mitchel (CA)	NS	452	Bialer, Martin (NY)	CG	153

Name	Specialty	Pg	Name	Specialty	Pg
Biancaniello, Thomas (NY)	PCd	670	Blebea, John (OH)	VascS	1088
Bianchi, Diana (MA)	CG	152	Bleday, Ronald (MA)	CRS	164
Bichell, David (TN)	TS	1026	Bleiberg, Efrain (TX)	ChAP	828
Bickers, David (NY)	D	180	Blinder, Morey (MO)	Hem	295
Bieber, Eric (PA)	RE	927	Blitzer, Andrew (NY)	Oto	601
Biederman, Joseph (MA)	ChAP	822	Block, Susan (MA)	Psyc	804
Bierbrauer, Karin (OH)	NS	442	Bloom, David (MI)	U	1063
Bierman, Fredrick (NY)	PCd	670	Bloom, Patricia (NY)	Ger	246
Bierman, Philip (NE)	Onc	345	Bloomer, Joseph (AL)	Ge	225
Biermann, J Sybil (MI)	OrS	576	Bluemke, David (MD)	DR	900
Bigelow, Carolyn (MS)	Hem	293	Blum, Conrad (NY)	EDM	200
Biggs, David (DE)	Onc	310	Blumberg, Henry (GA)	Inf	378
Bigliani, Louis (NY)	OrS	560	Blume, Ralph (NY)	Rhu	941
Bilchik, Anton (CA)	S	1000	Blumenfeld, Hal (CT)	N	464
Bilezikian, John (NY)	EDM	200	Blumenfeld, Jon (NY)	Nep	417
Biller, Beverly (MA)	EDM	198	Blumenfield, Michael (CA)	Psyc	816
Billings, J Andrew (MA)	PM	634	Blumenkranz, Mark (CA)	Oph	543
Billmire, David (OH)	PlS	785	Blumenthal, David (NY)	Cv	95
Bilsky, Mark (NY)	NS	430	Blumenthal, Roger (MD)	Cv	95
Binder, Perry (CA)	Oph	543	Boachie-Adjei, Oheneba (NY)	OrS	560
Bird, Hector (NY)	ChAP	824	Bobrove, Arthur (CA)	Rhu	950
Bishop, Allen (MN)	HS	280	Bock, Samuel (CO)	PA&I	667
Bissell, Dwight (CA)	IM	391	Bockenstedt, Paula (MI)	Hem	295
Bitan, Fabien (NY)	OrS	560	Bockman, Richard (NY)	EDM	200
Bitran, Jacob (IL)	Onc	336	Boden, Scott (GA)	OrS	572
Bjorkman, David (UT)	Ge	235	Bodenheimer, Henry (NY)	Ge	217
Black, C Thomas (TX)	PS	740	Bogart, Jeffrey (NY)	RadRO	872
Black, Keith (CA)	NS	452	Boggan, James (CA)	NS	452
Black, Kevin (MO)	Psyc	812	Bogrov, Michael (MD)	ChAP	824
Black, Peter (MA)	NS	428	Bohlman, Henry (OH)	OrS	576
Black, William (NH)	DR	899	Boice, Charles (MD)	GO	260
Blackstock, A William (NC)	RadRO	877	Bojrab, Dennis (MI)	Oto	614
Blackwell, Richard (AL)	RE	931	Boland, C Richard (TX)	Ge	236
Blaha, John (MI)	OrS	576	Boles, Richard (CA)	CG	157
Blaivas, Jerry (NY)	U	1050	Bolger, Graeme (AL)	Onc	326
Blanchard, Daniel (CA)	Cv	112	Bolger, William (FL)	Oto	609
Bland, Kirby (AL)	S	977	Boling, Peter (VA)	Ger	247
Blaney, Susan (TX)	PHO	707	Bollen, Andrew (CA)	Path	655
Blatt, Julie (NC)	PHO	697	Bolman, Ralph Morton (MA)	TS	1016
Blazer, Dan (NC)	Psyc	811	Bolognia, Jean (CT)	D	178

Alphabetical Listing of Doctors

Name	Specialty	Pg	Name	Specialty	Pg
Bolton, John (LA)	S	995	Boxrud, Cynthia (CA)	Oph	544
Bolton, W Kline (VA)	Nep	419	Boyajian, Michael (DC)	PlS	774
Bolwell, Brian (OH)	Onc	336	Boyd, Stuart (CA)	U	1073
Bond, Sheldon (KY)	PS	736	Boyer, Thomas (AZ)	Ge	237
Bonner, James (AL)	A&I	84	Boyle, Robert (VA)	NP	409
Bonner, James (AL)	RadRO	877	Brackmann, Derald (CA)	Oto	624
Bonomi, Philip (IL)	Onc	336	Braddom, Randall (NJ)	PMR	759
Bonow, Robert (IL)	Cv	104	Bradford, Carol (MI)	Oto	614
Boone, Timothy (TX)	U	1070	Bradley, James (PA)	SM	954
Boop, Frederick (TN)	NS	437	Bradley, Jeffrey (MO)	RadRO	881
Booth, Robert (PA)	OrS	560	Bradley, John (CA)	PInf	716
Borchert, Mark (CA)	Oph	543	Brady, Charles (TX)	Ge	237
Borden, Ernest (OH)	Onc	336	Brady, Kathleen (SC)	AdP	821
Borer, Jeffrey (NY)	Cv	95	Braman, Sidney (RI)	Pul	844
Borgen, Patrick (NY)	S	966	Branch, Charles (NC)	NS	437
Borges, Lawrence (MA)	NS	428	Brandt, Fredric (NY)	D	181
Borkowsky, William (NY)	PInf	712	Brandt, Harry (MD)	Psyc	806
Boronow, John (MD)	Psyc	806	Brandt, Keith (MO)	PlS	785
Borowitz, Drucy (NY)	PPul	725	Brandt, Lawrence (NY)	Ge	217
Borson, Soo (WA)	GerPsy	832	Branham, Gregory (MO)	Oto	615
Borum, Marie (DC)	Ge	217	Brasington, Richard (MO)	Rhu	947
Borzak, Steven (FL)	Cv	101	Braun, Martin (DC)	D	181
Bos, Gary (WA)	OrS	584	Braunstein, Glenn (CA)	EDM	211
Bosl, George (NY)	Onc	310	Braunstein, Seth (PA)	IM	388
Boston, Barry (TN)	Onc	326	Brause, Barry (NY)	Inf	375
Bostwick, David (VA)	Path	648	Braverman, Alan (MO)	Cv	104
Boucek, Robert (WA)	PCd	676	Braylan, Raul (FL)	Path	648
Bourdette, Dennis (OR)	N	492	Brazer, Scott (NC)	Ge	225
Bourge, Robert (AL)	Cv	101	Brecher, Martin (NY)	PHO	692
Boushey, Homer (CA)	Pul	861	Breidenbach, Warren (KY)	HS	279
Bouvet, Michael (CA)	S	1000	Breitbart, William (NY)	Psyc	806
Bove, Alfred (PA)	Cv	95	Brem, Henry (MD)	NS	430
Bove, Edward (MI)	PS	738	Brem, Rachel (DC)	DR	900
Bowden, Charles (TX)	Psyc	815	Brem, Steven (FL)	NS	437
Bowen, Glen (UT)	D	191	Brems, John (IL)	S	984
Bowen, James (WA)	N	492	Brendler, Charles (IL)	U	1063
Bower, Charles (AR)	PO	724	Brener, Bruce (NJ)	VascS	1083
Boxer, Gary (MO)	ChAP	827	Brennan, Daniel (MO)	Nep	420
Boxer, Laurence (MI)	PHO	702	Brennan, Michael (MN)	EDM	206
Boxer Wachler, Brian (CA)	Oph	543	Brennan, Murray (NY)	S	967

Name	Specialty	Pg	Name	Specialty	Pg
Brennan, Stephen (TX)	Nep	422	Brooks, Ari (PA)	S	967
Brenner, Barry (MA)	Nep	416	Brooks, Benjamin (NC)	N	477
Brenner, Joel (MD)	PCd	670	Brooks, David (MA)	S	962
Brenner, Malcolm (TX)	Hem	300	Brooks, John (PA)	Path	643
Brenner, Michael (MA)	Rhu	940	Brooks, Stuart (FL)	Pul	851
Brent, Burton (CA)	PlS	792	Brown, Daniel (PA)	VIR	916
Brent, David (PA)	ChAP	824	Brown, Frederick (IL)	NS	442
Bresalier, Robert (TX)	Ge	237	Brown, Gary (PA)	Oph	520
Brescia, Frank (SC)	Onc	326	Brown, John (IN)	TS	1030
Bressler, Neil (MD)	Oph	520	Brown, Kevin (CO)	Pul	858
Bressman, Susan (NY)	N	466	Brown, Kimberly (MI)	Ge	230
Brewer, Molly (CT)	GO	258	Brown, Robert (NY)	Ge	218
Brewster, David (MA)	VascS	1082	Brown, Robert (MN)	N	482
Brick, Gregory (MA)	OrS	556	Browne, J Dale (NC)	Oto	609
Brick, John (WV)	N	467	Browner, Bruce (CT)	OrS	556
Bricker, John (KY)	PCd	672	Brozena, Susan (PA)	Cv	95
Bricker, Leslie (MI)	Onc	337	Bruce, Jeffrey (NY)	NS	430
Bridges, Charles (PA)	TS	1019	Brucker, Alexander (PA)	Oph	520
Bridwell, Keith (MO)	OrS	576	Bruera, Eduardo (TX)	Onc	348
Brien, Earl (CA)	OrS	584	Brufsky, Adam (PA)	Onc	310
Brindis, Ralph (CA)	Cv	112	Bruggers, Carol (UT)	PHO	706
Brink, Robert (CA)	PlS	792	Bruner, Janet (TX)	Path	653
Bristow, Robert (MD)	GO	260	Brunicardi, F Charles (TX)	S	995
Britt, L D (VA)	S	977	Brunsting, Louis (TN)	TS	1026
Brizel, David (NC)	RadRO	877	Brunstrom, Janice (MO)	ChiN	145
Brock, John (TN)	U	1058	Brunt, L Michael (MO)	S	984
Brockstein, Bruce (IL)	Onc	337	Brushart, Thomas (MD)	OrS	560
Broderick, Gregory (FL)	RE	931	Brust, John (NY)	N	467
Broderick, Joseph (OH)	N	482	Bryson, Yvonne (CA)	PInf	716
Brodkin, Edward (PA)	Psyc	806	Buatti, John (IA)	RadRO	881
Brodland, David (PA)	D	181	Bubley, Glenn (MA)	Onc	304
Brodman, Michael (NY)	ObG	508	Bucciarelli, Richard (FL)	NP	409
Brodsky, James (TX)	OrS	583	Buch, Jeffrey (TX)	U	1070
Brody, Fred (DC)	S	967	Buchanan, George (TX)	PHO	707
Brody, Harold (GA)	D	185	Buchbinder, Ellen (NY)	A&I	82
Bromberg, Jonathan (NY)	S	967	Buchholz, David (MD)	N	467
Bromberg, Mark (UT)	N	487	Buchholz, Thomas (TX)	RadRO	886
Bromfield, Edward (MA)	N	464	Buchman, Steven (MI)	PlS	785
Bronheim, Harold (NY)	Psyc	807	Buchman, Timothy (GA)	S	977
Bronson, Michael (NY)	OrS	560	Bucholz, Robert (TX)	OrS	583

Alphabetical Listing of Doctors

Name	Specialty	Pg	Name	Specialty	Pg
Buckley, Edward (NC)	Oph	529	Burton, Claude (NC)	D	185
Buckner, Jan (MN)	Onc	337	Burton, John (MD)	Ger	246
Buckwalter, Joseph (IA)	OrS	576	Bury, Robert (ND)	ObG	512
Bucky, Louis (PA)	PlS	775	Bushman, Wade (WI)	U	1063
Budd, George (OH)	Onc	337	Busse, William (WI)	A&I	85
Budenz, Donald (FL)	Oph	529	Bussel, James (NY)	PHO	692
Budoff, Matthew (CA)	Cv	113	Busuttil, Ronald (CA)	S	1000
Bueno, Raphael (MA)	TS	1016	Butler, Charles (TX)	PlS	790
Bukstein, Oscar (PA)	ChAP	824	Butler, David (TX)	D	191
Bull, David (UT)	TS	1035	Butler, John (CA)	S	1000
Bull, Marilyn (IN)	Ped	663	Butler, William (SC)	Onc	326
Buly, Robert (NY)	OrS	560	Buxton, Alfred (RI)	CE	115
Bumpous, Jeffrey (KY)	Oto	609	Buyon, Jill (NY)	Rhu	942
Bunchman, Timothy (MI)	PNep	718	Buys, Saundra (UT)	Onc	346
Bunn, Paul (CO)	Onc	345	Buysse, Daniel (PA)	Psyc	807
Bunning, Robert (DC)	Rhu	942	Buzdar, Aman (TX)	Onc	348
Burchiel, Kim (OR)	NS	452	Byrd, Benjamin (TN)	Cv	101
Burger, Peter (MD)	Path	643	Byrd, David (WA)	S	1000
Burgess, David (NJ)	Ped	662	Byrd, H Stephenson (TX)	PlS	790
Burke, Allan (IL)	N	482	Byrd, John (OH)	Hem	295
Burke, Charles (PA)	SM	954	Byrne, Janice (UT)	ObG	512
Burke, Dennis (MA)	OrS	556	Bystritsky, Alexander (CA)	Psyc	816
Burke, Miles (OH)	Oph	534	Bystryn, Jean-Claude (NY)	D	181
Burke, Peter (MA)	S	962			
Burke, William (NE)	GerPsy	831			
Burket, Mark (OH)	Cv	105			
Burkey, Brian (OH)	Oto	615			
			## C		
Burks, Arvil Wesley (NC)	PA&I	666	Cabin, Henry (CT)	Cv	92
Burnett, Alexander (AR)	GO	268	Cagle, Philip (TX)	Path	653
Burnett, Arthur (MD)	U	1050	Cahill, John (NY)	PrM	800
Burns, A Jay (TX)	PlS	789	Cahill, Kevin (NY)	PrM	801
Burns, Richard (AZ)	N	488	Cain, Joanna (RI)	GO	258
Burris, Howard (TN)	Onc	326	Cairo, Mitchell (NY)	PHO	692
Burstein, Fernando (GA)	PlS	781	Calabrese, Joseph (OH)	Psyc	813
Burstein, Harold (MA)	Onc	304	Caldamone, Anthony (RI)	U	1048
Burt, Randall (UT)	Ge	235	Caldarelli, David (IL)	Oto	615
Burt, Richard (IL)	Onc	337	Caldwell, Randall (IN)	PCd	673
Burt, Vivien (CA)	Psyc	816	Calhoon, John (TX)	TS	1036
Burton, Allen (TX)	PM	638	Califf, Robert (NC)	Cv	101
Burton, Barbara (IL)	CG	155	Callaghan, John (IA)	OrS	577
			Callans, David (PA)	CE	115

Alphabetical Listing of Doctors

Alphabetical Listing of Doctors

Name	Specialty	Pg	Name	Specialty	Pg
Cassisi, Nicholas (FL)	Oto	609	Chang, Helena (CA)	S	1000
Castell, Donald (SC)	Ge	225	Chang, James (CA)	PlS	792
Castellino, Sharon (NC)	PHO	697	Chang, Jenny (TX)	Onc	349
Caster, Andrew (CA)	Oph	544	Chang, Karen (CA)	Path	656
Castle, Valerie (MI)	PHO	702	Chang, Kenneth (CA)	Ge	239
Catalona, William (IL)	U	1063	Chang, R Jeffrey (CA)	RE	936
Catanzaro, Antonino (CA)	Pul	861	Chang, Rowland (IL)	Rhu	947
Catherwood, Edward (NH)	Cv	92	Chang, Sam (TN)	U	1059
Caushaj, Fillor Philip (NY)	CRS	165	Chang, Stanley (NY)	Oph	520
Cederbaum, Stephen (CA)	CG	158	Chang-Miller, April (AZ)	Rhu	949
Cederna, Paul (MI)	PlS	786	Chao, Nelson (NC)	Onc	327
Celli, Bartolome (MA)	Pul	844	Chap, Linnea (CA)	Onc	354
Cello, John (CA)	Ge	239	Chapman, Paul (NY)	Onc	311
Cerfolio, Robert (AL)	TS	1026	Chapman, Robert (MI)	Onc	337
Cerqueira, Manuel (OH)	Cv	105	Chapman, William (MO)	S	985
Cetta, Frank (MN)	PCd	673	Char, Devron (CA)	Oph	544
Cha, Soonmee (CA)	NRad	914	Charboneau, J William (MN)	RadRO	881
Chabner, Bruce (MA)	Onc	305	Chari, Ravi (TN)	S	977
Chabot, John (NY)	S	967	Chari, Suresh (MN)	Ge	230
Chachoua, Abraham (NY)	Onc	311	Charles, Andrew (CA)	N	492
Chaikof, Elliot (GA)	VascS	1086	Charney, Jonathan (NY)	N	467
Chaisson, Richard (MD)	Inf	375	Charrow, Joel (IL)	CG	155
Chaitman, Bernard (MO)	Cv	105	Chatham, Walter (AL)	Rhu	945
Chakravarthy, Anuradha (TN)	RadRO	877	Chatterjee, Kanu (CA)	Cv	113
Chalian, Ara (PA)	Oto	601	Chen, Allen (MD)	PHO	692
Chamberlain, Marc (WA)	ChiN	147	Chen, Chun (NY)	NS	430
Chambers, Richard (CA)	OrS	585	Chen, David (IL)	PMR	762
Chambers, Setsuko (AZ)	GO	269	Chen, Thomas (CA)	NS	452
Champlin, Richard (TX)	Hem	300	Cheng, Edward (MN)	OrS	577
Chan, John (CA)	GO	270	Cherny, W Bruce (ID)	NS	447
Chan, Kenny (CO)	PO	723	Cherry, Kenneth (VA)	VascS	1086
Chanan-Khan, Asher (NY)	Onc	311	Chervenak, Francis (NY)	MF	395
Chancellor, Michael (MI)	U	1064	Chesney, Carolyn (TN)	Path	648
Chand, Bipan (OH)	S	984	Cheson, Bruce (DC)	Hem	289
Chandar, Jayanthi (FL)	PNep	717	Cheville, Andrea (MN)	PMR	763
Chandler, James (IL)	NS	443	Chey, William (MI)	Ge	230
Chandler, Michael (NY)	A&I	82	Childs, Stacy (CO)	U	1069
Chandler, William (MI)	NS	443	Chinitz, Larry (NY)	CE	115
Chandrasoma, Parakrama (CA)	Path	655	Chiocca, E Antonio (OH)	NS	443
Chang, Alfred (MI)	S	984	Chitambar, Christopher (WI)	Onc	337

Alphabetical Listing of Doctors

Alphabetical Listing of Doctors

Name	Specialty	Pg	Name	Specialty	Pg
Cohen, Mark (IL)	HS	280	Connolly, Heidi (MN)	Cv	105
Cohen, Martin (NY)	CE	116	Connolly, James (MA)	Path	642
Cohen, Michael (IA)	Path	651	Connolly, Suzanne (AZ)	D	191
Cohen, Mitchell (OH)	PGe	687	Conrad, Ernest (WA)	OrS	585
Cohen, Mitchell (PA)	Psyc	807	Conry, Robert (AL)	Onc	327
Cohen, Myron (NC)	Inf	379	Constantian, Mark (NH)	PlS	772
Cohen, Philip (DC)	Onc	311	Constine, Louis (NY)	RadRO	872
Cohen, Robbin (CA)	TS	1038	Conte, John (MD)	TS	1019
Cohen, Roger (PA)	Onc	311	Conti, David (NY)	S	968
Cohen, Seymour (NY)	Onc	312	Cook, Jonathan (NC)	D	186
Cohen, Steven (CA)	PlS	792	Cook, Stuart (NJ)	N	467
Cohn, David (CO)	Inf	382	Cookson, Michael (TN)	U	1059
Cohn, John (PA)	A&I	82	Cooney, Leo (CT)	Ger	246
Cohn, Richard (IL)	PNep	718	Cooper, Barry (TX)	Hem	300
Cohn, Susan (IL)	PHO	702	Cooper, Christopher (OH)	Cv	105
Coit, Daniel (NY)	S	967	Cooper, Dan (CA)	PPul	729
Colachis, Samuel (OH)	PMR	763	Cooper, Daniel (TX)	OrS	583
Colberg, John (CT)	U	1048	Cooper, David (MD)	EDM	200
Cole, Andrew (MA)	N	464	Cooper, Joel (PA)	TS	1019
Cole, Brian (IL)	SM	956	Cooper, John (AL)	Pul	851
Cole, David (SC)	S	978	Cooper, Michael (CO)	VascS	1090
Cole, Francis (MO)	NP	410	Cooper, Rubin (NY)	PCd	670
Coleman, Beverly (PA)	DR	900	Cooper, William (VA)	Pul	852
Coleman, John (IN)	PlS	786	Cope, Doris (PA)	PM	634
Coleman, Morton (NY)	Onc	312	Copel, Joshua (CT)	MF	394
Coleman, R Edward (NC)	NuM	504	Copelan, Edward (OH)	Hem	295
Collea, Joseph (DC)	MF	395	Copeland, Jack (AZ)	TS	1036
Coller, Barry (NY)	Hem	290	Copeland, Larry (OH)	GO	266
Collins, Dale (NH)	PlS	772	Coplen, Douglas (MO)	U	1064
Colombani, Paul (MD)	PS	733	Copp, Steven (CA)	OrS	585
Colon-Otero, Gerardo (FL)	Onc	327	Copperman, Alan (NY)	RE	927
Colquhoun, Steven (CA)	S	1000	Coppola, John (NY)	Cv	95
Colvin, Edward (AL)	PCd	672	Coran, Arnold (MI)	PS	738
Come, Steven (MA)	Onc	305	Corbett, James (MS)	N	477
Comenzo, Raymond (MA)	Hem	288	Cordeiro, Peter (NY)	PlS	775
Comerota, Anthony (OH)	VascS	1088	Corey, G Ralph (NC)	Inf	379
Comi, Anne (MD)	ChiN	143	Corey, Jacquelynne (IL)	Oto	615
Comi, Richard (NH)	EDM	198	Corey, Lawrence (WA)	Inf	383
Cominelli, Fabio (OH)	Ge	230	Corey, Seth (IL)	PHO	702
Conant, Emily (PA)	DR	900	Corey-Bloom, Jody (CA)	N	492

Alphabetical Listing of Doctors

Name	Specialty	Pg	Name	Specialty	Pg
Currie, John (CT)	GO	258	Darras, Basil (MA)	ChiN	142
Curry, Cynthia (CA)	CG	158	Darrow, David (VA)	PO	722
Curtin, Hugh (MA)	NRad	909	Darwin, Christine (CA)	EDM	211
Curtin, John (NY)	GO	261	Das, Ananya (AZ)	Ge	237
Curtis, Anne (FL)	CE	116	Daspit, C Phillip (AZ)	Oto	622
Cushing, Brad (ME)	S	962	Daud, Adil (CA)	Onc	355
Cushman, William (TN)	IM	389	Daugherty, Christopher (IL)	Onc	338
Cutrer, F Michael (MN)	N	482	David, Carlos (MA)	NS	428
Cutting, Court (NY)	PlS	775	Davidoff, Andrew (TN)	PS	736
Czuczman, Myron (NY)	Onc	312	Davidson, Bruce (DC)	Oto	602
			Davidson, Dennis (NY)	NP	406
			Davidson, Joyce (TX)	Psyc	815
			Davidson, Nancy (PA)	Onc	312

D

Name	Specialty	Pg
D'Alton, Mary (NY)	MF	396
D'Amico, Anthony (MA)	RadRO	870
D'Amico, Donald (NY)	Oph	520
D'Amico, Thomas (NC)	TS	1026
Daar, Eric (CA)	Inf	383
Dabbagh, Shermine (DE)	PNep	716
Dacey, Ralph (MO)	NS	443
Dae, Michael (CA)	NuM	505
Dagum, Alexander (NY)	PlS	775
Dakhil, Shaker (KS)	Onc	346
Dalakas, Marinos (PA)	N	467
Dale, Lowell (MN)	Ger	248
Dalinka, Murray (PA)	DR	901
Dalkin, Alan (VA)	EDM	204
Dalsing, Michael (IN)	VascS	1088
Daly, Mary (PA)	Onc	312
Damewood, Marian (PA)	RE	928
Damiano, Ralph (MO)	TS	1031
Damon, Lloyd (CA)	Hem	302
Dana, Reza (MA)	Oph	518
Daneshmand, Siamak (OR)	U	1073
Dang, Michael (HI)	TS	1038
Daniel, Rollin (CA)	PlS	792
Daniels, Gilbert (MA)	EDM	198
Danoff, Dudley (CA)	U	1073
Darcy, Michael (MO)	VIR	919
Darling, R Clement (NY)	VascS	1084

Name	Specialty	Pg
Davidson, Richard (PA)	OrS	561
Davidson, Susan (CO)	GO	268
Davies, Stella (OH)	PHO	702
Davies, Terry (NY)	EDM	200
Davis, Bradley (KS)	U	1069
Davis, Gary (TX)	Ge	237
Davis, Jessica (NY)	CG	153
Davis, Jonathan (MA)	NP	406
Davis, Mellar (OH)	Onc	338
Davis, William (LA)	Rhu	949
Dawson, Nancy (DC)	Onc	312
Day, Arthur (MA)	NS	428
Day, Susan (CA)	Oph	544
Day, Terrence (SC)	Oto	610
Dayton, Merril (NY)	S	968
De Angelis, Lisa (NY)	N	468
De Cherney, Alan (MD)	ObG	509
De Geest, Koen (IA)	GO	266
De Juan, Eugene (CA)	Oph	544
de Kernion, Jean (CA)	U	1073
De la Cruz, Antonio (CA)	Oto	625
De Lateur, Barbara (MD)	PMR	759
De Leon-Casasola, Oscar (NY)	PM	634
De Lia, Julian (WI)	ObG	511
De Long, Mahlon (GA)	N	477
De Luca, Francesco (PA)	PEn	679
De Masters, Bette (CO)	Path	653

Name	Specialty	Pg	Name	Specialty	Pg
De Meester, Tom (CA)	TS	1038	Dempsey, Robert (WI)	NS	443
De Monte, Franco (TX)	NS	449	Denenberg, Steven (NE)	Oto	621
De Simone, Philip (KY)	Onc	327	Denny, Donald (NJ)	VIR	916
De Vivo, Darryl (NY)	ChiN	143	Denson, Susan (TX)	NP	411
Dean, Jonathan (UT)	PCCM	677	DeOrio, James (NC)	OrS	572
Deas, Deborah (SC)	ChAP	826	DePaulo, J Raymond (MD)	Psyc	807
DeBaun, Michael (MO)	PHO	702	DePompolo, Robert (MN)	PMR	763
DeCamp, Malcolm (MA)	TS	1016	DePriest, Paul (KY)	GO	263
Deeg, H. Joachim (WA)	Onc	355	Derman, Gordon (IL)	HS	280
DeFilippi, Vincent (CA)	TS	1038	DeRose, Joseph (NY)	TS	1019
DeGiorgio, Christopher (CA)	N	492	Dershaw, D David (NY)	DR	901
Deitch, Edwin (NJ)	S	968	Deschamps, Claude (MN)	TS	1031
Deitz, Joel (PA)	Pul	847	Deschler, Daniel (MA)	Oto	599
DeKosky, Steven (VA)	N	477	DeShazo, Richard (MS)	A&I	84
Del Giudice, Stephen (NH)	D	178	DeSilva, Stephen (MI)	HS	281
Del Monte, Monte (MI)	Oph	534	Desnick, Robert (NY)	CG	153
Del Negro, Albert (VA)	CE	116	Desposito, Franklin (NJ)	CG	153
Del Priore, Lucian (NY)	Oph	521	DeVane, Gary (FL)	RE	931
Delahay, John (DC)	OrS	561	DeVault, Kenneth (FL)	Ge	226
Delamarter, Rick (CA)	OrS	585	Devereux, Richard (NY)	Cv	95
DeLancey, John (MI)	ObG	511	Devinsky, Orrin (NY)	N	468
Deland, Jonathan (NY)	OrS	561	DeVita, Vincent (CT)	Onc	305
Delaney, Conor (OH)	CRS	168	Dewberry, Robert (MD)	N	468
DeLaney, Thomas (MA)	RadRO	870	DeWeese, Theodore (MD)	RadRO	872
DeLellis, Ronald (RI)	Path	642	Deziel, Daniel (IL)	S	985
Deleo, Vincent (NY)	D	181	Dezube, Bruce (MA)	Hem	288
Deleyiannis, Frederic (PA)	PlS	775	Dhanireddy, Ramasubbareddy (TN)	NP	409
Delivoria-Papadopoulos, Maria (PA)		NP 407	Di Bisceglie, Adrian (MO)	Ge	231
			Di Cesare, Paul (CA)	OrS	585
Dell, Diana (NC)	Psyc	811	Di Giacinto, George (NY)	NS	431
Della Rocca, Robert (NY)	Oph	521	Di Marino, Anthony (PA)	Ge	218
Delmez, James (MO)	Nep	420	Di Persio, John (MO)	Hem	295
DeLurgio, David (GA)	CE	117	Di Saia, Philip (CA)	GO	271
Demarest, Gerald (NM)	S	995	Diamond, Frank (FL)	PEn	680
DeMars, Leslie (NH)	GO	258	Diamond, Michael (MI)	RE	933
Demer, Joseph (CA)	Oph	545	Diamond, Paul (VA)	PMR	761
Demetri, George (MA)	Onc	305	Dias, Mark (PA)	NS	431
Demetris, Anthony (PA)	Path	644	Diaz, Angela (NY)	AM	76
Demmy, Todd (NY)	TS	1019	Diaz, Fernando (MI)	NS	443
Dempsey, Daniel (PA)	S	968	Dichek, David (WA)	Cv	113

Alphabetical Listing of Doctors

Name	Specialty	Pg	Name	Specialty	Pg
Dromerick, Alexander (DC)	N	468	Eagle, Ralph (PA)	Oph	521
Drossman, Douglas (NC)	Ge	226	Earp, H Shelton (NC)	EDM	204
Druker, Brian (OR)	Onc	355	Eason, James (TN)	S	978
Druzin, Maurice (CA)	MF	402	Easter, David (CA)	S	1001
Dubeau, Louis (CA)	Path	656	Eaton, James (DC)	Psyc	807
Dubinsky, Marla (CA)	PGe	689	Eavey, Roland (TN)	PO	722
Dubois, Michel (NY)	PM	635	Eberlein, Timothy (MO)	S	985
Ducore, Jonathan (CA)	PHO	709	Ebraheim, Nabil (OH)	OrS	577
Duff, W Patrick (FL)	MF	510	Echeverri, Luis (TX)	TS	1036
Duffner, Patricia (NY)	ChiN	143	Eckardt, Jeffrey (CA)	OrS	586
Duffy, Thomas (CT)	Hem	288	Eckel, Robert (CO)	EDM	209
Dufresne, Craig (MD)	PlS	775	Eckhardt, S (CO)	Onc	346
Dugoff, Lorraine (CO)	MF	400	Eckhoff, Devin (AL)	S	978
Duh, Quan-Yang (CA)	S	1001	Econs, Michael (IN)	EDM	206
Duhaime, Ann (NH)	NS	428	Edelman, Martin (MD)	Onc	313
Duker, Jay (MA)	Oph	518	Edelman, Robert (IL)	DR	905
Dulcan, Mina (IL)	ChAP	827	Edelson, Richard (CT)	D	178
Dumesic, Daniel (MN)	RE	933	Edelstein, Barbara (NY)	DR	901
Dumitru, Daniel (TX)	PMR	766	Edelstein, David (NY)	Oto	602
Duncan, Brian (OH)	PS	738	Edgar, Terence (WI)	ChiN	146
Duncan, Newton (TX)	PO	724	Edge, Stephen (NY)	S	968
Dunkel, Ira (NY)	PHO	693	Edington, Howard (PA)	S	969
Dunlap, Nancy (AL)	Pul	852	Edmond, Michael (VA)	Inf	379
Dunphy, Frank (NC)	Onc	327	Edmundowicz, Daniel (PA)	Cv	96
Dunton, Charles (PA)	GO	261	Edmundowicz, Steven (MO)	Ge	231
DuPont, Herbert (TX)	Inf	382	Edney, James (NE)	S	993
Durbin, William (MA)	PInf	712	Edwards, John (CA)	Inf	383
Dure, Leon (AL)	N	477	Edwards, Kathryn (TN)	PInf	713
Durham, Janette (CO)	VIR	920	Edwards, Michael (OH)	S	985
Durham, Samuel (OH)	TS	1031	Edwards, Michael (CA)	NS	452
Durrie, Daniel (KS)	Oph	540	Edwards, Robert (PA)	GO	261
Duthie, Edmund (WI)	Ger	249	Edye, Michael (NY)	S	969
Dutton, Jonathan (NC)	Oph	529	Efron, Jonathan (AZ)	CRS	171
Duvic, Madeleine (TX)	D	191	Eggers, Howard (NY)	Oph	521
Dyer, Carmel (TX)	Ger	250	Ehrenkranz, Richard (CT)	NP	406
Dzubow, Leonard (PA)	D	181	Ehresmann, Glenn (CA)	Rhu	950
			Ehrlich, Paul (NY)	PA&I	665
			Ehrlich, Peter (MI)	PS	738
E			Ehrmann, David (IL)	EDM	206
			Ehya, Hormoz (PA)	Path	644
Eagle, Kim (MI)	Cv	105			

Alphabetical Listing of Doctors

Name	Specialty	Pg	Name	Specialty	Pg
Eichelberger, Martin (DC)	PS	734	Ellis, William (WA)	U	1073
Eichenfield, Lawrence (CA)	D	193	Ellison, David (OR)	Nep	424
Eichler, Craig (FL)	D	186	Ellison, E Christopher (OH)	S	985
Eidt, John (AR)	VascS	1090	Ellison, James (MA)	Psyc	804
Eifel, Patricia (TX)	RadRO	886	Ellman, Leonard (MA)	Hem	288
Eilber, Frederick (CA)	S	1001	Elmets, Craig (AL)	D	186
Ein, Daniel (DC)	A&I	83	Elner, Victor (MI)	Oph	534
Einhorn, Lawrence (IN)	Onc	338	Eloubeidi, Mohamad (AL)	Ge	226
Einhorn, Thomas (MA)	OrS	556	Elster, Allen (NC)	DR	904
Eisele, David (CA)	Oto	625	Elta, Grace (MI)	Ge	231
Eisen, Howard (PA)	Cv	96	Emami, Bahman (IL)	RadRO	882
Eisenberg, Burton (NH)	S	962	Emans, Sarah (MA)	AM	76
Eisenberg, Howard (MD)	NS	431	Emanuel, Peter (AR)	Hem	300
Eisenberger, Mario (MD)	Onc	313	Emanuele, Mary Ann (IL)	EDM	207
Eisendrath, Stuart (CA)	Psyc	817	Emanuele, Nicholas (IL)	EDM	207
Eisenstat, Theodore (NJ)	CRS	165	Emery, Helen (WA)	PRhu	732
Eismont, Frank (FL)	OrS	572	Emhoff, Timothy (MA)	S	963
El-Galley, Rizk (AL)	U	1059	Emmanuel, Patricia (FL)	PInf	714
El-Youssef, Mounif (MN)	PGe	687	Emond, Jean (NY)	S	969
Elder, Jack (MI)	U	1064	Emre, Sukru (CT)	S	963
Elefteriades, John (CT)	TS	1016	Emslie, Graham (TX)	ChAP	828
Elias, Anthony (CO)	Onc	346	Endrizzi, Donald (ME)	OrS	556
Elias, Sherman (IL)	CG	155	Enelow, Richard (NH)	Pul	844
Elias, Stanton (MI)	N	482	Eng, Charis (OH)	Onc	339
Elkayam, Uri (CA)	Cv	113	Eng, Kenneth (NY)	S	969
Ellenbogen, Kenneth (VA)	CE	117	Engel, William King (CA)	N	492
Ellenbogen, Richard (WA)	NS	452	Engstrom, John (CA)	N	493
Ellenhorn, Joshua (CA)	S	1001	Engstrom, Paul F (PA)	Onc	313
Elliott, C Gregory (UT)	Pul	858	Ennis, Ronald (NY)	RadRO	873
Elliott, David (IA)	Ge	231	Ensminger, William (MI)	Onc	339
Elliott, John (AZ)	MF	401	Epstein, Jeffrey (FL)	D	186
Elliott, Norman (GA)	Ge	226	Epstein, Jonathan (MD)	Path	644
Ellis, David (TX)	U	1070	Epstein, Leon (IL)	ChiN	146
Ellis, Demetrius (PA)	PNep	716	Epstein, Michael (FL)	PCd	672
Ellis, George (LA)	Oph	540	Epstein, Stuart (CA)	PA&I	668
Ellis, Georgiana (WA)	Onc	355	Erasmus, Jeremy (TX)	DR	907
Ellis, Jonathan (CA)	Ge	239	Erba, Harry (MI)	Hem	295
Ellis, Lee (TX)	S	995	Erban, John (MA)	Onc	305
Ellis, Matthew (MO)	Onc	339	Eriksson, Elof (MA)	PlS	772
Ellis, Stephen (OH)	IC	124	Ernst, Armin (MA)	Pul	845

Alphabetical Listing of Doctors

Name	Specialty	Pg	Name	Specialty	Pg
Feldman, Joel (MA)	PlS	772	Finger, Paul (NY)	Oph	521
Feldman, Joseph (IL)	PMR	763	Fink, Matthew (NY)	N	468
Feldman, Kenneth (WA)	Ped	664	Finkel, Alan (NC)	N	477
Feldman, Mark (TX)	Ge	237	Finkel, Michael (FL)	N	477
Feldman, Ted (IL)	IC	124	Finkel, Richard (PA)	ChiN	144
Feldmann, Edward (RI)	N	464	Finkel, Terri (PA)	PRhu	730
Feldon, Steven (NY)	Oph	521	Finklestein, Jerry (CA)	PHO	709
Feldstein, Neil (NY)	NS	431	Finlay, Jonathan (CA)	PHO	709
Feliciano, David (GA)	S	978	Finlayson, Christina (CO)	S	993
Felig, Philip (NY)	EDM	201	Finucane, Thomas (MD)	Ger	246
Felix, Carolyn (PA)	PHO	693	Fiorica, James (FL)	GO	264
Fenichel, Gerald (TN)	ChiN	144	Firlit, Casimir (MO)	U	1064
Fennerty, Brian (OR)	Ge	239	First, Michael (NY)	Psyc	808
Fenske, Neil (FL)	D	186	Fisch, Harry (NY)	U	1051
Ferber, Richard (MA)	Ped	662	Fischbein, Lewis (MO)	Rhu	947
Ferguson, James (VA)	MF	397	Fischer, Thomas (IN)	HS	281
Ferguson, Mark (IL)	TS	1031	Fish, Frank (TN)	PCd	672
Fernhoff, Paul (GA)	CG	154	Fishbein, Daniel (WA)	Cv	113
Ferrante, F Michael (CA)	PM	639	Fishbein, Michael (CA)	Path	656
Ferrara, James (MI)	PHO	703	Fisher, Garth (CA)	PlS	793
Ferrell, Linda (CA)	Path	656	Fisher, George (CA)	Onc	356
Ferrendelli, James (TX)	N	489	Fisher, Mark (CA)	N	493
Ferriero, Donna (CA)	ChiN	148	Fisher, Paul (CA)	ChiN	148
Ferris, Frank (CA)	IM	391	Fisher, Richard (NY)	Onc	314
Fessler, Richard (IL)	NS	443	Fisher, Robert (PA)	Ge	218
Fewkes, Jessica (MA)	D	178	Fisher, Robert (CA)	N	493
Fidler, Jeff (MN)	DR	905	Fisher, William (TX)	S	996
Fields, Abbie (DC)	GO	261	Fishman, David (NY)	GO	261
Fields, Theodore (NY)	Rhu	942	Fishman, Elliot (MD)	DR	901
Figlin, Robert (CA)	Onc	356	Fishman, Henry (DC)	A&I	83
Files, Joe (MS)	Hem	293	Fishman, Scott (CA)	PM	639
Filip, Stanley (NC)	ObG	510	Fitch, Tom (AZ)	Onc	349
Filley, Christopher (CO)	N	487	Fitzgerald, Paul (CA)	EDM	211
Filly, Roy (CA)	DR	908	Fitzgibbon, Dermot (WA)	PM	640
Finan, Michael (AL)	GO	263	Fitzgibbons, Robert (NE)	S	993
Fine, Howard (MD)	Onc	313	Fitzpatrick, Richard (CA)	D	193
Fine, Perry (UT)	PM	638	Fivenson, David (MI)	D	188
Fine, Robert (NY)	Onc	314	Fivush, Barbara (MD)	PNep	717
Fine, Robert (TX)	IM	390	Fix, R Jobe (AL)	PlS	781
Finerman, Gerald (CA)	OrS	586	Flaherty, Alice (MA)	N	464

Name	Specialty	Pg	Name	Specialty	Pg
Flaherty, John (IL)	Inf	380	Forbess, Joseph (TX)	TS	1036
Flake, Alan (PA)	PS	734	Ford, Carol Ann (NC)	AM	76
Flamm, Scott (OH)	DR	905	Ford, Charles (WI)	Oto	615
Flanagan, Steven (NY)	PMR	760	Ford, Henri (CA)	PS	741
Flanders, Adam (PA)	NRad	910	Ford, James (CA)	Onc	356
Flanigan, D Preston (CA)	VascS	1091	Forero, Andres (AL)	Onc	327
Flanigan, Robert (IL)	U	1064	Forget, Bernard (CT)	Hem	288
Flanigan, Timothy (RI)	Inf	374	Forman, Jeffrey (MI)	RadRO	882
Flatow, Evan (NY)	OrS	562	Forman, Stephen (CA)	Hem	302
Fleischer, David (AZ)	Ge	238	Formenti, Silvia (NY)	RadRO	873
Fleischer, Norman (NY)	EDM	201	Fornari, Victor (NY)	ChAP	824
Fleisher, Gary (MA)	PCCM	676	Forscher, Charles (CA)	Onc	356
Fleming, Gini (IL)	Onc	339	Forsmark, Christopher (FL)	Ge	226
Fleshman, James (MO)	CRS	168	Forster, Richard (FL)	Oph	529
Fletcher, Christopher (MA)	Path	642	Fortenberry, J Dennis (IN)	AM	76
Fletcher, Eugene (IN)	Pul	855	Foss, Francine (CT)	Onc	305
Flickinger, John (PA)	RadRO	873	Fossella, Frank (TX)	Onc	349
Flinn, Ian (TN)	Onc	327	Fost, Norman (WI)	Ped	664
Flint, Paul (OR)	Oto	625	Foster, C Stephen (MA)	Oph	518
Flomenberg, Neal (PA)	Onc	314	Foster, Carol (UT)	PEn	683
Flowers, Franklin (FL)	D	186	Foster, Harris (CT)	U	1048
Flynn, Harry (FL)	Oph	529	Foster, Mark (NC)	OrS	572
Flynn, Joseph (WA)	PNep	720	Foster, Richard (IN)	U	1064
Flynn, Michael (KY)	S	978	Foucar, M Kathryn (NM)	Path	653
Flynn, Patrick (MN)	Hem	296	Fowble, Barbara (CA)	RadRO	888
Flynn, Timothy (FL)	VascS	1086	Fowl, Richard (AZ)	VascS	1090
Fodor, Peter (CA)	PlS	793	Fowler, Jeffrey (OH)	GO	266
Foglia, Robert (TX)	PS	741	Fowler, Wesley (NC)	GO	264
Fogt, Franz (PA)	Path	644	Fox, Harold (MD)	MF	396
Foley, Carmel (NY)	ChAP	824	Fox, James W (PA)	PlS	776
Foley, Eugene (WI)	CRS	168	Fox, Kevin (PA)	Onc	314
Foley, Kevin (TN)	NS	438	Fox, Peter (TX)	N	489
Follansbee, William (PA)	Cv	96	Fracasso, Paula (VA)	Onc	328
Follen, Michele (TX)	GO	269	Fraker, Douglas (PA)	S	969
Fonarow, Gregg (CA)	Cv	113	Frances, Richard (NY)	AdP	820
Fong, Yuman (NY)	S	969	Francisco, Gerard (TX)	PMR	766
Fonseca, Rafael (AZ)	Hem	301	Frangoul, Haydar (TN)	PHO	697
Fontana, Gregory (CA)	TS	1039	Frank, Ian (PA)	Inf	375
Foo, Sun-Hoo (NY)	N	469	Franklin, Morris (TX)	S	996
Forastiere, Arlene (MD)	Onc	314	Franks, Andrew (NY)	D	182

Alphabetical Listing of Doctors

Name	Specialty	Pg	Name	Specialty	Pg
Frantz, Christopher (DE)	PHO	693	Friedman, Matthew (VT)	Psyc	804
Frantzides, Constantine (IL)	S	986	Friedman, Michael (IL)	Oto	615
Fraser, Charles (TX)	TS	1036	Friedman, Nancy (NC)	PEn	681
Fraser, Lionel (MS)	U	1059	Friedman, Richard (TX)	PCd	675
Frassica, Frank (MD)	OrS	562	Friedman, Sanford (NY)	Cv	96
Frazee, John (CA)	NS	452	Friedman, Stuart (FL)	A&I	84
Frazier, Oscar (TX)	TS	1036	Frim, David (IL)	NS	444
Frazier, Thomas (PA)	S	970	Fritz, Gregory (RI)	ChAP	822
Freedman, Barry (NC)	Nep	419	Fritz, Marc (NC)	RE	931
Freedman, Gary (PA)	RadRO	873	Fromm, Geri-Lynn (TX)	GO	269
Freedman, Michael (NY)	Ger	247	Fronek, Jan (CA)	SM	957
Freedman, Robert (CO)	Psyc	814	Frost, Frederick (OH)	PMR	763
Freedman, Sharon (NC)	Oph	529	Fruchtman, Steven (NY)	Hem	290
Freeman, Gregory (TX)	Cv	110	Fry, Robert (PA)	CRS	165
Freeman, Leonard (NY)	NuM	502	Fu, Freddie (PA)	OrS	562
Freeman, Theodore (TX)	A&I	87	Fuchs, Charles (MA)	Onc	306
Freeman, Thomas (FL)	NS	438	Fuchs, Eugene (OR)	U	1073
Freemark, Michael (NC)	PEn	681	Fuchs, Wayne (NY)	Oph	522
Freiman, Hal (NY)	Ge	219	Fuhrman, Bradley (NY)	PCCM	676
Freischlag, Julie (MD)	VascS	1085	Fuhrman, Carl (PA)	DR	901
French, Jacqueline (NY)	N	469	Fulkerson, John (CT)	OrS	557
Friberg, Thomas (PA)	Oph	521	Fulkerson, William (NC)	Pul	852
Fricker, Frederick (FL)	PCd	672	Fullerton, David (CO)	TS	1035
Friebert, Sarah (OH)	PHO	703	Fung, John (OH)	S	986
Fried, Guy (PA)	PMR	760	Funk, Gerry (IA)	Oto	616
Fried, Marvin (NY)	Oto	602	Furie, Karen (MA)	N	465
Friedberg, Jonathan (NY)	Onc	314	Furlan, Anthony (OH)	N	483
Friedberg, Joseph (PA)	TS	1019	Furman, Wayne (TN)	PHO	698
Frieden, Ilona (CA)	D	193	Furukawa, Satoshi (PA)	TS	1020
Friedlaender, Gary (CT)	OrS	556	Fuster, Valentin (NY)	Cv	96
Friedland, Jack (AZ)	PlS	790	Futran, Neal (WA)	Oto	625
Friedlander, Sheila (CA)	D	193	Fyer, Abby (NY)	Psyc	808
Friedman, Aaron (MN)	PNep	719			
Friedman, Allan (NC)	NS	438			
Friedman, Barry (CA)	Psyc	817			
Friedman, Debra (TN)	PHO	698			
Friedman, Ellen (TX)	PO	724			
Friedman, Henry (NC)	PHO	698			
Friedman, Lawrence (MA)	Ge	216			
Friedman, Lloyd (CT)	Pul	845			

G

Name	Specialty	Pg
Gaasterland, Douglas (MD)	Oph	522
Gabbard, Glen (TX)	Psyc	816
Gabram, Sheryl (GA)	S	978
Gabrilove, Janice (NY)	Onc	314
Gaffney, David (UT)	RadRO	885

Name	Specialty	Pg	Name	Specialty	Pg
Gagner, Michel (FL)	S	978	Gearhart, John (MD)	U	1051
Gaissert, Henning (MA)	TS	1016	Gebhardt, Mark (MA)	OrS	557
Gajjar, Amar (TN)	PHO	698	Geffner, Mitchell (CA)	PEn	683
Galandiuk, Susan (KY)	CRS	167	Gefter, Warren (PA)	DR	901
Galanter, Marc (NY)	AdP	820	Geisler, Daniel (OH)	CRS	168
Galati, Joseph (TX)	Ge	238	Gejerman, Glen (NJ)	RadRO	873
Galetta, Steven (PA)	N	469	Gelb, Bruce (NY)	PCd	670
Galland, Leo (NY)	IM	388	Gelberman, Richard (MO)	HS	281
Gallico, G Gregory (MA)	PlS	772	Gelenberg, Alan (WI)	Psyc	813
Gallin, Pamela (NY)	Oph	522	Gelfand, Erwin (CO)	PA&I	668
Galloway, Aubrey (NY)	TS	1020	Geller, Kenneth (CA)	PO	724
Gambardella, Ralph (CA)	SM	957	Gelmann, Edward (NY)	Onc	314
Gambert, Steven (MD)	Ger	247	Geltman, Edward (MO)	Cv	105
Gambetti, Pierluigi (OH)	Path	651	Gendelman, Seymour (NY)	N	469
Gamble, Gail (IL)	PMR	763	Genden, Eric (NY)	Oto	602
Gamelli, Richard (IL)	S	986	Gentile, Ronald (NY)	Oph	522
Gandara, David (CA)	Onc	356	Georgeson, Keith (AL)	PS	736
Gandy, Winston (GA)	Cv	102	Georgiade, Gregory (NC)	PlS	782
Gang, Eli (CA)	CE	119	Gerdes, Hans (NY)	Ge	219
Ganguli, Rohan (PA)	Psyc	808	Geronemus, Roy (NY)	D	182
Gantz, Bruce (IA)	Oto	616	Gershenson, David (TX)	GO	269
Ganz, Patricia (CA)	Onc	356	Gershwin, Merrill (CA)	Rhu	950
Garber, Judy (MA)	Onc	306	Gerson, Lauren (CA)	Ge	239
Garcia-Prats, Joseph (TX)	NP	412	Gerson, Stanton (OH)	Onc	339
Garden, Jerome (IL)	D	188	Gertz, Morie (MN)	Hem	296
Garfin, Steven (CA)	OrS	586	Geschwind, Jean-Francois (MD)	VIR	917
Garin, Eduardo (FL)	PNep	717	Gewertz, Bruce (CA)	VascS	1092
Garner, Warren (CA)	PlS	793	Gewirtz, Alan (PA)	Hem	290
Garnick, Marc (MA)	Onc	306	Gewitz, Michael (NY)	PCd	670
Garrett, Algin (VA)	D	186	Gewolb, Ira (MI)	NP	410
Garrett, William (NC)	OrS	573	Gewurz, Anita (IL)	A&I	86
Garrity, Edward (IL)	Pul	855	Geyer, Charles (PA)	Onc	315
Garst, Jennifer (NC)	Onc	328	Geyer, J Russell (WA)	PHO	709
Garth, William (AL)	SM	956	Ghamande, Sharad (GA)	GO	264
Gartner, J Carlton (DE)	Ped	662	Gharagozloo, Farid (DC)	TS	1020
Garver, Robert (AL)	Pul	852	Gharibo, Christopher (NY)	PM	635
Garvin, James (NY)	PHO	693	Giannotta, Steven (CA)	NS	453
Garvin, Kevin (NE)	OrS	581	Gianoli, Gerard (LA)	Oto	622
Gater, David (VA)	PMR	762	Gianopoulos, John (IL)	MF	398
Gaynor, Ellen (IL)	Hem	296	Giardiello, Francis (MD)	Ge	219

Alphabetical Listing of Doctors

Name	Specialty	Pg	Name	Specialty	Pg
Giardina, Patricia (NY)	PHO	693	Glass, Jon (PA)	N	469
Gibbons, Raymond (MN)	Cv	106	Glass, Jonathan (GA)	N	478
Gibbs, John (NY)	S	970	Glassberg, Kenneth (NY)	U	1051
Gibbs, Ronald (CO)	MF	400	Glassburn, John (PA)	RadRO	873
Gibralter, Richard (NY)	Oph	522	Glassford, David (TN)	TS	1027
Gibson, C Michael (MA)	IC	120	Glat, Paul (PA)	PlS	776
Gigantelli, James (NE)	Oph	540	Glatstein, Eli (PA)	RadRO	873
Gilbert, Mark (TX)	N	489	Glenn, Mel (MA)	PMR	758
Gilchrest, Barbara (MA)	D	179	Glick, John (PA)	Onc	315
Gill, Harcharan (CA)	U	1074	Glick, Philip (NY)	PS	734
Gill, Inderbir (CA)	U	1074	Glickel, Steven (NY)	HS	277
Gillette, Paul (TX)	PCd	675	Gliklich, Jerry (NY)	Cv	96
Gillman, Matthew (MA)	IM	388	Gliklich, Richard (MA)	Oto	599
Gilman, Sid (MI)	N	483	Glisson, Bonnie (TX)	Onc	349
Gilsanz, Vicente (CA)	DR	908	Glode, L Michael (CO)	Onc	346
Gingold, Bruce (NY)	CRS	165	Glogau, Richard (CA)	D	193
Ginsberg, David (CA)	U	1074	Glombicki, Alan (TX)	Ge	238
Ginsberg, Gregory (PA)	Ge	219	Gloviczki, Peter (MN)	VascS	1088
Ginsburg, Elizabeth (MA)	RE	926	Gluck, Stephen (CA)	Nep	424
Ginsburg, Howard (NY)	PS	734	Gluckman, Gordon (IL)	U	1064
Ginsburg, Kenneth (PA)	AM	76	Gochfeld, Michael (NJ)	OM	800
Ginsburg, Mark (NY)	TS	1020	Gockerman, Jon (NC)	Onc	328
Ginzler, Ellen (NY)	Rhu	942	Godder, Kamar (VA)	PHO	698
Girardi, Leonard (NY)	TS	1020	Godine, John (MA)	EDM	198
Gish, Robert (CA)	Ge	239	Godley, Paul (NC)	Onc	328
Gitelis, Steven (IL)	OrS	577	Godwin, John (IL)	Hem	296
Gitlin, Michael (CA)	Psyc	817	Godzik, Cathleen (CA)	HS	283
Gittes, George (PA)	PS	734	Goebel, Joel (MO)	Oto	616
Gittler, Michelle (IL)	PMR	763	Goetz, Christopher (IL)	N	483
Giuliano, Armando (CA)	S	1002	Goff, Barbara (WA)	GO	271
Giuntoli, Robert (MD)	GO	261	Goff, Donald (MA)	Psyc	804
Giustra, Lawrence (GA)	Psyc	811	Goggins, Michael (MD)	Ge	219
Givan, Deborah (IN)	PPul	727	Goitz, Henry (MI)	OrS	577
Givner, Laurence (NC)	PInf	714	Gokaslan, Ziya (MD)	NS	431
Gizzi, Martin (NJ)	N	469	Golbe, Lawrence (NJ)	N	469
Glader, Bertil (CA)	PHO	709	Gold, Philip (WA)	Onc	357
Gladstone, James (NY)	OrS	562	Gold, Scott (NY)	Oto	602
Glaser, Joel (FL)	Oph	530	Gold, Stuart (NC)	PHO	698
Glashow, Jonathan (NY)	OrS	563	Goldberg, Jack (NJ)	Hem	290
Glaspy, John (CA)	Onc	356	Goldberg, James (CA)	MF	402

Name	Specialty	Pg	Name	Specialty	Pg
Goldberg, Michael (IL)	Ge	231	Goodrich, James (NY)	NS	431
Goldberg, Morton (MD)	Oph	522	Goodson, William (CA)	S	1002
Goldberg, Nieca (NY)	Cv	96	Goodwin, Scott (CA)	VIR	921
Goldberg, Richard (NC)	Onc	328	Goodwin, W Jarrard (FL)	Oto	610
Goldberg, Victor (OH)	OrS	577	Gorbien, Martin (IL)	Ger	249
Goldblum, John (OH)	Path	651	Gordon, Catherine (MA)	PEn	678
Golden, Michael (PA)	VascS	1085	Gordon, Leo (IL)	Hem	296
Goldenberg, David (PA)	Oto	602	Gordon, Marsha (NY)	D	182
Goldman, Allan (FL)	Pul	852	Gorensek, Margaret (FL)	Inf	379
Goldman, Stanton (TX)	PHO	708	Gorevic, Peter (NY)	Rhu	942
Goldman, Stewart (IL)	PHO	703	Gorfine, Stephen (NY)	CRS	166
Goldner, Richard (NC)	OrS	573	Gorin, Michael (CA)	Oph	545
Goldsmith, Ari (NY)	PO	721	Gorovoy, Mark (FL)	Oph	530
Goldsmith, Donald (PA)	PRhu	730	Gostout, Christopher (MN)	Ge	231
Goldsmith, Stanley (NY)	NuM	502	Gottdiener, John (MD)	Cv	96
Goldstein, Edward (GA)	ChiN	145	Gottlieb, Alice (MA)	D	179
Goldstein, Jeffrey (NY)	OrS	563	Gottlieb, Geoffrey (NY)	Path	644
Goldstein, Larry (NC)	N	478	Gottlieb, Stephen (MD)	Cv	97
Goldstein, Lori (PA)	Onc	315	Gould, K Lance (TX)	Cv	111
Goldstein, Marc (NY)	U	1051	Goulet, Robert (IN)	S	986
Goldstein, Martin (NY)	ObG	509	Goumnerova, Liliana (MA)	NS	428
Goldstein, Richard (KY)	S	979	Gourley, Mark (MD)	Rhu	942
Goldstein, Scott (PA)	CRS	165	Govindarajan, Sugantha (CA)	Path	656
Goldstein, Wayne (IL)	OrS	577	Gower, Roland (AK)	S	1002
Golfinos, John (NY)	NS	431	Goy, Andre (NJ)	Onc	315
Golomb, Harvey (IL)	Onc	339	Gradishar, William (IL)	Onc	339
Golub, Richard (FL)	CRS	167	Grado, Gordon (AZ)	RadRO	886
Gomella, Leonard (PA)	U	1052	Grady, M Sean (PA)	NS	432
Gomery, Pablo (MA)	U	1048	Graf, Ben (WI)	OrS	578
Gomes, Antoinette (CA)	VIR	920	Graham, John (CA)	CG	158
Gonik, Bernard (MI)	ObG	511	Graham, Mark (NC)	Onc	328
Gonzales, Edmond (TX)	U	1070	Graham, Michael (AZ)	PHO	708
Goodgold, Albert (NY)	N	469	Graham, Thomas (MD)	HS	277
Goodin, Douglas (CA)	N	493	Gralow, Julie (WA)	Onc	357
Goodman, Lawrence (WI)	DR	905	Grammer, Leslie (IL)	A&I	86
Goodman, Neil (FL)	RE	931	Grana, Generosa (NJ)	Onc	315
Goodman, Robert (NJ)	RadRO	873	Granai, Cornelius (RI)	GO	258
Goodman, Robert (NY)	NS	431	Grandis, Jennifer (PA)	Oto	602
Goodman, Stuart (CA)	OrS	586	Granet, David (CA)	Oph	545
Goodnight, James (CA)	S	1002	Grannis, Frederic (CA)	TS	1039

Alphabetical Listing of Doctors

Name	Specialty	Pg	Name	Specialty	Pg
Granstein, Richard (NY)	D	182	Greenwald, Mark (IL)	Oph	535
Grant, Clive S (MN)	S	986	Greenway, Hubert (CA)	D	193
Grant, Michael (TX)	S	996	Greenwood, Robert (NC)	ChiN	145
Grant, Richard (OH)	OrS	578	Greer, Benjamin (WA)	GO	271
Grasso, Michael (NY)	U	1052	Greer, John (TN)	Hem	293
Graver, L Michael (NY)	TS	1020	Greganti, Mac (NC)	Ger	248
Graves, Michael (CA)	N	493	Gregory, Richard (FL)	PlS	782
Gravett, Michael (WA)	MF	402	Gregory, Stephanie (IL)	Hem	296
Gray, Richard (AZ)	S	996	Greiner, Carl (NE)	Psyc	814
Gray, William (NY)	IC	121	Greipp, Philip (MN)	Hem	296
Grazi, Richard (NY)	RE	928	Greisler, Howard (IL)	VascS	1089
Greco, F Anthony (TN)	Onc	328	Grelsamer, Ronald (NY)	OrS	563
Greden, John (MI)	Psyc	813	Grem, Jean (NE)	Onc	346
Green, Andrew (RI)	OrS	557	Gress, Daryl (VA)	N	478
Green, Barth (FL)	NS	438	Grever, Michael (OH)	Hem	297
Green, Carmen (MI)	PM	637	Gribetz, Michael (NY)	U	1052
Green, Daniel (TN)	PHO	698	Grichnik, James (FL)	D	187
Green, Howard (FL)	D	187	Griepp, Randall (NY)	TS	1020
Green, Michael (PA)	PInf	712	Grier, Holcombe (MA)	PHO	690
Green, Peter (NY)	Ge	219	Griffin, John (MD)	N	469
Green, Richard (NY)	VascS	1085	Griffith, Bartley (MD)	TS	1020
Green, Thomas (IL)	PPul	727	Grifo, James (NY)	RE	928
Greenberg, Donna (MA)	Psyc	804	Grigsby, Perry (MO)	RadRO	882
Greenberg, Harly (NY)	Pul	847	Grillone, Gregory (MA)	Oto	599
Greenberg, Mark (NY)	Cv	97	Grimes, Pearl (CA)	D	193
Greenberg, Richard (PA)	U	1052	Griswold, John (TX)	S	996
Greenberger, Joel (PA)	RadRO	874	Grobelny, Thomas (IL)	NRad	912
Greenberger, Paul (IL)	A&I	86	Grody, Wayne (CA)	CG	158
Greene, Clarence (MO)	NS	444	Groene, Linda (FL)	Ger	248
Greene, Frederick (NC)	S	979	Grogan, Thomas (AZ)	Path	653
Greene, Graham (AR)	U	1070	Grosh, William (VA)	Onc	328
Greene, Loren Wissner (NY)	EDM	201	Gross, Ian (CT)	NP	406
Greene, Michael (MA)	MF	394	Grossbard, Michael (NY)	Onc	315
Greene, Thomas (FL)	HS	279	Grossberg, George (MO)	GerPsy	831
Greenhalgh, David (CA)	S	1002	Grossi, Eugene (NY)	TS	1021
Greenson, Joel (MI)	Path	651	Grossman, H Barton (TX)	U	1070
Greenspan, Stanley (MD)	ChAP	825	Grossman, John (CO)	PlS	789
Greenspan, Susan (PA)	EDM	201	Grossman, Melanie (NY)	D	182
Greenwald, Blaine (NY)	GerPsy	830	Grossman, Robert (NY)	NRad	910
Greenwald, Bruce (MD)	Ge	219	Grossman, Stuart (MD)	Onc	315

Name	Specialty	Pg
Grossniklaus, Hans (GA)	Oph	530
Grotta, James (TX)	N	489
Grotting, James (AL)	PlS	782
Grubb, Blair (OH)	Cv	106
Grubb, Robert (MO)	NS	444
Gruber, Scott (MI)	S	987
Gruber, Stephen (MI)	Onc	339
Gruchalla, Rebecca (TX)	A&I	87
Grum, Cyril (MI)	Pul	855
Grunberg, Steven (VT)	Onc	306
Grundfast, Kenneth (MA)	Oto	599
Grunfeld, Lawrence (NY)	RE	928
Grupp, Stephan (PA)	PHO	693
Gruss, Joseph (WA)	PlS	793
Guarda, Angela (MD)	Psyc	808
Guarini, Ludovico (NY)	PHO	693
Guerrant, Richard (VA)	Inf	379
Gugenheim, Joseph (TX)	OrS	583
Guidry, George (LA)	Pul	860
Guillem, Jose (NY)	CRS	166
Guilleminault, Christian (CA)	Psyc	817
Gujral, Saroj (MN)	U	1065
Gulley, James (MD)	Onc	315
Gullquist, Scott (VA)	PCd	672
Gumprecht, Jeffrey (NY)	Inf	375
Gunasekaran, T S (IL)	PGe	687
Gunderson, John (MA)	Psyc	804
Gunderson, Leonard (AZ)	RadRO	886
Gundry, Steven (CA)	TS	1039
Gunter, Jack (TX)	PlS	790
Gupta, Nalin (CA)	NS	453
Gupta, Prabodh (PA)	Path	644
Gupta, Rajan (NH)	S	963
Gusberg, Richard (CT)	VascS	1082
Gutai, James (MI)	PEn	682
Guthikonda, Murali (MI)	NS	444
Guthrie, Barton (AL)	NS	438
Gutierrez, Francisco (IL)	NS	444
Gutin, Philip (NY)	NS	432
Guyton, David (MD)	Oph	522

Name	Specialty	Pg
Guyton, Robert (GA)	TS	1027

H

Name	Specialty	Pg
Haas, Naomi (PA)	Onc	316
Haas, Richard (CA)	ChiN	148
Haas, Steven (NY)	OrS	563
Haber, Gregory (NY)	Ge	219
Habermann, Thomas (MN)	Hem	297
Hackney, David (MA)	NRad	909
Haddad, Joseph (NY)	PO	721
Hadler, Nortin (NC)	Rhu	945
Hadley, Mark (AL)	NS	438
Hadlock, Theresa (MA)	Oto	599
Haffty, Bruce (NJ)	RadRO	874
Hafler, David (MA)	N	465
Hagan, Kevin (TN)	PlS	782
Hager, W David (KY)	ObG	510
Hagman, Jennifer (CO)	ChAP	828
Hahn, Stephen (PA)	RadRO	874
Haid, Regis (GA)	NS	438
Haig, Andrew (MI)	PMR	764
Haik, Barrett (TN)	Oph	530
Hain, Timothy (IL)	N	483
Haines, Kathleen (NJ)	PRhu	730
Hakaim, Albert (FL)	VascS	1087
Halberg, Francine (CA)	RadRO	888
Hale, Douglass (IN)	ObG	511
Haley, Barbara (TX)	Onc	349
Haley, Elliott (VA)	N	478
Halff, Glenn (TX)	S	996
Hall, Jesse (IL)	Pul	855
Hall, Lisabeth (NY)	Oph	522
Hall, Simon (NY)	U	1052
Halle, Jan (NC)	RadRO	877
Haller, Daniel (PA)	Onc	316
Haller, Julia (PA)	Oph	523
Hallett, John (SC)	VascS	1087
Hallisey, Michael (CT)	VIR	916
Halperin, Jonathan (NY)	Cv	97

Alphabetical Listing of Doctors

Name	Specialty	Pg	Name	Specialty	Pg
Halpern, Allan (NY)	D	182	Haque, Waheedul (TX)	Psyc	816
Halpern, Howard (IL)	RadRO	882	Har-El, Gady (NY)	Oto	603
Halpern, Steven (NJ)	PHO	693	Haraf, Daniel (IL)	RadRO	882
Haluszka, Oleh (PA)	Ge	220	Harari, Paul (WI)	RadRO	882
Hamilton, Stanley (TX)	Path	654	Harati, Yadollah (TX)	N	489
Hammar, Samuel (WA)	Path	656	Harbaugh, Robert (PA)	NS	432
Hammer, Glenn (NY)	Inf	376	Harber, Philip (CA)	OM	800
Hammer, Scott (NY)	Inf	376	Harbour, J William (MO)	Oph	535
Hammerschlag, Paul (NY)	Oto	603	Harden, R Norman (IL)	PM	637
Hammill, Stephen (MN)	CE	118	Hardesty, Robert (CA)	PlS	793
Hammond, Charles (NC)	RE	932	Hardin, Joel (IL)	PCd	674
Hammond, Denis (NH)	Onc	306	Hare, Joshua (FL)	Cv	102
Hammond, Dennis (MI)	PlS	786	Hargrove, W Clark (PA)	TS	1021
Hamra, Sameer (TX)	PlS	790	Harken, Alden (CA)	TS	1039
Hamvas, Aaron (MO)	NP	410	Harley, Earl (DC)	PO	721
Han, Steven-Huy B (CA)	Ge	239	Harman, Eloise (FL)	Pul	852
Hanauer, Stephen (IL)	Ge	231	Harner, Christopher (PA)	SM	955
Hancock, Steven (CA)	RadRO	888	Harnsberger, Jeffrey (NH)	CRS	164
Handa, James (MD)	Oph	523	Harolds, Jay (OK)	DR	907
Hande, Kenneth (TN)	Onc	329	Harper, Richard (TX)	NS	449
Handy, John (OR)	TS	1039	Harpole, David (NC)	TS	1027
Hanel, Douglas (WA)	HS	283	Harrell, James (TX)	TS	1037
Haney, Arthur (IL)	RE	933	Harrington, Elizabeth (NY)	VascS	1085
Hanifin, Jon (OR)	D	193	Harris, David (TX)	PMR	766
Hanke, C William (IN)	D	189	Harris, Gerald (IL)	HS	281
Hankins, Gary (TX)	MF	401	Harris, Jay (MA)	RadRO	870
Hankinson, Hal (NM)	NS	449	Harris, Jeffrey (CA)	Oto	625
Hanks, John (VA)	S	979	Harris, Michael (NJ)	PHO	694
Hanley, Frank (CA)	TS	1039	Harris, Nancy (MA)	Path	642
Hann, Lucy (NY)	DR	901	Harrison, J Kevin (NC)	Cv	102
Hanna, Ehab (TX)	Oto	623	Harrison, Louis (NY)	RadRO	874
Hanna, Nader (MD)	S	970	Harsh, Griffith (CA)	NS	453
Hannafin, Jo (NY)	OrS	563	Hart, Robert (TX)	N	489
Hansen, Juliana (OR)	PlS	793	Hartig, Gregory (WI)	Oto	616
Hansen, Kimberley (NC)	VascS	1087	Hartl, Roger (NY)	NS	432
Hansen, Nora (IL)	S	987	Hartman, Barry (NY)	Inf	376
Hansen, Ronald (AZ)	D	192	Hartmann, Lynn (MN)	Onc	340
Hansen, Sigvard (WA)	OrS	586	Hartmann, Rene (FL)	CRS	167
Hansen-Flaschen, John (PA)	Pul	847	Harty, James (KY)	U	1059
Hanson, Laura (NC)	Ger	248	Hashim, Sabet (CT)	TS	1016

Alphabetical Listing of Doctors

Name	Specialty	Pg	Name	Specialty	Pg
Haskal, Ziv (MD)	VIR	917	Heldman, Alan (FL)	IC	123
Haskett, Roger (PA)	Psyc	808	Helfet, David (NY)	OrS	564
Hastings, Hill (IN)	HS	281	Hellenbrand, William (NY)	PCd	670
Hatch, Kenneth (AZ)	GO	269	Heller, Debra (NJ)	Path	644
Haughey, Bruce (MO)	Oto	616	Hellstrom, Wayne (LA)	U	1070
Haughton, Victor (WI)	NRad	913	Helman, Lee (MD)	PHO	694
Hauke, Ralph (NE)	Onc	347	Helvie, Mark (MI)	DR	906
Hauptman, Paul (MO)	Cv	106	Hemal, Ashok (NC)	U	1059
Hauser, Stephen (CA)	N	493	Hemming, Alan (CA)	S	1002
Hausman, Michael (NY)	OrS	563	Henderson, Victor (CA)	N	493
Haut, Paul (IN)	PHO	703	Henderson, William (WA)	A&I	87
Hawes, Robert (SC)	Ge	226	Hendricks-Munoz, Karen (NY)	NP	407
Hawkins, Douglas (WA)	PHO	709	Hendrickson, Michael (CA)	Path	656
Hawkins, Irvin (FL)	VIR	918	Heney, Niall (MA)	U	1048
Hayani, Ammar (IL)	PHO	703	Henke, David (NC)	Pul	853
Hayashi, Robert (MO)	PHO	703	Henry, Timothy (MN)	IC	124
Hayden, Richard (AZ)	Oto	623	Henschke, Claudia (NY)	DR	901
Hayes, Daniel (MI)	Onc	340	Hensinger, Robert (MI)	OrS	578
Hayes, David (MN)	CE	118	Hensle, Terry (NY)	U	1052
Hayes, Sharonne (MN)	Cv	106	Hentz, Vincent (CA)	HS	284
Hayman, James (MI)	RadRO	882	Heppell, Jacques (AZ)	CRS	171
Haynes, Johnson (AL)	Pul	853	Herbst, Roy (TX)	Onc	349
Healey, John (NY)	OrS	563	Hergenroeder, Albert (TX)	AM	77
Healy, Gerald (MA)	PO	720	Hering, Bernhard (MN)	S	987
Heber, David (CA)	EDM	211	Herling, Irving (PA)	Cv	97
Hebert, James (VT)	S	963	Herman, John (MA)	Psyc	804
Hecht, Andrew (NY)	OrS	564	Herman, Terence (OK)	RadRO	886
Heck, Christianne (CA)	N	493	Herman, William (MI)	EDM	207
Heckenlively, John (MI)	Oph	535	Heros, Roberto (FL)	NS	438
Hecox, Kurt (WI)	N	483	Heroux, Alain (IL)	Cv	106
Hedges, Thomas (MA)	Oph	518	Herr, Harry (NY)	U	1052
Heffner, John (OR)	Pul	861	Herring, Stanley (WA)	PMR	767
Heffner, Linda (MA)	MF	394	Herrmann, Howard (PA)	IC	121
Heidary, Dariush (GA)	TS	1027	Herrmann, Virginia (SC)	S	979
Heilman, Carl (MA)	NS	429	Hersh, Peter (NJ)	Oph	523
Heilman, Kenneth (FL)	N	478	Hershman, Elliott (NY)	SM	955
Heimburger, Douglas (AL)	IM	389	Hershorin, Eugene (FL)	Ped	663
Heinrich, Michael (OR)	Hem	302	Hertz, Marshall (MN)	Pul	855
Heitmiller, Richard (MD)	TS	1021	Hertzig, Margaret (NY)	ChAP	825
Helderman, J Harold (TN)	Nep	419	Herzenberg, John (MD)	OrS	564

Alphabetical Listing of Doctors

Name	Specialty	Pg	Name	Specialty	Pg
Herzog, David (MA)	ChAP	823	Hodges, David (TX)	Ge	238
Herzog, Thomas (NY)	GO	261	Hodgson, Kim (IL)	VascS	1089
Heslin, Martin (AL)	S	979	Hoefflin, Steven (CA)	PlS	793
Hess, David (GA)	N	478	Hoffenberg, Edward (CO)	PGe	688
Hess, J Bruce (FL)	Oph	530	Hoffman, Andrew (CA)	EDM	212
Hesselink, John (CA)	NRad	915	Hoffman, Brenda (SC)	Ge	227
Hester, T Roderick (GA)	PlS	782	Hoffman, Daniel (CO)	Psyc	814
Heston, Jerry (TN)	ChAP	826	Hoffman, Henry (IA)	Oto	616
Hetherington, Maxine (MO)	PHO	703	Hoffman, John (PA)	S	970
Heuer, Dale (WI)	Oph	535	Hoffman, Lloyd (NY)	PlS	776
Heyman, Melvin (CA)	PGe	689	Hoffman, Philip (IL)	Onc	340
Hibbard, Judith (IL)	MF	398	Hoffman, Robert (NY)	PrM	801
Hicks, Wesley (NY)	Oto	603	Hoffman, Ronald (NY)	Oto	603
Hidalgo, David (NY)	PlS	776	Hoffman, William (CA)	PlS	794
Hiesiger, Emile (NY)	N	470	Hofkosh, Dena (PA)	Ped	663
Higano, Celestia (WA)	Onc	357	Hogan, Thomas (WV)	Onc	316
Higashida, Randall (CA)	NRad	915	Hogikyan, Norman (MI)	Oto	616
Hijazi, Ziyad (IL)	PCd	674	Holden, Stuart (CA)	U	1074
Hilden, Joanne (IN)	PHO	704	Holinger, Lauren (IL)	PO	723
Hilfiker, Mary (CA)	PS	741	Holladay, Jack (TX)	Oph	541
Hilger, Peter (MN)	Oto	616	Holland, Edward (OH)	Oph	535
Hilibrand, Alan (PA)	OrS	564	Holland, James (NY)	Onc	316
Hill, Ivor (NC)	PGe	686	Hollander, Eric (NY)	Psyc	808
Hill, Joseph (NH)	RE	926	Holliday, James (TN)	Oph	530
Hillebrand, Donald (CA)	Ge	240	Holliday, Michael (MD)	Oto	603
Hillemeier, A Craig (PA)	PGe	685	Holliday, Roy (NY)	DR	902
Himelstein, Andrew (DE)	Onc	316	Hollier, Larry (LA)	VascS	1091
Hinkle, Andrea (NY)	PHO	694	Holmes, David (MN)	IC	124
Hinshaw, Daniel (MI)	S	987	Holmes, Gregory (NH)	ChiN	142
Hirsch, Barry (PA)	Oto	603	Holmes, Lewis (MA)	CG	152
Hirsch, Glenn (NY)	ChAP	825	Holroyd, Suzanne (VA)	GerPsy	831
Hirsch, Irl (WA)	EDM	212	Holterman, Mark (IL)	PS	738
Hirsch, Joshua (MA)	NRad	909	Holtzman, Ronald (NC)	NP	409
Hirschfeld, Robert (TX)	Psyc	816	Holzman, Ian (NY)	NP	407
Ho, Allen (PA)	Oph	523	Homans, Alan (VT)	PHO	690
Ho, Sherwin (IL)	SM	956	Hong, Waun (TX)	Onc	350
Hochberg, Marc (MD)	Rhu	943	Hoogwerf, Byron (OH)	EDM	207
Hochschuler, Stephen (TX)	OrS	583	Hoops, Timothy (PA)	Ge	220
Hochster, Howard (NY)	Onc	316	Hoots, William (MD)	PHO	694
Hoda, Syed (NY)	Path	644	Hopewell, Philip (CA)	Pul	862

Name	Specialty	Pg	Name	Specialty	Pg
Hopkins, L Nelson (NY)	NS	432	Hudes, Gary (PA)	Onc	316
Hoppe, Richard (CA)	RadRO	889	Hudgins, Louanne (CA)	CG	158
Hopping, Steven (DC)	Oto	603	Hudis, Clifford (NY)	Onc	317
Horbar, Jeffrey (VT)	NP	406	Hudson, Leonard (WA)	Pul	862
Hord, Jeffrey (OH)	PHO	704	Hudson, Melissa (TN)	PHO	698
Horn, Biljana (CA)	PHO	710	Hudziak, James (VT)	ChAP	823
Horn, Evelyn (NY)	Cv	97	Hughes, Kevin (MA)	S	963
Hornicek, Francis (MA)	OrS	557	Huitt, Gwen (CO)	Inf	382
Horning, Sandra (CA)	Onc	357	Hultman, C Scott (NC)	PlS	782
Hornstein, Mark (MA)	RE	926	Humayun, Mark (CA)	Oph	545
Horowitz, Ira (GA)	GO	264	Hume, Eric (NJ)	OrS	564
Horowitz, Jed (CA)	PlS	794	Hungerford, Marc (MD)	OrS	564
Horsager, Robyn (TX)	MF	401	Hunninghake, Gary (IA)	Pul	855
Hortobagyi, Gabriel (TX)	Onc	350	Hunstad, Joseph (NC)	PlS	782
Horvath, Keith (MD)	TS	1021	Hunt, John (TX)	S	996
Horwitz, Eric (PA)	RadRO	874	Hunt, Kelly (TX)	S	996
Horwitz, Steven (NY)	Onc	316	Hunt, Sharon (CA)	Cv	113
Hotaling, Andrew (IL)	Oto	617	Hunt, Thomas (AL)	HS	280
Hotchkiss, Robert (NY)	OrS	564	Hunter, David (MA)	Oph	518
Hovsepian, David (CA)	VIR	921	Hunter, Ellen (ID)	Ge	236
Howard, Richard (FL)	S	979	Hunter, Jill (TX)	NRad	914
Howard, Thomas (NE)	VascS	1090	Hunter, John (OR)	S	1002
Howe, James (IA)	S	987	Huntoon, Marc (MN)	PM	637
Howell, Elizabeth (UT)	AdP	822	Hura, Claudia (TX)	Nep	423
Howerton, Russell (NC)	S	979	Hurd, David (NC)	Onc	329
Howington, John (IL)	TS	1031	Hurst, Michael (WV)	Oto	603
Hoyme, H Eugene (SD)	CG	156	Hurst, Robert (PA)	NRad	910
Hoyt, David (CA)	S	1002	Hurt, Hallam (PA)	NP	407
Hozack, William (PA)	OrS	564	Hurtig, Howard (PA)	N	470
Hrebinko, Ronald (PA)	U	1052	Hurwitz, Barrie (NC)	N	478
Hricak, Hedvig (NY)	DR	902	Hurwitz, Dennis (PA)	PlS	776
Hruban, Ralph (MD)	Path	645	Hussain, Maha (MI)	Onc	340
Hruska, Keith (MO)	Nep	421	Hussey, Michael (IL)	MF	399
Hruza, George (MO)	D	189	Hutchins, Laura (AR)	Onc	350
Hsu, Daphne (NY)	PCd	671	Hutchinson, Raymond (MI)	PHO	704
Hsueh, Willa (CA)	EDM	212	Hutter, Adolph (MA)	Cv	92
Huang, Laurence (CA)	Pul	862	Huynh, Phan Tuong (TX)	DR	907
Huben, Robert (NY)	U	1053	Hyers, Thomas (MO)	Pul	855
Huber, Philip (TX)	CRS	172	Hyman, Neil (VT)	CRS	164
Huddleston, Charles (MO)	TS	1031			

Alphabetical Listing of Doctors

Name	Specialty	Pg	Name	Specialty	Pg
I			**J**		
Iannaccone, Susan (TX)	ChiN	147	Jaafar, Mohamad (DC)	Oph	523
Iannettoni, Mark (IA)	TS	1031	Jablons, David (CA)	TS	1039
Iannotti, Joseph (OH)	OrS	578	Jabs, Douglas (NY)	Oph	523
Idler, Richard (CO)	HS	283	Jackler, Robert (CA)	Oto	625
Iglehart, J Dirk (MA)	S	963	Jackman, Stephen (PA)	U	1053
Ikramuddin, Sayeed (MN)	S	987	Jackson, Amie (AL)	PMR	762
Ilbawi, Michel (IL)	PS	738	Jackson, Gilchrist (TX)	S	996
Iliff, Nicholas (MD)	Oph	523	Jackson, Richard (TX)	PS	741
Ilowite, Norman (NY)	PRhu	730	Jackson, Valerie (IN)	DR	906
Ilson, David (NY)	Onc	317	Jackson, Vicki (MA)	IM	388
Imber, Gerald (NY)	PlS	776	Jacob, Molly (IL)	Ped	664
Imbriglia, Joseph (PA)	HS	277	Jacobs, Alice (MA)	IC	120
Infante, Anthony (TX)	Ped	664	Jacobs, Charlotte (CA)	Onc	357
Infante, Ernesto (TX)	N	490	Jacobs, Joseph (NY)	Oto	604
Ingle, James (MN)	Onc	340	Jacobs, Laurence (IL)	RE	933
Inglis, Andrew (WA)	PO	724	Jacobs, Richard (AR)	PInf	715
Ingram, David (NC)	PInf	714	Jacobs, Thomas (NY)	EDM	201
Inra, Lawrence (NY)	Cv	97	Jacobson, Alan (MA)	Psyc	804
Interian, Alberto (FL)	CE	117	Jacobson, Ira (NY)	Ge	220
Inzucchi, Silvio (CT)	EDM	199	Jacoby, David (OR)	Pul	862
Ipp, Eli (CA)	EDM	212	Jaffe, Allan (MN)	Cv	106
Irby, Pierce (NC)	U	1059	Jaffe, Elaine (MD)	Path	645
Irvine, John (CA)	Oph	545	Jaffe, Kenneth (WA)	PMR	767
Irwin, Charles (CA)	AM	77	Jahanzeb, Mohammad (FL)	Onc	329
Irwin, Richard (MA)	Pul	845	Jain, Subhash (NY)	PM	635
Irwin, Ronald (MI)	OrS	578	Jakacki, Regina (PA)	PHO	694
Isaacs, Claudine (DC)	Onc	317	Jallo, George (MD)	NS	432
Isaacs, Kim (NC)	Ge	227	James, William (PA)	D	182
Isaacson, Keith (MA)	RE	926	Jamieson, Stuart (CA)	TS	1039
Isaacson, Steven (NY)	RadRO	874	Janeiro, John (NH)	U	1048
Iseman, Michael (CO)	Pul	858	Janicak, Philip (IL)	Psyc	813
Isenberg, Sherwin (CA)	Oph	545	Jankovic, Joseph (TX)	N	490
Isik, Ferda (WA)	PlS	794	Janss, Anna (GA)	N	478
Iskandrian, Ami (AL)	Cv	102	Jaramillo, Diego (PA)	DR	902
Ismail, Mahmoud (IL)	MF	399	Jarnagin, William (NY)	S	970
Isom, O Wayne (NY)	TS	1021	Jarow, Jonathan (MD)	U	1053
Itzkowitz, Steven (NY)	Ge	220	Jarvik, Jeffrey (WA)	NRad	915
Ivanhoe, Cindy (TX)	PMR	766	Jeevanandam, Valluvan (IL)	TS	1031
Iwach, Andrew (CA)	Oph	545	Jenike, Michael (MA)	Psyc	805

Alphabetical Listing of Doctors

Name	Specialty	Pg	Name	Specialty	Pg
Kawachi, Mark (CA)	U	1074	Kenan, Samuel (NY)	OrS	565
Kawamoto, Henry (CA)	PlS	794	Kenkel, Jeffrey (TX)	PlS	790
Kay, Dennis (LA)	VIR	920	Kennedy, David (PA)	Oto	604
Kay, G Neal (AL)	CE	117	Kennedy, Gary (NY)	GerPsy	830
Kay, Jonathan (MA)	Rhu	940	Kennelly, Michael (NC)	U	1060
Kaye, Mitchell (MN)	Pul	856	Kent, Kenneth (WI)	VascS	1089
Kaysen, George (CA)	Nep	424	Kent, Thomas (TX)	N	490
Kazahaya, Ken (PA)	PO	721	Kereiakes, Dean (OH)	Cv	106
Kazanjian, Powel (MI)	Inf	381	Kern, Robert (IL)	Oto	617
Kazer, Ralph (IL)	RE	934	Kernstine, Kemp (CA)	TS	1040
Keane, Thomas (SC)	U	1060	Kerr, Natalie (TN)	Oph	530
Keane, William (PA)	Oto	604	Kerrihard, Thomas (CA)	Psyc	817
Keating, Michael (TX)	Hem	301	Kesser, Bradley (VA)	Oto	610
Keefe, David (FL)	RE	932	Kessler, Craig (DC)	Hem	290
Keen, Mary (IL)	PMR	764	Kestle, John RW (UT)	NS	448
Keenan, Mary Ann (PA)	OrS	565	Ketcham, Douglas (MN)	VIR	919
Keenan, Robert (PA)	TS	1022	Kevorkian, Charles (TX)	PMR	766
Keens, Thomas (CA)	PPul	729	Key, L Lyndon (SC)	PEn	681
Keepers, George (OR)	Psyc	817	Khan, Agha (MD)	NS	433
Keiser, Philip (TX)	Inf	382	Khandji, Alexander (NY)	NRad	910
Kelepouris, Ellie (PA)	Nep	418	Khawaja, Shazib (GA)	IC	123
Keller, Frank (GA)	PHO	699	Khosla, Sundeep (MN)	EDM	207
Keller, Frederick (OR)	VIR	921	Khuri, Fadlo (GA)	Onc	329
Keller, Gregory (CA)	Oto	626	Kibel, Adam (MO)	U	1065
Keller, Steven (NY)	TS	1022	Kidwell, Earl (DC)	Oph	524
Kelley, Joseph (PA)	GO	262	Kiel, Krystyna (GA)	RadRO	878
Kelley, Mark (TN)	S	979	Kieran, Mark (MA)	PHO	690
Kelly, Cynthia (VA)	PA&I	666	Kiernan, Paul (VA)	TS	1027
Kelly, James (CO)	N	488	Kies, Merrill (TX)	Onc	350
Kelly, John (OK)	PlS	790	Kiev, Jonathan (MD)	TS	1022
Kelly, Karen (KS)	Onc	347	Kilmer, Suzanne (CA)	D	193
Kelly, Kevin (TN)	PlS	782	Kim, Daniel (TX)	NS	449
Kelly, Thomas (CA)	MF	402	Kim, Edward (TN)	U	1060
Kelly, William (CT)	Onc	307	Kim, Jae (MI)	RadRO	882
Kelsen, David (NY)	Onc	317	Kim, Jonathan (CA)	Oph	545
Kelts, K Alan (SD)	N	488	Kim, Julian (OH)	S	987
Kemeny, Nancy (NY)	Onc	317	Kim, Lawrence (AR)	S	997
Kemp, James (MO)	PPul	727	Kim, Youn-Hee (CA)	D	194
Kempin, Sanford (NY)	Hem	290	Kim, Young-Jee (IN)	PPul	728
Kempson, Richard (CA)	Path	657	Kimberly, Robert (AL)	Rhu	946

Alphabetical Listing of Doctors

Name	Specialty	Pg	Name	Specialty	Pg
Kimmey, Michael (WA)	Ge	240	Kline, Mark (TX)	PInf	715
Kincaid, John (IN)	N	484	Klingensmith, Georgeanna (CO)	PEn	683
Kindler, Hedy (IL)	Onc	341	Kloos, Richard (OH)	EDM	207
King, Andrew (CA)	Nep	424	Klutke, Carl (MO)	U	1065
King, Bryan (WA)	ChAP	829	Knechtle, Stuart (GA)	S	979
King, Earl (PA)	Pul	847	Kneisl, Jeffrey (NC)	OrS	573
King, John (TX)	PMR	766	Knisely, Jonathan (CT)	RadRO	870
King, Richard (GA)	PMR	762	Knoefel, Janice (NM)	N	490
King, Robert (CT)	ChAP	823	Knopf, William (GA)	IC	123
King, Talmadge (CA)	Pul	862	Knowles, Daniel (NY)	Path	645
Kingdom, Todd (CO)	Oto	621	Knudson, Mary (CA)	S	1003
Kinney, Marsha (TX)	Path	654	Kobashigawa, Jon (CA)	Cv	114
Kipps, Thomas (CA)	Hem	302	Kobrin, Sidney (PA)	Nep	418
Kirklin, James (AL)	TS	1027	Kobrine, Arthur (DC)	NS	433
Kirkwood, John (PA)	Onc	317	Koch, Christian (MS)	EDM	204
Kirschenbaum, Alexander (NY)	U	1053	Koch, Douglas (TX)	Oph	541
Kirschner, Barbara (IL)	PGe	687	Koch, Wayne (MD)	Oto	604
Kirschner, Kristi (IL)	PMR	764	Kocher, Mininder (MA)	OrS	557
Kirshblum, Steven (NJ)	PMR	760	Kochman, Michael (PA)	Ge	221
Kirshenbaum, James (MA)	Cv	92	Koczywas, Marianna (CA)	Onc	357
Kirshner, Howard (TN)	N	479	Kodner, Ira (MO)	CRS	169
Kirsner, Robert (FL)	D	187	Koeller, Kelly (MN)	NRad	913
Klagsbrun, Samuel (NY)	Psyc	808	Koff, Stephen (OH)	U	1065
Klapheke, Martin (KY)	Psyc	812	Koh, Wui-Jin (WA)	RadRO	889
Kleber, Herbert (NY)	AdP	821	Kohler, Matthew (SC)	GO	264
Kleiman, Martin (IN)	PInf	715	Kokotailo, Patricia (WI)	AM	77
Kleiman, Neal (TX)	IC	125	Koller, Harold (PA)	Oph	524
Klein, Andrew (CA)	S	1003	Kolodny, Edwin (NY)	N	470
Klein, Eric (OH)	U	1065	Komaki, Ritsuko (TX)	RadRO	887
Klein, Lloyd (IL)	Cv	107	Koman, L Andrew (NC)	HS	280
Klein, Robert (RI)	PA&I	665	Kondziolka, Douglas (PA)	NS	433
Klein-Gitelman, Marisa (IL)	PRhu	731	Konicek, Frank (IL)	Ge	232
Kleinberg, David (NY)	EDM	201	Konski, Andre (MI)	RadRO	882
Kleinberg, Lawrence (MD)	RadRO	874	Konstam, Marvin (MA)	Cv	93
Kleinerman, Eugenie (TX)	Ped	664	Konstan, Michael (OH)	PPul	728
Kleinman, Ronald (MA)	PGe	684	Koo, John (CA)	D	194
Kleinman, William (IN)	HS	281	Koos, Brian (CA)	MF	402
Klibanski, Anne (MA)	EDM	199	Kopans, Daniel (MA)	DR	899
Kliger, Alan (CT)	Nep	416	Kopel, Samuel (NY)	Hem	290
Klimberg, Vicki (AR)	S	997	Kopf, Gary (CT)	TS	1017

Name	Specialty	Pg	Name	Specialty	Pg
Koplin, Lawrence (CA)	PlS	794	Kraut, Eric (OH)	Hem	297
Kopp, Peter (IL)	EDM	207	Krebs, Nancy (CO)	PGe	688
Korenblat, Phillip (MO)	A&I	86	Kreissman, Susan (NC)	PHO	699
Korf, Bruce (AL)	CG	154	Kreitzer, Joel (NY)	PM	635
Kormos, Robert (PA)	TS	1022	Krellenstein, Daniel (NY)	TS	1022
Kornmehl, Ernest (MA)	Oph	518	Krespi, Yosef (NY)	Oto	605
Korones, David (NY)	PHO	694	Kress, Douglas (PA)	D	183
Korsten, Mark (NY)	Ge	221	Kress, Kenneth (GA)	OrS	573
Koruda, Mark (NC)	S	980	Kretschmar, Cynthia (MA)	PHO	691
Korytkowski, Mary (PA)	EDM	201	Kriegel, David (NY)	D	183
Koss, Michael (CA)	Path	657	Krieger, Karl (NY)	TS	1022
Kosten, Thomas (TX)	AdP	822	Krilov, Leonard (NY)	PInf	712
Kostis, John (NJ)	Cv	97	Kris, Mark (NY)	Onc	318
Kotagal, Suresh (MN)	ChiN	146	Krisht, Ali (AR)	NS	450
Kotapka, Mark (PA)	NS	433	Kron, Irving (VA)	TS	1028
Kotler, Donald (NY)	Ge	221	Krouse, Robert (AZ)	S	997
Kotloff, Karen (MD)	PInf	712	Krowka, Michael (MN)	Pul	856
Kotloff, Robert (PA)	Pul	847	Krueger, Gerald (UT)	D	191
Koufman, Jamie (NY)	Oto	604	Krueger, Ronald (OH)	Oph	536
Kougias, Panagiotis (TX)	VascS	1091	Krumholz, Allan (MD)	N	470
Koulos, John (NY)	GO	262	Krummel, Thomas (CA)	PS	742
Kovac, S Robert (GA)	ObG	510	Kucuk, Omer (GA)	Onc	329
Kovitz, Kevin (IL)	Pul	856	Kuettel, Michael (NY)	RadRO	874
Kovnar, Edward (WI)	ChiN	146	Kuhel, William (NY)	Oto	605
Kowalski, Thomas (PA)	Ge	221	Kuhn, Frederick (GA)	Oto	610
Koyle, Martin (WA)	U	1074	Kuhn, Joseph (TX)	S	997
Kozarek, Richard (WA)	Ge	240	Kuiken, Todd (IL)	PMR	764
Kozin, Scott (PA)	HS	277	Kula, Roger (NY)	N	470
Kozlowski, James (IL)	U	1065	Kulick, Roy (NY)	HS	277
Krachmer, Jay (MN)	Oph	535	Kumpe, David (CO)	VIR	920
Krackow, Kenneth (NY)	OrS	565	Kun, Larry (TN)	RadRO	878
Kraft, Andrew (SC)	Onc	329	Kunkel, Elisabeth (PA)	Psyc	809
Kraft, George (WA)	PMR	767	Kunschner, Lara (PA)	N	470
Krag, David (VT)	S	963	Kupersmith, Mark (NY)	Oph	524
Krajcer, Zvonimir (TX)	Cv	111	Kupfer, David (PA)	Psyc	809
Kramer, Barry (CA)	GerPsy	832	Kupper, Thomas (MA)	D	179
Krasna, Mark (MD)	TS	1022	Kurachek, Stephen (MN)	PPul	728
Kraus, Dennis (NY)	Oto	604	Kuriakose, Philip (MI)	Hem	297
Kraus, Michael (IN)	Nep	421	Kurland, Geoffrey (PA)	PPul	725
Krauss, Gregory (MD)	N	470	Kurman, Robert (MD)	Path	645

Alphabetical Listing of Doctors

Name	Specialty	Pg	Name	Specialty	Pg
Kurtin, Paul (MN)	Path	651	Lambert, Scott (GA)	Oph	530
Kurtz, Alfred (PA)	DR	902	Lamberti, John (CA)	TS	1040
Kurtz, Robert (NY)	Ge	221	Lambiase, Louis (FL)	Ge	227
Kurtzberg, Joanne (NC)	PHO	699	Lamonica, Dominick (NY)	NuM	502
Kurtzke, Robert (VA)	N	479	LaMuraglia, Glenn M (MA)	VascS	1082
Kushner, Brian (NY)	PHO	694	Lancaster, Johnathan (FL)	GO	264
Kushner, Burton (WI)	Oph	536	Landefeld, Charles (CA)	Ger	251
Kuske, Robert (AZ)	RadRO	887	Landers, Daniel (MN)	MF	399
Kutner, Jean (CO)	Ger	249	Landrigan, Philip (NY)	OM	800
Kutteh, William (TN)	RE	932	Landry, Jerome (GA)	RadRO	878
Kuttesch, John (TN)	PHO	699	Landy, Helain (DC)	MF	396
Kuzel, Timothy (IL)	Hem	297	Landy, Howard (FL)	NS	439
Kuzniecky, Ruben (NY)	N	471	Lane, Dorothy (NY)	PrM	801
Kuzon, William (MI)	PlS	786	Lane, Joseph (NY)	OrS	565
Kveton, John (CT)	Oto	599	Lane, Lewis (NY)	HS	278
Kvols, Larry (FL)	Onc	330	Lane, Stephen (MN)	Oph	536
Kwak, Larry (TX)	Onc	350	Lang, Frederick (TX)	NS	450
Kwo, Paul (IN)	Ge	232	Lang, Peter (MA)	PCd	669
Kwolek, Christopher (MA)	VascS	1082	Lang, Samuel (NY)	TS	1022
			Lange, Beverly (PA)	PHO	695
			Lange, Paul (WA)	U	1074
			Langer, Corey (PA)	Onc	318
L			Langford, Carol (OH)	Rhu	947
			Langman, Craig (IL)	PNep	719
La Ban, Myron (MI)	PMR	764	Langston, J William (CA)	N	493
La Gamma, Edmund (NY)	NP	407	Lannin, Donald (CT)	S	964
La Quaglia, Michael (NY)	PS	734	Lansman, Steven (NY)	TS	1023
La Russo, Nicholas (MN)	Ge	232	Lanteri, Vincent (NJ)	U	1053
Labar, Douglas (NY)	N	471	Lantos, John (MO)	Ped	664
Labiner, David (AZ)	N	490	Lanza, Donald (FL)	Oto	611
Lachs, Mark (NY)	Ger	247	Lanza, Louis (AZ)	TS	1037
Lackman, Richard (PA)	OrS	565	Lapey, Allen (MA)	PPul	725
Lacomis, David (PA)	N	471	Laramore, George (WA)	RadRO	889
Lacy, Jill (CT)	Onc	307	Larner, James (VA)	RadRO	878
Ladenson, Paul (MD)	EDM	202	Larrabee, Wayne (WA)	Oto	626
Lage, Janice (SC)	Path	649	Larsen, Christian (GA)	S	980
Laham, Roger (MA)	IC	120	Larsen, Donald (CA)	NRad	915
Lahita, Robert (NJ)	Rhu	943	Larsen, Gary (CO)	PPul	728
Laks, Hillel (CA)	TS	1040	Larson, David (CA)	RadRO	889
Lalwani, Anil (NY)	Oto	605	Larson, Richard (IL)	Hem	297
Lambert, H Michael (TX)	Oph	541			
Lambert, Paul (SC)	Oto	610			

Name	Specialty	Pg	Name	Specialty	Pg
Larson, Steven (NY)	NuM	502	Lee, Chung (MN)	RadRO	883
Lashner, Bret (OH)	Ge	232	Lee, Francis (NY)	OrS	566
Lask, Gary (CA)	D	194	Lee, Jeffrey (TX)	S	997
Laske, Douglas (PA)	NS	433	Lee, Kenneth (PA)	S	971
Latchaw, Laurie (NH)	PS	732	Lee, Patrick (OR)	CRS	172
Laterra, John (MD)	N	471	Lee, Paul (NC)	Oph	531
Latov, Norman (NY)	N	471	Lee, Raphael (IL)	PlS	786
Latson, Larry (OH)	PCd	674	Lee, W P Andrew (PA)	HS	278
Lauerman, William (DC)	OrS	566	Lee, W Robert (NC)	RadRO	878
Laufer, Marc (MA)	ObG	508	Leffell, David (CT)	D	179
Laughlin, Mary (OH)	Hem	297	Lefrak, Stephen (MO)	Pul	856
Laurencin, Cato (CT)	OrS	558	Legare, Robert (RI)	Onc	307
Lavenstein, Bennett (VA)	ChiN	145	Legato, Marianne (NY)	IM	388
Laver, Joseph (TN)	PHO	699	Legro, Richard (PA)	RE	928
Lavertu, Pierre (OH)	Oto	617	Lehman, Constance (WA)	DR	908
Lavery, Ian (OH)	CRS	169	Lehman, Thomas (NY)	PRhu	730
Lavin, Patrick (TN)	N	479	Leighton, Jonathan (AZ)	Ge	238
Lavis, Victor (TX)	EDM	210	Leipziger, Lyle (NY)	PlS	776
Lavyne, Michael (NY)	NS	433	Leitch, A Marilyn (TX)	S	997
Lawrence, Theodore (MI)	RadRO	883	Lele, Shashikant (NY)	GO	262
Lawry, George (IA)	Rhu	947	Lem, Vincent (MO)	Pul	856
Lawson, David (GA)	Onc	330	Lemanske, Robert (WI)	PA&I	667
Lawson, Edward (MD)	NP	407	Lemons, James (IN)	NP	410
Lawson, William (NY)	Oto	605	Lenke, Lawrence (MO)	OrS	578
Lawson, William (DC)	Psyc	809	Lentz, Christopher (NY)	S	971
Lazarus, Hillard (OH)	Hem	298	Lentz, Samuel (NC)	GO	264
Le, Quynh-Thu Xuan (CA)	RadRO	889	Lenz, Heinz J (CA)	Ge	240
Le Boit, Philip (CA)	Path	657	Leon, Martin (NY)	IC	121
Lea, Janice (GA)	Nep	419	Leonard, James (MI)	PMR	764
Leadbetter, Wayne (MD)	OrS	566	Leonetti, John (IL)	Oto	617
Leaf, Norman (CA)	PlS	794	Leopold, Donald (NE)	Oto	621
LeBoff, Meryl (MA)	EDM	199	Lepanto, Philip (WV)	RadRO	875
Lebwohl, Mark (NY)	D	183	Lepor, Herbert (NY)	U	1053
Lebwohl, Oscar (NY)	Ge	221	Lerman, Bruce (NY)	CE	116
Lechan, Ronald (MA)	EDM	199	Lerner, Seth (TX)	U	1071
Leckman, James (CT)	ChAP	823	Lesavoy, Malcolm (CA)	PlS	795
Ledford, Dennis (FL)	A&I	84	Leshin, Barry (NC)	D	187
Lee, Andrew (TX)	RadRO	887	Leslie, Donald (GA)	PMR	762
Lee, Andrew (TX)	Oph	541	Leslie, Kevin (AZ)	Path	654
Lee, Cheryl (MI)	U	1065	Leslie, Kimberly (IA)	MF	399

Alphabetical Listing of Doctors

Alphabetical Listing of Doctors

Name	Specialty	Pg	Name	Specialty	Pg
Lindsay, Bruce (OH)	CE	118	Locala, Joseph (OH)	Psyc	813
Lindsey, Stephen (LA)	Rhu	949	Lock, James (MA)	PCd	669
Lindstrom, Richard (MN)	Oph	536	Lock, Terrence (MI)	OrS	578
Linenberger, Michael (WA)	Hem	303	Lockey, Richard (FL)	A&I	85
Link, Michael (MN)	NS	445	Lockhart, Jorge (FL)	U	1060
Link, Michael (CA)	PHO	710	Lockshin, Michael (NY)	Rhu	943
Linker, Charles (CA)	Hem	303	Lockwood, Charles (CT)	MF	394
Linsenmeyer, Todd (NJ)	U	1054	Loder, Elizabeth (MA)	PM	634
Linskey, Mark (CA)	NS	453	Loeffler, Jay (MA)	RadRO	870
Linstrom, Christopher (NY)	Oto	605	Loehrer, Patrick (IN)	Onc	341
Linton, MacRae (TN)	Cv	102	Loevner, Laurie (PA)	NRad	910
Lipkowitz, George (MA)	S	964	Loewenstein, Richard (MD)	Psyc	809
Liporace, Joyce (PA)	N	471	Loftus, Christopher (PA)	NS	434
Lippman, Marc (FL)	Onc	330	Loftus, Edward (MN)	Ge	232
Lippman, Scott (TX)	Onc	350	Logan, William (MO)	N	484
Lipschitz, David (AR)	Ger	250	Loggie, Brian (NE)	S	993
Lipscomb, Gary (IL)	ObG	512	Logigian, Eric (NY)	N	472
Lipshultz, Larry (TX)	U	1071	Logothetis, Christopher (TX)	Onc	351
Lipshutz, William (PA)	Ge	222	Long, Sarah (PA)	PInf	713
Lipsitz, Lewis (MA)	Ger	246	Longo, Walter (CT)	CRS	164
Lipstate, James (LA)	Rhu	949	Longworth, David (MA)	Inf	374
Lipton, Jeffrey (NY)	PHO	695	Loprinzi, Charles (MN)	Onc	341
Lipton, Richard (NY)	N	472	Lorber, Bennett (PA)	Inf	376
Lisak, Robert (MI)	N	484	Loree, Thom (NY)	PlS	777
Lisman, Richard (NY)	Oph	524	LoRusso, Thomas (VA)	Pul	853
List, Alan (FL)	Hem	294	Loscalzo, Joseph (MA)	Cv	93
Litt, Andrew (NY)	NRad	910	Losee, Joseph (PA)	PlS	777
Little, Alex (OH)	TS	1032	Losordo, Douglas (IL)	IC	124
Little, John (DC)	PlS	777	Lossos, Izidore (FL)	Onc	330
Litzow, Mark (MN)	Hem	298	Lott, Ira (CA)	ChiN	148
Liu, Charles (CA)	NS	453	Loughlin, Gerald (NY)	PPul	726
Liu, Donald (IL)	PS	739	Loughlin, Kevin (MA)	U	1049
Liu, Grant (PA)	N	472	Louie, Eddie (NY)	Inf	376
Livingston, Edward (TX)	S	997	Loulmet, Didier (NY)	TS	1023
Livingston, Philip (NY)	Onc	318	Love, Charles (OH)	CE	118
Livingston, Robert (AZ)	Onc	350	Love, Robert (IL)	TS	1032
Livingstone, Alan (FL)	S	980	Low, David (PA)	PlS	777
Ljung, Britt-Marie (CA)	Path	657	Lowe, Franklin (NY)	U	1054
Lloyd, L Keith (AL)	U	1060	Lowe, Lori (MI)	D	189
Lobe, Thom (IA)	PS	739	Lowenberg, David (CA)	OrS	586

Alphabetical Listing of Doctors

M

Name	Specialty	Pg	Name	Specialty	Pg
Mahmud, Ehtisham (CA)	IC	125	Mapstone, Timothy (OK)	NS	450
Mahon, Kathleen (NV)	Oph	546	Maraganore, Demetrius (IL)	N	484
Mahoney, Maurice (CT)	CG	152	Marcet, Jorge (FL)	CRS	167
Mahony, Lynn (TX)	PCd	675	Marchlinski, Francis (PA)	CE	116
Mahowald, Mark (MN)	N	484	Marcom, Paul (NC)	Onc	331
Majd, Massoud (DC)	NuM	502	Marcus, Carole (PA)	PPul	726
Makaroun, Michel (PA)	VascS	1085	Marcus, Robert (FL)	RadRO	878
Make, Barry (CO)	Pul	859	Marder, Stephen (CA)	Psyc	818
Makhija, Sharmila (GA)	GO	265	Marentette, Lawrence (MI)	Oto	617
Maki, Dennis (WI)	Inf	381	Margolin, Kim (WA)	Onc	358
Malawer, Martin (DC)	OrS	566	Margolis, James (FL)	IC	123
Malik, Ghaus (MI)	NS	445	Marin, Deborah (NY)	Psyc	809
Malkowicz, S Bruce (PA)	U	1054	Marin, Michael (NY)	VascS	1085
Maloney, David (WA)	Onc	358	Marina, Neyssa (CA)	PHO	710
Maloney, Mary (MA)	D	179	Marini, John (MN)	Pul	856
Maloney, Robert (CA)	Oph	546	Marino, Ralph (PA)	PMR	760
Mamelak, Adam (CA)	NS	454	Marion, Robert (NY)	CG	153
Mamounas, Eleftherios (OH)	S	988	Maris, John (PA)	PHO	695
Manche, Edward (CA)	Oph	546	Mark, Eugene (MA)	Path	642
Manco-Johnson, Marilyn (CO)	PHO	707	Markert, James (AL)	NS	439
Mancuso, Anthony (FL)	DR	904	Markman, Maurie (TX)	Onc	351
Mandel, Eric (NY)	Oph	525	Markoe, Arnold (FL)	RadRO	879
Mandel, Susan (PA)	EDM	202	Markowitz, Bernard (CA)	PlS	795
Mandelbaum, Bert (CA)	OrS	587	Markowitz, David (NY)	Ge	222
Mandelbaum, David (RI)	ChiN	142	Markowitz, Sanford (OH)	Onc	341
Manders, Ernest (PA)	PlS	777	Marks, Lawrence (NC)	RadRO	879
Manera, Ricarchito (IL)	PHO	704	Marks, Stanley (PA)	Hem	291
Manevitz, Alan (NY)	Psyc	809	Marmar, Charles (CA)	Psyc	818
Mangan, Kenneth (PA)	Hem	291	Marmor, Michael (CA)	Oph	546
Manganiello, Paul (NH)	RE	927	Maroon, Joseph (PA)	NS	434
Mangat, Devinder (KY)	Oto	611	Marrs, Richard (CA)	RE	936
Mann, J John (NY)	Psyc	809	Marsh, Christopher (CA)	U	1074
Manning, Warren (MA)	Cv	93	Marsh, James (PA)	S	971
Mannis, Mark (CA)	Oph	546	Marsh, James (CT)	OrS	558
Manoli, Arthur (MI)	OrS	579	Marsh, Jeffrey (MO)	PlS	787
Mansfield, Paul (TX)	S	998	Marshall, Fray (GA)	U	1060
Manske, Paul (MO)	HS	282	Marshall, John (VA)	EDM	205
Manson, Paul (MD)	PlS	777	Marshall, John (DC)	Onc	318
Mantyh, Christopher (NC)	CRS	167	Marshall, Lawrence (CA)	NS	454
Manzi, Susan (PA)	Rhu	943	Marshall, Margaret Blair (DC)	TS	1023

Alphabetical Listing of Doctors

Alphabetical Listing of Doctors

Name	Specialty	Pg	Name	Specialty	Pg
Menezes, Arnold (IA)	NS	445	Mih, Alexander (IN)	HS	282
Menick, Frederick (AZ)	PIS	791	Mihm, Martin (MA)	D	179
Menon, Mani (MI)	U	1066	Mikkelsen, Tommy (MI)	N	484
Menon, Ram (MI)	PEn	682	Milad, Magdy (IL)	RE	934
Menter, M Alan (TX)	D	192	Milam, Douglas (TN)	U	1060
Merchant, Thomas (TN)	RadRO	879	Mildvan, Donna (NY)	Inf	376
Meredith, Ruby (AL)	RadRO	879	Miles, Brian (TX)	U	1071
Meredith, Travis (NC)	Oph	531	Millenson, Michael (PA)	Hem	291
Merkel, Peter (MA)	Rhu	940	Miller, Aaron (NY)	N	472
Merrick, Hollis (OH)	S	988	Miller, Antonius (NC)	Onc	331
Merrick, Scot (CA)	TS	1040	Miller, Charles (IL)	RE	934
Merrill, Walter (OH)	TS	1032	Miller, D Douglas (GA)	Cv	102
Merritt, Diane (MO)	ObG	512	Miller, Daniel (GA)	TS	1028
Mersey, James (MD)	EDM	202	Miller, David (CA)	TS	1040
Mertz, Howard (TN)	Ge	227	Miller, Donald (KY)	Onc	331
Mesrobian, Hrair-George (WI)	U	1066	Miller, Franklin (KY)	MF	397
Mesulam, Marel (IL)	N	484	Miller, Joan (MA)	Oph	519
Metcalfe, Dean (MD)	A&I	83	Miller, Joseph (AZ)	Oph	541
Metersky, Mark (CT)	Pul	845	Miller, Joseph (GA)	TS	1028
Mets, Marilyn (IL)	Oph	536	Miller, Kenneth (MA)	Hem	289
Metson, Ralph (MA)	Oto	600	Miller, Mark (VA)	OrS	573
Metz, David (PA)	Ge	222	Miller, Neil (MD)	Oph	525
Metzl, Jordan (NY)	SM	955	Miller, Robert (IL)	PO	723
Meyer, Anthony (NC)	S	981	Miller, Stanley (MD)	D	183
Meyer, Fredric (MN)	NS	445	Miller, Thomas (AZ)	Onc	351
Meyer, William (OK)	PHO	708	Miller, Timothy (CA)	PIS	795
Meyers, Bryan (MO)	TS	1032	Miller, Vincent (NY)	Onc	319
Meyers, Paul (NY)	PHO	695	Millett, Peter (CO)	OrS	582
Meyers, Rebecka (UT)	PS	740	Milley, J Ross (UT)	NP	411
Meyers, William (PA)	S	971	Millis, J Michael (IL)	S	988
Meyskens, Frank (CA)	Onc	358	Millman, Richard (RI)	Pul	845
Michaels, Marian (PA)	PInf	713	Mills, Monte (PA)	Oph	525
Michalska, Margaret (IL)	Rhu	948	Mills, Stacey (VA)	Path	649
Michalski, Jeff M (MO)	RadRO	883	Milsom, Jeffrey (NY)	CRS	166
Michelassi, Fabrizio (NY)	S	971	Mims, James (TX)	Oph	542
Micheli, Lyle (MA)	SM	954	Minaker, Kenneth (MA)	Ger	246
Mickey, Bruce (TX)	NS	450	Minckler, Donald (CA)	Oph	546
Mieler, William (IL)	Oph	537	Miniaci, Anthony (OH)	SM	957
Mieres, Jennifer (NY)	Cv	98	Minich, Lois (UT)	PCd	675
Mies, Carolyn (PA)	Path	646	Mink, Jonathan (NY)	ChiN	144

Name	Specialty	Pg	Name	Specialty	Pg
Minkoff, Howard (NY)	ObG	509	Moneim, Moheb (NM)	HS	283
Minor, Lloyd (MD)	Oto	605	Money, Samuel (AZ)	VascS	1091
Minsky, Bruce (IL)	RadRO	883	Monk, Bradley (CA)	GO	271
Mintzer, David (PA)	Onc	319	Monsees, Barbara (MO)	DR	906
Mirmira, Raghu (IN)	PEn	682	Montague, Drogo (OH)	U	1066
Miro-Quesada, Miguel (TX)	Hem	301	Montanaro, Anthony (OR)	A&I	88
Mirvis, Stuart (MD)	DR	902	Montgomery, Elizabeth (MD)	Path	646
Mirzayan, Raffy (CA)	SM	957	Montgomery, Erwin (AL)	N	479
Mischel, Paul (CA)	Path	657	Montgomery, Robert (MD)	S	971
Miskovitz, Paul (NY)	Ge	222	Montie, James (MI)	U	1066
Mitch, William (TX)	Nep	423	Moodie, Douglas (LA)	PCd	675
Mitchell, Beverly (CA)	Hem	303	Moore, Anne (NY)	Onc	319
Mitchell, Charles (FL)	PInf	714	Moore, Joseph (NC)	Onc	331
Mitchell, James (ND)	Psyc	815	Moore, Thomas (CA)	MF	402
Mitchell, John (CO)	TS	1035	Moore, Walter (GA)	Rhu	946
Mitchell, Marc (MS)	VascS	1087	Moossa, AR (CA)	S	1003
Mitchell, Max (CO)	TS	1035	Morady, Fred (MI)	CE	118
Mitchell, Michael (WI)	U	1066	Moran, Cesar (TX)	Path	654
Mitchell, Paul (CT)	Oph	519	Moran, Christopher (MO)	NRad	913
Mitchell, Wendy (CA)	ChiN	148	Moran, John (IL)	Cv	107
Mitnick, Hal (NY)	Rhu	943	Morgan, Elaine (IL)	PHO	704
Mitnick, Julie (NY)	DR	902	Morgan, Linda (FL)	ObG	510
Mitros, Frank (IA)	Path	651	Morgan, Mark (PA)	GO	262
Mitsumoto, Hiroshi (NY)	N	472	Morgan, Raymond (VA)	PlS	783
Mitsuyasu, Ronald (CA)	Onc	358	Morgan, Walter (TN)	PS	736
Mittal, Bharat (IL)	RadRO	883	Morgan, Wayne (AZ)	PPul	729
Miyamoto, Richard (IN)	Oto	617	Morgenlander, Joel (NC)	N	479
Mizen, Thomas (IL)	Oph	537	Morley, John (MO)	Ger	249
Moder, Kevin (MN)	Rhu	948	Morrell, Martha (CA)	N	494
Modic, Michael (OH)	NRad	913	Morris, Colleen (NV)	CG	159
Moench, Louis (UT)	Psyc	815	Morris, Douglas (GA)	IC	123
Mohammad, Yousef (IL)	N	484	Morris, John (MO)	N	485
Mohl, Paul (TX)	Psyc	816	Morris, P Pearse (NC)	NRad	912
Mohler, James (NY)	U	1054	Morris, Robert (CA)	AM	78
Mohr, JP (NY)	N	473	Morris, Rohinton (PA)	TS	1023
Moley, Jeffrey (MO)	S	988	Morrison, Glenn (FL)	NS	439
Molleston, Jean (IN)	PGe	688	Morrow, Monica (NY)	S	972
Molnar, Joseph (NC)	PlS	783	Mortimer, Joanne (CA)	Onc	358
Molo, Mary (IL)	RE	934	Morton, D Holmes (PA)	Ped	663
Mondino, Bartly (CA)	Oph	547	Morton, John (CA)	S	1003

Alphabetical Listing of Doctors

Name	Specialty	Pg	Name	Specialty	Pg
Mosca, Lori (NY)	Cv	98	Muschler, George (OH)	OrS	579
Moscatello, Augustine (NY)	Oto	605	Muss, Hyman (NC)	Onc	331
Moscow, Jeffrey (KY)	PHO	699	Mustoe, Thomas (IL)	PlS	787
Mosenifar, Zab (CA)	Pul	862	Mutch, David (MO)	GO	267
Moses, Jeffrey (NY)	IC	121	Muto, Michael (MA)	GO	259
Mosher, Deane (WI)	Hem	298	Myer, Charles (OH)	PO	723
Moskowitz, William (VA)	PCd	672	Myerburg, Robert (FL)	Cv	102
Moss, R Lawrence (CT)	PS	733	Myers, Jeffrey (MI)	Path	652
Mostwin, Jacek (MD)	U	1054	Myers, Jeffrey (TX)	Oto	623
Mott, Michael (MI)	OrS	579	Myers, Jonathan (PA)	Oph	525
Motzer, Robert (NY)	Onc	319	Myers, Robert (MN)	U	1067
Moul, Judd (NC)	U	1061	Myerson, Mark (MD)	OrS	567
Mountz, James (PA)	NuM	503	Myerson, Robert (MO)	RadRO	884
Movsas, Benjamin (MI)	RadRO	884	Myones, Barry (TX)	PRhu	732
Muggia, Franco (NY)	Onc	319	Myseros, John (VA)	NS	439
Mukherjee, Tanmoy (NY)	RE	929	Mysiw, W Jerry (OH)	PMR	764
Mukherji, Suresh (MI)	NRad	913			
Muldoon, Thomas (NY)	Oph	525			
Mulhall, John (NY)	U	1054			
Mullett, Timothy (KY)	TS	1028			

N

Name	Specialty	Pg
Mulliken, John (MA)	PlS	773
Mulvihill, John (OK)	CG	157

Name	Specialty	Pg
Nabell, Lisle (AL)	Onc	331
Nabors, Louis (AL)	N	479
Naccarelli, Gerald (PA)	Cv	98
Nachman, James (IL)	PHO	704
Naclerio, Robert (IL)	Oto	618
Nademanee, Auayporn (CA)	Hem	303
Nadler, Lee (MA)	Onc	307
Nadol, Joseph (MA)	Oto	600
Nagel, Theodore (MN)	RE	934
Nagib, Mahmoud (MN)	NS	445
Nagle, Daniel (IL)	HS	282
Nagle, Deborah (MA)	CRS	164
Nagler, Harris (NY)	U	1054
Nagorney, David (MN)	S	989
Nagueh, Sherif (TX)	Cv	111
Nahass, Ronald (NJ)	Inf	377
Naka, Yoshifumi (NY)	TS	1023
Nakakura, Eric (CA)	S	1003
Nakayama, Don (GA)	PS	736
Nance, Michael (PA)	PS	735
Nand, Sucha (IL)	Hem	298

Name	Specialty	Pg
Mulvihill, Sean (UT)	S	993
Mundt, Arno (CA)	RadRO	889
Munin, Michael (PA)	PMR	760
Munker, Reinhold (LA)	Hem	301
Munoz, Jose (NY)	PInf	713
Munoz, Santiago (PA)	Ge	223
Muntz, Howard (WA)	GO	271
Murali, Raj (NY)	NS	434
Muraskas, Jonathan (IL)	NP	410
Murphree, A Linn (CA)	Oph	547
Murphy, Ana (GA)	RE	932
Murphy, Douglas (GA)	TS	1028
Murphy, Thomas (NC)	PPul	727
Murphy, Timothy (RI)	VIR	916
Murray, Joseph (MN)	Ge	233
Murray, Pamela (PA)	AM	76
Murray, Timothy (FL)	Oph	531
Murtagh, F Reed (FL)	NRad	912

Name	Specialty	Pg	Name	Specialty	Pg
Napoli, Joseph (DE)	PlS	778	Neumann, Ronald (MD)	NuM	503
Nardell, Edward (MA)	Pul	846	Neumeister, Michael (IL)	PlS	787
Narkewicz, Michael (CO)	PGe	689	Neuwelt, Edward (OR)	NS	454
Nascimento, Antonio (MN)	Path	652	Neuwirth, Michael (NY)	OrS	567
Nash, Martin (NY)	PNep	717	Neville, Richard (DC)	VascS	1085
Nash, Thomas (NY)	Pul	848	Nevins, Thomas (MN)	PNep	719
Naslund, Michael (MD)	U	1055	New, Maria (NY)	PEn	680
Natale, Ronald (CA)	Onc	358	Newburger, Jane (MA)	PCd	669
Nath, Avindra (MD)	N	473	Newell, Kenneth (GA)	S	981
Nathanson, S David (MI)	S	989	Newman, Lawrence (NY)	N	473
Nathwani, Bharat (CA)	Path	657	Newman, Leonard (NY)	PGe	685
Naunheim, Keith (MO)	TS	1033	Newman, Lisa (MI)	S	989
Nava-Villarreal, Hector (NY)	S	972	Newman, Nancy (GA)	N	479
Nazzaro, Jules (KS)	NS	448	Newton, Herbert (OH)	N	485
Neel, Victor (MA)	D	180	Ngeow, Jeffrey (NY)	PM	635
Neglia, Joseph (MN)	PHO	705	Nguyen, Ninh (CA)	S	1003
Negrin, Robert (CA)	Hem	303	Nicholas, Stephen (NY)	OrS	567
Nehra, Ajay (MN)	U	1067	Nicholl, Jeffrey (LA)	N	490
Neiberger, Richard (FL)	PNep	718	Nichols, Craig (OR)	Onc	358
Neifeld, James (VA)	S	981	Nicholson, Henry (OR)	PHO	710
Nelson, Edward (UT)	S	993	Nichter, Larry (CA)	PlS	795
Nelson, Heidi (MN)	CRS	169	Nicolaou, Nicos (PA)	RadRO	875
Nelson, James (CA)	Psyc	818	Nicosia, Santo (FL)	Path	649
Nelson, Joel (PA)	U	1055	Nieder, Michael (FL)	PHO	700
Nelson, Judith (NY)	Pul	848	Niederman, Michael (NY)	Pul	848
Nelson, Leonard (PA)	Oph	525	Nigra, Thomas (DC)	D	183
Nelson, Maureen (NC)	PMR	762	Nimer, Stephen (NY)	Hem	291
Nemcek, Albert (IL)	VIR	919	Ninan, Mathews (TN)	TS	1028
Nemickas, Rimgaudas (IL)	Cv	107	Niparko, John (MD)	Oto	605
Nemunaitis, John (TX)	Onc	351	Nishimura, Rick (MN)	Cv	107
Neppe, Vernon (WA)	Psyc	818	Nisonson, Barton (NY)	SM	955
Nerad, Jeffrey (OH)	Oph	537	Nissen, Nicholas (CA)	S	1004
Nesbitt, Jonathan (TN)	TS	1028	Nissen, Steven (OH)	Cv	107
Ness, John (MN)	PlS	787	Nissenblatt, Michael (NJ)	Onc	319
Nestler, John (VA)	EDM	205	Nitti, Victor (NY)	U	1055
Netterville, James (TN)	Oto	611	Nobunaga, Austin (OH)	PMR	764
Neu, Josef (FL)	NP	409	Nocero, Michael (FL)	Cv	102
Neuberg, Ronnie (SC)	PHO	700	Noetzel, Michael (MO)	ChiN	146
Neuburg, Marcelle (WI)	D	189	Nogee, Lawrence (MD)	NP	407
Neumann, Donald (OH)	NuM	504	Nogueras, Juan (FL)	CRS	167

Alphabetical Listing of Doctors

Name	Specialty	Pg	Name	Specialty	Pg
Nolan, Bruce (FL)	N	479	O'Donnell, Michael (IA)	U	1067
Noller, Kenneth (MA)	ObG	508	O'Donnell, Richard (CA)	OrS	587
Noone, R Barrett (PA)	PlS	778	O'Dorisio, M Sue (IA)	PHO	705
Norbash, Alexander (MA)	NRad	909	O'Driscoll, Shawn (MN)	OrS	579
Nordli, Douglas (IL)	ChiN	146	O'Gara, Patrick (MA)	Cv	93
Norenberg, Michael (FL)	Path	649	O'Hea, Brian (NY)	S	972
Nori, Dattatreyudu (NY)	RadRO	875	O'Keefe, J Paul (IL)	Inf	381
Norman, David (CA)	NRad	915	O'Keefe, Regis (NY)	OrS	567
Norman, Kim (CA)	Psyc	818	O'Laughlin, Martin (MO)	PCd	674
Northfelt, Donald (AZ)	Onc	351	O'Leary, Michael P (MA)	U	1049
Northrup, Hope (TX)	CG	157	O'Leary, Patrick (NY)	OrS	567
Norton, Jeffrey (CA)	S	1004	O'Malley, Bert (PA)	Oto	606
Norton, Karen (NJ)	DR	903	O'Neill, William (FL)	Cv	103
Norton, Larry (NY)	Onc	320	O'Regan, Ruth (GA)	Onc	332
Nour, Nawal (MA)	ObG	508	O'Reilly, Eileen (NY)	Onc	320
Novak, Donald (FL)	PGe	686	O'Reilly, Richard (NY)	PHO	695
Novotny, Edward (CT)	ChiN	142	O'Rourke, Donald (PA)	NS	434
Nowak, Eugene (NY)	S	972	O'Shaughnessy, Joyce (TX)	Onc	351
Noyes, Nicole (NY)	RE	929	Oakes, W Jerry (AL)	NS	439
Nuber, Gordon (IL)	OrS	579	Oaks, Timothy (NC)	TS	1029
Nuchtern, Jed (TX)	PS	741	Oates, Robert (MA)	U	1049
Nugent, William (NH)	TS	1017	Oberfield, Sharon (NY)	PEn	680
Nunery, William (IN)	Oph	537	Oberholzer, Jose (IL)	S	989
Nunley, James (NC)	OrS	574	Oddis, Chester (PA)	Rhu	943
Nurnberger, John (IN)	Psyc	814	Odel, Jeffrey (NY)	Oph	526
Nuss, Daniel (LA)	Oto	623	Odem, Randall (MO)	RE	934
Nuss, Donald (VA)	PS	736	Odom, Lorrie (CO)	PHO	707
Nussbaum, Julian (GA)	Oph	531	Odom, Michael (TX)	NP	412
Nussbaum, Robert (CA)	CG	159	Odunsi, Adekunle (NY)	GO	262
Nutt, John (OR)	N	494	Odze, Robert (MA)	Path	642
			Oeffinger, Kevin (NY)	Ped	663
			Offit, Kenneth (NY)	Onc	320
			Offit, Paul (PA)	PInf	713
O			Oh, Shin (AL)	N	480
O'Brien, Joan (CA)	Oph	547	Oh, William (NY)	Onc	320
O'Brien, John (MI)	Ge	233	Ohl, Dana (MI)	U	1067
O'Brien, Susan (TX)	Onc	351	Ohman, E Magnus (NC)	Cv	103
O'Connor, Christopher (NC)	Cv	103	Okolo, Patrick (MD)	Ge	223
O'Day, Steven (CA)	Onc	358	Okusa, Mark (VA)	Nep	419
O'Dell, James (NE)	Rhu	948	Olanow, C Warren (NY)	N	473
O'Donnell, Margaret (CA)	Hem	303			

Name	Specialty	Pg	Name	Specialty	Pg
Olbricht, Suzanne (MA)	D	180	Ostroff, James (CA)	Ge	240
Oldham, Keith (WI)	PS	739	Ostrom, Nancy (CA)	A&I	88
Olitsky, Scott (MO)	Oph	537	Otley, Clark (MN)	D	189
Oliva-Hemker, Maria (MD)	PGe	685	Ott, David (TX)	TS	1037
Olivero, Juan (TX)	Nep	423	Ott, Kenneth (CA)	NS	454
Olopade, Olufunmilayo (IL)	Onc	341	Ott, Susan (WA)	Nep	424
Olsen, Elise (NC)	D	187	Otto, Pamela (TX)	DR	907
Olsen, Kerry (MN)	Oto	618	Otto, Randal (TX)	Oto	623
Olson, Jack (IL)	Ger	249	Ovalle, Fernando (AL)	EDM	205
Olson, Jeffrey (GA)	NS	439	Ownby, Dennis (GA)	PA&I	667
Olson, Thomas (GA)	PHO	700	Owyang, Chung (MI)	Ge	233
Olthoff, Kim (PA)	S	972	Oz, Mehmet (NY)	TS	1023
Onders, Raymond (OH)	S	989	Ozer, Enver (OH)	Oto	618
Ontjes, David (NC)	EDM	205			
Oommen, Kalarickal (TX)	N	490			
Oparil, Suzanne (AL)	Cv	103	**P**		
Opitz, John (UT)	CG	156			
Oppenheim, William (CA)	OrS	587	Pachter, H Leon (NY)	S	972
Oquendo, Maria (NY)	Psyc	809	Pacin, Michael (FL)	A&I	85
Oratz, Ruth (NY)	Onc	320	Pack, Allan (PA)	Pul	848
Orazi, Attilio (NY)	Path	646	Packer, Roger (DC)	ChiN	144
Orengo, Ida (TX)	D	192	Padgett, Douglas (NY)	OrS	567
Orenstein, David (PA)	PPul	726	Pagani, Francis (MI)	TS	1033
Orgill, Dennis (MA)	PlS	773	Page, David (TN)	Path	650
Origitano, Thomas (IL)	NS	445	Paget, Stephen (NY)	Rhu	944
Orlow, Seth (NY)	D	183	Pagon, Roberta (WA)	CG	159
Orlowski, Robert (TX)	Onc	351	Pahl, Elfriede (IL)	PCd	674
Orobello, Peter (FL)	PO	722	Paidas, Charles (FL)	PS	736
Orringer, Mark B (MI)	TS	1033	Paidas, Michael (CT)	MF	395
Ortel, Thomas (NC)	Hem	294	Palacios, Igor (MA)	Cv	93
Orwoll, Eric (OR)	EDM	212	Palascak, Joseph (OH)	Hem	298
Ory, Steven (FL)	RE	932	Palefsky, Joel (CA)	Inf	384
Osborn, Anne (UT)	NRad	914	Paletta, George (MO)	SM	957
Osborne, Charles (TX)	Onc	352	Palevsky, Harold (PA)	Pul	848
Osborne, Michael (NY)	S	972	Paley, Dror (FL)	OrS	574
Osguthorpe, John (SC)	Oto	611	Palfrey, Judith (MA)	Ped	662
Osher, Robert (OH)	Oph	537	Paller, Amy (IL)	D	190
Oster, Martin (NY)	Onc	320	Palmberg, Paul (FL)	Oph	531
Osterman, A Lee (PA)	HS	278	Palmer, Earl A (OR)	Oph	547
Ostrer, Harry (NY)	CG	153	Palmer, Robert (PA)	Ger	247
			Palmer, William (MA)	DR	899

Alphabetical Listing of Doctors

Name	Specialty	Pg	Name	Specialty	Pg
Panicek, David (NY)	DR	903	Patterson, Anthony (TN)	U	1061
Panitch, Howard (PA)	PPul	726	Patterson, G Alexander (MO)	TS	1033
Pantilat, Steven (CA)	IM	391	Patterson, James (OR)	Pul	863
Papadopoulos, Nicholas (TX)	Onc	352	Patterson, Jan E Evans (TX)	Inf	383
Papadopoulos, Stephen (AZ)	NS	450	Patterson, Marc (MN)	ChiN	146
Paparella, Michael (MN)	Oto	618	Patterson, Thomas (TX)	Inf	383
Papel, Ira (MD)	Oto	606	Paty, Philip (NY)	S	972
Pappas, Theodore (NC)	S	981	Patz, Edward (NC)	DR	905
Parent, Andrew (MS)	NS	439	Patzakis, Michael (CA)	OrS	587
Parisier, Simon (NY)	Oto	606	Paul, Malcolm (CA)	PlS	795
Park, Adrian (MD)	S	972	Paul, T Otis (CA)	Oph	547
Park, Catherine (CA)	RadRO	889	Paulson, Richard (CA)	RE	936
Park, Tae Sung (MO)	NS	445	Payne, Christopher (CA)	U	1075
Parker, Barbara (CA)	Onc	359	Paz, Isaac (CA)	S	1004
Parker, Robert (NY)	PHO	695	Peabody, Terrance (IL)	OrS	580
Parness, Ira (NY)	PCd	671	Pearce, William (IL)	VascS	1089
Parrillo, Joseph (NJ)	Cv	98	Pearlman, Nathan (CO)	S	993
Parrish, Richard (FL)	Oph	531	Pearson, Richard (VA)	Inf	379
Parry, Samuel (PA)	MF	396	Pearson, Thomas (NY)	PrM	801
Parsons, Polly (VT)	Pul	846	Pecora, Andrew (NJ)	Onc	320
Parsons, Rosaleen (PA)	DR	903	Pedley, Timothy (NY)	N	473
Parsons, Theodore (MI)	OrS	579	Peereboom, David (OH)	Onc	341
Partain, Clarence (TN)	DR	904	Pegram, P Samuel (NC)	Inf	379
Partin, Alan (MD)	U	1055	Peikin, Steven (NJ)	Ge	223
Pasche, Boris (AL)	Onc	332	Peitzman, Andrew (PA)	S	973
Pascuzzi, Robert (IN)	N	485	Pellegrini, Carlos (WA)	S	1004
Pasmantier, Mark (NY)	Onc	320	Pellicci, Paul (NY)	OrS	567
Pasricha, Pankaj (CA)	Ge	240	Pelzer, Harold (IL)	Oto	618
Pass, Harvey (NY)	TS	1024	Pemberton, John (MN)	CRS	169
Passo, Murray (SC)	PRhu	731	Pena, Alberto (OH)	PS	739
Patchefsky, Arthur (PA)	Path	646	Penalver, Manuel (FL)	GO	265
Patchell, Roy (KY)	N	480	Penar, Paul (VT)	NS	429
Patel, Pravin (IL)	PlS	787	Pendergrass, Thomas (WA)	PHO	710
Patel, Shreyaskumar (TX)	Onc	352	Pensak, Myles (OH)	Oto	618
Patel, Sunil (SC)	NS	439	Penson, David (CA)	U	1075
Patel, Vipul (FL)	U	1061	Pepine, Carl (FL)	Cv	103
Pathria, Mini (CA)	DR	908	Pepose, Jay (MO)	Oph	537
Patrinely, James (FL)	Oph	531	Perez, Edith (FL)	Onc	332
Patrizio, Pasquale (CT)	RE	927	Perez, Victor (FL)	Oph	532
Patt, Yehuda (NM)	Onc	352	Perez Fontan, J Julio (TX)	PCCM	677

Name	Specialty	Pg	Name	Specialty	Pg
Pergament, Eugene (IL)	CG	155	Pfeifer, Samantha (PA)	RE	929
Perin, Emerson (TX)	IC	125	Pfister, David (NY)	Onc	321
Perkash, Inder (CA)	U	1075	Pflugfelder, Stephen (TX)	Oph	542
Perkins, James (WA)	S	1004	Philippon, Marc (CO)	OrS	582
Perler, Bruce (MD)	VascS	1085	Philipson, Elliot (OH)	MF	399
Perlman, David (NY)	Inf	377	Phillips, Edward (CA)	S	1004
Perlman, Jeffrey (NY)	NP	408	Phillips, Harry (NC)	Cv	103
Perlmutter, Joel (MO)	N	485	Phillips, Katharine (RI)	Psyc	805
Perret, Philip (LA)	Pul	860	Phillips, Peter (PA)	ChiN	144
Perrone, Ronald (MA)	Nep	416	Phillips, Robert (MA)	Cv	94
Perry, Arie (MO)	Path	652	Phuphanich, Surasak (CA)	N	494
Perry, David (DC)	Onc	321	Pi, Edmond (CA)	Psyc	818
Perry, Michael (MO)	Onc	341	Piatt, Joseph (PA)	NS	434
Perry, Stanton (CA)	PCd	676	Piccirillo, Jay (MO)	Oto	618
Persing, John (CT)	PlS	773	Piccoli, David (PA)	PGe	685
Persky, Mark (NY)	Oto	606	Pichard, Augusto (DC)	IC	121
Peschel, Richard (CT)	RadRO	871	Picken, Catherine (DC)	Oto	606
Pestronk, Alan (MO)	N	485	Picozzi, Vincent (WA)	Onc	359
Petelin, Joseph (KS)	S	993	Picus, Joel (MO)	Onc	342
Peters, Glenn (AL)	Oto	611	Pienta, Kenneth (MI)	Onc	342
Peters, Jeffrey (NY)	S	973	Piepgras, David (MN)	NS	446
Petersdorf, Stephen (WA)	Onc	359	Piepmeier, Joseph (CT)	NS	429
Petersen, Ronald (MN)	N	485	Pierce, Lori (MI)	RadRO	884
Peterson, Bruce (MN)	Onc	341	Pierson, Richard (MD)	TS	1024
Peterson, Davis (AK)	OrS	587	Pile-Spellman, John (NY)	NRad	910
Peterson, Laura (HI)	S	1004	Pillsbury, Harold (NC)	Oto	612
Petito, Carol (FL)	Path	650	Pinckert, Thomas (MD)	MF	396
Petito, Frank (NY)	N	473	Pinson, C Wright (TN)	S	981
Petras, Robert (OH)	Path	652	Pinto, Harlan (CA)	Onc	359
Petrelli, Nicholas (DE)	S	973	Pinzur, Michael (IL)	OrS	580
Petri, Michelle (MD)	Rhu	944	Piraino, Beth (PA)	Nep	418
Petrossian, George (NY)	IC	121	Pisters, Katherine (TX)	Onc	352
Petru, Ann (CA)	PInf	716	Pisters, Louis (TX)	U	1071
Petruzzelli, Guy (IL)	Oto	618	Pisters, Peter (TX)	S	998
Petrylak, Daniel (NY)	Onc	321	Pitman, Gerald (NY)	PlS	778
Pettrone, Frank (VA)	OrS	574	Pitman, Karen (MS)	Oto	612
Pevec, William (CA)	VascS	1092	Plager, David (IN)	Oph	537
Pezner, Richard (CA)	RadRO	889	Plancher, Kevin (NY)	SM	955
Pezzone, Michael (PA)	Ge	223	Plante, Lauren (PA)	ObG	509
Pfeffer, Marc (MA)	Cv	93	Platt, Lawrence (CA)	MF	402

Alphabetical Listing of Doctors

Name	Specialty	Pg	Name	Specialty	Pg
Platzker, Arnold (CA)	PPul	729	Poppas, Dix (NY)	U	1055
Plautz, Gregory (OH)	PHO	705	Porayko, Michael (TN)	Ge	228
Plaxe, Steven (CA)	GO	271	Porcu, Pierluigi (OH)	Hem	298
Plehn, Jonathan (MD)	Cv	98	Porrazzo, Michael (DC)	RadRO	875
Plevy, Scott (NC)	Ge	228	Portenoy, Russell (NY)	PM	635
Plon, Sharon (TX)	CG	157	Porter, Co-burn (MN)	PCd	674
Plotnick, Leslie (MD)	PEn	680	Porter, David (PA)	Hem	291
Plotz, Paul (MD)	Rhu	944	Posey, James (AL)	Onc	332
Pochapin, Mark (NY)	Ge	223	Posner, Jerome (NY)	N	473
Pochettino, Alberto (PA)	TS	1024	Posner, Marshall (MA)	Onc	307
Pockaj, Barbara (AZ)	S	998	Posner, Mitchell (IL)	S	989
Podoloff, Donald (TX)	NuM	505	Posnick, Jeffrey (MD)	PlS	778
Poehling, Gary (NC)	OrS	574	Postier, Russell (OK)	S	998
Pohl, Marc (OH)	Nep	421	Postma, Gregory (GA)	Oto	612
Pohlman, Brad (OH)	Onc	342	Potenza, Bruce (CA)	S	1004
Poliakoff, Steven (FL)	GO	265	Potkul, Ronald (IL)	GO	267
Polin, Richard (NY)	NP	408	Potter, Hollis (NY)	DR	903
Polisson, Richard (MA)	Rhu	940	Pow-Sang, Julio (FL)	U	1061
Pollack, Alan (FL)	RadRO	879	Powell, Bayard (NC)	Hem	294
Pollack, Ian (PA)	NS	435	Powell, Catherine (CA)	GO	271
Pollard, Zane (GA)	Oph	532	Powell, Nelson (CA)	Oto	626
Polley, John (IL)	PlS	787	Powers, Alvin (TN)	EDM	205
Pollock, Raphael (TX)	S	998	Powers, Eric (SC)	Cv	103
Polly, David (MN)	OrS	580	Powers, Pauline (FL)	Psyc	812
Polonsky, Kenneth (MO)	EDM	208	Prados, Michael (CA)	Onc	359
Polsky, Bruce (NY)	Inf	377	Prager, Joshua (CA)	PM	640
Pomeroy, John (NY)	ChAP	825	Prakash, Udaya (MN)	Pul	857
Pomeroy, Scott (MA)	ChiN	142	Preminger, Glenn (NC)	U	1061
Pomp, Alfons (NY)	S	973	Press, Joel (IL)	PMR	765
Pomposelli, Frank (MA)	VascS	964	Press, Oliver (WA)	Onc	359
Pongracic, Jacqueline (IL)	PA&I	667	Presti, Joseph (CA)	U	1075
Ponn, Teresa (NH)	S	964	Price, Lawrence (RI)	Psyc	805
Ponsky, Jeffrey (OH)	S	989	Pridjian, Gabriella (LA)	MF	401
Ponton, Lynn (CA)	ChAP	829	Prieto, Victor (TX)	Path	654
Poole, Michael (GA)	Oto	612	Prinz, Richard (IL)	S	989
Poon, Michael (NY)	Cv	98	Prosnitz, Leonard (NC)	RadRO	879
Poordad, Fred (CA)	Ge	240	Provenzale, James (NC)	NRad	912
Pope, John (TN)	U	1061	Pruitt, David (MD)	ChAP	825
Pope, Richard (IL)	Rhu	948	Prystowsky, Eric (IN)	CE	118
Popovich, John (MI)	Pul	857	Puccetti, Diane (WI)	PHO	705

Name	Specialty	Pg
Puckett, Charles (MO)	PlS	787
Pui, Ching-Hon (TN)	PHO	700
Pula, Thaddeus (MD)	N	473
Puliafito, Carmen (CA)	Oph	547
Pulido, Jose (MN)	Oph	538
Purdue, Gary (TX)	S	998
Putnam, Joe (TN)	TS	1029
Putnam, Matthew (MN)	HS	282
Putterman, Allen (IL)	Oph	538
Pyeritz, Reed (PA)	CG	154
Pynoos, Robert (CA)	Psyc	818

Q

Name	Specialty	Pg
Quaegebeur, Jan (NY)	PS	735
Quagliarello, Vincent (CT)	Inf	374
Quatela, Vito (NY)	Oto	606
Quencer, Robert (FL)	NRad	912
Quigley, Harry (MD)	Oph	526
Quill, Timothy (NY)	IM	389
Quinn, David (CA)	Onc	359
Quinn, Graham (PA)	Oph	526
Quinn, Suzanne (FL)	EDM	205
Quinones, Miguel (TX)	Cv	111
Quintessenza, James (FL)	TS	1029
Quittell, Lynne (NY)	PPul	726
Quivey, Jeanne (CA)	RadRO	889

R

Name	Specialty	Pg
Rabinovitch, Rachel (CO)	RadRO	885
Rabow, Michael (CA)	IM	391
Racz, Gabor (TX)	PM	639
Rader, Daniel (PA)	IM	389
Rader, Janet (MO)	GO	267
Radtke, Wolfgang (DE)	PCd	671
Raffel, Corey (OH)	NS	446
Rafferty, Janice (OH)	CRS	169
Raghavan, Derek (OH)	Onc	342

Name	Specialty	Pg
Raghu, Ganesh (WA)	Pul	863
Ragnarsson, Kristjan (NY)	PMR	761
Rahal, James (NY)	Inf	377
Rahko, Peter (WI)	Cv	107
Rai, Kanti (NY)	Hem	291
Raiford, David (TN)	Ge	228
Raja, Srinivasa (MD)	PM	635
Rajfer, Jacob (CA)	U	1075
Rakowski, Thomas (VA)	Nep	419
Ramamoorthy, Sonia (CA)	CRS	172
Ramamurthy, Somayaji (TX)	PM	639
Raman, Jai (IL)	TS	1033
Ramanathan, Ramesh (PA)	S	973
Ramee, Stephen (LA)	Cv	111
Ramirez, Oscar (FL)	PlS	783
Ramsay, David (NY)	D	183
Ramsey, Bonnie (WA)	PPul	729
Ramsey, Matthew (PA)	OrS	568
Ranawat, Chitranjan (NY)	OrS	568
Rand, Jacob (NY)	Hem	291
Rand, Richard (WA)	PlS	795
Randall, Marcus (KY)	RadRO	880
Randall, R Lor (UT)	OrS	582
Randall, Thomas (PA)	GO	262
Randolph, Gregory (MA)	Oto	600
Randolph, Linda (CA)	CG	159
Rao, Nalini (PA)	Inf	377
Rao, Narsing (CA)	Oph	547
Rao, Satish (IA)	Ge	233
Rao, Vijay (PA)	DR	903
Raphael, Bruce (NY)	Hem	292
Rapoport, Judith (DC)	ChAP	825
Rappaport, Leonard (MA)	Ped	662
Rappaport, Norman (TX)	PlS	791
Raptis, George (NY)	Onc	321
Rashid, Asif (TX)	Path	654
Raskin, Keith (NY)	HS	278
Raskin, Neil (CA)	N	494
Raskin, Philip (TX)	EDM	210
Raskind, Murray (WA)	Psyc	818

Alphabetical Listing of Doctors

Name	Specialty	Pg	Name	Specialty	Pg
Rasmussen, Steven (RI)	Psyc	805	Reich, Stephen (MD)	N	473
Rassekh, Christopher (WV)	Oto	606	Reichelderfer, Mark (WI)	Ge	233
Rassman, William (CA)	S	1004	Reid, Tony (CA)	Onc	359
Raszka, William (VT)	PInf	712	Reid, William (TN)	NS	440
Ratain, Mark (IL)	Onc	342	Reilly, Donald (MA)	OrS	558
Ratts, Valerie (MO)	RE	934	Reilly, John (PA)	Pul	848
Ratzan, Kenneth (FL)	Inf	380	Reilly, Raymond (MA)	ObG	508
Rauch, Paula (MA)	Psyc	805	Reiner, Jonathan (DC)	IC	121
Rauch, Steven (MA)	Oto	600	Reiner, Mark (NY)	S	973
Rauck, Richard (NC)	PM	636	Reinisch, John (CA)	PlS	795
Rausen, Aaron (NY)	PHO	696	Reinus, William (PA)	DR	903
Ravich, William (MD)	Ge	223	Reis, Steven (PA)	Cv	98
Rayan, Ghazi (OK)	HS	283	Reisberg, Barry (NY)	GerPsy	830
Raz, Shlomo (CA)	U	1075	Reisman, Robert (NY)	A&I	83
Razzouk, Bassem (IN)	PHO	705	Reiss, Craig (MO)	Cv	108
Read, Thomas (MA)	CRS	164	Reitz, Bruce (CA)	TS	1040
Ready, John (MA)	OrS	558	Relkin, Norman (NY)	N	474
Ready, L Brian (WA)	PM	640	Remick, Scot (WV)	Onc	321
Ready, Neal (NC)	Onc	332	Remmenga, Steven (NE)	GO	268
Reaman, Gregory (DC)	PHO	696	Remzi, Feza (OH)	CRS	170
Reardon, Michael (TX)	TS	1037	Rennard, Stephen (NE)	Pul	859
Reasner, Charles (TX)	EDM	210	Rennke, Helmut (MA)	Path	643
Rebeiz, Elie (MA)	Oto	600	Repke, John (PA)	MF	396
Reber, Howard (CA)	S	1005	Resar, Jon (MD)	IC	122
Recht, Abram (MA)	RadRO	871	Rescorla, Frederick (IN)	PS	739
Rechtine, Glenn (NY)	OrS	568	Resnick, Neil (PA)	Ger	247
Recker, Robert (NE)	EDM	209	Reuben, David (CA)	Ger	251
Redberg, Rita (CA)	Cv	114	Reus, Victor (CA)	Psyc	819
Redding, Gregory (WA)	PPul	729	Reuter, Victor (NY)	Path	646
Reddy, Bhagat (GA)	IC	123	Rex, Douglas (IN)	Ge	234
Reddy, K Rajender (PA)	Ge	223	Reynolds, James (PA)	Ge	223
Reder, Anthony (IL)	N	485	Reynolds, James (NY)	Oph	526
Redlich, Carrie (CT)	Pul	846	Reynolds, Marleta (IL)	PS	739
Reed, Carolyn (SC)	TS	1029	Reynolds, R Kevin (MI)	GO	267
Reed, Kathryn (AZ)	MF	401	Rezai, Ali (OH)	NS	446
Reed, Robert (OH)	N	485	Rheingold, Susan (PA)	PHO	696
Rees, Riley (MI)	PlS	788	Rhoads, J Marc (TX)	PGe	689
Regillo, Carl (PA)	Oph	526	Rhodes, Arthur (IL)	D	190
Regine, William (MD)	RadRO	875	Riba, Michelle (MI)	Psyc	814
Reich, David (PA)	S	973	Rice, Dale (CA)	Oto	626

Name	Specialty	Pg	Name	Specialty	Pg
Rice, Henry (NC)	PS	737	Riviello, James (TX)	ChiN	147
Rice, Laurel (WI)	GO	267	Rivkees, Scott (CT)	PEn	678
Rice, Thomas (OH)	TS	1033	Rivlin, Richard (NY)	IM	389
Rich, Keith (MO)	NS	446	Rizk, Norman (CA)	Pul	863
Rich, Stuart (IL)	Cv	108	Rizza, Robert (MN)	EDM	208
Rich, Tyvin (VA)	RadRO	880	Rizzo, Joseph (MA)	Oph	519
Richard, James (OK)	Oph	542	Roach, Mack (CA)	RadRO	890
Richards, Jon (IL)	Onc	342	Robb, Geoffrey (TX)	PlS	791
Richardson, Marilyn (KS)	RE	935	Robbins, Lawrence (IL)	PM	637
Richardson, Mark (OR)	PO	725	Robbins, Richard (TX)	EDM	210
Richardson, William (NC)	OrS	574	Robbins, Robert (CA)	TS	1040
Richie, Jerome (MA)	U	1049	Robert, Nicholas (VA)	Onc	332
Richman, Douglas (CA)	Inf	384	Robert-Vizcarrondo, Francisco (AL)	Onc	332
Richter, Edwin (CT)	PMR	758	Roberts, Barbara (RI)	Cv	94
Richter, Joel (PA)	Ge	224	Roberts, John (CA)	S	1005
Ricketts, Richard (GA)	PS	737	Roberts, Kenneth (CT)	RadRO	871
Ricotta, John (DC)	VascS	1086	Roberts, Michelle (PA)	EDM	202
Riddle, Mark (MD)	ChAP	825	Roberts, Patricia (MA)	CRS	164
Riddle, Matthew (OR)	EDM	213	Roberts, William (TX)	Path	654
Ridge, John Andrew (PA)	S	973	Robertson, Cary (NC)	U	1061
Ridgway, E (CO)	EDM	209	Robins, Perry (NY)	D	184
Ridker, Paul (MA)	Cv	94	Robinson, Julian (MA)	MF	395
Ried, Stephanie (PA)	PMR	761	Robinson, Lary (FL)	TS	1029
Riew, K Daniel (MO)	OrS	580	Robinson, Lawrence (WA)	PMR	767
Rigamonti, Daniele (MD)	NS	435	Rocchini, Albert (MI)	PCd	674
Rigel, Darrell (NY)	D	183	Rochester, Carolyn (CT)	Pul	846
Riina, Howard (NY)	NS	435	Rock, Jack (MI)	NS	446
Rikkers, Layton (WI)	S	989	Rodby, Roger (IL)	Nep	421
Riles, Thomas (NY)	VascS	1086	Roddy, Sarah (CA)	ChiN	148
Riley, Laura (MA)	MF	395	Rodeo, Scott (NY)	SM	956
Rilling, William (WI)	VIR	919	Rodgers, Bradley (VA)	PS	737
Rimoin, David (CA)	CG	159	Rodgers, George (UT)	Path	653
Ring, W Steves (TX)	TS	1037	Rodosky, Mark (PA)	OrS	568
Ringel, Steven (CO)	N	488	Rodts, Gerald (GA)	NS	440
Rink, Richard (IN)	U	1067	Roehrborn, Claus (TX)	U	1071
Riordan, John (CA)	Nep	424	Rogers, Douglas (OH)	PEn	682
Ristow, Brunno (CA)	PlS	796	Rogers, Gary (OH)	Oph	538
Ritch, Robert (NY)	Oph	526	Rogers, James (TX)	PCd	675
Ritchey, A Kim (PA)	PHO	696	Rogers, Joseph (NC)	Cv	103
Ritchie, Christine (AL)	Ger	248	Rogers, Lisa (MI)	N	486

Alphabetical Listing of Doctors

Name	Specialty	Pg	Name	Specialty	Pg
Rogers, Stanley (CA)	S	1005	Rosenbush, Stuart (IL)	Cv	108
Roh, Mark (PA)	S	973	Rosenfeld, Myrna (PA)	N	474
Rohrich, Rod (TX)	PlS	791	Rosenfeld, Philip (FL)	Oph	532
Roland, J Thomas (NY)	Oto	606	Rosenfeld, Richard (NY)	PO	721
Romagnoli, Mario (NY)	Inf	377	Rosenfeld, Steven (NY)	N	474
Romaguera, Jorge (TX)	Onc	352	Rosenfield, Kenneth (MA)	IC	120
Romano, James (CA)	PlS	796	Rosenfield, Robert (IL)	PEn	682
Rombeau, John (PA)	CRS	166	Rosengart, Todd (NY)	TS	1024
Romond, Edward (KY)	Onc	332	Rosenman, Julian (NC)	RadRO	880
Roodman, G David (PA)	Hem	292	Rosenquist, Richard (IA)	PM	637
Rook, Alain (PA)	D	184	Rosenthal, David (GA)	VascS	1087
Roos, Karen (IN)	N	486	Rosenthal, Joseph (CA)	PHO	711
Roos, Raymond (IL)	N	486	Rosenthal, Richard (NY)	Psyc	810
Roose, Steven (NY)	Psyc	810	Rosenwaks, Zev (NY)	RE	929
Ropper, Allan (MA)	N	465	Rosenwasser, Melvin (NY)	HS	278
Rosato, Ernest (PA)	S	974	Rosenwasser, Robert (PA)	NS	435
Rosbe, Kristina (CA)	PO	725	Roses, Daniel (NY)	S	974
Rose, Cecile (CO)	Pul	859	Rosier, Randy (NY)	OrS	568
Rose, Christopher (CA)	RadRO	890	Roskes, Saul (MD)	PNep	717
Rose, Peter (OH)	GO	267	Rosner, Howard (CA)	PM	640
Rosemurgy, Alexander (FL)	S	981	Rosoff, Philip (NC)	PHO	700
Rosen, Antony (MD)	Rhu	944	Ross, Edgar (MA)	PM	634
Rosen, Charles (MN)	S	990	Ross, Helen (AZ)	Onc	352
Rosen, Clark (PA)	Oto	607	Ross, Jeffrey (NY)	Path	647
Rosen, Jules (PA)	GerPsy	830	Ross, Lawrence (IL)	U	1067
Rosen, Paul (NY)	Path	646	Ross, Merrick (TX)	S	998
Rosen, Steven (IL)	Onc	342	Rosse, Richard (DC)	Psyc	810
Rosenbaum, Jerrold (MA)	Psyc	805	Rosser, Tena (CA)	ChiN	148
Rosenbaum, Kenneth (DC)	CG	154	Rossi, Carl (CA)	RadRO	890
Rosenbaum, Richard (OR)	N	494	Rossman, Milton (PA)	Pul	849
Rosenberg, Aaron (IL)	OrS	580	Rostain, Anthony (PA)	ChAP	825
Rosenberg, Howard (CA)	PlS	796	Roth, Andrew (NY)	Psyc	810
Rosenberg, Michael (IL)	Oph	538	Roth, Bennett (CA)	Ge	240
Rosenberg, Steven (MD)	S	974	Roth, Bruce (TN)	Onc	333
Rosenberg, Thomas (UT)	OrS	582	Roth, David (FL)	Nep	420
Rosenblatt, Joseph (FL)	Hem	294	Roth, Elliot (IL)	PMR	765
Rosenblum, Marc (NY)	Path	647	Roth, Jack (TX)	TS	1037
Rosenblum, Mark (MI)	NS	446	Roth, Susan (PA)	DR	903
Rosenblum, Norman (PA)	GO	262	Rothbaum, Robert (MO)	PGe	688
Rosenbluth, Daniel (MO)	Pul	857	Rothenberg, Russell (MD)	Rhu	944

Name	Specialty	Pg
Rothenberger, David (MN)	CRS	170
Rothman, Richard (PA)	OrS	568
Rothrock, John (AL)	N	480
Rothstein, Richard (NH)	Ge	216
Rotman, Marvin (NY)	RadRO	875
Rotmensch, Jacob (IL)	GO	267
Roubin, Gary (NY)	IC	122
Routes, John (WI)	A&I	86
Rovner, Barry (PA)	GerPsy	830
Rowbotham, Michael (CA)	PM	640
Rowland, Randall (KY)	U	1061
Rowley, Howard (WI)	NRad	913
Rowley, Scott (NJ)	Hem	292
Roy-Byrne, Peter (WA)	Psyc	819
Roye, David (NY)	OrS	568
Rozbruch, S Robert (NY)	OrS	568
Rubenfeld, Sheldon (TX)	EDM	210
Rubin, Brian (OH)	Path	652
Rubin, Bruce (NC)	PPul	727
Rubin, Geoffrey (CA)	DR	908
Rubin, Lewis (CA)	Pul	863
Rubin, Mark (CA)	D	194
Rubin, Peter (MA)	Oph	519
Rubin, Raymond (GA)	Ge	228
Rubin, Robert (MA)	Inf	374
Rubin, Stephen (PA)	GO	263
Rubin, Susan (IL)	N	486
Rubino, Francesco (NY)	S	974
Rubinstein, Wendy (IL)	CG	156
Ruckdeschel, John (MI)	Onc	342
Rudnick, Michael (PA)	Nep	418
Rudolph, Colin (WI)	PGe	688
Ruff, Robert (OH)	N	486
Ruge, John (IL)	NS	446
Ruggiero, Joseph (NY)	Onc	321
Rugo, Hope (CA)	Onc	360
Rushton, H Gil (DC)	U	1055
Ruskin, Jeremy (MA)	CE	115
Russell, Andrew (CA)	ChAP	829
Russell, Christy (CA)	Onc	360

Name	Specialty	Pg
Russell, Kenneth (WA)	RadRO	890
Russell, Stuart (MD)	Cv	99
Russo, Carolyn (CA)	PHO	711
Rutgers, Joanne (CA)	Path	657
Rutherford, Thomas (CT)	GO	259
Ryan, Colleen (MA)	S	964
Ryken, Timothy (IA)	NS	446

S

Saag, Michael (AL)	Inf	380
Saal, Howard (OH)	CG	156
Saal, Jeffrey (CA)	PMR	767
Sacchi, Terrence (NY)	Cv	99
Sacco, Ralph (FL)	N	480
Sachs, Greg (IN)	Ger	249
Saclarides, Theodore (IL)	CRS	170
Sadock, Virginia (NY)	Psyc	810
Sadowsky, Carl (FL)	N	480
Saffle, Jeffrey (UT)	S	994
Safi, Hazim (TX)	TS	1037
Safian, Robert (MI)	Cv	108
Sagalowsky, Arthur (TX)	U	1071
Sage, Jacob (NJ)	N	474
Sagel, Stuart (MO)	DR	906
Saha, Sukamal (MI)	S	990
Sahin, Aysegul (TX)	Path	654
Sahin, Mustafa (MA)	ChiN	142
Sahn, Steven (SC)	Pul	853
Saiki, John (NM)	Onc	352
Sailer, Scott (NC)	RadRO	880
Saiman, Lisa (NY)	PInf	713
Saint-Phard, Deborah (CO)	SM	957
Sakamoto, Kathleen (CA)	PHO	711
Salant, David (MA)	Nep	416
Salem, Riad (IL)	VIR	919
Salem, Ronald (CT)	S	964
Salgia, Ravi (IL)	Onc	343
Salky, Barry (NY)	S	974
Sallan, Stephen (MA)	PHO	691

Alphabetical Listing of Doctors

Name	Specialty	Pg	Name	Specialty	Pg
Sallent, Jorge (FL)	PPul	727	Santana, Victor (TN)	PHO	700
Salo, Jonathan (NC)	S	982	Santin, Alessandro (CT)	GO	259
Saltz, Leonard (NY)	Onc	321	Santos, Cesar (NC)	ChiN	145
Saltzman, Charles (UT)	OrS	582	Sanz, Luis (VA)	ObG	511
Salvati, Eduardo (NY)	OrS	569	Saper, Clifford (MA)	N	465
Salvi, Sharad (IL)	PHO	705	Saper, Joel (MI)	N	486
Salz, James (CA)	Oph	547	Sargent, Albert (TX)	ChAP	828
Salzman, Carl (MA)	Psyc	805	Sarnaik, Ashok (MI)	PCCM	677
Samadi, David (NY)	U	1055	Sarnoff, Deborah (NY)	D	184
Samberg, Eslee (NY)	Psyc	810	Sarr, Michael (MN)	S	990
Samlowski, Wolfram (NV)	Onc	360	Sartor, R Balfour (NC)	Ge	228
Sampson, Christian (MA)	HS	276	Sasaki, Clarence (CT)	Oto	600
Sampson, Hugh (NY)	PA&I	665	Sasson, Aaron (NE)	S	994
Sampson, John (NC)	NS	440	Sataloff, Robert (PA)	Oto	607
Samson, Duke (TX)	NS	450	Satava, Richard (WA)	S	1005
Samuels, Brian (ID)	Onc	347	Sato, Thomas (WI)	PS	740
Samuels, Louis (PA)	TS	1024	Saudek, Christopher (MD)	EDM	202
Samuels, Martin (MA)	N	465	Sauer, Mark (NY)	RE	929
Samuelson, Thomas (MN)	Oph	538	Saul, Robert (SC)	CG	155
Sanborn, Timothy (IL)	Cv	108	Saunders, Elijah (MD)	Cv	99
Sanchez, Luis (MO)	VascS	1089	Savage, David (NY)	Hem	292
Sanchez, Miguel (NJ)	Path	647	Saven, Alan (CA)	Hem	303
Sanda, Martin (MA)	U	1049	Saver, Jeffrey Lawrence (CA)	N	494
Sandborn, William (MN)	Ge	234	Savino, Peter (CA)	Oph	547
Sanders, Georgiana (MI)	A&I	86	Sawaya, Raymond (TX)	NS	450
Sanders, William (GA)	U	1061	Sawczuk, Ihor (NJ)	U	1055
Sandhu, Harvinder (NY)	OrS	569	Sawin, Robert (WA)	PS	742
Sandler, Alan (OR)	Onc	360	Sax, Paul (MA)	Inf	374
Sandler, Eric (FL)	PHO	700	Saxena, Sanjaya (CA)	Psyc	819
Sandler, Howard (CA)	RadRO	890	Scandling, John (CA)	Nep	425
Sandler, Martin (TN)	NuM	504	Scantlebury, Velma (DE)	S	974
Sandlow, Jay (WI)	U	1067	Scarborough, Mark (FL)	OrS	574
Sandlund, John (TN)	PHO	700	Scardino, Peter (NY)	U	1056
Sanfilippo, Joseph (PA)	RE	929	Schachat, Andrew (OH)	Oph	538
Sanford, Robert (TN)	NS	440	Schaefer, Steven (NY)	Oto	607
Sangeorzan, Bruce (WA)	OrS	587	Schaeffer, Anthony (IL)	U	1067
Sanger, James (WI)	PlS	788	Schafer, Michael (IL)	OrS	580
Sanger, Joseph (NY)	NuM	503	Schaff, Hartzell (MN)	TS	1033
Sankar, Raman (CA)	ChiN	148	Schanberg, Laura (NC)	PRhu	731
Santa-Emma, Philip (OH)	IM	390	Schantz, Stimson (NY)	Oto	607

Name	Specialty	Pg	Name	Specialty	Pg
Schatz, Lisa (CO)	CRS	170	Schluger, Neil (NY)	Pul	849
Schatz, Norman (FL)	N	480	Schmalzried, Thomas (CA)	OrS	587
Schatzberg, Alan (CA)	Psyc	819	Schmidt, Richard (PA)	OrS	569
Schauer, Philip (OH)	S	990	Schnabel, Freya (NY)	S	974
Schechter, David (CA)	SM	957	Schnipper, Lowell (MA)	Onc	308
Scheff, Alice (CA)	NuM	505	Schnitt, Stuart (MA)	Path	643
Schein, Oliver (MD)	Oph	526	Schnittger, Ingela (CA)	Cv	114
Scheinberg, David (NY)	Onc	321	Schoen, Robert (CT)	Rhu	941
Scheinman, Steven (NY)	Nep	418	Schoenberg, Mark (MD)	U	1056
Scheithauer, Bernd (MN)	Path	652	Schoetz, David (MA)	CRS	165
Schelbert, Heinrich (CA)	NuM	505	Schomberg, Paula (MN)	RadRO	884
Scheld, W Michael (VA)	Inf	380	Schooley, Robert (CA)	Inf	384
Scheller, Arnold (MA)	SM	954	Schottenfeld, Richard (CT)	AdP	820
Schenken, Robert (TX)	RE	935	Schraut, Wolfgang (PA)	S	974
Schepsis, Anthony (MA)	SM	954	Schreiber, Theodore (MI)	IC	124
Scher, Charles (LA)	PHO	708	Schrier, Robert (CO)	Nep	422
Scher, Howard (NY)	Onc	322	Schubert, Mark (AZ)	A&I	87
Scher, Jonathan (NY)	ObG	509	Schuberth, Kenneth (MD)	PA&I	666
Scherr, Douglas (NY)	U	1056	Schuchter, Lynn (PA)	Onc	322
Schiano, Thomas (NY)	Ge	224	Schuckit, Marc (CA)	AdP	822
Schiff, David (VA)	N	480	Schuger, Claudio (MI)	CE	118
Schiff, Eugene (FL)	Ge	228	Schulak, James (OH)	S	990
Schiff, Peter (NY)	RadRO	876	Schulick, Richard (MD)	S	974
Schiff, William (NY)	Oph	526	Schulman, Steven (MD)	Cv	99
Schiffer, Charles (MI)	Onc	343	Schultz, Neal (NY)	D	184
Schiffman, Fred (RI)	Hem	289	Schulze, Konrad (IA)	Ge	234
Schiffman, Jade (TX)	Oph	542	Schuman, Joel (PA)	Oph	527
Schild, Steven (AZ)	RadRO	887	Schurman, David (CA)	OrS	588
Schilder, Russell (PA)	Onc	322	Schuster, Michael (NY)	Hem	292
Schiller, Alan (NY)	Path	647	Schusterman, Mark (TX)	PlS	791
Schiller, Gary (CA)	Hem	304	Schwab, Richard (PA)	Pul	849
Schiller, Joan (TX)	Onc	352	Schwartz, Allan (NY)	Cv	99
Schiller, Lawrence (TX)	Ge	238	Schwartz, Burton (MN)	Onc	343
Schilsky, Richard (IL)	Onc	343	Schwartz, Cindy (RI)	PHO	691
Schink, Julian (IL)	GO	267	Schwartz, Gary (MN)	Nep	421
Schirmer, Bruce (VA)	S	982	Schwartz, Herbert (TN)	OrS	574
Schlaff, William (CO)	RE	935	Schwartz, L Matthew (PA)	PMR	761
Schlegel, Peter (NY)	U	1056	Schwartz, Marshall (PA)	PS	735
Schley, W Shain (NY)	Oto	607	Schwartz, Michael (FL)	Onc	333
Schlinkert, Richard (AZ)	S	998	Schwartz, Peter (CT)	GO	259

Alphabetical Listing of Doctors

Name	Specialty	Pg	Name	Specialty	Pg
Schwartz, Robert (CO)	Ger	250	Seltzer, Dana (AZ)	OrS	584
Schwartz, Robert (NC)	PEn	681	Selvaggi, Kathy (PA)	Onc	322
Schwartz, Stanley (PA)	EDM	202	Selwyn, Peter (NY)	IM	389
Schwartz, William (NY)	Cv	99	Semenkovich, Clay (MO)	EDM	208
Schwartzberg, Lee (TN)	Hem	294	Semrad, Carol (IL)	Ge	234
Schwartzentruber, Douglas (IN)	S	990	Sen, Chandranath (NY)	NS	435
Schwartzman, Robert (PA)	N	474	Senagore, Anthony (MI)	CRS	170
Schwarz, Adam (CA)	PCCM	678	Sencer, Susan (MN)	PHO	705
Schwarz, Kathleen (MD)	PGe	685	Senders, Craig (CA)	Oto	626
Schwarz, Marvin (CO)	Pul	859	Sener, Stephen (CA)	S	1005
Schwarz, Steven (NY)	PGe	686	Senior, Brent (NC)	Oto	612
Scott, C Paul (PA)	Psyc	810	Senzer, Neil (TX)	RadRO	887
Scott, Gwendolyn (FL)	PInf	714	Sepkowitz, Kent (NY)	Inf	377
Scott, Richard (MA)	OrS	558	Serafano, Donald (CA)	Oph	548
Scott, W Norman (NY)	OrS	569	Sergent, John (TN)	Rhu	946
Scott, Walter (PA)	TS	1024	Sergott, Robert (PA)	Oph	527
Scott-Conner, Carol (IA)	S	990	Serletti, Joseph (PA)	PlS	778
Scudera, Peter (VA)	Ge	228	Serody, Jonathan (NC)	Onc	333
Sculco, Thomas (NY)	OrS	569	Serota, Ronald (PA)	AdP	821
Scully, Sean (FL)	OrS	574	Service, Frederick (MN)	EDM	208
Seashore, Margretta (CT)	CG	152	Session, Donna (GA)	RE	932
Seaver, Laurie (HI)	CG	159	Sessoms, Sandra (TX)	Rhu	949
See, William (WI)	U	1067	Sethi, Kapil (GA)	N	480
Seeger, James (FL)	VascS	1087	Seton, Margaret (MA)	Rhu	941
Seely, Ellen (MA)	EDM	199	Setzen, Michael (NY)	Oto	607
Seftel, Allen (OH)	U	1068	Seung, Steven (OR)	RadRO	890
Segal, Brahm (NY)	Inf	377	Sewell, C Whitaker (GA)	Path	650
Seibel, Barry (CA)	Oph	548	Sexson, Sandra (GA)	ChAP	826
Seidner, Douglas (TN)	Ge	228	Seyfer, Alan (MD)	PlS	779
Seidner, Steven (TX)	NP	412	Sha, Beverly (IL)	Inf	381
Seifer, David (NY)	RE	930	Shaban, Stephen (NC)	U	1062
Seiff, Stuart (CA)	Oph	548	Shabto, Uri (NY)	Oph	527
Seifter, Julian (MA)	Nep	417	Shadick, Nancy (MA)	Rhu	941
Seitz, William (OH)	HS	282	Shafer, Frank (PA)	PHO	696
Sekhar, Laligam (WA)	NS	454	Shaffrey, Christopher (VA)	NS	440
Selby, Robert (CA)	S	1005	Shaffrey, Mark (VA)	NS	440
Selden, Nathan (OR)	NS	455	Shah, Jatin (NY)	S	975
Selkoe, Dennis (MA)	N	465	Shah, Prediman (CA)	Cv	114
Sellke, Frank (RI)	TS	1017	Shaker, Reza (WI)	Ge	234
Selman, Warren (OH)	NS	447	Shalita, Alan (NY)	D	184

Name	Specialty	Pg	Name	Specialty	Pg
Shamberger, Robert (MA)	PS	733	Sherman, Carol (SC)	Onc	333
Shani, Jacob (NY)	IC	122	Sherman, James (VA)	PPul	727
Shannon, John (TX)	Pul	860	Sherman, Orrin (NY)	OrS	569
Shapiro, Amy (IN)	PHO	705	Sherman, Randolph (CA)	PlS	796
Shapiro, Charles (OH)	Onc	343	Sherman, Steven (TX)	EDM	210
Shapiro, Edward (MA)	Psyc	805	Sherman, Stuart (IN)	Ge	234
Shapiro, Eugene (CT)	PInf	712	Sherry, David (PA)	PRhu	731
Shapiro, Jerrold (IL)	Cv	108	Sherwin, Robert (CT)	EDM	199
Shapiro, Lawrence (NY)	CG	154	Sherwood, Mark (FL)	Oph	532
Shapiro, Ron (PA)	S	975	Shibata, Stephen (CA)	Onc	360
Shapiro, Scott (IN)	NS	447	Shields, Carol (PA)	Oph	527
Shapiro, William (AZ)	N	490	Shields, Jerry (PA)	Oph	527
Shapshay, Stanley (NY)	Oto	607	Shields, Peter (DC)	Onc	322
Sharlip, Ira (CA)	U	1075	Shields, William (CA)	ChiN	149
Sharma, Om Prakash (CA)	Pul	863	Shiffman, Mitchell (VA)	Ge	229
Sharp, Gregory (AR)	ChiN	147	Shike, Moshe (NY)	Ge	224
Sharp, Kenneth (TN)	S	982	Shikora, Scott (MA)	S	964
Shaw, Byers (NE)	S	994	Shin, Dong Moon (GA)	Onc	333
Shaw, Edward (NC)	RadRO	880	Shina, Donald (NM)	RadRO	887
Shaywitz, Bennett (CT)	ChiN	142	Shindo, Maisie (OR)	Oto	626
Shaywitz, Sally (CT)	Ped	662	Shingleton, Bradford (MA)	Oph	519
Shea, Thomas (NC)	Onc	333	Shinnar, Shlomo (NY)	ChiN	144
Shear, M Katherine (NY)	Psyc	810	Shipley, William (MA)	RadRO	871
Shearer, Patricia (FL)	PHO	701	Shlansky-Goldberg, Richard (PA)	VIR	917
Shearer, William (TX)	PA&I	668	Shlasko, Edward (NY)	PS	735
Sheehan, Myles (IL)	Ger	249	Shlofmitz, Richard (NY)	Cv	99
Shefner, Jeremy (NY)	N	474	Shochat, Stephen (TN)	PS	737
Sheinfeld, Joel (NY)	U	1056	Shockley, William (NC)	Oto	612
Shelbourne, K Donald (IN)	OrS	580	Shore, Bernard (MO)	Pul	857
Sheldon, Curtis (OH)	U	1068	Shorofsky, Stephen (MD)	IC	122
Shellito, Judd (LA)	Pul	860	Short, Billie (DC)	NP	408
Shellito, Paul (MA)	CRS	165	Shortliffe, Linda (CA)	U	1076
Shelton, Clough (UT)	Oto	621	Shoulson, Ira (NY)	N	474
Shemin, Richard (CA)	TS	1040	Shrager, Joseph (CA)	TS	1041
Shen, Perry (NC)	S	982	Shrieve, Dennis (UT)	RadRO	885
Shenk, Robert (OH)	S	990	Shuer, Lawrence (CA)	NS	455
Shenot, Patrick (PA)	U	1056	Shuldiner, Alan (MD)	EDM	203
Shepard, Alexander (MI)	VascS	1089	Shulman, Lawrence (MA)	Onc	308
Shepherd, Gillian (NY)	A&I	83	Shulman, Lee (IL)	ObG	512
Sherertz, Elizabeth (NC)	D	187	Shulman, Lisa (MD)	N	474

Alphabetical Listing of Doctors

Name	Specialty	Pg	Name	Specialty	Pg
Shulman, Stanford (IL)	PInf	715	Simeone, Diane (MI)	S	991
Shupack, Jerome (NY)	D	184	Simms, Robert (MA)	Rhu	941
Siatkowski, R Michael (OK)	Oph	542	Simon, George (PA)	Onc	322
Sibley, Richard (CA)	Path	657	Simon, James (DC)	RE	930
Sicard, Gregorio (MO)	VascS	1089	Simon, John (NY)	Oph	527
Sicherer, Scott (NY)	PA&I	666	Simon, Richard (MI)	Pul	857
Siddique, Teepu (IL)	N	486	Simons, Michael (CT)	Cv	94
Siebert, John (NY)	PlS	779	Simpson, Joe Leigh (FL)	ObG	511
Siegel, Barry (MO)	NuM	504	Sinanan, Mika (WA)	S	1005
Siegel, Corey (NH)	Ge	216	Sinatra, Frank (CA)	PGe	690
Siegel, Gordon (IL)	Oto	619	Singer, Carlos (FL)	N	481
Siegel, Herrick (AL)	OrS	575	Singer, Daniel (HI)	OrS	588
Siegel, Stuart (CA)	PHO	711	Singer, Mark (CA)	Oto	627
Sielaff, Timothy (MN)	S	991	Singer, Peter (CA)	EDM	213
Siemionow, Maria (OH)	PlS	788	Singer, Robert (CA)	PlS	796
Sigman, Mark (RI)	U	1049	Singer, Samuel (NY)	S	975
Sigurdson, Elin (PA)	S	975	Singh, Arun (RI)	TS	1017
Sikic, Branimir (CA)	Onc	360	Singh, Nalini (DC)	PInf	713
Silber, Sherman (MO)	U	1068	Singhal, Seema (IL)	Hem	299
Silbergeld, Daniel (WA)	NS	455	Singletary, S (TX)	S	998
Silberstein, Stephen (PA)	N	475	Sinha, Uttam (CA)	Oto	627
Sillers, Michael (AL)	Oto	612	Siperstein, Allan (OH)	S	991
Sills, Allen (TN)	NS	440	Sirdofsky, Michael (DC)	N	475
Sills, Edward (MD)	PRhu	731	Siris, Ethel (NY)	EDM	203
Silva, Elvio (TX)	Path	655	Sison, Joseph (NJ)	NP	408
Silver, Julie (MA)	PMR	758	Sisti, Michael (NY)	NS	435
Silver, Lester (NY)	PlS	779	Sisung, Charles (IL)	PMR	765
Silver, Michael (IL)	Pul	857	Sivina, Manuel (FL)	VascS	1087
Silver, Richard (SC)	Rhu	946	Sivit, Carlos (OH)	DR	906
Silver, Samuel (MI)	Onc	343	Skibber, John (TX)	S	999
Silverberg, Steven (MD)	Path	647	Skinner, Eila (CA)	U	1076
Silverman, Gary (PA)	NP	408	Skinner, Kristin (NY)	S	975
Silverman, Jan (PA)	Path	647	Skinner, Michael (TX)	PS	741
Silverman, Lewis (NY)	Onc	322	Sklar, Charles (NY)	PEn	680
Silverman, Paula (OH)	Onc	343	Sklar, Frederick (TX)	NS	451
Silverman, William (IA)	Ge	234	Skoner, David (PA)	PA&I	666
Silverstein, Herbert (FL)	Oto	612	Skyler, Jay (FL)	EDM	205
Silverstein, Janet (FL)	PEn	681	Slama, Thomas (IN)	Inf	381
Silverstein, Melvin (CA)	S	1005	Slankard, Marjorie (NY)	A&I	83
Silverstein, Roy (OH)	Hem	299	Slatkin, Neal (CA)	PM	640

Name	Specialty	Pg	Name	Specialty	Pg
Slaughter, Mark (KY)	TS	1029	Smythe, W Roy (TX)	TS	1037
Slavin, Sumner (MA)	PlS	773	Snyder, David (CA)	Hem	304
Slawin, Kevin (TX)	U	1071	Snyder, Howard (PA)	U	1056
Slease, Robert (DE)	Hem	292	Snyder, Peter (PA)	EDM	203
Sleasman, John (FL)	PA&I	667	Snyderman, Carl (PA)	Oto	607
Sledge, George (IN)	Onc	343	Sobel, Jack (MI)	Inf	381
Slezak, Sheri (MD)	PlS	779	Sobel, Michael (WA)	S	1005
Slingluff, Craig (VA)	S	982	Sobel, Stuart (FL)	D	188
Slivka, Adam (PA)	Ge	224	Sober, Arthur (MA)	D	180
Sliwa, James (IL)	PMR	765	Socinski, Mark (NC)	Onc	333
Slomowitz, Marcia (IL)	ChAP	828	Socol, Michael (IL)	MF	399
Slutsky, David (CA)	HS	284	Soiffer, Robert (MA)	Onc	308
Sly, R Michael (DC)	PA&I	666	Soisson, Andrew (UT)	GO	268
Small, Eric (CA)	Onc	360	Sokol, Thomas (CA)	CRS	172
Small, Gary (CA)	GerPsy	832	Sokoloff, Daniel (FL)	D	188
Small, William (IL)	RadRO	884	Solberg, Lawrence (FL)	Hem	294
Smalley, Stephen (KS)	RadRO	885	Solin, Lawrence (PA)	RadRO	876
Smalling, Richard (TX)	IC	125	Solomon, Gary (NY)	Rhu	944
Smart, Frank (NJ)	Cv	99	Solomon, Robert (NY)	NS	435
Smedira, Nicholas (OH)	TS	1033	Soloway, Mark (FL)	U	1062
Smith, Barbara (MA)	S	964	Somerville, James (MN)	Nep	421
Smith, Craig (NY)	TS	1024	Sondak, Vernon (FL)	S	982
Smith, David (FL)	PlS	783	Sondel, Paul (WI)	PHO	706
Smith, Donna (IL)	GO	268	Sondheimer, Steven (PA)	RE	930
Smith, Joanne (IL)	PMR	765	Sonett, Joshua (NY)	TS	1024
Smith, John (OH)	TS	1034	Song, John (CO)	Oto	622
Smith, Joseph (TN)	U	1062	Sonntag, Volker (AZ)	NS	451
Smith, Lloyd (CA)	GO	272	Sontheimer, Richard (UT)	D	191
Smith, Matthew (MA)	Onc	308	Sood, Anil (TX)	GO	270
Smith, Mitchell (PA)	Onc	322	Sood, Rajiv (IN)	PlS	788
Smith, Paul (FL)	PlS	784	Soparkar, Charles (TX)	Oph	542
Smith, Peter (NC)	TS	1029	Soper, John (NC)	GO	265
Smith, Ronald (CA)	Oph	548	Soper, Nathaniel (IL)	S	991
Smith, Sidney (NC)	Cv	104	Sorrell, Michael (NE)	Ge	236
Smith, Steven (IL)	VIR	919	Sorrentino, Matthew (IL)	Cv	108
Smith, Thomas (VA)	Onc	333	Sorrentino, Robert (GA)	CE	117
Smith, Thomas (MA)	Path	643	Sosa, R Ernest (NY)	U	1056
Smith, Wade (CA)	N	494	Sosman, Jeffrey (TN)	Onc	334
Smith, Yolanda (MI)	RE	935	Soter, Nicholas (NY)	D	184
Smoot, Duane (DC)	Ge	224	Sotereanos, Dean (PA)	HS	279

Alphabetical Listing of Doctors

Name	Specialty	Pg	Name	Specialty	Pg
Sotomayor, Eduardo (FL)	Onc	334	Stahl, Donna (OH)	S	991
Soulen, Michael (PA)	VIR	917	Stahl, Richard (CT)	PlS	773
Soules, Michael (WA)	RE	936	Stainback, Raymond (TX)	Cv	111
Souryal, Tarek (TX)	OrS	584	Stal, Samuel (TX)	PlS	791
Sowers, James (MO)	EDM	209	Stamos, Michael (CA)	CRS	172
Spack, Norman (MA)	PEn	679	Stangel, John (NY)	RE	930
Spann, Cyril (GA)	GO	265	Stankiewicz, James (IL)	Oto	619
Speeg, Kermit (TX)	Ge	238	Stanley, Charles (PA)	PEn	680
Speer, Kevin (NC)	SM	956	Stanley, James (MI)	VascS	1090
Spence, Robert (MD)	PlS	779	Stanley, John (PA)	D	184
Spencer, Dennis (CT)	NS	429	Staples, Edward (FL)	TS	1030
Spencer, Susan (CT)	N	466	Staren, Edgar (IL)	S	991
Spencer, Thomas (MA)	ChAP	823	Stark, Walter (MD)	Oph	527
Spengler, Dan (TN)	OrS	575	Starnes, Vaughn (CA)	TS	1041
Spergel, Jonathan (PA)	PA&I	666	Starr, Arnold (CA)	N	494
Sperling, Mark (PA)	PEn	680	Starz, Terence (PA)	Rhu	944
Sperling, Michael (PA)	N	475	Stasney, C Richard (TX)	Oto	624
Spetzler, Robert (AZ)	NS	451	Staton, Gerald (GA)	Pul	853
Speyer, James (NY)	Onc	323	Stea, Baldassarre (AZ)	RadRO	887
Spiegel, David (CA)	Psyc	819	Steadman, J Richard (CO)	OrS	582
Spiera, Harry (NY)	Rhu	944	Steed, David (PA)	VascS	1086
Spindler, Kurt (TN)	OrS	575	Steege, John (NC)	ObG	511
Spinelli, Henry (NY)	PlS	779	Steen, Virginia (DC)	Rhu	945
Spirtos, Nicola (NV)	GO	272	Steers, William (VA)	U	1062
Spitzer, Thomas (MA)	Hem	289	Stefanyszyn, Mary (PA)	Oph	527
Spivak, Jeffrey (NY)	OrS	569	Stehman, Frederick (IN)	GO	268
Spivak, Jerry (MD)	Hem	292	Steiger, David (NY)	Pul	849
Spivak, William (NY)	PGe	686	Stein, David (PA)	CRS	166
Sponseller, Paul (MD)	OrS	569	Stein, Elliott (FL)	GerPsy	831
Spray, Thomas (PA)	PS	735	Stein, James (CA)	PS	742
Spriggs, David (NY)	Onc	323	Stein, James (WI)	Cv	109
Springfield, Dempsey (MA)	OrS	558	Stein, Murray (CA)	Psyc	819
Squires, Robert (PA)	PGe	686	Steinberg, Gary (CA)	NS	455
Srivastava, Sudhir (GA)	TS	1029	Steinberg, Gary (IL)	U	1068
Staats, Peter (NJ)	PM	636	Steinberg, Harry (NY)	Pul	849
Stadelmann, Wayne (NH)	PlS	773	Steiner, Hans (CA)	ChAP	829
Stadler, Walter (IL)	Onc	344	Steiner, Mark (MA)	SM	954
Stadtmauer, Edward (PA)	Onc	323	Steinert, Roger (CA)	Oph	548
Staffenberg, David (NY)	PlS	779	Steingart, Richard (NY)	Cv	100
Staggers, Barbara (CA)	AM	78	Steinhagen, Randolph (NY)	CRS	166

Alphabetical Listing of Doctors

Name	Specialty	Pg	Name	Specialty	Pg
Stuzin, James (FL)	PlS	784	Swanstrom, Lee (OR)	S	1006
Stylianos, Steven (FL)	PS	737	Swarm, Robert (MO)	PM	638
Suarez, Jose (TX)	N	491	Swartz, Richard (MI)	Nep	422
Suchy, Frederick (NY)	PGe	686	Sweeney, John (GA)	S	982
Suen, James (AR)	Oto	624	Sweet, Richard (CA)	ObG	513
Sugarbaker, David (MA)	TS	1017	Sweetenham, John (OH)	Hem	299
Sugarbaker, Paul (DC)	S	975	Swensen, Stephen (MN)	DR	906
Suh, John (OH)	RadRO	884	Swerdloff, Ronald (CA)	EDM	213
Suki, Wadi (TX)	Nep	423	Swerdlow, Charles (CA)	CE	119
Sulica, Radu Lucian (NY)	Oto	608	Swerdlow, Michael (NY)	N	475
Sullivan, Patrick (RI)	PlS	773	Swerdlow, Steven (PA)	Path	647
Sullivan, Timothy (GA)	A&I	85	Swetter, Susan (CA)	D	194
Sultan, Mark (NY)	PlS	779	Swiontkowski, Marc (MN)	OrS	581
Summer, Warren (LA)	Pul	860	Swisher, Stephen (TX)	TS	1038
Summers, C Gail (MN)	Oph	538	Swistel, Alexander (NY)	S	975
Sumpio, Bauer (CT)	VascS	1083	Szabo, Robert (CA)	HS	284
Sun, Peter (CA)	NS	455	Szachowicz, Edward (MN)	Oto	619
Sun, Weijing (PA)	Onc	323			
Sundaram, Magesh (WV)	S	975			
Sundt, Thoralf (MN)	TS	1034			
Sundy, John (NC)	Rhu	946	**T**		
Supiano, Mark (UT)	Ger	250			
Surawicz, Christina (WA)	Ge	241	Tabbal, Nicolas (NY)	PlS	780
Suresh, Santhanam (IL)	PM	638	Tabsh, Khalil (CA)	MF	402
Surks, Martin (NY)	EDM	203	Tafra, Lorraine (MD)	S	975
Surrey, Eric (CO)	RE	935	Taft, Timothy (NC)	OrS	575
Sussman, Norman (NY)	Psyc	811	Taghian, Alphonse (MA)	RadRO	871
Suster, Saul (WI)	Path	652	Tajik, A Jamil (AZ)	Cv	112
Sutherland, David (MN)	S	991	Talamonti, Mark (IL)	S	991
Sutphen, Rebecca (FL)	CG	155	Tallman, Martin (IL)	Hem	299
Sutton, John (NH)	S	964	Tamargo, Rafael (MD)	NS	436
Sutton, Leslie (PA)	NS	436	Tamaroff, Marc (CA)	A&I	88
Sutton, Linda (NC)	Onc	334	Tamborlane, William (CT)	PEn	679
Svensson, Lars (OH)	TS	1034	Tanabe, Kenneth (MA)	S	965
Swaid, Swaid (AL)	NS	440	Taneja, Samir (NY)	U	1057
Swain, Sandra (DC)	Onc	323	Tanner, Caroline (CA)	N	495
Swanson, David (TX)	U	1072	Tannous, Raymond (IA)	PHO	706
Swanson, Jerry (MN)	N	486	Taplin, Mary-Ellen (MA)	Onc	308
Swanson, Neil (OR)	D	194	Tapson, Victor (NC)	Pul	854
Swanson, Scott (MA)	TS	1017	Tarbell, Nancy (MA)	RadRO	871
			Targan, Stephan (CA)	Ge	241
			Tarraza, Hector (ME)	GO	259

Alphabetical Listing of Doctors

Name	Specialty	Pg	Name	Specialty	Pg
Tomlinson, Gail (TX)	PHO	708	Trump, Donald (NY)	Onc	324
Toonkel, Leonard (FL)	RadRO	880	Tsai, James (CT)	Oph	519
Toriumi, Dean (IL)	Oto	619	Tsangaris, Theodore (MD)	S	976
Tornetta, Paul (MA)	OrS	558	Tse, David (FL)	Oph	532
Tornos, Carmen (NY)	Path	648	Tsokos, George (MA)	Rhu	941
Torres, Vicente (MN)	Nep	422	Tucci, Debara (NC)	Oto	613
Torti, Frank (NC)	Onc	334	Tucker, Rodney (AL)	IM	390
Tortolani, Anthony (NY)	TS	1025	Tulsky, James (NC)	IM	390
Toskes, Phillip (FL)	Ge	229	Tune, Larry (GA)	GerPsy	831
Toth, Thomas (MA)	RE	927	Tunkel, David (MD)	PO	722
Toto, Robert (TX)	Nep	423	Tureck, Richard (PA)	RE	930
Townsend, Raymond (PA)	Nep	418	Turecki, Stanley (NY)	ChAP	826
Traboulsi, Elias (OH)	Oph	539	Turek, Paul (CA)	U	1076
Tracy, Thomas (RI)	PS	733	Turner, William (TX)	TS	1038
Tranbaugh, Robert (NY)	TS	1025	Turrentine, Mark (IN)	TS	1034
Trauner, Doris (CA)	ChiN	149	Turtz, Alan (NJ)	NS	436
Traverso, L William (WA)	S	1006	Tuttle, R Michael (NY)	EDM	203
Travis, William (NY)	Path	648	Tuttle, Todd (MN)	S	992
Traynelis, Vincent (IL)	NS	447	Twardowski, Przemyslaw (CA)	Onc	361
Treadwell, Marjorie (MI)	MF	400	Tychsen, Lawrence (MO)	Oph	539
Treadwell, Patricia (IN)	D	190	Tyler, Douglas (NC)	S	983
Treem, William (NY)	PGe	686	Tyson, Jon (TX)	NP	412
Tremaine, William (MN)	Ge	234	Tzakis, Andreas (FL)	S	983
Trenholme, Gordon (IL)	Inf	381			
Trento, Alfredo (CA)	TS	1041			
Treon, Steven (MA)	Onc	308			
Trerotola, Scott (PA)	VIR	917	**U**		
Trese, Michael (MI)	Oph	539	Uberti, Joseph (MI)	Hem	299
Triche, Timothy (CA)	Path	658	Udelsman, Robert (CT)	S	965
Trick, Lorence (TX)	OrS	584	Ulbright, Thomas (IN)	Path	652
Triozzi, Pierre (OH)	Onc	344	Ulshen, Martin (NC)	PGe	687
Tripathy, Debasish (CA)	Onc	361	Umetsu, Dale (MA)	A&I	82
Tripuraneni, Prabhakar (CA)	RadRO	890	Underwood, Paul (SC)	ObG	511
Trisal, Vijay (CA)	S	1006	Unger, Michael (PA)	Pul	850
Trobe, Jonathan (MI)	Oph	539	Ungerleider, Ross (OH)	TS	1034
Troner, Michael (FL)	Onc	334	Urata, Mark (CA)	PlS	796
Trudel, Judith (MN)	CRS	170	Urba, Susan (MI)	Onc	344
True, Lawrence (WA)	Path	658	Urba, Walter (OR)	Onc	361
Trulock, Elbert (MO)	Pul	858	Uribe, John (FL)	OrS	575
Trumble, Thomas (WA)	HS	284	Urist, Marshall (AL)	S	983
			Urken, Mark (NY)	Oto	608

Name	Specialty	Pg
Uzzo, Robert (PA)	U	1057

V

Name	Specialty	Pg
Vaccaro, Alexander (PA)	OrS	570
Vachharajani, Tushar (NC)	Nep	420
Vaezi, Michael (TN)	Ge	229
Vail, Thomas (CA)	OrS	588
Valenstein, Edward (FL)	N	481
Valentine, Alan (TX)	Psyc	816
Valentino, Joseph (KY)	Oto	613
Valentino, Leonard (IL)	PHO	706
Valero, Vicente (TX)	Onc	353
Valji, Karim (WA)	VIR	921
Vallieres, Eric (WA)	TS	1041
Van Arsdalen, Keith (PA)	U	1057
van Besien, Koen (IL)	Hem	299
van der Horst, Charles (NC)	Inf	380
Van Dorsten, J Peter (SC)	MF	397
Van Heertum, Ronald (NY)	NuM	503
van Hoff, Jack (NH)	PHO	691
Van Loveren, Harry (FL)	NS	441
Van Marter, Linda (MA)	NP	406
Van Nagell, John (KY)	GO	265
Van Thiel, David (IL)	Ge	235
Vance, Mary Lee (VA)	EDM	205
Vance, Ralph (MS)	Onc	334
Vander, James (PA)	Oph	528
Vander Kolk, Craig (MD)	PlS	780
Vander Salm, Thomas (MA)	TS	1017
Vanderhoof, Jon (NE)	PGe	689
Vanderkolk, Bessel (MA)	Psyc	806
Vapnek, Jonathan (NY)	U	1057
Varadhachary, Gauri (TX)	Onc	353
Vargo, John (OH)	Ge	235
Vas, George (NY)	N	475
Vasconez, Henry (KY)	PlS	784
Vasconez, Luis (AL)	PlS	784
Vaughan, Edwin (NY)	U	1057
Vaughan, William (AL)	Onc	335

Name	Specialty	Pg
Vaughey, Ellen (VA)	Pul	854
Vaughn, David (PA)	Onc	324
Vauthey, Jean (TX)	S	999
Vege, Santhi (MN)	Ge	235
Veith, Richard (WA)	GerPsy	832
Velcek, Francisca (NY)	PS	735
Veldhuis, Johannes (MN)	EDM	209
Velvis, Harm (NY)	PCd	671
Venkat, K K (MI)	Nep	422
Venook, Alan (CA)	Onc	361
Vernava, Anthony (FL)	CRS	168
Verrier, Edward (WA)	TS	1041
Verschraegen, Claire (NM)	Onc	353
Vescio, Robert (CA)	Onc	361
Vetrovec, George (VA)	Cv	104
Vetto, John (OR)	S	1006
Vezina, L Gilbert (DC)	NRad	911
Vicini, Frank (MI)	RadRO	884
Vick, Nicholas (IL)	N	487
Vickers, Selwyn (MN)	S	992
Videtic, Gregory (OH)	RadRO	885
Vierling, John (TX)	Ge	239
Vigneswaran, Wickii (IL)	TS	1034
Vignola, Paul (FL)	Cv	104
Vijayakumar, Srinivasan (MS)	RadRO	880
Vik, Terry (IN)	PHO	706
Vining, Eileen (MD)	Ped	663
Vining, Eugenia (CT)	Oto	600
Vinuela, Fernando (CA)	NRad	915
Vitek, Jerrold (OH)	N	487
Vivino, Frederick (PA)	Rhu	945
Vlahakes, Gus (MA)	S	965
Voelkel, Norbert (VA)	Pul	854
Vogelzang, Nicholas (NV)	Onc	362
Vogelzang, Robert (IL)	VIR	920
Vogt, Peter (MN)	PlS	788
Volberding, Paul (CA)	Onc	362
Volgman, Annabelle (IL)	Cv	109
Volkmar, Fred (CT)	ChAP	823
Vollmer, Timothy (CO)	N	488

Alphabetical Listing of Doctors

Name	Specialty	Pg	Name	Specialty	Pg
Volpe, Joseph (MA)	ChiN	143	Wallace, Richard (TX)	Inf	383
Volshteyn, Oksana (MO)	PMR	765	Wallace, Robert (LA)	Oph	542
Von Burton, Gary (LA)	Onc	353	Wallach, Edward (MD)	RE	930
von der Lohe, Elisabeth (IN)	Cv	109	Wallach, Frances (NY)	Inf	378
von Gunten, Charles (CA)	Onc	362	Walling, Arthur (FL)	OrS	575
Von Hoff, Daniel (AZ)	Onc	353	Walmer, David (NC)	RE	932
von Mehren, Margaret (PA)	Onc	324	Walsh, B Timothy (NY)	Psyc	811
Von Roenn, Jamie (IL)	Onc	344	Walsh, Christine (NY)	PCd	671
Voorhees, John (MI)	D	190	Walsh, Edward (MA)	PCd	669
Vose, Julie (NE)	Hem	300	Walsh, John (LA)	NS	451
			Walsh, Joseph (NY)	Oph	528
			Walsh, Mary (IN)	Cv	109
			Walsh, Nicolas (TX)	PM	639
W			Walsh, Patrick (MD)	U	1057
			Walsh, R Matthew (OH)	S	992
Wackym, P Ashley (WI)	Oto	619	Walton, David (MA)	Oph	519
Wade, James (WI)	Onc	344	Walton, Robert (IL)	PIS	788
Waggoner, Steven (OH)	GO	268	Wamboldt, Marianne (CO)	ChAP	828
Wagman, Lawrence (CA)	S	1006	Waner, Milton (NY)	Oto	608
Wagner-Weiner, Linda (IL)	PRhu	731	Wang, Frederick (NY)	Oph	528
Wagoner, Lynne (OH)	Cv	109	Wang, Jeffrey (CA)	OrS	588
Waguespack, Steven (TX)	EDM	211	Wang, Ming (TN)	Oph	532
Wahl, Richard (MD)	NuM	503	Wang, Winfred (TN)	PHO	701
Wain, John (MA)	TS	1018	Wanner, Adam (FL)	Pul	854
Waintraub, Stanley (NJ)	Onc	324	Wapner, Keith (PA)	OrS	570
Wait, Susan (MD)	Psyc	811	Wapner, Ronald (NY)	MF	396
Wakefield, Thomas (MI)	S	992	Wara, Diane (CA)	PA&I	669
Wald, Arnold (WI)	Ge	235	Wara, William (CA)	RadRO	891
Wald, Ellen (WI)	PInf	715	Warady, Bradley (MO)	PNep	719
Waldo, Albert (OH)	CE	119	Ward, Barbara (CT)	S	965
Walker, Alonzo (WI)	S	992	Ward, John (UT)	Onc	347
Walker, David (TX)	Path	655	Ward, Robert (NY)	PO	722
Walker, Joan (OK)	GO	270	Ward, William (NC)	OrS	575
Walker, Marion (UT)	NS	448	Waring, George (GA)	Oph	533
Walker, R Dale (OR)	AdP	822	Warner, Ann (MO)	Rhu	948
Walkup, John (MD)	ChAP	826	Warner, Brad (MO)	PS	740
Wall, Michael (OR)	PPul	729	Warnick, Ronald (OH)	NS	447
Wallace, Anne Marie (CA)	S	1006	Warnke, Roger (CA)	Path	658
Wallace, Daniel (CA)	Rhu	950	Warnock, David (AL)	Nep	420
Wallace, Jeanne (CA)	Pul	863	Warren, Robert (AR)	PPul	729
Wallace, Mark (FL)	Inf	380			
Wallace, Mark (CA)	PM	640			

Name	Specialty	Pg	Name	Specialty	Pg
Warren, Robert (TX)	PRhu	732	Weinblatt, Mark (NY)	PHO	696
Warren, Robert (CA)	S	1006	Weinblatt, Michael (MA)	Rhu	941
Warren, Russell (NY)	OrS	570	Weiner, George (IA)	Onc	344
Warshaw, Andrew (MA)	S	965	Weiner, Howard (NY)	NS	436
Wartofsky, Leonard (DC)	EDM	203	Weiner, Howard (MA)	N	466
Wasserman, Stephen (CA)	A&I	88	Weiner, I David (FL)	Nep	420
Watchko, Jon (PA)	NP	408	Weiner, Kenneth (CO)	Psyc	815
Waters, Peter (MA)	HS	276	Weiner, Leslie (CA)	N	495
Watkins, Robert (CA)	OrS	588	Weiner, Louis (DC)	Onc	324
Watson, Thomas (NY)	TS	1025	Weiner, Michael (NY)	PHO	696
Watts, Nelson (OH)	EDM	209	Weiner, Myron (TX)	Psyc	816
Watts, Ray (AL)	N	481	Weiner, Richard (NC)	Psyc	812
Wax, Mark (OR)	Oto	627	Weiner, Richard (FL)	OrS	576
Waxman, Alan (CA)	NuM	505	Weiner, William (MD)	N	476
Waxman, Harvey (PA)	Cv	100	Weinfeld, Steven (NY)	OrS	570
Waxman, Irving (IL)	Ge	235	Weingeist, Thomas (IA)	Oph	539
Waye, Jerome (NY)	Ge	224	Weinreb, Jeffrey (CT)	DR	899
Wazen, Jack (FL)	Oto	613	Weinstein, Arthur (DC)	Rhu	945
Wazer, David (RI)	RadRO	871	Weinstein, Gregory (PA)	Oto	608
Weaver, David (IN)	CG	156	Weinstein, Howard (MA)	PHO	691
Weaver, W Douglas (MI)	Cv	109	Weinstein, James (NH)	OrS	559
Webb, Gary (PA)	Cv	100	Weinstein, Sharon (UT)	PM	638
Webb, Lawrence (NC)	OrS	575	Weinstein, Stuart (IA)	OrS	581
Weber, Jeffrey (FL)	Onc	335	Weinstock, Robert (CA)	Psyc	819
Weber, Randal (TX)	Oto	624	Weisberg, Tracey (ME)	Onc	308
Weber, Samuel (TX)	Oto	624	Weisenburger, Dennis (NE)	Path	653
Webster, George (NC)	U	1062	Weisler, Richard (NC)	Psyc	812
Webster, Harry (MA)	PMR	758	Weisman, Robert (CA)	Oto	627
Wechsler, Lawrence (PA)	N	475	Weisman, Steven (WI)	PM	638
Weder, Alan (MI)	IM	390	Weiss, Arnold (RI)	HS	276
Wei, Jeanne (AR)	Ger	250	Weiss, Avery (WA)	Oph	548
Weichselbaum, Ralph (IL)	RadRO	885	Weiss, Geoffrey (VA)	Onc	335
Weigel, Ronald (IA)	S	992	Weiss, Gerson (NJ)	RE	930
Weiland, Andrew (NY)	HS	279	Weiss, Lawrence (CA)	Path	658
Weiman, Darryl (TN)	TS	1030	Weiss, Marisa (PA)	RadRO	876
Wein, Alan (PA)	U	1057	Weiss, Robert (NJ)	U	1058
Weinberg, David (PA)	Ge	225	Weiss, Robert (CT)	U	1050
Weinberg, Harold (NY)	N	475	Weiss, Sharon (GA)	Path	650
Weinberg, Paul (PA)	PCd	671	Weiss, Stanley (NJ)	PrM	801
Weinberger, Michael (NY)	PM	636	Weissler, Jonathan (TX)	Pul	860

Alphabetical Listing of Doctors

Name	Specialty	Pg	Name	Specialty	Pg
Weissler, Mark (NC)	Oto	613	White, Neil (MO)	PEn	682
Weissman, David (WI)	Onc	344	White, Richard (NC)	S	983
Weissman, Peter (FL)	EDM	206	White, Richard (FL)	DR	905
Weitz, Howard (PA)	Cv	100	White, Robert (CT)	VIR	916
Weitzel, Jeffrey (CA)	CG	159	White, Rodney (CA)	VascS	1092
Weksler, Benny (PA)	TS	1025	Whiting, Donald (PA)	NS	436
Welch, Peter (NY)	Inf	378	Whitington, Peter (IL)	PGe	688
Welch, William (PA)	NS	436	Whitlock, James (TN)	PHO	701
Weller, Elizabeth (PA)	ChAP	826	Whitlow, Patrick (OH)	IC	124
Wells, Gretchen (NC)	Cv	104	Whitsett, Jeffrey (OH)	NP	411
Wells, James (CA)	PIS	796	Whitworth, Pat (TN)	S	983
Wells, Robert (WI)	DR	906	Whyte, Richard (CA)	TS	1041
Wells, Winfield (CA)	TS	1041	Wicha, Max (MI)	Onc	344
Welton, Mark (CA)	CRS	173	Wickiewicz, Thomas (NY)	OrS	571
Wener, Mark (WA)	Rhu	950	Wiebke, Eric (IN)	S	992
Wenstrom, Katharine (TN)	MF	398	Wiedel, Jerome (CO)	OrS	582
Wenzel, Sally (PA)	Pul	850	Wiedemann, Herbert (OH)	Pul	858
Werner, Phillip (IL)	EDM	209	Wierman, Ann (NV)	Onc	362
Werner-Wasik, Maria (PA)	RadRO	876	Wiesel, Sam (DC)	OrS	571
Werth, Victoria (PA)	D	185	Wiesenfeld, Harold (PA)	ObG	509
West, Sterling (CO)	Rhu	949	Wiesner, Russell (MN)	Ge	235
Westrich, Geoffrey (NY)	OrS	570	Wiet, Richard (IL)	Oto	620
Wetzel, F Todd (PA)	OrS	570	Wigley, Frederick (MD)	Rhu	945
Wetzler, Meir (NY)	Onc	324	Wilansky, Susan (AZ)	Cv	112
Wexler, Leonard (NY)	PHO	697	Wilber, David (IL)	CE	119
Wexner, Steven (FL)	CRS	168	Wilcox, C Mel (AL)	Ge	229
Weymuller, Ernest (WA)	Oto	627	Wilcox, Christopher (DC)	Nep	418
Wharam, Moody (MD)	RadRO	876	Wilcox, William (CA)	CG	160
Wharen, Robert (FL)	NS	441	Wilczynski, Sharon (CA)	Path	658
Wheeland, Ronald (MO)	D	190	Wilding, George (WI)	Onc	345
Wheeler, Arthur (TN)	Pul	854	Wilens, Timothy (MA)	ChAP	823
Wheeler, Thomas (TX)	Path	655	Wilhelmi, Bradon (KY)	PIS	784
Whelan, Alison (MO)	CG	156	Wilhelmus, Kirk (TX)	Oph	542
Whelan, Richard (NY)	CRS	166	Wilking, Andrew (TX)	PRhu	732
Wheless, James (TN)	ChiN	145	Wilkins, Edwin (MI)	PIS	788
Whitaker, Linton (PA)	PIS	780	Wilkins, Isabelle (IL)	MF	400
White, Charles (MD)	DR	903	Wilkins, Ross (CO)	OrS	582
White, David (MA)	Pul	846	Wilkinson, Robert (HI)	PHO	711
White, Dorothy (NY)	Pul	851	Wilkoff, Bruce (OH)	Cv	109
White, Jocelyn (OR)	IM	391	Willerson, James (TX)	Cv	112

Name	Specialty	Pg	Name	Specialty	Pg
Willett, Christopher (NC)	RadRO	880	Wise, Christopher (VA)	Rhu	946
Willey, Shawna (DC)	S	976	Wiseman, Gregory (MN)	NuM	504
Williams, David (MA)	IC	120	Wisoff, Jeffrey (NY)	NS	436
Williams, George (MI)	Oph	539	Witt, Thomas (IL)	S	992
Williams, Gerald (PA)	OrS	571	Witter, Frank (MD)	ObG	510
Williams, Kim (IL)	Cv	110	Wittig, James (NY)	OrS	571
Williams, Michael (VA)	Onc	335	Wityk, Robert (MD)	N	476
Williams, Richard (IA)	U	1068	Wiviott, Lory (CA)	Inf	384
Williams, Riley (NY)	OrS	571	Wixson, Richard (IL)	OrS	581
Williams, Ronald (TX)	OrS	584	Wiznitzer, Max (OH)	ChiN	146
Williams, Shauna (ID)	CRS	171	Woeber, Kenneth (CA)	EDM	213
Willis, Irvin (FL)	S	983	Wofsy, David (CA)	Rhu	950
Willson, James (TX)	Onc	353	Wolf, Gregory (MI)	Oto	620
Wilson, Daniel (NE)	Psyc	815	Wolf, Raoul (IL)	PA&I	667
Wilson, Darrell (CA)	PEn	683	Wolfe, Lawrence (NY)	PHO	697
Wilson, David (OR)	Oph	548	Wolfe, M Michael (MA)	Ge	217
Wilson, J Frank (WI)	RadRO	885	Wolfe, S Anthony (FL)	PlS	784
Wilson, John (NC)	NS	441	Wolfe, Scott (NY)	HS	279
Wilson, Keith (OH)	Oto	620	Wolff, Antonio (MD)	Onc	325
Wilson, Lynn (CT)	RadRO	871	Wolff, Bruce (MN)	CRS	170
Wilson, Marion (SC)	Oph	533	Wolff, Robert (TX)	IM	390
Wilson, Matthew (TN)	Oph	533	Wolfson, Aaron (FL)	RadRO	881
Wilson, Steven (OH)	Oph	539	Wolinsky, Jerry (TX)	N	491
Wilson, Timothy (CA)	U	1076	Woltering, Eugene (LA)	S	999
Wilson, Walter (MN)	Inf	382	Wong, Jeffrey (CA)	RadRO	891
Wilson, Wyndham (MD)	Onc	324	Wong, Johnson (MA)	A&I	82
Winawer, Sidney (NY)	Ge	225	Wong, Ronald (HI)	CRS	173
Winchell, Robert (ME)	S	965	Wong, W Douglas (NY)	CRS	167
Windebank, Anthony (MN)	N	487	Woo, Howard (LA)	U	1072
Winer, Eric (MA)	Onc	309	Woo, Peak (NY)	Oto	608
Winer, Sharon (CA)	RE	936	Woo, Shiao (TX)	RadRO	888
Winfield, Howard (AL)	U	1063	Woo, Y Joseph (PA)	TS	1025
Wingard, John (FL)	Onc	335	Wood, Beverly (CA)	DR	908
Winick, Naomi (TX)	PHO	708	Wood, Bradford (MD)	VIR	917
Winn, Hung (MO)	MF	400	Wood, David (MI)	U	1068
Winston, Ken (CO)	NS	448	Wood, Douglas (WA)	TS	1042
Winter, Jane (IL)	Hem	299	Wood, Gary (WI)	D	190
Winters, Jack (LA)	U	1072	Wood, John (MO)	A&I	86
Wirth, Michael (TX)	OrS	584	Wood, R Patrick (TX)	S	999
Wisch, Nathaniel (NY)	Hem	292	Wood, Robert (MD)	PA&I	666

Alphabetical Listing of Doctors

Name	Specialty	Pg	Name	Specialty	Pg
Wood, William (GA)	S	983	Yeh, John (MA)	RE	927
Woods, William (GA)	PHO	701	Yen, Yun (CA)	Onc	362
Woodson, B Tucker (WI)	Oto	620	Yeo, Charles (PA)	S	976
Woodson, Gayle (IL)	Oto	620	Yetman, Randall (OH)	PlS	788
Wooten, George (VA)	N	481	Yeung, Alan (CA)	IC	125
Wooten, Virgil (OH)	Psyc	814	Yeung, Raymond (WA)	S	1006
Worden, Francis (MI)	Onc	345	Yonas, Howard (NM)	NS	451
Wormser, Gary (NY)	Inf	378	Yoo, Jung (OR)	OrS	589
Worsey, Michael (CA)	CRS	173	Yoon, Sydney (FL)	DR	905
Wright, Cameron (MA)	TS	1018	Yoshikawa, Thomas (CA)	Inf	384
Wright, Harry (SC)	ChAP	826	Young, Amy (TX)	ObG	513
Wright, Jackson (OH)	IM	390	Young, Anne (MA)	N	466
Wright, Kenneth (CA)	Oph	549	Young, Bruce (NY)	ObG	510
Wright, Robert (IL)	N	487	Young, Byron (KY)	NS	441
Wunderink, Richard (IL)	Pul	858	Young, Iven (NY)	EDM	203
Wyatt, Robert (TN)	PNep	718	Young, James (OH)	Cv	110
Wyllie, Elaine (OH)	ChiN	147	Young, K Randall (AL)	Pul	854
Wyllie, Robert (OH)	PGe	688	Young, Ming-Lon (FL)	PCd	672
			Young, Nancy (IL)	Oto	620
			Young, Renee (NE)	Ge	236
Y			Young, Robert (MA)	Path	643
			Young, Vernon (MO)	PlS	789
Yaddanapudi, Ravindranath (MI)	PHO	706	Younge, Brian (MN)	Oph	539
Yaffe, Bruce (NY)	IM	389	Younossi, Zobair (VA)	Ge	229
Yahalom, Joachim (NY)	RadRO	876	Yousem, David (MD)	NRad	911
Yakes, Wayne (CO)	VIR	920	Yousem, Samuel (PA)	Path	648
Yamaguchi, Ken (MO)	OrS	581	Yu, George (MD)	U	1058
Yan, Albert (PA)	D	185	Yu, Jack (GA)	PlS	785
Yancovitz, Stanley (NY)	Inf	378	Yu, John (CA)	NS	455
Yanda, Randy (GA)	Ge	229	Yu, Victor (PA)	Inf	378
Yang, James (MD)	S	976	Yueh, Bevan (MN)	Oto	620
Yang, Stephen (MD)	TS	1025	Yuen, James (AR)	PlS	792
Yankelevitz, David (NY)	DR	904	Yung, Wai-Kwan (TX)	N	491
Yannuzzi, Lawrence (NY)	Oph	528	Yunus, Furhan (TN)	Onc	335
Yarbrough, Wendell (TN)	Oto	613	Yurt, Roger (NY)	S	976
Yasko, Alan (IL)	OrS	581			
Yeager, Andrew (AZ)	Hem	302			
Yeatman, Timothy (FL)	S	983	**Z**		
Yeatts, R Patrick (NC)	Oph	533			
Yee, Billy (CA)	RE	936	Zach, Terence (NE)	NP	411
Yee, Douglas (MN)	Onc	345	Zackai, Elaine (PA)	CG	154

Alphabetical Listing of Doctors

Name	Specialty	Pg	Name	Specialty	Pg
Zacur, Howard (MD)	RE	930	Zoghbi, William (TX)	Cv	112
Zafonte, Ross (MA)	PMR	758	Zorumski, Charles (MO)	Psyc	814
Zager, Eric (PA)	NS	437	Zubrow, Alan (PA)	NP	408
Zagoria, Ronald (NC)	DR	905	Zuckerman, Joseph (NY)	OrS	571
Zagzag, David (NY)	Path	648	Zuckerman, Kenneth (FL)	Hem	294
Zahn, Evan (FL)	PCd	673	Zusman, Randall (MA)	Cv	94
Zaidman, Gerald (NY)	Oph	528	Zwischenberger, Joseph (KY)	TS	1030
Zalusky, Ralph (NY)	Hem	293			
Zalzal, George (DC)	Oto	609			
Zannis, Victor (AZ)	S	999			
Zaret, Barry (CT)	Cv	94			
Zarins, Bertram (MA)	OrS	559			
Zarins, Christopher (CA)	VascS	1092			
Zdeblick, Thomas (WI)	OrS	581			
Zeanah, Charles (LA)	ChAP	828			
Zeitels, Steven (MA)	Oto	600			
Zeitlin, Pamela (MD)	PPul	726			
Zelefsky, Michael (NY)	RadRO	877			
Zelenetz, Andrew (NY)	Onc	325			
Zelickson, Brian (MN)	D	190			
Zeltzer, Lonnie (CA)	Ped	665			
Zerbe, Kathryn (OR)	Psyc	820			
Zide, Barry (NY)	PlS	780			
Ziedonis, Douglas (MA)	AdP	820			
Ziegler, Moritz (CO)	PS	740			
Zietman, Anthony (MA)	RadRO	872			
Zilleruelo, Gaston (FL)	PNep	718			
Zimmerman, Christian (ID)	NS	449			
Zimmerman, Donald (IL)	PEn	683			
Zimmerman, Earl (NY)	N	476			
Zimmerman, Jerry (WA)	PCCM	678			
Zimmerman, Robert (PA)	NRad	911			
Zinaman, Michael (MA)	RE	927			
Zinner, Michael (MA)	S	965			
Zinreich, S James (MD)	NRad	911			
Zins, James (OH)	PlS	789			
Zippe, Craig (OH)	U	1068			
Zisook, Sidney (CA)	Psyc	820			
Zitelli, Basil (PA)	Ped	663			
Zitelli, John (PA)	D	185			

Acknowledgments

The publishers would like to thank the entire staff for their many hours and days of intense and precise work on this guide in order to further its goal of assisting consumers in making the best healthcare choices.

Castle Connolly Executive Management:

Chairman	John K. Castle
President & CEO	John J. Connolly, Ed.D.
Vice President, Chief Medical & Research Officer	Jean Morgan, M.D.
Vice President, Chief Strategy & Operations Officer	William Liss-Levinson, Ph.D.

Research Coordinators

Maryann Hynd, RN
Sara Sezer
Mandy Guerrero
Jerville Weekes
Terysia Herbert
Stephanie Sanchez

Book Layout, Database Management

Russell Hodgson
Tara Rolandelli
Krista Feierabend

Office Manager, Book Coordination
Corporate Services Manager

Marcie Samartino
Jennifer Mojave

We also would like to extend our gratitude to the American Board of Medical Specialties (ABMS) for allowing us to use excerpts, especially the descriptions of medical specialties and subspecialties, from the text of their publication "Which Medical Specialist for You?"

Other Publications from Castle Connolly Medical Ltd.:
America's Top Doctors® for Cancer; Top Doctors: New York Metro Area; Top Doctors: Chicago Metro Area; Cancer Made Easier: New York Metro Area, and others...
Order online at http://www.castleconnolly.com/books

Doctor-Patient Advisor

Doctor-Patient Advisor is a Castle Connolly Medical Ltd. service providing one-on-one consultations with a physician or nurse to individuals who have serious or complex medical problems or to anyone who feels he/she needs assistance finding the right physician for any purpose. Each client will receive personalized assistance in identifying the appropriate specialists for his/her condition, utilizing the Castle Connolly Medical Ltd. database of physicians and hospitals, as well as individual searches, to locate the best resources to meet the client's needs.

Fee: $375. For further information call (212) 367-8400 x 16.